W9-DHT-572

UROLOGIC SURGICAL PATHOLOGY

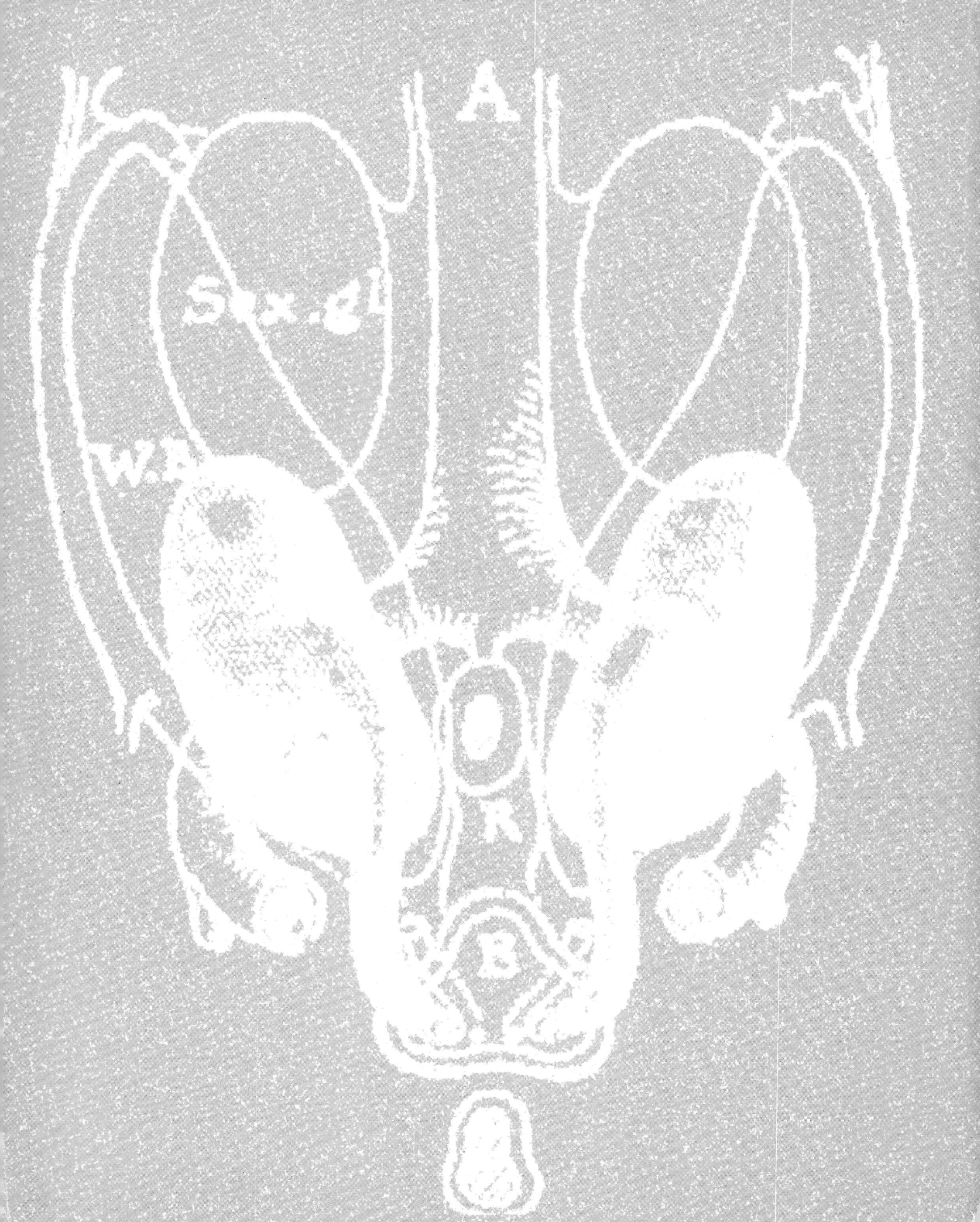
A
Sex.gl
O
R
B

UROLOGIC SURGICAL PATHOLOGY

EDITED BY

David G. Bostwick, M.D.
Professor of Pathology
Mayo Medical School
Consultant
Department of Laboratory Medicine and Pathology
Mayo Clinic
Rochester, Minnesota

John N. Eble, M.D.
Professor of Pathology and Experimental Oncology
Indiana University School of Medicine
Chief Pathologist
Richard L. Roudebush Veterans Affairs Medical Center
Indianapolis, Indiana

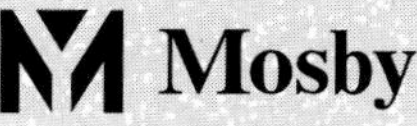

St. Louis Baltimore Boston
Carlsbad Chicago Naples New York Philadelphia Portland
London Madrid Mexico City Singapore Sydney Tokyo Toronto Wiesbaden

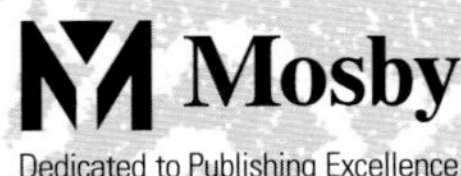

A Times Mirror
Company

Publisher: Anne S. Patterson
Senior Managing Editor: Lynne Gery
Project Manager: Linda Clarke
Production Editor: Julie Cullen
Composition Specialist: Pamela Merritt
Designer: Carolyn O'Brien
Manufacturing Supervisor: Andrew Christensen

Composition by Mosby Electronic Production, Philadelphia
Lithography/color film by Lehigh Press Colortronics
Printed in Canada by Friesens

Mosby–Year Book, Inc.
11830 Westline Industrial Drive
St. Louis, Missouri 63146

Library of Congress Cataloging-in-Publication Data

Urologic surgical pathology / edited by David G. Bostwick, John N. Eble.—1st ed.
p. cm.
Includes bibliographical references and index.
ISBN 0-8016-7503-0
1. Genitourinary organs—Histopathology. 2. Pathology, Surgical.
I. Bostwick, David G. II. Eble, John N.
[DNLM: 1. Urologic Diseases—pathology. 2. Genital Diseases, Male—pathology. 3. Pathology, Surgical. WJ 101 U78 1997]
RD571.U735 1997
617.4'607—dc20
DNLM/DLC
for Library of Congress 96-13923
CIP

98 99 00 01 / 9 8 7 6 5 4 3 2

CONTRIBUTORS

Mahul B. Amin, M.D.
Assistant Professor of Pathology
Case Western Reserve University School of Medicine
Cleveland Ohio
Clinical Assistant Professor of Pathology
Wayne State University School of Medicine
Senior Staff
Department of Pathology and Bone and Joint Centre
Henry Ford Hospital
Detroit, Michigan

Alberto G. Ayala, M.D.
Professor and Deputy Chairman
Department of Pathology
University of Texas—Houston Medical School
Director
Surgical Pathology
University of Texas M.D. Anderson Cancer Center
Houston, Texas

Stephen M. Bonsib, M.D.
Professor
Department of Pathology
University of Iowa Hospital and Clinics
Iowa City, Iowa

David G. Bostwick, M.D.
Professor of Pathology
Mayo Medical School
Consultant
Department of Laboratory Medicine and Pathology
Mayo Clinic
Rochester, Minnesota

John A. Bryan, M.D.
Resident
Department of Pathology
Georgetown University Medical Center
Washington, D.C.

John N. Eble, M.D.
Professor and Associate Chairman
Department of Pathology and Laboratory Medicine
Professor of Experimental Oncology
Indiana University School of Medicine
Chief Pathologist
Richard L. Roudebush Veterans Affairs Medical Center
Indianapolis, Indiana

Jonathan I. Epstein, M.D.
Professor
Departments of Pathology and Urology
The Johns Hopkins Medical Institutions
Associate Director of Surgical Pathology
Johns Hopkins Hospital
Baltimore, Maryland

David J. Grignon, M.D.
Associate Professor
Department of Pathology
Wayne State University School of Medicine
Director of Anatomical Pathology
Harper Hospital
Detroit, Michigan

Ernest E. Lack, M.D.
Director of Anatomic Pathology
Professor
Department of Pathology
Georgetown University School of Medicine
Washington, D.C.

Michael Richard Lewin-Smith, B.Sc., M.B., B.S.
Fellow in Surgical Pathology and Cytology
Department of Pathology
The George Washington University Medical Center
Washington, D.C.

Manuel Nistal, M.D.
Head of Service
Department of Pathology
La Paz Hospital
Madrid, Spain

Ricardo Paniagua, Ph.D.
Professor of Cell Biology
Department of Cell Biology and Genetics
University of Alcalá de Henares
Alcalá de Henares (Madrid), Spain

Victor E. Reuter, M.D.
Associate Professor of Pathology
Cornell University Medical College
Associate Attending Pathologist
Memorial Sloan-Kettering Cancer Center
New York, New York

Jae Y. Ro, M.D., Ph.D.
Professor and Pathologist
Department of Pathology
The University of Texas M.D. Anderson Cancer Center
Houston, Texas

Thomas M. Ulbright, M.D.
Professor of Pathology and Laboratory Medicine
Indiana University School of Medicine
Director of Anatomic Pathology
Indiana University Medical Center
Indianapolis, Indiana

Robert H. Young, M.D., M.R.C.Path
Associate Professor of Pathology
Harvard Medical School
Pathologist and Director of Surgical Pathology
Massachusetts General Hospital
Boston, Massachusetts

PREFACE

Recent years have seen tremendous progress in urologic surgical pathology. Among the most important advances have been the recognition of precursors of prostatic adenocarcinoma and its histologic mimics, dramatic growth in the number of prostate biopsies afforded by the 18-gauge needle, new classification of renal cell neoplasms and its genetic correlation, resurgence of the urothelial carcinoma/papilloma controversy, new concepts of the origin and relationships of the different types of testicular germ cell neoplasms, and the recognition that not all kidney tumors in children are Wilms' tumors. For today's surgical pathologist, urologic specimens are an important part of everyday sign-out, and the expectation for excellence in diagnosis, staging, and consultation is very high. It was with this in mind that we planned this book.

As the title *Urologic Surgical Pathology* indicates, this book is primarily intended for use by surgical pathologists in their daily practice. The emphasis is on practical diagnostic and differential diagnostic considerations; these are addressed with more than 1000 illustrations of gross and microscopic pathology and with an abundance of tables and boxes summarizing key points. Our purpose has been to provide a framework in which evolving diagnostic criteria can be compared, evaluated, and integrated. While there are extensive references to guide the reader to the original literature, the authors have also been encouraged to share practical tips from their own experience as diagnostic consultants. We have attempted to strike a balance between encyclopedic coverage and the physical constraint of a single volume. Practical ancillary techniques are presented as appropriate, including histochemistry, electron microscopy, immunohistochemistry, and molecular biology.

The fourteen chapters are defined anatomically, beginning with the kidney and ending with the adrenal. Two chapters each are accorded to the kidney, prostate, testis, and urinary bladder, and these are devoted to neoplastic and non-neoplastic diseases. The authors and editors have striven for uniformity of style among the chapters. The graciousness of some of the authors in acceding to editorial decisions concerning usage will be obvious to some readers and is testimony to the teamwork that has gone into this book.

In Indianapolis, we thank Karen Miller and James Bogue who helped prepare some of the color illustrations, and Carol Johns who helped with bibliographic work. In Rochester, we thank Annette Bjorheim who helped with secretarial work. At Mosby–Year Book, thanks go to Susan Gay, who carried the flag for color illustrations and the size of the book in the initial stages; to Lynne Gery and Julie Cullen, who saw it through; and to Carolyn O'Brien, the designer, and Pamela Merritt, composition specialist, who put the parts together into a whole.

David G. Bostwick
Rochester

John N. Eble
Indianapolis

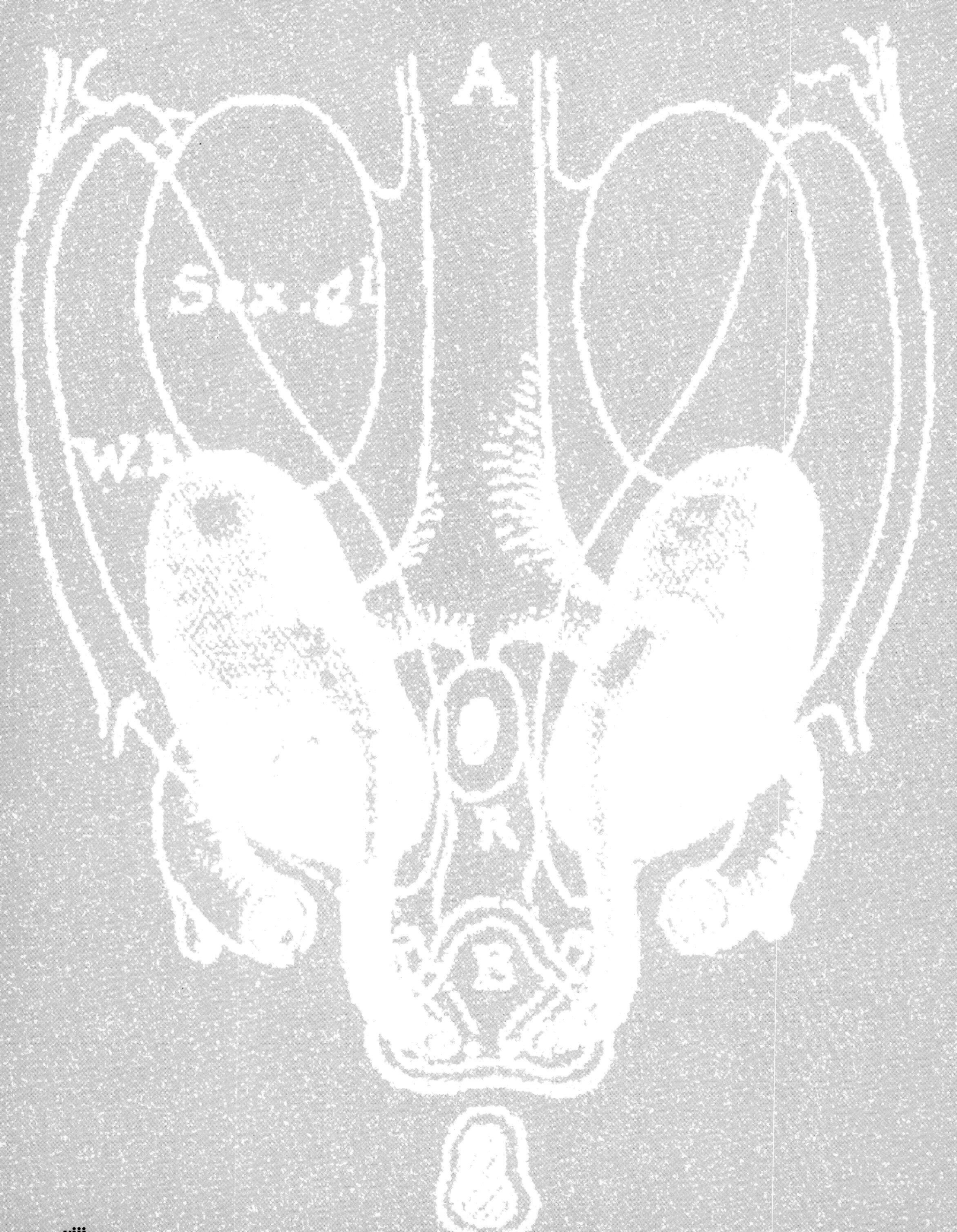
A
Sex.gl
R
B

CONTENTS

Embryologic Development and Normal Structure

- Pronephros
- Mesonephros
- Metanephros
- Nephron differentiation
- Gross anatomy
- Microscopic anatomy

Congenital Anomalies and Cystic Diseases

- Abnormalities in form and position
- Abnormalities in mass and number
- Parenchymal maldevelopment and cystic diseases

Vascular Diseases

- Hypertension-associated renal disease
- Thrombotic microangiopathy
- Renal artery stenosis
- Renal artery dissection
- Renal artery aneurysm
- Arteriovenous malformation and fistula
- Renal emboli and infarcts
- Renal cortical necrosis
- Renal cholesterol microembolism syndrome
- Renal artery thrombosis
- Renal vein and renal venous thrombosis
- Bartter's syndrome
- Vasculitis

Tubulointerstitial Diseases

- Infection-related tubulointerstitial nephritis
- Chronic pyelonephritis
- Xanthogranulomatous pyelonephritis
- Malakoplakia
- Tuberculosis
- Acute tubulointerstitial disease
- Chronic interstitial nephritis
- Metabolic abnormalities and tubulointerstitial diseases
- Miscellaneous conditions

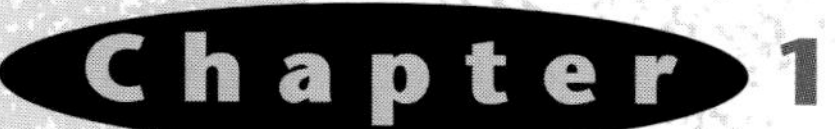

NON-NEOPLASTIC DISEASES OF THE KIDNEY

STEPHEN M. BONSIB

Study with me, then, a few things in the spirit of truth alone so we may establish the manner of Nature's operation. For this essay which I plan, will shed light upon the structure of the kidney. Do not stop to question whether these ideas are new or old, but ask, more properly, whether they harmonize with Nature. I never reached my idea of the structure of the kidney by the aid of books, but by the long and varied use of the microscope. I have gotten the rest by the deductions of reason, slowly, and with an open mind, as is my custom.[1]

Marcello Malpighi
1666

In keeping with the spirit of Marcello Malpighi, this chapter also aspires to reveal "the manner of Nature's operations" as it affects the kidney.[1] However, unlike Malpighi today's knowledge draws extensively upon the labors, discoveries, and insights of investigators of the last 4 centuries.

Knowledge of the normal structure and function of the kidney has been acquired over centuries of scholarly effort. We have come a long way since Aristotle taught that urine was formed by the bladder and that kidneys were present "not of actual necessity, but as matters of greater finish and perfection."[1] The foundation of urology was established in the sixteenth century by Leonardo da Vinci and Vesalius who provided the first accurate and detailed drawings of the female and male genitourinary tracts (Fig. 1-1).[2,3] Over 300 years passed before William Bowman, in 1842, coupled intravascular dye injection with microscopic examination to demonstrate the structural organization of the nephron and its vascular supply (Fig. 1-2).[4,5] Bowman's observations provided morphologic support for Malpighi's seventeenth-century speculation of a filtration function for the Malpighian body (the glomerulus).[1] Sixty years later the embryologic development of the nephron was demonstrated by Huber in a thin-section serial reconstruction study of embryos (Fig. 1-3). Huber's observations were refined and elegantly illustrated by Brödel in 1907.[6,7] Potter and Osathanondh validated the findings in a series of microdissection studies of developing kidneys, which were published in the 1960s.[8-11]

The ultrastructural features and immunohistochemical profiles of the normal kidney and many diseases were elucidated in the 1970s and 1980s following refinement of the percutaneous biopsy technique and advances in morphologic analyses. Today, science is on the threshold of discovering the genetic basis of many mechanisms that mediate normal and abnormal renal development and physiology.

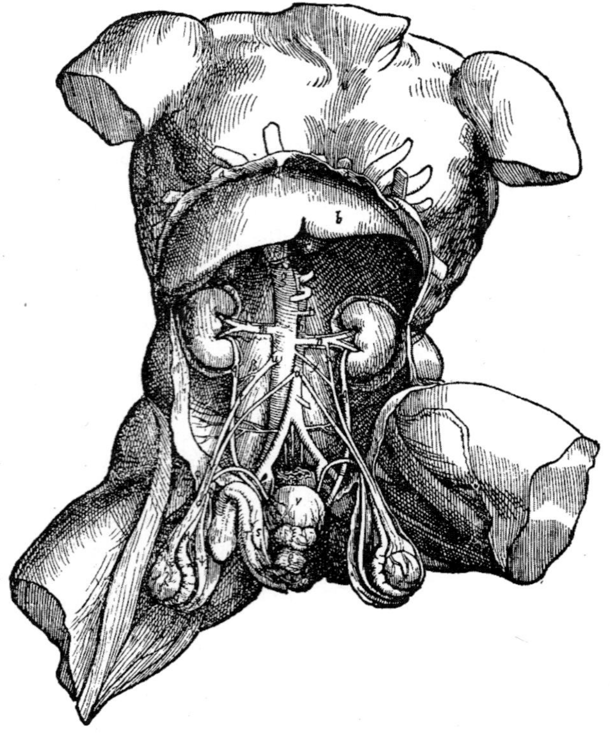

1-1. Vesalius' anatomic illustration of the male genitourinary tract published in 1543. Notice the left kidney is placed lower than the right kidney. *(From Murphy LJT: The history of urology, Springfield, Mass, 1972, Charles C. Thomas; with permission.)*

EMBRYOLOGIC DEVELOPMENT AND NORMAL STRUCTURE

This chapter begins with a brief review of the embryology and normal gross and microscopic structure of the kidney. For a more in-depth coverage of these topics several excellent resources are available.[12-15]

The development of the urinary and genital tracts is closely related (Fig. 1-4). They both develop from paired longitudinal cords of tissue lateral to the aorta, known as the intermediate mesoderm.[12-13] From the portion caudal to the seventh somite, known as the nephrogenic mesoderm (or nephrogenic cord), three nephronic structures develop in quick succession: the pronephros, the mesonephros, and the metanephros. Although the pronephros and the mesonephros are transient organs, they are crucial for the proper development of both the urinary and reproductive tracts.

PRONEPHROS

The first embryologic derivative of the nephrogenic cord is the pronephros, a structure functional only in the lowest forms of fish. It arises from the cranial portion of the mesonephric cord during the third week of gestation (1.7 mm stage). Approximately seven pairs of tubules form, only to regress 2 weeks later (Fig. 1-4). The pronephros is important because the pronephric tubules grow caudally and fuse with the next pronephric unit, giving rise to the pronephric duct, now called the mesonephric duct.

MESONEPHROS

Cells of the mesonephric duct continue to proliferate caudally (Fig. 1-4) and begin to form the mesonephric kidney during the fourth week of gestation (4 mm). The mesonephros is a highly differentiated structure and is the functional kidney of higher fishes and amphibians. Portions of the mesonephric kidney can be easily identified in small embryos (1–3 cm in size), which are occasionally encountered in surgical specimens such as those from ectopic pregnancies (Fig. 1-5).

The mesonephric kidney consists of approximately 40 pairs of nephrons. The cranial nephrons sequentially regress while caudal nephrons form, with 7 to 15 nephrons functional at all times (Fig. 1-4). The nephrons are induced in a fashion analogous to their metanephric counterparts. A fully developed mesonephric nephron consists of a glomerulus connected to the mesonephric duct by a convoluted proximal tubule (Fig. 1-6*A*). The glomerulus is vascularized by capillaries that branch from

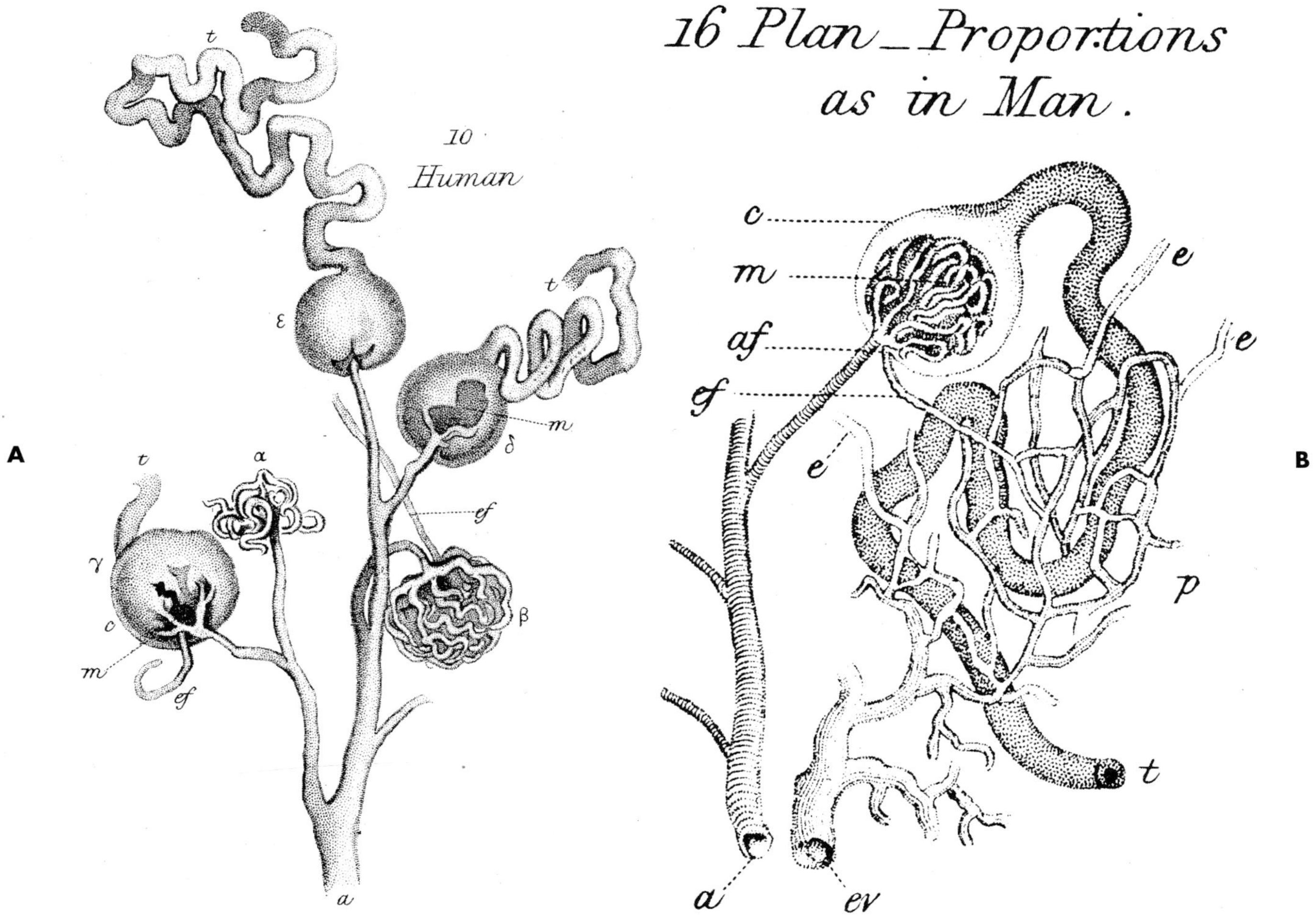

1-2. **A and B,** William Bowman's illustration of the vascular supply to glomeruli and the relationship of the efferent arteriole to the convoluted tubules. *(From Bowman W: On the structure and use of the malphigian bodies of the kidney, with observations on the circulation through that gland, Philos Trans R Soc Lond Biol 132:57, 1842; with permission.)*

small arterioles originating from the aorta and its efferent arteriole empties into the posterior cardinal vein. The glomerulus appears to filter plasma. Its tubule possesses a brush border and appears capable of nutrient resorption, concentration, and dilution of urine. The mesonephric kidney remains functional until the end of the fourth month of gestation.

METANEPHROS

The metanephric kidney is the result of a complex orchestration of embryologic processes. Although discussed separately, it must be appreciated that while the collecting system and renal pyramids are forming there is a simultaneous induction of thousands of nephrons, and neurovascular and lymphatic components ramify in a carefully organized architecture throughout the cortex and medulla.

While the metanephric kidney forms, substantial changes also are occurring in the adjacent müllerian duct and the mesonephric duct (Fig. 1-4) proximal to the origin of the ampullary bud.[12] Following the degeneration of the mesonephric nephrons in males the persisting mesonephric duct develops into male genital secretory structures: epididymis, vas deferens, seminal vesicle, and ejaculatory duct. In females, the müllerian ducts form the fallopian tubes, uterus, and proximal vagina while the mesonephric ducts largely regress, although several embryologic remnant structures persist: epoöphoron, the paroöphoron, and Gartner's ducts.

The formation of the adult metanephric kidney begins during the fifth and sixth weeks of gestation (4–5 mm), after the mesonephric duct has established communication with the urogenital sinus. A diverticulum, known as the ampullary (or ureteric) bud, forms on its posterior medial aspect (Fig. 1-4), establishing contact with the sacral portion of the nephrogenic mesoderm, the nephrogenic blastema. A complex reciprocal inductive process occurs resulting in dichotomous ampullary bud branching and nephron induction eventually culminating in the adult metanephric kidney. The metanephros is therefore a product of two embryonic derivatives; the nephrons are of blastemal origin while the ureter, pelvis,

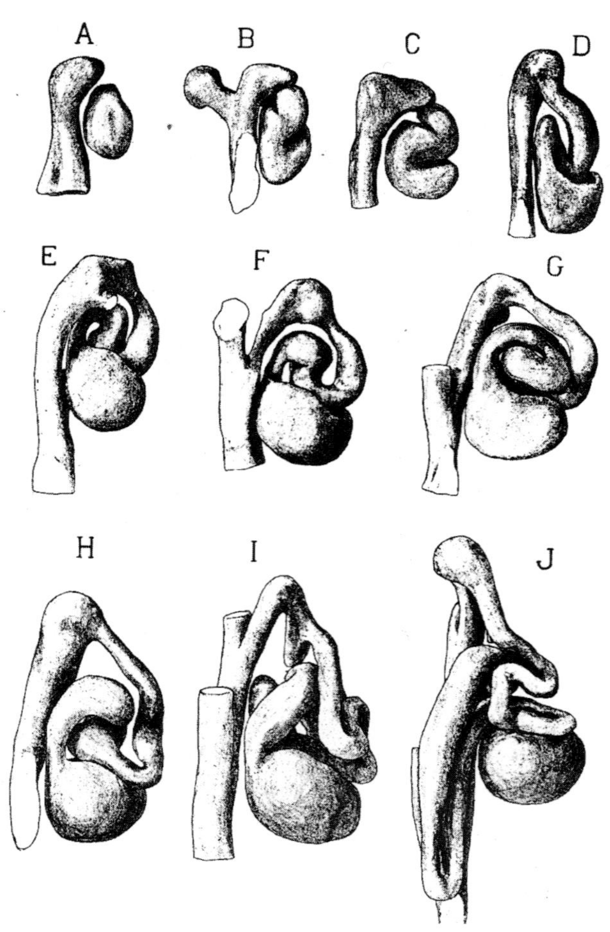

1-3. Wax model serial reconstruction of nephron differentiation by Huber. *(From Huber GC: On the development and shape of uriniferous tubules of certain of the higher mammals, Am J Anat Suppl 4:29, 1905; with permission.)*

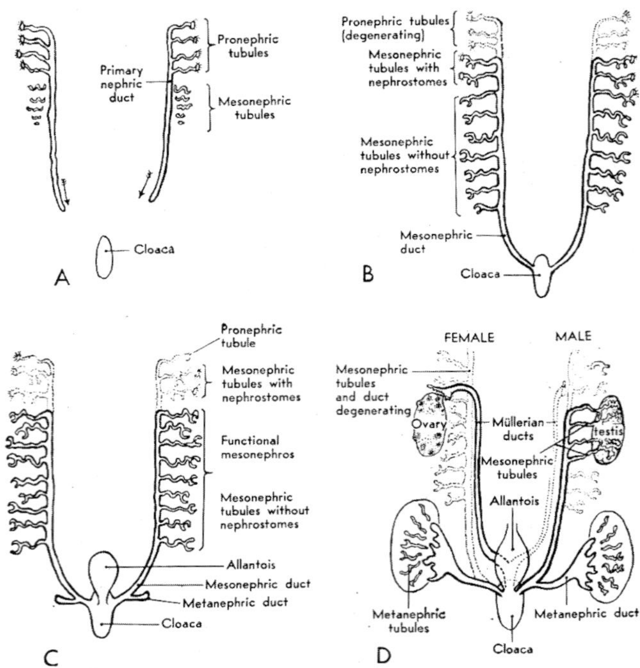

1-4. Diagram illustrating the relationship between reproductive tract and urinary tract development. *(From Patton BM: Human embryology, New York, 1968, McGraw Hill Book Co; with permission.)*

calyces, cortical, and medullary collecting ducts are derived from the ampullary bud.

Upon contact with metanephric blastema, the ampullary bud undergoes a rapid sequence of dichotomous branching and fusion forming the renal collecting system by the fourteenth week.[8] The initial two branches form the renal pelvis, the third to sixth branches form the major and minor calyces, and the sixth to eleventh branches form the papillary ducts (Fig. 1-7). Ampullary bud branching is more rapid in the upper and lower poles, resulting in more numerous calyces and papillae in those regions.

While the collecting system is forming, nephron induction has already begun (Fig. 1-5). The kidneys have moved into the flanks, due to a combination of migration out of the pelvis and rapid caudal growth of the embryo (Fig. 1-8). The kidney also has rotated from its original position with the pelvis anterior to its final position with the pelvis medial.[7] By week 13 or 14, the minor calyces and renal pyramids are well formed and the lobar architecture can be appreciated grossly (Fig. 1-9, 1-10). At this time, the cortex contains several generations of nephrons and the lateral portions of adjacent lobes begin to merge to form the columns of Bertin.

By week 20 to 22 the renal lobes are well formed and the kidney is a miniature of the adult kidney (Fig. 1-11). The ampullae (or collecting ducts at this time) have ceased branching but continue to lengthen.[9,10] As they lengthen, they induce arcades of four to seven nephrons, which are connected to the collecting duct by a connecting tubule (Fig. 1-12). Additional groups of three to seven nephrons then form, each attached directly to a collecting duct without a connecting tubule. Therefore, each cortical collecting duct will have 10 to 14 generations of nephrons attached, with the most recently formed and least mature nephrons located beneath the renal capsule.

NEPHRON DIFFERENTIATION

The formation of individual nephrons begins as early as 7 weeks gestation resulting in a limited degree of "renal function" by 9 weeks. In the subcapsular nephrogenic zone of any immature kidney (Fig. 1-13) the sequence of nephron induction can be observed in its various stages of completion. The wax models made by Huber and the drawing by Brödel (Fig. 1-3, 1-14) provide a three-dimensional perspective useful in understanding the cellular events visible in Fig. 1-13.

An individual nephron begins to form when the metanephric blastema aggregates adjacent to the ampullary bud to form a hollow vesicle.[9-11] The molecular basis for this event is complex and appears to involve growth factors, adhesion molecules, matrix components, and other regulatory proteins.[16,17] The cells within the vesicle grow differentially, resulting in elongation and

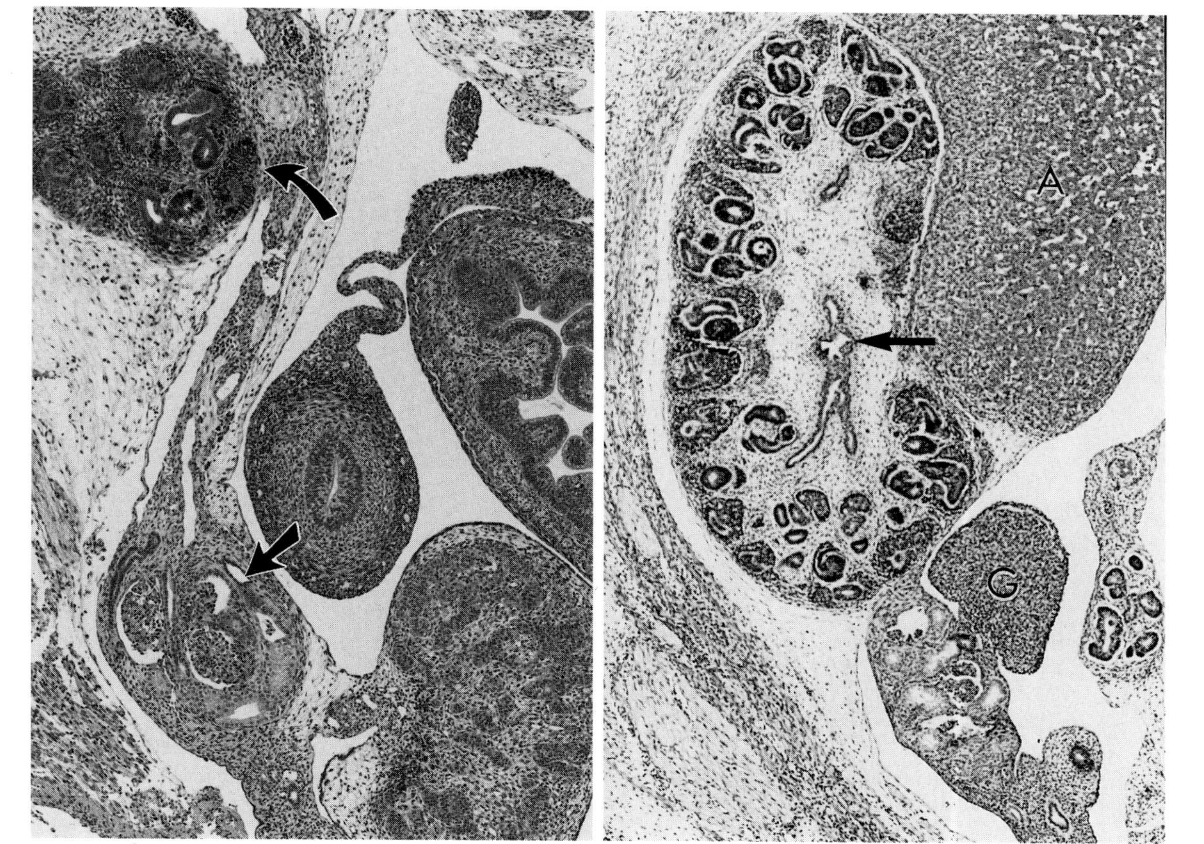

1-5. **A**, An embryo of 7 weeks gestation showing initial induction of the metanephric kidney (*curved arrow*) and glomeruli of the mesonephric kidney (*arrow*). **B**, Embryo of 12 weeks gestation showing a metanephric kidney with a rudimentary collecting system (*arrow*) and active nephrogenesis. The adrenal gland (*A*), gonad (*G*), and mesonephric kidney are also visible.

formation of two indentations creating an S-shaped structure with three segments. The upper and middle segments are destined to become the proximal and distal tubules. They form tubular structures and establish communication with themselves and with the collecting duct. A capillary grows into the lower indentation and branches, and there is broadening and separation of the lower segment into two cell layers, forming a podocyte-invested and vascularized glomerular tuft within Bowman's capsule.

Cells of the upper layer continue to proliferate to form a connecting duct and the distal convoluted tubule while cells of the middle limb produce the proximal convoluted tubule and the limb of Henle. Finally the limb of Henle grows down along the collecting duct to form the medullary rays. Nephrogenesis is usually complete by 32 to 36 weeks gestation. Maturation occurs beyond this period and continues until adulthood, resulting in renal enlargement that reflects elongation and enlargement of the tubular portions of the nephron.

GROSS ANATOMY

The kidneys are paired retroperitoneal organs that normally extend from the twelfth thoracic vertebrae to the third lumbar vertebrae. The upper poles are tilted slightly toward the midline, and the right kidney is slightly lower and shorter than the left kidney. The average adult kidney is 11 to 12 cm long, 5 to 7 cm wide, 2.5 to 3 cm thick, and weighs 125 to 170 g in males and 115 to 155 g in females.[7,12,15] The combined mass of the kidneys correlates with body surface area. Its volume can increase or decrease by 15% to 40% with major fluctuations in blood pressure, hydration, or interstitial expansion by edema.

The posterior surfaces are flatter than the anterior and the medial surface is concave with a 3 cm slit-like space, called the hilum. The hilum is the vestibule through which pass the collecting system, nerves, and vessels. In the adult, these structures are invested by fat within the renal sinus.

The subcapsular surface of the renal cortex may be smooth and featureless or may show grooves corresponding to the individual renal lobes (Fig. 1-15). The persistence of distinct fetal lobes is common and is a normal anatomic variant. In some kidneys, three zones are created by two shallow superficial grooves that radiate from the hilum to the lateral border (Fig. 1-16). The three regions are the upper pole, middle zone, and lower pole and usually reflect regions drained by the three lobar veins.

Text continued on p. 12.

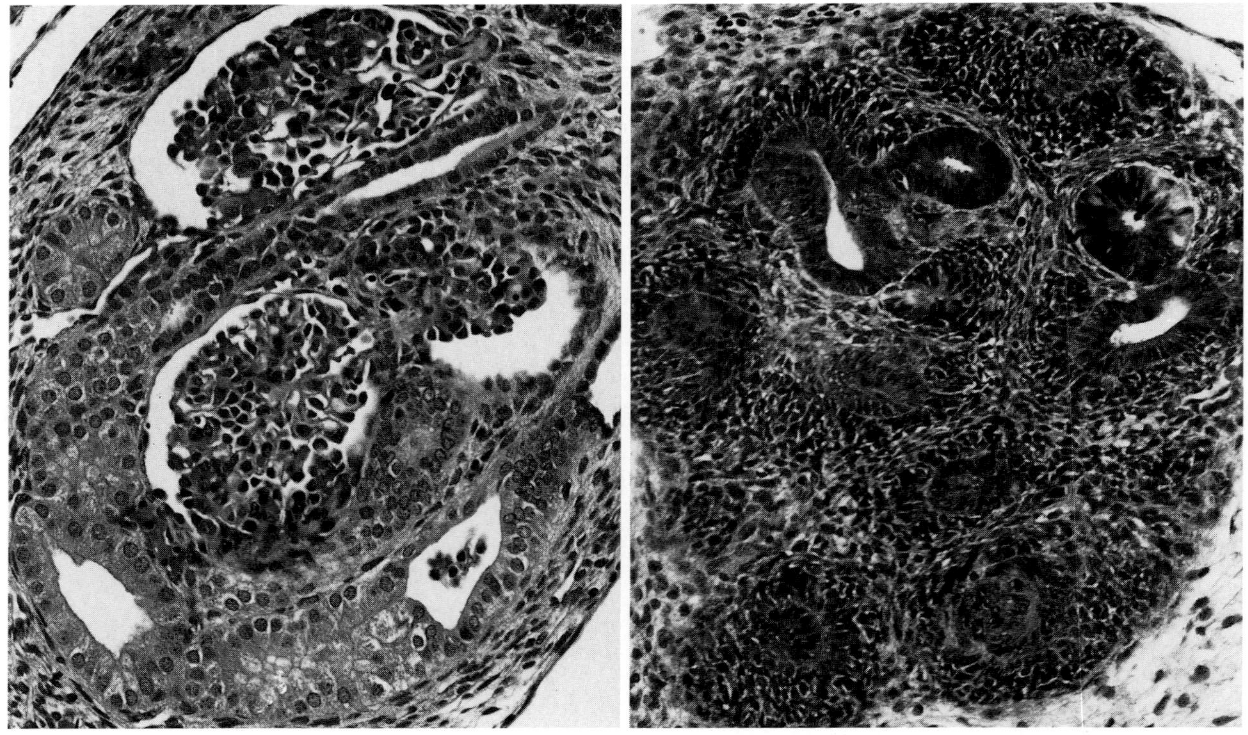

1-6. A, A portion of the mesonephric kidney (*from Fig 1-5A*) showing well developed glomeruli and proximal tubules. **B**, Metanephric kidney (*from Fig 1-5B*) beginning to form, showing condensations of cells destined to form glomeruli.

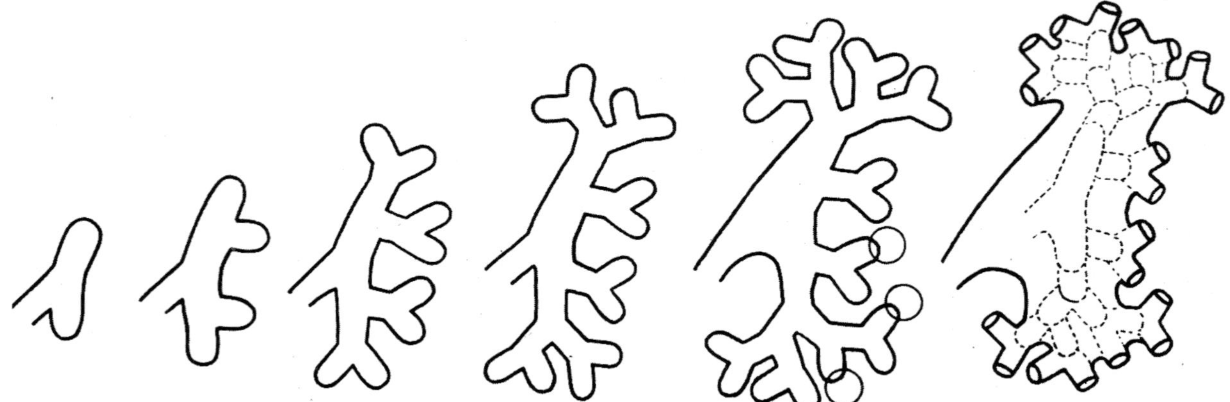

1-7. Development of renal pelvis. Diagram showing branches of ureteral bud. Circles indicate possible locations of minor calyces at level of third, fourth, or fifth generation branches. Figure at right indicates ureteral bud branches that may dilate to form renal pelvis. *(From Osathanondth V, Potter EL: Development of the human kidney as shown by microdissection III. Formation and interrelationship of collecting tubules and nephrons, Arch Pathol 76:61,1963; with permission.)*

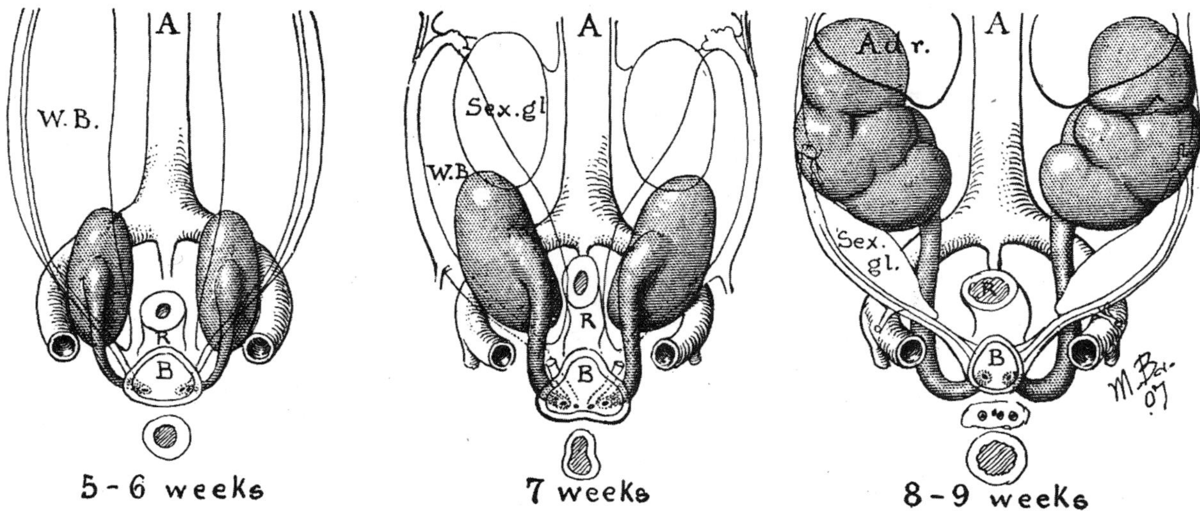

1-8. A 1907 diagram by Max Brödel showing the ascent and medial rotation of the kidney. *(From Kelly HA, Burnam CF: Diseases of kidneys, ureters and bladder, New York, 1914, Appleton, Century and Crofts; with permission.)*

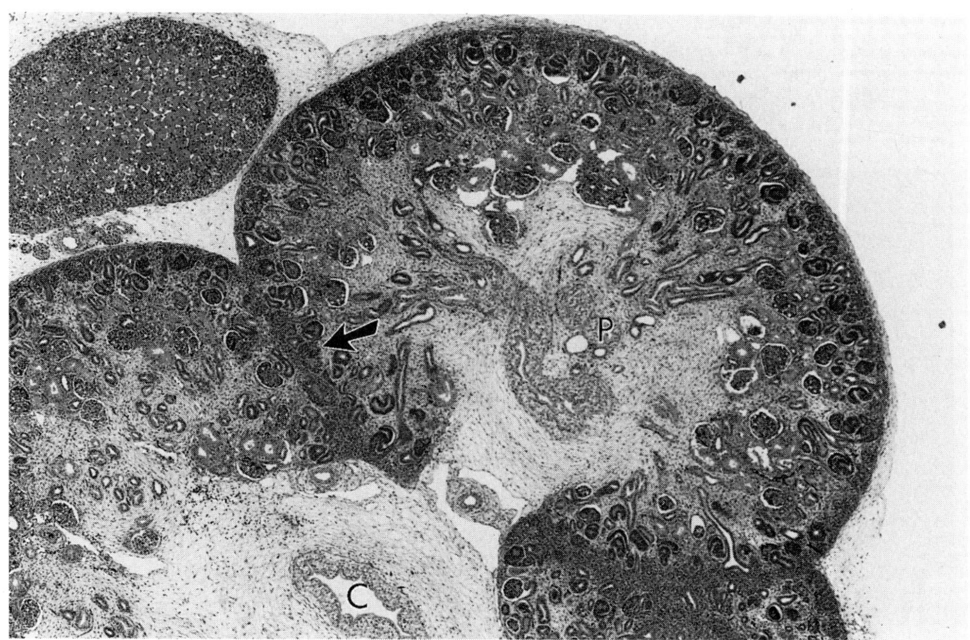

1-9. Kidney from a 13 week fetus (*compare with Fig 1-10*) showing a renal lobe with a pyramid (*P*) and the collecting system (*C*). There is fusion of adjacent lobes forming columns of Bertin (*arrow*).

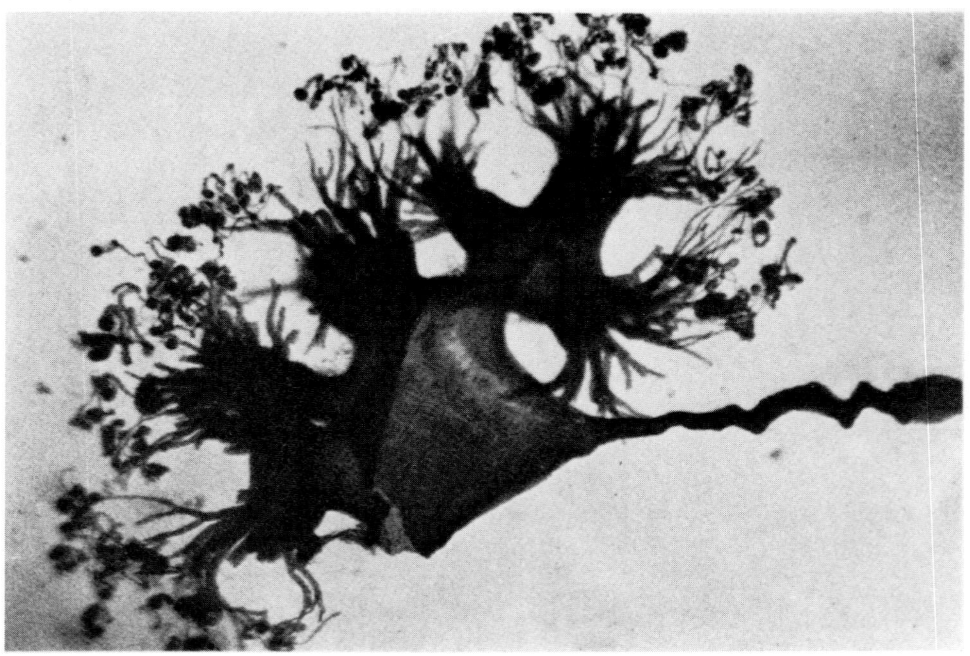

1-10. Microdissected 13 week kidney showing collecting system, renal pyramids, and several generations of glomeruli. Most of the tubules have been removed. *(From Osathanondth V, Potter EL: Development of the human kidney as shown by microdissection III. Formation and interrelationship of collecting tubules and nephrons, Arch Pathol 76:61,1963; with permission.)*

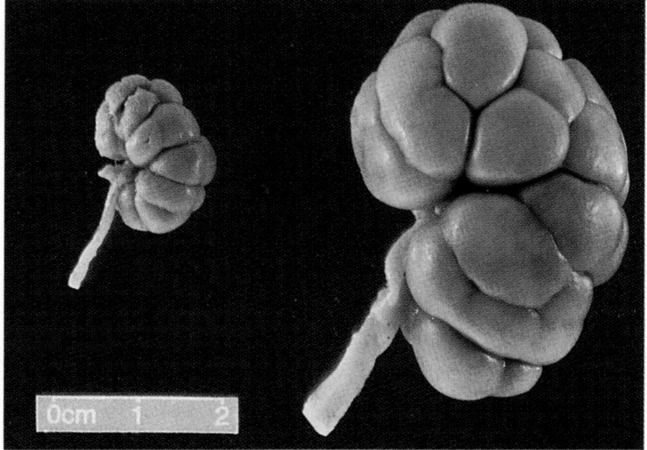

1-11. A 22 week fetal kidney (*left*) and a 40 week term kidney (*right*) showing distinct fetal lobes.

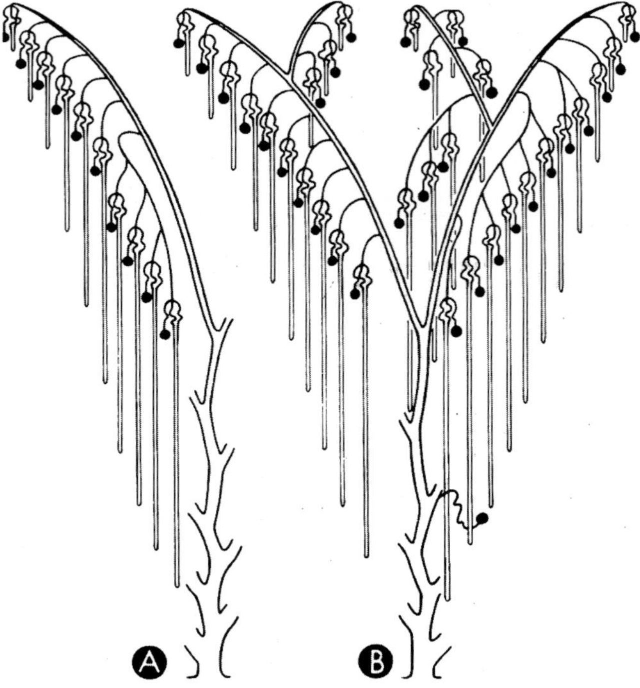

1-12. Kidney showing arrangement of nephrons at birth. **A**, usual pattern; **B**, possible variations. *(From Osathanondth V, Potter EL: Development of the human kidney as shown by microdissection III. Formation and interrelationship of collecting tubules and nephrons, Arch Pathol 76:295, 1963; with permission.)*

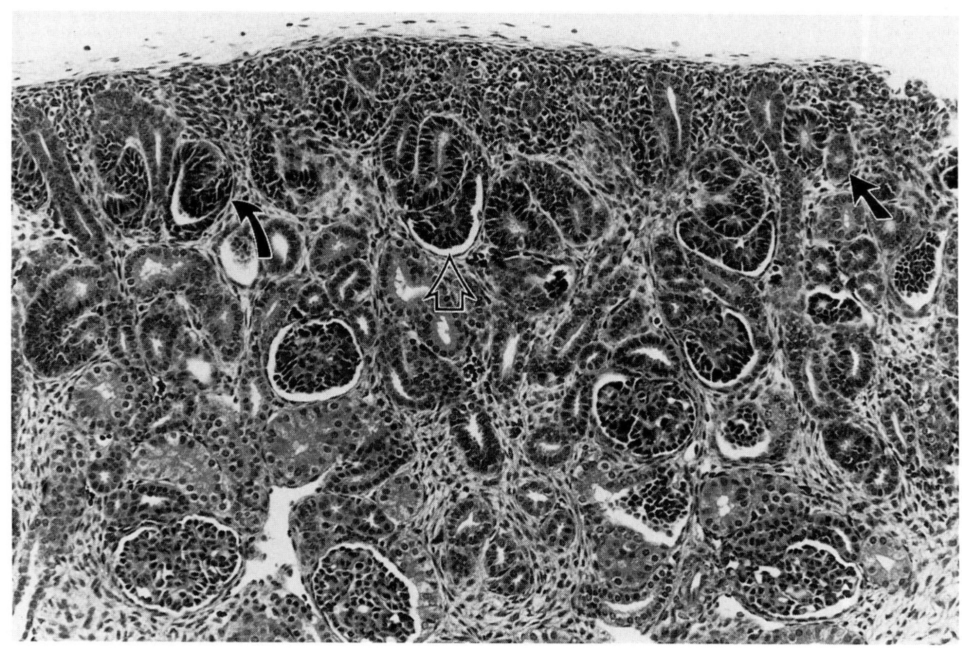

1-13. Nephrogenic zone of a 14 week kidney. Notice ampullary bud and hollow vesicles (*arrow*), early S-phase (*curved arrow*), primitive glomerular tuft (*open arrow*), and increasingly mature glomeruli.

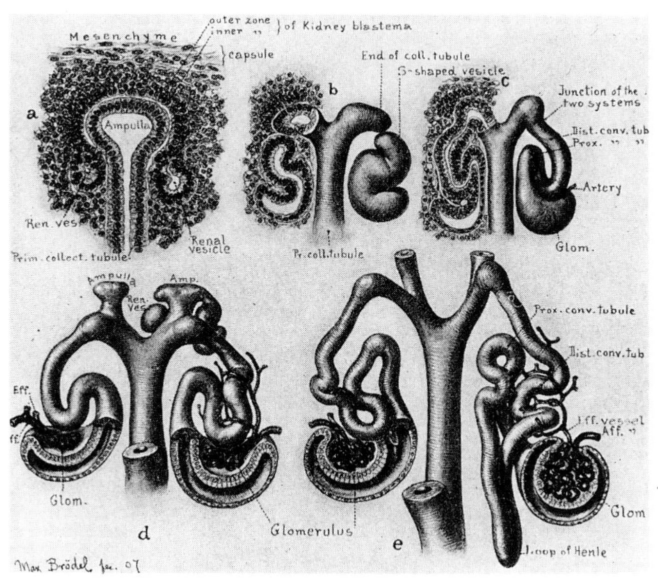

1-14. A 1907 illustration by Max Brödel showing the sequence of nephron induction. *(From Kelly HA, Burnam CF: Diseases of kidneys, ureters and bladder, New York, 1914, Appleton, Century and Crofts; with permission.)*

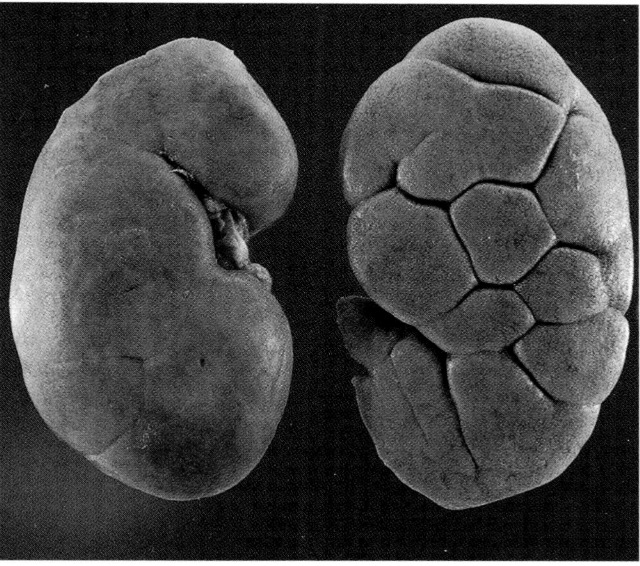

1-15. Two adult kidneys with capsules removed showing subtle fetal lobation (*left*) and prominent fetal lobation (*right*).

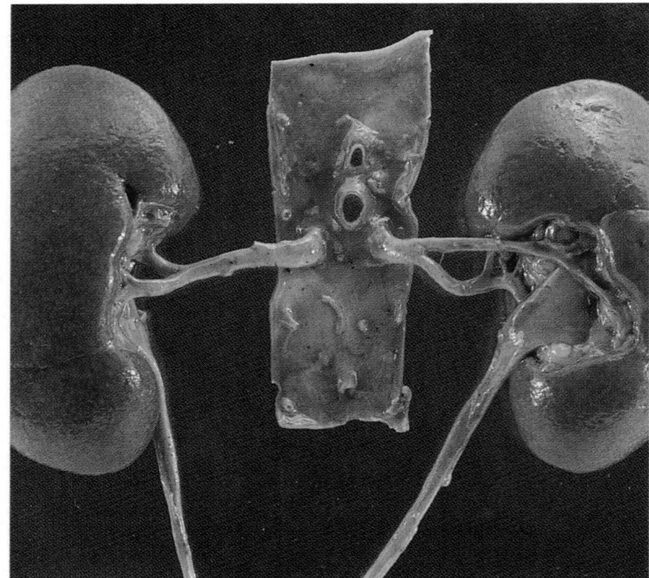

1-16. Kidneys showing two grooves defining renal poles. In each kidney an anterior and posterior division of the renal artery is visible. The left kidney (*right side*) is incompletely rotated.

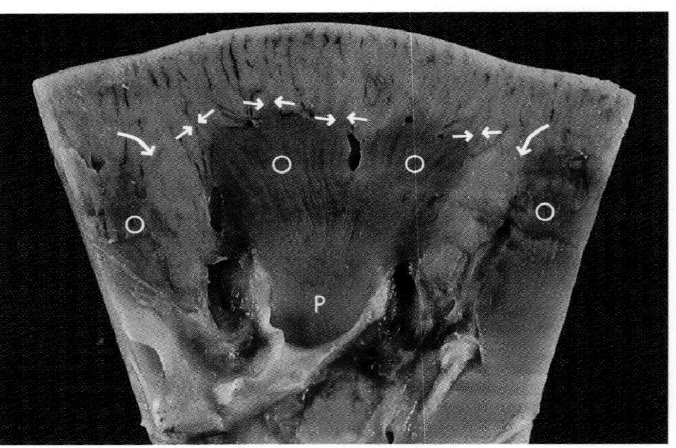

1-17. This renal lobe shows the cortical medullary rays (*arrows*). The columns of Bertin (*curved arrows*) invest the outer medulla (*O*), while the papilla (*P*) or inner medulla is nestled within a minor calyx.

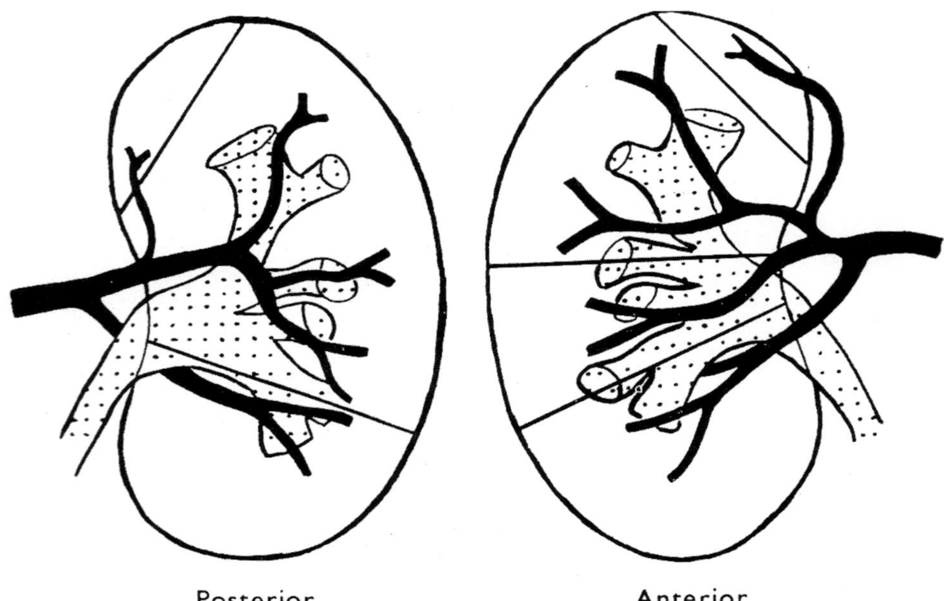

1-18. A diagram of the most common arterial pattern of the kidney showing main renal artery, anterior and posterior divisions, segmental, interlobar, and arcuate arteries. *(From Graves FT: The anatomy of the intrarenal arteries and its application to segmental resection of the kidney, Br J Surg 42:133, 1954; with permission.)*

The normal adult kidney has a minimum of 10 to 14 lobes, each composed of a central conical medullary pyramid surrounded by a cap of cortex (Fig. 1-17). Often there are six lobes in the upper pole and four lobes each in the middle zone and lower pole. However, there is substantial variability both in the number of lobes in the adult kidney and their visibility when the renal capsule is removed.

The renal parenchyma consists of cortex and medulla that are grossly quite distinct (Fig. 1-17). The renal cortex is the nephron containing parenchyma. It forms a 1.0 cm layer beneath the renal capsule and extends down between the renal pyramids forming the columns of Bertin. The midplane of a column of Bertin is the line of fusion of two renal lobes. The medulla consists of renal pyramids and is divided into an outer medulla and the

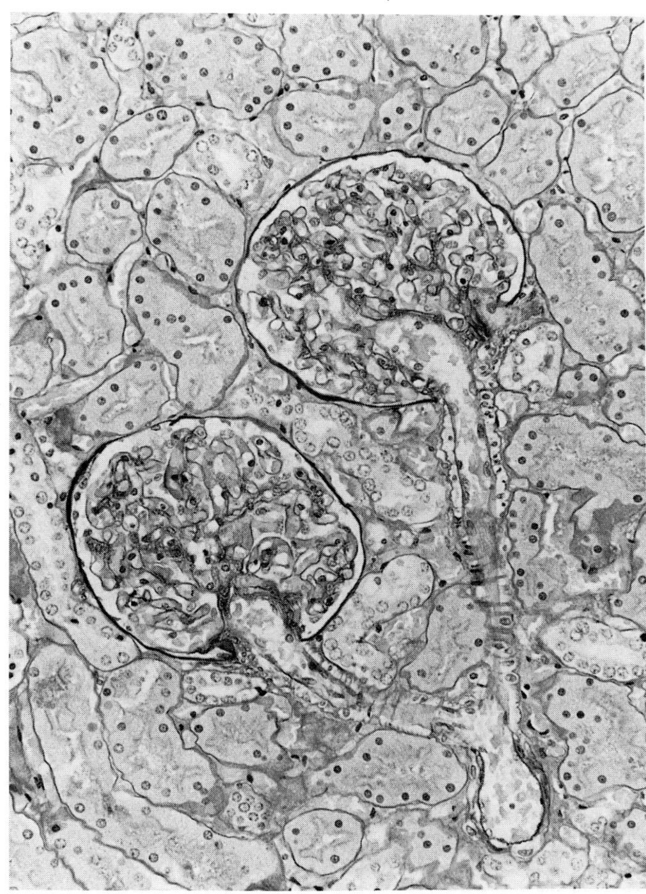

1-19. The interlobular artery supplies arterioles to glomeruli. PAS stain.

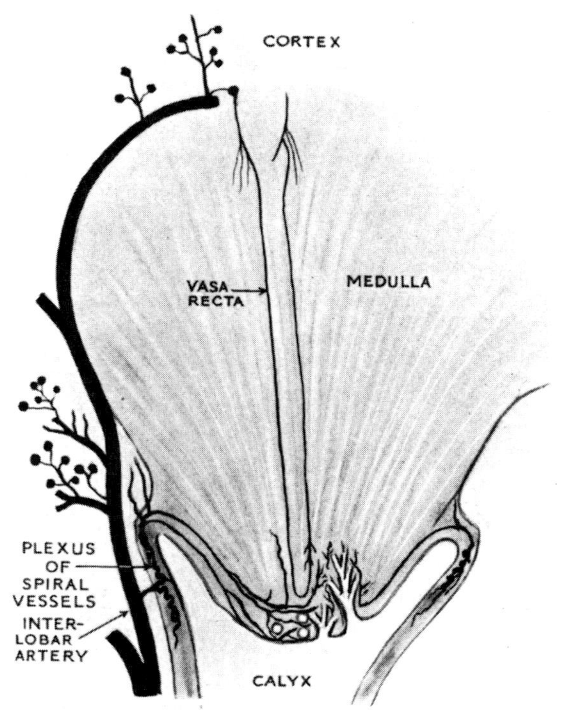

1-20. Diagram of the dual blood supply to the papillae. *(From Baker SB: The blood supply to the renal papillae, Br J Urol 31:57, 1959; with permission.)*

inner medulla or papilla (Fig. 1-17). The outer medulla receives input from nephrons in the overlying cortex and nephrons in the adjacent half of a column of Bertin. The papilla protrudes into a minor calyx. Its tip has from 20 to 70 openings of the papillary collecting ducts (Bellini's ducts).[14,15]

The arterial supply to the kidney follows a general overall blueprint, and knowledge of its details is useful when evaluating lesions in a kidney affected by vascular abnormalities.[18-20] In 1901, Brödel first appreciated the distinctive renovascular segmentation of the kidney.[18] (The nomenclature used here was established by Graves in 1954.[19]) The main renal artery arises from the aorta and divides into an anterior and a posterior division and five segmental arteries are usually derived from these two divisions (Fig. 1-16, 1-18).

The anterior division supplies most of the kidney and often divides into four segmental arteries: the apical, upper, middle, and lower segmental branches. The apical and lower segmental arteries supply the anterior and posterior aspects of the upper and lower poles, respectively (Fig. 1-18). In 20% to 30% of kidneys one or both of these arteries arise separately from the aorta forming supernumerary arteries (also known as aberrant, accessory, or polar arteries). The posterior division becomes the posterior segmental artery. It passes behind the pelvis and supplies the middle two thirds of the posterior surface. The five segmental arteries and all of their branches are end arteries with no collateral blood flow. Thus, occlusion of a segmental artery or any of its subsequent branches results in infarction of the zone of parenchyma it supplies.[20]

From segmental arteries, the interlobar arteries, arcuate arteries, interlobular arteries, and arterioles are sequentially derived. A segmental artery branches within the renal sinus, giving rise to several interlobar arteries. An interlobar artery enters the parenchyma in a column of Bertin between two renal pyramids (i.e., at the junction of two lobes) and forms a splay of six to eight arcuate arteries. The arcuate arteries course along the corticomedullary junction and terminate at the mid-point of a renal lobe. At perpendicular or slightly oblique angles, the interlobular arteries arise from an arcuate artery and may branch as they pass through the cortex toward the renal capsule. The interlobular arteries course between medullary rays and are encircled by tiers of five to six glomeruli, which they supply with afferent arterioles (Fig. 1-19). The glomerular efferent arteriole forms a portal system of capillaries, which supplies the adjacent tubules that arise from more than one glomerulus (see Fig. 1-2*B*).

The renal medulla has a dual blood supply.[21] Its principal blood supply arises from the efferent arterioles of the juxtamedullary glomeruli, which course directly into the medulla forming the vasa rectae (Fig. 1-20). In addition, as an interlobar artery courses along a minor calyx it gives rise to several spiral arteries, which supply arterioles to the papillary tip. These arterioles anastomose freely with arterioles from the opposite side, forming a plexus around the ducts of Bellini.

The interlobular, arcuate, and interlobar veins parallel the arteries. Unlike the arcuate arteries, the arcuate veins have abundant anastomoses. They combine to form three large lobar veins that drain the three poles of the kidney.[18] These veins lie anterior to the pelvis and unite to form the main renal vein.

The lymphatic drainage is a dual system. The major lymphatic drainage follows the blood vessels from parenchyma to the renal sinus, to the hilum, and terminates in lateral para-aortic lymph nodes. There also is a capsular lymphatic drainage from the superficial cortex, which courses into the capsule and then around to the hilum to join the major lymphatic flow.

MICROSCOPIC ANATOMY

The cortex is organized into two regions: the cortical labyrinth and the medullary rays (Fig. 1-21). The labyrinth contains glomeruli, proximal and distal convo-

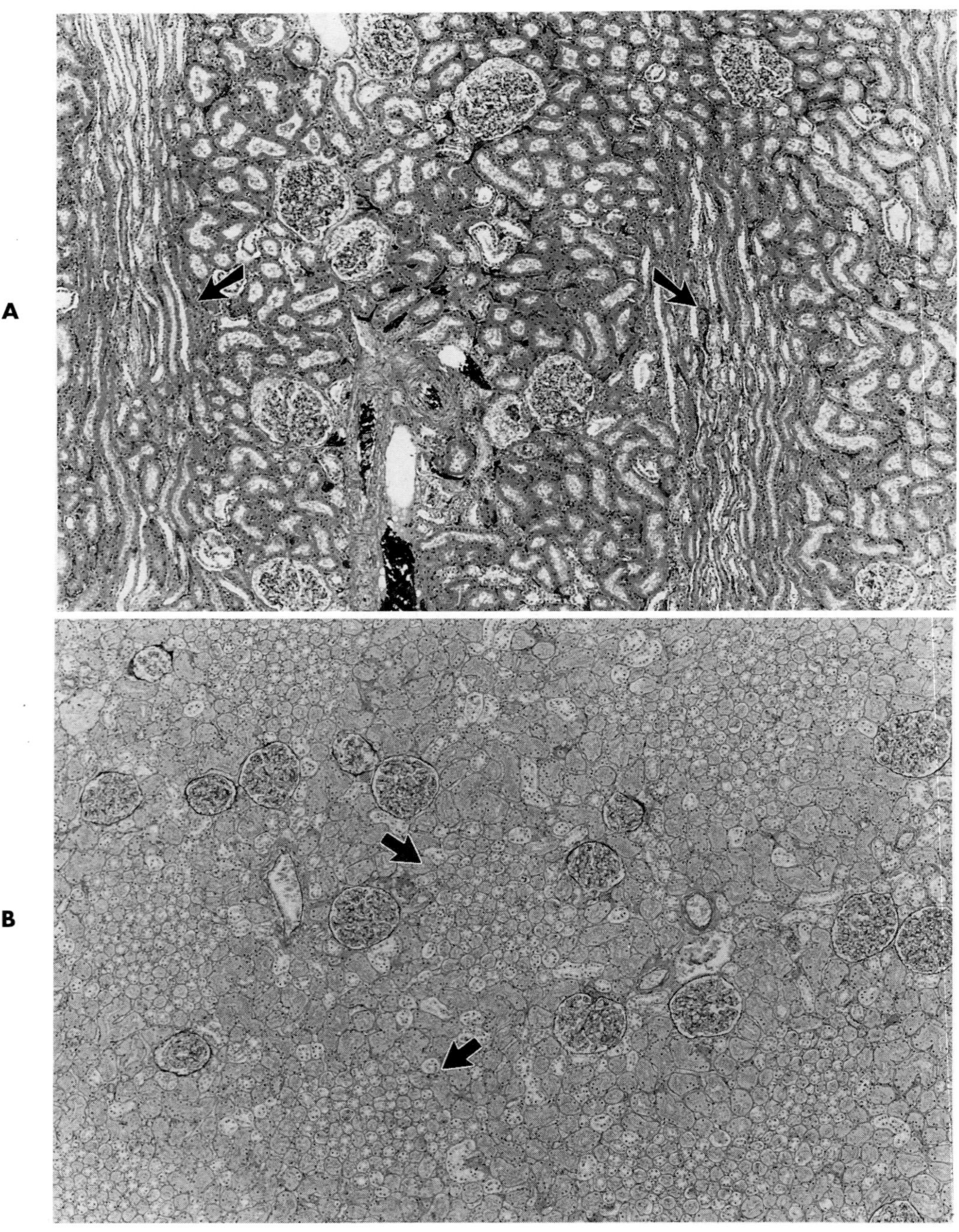

1-21. Renal cortex sectioned perpendicular (**A**) and parallel (**B**) to the renal capsule showing medullary rays (*arrow*) and the cortical labyrinth. B-PAS stain.

luted tubules, connecting tubules, the initial portion of the collecting ducts as well as interlobular vessels, arterioles, capillaries, and lymphatics. The principal components of the labyrinth are mostly proximal tubules. In the normal cortex the tubules are closely packed with basement membranes in close contact (Fig. 1-19, 1-21). The interstitial space is scant. It contains the peritubular capillary plexus and lymphatic capillaries. A medullary ray consists of collecting ducts and the proximal and distal straight tubules that course down into and back up from the medulla. The nephrons that empty into the collecting ducts of a single medullary ray comprise a renal lobule, the functional unit of the kidney.

The medulla is divided into an outer medulla composed of an outer stripe and an inner stripe and the inner medulla or papilla. Each zone contains specific tubular segments arranged in an elaborate architecture to create the countercurrent concentration system. For further details of the microscopic anatomy of the medulla or for the ultrastructural features of the nephron components, Clapp[14] and Venkatachalam and Kris[15] are two excellent resources.

CONGENITAL ANOMALIES AND CYSTIC DISEASES

> The more complicated an organ in its development, the more subject it is to maldevelopment, and in this respect the kidney outranks most other organs.[13]
>
> Edith Potter

Abnormalities of development of the genitourinary tract occur in approximately 10% of the population.[22] As captured in the quote by Potter, this is not surprising in light of the complicated organogenesis of these systems.[13]

It is difficult to develop a completely satisfactory classification of the diverse array of anomalies that affect the urinary tract (see box on this page). The ideal schema would account for morphologic features and clinical importance as well as pathogenesis. The occurrence of multiple malformations in a single patient and the occurrence of a specific malformation in multiple hereditary and nonhereditary syndromes, coupled with limitations in our understanding of pathogenesis, make classification extremely difficult. Although knowledge of the embryologic development of the kidney provides a tempting basis for explaining departures from the normal renal development, it must be accepted that there is little experimental evidence to defend most such conjectures. This section, therefore, emphasizes diagnostic features and their clinical importance.

DEVELOPMENTAL ABNORMALITIES AND CYSTIC DISEASES OF THE KIDNEY

Abnormalities in form and position
- Rotation anomaly
- Ectopia
- Fusion

Abnormalities of mass and number

Supernumerary kidney

Renal hypoplasia
- Simple hypoplasia
- Oligomeganephronia

Renal agenesis
- Unilateral agenesis
- Potter's syndrome
- Syndromic agenesis

Parenchymal maldevelopment and cystic diseases

Renal dysplasia
- Multicystic and aplastic dysplasia
- Segmented dysplasia
- Dysplasia associated with lower tract obstruction
- Dysplasia associated with hereditary syndromes
- Hereditary renal dysplasia and urogenital dysplasia

Polycystic kidney disease
- Infantile (recessive) polycystic kidney disease
- Adult (dominant) polycystic kidney disease

Cysts (without dysplasia) in hereditary syndromes
- Medullary cystic disease/nephronophthisis
- von Hippel-Lindau disease
- Tuberous sclerosis
- Glomerulocystic kidney disease
- Congenital nephrotic syndrome of the Finnish type

Miscellaneous
- Renal tubular dysgenesis
- Acquired cystic disease
- Segmental cystic disease
- Medullary sponge kidney
- Simple cortical cyst
- Pyelocalyceal ectasia and diverticuli

ABNORMALITIES IN FORM AND POSITION

It is useful to group abnormalities of form and position because they often occur in combination. For instance, fused kidneys are always ectopic and most ectopic or fused kidneys also are abnormally rotated. Each anomaly may occur in isolation or may represent one component of a more serious complex of malformations affecting other urologic sites or other organ systems. Each may be completely innocent and asymptomatic; however, if urinary tract symptoms develop, they invariably result from impaired urinary drainage, which may cause hydronephrosis or pain and may be complicated by infection or nephrolithiasis.

Rotation anomaly

During ascent of the kidney to a lumbar location, the renal pelvis rotates 90 degrees from an anterior to a medial position (Fig. 1-8). Failure of the pelvis to assume a medial orientation, reverse rotation, or over rotation to a posterior or even lateral location, comprise a spectrum of orientation abnormalities known as rotation

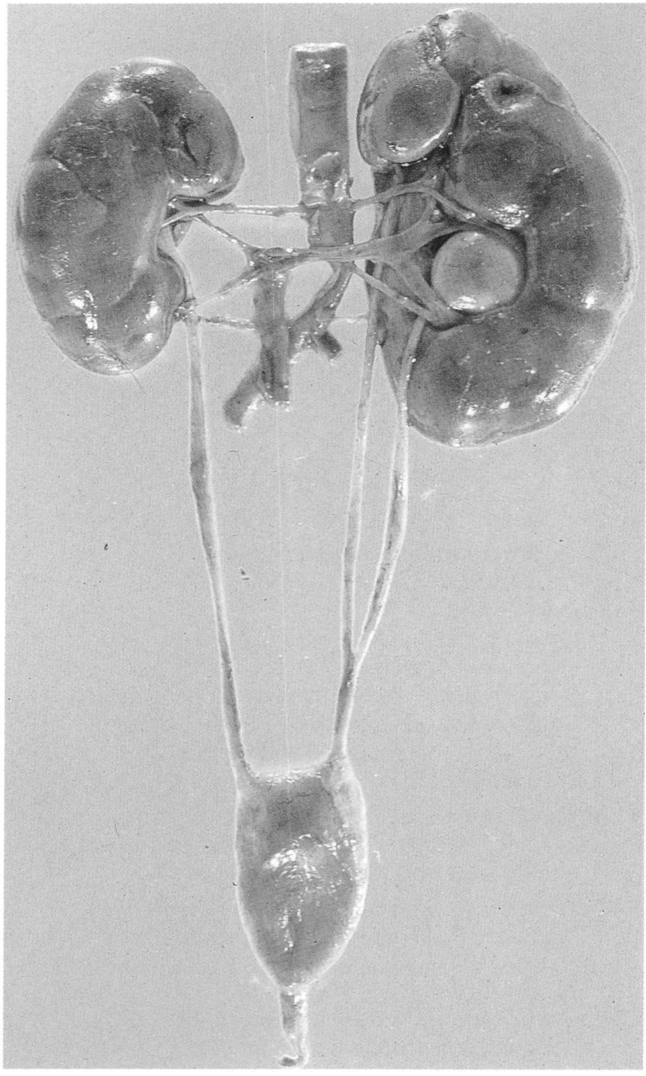

1-22. A duplex left kidney with a bifid ureter and a nonrotated (anterior) lower pelvis. An inferior supernumerary artery and a normal vein cross the ureter resulting in ureteropelvic junction obstruction.

anomalies.[23] Some degree of malrotation occurs in 1:400 to 1:1000 individuals.[22] The most common rotation anomaly is nonrotation or incomplete medial rotation resulting in an anterior location of the pelvis and ureter (Fig. 1-16, 1-22). This may occur as an isolated abnormality in an otherwise normal kidney. It always accompanies renal ectopia or renal fusion. Ureteropelvic obstruction may on occasion result from a crossing vessel (Fig. 1-22). Excess rotation or reverse rotation with the pelvis posterior or lateral pelvis are very rare.[23]

Renal ectopia

Failure of the kidney to assume its proper location in the renal fossa is known as renal ectopia.[24-29] There are several varieties named according to location (see box on this page). Renal ectopia should be distinguished from renal ptosis in which a normally situated kidney shifts to a lower position. The origin of the renal artery from a normal aortic location identifies a lower situated kidney as ptotic rather than ectopic. The incidence of ectopia at autopsy ranges from 1:660 to 1:1200.[24,25] Renal ectopia is bilateral in 10% of cases.

The three most common forms of renal ectopia are inferiorly located kidneys.[24,25] The kidney may be nonreniform in shape, its pelvis and ureter are anterior (nonrotated), and the ureter is short and usually placed in the bladder, but may have a high insertion on the pelvis leading to obstruction. The vascular supply is influenced by the final location of the kidney, arising from the aorta, common iliac, internal or external iliac, or inferior mesenteric arteries (Fig. 1-23). The contralateral kidney may be normal or occasionally may be absent or even dysplastic. Other anomalies of urologic organs and cardiovascular, skeletal, and gastrointestinal systems are frequent in both males and females.[24,25]

Cephaloid ectopia is usually associated with an omphalocele.[26] The kidney appears to continue its ascent when the abdominal organs herniate into the omphalo-

TYPES OF RENAL ECTOPIA

- Pelvic—opposite sacrum
- Iliac—opposite sacral prominence
- Abdominal—above iliac crest
- Cephaloid—subdiaphragmatic
- Thoracic—supradiaphragmatic
- Crossed—contralateral
  - with fusion (90%)
  - without fusion (10%)
  - solitary crossed (rare)
  - bilateral crossed (rarest)

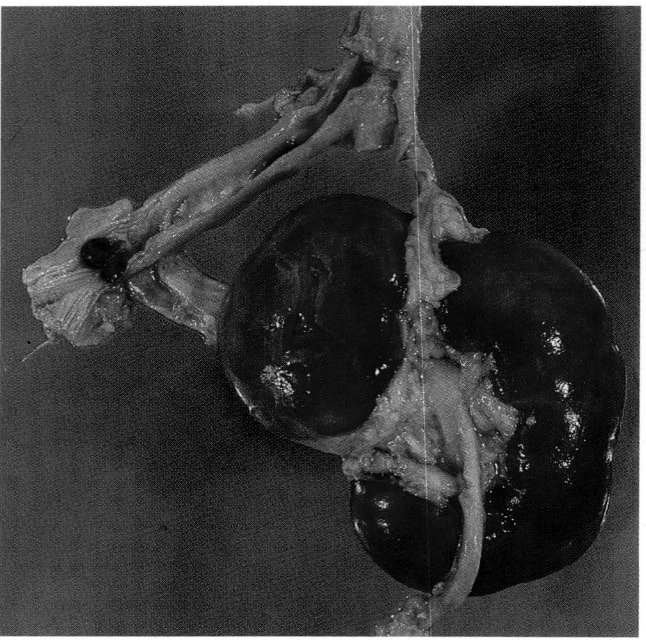

1-23. A hypertrophic pelvic kidney with an anterior ureter in an asymptomatic patient with unilateral agenesis.

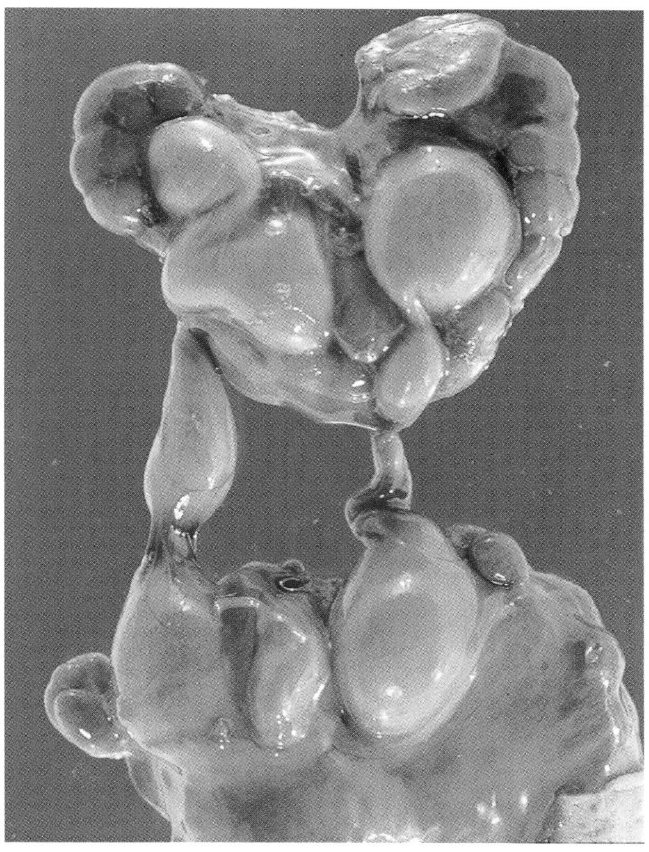

1-24. Horseshoe kidney showing hydroureteronephrosis from a neonate with trisomy 18 and multiple congenital anomalies.

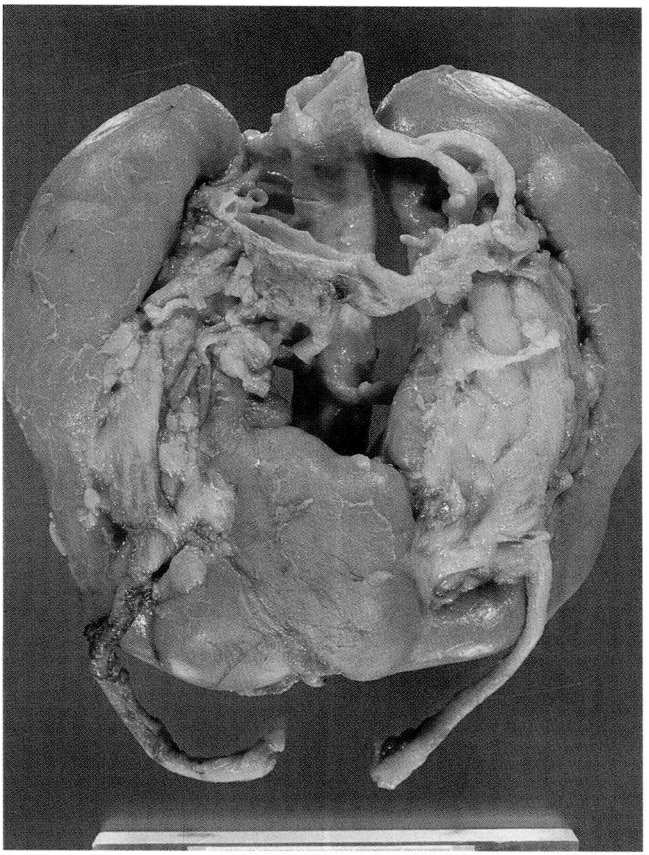

1-25. Horseshoe kidney as an incidental autopsy finding in an adult.

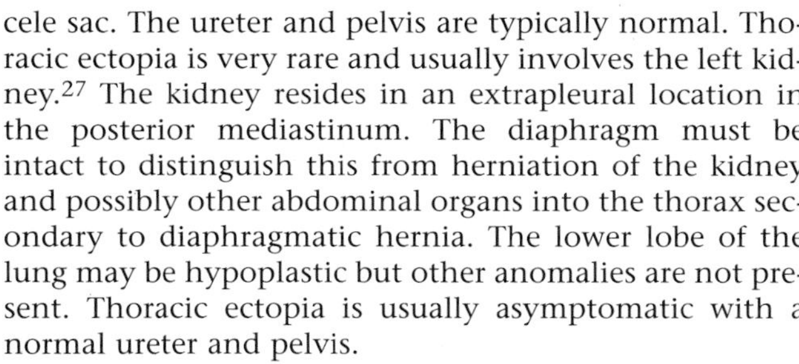

cele sac. The ureter and pelvis are typically normal. Thoracic ectopia is very rare and usually involves the left kidney.[27] The kidney resides in an extrapleural location in the posterior mediastinum. The diaphragm must be intact to distinguish this from herniation of the kidney and possibly other abdominal organs into the thorax secondary to diaphragmatic hernia. The lower lobe of the lung may be hypoplastic but other anomalies are not present. Thoracic ectopia is usually asymptomatic with a normal ureter and pelvis.

In crossed ectopia the kidney is situated opposite the side of insertion of its ureter in the trigone.[28,29] Four combinations are possible as listed in the box on page 16. In 90% of cases there is also fusion to the other kidney. In crossed fused ectopia the kidneys may assume a variety of shapes and positions giving rise to six "types": inferior, superior, lump, sigmoid, disc, L-shaped.[28] The kidneys function normally and their ureters are normally located within the bladder, but their pelves are nonrotated. Extrarenal anomalies (genital, skeletal, and anal-rectal) occur in 20% to 25% of patients.[28,29]

Horseshoe kidney

Horseshoe kidney is the most common form of renal fusion.[30,31] It is the midline fusion of two distinct renal masses, each with its own ureter and pelvis (Fig. 1-24, 1-25). Horseshoe kidney is relatively common (1:400-2000) with a 2:1 male predominance.[30] The fusion is typically at the lower poles but can vary greatly in the quantity of fused parenchyma. A horseshoe kidney is ectopic and usually situated anterior to the aorta and vena cava. Occasionally the fusion will be posterior to the vena cava or posterior to both the aorta and vena cava. The ureters and pelves are always anterior. This coupled with commonly encountered high insertion of the ureter on the pelvis can result in obstruction (Fig. 1-24). Approximately 30% of patients will also have other anomalies of the urinary tract, central nervous system, heart, gastrointestinal tract, or skeletal system.[30,31]

ABNORMALITIES IN MASS AND NUMBER

In contrast to those anomalies listed in the preceding section, the following group of anomalies is much less common and they are unrelated abnormalities. Hypoplasia is usually bilateral while supernumerary kidney is usually unilateral and neither is hereditary. The renal parenchyma in each is normally formed. In contrast renal agenesis can be either unilateral or bilateral and may be hereditary.

Supernumerary kidney

Supernumerary or duplicated kidney is one of the rarest disorders.[32,33] It has been defined as "a free accessory

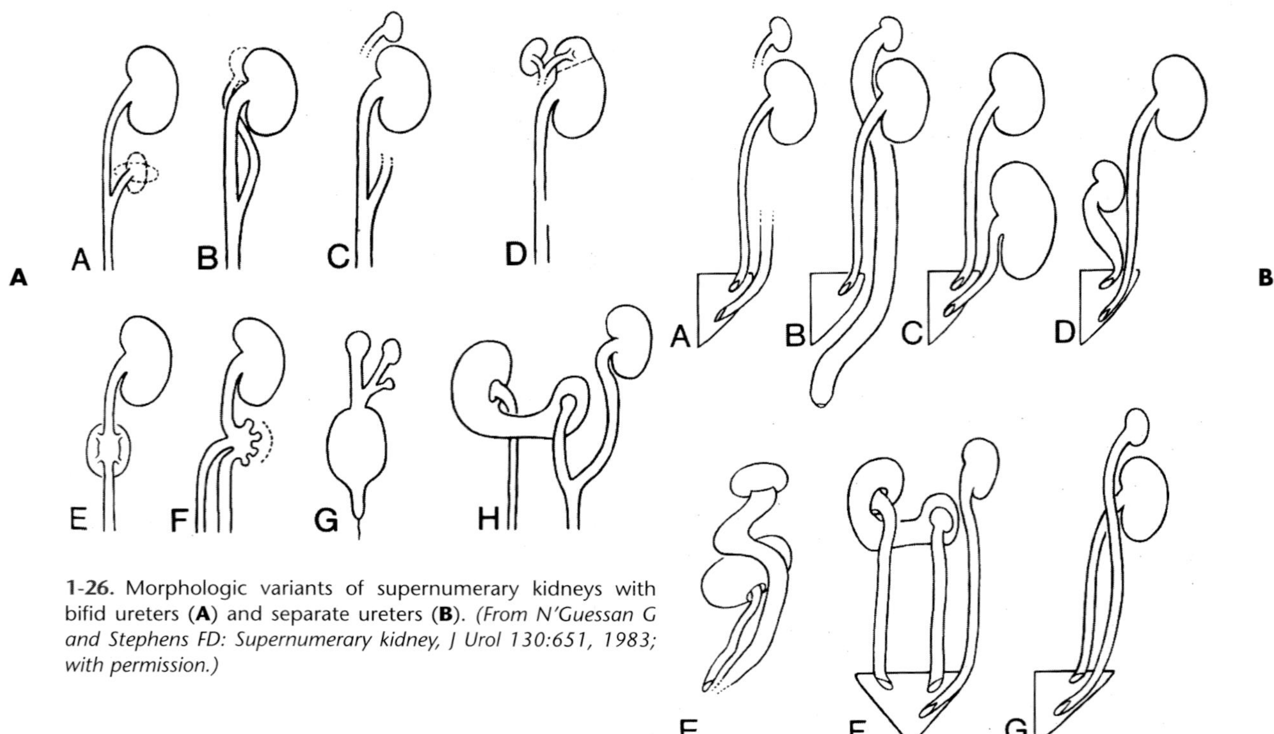

1-26. Morphologic variants of supernumerary kidneys with bifid ureters (**A**) and separate ureters (**B**). *(From N'Guessan G and Stephens FD: Supernumerary kidney, J Urol 130:651, 1983; with permission.)*

organ, which is a distinct, encapsulated, large or small parenchymatous mass topographically related to the usual kidney by a loose, cellular attachment at most and often by no attachment whatsoever."[32] It may be located below (most common), above, or adjacent to the kidney and is rarely bilateral. It is connected to the lower urinary tract by either a bifid ureter or its own completely separate ureter (Fig. 1-26). In half the reported cases, complications have developed related to obstruction and infection.[32,33]

Hypoplasia

Hypoplasia refers to a small (less than 50% of normal) but otherwise normally developed kidney.[20,34] By definition, dysplastic elements are absent. There are two types of hypoplasia: simple hypoplasia and oligomeganephronia. Previously included in this category was the so-called segmental hypoplasia or Ask-Upmark kidney, which is now regarded as an acquired lesion secondary to vesicoureteral reflux.

Simple hypoplasia. Simple hypoplasia is a rare, usually bilateral, nonhereditary disease in which the small size of the kidney usually reflects a marked reduction in the number of renal lobes.[34,35] Frequently only one to five lobes are present. Occasionally the small size reflects a decrease in the number of cortical glomeruli. Hypertrophic nephrons and dysplastic elements are absent. When bilateral, the small kidneys may eventually fail to provide renal function with body growth and renal insufficiency or renal failure may develop, the severity determined by the degree of hypoplasia.

Oligomeganephronia. Oligomeganephronia, the most common form of renal hypoplasia, is a bilateral nonhereditary disorder.[36-38] The kidneys are small due to a reduction in the number of renal lobes and in the number of nephrons within each lobe. Microscopically the nephrons present are tremendously enlarged (Fig. 1-27). Glomerular and tubular volumes have been measured to be 12-times and 17-times normal, respectively.[37]

Children with oligomeganephronia present with a concentration defect causing polyuria, polydipsia, and salt wasting, resembling patients with juvenile nephronophthisis. Renal insufficiency and proteinuria gradually develop with body growth as progressive glomerular and tubulointerstitial scarring develops. The absence of a family history of renal disease, the presence

RENAL AGENESIS

Sporadic forms of renal agenesis
- Unilateral renal agenesis
- Bilateral renal agenesis (Potter's syndrome)

Syndromic renal agenesis
- Chromosomal anomalies (Trisomy 13 and 18)
- VATER association
- Müllerian aplasia syndrome (MURCS)
- Sirenomelia (caudal regression syndrome)
- Cloacal exstrophy
- Fraser's syndrome
- Williams syndrome
- Multiple malformation syndromes, NOS
- Hereditary renal adysplasia

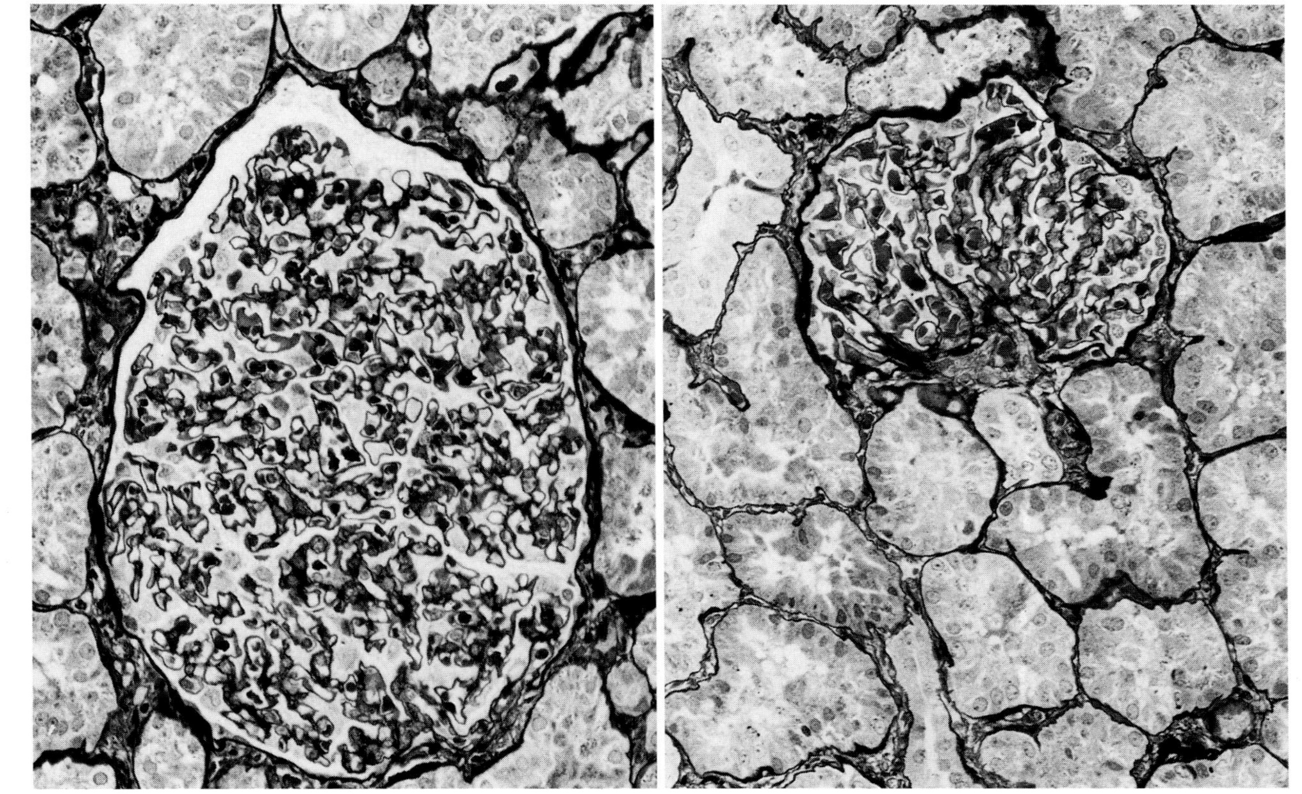

1-27. **A**, Oligomeganephronia in a 22-month-old with an enlarged glomerulus. **B**, Glomerulus of normal size in a 2-year-old.

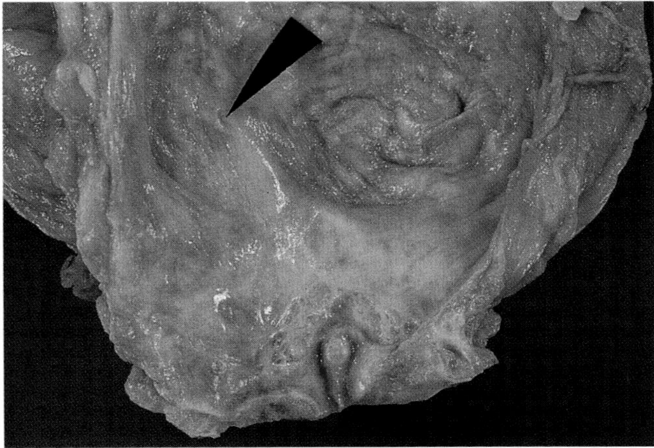

1-28. Bladder showing absent left hemitrigone in an adult with a sporadic form of unilateral renal agenesis. The right hemitrigone is indicated with arrow.

of proteinuria, and imaging studies revealing symmetrically small noncystic kidneys, usually permit separation from nephronophthisis.

Renal agenesis

Absence of the kidney and its corresponding ureter is known as renal agenesis (see box on this page).[39-43] The corresponding hemitrigone is also absent because it represents the distal continuation of the ureteral smooth muscle (Fig. 1-28).[42]

OLIGOHYDRAMNIOS PHENOTYPE

- Potter facies
- Increased interocular distance
- Broad flattened nose
- Prominent inner canthic folds (sweep downward and lateral)
- Receding chin
- Large, low-set ears with little cartilage
- Positional deformities (flexion of hips and knees, clubbed feet)
- Dry skin
- Hypoplastic lungs
- Small bladder with absent trigone
- Placenta—amnion nodosum

Unilateral renal agenesis. In unilateral renal agenesis the contralateral kidney may be hypertrophic up to twice the normal size. The overall renal function may be normal and the condition may be entirely asymptomatic (Fig. 1-23). In up to 70% of patients, agenesis is associated with additional anomalies most often affecting the genital tracts.[41-46] This presumably reflects a common abnormality affecting development of both the mesonephric duct–and müllerian duct–derived structures. The genital

1-29. A fetus born with oligohydramnios showing the characteristic Potter's facies in anterior (**A**) and lateral (**B**) views.

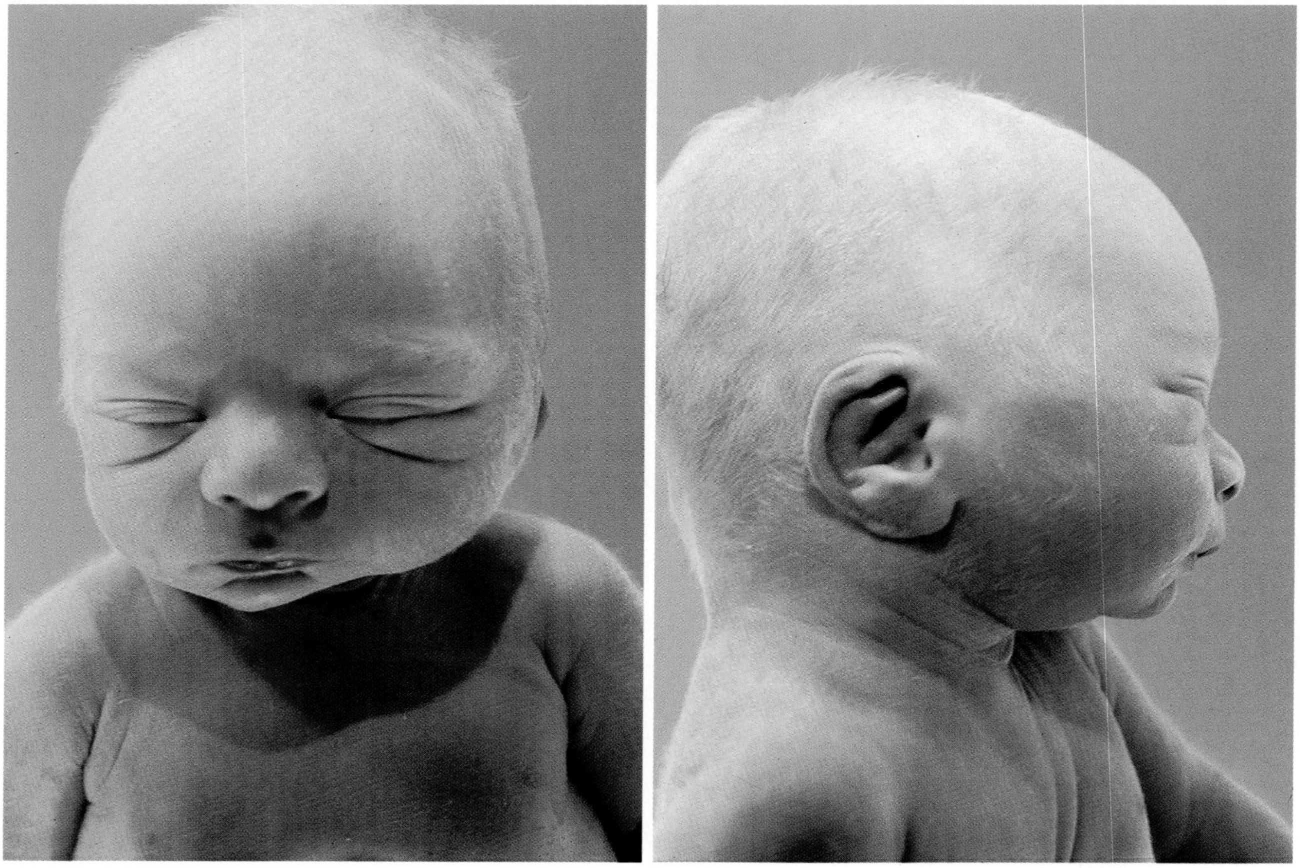

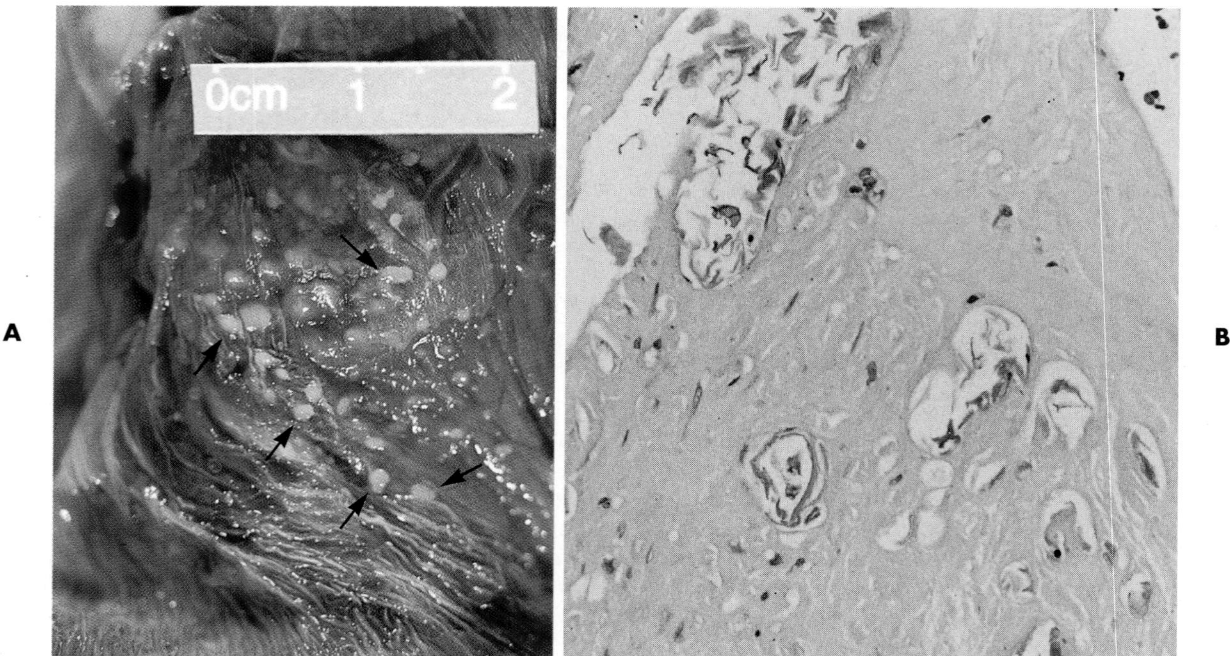

1-30. A, Placenta with plaques of amnion nodosum (*arrow*). **B**, Plaques of amnion nodosum contain clumps of fetal squames embedded in dense collagen.

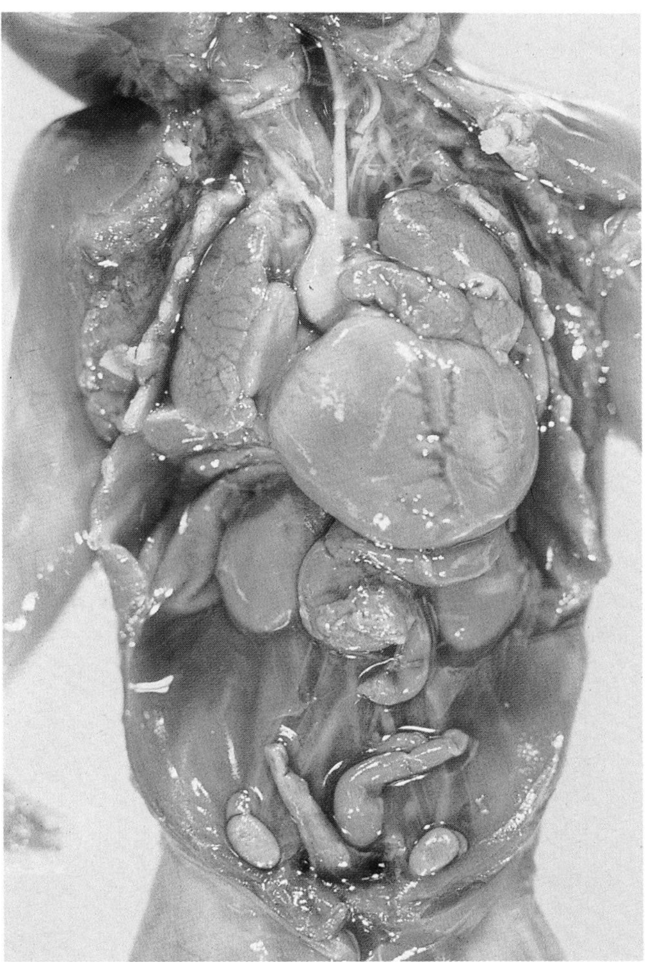

1-31. The third consecutive fetus affected with bilateral renal-ureteral agenesis in familial renal adysplasia. The small and large bowel have been removed to reveal adrenal glands but absent kidneys.

anomalies in females include absence of the ipsilateral fallopian tube, uterine horn, and proximal vagina or uterine didelphia or vaginal septum.[43-46] In males there may be absence of the ipsilateral epididymis, vas deferens, or seminal vesicle or a seminal vesicle cyst may be encountered.[41-42] Identification of a patient with a unilateral genital anomaly or renal agenesis should therefore prompt evaluation of the other organ system.

Potter's syndrome (bilateral renal agenesis). Bilateral renal agenesis is a uniformly fatal disorder known as Potter's syndrome.[39] Approximately 40% of affected fetuses are stillbirths and those born alive die of pulmonary failure within 48 hours. Mothers present with severe oligohydramnios because fetal urine normally accounts for most of the amniotic fluid in the second half of gestation. Oligohydramnios impairs pulmonary development resulting in pulmonary hypoplasia and produces a variety of distinctive gross features known as the Potter's or oligohydramnios phenotype[40,47,48] (see box on this page). (Figures 1-29 through 1-31 demonstrate some of these characteristic findings.)

CAUSES OF OLIGOHYDRAMNIOS

Major causes
- Potter's syndrome (bilateral renal agenesis)
- Bilateral renal dysplasia
- Distal (complete) urinary tract obstruction

Rare causes
- Infantile polycystic kidney disease
- Glomerulocystic kidney disease
- Renal tubular dysgenesis
- Chronic amniotic fluid leak
- In utero acute renal failure
- Idiopathic

Some doctors refer to any fetus born with the oligohydramnios phenotype as having Potter's syndrome, rather than reserving the term for the entity of bilateral renal-ureteral agenesis as initially described. This can be confusing because oligohydramnios has several other causes[49,50] (see box on this page).

Syndromic renal agenesis. A large number of syndromes have absence of one (or rarely both) kidney as a component of a constellation of congenital anomalies.[41,46,49-62] This includes chromosomal anomalies, several malformation complexes, and multiple malformation events affecting the gastrointestinal, cardiac, central nervous system, or skeletal system, which do not conform to a specific syndrome. Finally it may also occur in a familial disorder with renal dysplasia (see Hereditary Renal Adysplasia later in this chapter).[58-62] In each disorder, identification of extrarenal components and a detailed family history are essential for proper classification and appropriate genetic counseling. The extrarenal anomalies are responsible for many complications and for the lethal nature of many of the syndromes.

PARENCHYMAL MALDEVELOPMENT AND CYSTIC DISEASES

Abnormalities of development and cystic diseases are a challenging group of anomalies that are important because several forms have hereditary implications. They are difficult to clarify because of inconsistent use of terminology, a failure to understand existing classifications, and the rarity of certain forms.

When a cystic kidney is encountered, the initial task is classification. Potter's classification of congenital cystic diseases (Table 1-1) first introduced some order into this perplexing field.[13] The classification is based on microdissection of cystic kidneys, which localized the cysts to specific segments of the nephron. Unfortunately this approach did not translate into a clinically useful formulation because hereditary and nonhereditary forms were not separated and dysplasia appeared in three of the four types (see box on page 15). A more practical formulation separates the two hereditary polycystic kidney diseases (infantile and adult) from renal dysplasia, and divides dysplasia into sporadic forms and those occurring in hereditary syndromes with multiple malformations.[63-65]

TABLE 1-1.
CLINICOPATHOLOGIC ENTITIES AND THEIR RELATIONSHIP TO POTTER'S CLASSIFICATION OF CYSTIC DISEASES

Potter's Classification	Clinicopathologic Entities
Type I	Infantile (autosomal recessive) polycystic kidney disease, perinatal, and neonatal form
Type IIa	Multicystic renal dysplasia
IIb	Aplastic renal dysplasia
Type III	Adult (autosomal dominant) polycystic kidney disease Focal renal dysplasia Dysplasia in hereditary syndromes Infantile polycystic kidney disease, infantile and juvenile form
Type IV	Dysplasia associated with lower tract obstruction

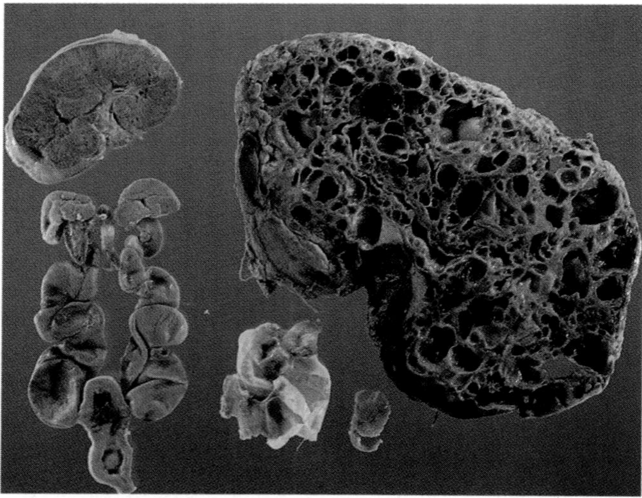

1-32. Infantile polycystic kidney and adult polycystic kidney (*upper left and right*) and three forms of renal dysplasia: aplastic dysplasia from a 35-year-old, multicystic dysplasia from a neonate, and bilateral dysplasia associated with lower tract obstruction (*lower left*).

TABLE 1-2.
CONGENITAL CYSTIC DISEASES

	Dysplasia	IPKD	APKD
Incidence	1:1000-2000	1:50,000	1:500-1000
Bilateral	+/-	+	+
Segmental	+/-	-	-
Ureter abnormal	+	-	-
Reniform shape	+/-	+	+
Uniform cysts	-	+	-
Liver abnormal	-	+	+
Other malformations	+/-	-	-

IPKD=Infantile polycystic kidney disease; *APKD*=Adult polycystic kidney disease.

MULTIPLE MALFORMATION SYNDROMES IN WHICH RENAL DYSPLASIA MAY OCCUR

Common Occurrence

- VATER (VACTERL) association
- MURC syndrome
- Prune-belly syndrome
- Caudal regression syndrome
- Cloacal exstrophy
- Urogenital sinus syndrome
- Urorectal septum syndrome sequence
- Meckel-Gruber syndrome*
- Dandy-Walker syndrome*
- Short rib-polydactyly syndrome*
- Elejalde's syndrome*

Occasional Occurrence

- Trisomy C
- Trisomy 13
- Trisomy 18
- Persisting mesonephric duct syndrome
- Zellweger syndrome*
- Jeune's syndrome*
- Smith-Lemli-Opitz syndrome*
- Beckwith-Wiedemann syndrome*
- Laurence-Moon-Bardet-Biedl syndrome*

*Autosomal recessive inheritance

Although there are numerous conditions that can give rise to cystic kidneys, three are of greatest importance: renal dysplasia, infantile polycystic kidney disease, and adult polycystic kidney disease. Although subtle versions of each occur, most cases encountered are sufficiently distinctive that they can be recognized by gross examination (Fig. 1-32 and Table 1-2).

Both polycystic kidney diseases are hereditary and result in enormous, bilateral, diffusely cystic kidneys with reniform shapes and normal ureters (Fig. 1-32). Although cystic, parenchymal maldevelopment is not present. Each has an associated hepatic lesion, but other visceral malformations are absent. In contrast, dysplastic kidneys are by definition maldeveloped (Fig. 1-32). They are usually not reniform, they vary greatly in size and appearance, and they occur in several patterns: unilateral, bilateral, or confined to the upper pole of a duplex kidney. Approximately 90% of cases have a ureteral abnormality or are associated with distal obstruction resulting in ureteral stenosis or dilation and megacystis or bladder hypertrophy. Renal dysplasia most commonly is sporadic but may be familial, part of a multiple mal-

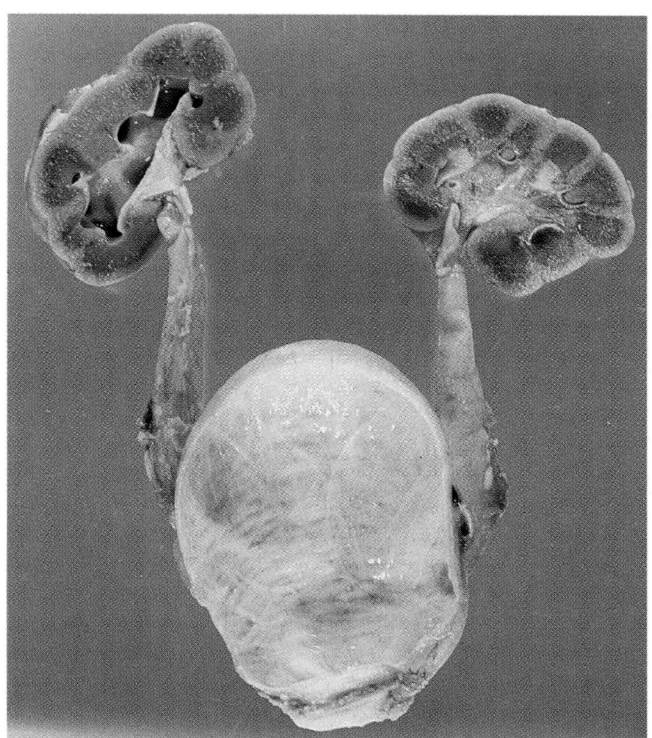

1-33. Megacystis and hydroureteronephrosis without renal dysplasia in a term infant with complete urinary tract obstruction secondary to urethral atresia.

formation complex, or a component of an hereditary malformation syndrome (see box on p. 22).

Renal dysplasia

A dysplastic kidney is a metanephric structure with aberrant nephronic differentiation.[13,63-66] The term *dysplasia* is used in a developmental sense and does not connote any relationship to neoplasia. Dysplastic kidneys should not be confused with hypoplastic kidneys, which are small but otherwise normally developed, nor with polycystic kidney diseases, which although cystic do not contain dysplastic elements.

The pathogenesis of renal dysplasia has not been established. There are two major theories that are not mutually exclusive. Dysplasia has traditionally been attributed to "in utero" urinary tract obstruction, a reasonable concept in light of the common association between obstruction and dysplasia.[64,65] However, normal renal development can occur in the face of complete urinary tract obstruction (Fig. 1-33) and dysplasia resembling the human disease has been very difficult to produce in experimental animals by early in utero urinary tract obstruction.[67]

The second theory implicates a fundamental defect in inducer tissue (ampullary bud) or responding tissue (blastema).[16,17,67,68] This postulate can also account for the combination of ureteral and renal maldevelopment and can accommodate the occurrence of dysplasia in hereditary syndromes and malformation complexes where diverse genetic, teratogenic, and developmental field defects have been implicated.

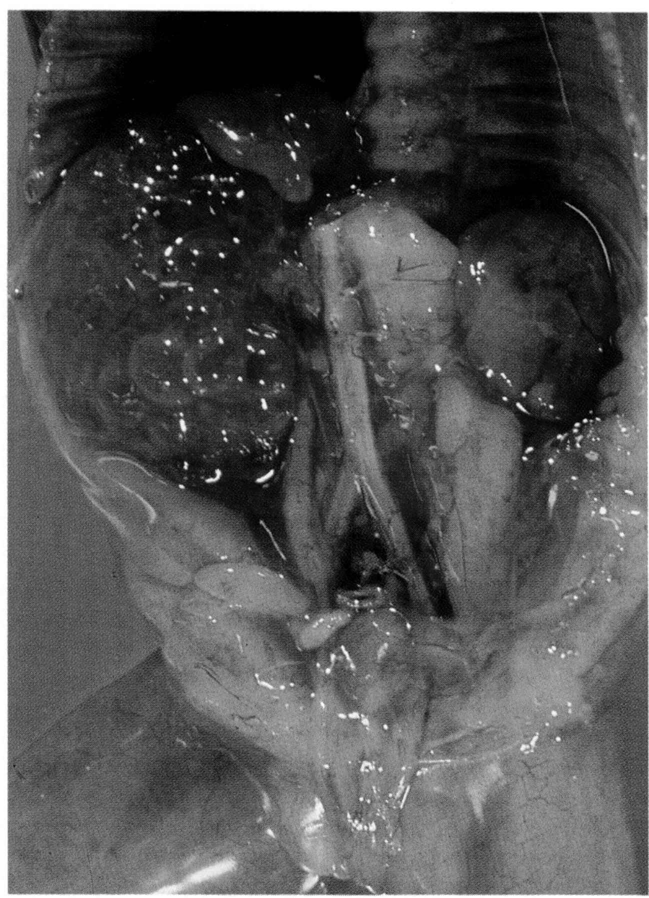

1-34. Unilateral multicystic dysplasia shown in situ.

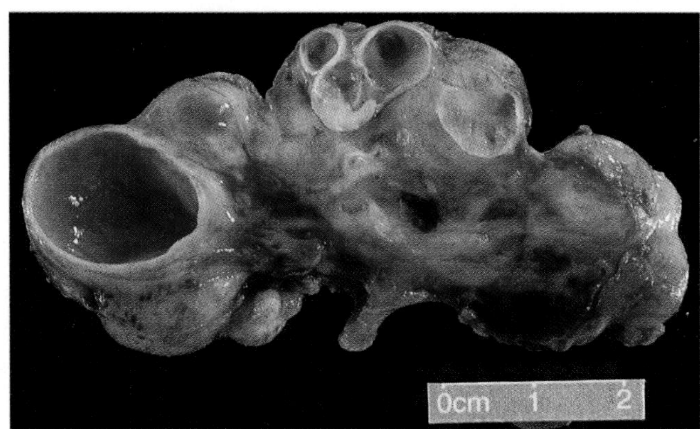

1-35. Transverse section of a multicystic dysplastic kidney.

Multicystic and aplastic dysplasia. Dysplastic kidneys vary tremendously in gross appearance, ranging from the large multicystic kidney to the small aplastic kidney (Fig. 1-32). These represent a morphologic continuum and differ only in the extent of cyst formation. When multicystic dysplasia or aplastic dysplasia is bilateral the infant presents with Potter's syndrome and dies of pulmonary hypoplasia. The multicystic kidney is the most common cause of a renal mass in a child and is usually unilateral (Fig. 1-34, 1-35).

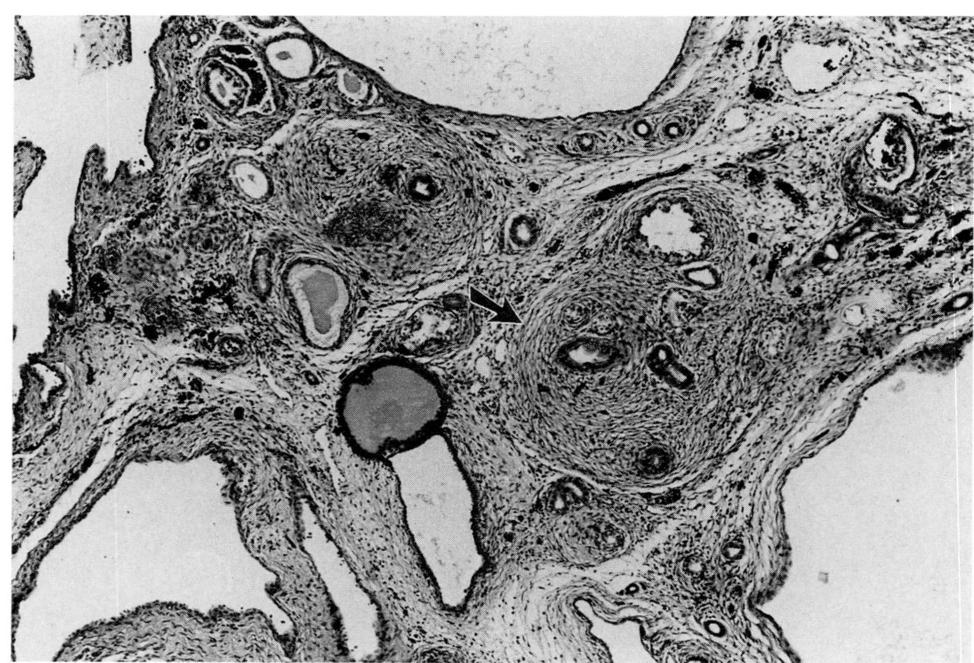

1-36. A dysplastic kidney composed of cysts, dysplastic ducts (*arrow*), and primitive tubules.

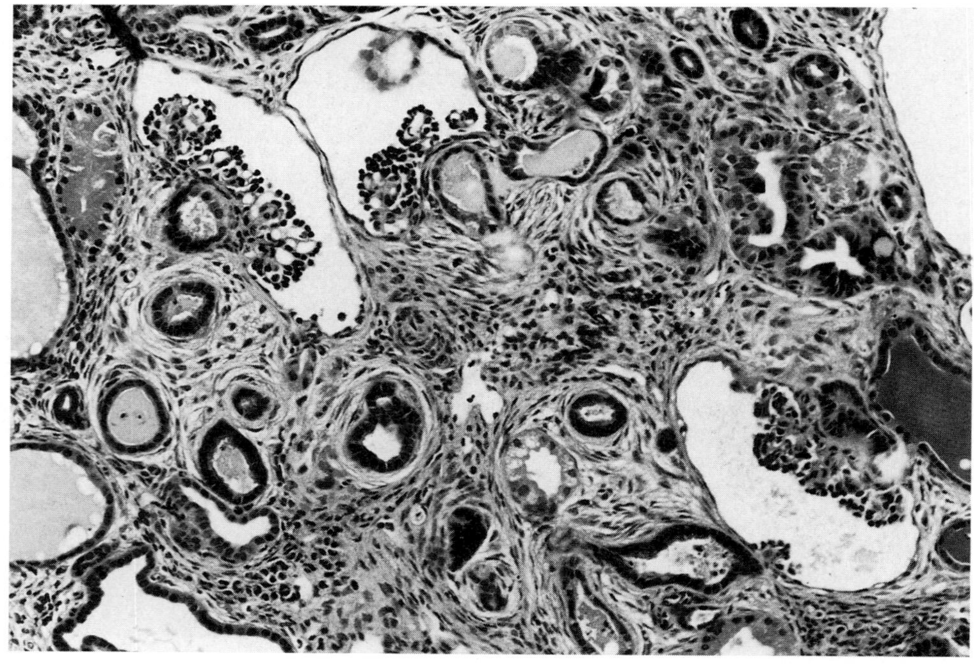

1-37. A dysplastic kidney containing abnormally formed glomeruli and immature tubules.

The histologic appearance of a dysplastic kidney can be quite varied.[13,64-70] Primitive or dysplastic ducts and fetal or immature appearing cartilage often are present (Fig. 1-36, 1-37, 1-38, 1-39). Dysplastic ducts are lined with columnar epithelium and surrounded by collars of spindle cells (Fig. 1-36). They are thought to originate from the ampullary buds while the immature cartilage is believed to be derived from blastema.[71] The number of ducts is variable and they may be rare (Fig. 1-38). Cysts lined by flattened cells, immature tubules, and aberrantly formed glomeruli may predominate or more normal tubules and well-formed glomeruli also may be present (Fig. 1-37).

Occasionally an infant will present with renal insufficiency and small reniform kidneys with normal ureters and pelves. Simple hypoplasia may be suspected but biopsy reveals a focal form of dysplasia characterized by

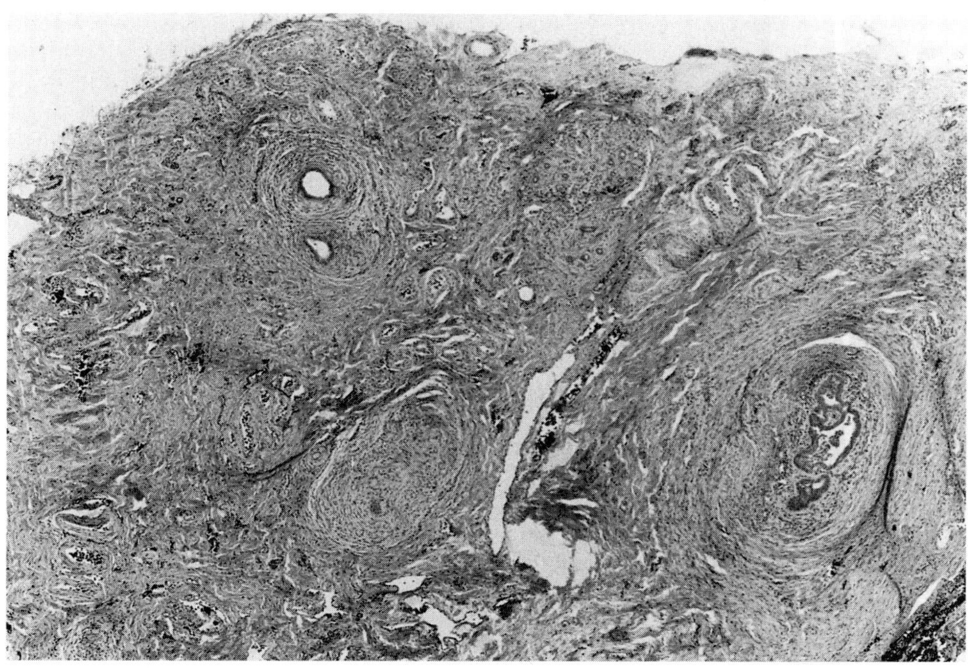

1-38. Aplastic dysplasia showing collagenous tissue with a few dysplastic ducts.

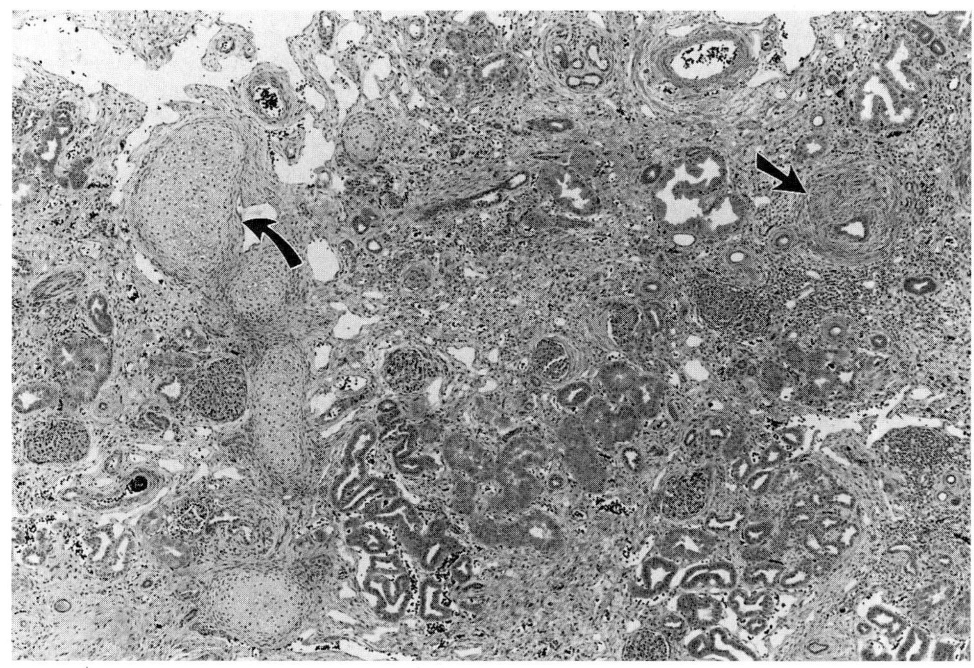

1-39. A focal form of renal dysplasia from a 1-year-old with renal insufficiency and bilateral small kidneys. Cartilage (*curved arrow*) and a dysplastic duct (*arrow*) are present.

an admixture of normal nephrons and aberrantly formed nephrons usually with microcysts and cartilage or dysplastic ducts (Fig. 1-39). The renal prognosis is bleak, and the infant usually develops progressive renal failure as it grows.

Segmental dysplasia. Segmental dysplasia occurs only in kidneys with duplication of the collecting system (duplex kidney).[65,72] Usually the duplication is complete with two separate ureters. The upper pole moiety is affected and histologically shows the same range of aberrant nephrogenesis encountered in aplastic and multicystic dysplasia. The upper pole ureter is usually ectopic, in a more cranial or caudal location relative to the normally situated lower pole ureter. The incidence of dysplasia increases with the severity of the ectopia.[73]

Dysplasia associated with lower tract obstruction. Bilateral renal dysplasia can be associated with distal obstruction due to urethral stenosis, posterior urethral valves, or bladder neck obstruction. This form of dysplasia has a distinctive gross appearance. The kidneys are typically reniform, may be large or small, but show distinct corticomedullary differentiation. The bladder is either hypertrophic or greatly dilated and the ureters are dilated and tortuous (Fig. 1-32, 1-40). There may be a severe degree of dysplasia with scant nephronic elements (Fig. 1-40) or only a peripheral zone of dysplastic elements with normal deeper nephrons.

Dysplasia associated with malformation syndromes. Renal dysplasia may develop in a large number of multiple malformation syndromes, chromosomal anomalies, and hereditary malformation syndromes[49-62,74-79] (see the box on p. 22). When multiple malformations are encountered in a pediatric autopsy, it is important to obtain tissue for karyotype analysis and to meticulously document all anomalies. Consultation with specialists in pediatrics and genetics is advisable to provide the proper classification of the disease so that appropriate family counseling can be provided.

Hereditary renal adysplasia and urogenital adysplasia. Renal agenesis, aplastic dysplasia, and multicystic dysplasia are the most severe forms of metanephric kidney maldevelopment. When not associated with extrarenal anomalies of a multiple malformation syndrome, they usually are sporadic events with little risk of a subsequently affected sibling. Rarely, however, renal agenesis or renal dysplasia, either unilateral or bilateral (Fig. 1-31), or combined agenesis and dysplasia may be familial (usually autosomal dominant); this is known as hereditary renal adysplasia.[59-62] There may also be concomitant malformation of müllerian structures, a condition referred to as hereditary urogenital adysplasia.[58] Unfortunately neither syndrome can be anticipated until a second family member is identified with either agenesis or dysplasia.

A

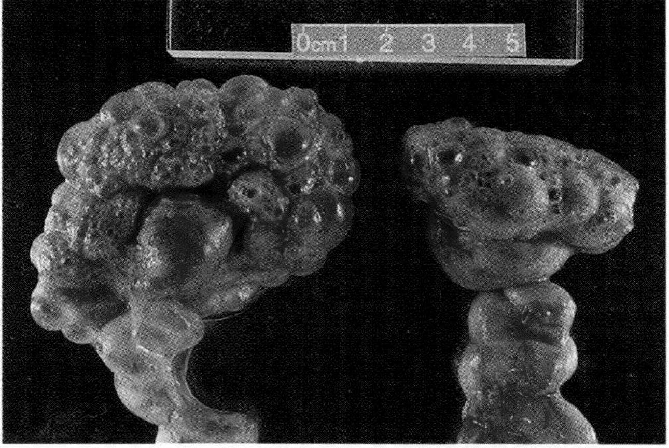

B

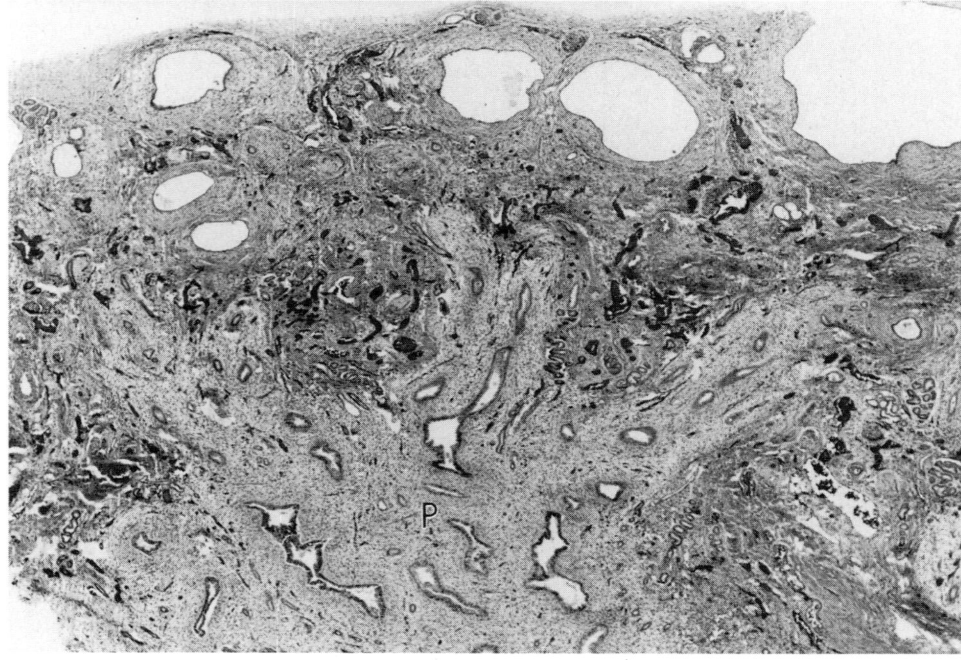

1-40. **A**, Renal dysplasia associated with urinary tract obstruction. **B**, Cortical medullary development is present, however, few differentiated elements are present (*P-pyramid*).

Polycystic kidney diseases

Infantile polycystic kidney disease. Infantile polycystic kidney disease is an autosomal recessive disorder.[13,80-83] While its pathogenesis is not known, organogenesis appears normal based on microdissection studies of severe neonatal forms.[13] There is ectasia of cortical and medullary collecting ducts, which often is accompanied by a liver lesion that in older patients is identical to congenital hepatic fibrosis.

Infantile polycystic kidney disease was originally believed to be an invariably lethal neonatal disorder.[80] Observation of some cases that survived into childhood prompted Blyth and Ockenden[81] to propose a subclassification of patients into forms: perinatal, neonatal, infantile, and juvenile. These forms vary in the degree of cyst formation. Although conceptually useful, it is often difficult to place a patient into a given category. It appears that as the extent of cyst formation decreases, there is better pulmonary development and a greater likelihood of survival. Unfortunately, with increasing duration of survival there is worsening of the liver disease, which in some patients culminates in congenital hepatic fibrosis.[81-83] If one examines the kidneys of children with congenital hepatic fibrosis, two thirds have some degree of medullary cyst formation and a concentrating defect similar to that of infantile polycystic kidney disease is present in almost all. This has led to the suggestion that infantile polycystic kidney disease and congenital hepatic fibrosis may be different manifestations of a single entity.[83]

Most cases of infantile polycystic kidney disease result in stillbirth or early neonatal death. Affected neonates have massively enlarged and diffusely cystic kidneys that produce abdominal distension and compress thoracic organs (Fig. 1-41). The lungs cannot develop normally and death is from pulmonary hypoplasia. Despite the impressive cyst formation the kidneys may be functional. If they are nonfunctional, oligohydramnios and a Potter's phenotype may develop.

The cysts extend through the cortex and medulla in a distinctive radiating pattern imparting a spongy quality (Fig. 1-41). Histologically, the cysts consist of dilated collecting ducts lined with uniform cuboidal cells (Fig. 1-42, 1-43). The nephrons between the collecting ducts appear normal.

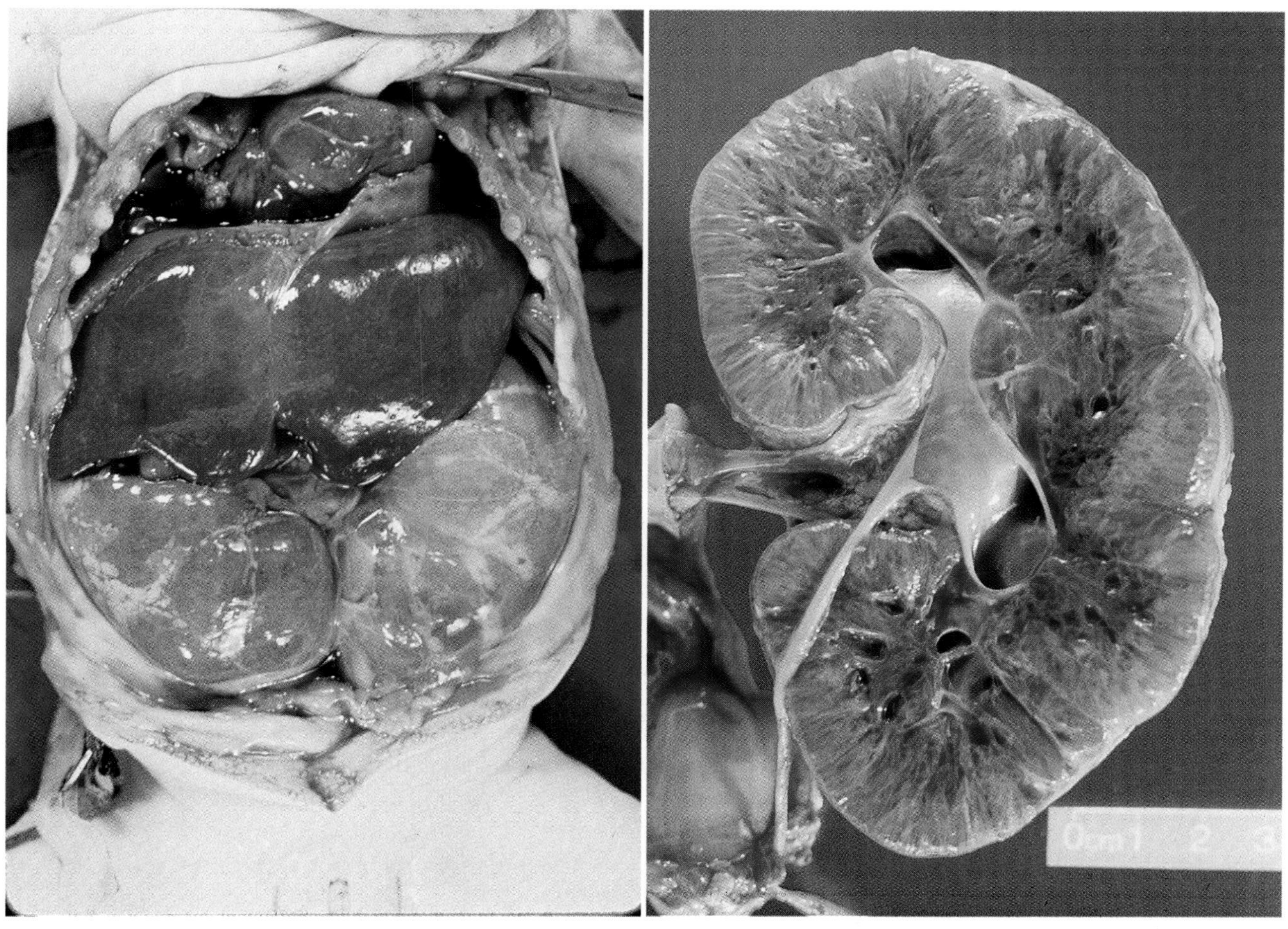

1-41. A, Infantile polycystic kidney disease showing massive kidneys that distend the abdomen, elevate the diaphragm, and compromise the thoracic cavity. **B,** The bivalved kidney shows a reniform shape and normal collecting system. The cortex and medulla contain diffuse relatively uniform cysts.

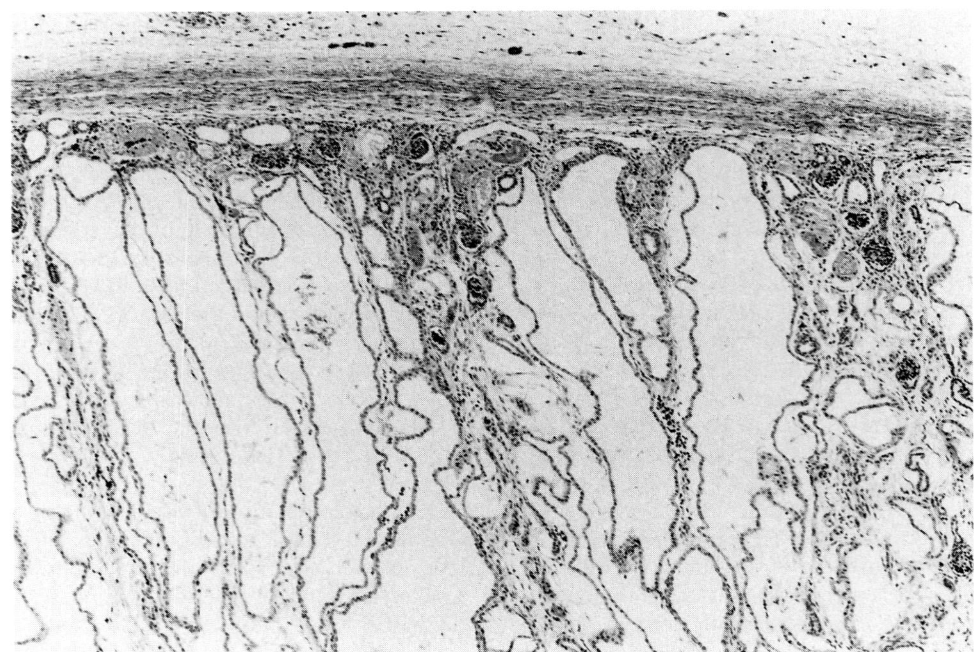

1-42. The cysts in infantile polycystic kidney disease are elongated and involve the cortical and medullary collecting ducts.

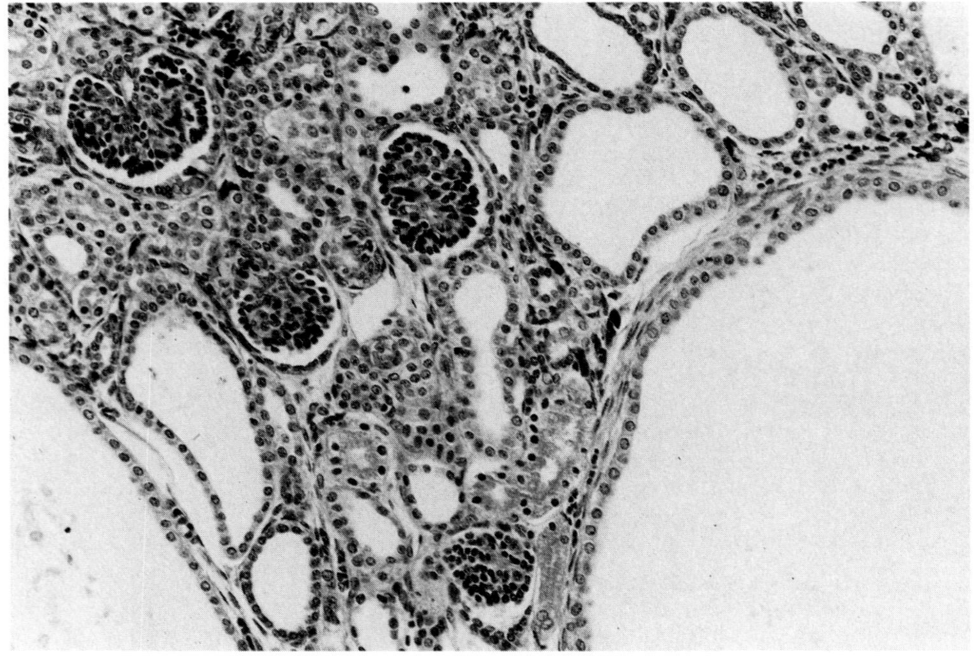

1-43. The cysts in infantile polycystic kidney disease are lined with uniform cuboidal epithelium with normal nephron elements in between.

In the hepatic lesion in patients dying in the neonatal period, the portal bile ducts proliferate and assume a dilated and irregular pattern of anastomosing channels at the periphery of portal triads (Fig. 1-44). There is a marked increase in the size of portal areas with increased fibrous tissue. In older patients, congenital hepatic fibrosis develops resulting in portal hypertension and hepatosplenomegaly.

In less severely affected kidneys of older children the appearance is variable, and the diagnosis may be less obvious. The kidneys are smaller and the cysts are fewer. Medullary cysts are always present and tend to be elon-

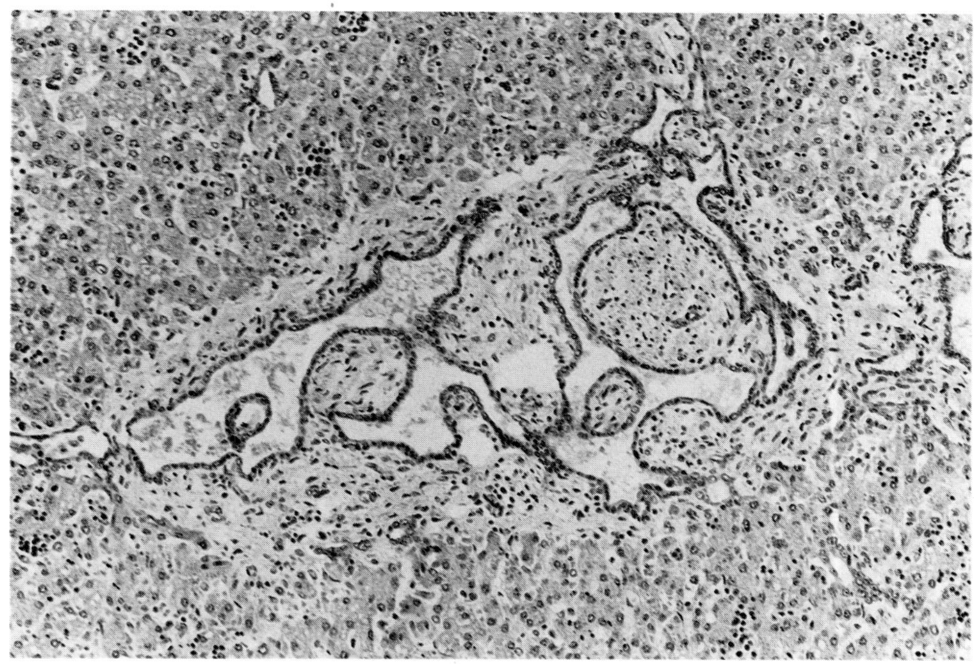

1-44. The liver in perinatal infantile polycystic kidney disease showing the irregular architecture of portal bile ducts and portal fibrosis.

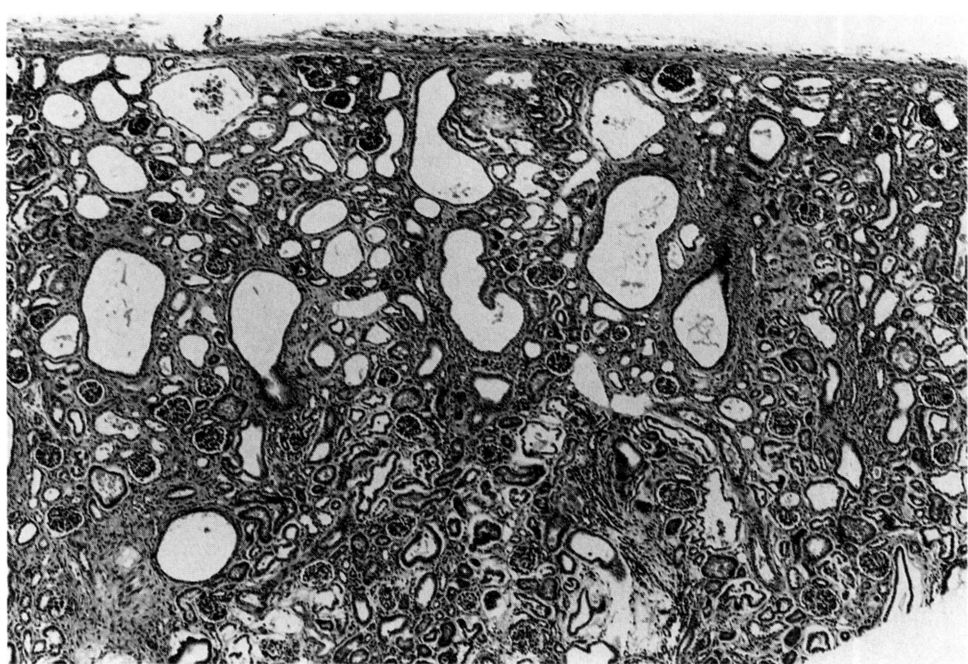

1-45. An infantile form of infantile polycystic kidney disease in a 4-year-old showing less prominent collecting duct ectasia. Interstitial fibrosis is developing.

gated. The cortical cysts are often rounded and variably distributed (Fig. 1-45). The parenchyma adjacent to the cysts eventually develops atrophic changes with tubulointerstitial scarring and glomerulosclerosis. This may create a resemblance to adult polycystic kidney disease. The liver lesion of congenital hepatic fibrosis therefore is a useful diagnostic feature. However, a number of diseases may be associated with renal cysts and liver disease, which require awareness of additional anomalies for proper classification[74] (see box on p. 30).

Adult (autosomal dominant) polycystic kidney disease. Adult polycystic kidney disease is the most

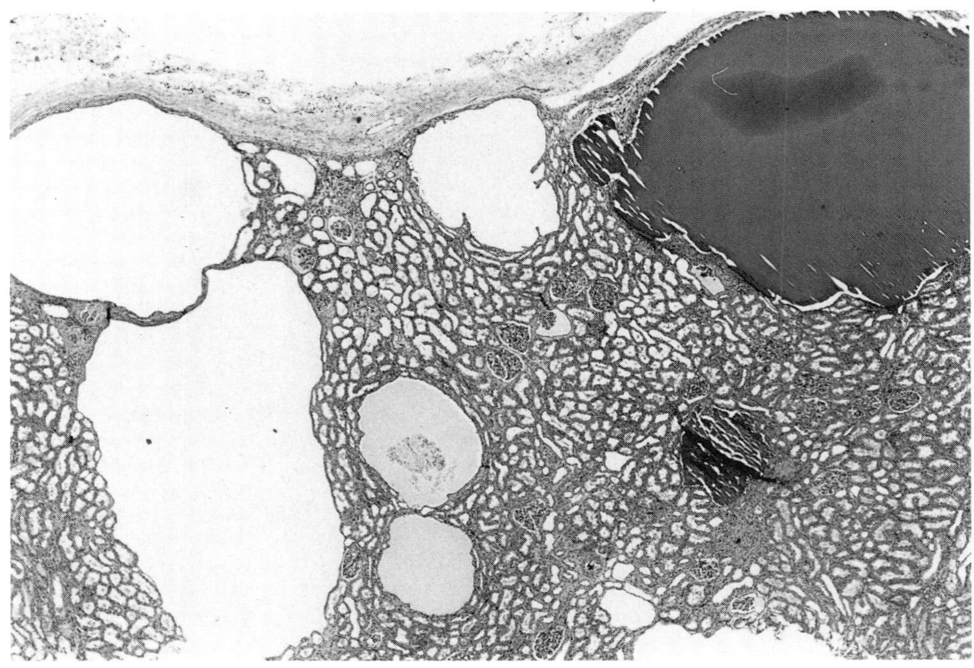

1-46. Infantile onset of adult polycystic kidney disease at age 7 years showing a largely intact cortex and multiple cysts.

CYSTIC RENAL DISEASE ASSOCIATED WITH CONGENITAL HEPATIC FIBROSIS OR BILIARY DYSGENESIS

- Infantile polycystic kidney disease
- Adult polycystic kidney disease
- Juvenile nephronophthisis
- Meckel-Gruber syndrome*
- Zellweger syndrome*
- Ivemark's syndrome*
- Chondrodysplastic syndromes*
- Trisomy C*
- Trisomy D*

*Additional malformations are present

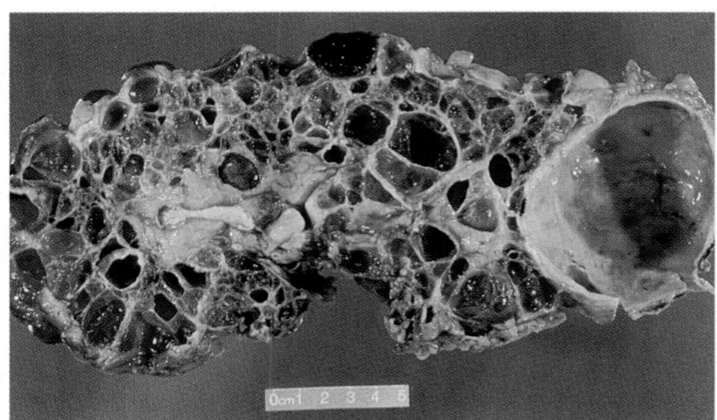

1-47. Transverse section of an adult polycystic kidney.

common cystic renal disease and the most common genetically transmitted disease.[84-86] It occurs with an estimated frequency of between 1:500 to 1:1000. It is the third to fourth leading cause of end-stage renal disease and patients comprise 5% to 10% of dialysis patients. Although patients vary greatly in the age of onset of symptoms, most present in their 30s to 50s. There is nearly 100% penetrance if the individual survives to age 80. Approximately 25% of affected patients lack a family history and presumably represent a new mutation. The principal gene associated with adult polycystic kidney disease has been localized to chromosome 16 in 90% of patients.[85,86] In addition, another genetic locus on chromosome 4 has recently been identified.

Patients present with a variety of symptoms, most referable to the urinary tract.[84-86] Chronic flank pain is the most common and correlates with renal weight and cyst size greater than 3 cm. Acute flank pain often reflects hemorrhage into a cyst. Hematuria is the second most common symptom. This may be gross, resulting in clot formation and urinary tract obstruction. Hypertension often develops early in the disease and activation of the renin-angiotensin system secondary to intrarenal vascular occlusion by expanding cysts has been implicated. Urinary tract infection develops in 50% to 75% of patients and affects women more often than men. The infection may be confined to the collecting system or a cyst, or may involve the parenchyma. Perinephric extension with abscess is a serious complication with a 60% mortality rate. Urate or calcium oxalate nephrolithiasis develops in 10% of patients and renal cell carcinoma develops in 1% to 5%.

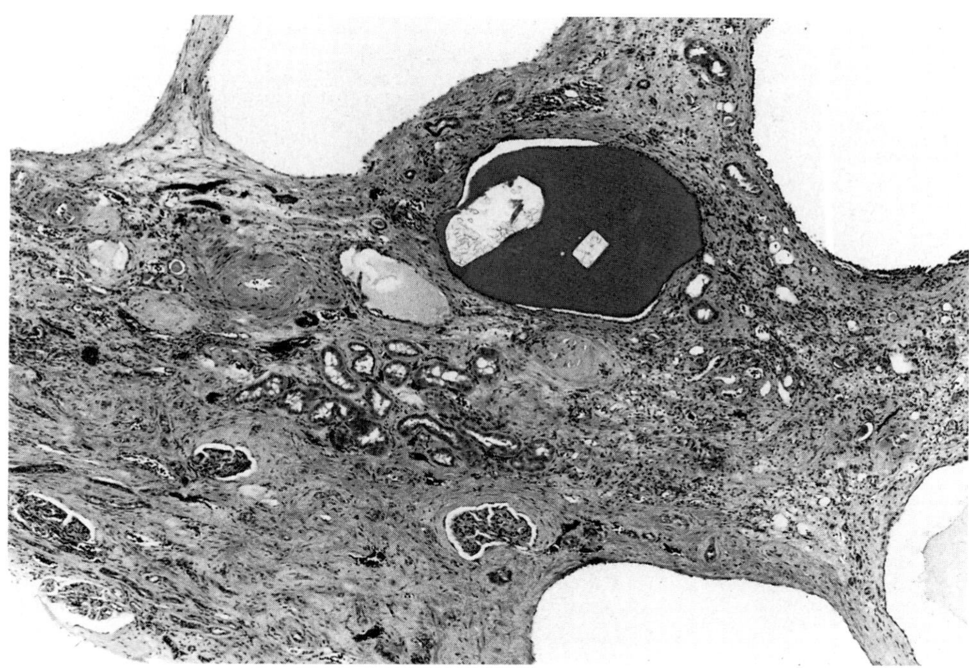

1-48. Advanced adult polycystic kidney disease showing severe interstitial scarring and cysts that contain proteinaceous fluid and calcium oxalate crystals, from an adult in renal failure.

Extrarenal complications related to hypertension and berry aneurysms develop in 5% to 15%.

Early in the disease (Fig. 1-46), the kidney may appear nearly normal with only scattered cysts in the cortex and medulla and normal intervening parenchyma.[87-89] The cysts initially are small and develop in only about 1% of nephrons. Microdissection studies have shown that the cysts develop in all segments of the nephron.[89] Scanning electron microscopy and immunohistochemistry of cyst lining cells have confirmed these observations.[90,91]

As the disease progresses, the cysts grow in size and number resulting in massive renal enlargement (Fig. 1-47). Despite the cystic transformation, the kidneys retain a reniform shape and preserve their collecting systems. The cysts range in size from a few millimeters to several centimeters, and cyst contents vary from transparent to opaque to hemorrhagic fluid.

Most of the cysts are lined with a single layer of flattened to cuboidal epithelium (Fig. 1-48). Hyperplastic foci or polyp formation (Fig. 1-49) are detectable in some cysts and renal neoplasms, often of a papillary architecture, may also be present.[92,93] The cyst contents may be proteinaceous or contain red cells or calcific deposits. The intervening parenchyma shows interstitial fibrosis with a lymphoid infiltrate, tubular atrophy, glomerular, and vascular sclerosis.

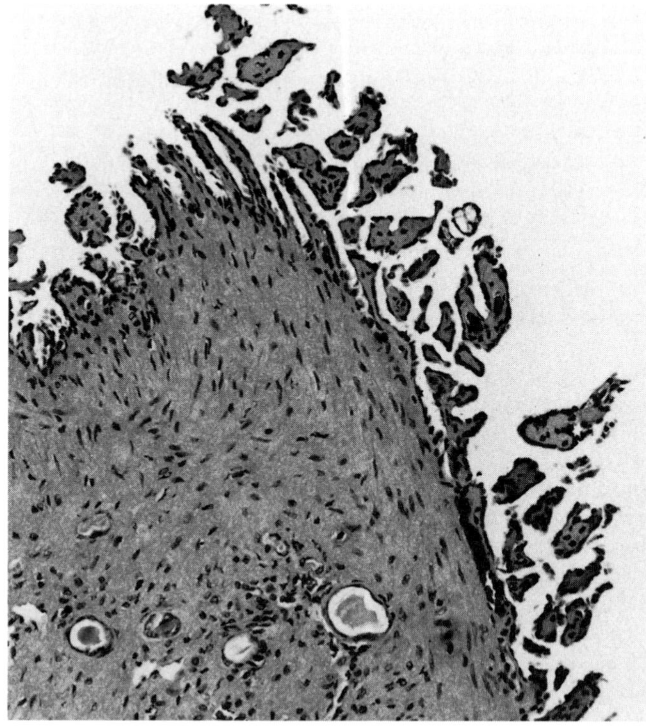

1-49. Papillary tufts lining a cyst in adult polycystic kidney disease.

Cysts (without dysplasia) in hereditary syndromes

Juvenile nephronophthisis/medullary cystic disease. Juvenile nephronophthisis/medullary cystic disease is a hereditary form of progressive renal disease.[94-97] Although fundamentally a tubulointerstitial disease, it is usually classified as a cystic disease because 75% of cases are accompanied by medullary cysts. Affected individuals present with polyuria and polydipsia due to salt wasting, a concentration defect, anemia disproportionately severe for the level of renal insufficiency, and growth retardation.

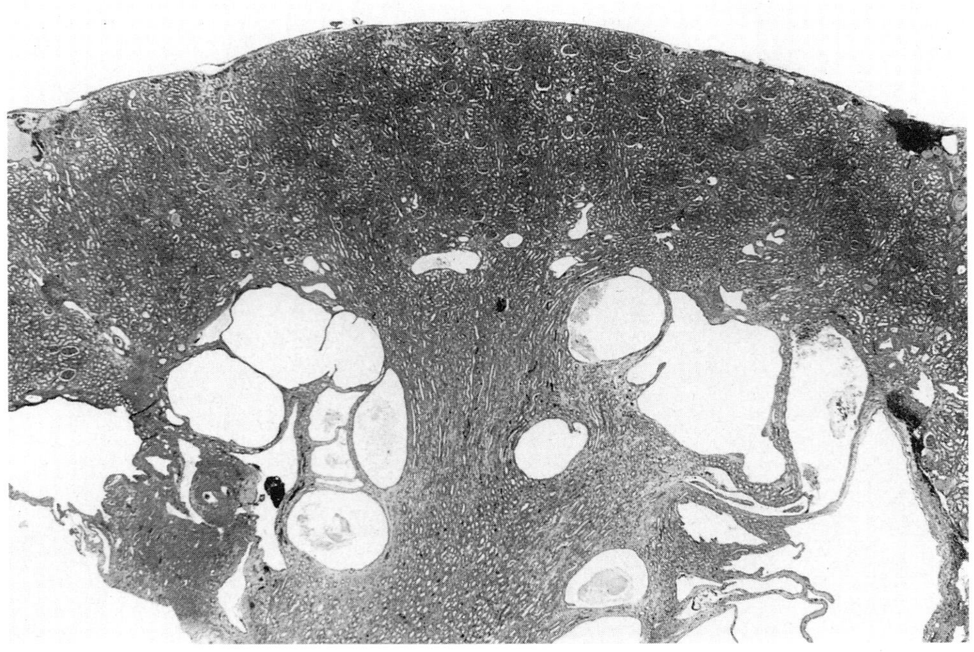

1-50. Early stage of juvenile nephronophthisis showing cysts along the outer medulla.

JUVENILE NEPHRONOPHTHISIS/MEDULLARY CYSTIC DISEASE

- Familial juvenile nephronophthisis—autosomal recessive
- Renal-retinal dysplasia—autosomal recessive
- Medullary cystic disease—autosomal dominant
- Sporadic medullary cystic disease—nonfamilial

Four morphologically indistinguishable forms are recognized (see box on this page). The two autosomal recessive forms account for 70% of cases while the remaining two forms each account for 15% of cases. The dominant form presents in young adults while the other forms present in childhood.

The kidneys are usually small at the time of clinical presentation due to cortical atrophy. Although medullary cysts are common, within a given family not all affected individuals have cysts. The cysts congregate at the corticomedullary junction and range up to 1 cm in size (Fig. 1-50). Cyst formation does not appear to increase as the disease progresses. Microscopically, the appearance is that of a nonspecific chronic interstitial nephritis with tubular atrophy, interstitial fibrosis, and periglomerular fibrosis. A prominent lymphoid infiltrate is usually present. The tubulointerstitial nephritis worsens over time. Eventually glomerulosclerosis develops. If cysts are present, they are lined with a flattened to cuboidal epithelium.

Von Hippel-Lindau disease. Von Hippel-Lindau disease is an uncommon autosomal dominant disorder in which renal and extrarenal cysts and neoplasms develop.[98-100] The syndrome includes retinal, cerebellar, and spinal hemangioblastomas, pheochromocytoma, and epididymal and pancreatic cysts and cystadenomas. In addition, multiple and bilateral renal cysts develop in 75% of patients and renal cell carcinomas develop in approximately 50% of patients, often bilateral and multicentric (Fig. 1-51).

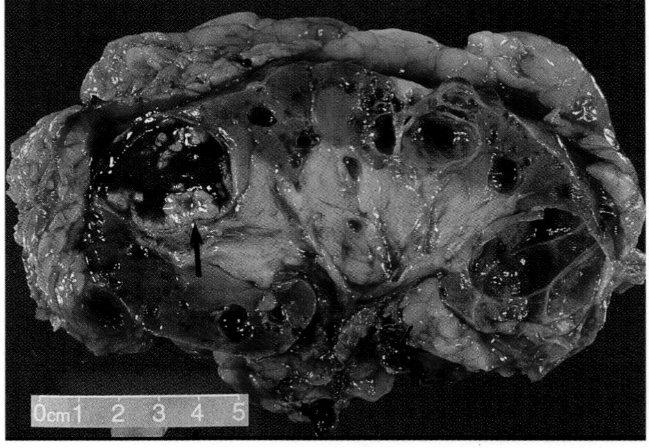

1-51. Nephrectomy in von Hippel-Lindau disease showing multiple cysts. One cyst side contains a mural nodule (*arrow*) of renal cell carcinoma.

The renal cysts are lined with glycogen-rich cells similar to those of grade 1 clear cell renal cell carcinoma (Fig. 1-52).[98-100] These range from a benign-appearing lining of one to two cell layers of clear cells to multiple layers of cells. Papillary tufts of mildly atypical cells, solid mural nodules, and cystic masses that are clearly neoplastic in nature also develop.[99,100] Deoxyribonucleic acid (DNA) analysis has shown aneuploidy in both the cells of cysts and cells of solid

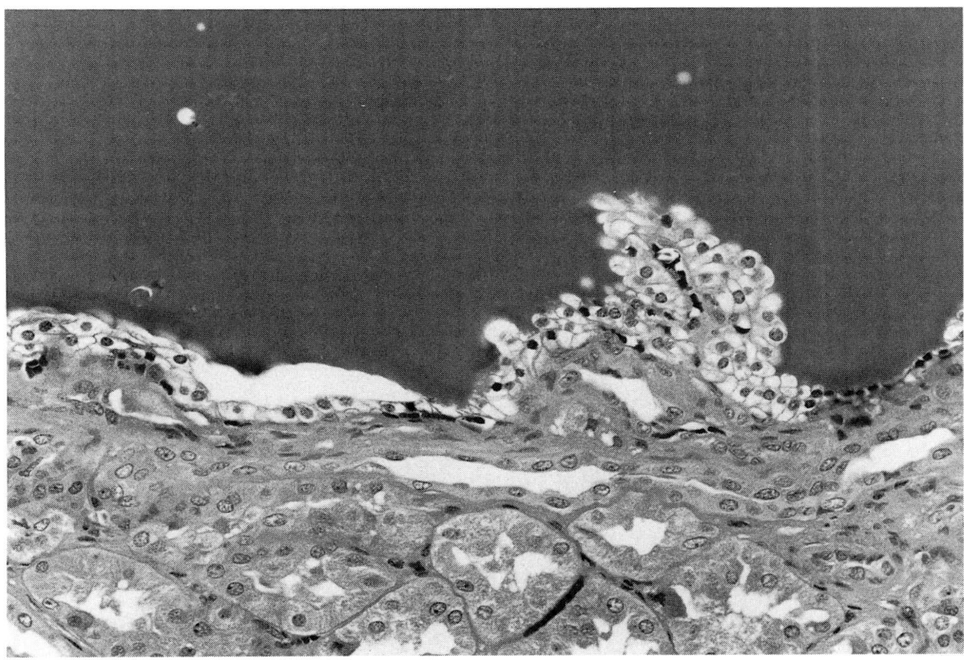

1-52. A cyst (*from Fig 1-51*) in von Hippel-Lindau disease lined with clear cells with a papillary tuft.

tumors.[100] This morphologic spectrum represents a challenge in the classification of lesions in biopsy and nephrectomy material. The appropriate morphologic threshold for a malignant diagnosis has yet to be established.

Tuberous sclerosis. Tuberous sclerosis is an autosomal dominant disorder characterized by mental retardation, epilepsy, angiofibromas, cardiac rhabdomyomas, renal angiomyolipomas, and renal cysts.[101,102] While renal cysts are uncommon and usually not extensive, some individuals, usually children, develop a diffuse cystic renal disease with numerous large cortical and medullary cysts that resemble autosomal dominant polycystic disease.[101]

The cysts in tuberous sclerosis are distinctive and appear to have diagnostic specificity in the recognition of this disorder.[101] The cysts are lined with large eosinophilic cells with large hyperchromatic nuclei. They may form papillary or polyploid masses and may show occasional mitotic activity. Renal cell carcinomas have rarely developed but this is far less common than in von Hippel-Lindau disease.[102]

Glomerulocystic kidney diseases. Glomerular cysts develop in several forms of pediatric and adult cystic disease (see box on this page), either as the predominant abnormality or accompanied by renal dysplasia or extrarenal abnormalities of a congenital syndrome.[103-107] Glomerulocystic kidney disease comprises the subgroup in which glomerular cysts constitute the principal abnormality and other abnormalities outside of the kidney are absent. Several genetic diseases occur within the glomerulocystic kidney disease category.

Most glomerulocystic kidney diseases are autosomal dominant disorders. Approximately half of all cases will be found to have a family history typical of adult polycystic kidney disease. The patient is usually an infant and appears to have early onset of severe adult polycystic kidney disease, which begins with glomerular cysts as the major finding.[103] Other kindreds have a strong family history of renal disease that is not consistent with adult polycystic kidney disease and in which biopsies of siblings or parents consistently show only glomerular

GLOMERULOCYSTIC KIDNEYS

Glomerulocystic Kidney Disease

- Autosomal dominant glomerulocystic kidney disease
- Familial hypoplastic glomerulocystic kidney disease
- "Sporadic" glomerulocystic kidney disease

Syndromes with Glomerular Cysts

- Tuberous sclerosis
- Familial juvenile nephronophthisis with hepatic fibrosis
- Zellweger cerebral-renal-hepatic syndrome
- Trisomy 13 syndrome
- Oral-facial-digital syndrome, type I
- Brachymesomelia-renal syndrome
- Short rib-polydactyly syndrome, Majewski type

Dysplastic glomerulocystic kidneys

- Hereditary and syndromal renal dysplasia

From Bernstein J, Landing BH: Genetics of kidney disorders, 1989, New York, Alan R. Liss; with permission.

cysts.[105,106] Several kindreds have also been found to have small kidneys with reduced or absent renal pyramids, called familial hyperplastic glomerulocystic kidney disease.[104] Finally, rare sporadic forms have been reported.[107] However, in situations in which a family history is absent, the prospect of a new mutation with early onset of a genetic form should always be entertained.

The glomerular cysts in glomerulocystic kidney diseases may be microscopic or sufficiently large to be grossly visible and result in nephromegaly (Fig. 1-53). The cysts may be confined to a subcapsular zone, affect the entire cortex, or be confined to the inner cortex. Tubulointerstitial scarring may also develop or be absent. Once glomerular cysts are recognized, additional morphologic

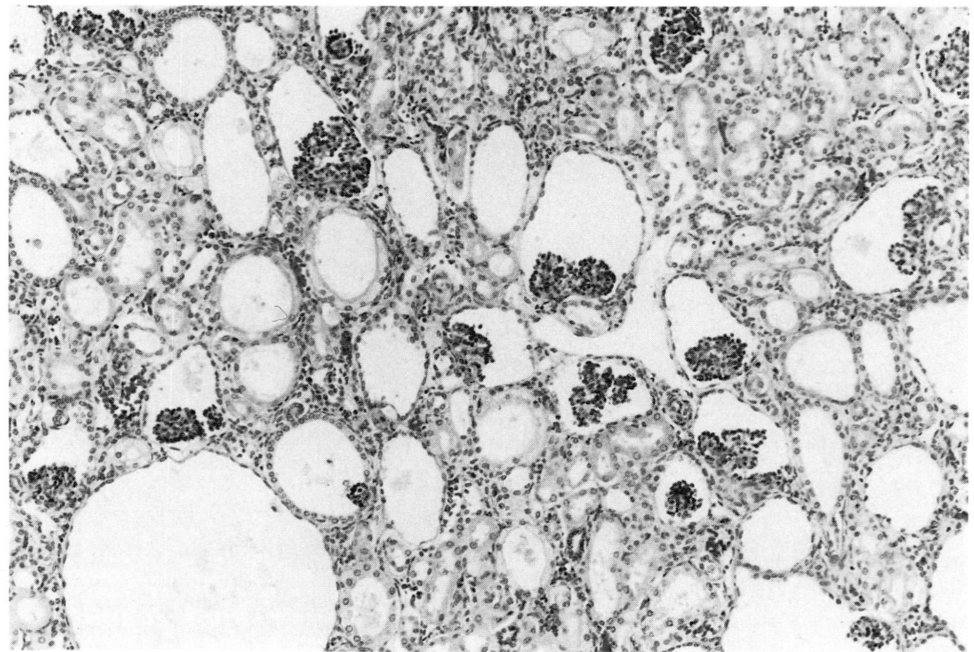

1-53. Glomerulocystic kidney disease showing microcysts principally involving Bowman's capsules.

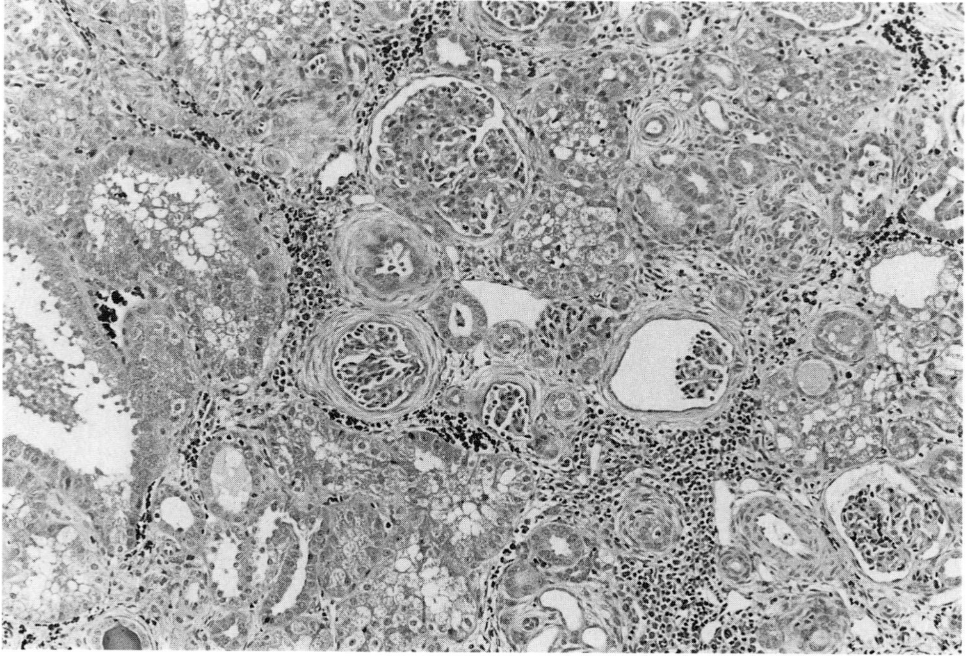

1-54. Congenital nephrotic syndrome of the Finnish type in a 2-year-old at the time of renal transplantation. There is mild ectasia of tubules and Bowman's capsule, glomerular sclerosis, and tubular atrophy.

and clinical data are required to resolve the differential possibilities. If extrarenal anomalies are present or if features of renal dysplasia are present, then this is not a primary glomerulocystic kidney disease.

Congenital nephrotic syndrome of the Finnish type. Congenital nephrotic syndrome of the Finnish type is an autosomal recessive disease.[108-111] Although rare, it is the most common cause of nephrotic syndrome in the first 3 months of life. It is included in this section because it is also known as "microcystic disease." Although most prevalent in Finland, it has been recognized throughout the world.

The affected fetus is born prematurely with a low birth weight and a large placenta. The kidneys may be grossly enlarged due to edema and microcysts resulting from mild ectasia of tubules, especially collecting ducts, and often of Bowman's capsule. Progressive nephrotic syndrome, poor growth, and renal insufficiency develop. As the nephrotic syndrome continues, progressive glomerulosclerosis and tubular atrophy develop and renal failure ensues (Fig. 1-54). Most infants die of infection by three years of age unless transplantation is successful.

Miscellaneous conditions

Renal tubular dysgenesis. Failure of differentiation of normal-appearing tubules is known as renal tubular dysgenesis.[112-114] It results in neonatal renal failure with the oligohydramnios sequence, a Potter's syndrome phenotype, and may result in death due to pulmonary hypoplasia. The kidneys are usually grossly normal although they may be increased in weight. The glomeruli are close together and appear increased in number. The intervening tubules are small and appear undifferentiated in routine section (Fig. 1-55). Ultrastructurally and with lectin staining, they exhibit features of the distal tubule and collecting duct.

The original reports of renal tubular dysgenesis indicated a hereditary pattern consistent with an autosomal recessive disorder.[112] However, the same lesion has been reported in other contexts. It has recently been described in monochorionic twins with twin-twin transfusions in which only the donor twin was affected.[113] It has also been reported to be associated with hypocalvaria as a complication of maternal use of angiotensin-converting enzyme inhibitors.[114]

Acquired cystic kidney disease. Acquired cystic kidney disease refers to the development of multiple and bilateral renal cysts in patients whose chronic renal failure cannot be attributed to an hereditary cystic disease.[115-119] Although identified as long ago as 1847 by Simon,[115] in 1977 Dunnill[116] revived interest in this phenomenon when in an autopsy study of hemodialysis patients he observed not only a high prevalence of renal cysts but also found renal tumors in 20% of the patients. One patient died of metastatic renal cell carcinoma. The development of both cysts and tumors appears to be related to the uremic state because it is independent of the type of dialysis and the cause of original renal disease.[117,118]

Acquired cystic kidney disease is bilateral and asymptomatic in its early stages.[116-118] Cysts are present in 8% of patients at the time dialysis is initiated and increase in incidence, number, and size proportional to the duration of dialysis. After 3 to 5 years of dialysis, approximately 50% of patients develop cysts while by 10 years almost 90% have cysts. The complications of acquired cystic

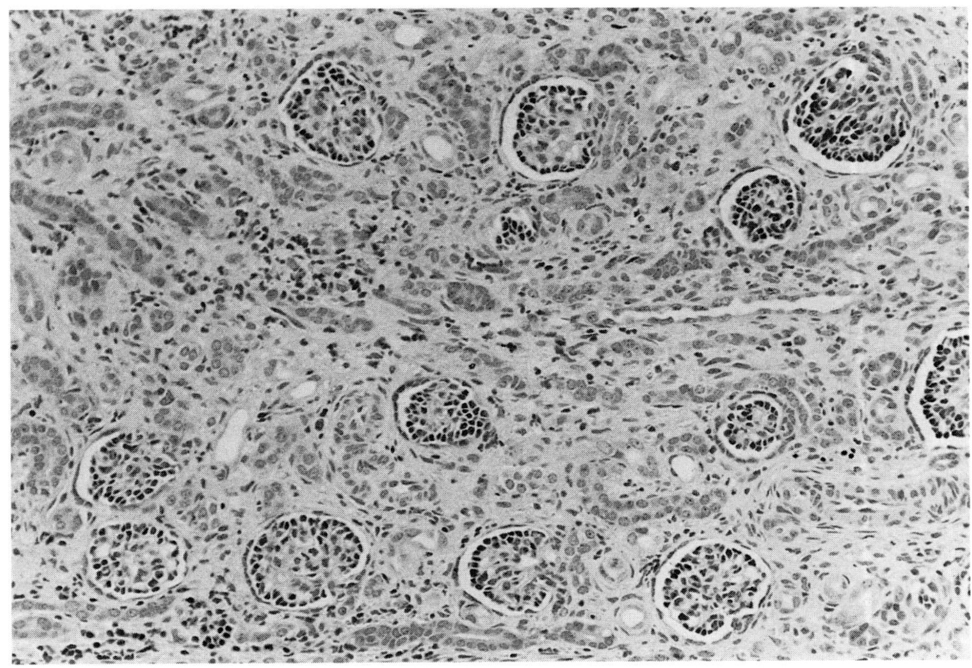

1-55. Congenital renal tubular dysgenesis presenting with oliguric acute renal failure. No normal proximal tubules are present.

kidney disease include intrarenal and retroperitoneal hemorrhage, cyst infection, and renal cell carcinoma.[118-119] Although improvement in the cystic disease occurs in many patients following a successful transplantation, the influence of transplantation on neoplastic complications remains unclear. As the number of dialysis patients increases and their survivals improve, the occurrence of cystic disease and neoplastic complications can also be expected to increase.

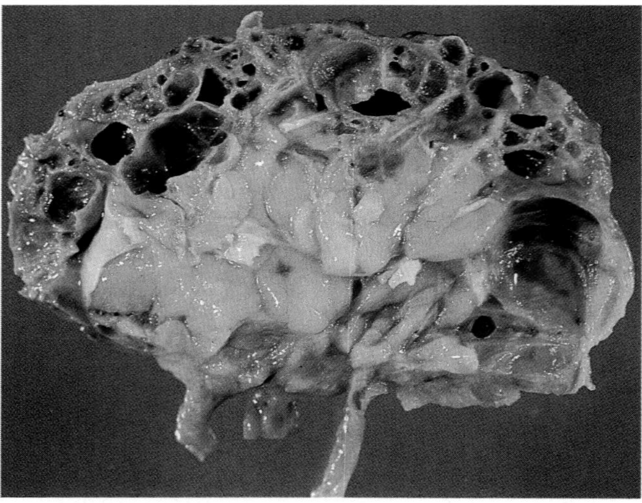

1-56. Acquired cystic disease of the kidney. Although diffusely cystic, the kidney is small and the renal sinus fat is prominent.

The cysts initially form in the proximal tubules of end stage kidneys. Most cysts are less than 0.5 cm in size, but cysts 2 to 3 cm in size can develop. Initially the cysts are cortical, but in advanced cases medullary cysts form and the entire kidney may be replaced by cysts and resemble a smaller version of adult polycystic kidney disease (Fig. 1-56).

The cysts are lined with flattened, cuboidal, or columnar epithelium and may contain a proteinaceous to hemorrhagic fluid. Foci of epithelial hyperplasia are common in the cysts and tubules. Solid and papillary tumors also develop, some of which have metastasized.[118-119]

Segmental cystic disease. The literature contains several cases of a unilateral and segmental form of cystic disease that histologically resembles adult polycystic kidney disease but lacks the progression, extrarenal complications, and familial nature.[120] An early stage of adult polycystic kidney disease is often entertained because early on one kidney may be more severely affected. Careful imaging of the opposite kidney and inquiry into family history is required.

The differential includes a broad range of other diseases: multiple simple cysts, cystic dysplasia, cystic nephroma, and cystic carcinoma. In multiple simple cysts, the cysts are widely separated and do not congregate in a single region. In segmental forms of dysplasia, ureteral duplication is present. Cystic nephromas are more circumscribed and well demarcated, and cystic carcinomas will show a neoplastic vascular pattern and usually have solid areas. Despite these differences, excision and follow-up may be required to confidently establish the disease's nature and hereditary implications.

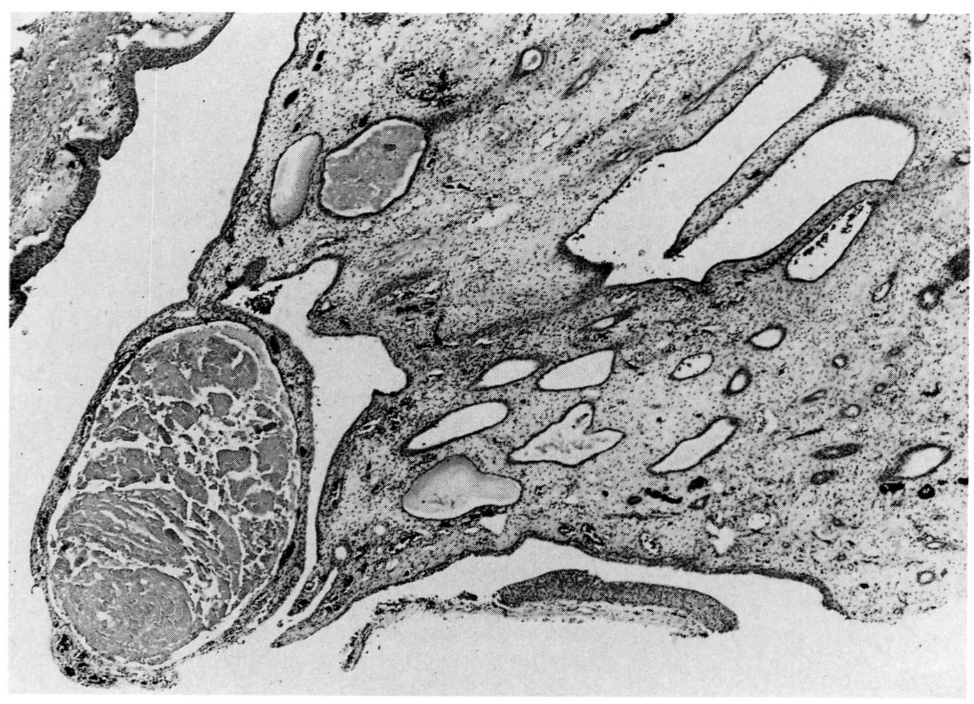

1-57. Medullary sponge kidney showing prominent ectasia and a microlith within a papillary collecting duct.

Medullary sponge kidney. In medullary sponge kidney there is ectasia of the papillary collecting ducts of one or more renal pyramids.[121] Usually bilateral and more common in males, medullary sponge kidney is usually detected radiographically in adults evaluated for nephrolithiasis. The kidneys are not enlarged and renal function is normal although a concentrating defect may be present in more severely affected patients.

Microscopically, the collecting ducts are dilated and lined with cuboidal or flattened epithelium[121] (Fig. 1-57). Intratubular calcifications are common. If stones have obstructed the ducts, localized scarring may be present. Medullary sponge kidney can be distinguished from medullary cystic disease and infantile polycystic kidney disease by patient age and by cyst locations. In medullary cystic disease the cysts are located at the corticomedullary junction, while in the juvenile form of infantile polycystic kidney disease the cysts are in the cortex and medulla and do not congregate at the papillary tips.

Simple cortical cyst. Simple cortical cysts are the most common cystic renal lesion.[122,123] They are rare before the age of 40, so cysts in a child or young adult, especially if bilateral, can be an important clue to the presence of a cystic renal disease. Simple cysts increase in frequency with advancing age. In older patients the cysts may be multiple and large (Fig. 1-58). The cysts are lined with a flattened layer of cells or lack an epithelial lining. The cyst wall may occasionally calcify, a radiographic finding mimicking infection or malignancy.[122-123]

Pyelocalyceal ectasia and diverticula. There are several lesions (hydrocalyx, megacalycosis, and calyceal diverticulum) that have in common a cavity lined with urothelium which communicates with the collecting system and is associated with recurrent infections and nephrolithiasis.[124-126] In hydrocalyx there is calyectasis secondary to infundibular stenosis. The stenosis may be congenital or the sequela of inflammation. In contrast, in megacalycosis obstruction is not evident.[124] In both lesions the renal pyramid is flattened or concave and in cases complicated by infection, parenchymal inflammation and scarring may be present.

In calyceal diverticulum the cavity communicates with a minor calyx via a narrow isthmus[125,126] and no obstruction is present. The upper pole calyx is involved in 54% of cases and parenchymal inflammation and scarring usually are absent unless the case is complicated by infections.

VASCULAR DISEASES

HYPERTENSION-ASSOCIATED RENAL DISEASE

Vascular disease, in its various forms (see box on this page), is the most common cause of renal injury

VASCULAR DISEASES OF THE KIDNEY

- Hypertension-associated renal disease
  - Benign nephrosclerosis
  - Malignant nephrosclerosis
- Thrombotic microangiopathy
- Renal artery stenosis
  - Atherosclerosis
  - Fibromuscular dysplasia
- Renal artery dissection
- Renal artery aneurysm
- Arteriovenous malformation and fistula
- Renal emboli and infarcts
- Renal cortical necrosis
- Renal cholesterol microembolism syndrome
- Renal artery thrombosis
- Renal vein and renal venous thrombosis
- Bartter's syndrome
- Vasculitis

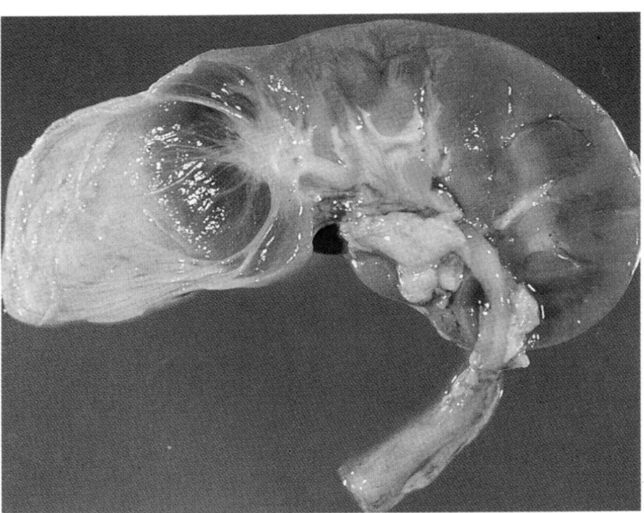

1-58. A large simple cortical cyst as an incidental autopsy finding.

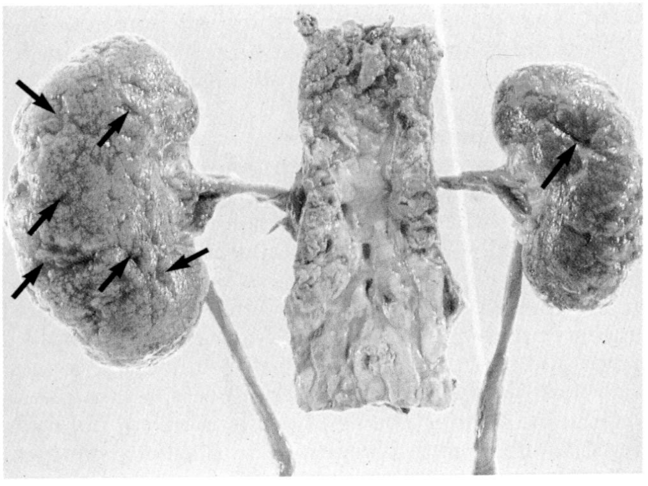

1-59. Complicated atherosclerotic vascular disease showing arterial nephrosclerosis, small atheroembolic infarcts (*arrow*), and an atrophic right kidney from renal artery stenosis.

TYPES AND CAUSES OF HYPERTENSION

Primary
- Benign (essential) hypertension
- Malignant hypertension

Secondary
- Renal artery stenosis
- Acute glomerulonephritis
- Chronic renal diseases
- Neoplasms
  - Renin producing tumors
  - Adrenal cortical tumors
  - Pheochromocytoma
- Endocrine abnormalities
  - Thyrotoxicosis
  - Adrenal cortical hyperplasia
  - Hyperparathyroidism
  - Oral contraceptives
- Neurogenic
- Miscellaneous vascular
  - Preeclampsia
  - Thrombotic microangiopathy
  - Vasculitis
  - Coarctation of aorta

encountered at autopsy due to the high incidence of atherosclerosis and hypertension (Fig. 1-59).[127-129] A connection between hypertension and renal and cardiovascular diseases has been recognized for over 100 years.[130-132] Hypertension-associated renal disease was first separated from other forms of renal disease in 1914 by Volhard and Fahr, who first recognized the existence of two forms.[133] The most common form, which they called *benign nephrosclerosis*, occurred in elderly individuals who had mild hypertension and little renal impairment. The second form, which they called *malignant nephrosclerosis*, occurred in younger patients with severe hypertension and renal failure. Although most patients with hypertension (90% to 95%) have idiopathic disease, there are numerous secondary causes that can produce either benign or malignant nephrosclerosis (see box on this page).

Benign nephrosclerosis

Benign (or essential) hypertension is an asymptomatic disorder affecting approximately 50 million Americans.[128,129] Its pathogenesis is unknown but is probably multifactorial. Genetic factors appear important, however no specific genetic marker has been identified. It is more common in blacks. Hypertension usually first appears around age 45 to 54 years and if unchecked places the patient at risk for renal insufficiency, congestive heart failure, coronary artery disease, and stroke in later years. Although benign hypertension will not cause renal failure in most patients, it is sufficiently prevalent to account for approximately 15% to 30% of patients with end stage renal disease.[128]

In benign nephrosclerosis, the kidneys are symmetrically reduced in size and weigh between 60 and 100 g

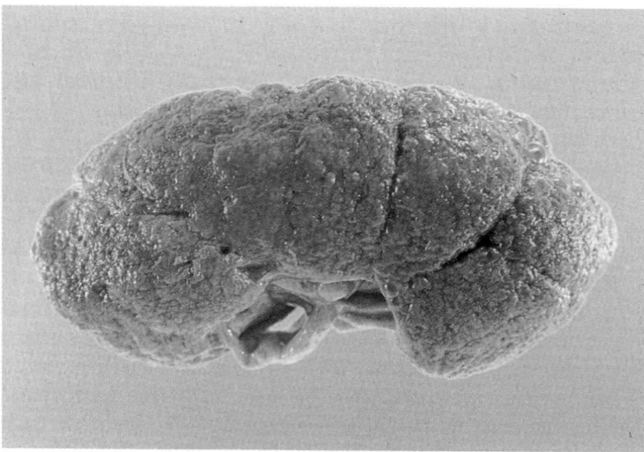

1-60. Granular subcapsular surface of benign hypertension-associated arterial nephrosclerosis.

(Fig. 1-60). They have granular subcapsular surfaces and thin cortices, the extent of which is influenced by the severity and duration of the hypertension.[129] Microscopically, arteries of intralobular size or greater show fibrous intimal thickening with reduplication or fragmentation of the elastic lamina.[127,134] Lipid and calcification are not usually present. The grossly visible subcapsular granularity corresponds to shallow subcapsular scars that contain sclerotic glomeruli, atrophic tubules, and thick-walled hyalinized or hyperplastic arterioles (Fig. 1-61).[127,135,136] Similar hyaline arteriolar thickening also occurs in diabetes mellitus and develops to a mild degree in individuals over the age of 60 in the absence of hypertension.

Malignant nephrosclerosis

Malignant nephrosclerosis develops as a consequence of malignant hypertension.[137] Malignant hypertension usually arises in a patient with preexisting benign hypertension but may develop as a de novo disorder. Patients present with headache, dizziness, and impaired vision. Their diastolic blood pressure exceeds 120 to 140 mm Hg and retinal hemorrhages and exudates and papilledema are present. Hematuria, proteinuria, and a microangiopathic hemolytic anemia develop. Without treatment, the patient will develop renal failure and may die suddenly from heart failure, myocardial infarct, or cerebral hemorrhage.

The kidney in malignant nephrosclerosis often has petechial subcapsular hemorrhages or a mottled red and yellow cortex if infarcts are present. Microscopically, a range of lesions is encountered depending on whether the lesions are acute or chronic.

In the acute phase of malignant hypertension an acute thrombotic microangiopathy develops (Fig. 1-62). The glomeruli show capillary loop thrombosis and mesangiolysis reflecting necrosis of endothelial and mesangial cells and may develop segmental capillary loop necrosis with crescent formation. The arterioles develop fibrinoid necrosis (necrotizing arteriolitis) and thrombosis reflecting necrosis of endothelium and medial smooth muscle cells. The intralobular arteries and arcuate arteries show a

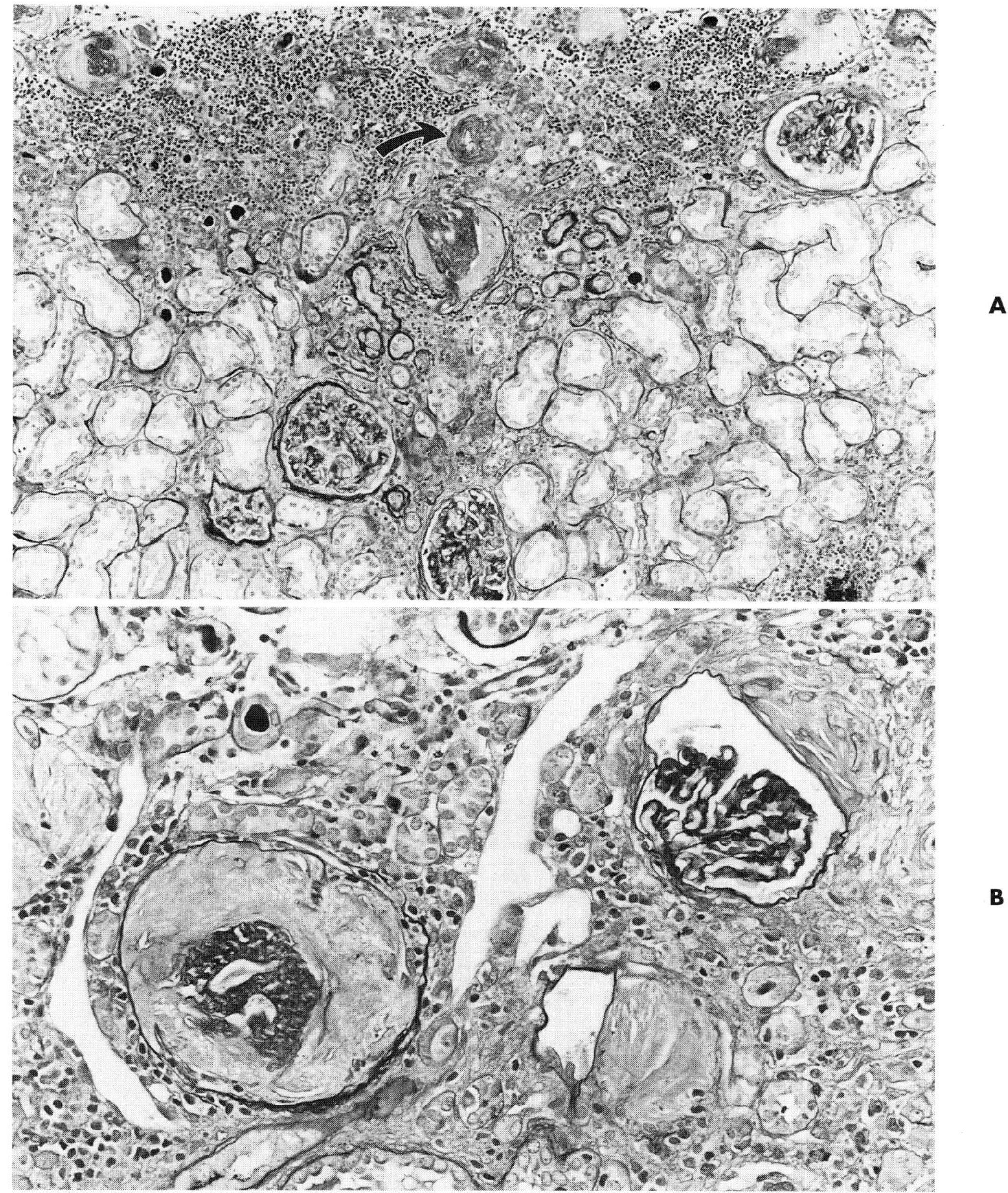

1-61. **A**, The shallow subcapsular scars contain sclerotic glomeruli and atrophic tubules and thickened arterioles (*arrow*). PAS stain. **B**, Glomerular injury in hypertension showing ischemic glomerular basement membrane wrinkling and end-stage ischemic obsolescence. PAS stain.

distinctive mucoid or edematous appearing intimal thickening and may also contain subendothelial fibrin and fragmented red blood cells.

In the more protracted case, chronic or reparative changes are present alone or superimposed upon the acute thrombotic microangiopathy. At this stage, with basement membrane stains such as periodic acid-Schiff (PAS) or a silver stain, the glomeruli may either show ischemic wrinkling and collapse (Fig. 1-63) or may show an impressive lucent subendothelial expansion and capillary loop basement membrane reduplication. The arterioles and arteries show concentric (onion-skin) myointimal proliferation resulting in severe luminal occlusion (Fig. 1-63).

THROMBOTIC MICROANGIOPATHY

The two classic syndromes dominated by thrombotic microangiopathy are thrombotic thrombocytopenic purpura described by Moschcowitz[138] in 1925 and hemolytic uremic syndrome described by Gasser et al[139] in 1955. Thrombotic microangiopathy is a term coined by Symmers[140] in 1952 for the microvascular lesions that develop in thrombotic thrombocytopenic purpura. Since that time, use of the term has been expanded (see box

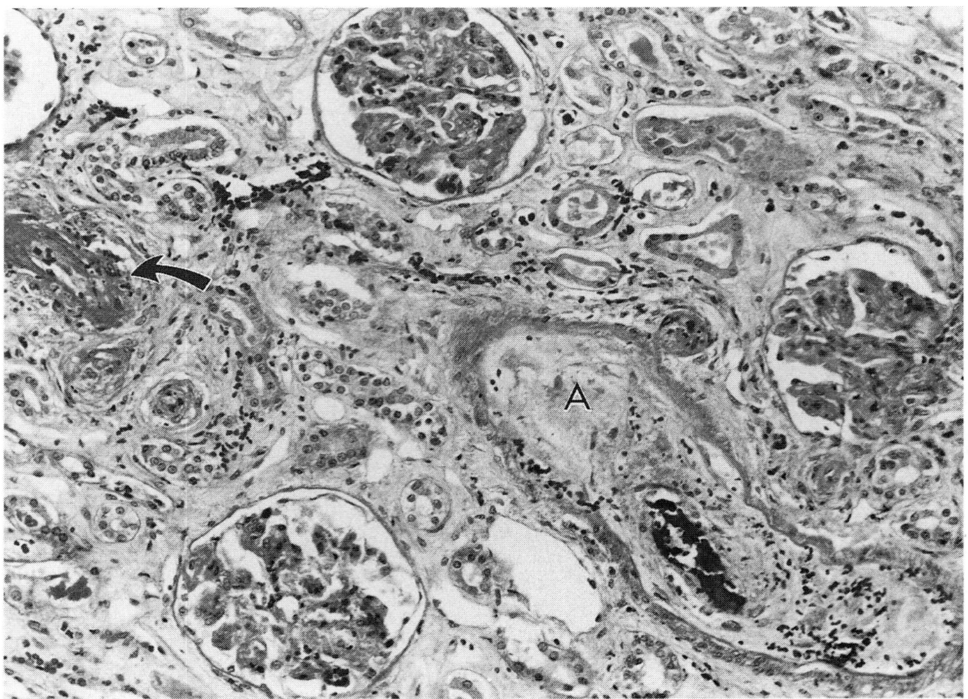

1-62. Necrotizing arteriolitis (*arrow*), glomerular thrombosis, and intralobular arterial (*A*) intimal thickening with extravasated red cells in malignant hypertension.

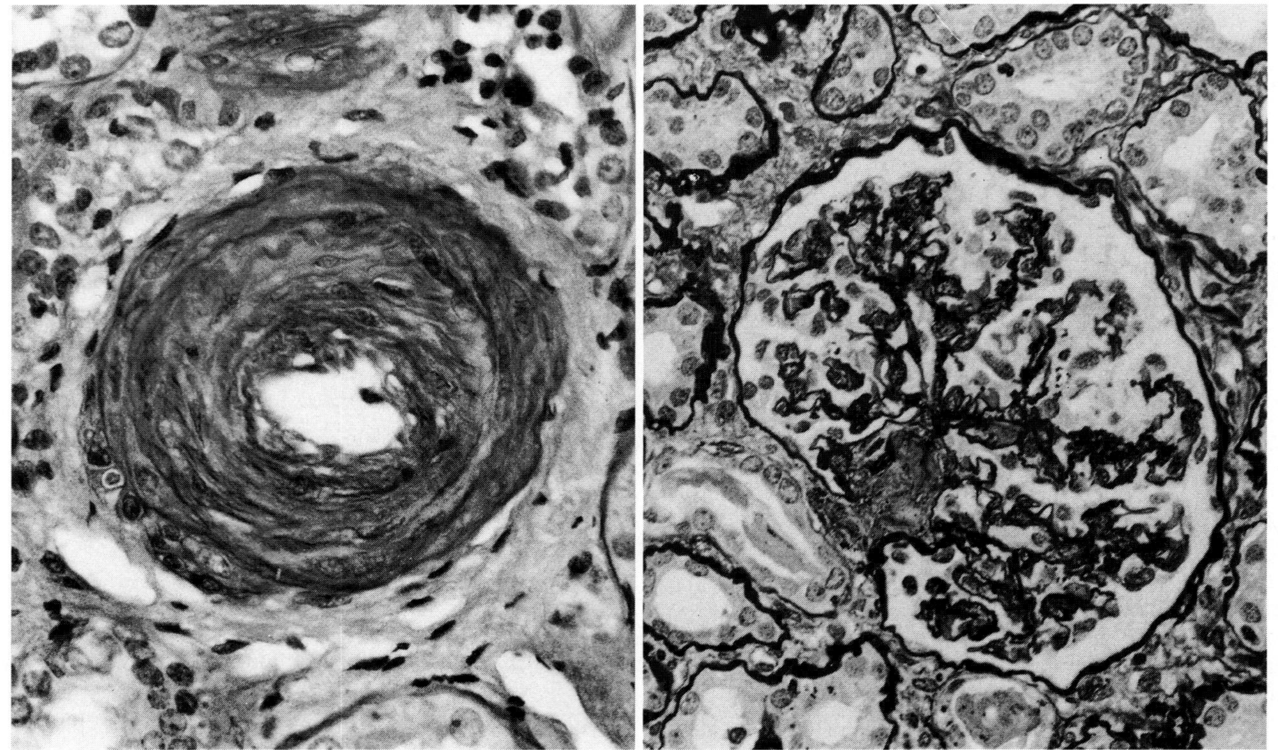

1-63. Hyperplastic arteriolitis (**A**) and ischemic capillary loop wrinkling (**B**) in malignant hypertension. A-PAS stain, B-silver stain.

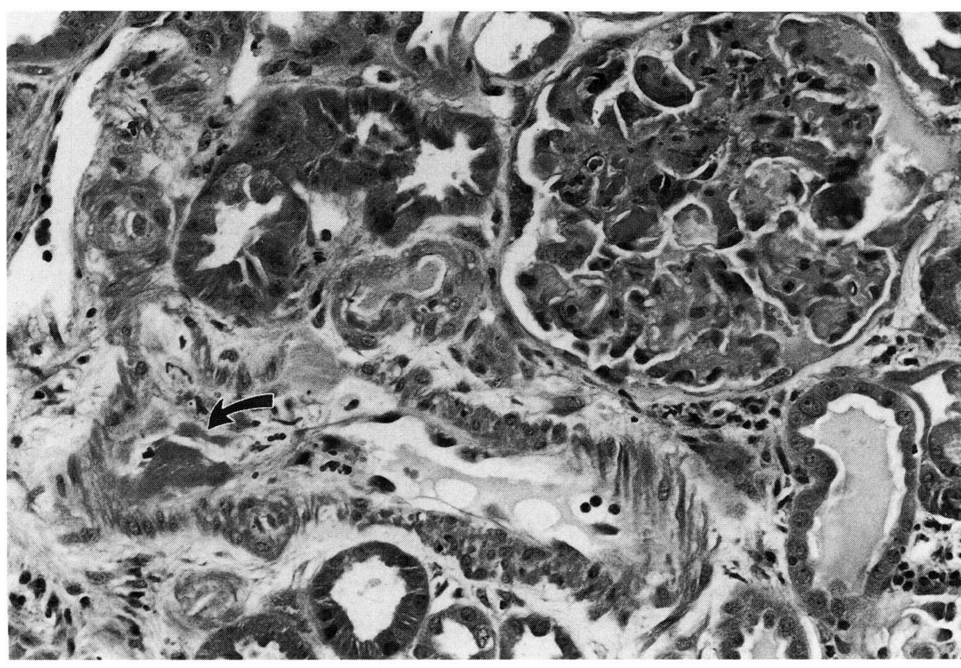

1-64. Hemolytic-uremic syndrome showing an artery with subendothelial fibrin (*arrow*) and glomerular capillary thrombosis.

THROMBOTIC MICROANGIOPATHY

- Thrombotic thrombocytopenic purpura
- Hemolytic uremic syndrome
- Malignant hypertension
- Disseminated intravascular coagulation
- Scleroderma renal crisis
- Postpartum acute renal failure
- Irradiation
- Drugs
  - Oral contraceptives
  - Chemotherapeutic agent
  - Cyclosporine

on this page) and now includes a group of largely noninflammatory microvascular thrombotic diseases accompanied by renal disease, hemolytic anemia, and thrombocytopenia.[141-146]

The relationship between the two classic forms of primary thrombotic microangiopathy, thrombotic thrombocytopenic purpura and hemolytic uremic syndrome, remains controversial.[147-149] In thrombotic thrombocytopenic purpura the clinical picture is dominated by central nervous system involvement with only mild renal disease.[138,140,147,148] It usually develops in adults and has a fulminant course. It has a high fatality rate if not promptly diagnosed and treated by plasma exchange or plasma infusion.

In contrast, the clinical picture of hemolytic uremic syndrome is dominated by acute renal failure, and patients are usually children.[139,148,149] It has an acute usually gastrointestinal diarrhea prodrome (occasionally upper respiratory infection prodrome), which has been shown to result from infection by verotoxin-producing stains of *Escherichia coli* in 80% to 90%.[150,151] It is the most common cause of pediatric acute renal failure, but most children recover. Children over the age of 4 years and those lacking the diarrhea prodrome have a poorer prognosis.

The histopathologic spectrum of the microvascular lesions in thrombotic microangiopathy is similar regardless of cause and identical to those described for malignant hypertension. Therefore clinical correlation is required to distinguish thrombotic thrombocytopenic purpura from hemolytic uremic syndrome or to implicate one of the secondary forms. Unfortunately, even when a secondary form is excluded not all patients are readily classified as either primary thrombotic thrombocytopenic purpura or hemolytic uremic syndrome because an insidious onset can occur with milder forms of both central nervous system and renal disease. Furthermore, acute renal failure and severe hypertension may both be present, making separation between hemolytic uremic syndrome and primary malignant hypertension difficult if not impossible.

In acute thrombotic microangiopathy, glomeruli, arterioles and arteries may each be affected (Fig. 1-64, 1-65). Glomeruli show endothelial cell and often mesangial cell necrosis with capillary loop thrombosis and mesangiolysis. The arterioles show luminal thrombosis and fibrin extravasation beneath the endothelium and into the media. The arteries show severe intimal edema or so-called mucoid intimal thickening and may also contain fibrin and red cells. Fragmented red cells can be seen in all structures and cortical infarcts may develop.

In the chronic phase observed in treated patients or in patients with a more insidious onset of the disease, the

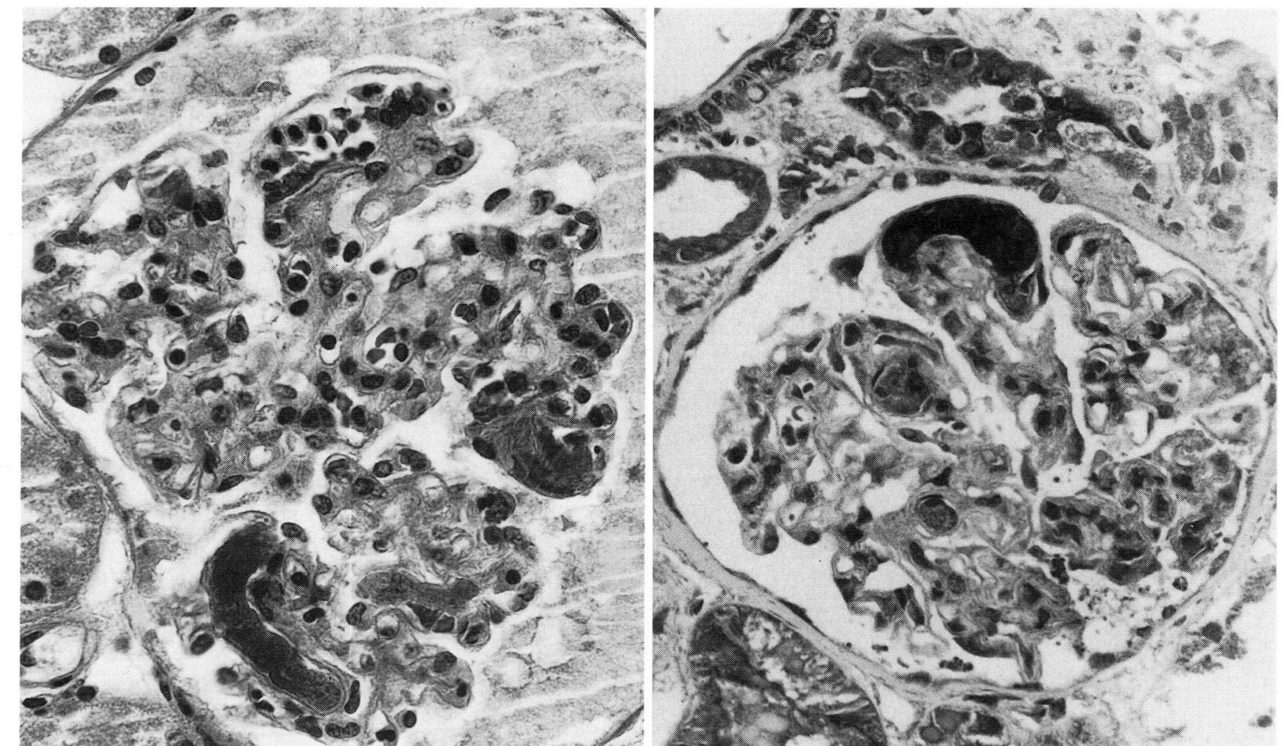

1-65. **A**, Disseminated intravascular coagulation showing glomerular capillary thrombi. **B**, Cyclosporine toxicity showing glomeruli capillary loop thrombi in a renal allograft.

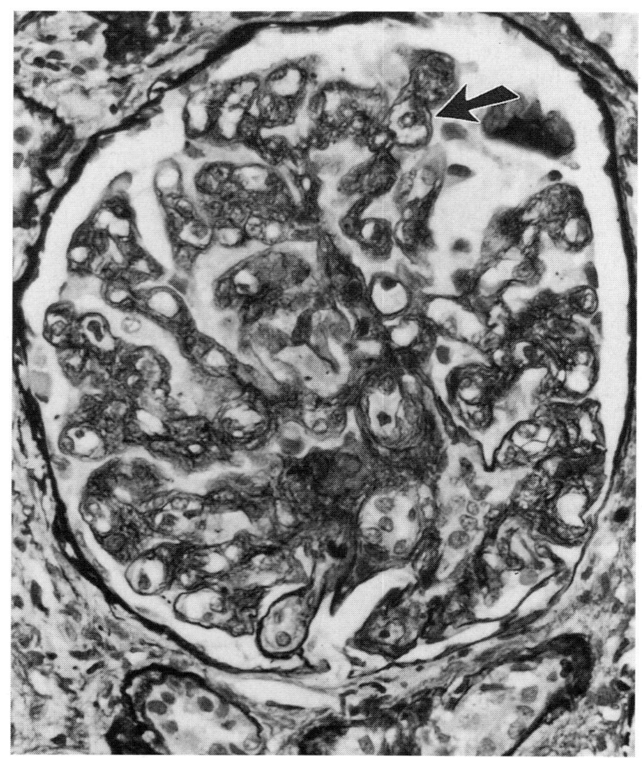

1-66. Chronic therapy-related thrombotic microangiopathy showing basement membrane reduplication (*arrow*) in a bone marrow transplant patient. Silver stain.

glomeruli show prominent mesangial expansion, microaneurysms, and reduplication of the capillary loop basement membranes (Fig. 1-66). Arterioles may show hyaline luminal occlusion, or both arterioles and arteries may show hyperplastic concentric myointimal proliferation resulting in severe luminal occlusion.

RENAL ARTERY STENOSIS

In 1934 Goldblatt et al[152] established a role for decreased renal perfusion in the generation of systemic hypertension by partially occluding one renal artery of a dog, producing hypertension that was reversed after restoration of blood flow. Hypertension resulting from

CAUSES OF RENAL ARTERY STENOSIS

- Atherosclerosis
- Fibromuscular dysplasia
- Rare other causes
  - renal artery dissection
  - renal artery aneurysm
  - renal artery thrombosis
  - renal artery emboli
  - arterial—venous malformation
  - arteritis
  - radiation injury
  - transplant artery stenosis
  - neurofibromatosis

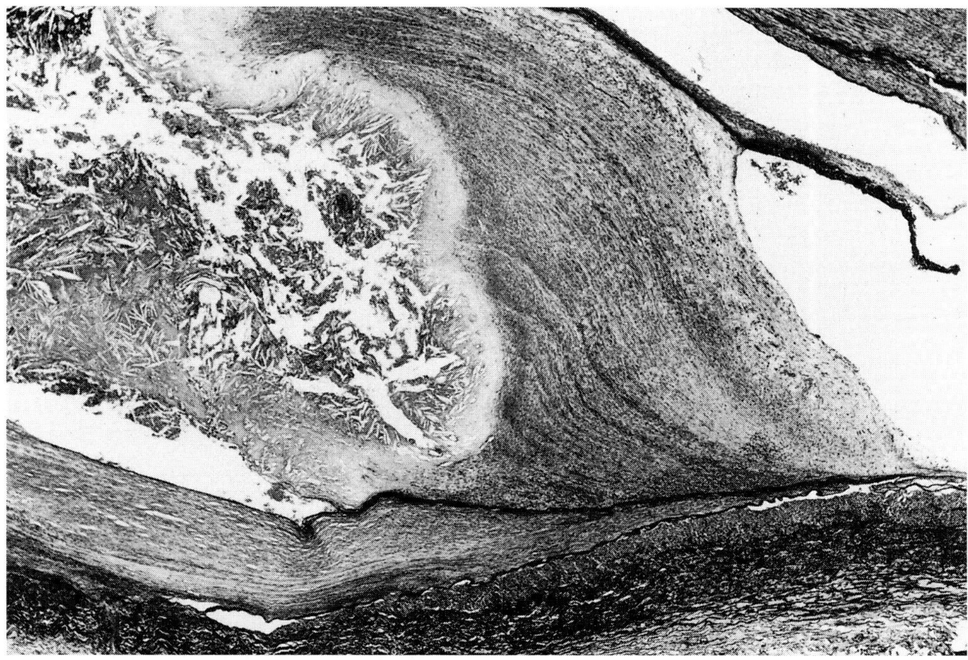

1-67. Atherosclerotic renal artery stenosis with a plaque at the renal artery ostium. Elastic stain.

TABLE 1-3.
LARGE VESSEL DISEASES AND POSSIBLE COMPLICATIONS

Primary Disorder	Hypertension	Dissection	Aneurysm	Infarct	Rupture
Renal artery stenosis	+	+	+	+	-
Renal artery dissection	+	+	+	+	+
Renal artery aneurysms	+	+	+	+	+
Renal artery thrombosis	+	-	-	+	-
Renal artery emboli	+	-	-	+	-
AV malformation fistula	+	-	-	-	+
Renal arteritis	+	-	+	+	-
Renal vein thrombosis	+	-	-	-	-

decreased renal perfusion and relieved by restoration of flow is known as renovascular hypertension. Renal artery stenosis is the most common cause.[153,154] The two major etiologies of renal artery stenosis (see box on p. 42) are atherosclerosis (66% of cases) and fibromuscular dysplasia (33% of cases). The remaining causes of renal artery stenosis, although numerous, comprise less than 1% of cases. Renal artery stenosis may result in several complications (Table 1-3).

Atherosclerosis-related renal artery stenosis

Atherosclerosis causes 60% to 70% of cases of renal artery stenosis. There is a male predominance and patients usually present from age 50 to 70 and have significant atherosclerosis of the aorta and other major arteries, which influences the management of the disease and its prognosis. Because atherosclerosis develops over many years and is a complication of prolonged essential hypertension, the kidney may exhibit benign nephrosclerosis or may contain remote infarcts from aortic atheroemboli (Fig. 1-59). Bilateral disease occurs in 30% of cases and if severe causes ischemic chronic renal failure. Revascularization can improve renal function in some patients; however, because these patients have a long history of hypertension, arterial nephrosclerosis is usually implicated in the renal failure and renal artery stenosis is not recognized.

The renal artery is occluded by eccentrically thickened intima at its aortic ostium or in its proximal portion (Fig. 1-67). Intimal thickening begins when myointimal cells enter the media and synthesize connective tissue components and mucopolysaccharides.[135] Lipid and foam cells accumulate and fibrosis develops. The advanced lesion contains atheromatous material in the

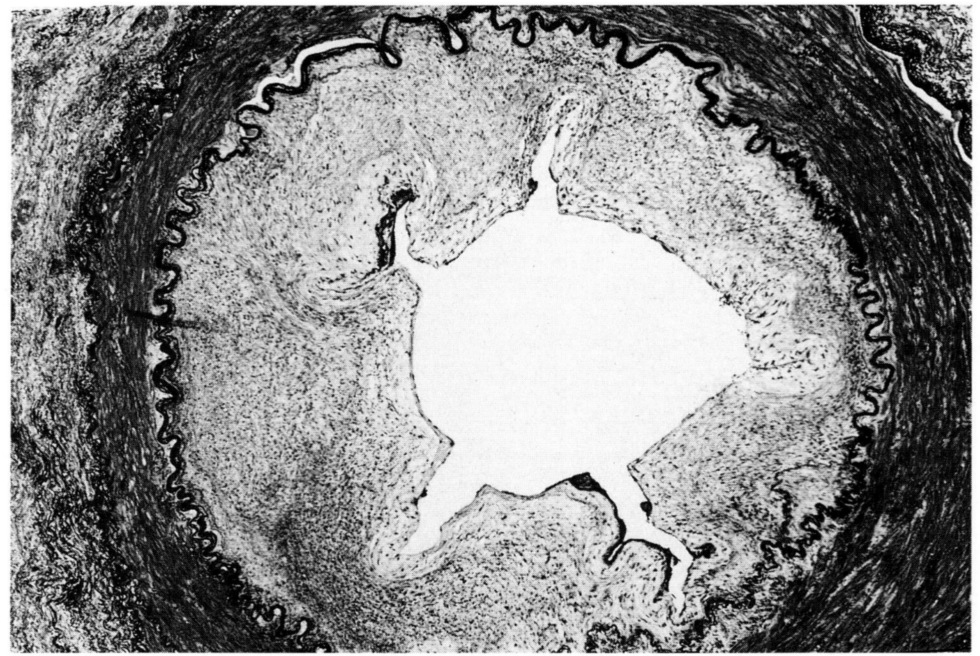

1-68. Intimal fibromuscular dysplasia showing fibroblastic intimal thickening and intact internal elastic lamina. Elastic stain.

FIBROMUSCULAR DYSPLASIA
- Intimal fibroplasia
- Medial fibroplasia
  - Medial hyperplasia
  - Medial fibroplasia with aneurysms
  - Perimedial fibroplasia
- Periarterial fibroplasia

form of acingulate cholesterol clefts, foamy macrophages, and calcification. Irregular reduplication of elastica with sclerosis and atrophy of medial smooth muscle is present.

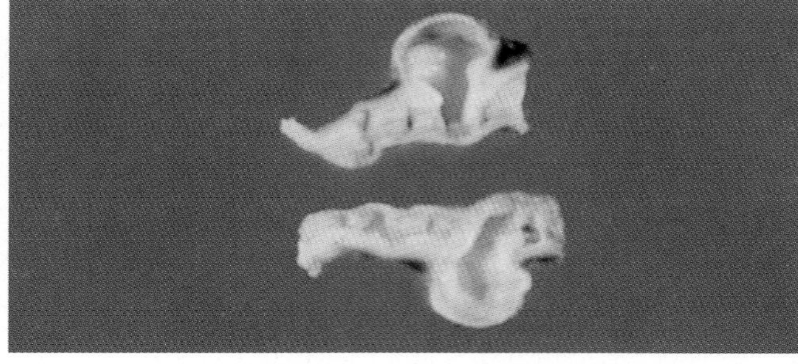

1-69. A segment of the main renal artery showing medial fibroplasia complicated by a saccular aneurysm.

Fibromuscular dysplasia

Fibromuscular dysplasia is the second most common cause of renal artery stenosis in adults and is the most common cause in children.[155-157] It consists of a group of lesions (see box on this page), which despite histological differences, have a similar clinical presentation, affecting women in their 20s to 40s. The prognosis for fibromuscular dysplasia is much better than for atherosclerosis-associated renal artery stenosis because the patient is younger, the hypertension is of recent onset, and hypertension and atherosclerosis-related diseases in other sites are absent. There are five subtypes (dissection is discussed later in this chapter).

Intimal fibroplasia. Intimal fibroplasia is a rare (<1% of cases) form of fibromuscular dysplasia. It produces circumferential intimal thickening in a substantial segment of the renal artery and may also extend into its segmental branches. The thickened intima is composed of fibroblastic tissue (Fig. 1-68). It is distinguished from atherosclerotic intimal thickening by the absence of lipids and calcification and the presence of an intact internal elastic lamina. It is prone to develop thrombosis and dissection.

Medial hyperplasia. Medial hyperplasia consists of a localized segment of disorganized medial smooth muscle thickening. Radiographically it resembles the intimal form and is also prone to develop thrombosis and dissection. The intima is not thickened and the internal elastic lamina is intact.

Medial fibroplasia with aneurysms. Medial fibroplasia with aneurysms is the most frequent and distinctive form of fibromuscular dysplasia. It tends to involve the distal main renal artery and its segmental branches and is commonly bilateral. It is characterized by ridges of medial thickening without fibrosis, alternating with areas of extreme medial thinning in which there is close approximation of the internal and external elastic lamina (Fig. 1-69, 1-70). These areas of thinning represent

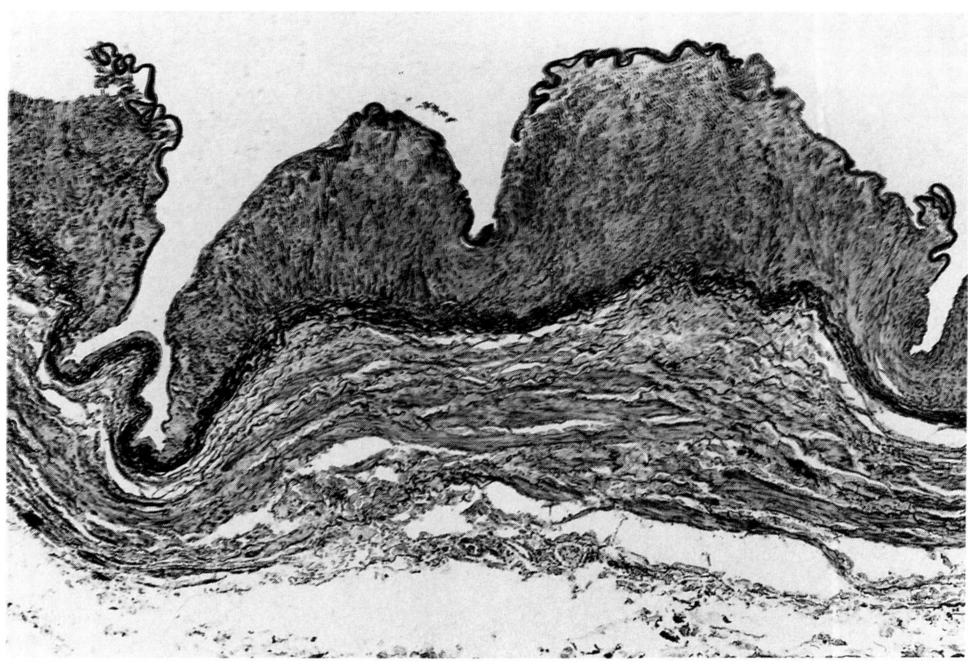

1-70. Medial fibroplasia. Elastic stain.

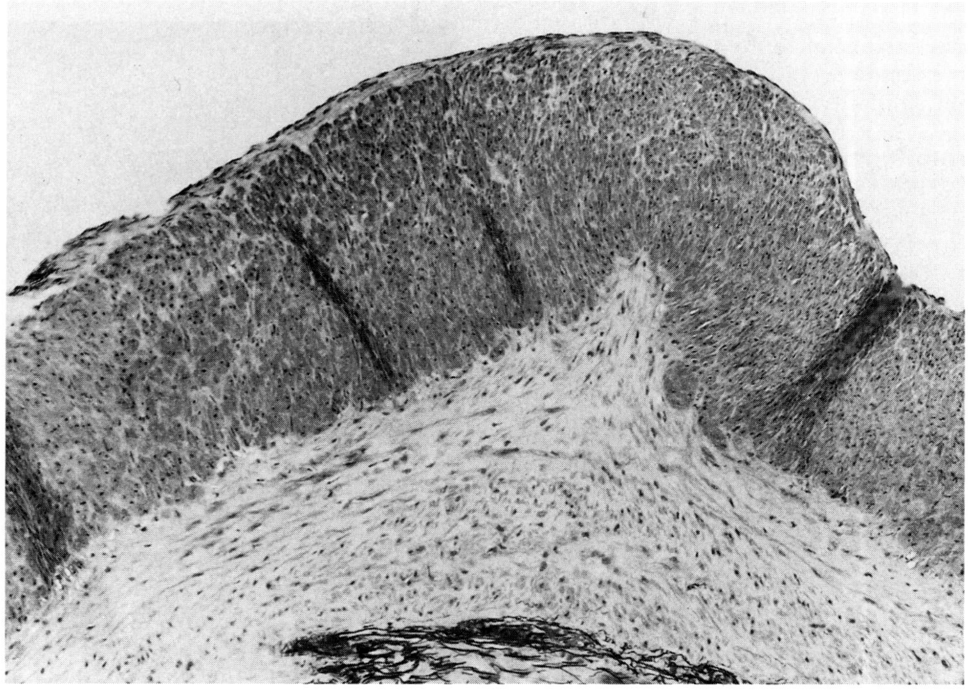

1-71. Perimedial fibroplasia. Trichrome stain.

the "aneurysms" and result in a characteristic pattern (string of pearls) on angiogram.

Perimedial fibroplasia. Perimedial fibroplasia is the second most common form of fibromuscular dysplasia. It is characterized by an irregular pattern of fibrosis that replaces the outer one half to two thirds of the media by fibrous tissue (Fig. 1-71). It can lead to severe stenosis and the development of thrombosis and renal infarcts.

Periarterial fibroplasia. Periarterial fibroplasia is the rarest form of fibromuscular dysplasia. It consists of dense collagenous tissue that forms within the adventitia

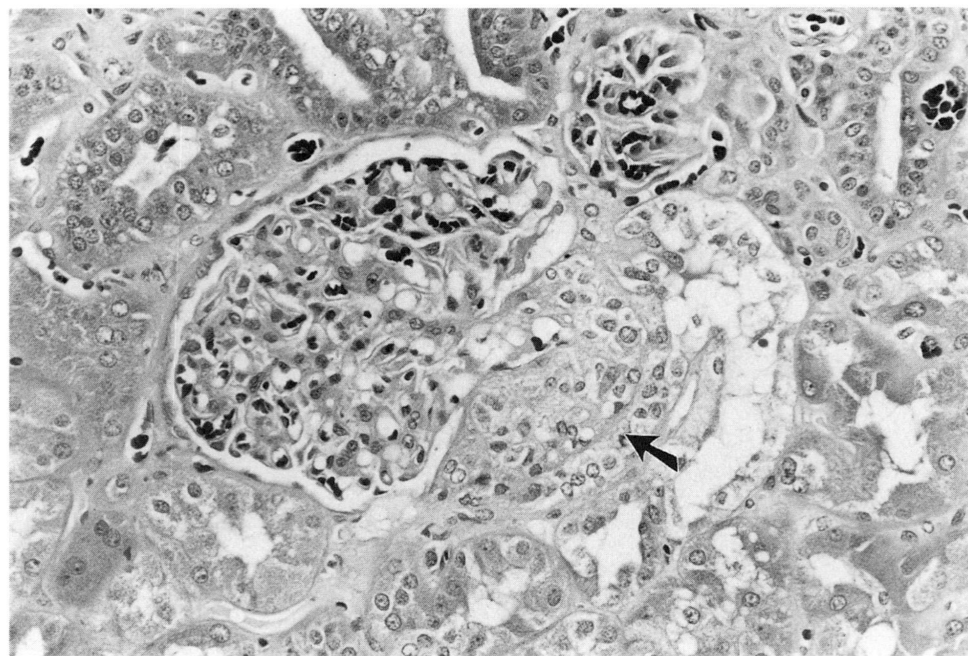

1-72. Acute renal artery stenosis in a renal transplant showing prominent enlargement of the juxtaglomerular apparatus (*arrow*).

and restricts arterial expansion during systole. The collagenous tissue can extend into the adjacent fibrofatty tissue, creating a vague similarity to retroperitoneal fibrosis.

The kidney in renal artery stenosis

In renal artery stenosis of recent onset there is initial enlargement of the juxtaglomerular apparatus resulting from an increase in the number of the extraglomerular mesangial cells, or lacis cells (Fig. 1-72). There is metaplasia of smooth muscle cells of the afferent arteriole to form contractile filament poor, renin synthesizing cells. Distinctive renin protogranules and mature renin granules can be detected in increased quantities in these cells by the Bowie stain, immunocytochemistry, or electron microscopy.

After several weeks of renal artery stenosis the juxtaglomerular apparatus shrinks, again becoming inconspicuous. At this time the parenchyma supplied by the stenotic artery shows a very distinctive alteration. Grossly there is uniform cortical thinning (Fig. 1-73) resulting from diffuse atrophy of tubules and causing close approximation of glomeruli due to loss of tubular volume (Fig. 1-74). The glomeruli appear slightly contracted but remain viable. If the main renal artery is the site of stenosis then the entire kidney becomes small (40 to 70 g) and uniformly contracted with a smooth subcapsular surface. If a segmental artery is stenotic, or conversely, if it is free of stenosis while the main renal artery is stenotic (Fig. 1-75), then a characteristic line of transition from a thinned cortex to a thicker cortex will be grossly apparent.

RENAL ARTERY DISSECTION

Dissection of the renal artery refers to a disruption of the intima that extends into the media (Fig. 1-76, 1-77)

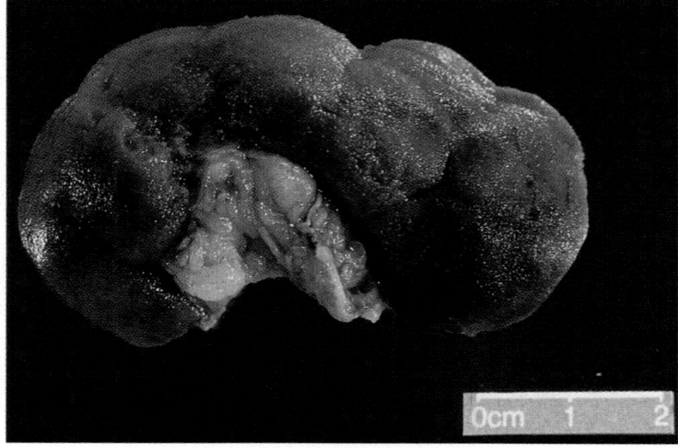

1-73. A small contracted kidney with a smooth surface in chronic renal artery stenosis secondary to fibromuscular dysplasia.

with creation of a false lumen or a double channel or results in a complete vascular occlusion causing renal infarction.[158-160] Dissection is associated with hypertension, flank pain, and hematuria. The hypertension may not always precede the dissection but is invariably present following the dissection. Renal artery dissection has several etiologies[158-160] (see box on p. 47).

The most common cause of renal artery dissection is extension from an aortic dissection. Primary renal artery dissection is much rarer and in the past was usually a complication of preexisting fibromuscular dysplasia. Catheter-related causes are increasing with more frequent use of that procedure to correct renal artery stenosis. Dissection due to blunt trauma is rare and is usually the consequence of an automobile accident.

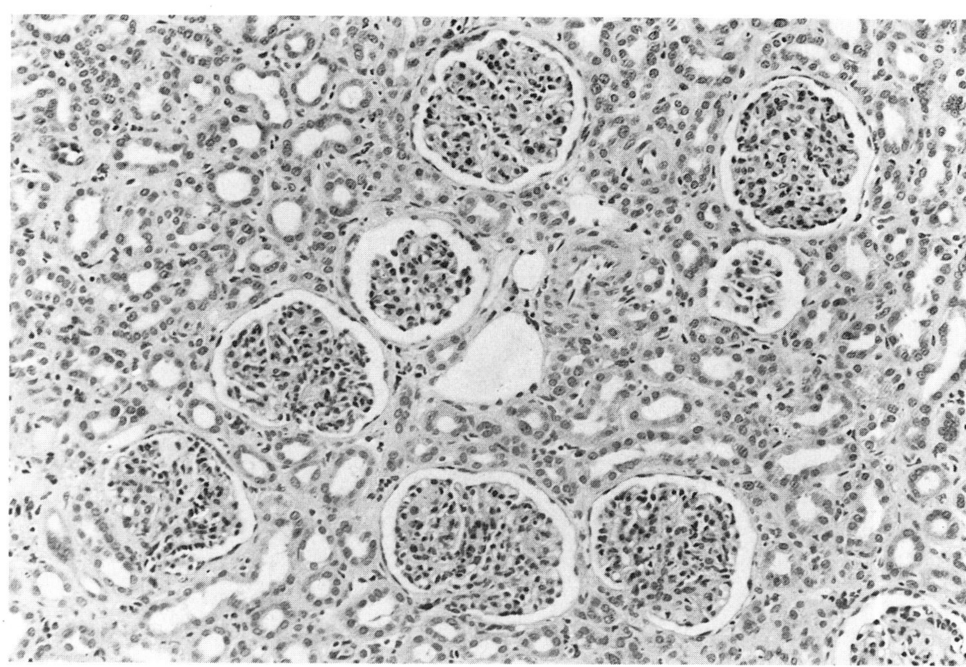

1-74. The thin cortex in chronic renal artery stenosis shows diffuse small atrophic tubules and crowding of nonsclerotic glomeruli.

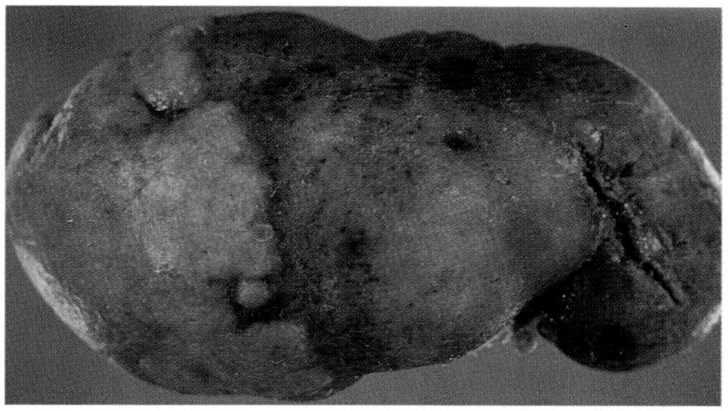

1-75. Chronic renal artery stenosis affecting the middle and lower poles. The upper pole was supplied by a patent supernumerary (polar segmental) artery.

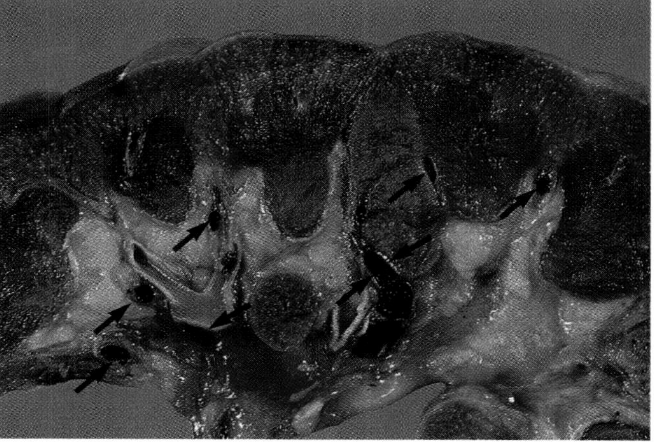

1-76. Extensive renal artery dissection (*arrows*) following an unsuccessful angioplasty.

CAUSES OF RENAL ARTERY DISSECTION
- Extension from aortic dissection
- Fibromuscular dysplasia
- Blunt abdominal trauma
- Catheter injury
- Spontaneous or idiopathic

RENAL ARTERY ANEURYSM

Aneurysms of the main renal artery or one of its tributaries are rare, found in 0.01% of autopsies.[160-164] They may be classified as true aneurysms, which may be either congenital or acquired, or false aneurysms, which are usually the result of trauma. Most are small and asymptomatic. If a large vessel is involved, renal artery aneurysms may be associated with thrombosis and vascular occlusion leading to infarction or hypertension (see box on p. 43). Pain is an ominous symptom that usually indicates impending rupture or dissection. The risk of rupture is greatest during pregnancy and parturition and is usually fatal. Three categories of aneurysms have been identified: saccular, fusiform, and intrarenal. Dissecting aneurysm is not included in this list because aneurysmal enlargement is not a feature of renal arterial dissection.

Saccular aneurysm

Saccular aneurysms develop in the main renal artery at the bifurcation of the anterior and posterior divisions or

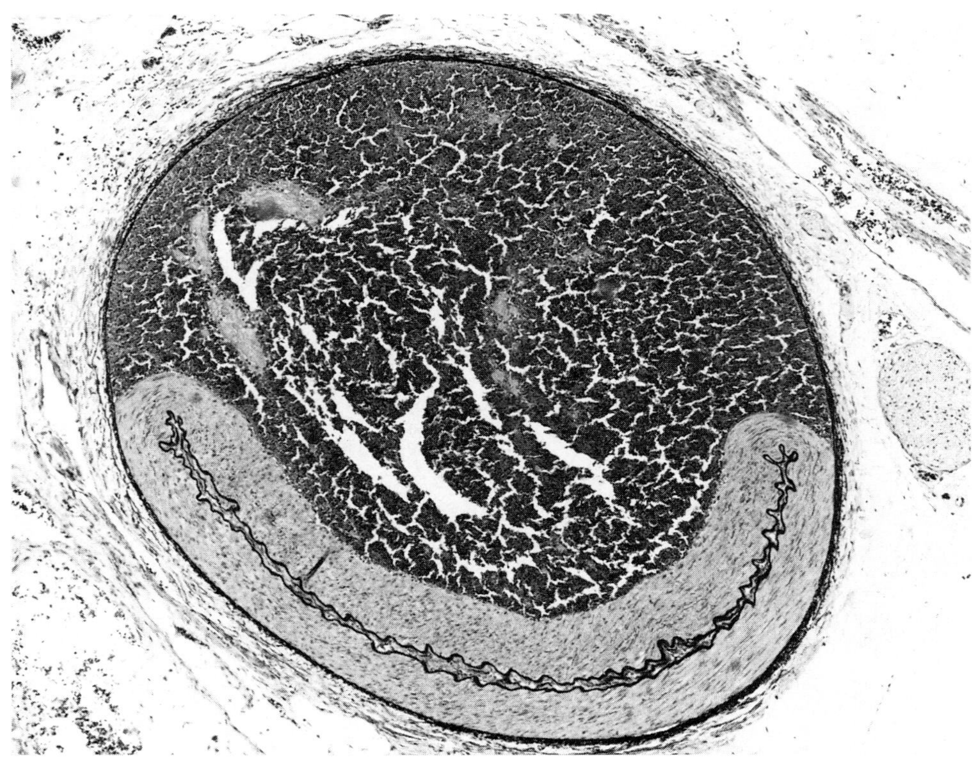

1-77. The dissection (*from Fig 1-76*) developed at the interface of the media and adventitia.

at a branch point of a segmental artery. Although they are frequently calcified or show atherosclerotic changes, they are usually regarded as congenital with the atherosclerosis considered a secondary event. They may be small or enlarge to 4 to 5 cm. Especially if noncalcified, the large aneurysms are prone to rupture or may erode into an adjacent vein producing an arteriovenous fistula.

Fusiform aneurysm

Fusiform aneurysms usually occur in young patients and represent a poststenotic dilation that develops distal to renal artery stenosis, often secondary to fibromuscular dysplasia. Thrombosis with secondary renal infarction is a serious potential complication.

Intrarenal aneurysm

Intrarenal aneurysms are usually false aneurysms.[164] They have many causes: trauma (biopsy, surgery), arteritis (polyarteritis nodosa), postinflammatory injury (tuberculosis or transplant rejection), and neurofibromatosis.[164] Rarely, intrarenal aneurysms may be congenital.

ARTERIOVENOUS MALFORMATION AND FISTULA

Direct communication between renal arteries and veins may either be congenital or acquired.[165-167] Congenital lesions are referred to as arteriovenous malformations while acquired lesions are called arteriovenous fistulas. High output heart failure, hypertension, and hematuria may develop depending upon the size of the shunt and location of the lesion. The most common type is an acquired fistula (65% to 75% of cases). It usually has a single point of communication between an artery and a vein.[165] It may have several causes; the most common is iatrogenic[167] (see box on this page).

CAUSES OF ACQUIRED ARTERIOVENOUS FISTULA

- Surgical injury
- Needle biopsy
- Penetrating injury
- Neoplasia
- Arterial aneurysm erosion
- Inflammation

Congenital arteriovenous malformations are rare. Most consist of circoid arteriovenous communications in which there are multiple points of communication between artery and vein. Most are located within the medulla or in the calyceal or pelvic mucosa and usually cause gross hematuria. Hilar vessels may also be affected. When a single cavernous channel connects an artery with a vein, an abdominal bruit may be heard.

RENAL EMBOLI AND INFARCTS

Renal artery emboli invariably cause infarction because of the end artery organization of the renal blood flow.[18-20] If the infarct is small, it may be clinically and functionally asymptomatic. Larger infarcts cause flank

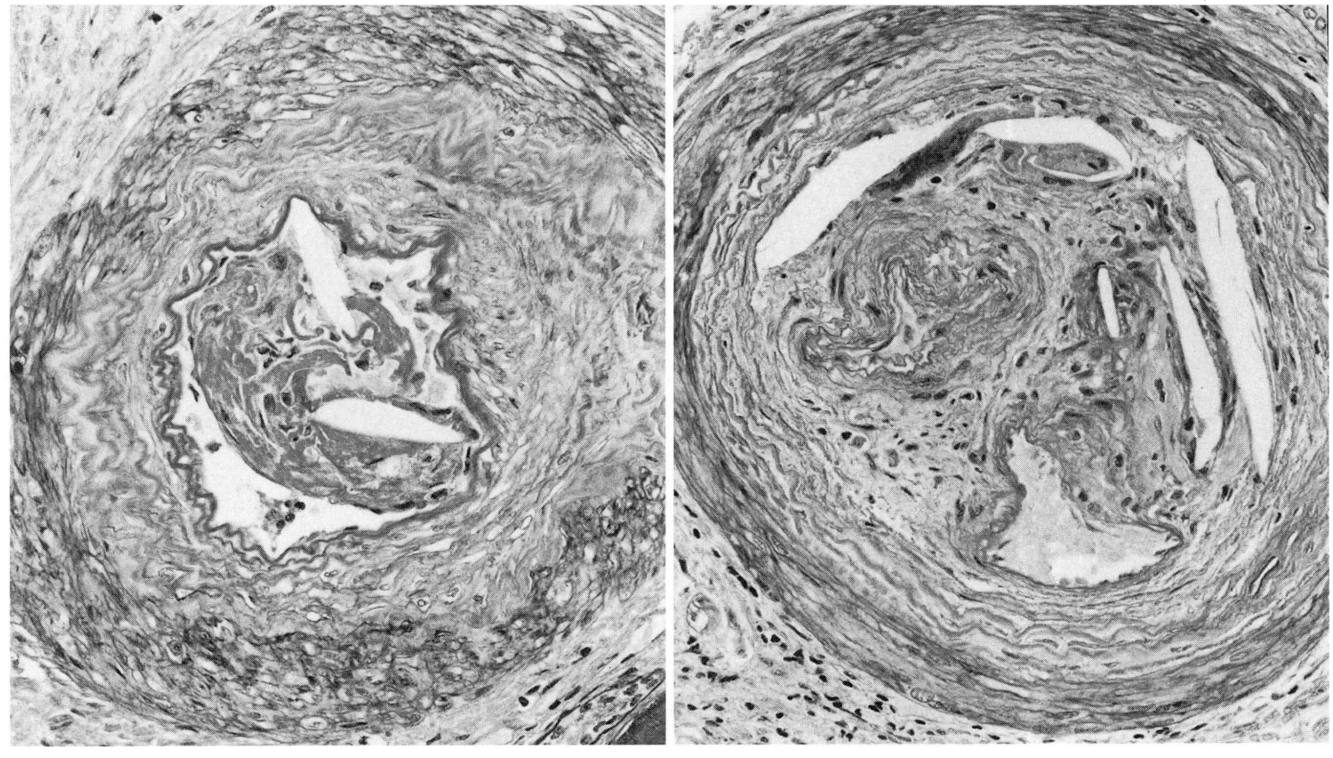

1-78. Recent (**A**) and remote (**B**) atheroemboli showing a fibrin thrombus and recanalization with giant cells, respectively.

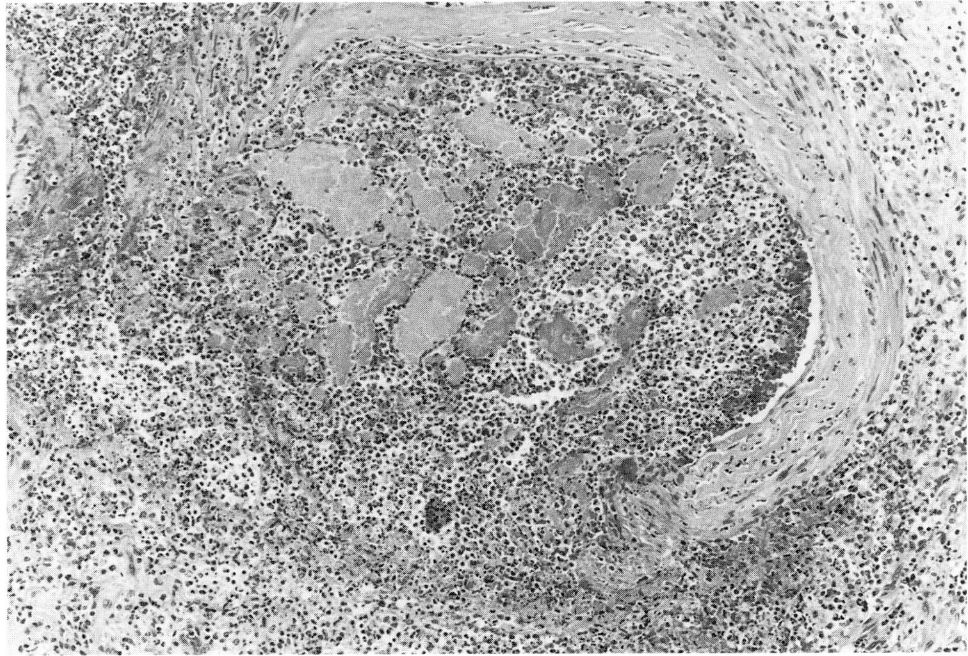

1-79. This thromboembolus from a patient with infective endocarditis contains gram-positive cocci and has destroyed a portion of the arterial wall.

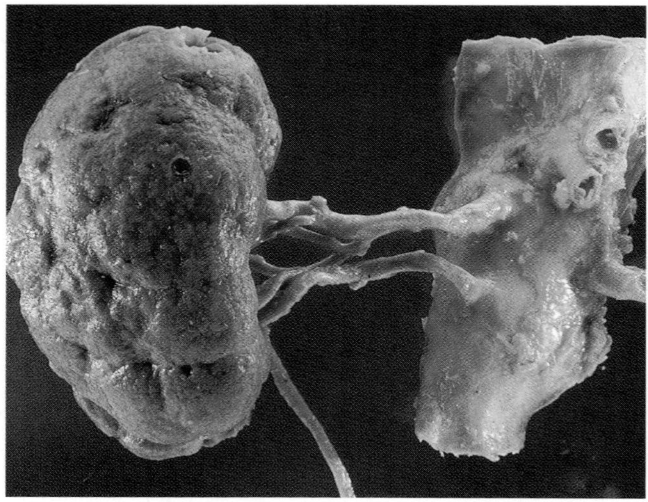

1-80. Multiple depressed scars resulting from arcuate and interlobular atheroembolic infarcts.

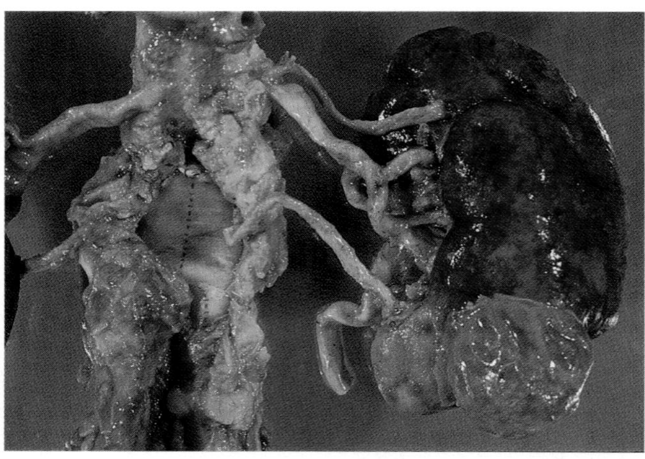

1-81. A remote lower pole infarct and cyst resulting from occlusion of a supernumerary (lower pole segmental) artery during aortic aneurysm repair.

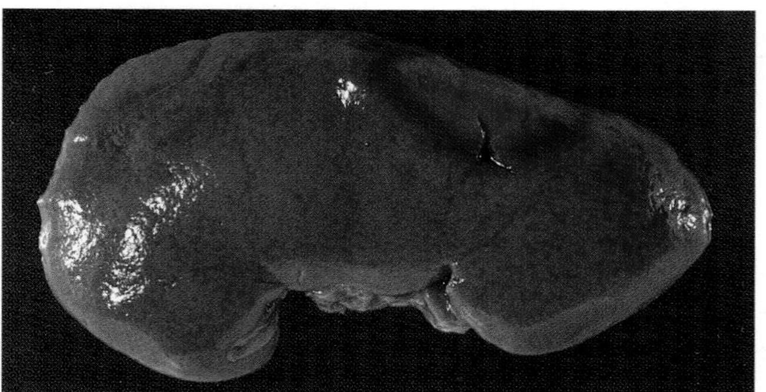

1-82. An acute infarct resulting from an interlobar artery occlusion.

TABLE 1-4
RELATIONSHIP BETWEEN ARTERY OCCLUDED AND INFARCT

Artery	Size of Infarct	Relationship to Lobes
Segmental	4-5 cm	entire lobe and portion of adjacent lobe
Interlobar	2-3 cm	columns of Bertin and portions of adjacent lobes
Arcuate	0.5-1.0 cm	⅙-⅛ of a lobe extending to the middle of the lobe
Interlobular	0.1-0.2 cm	small portion of a lobe

pain, hematuria, and hypertension.[168-173] If bilateral and widespread, renal insufficiency results. Emboli originate either from the heart in patients with valvular disease or atrial fibrillation or from the aorta.[168-173] Aortic atheroemboli are by far the most frequent (Fig. 1-78). If an infected vegetation is responsible, a more complicated picture develops with hematogenous pyelonephritis and microabscesses (Fig. 1-79).

Familiarity with the arterial supply to the kidney often enables one, on gross examination, to infer the caliber of vessel occluded by virtue of the size of infarct and its relationship to the renal lobes (Fig. 1-80, 1-81 and Table 1-4).

The acute infarct shows a sharply demarcated zone of transcortical coagulation necrosis, which will also involve the medulla if an arcuate or larger artery is involved (Fig. 1-82, 1-83). The margins of the infarct are hemorrhagic and contain many neutrophils and histiocytes. Cholesterol clefts or infected material in the arteries may reveal the source of the embolus (Fig. 1-78, 1-79).

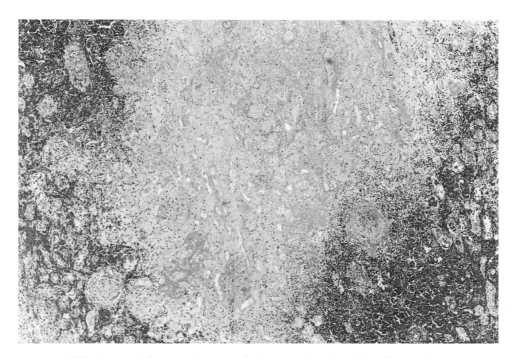

1-83. An acute infarct showing coagulation necrosis with peripheral hemorrhage.

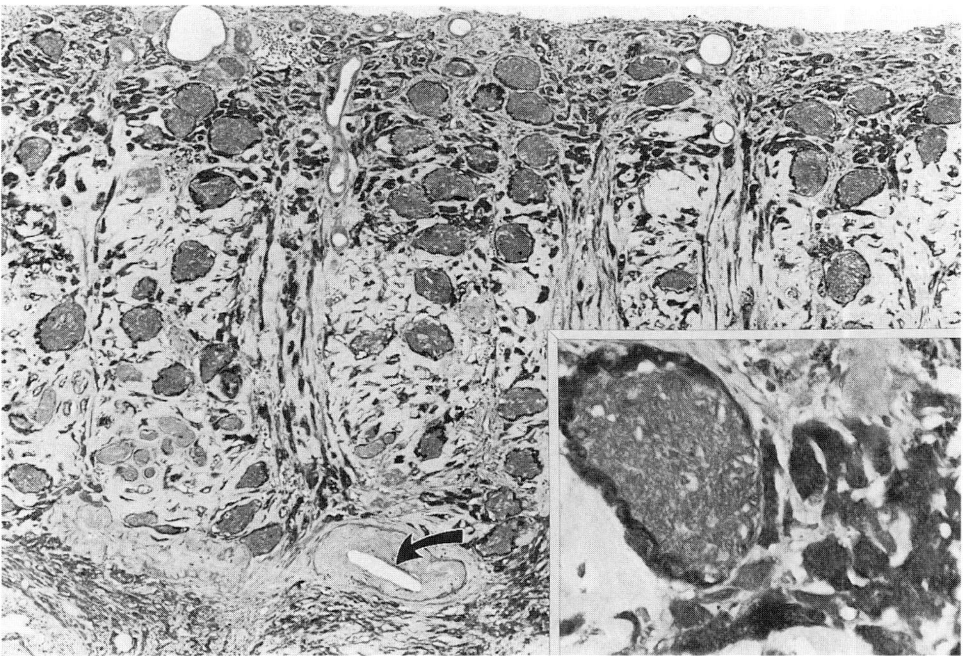

1-84. Remote atheroembolic (*arrow*) cortical infarct. PAS stain. Inset: Note solid PAS-positive glomeruli and tubules.

Eventually, infarcts become depressed cortical scars (Fig. 1-80, 1-81, 1-84). Within them, ghost-like remnants of glomeruli and tubules are present (Fig. 1-84). A PAS stain is helpful in determining whether a scar is an infarct or a more chronic form of injury because infarcted glomeruli contain condensed masses of capillary loop basement membranes without the collagenous tissue in Bowman's space that forms with other causes of glomerulosclerosis.

RENAL CORTICAL NECROSIS

Renal cortical necrosis is a serious bilateral ischemic injury that can complicate a variety of extrarenal diseases[174-176] (see box on p. 52). Obstetric causes are most frequent. Patients develop acute renal failure, usually associated with anuria and hematuria, which may be gross. The condition has a high fatality rate related to extrarenal complications.

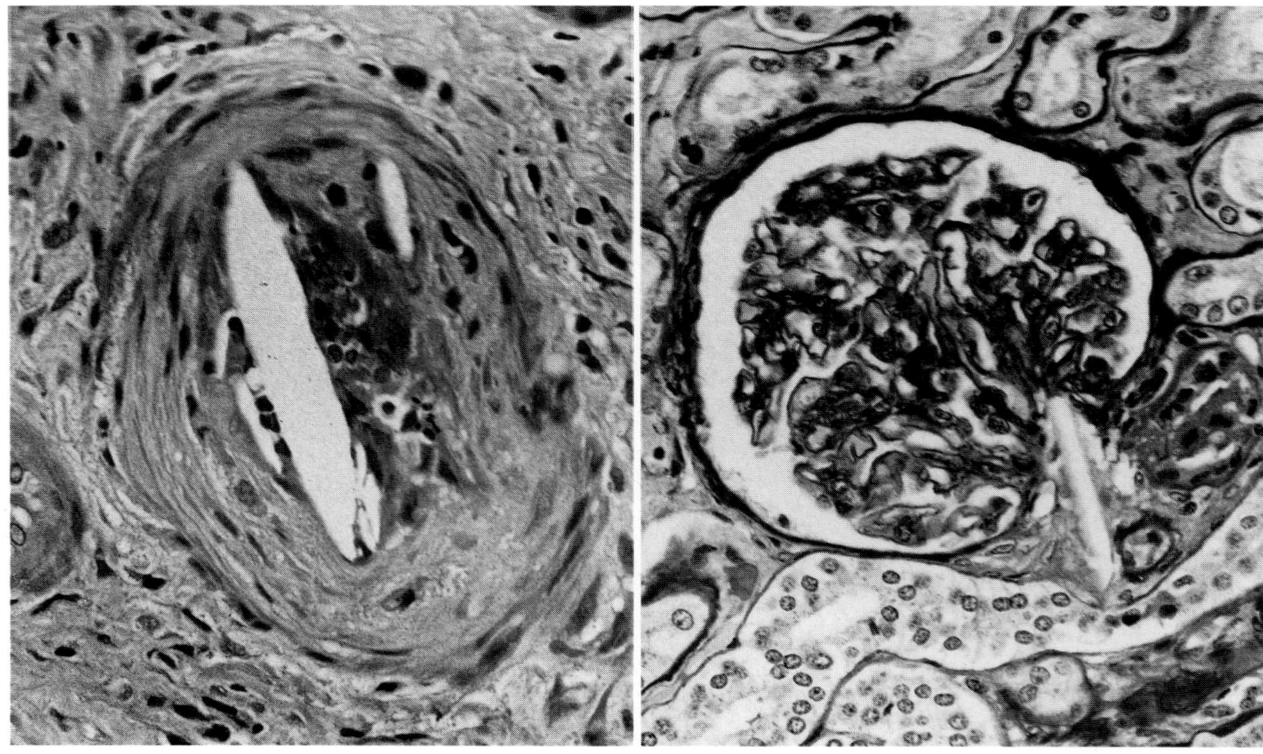

1-85. Renal cholesterol microembolism syndrome with cholesterol emboli in an arteriole (**A**) and in the glomerular hilum (**B**).

CAUSES OF RENAL CORTICAL NECROSIS

- Obstetric complications
  - Abruptio placentae
  - Septic abortion
  - Intrauterine fetal demise
- Infections
  - Sepsis
  - Peritonitis
- Burns
- Gastrointestinal hemorrhage
- Transfusion reactions
- Toxins
- Hemolytic uremic syndrome

The kidneys develop diffuse or patchy sharply demarcated zones of cortical pallor with hyperemic rims that also involve the column's of Bertin. The renal pyramids and a thin subcapsular rim of cortex are spared. There is coagulation necrosis of glomeruli and tubules, usually with widespread thrombosis.

RENAL CHOLESTEROL MICROEMBOLISM SYNDROME

In recent years, a syndrome characterized by systemic microembolization of atheromatous material has been recognized as the cholesterol microembolism syndrome.[172,173,177] This syndrome usually develops following a vascular procedure such as catheterization or aneurysm surgery but occasionally arises spontaneously. Emboli shower the microvasculature of multiple organs including kidneys, skin, brain, and gastrointestinal tract.

Renal involvement manifests with slowly progressive renal insufficiency, often leading to renal failure over a period of weeks to months. In 80% of cases it is associated with peripheral blood eosinophilia.[178] It is not clear why the renal complication should evolve so insidiously or why eosinophilia is so common. Kidney biopsies are often obtained to confirm the clinical diagnosis of an allergic reaction only to show numerous cholesterol crystals within small arteries, arterioles, and even glomeruli (Fig. 1-85). The patient's prognosis is grave and depends upon the severity of the extrarenal disease.

CAUSES OF RENAL ARTERY THROMBOSIS

- Umbilical artery catheters in neonates
- Blunt abdominal trauma
- Intraaortic balloons in adults
- Renal transplantation
- Electrical injury

RENAL ARTERY THROMBOSIS

Thombosis of the renal artery is an uncommon event that usually follows a traumatic injury to the renal artery or to the aorta[171,179] (see box on this page). Renovascular hypertension and renal infarction are the major complications (see Table 1-3).

RENAL VEIN AND RENAL VENOUS THROMBOSIS

In the past renal vein thrombosis was believed to cause nephrotic syndrome.[180,181] With the increased utilization of the renal biopsy and advances in understanding of the physiologic consequences of nephrotic syndrome, it is now clear that renal vein thrombosis is a complication of the hypercoagulable state that develops in patients with nephrotic syndrome. Patients with renal vein thrombosis present with flank pain or tenderness and hematuria and often have hypertension. Renal failure and pulmonary emboli are serious complications. Although there are no pathognomonic histologic findings, interstitial edema and marginating neutrophils within dilated glomerular capillaries have been described in acute cases. Organizing thrombi are seen in veins at autopsy.[182,183]

Renal venous thrombosis differs from renal vein thrombosis in that smaller intrarenal vessels are affected, such as interlobular and arcuate veins, rather than the main renal vein.[183,184] Infants are usually affected and the condition is associated with serious illnesses such as diarrhea, congenital heart disease, maternal diabetes mellitus, seizures, and birth trauma. Hemorrhagic cortical infarcts may develop if the thrombosis is sufficiently widespread to interfere with collateral blood flow.

BARTTER'S SYNDROME

Bartter's syndrome is characterized by hyperplasia of the juxtaglomerular apparatus, hyperaldosteronism, and hypokalemic alkalosis.[185] Despite the impressive enlargement of the juxtaglomerular apparatus and hyperreninemia, both renal artery stenosis and systemic hypertension are absent. It is most commonly identified in children and in many cases it appears to be familial with an autosomal recessive inheritance.

VASCULITIS

Vasculitis comprises a large and heterogeneous group of disorders that have in common inflammatory injury to vascular structures. The first major description of vasculitis dates to the 1866 description of periarteritis (polyarteritis) nodosa by Küssmaul and Maier (Fig. 1-86).[186] The seriousness of systemic vasculitis with major visceral involvement was graphically captured in their report. They stated, "He was one of those patients for whom one could make the prognosis even before making the diagnosis, he gave the impression of being one whose days were numbered."[186]

A major advance in the diagnosis and management of patients with vasculitis was the discovery of a serologic marker for certain forms of vasculitis, the antineutrophil cytoplasmic antibody.[185,187,188] Antineutrophil cytoplasmic antibody (ANCA) refers to a family of autoantibodies detectable in the serum of patients with the major forms of systemic vasculitis involving the kidney and in idiopathic (immune complex negative or "pauci-immune") crescentic glomerulonephritis (Table 1-5).[189,190] ANCA has specificity of one of several proteases in lysosomal enzymes of neutrophils and monocytes and is detected by indirect immunofluorescence on alcohol fixed neutrophils. Two principal patterns are detected, a cytoplasmic pattern (C-ANCA) and a perinuclear pattern (P-ANCA). The former is principally due to anti-proteinase 3 specificity while the latter is principally due to anti-myeloperoxidase specificity.

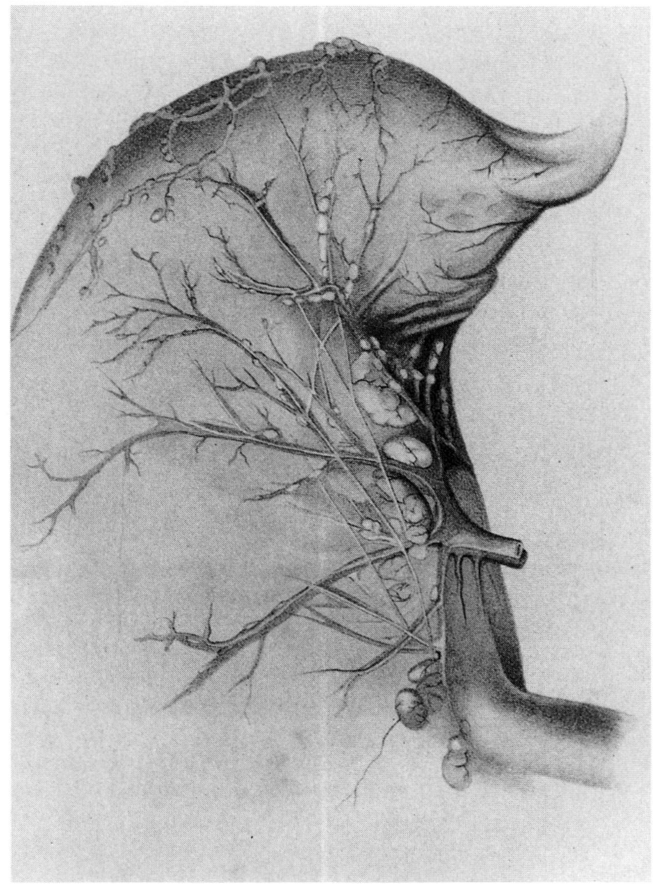

1-86. Nodules along renal arteries in polyarteritis nodosa, from the 1866 description by Kussmaul and Maier. *(From Küssmaul A and Maier R: Ueber eine bisher niche beschriebene eigenthumliche arterienerkrankung (periarteritis nodosa), die mit morbus Brightii und rapid fortschreitender ailgemeiner muskellahmung, Dtsch Arch Klin Med 1:484, 1866; with permission.)*

Although C-ANCA correlates with Wegener's granulomatosis and P-ANCA correlates with polyarteritis and idiopathic crescentic glomerulonephritis, there are sufficient exceptions to indicate that it is the presence of a positive antineutrophil cytoplasmic antibody test that is important rather than its subtype. Antineutrophil cytoplasmic antibody is useful because it simplifies the morphologic and clinical differential (Table 1-5). It can also be used to monitor response to therapy (insensitive due to slow decline in titer with remission) and to distinguish a clinical relapse (rising titer) from a therapeutic complication (falling titer).

The kidney is the most commonly affected organ in systemic vasculitis.[191-193] Either a necrotizing and crescentic glomerulonephritis (most common) or a true arteritis may develop. Crescentic glomerulonephritis is the most common pattern of renal involvement by vasculitis.[191-194] A crescent forms following necrosis of the glomerular capillary wall.[195] Extravasation of fibrin,

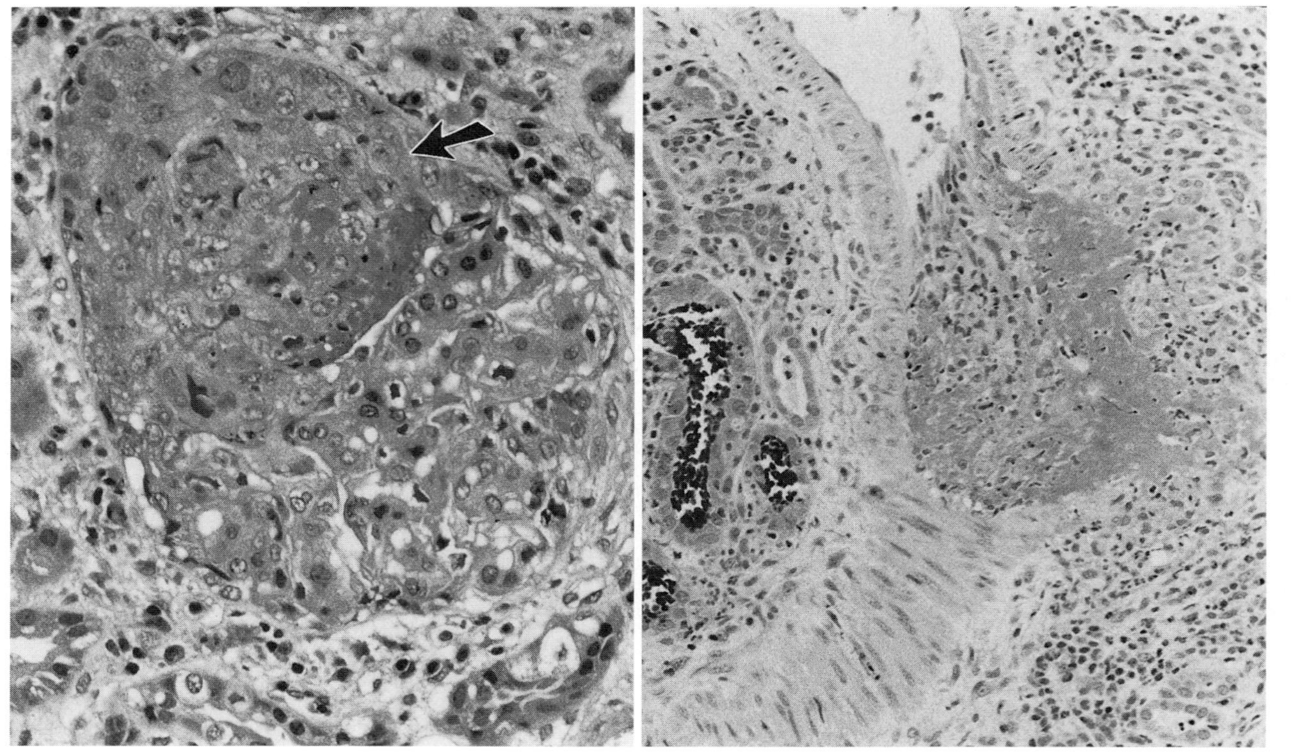

1-87. **A**, A cellular crescent (*arrow*) in a patient with classic Wegener's granulomatosis. **B**, Segmental fibrinoid necrosis of an artery in a patient with polyarteristic nodosa.

TABLE 1-5.
VASCULITIS AND ANCA ANTIBODY

ANCA positive vasculitis	(% positive)	ANCA negative vasculitis
Wegener's granulomatosis	(>90%)	Temporal arteritis
Microscopic polyarteritis	(>90%)	Takayasu's arteritis
Polyarteritis nodosa	(30-50%)	Henoch-Schönlein purpura*
Idiopathic crescentic	(>90%)	Connective tissue diseases*
Glomerulonephritis		Cryoglobulenemia
Kawasaki disease	(50%)	Drug reaction*
Churg-Strauss syndrome	(50-60%)	Infectious arteritis

*Very rare positive cases.
ANCA=Antineutrophil cytoplasmic antibody.

protein, and red cells ensues and epithelial cell proliferation occurs in the area of damage (Fig. 1-87). If healing occurs, a segmental to circumferential scar (fibrous crescent) forms, the size of which varies with the size of the initial necrosis. If the percentage of glomeruli affected by necrosis exceeds 50%, the patients present with rapidly progressive renal failure. Their urine contains protein, red cells, and often red cell casts.

The process of crescent formation is not specific for vasculitis. Crescents also form in other types of glomerulonephritis. The process is subclassified by the findings on direct immunofluorescence[194] (see box on p. 55). Vasculitis is distinctive because of the absence of appreciable detectable immune reactants by direct immunofluorecence. Most are antineutrophil cytoplasmic antibody positive.

Necrotizing arteritis and arteriolitis is a less common lesion than crescentic glomerulonephritis when vasculitis affects the kidney.[193,194] It is characterized by fibrinoid necrosis of vessel wall, karyorrhexis, and a mixed inflammatory cell response rich in neutrophils (Fig. 1-87). The prominent inflammatory component distinguishes vasculitis from acute thrombotic microangio-

DIRECT IMMUNOFLUORESCENCE IN CRESCENTIC GLOMERULONEPHRITIS

- Linear immunofluorescence
  - Goodpasture's syndrome
  - Antiglomerular basement membrane disease
- Granular immunofluorescence
  - Immune complex glomerulonephritis
- Negative immunofluorescence
  - Systemic vasculitis
  - Idiopathic ("pauci-immune") crescentic glomerulonephritis

pathy. Although necrotizing arteritis is most common in classic polyarteritis nodosa and Wegener's granulomatosis, necrotizing arteritis can develop in other forms of vasculitis (see Table 1-5). Serologic data and clinical correlation are crucial to proper classification.[196]

TUBULOINTERSTITIAL DISEASES

Disorders of tubules and interstitium are discussed together because they rarely occur in isolation. Any alteration in one affects the other. Tubules make up 90% of the renal cortex while the renal interstitium consists of a slender zone separating the cortical tubules. The renal interstitium contains peritubular capillaries, collagen fibers, and a few interstitial cells (Fig. 1-19, 1-21). Although normally scant the interstitium can expand rapidly following an acute tubular or interstitial disease. This is the principal nonneoplastic manner in which gross renal expansion can occur. Conversely, because tubules comprise 90% of the cortical mass, tubular atrophy is responsible for most of the cortical thinning that occurs in any form of chronic renal disease. Interstitial expansion is also the parameter that is most closely linked to the level of renal insufficiency, even in those diseases primarily affecting vessels or glomeruli.[196,197]

In no other area of renal disease is clinical information more crucial in establishing the etiology of an abnormality than in a tubulointerstitial disease. This is a consequence of the limited spectrum of histologic abnormalities that may result from a large number of different injuries. Because tubulointerstitial alterations correlate with renal dysfunction, most forms of tubulointerstitial disease present with some degree of renal insufficiency. The rate of development of renal insufficiency can be used to formulate a classification of tubulointerstitial diseases. This is useful because it separates entities with the greatest potential for recovery of renal function (acute forms) from those in which some irreversible injury is present (chronic forms). It also is convenient to separate infection-related entities into a third group (see box on this page) because their etiology is usually more obvious and many forms are interrelated.

Acute tubulointerstitial diseases have a rapid clinical onset and are associated with edema and variable inflammation and are potentially reversible.[198] The inflammation is neutrophilic in acute pyelonephritis and is principally lymphohistiocytic in acute interstitial nephritis. Chronic tubulointerstitial diseases have a gradual or insidious onset and are associated with irreversible tubular atrophy and interstitial fibrosis. A lymphocytic infiltrate is also present, even in forms not associated with infection.

INFECTION-RELATED TUBULOINTERSTITIAL NEPHRITIS

Acute infection

- Acute pyelonephritis
- Pyonephrosis
- Perinephric abscess
- Emphysematous pyelonephritis
- Renal papillary necrosis
- Fungal infections
- Viral infections

Chronic infection

- Chronic pyelonephritis
- Xanthogranulomatous pyelonephritis
- Malakoplakia
- Tuberculosis

INFECTION-RELATED TUBULOINTERSTITIAL NEPHRITIS

Acute pyelonephritis

Acute pyelonephritis is a bacterial infection of the kidney.[199] Patients present with fever, leukocytosis, and flank tenderness and may suffer a variety of complications (see box on p. 56). Pyuria and urinary white blood cell casts usually are present. The kidneys may be seeded by organisms via two major pathways: ascending infection and hematogenous route.

The most common avenue of infection is an ascent from a lower urinary tract infection. *Escherichia coli* is the most frequent organism followed by other enteric organisms such as *Proteus, Klebsiella*, and *Enterobacter*. In most individuals with bacterial cystitis the infection remains localized to the bladder. In susceptible individuals, vesicoureteral reflux occurs, permitting colonization of the upper tracts.[200-202] This most often occurs in children with primary vesicoureteral reflux, a congenital (often hereditary) abnormality in the anatomy of the ureterovesical junction.[203] Reflux can also develop in nonrefluxing systems if the cystitis is severe or if there is distal obstruction or a neurogenic bladder.

Even with an upper tract infection, parenchymal infection is not inevitable. The organisms must first gain access to the papillary collecting ducts, a process known as intrarenal reflux.[200-202,204] The architecture of the renal pyramids influences their susceptibility to intrarenal reflux (see Reflux Nephropathy later in this chapter). Following initial infection of the pyramids, the infection extends up the medullary rays prior to more generalized cortical spread.

Acute pyelonephritis in surgical and autopsy specimens represents the most severe examples. The collecting system is thickened and yellow-white suppurative foci or

COMPLICATIONS OF ACUTE PYELONEPHRITIS

- Renal abscess
- Pyonephrosis
- Perinephric abscess
- Emphysematous pyelonephritis
- Sepsis

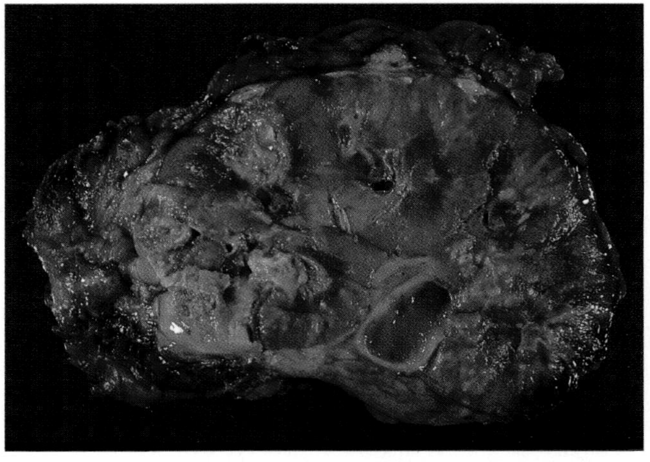

1-88. Ascending acute pyelonephritis complicated by abscess formation most severely affecting the lower pole (*left*).

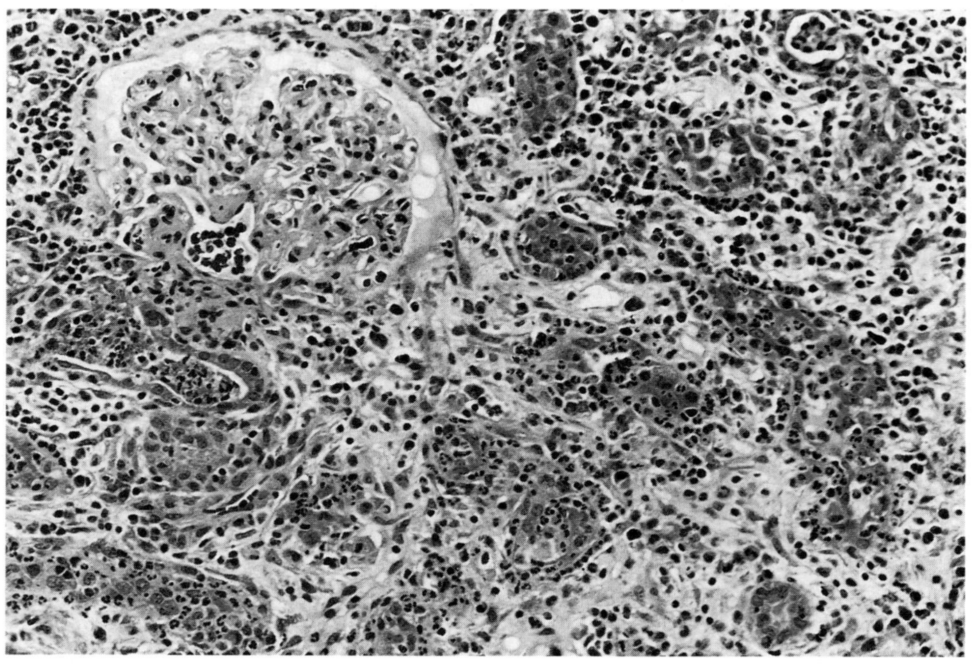

1-89. Acute pyelonephritis showing numerous neutrophils adjacent to and within renal tubules (destined to form urinary white blood cell casts).

overt abscesses are present in both pyramids and cortex (Fig. 1-88). Microscopically, there is mucosal ulceration and an intense neutrophilic response within the tubules and interstitium (Fig. 1-89). Occasionally, in sites of early involvement, bacteria or neutrophils can be seen within collecting ducts of the cortex and medulla (Fig. 1-90). Glomeruli may be spared initially but with increasing severity generalized parenchymal destruction occurs, which may liquefy, resulting in abscess formation.

Hematogenous pyelonephritis usually complicates prolonged sepsis or infectious endocarditis. The kidneys are usually peppered with abscesses, which are more numerous in the cortex than the medulla (Fig. 1-91, 1-92). The organisms responsible are more often gram-positive bacteria or fungi.

Pyonephrosis. Pyonephrosis refers to the near total destruction of an obstructed kidney by acute pyelonephritis. The parenchyma is replaced by suppurative inflammation transforming the kidney into a large abscess. The patient is typically septic. Urine cultures may be negative because of the urinary tract obstruction.

Perinephric abscess. A perinephric abscess is the accumulation of infectious material and neutrophils within perinephric fat (Fig. 1-93). It usually originates from rupture of a renal abscess or from pyonephrosis but can develop following a surgical procedure such as renal

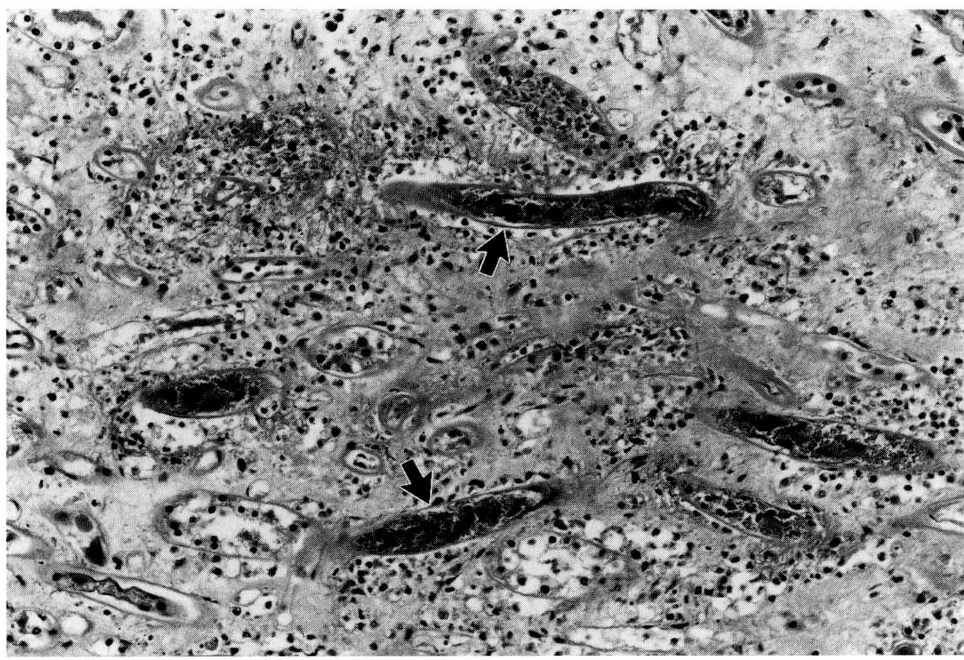

1-90. Ascending acute pyelonephritis with colonies of bacteria in papillary collecting ducts (*arrow*).

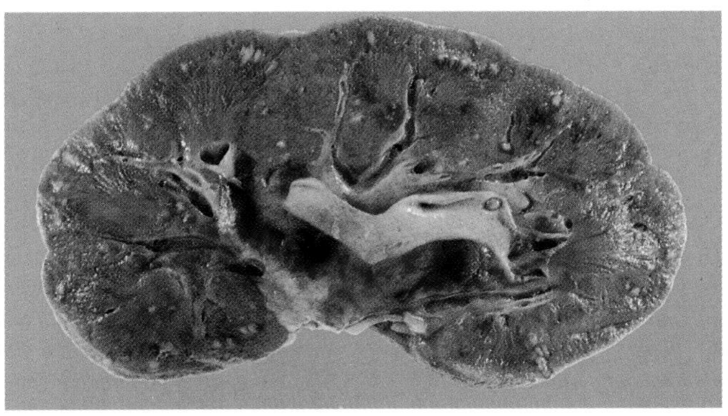

1-91. Hematogenous pyelonephritis showing miliary abscesses in a patient with bacterial sepsis.

CAUSES OF RENAL PAPILLLARY NECROSIS

- Diabetes mellitus
- Urinary tract obstruction
- Acute pyelonephritis
- Analgesic abuse
- Sickle cell disease
- Hypoxia
- Dehydration

Combination of above = 55%.

transplantation or surgery for calculi. Rarely, it may originate from an infected nidus extrinsic to the kidney, such as the gastrointestinal tract in diverticulitis and Crohn's disease, or from bone in osteomyelitis.[199,205,206] Either Gram-negative or Gram-positive organisms can be responsible.

Emphysematous pyelonephritis. Emphysematous pyelonephritis is an uncommon but potentially life threatening complication of acute suppurative bacterial (rarely fungal) infection of the kidney.[207,208] In emphysematous pyelonephritis gas bubbles develop within the renal parenchyma and may extend into perinephric and even retroperitoneal sites. It should be distinguished from emphysematous pyelitis and ureteritis, which are far less dangerous conditions. Approximately 90% of patients with this infection have diabetes mellitus and urinary tract obstruction is present in approximately 40%. Women outnumber men by a 2:1 ratio. *Escherichia coli* is the responsible organism in 68% of cases and *Klebsiella* in 9% of cases, with a mixed infection in 19% of cases. No reported cases have been attributed to *Clostridium*.

The kidney of a patient with emphysematous pyelonephritis grossly shows widespread abscesses with papillary necrosis and cortical infarcts. It may have a cystic appearance due to gas bubbles. Microscopically, the characteristic feature is empty spaces lacking epithelial cell linings and distorting the parenchyma (Fig. 1-94). Adjacent areas show vascular thrombosis, ischemic necrosis, suppurative inflammation, and abscesses.

Renal papillary necrosis

Necrosis of portions of the renal medulla is known as renal papillary necrosis.[209-213] A number of diseases are associated with papillary necrosis (see box on this page). When bilateral and diffuse, it presents as an acute devastating illness with renal failure, fever, chills, flank pain, and hematuria. Alternately, it may be an insidious process

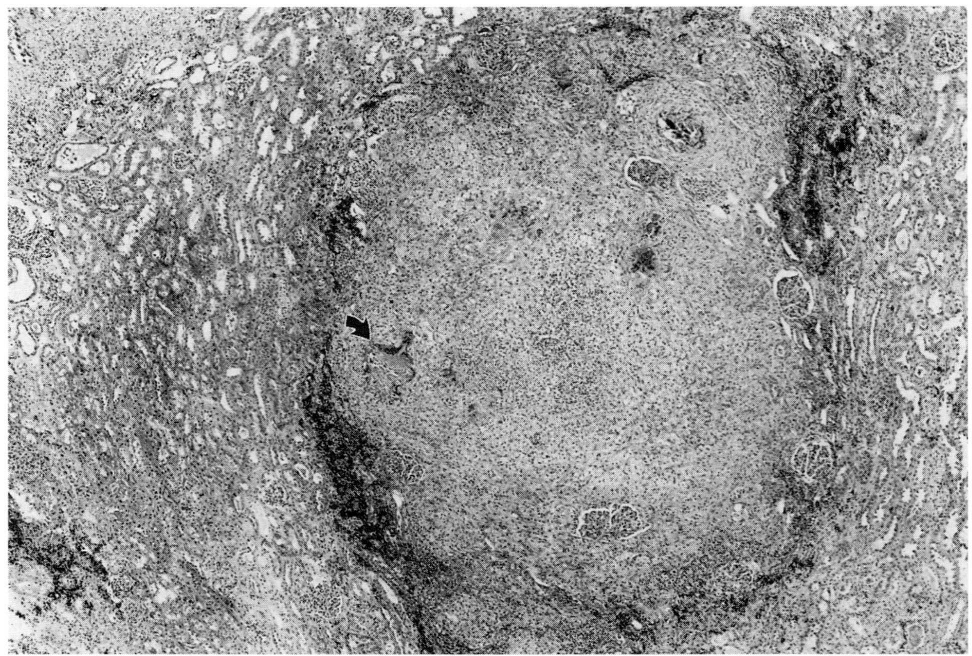

1-92. A cortical microabscess in a patient with fungal endocarditis. Notice the multinucleated giant cells (*arrow*).

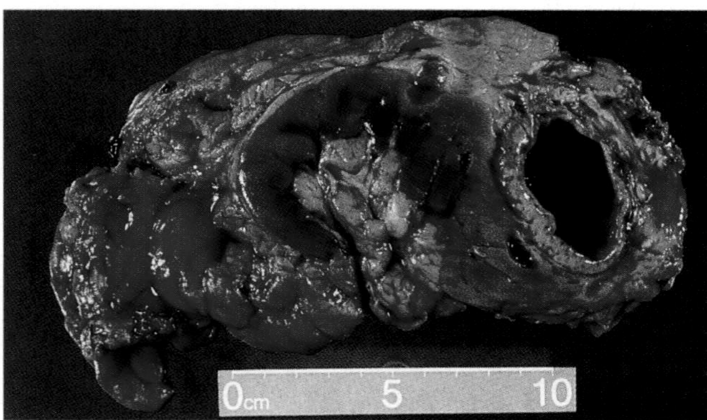

1-93. A perinephric abscess.

that manifests as a urinary concentrating defect or with the gradual development of renal failure. Renal papillary necrosis is always the complication of some other disease process and most patients have more than one risk factor present. In the United States, diabetes is the most prevalent underlying disorder.

Because of the strong association with infection, renal papillary necrosis is often included in discussions of pyelonephritis. However, its pathogenesis is ischemia related to the marginal medullary blood supply. This accounts for its association with disorders that compromise medullary blood flow.

Renal papillary necrosis is usually a disease of adults; however, infants can also develop renal papillary necrosis. Although often referred to in the pediatric literature as renal medullary necrosis, approximately 25% to 30% of patients will also develop focal cortical infarcts.[212] Infants with renal papillary necrosis are usually less than 1 month old and have perinatal asphyxia or a severe infantile disease associated with vascular collapse and dehydration such as gastroenteritis.

In the 1950s and 1960s renal papillary necrosis became a serious problem, particularly in Australia and in Scandinavian countries where analgesic combinations were in widespread use.[214-217] Analgesic nephropathy, as it came to be known, rapidly became the leading cause of chronic renal failure and renal papillary necrosis in those regions. (See Analgesic Nephropathy later in this chapter.)

In renal papillary necrosis, the necrosis usually does not involve the entire medulla. The papillary tip is most vulnerable while the outer medulla is often preserved. A medullary form and a papillary form have been described.[212,213] In the medullary form, the calyceal spiral arteries are patent and peripheral or fornical portions of the pyramid are intact with the central portions necrotic (Fig. 1-95). In the papillary form, the necrosis is more extensive and the entire papilla or inner medulla is necrotic (Fig. 1-96). In both forms, the necrosis is of a coagulation type, in keeping with its ischemic etiology.

Fungal infections

Acute fungal tubulointerstitial nephritis is usually encountered in immunocompromised or diabetic patients. Antibiotic therapy and urinary tract instrumentation are other major risk factors.[218-220] As with bacterial infections, the kidney may be seeded by either an ascending or hematogenous route. *Candida* species and *Torulopsis* are the most common organisms. In patients with acquired

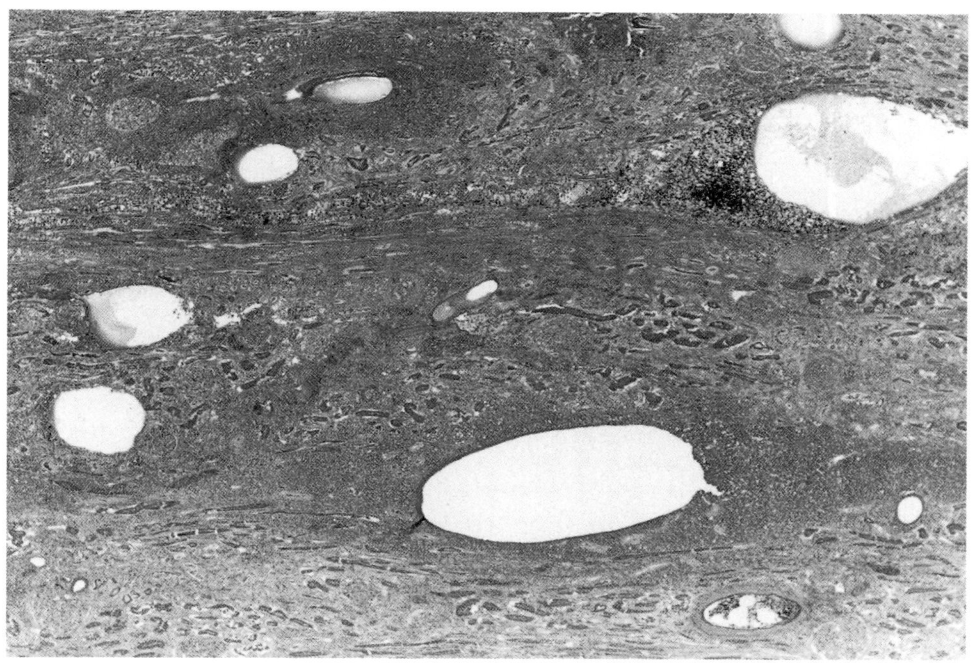

1-94. Emphysematous pyelonephritis showing silhouettes of gas bubbles within necrotic parenchyma.

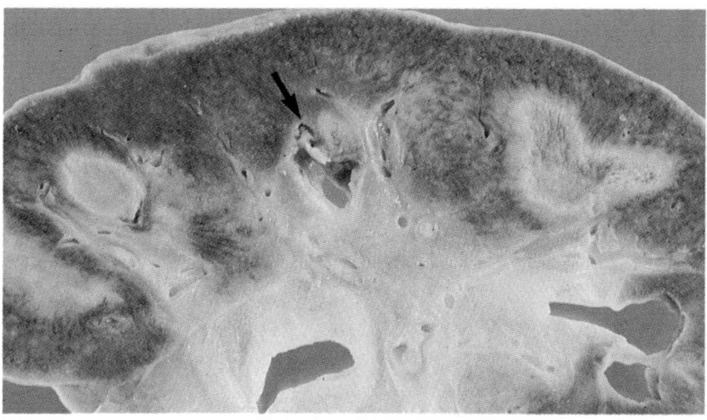

1-95. Renal papillary necrosis in a diabetic patient. Papilla in center has sloughed (*arrow*).

VIRAL RENAL DISEASES

Acute tubulointerstitial
- Nephritis
- Cytomegalovirus
- Adenovirus
- HIV
- Polyomavirus (BK type)

Glomerulonephritis
- Hepatitis B
- Hepatitis C
- HIV
- Rare others:
  - Mumps
  - Varicella
  - Echovirus
  - Cytomegalovirus

Arteritis
- Hepatitis B

immunodeficiency syndrome (AIDS) almost any fungus may be encountered. The kidney shows a mixed neutrophilic and granulomatous response and fungal elements are usually demonstrable (Fig. 1-92).

Viral infections

Viruses can produce a variety of renal diseases including acute tubulointerstitial nephritis, glomerulonephritis (most common), and arteritis (see box on this page)[220-231] Cytomegalovirus, adenovirus, and polyomavirus can cause a typical acute interstitial nephritis in which viral inclusions are visible within the kidney.[220-224] Both polyomavirus and adenovirus result in smudgy-appearing intranuclear inclusions within tubular cells. Cytomegalovirus produces the characteristic large intranuclear inclusions with halos and eosinophilic cytoplasmic inclusions in tubular cells, podocytes, and endothelial cells (Fig. 1-97).

Viral inclusions are not visible in the other viral renal diseases and most produce a glomerulonephritis, often with immune complex deposits.[225-227] Human immunodeficiency virus (HIV) causes a complex renal disease known as HIV nephropathy. This is characterized by a triad of interstitial nephritis with large tubular casts, glomerulonephritis due to focal-segmental

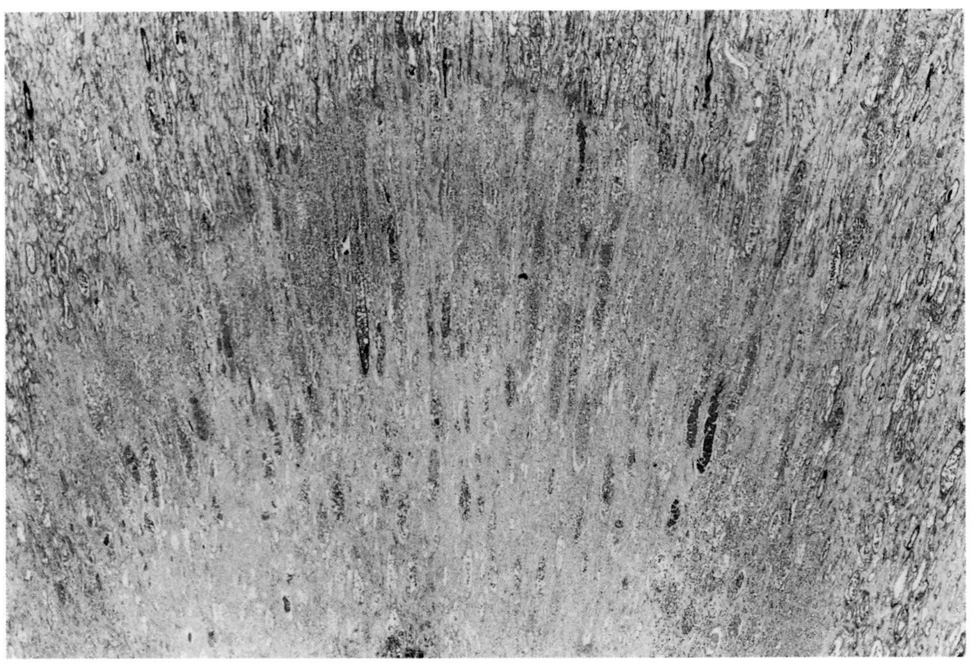

1-96. Papillary necrosis showing coagulation necrosis and peripheral inflammation.

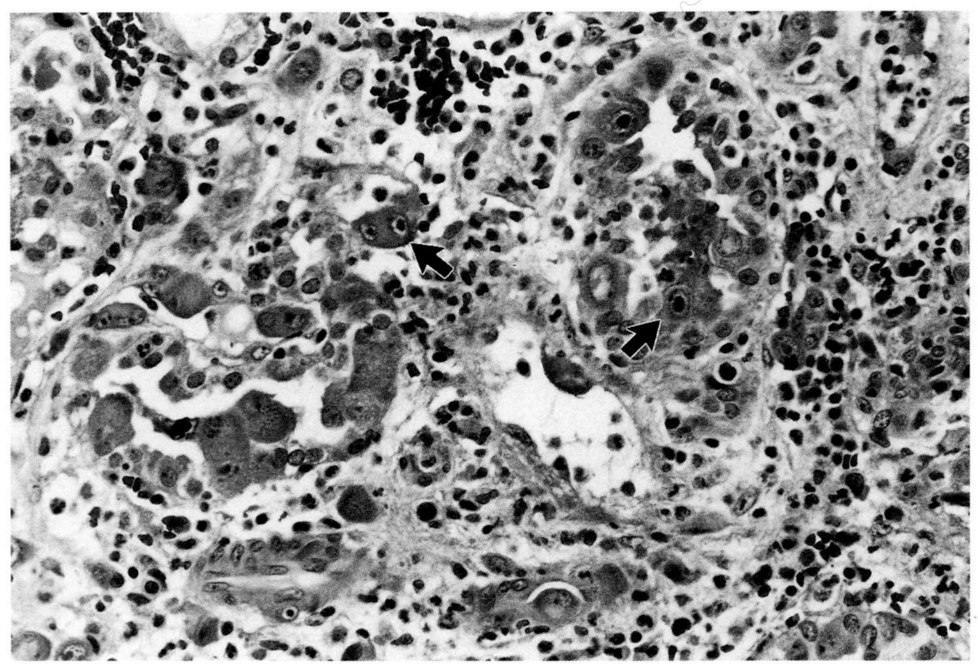

1-97. Cytomegaloviral (*arrows*) acute interstitial nephritis in an immunocompromised patient.

glomerulosclerosis, and numerous endothelial reticulotubular inclusions.[228,229] Hantavirus (nephropathica epidemica, hemorrhagic fever with renal syndrome) can produce an uncommon rodent-derived, acute, self-limited influenza-like illness with an acute interstitial nephritis.[230,231]

CHRONIC PYELONEPHRITIS

Chronic pyelonephritis is a chronic destructive tubulointerstitial disease usually regarded as a sequela of recurrent or persistent episodes of bacterial infection of the kidney. It is responsible for 5% to 15% of end-stage kidney disease. Usually it is subdivided into

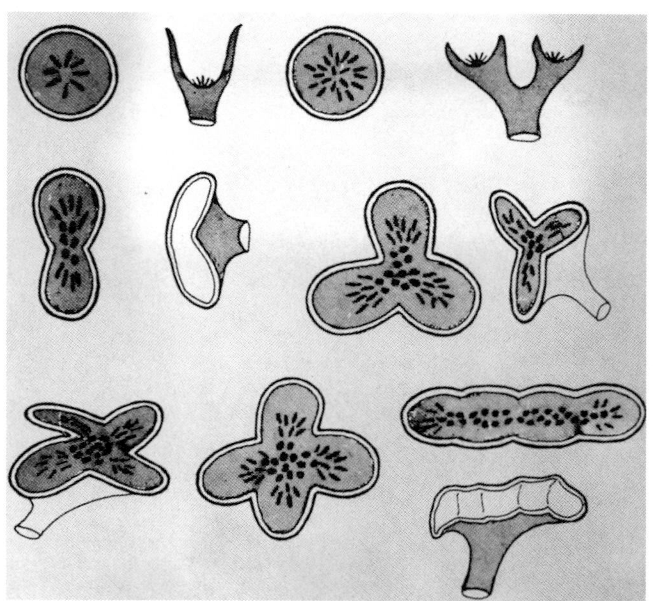

1-98. Various possible shapes of simple and compound pyramids. *(From Hodson CJ: Reflux nephropathy: a personal historical review, AJR Am J Roentgenol 137:456, 1981; with permission.)*

reflux nephropathy (or chronic nonobstructive pyelonephritis) and obstructive pyelonephritis.

Reflux nephropathy (chronic nonobstructive pyelonephritis)

In 1960 Hodson and Edwards[201] established a link between nonobstructive chronic pyelonephritis and vesicoureteral reflux. Appreciation of the nearly ubiquitous association between nonobstructive forms of chronic pyelonephritis and vesicoureteral reflux led Bailey, in 1973, to coin the term "reflux nephropathy."[232] Reflux nephropathy appears to be responsible for the majority of pyelonephritic scars.

Vesicoureteral reflux is a congenital disorder in which there is regurgitation of urine from the bladder into a ureter because of inadequate development of its musculature or because the submucosal portion of the ureter is too short.[203,233] Often it is a familial disorder and usually is detected following a urinary tract infection at an early age. Although reflux tends to decrease in frequency with increasing age as the submucosal ureteral segment matures or lengthens, the renal scars are already present, possibly developing at the time of the first infection.[200-202] Scars are usually noted in patients with the most severe degrees of reflux.

Not all patients with urinary tract infections and vesicoureteral reflux develop reflux nephropathy. This observation was explained by Ransley and Risdon[203] who identified two types of renal pyramids, simple and compound (Fig. 1-98). In simple pyramids Bellini's ducts open through a convex papilla at an oblique angle and close with an increase in intrapelvic pressure. However, compound pyramids that drain multiple lobes have concave surfaces and the orifices of Bellini's ducts fail to close, resulting in reflux. It is believed that reflux nephropathy represents the combined effect of recurrent or persistent vesicoureteral reflux and interrenal reflux, which permits infection within the urinary tract to gain access to the renal parenchyma. It also is possible that high pressures in absence of infection may also result in similar segmental scarring. Compound papillae are usually located in the polar regions of the kidney, the location of most scars in reflux nephropathy.

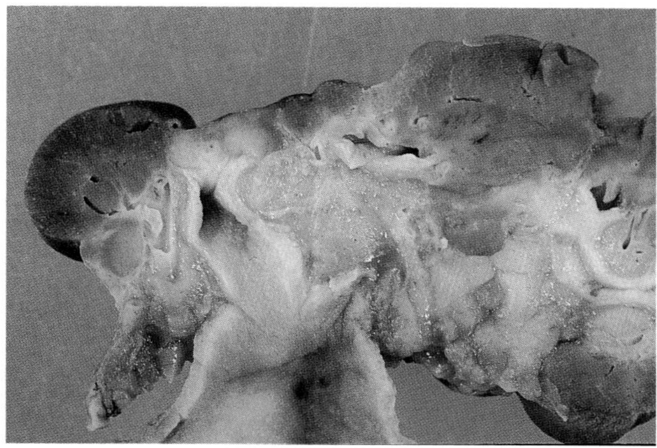

1-99. Reflux nephropathy showing slender transverse cortical grooves and dilated calices.

The kidneys are small and irregularly contracted, usually weighing from 30 to 50 gm. Their capsular surfaces show broad depressed scars, usually in polar regions. On cut surface, there is scalloping and loss of the renal pyramids beneath the cortical scars resulting in dilated calices (Fig. 1-99). The cortex adjacent to the scars may be unaffected or hypertrophic. The pelvicalyceal system and ureter usually are dilated and their walls thickened.

Microscopically, the cortical scars show chronic interstitial nephritis with a lymphoid interstitial infiltrate (Fig. 1-100). There is extensive tubular atrophy and tubules frequently contain eosinophilic casts (thyroidization). Periglomerular fibrosis and global glomerular sclerosis also are typical. The vessels show a striking intimal sclerosis, a finding not present in the adjacent cortex. The uninvolved cortex may appear essentially normal or show a compensatory hypertrophy of nephrons. The collecting system shows chronic pyelitis and ureteritis with lymphoid aggregates or germinal centers in the mucosa.

In some patients hypertension, proteinuria, and progressive renal failure develop. Proteinuria (often in the nephrotic range) is an important finding because it identifies patients at risk for renal failure. The glomerular lesion of focal segmental glomerulosclerosis (Fig. 1-100) is responsible for the proteinuria.[234,235] Unfortunately, correction of the reflux or prevention of recurrent infection does not prevent progression of the glomerular lesion.

Ask-Upmark kidney

Some patients, mostly children, develop hypertension leading to the identification of vesicoureteral reflux and small kidneys that have one or more circumferential cortical grooves with an underlying

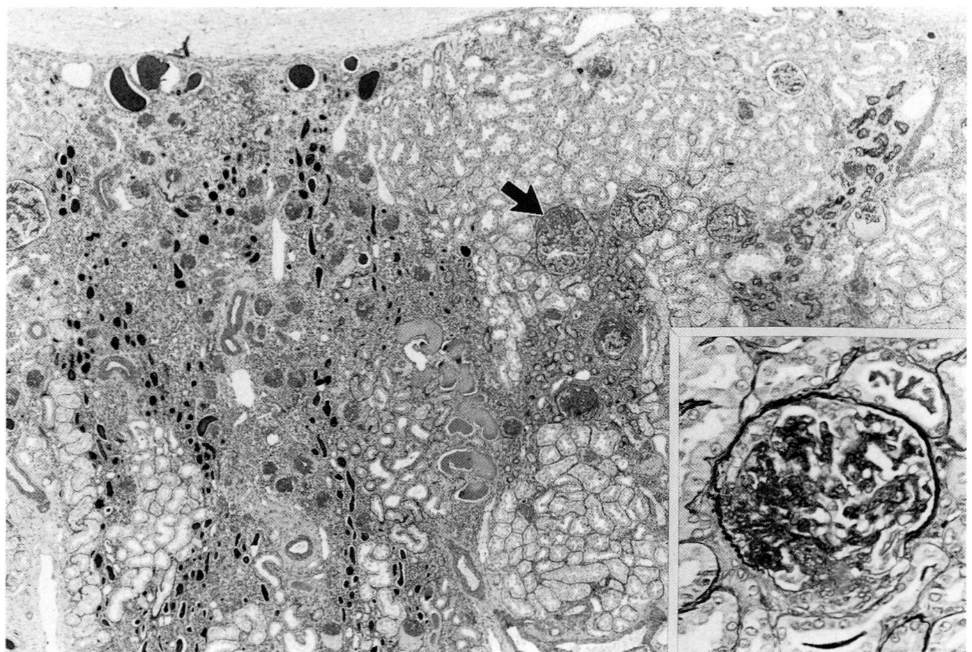

1-100. Reflux nephropathy showing focal chronic interstitial nephritis. In the adjacent intact cortex, several glomeruli show focal-segmental glomerulosclerosis (*arrow and inset*). PAS stain.

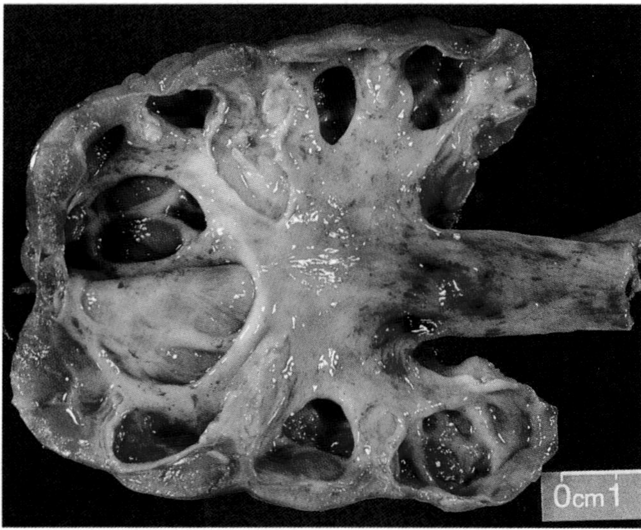

1-101. Chronic obstructive pyelonephritis showing a diffusely attenuated cortex, effaced pyramids, and dilated collecting system and ureter.

dilated calix.[236,237] These lesions were originally regarded as developmental, leading to the term segmental hypoplasia (or Ask-Upmark kidney). This condition is now regarded as a form of reflux nephropathy, possibly beginning in utero. The cortical scars are distinctive because the glomeruli have disappeared and there is a sharp junction between the uninvolved cortex and the scar, which in general lacks residual inflammation.

GRANULOMATOUS DISEASES OF THE KIDNEY

- Xanthogranulomatous pyelonephritis
- Malakoplakia
- Mycobacterial infection
- Fungal infection
- Parasitic infection
- Urate nephropathy
- Sarcoidosis
- Vasculitis
- Drug hypersensitivity

Chronic obstructive pyelonephritis

In chronic obstructive pyelonephritis the kidney is damaged by a combination of pressure-related atrophy and bacterial infection. In advanced cases, the kidney is hydronephrotic with diffuse caliceal dilation, blunting or effacement of papillae, and cortical thinning. This uniform alteration is in contrast to the irregular pattern of scarring characteristic of reflux nephropathy (Fig. 1-101). Microscopically, the picture is that of a diffuse chronic interstitial nephritis with tubular atrophy, interstitial fibrosis, and glomerular sclerosis (Fig. 1-102). Sections including renal pyramid may show mild blunting of papillary tip in mild cases or complete effacement of pyramid in advanced cases.

XANTHOGRANULOMATOUS PYELONEPHRITIS

A number of granulomatous diseases may affect the kidney and urinary tract[238-247] (see box on this page). Most are the result of infections. Xanthogranulomatous

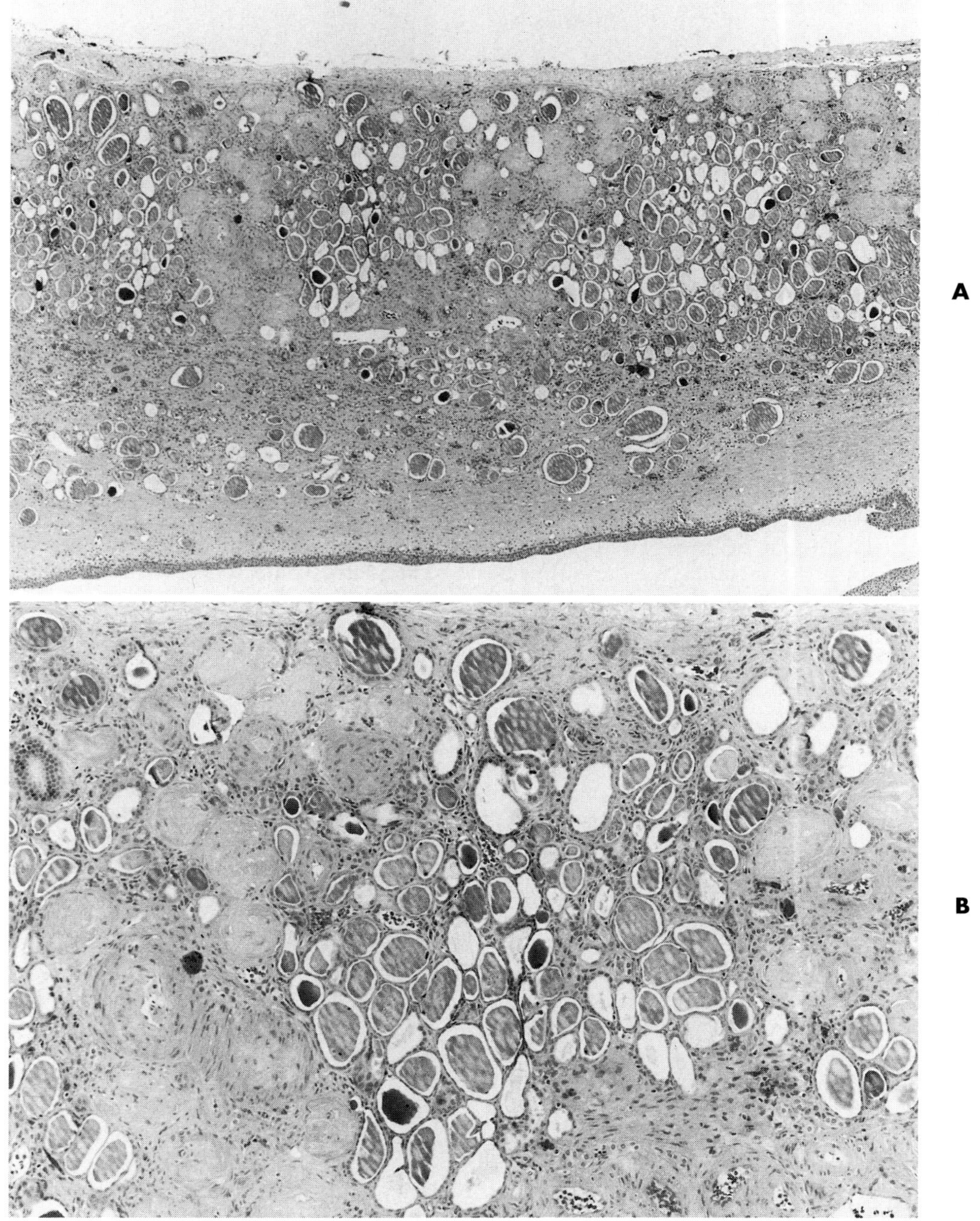

1-102. A, B, End-stage chronic obstructive pyelonephritis showing effaced pyramid, "thyroidization" of tubules, glomerulosclerosis, and secondary occlusive vascular changes.

pyelonephritis is the inflammatory sequela of chronic suppurative renal infections and usually develops in an obstructed kidney in which portions of the renal parenchyma are transformed into a xanthomatous and suppurative inflammatory mass.[238-241] Although a variety of theories of pathogenesis have been proposed, such as metabolic abnormalities, aberrant immune responses, lower virulence organisms, or ineffective antimicrobial therapy, the most plausible and simplest mechanism is renal outflow obstruction in the face of a pyogenic infection. This view accommodates the major clinical and pathologic features encountered in the majority of patients. The principal importance of xanthogranulomatous pyelonephritis relates to the difficulty in preoperative diagnosis and its ability to clinically, radiographically, and grossly mimic the destructive growth of a renal neoplasm.

Xanthogranulomatous pyelonephritis begins with suppurative inflammation and edema within the pelvic lamina propria and adjacent sinus fat resulting in

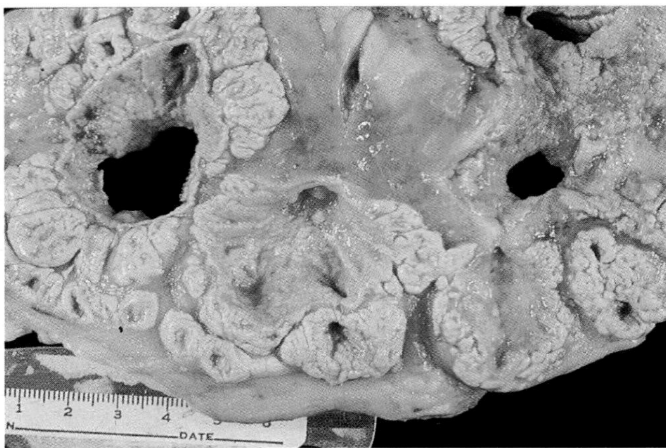

1-103. Xanthogranulomatous pyelonephritis showing xanthomatous nodules centered upon pyramids and xanthomatous thickening of collecting system.

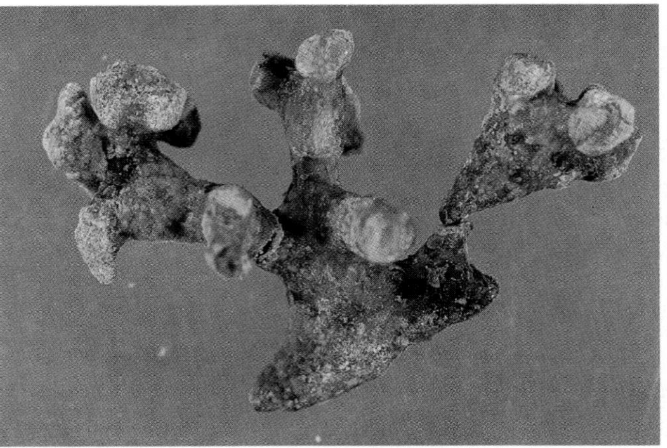

1-104. Staghorn calculus from a patient with xanthogranulomatous pyelonephritis.

pelvicalyceal ulceration and fat necrosis. The inflammatory process extends into the medulla, also resulting in necrosis. The cortex, perinephric fat, and even retroperitoneal tissue may eventually be involved. The gross extent of the process has been classified into three "stages."[238] In Stage I (nephric stage) the process is confined within the renal capsule. In Stage II (perinephric stage) the perinephric fat is involved. In Stage III (paranephric stage) there is extension outside Gerota's capsule.

Xanthogranulomatous pyelonephritis may involve all or only portions of the renal parenchyma giving rise to three general patterns: diffuse, segmental, and focal.[239] The diffuse form is most common (Fig. 1-103). It arises in a completely obstructed kidney, usually due to calculi, often of staghorn form (Fig. 1-104). The kidney is nonfunctional and nephrectomy is the treatment of choice. Preoperative diagnosis is most accurate in this form. The segmental and focal forms are more difficult to diagnose preoperatively and are more likely to be mistaken for neoplasms. They show the same microscopic features as diffuse xanthogranulomatous pyelonephritis but differ anatomically. Segmental xanthogranulomatous pyelonephritis is polar and is more common in children. The focal (or tumefactive) form is a cortical variant that lacks communication with the pelvis and is not associated with pyelitis or urinary tract obstruction. These two forms are amenable to partial nephrectomy.

Histologically, the xanthogranulomatous nodules show a zonal pattern. There is a central nidus of necrotic debris and neutrophils that is surrounded by the zone of foamy macrophages (Fig. 1-105). The most peripheral tissue show a fibroblastic response as the host attempts to confine or organize the inflammatory process.

The presence of the xanthogranulomatous mass, coupled with its histologic cellularity, can elicit concern regarding a neoplasm, particularly if a biopsy or frozen section is examined. The foam cells can resemble clear cell renal carcinoma, while the fibroblastic response can resemble a spindle cell neoplasm. The bubbly microvesicular fat of the foam cells contrasts with the cleared out cytoplasm characteristic of renal carcinoma. Additional features include a lack of cohesive growth on touch preps and the absence of cytologic atypia or mitoses. If diagnostic dilemma persist, glycogen stains or demonstration of epithelial markers by immunohistochemistry or electron microscopy can be used.

MALAKOPLAKIA

Malakoplakia is an uncommon chronic granulomatous disease most frequently observed in the urinary tracts of middle-aged women as a complication of recurrent infections.[241,242] Bladder involvement is 4 to 10 times as common as upper tract involvement and renal involvement is rare. Diverse extraurinary tract sites also are rarely affected, a situation often associated with a concomitant malignancy. In addition, similar to nephrogenic adenoma, increasing numbers of immunosuppressed patients have been reported to develop urinary tract malakoplakia.

The typical mucosal lesion of malakoplakia is characterized by a yellow-brown soft (*malakos*) plaque (*plakos*) that often has a central umbilication. The parenchymal lesions consist of similar soft yellow-brown nodules. Microscopically, masses of large eosinophilic histiocytes (von Hansemann histiocytes) are present, many of which contain basophilic inclusions (Michaelis-Gutmann bodies) (Fig. 1-106). PAS stain and special stains for calcium or iron enhance the target-like appearance of these cytoplasmic inclusions and indicate their mineralized nature. They have been shown by a variety of methods to represent incompletely digested bacilli.[242]

TUBERCULOSIS

Genitourinary tuberculosis is the most common extrapulmonary site of infection occurring in up to 5% of patients.[243,244] It is principally a disease of the young to middle aged with 75% of patients under the age of 50. Most patients will not have radiographic or clinical evidence of pulmonary disease at the time the genitourinary tract involvement is identified.[243]

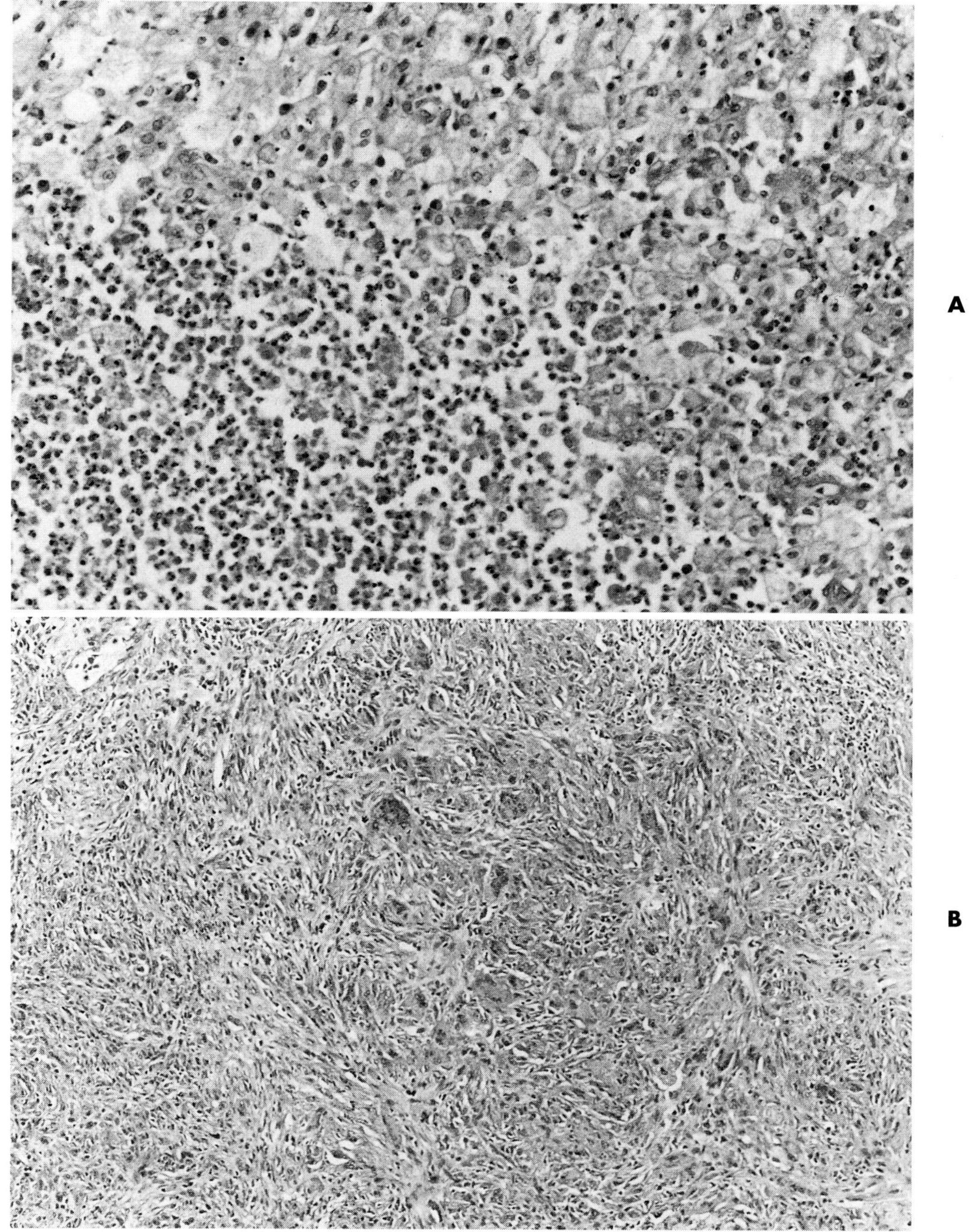

1-105. **A**, The center of a xanthogranulomatous nodule usually contains neutrophils and cell debris, and is surrounded by foamy macrophages. **B**, The peripheral areas show fibrosis, chronic inflammation, and giant cells.

The renal parenchyma initially becomes infected by hematogenous dissemination resulting in the bilateral development of small cortical neutrophilic microabscesses that gradually evolve into more typical granuloma and may caseate. Although progressive active disease may occur, in most patients the process is arrested. It may reactivate after a long latency period following a perturbation in the immune system.

Medullary involvement results with reactivation. The organisms appear to favor the thin limbs of Henle where they proliferate, causing destructive granulomatous lesions that caseate and cavitate (Fig. 1-107). Papillary necrosis follows, with seeding of the collecting system and lower urinary tract. Infection in these sites elicits granulomatous and fibrotic sequelae resulting in contraction of collection system, ureter, and bladder. The patient thus presents with a concentrating defect, dysuria, and hematuria. Cavitary lesions, calyceal deformity, and ureteral strictures are demonstrable by various imaging studies.

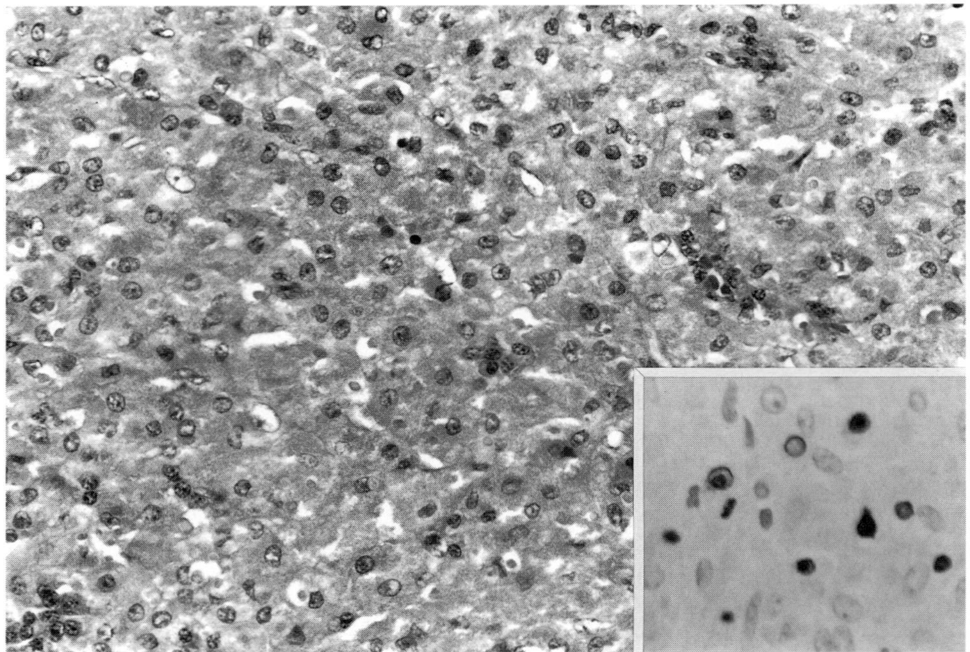

1-106. Malakoplakia showing von Hansemann histiocytes. Inset: Michaelis-Gutmann bodies revealed by von Kossa's stain for calcium.

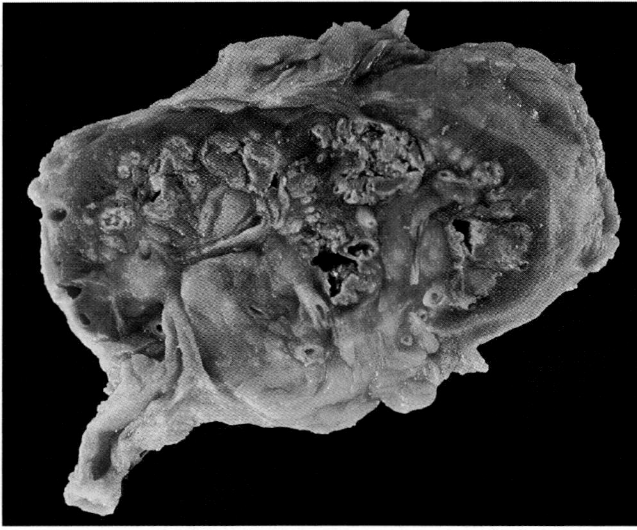

1-107. Renal tuberculosis with caseating granulomas and contracted renal pelvis and ureter.

ACUTE TUBULOINTERSTITIAL DISEASE

Acute tubulointerstitial disease usually causes a sudden deterioration in renal function and a rise in serum creatinine of 0.5-1.0 mg/dl/day. The urine may contain red cells, but red cell and white cell casts are absent, urinary protein is less than 2 g/day, and the urinary sodium concentration is increased. Many patients also are oliguric (<400 cc urine/day). The rapid evolution of renal failure correlates with the rapid expansion of the interstitial areas by edema. Tubular cell injury and edema, with or

CAUSES OF ACUTE TUBULAR NECROSIS

- Ischemia
- Antibiotics
  - Aminoglycosides
  - Amphotericin B
  - Polymixin B
  - Rifampicin
  - Cephalosporin
  - Colistin
- Radiographic contrast agents
- Nonsteroidal anti-inflammatory drugs
- Chemotherapeutic agents
  - Cis-platinum
- Organic solvents
  - Carbon tetrachloride
  - Ethylene glycol
  - Trichloroethylene
- Insecticides and herbicides
- Heavy metals
  - Mercury
  - Bismuth
  - Lead
  - Cadmium
  - Uranium
  - Arsenic
- Rhabdomyolysis
- Hemolysis
- Cocaine
- Toxins
  - Insect stings
  - Snake bites
  - Mushroom poisoning

without inflammation, are the principal morphologic findings, known as acute tubular necrosis and acute interstitial nephritis, respectively.

Acute tubular necrosis

Acute tubular necrosis is the most common renal parenchymal cause of acute renal failure.[248-255] It is characterized by morphologic evidence of tubular cell injury and is associated with interstitial edema.[249] There is little or no cortical inflammation although inflammatory cells may accumulate in the vasa recta of the outer medulla.[249] Glomeruli and other vessels are not affected. It usually is divided into ischemic and toxic forms.[248-255] Ischemic injury is more common. Although its etiology usually can be established because it results from decreased renal perfusion secondary to hemorrhage, hypotension, or dehydration, in some patients these are not observed directly but are inferred based on the clinical setting. The

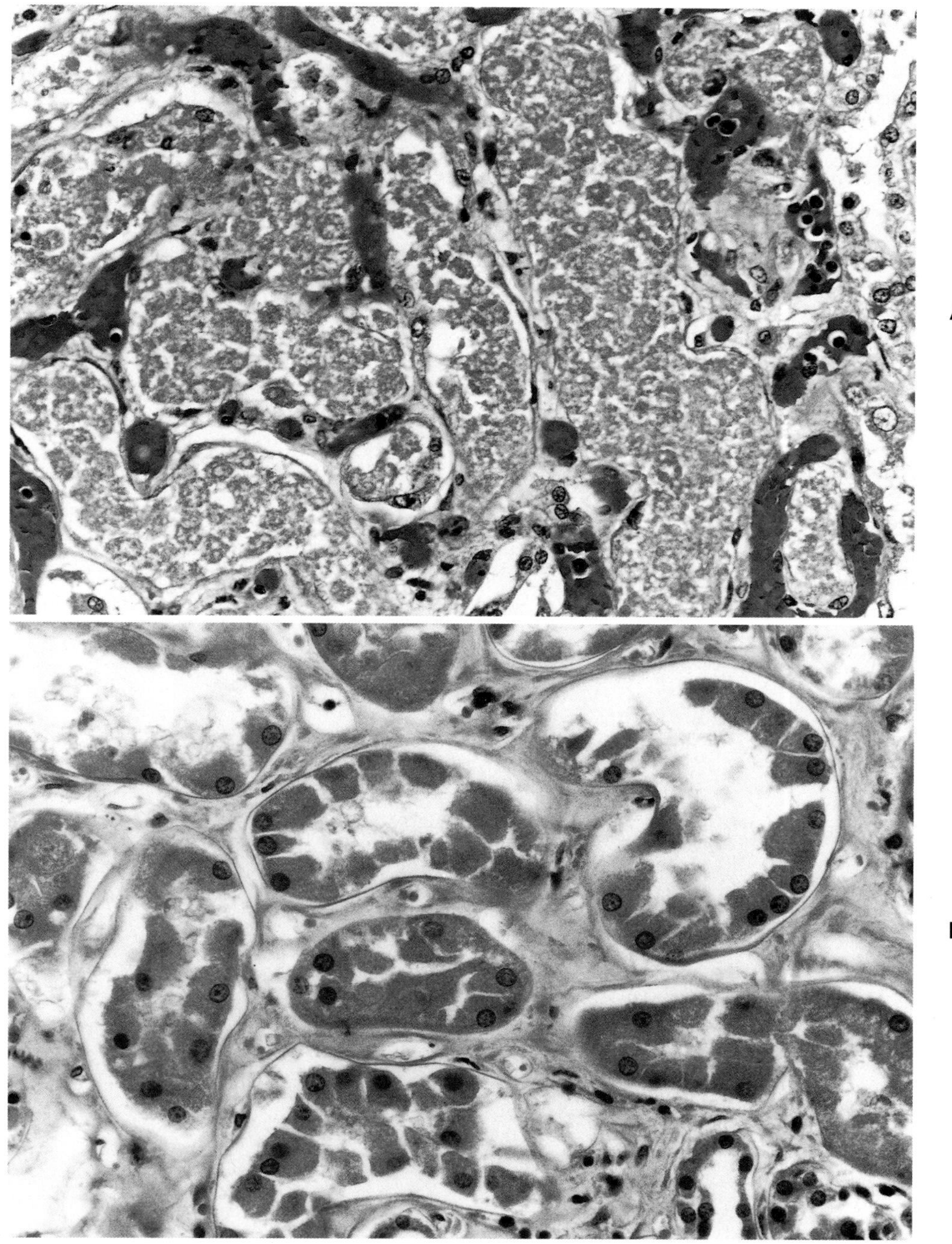

1-108. A, Acute tubular necrosis at autopsy showing coagulation necrosis. **B**, Autopsy autolysis showing cells with intact nuclei that are separating from the tubular basement membranes and from adjacent cells.

etiologies of toxic acute tubular necrosis are more diverse (see box on p. 64) and may be difficult to identify because they often develop in the context of therapy for other illnesses or may result from exogenous agents.[252-255] In heavy metal lesions such as those caused by bismuth, cadmium, and lead, proximal tubular intranuclear inclusions are present. Myeloid bodies detectable by electron microscopy are present in lesions caused by aminoglycoside antibiotics, although their presence does not correlate with toxicity.[252] Pigmented casts in distal tubules are present in lesions caused by hemolysis and rhabdomyolysis. Some agents can also produce an acute and a chronic interstitial nephritis.

For acute tubular necrosis to result in acute renal failure it must be diffuse and bilateral. If unilateral or even focal in one kidney, then renal insufficiency will not occur. The renal size and weight are increased as a consequence of interstitial edema. In certain situations (such as older patients with arterial nephrosclerosis) with underlying renal atrophy, acute tubular necrosis may result in normal renal size and weight. The cortex usually is pale and may bulge slightly compared to the medulla. The medulla, particularly the outer medulla, often is congested and dark, secondary to dilation of the vasa recta.

In acute tubular necrosis there is interstitial expansion without significant inflammation. If inflammation is present, it consists of a predominantly mononuclear cell infiltrate at the cortical-medullary junction or within the vessels in the vasa recta of the outer medulla. The tubules themselves can show two patterns of injury. In the more obvious and severe form, there is extensive coagulative necrosis of tubular cells, particularly in the proximal tubules, with loss of nuclei (Fig. 1-108*A*). This form is most common in toxic injuries and at autopsy. In autopsy material this alteration must be distinguished from autolysis. Autolytic tubules may be recognized by the tendency of their epithelium to separate from their tubular basement membranes and from each other, with preservation of their nuclei and intact cell membranes (Fig. 1-108*B*).

The second pattern of acute tubular necrosis is more subtle. It is characterized by attenuation or flattening of the tubular epithelium causing luminal enlargement and widely spaced nuclei (Fig. 1-109). At low magnification, this imparts a microcystic appearance to the cortex as a result of single cell necrosis and sloughing. The remaining cells lose their brush border and spread out to cover the basement membrane. There may be short segments of denuded tubular basement membranes. Mitotic figures may be present but are usually very infrequent. Distal tubules and collecting ducts may contain granular casts of sloughed cells.

Acute interstitial nephritis

Acute interstitial nephritis is an inflammatory cause of acute renal failure.[198,251-257] The term *acute* refers to the rapid development of renal failure rather than the character of the infiltrate, which actually consists of lymphocytes, plasma cells, histiocytes, and scattered eosinophils. Acute interstitial nephritis is a hypersensitivity reaction to a variety of stimuli (see box on p. 69) and most are cell-mediated reactions.[258] However, immune complex formation can occur in connective tissue diseases such as lupus and rarely in drug reactions.[258] Antitubular basement antibody may also develop in a rare drug reaction, in renal transplant rejection, associated with anti-

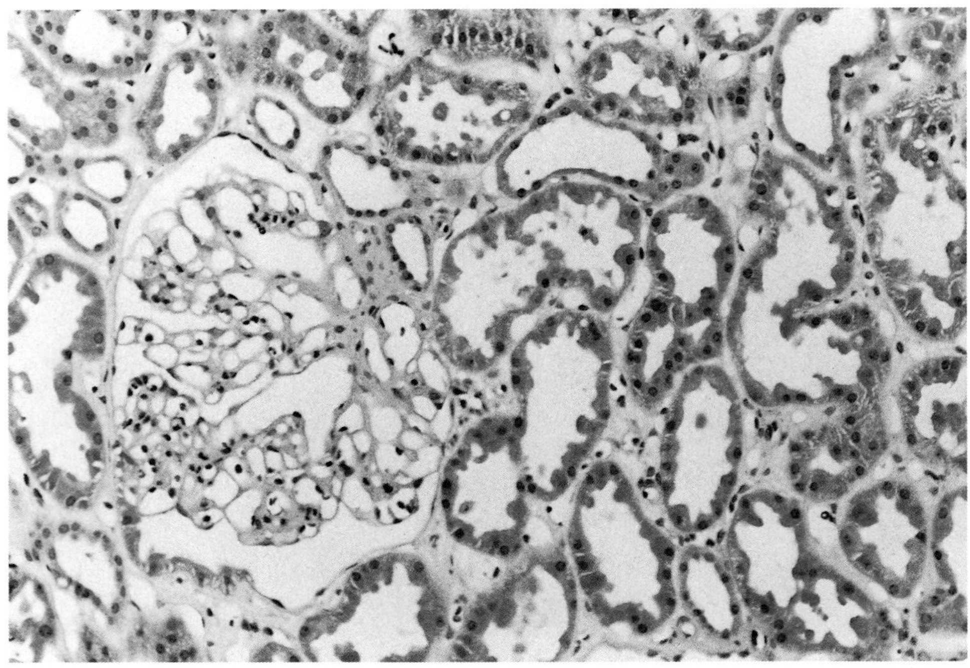

1-109. Mild acute tubular necrosis on renal biopsy showing attenuation of tubular epithelium and interstitial edema.

CAUSES OF ACUTE INTERSTITIAL NEPHRITIS

- Drug associated
  - Beta lactam and other antibiotics
  - Diuretics
  - Nonsteroidal anti-inflammatory drugs
  - Allopurinol
  - Rifampicin
  - Cimetidine
  - Sulfa drugs
  - Phenytoin
- Connective tissue diseases
  - Systemic lupus erythematosus
  - Sjögren's syndrome
- Transplant rejection
- Sarcoidosis
- Acute interstitial nephritis—uveitis syndrome
- Antitubular basement membrane disease
- Bacterial infections
  - Scarlet fever
  - Diphtheria
  - Typhoid fever
  - Brucellosis
  - Leptospiral infection
  - Rickettsia
- Viral infection
  - Cytomegalovirus
  - Epstein-Barr virus
  - Polyomavirus
  - HIV
  - Hantavirus

glomerular basement membrane disease (most common), and also as an idiopathic disorder.[258-260] Direct immunofluorescence is required to identify immune complex and antitubular basement membrane mediated lesions.

Patients often have enlarged tender kidneys secondary to edema. Morphologically, there is interstitial expansion by edema resulting in tubular separation.[198,256-261] There is a variably distributed mixed cell infiltrate consisting principally of lymphocytes and monocytes (Fig. 1-110). Smaller numbers of plasma cells and eosinophils may be present, however eosinophils are not required to implicate an allergic reaction. The lymphocytes infiltrate between tubular epithelial cells (tubulitis), which may themselves appear reactive or may show individual cell necrosis. In antibody-mediated cases immune complex deposits may be identified within tubular basement membranes or in peritubular capillaries, or a linear tubular basement membrane reaction can be demonstrated if antitubular basement membrane antibody is present. Occasionally a necrotizing vasculitis or granulomas may also develop in allergic reactions.[247,252]

The history and certain laboratory data are required to establish the cause because, except for identifying an infective agent or an antibody mediated lesion, there are no morphologic features to discriminate between the various possible causes. Prior to the use of antibiotics, acute interstitial nephritis was usually caused by infections, most often scarlet fever or diphtheria.[256] Today, an allergic drug reaction is clearly the first consideration.[252-257,260] The presence of a rash, fever, eosinophilia, or eosinophiluria can corroborate that impression, but often they are absent. Although the most frequently implicated drugs are listed in the box on p. 70, almost any drug can cause an allergic reaction. Fre-

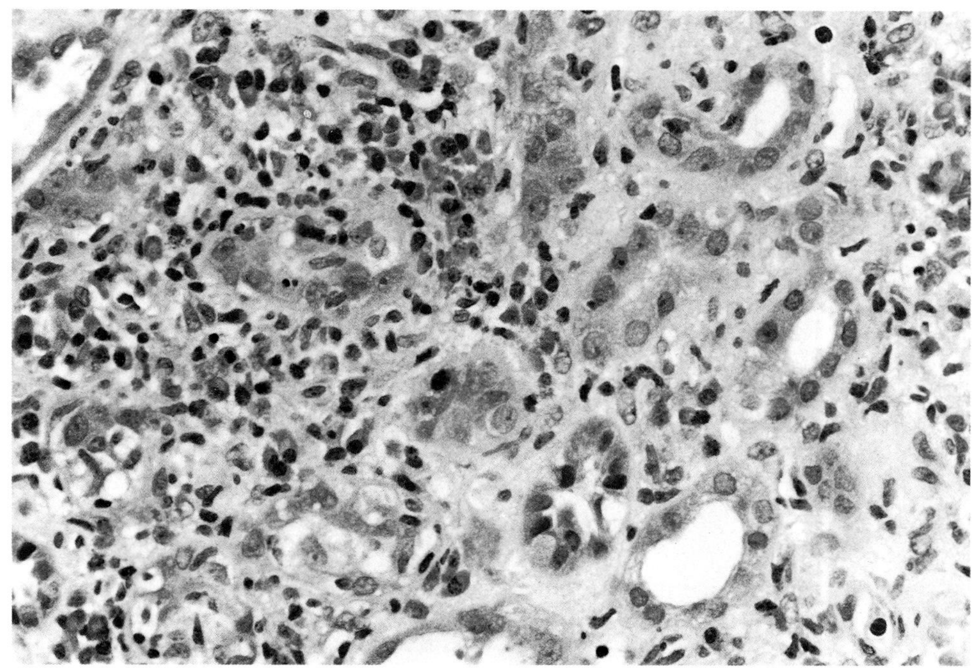

1-110. Allergic acute interstitial nephritis secondary to drug reaction.

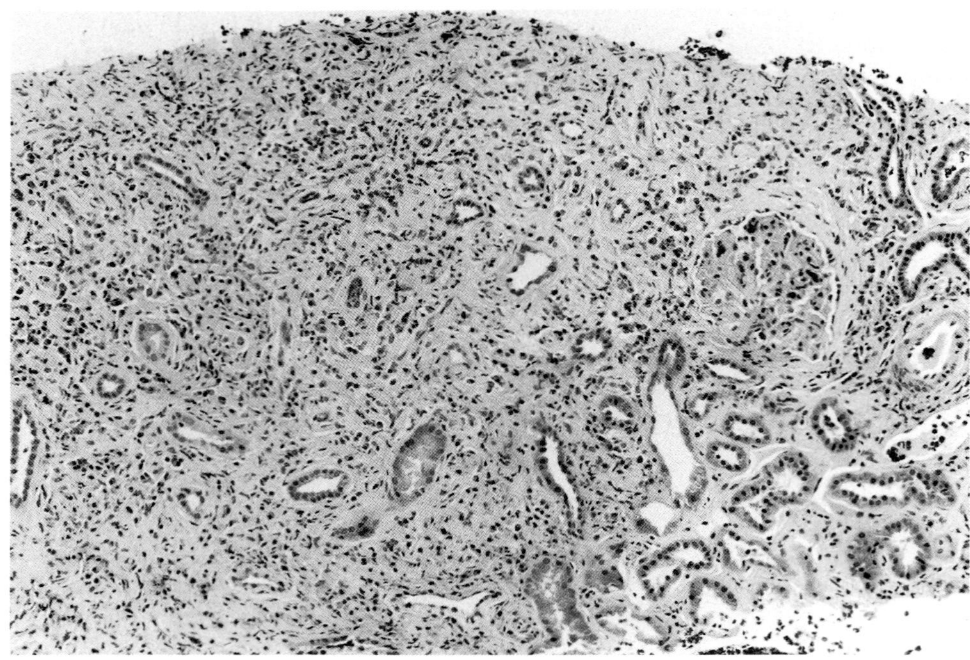

1-111. Idiopathic chronic interstitial nephritis showing interstitial fibrosis, tubules atrophy, and scant inflammation.

quently, the clinician will attribute it to the drug most recently taken. Proteinuria is usually less than 1 g per day, so the presence of significant proteinuria is very useful because it is most commonly associated with non-steroidal anti-inflammatory drugs (NSAIDS). In patients with a systemic disease that can be associated with acute interstitial nephritis, the underlying disease should be considered the cause.[253,257,261-264]

CHRONIC INTERSTITIAL NEPHRITIS

Chronic interstitial nephritis refers to the gradual development of renal failure due to tubulointerstitial disease.[198] As in acute interstitial nephritis, lymphocytes and histiocytes are the predominant inflammatory cells. However, the histologic picture is dominated by interstitial fibrosis and tubular atrophy (Fig. 1-111). Many of the same agents that cause acute tubular necrosis or acute interstitial nephritis also produce chronic interstitial nephritis (see box on this page), such as heavy metals, drugs, connective tissue diseases, and sarcoidosis.[252,253] Therefore, in a single patient there may be a combination of acute and chronic features. The lack of a specific cause of the histology requires careful clinical correlation to understand the cause of chronic interstitial nephritis. In some patients, no specific cause can be established and this is called idiopathic chronic interstitial nephritis.

Drugs and heavy metals

A variety of therapeutic agents and heavy metal exposures can cause the insidious development of chronic interstitial nephritis.[251,252,265-271] The tubulointerstitial scarring is irreversible, but if the toxic injury is recognized and the agent eliminated, some improvement in renal function often is possible. For most agents, no distinctive histologic features develop. However, in lead and cadmium toxicity intranuclear inclusions in tubular cells may be present and chronic lead toxicity often presents with gout and hypertension. Papillary necrosis is the principal underlying lesion in analgesic nephropathy.

EXOGENOUS CAUSES OF CHRONIC INTERSTITIAL NEPHRITIS

Drugs

- Analgesics
  - Combined analgesics
  - Nonsteroidal anti-inflammatory drugs
- Chemotherapeutic agents
  - Cis-platinum
  - Methyl CCMU
- Cyclosporine
- Lithium

Heavy Metals

- Lead
- Cadmium

Analgesic nephropathy. Analgesic nephropathy is characterized by renal papillary necrosis and cortical chronic interstitial nephritis resulting from the prolonged use (10 to 20 years) of phenacetin-containing compound analgesic preparations.[214-217] This association was first recognized following a marked increase in chronic interstitial nephritis and renal papillary necrosis in several geographic regions in Scandinavia and Australia. Originally the chronic interstitial nephritis was recognized, however,

Kincaid-Smith[214] demonstrated that papillary necrosis was the primary injury and the cortical scarring was secondary. Analgesic abuse has been implicated as the cause of 80% to 90% of renal papillary necrosis in nondiabetic Australians. In addition to chronic renal disease, approximately 34% of patients develop coronary artery disease and other atherosclerotic complications.[217] Furthermore, 8% of patients develop transitional cell carcinoma.

Phenacetin and aspirin combined with caffeine or codeine were the original offending preparations. The substitution of acetaminophen for phenacetin, control over marketing practices, and increasing recognition of the risk factors have substantially lowered the prevalence of analgesic nephropathy. However, a similar chronic renal disease has now been identified by chronic misuse of nonsteroidal anti-inflammatory drugs.[217]

The renal lesions of analgesic abuse begin in the inner medulla and have been divided into three stages.[214-216] In the first stage there is a yellowish radiating discoloration of the papillary tip. Microscopically, there is necrosis of loops of Henle and interstitial cells with thickening and sclerosis of small vessels. In the second stage, the process involves the entire inner medulla with widespread necrosis of collecting ducts, loops of Henle, and vasa recta. Interstitial calcification frequently is present.

During the third stage, cortical changes develop following necrosis of the renal pyramid. The cortex overlying the pyramid becomes thin and atrophic, histologically showing a nonspecific chronic interstitial nephritis with tubular atrophy, interstitial fibrosis, and a lymphoid infiltrate. The column's of Bertin may be spared producing an alternating pattern of atrophy and thickening of the cortex. The necrotic papillae often have been described as darkly colored and focally may detach and slough. In contrast to other forms of papillary necrosis, a neutrophilic response is not evident. A distinctive capillary sclerosis affects the small vessels of the papillary tip and the small mucosal vessels of the renal pelvis, ureter, and bladder characterized by extensive reduplication of the basal lamina best demonstrated by PAS stain.

METABOLIC ABNORMALITIES AND TUBULOINTERSTITIAL DISEASES

A variety of metabolic abnormalities may affect the kidney. The four most important involve calcium, uric acid, oxalate, and cystine. Each can exert its effect by parenchymal deposition or by formation of calculi.

Hypercalcemic Nephropathy

Hypercalcemia can result from many systemic diseases (see box on this page) and has several renal consequences.[272-274] The most common renal effects are a decrease in glomerular filtration rate and a decrease in concentrating capacity, which may lead to polyuria and, when severe and prolonged, to volume depletion and acute renal failure. Hypercalcemia also can have

MAJOR CAUSES OF HYPERCALCEMIA

- Primary and secondary hyperparathyroidism
- Vitamin D intoxication
- Milk alkali syndrome
- Sarcoidosis
- Malignant neoplasms
- Increased bone turnover
- Idiopathic

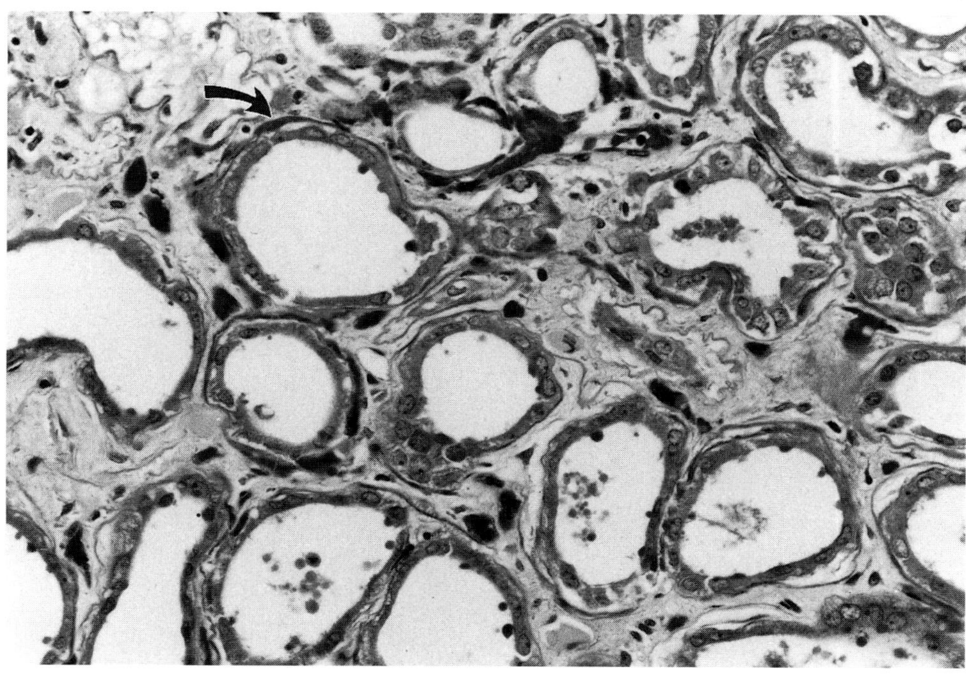

1-112. Nephrocalcinosis showing tubular basement membranes (*arrow*) encrusted with calcium.

direct morphologic effects: nephrolithiasis, calcium oxalate crystal formation in tubules, and calcium deposition along cortical tubular basement membranes (Fig. 1-112).

Nephrolithiasis

Nephrolithiasis is a common abnormality affecting 500,000 Americans each year.[275,276] It is not a single disease but rather a common end point with obstructive complications that may arise within the context of diverse abnormalities of metabolism, renal tubular cell function, or result from urinary tract diseases such as obstruction or bacterial infections. Nephrolithiasis is a dynamic process. In its early stages, there is potential for medical therapy to control or prevent its complications by modifying factors that permit crystallization. There are several types of stones, which may be pure or heterogeneous in composition (see box on this page). Each has multiple etiologies and clinical associations.[275,276]

Calcium-containing stones are the most common variety and can have a variable composition such as calcium oxalate or calcium phosphate (hydroxyapatite, carbonateapatite, or brushite). Most patients with calcium oxalate–containing stones do not have an abnormality of oxalate metabolism. Hypercalciuria is the most common underlying metabolic abnormality, encountered in 60% of patients.

Struvite stones (infection or triple phosphate stones) are a combination of struvite ($MgNH_4PO_4$-GH_2O) and carbonate-apatite ($CA_{10}[PO_4]_6$-CO_3). These form only in the presence of urea-splitting organisms such as *Proteus*, *Staphylococcus albus*, *Pseudomonas*, and *Klebsiella*.[277] Struvite stones can form very rapidly and form most staghorn calculi (Fig. 1-104).

Not all stones are heavily mineralized. Matrix stones are composed principally of a glycoprotein matrix with focal calcification.[278,279] Matrix stones form large casts of the collecting system and have a soft yellow to tan gross appearance and a laminated structure histologically. They are often associated with urinary tract infection.

Because nephrolithiasis can result from urinary tract obstruction or cause urinary tract obstruction, affected kidneys may show diverse changes such as hydronephrosis, acute or chronic pyelonephritis, or xanthogranulomatous pyelonephritis. Many will also contain small calcified plaques along the papillary tips known as Randall's plaques. In the 1950s Randall[280] noted that 20% of patients with stones had 2 to 4 mm of submucosal calcified plaques, which he felt represented precursor lesions in stone formation.[281] These plaques are derived from interstitial and tubular basement membrane calcification (Fig. 1-113), which in certain patients becomes a nucleation site for stone formation.

TYPES OF RENAL STONES

- Calcium phosphate
- Calcium oxalate
- Struvite
- Uric acid
- Cystine
- Matrix stone

Oxalate-associated renal disease

Oxalic acid is the simplest dicarboxylic acid found in nature.[282] It is a major constituent of many plants and a

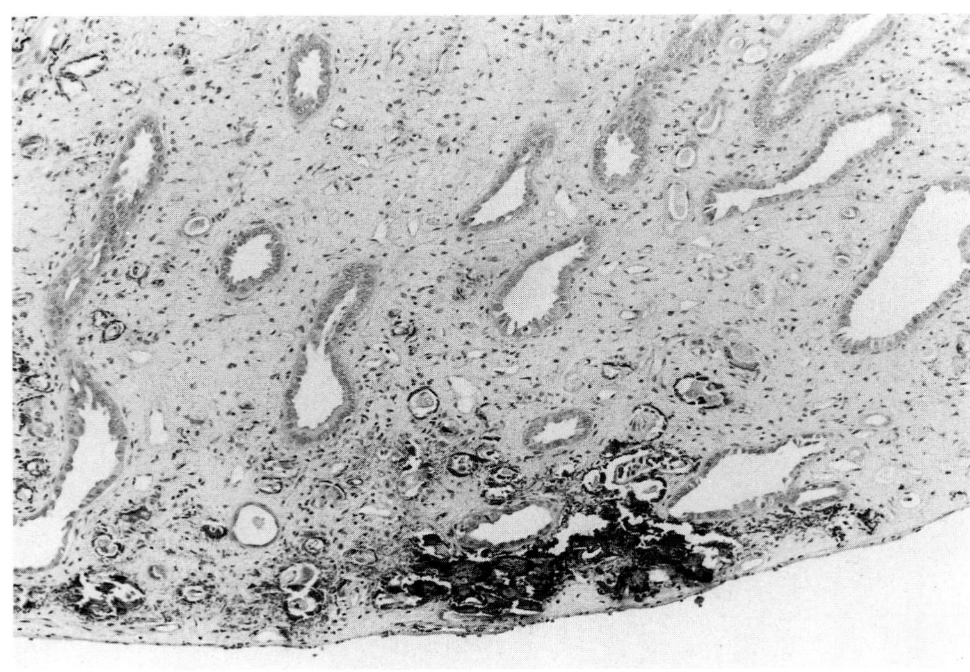

1-113. Randall's plaque in a papillary tip from a patient with nephrolithiasis.

metabolic by-product of endogenous and exogenous compounds. The kidneys may be confronted with an excessive oxalate load in several situations (see box on this page), and this results in oxalosis and calcium oxalate calculi.[282] However, most patients with calcium oxalate stones have none of these disorders but have abnormalities in calcium metabolism.[275,276]

Primary hyperoxaluria types I and II are autosomal recessive, inborn errors in metabolism, which result in excessive production of oxalate.[282,283] Calcium oxalate deposits form in vessels in several extrarenal tissues such as the heart, brain, eye, and bone marrow. Renal tubular oxalosis and calcium oxalate calculi form and result in renal failure at an early age.

Secondary hyperoxaluria and renal oxalosis may result from ethylene glycol (automobile antifreeze) ingestion or from methoxyflurane anesthesia and cause acute renal failure with renal tubular oxalosis.[282,284,285] In ethylene glycol intoxication, glycol is metabolized to oxalate, which precipitates in the distal tubules causing obstruction (Fig. 1-114). There also is a direct toxic effect of glycol on tubular epithelium, which contributes to the renal injury. The free fluoride in methoxyflurane appears to stimulate excessive oxalate production by the liver, causing a heavy acute oxalate load to the kidney. In renal tubular oxalosis, calcium oxalate crystals are found both within renal tubular lumina and within tubular epithelial cells. The crystals are strongly birefringent under polarized light (Fig. 1-114).

Secondary hyperoxaluria of a more chronic form, leading to stone formation, occurs in patients with small bowel or pancreatobiliary tract disease (enteric oxalosis).[281,286] Unabsorbed lipids bind intraintestinal calcium, leaving insufficient calcium to precipitate the oxalate within the gut, leading to increased oxalate absorption. Finally, it also is common to encounter scattered calcium oxalate crystals within renal tubules at autopsy in patients with chronic renal failure and in the absence of overt renal disease.[287]

CAUSES OF HYPEROXALURIA

- Primary hyperoxaluria, types I and II
- Secondary hyperoxaluria
  - Ethylene glycol ingestion
  - Methoxyflurane anesthesia
  - Gastrointestinal disease
  - Pancreatobiliary disease
  - Chronic renal failure
  - Idiopathic

Cystinosis

Cystinosis is an autosomal recessive storage disease characterized by impaired transport of the amino acid cystine across lysosomal membranes resulting in its excessive accumulation in several organs, including the kidney.[288] Three forms are recognized: an infantile nephropathic form, an adolescent form, and an adult form. In the infantile nephropathic form there is initial tubular dysfunction characterized by Fanconi's syndrome, which progresses to uremia and death by 9 to 10 years of age if untreated.[288-290] This is accompanied by growth retardation, photophobia, and hypothyroidism. Its progress can be arrested by treatment with cysteamine,

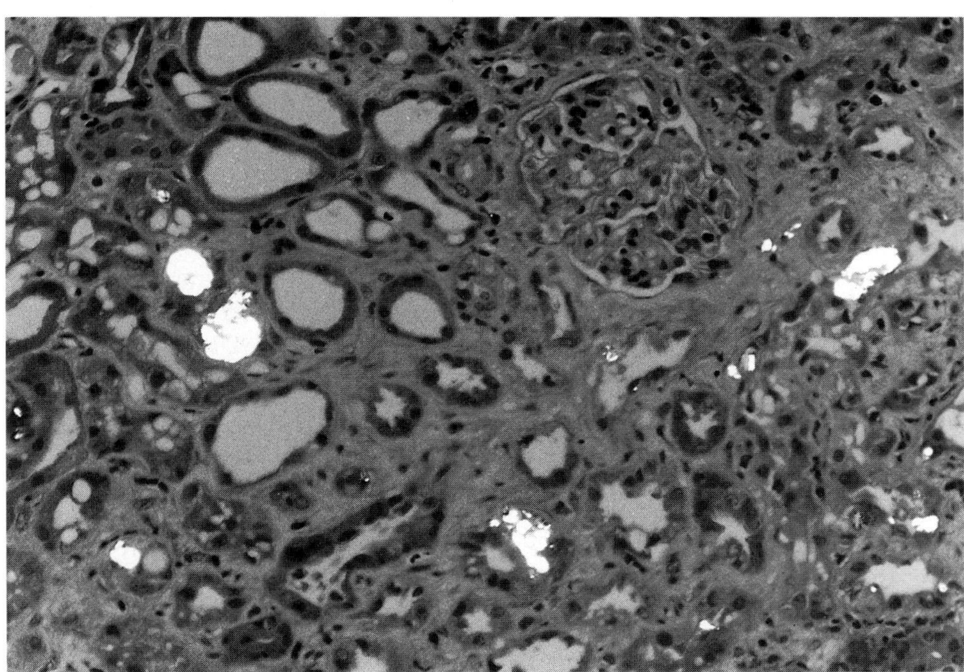

1-114. Calcium oxalate crystals under polarized light in a patient with acute renal failure secondary to ethylene glycol ingestion.

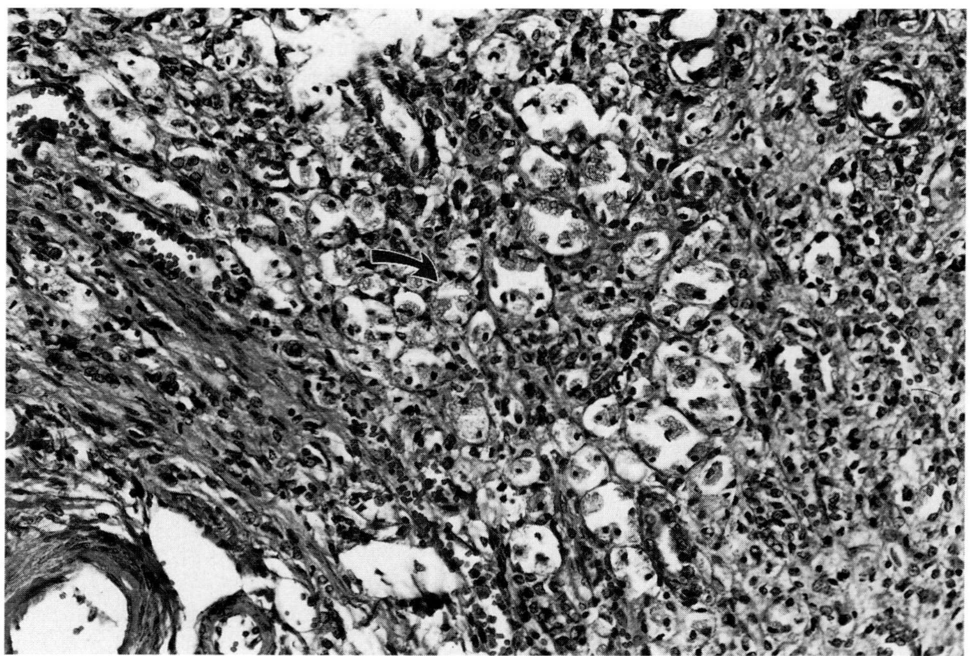

1-115. Infantile nephropathic cystinosis showing cystine crystals (*arrow*) in a 6-year-old.

which reduces intracellular cystine levels.[291] The adolescent form is rare and slowly progressive while the adult form causes only ocular disease.

In the early phase of nephropathic cystinosis the kidneys may have enlarged multinucleated podocytes (referred to as polykaryocytosis) and cystine crystals may be visible in macrophages within glomeruli or in interstitial areas.[289,290] With progression of the disease a chronic interstitial nephritis develops with tubulointerstitial scarring and clusters of crystal-containing macrophages in the interstitium (Fig. 1-115). Because cystine crystals are birefringent and soluble in water, alcohol fixation and polarization provide optimum demonstration and retention of the crystals.

CAUSES OF HYPERURICEMIA AND GOUT

- Lymphoproliferative disorders
- Myeloproliferative disorders
- Lead (saturnine gout)
- Diuretics
- Alcohol
- Aspirin
- Endocrine dysfunctions
- Starvation
- Hypoxanthine-guanine phosphoribosyltransferase deficiency
- Phosphoribosylpyrophosphate synthetase increase activity

Uric acid-associated renal disease

Uric acid is the final degradation product of purine metabolism in humans. It is poorly soluble in plasma and when symptomatic and deposited in tissues it is known as gout. Outside the joints, the kidney is the major site of clinically significant disease caused by hyperuricemia. Three forms of disease occur: acute uric acid nephropathy, uric acid lithiasis, and chronic gouty nephropathy.[292-294]

In acute uric acid nephropathy, there is acute renal failure due to intratubular uric acid crystals. It develops as a complication of rapid tumor lysis in lymphoproliferative and myeloproliferative disorders following initiation of chemotherapy.[292] The acidity and concentration in the collecting ducts favor uric acid crystal formation. The renal medulla, particularly the papilla, may have grossly visible yellow streaks. Uric acid crystals are very soluble in water and birefringent. Therefore, the histologic demonstration of uric acid crystals requires tissue fixed in absolute alcohol (or the use of touch smears or frozen sections) and viewing under polarized light. Crystals may also form within the collecting system and be detectable in the urine. Hydration, alkalization of urine, and pretreatment with allopurinol have greatly reduced the incidence of crystal formation.

Uric acid stones, which may be composed of pure uric acid, are radiolucent or mixed with calcium oxalate and radiopaque. Uric acid stones develop in 20% of patients with gout.[292,293] Stones become more prevalent with the increase in the amount of uric acid excreted. Stone formation can be inhibited by alkalinization of the urine and hydration.

Chronic gouty nephropathy develops in patients with sustained hyperuricemia (see box on this page). It is characterized by the interstitial deposition of sodium urate. Urate elicits a mononuclear cell and giant cell reaction resulting in microtophus formation (Fig. 1-116). These lesions develop mainly within the outer medulla. Small

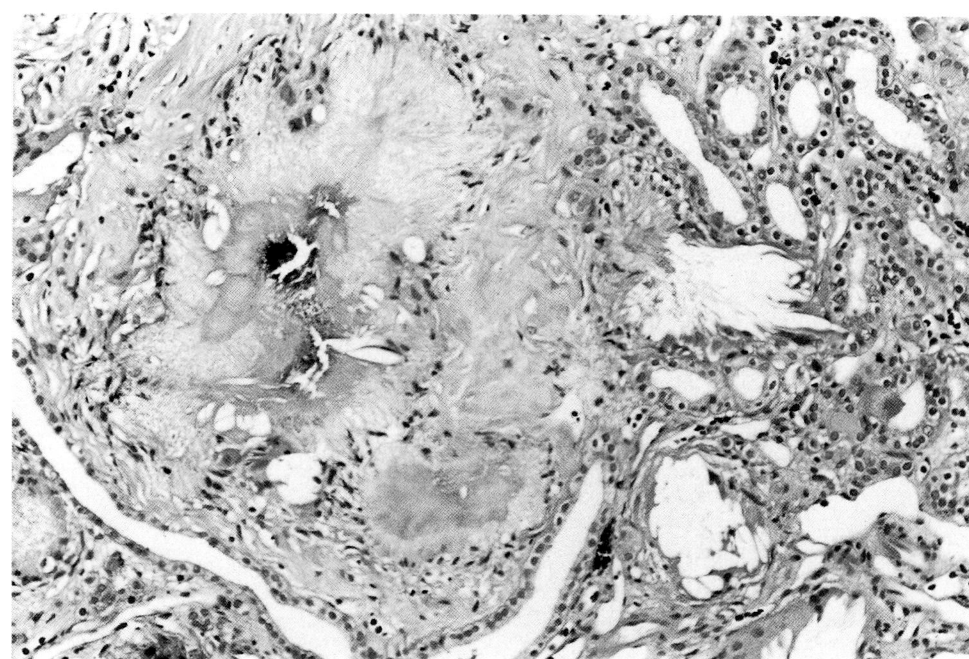

1-116. Medullary urate granuloma.

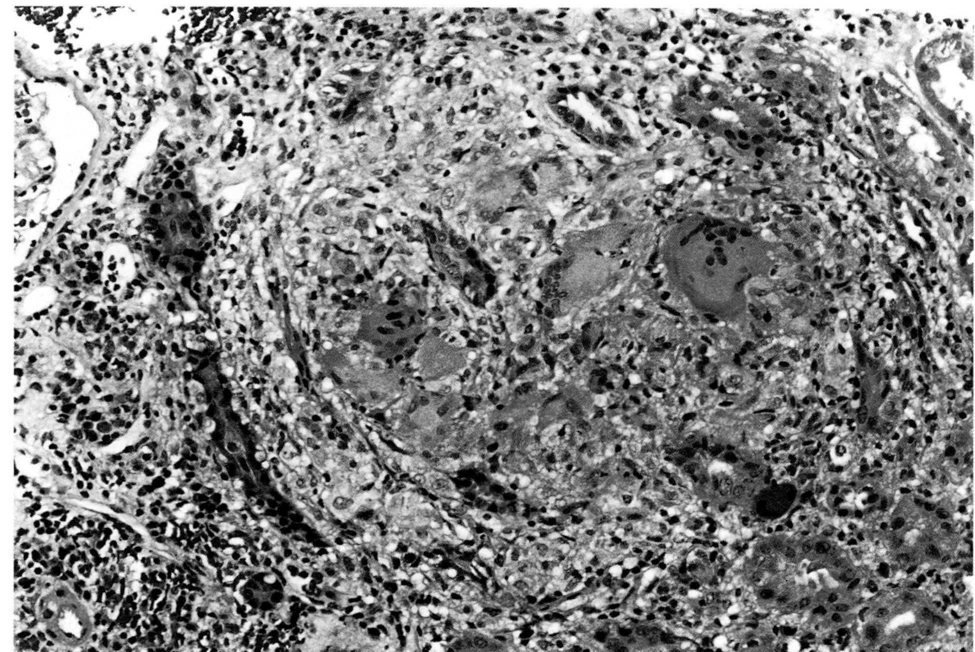

1-117. Sarcoid granuloma in patient with acute renal failure.

urate granulomas can also be seen in azotemia of other causes and occasionally in otherwise normal kidneys.[294] In patients with renal failure attributed to chronic gout, the cortex shows changes of hypertension-associated arterial nephrosclerosis and chronic interstitial nephritis. Tophi usually are not identified.

It was previously believed that primary gout caused renal failure in a substantial number of gouty patients. This concept has been challenged on the grounds that the gout in many of the patients in older reports was probably secondary, and that the renal disease was actually caused by lead toxicity and underlying diabetes and hypertension.[295-297] It is now known that chronic lead nephropathy causes clinical gout and hypertension and produces the same histologic findings previously regarded as typical of chronic gouty nephropathy.

MISCELLANEOUS CONDITIONS

Sarcoidosis

Sarcoidosis is a chronic disease of unknown cause in which multiple organ systems are affected, usually by

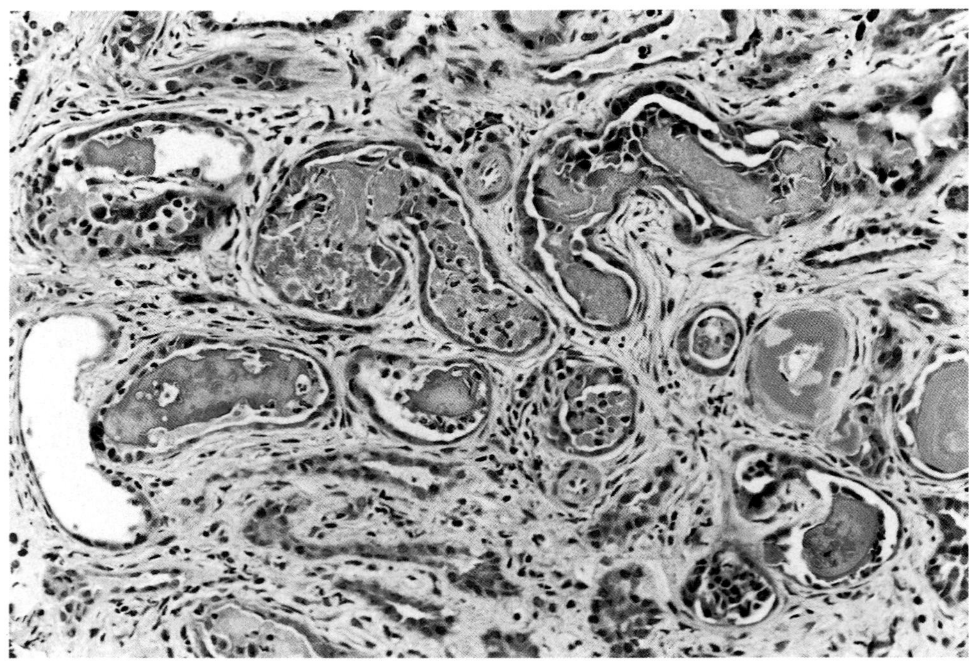

1-118. Light chain cast nephropathy causing renal failure.

RENAL LESIONS ASSOCIATED WITH HEMATOPOIETIC NEOPLASMS

- Light chain cast nephropathy
- Immunoglobulin deposition disease
- Amyloidosis
- Nephrocalcinosis
- Uric acid nephropathy
- Nephrolithiasis
- Neoplastic infiltration
- Acute tubular necrosis
- Acute interstitial nephritis

noncaseating granulomas. Symptomatic renal disease occurs in less than 10% of sarcoidosis patients.[246,298] The most frequent renal abnormalities result from hypercalcemia, which causes a reduction in glomerular filtration rate, a decrease in concentrating ability, renal tubular acidosis, nephrocalcinosis, or results in calcium stones. In addition, a granulomatous acute interstitial nephritis (Fig. 1-117) or chronic interstitial nephritis may develop.

Paraprotein-associated tubulointerstitial disease

Patients with multiple myeloma, lymphoma, or leukemia frequently develop renal disease either from a direct effect of the neoplasm or from a therapeutic complication (see box on this page). Either glomerular or tubulointerstitial lesions may develop and result in proteinuria and renal insufficiency.[299,300]

Light chain cast nephropathy (myeloma kidney) is the intratubular formation of large eosinophilic (often

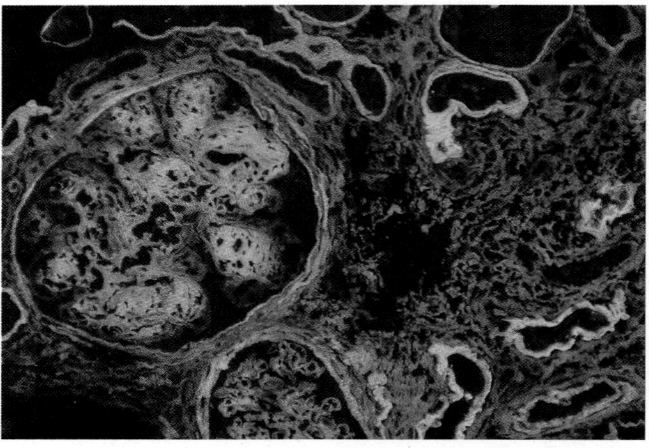

1-119. Direct immunofluorescence showing kappa light chain deposition along tubular and glomerular capillary basement membranes and within the mesangium.

cracked or fractured) casts composed of a Bence Jones protein and Tamm-Horsfall glycoprotein.[299,300] The casts form in the distal tubules and collecting ducts and may extend into the adjacent interstitium. They elicit an inflammatory response that includes neutrophils and histiocytes, which may form giant cells (Fig. 1-118).

Immunoglobulin deposition disease refers to the deposition of granular paraprotein deposits in glomeruli, tubulointerstitial areas, or both, causing nephrotic syndrome, Fanconi syndrome, and renal insufficiency (Fig. 1-119, 1-120). The glomerular lesion resembles amyloid; however, the deposits are granular rather than fibrillar in

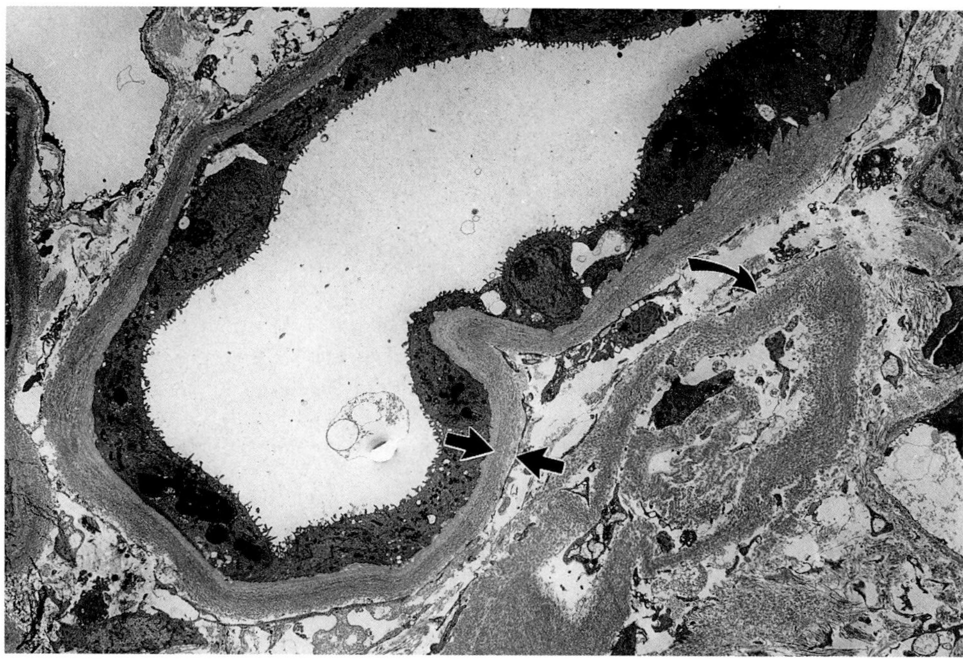

1-120. Granular paraprotein deposits of kappa light chains within the interstitium (*curved arrow*) and along the outer aspect of a tubular basement membrane (*between arrows*).

appearance by electron microscopy.[299,300] Similar tubulointerstitial deposits form along the outside of the tubular basement membrane, within the interstitium, and in small vessels. Similar to amyloidosis, systemic involvement also occurs.

ACKNOWLEDGEMENTS

The author greatly appreciates the assistance of Daniel Slagel, M.D. and Karen M. Fitzsimmons, M.D. in obtaining some of the gross specimens used to illustrate this chapter, the secretarial efforts of Marcia Wood, and photographic expertise of Joel Carl.

REFERENCES

1. Hayman JM Jr: Malpighi's "Concerning the structure of the kidneys." A translation and introduction. Ann Med Hist 7:242-263, 1925.
2. Clark W: The drawings of Leonardo Da Vinci in the collection of Her Majesty the Queen at Windsor Castle, Edinburgh, England, 1969, R & R Clark LTD.
3. Murphy LJT, ed: The history of urology. Springfield, Mass, 1972, Charles C. Thomas.
4. Bowman W: On the structure and use of the malpighian bodies of the kidney, with observations on the circulation through that gland, Philos Trans R Soc Lond Biol 132:57-80, 1842.
5. Fine LG: William Bowman's description of the glomerulus, Am J Nephrol 5:433-440, 1985.
6. Huber GC: On the development and shape of uriniferous tubules of certain of the higher mammals, Am J Anat Suppl 4:29, 1-98, 1905.
7. Kelly HA, Burnam CF: Diseases of the kidneys, ureters and bladder, New York, 1914, D. Appleton, Century and Crofts.
8. Osathanondh V, Potter EL: Development of the human kidney as shown by microdissection II. Renal pelvis, calyces and papillae, Arch Pathol 76:276-289, 1963.
9. Osathanondh V, Potter EL: Development of the human kidney as shown by microdissection III. Formation and interrelationship of collecting tubules and nephrons, Arch Pathol 76:290-302, 1963.
10. Osathanondh V, Potter EL: Development of the human kidney as shown by microdissection IV. Development of tubular portions of nephrons, Arch Pathol 82:391-402, 1966.
11. Osathanondh V, Potter EL: Development of the human kidney as shown by microdissection V. Development of vascular pattern of glomeruli, Arch Pathol 82:403-411, 1966.
12. Patten BM: Human embryology, New York, 1968, McGraw-Hill Book Co.
13. Potter EL: Normal and abnormal development of the kidney, Chicago, 1972, Year Book Medical Publishers, Inc.
14. Clapp WL: Adult kidney. In Sternberg SS, ed: Histology for the pathologist, New York, 1992, Raven Press.
15. Venkatachalam MA, Kris W: Anatomy. In Heptinstall RH, ed: Pathology of the kidney, Boston, 1992, Little, Brown and Company.
16. Brenner BM: Determinants of epithelial differentiation during early nephrogenesis, J Am Soc Nephrol 1:127-139, 1990.
17. Fouser L, Avner ED: Normal and abnormal nephrogenesis, Am J Kidney Dis 21:64-70, 1993.

18. Brodel M: The intrinsic blood vessels of the kidney and their significance in nephrotomy, Bull Johns Hopkins Hosp 12:10-13, 1901.
19. Graves FT: The anatomy of the intrarenal arteries and its application to segmental resection of the kidney, Br J Surg 42:132-139, 1954.
20. Hodson J: The lobar structure of the kidney, Br J Urol 44:246-261, 1972.
21. Baker SB: The blood supply to the renal papillae, Br J Urol 31:53-59, 1959.
22. Campbell MF: Urology, Philadelphia, 1986, WB Saunders.
23. Weyrauch HM Jr: Anomalies of renal rotation, Surg Gynecol Obstet 69:183-199, 1939.
24. Thompson GJ, Pace JM: Ectopic kidney: a review of 97 cases, Surg Gynecol Obstet 69:935-943, 1939.
25. Kelalis PP, Malek RS, Segura JW: Observations on renal ectopia and fusion in children, J Urol 110:588-593, 1973.
26. Aliotta PJ, Seidel FG, Karp M et al: Renal malposition in patients with omphalocele, J Urol 137:942-944, 1987.
27. Malter IJ, Stanley RJ: The intrathoracic kidney; with a review of the literature, J Urol 107:538-541, 1972.
28. McDonald JH, McClellan DS: Crossed renal ectopia, Am J Surg 93:995-1002, 1957.
29. Hendren WH, Donahoe PK, Pfister RC: Crossed renal ectopia in children, Urology 7:135-144, 1976.
30. Boatman DL, Kolln CP, Flocks RN: Congenital anomalies associated with horseshoe kidney, J Urol 107:205-207, 1972.
31. Zondek LH, Zondek T: Horseshoe kidney and associated congenital malformations, Urol Int 18:347-350, 1964.
32. Geisinger JF: Supernumerary kidney, J Urol 38:331-356, 1936.
33. N'Guessan G, Stephens FD: Supernumerary kidney, J Urol 130:649-653, 1983.
34. Risdon RA, Young LW, Chrispin AR: Renal hypoplasia and dysplasia: a radiological and pathological correlation, Pediatr Radiol 3:213-225, 1975.
35. Schwartz RD, Stephens RD, Cussen LJ: The pathogenesis of renal dysplasia. I. Quantitation of hyoplasia and dysplasia, Invest Urol 19:94-96, 1981.
36. Royer P, Habib R, Mathieu H et al: Bilateral congenital renal hypoplasia with reduction in number and hypertrophy of the nephrons in children, Ann Pediatr 38:753-766, 1962.
37. Fetterman GH, Habib R: Congenital bilateral oligomeganephronic renal hypoplasia with hypertrophy of nephrons (oligomeganephronie), Am J Clin Pathol 52:199-207, 1969.
38. Moerman PH, van Damme B, Proesmans W et al: Oligomeganephronic renal hypoplasia in two siblings, J Pediatr 105:75-77, 1984.
39. Potter EL: Bilateral absence of ureters and kidneys. A report of 50 cases, Obstet Gynecol 25:3-12, 1965.
40. Potter EL: Facial characteristics of infants with bilateral renal agenesis, Am J Obstet Gynecol 51:885-888, 1946.
41. Fitch N: Heterogeneity of bilateral renal agenesis, CMA Journal 116:381-382, 1977.
42. Rush WH Jr, Currie DP: Hemitrigone in renal agenesis or single ureteral ectopia, Urology 11:161-163, 1978.
43. Emanuel B, Nachman R, Aronson N et al: Congenital solitary kidney: a review of 74 cases, J Urol 111:394-397, 1974.
44. Thompson DP, Lynn HB: Genital anomalies associated with solitary kidney, Mayo Clin Proc 41:538-548, 1966.
45. Acien P, Ruiz JA, Hernandez JF et al: Renal agenesis in association with malformation of the female genital tract, Am J Obstet Gynecol 165:1368-1370, 1991.
46. Duncan PA, Shapiro LR, Stangel JJ et al: The MURCS association: müllerian duct aplasia, renal aplasia, and cervicothoracic somite dysplasia, J Pediatr 95:399-402, 1979.
47. Thomas IT, Smith DW: Oligohydramnios, causes of the nonrenal features of Potter's syndrome, including pulmonary hypoplasia, J Pediatr 84:811-814, 1974.
48. Salazar H, Kanbour AI, Pardo M: Amnion nodosum. Ultrastructure and histopathogenesis, Arch Pathol 98:39-46, 1974.
49. Bain AD, Scott JS: Renal agenesis and severe urinary tract dysplasia, Br Med J 1:841-846, 1960.
50. Curry CJR, Jensen K, Holland J et al: The Potter sequence: a clinical analysis of 80 cases, Am J Med Genet 19:679-702, 1984.
51. Escobar LF, Weaver DD, Bixler D et al: Urorectal septum malformation sequence, Am J Dis Child 141:1021-1024, 1987.
52. Ingelfinger JR, Newburger JW: Spectrum of renal anomalies in patients with Williams syndrome, J Pediatr 119:771-773, 1991.
53. Hurwitz RS, Manzoni GAM, Ransley PG et al: Cloacal extrophy: a report of 34 cases, J Urol 138:1060-1064, 1987.
54. Quan L, Smith DW: The VATER association, vertebral defects, and atresia, T-E fistula with esophageal atresia, radial and renal dysplasia: a spectrum of associated defects, J Pediatr 82:104-107, 1973.
55. Khoury MJ, Cordero JF, Greenberg F et al: A population based study of the VACTERL association: evidence for its etiologic heterogeneity, Pediatr 71:815-820, 1983.
56. Burn J, Marwood RP: Fraser syndrome presenting as bilateral renal agenesis, J Med Genet 19:360-361, 1982.
57. Rubenstein MA, Bucy JG: Caudal regression syndrome: the urologic implications, J Urol 114:934-937, 1975.
58. Biedel CW, Pagon RA, Zapata JO: Müllerian anomalies and renal agenesis: autosomal dominant urogenital adysplasia, J Pediatr 104:861-864, 1984.
59. Buchta RM, Viseskul C, Gilbert EF et al: Familial bilateral renal agenesis and hereditary renal adysplasia, Z Kinderheilkd 115:111-129, 1973.
60. Cain DR, Griggs D, Lackey DA et al: Familial renal agenesis and total dysplasia, Am J Dis Child 128:377-380, 1974.
61. Roodhooft AM, Birnholz JC, Holmes LB: Familial nature of congenital absence and severe dysgenesis of both kidneys, New Engl J Med 310:1341-1345, 1984.
62. Murugasu B, Cole BR, Hawkins EP et al: Familial renal adysplasia, Am J Kidney Dis 18:490-494, 1991.
63. Elkin M, Bernstein J: Cystic diseases of the kidney—radiological and pathological considerations, Clin Radiol 20:65-82, 1969.
64. Bernstein J: Renal cystic disease: classification and pathogenesis, Cong Anom 33:5-13, 1993.
65. Bernstein J: The morphogenesis of renal parenchymal maldevelopment (renal dysplasia), Pediatr Clin North Am 18:395-407, 1971.
66. Osathananth V, Potter EL: Pathogenesis of polycystic kidneys, Arch Pathol 77:459-465, 1964.
67. Berman DJ, Maizals M: The role of urinary obstruction in the genesis of renal dysplasia, J Urol 128:1091-1096, 1982.

68. Schwartz RD, Stephens FD, Cussen LJ: The pathogenesis of renal dysplasia II. The significance of lateral and medial ectopy of the ureteric orifice, Invest Urol 19:97-100, 1981.
69. Cussen LJ: Cystic kidneys in children with congenital urethral obstruction, J Urol 106:939-941, 1971.
70. Taxy JB: Renal dysplasia: a review. In Sommers SC, Rosen PP, Fechner RE, ed: Pathology annual, part 2, Norwalk, CT, 1985, Appleton-Century-Crofts.
71. Maizals M, Simpson SB Jr: Primitive ducts of renal dysplasia induced by culturing ureteral buds denuded of condensed renal blastema, Science 219:509-510, 1983.
72. Mackie GG, Stephens FD: Duplex kidneys: a correlation of renal dysplasia with position of the ureteral orifice, J Urol 114:274-280, 1975.
73. Bernstein J, Brough AJ, McAdams AJ: The renal lesion in syndromes of multiple congenital malformations, Birth Defects 10:35-43, 1974.
74. Bernstein J: Hepatic and renal involvement in malformation syndromes, Mt Sinai J Med (NY) 53:421-428, 1986.
75. Osler W: Congenital absence of abdominal muscles with distended and hypertrophied urinary bladder, Bull Johns Hopkins Hosp 12:331, 1901.
76. Manivel JC, Pettinato G, Reinberg Y et al: Prune belly syndrome: clinicopathological study of 29 cases, Pediatr Pathol 9:691-711, 1989.
77. Zerres K, Valpel M-C, Weib H: Cystic kidneys. Genetics, pathological anatomy clinical picture and prenatal diagnosis, Human Genet 68:104-135, 1984.
78. Kravtzova GI, Lazjuk GI, Lurie IW: The malformations of the urinary system in autosomal disorders, Virchows Arch [A] 368:167-178, 1975.
79. Duncan PA, Shapiro LR: Interrelationship of the hemifacial microsomia-VATER, VATER and sirenomelia phenotype, Am J Med Gen 47:75-84, 1993.
80. Lieberman E, Salinas-Madrigal L, Gwinn JL et al: Infantile polycystic disease of the kidneys and liver, Medicine 50:277-318, 1971.
81. Blyth H, Ockenden BG: Polycystic disease of kidneys and liver presenting in childhood, J Med Genet 8:257-284, 1971.
82. Vuthibhagdee A, Singleton EB: Infantile polycystic disease of the kidney, Am J Dis Child 125:167-170, 1973.
83. Gang DL, Herrin JT: Infantile polycystic disease of the liver and kidneys, Clin Nephrol 28:28-36, 1986.
84. Suki WN: Polycystic kidney disease, Kidney Int 22:571-580, 1982.
85. Gabow PA: Autosomal dominant polycystic kidney disease, N Engl J Med 329:332-342, 1993.
86. Lieske JC, Toback FG: Autosomal dominant polycystic kidney disease, J Am Soc Nephrol 3:1442-1450, 1993.
87. Porch P, Noe HN, Stapleton FB: Unilateral presentation of adult type polycystic kidney disease in children, J Urol 135:744-746, 1986.
88. Shokeir MHK: Expression of "adult" polycystic renal disease in the fetus and newborn, Clin Genet 14:61-72, 1978.
89. Baert L: Hereditary polycystic kidney disease (adult form): a microdissection study of two cases at an early stage of the disease, Kidney Int 13:519-525, 1978.
90. Grantham JJ, Geiser JL, Evan AP: Cyst formation and growth in autosomal dominant polycystic kidney disease, Kidney Int 31:1145-1152, 1987.
91. Verani RR, Silva FG: Histogenesis of the renal cysts in adult (autosomal dominant) polycystic kidney disease: a histochemical study, Mod Pathol 1:457-463, 1988.
92. Bernstein J, Evan AP, Gardner KD Jr: Epithelial hyperplasia in human polycystic kidney diseases, Am J Pathol 129:92-101, 1987.
93. Gregoiri JR, Torres VE, Holley KE et al: Renal epithelial hyperplasitc and neoplastic proliferation in autosomal dominant polycystic kidney disease, Am J Kidney Dis 9:27-38, 1987.
94. Mongeau JG, Worthen HG: Nephronophthisis and medullary cystic disease, Am J Med 43:345-355, 1967.
95. Herdman RC, Good RA, Vernier RL: Medullary cystic disease in two siblings, Am J Med 43:335-344, 1967.
96. Chamberlin BC, Hagge WW, Stickler GB: Juvenile nephronophthisis and medullary cystic disease, Mayo Clin Proc 52:485-491, 1971.
97. Waldherr R, Lennert T, Weber H-P et al: The nephronophthisis complex. A clinicopathologic study in children, Virchows Arch [A] 394:235-254, 1982.
98. Lamiell JM, Salazar FG, Hsia YEL: Von Hippel-Lindau disease affecting 43 members of a single kindred, Medicine 68:1-29, 1989.
99. Solomon O, Schwartz A: Renal pathology in von Hippel-Lindau disease, Hum Pathol 19:1072-1079, 1988.
100. Ibrahim RE, Weinberg DS, Weidner N: Atypical cysts and carcinomas of the kidneys in phacomatoses, Cancer 63:148-157, 1989.
101. Bernstein J, Robbins TO, Kissane JM: The renal lesions of tuberous sclerosis, Semin Diagn Pathol 3:97-105, 1986.
102. Ahuja S, Loffler W, Wegener O-H et al: Tuberous sclerosis with angiomyolipoma and metastasized hypernephroma, Urology 28:413-419, 1986.
103. Bernstein J, Landing BH: Glomerulocystic kidney diseases. In Bartsocas CS, ed: Genetics of kidney disorders, New York, 1989, Alan R. Liss Inc.
104. Kaplan BS, Gordon I, Pincott J et al: Familial hypoplastic glomerulocystic kidney disease: a definite entity with dominant inheritance, Am J Med Genet 34:569-573, 1989.
105. Romero R, Bonal J, Campo E et al: Glomerulocystic kidney disease: a single entity? Nephron 63:100-103, 1993.
106. Melnick SC, Brewer DB, Oldham JS: Cortical microcystic disease of the kidney with dominant inheritance: a previously undescribed syndrome, J Clin Pathol 37:494-499, 1984.
107. Dosa S, Thompson AM, Abraham A: Glomerulocystic kidney disease, report of an adult case, Am J Clin Pathol 82:619-621, 1984.
108. Hallman N, Hjelt L: Congenital nephrotic syndrome, J Pediatr 55:152-162, 1959.
109. Hallman N, Norio R, Rapola J: Congenital nephrotic syndrome, Nephron 11:101-110, 1973.
110. Fujinami M, Hane Y, Ito K et al: Congenital nephrotic syndrome (Finnish type), Acta Pathol Jpn 35:517-525, 1985.
111. Sibley RK, Mahan J, Mauer SM et al: A clinicopathologic study of forty-eight infants with nephrotic syndrome, Kidney Int 27:544-552, 1985.
112. Swinford AE, Bernstein J, Toriello HV et al: Renal tubular dysgenesis: delayed onset of oligohydrananios, Am J Med Genet 32:127-132, 1989.
113. Genest DC, Lage JM: Absence of normal appearing proximal tubules in the fetal and neonatal kidney: prevalence and significance, Hum Pathol 22:147-153, 1991.

114. Pryde PG, Sedman AB, Nugent CE et al: Angiotensin—converting enzyme inhibitor fetopathy, J Am Soc Nephrol 3:1575-1582, 1993.
115. Simon J: On subacute inflammation of the kidney, Medicochir Trans 30:141-164, 1847.
116. Dunnill MS, Millard PR, Oliver D: Acquired cystic disease of the kidneys: a hazard of long-term intermittent maintenance hemodialysis, J Clin Pathol 30:868-877, 1977.
117. Grantham JJ: Acquired cystic disease, Kidney Int 40:143-152, 1991.
118. Bretan PN Jr, Busch MP, Hricak H et al: Chronic renal failure: a significant risk factor in the development of acquired renal cysts and renal cell carcinoma, Cancer 57:1871-1879, 1986.
119. Matson MA, Cohen EP: Acquired cystic kidney disease: occurrence prevalence and renal cancers, Medicine 69:217-226, 1990.
120. Cho KJ et al: Localized cystic disease of the kidney: 'angiographic'—pathologic correlation, AJR Am J Roentgenol 132:891-895, 1979.
121. Pyrah LN: Medullary sponge kidney, J Urol 90:274-283, 1966.
122. Dalton D, Neiman H, Grayhack JT: The natural history of simple renal cysts: a preliminary study, J Urol 135:905-908, 1986.
123. Laucks SP Jr, McLachlan MSF: Aging and simple cysts of the kidney, Br J Radiol 54:12-14, 1981.
124. Kimche D, Lask D: Megacalycosis, Urology 19:478-481, 1978.
125. Timmons JW Jr, Malek RS, Hattery RR et al: Caliceal diverticulum, J Urol 114:6-9, 1975.
126. Mathieson AJM: Calyceal diverticulum: a case with a discussion and review of the condition, Br J Urol 25:147-154, 1953.
127. Sommers SC, Relman AS, Smithwick RH: Histologic studies of kidney biopsy specimens from patients with hypertension, Am J Pathol 34:685-701, 1958.
128. Walker WG: Hypertension-related renal injury: a major contributor to end stage renal disease, Am J Kidney Dis 22:164-173, 1993.
129. Schwartz GL, Strong CG: Renal parenchymal involvement in essential hypertension, Med Clin North Am 71:843-858, 1987.
130. Bright R: Tubular view of the morbid appearances in 100 cases connected with albuminous urine: with observations, Guy's Hosp Rep 1:380, 1836.
131. Johnson GI: On certain points in the anatomy and pathology of Bright's disease, Trans Med Chir Soc 51:57-78, 1868.
132. Mahomed FA: Some of the clinical aspects of Bright's disease, Guy's Hosp Rep 24:363, 1879.
133. Volhard F, Fahr T: Die Brightsche Nierenkrankheit: Klinik, pathologie und atlas, Berlin, 1914, Julius Springer.
134. Ratliff NB: Renal vascular disease: pathology of large blood vessel disease, Am J Kidney Dis 5:A93-A103, 1985.
135. Kashgarian M: Pathology small blood vessel disease in hypertension, Am J Kidney Dis 5:A104-A110, 1985.
136. McManus JFA, Lupton GH Jr: Ischemic obsolescence of renal glomeruli, Lab Invest 9:413-434, 1960.
137. MacMahon HE: Malignant nephrosclerosis—a reappraisal, Pathol Annu 3:297-334, 1968.
138. Moschcowitz E: An acute febrile pleiochromic anemia with hyalin thrombosis of the terminal arterioles and capillaries, Arch Int Med 36:89-93, 1925.
139. Gasser VC, Gautier E, Steek A et al: Hämolytisch-uramische syndrome: bilaterale Nierenyindennekrosen bei akuten erworbenen hamolytischen anamien, Schweiz Med Wochenschr 38:905-909, 1955.
140. Symmers WSC: Thrombotic microangiopathic hemolytic anemia (thrombotic microangiopathy), Br Med J 2:897-903, 1952.
141. Murgo AJ: Thrombotic microangiopathy in cancer patients including those induced by chemotherapeutic agents, Semin Hematol 24:161-177, 1987.
142. Churg J, Strauss L: Renal involvement in thrombotic microangiopathy, Semin Nephrol 5:46-56, 1985.
143. Donohoe JF: Scleroderma and the kidney, Kidney Int 41:462-477, 1992.
144. Stratta P, Canavese C, Colla L: Microangiopathic hemolytic anemia and postpartum acute renal failure, Nephron 44:253-255, 1986.
145. Hauglustaine D, van Damme B et al: Recurrent hemolytic uremic syndrome during oral contraception, Clin Nephrol 15:148-153, 1981.
146. Remuzzi G, Bertani T: Renal vascular and thrombotic effect of cyclosporine, Am J Kidney Dis 13:261-272, 1989.
147. Kwaan HC: Clinicopathologic features of thrombotic thrombocytopenic purpura, Semin Hematol 24:71-81, 1987.
148. Remuzzi G: HUS and TTP: variable expression of a single entity, Kidney Int 32:292-308, 1987.
149. Kaplan BS, Proesmans W: The hemolytic uremic syndrome of childhood and its variants, Semin Hematol 24:148-160, 1987.
150. Ashkenazi S: Role of bacterial cytotoxins in hemolytic uremic syndrome and thrombotic thrombocytopenic purpura, Ann Rev Med 44:11-18, 1993.
151. Richardon SE, Karmali MLA, Becker LE et al: The histopathology of the hemolytic uremic syndrome associated with verocytotoxin-producing Escherichia coli infections, Hum Pathol 19:1102-1108, 1988.
152. Goldblatt H, Lynch J, Hanzal RF et al: Studies in experimental hypertension I. The production of persistent elevation of systolic blood pressure by means of renal ischemia, J Exp Med 59:347-357, 1934.
153. Wise KL, McCann RL, Dunnick NR et al: Renovascular hypertension, J Urol 140:911-924, 1988.
154. Stimpel M, Groth H, Greminger P et al: The spectrum of renovascular hypertension, Cardiology 72 Suppl 1:1-9, 1985.
155. Harrison EG Jr, McCormack LJ: Pathologic classification of renal arterial disease in renovascular hypertension, Mayo Clin Proc 46:161-167, 1971.
156. Youngberg SP, Sheps SG, Strong CG: Fibromuscular disease of the renal arteries, Med Clin North Am 61:623-641, 1977.
157. Ingelfinger JR: Renovascular disease in children, Kidney Int 43:493-505, 1993.
158. Edwards BS, Stanton AW, Holley KE et al: Isolated renal artery dissection. Presentation, evaluation, management and pathology, Mayo Clin Proc 57:564-571, 1982.
159. Rao CW, Blaivas JG: Primary renal artery dissection: a review, J Urol 118:716-719, 1977.

160. Tynes WV II: Unusual renovascular disorders, Urol Clin North Am 11:529-542, 1984.
161. Poutasse EF: Renal artery aneurysms, J Urol 113:443-449, 1975.
162. Altebarmakian VK, Caldamone AA, Dachelet RJ et al: Renal artery aneurysm, Urology 13:257-260, 1979.
163. Harrow BR, Sloane JA: Aneurysm of renal artery: report of five cases, J Urol 81:35-39, 1956.
164. Smith JN, Hinman F Jr: Intrarenal arterial aneurysms, J Urol 97:990-996, 1967.
165. Maldonado JE, Sheps SG: Renal arteriovenous fistula, Postgrad Med 40:263-269, 1966.
166. Kopchick JH, Jacobson HA, Bourne NK et al: Congenital renal arteriovenous malformations, Urology 17:13-17, 1981.
167. Takaha M, Matsumoto A, Ochi K et al: Intrarenal arteriovenous malformations, J Urol 124:315-318, 1980.
168. Thurlbeck WM, Castleman B: Atheromatous emboli to the kidneys after aortic surgery, N Engl J Med 257:442-447, 1957.
169. Gasparini M, Hofman R, Stoller M: Renal artery embolism: clinical features and therapeutic options, J Urol 147:567-572, 1992.
170. Richards AM, Eliot RS, Kanjuh VL et al: Cholesterol embolism. A multiple-system disease masquerading as polyarteritis nodosa, Am J Cardio 15:696-707, 1965.
171. Hoxie HF, Coggin CB: Renal infarction, Arch Int Med 65:587-594, 1940.
172. Fine MJ, Kapoor W, Falanga V: Cholesterol crystal embolization: a review of 221 cases in the English literature, Angiology 38:769-784, 1987.
173. Colt HG, Begg RJ, Saporito J et al: Cholesterol emboli after cardiac catheterization, Medicine 67:389-400, 1988.
174. Wells JD, Margolin ELG, Gall EA: Renal cortical necrosis: clinical and pathologic features in 21 cases, Am J Med 29:257-267, 1960.
175. Kleinknecht D, Grunfeld JP, Gomez PC et al: Diagnostic procedures and long term prognosis in bilateral renal cortical necrosis, Kidney Int 4:390-400, 1973.
176. Grunfeld JP, Ganeval D, Bournerias F: Acute renal failure in pregnancy, Kidney Int 18:179-191, 1980.
177. Jones DB, Iannaccone PM: Atheromatous emboli in renal biopsies, Am J Pathol 78:261-276, 1975.
178. Kasinath BS, Corwin HL, Bidoni AK et al: Eosinophilia in the diagnosis of atheroembolic renal disease, Am J Nephrol 7:173-177, 1987.
179. Stables DP, Fouche RE, DeVillers JP et al: Traumatic renal artery occlusion: 21 cases, J Urol 115:229-233, 1976.
180. Llach F: Hypercoagulability, renal vein thrombosis, and other thrombotic complications of nephrotic syndrome, Kidney Int 28:429-439, 1985.
181. Rosenmann E, Pollack VE, Pirani CL: Renal vein thrombosis in the adult: a clinical and pathologic study based on renal biopsies, Medicine 47:269-335, 1968.
182. Llach F, Papper S, Massry SG: The clinical spectrum of renal vein thrombosis: acute and chronic, Am J Med 69:819-827, 1980.
183. Arneil GC, MacDonald AM, Murphy AV et al: Renal venous thrombosis, Clin Nephrol 1:119-131, 1973.
184. Ricci MA, Lloyd DA: Renal venous thrombosis in infants and children, Arch Surg 125:1195-1199, 1990.
185. Christensen JA, Bader H, Bohle A et al: The structure of the juxtaglomerular apparatus in Addison's disease, Bartter's syndrome and in Conn's syndrome, Virchows Arch [A] 370:103-112, 1976.
186. Küssmaul A, Maier R: Ueber eine bisher nicht beschriebene eigenthumliche arterienerkrankung (periarteritis nodosa), die mit morbus Brightii und rapid fortschreitender allgemeiner muskellahmung einherght, Dtsch Arch Klin Med 1:484-516, 1866.
187. Davies D, Moran ME, Niall JF et al: Segmental glomerulonephritis with antineutrophil antibody: possible arbovirus aetiology, Br J Med 285:606, 1982.
188. van der Woude FJ, Rasmussen N et al: Autoantibodies against neutrophils and monocytes: tool for diagnosis and marker of disease activity in Wegener's granulomatosis, Lancet 1:425-429, 1985.
189. Jennette JC, Falk RJ: Antineutrophil cytoplasmic autoantibodies and associated diseases: a review, Am J Kidney Dis 15:517-529, 1990.
190. Goeken JA: Anti-neutrophil cytoplasmic antibody—a useful serological marker for vasculitis, J Clin Immunol 11:161-174, 1991.
191. Balow JE: Renal vasculitis, Kidney Int 27:954-964, 1985.
192. Adu D, Howie AJ, Scott DGI et al: Polyarteritis and the kidney, Q J Med 62:221-237, 1987.
193. Churg J, Churg A: Idiopathic and secondary vasculitis: a review, Mod Pathol 2:144-160, 1989.
194. Couser WG: Rapidly progressive glomerulonephritis: classification, pathogenetic mechanisms and therapy, Am J Kidney Dis 11:449-464, 1988.
195. Bonsib SM: Glomerular basement membrane necrosis and crescent organization: a scanning electron microscopic study, Kidney Int 33:966-974, 1988.
196. Bohle A, Gise HV, Mackensen-Haen S et al: The obliteration of the postglomerular capillaries and its influence upon the function of both glomeruli and tubules, Klin Wochenschr 59:1043-1051, 1981.
197. Fine LG, Ong ACM, Norman JT: Mechanisms of tubulo-interstitial injury in progressive renal diseases, Eur J Clin Invest 23:259-265, 1993.
198. Heptinstall RH: Interstitial nephritis. A brief review, Am J Pathol 83:214-233, 1976.
199. Roberts JA: Pyelonephritis, cortical abscess and perinephric abscess, Urol Clin North Am 13:637-645, 1986.
200. Hodson CJ: Reflux nephropathy: a personal historical review, AJR Am J Roent 137:451-462, 1981.
201. Hodson CJ, Edwards O: Chronic pyelonephritis and vesicoureteral reflux, Clin Radiol 11:219-231, 1960.
202. Arant BS Jr: Vesicoureteral reflux and renal injury, Am J Kidney Dis 17:491-511, 1991.
203. Ransley PG, Risdon RA: Renal papillary morphology in infants and children, Urol Res 3:111-114, 1975.
204. Tamminen TE, Kaprio EA: The relation of the shape of papillae and of collecting duct openings to intrarenal reflux, Br J Urol 49:345-354, 1977.
205. Edelstein H, McCabe RE: Perinephric abscess: modern diagnosis and treatment in 47 cases, Medicine 67:118-131, 1988.
206. Sheinfeld J, Erturk E, Spataro RF et al: Perinephric abscess: current concepts, J Urol 137:191-194, 1987.
207. Michaeli J, Mogle P et al: Emphysematous pyelonephritis, J Urol 131:203-208, 1984.

208. Klein FA, Smith MJV, Vick CW III et al: Emphysematous pyelonephritis: diganosis and management, South Med J 79:41-46, 1986.
209. Eknoyan G, Qunibi WY, Grissom RT et al: Renal papillary necrosis: an update, Medicine 61:55-73, 1982.
210. Harvald B: Renal papillary necrosis. A clinical survey of sixty-six cases, Am J Med 35:481-486, 1963.
211. Pandya KK, Koshy M, Brown N et al: Renal papillary necrosis in sickle cell hemoglobinopathies, J Urol 115:497-501, 1976.
212. Davies DJ, Kennedy A, Roberts C: Renal medullary necrosis of infancy and childhood, J Pathol 99:125-130, 1969.
213. Kozlowski K, Brown RW: Renal medullary necrosis in infants and children, Pediatr Radiol 7:85-89, 1978.
214. Kincaid-Smith P: Pathogenesis of the renal lesion associated with the abuse of analgesics, Lancet 1:859-862, 1967.
215. Burry A: Pathology of analgesic nephropathy: an Australian experience, Kidney Int 13:34-40, 1978.
216. Gloor FJ: Changing concepts in pathogenesis and morphology of analgesic nephropathy as seen in Europe, Kidney Int 13:27-33, 1978.
217. Nanra RS: Analgesic nephropathy in the 1990's—an Australian experience, Kidney Int 44(Suppl 92):S86-S92, 1993.
218. Michigan S: Genitourinary fungal infections, J Urol 116:390-397, 1976.
219. Wise GJ, Silver D: Fungal infections of the genitourinary system, J Urol 149:1377-1388, 1993.
220. Sinniah R, Churg J, Sobin LH: Renal disease: classification and atlas of infectious and tropical diseases, Chicago, 1988, American Society of Clinical Pathologists Press.
221. Platt JL, Sibley RK, Michael AF: Interstitial nephritis associated with cytomegalovirus infection, Kidney Int 28:550-552, 1985.
222. Ito M, Hirabayashi N, Uno Y et al: Necrotizing tubulointerstitial nephritis associated with adenovirus infection, Hum Pathol 22:1225-1231, 1991.
223. Rosen S, Harmon W, Krensky AM et al: Tubulointerstitial nephritis associated with polyomavirus (BK type) infection, N Engl J Med 308:1192-1196, 1983.
224. Fetterman GH, Sherman FE, Fabrizio NS et al: Generalized cytomegalic inclusion disease, Arch Pathol 86:86-94, 1968.
225. Vas SI: Primary and secondary role of viruses in chronic renal failure, Kidney Int 401(Suppl 35):52-54, 1991.
226. Johnson RJ, Couser WG: Hepatitis B infection and renal disease: clinical, immunopathogenetic and therapeutic considerations, Kidney Int 37:663-676, 1990.
227. Johnson RJ, Gretch DR, Yamabe H et al: Membranoproliferative glomerulonephritis associated with hepatitis C virus infection, New Engl J Med 378:465-470, 1993.
228. D'Agati V, Suh J-I, Carbone L et al: Pathology of HIV-associated nephropathy: a detailed morphologic and comparative study, Kidney Int 35:1358-1370, 1989.
229. Cohen AH, Nast CC: HIV-associated nephropathy. A unique combined glomerular, tubular and interstitial lesion, Med Pathol 1:87-97, 1988.
230. Bruno P, Hassell LH, Brown J et al: The protean manifestations of hemorrhagic fever with renal syndrome, Ann Int Med 113:385-391, 1990.
231. Collan Y, Mihatsch MJ, Lahdevirta J et al: Nephropathia epidemica: mild variant of hemorrhagic fever with renal syndrome, Kidney Int 40 (Suppl 35):S62-S71, 1991.
232. Bailey RR: The relationship of vesico-ureteric reflux to urinary tract infection and chronic pyelonephritis-reflux nephropathy, Clin Nephrol 1:132-141, 1973.
233. Huland H, Buchardt P, Kollerman M et al: Vesicoureteral reflux in end stage renal disease, J Urol 121:10, 1979.
234. Torres VE, Velosa JA, Holley KE et al: The progression of vesicoureteral reflux nephropathy, Ann Int Med 92:766-784, 1980.
235. Cotran RS: Glomerulosclerosis in reflux nephropathy, Kidney Int 21:528-534, 1982.
236. Arant BS Jr, Sotelo-Avila C, Bernstein J: Segmental "hypoplasia" of the kidney (Ask-Upmark), J Pediatr 95:931-939, 1979.
237. Shindo S, Bernstein J, Arant BS Jr: Evolution of renal segmental atrophy (Ask-Upmark kidney) in children with vesicoureteral reflux: radiographic and morphologic studies, J Pediatr 102:847-854, 1983.
238. Malek RS, Elder JS: Xanthogranulomatous pyelonephritis: a clinical analysis of 26 cases and of the literature, J Urol 119:589, 1978.
239. Hartman DS, Davis CJ Jr, Goldman ST et al: Xanthogranulomatous pyelonephritis: sonographic-pathologic correlation of 16 cases, J Ultrasound Med 3:481, 1984.
240. Parsons MA, Harris SC, Longstaff AJ et al: Xanthogranulomatous pyelonephritis: a pathological clinical and aetiologic analysis of 87 cases, Diagn Hist 6:203, 1983.
241. Esparza AR, McKay DB, Cronan JJ et al: Renal parenchymal malakoplakia: histologic spectrum and its relationship to megalocytic interstitial nephritis and xanthogranulomatous pyelonephritis, Am J Surg Pathol 13:225-236, 1989.
242. Dobyan DC, Truong LD, Eknoyan G: Renal malacoplakia revisited, Am J Kidney Dis 22:243-252, 1993.
243. Narayana AS: Overview of renal tuberculosis, Urology 19:231-237, 1982.
244. Farer LS, Lowell AM, Meador MP: Extrapulmonary tuberculosis in the United States, Am J Epidemiol 109:205-217, 1979.
245. Cohen MS: Granulomatous nephritis, Urol Clin North Am 13:6477-6659, 1986.
246. Casella FJ, Allan M: The kidney in sarcoidosis, J Am Soc Nephrol 3:1555-1562, 1993.
247. Magil AB: Drug-induced acute interstitial nephritis with granulomas, Human Pathol 13:36-41, 1983.
248. Wilke BM, Mailloux LU: Acute renal failure: pathogenesis and prevention, Am J Med 80:1129-1135, 1986.
249. Solez K, Morel-Maroger L, Sraer JD: The morphology of "acute tubular necrosis" in man: analysis of 57 renal biopsies and a comparison with the glycerol model, Medicine 58:362-376, 1979.
250. Beaman M, Turney JH, Rodger RSC et al: Changing pattern of acute renal failure, Q J Med 62:15-23, 1987.
251. Schreiner GE, Maher FJ: Toxic nephropathy, Am J Med 38:409-449, 1965.
252. Jao W: Iatrogenic renal disease as revealed by renal biopsy, Semin Diagn Pathol 5:63-79, 1988.
253. Abuelo JG: Renal failure caused by chemicals, foods, plants, animal venoms and misuse of drugs. An overview, Arch Int Med 150:505-510, 1990.
254. Paller MS: Drug-induced nephropathies, Med Clin North Am 74:909-917, 1990.

255. Cooper K, Bennett WM: Nephrotoxicity of common drugs used in clinical practice, Arch Int Med 147:1213-1218, 1987.
256. Councilman WT: Acute interstitial nephritis, J Exp Med 3:393-418, 1898.
257. Laberke H-C, Bohle A: Acute interstitial nephritis. Correlations between clinical and morphological findings, Clin Nephrol 14:263-273, 1980.
258. McClusky RT: Immunologically mediated tubulointerstitial nephritis, Contemp Issues Nephrol 10:121-150, 1983.
259. Andres GA, McCluskey RT: Tubular and interstitial renal disease due to immunological mechanisms, Kidney Int 7:271-289, 1975.
260. Ten RM et al: Acute interstitial nephritis: immunologic and clinical aspects, Mayo Clin Proc 63:921-930, 1988.
261. Sibley RK, Payne W: Morphologic findings in the renal allograft biopsy, Semin Nephrol 5:294-306, 1985.
262. Dobrin RS, Vernier RL, Fish AJ: Acute esoinophilic interstitial nephritis and renal failure with bone marrow-lymph node granulomas and anterior uveitis, Am J Med 59:325-333, 1975.
263. Park MH, D'Agati V, Appel GB et al: Tubulointerstitial disease in lupus nephritis—relationship to immune deposits, interstitial inflammation, glomerular changes, renal function and prognosis, Nephron 44:309-319, 1986.
264. Winer RL, Cohen AH, Sawhney AS et al: Sjogren's syndrome with immune complex tubulointerstitial disease, Clin Immunol Immunopathol 8:494-503, 1977.
265. Gonzalez-Vitale JC, Hayes DM, Cuitovic E et al: The renal pathology in clinical trials of CIS-Platinum (II) diamminedichloride, Cancer 39:1362-1371, 1977.
266. Farnsworth A, Horvath JS, Hall BM et al: Renal biopsy morphology in renal transplantation, Am J Surg Pathol 8:243-252, 1984.
267. Myers BD, Ross J, Newton L et al: Cyclosporine-associated nephropathy, New Engl J Med 311:699-705, 1984.
268. Walker RG: Lithium toxicity, Kidney Int 44:593-598, 1993.
269. Richter GW, Kress Y, Cornwall CC: Another look at lead inclusions, Am J Pathol 53:189-207, 1968.
270. Beaver DL, Burr RE: Bismuth inclusions in the human kidney, Arch Pathol 76:89-94, 1963.
271. Fowler BA: Mechanisms of kidney cell injury from metals, Environ Health Perspect 100:57-73, 1992.
272. Benabe JE, Martinez-Maldonado M: Hypercalcemic nephropathy, Arch Int Med 138:777-779, 1978.
273. Ibels LS, Alfrey AC, Huffer WE et al: Calcifications in endstage kidneys, Am J Med 71:33-37, 1981.
274. Haggitt RC, Pitcock JA: Renal medullary calcifications: a light and electron microscopic study, J Urol 106:342-347, 1971.
275. Smith LH: Pathogenesis of renal stones, Miner Electrolyte Metab 13:214-219, 1987.
276. Pac CYC: Etiology and treatment of urolithiasis, Am J Kidney Dis 18:624-637, 1991.
277. Griffith DP: Struvite stones, Kidney Int 13:372-382, 1978.
278. Williams DI: Matrix calculi, Br J Urol 35:411-415, 1963.
279. Allen TD, Spence HM: Matrix stones, J Urol 95:284-290, 1966.
280. Randall A: Papillary pathology as a recursor of primary renal calculus, J Urol 44:580-589, 1940.
281. Prien EL Sr: The riddle of Randall's plaques, J Urol 114:500-507, 1975.
282. Williams HE: Oxalic acid and the hyperoxaluric syndrome, Kidney Int 13:410-417, 1978.
283. Scheinman JI: Primary hyperoxaluria: therapeutic strategies for the 90's, Kidney Int 40:389-399, 1991.
284. Case Records 38-1979, N Engl J Med 301:650-657,1979.
285. Hollenberg NK, McDonald FD, Cotran R: Irreversible acute oliguric renal failure. A complication of methoxyflurane anesthesia, New Engl J Med 296:877-879, 1972.
286. Drenik EJ, Stanley TM, Border WA et al: Renal damage with intestinal bypass, Ann Int Med 89:594-599, 1978.
287. Salzer WR, Keren D: Oxalosis as a complication of chronic renal failure, Kidney Int 4:61-66, 1973.
288. Foreman JW: Cystinosis, Semin Nephrol 9:62-64, 1989.
289. Spear GS, Slusser RJ, Schulman JD et al: Polykaryocytosis of the visceral glomerular epithelium in cystinosis with description of an unusual clinical variant, Johns Hopkins Med J 129:83-99, 1971.
290. Spear GS, Slusser RJ, Tonsimis AJ et al: Cystinosis: an ultrastructural and electron-probe study of the kidney with unusual findings, Arch Pathol 21:206-221, 1971.
291. Markello TC, Bernardini IM, Gahl WA: Improved renal function in children with cystinosis treated with cysteamine, N Engl J Med 328:1157-1162, 1993.
292. Boss GR, Seegmiller JE: Hyperuricemia and gout, New Engl J Med 300:1459-1468, 1979.
293. Talbot JH, Terplan KL: The kidney in gout, Medicine 39:405-463, 1960.
294. Linnane JW, Burry AF, Emmerson BT: Urate deposits in the renal medulla. Prevalence and association, Nephron 29:216-222, 1981.
295. Batuman V: Lead nephropathy, gout and hypertension, Am J Med Sci 305:241-247, 1993.
296. Bennett WM: Lead nephropathy, Kidney Int 28:212-220, 1985.
297. Beck LH: Requiem for gouty nephropathy, Kidney Int 30:280-287, 1986.
298. McCurley T, Salter J, Glick A: Renal insufficiency in sarcoidosis, Arch Pathol Lab Med 114:488-492, 1990.
299. Silva FG, Pirani CL, Mesa-Tejada R et al: The kidney in plasma cell dyscrasias: a review and a clinicopathologic study of 50 patients, Prog Surg Pathol 5:131-176, 1983.
300. Sanders PN, Herrera GA, Kirk KA et al: Spectrum of glomerular and tubulointerstitial renal lesions associated with monotypical immunoglobulin light chain deposition, Lab Invest 64:527-537, 1991.

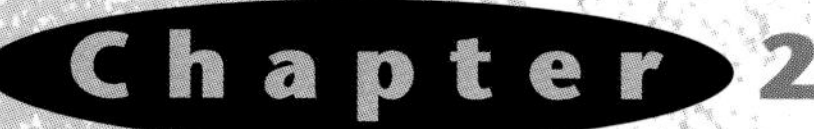

NEOPLASMS OF THE KIDNEY

JOHN N. EBLE

A remarkable variety of benign and malignant neoplasms arise in the kidneys of adults and children. The diagnostic challenges that these pose to surgical pathologists are made greater by the wide spectrum of appearances of renal cell carcinoma and nephroblastoma, the most common renal tumors of adults and children. Adding to the potential for confusion is a number of tumorlike lesions of inflammatory and developmental origin, as well as a handful of lesions the nature of which, whether neoplastic or not, is uncertain. To a large extent the tumors most common in children are exceptional in adults and vice versa. In accord with this the first part of the chapter is devoted to renal cell carcinoma and other neoplasms typically found in adults and the second part to those found mainly in children. However, the chapter is not strictly divided by age, and discussion of the exceptions will be found in the relevant section covering the more common situation.

RENAL TUMORS IN ADULTS

RENAL ADENOMA

For decades controversy has raged concerning the relationship between small and large renal cortical epithelial neoplasms and the existence of "renal adenoma" and its relationship to renal cell carcinoma.[1] The prevalence of small cortical lesions at autopsy suggests that many proliferations of renal cortical epithelium lack the capacity to develop into clinical cancer. However, the search for means to distinguish between those lesions that have the potential to progress and those that do not has been unsuccessful.[2] Small examples of each of the cellular and architectural types of renal cell carcinoma recognized in current classifications are found in surgical and autopsy specimens.[3] Conversely there is no histologic pattern found among the small cortical tumors, which has no counterpart in clinical cancer. The recent dramatic increase in the incidental discovery of small renal tumors by ultrasonography and computed tomography conducted for other disorders[4,5] makes the definition of renal adenoma on the basis of size even less tenable than before, particularly since they are frequently of low stage.[6] It is inappropriate and dangerous to diagnose a small renal cell carcinoma that has been detected early and, in all probability, cured by surgery as an adenoma simply because the tumor is smaller than some arbitrarily chosen size. The study by Bell,[1] which is frequently cited as indicating that renal cortical neoplasms smaller than 3 cm in diameter rarely have metastasized, was an autopsy study. Neither that study nor surgical studies in which the tumors have been resected, is capable of showing, for example, that a tumor 1 cm in diameter can be safely left in place. Presently there is no evidence to suggest that if such small tumors, particularly if they are of the clear cell type, are left in place, they will not grow and progress (Fig. 2-1).

The tumor most frequently considered to be adenoma is small and located in the superficial cortex; it may be multiple and the term *adenomatosis* is sometimes applied to such cases (Fig. 2-2). It is composed of small cells with little cytoplasm and a papillary or tubular architecture.[7,8] Unfortunately, histologically similar tumors that present clinically have a rate of metastasis of approximately 20%.[9-11] It remains controversial whether clinically apparent chromophil carcinoma has a better or worse prognosis than clear cell carcinoma, but it is clear that metastasis and death result from them in a significant percentage of cases and that reports of "giant adenomas"[12] may reflect successful surgical treatment rather than inherent benignity.

RENAL CELL CARCINOMA

Clinically, the most common renal neoplasm is renal cell carcinoma. For nearly a century some thought that it was derived from adrenal rests, and the name *hypernephroma* still persists. Another frequently seen synonym is *renal adenocarcinoma*. Until recently renal cell carcinoma was regarded as a single entity with a wide variety of gross and histologic appearances and a highly variable clinical course. Today renal cell carcinoma is recognized

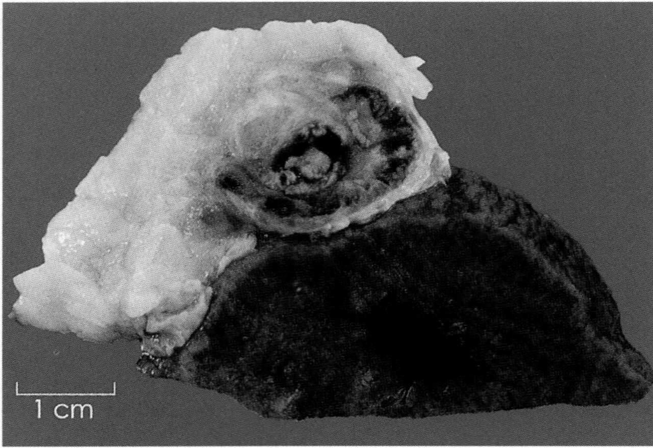

2-1. Small clear cell renal cell carcinoma with invasion of perirenal fat.

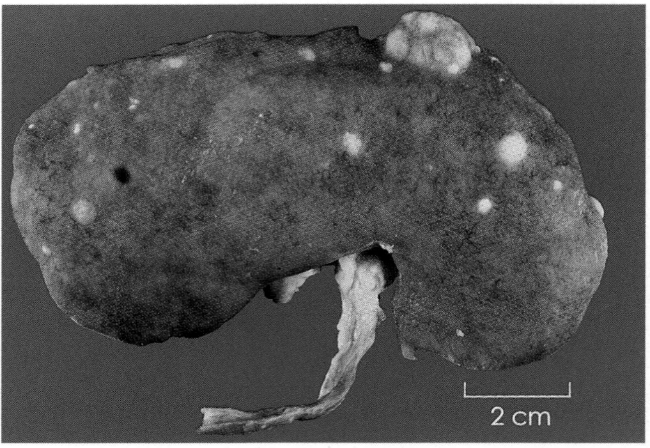

2-2. Renal adenomatosis: multiple small chromophil renal cell neoplasms.

as a family of cancers derived from the epithelium of the renal tubules but having distinct morphological features and resulting from different genetic abnormalities.

EPIDEMIOLOGY

Renal cell carcinoma is almost exclusively a cancer of adults, occurring at rates of 5.6 and 4.1 per 100,000 among males and females, respectively.[13] Approximately 23,000 new cases are diagnosed each year in the United States. Renal cell carcinoma is rare in the first 2 decades of life, comprising only 2% of pediatric renal tumors.[14] Few cases occur in patients younger than 40 years old but its incidence increases thereafter, reaching a peak in the sixth and seventh decades.[13] The ratio of males to females among patients with renal cell carcinoma is about 2:1.[13] A few dozen reports have been made of familial clustering of renal cell carcinoma outside recognized hereditary syndromes such as von Hippel-Lindau disease (see Associations and Syndromes), but it is not clear whether these represent hereditary renal cell carcinoma, shared exposure to carcinogens, or coincidence.[15]

ETIOLOGY AND PATHOGENESIS

Smoking is a major risk factor[16] accounting for as much as 30% of renal cell carcinoma.[17] Obesity,[18] especially in women,[19] also is important and up to 25% of cases are attributed to this risk factor.[20] Long-term phenacetin and acetaminophen use[21] and exposure to cadmium,[22] petroleum products,[23] and industrial chemicals[24] also are risk factors. The excess risk from exposure to gasoline is highest after a latent period of about 30 years.[25] Kidney stones also are a risk factor.[18] However, in most cases the carcinogenic influence is unknown.

SIGNS AND SYMPTOMS

Hematuria, pain, and flank mass are the classic triad of presenting symptoms, but nearly 40% of patients lack all of these and present with systemic symptoms (Table 2-1).[26] Other common presenting symptoms are weight loss, abdominal pain, and anorexia, and these may suggest a gastrointestinal cancer.[26] Fever without infection occurs in approximately 18% of patients[27] and is the presenting symptom in about 5% of cases.[28] Elevation of the erythrocyte sedimentation rate occurs in approximately 50% of cases.[29] Hypochromic anemia occurs in about one third of cases, appears to be unrelated to hematuria,[27,30] and is attributed to suppression of normal bone marrow activity. Elevation of serum alkaline phosphatase and transaminase, hepatosplenomegaly, coagulopathy, and elevation of alpha$_2$-globulin concentration may occur in the absence of liver metastases and may resolve when the renal tumor is resected.[28,31] Hepatic sinusoidal dilation may be the anatomical correlate of these functional abnormalities.[32] Systemic amyloidosis occurs in about 3% of patients with renal cell carcinoma and is of the AA type[33]; intercurrent chronic inflammatory disease may contribute to this.[34] A few cases of necrotizing myelopathy have been reported in association with renal cell carcinoma.[35,36]

Renal cell carcinoma may induce paraneoplastic endocrine syndromes,[28,37] including humoral hypercalcemia of malignancy (pseudohyperparathyroidism), erythrocytosis, hypertension, and gynecomastia (Table 2-1). Hypercalcemia without bone metastases (in some cases clinically significant) occurs in approximately 10% of patients with renal cell carcinoma and is more common with higher stage, approaching 20% in patients with disseminated carcinoma.[38] Erythropoietin concentration is elevated in almost two thirds of patients,[39] but erythrocytosis occurs in less than 4% of cases.[27] Molecular biologic techniques have shown that some renal cell carcinoma cells produce erythropoietin constitutively.[40] Hypertension is found in approximately one third of patients,[27,41] often associated with elevated renin concentrations in the renal vein from the kidney containing the tumor.[41] Immunohistochemical studies have shown renin in renal cell carcinoma cells from such patients.[41,42] Typically the blood pressure returns to normal after the tumor is resected. Production of biologically inactive renin may be more common; it was demonstrated immunohistochemically in 7 of 19 renal cell carcinomas from normotensive patients.[43] Gynecomastia may result from gonadotropin[44] or prolactin[45] production.

Renal cell carcinoma also is notorious for presenting as metastatic carcinoma of unknown primary, sometimes in unusual sites.[46-49] Together with malignant melanoma, renal cell carcinoma is considered one of the great mimics in medicine.

TABLE 2-1.
CLINICAL FINDINGS OF RENAL CELL CARCINOMA

Finding	Frequency (%)
Classical Triad	
Flank Pain	40
Hematuria	40
Mass	35
Endocrine	
Hypertension	33
Hypercalcemia	10
Erythrocytosis	4
Gynecomastia	Rare
Miscellaneous	
Sedimentation Rate Elevation	50
Anemia	33
Fever	18
Amyloidosis	3
Hepatic Dysfunction	Uncommon

ASSOCIATIONS AND SYNDROMES

Between one third and one half of patients with von Hippel-Lindau disease (an autosomal dominant constellation of lesions most frequently including central nervous system and retinal hemangioblastoma, pheochromocytoma, cystadenoma of the epididymis, cysts of the pancreas and kidney, and renal cell carcinoma) develop renal cell carcinoma.[50,51] In such patients, renal cell carcinoma is frequently bilateral, multiple, and occurs at an earlier age (mean age 41 years[52]) than sporadic renal cell carcinoma. Metastasis occurs in approximately 50% of cases and causes death in about one third.[52]

Tuberous sclerosis (an autosomal dominant[53] syndrome in which hamartomatous lesions occur in the brain, retina, skin, heart, bone, lung, and kidney[54]) is most prominently associated with renal cysts and multiple angiomyolipomas[55] (see later in this chapter); these patients also have increased risk for renal cell carcinoma.[56,57] Among 16 cases reviewed by Washecka and Hanna,[57] 43% had bilateral renal cell carcinoma and the median age was 28 years. Most such patients have no recurrence, but a few cases with metastases have been documented.[58,59]

The association of autosomal dominant polycystic kidney disease with renal cell carcinoma has been suspected for many years,[60] but it remains more controversial than the associations with von Hippel-Lindau disease and tuberous sclerosis. Evidence has recently emerged linking the two through a process of epithelial hyperplasia.[61,62]

Acquired renal cystic disease arising in patients with chronic renal failure also is strongly associated with renal cell carcinoma.[63-65] This was discussed in more detail in Chapter 1.

CLASSIFICATION

Until recently renal cell carcinoma was most often categorized on the basis of the character of the cytoplasm as clear cell and granular cell types. Tumors composed of mixtures of the two were regarded as common, as were tumors that fit imperfectly into either category. A number of studies explored the prognostic significance of these categories, but the results were inconclusive.[66] In 1979 Klein and Valensi[67] drew attention to a morphologically homogeneous subgroup of renal cell carcinoma with abundant finely granular eosinophilic cytoplasm, which had a remarkably good prognosis. Today these tumors are recognized as the benign renal oncocytoma (see later in this chapter). In 1985 Thoenes et al.[67a] reported the first cases of a morphologically distinct subtype of renal cell carcinoma, which they called the *chromophobe* type. While the chromophobe tumors originally described were extracted from the clear cell end of the spectrum, it was soon recognized that there is an eosinophilic variant of chromophobe renal cell carcinoma that emerged from the granular cell end of the spectrum. At about the same time it was recognized that some renal cell carcinomas arise from the distal nephron, and collecting duct carcinoma, which most often is composed of cells with granular cytoplasm, emerged from the granular end of the spectrum. In 1986 Thoenes, Störkel, and associates[67] at Johannes Gutenberg Universität proposed the Mainz classification of renal cell neoplasms (see box on this page), which recognized these new entities as well as chromophil renal cell carcinoma (which also is known as papillary renal cell carcinoma because it usually has a predominantly papillary architecture). Together these new entities comprise 25% to 30% of renal cell neoplasms in surgical series (Table 2-2).

The subtraction of so many of the new entities from the granular cell end of the spectrum, combined with the recognition that clear cell renal cell carcinoma may have areas in which the cells have eosinophilic cytoplasm, has made "granular cell renal cell carcinoma" obsolete as a diagnostic entity. The Mainz classification was based on morphological criteria, but subsequent genetic studies have confirmed its validity by showing characteristic genetic abnormalities in the groups.[68] The following sections discuss each of the currently recognized types of renal cell neoplasia.

CLEAR CELL RENAL CELL CARCINOMA

The most common type of renal cell carcinoma is clear cell renal cell carcinoma, so called because the cytoplasm usually contains abundant lipid and glycogen that dissolve in tissue processing, making the cytoplasm clear in routine sections. These tumors comprise approximately three quarters of the cases in clinical series. Their site of origin was controversial until 1960 when Oberling et al.[69] demonstrated apical brush borders of microvilli, which indicated origin from the proximal tubule. Subsequent immunohistochemical and lectin histochemical studies have supported this derivation.

Genetics

Over the past decade most cytogenetic studies of clear cell renal cell carcinoma have found that loss of genetic

CLASSIFICATION OF RENAL CELL TUMORS

Renal carcinoma
- Clear Cell
- Chromophil
  - Eosinophil
  - Basophil
- Chromophobe
  - Typical
  - Eosinophil

Carcinoma of Bellini's collecting ducts

Renal oncocytoma

TABLE 2-2. RELATIVE FREQUENCIES OF RENAL CELL NEOPLASMS IN SURGICAL SERIES

Neoplasm	Frequency (%)
Clear Cell Renal Cell Carcinoma	70
Chromophil Renal Cell Carcinoma	15
Chromophobe Renal Cell Carcinoma	5
Collecting Duct Carcinoma	2
Renal Oncocytoma	5
Other and Unclassified	3

material in the short arm of chromosome 3 (3p) is the most frequent and consistent abnormality.[70-75] Such losses have been found in tumors as small as 11 mm.[76] The abnormalities range from loss of the entire chromosome, to deletions of terminal or interstitial segments, to translocations, all resulting in a net loss of sequences in the region on 3p which extends from p11.2 to pter. A cluster of breakpoints in the region of 3p13 to 3p14 has been identified, and a common fragile site in 3p14 has been implicated.[77] A study of a family without von Hippel-Lindau disease with 10 cases of renal cell carcinoma found that 10 of 22 family members had a balanced reciprocal translocation between chromosomes 3 and 8.[78] This abnormality was present in all eight members who had renal cell carcinoma and whose karyotypes were known, while no family member without the translocation had a renal cancer. Renal cell carcinoma arising in patients with von Hippel-Lindau disease also commonly has deletion or partial deletion of chromosome 3p[79-81] with a breakpoint in the proximal short arm near the location of the von Hippel-Lindau gene.[82] These data suggest that a tumor suppressor gene located on 3p is involved in the genesis of clear cell renal cell carcinoma. This concept is supported epidemiologically by the "two-hit" kinetics of sporadic renal cell carcinoma and the "one-hit" kinetics of hereditary renal cell carcinoma.[83]

The success of the cytogenetic investigations has been followed by detailed studies at the molecular genetic level. In several laboratories,[71,84-86] DNA hybridization studies with gene probes for sequences in 3p have given similar results, showing loss of heterozygosity in the distal portion of 3p in clear cell renal cell carcinoma, suggesting the presence of a tumor suppressor gene in this region.[87] Gene probes have also been useful in localizing the breakpoint on 3p.[88] The finding that increasing immunoreactivity for the c-*myc* gene product correlates with increasing nuclear grade, suggests that activation of c-*myc* plays a role in progression.[89]

Gross pathology

The vivid chrome yellow or light orange color typical of clear cell renal cell carcinoma is the most distinctive aspect of its appearance (Fig. 2-3). It frequently has a variegated appearance, often mottled by scattered foci of hemorrhage and cream-colored areas of necrosis (Fig. 2-4). Sarcomatoid areas are often light-colored, almost white, solid, and firm. The tumors range in size from a centimeter in diameter, found by radiologists, to those weighing thousands of grams. Increasing numbers of tumors smaller than 3 cm are discovered incidentally by radiography during examinations for unrelated diseases.[90] Typically, clear cell renal cell carcinoma is solid, often lobulated, and bulges above the cut surface. Many are globular and well circumscribed with peripheral pseudocapsules, but some diffusely infiltrate and replace the kidney (Fig. 2-5). The centers of large tumors occasionally contain irregularly shaped areas of edematous gray connective tissue (see Fig. 2-3).

Cysts are common, ranging from a few millimeters to 1 or 2 cm in diameter (Fig. 2-6). Rarely, the tumors are nearly completely cystic with little or no solid component on gross inspection (Fig. 2-7).[91-93] The lining of the cysts usually is smooth, but may be finely granular. Occasionally, clear cell renal cell carcinoma arises in the wall of a preexisting simple cyst or develops a cystic character through necrosis and degeneration (see box on this page).

CYSTIC RENAL CELL CARCINOMA

15% of all renal cell carcinoma

- 6% Multilocular (mainly clear cell renal cell carcinoma)
- 5% Unilocular cystadenocarcinoma (mainly chromophil renal cell carcinoma)
- 3% Cystic necrosis
- 1% Arising in a preexisting simple cyst

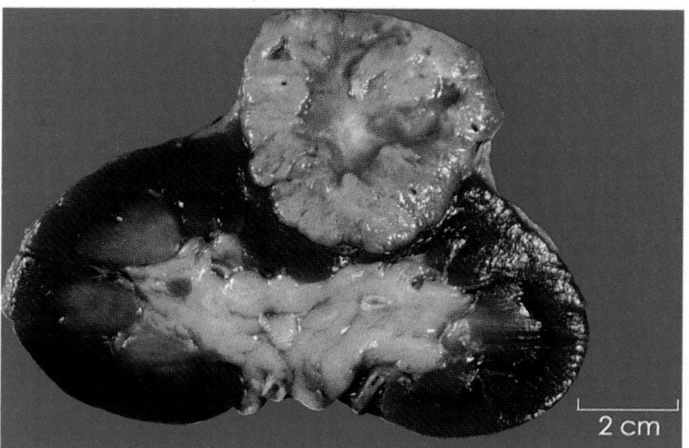

2-3. Clear cell renal cell carcinoma consisting of yellow parenchyma with a central area of edematous fibrous tissue.

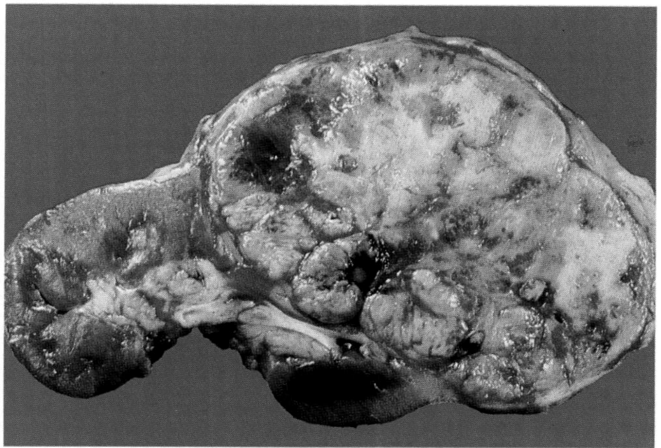

2-4. Clear cell renal cell carcinoma: a large tumor with a variegated cut surface.

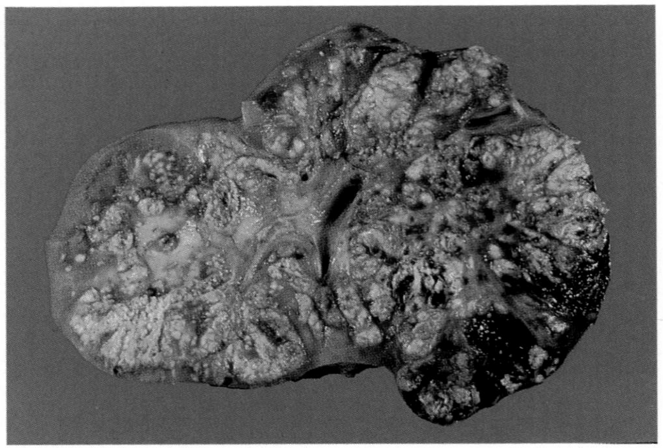

2-5. Clear cell renal cell carcinoma diffusely infiltrating the kidney.

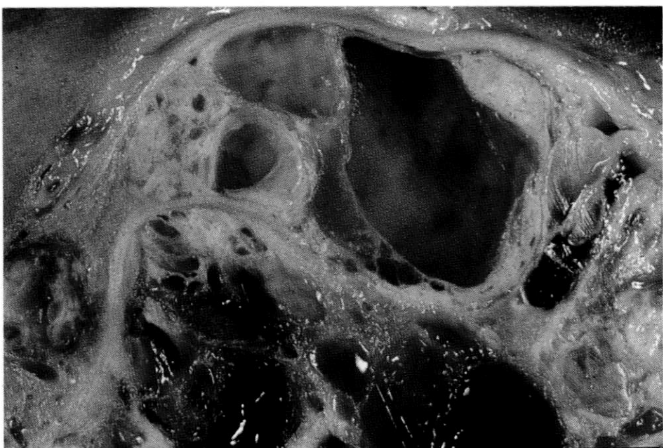

2-6. Clear cell renal cell carcinoma with small cysts.

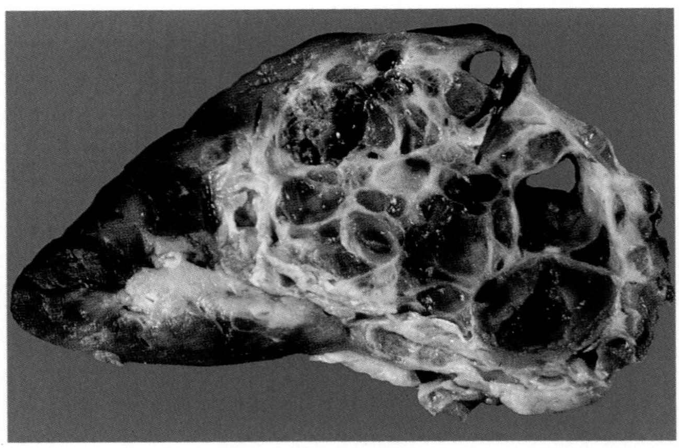

2-7. Multilocular cystic renal cell carcinoma.

Multicentricity occurs within the same kidney in up to 13% of cases[94] and carcinoma is present bilaterally in approximately 1% of patients.[2]

Microscopic pathology

The cytoplasm of clear cell renal cell carcinoma is usually abundant and strikingly clear, lacking the foamy appearance characteristic of the zona reticularis of the adrenal cortex. While this feature has given this carcinoma its name, it is not definitive and other features are important in making the diagnosis (see box on this page). Commonly, clear cell renal cell carcinoma contains scattered cells with eosinophilic cytoplasm or even areas in which the majority of cells have eosinophilic granular cytoplasm. Often this is associated with necrosis or degenerative changes nearby. Such areas are perfectly compatible with the diagnosis of clear cell renal cell carcinoma and should pose no diagnostic problem if the other features in the box are recognized. Hyaline globules[95] and extensive intracytoplasmic deposits of hemosiderin[96] are present occasionally.

The nuclei of clear cell renal cell carcinoma are usually nearly spherical and central, ranging from small and hyperchromatic without visible nucleoli to large and pleomorphic with prominent macronucleoli. The mitotic rate is highly variable and mitotic figures may be rare or absent even in lethal tumors. Multinucleated giant cells are uncommon.

CLEAR CELL RENAL CELL CARCINOMA: CHARACTERISTIC FEATURES

Delicate, interconnecting vasculature
Compact and tubulocystic architecture
Low nuclear/cytoplasmic ratio
Clear cytoplasm (most of the time)

The major architectural patterns of clear cell renal cell carcinoma are compact (alveolar) (Fig. 2-8), tubular, and cystic. These occur alone or commonly in combination. A prominent array of thin-walled blood vessels that may or may not contain red blood cells (Fig. 2-9) is a striking and diagnostically valuable feature of most clear cell renal cell carcinomas. The pattern of blood vessels is particularly apparent in tumors with an alveolar pattern of growth. Tubular structures range from small to large and dilated, merging with the cystic pattern. The tubules are usually round to oval but occasionally may be elongate. Small tubules often are empty, but large ones frequently contain eosinophilic fluid or blood. A few papillae are sometimes seen in clear cell renal cell carcinoma, but a predominance of papillae covered by cells with abundant clear cytoplasm is rare and it is uncertain whether such tumors are best classified as clear cell renal cell carcinoma or chromophil renal cell carcinoma (see later in this chapter).

A few clear cell renal cell carcinomas are grossly multilocular and consist mainly of fibrous septa containing only a small population of carcinoma cells lining the cysts and in aggregates within the septa.[92] These are termed *multilocular cystic renal cell carcinoma*. Typically the cells with clear cytoplasm have small darkly staining nuclei. Small papillae sometimes extend into the cysts of the multilocular cystic renal cell carcinoma. Although this tumor is considered a variant of clear cell renal cell

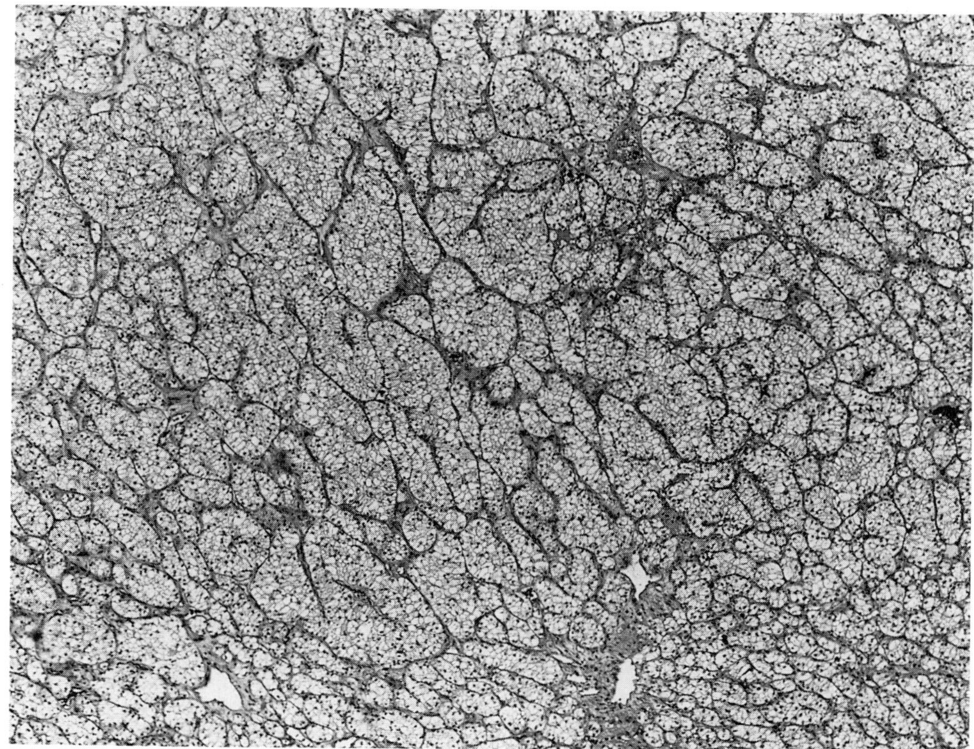

2-8. Clear cell renal cell carcinoma composed of compact alveolar structures bounded by delicate vascular septa.

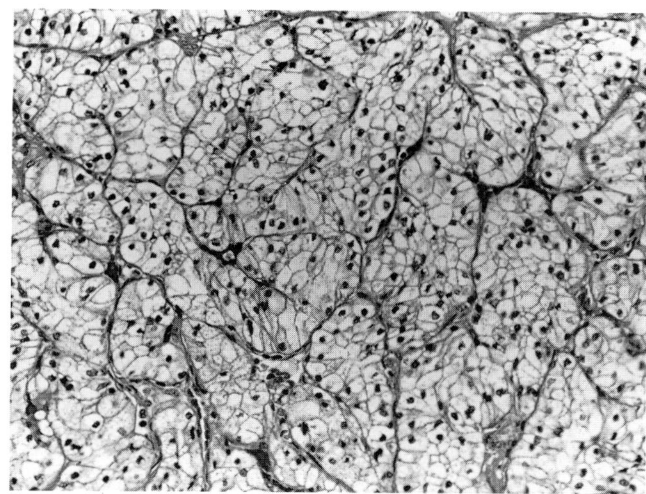

2-9. Clear cell renal cell carcinoma.

carcinoma,[92,97,98] it has a very low potential for recurrence or metastasis.[99]

Tumors of any architectural pattern may exhibit varying degrees of necrosis and hemorrhage. Other degenerative changes, including edema, fibrosis, hemosiderin, cholesterol clefts, and calcification are common.

Differential diagnosis

Urothelial carcinoma of the renal pelvis may be confused with clear cell renal cell carcinoma, especially when the tumor is large and extensively infiltrates the kidney. Urothelial carcinoma sometimes consists mainly of large cells with clear or pale cytoplasm, further confusing the diagnosis. Attention to the vascular pattern is often helpful in such cases. The diagnosis also may be difficult when the urothelial carcinoma is predominantly sarcomatoid.[100] Extensive sampling may be necessary to find small areas of typical urothelial carcinoma, even in situ, or of renal cell carcinoma. Immunohistochemical demonstration of high molecular weight cytokeratin or carcinoembryonic antigen indicate that such a tumor is probably of urothelial origin.[101]

Multilocular cystic renal cell carcinoma containing only small populations of clear cells may be difficult to distinguish from cystic nephroma. The presence of even a small amount of epithelium with clear cells is presently taken to indicate that these are renal cell carcinoma.[92] Cystic renal masses should be rigorously examined with extensive sampling before a benign cystic lesion is diagnosed.

In children and adolescents, renal cell carcinoma must be distinguished from Wilms' tumor with epithelial predominance. Beckwith[102] emphasized the similarity of some Wilms' tumors to renal cell carcinoma. Thorough sampling of such tumors usually reveals blastema or differentiated stroma (e.g., skeletal muscle) and the diagnosis of Wilms' tumor can be made with relative ease. Nuclei tend to be elongate with tapered ends in the epithelium of Wilms' tumor and spherical in renal cell carcinoma.

Xanthogranulomatous pyelonephritis is an unusual inflammatory disorder that clinically and pathologically can be confused with renal cell carcinoma.[103,104] The presenting symptoms overlap with those of renal cell carcinoma; patients present with a variety of symptoms, including flank pain, fever, malaise, weight loss, and hematuria.[105,106] The preoperative diagnosis is further confused by the frequent finding of a flank mass. The gross appearance also is confusing because the inflammation may produce a tumorlike mass of yellow tissue that may infiltrate the perinephric fat. The renal outflow is almost always obstructed, usually by a calculus, but sometimes by narrowing of the ureteropelvic junction.[107] Xanthogranulomatous pyelonephritis may also be confusing microscopically since an infiltrate of foamy histiocytes, which may be misconstrued as the clear cells of renal cell carcinoma, is usually the predominant element.[108] Close attention to the cytoplasm reveals its foamy character, which is unlike that of clear cell renal cell carcinoma. The vascular pattern typical of clear cell renal cell carcinomas is lacking. Furthermore, the presence of other inflammatory cells, principally lymphocytes and plasma cells, should assist in its recognition.

Malakoplakia is another inflammatory process which may resemble a primary renal tumor.[109] Grossly, it consists of large yellowish masses that may infiltrate perinephric fat. Microscopically, the large eosinophilic histiocytes (von Hansemann cells) characteristic of malakoplakia may be confused with the eosinophilic cells of renal cell carcinoma. The presence of Michaelis-Gutmann bodies is important in establishing the correct diagnosis, as are the lack of cytologic atypia and architectural patterns characteristic of renal cell carcinoma but inconsistent with malakoplakia.

Sarcomatoid renal cell carcinoma may closely resemble sarcoma. This problem is well known, however, and, because of the rarity of renal sarcoma, it should be diagnosed with caution. Extensive sampling may be helpful since sarcomatoid renal cell carcinoma frequently has foci, albeit sometimes small, of typical renal cell carcinoma that make the correct diagnosis apparent. Ultrastructural and immunohistochemical studies[110-112] may demonstrate epithelial features in cells that appear sarcomatous in sections stained with hematoxylin and eosin.

CHROMOPHIL RENAL CELL CARCINOMA

The second most common carcinoma arising from the renal tubular epithelium is chromophil renal cell carcinoma, also called papillary renal cell carcinoma. While most of these carcinomas consist entirely or partially of a papillary proliferation, many also have areas of tubular architecture and areas in which the papillae are packed so tightly as to appear solid at first inspection.[113] The tubular architecture may be prominent and has led some to call this *tubulopapillary carcinoma*.[9] For this reason the name *chromophil*, which was proposed in the Mainz classification[67] and indicates that the definition is not based solely on the papillary architecture, is preferred.

Chromophil renal cell carcinoma makes up approximately 10% to 15% of renal cell carcinoma in surgical series[11,114-119] (Table 2-3). There is a predominance of males of approximately 2:1. The age range is wide, from early adulthood to old age, and the mean is between 50 and 55 years. It is uncertain whether the prognosis for chromophil renal cell carcinoma is better or worse than for clear cell renal cell carcinoma.[66] However, it is clear that these carcinomas have a mortality of at least 16% at 10 years[119] and may present with regional or distant spread.[113]

Genetics

Chromophil renal cell carcinoma has a characteristic pattern of cytogenetic abnormalities that is different from that of clear cell renal cell carcinoma. Chromophil renal cell carcinoma has a gain of chromosomes, most typically trisomy or tetrasomy of 17 and 7.[120,121] Trisomy 7 can be detected by fluorescent in situ hybridization.[113] The Y chromosome is lost in most of these tumors that arise in men.[121] Loss of DNA on 3p (the hallmark of clear cell renal cell carcinoma) is not found in chromophil renal cell carcinoma.[122] These results have been consistently observed in several laboratories.[123-127] Gain of 5q, which often occurs in clear cell renal cell carcinoma, is not found in chromophil renal cell carcinoma.[121] There is some evidence that trisomy or tetrasomy only of chromosomes 7 and 17 correlates with low grade and that acquisition of additional trisomies correlates with progression.[121]

**TABLE 2-3.
CHROMOPHIL RENAL CELL CARCINOMA IN SURGICAL SERIES**

Institution	No. in Series	No. Chromophil (%)	M:F	Age (Mean)
Barnes Hospital[11]	221	31 (14)	23:11	27–78 (52)
Montefiore Hospital[113]	NA	10 (NA)	5:5	44–76 (61)
Mainz, Germany[114]	797	92 (11)	NA	NA
Santander, Spain[115]	199	12 (6)	10:2	11–78 (55)
M.D. Anderson[116]	238	22 (9.2)	13:9	23–79 (52)
Brigham & Womens[117]	NA	36 (NA)	25:11	38–75 (NA)

NA = Not Available

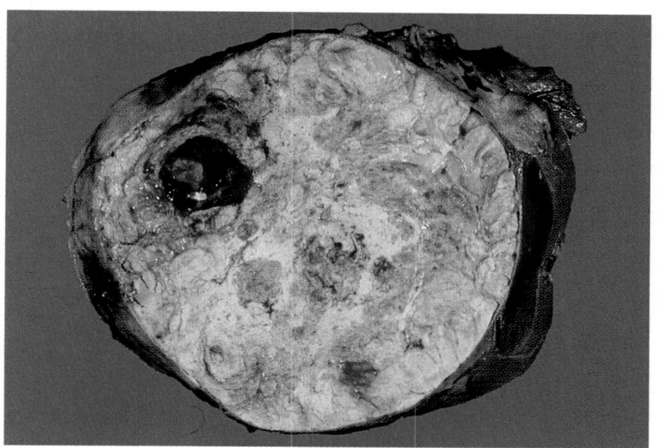

2-10. Chromophil renal cell carcinoma.

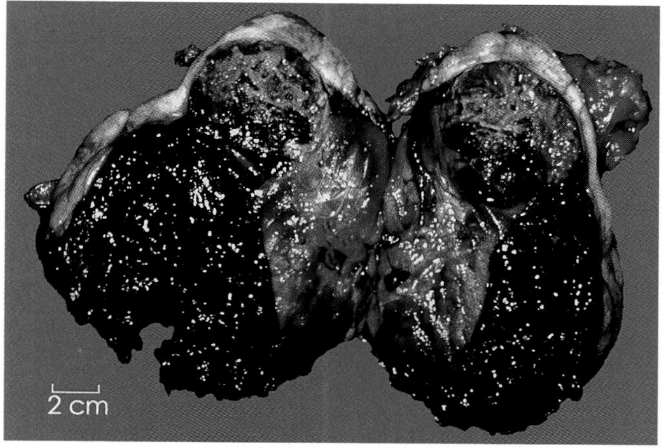

2-11. Chromophil renal cell carcinoma; hemorrhage and necrosis within pseudocapsule give the appearance of cystadenocarcinoma.

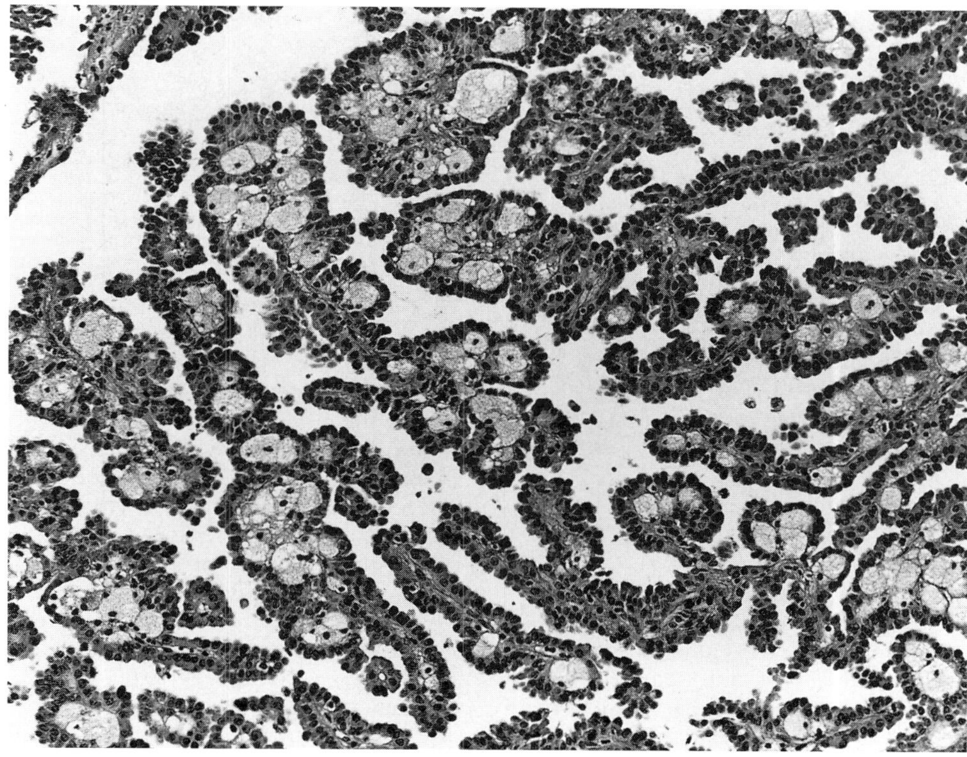

2-12. Chromophil renal cell carcinoma consisting of branching papillae covered by a single layer of cells with inconspicuous cytoplasm. Note foamy macrophages in papillary cores.

Gross pathology

Chromophil renal cell carcinoma is typically well circumscribed, globular, and tan or brown (Fig. 2-10). Hemorrhage and necrosis are present in approximately two thirds of cases and may be extensive, causing the tumor to appear hypovascular by angiography.[11,114] Sizes range widely and many are large. The cut surface frequently has a friable granular character, reflecting the papillary architecture seen microscopically. A rim of dense fibrous tissue commonly encapsulates the larger tumors, giving an appearance of cystadenocarcinoma (Fig. 2-11).[128,129] Calcifications are present in approximately one third of cases.[11,114]

While it has not been validated for chromophil renal cell carcinoma, the AJCC staging system (see Table 2-6) is recommended at present.

Microscopic pathology

The diagnosis of chromophil renal cell carcinoma is based on architectural and cytoplasmic features (see box

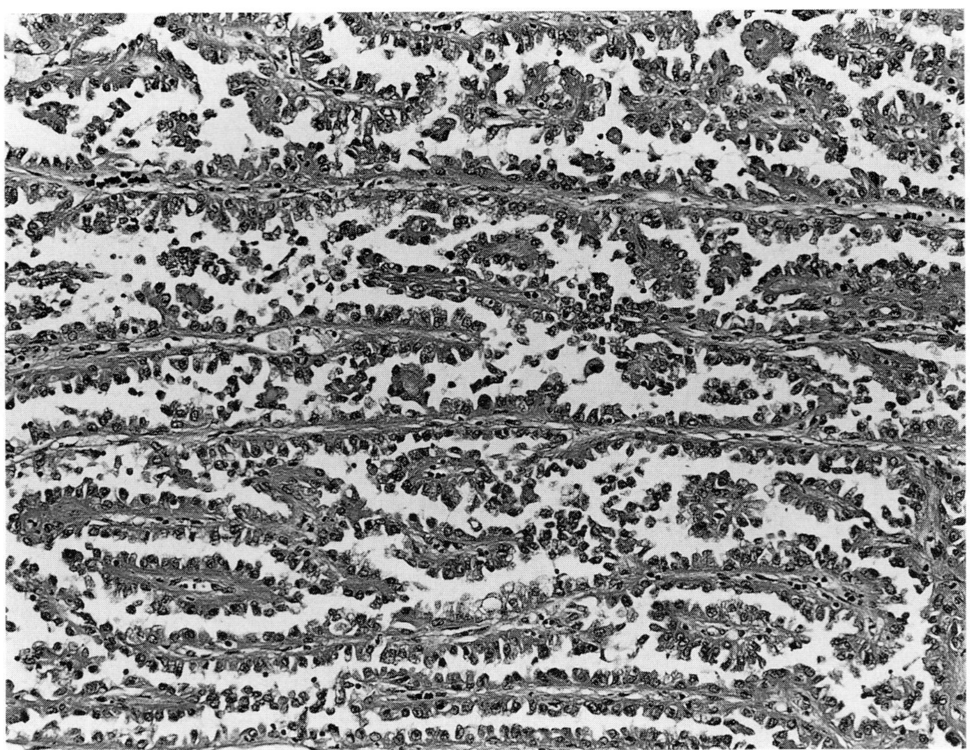

2-13. Chromophil renal cell carcinoma consisting of parallel papillae covered by a single layer of cells with inconspicuous cytoplasm.

CHROMOPHIL RENAL CELL CARCINOMA: CHARACTERISTIC FEATURES

- Papillary architecture
- Low cytoplasmic volume and high nuclear/cytoplasmic ratio
- Variable cytoplasmic staining

on this page). More than 90% of chromophil renal cell carcinomas have predominantly papillary or tubulopapillary architecture.[115] The remainder have a compact growth pattern that often appears to be the result of tight packing of papillary structures. The papillae usually consist of delicate fibrovascular cores covered by a single layer of carcinoma cells (Fig. 2-12). The pattern of the papillae is variable, ranging from complicated branching to parallel arrays of long papillae (Fig. 2-13), which has been termed the *trabecular pattern*.[118] Occasionally the papillary cores are expanded by numerous foamy macrophages. Psammoma bodies are less common and are found within the cores or between the papillae.[9] In some cases the papillary cores are wide and sclerotic.[118] The tubular architecture consists of small tubules lined by a single layer of cells identical to those covering the papillae.

The cells of chromophil renal cell carcinoma range from small cells with inconspicuous cytoplasm (Fig. 2-12, 2-13) to ones with abundant eosinophilic cytoplasm (Fig. 2-14). Although intermediate forms occur, the cells of most tumors are at one end or the other of this morphologic continuum. Tumors composed of small cells are more common. The small cells are called *basophil*[67] (or *dark cells*[130]) because their high nuclear/cytoplasmic ratio makes the tumors appear blue in routine sections. The high nuclear/cytoplasmic ratio results from the small volume of cytoplasm rather than from nuclear enlargement. The cytoplasm of these cells typically is pale and nearly clear.

The nuclei of chromophil renal cell carcinoma are typically uniform, spherical (or nearly so), and small, and they lack visible nucleoli. In some cases the nuclei are larger and more variable in size and have prominent nucleoli (Fig. 2-15). Lager et al. found that nuclear morphology correlated with stage at the time of diagnosis and with outcome in a series of 39 cases.[113] Thus, although it has not been validated in detail in large series for chromophil renal cell carcinoma, the nuclear grading system of Fuhrman et al.[131] (see Table 2-5) is recommended at this time. Sarcomatoid morphology occurs occasionally and probably has the same adverse significance that it does when it occurs in clear cell renal cell carcinoma.

CHROMOPHOBE RENAL CELL CARCINOMA

Chromophobe renal cell carcinoma has been recognized only recently. It was discovered by Bannasch[132] in experimentally induced tumors in rats in 1974, but Thoenes et al.[133] described the first cases in humans in 1985. Since then, more than 100 cases have been reported[134-138] (Table 2-4). Chromophobe renal cell

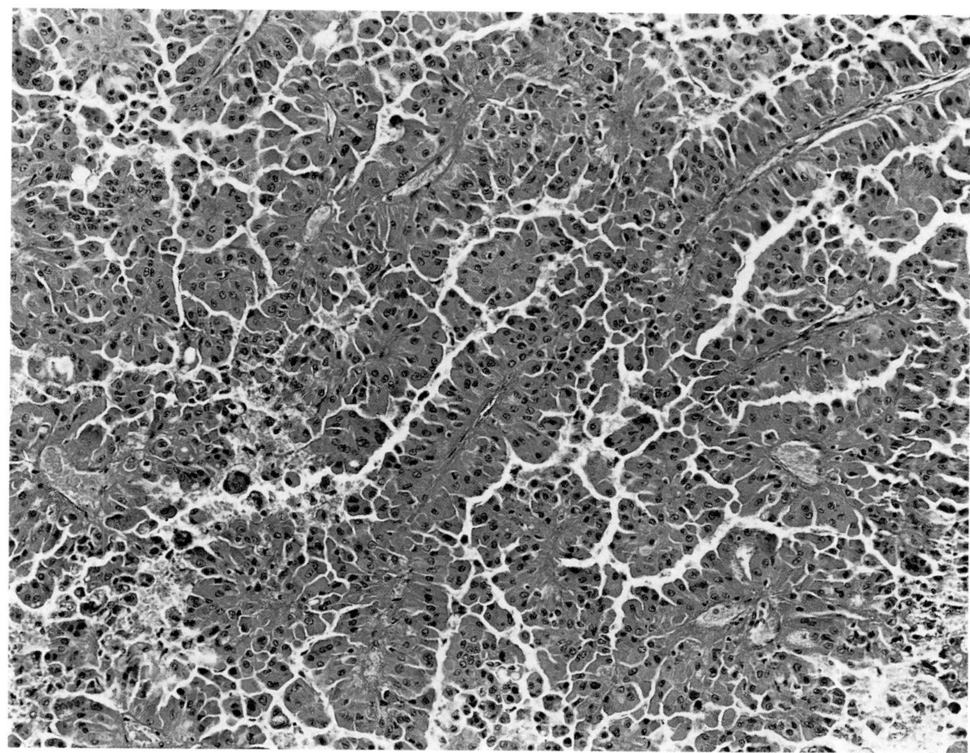

2-14. Chromophil renal cell carcinoma composed of branching papillae are covered by pseudostratified cells with abundant eosinophilic cytoplasm.

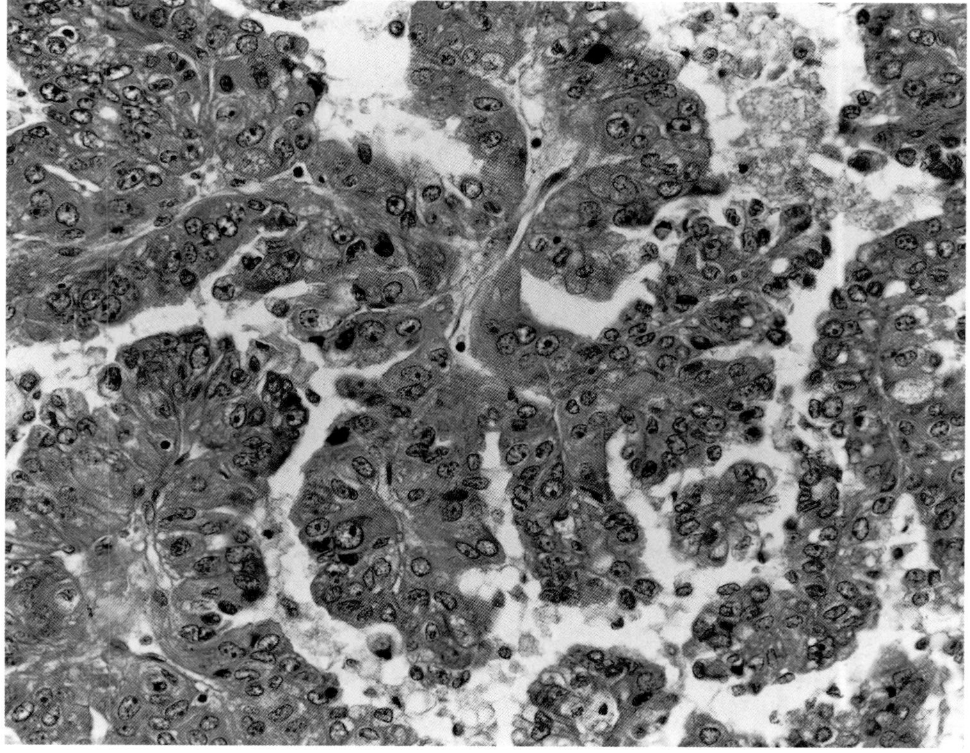

2-15. Chromophil renal cell carcinoma with prominent nucleoli and moderate nuclear pleomorphism.

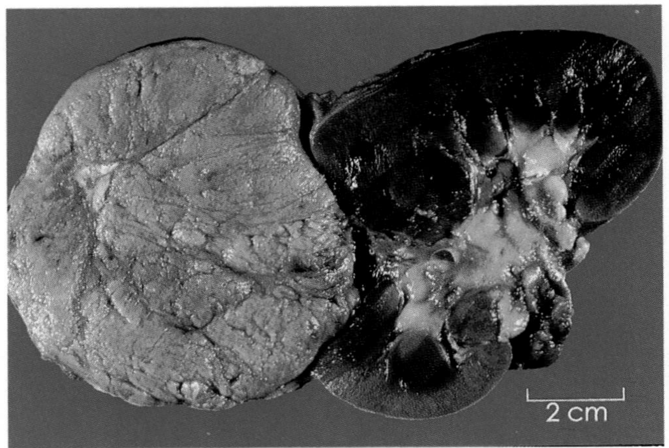

2-16. Chromophobe renal cell carcinoma forming a well-circumscribed mass with tan parenchyma.

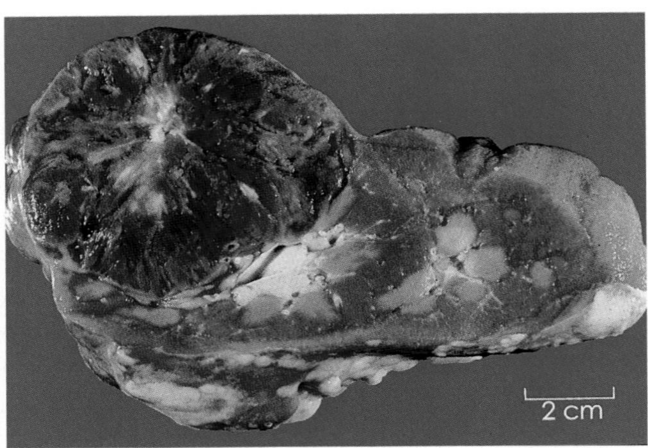

2-17. Chromophobe renal cell carcinoma with a brown cut surface, similar in appearance to renal oncocytoma.

TABLE 2-4.
CHROMOPHOBE RENAL CELL CARCINOMA

Institution	No. in Series	No. Chromophobe (%)	Typical/Eosinophil	Male:Female	Age (Mean)
Mainz[133]	697	32 (5)	22/10	17:15	31–75 (55)
Iowa[134]	NA	5 (NA)	3/2	4:1	26–64 (43)
Mayo Clinic[135]	1159	50 (4)	NA	26:24	27–86 (59)
Victoria Hospital[136]	363	23 (6)	6/5	NA	NA

NA = Not Available

carcinoma is not rare, and in surgical series comprises about 5% of neoplasms of the renal tubular epithelium.[119,136,137] Unlike clear cell renal cell carcinoma and chromophil renal cell carcinoma, chromophobe renal cell carcinoma affects men and women equally.[134,136] Patients range in age from 27 to 86 years, with a mean of approximately 55 years.

Chromophobe renal cell carcinoma may have a slightly better prognosis than clear cell renal cell carcinoma, but outcome data are limited.[134,136] Although it has not been validated for chromophobe renal cell carcinoma, the AJCC staging system (see Table 2-6) is recommended at this time.

Genetics

Chromophobe renal cell carcinoma is characterized genetically by chromosomal losses.[139,140] Losses of multiple entire chromosomes, most often chromosomes 1, 2, 10, 13, 6, 21, and 17, occur in 90% of cases. Loss of 3p, typical of clear cell renal cell carcinoma, and trisomy and tetrasomy of chromosomes 17 and 7 with loss of the Y chromosome, typical of chromophil renal cell carcinoma, are not observed.

Gross pathology

Chromophobe renal cell carcinoma is typically solitary, solid, beige or light brown, globular, and circumscribed (Fig. 2-16, 2-17). A minority of tumors have small foci of hemorrhage or necrosis. A few small cysts occasionally are present. The tumors vary in size from less than 2 cm to more than 20 cm. Renal vein invasion occurs in some cases.[136]

CHROMOPHOBE RENAL CELL CARCINOMA: CHARACTERISTIC FEATURES OF TYPICAL TYPE

- Compact architecture
- Prominent cytoplasmic membranes
- Pale flocculent cytoplasm
- Variable cell size (mainly large)
- Positive hale's colloidal iron stain
- EM: Cytoplasmic microvesicles

Microscopic pathology

Chromophobe renal cell carcinoma has two histologic variants: typical and eosinophilic. The typical type was the first to be recognized[133] and its characteristic features are listed in the box on this page. The growth pattern is usually solid, but tubular structures also may be present. It is composed of cells that are large and generally polygonal, although there is considerable variation in size and

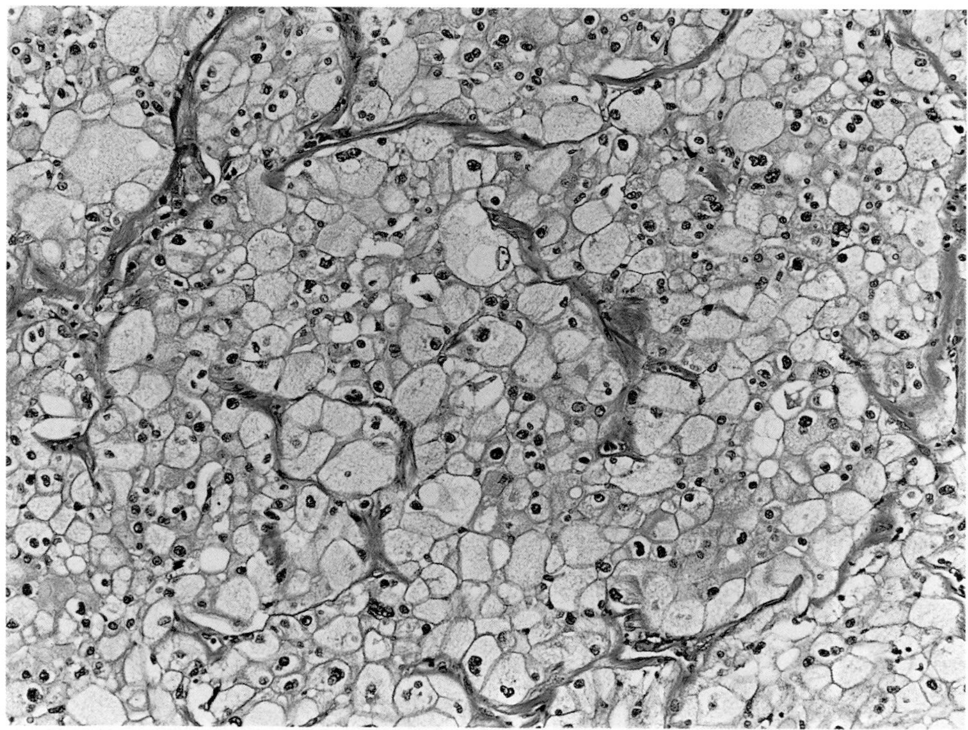

2-18. Chromophobe renal cell carcinoma, typical type consisting of large cells with pale cytoplasm. Note variability of cell size and prominence of cytoplasmic membranes.

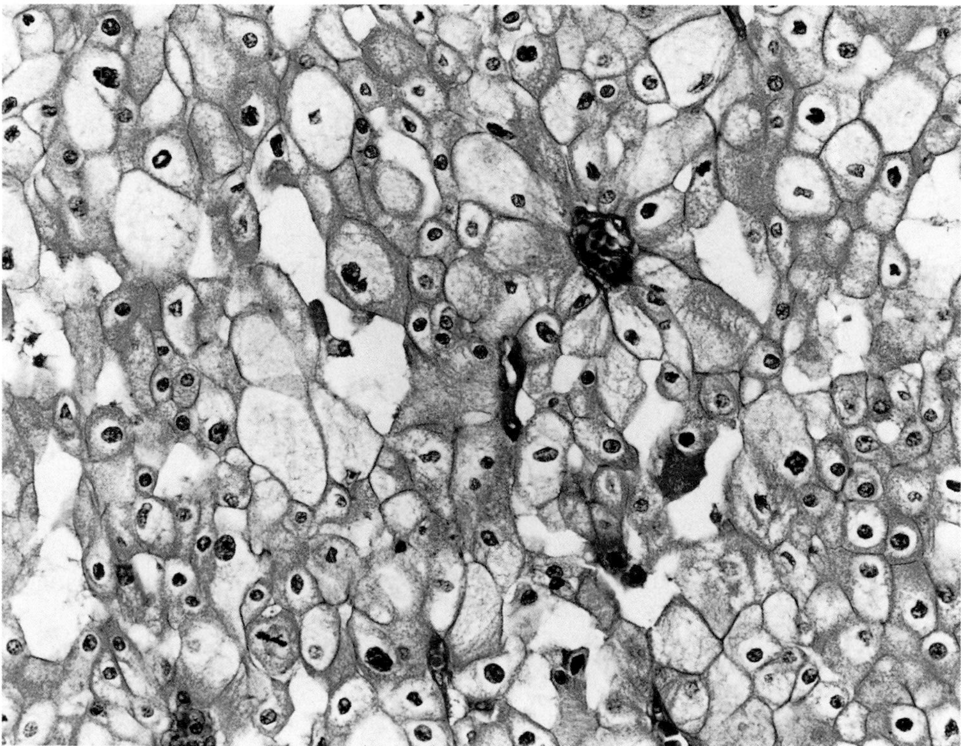

2-19. Chromophobe renal cell carcinoma, typical type. The cytoplasm is finely granular or flocculent and of variable density.

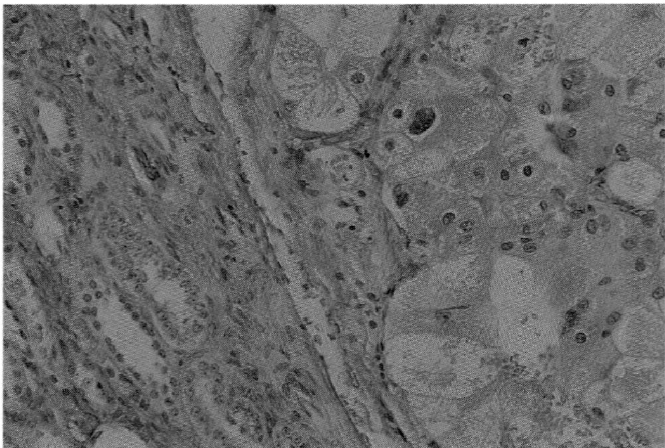

2-20. Chromophobe renal cell carcinoma, typical type. Hale's colloidal iron procedure staining cytoplasm blue.

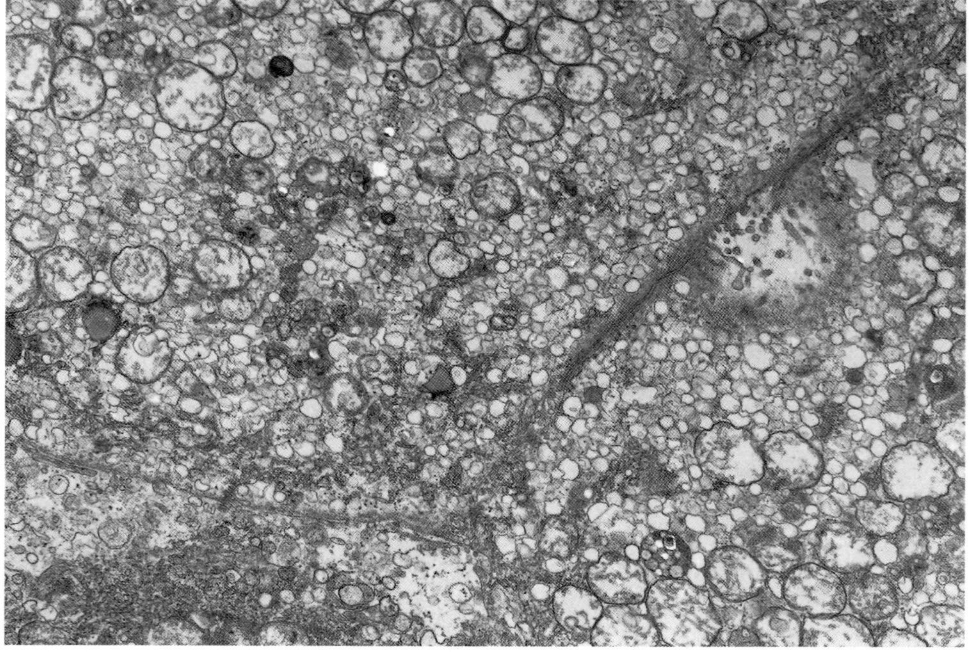

2-21. Chromophobe renal cell carcinoma. Electron micrograph showing the characteristic cytoplasmic vesicles.

shape (Fig. 2-18). These cells contain abundant pale reticular or flocculent cytoplasm in routine sections (Fig. 2-19). Cytoplasmic constituents are denser at the periphery, making the cytoplasmic membranes appear thick and distinct. Cells with eosinophilic cytoplasm may be present in small numbers. The nuclei are central or slightly eccentric and of moderate size, with small or medium-sized nucleoli. Mitotic figures are infrequent or rare.

Hale's colloidal iron stain[141] is diagnostically helpful and stains the cytoplasm of chromophobe cells a vivid blue (Fig. 2-20). It is useful to select a block that contains some renal cortex as an internal control. Glomeruli will stain, while the cytoplasm of the tubular epithelium should not. Clear cell renal cell carcinoma does not react with this stain. Hale's colloidal iron stain probably reacts with acid mucosubstances from the vesicles.[142]

Ultrastructurally the cytoplasm is filled with round-to-oval vesicles 150 to 300 nm in diameter (Fig. 2-21).[134,138] The vesicles often are invaginated, resembling vesicles seen in the intercalated cells of the collecting duct.[143,144] These vesicles are not found in other renal cell neoplasms. Bonsib et al.[145] have shown that the vesicles disintegrate in routine processing for paraffin embedding, so it is crucial that tissue for electron microscopy be primarily fixed in glutaraldehyde or recovered from formalin.

The eosinophilic variant of chromophobe cell renal cell carcinoma was recognized later.[134] It is composed of cells with abundant brightly eosinophilic granular cyto-

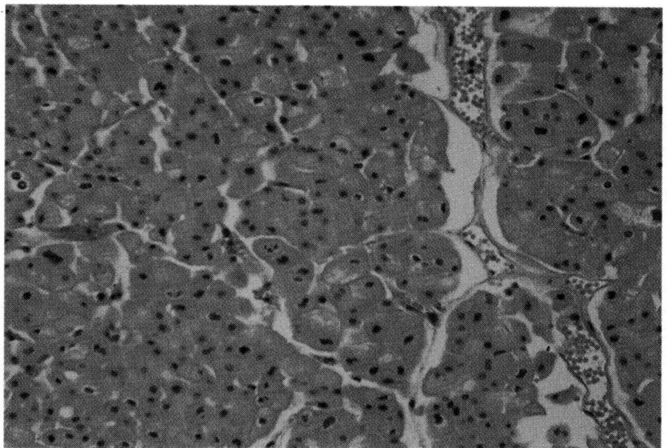

2-22. Chromophobe renal cell carcinoma, eosinophil type. The cytoplasm is finely granular and brightly eosinophilic.

plasm (Fig. 2-22). The cytoplasm surrounding the nucleus may be pale, creating a halo. The cells average somewhat smaller than those of the typical variant and areas of tubular architecture are more prevalent. Ultrastructurally, there are numerous mitochondria mixed with the cytoplasmic vesicles. Hale's colloidal iron stain is strongly positive. In hematoxylin and eosin-stained sections, the eosinophilic variant often closely resembles renal oncocytoma.[135] This is important because the limited information available indicates that this tumor behaves similarly to other types of renal cell carcinoma, while renal oncocytoma is benign (see later in this chapter). Thus it is worthwhile to routinely collect from renal tumors samples that are properly fixed for electron microscopy. It is important to do colloidal iron staining on any tumor for which the differential diagnosis is renal oncocytoma and the eosinophil variant of chromophobe renal cell carcinoma.

Although grading has not been validated for chromophobe renal cell carcinoma, most are nuclear grade 2.[131,135,136]

COLLECTING DUCT CARCINOMA

The collecting ducts begin in the renal cortex and descend through the medulla to the renal papillae; the short segments just above the papillary orifices are called Bellini's ducts.[146] There is evidence that the intercalated cells of the collecting duct may be the source of renal oncocytoma[147] and chromophobe renal cell carcinoma.[143] Additionally, Rumpelt et al.,[148] Fleming and Lewi,[149] Aizawa et al.,[150] and Kennedy et al.[151] have described a different and heterogeneous group of tumors to which they attribute collecting duct origin. The criteria for this diagnosis (see box on this page) are presently evolving and the prognosis of these tumors remains unclear. Davis et al.[152] reported a subgroup of collecting duct carcinoma that occurs in young adults with sickle cell anemia. Little information is available about the genetics of collecting duct carcinoma; a study of three cases showed consistent loss of chromosomes 1, 6, 14, 15, and 22.[153]

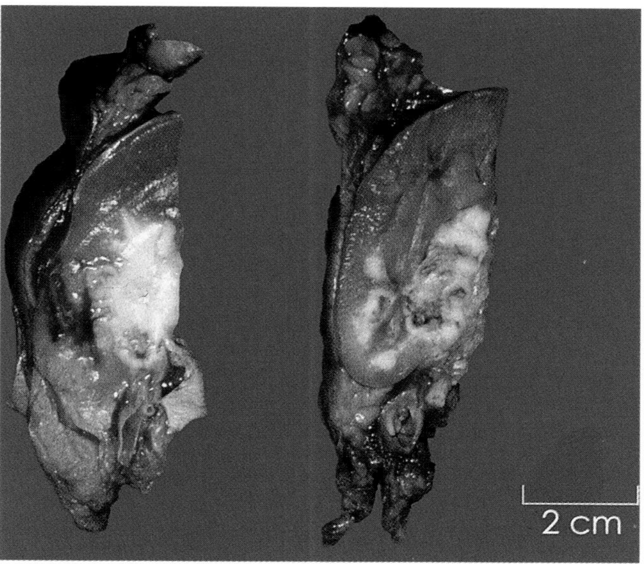

2-23. Collecting duct carcinoma replacing the renal medulla.

COLLECTING DUCT CARCINOMA: CHARACTERISTIC FEATURES

- Appears to arise in medulla
- Irregular tubular/glandular architecture
- Hobnail cells
- Abundant stroma with desmoplasia

Gross pathology

While the collecting ducts extend from the cortex to the medulla, the gross pathologic finding of a tumor arising in the medulla (Fig. 2-23) where other parts of the renal tubular system are absent, can be an important aid to the diagnosis.[150] Unfortunately, precise localization to the medulla is only possible with small tumors. Collecting duct carcinoma is usually centered in the medulla, often with extensions into the cortex or hilar tissues.[149,151] Infiltrative borders and white or gray cut surfaces with central necrosis are typical.[148] Connection with the renal pelvis is common.

Microscopic pathology

Collecting duct carcinoma is a histologically distinctive tumor with features of adenocarcinoma and urothelial carcinoma.[148,154-156] It consists of irregular ductlike structures, nests, and cords of cells in an abundant, loose, slightly basophilic stroma (Fig. 2-24). The cells lining the lumens have small or moderate amounts of cytoplasm and pleomorphic nuclei with thick nuclear membranes. An especially useful feature, rarely found in other types of renal cell carcinoma and not found in urothelial carcinoma, is the hobnail appearance sometimes seen in the cells lining duct lumens (Fig. 2-25). Some reported cases have a different pattern, consisting of papillary fronds covered by cells with small amounts of cytoplasm, similar to chromophil renal cell carcinoma.[150,151] Atypical

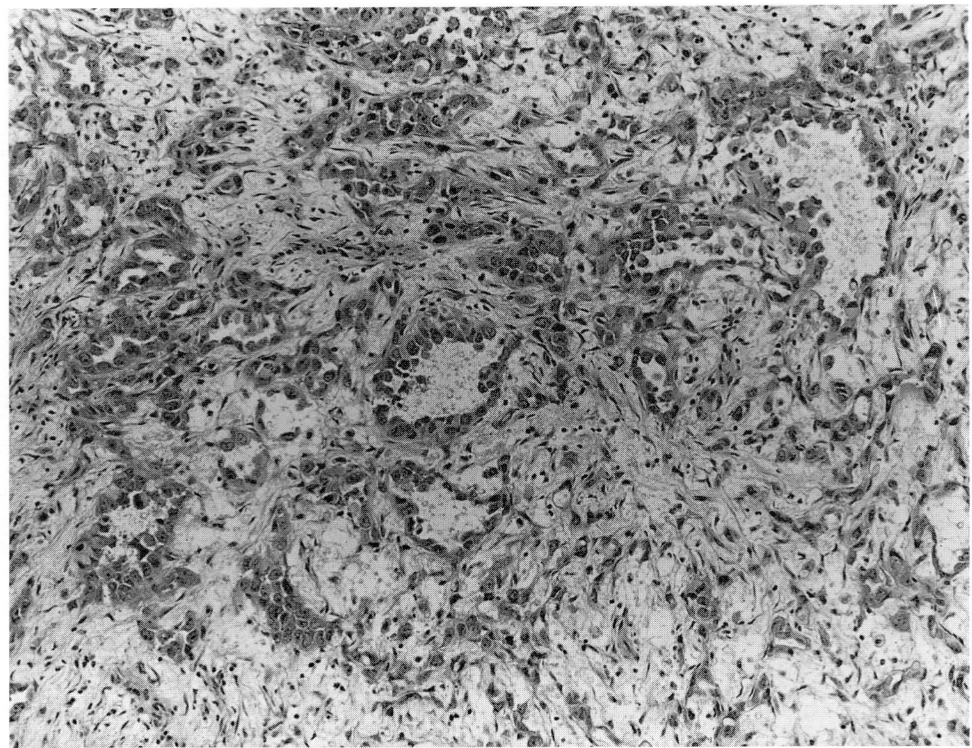

2-24. Collecting duct carcinoma consisting of irregular glands and ducts in chronically inflamed desmoplastic stroma.

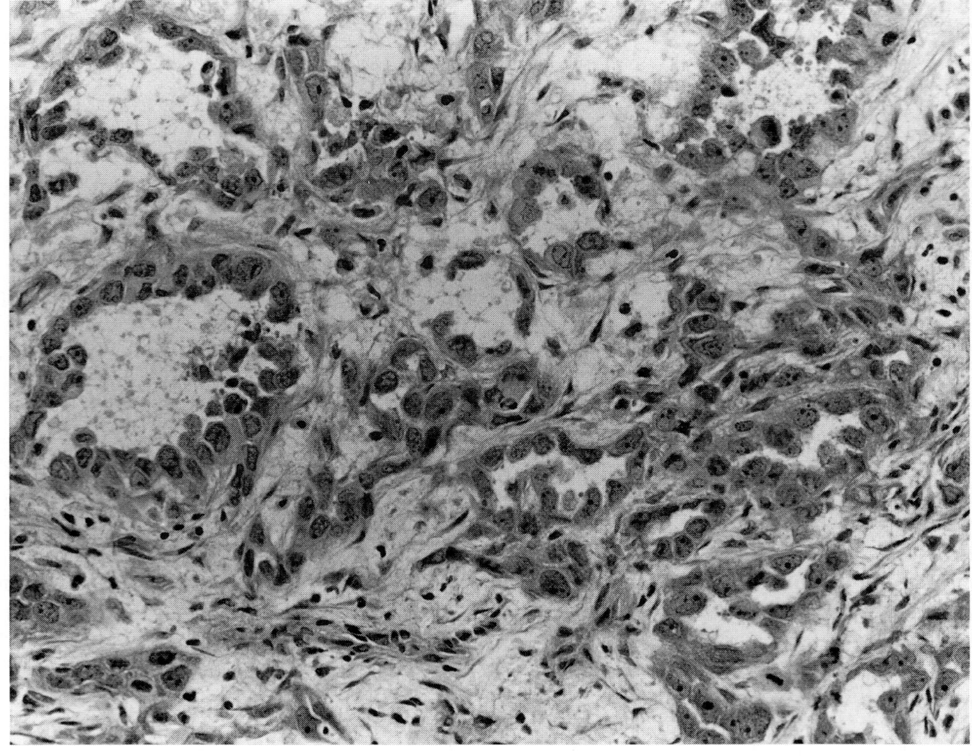

2-25. Collecting duct carcinoma. Hobnail cells lining irregular channels.

epithelium has been seen in some cases in the medullary tubules adjacent to the carcinoma and is a valuable clue to the collecting duct origin of the tumor.[11,151] Sarcomatoid dedifferentiation occurs occasionally.[157]

Differential diagnosis

Awareness of the entity and appreciation of the differences between the above microscopic features and those of other renal cancers should establish the diagnosis in most cases. In a small series, Rumpelt et al.[148] found immunohistochemical differences in cytokeratin patterns and lectin binding between collecting duct carcinoma and urothelial carcinomas and other types of renal cell carcinoma. Collecting duct carcinoma stained strongly positively for cytokeratin 19 and *Ulex europaeus* lectin, but moderately for vimentin while failing to stain for cytokeratin 13. Urothelial carcinoma uniformly failed to stain for vimentin and the renal cell carcinomas failed to stain with *U. europaeus* lectin. If these differences prove consistent in larger series, immunohistochemistry will be valuable in the diagnosis of collecting duct carcinoma. Until this is better understood, it is advisable to restrict the diagnosis of collecting duct carcinoma to those tumors in which the gross pathologic findings indicate this origin or that have the characteristic histopathologic appearance described above and illustrated in Fig. 2-24 and 2-25. Borderline cases should be diagnosed as renal cell carcinoma of unclassified type.

GRADING RENAL CELL CARCINOMA

Since Hand and Broders[158] introduced grading of renal cell carcinomas in 1932, several different systems have been proposed, with variable success. In addition to nuclear characteristics, cytoplasmic and architectural features have been incorporated, leading to a long controversy and considerable frustration for practicing surgical pathologists. In 1971 Skinner et al.[159] redirected attention to the correlation between nuclear features and survival. These observations were confirmed and refined into a system of practically applicable criteria by Fuhrman et al.[131] The Fuhrman system consists of four grades based on the size, contour, and conspicuousness of nucleoli (Table 2-5). Less than 10% of cases are grade 1 and about 20% are grade 4.[160] Grades 2 and 3 are approximately equally frequent, each accounting for about 35% of cases.[160] Medeiros et al.[160] showed that the Fuhrman system correlated well with survival in a large population of patients with renal cell carcinoma and in a smaller population of patients with stage I tumors. Actuarial five-year disease-free survival ranged from 86% for patients with grade 1 tumors to 24% for those with grade 4 tumors. The grade assigned is that of the highest grade found, regardless of extent.[161] Green et al.[162] studied 55 patients with stage I renal cell carcinoma and found a significant decrease in 5-year survival of patients with grade 4 tumors. The importance of nucleolar morphology also has been confirmed by Helpap et al.[163] Mitotic figures are not a part of this system but typically are rare in grade 1 and 2 tumors and the finding of more than 1 per 10 high-power fields has adverse prognostic significance.[161] Störkel and associates have proposed reducing the nuclear grades to three to improve the discriminatory power of the grades.[164]

Less than 5% of renal cell carcinomas contain areas histologically resembling sarcoma.[165,166] Grossly, these areas are often white, contrasting with the rest of the carcinoma (Fig. 2-26). Transition from typical renal cell carcinoma to sarcomatoid morphology can sometimes be found (Fig. 2-27). Usually sarcomatoid areas resemble malignant fibrous histiocytoma, fibrosarcoma, or an undifferentiated spindle cell sarcoma[167] (Fig. 2-28, 2-29). Less common are areas resembling osteogenic sarcoma or rhabdomyosarcoma.[168,169] Malignant bone should be distinguished

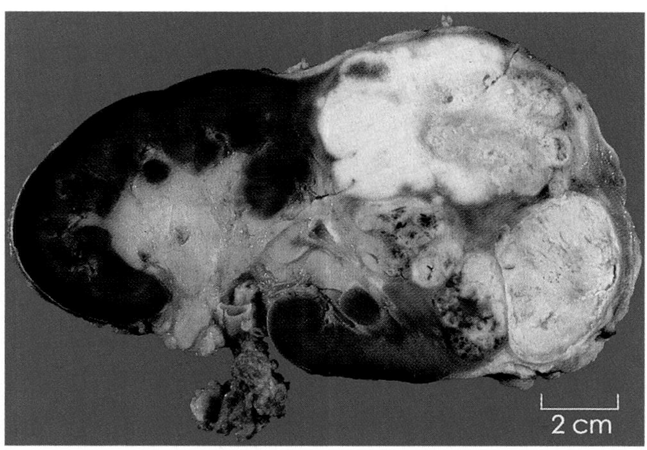

2-26. Sarcomatoid renal cell carcinoma. The white area is sarcomatoid.

TABLE 2-5.
NUCLEAR GRADING OF RENAL CELL CARCINOMA

Grade	Characteristics
Grade 1	Round, uniform nuclei approximately 10 µm in diameter with minute or absent nucleoli
Grade 2	Slightly irregular nuclear contours and diameters of approximately 15 µm with nucleoli visible at 400 x
Grade 3	Moderately to markedly irregular nuclear contours and diameters of approximately 20 µm with large nucleoli visible at 100 x
Grade 4	Nuclei similar to those of grade 3 but also multilobular or multiple nuclei or bizarre nuclei and heavy clumps of chromatin

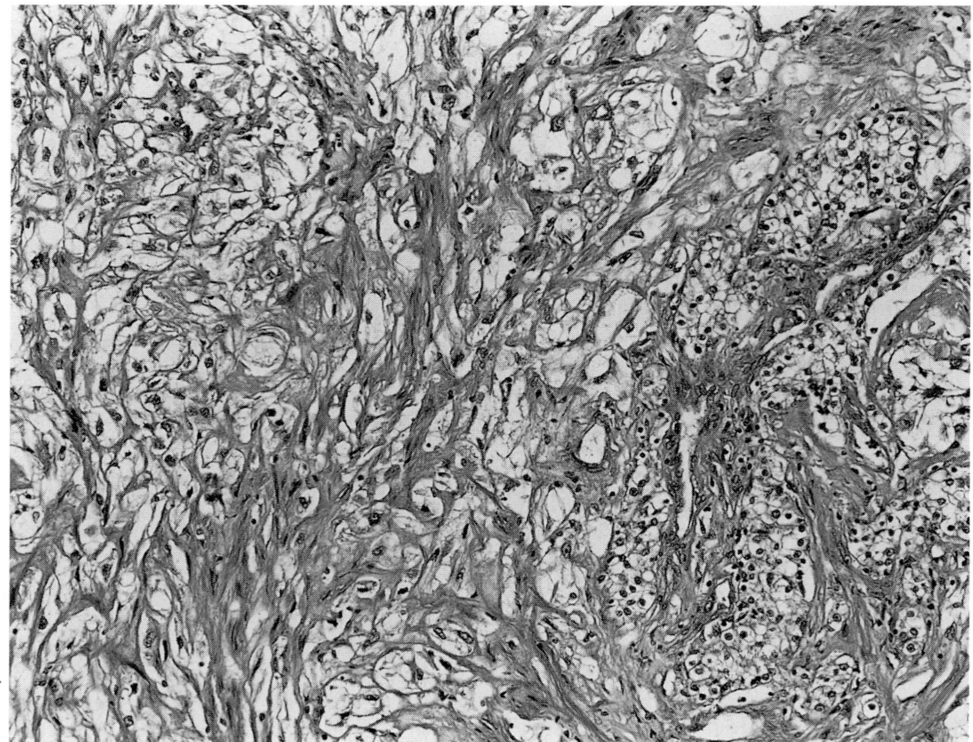

2-27. Sarcomatoid renal cell carcinoma. There is a transition from clear cell renal cell carcinoma (*lower right*) to spindle cells with clear cytoplasm.

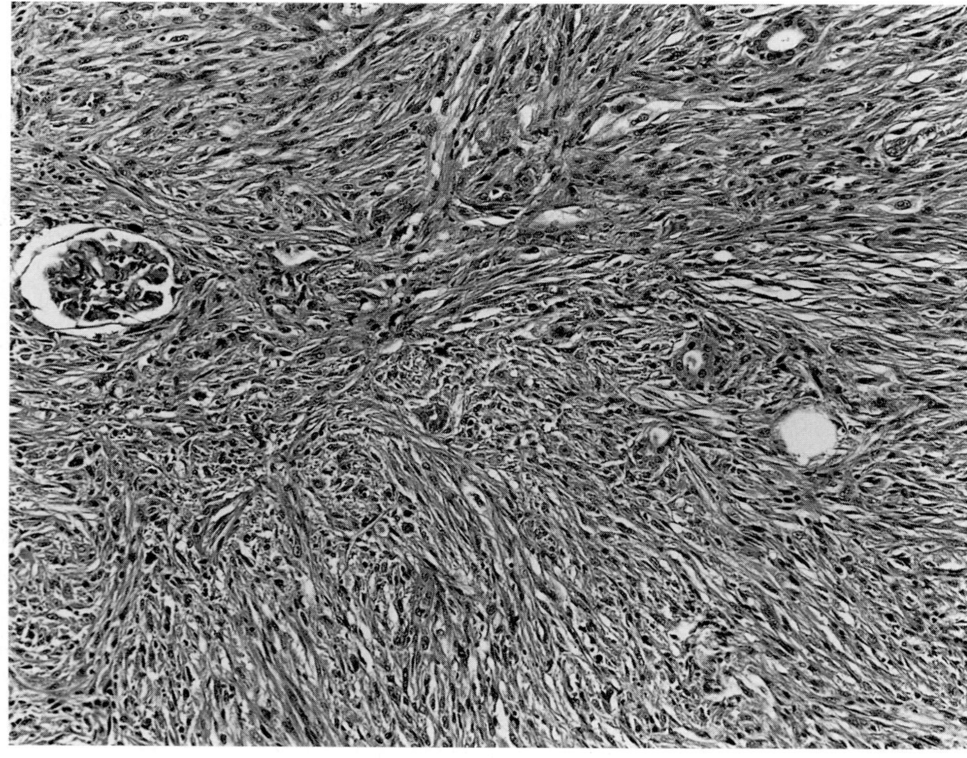

2-28. Sarcomatoid renal cell carcinoma infiltrating the renal parenchyma as fascicles of spindle cell sarcoma.

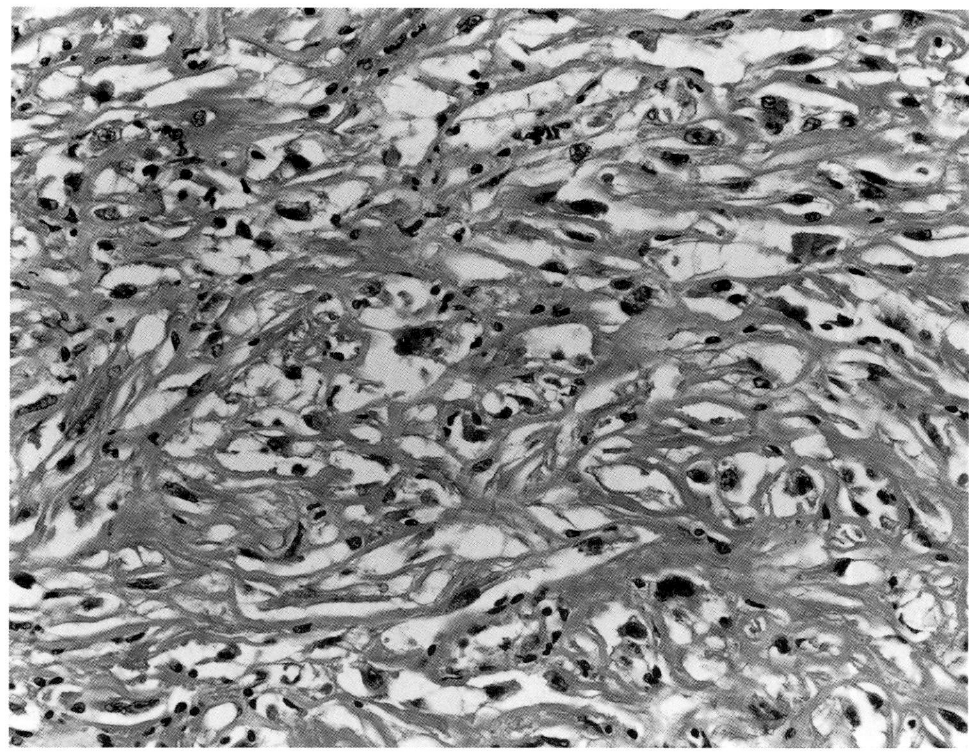

2-29. Sarcomatoid renal cell carcinoma typically consists of undifferentiated spindle cells with pleomorphic nuclei and a collagenous matrix.

from the benign metaplastic bone seen occasionally in the stroma of renal cell carcinoma, as it is in many tumors.[170] Patients with even small foci of sarcomatoid carcinoma have a much worse prognosis than those whose tumors do not.[111,165,167,171-175] Thus generous histologic sampling of renal cell carcinoma is imperative.

SPREAD AND OUTCOME

Staging

The extent of spread of renal cell carcinoma is the dominant factor in prognosis.[176] Two staging systems are widely used for renal cell carcinoma. The system proposed by Robson et al.[177,178] is compared with the tumor, nodes, metastases (TNM) system[179-182] in Table 2-6. These systems are roughly parallel, and comparable stage groups have been set off by horizontal lines. Surgery is the principal therapy for renal cell carcinoma; consequently, both systems include tumors confined within the renal capsule in the most favorable category. Unlike the Robson system, the TNM system takes size into account. Stage III is more complicated and controversial; renal cell carcinoma frequently invades the renal venous system and this is the criterion for stage IIIA (Fig. 2-30). The prognostic significance of venous invasion has been difficult to establish because many tumors with venous invasion have other features of high stage, such as metastases. Medeiros et al.[160,183] compared stage I tumors with stage III tumors, which would have been stage I but for venous invasion, and found that it was an independent prognostic factor among high-grade tumors but did not affect prognosis in low-grade tumors. Invasion of small veins within the main tumor does not indicate that the tumor is stage III; rather, invasion must occur in large veins with smooth muscle in their walls and must be at the edge or outside of the main tumor. Metastasis to regional lymph nodes without distant metastasis occurs in approximately 10% to 15% of cases,[184,185] but more than 50% of patients with enlarged regional lymph nodes have only inflammatory or hyperplastic changes.[186] Radical nephrectomy with regional lymph node dissection has been the standard operation for renal cell carcinoma for more than 3 decades,[177] but the therapeutic contribution of the lymph node dissection remains controversial.[187] Occasionally metastasis occurs via periureteral veins or lymphatics,[188] and for this reason the end of the ureter and its adventitial tissues are a surgical margin that should be examined histologically in radical nephrectomy specimens. Direct invasion of or metastasis to the ipsilateral adrenal (Fig. 2-31) is seen in approximately 5% of radical nephrectomy specimens,[189-191] almost always in cases with lymph node or distant metastases. The prognostic significance of involvement of the ipsilateral adrenal is unclear.

Metastases

Clinically, occult renal cell carcinoma may present at distant sites with unknown primary or recur years after an apparently successful radical nephrectomy, posing

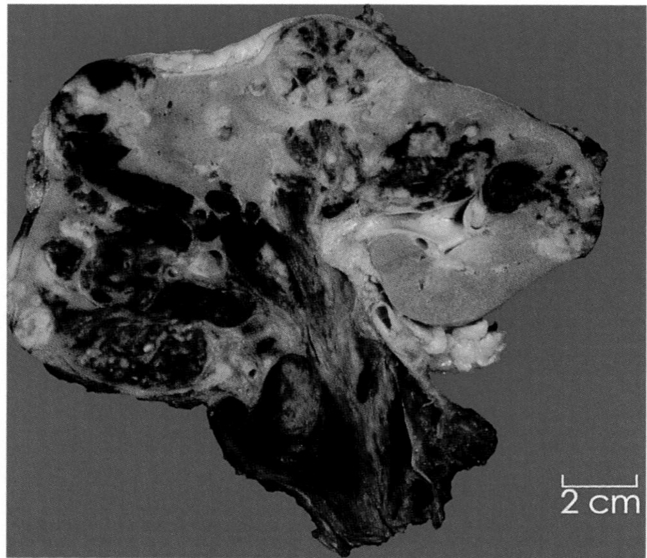

2-30. Renal cell carcinoma extending into the renal vein and distending it.

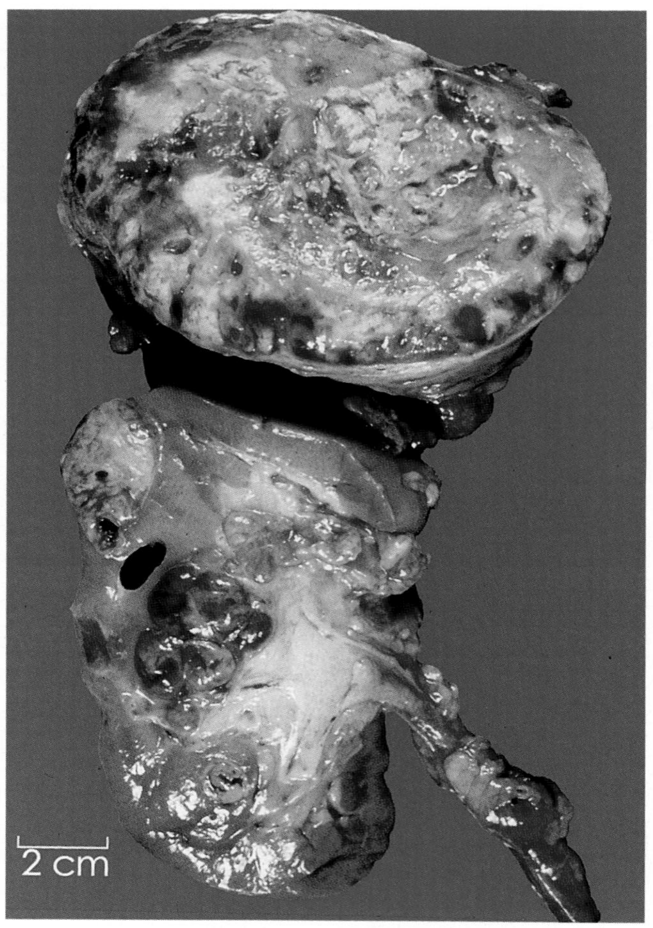

2-31. Renal cell carcinoma metastatic to the ipsilateral adrenal gland.

TABLE 2-6.
STAGING OF RENAL CELL CARCINOMA

Robson System	TNM System
Stage I	T1 Tumor size ≤ 25 mm
Confined within the renal capsule	T2 Tumor size > 25 mm
Stage II	T3 Local invasion
Confined by Gerota's fascia	
Stage III	T3a
A Grossly visible extension into renal vein or vena cava	T3b
B Lymphatic metastasis	N1 Single and size ≤ 20 mm
	N2 Multiple or single 20-50 mm
	N3 Fixed or any node > 50 mm
C Both vascular extension and metastasis to nodes	
Stage IV	
Invasion of adjacent organs (except adrenal)	T4 Extension beyond Gerota's fascia
Hematogenous metastases	M1

special diagnostic problems. The co-expression of cytokeratin and vimentin, which occurs in a majority of renal cell carcinomas,[192] is unusual among carcinomas and is suggestive of a renal primary when found in a metastasis of unknown origin.[101] Ultrastructurally, dense arrays of microvilli in intercellular spaces or on lumenal surfaces, together with abundant glycogen in the cytoplasm, are suggestive of renal cell carcinoma.[193] Solitary metastasis to the contralateral adrenal can resemble primary adrenal cortical carcinoma.[194] In such cases immunohistochemical reactions for epithelial membrane antigen and cytokeratins can be helpful since renal cell carcinoma almost always stains for one or both, while adrenal cortical carcinoma does not contain epithelial membrane antigen[195] and stains for cytokeratin only weakly and after a protease digestion.[101] Metastasis to the thyroid can mimic clear cell carcinoma of the thyroid[196]; thyroglobulin immunohistochemistry and ultrastructural detection of intracytoplasmic glycogen (which is not found in clear cell carcinoma of the thyroid) can be helpful in making the distinction. Metastases to the ovary can be confused with primary ovarian clear cell adenocarcinoma.[197] Capillary hemangioblastoma of the central nervous system may closely resemble clear cell renal cell carcinoma in sections stained with hematoxylin and eosin and poses a particular problem because both neoplasms are associated with von Hippel-Lindau disease. This problem can usually be resolved by staining for epithelial membrane antigen, which is present in clear cell renal cell carcinoma and absent from capillary hemangioblastoma.[198]

The clinical course of renal cell carcinoma is notoriously unpredictable, with documented cases of spontaneous regression of metastases[199-202] and prolonged course.[203] Recurrence 10 years or more after nephrectomy occurs in more than 10% of patients who survive that long.[204] There is some evidence that resection of solitary metastases improves survival,[205] while the presence of multiple metastases indicates a worse prognosis.[206] However, the resistance of renal cell carcinoma to radiation and chemotherapy gives most patients with remote metastases a poor prognosis.[207,208] Metastases to bone occur frequently and more than one third of these are to the scapula.[209]

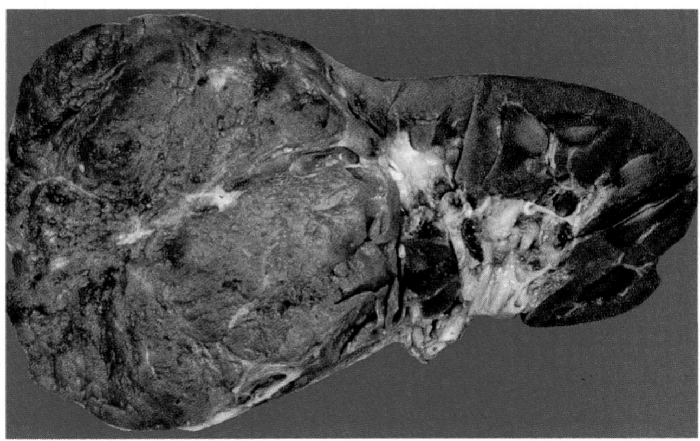

2-32. Renal oncocytoma. The parenchyma is dark brown.

RENAL ONCOCYTOMA

Renal oncocytoma is a neoplasm of the renal cortex, which often is discovered incidentally by radiologic examinations of the kidneys for other reasons, but may also present with a palpable mass or hematuria.[210] In 1976 Klein and Valensi[67] drew attention to renal oncocytoma as a renal tumor previously classified as granular cell renal cell carcinoma but distinguishable from it by gross and microscopic findings and having a benign course. There is a 2:1 incidence ratio of males to females and almost all cases have occurred in adults, most older than 50 years. Resection of the tumor is curative. A striking spoke-and-wheel appearance on radiography was initially thought to be diagnostic of oncocytoma, but greater experience has indicated that this is not specific because renal cell carcinoma may have a similar appearance.[212] The tumor often cannot reliably be distinguished preoperatively from renal cell carcinoma by biopsy. Thus radical nephrectomy is the usual operation. Some patients have had multicentric or bilateral tumors[213] and conservative operations.[214]

Gross pathology

The most characteristic macroscopic feature of renal oncocytoma is its mahogany-brown color (Fig. 2-32), which contrasts with the bright yellow color of clear cell renal cell carcinoma. Many oncocytomas have central stellate zones of white or pale gray stroma that may connect with the periphery (Fig. 2-33), giving the subcapsular surface a bosselated contour. Occasional tumors exhibit foci of hemorrhage, but necrosis is rare and often related to concurrent conditions such as vasculitis, sickle cell anemia, or sepsis.[210] The presence of gross necrosis or hemorrhage suggests caution in making the diagnosis of oncocytoma. Bilaterality or multicentricity occur in approximately 3.6% of cases. Rarely,

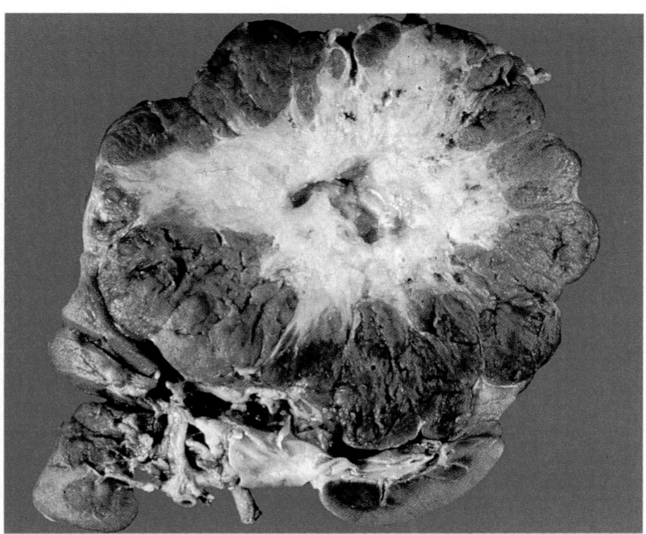

2-33. Renal oncocytoma. In this large tumor there is a central area of edematous connective tissue that connects with the periphery to give a hub-and-spoke appearance.

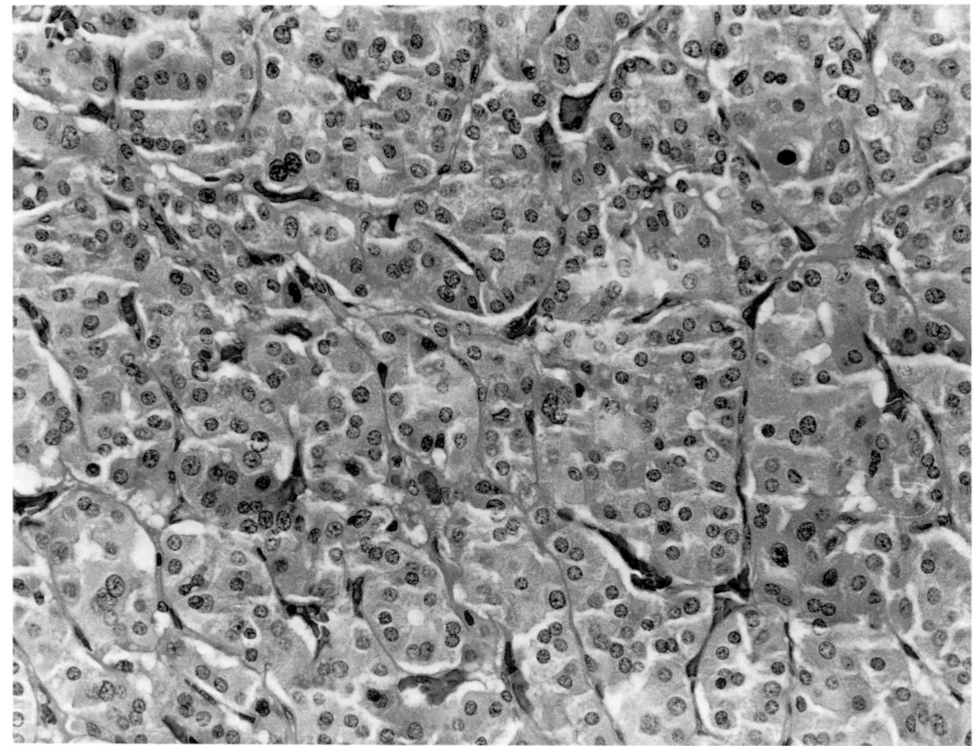

2-34. Renal oncocytoma. Diffuse pattern consisting of cells with abundant eosinophilic cytoplasm and delicate vasculature.

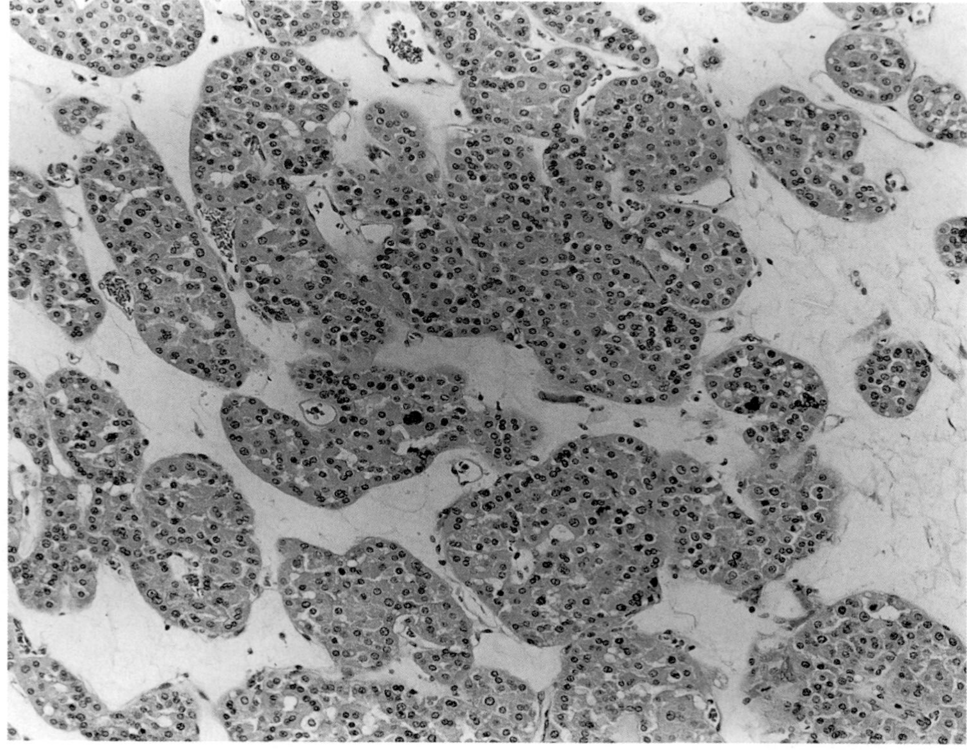

2-35. Renal oncocytoma. Insular pattern consisting of clusters of cells in an edematous stroma.

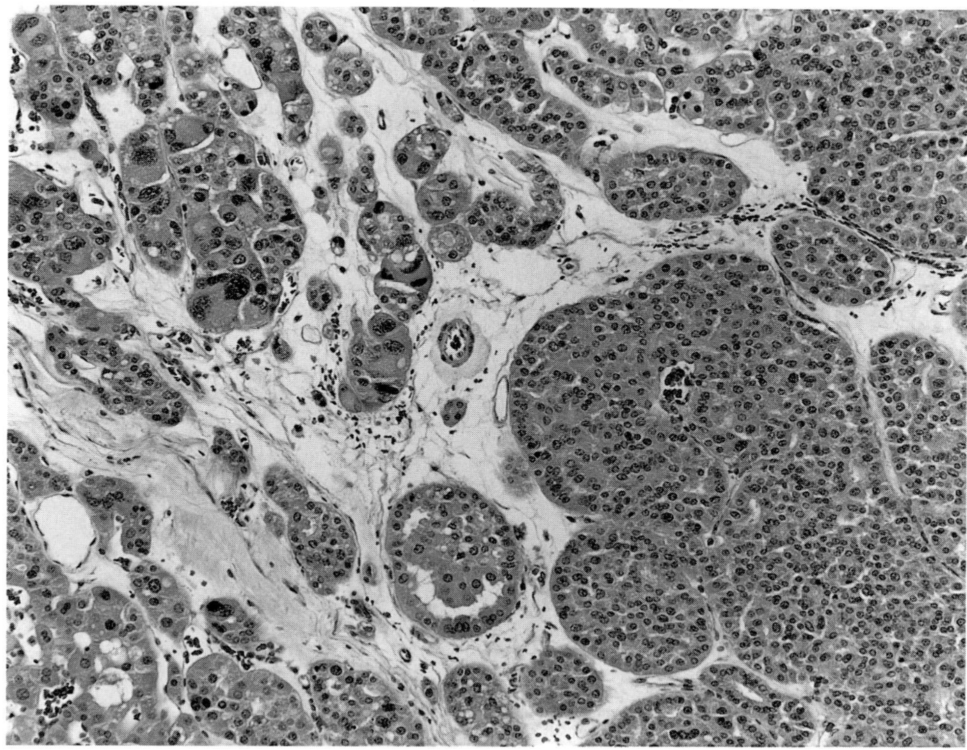

2-36. Renal oncocytoma with nuclear pleomorphism and scattered tubular structures.

RENAL ONCOCYTOMA: CHARACTERISTIC FEATURES

Compact and archipelaginous architecture
Abundant eosinophilic cytoplasm
Negative Hale's colloidal iron stain
EM: Cytoplasm packed with mitochondria

there are large numbers of small oncocytomas in the cortices of both kidneys, a condition referred to as *oncocytomatosis*.[215]

Microscopic pathology

The histologic features of renal oncocytoma are summarized in the box on this page. The cells usually are arranged either in diffuse sheets (Fig. 2-34) or as cellular islands in a background of loose edematous connective tissue (Fig. 2-35). Tubules, often mildly dilated, also are common. Occasionally the groups of cells contain hyaline deposits of type IV collagen, giving a cylindromatous appearance.[216] In sections stained with hematoxylin and eosin, the cytoplasm is intensely eosinophilic and finely granular. Cytoplasmic volume ranges from moderate to abundant. The nuclei are mainly round with small clumps of chromatin and inconspicuous nucleoli, but occasional bizarre, enlarged nuclei, sometimes containing cytoplasmic invaginations, may be seen (Fig. 2-36). Mitotic figures are absent or very rare. Since it is benign, oncocytoma is not graded. Ultrastructurally, the cytoplasm is filled with mitochondria and other organelles are scant (Fig. 2-37). Microvilli are sparse and completely formed brush borders usually are absent.[217]

Extension into small veins is seen microscopically in 5% to 10% of cases and appears to have no adverse prognostic significance.[210] Superficial extension into perirenal fat is seen in almost 10% of cases and also appears to have no adverse effect.[210]

Differential diagnosis

The principal consideration is the eosinophilic variant of chromophobe renal cell carcinoma. Hale's colloidal iron stain or electron microscopic examination is helpful in such cases. Since oncocytoma often has scattered large pleomorphic nuclei, and nucleoli are often visible at medium magnification, the incorrect diagnosis of carcinoma will be compounded by assignment of grade 2 or 3. However, the presence of nuclei with features of nuclear grade 4 in an apparent oncocytoma strongly suggests that the tumor is a carcinoma.

Prognosis

Renal oncocytoma has achieved acceptance as a clinically relevant entity distinct from renal cell carcinoma because it is benign. A few reports have suggested that oncocytoma may metastasize.[218] Typically these reports have been based on hematoxylin and eosin examinations without ultrastructural or histochemical studies to rule out the eosinophilic variant of chromophobe renal cell carcinoma. No oncocytoma meeting the criteria set forth in the top section and lacking those in the bottom

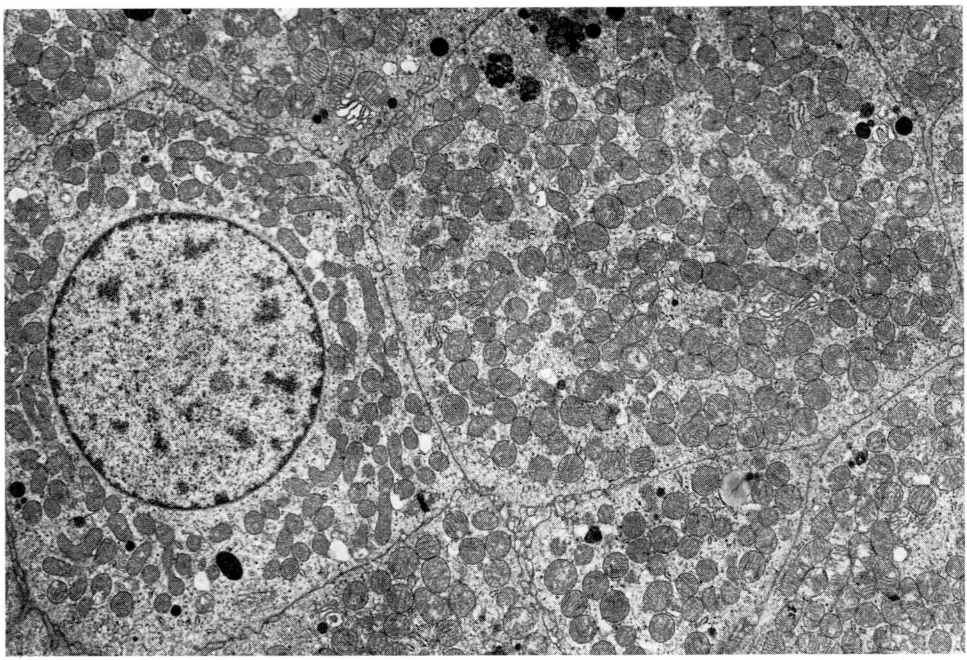

2-37. Renal oncocytoma. Electron micrograph showing the cytoplasm is filled with mitochondria.

DIAGNOSTIC FEATURES OF RENAL ONCOCYTOMA

Features of renal oncocytoma
- Finely granular, strongly eosinophilic cytoplasm
- Sheet, insular, or tubulocystic architectural patterns
- Mitochondria filling cytoplasm with other organelles and microvilli sparse

Features of atypical renal oncocytoma
- Microscopic vascular invasion
- Microscopic extension into perirenal fat

Features impermissible in renal oncocytoma
- Mitotic figures
- Papillary architecture
- Clear or spindle cells
- Positive colloidal iron stain
- Chromophobe-type vesicles seen by electron microscopy
- Gross vascular invasion
- Gross extension into perirenal fat

two sections of the box on this page has metastasized or recurred. The success of the strict criteria and the discovery of variants meeting them but having atypical features have led to the development of a working category with slightly more liberal criteria for which the prognosis is less certain. This category, originally described as "congeners" of oncocytoma by Barnes and Beckman[219] and as "atypical" oncocytoma by Davis et al.,[210] includes otherwise typical oncocytomas with one or more of the features listed in the middle section of the box. As more cases are studied, it is likely that some of the features now considered atypical will be shown to have no unfavorable consequences. This can occur only when there is convincing evidence because it is important that the diagnosis of typical oncocytoma remain associated with a benign course. The features listed in the third part of the box remain impermissible in renal oncocytoma. Obviously, some of the features depend on substantial sampling of the tumor. This implies that needle biopsies, by both core and aspirate techniques, are better instruments for excluding the diagnosis of oncocytoma than for making it.

NEUROENDOCRINE TUMORS OF THE KIDNEY

More than two dozen neuroendocrine neoplasms in the spectrum from carcinoid to small cell carcinoma have been described in the kidney.[156] Equally common in males and females, the patients' ages have ranged from adolescence to the ninth decade of life, with a mean age of approximately 50 years. A variety of endocrine manifestations have been reported, including cases of the carcinoid syndrome[220] and excess secretion of glucagon.[221] Metastases have been common, even among the cases of carcinoid.[222,223]

Pheochromocytoma arising in the renal sinus and compressing the renal artery appears to be more common than pheochromocytoma within the renal capsule.[224-226] Intrarenal pheochromocytoma does occur[227-231] and is associated with hypertension. Neuroblastoma rarely arises in the kidneys of adults.[232]

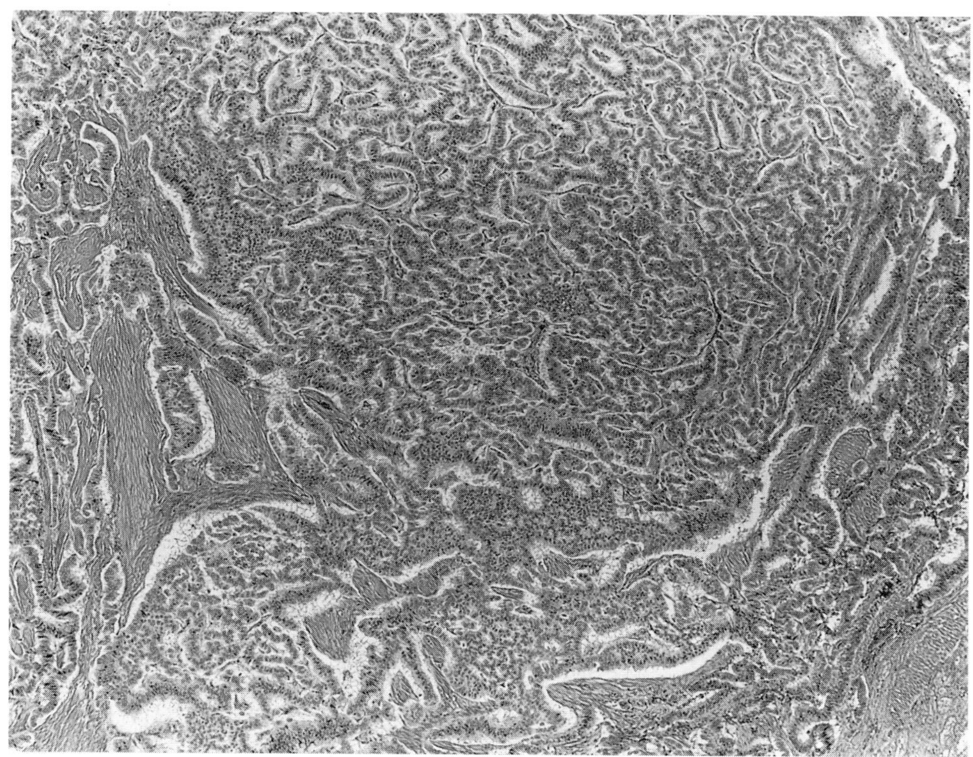

2-38. Renal carcinoid tumor with ribbon architecture.

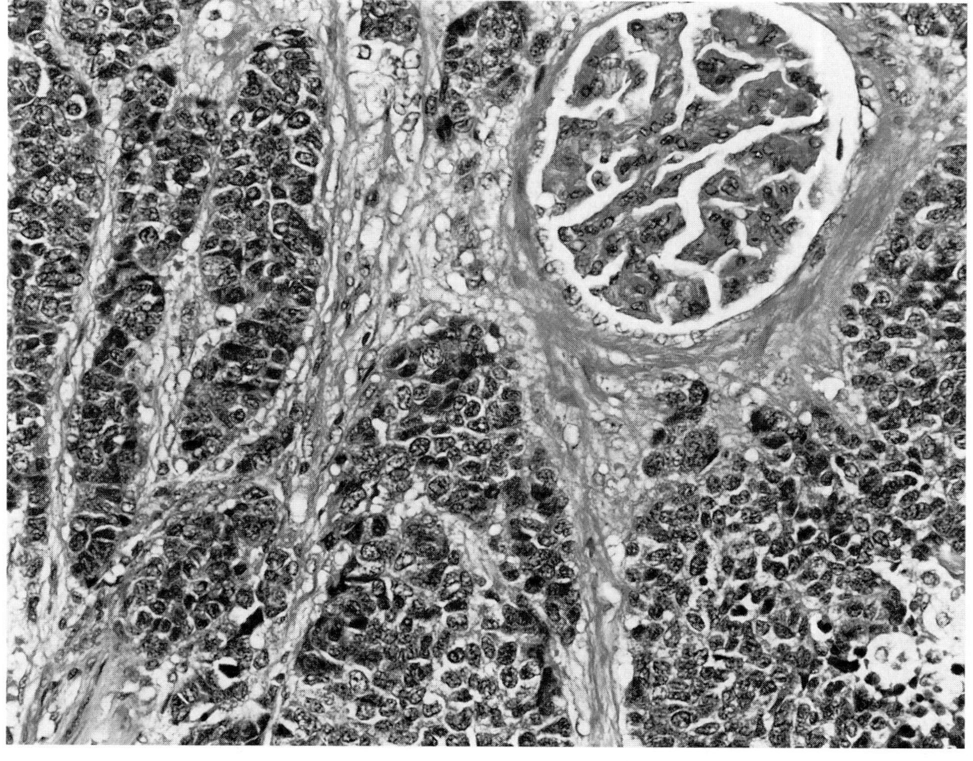

2-39. Renal small cell carcinoma.

Gross pathology

Renal carcinoid tumor often is well circumscribed[222,233,234] and consists of red or tan tissue with areas of hemorrhage[235] and necrosis.[236] Two cases have been described in which dysplastic or teratoid elements were associated with renal carcinoid.[237,238] Renal small cell carcinoma often is large and infiltrates retroperitoneal soft tissues; regional lymph node metastases are common.[239,240] Renal neuroblastoma often is large and firm, with a yellow-red cut surface mottled with hemorrhage.[232] Intrarenal pheochromocytoma has ranged from 2.5 to 9 cm in diameter[227,229] and consists of yellow-brown or brown tissue, often containing cysts.[228,229]

Microscopic pathology

Histopathologically, the tumors in the spectrum from carcinoid to small cell carcinoma resemble their counterparts arising elsewhere. Carcinoid (Fig. 2-38) consists of cords or nests of cells. At the other end of the spectrum of differentiation, small cell carcinoma (Fig. 2-39) consists of sheets of poorly differentiated cells with darkly staining nuclei and inconspicuous cytoplasm. Necrosis is common and two studies[239,240] noted the Azzopardi phenomenon (deposition of DNA in the walls of blood vessels).

Neuroblastoma is diagnosed using the same criteria applied in the adrenal gland; the presence of neuropil or Homer-Wright rosettes is helpful in distinguishing it from small cell carcinoma and neuron-specific enolase is usually demonstrable by immunohistochemistry.[232] Intrarenal pheochromocytoma resembles its adrenal counterpart histologically.

ANGIOMYOLIPOMA

Angiomyolipoma is a benign tumor of the kidney composed of variable amounts of mature fat, smooth muscle, and thick-walled blood vessels.[241,242] It occurs in two distinct clinical settings: approximately half are associated with tuberous sclerosis and half occur sporadically. In patients with tuberous sclerosis, angiomyolipoma is usually asymptomatic, multiple, bilateral, and small (Fig. 2-40), while in the general population it is often symptomatic, solitary, and large (Fig. 2-41).[243] Angiomyolipoma is uncommon in the general population, but more than 50% of patients with tuberous sclerosis develop them.[56] There is a strong female predominance.

Hemorrhage is the most common serious complication of angiomyolipoma.[244] This is more likely with tumors larger than 4 cm and these usually should be removed; smaller tumors often are followed radiographically.[245] Local invasion has been reported occasionally and in rare instances has been lethal.[246] In only two instances has a well-documented sarcoma arisen from an angiomyolipoma.[247,248] Invasion of the vena cava occurs rarely but has no prognostic significance beyond the greater surgical morbidity associated with the more complex procedure necessary for its removal.[249,250] Deposits of angiomyolipoma in regional lymph nodes occur rarely and also have no prognostic significance.[251,252]

Gross pathology

Ranging from less than 1 cm to 20 cm or more in diameter, most symptomatic tumors average about 9 cm.[241,242] Angiomyolipoma is typically golden yellow, but the color varies according to the proportions of smooth muscle and blood vessels. It is not encapsulated but is usually well demarcated and uncommonly may be locally infiltrative. The cut surface may resemble a lipoma.

Microscopic pathology

Angiomyolipoma varies histologically according to the relative proportions of fat, smooth muscle, and blood vessels. The smooth muscle component is variable in appearance. A frequent finding is radial arrays of smooth muscle fibers about blood vessels, but smooth muscle also occurs in bundles and scattered as individual fibers (Fig. 2-42). The smooth muscle cells are typically spindle-shaped but occasionally are epithelioid and have abundant eosinophilic cytoplasm (Fig. 2-43). The blood vessels are often abnormal, with thick

2-40. Multiple small angiomyolipomas in the kidney of a patient with tuberous sclerosis. Arrows indicate angiomyolipomas. Arrowheads indicate cysts.

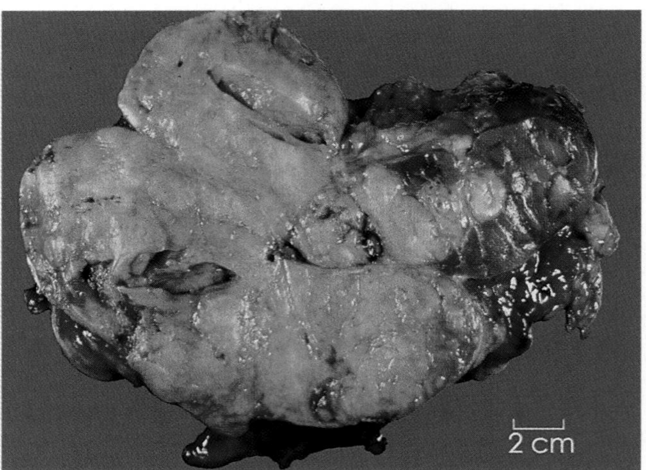

2-41. Angiomyolipoma. A large mass of yellow tissue resembling fat.

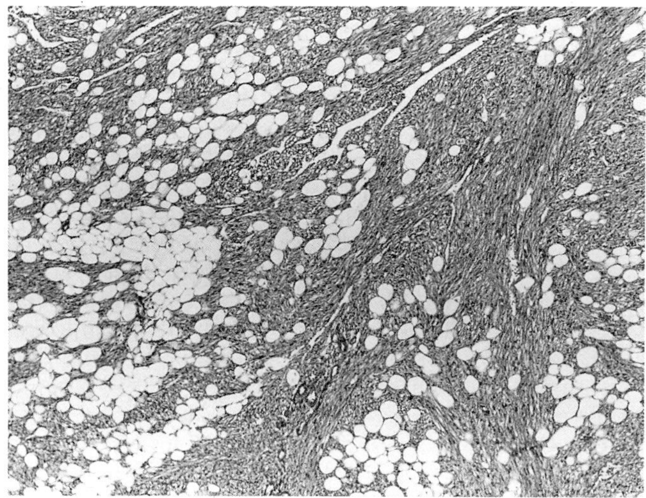

2-42. Angiomyolipoma. Smooth muscle and fat are mingled.

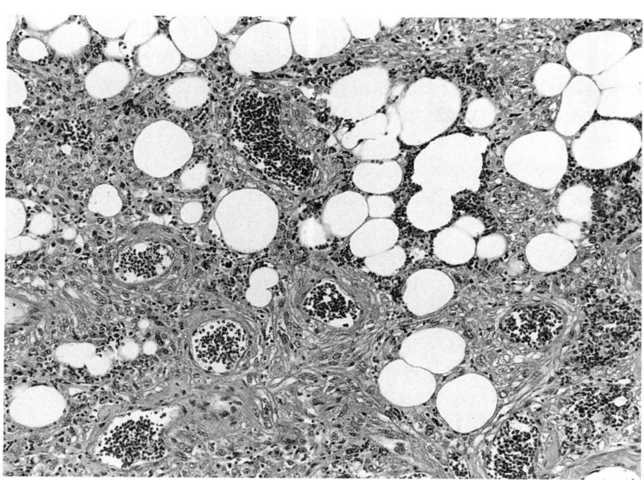

2-43. Angiomyolipoma. Thick-walled blood vessels with cuffs of epithelioid smooth muscle cells mingle with fat cells.

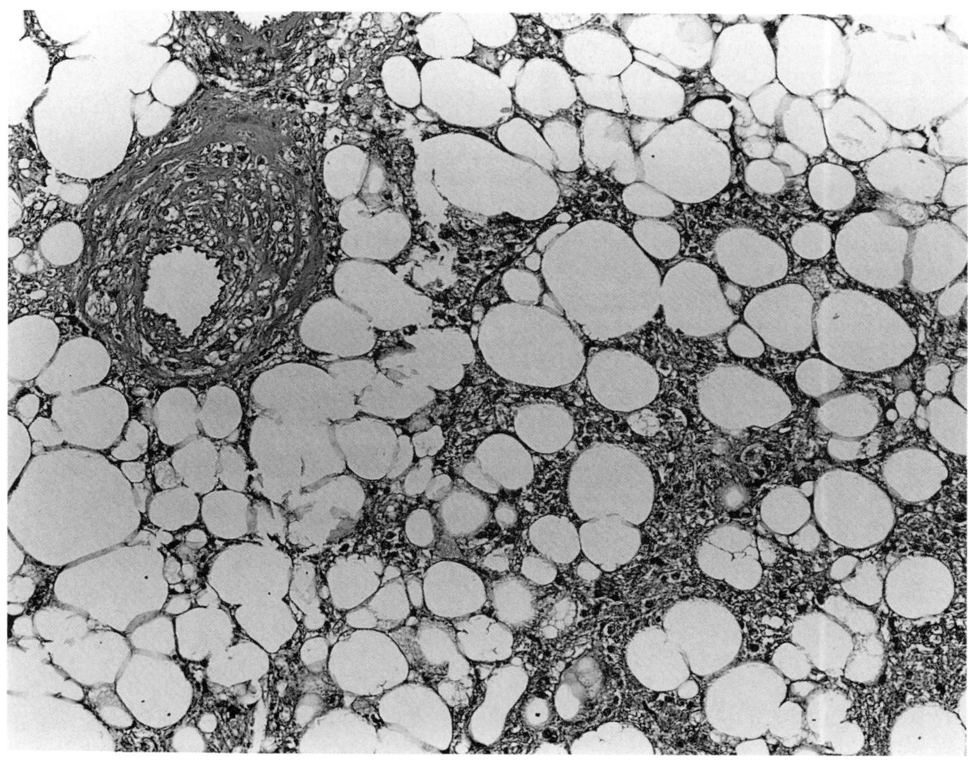

2-44. Angiomyolipoma. A thick-walled blood vessel with an eccentric lumen is in the upper left corner.

walls resembling those of arteries but with eccentric or very small lumens (Fig. 2-44). Nuclear pleomorphism may be pronounced and mitotic figures may be present. These findings have no prognostic significance. In some cases angiomyolipomatous tissue has been found in regional lymph nodes[253-255] and spleen.[256] This should not be misinterpreted as metastatic sarcoma. The smooth muscle cells of angiomyolipoma usually react with antibodies to the melanoma-associated antigen HMB-45.[257-259] This reaction can be useful in distinguishing angiomyolipoma from other spindle cell tumors in the kidney.

Differential diagnosis

In cases with an extreme predominance of fat, angiomyolipoma can be confused with lipoma; extensive sampling may be necessary to identify the vascular and smooth muscle components of the tumor. Tumors with scant fat may be confused with other mesenchymal tumors, such as leiomyoma. Tumors with epithelioid features may mimic epithelial tumors of the kidney and the possibility should be considered when examining an epithelial-like renal tumor that is hard to classify, particularly if the patient has tuberous sclerosis.

HEMANGIOMA

Hemangioma of the kidney usually occurs in adults and equally in men and women.[260,261] Solitary lesions are the most frequent, but more than 10% are multiple and bilaterality has been reported. Rarely, it is associated with the Klippel-Trenaunay and Sturge-Weber syndromes.[262] Many are asymptomatic and found only at autopsy. In symptomatic patients recurrent hematuria is the usual complaint, frequently associated with anemia.[263]

Gross pathology

Most renal hemangiomas are less than one centimeter in diameter and unimpressive to the naked eye. Larger lesions, up to 18 cm in diameter, have a spongy reddish appearance. Hemangioma may arise anywhere in the kidney, but the medulla and papilla are the sites of the majority of symptomatic lesions.[263]

Microscopic pathology

Microscopically, renal hemangioma is composed of vascular spaces of variable size (Fig. 2-45), some of which may have smooth muscle and elastic tissue in their walls. Thrombosis and organization are common. While it often has irregular borders and merges with the surrounding renal parenchyma, the lack of nuclear atypia and mitotic figures should make recognition of the benign nature easy in most cases. They are distinguished from angiosarcomas using the same criteria applied in soft tissue.

LYMPHANGIOMA

Renal lymphangioma is much less common than renal hemangioma. Fewer than 50 cases have been described. Patients range from infancy[264] to old age, about one third of the cases occurring in children and two thirds in adults.[265,266] Grossly, renal lymphangioma is usually a solitary encapsulated mass composed of small cysts containing clear fluid. Microscopic examination shows spaces lined by benign endothelial cells with septa that are generally fibrous but may contain smooth muscle. Lesions in the renal sinus may infiltrate the renal medulla,[264] obstructing the flow of urine.

LEIOMYOMA

Symptomatic renal leiomyoma is rare.[267] Rarely, it forms large masses as great as 37 kg[268]; small ones are usually found incidentally at autopsy. Most occur in adults.[269] Grossly, it is well circumscribed, solid, and rubbery with a whorled cut surface. As in the uterus, it consists of bundles of smooth muscle fibers that may focally calcify and show other degenerative changes.

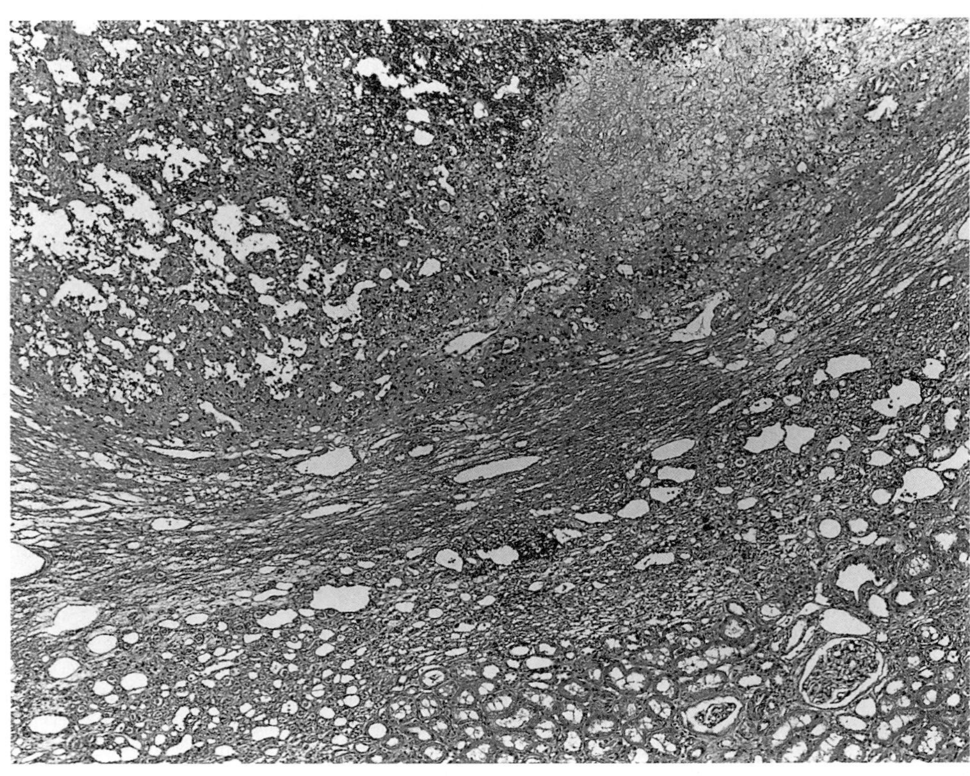

2-45. Renal hemangioma consisting of irregular anastomosing vascular channels.

Necrosis, nuclear atypia, or more than rare mitotic figures strongly suggest that the tumor is a leiomyosarcoma. Since smooth muscle may predominate in angiomyolipoma, it should be ruled out before leiomyoma is diagnosed. Immunohistochemistry for the melanoma-associated antigen HMB-45 is useful since angiomyolipoma contains this antigen and leiomyoma does not.[257-259]

LIPOMA

Symptomatic renal lipoma is rare and occurs almost exclusively in middle-aged women.[270] Patients usually present with abdominal or flank pain. Grossly, renal lipoma is a yellow lobulated and encapsulated mass; histopathologically, it consists entirely of mature fat (Fig. 2-46). Generous sampling is indicated since angiomyolipoma may consist predominantly of fat. Rarely, renal sinus fat around the renal pelvis may proliferate excessively, mimicking a neoplasm.[271]

LEIOMYOSARCOMA

Leiomyosarcoma is the most common primary renal sarcoma, with more than 100 reported cases.[272] Patients' ages range from childhood to old age, but most have occurred in patients older than 40, with a peak in the fifth and sixth decades. It appears in approximately twice as many women as men. Mass and flank pain are the most common presentation.

Gross pathology

The gross appearance often resembles that of leiomyoma: a firm, solid tumor with well-circumscribed margins and whorled cut surfaces, but necrosis and hemorrhage are more common.[273] Leiomyosarcoma may also arise from the renal capsule[273] or renal vein and the bulk of the tumor may be in the renal sinus.[274] Renal and perirenal infiltration are frequent.

Microscopic pathology

Microscopically, renal leiomyosarcoma is composed of fascicles of spindle-shaped cells with features resembling smooth muscle (Fig. 2-47). A myxoid variant has been described.[275] The degree of nuclear pleomorphism and the prevalence of mitotic figures vary over a wide range and no clear minimum criteria of malignancy have been established.[276] Necrosis, nuclear pleomorphism, or more than rare mitotic figures indicate that a renal smooth muscle tumor is probably leiomyosarcoma. Suspicion of leiomyosarcoma should be high, especially in large smooth muscle tumors, because metastasis and death have occasionally been caused by tumors with very low mitotic counts.[277]

LIPOSARCOMA

Liposarcoma is common in retroperitoneal soft tissue but rare in the kidney.[278,279] Careful gross examination is important to establish the intrarenal origin of this tumor since liposarcoma of retroperitoneal soft tissue invading or compressing the kidney is more common than renal

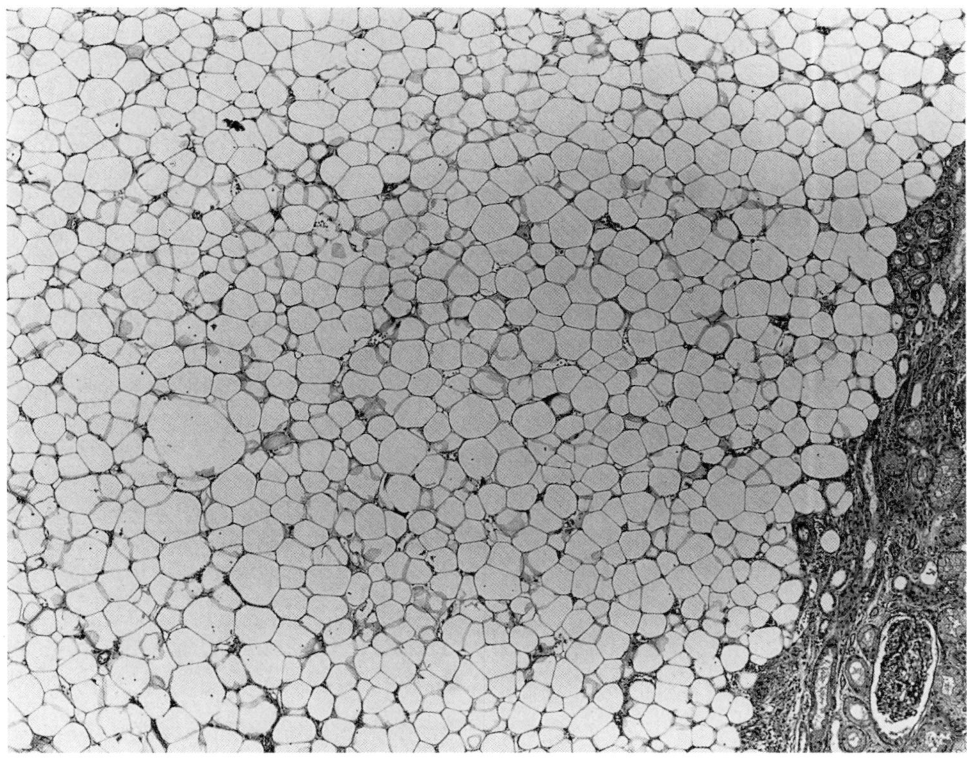

2-46. Renal lipoma. *(Courtesy of D. Grignon, M.D.)*

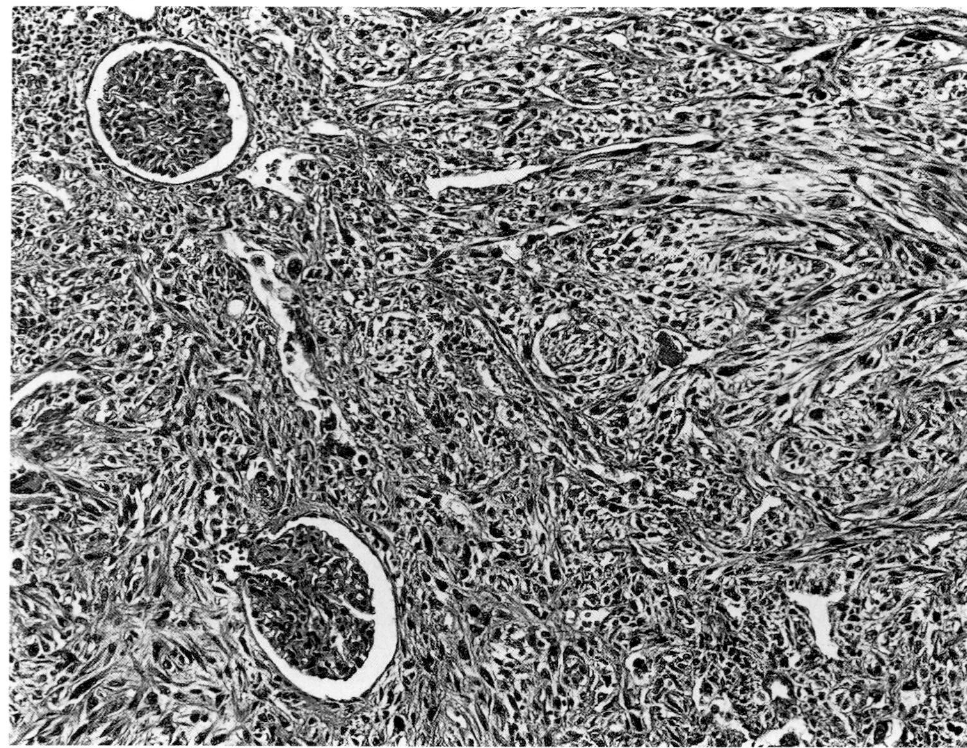

2-47. Leiomyosarcoma infiltrating the kidney.

liposarcoma invading retroperitoneal soft tissue.[273] In cases in which the origin is unclear (the larger and more infiltrative ones), the presumption should be in favor of a primary in retroperitoneal soft tissue. Some of the reported cases have, in retrospect, been large solitary angiomyolipomas. Grossly, the renal liposarcoma is usually a relatively well-circumscribed yellow lobulated mass. Histologically, it displays the variety of patterns found in soft tissue; 80% of the tumors described by Farrow et al.[273] were myxoid.

MALIGNANT FIBROUS HISTIOCYTOMA

Malignant fibrous histiocytoma may arise from the renal parenchyma or from the renal capsule.[280,281] Because the retroperitoneal soft tissues are a common site for malignant fibrous histiocytoma (Fig. 2-48), the recommendations made above for the attribution of primary site for liposarcoma involving the kidney also apply here. Renal malignant fibrous histiocytoma occurs mainly in adults and there has been a strong male predominance. It is usually large and infiltrative. Most have been of the storiform-pleomorphic and inflammatory types. The former may be difficult to distinguish from sarcomatoid renal cell carcinoma and the latter may resemble xanthogranulomatous pyelonephritis.

RHABDOMYOSARCOMA

Rhabdomyosarcoma rarely arises in the kidney[282-284]; Grignon et al. reviewed the literature and found only eight convincing cases, evenly divided between the genders and occurring in patients from 36 to 70 years old.[285] Four died of sarcoma within 14 months and the other four had less than 12 months of follow-up. In light of its rarity and the existence of other tumors that can be confused with it, the diagnosis of rhabdomyosarcoma should be made reluctantly. In children Wilms' tumors may grossly resemble sarcoma botryoides protruding into the renal pelvis and may contain extensive skeletal muscle (fetal rhabdomyomatous nephroblastoma).[286,287] The existence of rhabdomyosarcoma distinct from Wilms' tumor in children is questionable. Rhabdoid tumor of the

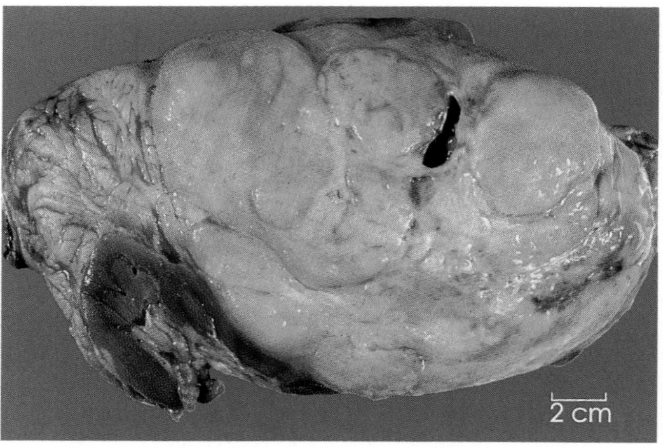

2-48. Retroperitoneal malignant fibrous histiocytoma.

kidney may also mimic rhabdomyosarcoma, as may sarcomatoid renal cell carcinoma.

OTHER SARCOMAS

Hemangiopericytoma primary in the kidney is rare[288,289] and subject to the confusion between intrarenal and extrarenal origin discussed in the section on liposarcoma.[273,290] It is usually large and cysts and foci of hemorrhage are common.[289] Osteogenic sarcoma rarely arises from the renal parenchyma or pelvis,[291,292] and a few examples of chondrosarcoma,[293,294] angiosarcoma,[295-297] and malignant mesenchymoma[298] have been reported.

JUXTAGLOMERULAR CELL TUMOR

Juxtaglomerular cell tumor, also called *reninoma*, was recognized independently by Robertson et al.[299] and Kihara et al.[300] More than 50 examples have been reported.[156,301] While all the patients have been hypertensive, it is a rare cause of hypertension, and Corvol et al.[302] found only seven tumors in 30,000 new hypertensive patients. Elevation of the plasma renin level is typical, and selective catheterization of the renal veins is an important guide to the resection of small tumors.[303] Most patients are young adults and adolescents, averaging 27 years of age at the time of resection.[156] Many are hypertensive for years before resection. Female cases exceed male cases by almost 2:1. Resection cures the hypertension in most cases and conservative resection has been effective in several cases. In no case has there been metastasis, local invasion, recurrence, multifocality, or bilaterality.

Gross pathology

Juxtaglomerular cell tumor is usually smaller than 3 cm and may not be visible when the renal capsule is stripped. Thus when a juxtaglomerular cell tumor is suspected, the specimen must be carefully dissected and any abnormal foci submitted for histopathologic examination. Larger tumors are sharply circumscribed and composed of rubbery gray-white tissue, sometimes containing small cystlike, smooth-walled cavities (Fig. 2-49).

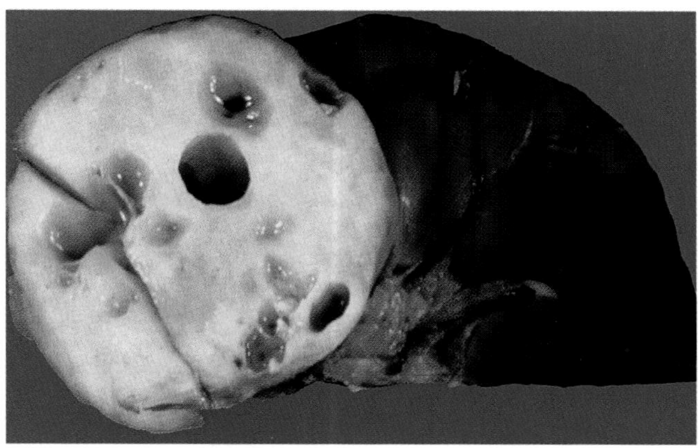

2-49. Juxtaglomerular cell tumor. A well-circumscribed nodule with scattered cysts.

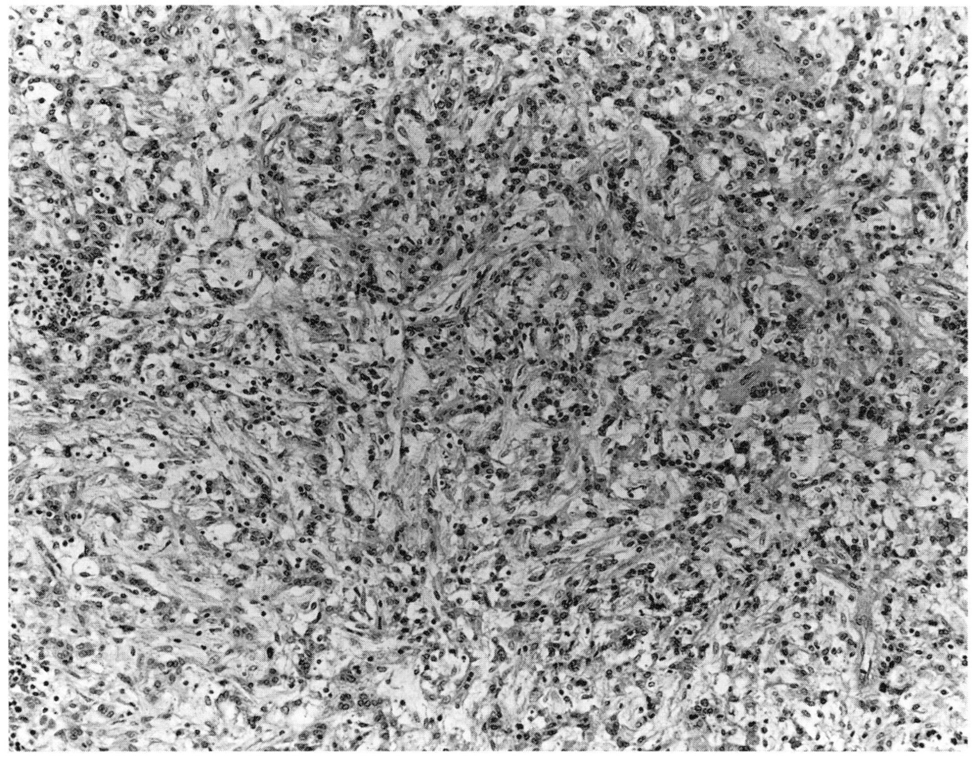

2-50. Juxtaglomerular cell tumor. Cords of cells in a loose stroma containing scattered lymphocytes.

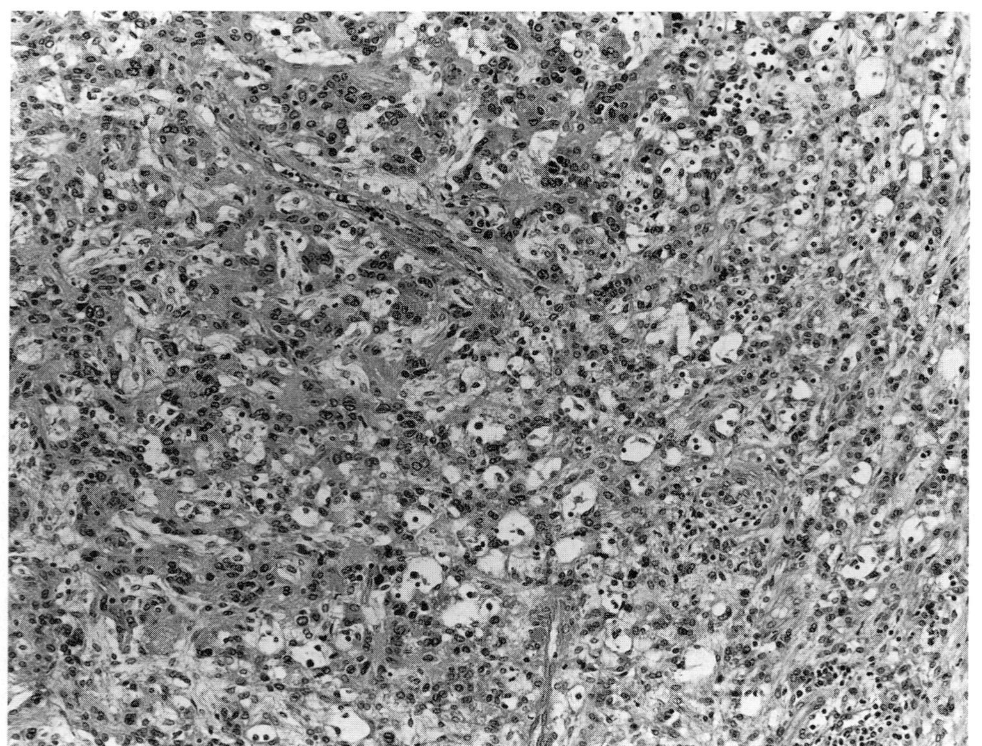

2-51. Juxtaglomerular cell tumor composed of cords of cells with lightly eosinophilic cytoplasm, numerous blood vessels, and scattered cells with clear cytoplasm.

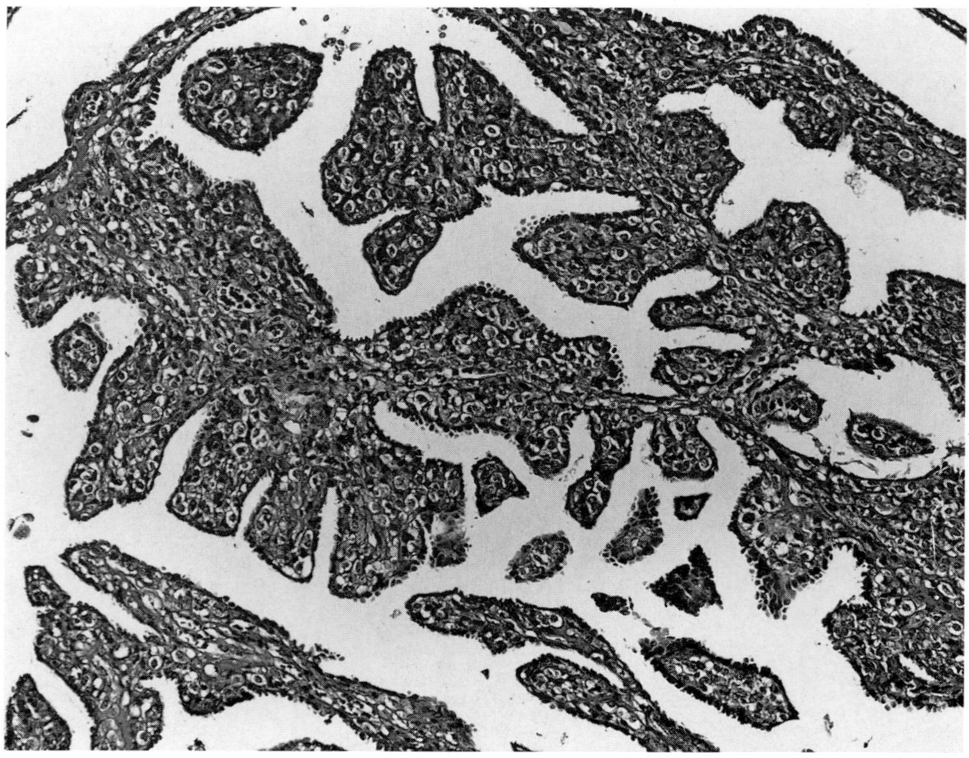

2-52. Juxtaglomerular cell tumor with papillary architecture and epithelioid cells with clear cytoplasm in the papillae.

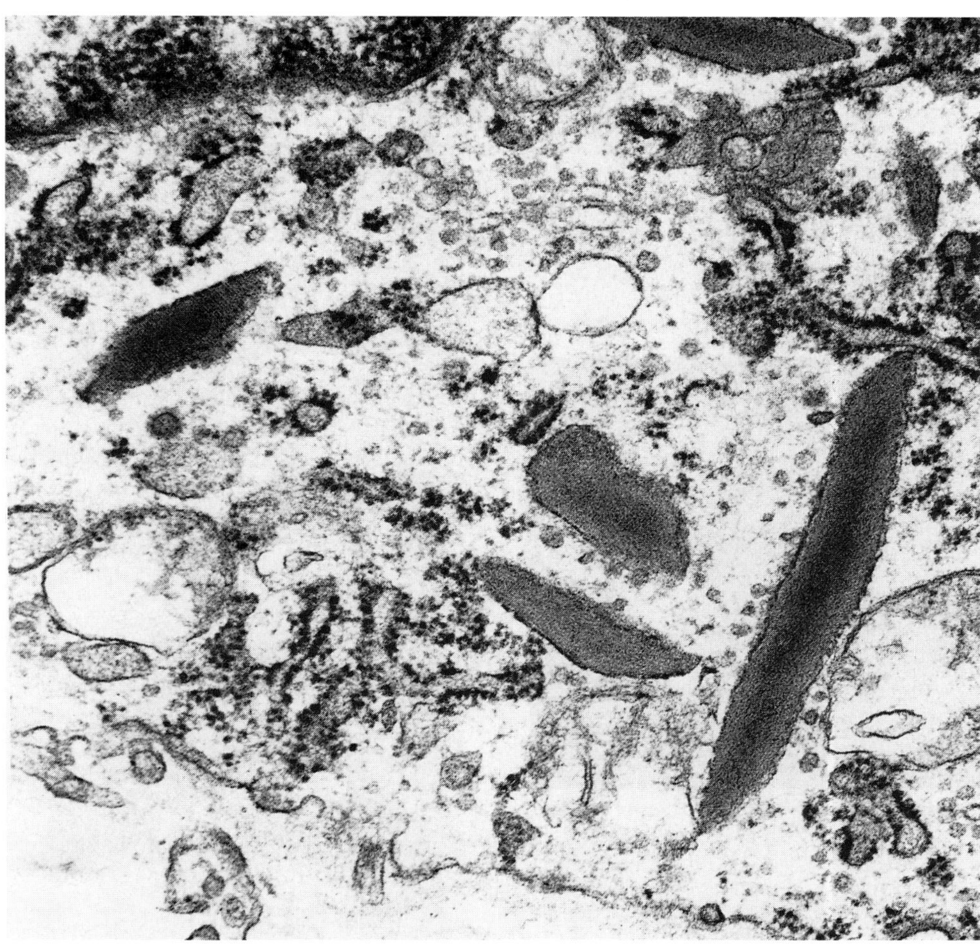

2-53. Juxtaglomerular cell tumor. Electron micrograph showing characteristic inclusions.

Microscopic pathology

The microscopic appearance of juxtaglomerular cell tumor is varied, and, without the history of hypertension in a young person, the diagnosis can be extremely difficult in routine sections. A common pattern is one of irregular trabeculae of polygonal cells in a loose myxoid stroma (Fig. 2-50, 2-51). Tubules and cysts often are present. There is frequently prominent vascularity and a lymphocytic infiltrate may be conspicuous. Islands of medium-sized round cells with pale cytoplasm and central nuclei, called *Spiegelei cells*, are often present and are diagnostically valuable (Fig. 2-51, 2-52). In a few cases, there have been broad papillae covered by epithelioid cells (Fig. 2-52).

The modified Bowie stain reveals intracytoplasmic granules and immunohistochemistry often demonstrates intracytoplasmic renin.[304,305] Electron microscopy is helpful in demonstrating the striking rhomboid granules of juxtaglomerular cell tumor (Fig. 2-53).[306]

Differential diagnosis

As it is almost invariably discovered in the investigation of hypertension, the nature of the tumor is often suspected preoperatively. The gross finding of a small light-colored rubbery tumor narrows the differential diagnosis. Since immunoreactive renin has been found in renal cell carcinoma and Wilms' tumor,[42,43,307] sometimes causing hypertension, these may rarely cause diagnostic confusion.

RENOMEDULLARY INTERSTITIAL CELL TUMOR

This small tumor of the renal medulla is a frequent finding at autopsy.[308] Ultrastructural and other studies have shown that it is composed of renomedullary interstitial cells that contain vasoactive substances important in the regulation of blood pressure.[309-311] Whether it is a neoplasm or a hyperplastic nodule that arises in response to hypertension remains controversial. It is rare in patients younger than 20 years, but in a large series of carefully dissected autopsy kidneys almost half the patients over 20 had at least one lesion and 57% of the patients with renomedullary interstitial cell tumor had more than one.[308]

Because this tumor is usually small, it rarely causes symptoms or diagnostic difficulty in surgical specimens. Most problems arise when the tumor is an unexpected finding in a kidney resected for other reasons, such as transplantation. The few symptomatic tumors have usually been pedunculated masses in the renal pelvis, and the early reports called them *renal pelvic fibroma*.[156]

Gross pathology

Renomedullary interstitial cell tumor is a well-circumscribed white nodule that occurs anywhere in the renal medulla (Fig. 2-54). The great majority are less than 5 mm in diameter.[312]

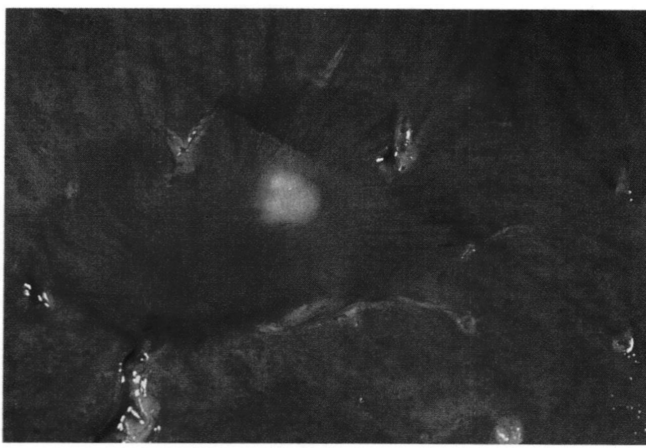

2-54. Renomedullary interstitial cell tumor consisting of a well-circumscribed white nodule in the renal medulla.

Microscopic pathology

Microscopically, small stellate cells lie in a faintly basophilic loose stroma, reminiscent of the stroma of the renal medulla. Bundles of loose fibers arranged in an interlacing pattern frequently are present (Fig. 2-55). The stromal matrix often entraps medullary tubules at the periphery of the nodules. The term *fibroma* is a misnomer since most of these lesions contain little collagen. Some do contain amyloid,[311] which may be deposited in irregular clumps, obscuring the characteristic delicate stroma.

CYSTIC NEPHROMA

Cystic nephroma, also called multilocular cyst[98] and multilocular cystic nephroma,[313,314] is an uncommon and controversial renal lesion that occurs both in adults and children.[315] Early criteria were designed to exclude developmental and other non-neoplastic lesions (see the box on this page).[313] With increasing recognition of cystic renal

CYSTIC NEPHROMA: DIAGNOSTIC CRITERIA

- Lesion must be multilocular
- Cysts are mostly lined by epithelium
- Cysts do not communicate with the renal pelvis
- Residual renal tissue is essentially normal
- Mature nephronic elements should be absent from septa

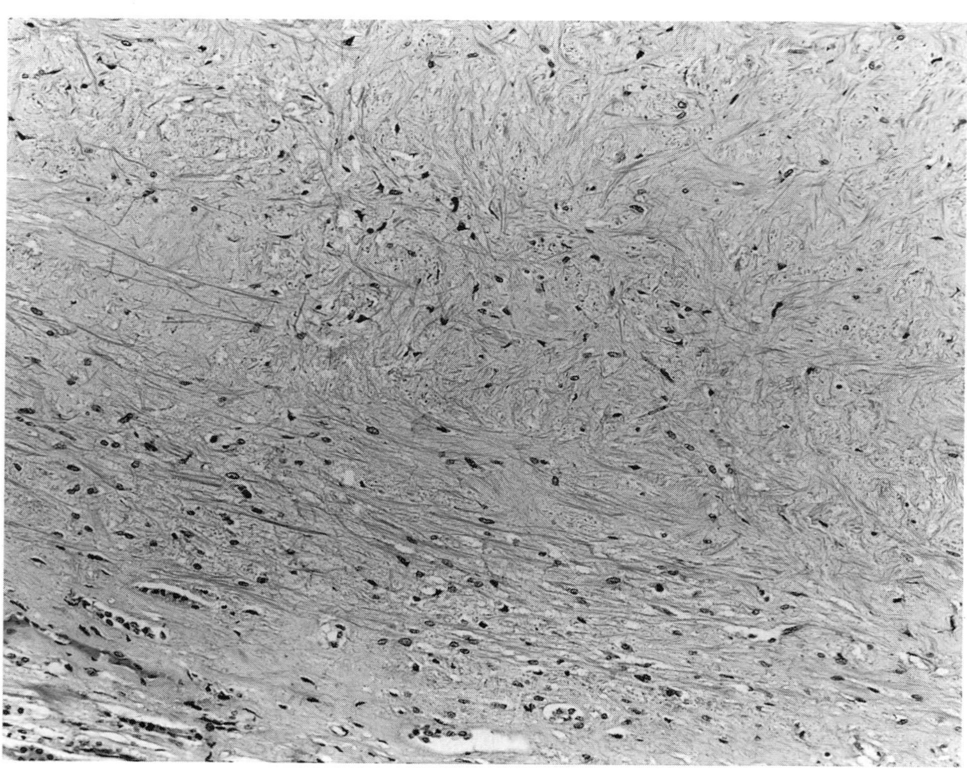

2-55. Renomedullary interstitial cell tumor consisting of delicate fibers containing scattered cells with elongate cytoplasmic processes.

cell carcinoma and cystic partially differentiated nephroblastoma, cystic nephroma has become rarer. Cystic nephroma is benign and effectively treated by conservative surgery.[316] Castillo et al.[316] reviewed 187 cases, including 29 from their own institution, and found a male predominance of almost 2:1 in patients younger than 2 years and a female predominance of more than 3:1 among adults (Table 2-7). Other studies have confirmed this.[93,317,318] Although the original definitions of this entity required unilaterality, bilateral lesions occur rarely.[319]

Gross pathology

Cystic nephroma is well circumscribed by a fibrous capsule and is composed of multiple noncommunicating locules that have smooth inner surfaces and contain clear yellow fluid (Fig. 2-56). Solid areas are absent or scant and the septa range from paper-thin to a few millimeters thick.

Microscopic pathology

Microscopically, the septa are composed of fibrous tissue that may contain foci of calcification (Fig. 2-57). Often the septa are densely collagenous, but they may be more cellular with a resemblance to ovarian stroma. The septa may contain differentiated tubules (as opposed to tubules with the morphology characteristic of Wilms' tumor), inflammatory cells, and reactive fibroblasts.[317] The cysts are usually lined by flattened or low cuboidal epithelium with small amounts of cytoplasm; occasionally the lining cells have a hobnail appearance.

Differential diagnosis

Cystic Wilms' tumor and cystic renal cell carcinoma are the principal differential diagnostic considerations clinically, radiographically, and pathologically. Although some authors consider tumors with intraseptal foci of immature renal tissues, including blastema and tubules, to be cystic nephroma, Joshi and Beckwith[317] designate these cystic partially differentiated nephroblastoma and when nodular solid areas of immature tissue are present, the tumor is a Wilms' tumor with multifocal cystic change. Review of the largest series of cystic nephroma and cystic partially differentiated nephroblastoma (Table

TABLE 2-7.
AGE AND GENDER DISTRIBUTION OF CYSTIC NEPHROMA

	0–4 Years		5–30 years		>30 years	
	Males	Females	Males	Females	Males	Females
Kajani[318]	4	5	1	0	2	9
Madewell[93]	22	8	0	4	2	18
Castillo[316]	38	25	0	4	2	18
Joshi[317]	16	4	0	1	0	0
Total	80	42	1	9	6	45

Excludes 59-year-old male from Kajani who had renal cell carcinoma.
Excludes four cases of sarcoma from Madewell.

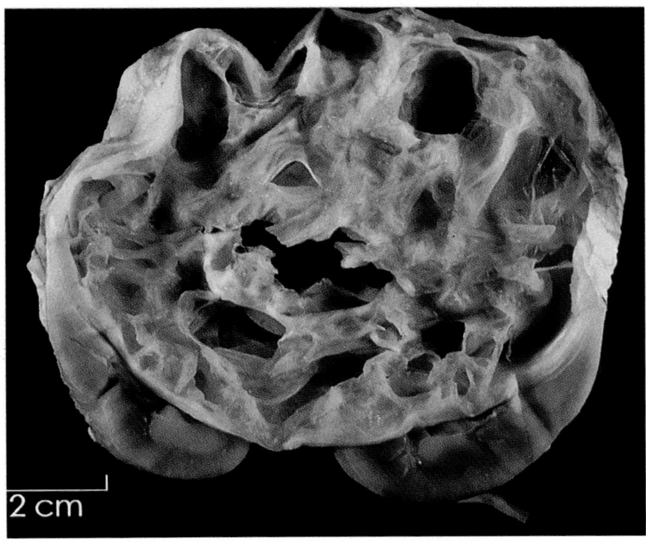

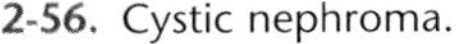
2-56. Cystic nephroma.

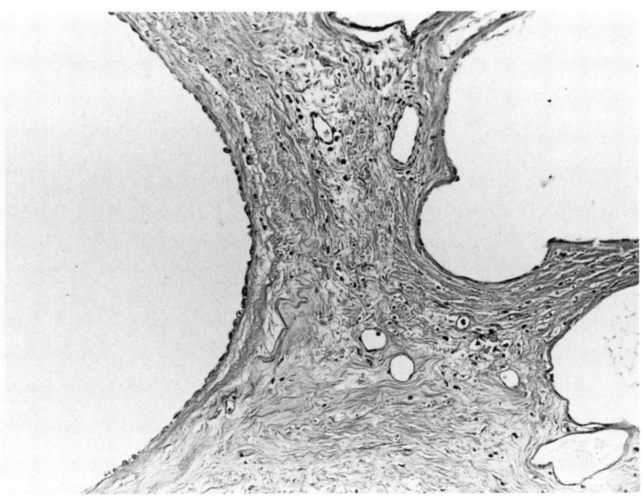

2-57. Cystic nephroma composed of multiple cysts separated by fibrous septa. The cysts are lined by atrophic and hobnail epithelium.

TABLE 2-8.
CYSTIC NEPHROMA AND CYSTIC PARTIALLY DIFFERENTIATED NEPHROBLASTOMA: BLASTEMA IN SEPTA

	0–4 Years Male	0–4 Years Female	5–30 Years Male and Female	>30 Years Male and Female
Kajani[318]	2/4	2/5	1/1	1/11
Madewell[93]	6/22	0/8	0/4	0/20
Castillo[316]	16/38	12/25	0/4	8/20
Joshi[317]	12/16	4/4	0/1	0/0
Total	36/80	18/42	1/10	9/51

2-8) shows that intraseptal blastema is rare in adults. If the single cases from the Castillo review of the literature[316] are excluded, then intraseptal blastema is almost unknown in adults. This, together with the predominance of females among adult patients, is strong evidence that cystic nephroma is a different entity from cystic partially differentiated nephroblastoma.

Multilocular cystic renal cell carcinoma differs from cystic nephroma in containing clear cells identical to those of clear cell renal cell carcinoma. These cells typically line some of the locules and may form small collections in the septa.[92]

The relationship of Wilms' tumor, cystic partially differentiated nephroblastoma, cystic nephroma, and multilocular cystic renal cell carcinoma remains incompletely understood and controversial.[315] A unifying concept links Wilms' tumor, cystic partially differentiated nephroblastoma, and cystic nephroma in a spectrum of differentiation within a family of tumors analogous to that of neuroblastoma, ganglioneuroblastoma, and ganglioneuroma.[317] Knowing that renal cell carcinoma arises in a variety of longstanding cystic diseases of the kidney, by analogy it is possible that renal cell carcinoma may in the same way occasionally arise in the cysts of cystic nephroma, accounting for some cases of multilocular cystic renal cell carcinoma.

METANEPHRIC ADENOMA AND NEPHROGENIC ADENOFIBROMA

Metanephric adenoma is a rare epithelial tumor of the kidney with features resembling the epithelial component of Wilms' tumor and the basophil end of the continuum of chromophil renal cell carcinoma. Individual cases and small series have been described under various names: metanephric adenoma,[320-322] néphrome néphrogène (nephrogenic nephroma),[323-325] metanephroider Nierentumor (metanephroid renal tumor),[326] and nephroblastomartiges Nierenadenom (nephroblastoma-like adenoma of the kidney).[327] Other examples have been described without offering a nosological innovation.[328,329] The tumors occur in children and adults and appear to be benign. Association with polycythemia has been observed in some cases.[329] A similar tumor with a fibromatous component has been called nephrogenic adenofibroma.[330]

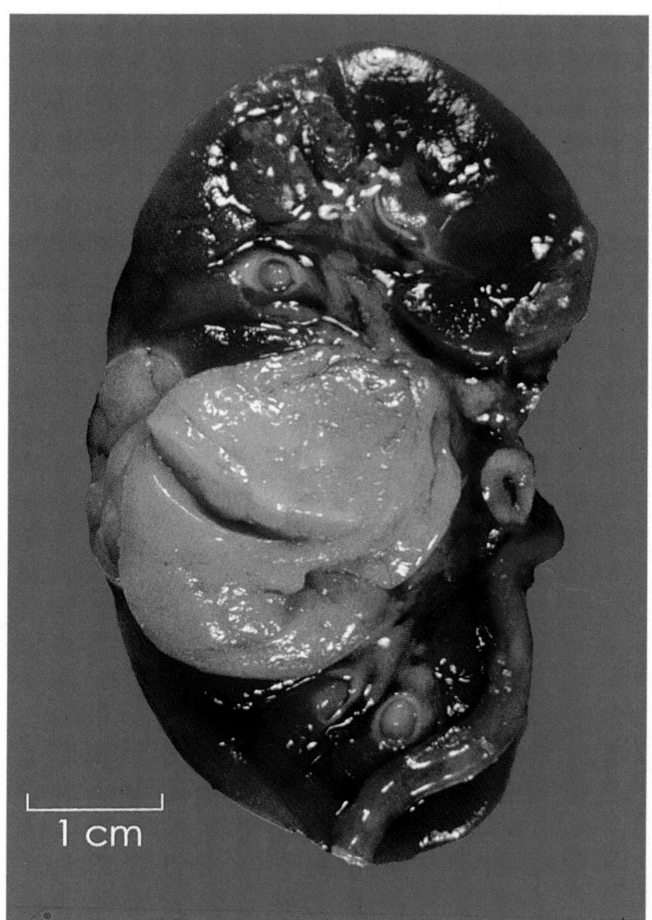

2-58. Metanephric adenoma.

Gross pathology

Metanephric adenoma is typically a sharply circumscribed solid mass, sometimes lobulated. The cut surface is tan, gray, or yellow (Fig. 2-58). Cysts are sometimes present, as are foci of hemorrhage and necrosis.

Microscopic pathology

This tumor is highly cellular and the dominant histologic feature is tightly packed small acini (Fig. 2-59). The cells have little cytoplasm (Fig. 2-60). The nuclei are

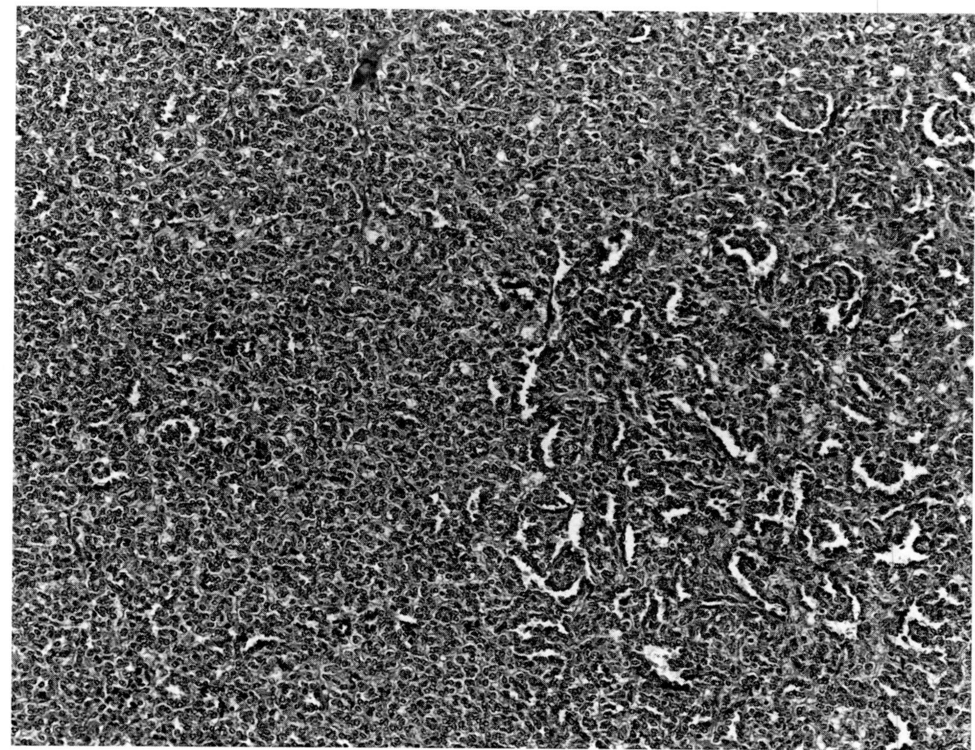

2-59. Metanephric adenoma composed of small tubules, some of which are tightly packed and appear solid.

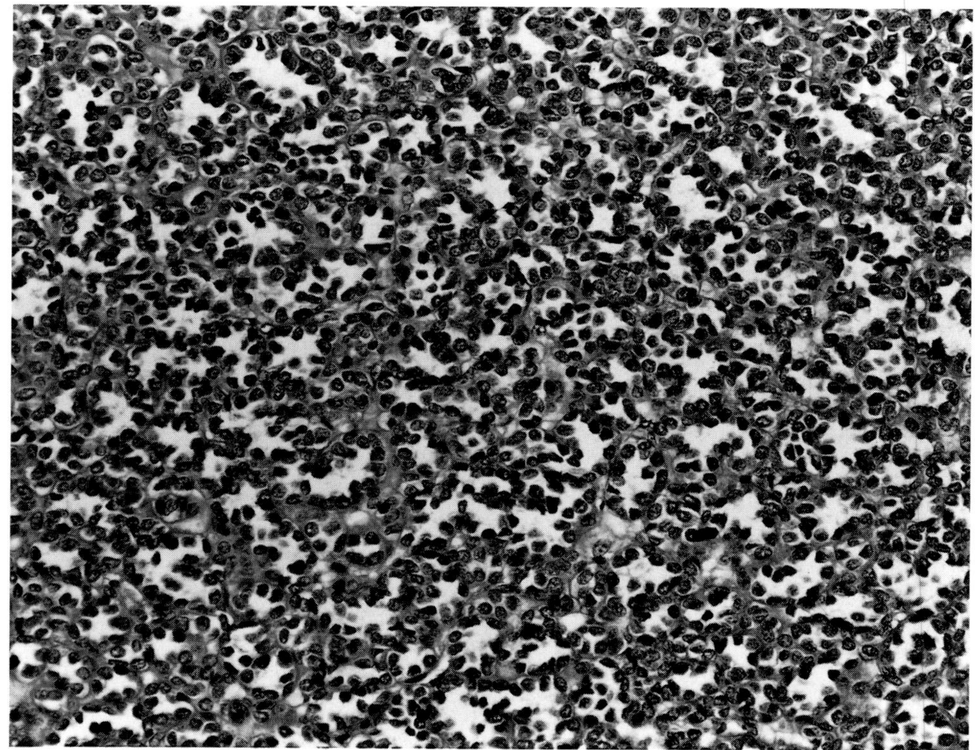

2-60. Metanephric adenoma. The cells have regular round nuclei and inconspicuous cytoplasm.

comparable in size to those of small lymphocytes and are oval with delicate chromatin. Nucleoli are small and inconspicuous. Papillary structures reminiscent of glomeruli are common and psammoma bodies are common. The border with the surrounding kidney is typically sharp.

LYMPHOMA

Secondary involvement of the kidney in cases of disseminated malignant lymphoma occurs in as many as 50% of cases. However, whether or not lymphoma occurs as a primary tumor in the kidney is controversial.[331] Rarely, lymphoma presents as a renal mass,[332-334] but in most cases extrarenal lymphoma has been discovered shortly thereafter.[331] The symptoms resemble those of renal cell carcinoma.[333]

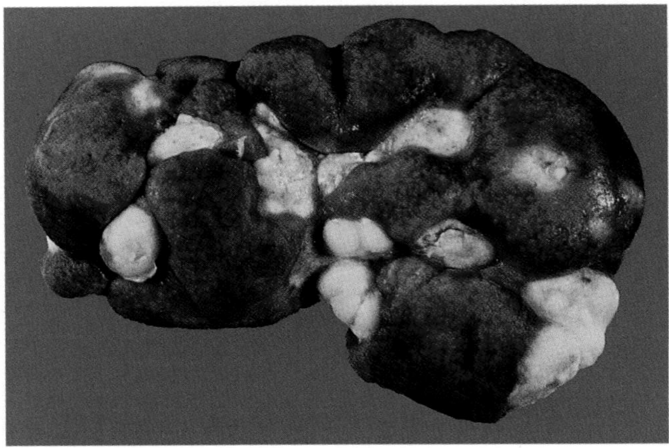

2-61. Renal lymphoma.

Gross pathology

The gross appearance of lymphoma in the kidney is variable. Frequently, the mass is parenchymal and circumscribed; less frequently, it is diffuse.[334] In the former case the lesions consist of whitish nodules in the kidney, typically visible on the cortical surface (Fig. 2-61). In the latter case the renal volume is expanded, and the cortex and medulla are pale and their junctions are obscured by the infiltrate. Lymphoma presenting as a renal mass often arises in the renal sinus, surrounding and invading the hilar structures.[334]

Microscopic pathology

The microscopic appearance varies according to the gross appearance and histologic type of lymphoma. Grossly, nodular lesions consist almost entirely of lymphoma cells microscopically. When there is diffuse infiltration, the renal interstitium is infiltrated by a monomorphous population of atypical lymphoid cells and there may be sparing of the glomeruli and tubules (Fig. 2-62). Among lymphomas presenting as renal primaries, large cell lymphoma is more common than small cell lymphoma[333,334] and Hodgkin's disease is unusual.[334] Plasmacytoma also occurs in the kidney.[335,336]

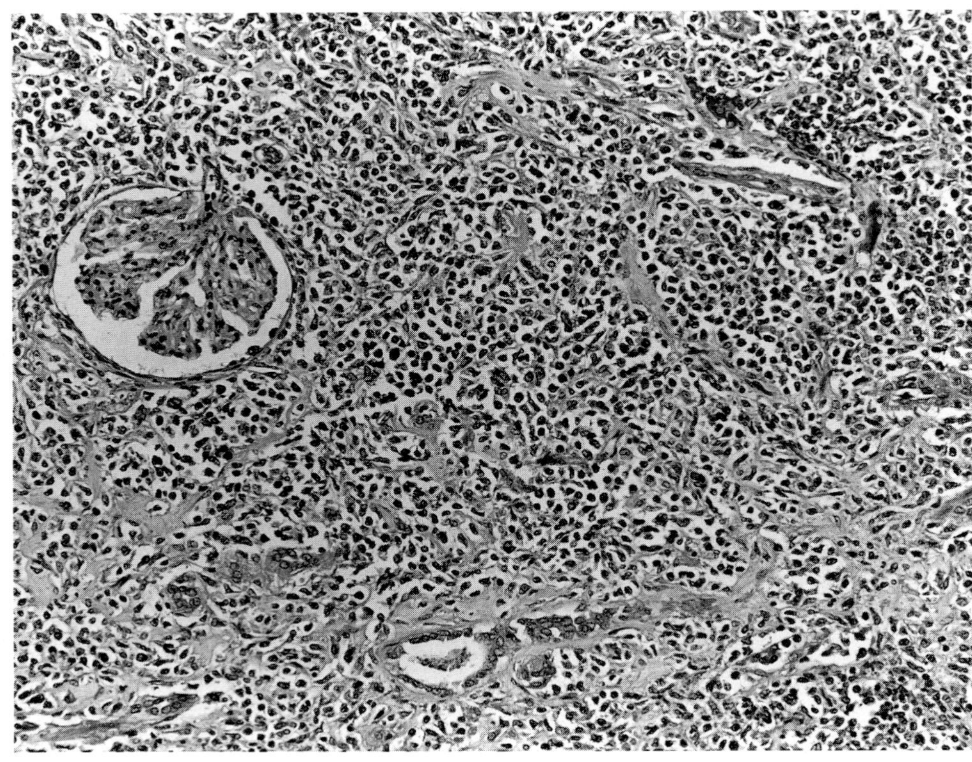

2-62. Small cell lymphoma infiltrating and expanding the renal interstitium with partial sparing of glomeruli and tubules.

METASTASIS TO THE KIDNEY

In a study of 11,328 autopsies of cancer patients, Bracken et al.[337] found that 7.2% of patients had metastases to the kidneys. These findings are supported by other studies.[338-341] Bronchogenic carcinomas are the most frequent source of metastatic carcinoma.[337,340] Rarely, metastases present as primary renal tumors and may be treated surgically for that mistaken diagnosis.[339] Solitary metastases may closely mimic primary renal neoplasms grossly,

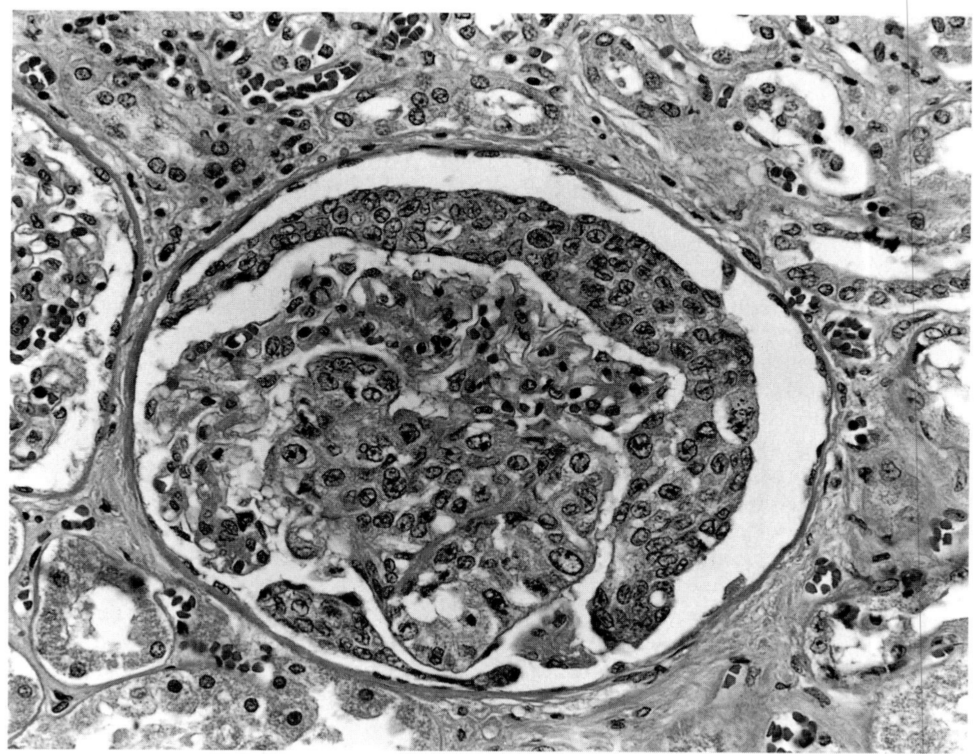

2-63. Pulmonary carcinoid metastatic to a glomerulus.

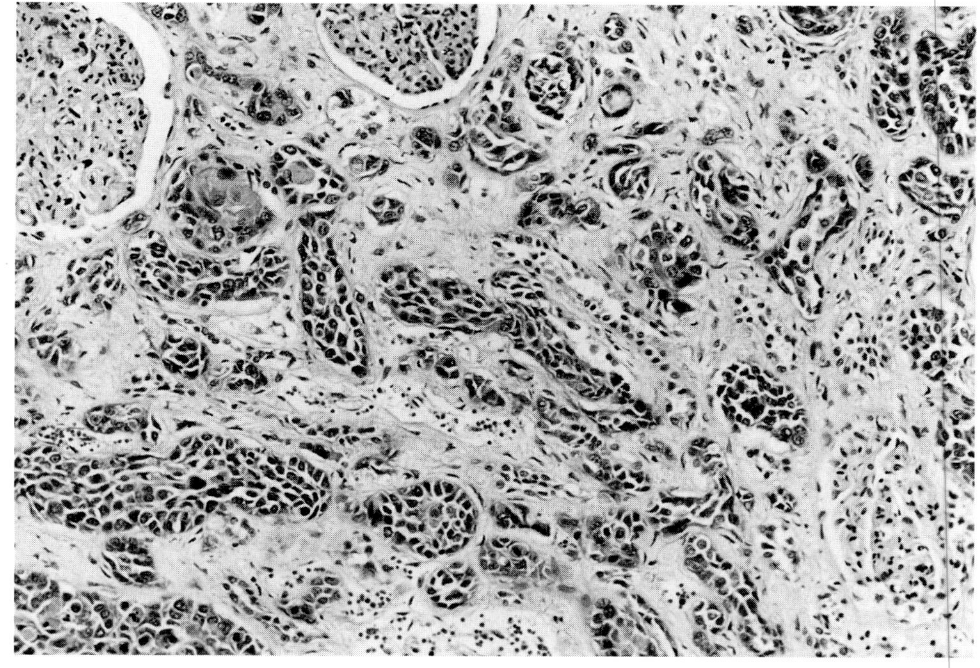

2-64. Pulmonary squamous cell carcinoma diffusely metastatic to renal lymphatics.

but microscopic examination usually clarifies the situation. Occasionally carcinoma metastatic to the kidney is found only as widespread microscopic metastases to the glomeruli[342] (Fig. 2-63) or diffusely to renal lymphatics[343] (Fig. 2-64).

RENAL TUMORS IN CHILDREN

Primary renal neoplasms are uncommon in children, with fewer than 500 new cases in the United States annually. However, they constitute the fifth most common group of pediatric cancers and are the second most frequent abdominal malignancy of children. The correct diagnosis and staging of pediatric renal neoplasms is of great clinical importance, particularly given the progress that has been made in the treatment of Wilms' tumor.[344-347] The variable and overlapping appearances of the tumors and their rarity make them an especially challenging group of lesions for the surgical pathologist.

The most common pediatric kidney tumor is Wilms' tumor, also called nephroblastoma. Clear cell sarcoma and rhabdoid tumor are important because of their poor response to therapy and consequent morbidity and mortality. In children younger than 3 months of age, mesoblastic nephroma is the most common renal neoplasm and usually has a favorable prognosis. A final rare tumor, ossifying renal tumor of infancy, is mentioned briefly in this section. Tumors that usually are found in adult kidneys (such as renal cell carcinoma, lymphoma, sarcoma, neuroendocrine tumors, and angiomyolipoma) occur rarely in children and do not in most instances differ pathologically from their counterparts in adults.

WILMS' TUMOR (NEPHROBLASTOMA)

Wilms' tumor comprises more than 80% of renal tumors of childhood.[348] It occurs most frequently in children 2 to 4 years old (median ages for boys and girls, respectively, are 36.5 and 42.5 months)[349] and is relatively uncommon in the first 6 months of life and in children older than 6 years.[350] Wilms' tumor is rare in the neonatal period.[351] The incidence of Wilms' tumor is about the same worldwide.[352] There is a slight preponderance of girls.[349] Wilms' tumor is bilateral in 4.4% of cases[353] and patients with bilateral tumors average more than a year younger than patients with unilateral tumors.[349] Associations with congenital anomalies, including cryptorchidism, hypospadias, other genital anomalies, hemihypertrophy, and aniridia, are recognized.[354] As many as 5% of patients with Beckwith-Wiedemann syndrome develop Wilms' tumor.[355] Patients with the Drash syndrome also have an increased risk of developing Wilms' tumor.[356] A variety of other malformations are less frequently associated with Wilms' tumor.[350,357] Uncommonly, Wilms' tumor has a familial association.[349] Wilms' tumors are rare in adults, and the stage at presentation and frequency of anaplasia are higher than in children and response to therapy correspondingly less.[358,359]

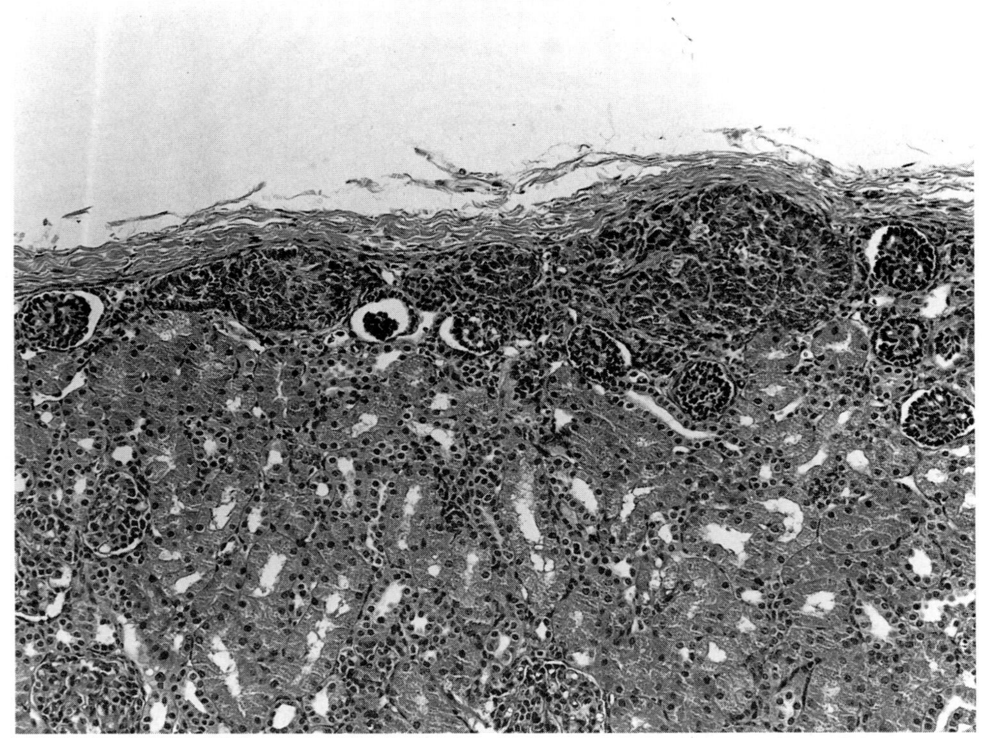

2-65. Nascent perilobar nephrogenic rest.

Nephrogenic rests and nephroblastomatosis

Aggregates of cells resembling blastema have been found in pediatric autopsies and in kidneys resected from patients with Wilms' tumors for decades.[360] Bove and McAdams[361] studied 69 kidneys resected for Wilms' tumors and observed microscopic nodules of blastemal cells in one third of the cases. From these observations they proposed a classification based on histologic features, including categories of nodular renal blastema, metanephric hamartoma, and others. Additional terminology accreted and the nomenclature became confusing.[348] Subsequently, Beckwith et al.[362] proposed a new classification based on the extensive case material of the National Wilms' Tumor Study Pathology Center (NWTS); the following discussion is based on that work.

Nephrogenic rests are foci of persistent nephrogenic cells resembling those of the developing kidney. These are divided into two categories: perilobar nephrogenic rests, which are located at the periphery of the renal lobes (the cortical surfaces, the centers of the Bertin's columns, and the tissue abutting the renal sinus), and intralobar nephrogenic rests, which are located in the cortex or medulla within the renal lobe. In addition to the location, perilobar nephrogenic rests differ from intralobar nephrogenic rests in having well-defined smooth borders, a predominance of blastema, and being often numerous or diffuse. Intralobar nephrogenic rests usually are single and mingle irregularly with renal parenchyma; stroma is usually the predominant element. Nephrogenic rests are subclassified histologically as dormant or nascent (Fig. 2-65); maturing, sclerosing, and obsolescent; hyperplastic; and neoplastic

TABLE 2-9.
CLASSIFICATION OF NEPHROGENIC RESTS

Type	Features
Dormant or nascent	Microscopic size, blastema predominant, mitotic figures rare
Maturing, sclerosing, and obsolescent	Differentiating stromal and epithelial cells, collagenization of stroma
Hyperplastic	Visible to naked eye, mixture of blastema with stromal and epithelial elements
Neoplastic	Visible to naked eye, appear to arise in a rest
Adenomatous	Mitotic figures uncommon
Nephroblastomatous	Mitotic figures common

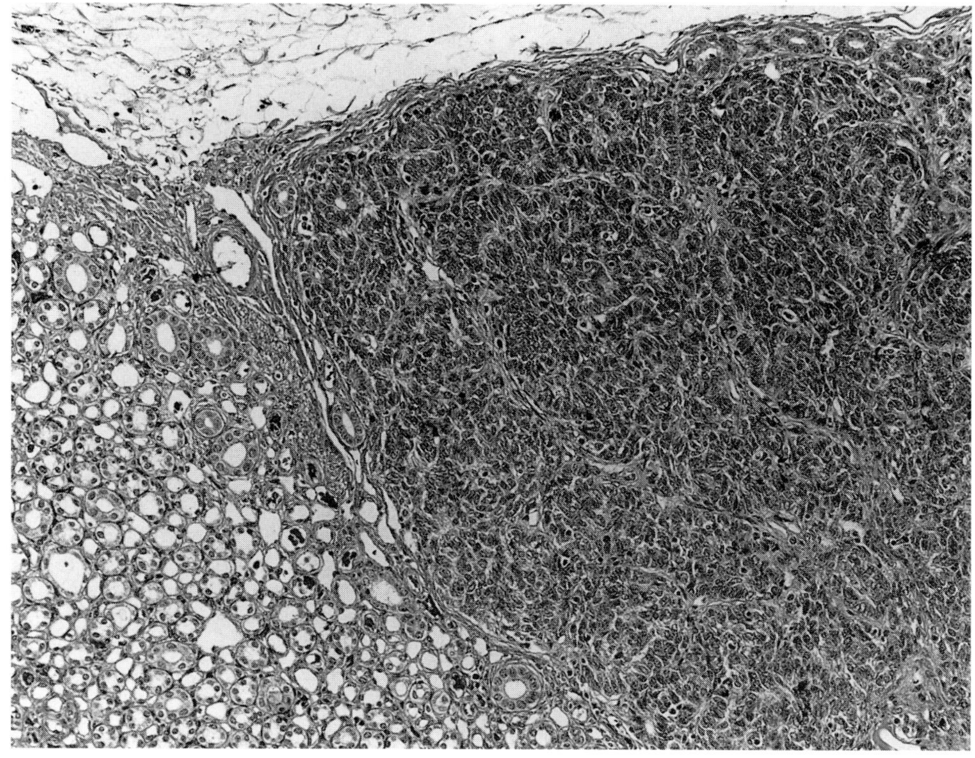

2-66. Hyperplastic perilobar nephrogenic rest.

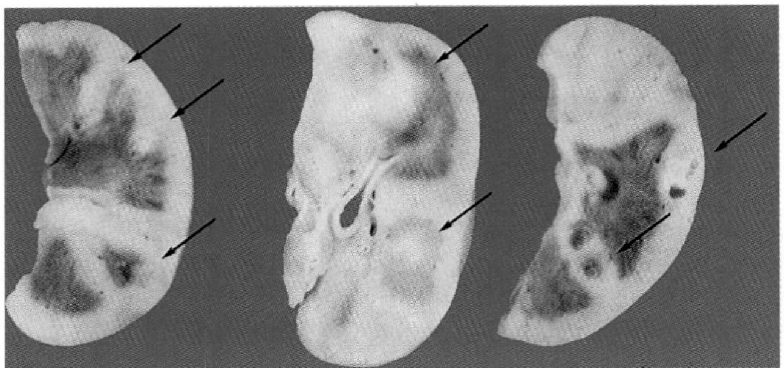

2-67. Nephroblastomatosis.

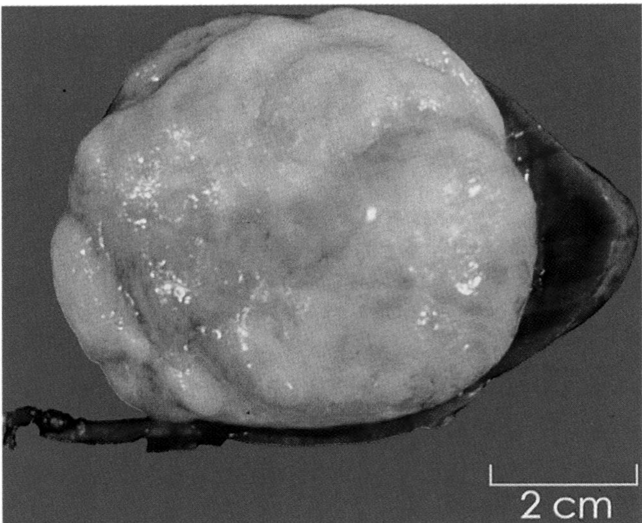

2-68. Wilms' tumor. A well-circumscribed spherical mass composed of tan tissue.

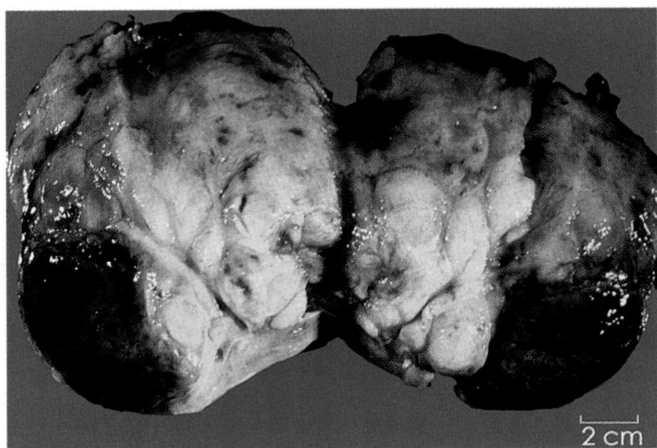

2-69. Wilms' tumor.

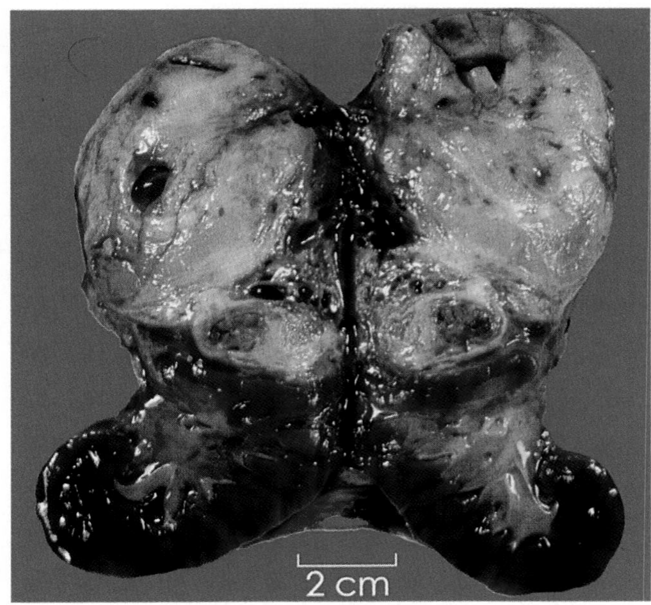

2-70. Wilms' tumor with scattered cysts.

(Fig. 2-66) (Table 2-9). Uncommonly, hyperplastic rests may diffusely replace much of the renal parenchyma. Nephroblastomatosis is defined as the diffuse or multifocal presence of nephrogenic rests (Fig. 2-67), or multicentric or bilateral Wilms' tumor.

Perilobar nephrogenic rests are present in approximately 1% of infants younger than 3 months,[2] a frequency two orders of magnitude greater than that of Wilms' tumor (1 per 10,000), while intralobar nephrogenic rests are almost never seen except with Wilms' tumor. Nephrogenic rests are extremely rare in adults.[363] In patients with unilateral Wilms' tumor, the NWTS found that perilobar and intralobar nephrogenic rests occur approximately equally frequently and are present in 41% of cases. However, nephrogenic rests are present in more than 95% of patients with synchronous or metachronous bilateral Wilms' tumor. Thus careful examination of the grossly uninvolved renal tissue is important in cases of Wilms' tumor, for the presence of nephrogenic rests indicates a greater probability of synchronous or metachronous bilaterality.

Gross pathology

Wilms' tumor is usually large, more than 5 cm in diameter, and one third or more are larger than 10 cm.[350] Often it weighs more than 500 g. The cut surface is typically solid, soft, and gray or pink resembling brain tissue (Fig. 2-68, 2-69). Foci of hemorrhage and necrosis are often present and cysts are common (Fig. 2-70). Rarely, it is extensively cystic (Fig. 2-71). The tumor usually is enclosed by a prominent pseudocapsule composed of compressed renal and perirenal tissues, giving an appearance of circumscription and even true encapsulation. Polypoid growth in the renal pelvic cavity, mimicking sarcoma botryoides, is a feature associated with extensive skeletal muscle differentiation[286,287,364,365] and may be mistaken for rhabdomyosarcoma.

Microscopic pathology

Wilms' tumor is typically composed of a variable mixture of blastema, epithelium, and stroma (Fig. 2-72, 2-73),

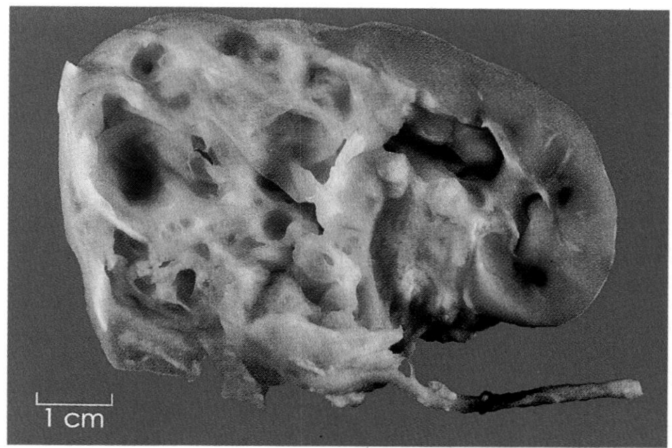

2-71. Cystic partially differentiated nephroblastoma.

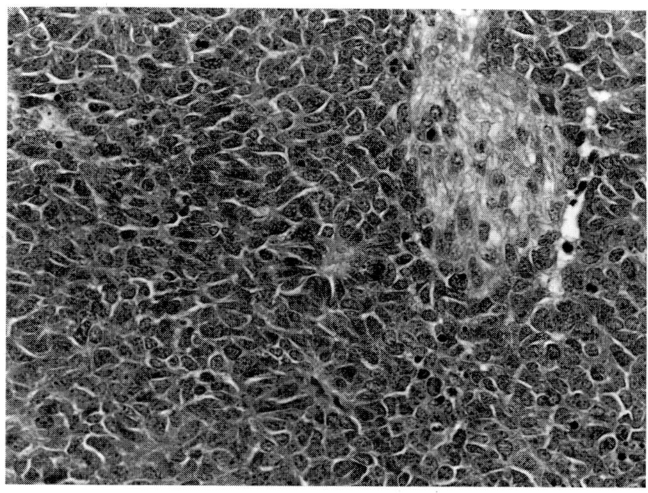

2-72. Wilms' tumor. Blastema and stroma.

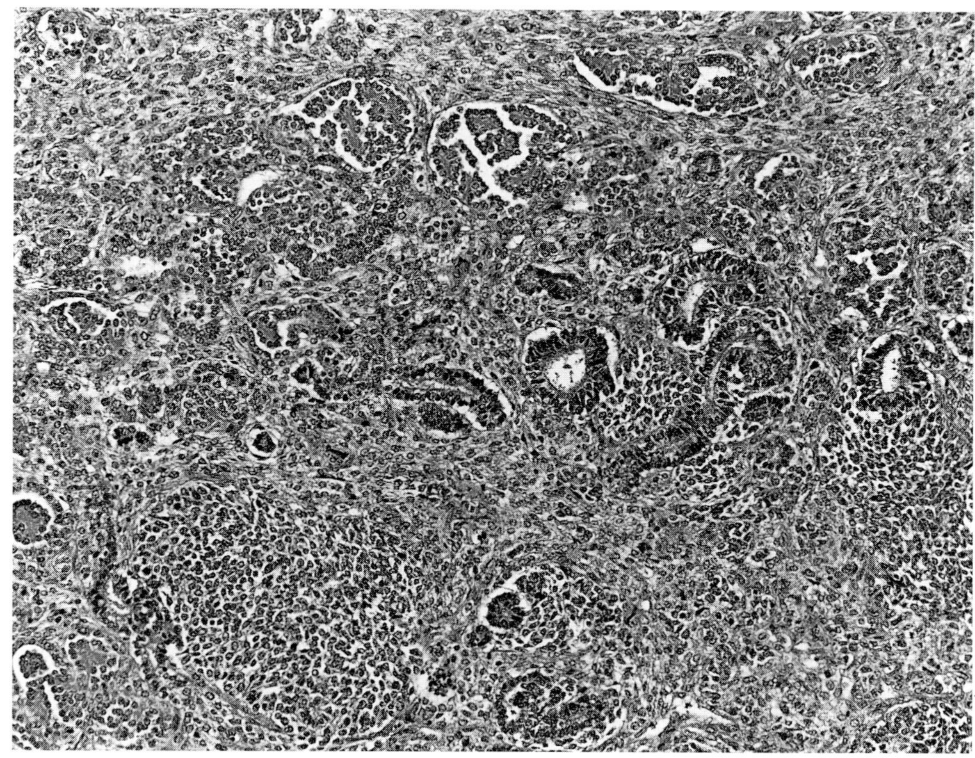

2-73. Wilms' tumor. Tubular and glomeruloid epithelial structures.

although in some tumors only one or two components are present. Blastema consists of sheets of randomly arranged, densely packed small cells with darkly staining nuclei, frequent mitotic figures, and inconspicuous cytoplasm, resembling other "small blue cell tumors" of childhood. Blastema is commonly arranged in three patterns: serpentine, nodular, and diffuse (Fig. 2-74). Serpentine and nodular are most common and diagnostically helpful, consisting of anastomosing serpiginous or spheroidal aggregates of blastema that are sharply circumscribed from the surrounding stromal elements.

The epithelial component usually consists of small tubules or cysts lined by primitive columnar or cuboidal cells (Fig. 2-73). The epithelium of Wilms' tumor may also form structures resembling glomeruli, or may display mucinous, squamous, neural,[366] or endocrine[367,368] differentiation.[102] Predominantly cystic Wilms' tumor (Fig. 2-71), which contain blastema and other Wilms' tumor tissues in their septa, are designated *cystic partially differentiated nephroblastoma*.[369,370]

The stroma of Wilms' tumor may differentiate along the lines of almost any type of soft tissue. Loose myxoid and

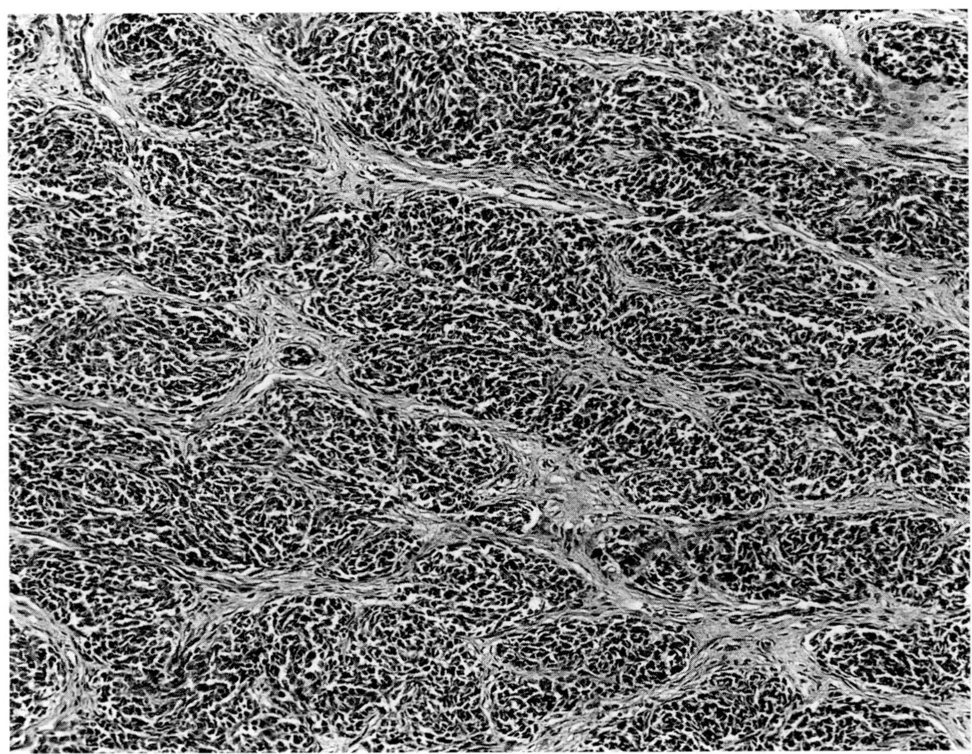

2-74. Wilms' tumor. Serpentine blastema.

fibroblastic spindle cell stroma are most common (Fig. 2-72), but smooth muscle, skeletal muscle, fat, cartilage, bone, and neural components also are present in some tumors.[102] Uncommonly, differentiation toward more mature soft tissue types is diffuse and predominant and such tumors have sometimes been given special names, such as *fetal rhabdomyomatous nephroblastoma*.[286,371] When complex combinations of differentiated epithelium and stroma are present, the term *teratoid Wilms' tumor* has been applied.[372-375]

Differential diagnosis

Cystic partially differentiated nephroblastoma grossly resembles cystic nephroma. Since the elements typical of Wilms' tumor may be inconspicuous, cystic renal tumors in children should be sampled extensively before cystic partially differentiated nephroblastoma is excluded.

Fetal rhabdomyomatous nephroblastoma has a favorable prognosis and should not be misinterpreted as rhabdomyosarcoma. This tumor contains extensive areas of relatively mature skeletal muscle but lacks the malignant small cells and rhabdomyoblasts found in rhabdomyosarcoma.

Monophasic epithelial Wilms' tumor can be difficult to distinguish from renal cell carcinoma, especially in adolescents and adults. Recognition of the nuclear characteristics typical of the epithelium of Wilms' tumor is often helpful. The epithelial nuclei in Wilms' tumor are often elongate or ovoid with molded, sometimes wedged shapes, which differ from those of renal cell carcinoma, which are usually nearly spherical.

The distinction of Wilms' tumor from rhabdoid tumor and clear cell sarcoma is discussed later in this chapter.

Grading, staging, and prognostic factors

Based on the results of the NWTS, Wilms' tumor is divided into categories of favorable and unfavorable histology, depending on the absence or presence of anaplasia. Anaplasia is found in approximately 6% of cases of Wilms' tumor. It is rare in patients younger than 1 year, and more than 80% of patients with anaplasia are older than 2 years.[376] Early in the NWTS, the presence of anaplasia was found to be predictive of treatment failure and death.[377] Even small foci of anaplasia can be associated with a poor response to therapy.[378] Thus it is important to sample Wilms' tumor specimens extensively. The NWTS recommends a minimum of one block of tumor for each centimeter of the largest diameter of the tumor, but this approach systematically samples small tumors much better than large ones. A better method is to sample in proportion to the weight of the tumor, and we suggest that one block be examined for every 20 grams of tumor.

Anaplasia has been defined by the NWTS as the combination of cells with very large hyperchromatic nuclei and multipolar mitotic figures. Correct recognition of anaplasia demands good histological preparations, including proper fixation, sectioning, and staining. The enlarged nuclei must be at least three times as large as typical blastemal nuclei in both axes, and the hyperchromasia must be obvious (Fig. 2-75). In addition to the

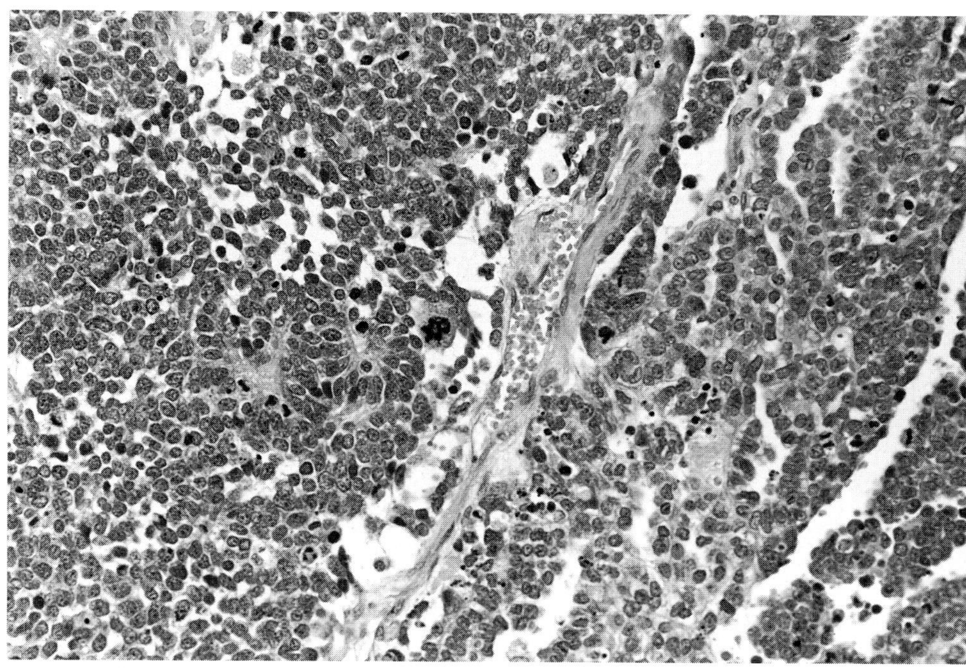

2-75. Wilms' tumor. Anaplasia.

enlarged nuclei, hyperdiploid mitotic figures must be present.

Several points should be borne in mind when evaluating a Wilms' tumor for anaplasia. First, enlarged nuclei in skeletal muscle fibers in the stroma of Wilms' tumors are not evidence of anaplasia. Second, the criteria for abnormal hyperdiploid mitotic figures are quite strict, demanding not only structural abnormalities but also enlargement of the mitotic figure as evidence of hyperploidy. Occasionally, mitotic figures of normal ploidy appear multipolar due to artifact, but these are much smaller than the hyperploid mitotic figures of anaplasia; comparison with the normal-sized mitotic figures in blastema elsewhere in the tumor facilitates this determination.

The NWTS has established a staging scheme for Wilms' tumor and other pediatric renal malignancies (Table 2-10). The tabular presentation, however, does not do justice to the challenges that staging presents to the surgical pathologist. Stage I requires assessment of the renal sinus and capsule. The renal sinus is the space within the kidney extending from the plane defined by the medial-most limits of the cortex (the hilar plane) laterally to the limits of the space between the medullary pyramids and contains the major branches of the renal artery and vein and the bulk of the renal pelvis. Unfortunately, Wilms' tumor usually distorts the renal contour to such an extent that the hilar plane is not readily discernible. In this situation microscopic recognition of renal sinus invasion in multiple blocks is justification for assuming that the hilar plane has been crossed and assigning stage II. On the other hand, sinus invasion must be true infiltration; bulging or herniation of encapsulated tumor into the sinus or renal pelvis does not constitute sinus invasion. Stage I also requires evaluation of the renal capsule, but this is often difficult, because, as a renal neoplasm grows, it sequentially is surrounded by an intrarenal pseudocapsule, the renal capsule, a pseudocapsule external to the kidney, Gerota's fascia, and the ultimate limits of the specimen. These layers frequently fuse, confusing the identification of the true renal capsule. When Wilms' tumor invades perirenal fat, it may destroy the fat cells and a fibrous response may give the appearance of stage I limitation by the renal capsule. If the renal capsule can be identified, it is the structure that must be used for staging. When the renal capsule is continuous with the soft tissue of Gerota's fascia, this layer must be used for staging. The presence of an inflammatory pseudocapsule beyond the renal capsule is currently not sufficient justification for assigning stage II but has been shown to be associated with an increase in the rate of relapse.[379] Stages II and IV are more straightforward as shown in Table 2-10. For stage V the most advanced individual tumor should be assigned a substage according to the stage it would have been assigned had it occurred alone, for example Stage V, Substage I.

MESOBLASTIC NEPHROMA

Although comprising less than 3% of primary renal tumors in children, mesoblastic nephroma is the predominant renal neoplasm in the first 3 months of life and is uncommon after 6 months.[351,380] Polyhydramnios and prematurity are associated with this tumor.[381,382] An abdominal mass is almost always the presenting finding. First recognized in 1966,[383] subsequent studies[384] have shown mesoblastic nephroma to be a morphologically distinct tumor with a good prognosis. The vast majority of patients are cured by surgical resection.[385-387] A few recurrences and adverse outcomes have been recorded, principally in patients older than 3 months at presentation.[388,389]

TABLE 2-10.
NATIONAL WILMS' TUMOR STUDY SYSTEM FOR STAGING PEDIATRIC RENAL TUMORS

Stage	Extent of Tumor
STAGE I	Tumor is confined to kidney and completely resected. **Specific Criteria:** The renal capsule is not penetrated by the tumor. Extension into the renal sinus does not go beyond the hilar plane. There is no lymphatic or hematogenous spread.
STAGE II	Tumor extends locally outside the kidney but is completely resected. **Specific Criteria:** The renal capsule is penetrated by tumor. Extension into the renal sinus goes beyond the hilar plane. The renal vein contains tumor. Local spillage or biopsy involves only the flank. Specimen margins are free of tumor and no residual tumor remains after surgery.
STAGE III	There is residual tumor confined to the abdomen without hematogenous spread. **Specific Criteria:** Spillage diffusely contaminates the peritoneum. There are tumor implants on the peritoneal surface. The specimen margins contain tumor. Abdominal lymph nodes contain tumor.
STAGE IV	There are blood-borne metastases.
STAGE V	Tumors are present in both kidneys.

This tumor is very rare in adults.[390-392] Mesoblastic nephroma has infiltrative borders that must be studied carefully by the surgical pathologist, because the risk of recurrence appears to be dependent on the completeness of the resection.[393,394] Metastasis is rare.[395]

Gross pathology

Mesoblastic nephroma is usually large relative to the infant's kidney. Externally, the surface of the tumor and kidney is smooth and the renal capsule and calyceal systems are stretched over the tumor. The surface may be bosselated. The cut surface resembles that of a leiomyoma: firm, whorled or trabeculated, and light colored (Fig. 2-76).[396] The tumor is unencapsulated, typically interdigitates with the surrounding kidney, and may extend into surrounding tissues. Renal vein invasion also occurs occasionally.[396] Cysts, hemorrhage, and necrosis are present in a minority of cases, particularly those that are cellular on microscopic examination.[396]

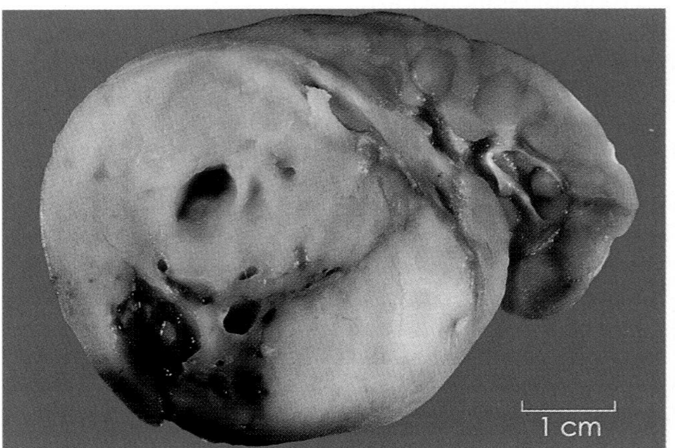

2-76. Mesoblastic nephroma.

Microscopic pathology

The classical pattern of mesoblastic nephroma described by Bolande et al.[384] is a moderately cellular proliferation of thick interlacing bundles of spindle cells with elongate nuclei that usually infiltrate renal and perirenal tissues (Fig. 2-77, 2-78). Entrapment of glomeruli and renal tubules is common. Mitotic figures are usually in the range of 0 to 1 per 10 high power

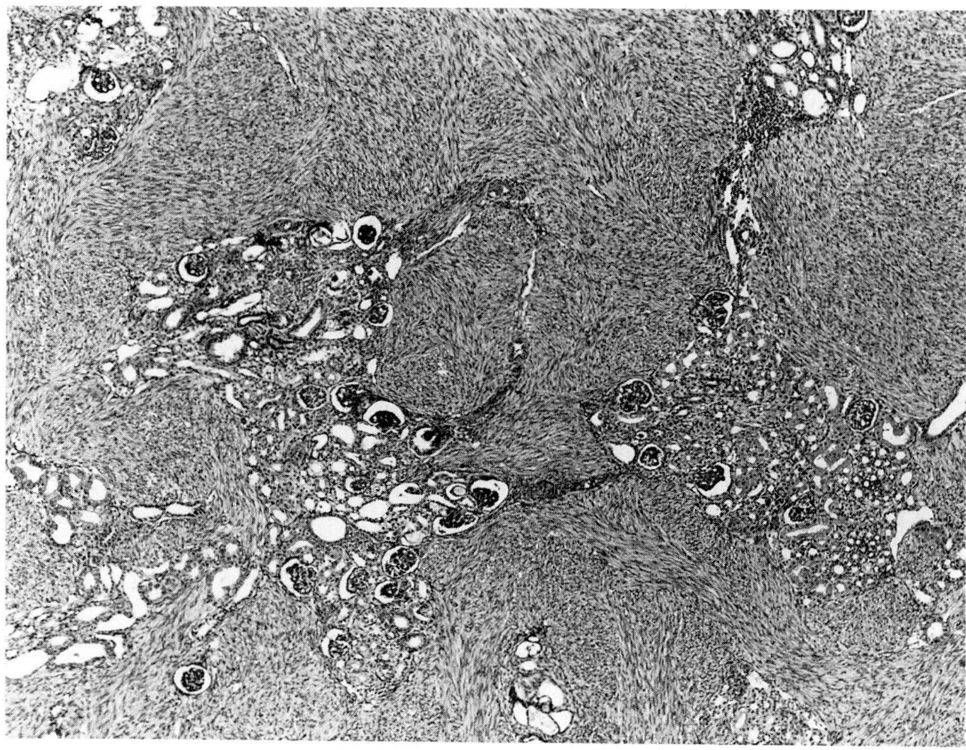

2-77. Mesoblastic nephroma. Classic type, composed of elongate spindle cells and infiltrating between renal structures.

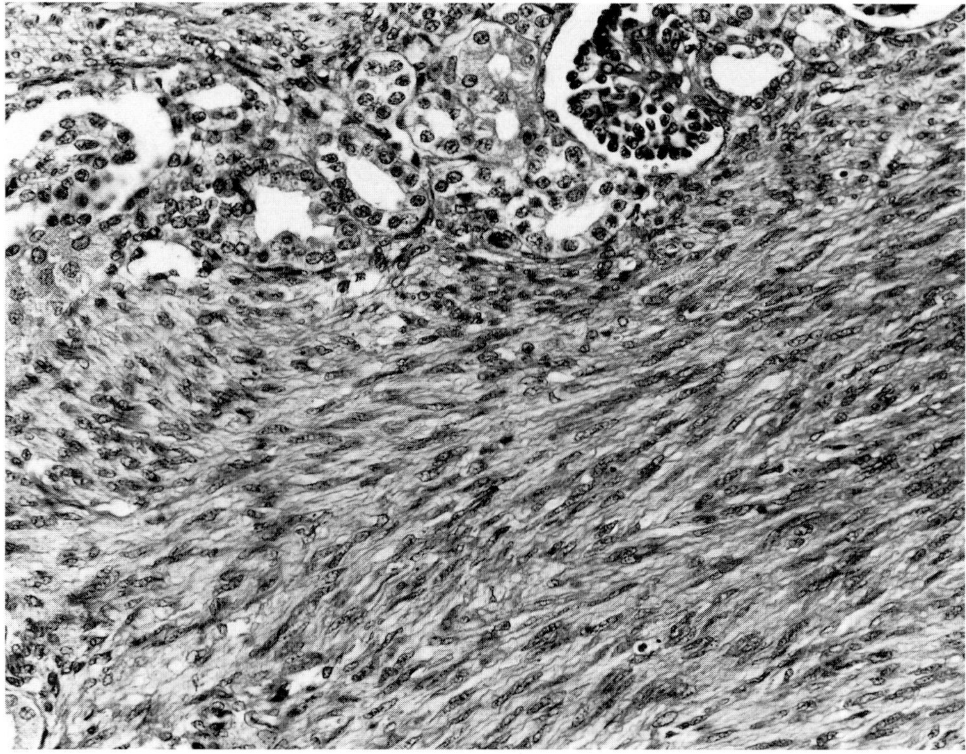

2-78. Mesoblastic nephroma, classic type. The spindle cells have elongate nuclei and delicate fibrillar cytoplasm.

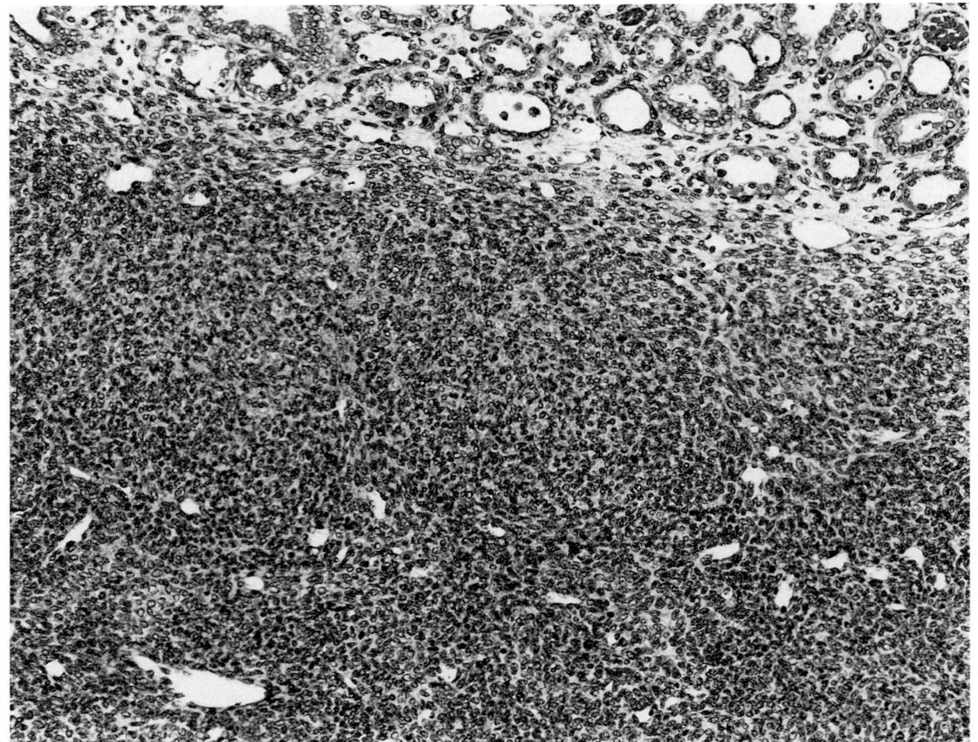

2-79. Mesoblastic nephroma, cellular type. The cells are polygonal and the border with the kidney is less infiltrative than is typical of the classic type.

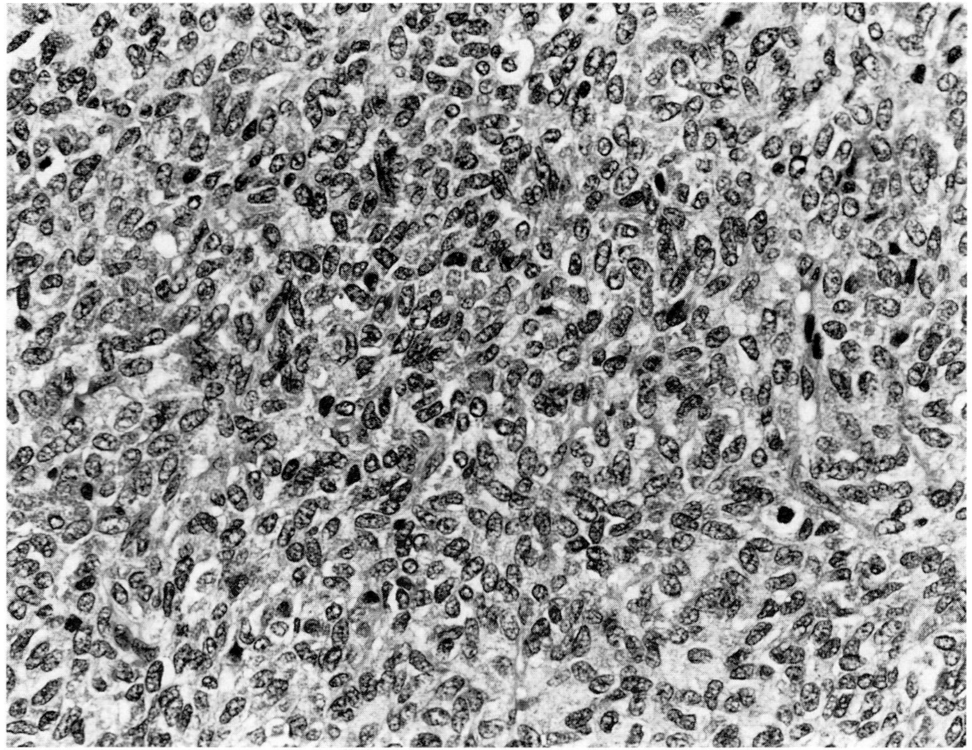

2-80. Mesoblastic nephroma, cellular type. The cells are densely packed, have short spindle shapes or are polygonal.

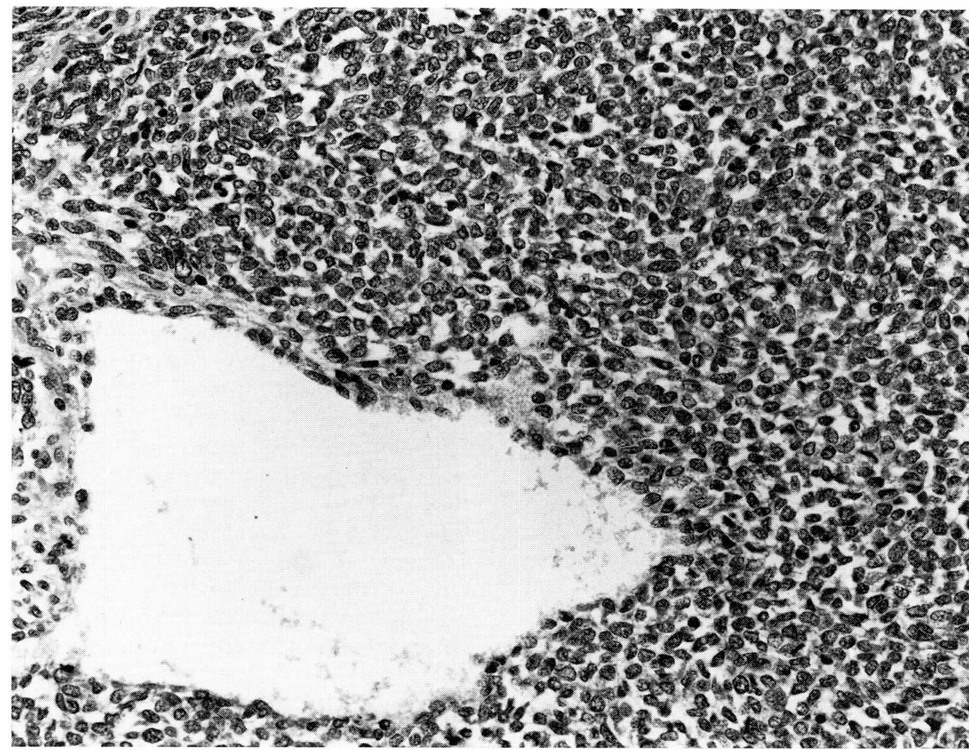

2-81. Mesoblastic nephroma, cellular type. A small cyst arises abruptly, without lining epithelium, in the midst of the tumor.

fields.[396] Islands of cartilage and foci of extramedullary hematopoiesis are present in some tumors.

Another more common pattern was recognized later and consists of a densely cellular proliferation of polygonal cells with mitotic figures in the range of 8 to 30 per 10 high power fields, and often pushing borders (Fig. 2-79, 2-80). This pattern has been called *cellular mesoblastic nephroma*.[397] Cysts are common in this pattern (Fig. 2-81). The classical and cellular patterns often are mixed in the same tumor. Some reports have suggested that the cellular pattern is prone to recurrence, but, as noted above, age and completeness of resection appear to be the primary risk factors for adverse outcome. In view of the generally favorable outcome for patients with mesoblastic nephroma and the predominance of lesions containing the cellular pattern, the histological pattern should not be a primary indication for therapy beyond adequate surgical resection. In adults, mesoblastic nephroma is virtually always of the classical pattern.

Differential diagnosis

Mesoblastic nephroma usually is easily diagnosed when the histology and patient age are considered. Wilms' tumor with stromal predominance may be confused with mesoblastic nephroma, particularly Wilms' tumor that has been treated preoperatively. This problem can usually be resolved by the identification of blastema that is not found in mesoblastic nephroma; also, Wilms' tumor usually has sharply circumscribed borders, whereas those of mesoblastic nephroma often are infiltrative. Age assists in making the correct diagnosis, and bilaterality favors Wilms' tumor. Although both occur in the same age group, mesoblastic nephroma, even the cellular variant, and rhabdoid tumor are usually easily distinguished.

CLEAR CELL SARCOMA OF KIDNEY

Originally called *bone-metastasizing renal tumor of childhood* by Marsden et al.,[398] clear cell sarcoma[399] is a highly malignant neoplasm resistant to conventional therapy for Wilms' tumor but often responsive to doxorubicin-containing regimens. Thus it is of considerable therapeutic importance that clear cell sarcoma be correctly diagnosed. Occurring in the same general age range as Wilms' tumor, clear cell sarcoma comprises approximately 6% of pediatric renal tumors.[400] Most are diagnosed in patients between 12 and 36 months of age. Approximately 66% of the patients are male. The propensity for metastasis to bone is marked; it is at least 10 times more likely to metastasize to bone than other pediatric renal cancers.

Gross pathology

The appearance of the cut surface of this tumor is variable: it may be homogeneous, gray and lobular or variegated, including firm gray whorled tissue and light pink soft areas (Fig. 2-82).[401] Occasionally the tumor may produce abundant mucin, which gives a slimy, glistening appearance. Most appear well circumscribed. Cysts ranging from a few millimeters to centimeters in diameter are present in approximately one third of cases.[401] Often the tumor weighs more than 500 g.[401] Bilaterality has not been reported.[348]

Microscopic pathology

At low magnification, clear cell sarcoma of kidney usually consists of a monotonous sheet of cells with lightly staining cytoplasm. At higher magnification, it is apparent that the cells are arranged in cords separated by septa composed of spindle cells with dark nuclei and a distinctive branching pattern of small blood vessels (Fig. 2-83).[402] The cells in the cords have pale or vacuolated cytoplasm and indistinct borders (Fig. 2-83). Despite the name, the cytoplasm of clear cell sarcoma is usually much less clear than that of clear cell renal cell carcinoma and cytoplasmic clarity should not be relied on to establish the diagnosis. The nuclei contain finely dispersed chromatin and the nucleoli are small. These nuclear characteristics are helpful in distinguishing clear cell sarcoma from rhabdoid tumor (see later in this chapter). A characteristic feature is the infiltrative border between the clear cell sarcoma and the surrounding renal parenchyma; renal tubules are frequently seen surrounded by the sarcoma.[401] Confusing variations on the classical appearance occur, including spindle cell, cystic, hyaline sclerosis, and palisade (Fig. 2-84, 2-85, 2-86).[102] The tumor should be sampled generously to find areas in which the septal vascular pattern and finely dispersed chromatin and small nucleoli in the nuclei of the cord cells indicate the correct diagnosis.

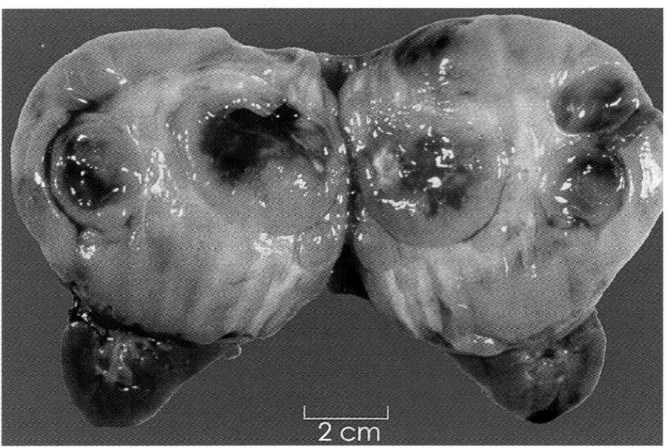

2-82. Clear cell sarcoma of kidney.

Differential diagnosis

In distinguishing clear cell sarcoma of kidney from Wilms' tumor, some pertinent negatives are important: blastema is not found in clear cell sarcoma; nonrenal elements such as cartilage or muscle are not found in

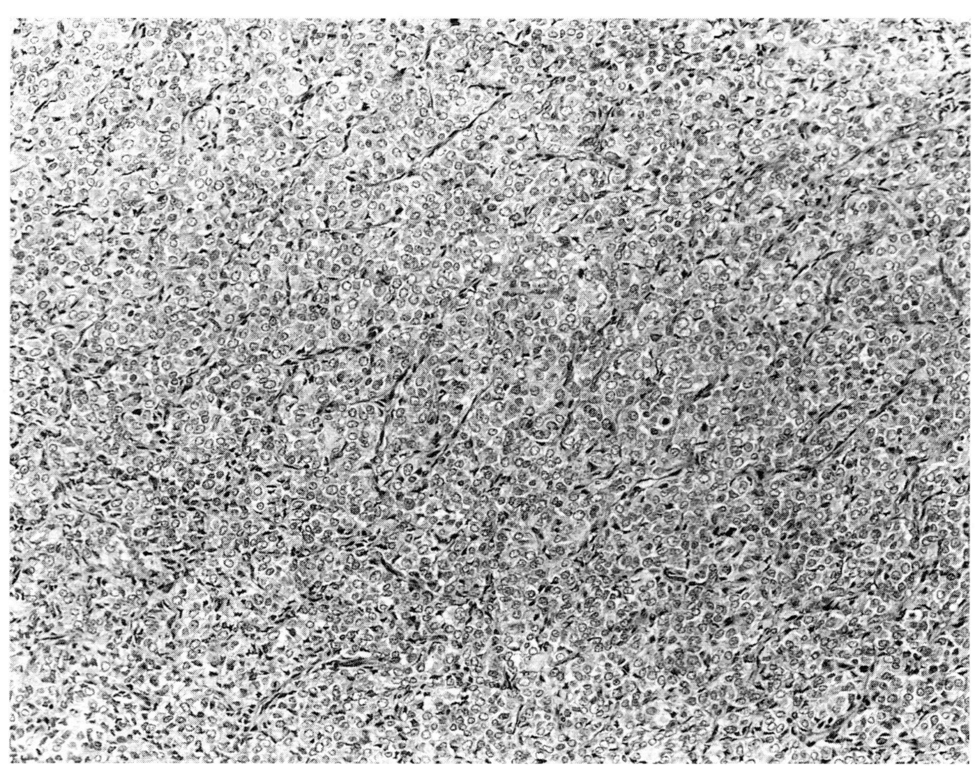

2-83. Clear cell sarcoma of kidney. The typical pattern is composed of cords of cells with pale cytoplasm divided by a "chicken wire" pattern of septa composed of spindle cells with dark nuclei and small blood vessels.

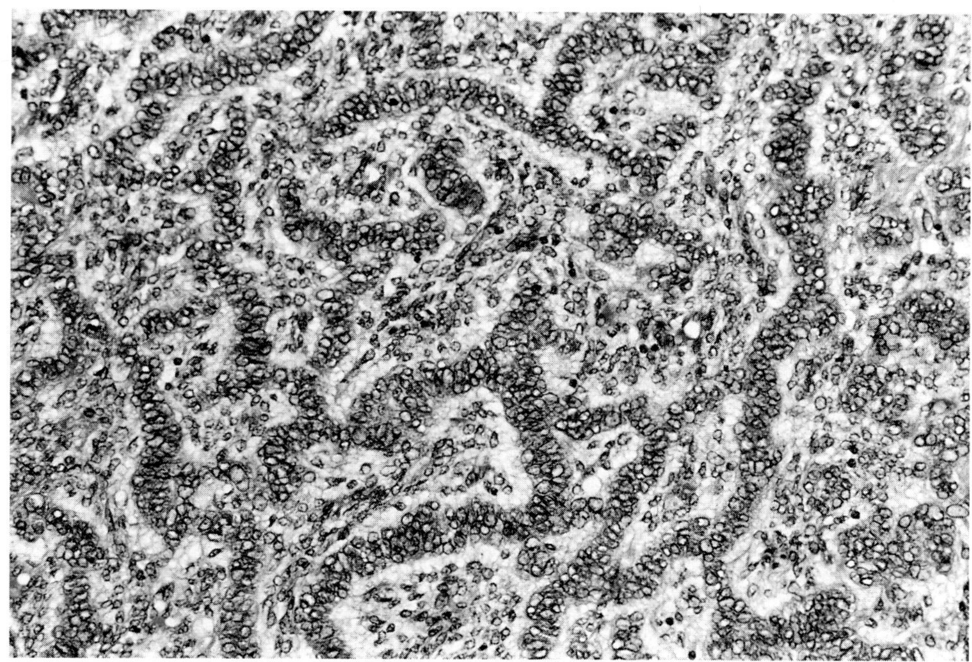

2-84. Clear cell sarcoma of kidney. The septa are expanded and more cellular, compressing the cords into ribbons.

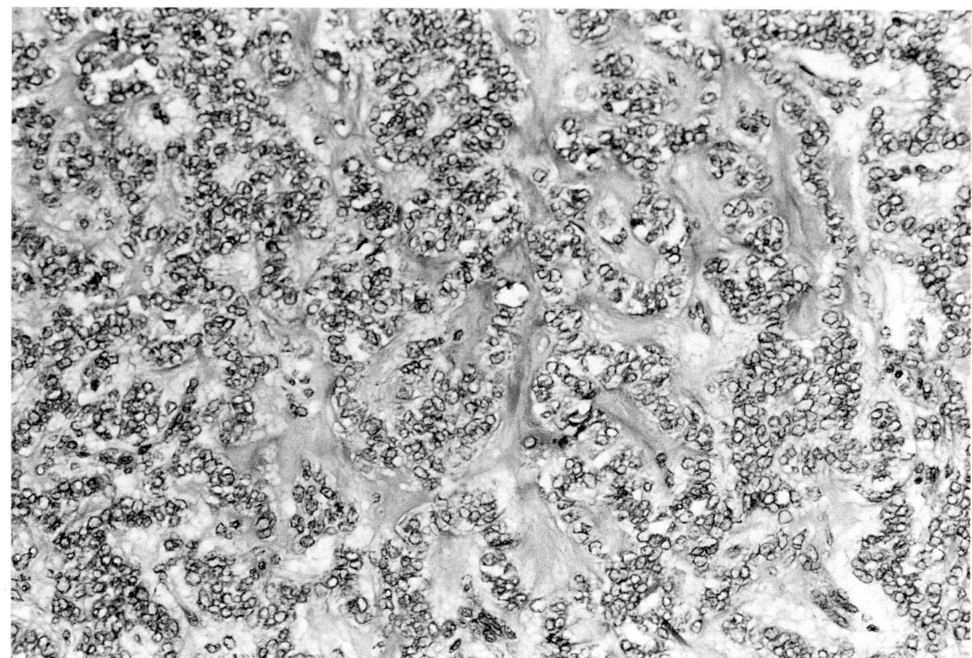

2-85. Clear cell sarcoma of kidney. The septa are hyalinized.

clear cell sarcoma; clear cell sarcoma is unilateral and unicentric, and sclerotic stroma is uncommon in Wilms' tumor before therapy. The distinctive vascular pattern of clear cell sarcoma is often helpful in distinguishing it from Wilms' tumor. The border with the kidney is usually infiltrative while the border of Wilms' tumor is typically "pushing." Exceptionally, clear cell sarcoma of kidney may contain foci in which the cells have prominent nucleoli, similar to those of rhabdoid tumor of kidney; other areas with patterns typical of clear cell sarcoma usually will clarify the diagnosis.

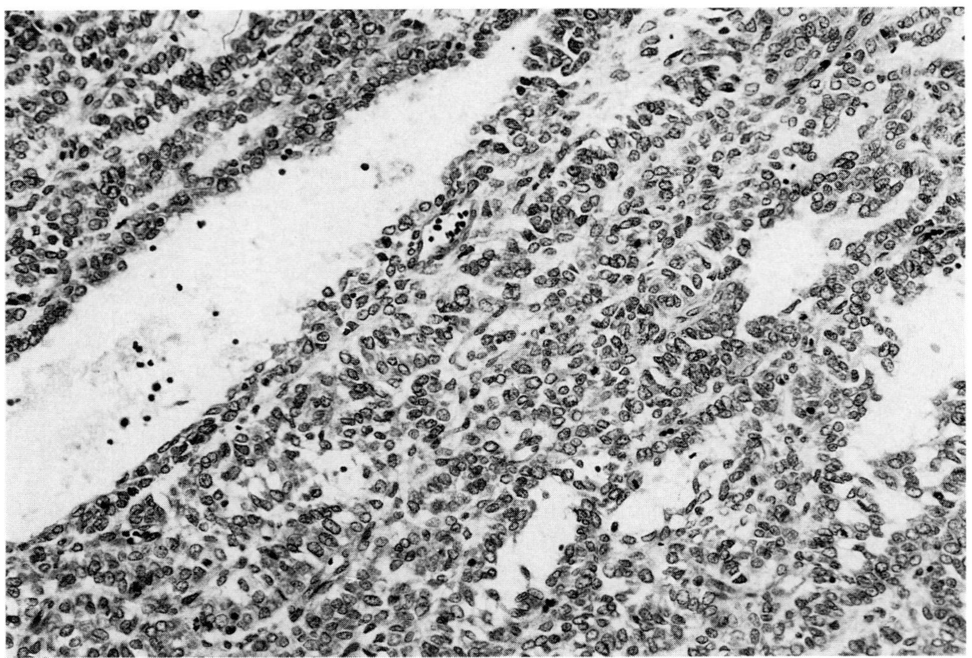

2-86. Clear cell sarcoma of kidney. Multiple cysts disrupt the typical architecture.

RHABDOID TUMOR OF KIDNEY

The most malignant renal neoplasm of childhood, rhabdoid tumor usually metastasizes widely and causes death within 12 months of diagnosis.[403] The patients usually are very young at the time of diagnosis (NWTS median age 11 months and rare after 3 years) and there is a 1.5:1 predominance of boys to girls.[404] Associations with embryonal tumors of the central nervous system[405] and paraneoplastic hypercalcemia [406,407] have been reported.

Gross pathology

Rhabdoid tumor lacks the appearance of encapsulation often seen in cases of Wilms' tumor or clear cell sarcoma. The tumors usually are located medially in the kidney[404] and the renal sinus and pelvis are almost always infiltrated. They are typically yellow-gray or light tan easily fragmented tumors with indistinct borders (Fig. 2-87). Necrosis and hemorrhage are common.

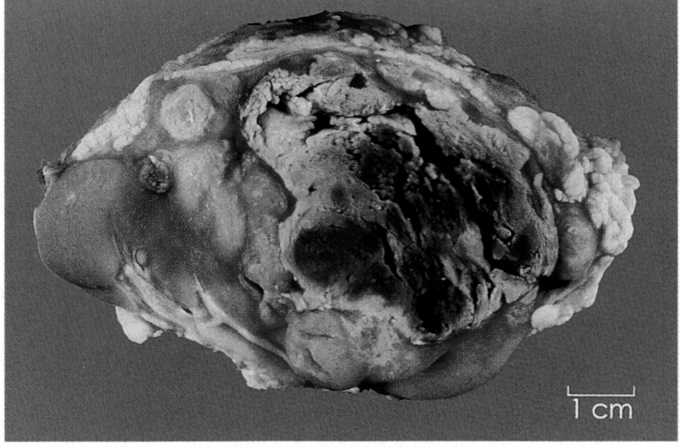

2-87. Rhabdoid tumor of kidney.

Microscopic pathology

Rhabdoid tumor of kidney is typically diffuse and monotonous, consisting of medium or large polygonal cells with abundant eosinophilic cytoplasm and round nuclei with thick nuclear membranes and large nucleoli (Fig. 2-88). It is the resemblance of the cytoplasm of these cells to differentiating rhabdomyoblasts that gave the tumor its name.[399] However, the resemblance to skeletal muscle is merely superficial, and if definite evidence of differentiation toward skeletal muscle is present, the tumor is not a rhabdoid tumor. Often the cytoplasm contains a large eosinophilic globular inclusion that displaces the nucleus (Fig. 2-89). Electron microscopy has shown that these consist of aggregates of whorled filaments (Fig. 2-90).[408] As more cases have accrued to the NWTS, a wide range of patterns has been appreciated, including sclerosing, epithelioid, spindle cell, lymphomatoid, vascular, pseudopapillary, and cystic.[404] Typically these patterns are mixed with the common pattern and with each other. The characteristic nuclear features of large centrally placed nucleoli and thick nuclear membranes are usually retained.

Differential diagnosis

A wide variety of renal and extrarenal tumors may mimic rhabdoid tumor in routine sections. The NWTS has received cases of Wilms' tumor, congenital mesoblastic nephroma, renal cell carcinoma, urothelial carcinoma, collecting duct carcinoma, oncocytoma, rhabdomyosarcoma, neuroendocrine carcinoma, and lymphoma that

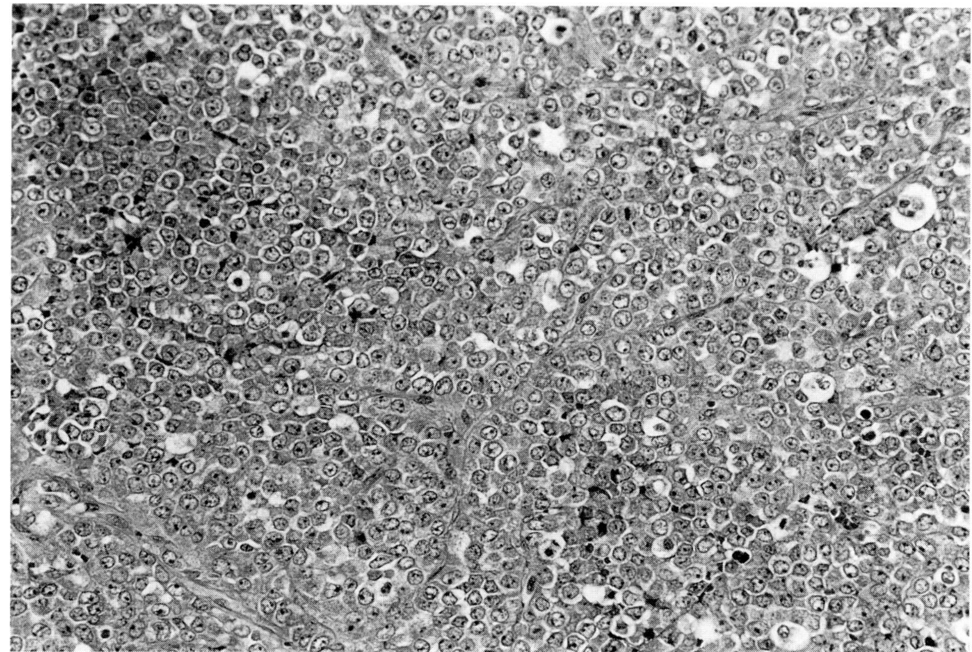

2-88. Rhabdoid tumor of kidney. Anaplastic cells with prominent nucleoli grow in diffuse sheets.

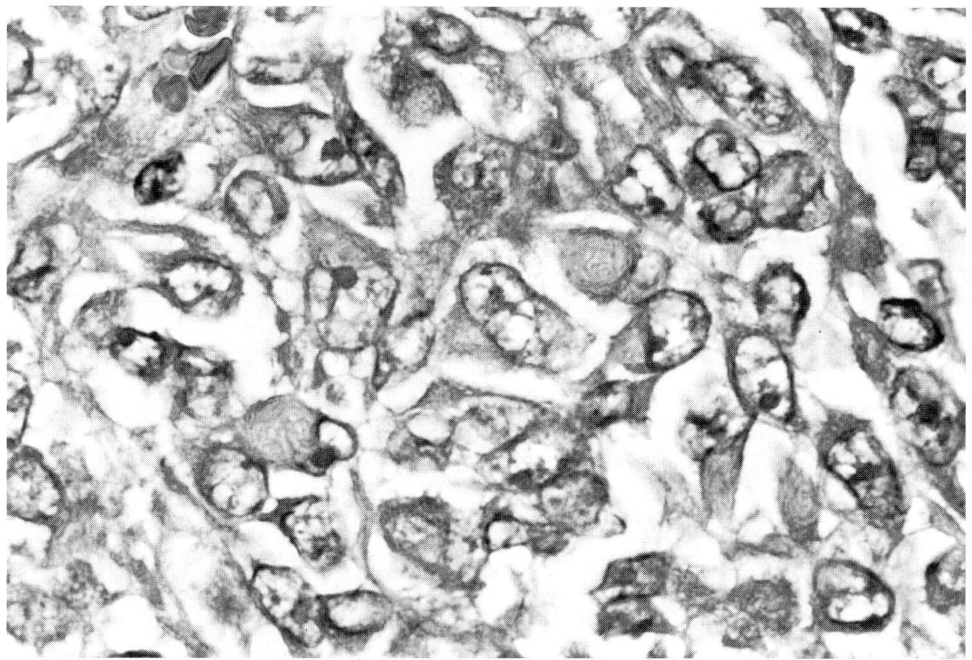

2-89. Rhabdoid tumor of kidney. Cytoplasmic inclusions displace the nuclei. Note prominent nucleoli.

have been confused with rhabdoid tumor of kidney.[409] Filamentous cytoplasmic inclusions or conspicuous macronucleoli are the misleading features in most cases. Conventional light microscopy is able to clarify most cases, but electron microscopy and immunohistochemistry are sometimes necessary to show the characteristic features of the mimics and exclude rhabdoid tumor. Occasionally, blastemal cells contain inclusions suggestive of rhabdoid tumor, but the presence of characteristic aggregates of blastema, such as nodules or serpentine groupings, clarifies the diagnosis.

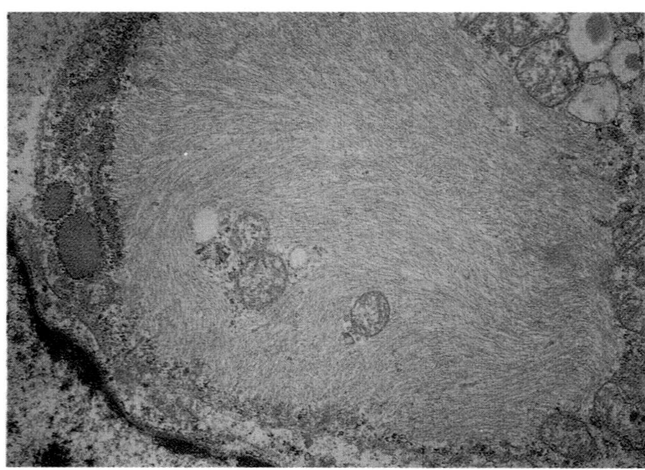

2-90. Rhabdoid tumor of kidney. Electron micrograph showing cytoplasmic inclusion of whorled microfilaments.

OSSIFYING RENAL TUMOR OF INFANCY

This rare tumor of uncertain histogenesis has been reported only in four boys younger than 6 months[410-412] and hematuria has been the presenting symptom in each case. Radiography often reveals a calcified mass in the renal collecting system or pelvis. Although there is an irregular infiltrative border, the limited information available suggests that the clinical course is benign.

Grossly, the tumor is typically stone-hard and projects into the lumen of the renal pelvis. The margins with the underlying medullary tissue are ill defined. Microscopically, the bulk of the tumor consists of sparsely cellular calcified osteoid containing nests of cells with small vesicular ovoid nuclei (Fig. 2-91, 2-92). These plump cells are larger than osteocytes and are more populous at the periphery of the lesion.[411] Mitotic figures are uncommon. Osteoclasts and cartilaginous tissues are absent.

GERM CELL NEOPLASMS

Renal teratoma is a rare and controversial lesion that may be difficult to distinguish from Wilms' tumor because it can contain areas of immature renal tissue with primitive glomerulogenesis and tubule formation.[413] The presence of a wide variety of tissue types representing all three germ cell layers is important in the diagnosis. Structures not ordinarily found in Wilms' tumor, such as lymph node or gutlike structures combining epithelium with smooth muscle[414] or hair follicle and sweat glands,[415] are

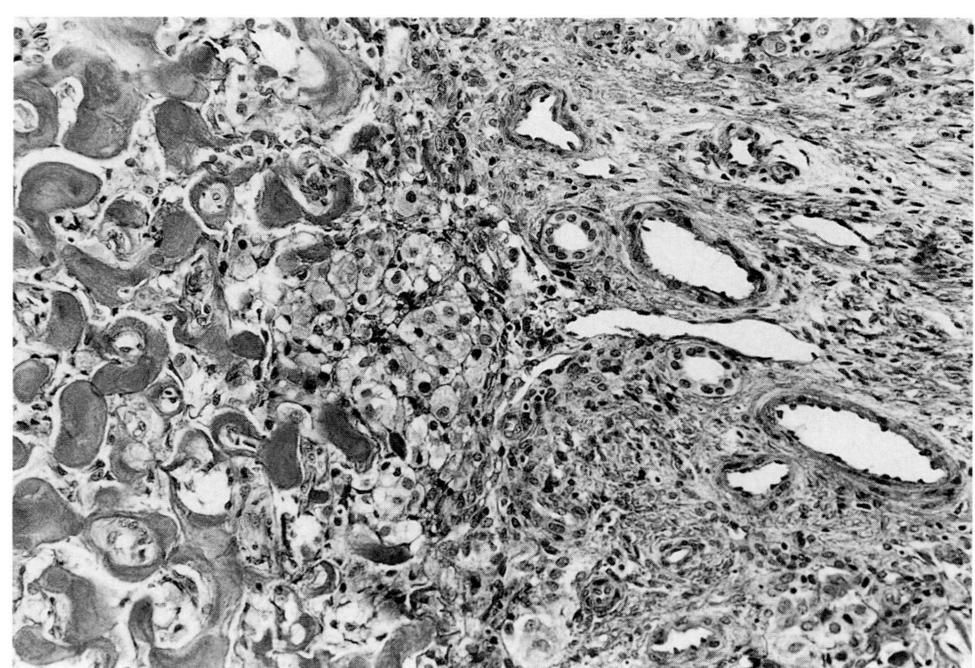

2-91. Ossifying renal tumor of infancy. Spicules of osteoid are separated by cords of epithelioid cells with abundant pale cytoplasm. *(Courtesy of Dr. B. Beckwith and the National Wilms' Tumor Study Pathology Center.)*

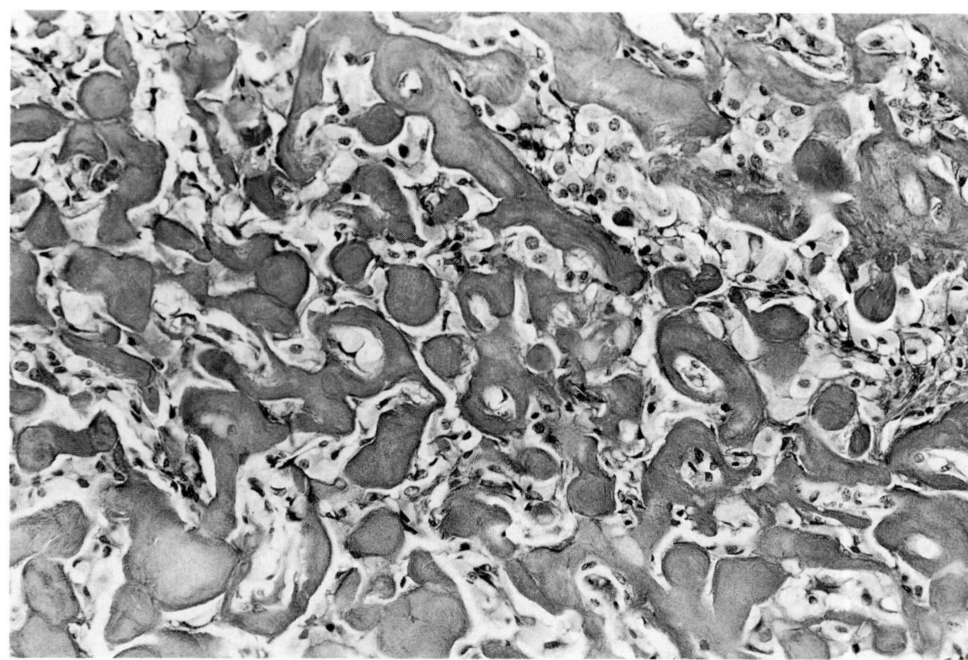

2-92. Ossifying renal tumor of infancy. At the border with the kidney, there is an aggregate of large round epithelioid cells with pale cytoplasm. *(Courtesy of Dr. B. Beckwith and the National Wilms' Tumor Study Pathology Center.)*

most helpful.[414] However, most renal tumors consisting of a variety of epithelial and mesenchymal elements are Wilms' tumor.

Choriocarcinoma has been reported to arise in the kidney.[416] Because differentiation toward choriocarcinoma is seen in some high grade urothelial carcinoma,[417] a thorough search for recognizable urothelial carcinoma should be made in all such cases.

REFERENCES

1. Bell ET: Renal diseases, ed 2, Philadelphia, 1950, Lea & Febiger.
2. Bennington JL, Beckwith JB: Atlas of tumor pathology, second series, fasicle 12, tumors of the kidney, renal pelvis, and ureter, Bethesda, 1975, Armed Forces Institute of Pathology.
3. Eble JN, Warfel K: Early human renal cortical epithelial neoplasia, Mod Pathol 4:45A, 1991.
4. Thompson IM, Peek M: Improvement in survival of patients with renal cell carcinoma—the role of the serendipitously detected tumor, J Urol 140:487-490, 1988.
5. Aso Y, Homma Y: A survey on incidental renal cell carcinoma in Japan, J Urol 147:340-343, 1992.
6. Dal Bianco M, Artibani W, Bassi PF et al: Prognostic factors in renal cell carcinoma, Eur Urol 15:73-76, 1988.
7. Murphy GP, Mostofi FK: Histologic assessment and clinical prognosis of renal adenoma, J Urol 103:31-36, 1970.
8. Pfannkuch F, Leistenschneider W, Nagel R: Problems of assessment in the surgery of renal adenomas, J Urol 125:95-98, 1981.
9. Orain I, Buzelin F, Ferry N: Les tumeurs tubulo-papillaires du rein, à propos de 20 nouveaux et d'une revue de la littérature, J Urol (Paris) 93:1-9, 1987.
10. Mydlo JH, Bard RH: Analysis of papillary renal adenocarcinoma, Urology 30:529-534, 1987.
11. Mancilla-Jimenez R, Stanley RJ, Blath RA: Papillary renal cell carcinoma, a clinical, radiologic, and pathologic study of 34 cases, Cancer 38:2469-2480, 1976.
12. Tobenkin MI, Frazier TH: Giant renal papillary tubular adenoma: case report in a 7-year-old boy, J Urol 91:141-144, 1964.
13. Kantor AF: Current concepts in the epidemiology and etiology of primary renal cell carcinoma, J Urol 117:415-417, 1977.
14. Leuschner I, Harms D, Schmidt D: Renal cell carcinoma in children: histology, immunohistochemistry, and follow-up of 10 cases, Med Pediatr Oncol 19:33-41, 1991.
15. Levinson AK, Johnson DE, Strong LC et al: Familial renal cell carcinoma: hereditary or coincidental? J Urol 144:849-851, 1990.
16. La Vecchia C, Negri E, D'Avanzo B et al: Smoking and renal cell carcinoma, Cancer Res 50:5231-5233, 1990.
17. McLaughlin JK, Mandel JS, Blot WJ et al: A population-based case-control study of renal cell carcinoma, J Natl Cancer Inst 72:275-284, 1984.
18. Maclure M, Willett W: A case-control study of diet and risk of renal adenocarcinoma, Epidemiology 1:430-440, 1990.
19. Wynder EL, Mabuchi K, Whitmore WF Jr: Epidemiology of adenocarcinoma of the kidney, J Natl Cancer Inst 53:1619-1634, 1974.
20. Asal NR, Risser DR, Kadamani S et al: Risk factors in renal cell carcinoma, I. Methodology, demographics, tobacco, beverage use, and obesity, Cancer Detect Prev 11:359-377, 1988.

21. McLaughlin JK, Blot WJ, Mehl ES et al: Relation of analgesic use to renal cancer: population-based findings, NCI Monogr 69:217-222, 1985.
22. Kolonel LN: Association of cadmium with renal cancer, Cancer 37:1782-1787, 1976.
23. McLaughlin JK, Blot WJ, Mehl ES et al: Petroleum-related employment and renal cell cancer, J Occup Med 27:672-674, 1985.
24. Sharpe CR, Rochon JE, Adam JM et al: Case-control study of hydrocarbon exposures in patients with renal cell carcinoma, Can Med Assoc J 140:1309-1318, 1989.
25. Partanen T, Heikkilä P, Hernberg S et al: Renal cell cancer and occupational exposure to chemical agents, Scand J Work Environ Health 17:231-239, 1991.
26. Gibbons RP, Montie JE, Correa RJ Jr et al: Manifestations of renal cell carcinoma, Urology 8:201-206, 1976.
27. Chisholm GD, Roy RR: The systemic effects of malignant renal tumours, Br J Urol 43:687-700, 1971.
28. Laski ME, Vugrin D: Paraneoplastic syndromes in hypernephroma, Semin Nephrol 7:123-130, 1987.
29. Dönmez T, Kale M, Özyürek Y et al: Erythrocyte sedimentation rates in patients with renal cell carcinoma, Eur Urol 21(suppl):51-52, 1992.
30. Cherukuri SV, Johenning PW, Ram MD: Systemic effects of hypernephroma, Urology 10:93-97, 1977.
31. Delpre G, Ilie B, Papo J et al: Hypernephroma with non-metastastic liver dysfunction (Stauffer's syndrome) and hypercalcemia, case report and review of the literature, Am J Gastroenterol 72:239-247, 1979.
32. Aoyagi T, Mori I, Ueyama Y et al: Sinusoidal dilatation of the liver as a paraneoplastic manifestation of renal cell carcinoma, Hum Pathol 20:1193-1197, 1989.
33. Vanatta PR, Silva FG, Taylor WE et al: Renal cell carcinoma and systemic amyloidosis, demonstration of AA protein and review of the literature, Hum Pathol 14:195-201, 1983.
34. Somer TP, Törnroth TS: Renal adenocarcinoma and systemic amyloidosis, immunohistochemical and histochemical studies, Arch Pathol Lab Med 109:571-574, 1985.
35. Wilson JWL, Morales A, Sharp D: Necrotizing myelopathy associated with renal cell carcinoma, Urology 21:390-392, 1983.
36. Herrera GA, Reimann BEF, Turbat EA et al: Hormone-producing capabilities of renal cell carcinomas, correlation with ultrastructural findings, Urology 22:421-428, 1983.
37. Sufrin G, Chasan S, Golio A et al: Paraneoplastic and serologic syndromes of renal adenocarcinoma, Semin Urol 7:158-171, 1989.
38. Fahn H-J, Lee Y-H, Chen M-T et al: The incidence and prognostic significance of humoral hypercalcemia in renal cell carcinoma, J Urol 145:248-250, 1991.
39. Sufrin G, Mirand EA, Moore RH et al: Hormones in renal cancer, J Urol 117:433-438, 1977.
40. Da Silva J-L, Lacombe C, Bruneval P et al: Tumor cells are the site of erythropoietin synthesis in human renal cancers associated with polycythemia, Blood 75:577-582, 1990.
41. Steffens J, Girardot P, Bock R et al: Les carcinomes du rein avec production de rénine, une forme spéciale de l'hypertension, Ann Urol 26:5-9, 1992.
42. Steffens J, Bock R, Braedel HU et al: Renin-producing renal cell carcinoma, Eur Urol 18:56-60, 1990.
43. Lindop GBM, Fleming S: Renin in renal cell carcinoma—an immunocytochemical study using an antibody to pure human renin, J Clin Pathol 37:27-31, 1984.
44. Golde DW, Schambelan M, Weintraub BD et al: Gonadotropin-secreting renal carcinoma, Cancer 33:1048-1053, 1974.
45. Stanisic TH, Donovan J: Prolactin secreting renal cell carcinoma, J Urol 136:85-86, 1986.
46. Serretta V, Pavone C, Messina G et al: Vaginal metastasis from renal cell carcinoma: the role of electron microscopy, Eur Urol 16:78-79, 1989.
47. Melnick SJ, Amazon K, Dembrow V: Metastatic renal cell carcinoma presenting as a parotid tumor: a case report with immunohistochemical findings and review of the literature, Hum Pathol 20:195-197, 1989.
48. Daniels GF Jr, Schaeffer AJ: Renal cell carcinoma involving penis and testis: unusual initial presentations of metastatic disease, Urology 37:369-373, 1991.
49. Leiman G, Markowitz S, Veiga-Ferreira MM et al: Renal adenocarcinoma presenting with bilateral metastases to Bartholin's glands: Primary diagnosis by aspiration cytology, Diagn Cytopathol 2:252-255, 1986.
50. Solomon D, Schwartz A: Renal pathology in von Hippel-Lindau disease, Hum Pathol 19:1072-1079, 1988.
51. Maher ER, Yates JRW, Harries R et al: Clinical features and natural history of von Hippel-Lindau disease, Q J Med 77:1151-1163, 1990.
52. Horton WA, Wong V, Eldridge R: Von Hippel-Lindau disease, clinical and pathological manifestations in nine families with 50 affected members, Arch Intern Med 136:769-777, 1976.
53. Nevin NC, Pearce WG: Diagnostic and genetical aspects of tuberous sclerosis, J Med Genet 5:273-280, 1968.
54. Bender BL, Yunis EJ: The pathology of tuberous sclerosis, Pathol Annu 17:339-382, 1982.
55. Stillwell TJ, Gomez MR, Kelalis PP: Renal lesions in tuberous sclerosis, J Urol 138:477-481, 1987.
56. Bernstein J, Robbins TO: Renal involvement in tuberous sclerosis, Ann N Y Acad Sci 615:36-49, 1991.
57. Washecka R, Hanna M: Malignant renal tumors in tuberous sclerosis, Urology 37:340-343, 1991.
58. Gutierrez OH, Burgener FA, Schwartz S: Coincidental renal cell carcinoma and renal angiomyolipoma in tuberous sclerosis, AJR Am J Roentgenol 132:848-850, 1979.
59. Ahuja S, Loffler W, Wegener O-H et al: Tuberous sclerosis with angiomyolipoma and metastasized hypernephroma, Urology 28:413-419, 1986.
60. Melicow MM, Gile HH: An hypernephroma in a polycystic kidney: review of literature and report of a case, J Urol 43:767-773, 1940.
61. Gregoire JR, Torres VE, Holley KE et al: Renal epithelial hyperplastic and neoplastic proliferation in autosomal dominant polycystic kidney disease, Am J Kidney Dis 9:27-38, 1987.
62. Bernstein J, Evan AP, Gardner KD, Jr: Epithelial hyperplasia in human polycystic kidney diseases, its role in pathogenesis and risk of neoplasia, Am J Pathol 129:92-101, 1987.
63. Fallon B, Williams RD: Renal cancer associated with acquired cystic disease of the kidney and chronic renal failure, Semin Urol 7:228-236, 1989.

64. Matson MA, Cohen EP: Acquired cystic kidney disease: occurrence, prevalence and renal cancers, Medicine 69:217-226, 1990.
65. Ishikawa I: Development of adenocarcinoma and acquired cystic disease of the kidney in hemodialysis patients, Int Symp Princess Takamatsu Cancer Res Fund 18:77-86, 1987.
66. Medeiros LJ, Weiss LM: Renal adenocarcinoma. In Eble JN, ed: Tumors and tumor-like conditions of the kidneys and ureters, New York, 1990, Churchill Livingstone.
67. Klein MJ, Valensi QJ: Proximal tubular adenomas of kidney with so-called oncocytic features, a clinicopathologic study of 13 cases of a rarely reported neoplasm, Cancer 38:9096-914, 1976.
67a. Thoenes W, Störkel S, Rumpelt H-J: Histopathology and classification of renal cell tumors (adenomas, oncocytomas and carcinomas) the basic cytological and histopathological elements and their use for diagnostics, Pathol Res Pract 181:125-143, 1986.
68. Kovacs G: Molecular differential pathology of renal cell tumours, Histopathology 22:1-8, 1993.
69. Oberling C, Rivière M, Hagueneau F: Ultrastructure of the clear cells in renal carcinomas and its importance for the demonstration of their renal origin, Nature 186:402-403, 1960.
70. Yoshida MA, Ohyashiki K, Ochi H et al: Cytogenetic studies of tumor tissue from patients with nonfamilial renal cell carcinoma, Cancer Res 46:2139-2147, 1986.
71. Kovacs G, Erlandsson R, Boldog F et al: Consistent chromosome 3p deletion and loss of heterozygosity in renal cell carcinoma, Proc Natl Acad Sci USA 85:1571-1575, 1988.
72. Nordenson I, Ljungberg B, Roos G: Chromosomes in renal carcinoma with reference to intratumor heterogeneity, Cancer Genet Cytogenet 32:35-41, 1988.
73. Kovacs G, Szücs S, De Riese W et al: Specific chromosome aberration in human renal cell carcinoma, Int J Cancer 40:171-178, 1987.
74. Teyssier JR, Ferre D: Chromosomal changes in renal cell carcinoma, no evidence for correlation with clinical stage, Cancer Genet Cytogenet 45:197-205, 1990.
75. Walter TA, Berger CS, Sandberg AA: The cytogenetics of renal tumors, where do we stand, where do we go? Cancer Genet Cytogenet 43:15-34, 1989.
76. Bergerheim USR, Frisk B, Stellan B et al: del(3p)(p13p21) in renal cell adenoma and del(4p)(p14) in bilateral renal cell carcinoma in two unrelated patients with von Hippel-Lindau disease, Cancer Genet Cytogenet 49:125-131, 1990.
77. Tajara EH, Berger CS, Hecht BK et al: Loss of common 3p14 fragile site expression in renal cell carcinoma with deletion breakpoint at 3p14, Cancer Genet Cytogenet 31:75-82, 1988.
78. Cohen AJ, Li FP, Berg S et al: Hereditary renal-cell carcinoma associated with a chromosomal translocation, N Engl J Med 301:592-595, 1979.
79. King CR, Schimke RN, Arthur T et al: Proximal 3p deletion in renal cell carcinoma cells from a patient with von Hippel Lindau disease, Cancer Genet Cytogenet 27:345-348, 1987.
80. Jordan DK, Patil SR, Divelbiss JE et al: Cytogenetic abnormalities in tumors of patients with von-Hippel-Lindau disease, Cancer Genet Cytogenet 42:227-241, 1989.
81. Goodman MD, Goodman BK, Lubin MB et al: Cytogenetic characterization of renal cell carcinoma in von Hippel-Lindau syndrome, Cancer 65:1150-1154, 1990.
82. Seizinger BR, Rouleau GA, Ozelius LJ et al: Von Hippel-Lindau disease maps to the region of chromosome 3 associated with renal cell carcinoma, Nature 332:268-269, 1988.
83. Erlandsson R, Boldog F, Sümegi J et al: Do human renal cell carcinomas arise by a double-loss mechanism? Cancer Genet Cytogenet 36:197-202, 1988.
84. Zbar B, Brauch H, Talmadge C et al: Loss of alleles of loci on the short arm of chromosome 3 in renal cell carcinoma, Nature 327:721-724, 1987.
85. van der Hout AH, Kok K, van den Berg A et al: Direct molecular analysis of a deletion of 3p in tumors from patients with sporadic renal cell carcinoma, Cancer Genet Cytogenet 32:281-285, 1988.
86. Anglard P, Tory K, Brauch H et al: Molecular analysis of genetic changes in the origin and development of renal cell carcinoma, Cancer Res 51:1071-1077, 1991.
87. Ogawa O, Kakehi Y, Ogawa K et al: Allelic loss at chromosome 3p characterizes clear cell phenotype of renal cell carcinoma, Cancer Res 51:949-953, 1991.
88. van der Hout AH, Brown RS, Li FP et al: Localization by in situ hybridization of three 3p probes with respect to the breakpoint in a t(3;8) in hereditary renal cell carcinoma, Cancer Genet Cytogenet 51:121-124, 1991.
89. Kinouchi T, Saiki S, Naoe T et al: Correlation of c-*myc* expression with nuclear pleomorphism in human renal cell carcinoma, Cancer Res 49:3627-3630, 1989.
90. Smith SJ, Bosniak MA, Megibow AJ et al: Renal cell carcinoma: earlier discovery and increased detection, Radiology 170:699-703, 1989.
91. Hartman DS, Davis CJ Jr, Johns T et al: Cystic renal cell carcinoma, Urology 28:145-153, 1986.
92. Murad T, Komaiko W, Oyasu R et al: Multilocular cystic renal cell carcinoma, Am J Clin Pathol 95:633-637, 1991.
93. Madewell JE, Goldman SM, Davis CJ Jr et al: Multilocular cystic nephroma: a radiographic-pathologic correlation of 58 patients, Radiology 146:309-321, 1983.
94. Cheng WS, Farrow GM, Zincke H: The incidence of multicentricity in renal cell carcinoma, J Urol 146:1221-1223, 1991.
95. Jagirdar J, Irie T, French SW et al: Globular mallory-like bodies in renal cell carcinoma: report of a case and review of cytoplasmic eosinophilic globules, Hum Pathol 16:949-952, 1985.
96. Weaver MG, Al-Kaisi N, Abdul-Karim FW: Fine-needle aspiration cytology of a renal cell adenocarcinoma with massive intracellular hemosiderin accumulation, Diagn Cytopathol 7:147-149, 1991.
97. Koga S, Yamasaki A, Nishikido M et al: Multiloculated renal cell carcinoma, Int Urol Nephrol 23:423-427, 1991.
98. Taxy JB, Marshall FF: Multilocular renal cysts in adults, possible relationship to renal adenocarcinoma, Arch Pathol Lab Med 107:633-637, 1983.
99. Sherman ME, Silverman ML, Balogh K et al: Multilocular renal cyst, Arch Pathol Lab Med 111:732-736, 1987.
100. Wick MR, Perrone TL, Burke BA: Sarcomatoid transitional cell carcinoma of the renal pelvis, an ultrastructural and immunohistochemical study, Arch Pathol Lab Med 109:55-58, 1985.
101. Wick MR, Cherwitz DL, Manivel JC et al: Immunohistochemical findings in tumors of the kidney. In Eble JN, ed: Tumors and tumor-like conditions of the kidneys and ureters, New York, 1990, Churchill Livingstone.

102. Beckwith JB: Wilms' tumor and other renal tumors of childhood: a selective review from the National Wilms' Tumor Study Pathology Center, Hum Pathol 14:481-492, 1983.
103. Kimura I, Takahashi N, Okumura R et al: Perinephric xanthogranulomatous pyelonephritis simulating a renal or retroperitoneal tumor on x-ray CT and angiography, Radiat Med 7:111-117, 1989.
104. Malek RS, Greene LF, DeWeerd JH et al: Xanthogranulomatous pyelonephritis, Br J Urol 44:296-308, 1972.
105. Goodman M, Curry T, Russell T: Xanthogranulomatous pyelonephritis (XGP): a local disease with systemic manifestations, report of 23 patients and review of the literature, Medicine 58:171-181, 1979.
106. Rosi P, Selli C, Carini M et al: Xanthogranulomatous pyelonephritis: clinical experience with 62 cases, Eur Urol 12:96-100, 1986.
107. Chuang C-K, Lai M-K, Chang P-L et al: Xanthogranulomatous pyelonephritis: experience in 36 cases, J Urol 147:333-336, 1992.
108. Parsons MA, Harris SC, Longstaff AJ et al: Xanthogranulomatous pyelonephritis: a pathological, clinical and aetiological analysis of 87 cases, Diagn Histopathol 6:203-219, 1983.
109. Esparza AR, McKay DB, Cronan JJ et al: Renal parenchymal malakoplakia, histologic spectrum and its relationship to megalocytic interstitial nephritis and xanthogranulomatous pyelonephritis, Am J Surg Pathol 13:225-236, 1989.
110. Deitchman B, Sidhu GS: Ultrastructural study of a sarcomatoid variant of renal cell carcinoma, Cancer 46:1152-1157, 1980.
111. Bonsib SM, Fischer J, Plattner S et al: Sarcomatoid renal tumors, clinicopathologic correlation of three cases, Cancer 59:527-532, 1987.
112. Lanzafame S: Carcinoma <<sarcomatode>> del rene, distribuzione dei filamenti intermedi di citocheratine e di vimentina nelle cellule carcinomatose e sarcomatose, Pathologica 79:323-337, 1987.
113. Lager DJ, Huston BJ, Timmerman TG et al: Papillary renal tumors, morphologic, cytochemical, and genotypic features, Cancer 76:669-673, 1995.
114. Bard RH, Lord B, Fromowitz F: Papillary adenocarcinoma of kidney, II. Radiographic and biologic characteristics, Urology 19:16-20, 1982.
115. Thoenes W, Störkel S, Rumpelt HJ et al: Cytomorphological typing of renal cell carcinoma—a new approach, Eur Urol 18(suppl):6-9, 1990.
116. Gutíerrez Baños JL, Martín García B, Hernández Rodríguez R et al: Adenocarcinoma papilar de riñon. Aportacion de 12 casos y puesta al dia, Actas Urol Esp 15:437-441, 1991.
117. El-Naggar AK, Ro JY, Ensign LG: Papillary renal cell carcinoma: clinical implication of DNA content analysis, Hum Pathol 24:316-321, 1993.
118. Renshaw AA, Corless CL: Papillary renal cell carcinoma, histology and immunohistochemistry, Am J Surg Pathol 19:842-849, 1995.
119. Thoenes W, Störkel S: Die Pathologie der benignen und malignen Nierenzelltumoren, Urologe [A] 30:W41-W50, 1991.
120. Kovacs G: Papillary renal cell carcinoma, a morphologic and cytogenetic study of 11 cases, Am J Pathol 134:27-34, 1989.
121. Kovacs G, Fuzesi L, Emanuel A et al: Cytogenetics of papillary renal cell tumors, Genes Chromosom Cancer 3:249-255, 1991.
122. Kovacs G, Wilkens L, Papp T et al: Differentiation between papillary and nonpapillary renal cell carcinomas by DNA analysis, J Natl Cancer Inst 81:527-530, 1989.
123. Presti JC Jr, Rao PH, Chen Q et al: Histopathological, cytogenetic, and molecular characterization of renal cortical tumors, Cancer Res 51:1544-1552, 1991.
124. Fournet JC, Béroud C, Austruy E et al: Aspects génétiques des tumeurs rénales de l'adulte, Arch Anat Cytol Pathol 40:301-306, 1992.
125. van der Hout AH, van den Berg E, van der Vlies P et al: Loss of heterozygosity at the short arm of chromosome 3 in renal-cell cancer correlates with the cytological tumour type, Int J Cancer 53:353-357, 1993.
126. Henn W, Zwergel T, Wullich B et al: Bilateral multicentric papillary renal tumors with heteroclonal origin based on tissue-specific karyotype instability, Cancer 72:1315-1318, 1993.
127. van den Berg E, van der Hout AH, Oosterhuis JW et al: Cytogenetic analysis of epithelial renal-cell tumors: relationship with a new histopathological classification, Int J Cancer 55:223-227, 1993.
128. Reznicek SB, Narayana AS, Culp DA: Cystadenocarcinoma of the kidney: a profile of 13 cases, J Urol 134:256-259, 1985.
129. Landier JF, Desligneres S, Debré B et al: Les cystadénocarcinomes papillaires du rein, Ann Urol 14:205-208, 1980.
130. Fryfogle JD, Dockerty MB, Clagett OT et al: Dark-cell adenocarcinomas of the kidney, J Urol 60:221-234, 1948.
131. Fuhrman SA, Lasky LC, Limas C: Prognostic significance of morphologic parameters in renal cell carcinoma, Am J Surg Pathol 6:655-663, 1982.
132. Bannasch P, Schacht U, Storch E: Morphogenese und Mikromorphologie epithelialer Nierentumoren bei Nitrosomorpholin-vergifteten Ratten, I. Induktion und Histologie der Tumoren, Z Krebsforsch 81:311-331, 1974.
133. Thoenes W, Störkel S, Rumpelt H-J: Human chromophobe cell renal carcinoma, Virchows Arch [B] 48:207-217, 1985.
134. Thoenes W, Störkel S, Rumpelt H-J et al: Chromophobe cell renal carcinoma and its variants—a report on 32 cases, J Pathol 155:277-287, 1988.
135. Bonsib SM, Lager DJ: Chromophobe cell carcinoma: analysis of five cases, Am J Surg Pathol 14:260-267, 1990.
136. Crotty TB, Farrow GM, Lieber MM: Chromophobe renal cell carcinoma: clinicopathologic features of 50 cases, J Urol 154:964-967, 1995.
137. DeLong WH, Sakr W, Grignon DJ: Chromophobe renal cell carcinoma: a comparative histochemical and immunohistochemical study, J Urol Pathol (in press).
138. Erlandson RA, Reuter VE: Renal tumor in a 62-year-old male, Ultrastruct Pathol 12:561-567, 1988.
139. Kovacs A, Kovacs G: Low chromosome number in chromophobe renal cell carcinomas, Genes Chromosom Cancer 4:267-268, 1992.

140. Speicher MR, Schoell B, du Manoir S et al: Specific loss of chromosomes 1, 2, 6, 10, 13, 17, and 21 in chromophobe renal cell carcinomas revealed by comparative genomic hybridization, Am J Pathol 145:356-364, 1994.
141. Vieillefond A, Paradis V, Gros P et al: Est-il utile d'isoler parmi les carcinomes du rein, une variante à cellules chromophobes? Arch Anat Cytol Pathol 40:250-254, 1992.
142. Bonsib SM: Renal chromophobe cell carcinoma: the relationship between cytoplasmic vesicles and colloidal iron stain, J Urol Pathol (in press).
143. Störkel S, Steart PV, Drenckhahn D et al: The human chromophobe cell renal carcinoma: its probable relation to intercalated cells of the collecting duct, Virchows Arch [B] 56:237-245, 1989.
144. Thoenes W, Baum H-P, Störkel S et al: Cytoplasmic microvesicles in chromophobe cell renal carcinoma demonstrated by freeze fracture, Virchows Arch [B] 54:127-130, 1987.
145. Bonsib SM, Bray C, Timmerman TG: Renal chromophobe cell carcinoma: limitations of paraffin-embedded tissue, Ultrastruct Pathol 17:529-536, 1993.
146. Kriz W, Bankir L: A standard nomenclature for structures of the kidney, Kidney Int 33:1-7, 1988.
147. Störkel S, Pannen B, Thoenes W et al: Intercalated cells as a probable source for the development of renal oncocytoma, Virchows Arch [B] 56:185-189, 1988.
148. Rumpelt HJ, Störkel S, Moll R et al: Bellini duct carcinoma: further evidence for this rare variant of renal cell carcinoma, Histopathology 18:115-122, 1991.
149. Fleming S, Lewi HJE: Collecting duct carcinoma of the kidney, Histopathology 10:1131-1141, 1986.
150. Aizawa S, Kikuchi Y, Suzuki M et al: Renal cell carcinoma of lower nephron origin, Acta Pathol Jpn 37:567-574, 1987.
151. Kennedy SM, Merino MJ, Linehan WM et al: Collecting duct carcinoma of the kidney, Hum Pathol 21:449-456, 1990.
152. Davis CJ Jr, Mostofi FK, Sesterhenn IA: Renal medullary carcinoma: the seventh sickle cell nephropathy, Am J Surg Pathol 19:1-11, 1995.
153. Füzesi L, Cober M, Mittermayer C: Collecting duct carcinoma: cytogenetic characterization, Histopathology 21:155-160, 1992.
154. Hai MA, Diaz-Perez R: Atypical carcinoma of kidney originating from collecting duct epithelium, Urology 19:89-92, 1982.
155. Cromie WJ, Davis CJ Jr: Atypical carcinoma of kidney possibly originating from collecting duct epithelium, Urology 13:315-317, 1979.
156. Eble JN: Unusual renal tumors and tumor-like conditions. In Eble JN, ed: Tumors and tumor-like conditions of the kidneys and ureters, New York, 1990, Churchill Livingstone.
157. Baer SC, Ro JY, Ordonez NG et al: Sarcomatoid collecting duct carcinoma: a clinicopathologic and immunohistochemical study of five cases, Hum Pathol 24:1017-1022, 1993.
158. Hand JR, Broders AC: Carcinoma of the kidney: the degree of malignancy in relation to factors bearing on prognosis, J Urol 28:199-216, 1932.
159. Skinner DG, Colvin RB, Vermillion CD et al: Diagnosis and management of renal cell carcinoma, a clinical and pathological study of 309 cases, Cancer 28:1165-1177, 1971.
160. Medeiros LJ, Gelb AB, Weiss LM: Renal cell carcinoma, prognostic significance of morphologic parameters in 121 cases, Cancer 61:1639-1651, 1988.
161. Grignon DJ, Ayala AG, El-Naggar A et al: Renal cell carcinoma, a clinicopathologic and DNA flow cytometric analysis of 103 cases, Cancer 64:2133-2140, 1989.
162. Green LK, Ayala AG, Ro JY et al: Role of nuclear grading in stage I renal cell carcinoma, Urology 34:310-315, 1989.
163. Helpap B, Knüpffer J, Essmann S: Nucleolar grading of renal cancer, correlation of frequency and localization of nucleoli to histologic and cytologic grading and stage of renal cell carcinomas, Mod Pathol 3:671-678, 1990.
164. Störkel S, Thoenes W, Jacobi GH et al: Prognostic parameters in renal cell carcinoma—a new approach, Eur Urol 16:416-422, 1989.
165. Tomera KM, Farrow GM, Lieber MM: Sarcomatoid renal carcinoma, J Urol 130:657-659, 1983.
166. Bernoni F, Ferri C, Benati A et al: Sarcomatoid carcinoma of the kidney, J Urol 137:25-28, 1987.
167. Ro JY, Ayala AG, Sella A et al: Sarcomatoid renal cell carcinoma: a clinicopathologic study of 42 cases, Cancer 59:516-526, 1987.
168. Macke RA, Hussain MB, Imray TJ et al: Osteogenic and sarcomatoid differentiation of a renal cell carcinoma, Cancer 56:2452-2457, 1985.
169. Menzies DW: Carcinoma and rhabdomyosarcoma in the same kidney, a study in the classification and histogenesis of mixed renal tumours, Aust N Z J Surg 25:214-224, 1955.
170. Fukuoka T, Honda M, Namiki M et al: Renal cell carcinoma with heterotopic bone formation, case report and review of tthe Japanese literature, Urol Int 42:458-460, 1987.
171. Veneziano S, Pavlica P, Busato F et al: Il nefrocarcinoma sarcomatoide, correlazione tra il quadro radiologico, istopatologico e prognostico, Radiol Med (Torino) 78:343-347, 1989.
172. Golomb J, Merimsky E, Baratz M et al: Le carcinome sarcomatoïde du rein, J Urol (Paris) 90:341-343, 1984.
173. Yoneda F, Kan M, Kagawa S et al: Clinicopathological observation on spindle cell type of renal cell carcinoma, Nippon Hinyokika Gakkai Zasshi 79:122-125, 1988.
174. Llarena Ibarguren R, Zabala Egurrola JA, Marin Lafuente JC et al: Carcinoma renal sarcomatoide, Arch Esp Urol 43:409-411, 1990.
175. Mucci B, Lewi HJE, Fleming S: The radiology of sarcomas and sarcomatoid carcinomas of the kidney, Clin Radiol 38:249-254, 1987.
176. Schouman M, Warter A, Roos M et al: Renal cell carcinoma: statistical study of survival based on pathological criteria, World J Urol 2:109-113, 1984.
177. Robson CJ: Radical nephrectomy for renal cell carcinoma, J Urol 89:37-42, 1963.
178. Robson CJ, Churchill BM, Anderson W: The results of radical nephrectomy for renal cell carcinoma, J Urol 101:297-301, 1969.
179. Bassil B, Dosoretz DE, Prout GR Jr: Validation of the tumor, nodes and metastasis classification of renal cell carcinoma, J Urol 134:450-454, 1985.
180. Brucher P, Brunier G, Ferrière JM et al: Étude critique du pronostic de l'adénocarcinome rénal et essai de classification, Ann Urol 24:504-511, 1990.

181. Nishio Y, Nishimura K, Hida S et al: Results of radical nephrectomy for renal cell carcinoma, report 1. Analysis according to the TNM staging system of the general rule for clinical and pathological studies on renal cell carcinoma, Acta Urol Jpn 33:337-343, 1987.
182. Hermanek P, Schrott KM: Evaluation of the new tumor, nodes and metastases classification of renal cell carcinoma, J Urol 144:238-242, 1990.
183. Medeiros LJ, Gelb AB, Weiss LM: Low-grade renal cell carcinoma, a clinicopathologic study of 53 cases, Am J Surg Pathol 11:633-642, 1987.
184. Giuliani L, Giberti C, Martorana G et al: Radical extensive surgery for renal cell carcinoma: long-term results and prognostic factors, J Urol 143:468-474, 1990.
185. Herrlinger A, Schrott KM, Sigel A et al: Results of 381 transabdominal radical nephrectomies for renal cell carcinoma with partial and complete en-bloc lymph-node dissection, World J Urol 2:114-121, 1984.
186. Studer UE, Scherz S, Scheidegger J et al: Enlargement of regional lymph nodes in renal cell carcinoma is often not due to metastases, J Urol 144:243-245, 1990.
187. Ramon J, Goldwasser B, Raviv G et al: Long-term results of simple and radical nephrectomy for renal cell carcinoma, Cancer 67:2506-2511, 1991.
188. Mitty HA, Droller MJ, Dikman SH: Ureteral and renal pelvic metastases from renal cell carcinoma, Urol Radiol 9:16-20, 1987.
189. Robey EL: The adrenal gland and renal cell carcinoma: is ipsilateral adrenalectomy a necessary component of radical nephrectomy? J Urol 135:453-455, 1986.
190. O'Brien WM, Lynch JH: Adrenal metastases by renal cell carcinoma, incidence at nephrectomy, Urology 29:605-607, 1987.
191. Haab F, Gattegno B, Duclos JM et al: Should adrenalectomy be performed systematically as part of radical nephrectomy for renal cancer? Prog Urol 1:889-893, 1991.
192. Waldherr R, Schwechheimer K: Co-expression of cytokeratin and vimentin intermediate-sized filaments in renal cell carcinoma, a comparative study of the intermediate-sized filaments in renal cell carcinoma and normal human kidney, Virchows Arch A Pathol Anat Histopathol 408:15-27, 1985.
193. Taxy JB: Renal adenocarcinoma presenting as a solitary metastasis: contribution of electron microscopy to diagnosis, Cancer 48:2056-2062, 1981.
194. Lemmers M, Ward K, Hatch T et al: Renal adenocarcinoma with solitary metastasis to the contralateral adrenal gland: report of 2 cases and review of the literature, J Urol 141:1177-1180, 1989.
195. Wick MR, Cherwitz DL, McGlennen RC et al: Adrenocortical carcinoma, an immunohistochemical comparison with renal cell carcinoma, Am J Pathol 122:343-352, 1986.
196. Green LK, Ro JY, Mackay B et al: Renal cell carcinoma metastatic to the thyroid, Cancer 63:1810-1815, 1989.
197. Young RH, Hart WR: Renal cell carcinoma metastatic to the ovary: a report of three cases emphasizing possible confusion with ovarian clear cell carcinoma, Int J Gynecol Pathol 1992.
198. Hufnagel TJ, Kim JH, True LD et al: Immunohistochemistry of capillary hemangioblastoma, immunoperoxidase-labeled antibody staining resolves the differential diagnosis with metastatic renal cell carcinoma, but does not explain the histogenesis of the capillary hemangioblastoma, Am J Surg Pathol 13:207-216, 1989.
199. Katz SE, Schapira HE: Spontaneous regression of genitourinary cancer—an update, J Urol 128:1-4, 1982.
200. Kavoussi LR, Levine SR, Kadmon D et al: Regression of metastatic renal cell carcinoma: a case report and literature review, J Urol 135:1005-1007, 1986.
201. De Riese W, Goldenberg K, Allhoff E et al: Metastatic renal cell carcinoma (RCC): spontaneous regression, long-term survival and late recurrence, Int Urol Nephrol 23:13-25, 1991.
202. Rodier JF, Rodier D, Janser JC et al: Régression spontanée de métastases pulmonaires de cancer du rein, J Chir 125:341-345, 1988.
203. Takáts LJ, Csapó Z: Death from renal carcinoma 37 years after its original recognition, Cancer 19:1172-1176, 1966.
204. McNichols DW, Segura JW, DeWeerd JH: Renal cell carcinoma: long-term survival and late recurrence, J Urol 126:17-23, 1981.
205. Hienert G, Latal D, Rummelhardt S: Urological aspects of surgical management for metastatic renal cell cancer, Semin Surg Oncol 4:137-138, 1988.
206. Neves RJ, Zincke H, Taylor WF: Metastatic renal cell cancer and radical nephrectomy: identification of prognostic factors and patient survival, J Urol 139:1173-1176, 1988.
207. Elson PJ, Witte RS, Trump DL: Prognostic factors for survival in patients with recurrent or metastatic renal cell carcinoma, Cancer Res 48:7310-7313, 1988.
208. Tobisu K-I, Kakizoe T, Takai K et al: Prognosis in renal cell carcinoma: analysis of clinical course following nephrectomy, Jpn J Clin Oncol 19:142-148, 1989.
209. Gurney H, Larcos G, McKay M et al: Bone metastases in hypernephroma, frequency of scapular involvement, Cancer 64:1429-1431, 1989.
210. Davis CJ Jr, Mostofi FK, Sesterhenn IA et al: Renal oncocytoma, clinicopathological study of 166 patients, J Urogenital Pathol 1:41-52, 1991.
211. Reference deleted in proofs.
212. Defossez SM, Yoder IC, Papanicolaou N et al: Nonspecific magnetic resonance appearance of renal oncocytomas: report of 3 cases and review of the literature, J Urol 145:552-554, 1991.
213. Mead GO, Thomas LR Jr, Jackson JG: Renal oncocytoma: report of a case with bilateral multifocal oncocytomas, Clin Imaging 14:231-234, 1990.
214. Takai K, Kakizoe T, Tobisu K et al: Renal oncocytoma treated by partial nephrectomy, a case report, Nippon Hinyokika Gakkai Zasshi 78:935-938, 1987.
215. Warfel KA, Eble JN: Renal oncocytomatosis, J Urol 127:1179-1180, 1982.
216. Kragel PJ, Williams J, Emory TS et al: Renal oncocytoma with cylindromatous changes: pathologic features and histogenetic significance, Mod Pathol 3:277-281, 1990.

217. Eble JN, Hull MT: Morphologic features of renal oncocytoma: a light and electron microscopic study, Hum Pathol 15:1054-1061, 1984.
218. Lieber MM, Tomera KM, Farrow GM: Renal oncocytoma, J Urol 125:481-485, 1981.
219. Barnes CA, Beckman EN: Renal oncocytoma and its congeners, Am J Clin Pathol 79:312-318, 1983.
220. Resnick ME, Unterberger H, McLoughlin PT: Renal carcinoid producing the carcinoid syndrome, Med Times 94:895-896, 1966.
221. Gleeson MH, Bloom SR, Polak JM et al: Endocrine tumour in kidney affecting small bowel structure, motility, and absorptive function, Gut 12:773-782, 1971.
222. Ghazi MR, Brown JS, Warner RS: Carcinoid tumor of kidney, Urology 14:610-612, 1979.
223. Stahl RE, Sidhu GS: Primary carcinoid of the kidney, light and electron microscopic study, Cancer 44:1345-1349, 1979.
224. Raghavaiah NV, Singh SM: Extra-adrenal pheochromocytoma producing renal artery stenosis, J Urol 116:243-245, 1976.
225. Naidich TP, Sprayregen S, Goldman AG et al: Renal artery alterations associated with pheochromocytoma, Angiology 23:488-499, 1972.
226. Van Way CW,III, Michelakis AM, Alper BJ et al: Renal vein renin studies in a patient with renal hilar pheochromocytoma and renal artery stenosis, Ann Surg 172:212-217, 1970.
227. Pengelly CDR: Phaeochromocytoma within the renal capsule, Br Med J 2:477-478, 1959.
228. Preger L, Gardner RE, Kawala BO et al: Intrarenal pheochromocytoma, preoperative angiographic diagnosis, Urology 8:194-196, 1976.
229. Simon H, Carlson DH, Hanelin J et al: Intrarenal pheochromocytoma: report of a case, J Urol 121:805-807, 1979.
230. Bezirdjian DR, Tegtmeyer CJ, Leef JL: Intrarenal pheochromocytoma and renal artery stenosis, Urol Radiol 3:121-122, 1981.
231. Rothwell DL, Vorstman B, Patton I et al: Intrarenal pheochromocytoma, Urology 21:175-177, 1983.
232. Gohji K, Nakanishi T, Hara I et al: Two cases of primary neuroblastoma of the kidney in adults, J Urol 137:966-968, 1987.
233. Zak FG, Jindrak K, Capozzi F: Carcinoidal tumor of the kidney, Ultrastruct Pathol 4:51-59, 1983.
234. Acconcia A, Miracco C, Mattei FM et al: Primary carcinoid tumor of kidney, light and electron microscopy, and immunohistochemical study, Urology 31:517-520, 1988.
235. Cauley JE, Almagro UA, Jacobs SC: Primary renal carcinoid tumor, Urology 32:564-566, 1988.
236. Huettner PC, Bird DJ, Chang YC et al: Carcinoid tumor of the kidney with morphologic and immunohistochemical profile of a hindgut endocrine tumor: report of a case, Ultrastruct Pathol 15:655-661, 1991.
237. Kojiro M, Ohishi H, Isobe H: Carcinoid tumor occurring in cystic teratoma of the kidney, a case report, Cancer 38:1636-1640, 1976.
238. Fetissof F, Benatre A, Dubois MP et al: Carcinoid tumor occurring in a teratoid malformation of the kidney, an immunohistochemical study, Cancer 54:2305-2308, 1984.
239. Capella C, Eusebi V, Rosai J: Primary oat cell carcinoma of the kidney, Am J Surg Pathol 8:855-861, 1984.
240. Têtu B, Ro JY, Ayala AG et al: Small cell carcinoma of the kidney, a clinicopathologic, immunohistochemical, and ultrastructural study, Cancer 60:1809-1814, 1987.
241. Hajdu SI, Foote FW Jr: Angiomyolipoma of the kidney: Report of 27 cases and review of the literature, J Urol 102:396-401, 1969.
242. Price EB Jr, Mostofi FK: Symptomatic angiomyolipoma of the kidney, Cancer 18:761-774, 1965.
243. Klapproth HJ, Poutasse EF, Hazard JB: Renal angiomyolipomas, report of four cases, Arch Pathol 67:400-411, 1959.
244. Corr P, Yang W, Tan I: Spontaneous haemorrhage from renal angiomyolipomata, Australas Radiol 38:132-134, 1994.
245. Oesterling JE, Fishman EK, Goldman SM et al: The management of renal angiomyolipoma, J Urol 135:1121-1124, 1986.
246. Kragel PJ, Toker C: Infiltrating recurrent renal angiomyolipoma with fatal outcome, J Urol 133:90-91, 1985.
247. Lowe BA, Brewer J, Houghton DC et al: Malignant transformation of angiomyolipoma, J Urol 147:1356-1358, 1992.
248. Ferry JA, Malt RA, Young RH: Renal angiomyolipoma with sarcomatous transformation and pulmonary metastases, Am J Surg Pathol 15:1083-1088, 1991.
249. Baert J, Vandamme B, Sciot R et al: Benign angiomyolipoma involving the renal vein and vena cava as a tumor thrombus: case report, J Urol 153:1205-1207, 1995.
250. Morris SB, Hampson SJ, Jackson P et al: Surgical management of an angiomyolipoma extending into the inferior vena cava, Br J Urol 74:383-385, 1994.
251. Brecher ME, Gill WB, Straus FH II: Angiomyolipoma with regional lymph node involvement and long-term follow-up study, Hum Pathol 17:962-963, 1986.
252. Ackerman TE, Levi CS, Lindsay DJ et al: Angiomyolipoma with lymph node involvement, Can Assoc Radiol J 45:52-55, 1994.
253. Taylor RS, Joseph DB, Kohaut EC et al: Renal angiomyolipoma associated with lymph node involvement and renal cell carcinoma in patients with tuberous sclerosis, J Urol 141:930-932, 1989.
254. McIntosh GS, Hamilton Dutoit S, Chronos NV et al: Multiple unilateral renal angiomyolipomas with regional lymphangioleiomyomatosis, J Urol 142:1305-1307, 1989.
255. Ro JY, Ayala AG, El-Naggar A et al: Angiomyolipoma of kidney with lymph node involvement, DNA flow cytometric analysis, Arch Pathol Lab Med 114:65-67, 1990.
256. Hulbert JC, Graf R: Involvement of the spleen by renal angiomyolipoma: metastasis or multicentricity, J Urol 130:328-329, 1983.
257. Pea M, Bonetti F, Zamboni G et al: Melanocyte-marker-HMB-45 is regularly expressed in angiomyolipoma of the kidney, Pathology 23:185-188, 1991.
258. Sturtz CL, Dabbs DJ: Angiomyolipomas: The nature and expression of the HMB45 antigen, Mod Pathol 7:842-845, 1994.
259. Kaiserling E, Kröber S, Xiao J-C et al: Angiomyolipoma of the kidney. Immunoreactivity with HMB-45. Light- and electron-microscopic findings, Histopathology 25:41-48, 1994.
260. Peterson NE, Thompson HT: Renal hemangioma, J Urol 105:27-31, 1971.

261. Edward HG, DeWeerd JH, Woolner LB: Renal hemangiomas, Mayo Clin Proc 37:545-566, 1962.
262. Schofield D, Zaatari GS, Gay BB: Klippel-Trenaunay and Sturge-Weber syndromes with renal hemangioma and double inferior vena cava, J Urol 136:442-445, 1986.
263. Moros Garcia M, Martinez Tello D, Ramon y Cajal Junquera S et al: Multiple cavernous hemangioma of the kidney, Eur Urol 14:90-92, 1988.
264. Pickering SP, Fletcher BD, Bryan PJ et al: Renal lymphangioma: a cause of neonatal nephromegaly, Pediatr Radiol 14:445-448, 1984.
265. Singer DRJ, Miller JDB, Smith G: Lymphangioma of kidney, Scott Med J 28:293-294, 1983.
266. Joost J, Schäfer R, Altwein JE: Renal lymphangioma, J Urol 118:22-24, 1977.
267. Di Palma S, Giardini R: Leiomyoma of the kidney, Tumori 74:489-493, 1988.
268. Clinton-Thomas CL: A giant leiomyoma of the kidney, Br J Surg 43:497-501, 1956.
269. Zollikofer C, Castaneda-Zuniga W, Nath HP et al: The angiographic appearance of intrarenal leiomyoma, Radiology 136:47-49, 1980.
270. Dineen MK, Venable DD, Misra RP: Pure intrarenal lipoma—report of a case and review of the literature, J Urol 132:104-107, 1984.
271. Hurwitz RS, Benjamin JA, Cooper JF: Excessive proliferation of peripelvic fat of the kidney, Urology 11:448-456, 1978.
272. Grignon DJ, Ro JY, Ayala AG: Mesenchymal tumors of the kidney. In Eble JN, ed: Tumors and tumor-like conditions of the kidneys and ureters, New York, 1990, Churchill Livingstone.
273. Farrow GM, Harrison EG Jr, Utz DC et al: Sarcomas and sarcomatoid and mixed malignant tumors of the kidney in adults—part I, Cancer 22:545-550, 1968.
274. Herman C, Morales P: Leiomyosarcoma of renal vein, Urology 18:395-398, 1981.
275. Yokose T, Fukuda H, Ogiwara A et al: Myxoid leiomyosarcoma of the kidney accompanying ipsilateral ureteral transitional cell carcinoma. A case report with cytological, immunohistochemical and ultrastructural study, Acta Pathol Jpn 41:694-700, 1991.
276. Krech RH, Loy V, Dieckmann K-P et al: Leiomyosarcoma of the kidney: immunohistological and ultrastructural findings with special emphasis on the growth fraction, Br J Urol 63:132-134, 1989.
277. Grignon DJ, Ayala AG, Ro JY et al: Primary sarcomas of the kidney, a clinicopathologic and DNA flow cytometric study of 17 cases, Cancer 65:1611-1618, 1990.
278. Mayes DC, Fechner RE, Gillenwater JY: Renal liposarcoma, Am J Surg Pathol 14:268-273, 1990.
279. Cano JY, D'Altorio RA: Renal liposarcoma: case report, J Urol 115:747-749, 1976.
280. Takashi M, Murase T, Kato K et al: Malignant fibrous histiocytoma arising from the renal capsule: report of a case, Urol Int 42:227-230, 1987.
281. Joseph TJ, Becker DI, Turton AF: Renal malignant fibrous histiocytoma, Urology 37:483-489, 1991.
282. Srinivas V, Sogani PC, Hajdu SI et al: Sarcomas of the kidney, J Urol 132:13-16, 1984.
283. Penchansky L, Gallo G: Rhabdomyosarcoma of the kidney in children, Cancer 44:285-292, 1979.
284. Gonzalez-Crussi F, Baum ES: Renal sarcomas of childhood, a clinicopathologic and ultrastructural study, Cancer 51:898-912, 1983.
285. Grignon DJ, McIsaac GP, Armstrong RF et al: Primary rhabdomyosarcoma of the kidney, a light microscopic, immunohistochemical, and electron microscopic study, Cancer 62:2027-2032, 1988.
286. Eble JN: Fetal rhabdomyomatous nephroblastoma, J Urol 130:541-543, 1983.
287. Losty P, Kierce B: Botryoid Wilms' tumour—an unusual variant, Br J Urol 72:251-252, 1993.
288. Ordóñez NG, Bracken RB, Stroehlein KB: Hemangiopericytoma of kidney, Urology 20:191-195, 1982.
289. Siniluoto TMJ, Päivänsalo M, Hellström PA et al: Hemangiopericytoma of the kidney: a case with preoperative ethanol embolization, J Urol 140:137-138, 1988.
290. Weiss JP, Pollack HM, McCormick JF et al: Renal hemangiopericytoma: surgical, radiological and pathological implications, J Urol 132:337-339, 1984.
291. Eble JN, Young RH, Störkel S et al: Primary osteosarcoma of the kidney: a report of three cases, J Urogenital Pathol 1:83-88, 1991.
292. O'Malley FP, Grignon DJ, Shepherd RR et al: Primary osteosarcoma of the kidney, report of a case studied by immunohistochemistry, electron microscopy, and DNA flow cytometry, Arch Pathol Lab Med 115:1262-1265, 1991.
293. Malhotra CM, Doolittle CH, Rodil JV et al: Mesenchymal chondrosarcoma of the kidney, Cancer 54:2495-2499, 1984.
294. Nativ O, Horowitz A, Lindner A et al: Primary chondrosarcoma of the kidney, J Urol 134:120-121, 1985.
295. Cason JD, Waisman J, Plaine L: Angiosarcoma of kidney, Urology 30:281-283, 1987.
296. Desai MB, Chess Q, Naidich JB et al: Primary renal angiosarcoma mimicking a renal cell carcinoma, Urol Radiol 11:30-32, 1989.
297. Terris D, Plaine L, Steinfeld A: Renal angiosarcoma, Am J Kidney Dis 8:131-133, 1986.
298. Mead JH, Herrera GA, Kaufman MF et al: Case report of a primary cystic sarcoma of the kidney, demonstrating fibrohistiocytic, osteoid, and cartilaginous components (malignant mesenchymoma), Cancer 50:2211-2214, 1982.
299. Robertson PW, Klidjian A, Harding LK et al: Hypertension due to a renin-secreting renal tumour, Am J Med 43:963-976, 1967.
300. Kihara I, Kitamura S, Hoshino T et al: A hitherto unreported vascular tumor of the kidney: a proposal of "juxtaglomerular cell tumor," Acta Pathol Jpn 18:197-206, 1968.
301. Remynse LC, Begun FP, Jacobs SC et al: Juxtaglomerular cell tumor with elevation of serum erythropoietin, J Urol 142:1560-1562, 1989.
302. Corvol P, Pinet F, Galen FX et al: Seven lessons from seven renin secreting tumors, Kidney Int 34(suppl. 25):S38-S44, 1988.
303. Valdés G, Lopez JM, Martinez P et al: Renin-secreting tumor, case report, Hypertension 2:714-718, 1980.
304. Tetu B, Totovic V, Bechtelsheimer H et al: Tumeur rénale à sécrétion de rénine, à propos d'un cas avec étude ultrastructurale et immunohistochimique, Ann Pathol 4:55-59, 1984.

305. Camilleri J-P, Hinglais N, Bruneval P et al: Renin storage and cell differentiation in juxtaglomerular cell tumors: an immunohistochemical and ultrastructural study of three cases, Hum Pathol 15:1069-1079, 1984.
306. Lindop GBM, Stewart JA, Downie TT: The immunocytochemical demonstration of renin in a juxtaglomerular cell tumour by light and electron microscopy, Histopathology 7:421-431, 1983.
307. Lindop GBM, Fleming S, Gibson AAM: Immunocytochemical localisation of renin in nephroblastoma, J Clin Pathol 37:738-742, 1984.
308. Warfel KA, Eble JN: Renomedullary interstitial cell tumors, Am J Clin Pathol 83:262, 1985.
309. Lerman RJ, Pitcock JA, Stephenson P et al: Renomedullary interstitial cell tumor (formerly fibroma of the renal medulla), Hum Pathol 3:559-568, 1972.
310. Stuart R, Salyer WR, Salyer DC et al: Renomedullary interstitial cell lesions and hypertension, Hum Pathol 7:327-332, 1976.
311. Zimmermann A, Luscieti P, Flury B et al: Amyloid-containing renal interstitial cell nodules (RICNs) associated with chronic arterial hypertension in older age groups, Am J Pathol 105:288-294, 1981.
312. Mai KT: Giant renomedullary interstitial cell tumor, J Urol 151:986-988, 1994.
313. Boggs LK, Kimmelstiel P: Benign multilocular cystic nephroma: report of two cases of so-called multilocular cyst of the kidney, J Urol 76:530-541, 1956.
314. Mostofi FK, Sesterhenn IA, Sobin LH: Histological typing of kidney tumours, Geneva, 1981, World Health Organization.
315. Eble JN: Cystic nephroma and cystic partially differentiated nephroblastoma: two entities or one? Adv Anat Pathol 1:33-42, 1994.
316. Castillo OA, Boyle ET Jr, Kramer SA: Multilocular cysts of kidney, a study of 29 patients and review of the literature, Urology 37:156-162, 1991.
317. Joshi VV, Beckwith JB: Multilocular cyst of the kidney (cystic nephroma) and cystic, partially differentiated nephroblastoma, terminology and criteria for diagnosis, Cancer 64:466-479, 1989.
318. Kajani N, Rosenberg BF, Bernstein J: Multilocular cystic nephroma, J Urol Pathol 1:33-42, 1993.
319. Chatten J, Bishop HC: Bilateral multilocular cysts of the kidneys, J Pediatr Surg 12:749-750, 1977.
320. Brisigotti M, Cozzutto C, Fabbretti G et al: Metanephric adenoma, Histol Histopathol 7:689-692, 1992.
321. Jones EC, Pins M, Dickersin GR et al: Metanephric adenoma of the kidney, a clinicopathological, immunohistochemical, flow cytometric, cytogenetic, and electron microscopic study of seven cases, Am J Surg Pathol 19:615-626, 1995.
322. Davis CJ Jr, Barton JH, Sesterhenn IA et al: Metanephric adenoma clinicopathological study of fifty patients, Am J Surg Pathol 19:1101-1114, 1995.
323. Saint-André JP, Guyetant S, Croué A et al: Le néphrome néphrogène, Arch Anat Cytol Pathol 40:266-271, 1992.
324. Cochand-Priollet B, Gariou G, de Baecque-Fontaine C: Une tumeur du rein à ne pas méconnaître, Ann Pathol 13:275-276, 1993.
325. Mottet N, Dagues F, Pignodel C et al: Le néphrome néphronogène rénal: une tumeur exceptionnelle peu connue. A propos d'un cas révélé par une pyélonéphrite xantho-granulomateuse, Prog Urol 4:251-255, 1994.
326. Störkel S, Husman G, Thoenes W: Zur Diagnose und Differentialdiagnose des metanephroiden Nierentumors des Erwachsenen—ein unbekannter Nierentumor, Verh Dtsch Ges Pathol 76:306, 1992.
327. Raess KM, Wegmann W, Huber AK: Nephroblastomartiges Nierenadenom: Fallbericht über einen extrem seltenen Nierentumor, Helv Chir Acta 60:581-586, 1994.
328. Nagashima Y, Arai N, Tanaka Y et al: Two cases of a renal epithelial tumour resembling immature nephron, Virchows Arch [A] 418:77-81, 1991.
329. Burnett AL, Epstein JI, Gearhart JP: Spectrum of differentiation in pediatric epithelial tumors of kidney: report of two cases, Urology 42:93-98, 1993.
330. Hennigar RA, Beckwith JB: Nephrogenic adenofibroma, a novel kidney tumor of young people, Am J Surg Pathol 16:325-334, 1992.
331. Kandel LB, McCullough DL, Harrison LH et al: Primary renal lymphoma, does it exist? Cancer 60:386-391, 1987.
332. Silber SJ, Chang CY: Primary lymphoma of kidney, J Urol 110:282-284, 1973.
333. Osborne BM, Brenner M, Weitzner S et al: Malignant lymphoma presenting as a renal mass: four cases, Am J Surg Pathol 11:375-382, 1987.
334. Farrow GM, Harrison EG Jr, Utz DC: Sarcomas and sarcomatoid and mixed malignant tumors of the kidney in adults—part II, Cancer 22:551-555, 1968.
335. Jaspan T, Gregson R: Extra-medullary plasmacytoma of the kidney, Br J Radiol 57:95-97, 1984.
336. Igel TC, Engen DE, Banks PM et al: Renal plasmacytoma: Mayo Clinic experience and review of the literature, Urology 37:385-389, 1991.
337. Bracken RB, Chica G, Johnson DE et al: Secondary renal neoplasms: an autopsy study, South Med J 72:806-807, 1979.
338. Klinger ME: Secondary tumors of the genito-urinary tract, J Urol 65:144-153, 1951.
339. Payne RA: Metastatic renal tumours, Br J Surg 48:310-315, 1960.
340. Wagle DG, Moore RH, Murphy GP: Secondary carcinomas of the kidney, J Urol 114:30-32, 1975.
341. Pascal RR: Renal manifestations of extrarenal neoplasms, Hum Pathol 11:7-17, 1980.
342. Melato M, Laurino L, Bianchi P et al: Intraglomerular metastases. A possibly maldiagnosed entity, Zentralbl Allg Pathol 137:90-92, 1991.
343. Naryshkin S, Tomaszewski JE: Acute renal failure secondary to carcinomatous lymphatic metastases to kidneys, J Urol 146:1610-1612, 1991.
344. Gonzalez-Crussi F (ed): Wilms' Tumor (Nephroblastoma) and Related Renal Neoplasms of Childhood, Boca Raton, 1984, CRC Press, Inc.
345. Beckwith JB: Wilms' tumor and other renal tumors of childhood. In Finegold M, ed: Pathology of neoplasia in children and adolescents, Philadelphia, 1986, W.B. Saunders.
346. Mierau GW, Beckwith JB, Weeks DA: Ultrastructure and histogenesis of the renal tumors of childhood: an overview, Ultrastruct Pathol 11:313-333, 1987.

347. Webber BL, Parham DM, Drake LG et al: Renal tumors in childhood, Pathol Annu 27, Part 1:191-232, 1992.
348. Sotelo-Avila C: Nephroblastoma and other pediatric renal cancers. In Eble JN, ed: Tumors and tumor-like conditions of the kidneys and ureters, New York, 1990, Churchill Livingstone.
349. Breslow N, Beckwith JB, Ciol M et al: Age distribution of Wilms' tumor: report from the National Wilms' Tumor Study, Cancer Res 48:1653-1657, 1988.
350. Lemerle J, Tournade M-F, Gerard-Marchant R et al: Wilms' tumor: natural history and prognostic factors, a retrospective study of 248 cases treated at the Institut Gustave-Roussy 1952-1967, Cancer 37:2557-2566, 1976.
351. Hrabovsky EE, Othersen HB Jr, deLorimier A et al: Wilms' tumor in the neonate: a report from the National Wilms' Tumor Study, J Pediatr Surg 21:385-387, 1986.
352. Innis MD: Nephroblastoma: index cancer of childhood, Med J Aust 2:322-323, 1973.
353. Blute ML, Kelalis PP, Offord KP et al: Bilateral Wilms tumor, J Urol 138:968-973, 1987.
354. Breslow NE, Beckwith JB: Epidemiological features of Wilms' tumor: results of the National Wilms' Tumor Study, J Natl Cancer Inst 68:429-436, 1982.
355. Sotelo-Avila C, Gonzalez-Crussi F, Fowler JW: Complete and incomplete forms of Beckwith-Wiedemann syndrome: their oncogenic potential, J Pediatr 96:47-50, 1980.
356. Heppe RK, Koyle MA, Beckwith JB: Nephrogenic rests in Wilms' tumor patients with Drash syndrome, J Urol 145:1225-1228, 1991.
357. Miller RW, Fraumeni JF Jr, Manning MD: Association of Wilms's tumor with aniridia, hemihypertrophy and other congenital malformations, N Engl J Med 270:922-927, 1964.
358. Huser J, Grignon DJ, Ro JY et al: Adult Wilms' tumor: a clinicopathologic study of 11 cases, Mod Pathol 3:321-326, 1990.
359. Arrigo S, Beckwith JB, Sharples K et al: Better survival after combined modality care for adults with Wilms' tumor, a report from the National Wilms' Tumor Study, Cancer 66:827-830, 1990.
360. Bove KE, Koffler H, McAdams AJ: Nodular renal blastema, definition and possible significance, Cancer 24:323-332, 1969.
361. Bove KE, McAdams AJ: The nephroblastomatosis complex and its relationship to Wilms' tumor: a clinicopathologic treatise, Perspect Pediatr Pathol 3:185-223, 1976.
362. Beckwith JB, Kiviat NB, Bonadio JF: Nephrogenic rests, nephroblastomatosis, and the pathogenesis of Wilms' tumor, Pediatr Pathol 10:1-36, 1990.
363. Scharfenberg JC, Beckman EN: Persistent renal blastema in an adult, Hum Pathol 15:791-793, 1984.
364. Mahoney JP, Saffos RO: Fetal rhabdomyomatous nephroblastoma with a renal pelvic mass simulating sarcoma botryoides, Am J Surg Pathol 5:297-306, 1981.
365. Gonzalez-Crussi F, Hsueh W, Ugarte N: Rhabdomyogenesis in renal neoplasia of childhood, Am J Surg Pathol 5:525-532, 1981.
366. Grimes MM, Wolff M, Wolff JA et al: Ganglion cells in metastatic Wilms' tumor, review of a histogenetic controversy, Am J Surg Pathol 6:565-571, 1982.
367. Fetissof F, Dubois MP, Robert M et al: Néphroblastome avec cellules endocrines, étude immunohistochimique, Ann Pathol 5:279-281, 1985.
368. Cummins GE, Cohen D: Cushing's syndrome secondary to ACTH-secreting Wilms' tumor, J Pediatr Surg 9:535-539, 1974.
369. Joshi VV, Banerjee AK, Yadav K et al: Cystic partially differentiated nephroblastoma, a clinicopathologic entity in the spectrum of infantile renal neoplasia, Cancer 40:789-795, 1977.
370. Joshi VV: Cystic partially differentiated nephroblastoma: an entity in the spectrum of infantile renal neoplasia, Perspect Pediatr Pathol 5:217-235, 1979.
371. Wigger HJ: Fetal rhabdomyomatous nephroblastoma—a variant of Wilms' tumor, Hum Pathol 7:613-623, 1976.
372. Fernandes ET, Parham DM, Ribeiro RC et al: Teratoid Wilms' tumor: The St. Jude experience, J Pediatr Surg 23:1131-1134, 1988.
373. Variend S, Spicer RD, MacKinnon AE: Teratoid Wilms' tumor, Cancer 53:1936-1942, 1984.
374. Magee JF, Ansari S, McFadden DE et al: Teratoid Wilms' tumour: a report of two cases, Histopathology 20:427-431, 1992.
375. Kotiloğlu E, Kale G, Sevinir B et al: Teratoid Wilms' tumor. A unilateral case, Tumori 80:61-63, 1994.
376. Bonadio JF, Storer B, Norkool P et al: Anaplastic Wilms' tumor: clinical and pathologic studies, J Clin Oncol 3:513-520, 1985.
377. Breslow NE, Palmer NF, Hill LR et al: Wilms' tumor: prognostic factors for patients without metastases at diagnosis, results of the National Wilms' Tumor Study, Cancer 41:1577-1589, 1978.
378. Zuppan CW, Beckwith JB, Luckey DW: Anaplasia in unilateral Wilms' tumor: a report from the National Wilms' Tumor Study Pathology Center, Hum Pathol 19:1199-1209, 1988.
379. Weeks DA, Beckwith JB, Luckey DW: Relapse-associated variables in stage I favorable histology Wilms' tumor, a report of the National Wilms' Tumor Study, Cancer 60:1204-1212, 1987.
380. Marsden HB, Lawler W: Primary renal tumours in the first year of life. A population based review, Virchows Arch [A] 399:1-9, 1983.
381. Blank E, Neerhout RC, Burry KA: Congenital mesoblastic nephroma and polyhydramnios, JAMA 240:1504-1505, 1978.
382. Favara BE, Johnson W, Ito J: Renal tumors in the neonatal period, Cancer 22:845-855, 1968.
383. Kay S, Pratt CB, Salzberg AM: Hamartoma (leiomyomatous type) of the kidney, Cancer 19:1825-1832, 1966.
384. Bolande RP: Congenital mesoblastic nephroma of infancy, Perspect Pediatr Pathol 1:227-250, 1973.
385. Howell CG, Othersen HB, Kiviat NE et al: Therapy and outcome in 51 children with mesoblastic nephroma: a report of the National Wilms' Tumor Study, J Pediatr Surg 17:826-831, 1982.
386. Chan HSL, Cheng M-Y, Mancer K et al: Congenital mesoblastic nephroma: a clinicoradiologic study of 17 cases representing the pathologic spectrum of the disease, J Pediatr 111:64-70, 1987.

387. Sandstedt B, Delemarre JFM, Krul EJ et al: Mesoblastic nephromas: a study of 29 tumours from the SIOP nephroblastoma file, Histopathology 9:741-750, 1985.
388. Joshi VV, Kasznica J, Walters TR: Atypical mesoblastic nephroma, Arch Pathol Lab Med 110:100-106, 1986.
389. Gonzalez-Crussi F, Sotelo-Avila C, Kidd JM: Malignant mesenchymal nephroma of infancy, report of a case with pulmonary metastases, Am J Surg Pathol 4:185-190, 1980.
390. Trillo AA: Adult variant of congenital mesoblastic nephroma, Arch Pathol Lab Med 114:533-535, 1990.
391. Van Velden DJJ, Schneider JW, Allen FJ: A case of adult mesoblastic nephroma: ultrastructure and discussion of histogenesis, J Urol 143:1216-1219, 1990.
392. Durham JR, Bostwick DG, Farrow GM et al: Mesoblastic nephroma of adulthood, report of three cases, Am J Surg Pathol 17:1029-1038, 1994.
393. Beckwith JB, Weeks DA: Congenital mesoblastic nephroma, when should we worry? Arch Pathol Lab Med 110:98-99, 1986.
394. Gormley TS, Skoog SJ, Jones RV et al: Cellular congenital mesoblastic nephroma: what are the options, J Urol 142:479-483, 1989.
395. Heidelberger KP, Ritchey ML, Dauser RC et al: Congenital mesoblastic nephroma metastatic to the brain, Cancer 72:2499-2502, 1993.
396. Pettinato G, Manivel JC, Wick MR et al: Classical and cellular (atypical) congenital mesoblastic nephroma: a clinicopathologic, ultrastructural, immunohistochemical, and flow cytometric study, Hum Pathol 20:682-690, 1989.
397. Beckwith JB: Mesenchymal renal neoplasms in infancy revisited, J Pediatr Surg 9:803-805, 1974.
398. Marsden HB, Lawler W: Bone-metastasizing renal tumour of childhood, Br J Cancer 38:437-441, 1978.
399. Beckwith JB, Palmer NF: Histopathology and prognosis of Wilms tumor, results from the First National Wilms' Tumor Study, Cancer 41:1937-1948, 1978.
400. Mierau GW, Weeks DA, Beckwith JB: Anaplastic Wilms' tumor and other clinically aggressive childhood renal neoplasms: ultrastructural and immunocytochemical features, Ultrastruct Pathol 13:225-248, 1989.
401. Sotelo-Avila C, Gonzalez-Crussi F, Sadowinski S et al: Clear cell sarcoma of the kidney: a clinicopathologic study of 21 patients with long-term follow-up evaluation, Hum Pathol 16:1219-1230, 1986.
402. Marsden HB, Lawler W: Bone metastasizing renal tumour of childhood, histopathological and clinical review of 38 cases, Virchows Arch [A] 387:341-351, 1980.
403. Palmer NF, Sutow W: Clinical aspects of the rhabdoid tumor of the kidney: a report of the National Wilms' Tumor Study Group, Med Pediatr Oncol 11:242-245, 1983.
404. Weeks DA, Beckwith JB, Mierau GW et al: Rhabdoid tumor of kidney, a report of 111 cases from the National Wilms' Tumor Study Pathology Center, Am J Surg Pathol 13:439-458, 1989.
405. Bonnin JM, Rubinstein LJ, Palmer NF et al: The association of embryonal tumors originating in the kidney and in the brain, a report of seven cases, Cancer 54:2137-2146, 1984.
406. Rousseau-Merck MF, Boccon-Gibod L, Nogues C et al: An original hypercalcemic infantile renal tumor without bone metastasis: heterotransplantaion to nude mice, report of two cases, Cancer 50:85-93, 1982.
407. Mayes LC, Kasselberg AG, Roloff JS et al: Hypercalcemia associated with immunoreactive parathyroid hormone in a malignant rhabdoid tumor of the kidney (rhabdoid Wilms' tumor), Cancer 54:882-884, 1984.
408. Haas JE, Palmer NF, Weinberg AG et al: Ultrastructure of malignant rhabdoid tumor of the kidney, a distinctive renal tumor of children, Hum Pathol 12:646-657, 1981.
409. Weeks DA, Beckwith JB, Mierau GW et al: Renal neoplasms mimicking rhabdoid tumor of kidney, a report from the National Wilms' Tumor Study Pathology Center, Am J Surg Pathol 15:1042-1054, 1991.
410. Küss MR: Un cas de néphroblastome calcifié simulant un calcul, J Urol Nephrol 73:653-655, 1966.
411. Chatten J, Cromie WJ, Duckett JW: Ossifying tumor of infantile kidney, report of two cases, Cancer 45:609-612, 1980.
412. Jerkins GR, Callihan TR: Ossifying renal tumor of infancy, J Urol 135:120-121, 1986.
413. Dehner LP: Intrarenal teratoma occurring in infancy: Report of a case with discussion of extragonadal germ cell tumors in infancy, J Pediatr Surg 8:369-378, 1973.
414. Aubert J, Casamayou J, Denis P et al: Intrarenal teratoma in a newborn child, Eur Urol 4:306-308, 1978.
415. Aaronson IA, Sinclair-Smith C: Multiple cystic teratomas of the kidney, Arch Pathol Lab Med 104:614, 1980.
416. Mihatsch MJ, Bleisch A, Six P et al: Primary choriocarcinoma of the kidney in a 49-year-old woman, J Urol 108:537-539, 1972.
417. Young RH, Eble JN: Unusual forms of carcinoma of the urinary bladder, Hum Pathol 22:948-965, 1991.

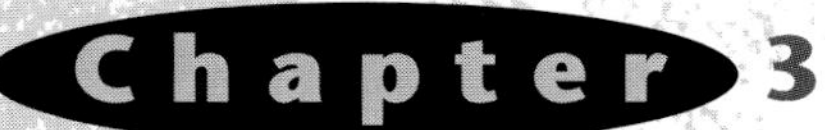

Chapter 3

RENAL PELVIS AND URETER

STEPHEN M. BONSIB
JOHN N. EBLE

The renal pelvis and ureter are muscular conduits lined by urothelium that function to propel urine from the renal calyceal system to the urinary bladder. The ureter and renal pelvis are affected by developmental, reactive, and neoplastic disorders. The developmental disorders are a group of closely related entities that include abnormalities in ureteral number, ureteral location, and structure and function of pelvic and ureteral muscularis propria. The mucosa is the site of the major reactive and neoplastic disorders.

DEVELOPMENT

The ureter and renal pelvis develop from the ampullary bud, which arises from the distal mesonephric duct during the fourth week of development.[1] Contact of the ampullary bud with metanephric blastema induces nephrogenesis. During the months that follow, the ampullary bud elongates and branches dichotomously in parallel with the development of the nephrons to create the adult metanephric kidney with its renal pelvis and ureter.[1] As the ureter elongates, there is a period of luminal obliteration followed by recanalization in the fifth week. Recanalization begins in the middle of the ureter and extends proximally and distally with the ureteropelvic and ureterovesical junctions, which are the last segments to recanalize.[2]

The mesonephric duct distal to the ampullary bud (the common nephric duct) is incorporated into the developing urogenital sinus, while the ureteral orifice migrates to the trigone of the urinary bladder.[1] The common nephric duct forms the trigone and contributes to the prostatic urethra in the male. Concomitant development of the male and female reproductive tract from the mesonephric (wolffian) and müllerian ducts, respectively, and division of the cloaca into bladder and hindgut, occur nearby as the ureter and kidney develop. Thus multiple malformations in these areas often occur together.

ANATOMY

The lumen of the renal pelvis and ureter is lined by urothelium (also called *transitional epithelium*), which rests on a basement membrane over a lamina propria composed of loose connective tissue that is highly vascular (Fig. 3-1*A*). The urothelium is composed of three to five layers of cells in the pelvis and four to seven layers of cells in the ureter (Fig. 3-1*B*). The pelvis and ureter have a continuous muscular wall that originates in the fornices of the minor calyces as small interlacing fascicles of

A
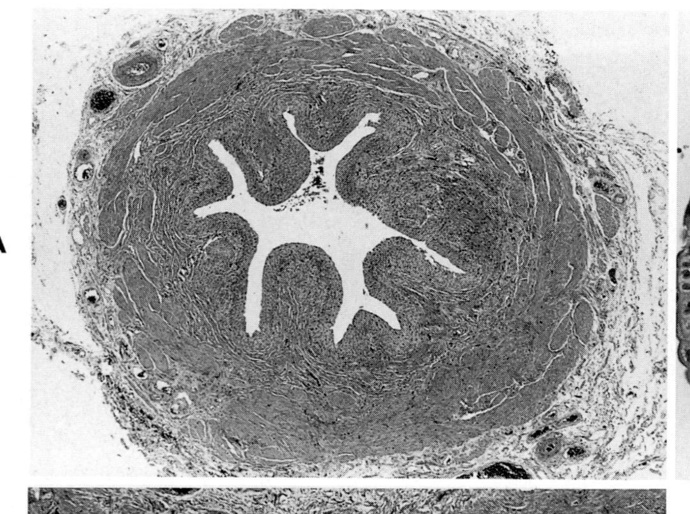

B
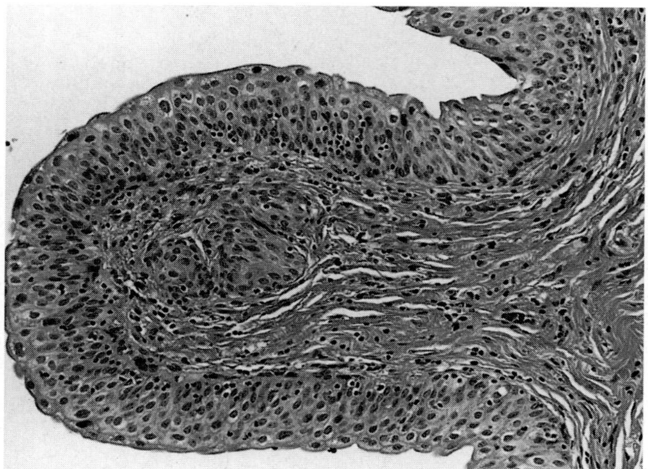

C
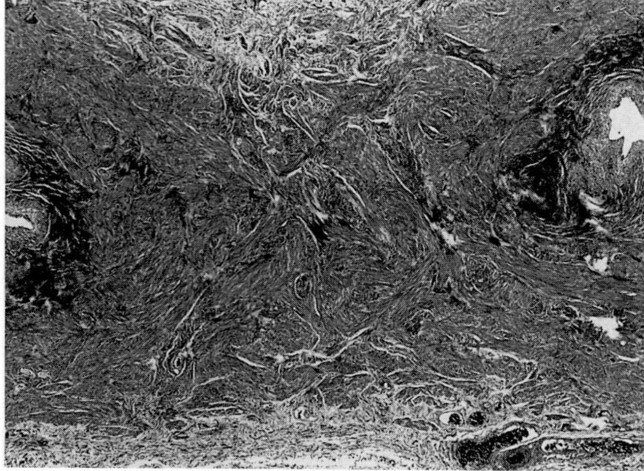

3-1. Adult ureter. **(A)** Cross section showing adventitia, muscularis propria, and irregular contour of relaxed mucosa. **(B)** The mucosa consists of a few layers of urothelial cells overlying loose connective tissue. No muscularis mucosae is visible. **(C)** A longitudinal section shows spiral arrangement of muscle fascicles.

smooth muscle cells.[3-5] These take on a spiral architecture in the pelvis and ureter, a structure necessary for effective peristalsis[3,4] (Fig. 3-1*C*). The muscularis propria is not divided into distinct layers. Near the bladder the ureter acquires an external sheath from the detrusor muscle, and the muscle fascicles become oriented longitudinally.[5,6] The longitudinal fibers continue through the wall of the bladder and into the submucosa, where they spread about the ureteral orifice to contribute to the trigone muscle. Ultimately they terminate near the bladder neck in the female and at the verumontanum in the male.

Peristalsis is initiated by "pace-maker" cells in the renal pelvic muscle near the calyces. These generate electrical impulses that propagate from cell to cell through gap junctions.[7,8] Effective peristalsis requires both continuity of gap junctions and appropriate quantity and organization of muscle fascicles. As will be discussed later in this chapter, disruption of this pattern, even focally, may cause ureteral incompetence or functional obstruction.

CONGENITAL MALFORMATIONS

Genitourinary tract malformations occur in 10% of the population and are the most common group of congenital anomalies.[9] Some, such as bifid ureters, are clinically insignificant.[10] Others are associated with ureteral incompetence or obstruction, carrying the risk of renal damage, or are associated with renal dysplasia.[1] Some are components of multiple malformation syndromes (e.g., VATER association or prune belly syndrome), are associated with chromosomal abnormalities (e.g., trisomy syndromes), or have a familial association.[11-18] The various congenital malformations of the ureters frequently occur together (Table 3-1).

Patients with ureteropelvic anomalies usually present with symptoms of ureteral or pelvic distention, such as flank pain or mass, or with complications such as infection, calculi, or renal insufficiency.[1,18] Ultrasound imaging permits the demonstration of ureteropelvic malformations in utero and in neonates. Most such lesions encountered in surgical pathology consist of intrinsic structural defects of the muscularis, usually involving the ends of the ureters, the last segments to recanalize during embryogenesis. These malformations are congenital and of developmental origin, but patients may present at any age, from newborn to adulthood. Surgical therapy usually consists of excision of the abnormal segment to preserve renal function. The surgical pathologist should define the anatomic basis of the functional deficit, which usually consists of a distinct but localized defect in smooth muscle quantity or organization (Table 3-2). Recognition of

TABLE 3-1.
COMMON ASSOCIATIONS BETWEEN URETERAL ANOMALIES

	Bifid/Duplex	Ectopia	Reflux	Obstruction of ureteropelvic junction	Ureterocele	Dysplasia
Bifid/duplex		+	+	+	+	+
Ectopia	+		+	+	+	+
Reflux	+	+		+	+	+
Obstruction of ureteropelvic junction	+	+	+		+	+
Ureterocele	+	+	+	+		+
Diverticulum	-	+	+	-	-	+
Primary Megaureter	-	-	-	-	-	+

TABLE 3-2.
URETERAL MUSCLE FINDINGS IN URETERAL ANOMALIES

	Muscle normal	Muscle deficient	Muscle dysplastic	Longitudinal fiber predominance	Circular fiber predominance	Sheath thick
Refluxing megaureter	+	+	+	-	-	-
Obstruction of ureteropelvic junction	+	+	+	+	-	-
Primary megaureter	-	-	+	-	+	+
Ureterocele	+	+	+	-	-	-
Paraureteral diverticulum	+	+	+	-	-	-

these lesions requires an appreciation of the normal muscle pattern, and their histologic demonstration requires well-oriented sections in which the pattern of the muscle fascicles is highlighted by a trichrome stain. For most lesions longitudinal orientation of the specimen best shows the deviation from the normal muscle pattern. Primary megaureter (see below) is an exception in which cross-sections display the predominance of circular fibers and thickening of the periureteral sheath.

ABNORMALITIES IN NUMBER OR LOCATION OF URETERS

Ureteral agenesis, ureteral duplication, and ureteral ectopia are a group of related malformations resulting from defective formation of the ampullary bud.[1] Isolated failure of ampullary bud formation causes ureteral agenesis with absence of the ipsilateral hemitrigone and kidney[1] (see Fig. 1-28). Another cause of agenesis of the ureter and kidney is wolffian duct failure. Wolffian duct failure can be recognized because of its associated genital tract malformations (e.g., absent testis or unicornuate uterus).[1,9] Unilateral agenesis of the kidney and ureter is associated with additional urologic malformations in 20% to 40% of patients.[19] Bilateral renal agenesis (Potter's syndrome) (see Fig. 1-34) is lethal because of its associated pulmonary hypoplasia.

Bifid ureter and duplex ureter, the most common (0.8 percent of all autopsies) ureteral anomalies, result from premature branching of the ampullary bud or development of two separate ampullary buds.[1,20] Premature branching results in two separate renal pelves and proximal ureters that join to form a single ureter at some point above the bladder[10] (Fig. 3-2). Duplex ureters (Fig. 3-3) have two separate ureteral orifices in the bladder.[20,21] The ureter from the lower pole usually has its orifice normally situated on the trigone or displaced laterally. The orifice of the ureter from the upper pole can be normally placed, but displacement toward the bladder neck or to an extravesical location is more typical.[21] Ureteral ectopia results from abnormally high or low origin of the ampullary bud from the mesonephric duct. Eighty percent of ureteral orifice ectopia is associated with the ureter from the upper pole of a duplicated system.[20,21] The ectopic ureteral orifice may be intravesical (lateral or caudal to the normal site) or extravesical in the urethra, vestibule, or genitalia. Symptoms are influenced by the patient's gender and the site of the ureteral orifice and may consist of urethral dribbling, vaginal "discharge," epididymo-orchitis, or pyelonephritis if reflux or obstruction are present.[9] The greater the degree of ectopia in a lateral or extravesical location, the more likely it is that the corresponding renal unit will be dysplastic.[21] The surgical pathology specimen thus may include a segmental or complete nephrectomy for dysplasia or pyelonephritis or a distal ureter excised for reflux, obstruction, or ureterocele.

REFLUXING MEGAURETER

Reflux from the bladder into the ureter is the most common ureteral problem requiring surgical intervention. Patients usually present in early childhood with urinary tract infections and often already have renal scars (reflux nephropathy).[22,23] Reflux may be unilateral or bilateral, and, in about one third of cases, the patients' siblings have similar urologic abnormalities.[17] Vesicoureteral reflux is caused by incompetence of the ureterovesical junction. There is a 5:1 predominance of females over males, possibly resulting from the additional mechanical support provided to the bladder by the prostate and seminal vesicles.

The affected ureters have abnormally short submucosal segments or deficiency of longitudinal fibers in the intramural segment or both.[1,18,22] Abnormally short submucosal segments are apparent to the urologist but difficult to demonstrate histologically. Deficiency of longitudinal fibers can be demonstrated in longitudinal sections of the intramural segment and may appear to the urologist as an abnormally thin and translucent segment of distal ureter (Fig. 3-4). Excision of the defective distal ureteral segment and reimplantation of the ureter is usually effective.[23]

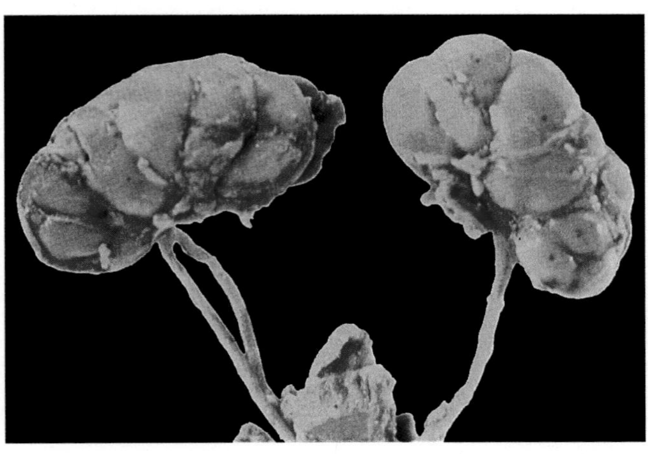

3-2. Bifid ureters joining to form a single ureter above the bladder.

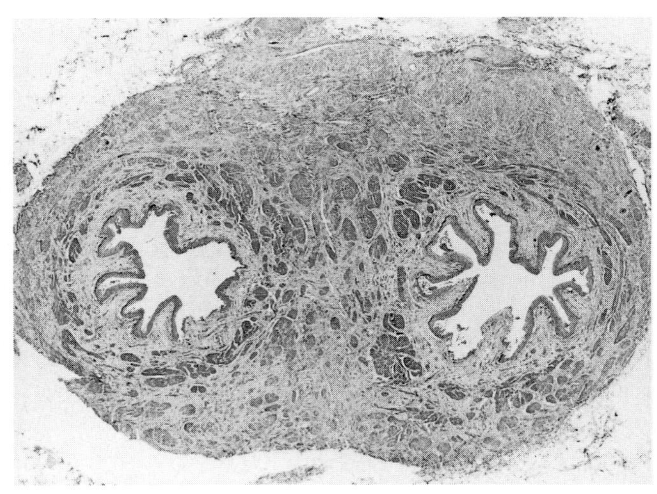

3-3. Duplex ureter near point of confluence.

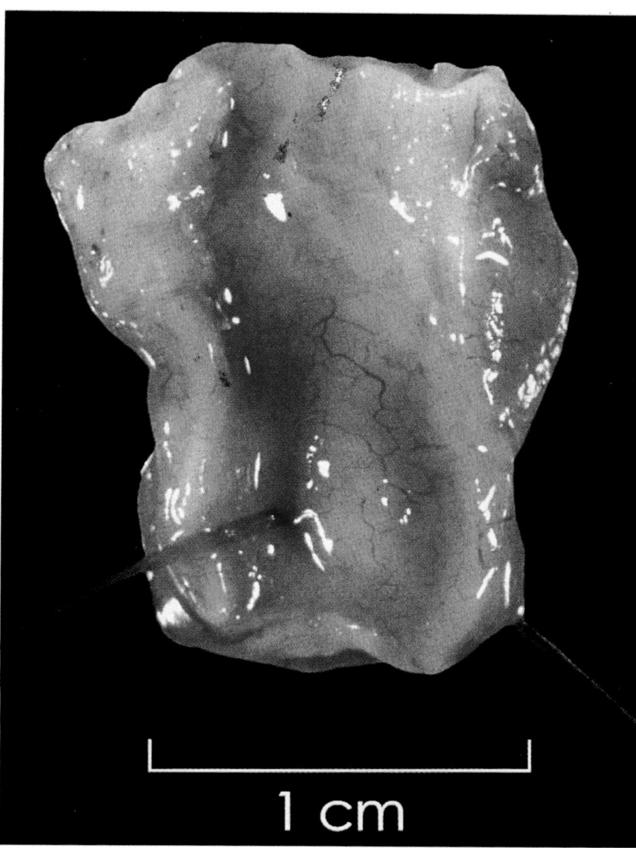

3-4. Longitudinal section showing mucosal aspect of distal ureter in reflux. Note the thin wall.

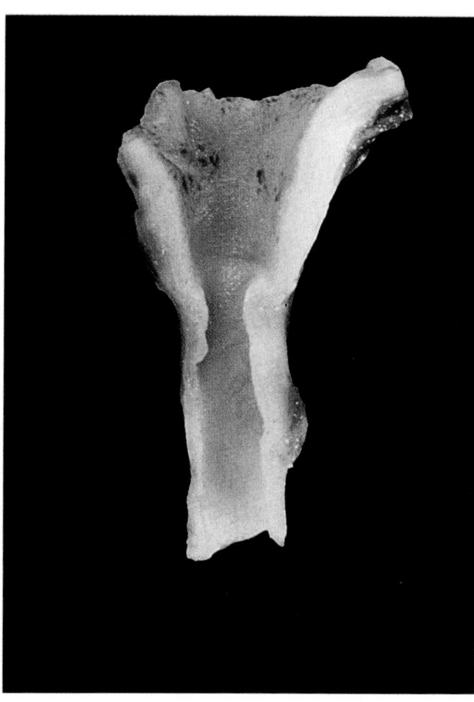

3-5. Funnel-shaped zone of ureteropelvic junction obstruction.

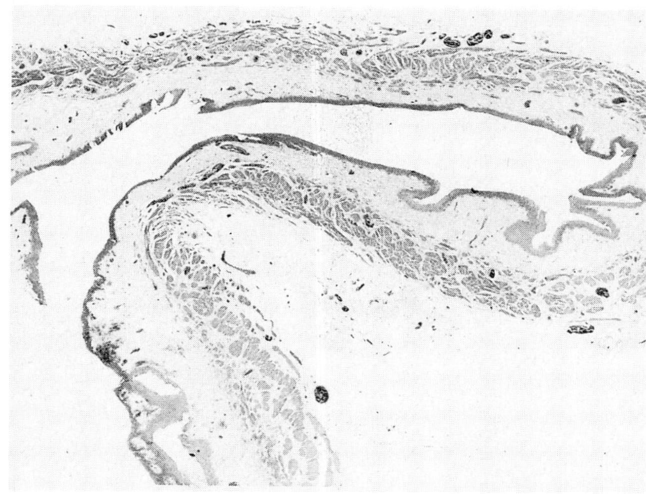

3-6. Ureteropelvic junction obstruction caused by an overlying vessel.

URETEROPELVIC JUNCTION OBSTRUCTION

Ureteropelvic junction obstruction is the most common cause of ureteral obstruction. It may present at any age. When presenting in childhood, it is frequently bilateral (16%), associated with other urologic malformations (15% to 20%), and predominantly on the left side and in boys.[15,24] When presenting in adulthood, ureteropelvic junction obstruction is most often unilateral and in women.[24] The two most common causes are defects in the muscularis (75%) and renal nonrotation associated with polar vessels (6% to 24%).[25-27]

The obstructed ureteropelvic junction is characteristically funnel-shaped (Fig. 3-5). It may have a grossly visible area of thin muscle, a valvelike intraluminal protrusion of edematous mucosa or muscularis or it may be stenotic. The histologic appearance of ureteropelvic junction obstruction is varied (Fig. 3-6, 3-7, 3-8). There may be segmental smooth muscle attenuation, often with a predominance of longitudinal fibers, diffuse lack of fascicular organization of pelvic muscles (i.e., dysplastic; see Ureteral Dysplasia, later in this chapter), segmental absence of smooth muscle, or a stenotic lumen with normal muscle.[25,26] "Valves" or "pleats" have also been described, which probably result from herniation at a site of muscle abnormality.[27]

Renal polar blood vessels are common anatomic variants of the renal vasculature that usually do not obstruct the ureter because of its medial origin at the renal hilum.[28] In congenitally nonrotated kidneys, the pelvis is anterior and polar vessels may cause significant ureteral obstruction[28] (see Fig. 1-22).

PRIMARY MEGAURETER

Primary megaureter is a nonrefluxing, nonobstructive form of ureteral dilation.[18] Its gross appearance is distinctive (Fig. 3-9). The ureters are narrow and straight immediately above the bladder and above that segment they are fusiform and markedly dilated. This fusiform dilation differs from the tortuous appearance of ureteral dilation secondary to reflux or obstruction. In 80% of

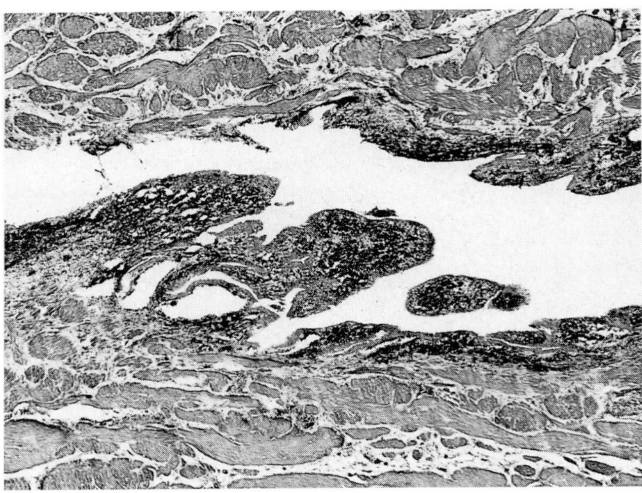

3-7. Ureteropelvic junction obstruction caused by a mucosal valve or pleat.

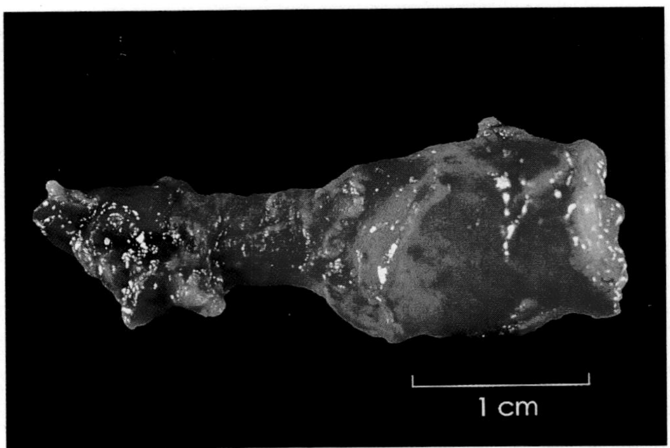

3-9. Primary megaureter with abrupt dilation at superior end.

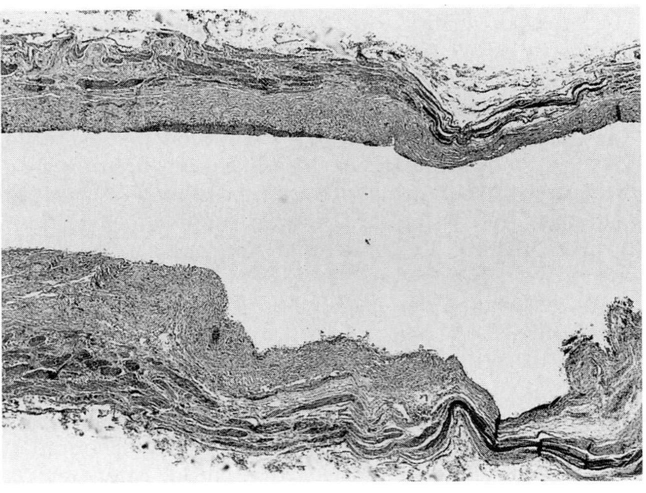

3-8. Ureteropelvic junction obstruction caused by a segment in which longitudinal muscle fibers predominate (*right*).

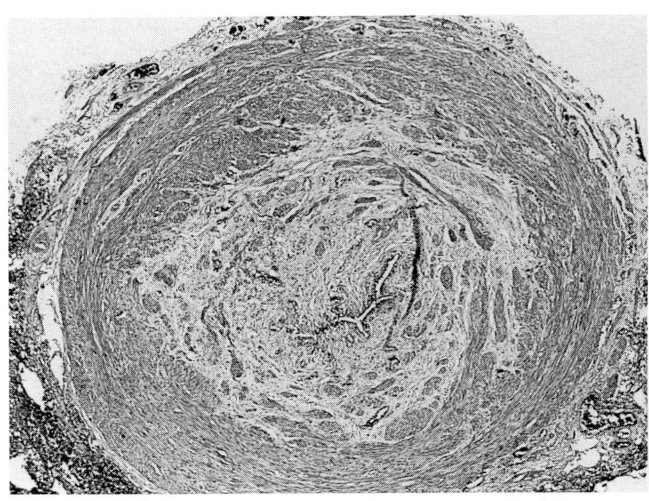

3-10. Primary megaureter: cross section of narrow segment showing thick periureteral sheath.

these patients there is functional obstruction at the level of the narrow segment and this must be excised.[29,30] Seen in cross-section (Fig. 3-10), the narrow segment shows either predominance of circular fibers, hypoplasia and fibrosis of the smooth muscle, or thickening of the periureteral sheath.[18] The only abnormality of the dilated segment is hypertrophy of the smooth muscle. In the other 20% of cases of primary megaureter, the narrow segment of ureter has normal muscle and the dilated ureter above it has an almost complete absence of muscle.[30] Such ureters have been called *dysplastic ureters* (see Ureteral Dysplasia, later in this chapter) and commonly are associated with a dysplastic kidney.[31,32]

URETEROCELE

Ureterocele is congenital dilation of the distal ureter within the bladder (Fig. 3-11). Ureterocele balloons into the bladder and occasionally protrudes into the urethra.[33-35] Most ureteroceles occur in the upper pole ureter of a duplicated system. In this situation the ureter usually passes dorsal to the lower pole ureter.[33] Its dilated portion may undermine and distort the trigone, often resulting in obstruction or reflux of the normally situated lower pole ureter, or, if the ureterocele is large, the contralateral ureter as well.[33] Ureterocele rarely affects a single ureter.

Microscopically, the muscle of the wall of the ureterocele varies from hypertrophic to atrophic or absent[34] (Fig. 3-12). Consistent with the usual ectopic location of the ureteral orifice associated with duplex kidneys, 70% of cases have segmental dysplasia of the upper pole of the kidney.[35]

PARAURETERAL DIVERTICULUM

Herniation of the urinary bladder involving the distal ureter is called *paraureteral diverticulum*. It is usually con-

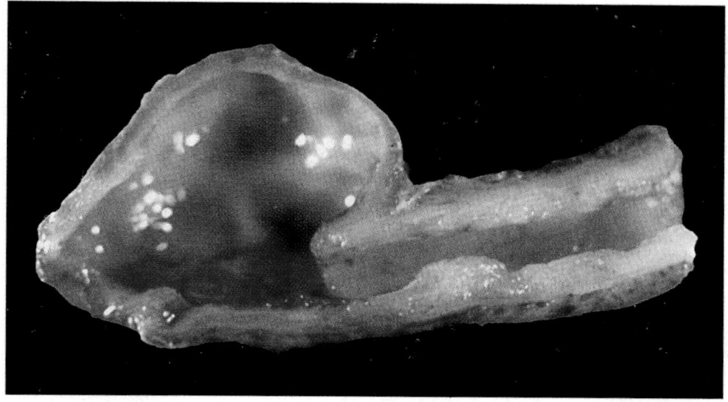

3-11. Ureterocele of upper pole ureter. Orifice was near bladder neck.

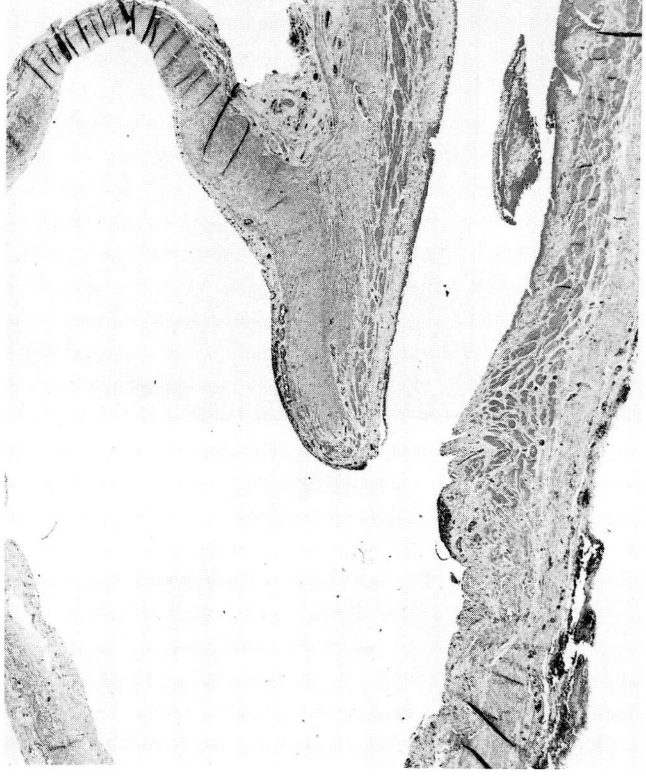

3-12. Ureterocele, showing lack of muscle in its wall (*upper left*).

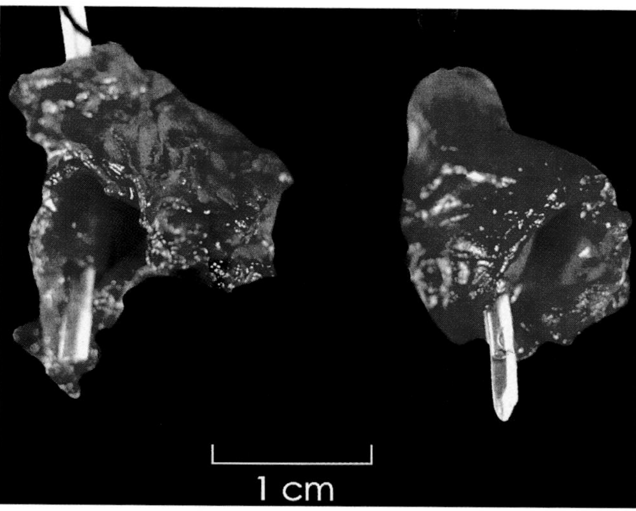

3-13. Bilateral paraureteral diverticula. Probes indicate ureteral orifices at the mouth of each diverticulum.

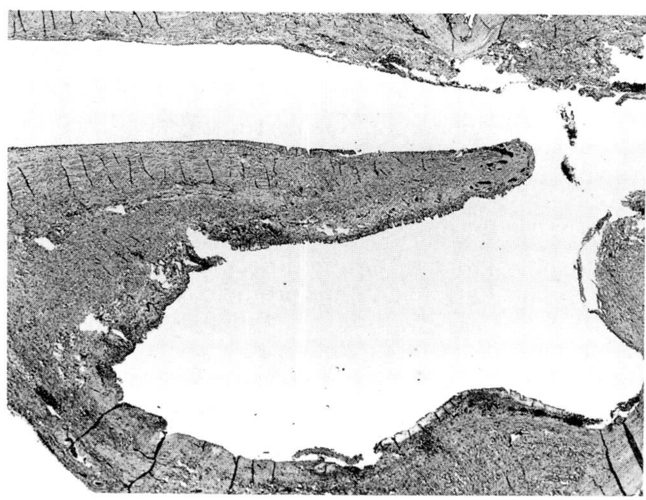

3-14. Paraureteral diverticulum showing deficient development of the muscular wall.

genital and detected in childhood but may result from urethral or bladder neck obstruction at any age.[36,37] Vesicoureteral reflux is commonly associated with paraureteral diverticulum. The location of the ureteral orifice within the diverticulum correlates with the risk of renal dysplasia[37] (Fig. 3-13). When the ureter opens into the dome of the diverticulum (a form of lateral ectopia) rather than near its orifice, the likelihood of renal dysplasia is great. There are few histologic studies of diverticula, but deficient ureteral muscle and sheath development have been reported[37] (Fig. 3-14).

URETERAL DYSPLASIA

Ureteral dysplasia refers to ureters composed of infrequent small muscle cells lacking organization and failing to form fascicles[25] (Fig. 3-15). Takunaka[32] showed that these small muscle cells possess thin actin filaments but lack the thick myosin filaments essential for normal muscle contractility. An alternative term, *ureteral maldevelopment*, was introduced by Hanna in 1979 for this condition. Recognition of dysplastic ureters is important because of their association with ipsilateral renal dysplasia in 56% to 70% of cases.[25,26]

Dysplastic ureters are variable in appearance, some appearing atretic (Fig. 1-40*A*) while others are dilated (Fig. 3-16) as well as anomalous in location. Recognition of their dysplastic nature is not possible with the naked eye, because ureters with normal muscle fascicle formation can have a similar appearance.

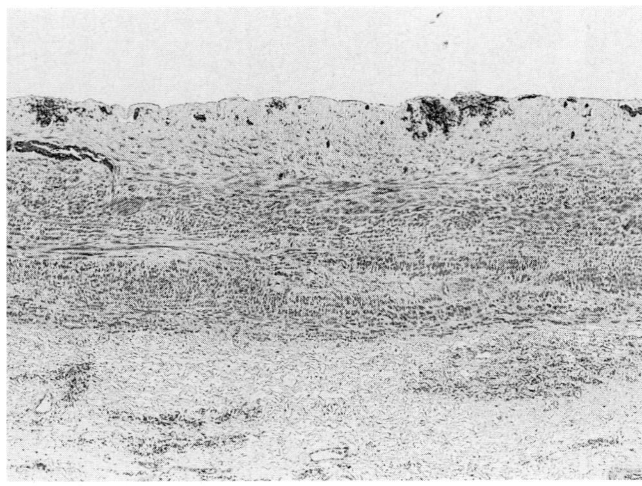

3-15. Ureteral dysplasia showing small muscle fibers.

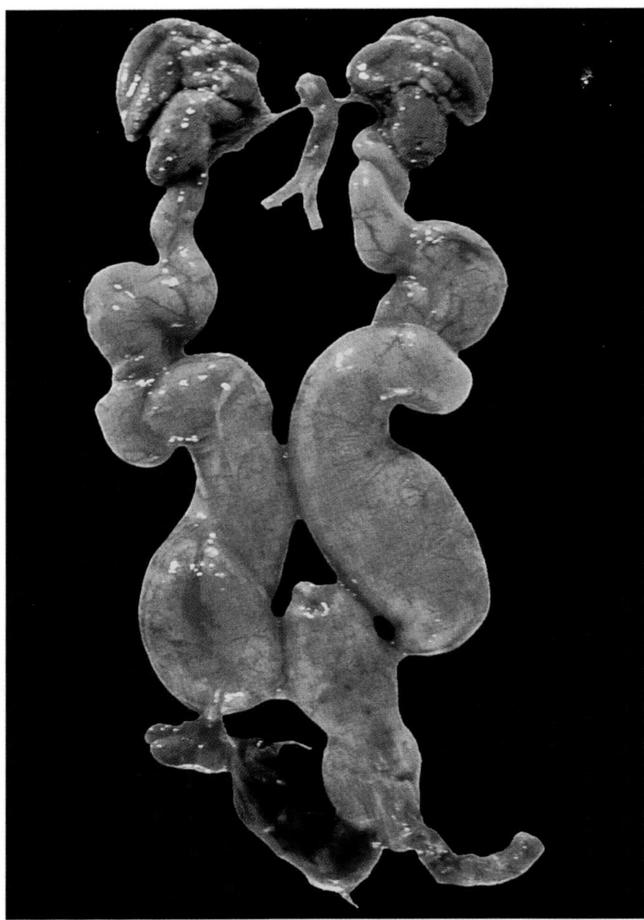

3-16. Dysplastic megaureter associated with bilateral renal dysplasia.

NON-NEOPLASTIC PROLIFERATIVE, METAPLASTIC, AND INFLAMMATORY LESIONS

HYPERPLASIA, VON BRUNN'S NESTS, URETEROPYELITIS CYSTICA, AND GLANDULARIS

The most common non-neoplastic urothelial proliferative lesions are simple hyperplasia, von Brunn's nests, and ureteropyelitis cystica and glandularis.[38,39] Simple hyperplasia is an increase in the number of layers of urothelial cells without cytologic atypia. It commonly accompanies inflammation and neoplasia. Von Brunn's nests are small nests of normal urothelial cells within the lamina propria. They are most common in the trigone of the bladder but are also found in 10% percent of normal ureters at autopsy.[39] When von Brunn's nests have central lumens lined by urothelium or columnar cells they are referred to as *ureteritis* or *pyelitis cystica* and *ureteritis* or *pyelitis glandularis*, respectively. Although usually of microscopic size, ureteritis and pyelitis cystica may rarely produce grossly visible fluid-filled cysts that elevate the urothelium[39-41] (Fig. 3-17, 3-18).

Von Brunn's nests and ureteropyelitis cystica are generally regarded as normal features of the urothelial mucosa. However, they may also be reactive lesions and they have arisen following experimental mucosal injury.[42] In that situation they develop within 24 to 48 hours and persist for months following removal of the inflammatory stimulus.

SQUAMOUS AND GLANDULAR METAPLASIA

Squamous metaplasia is the most common form of urothelial metaplasia.[39,40,43,44] It may be nonkeratinizing or show keratinization (Fig. 3-19) with or without atypia. When squamous metaplasia is encountered in the renal pelvis and ureter, it is often keratinizing. The keratin may be so copious that squames are seen in the urine or collect in the pelvis, forming a mass.[44] This sequence has prompted the use of terms such as *leukoplakia* and *cholesteatoma* when keratinization or keratin accumulation, respectively, are marked.[44] Keratinizing squamous metaplasia is usually the result of chronic irritation. Conditions such as chronic infection, indwelling catheters, and calculi are present in 60% to 70% of patients.[41] Keratinizing squamous metaplasia of the urothelial mucosa is associated with increased risk of squamous cell and urothelial carcinoma.[45,46]

Mucinous (glandular, enteric, intestinal, colonic) metaplasia indicates the presence of colonic-type mucinous epithelium, often containing enterochromaffin cells, in place of urothelium.[42,47-49] In the bladder these alterations may range from numerous minute foci to involvement of the entire mucosa, usually observed in bladder exstrophy.[48] Glandular metaplasia of the renal pelvis and ureter is rare, and most cases have been associated with adenocarcinoma.[42,49]

NEPHROGENIC ADENOMA

Nephrogenic adenoma is rare in the ureter and much more common in the urinary bladder, often appearing as an exophytic lesion which may cystoscopically mimic urothelial carcinoma. Microscopically, it is a benign papillary and tubular proliferation lined by cuboidal or hobnail epithelium.[50,51] Nephrogenic adenoma is discussed in detail in Chapter 4.

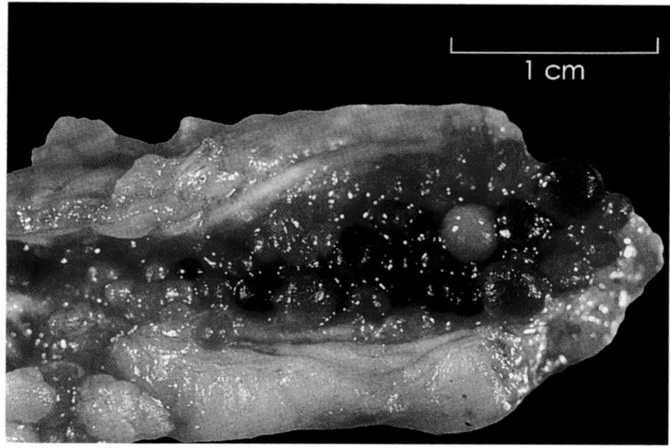

3-17. Ureteritis cystica with cobblestone appearance of vesicles protruding into the ureteral lumen.

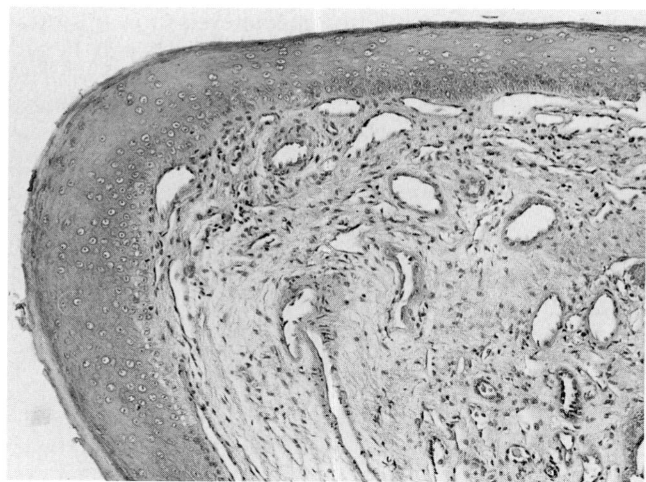

3-19. Keratinizing squamous metaplasia covering a renal papilla.

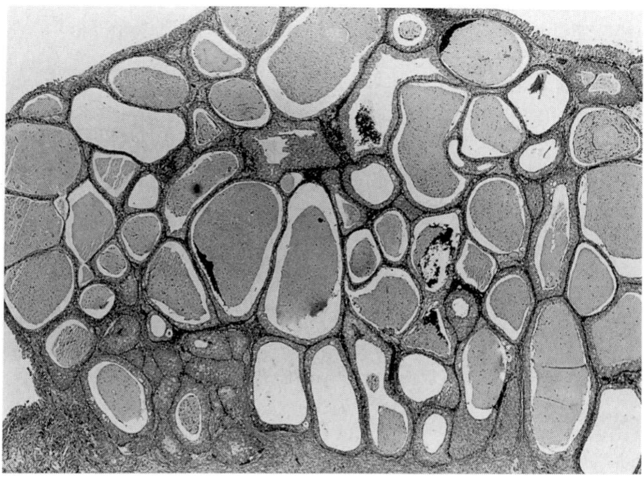

3-18. von Brunn's nests and ureteritis cystica forming a mass in the ureteral mucosa. *(Courtesy of Robert H. Young, M.D.)*

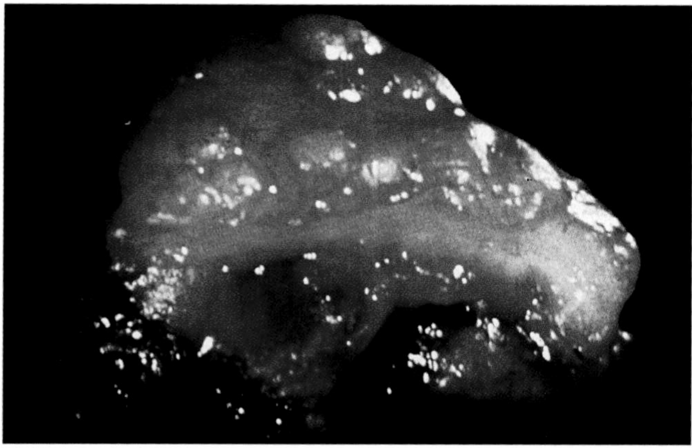

3-20. Malakoplakia of the ureter with yellow mucosal plaques. *(Courtesy of Robert H. Young, M.D.)*

REACTIVE ATYPIA

Reactive atypia may affect the urothelium and mimic urothelial carcinoma in situ. Thiotepa and mitomycin-C, intravesical chemotherapeutic agents used to treat noninvasive urothelial cancer, are most often implicated.[52,53] However, similar alterations can be produced by irradiation and catheterization. The resultant striking cytologic atypia characteristically affects superficial cells, which, although enlarged, have low nuclear cytoplasmic ratios, nuclear or cytoplasmic vacuoles, and smudged chromatin.[52,53] The mixture of normal urothelial cells with occasional large atypical cells is distinctive. Reactive atypia is characteristically encountered in the bladder but may also be encountered in the ureteral mucosa in patients who have vesicoureteral reflux.[53]

MALAKOPLAKIA

Malakoplakia is an uncommon chronic granulomatous disease originally described by Michaelis and Gutmann[54] in 1902 and elaborated upon by von Hansemann[55] in 1903. Malakoplakia is most frequently observed in the urinary tract of middle-aged women as a complication of recurrent infections. Bladder involvement is 4 to 10 times more common than involvement of the renal pelvis and ureter.[56-58]

The typical lesion of malakoplakia is a yellow-brown soft ("malakos") plaque ("plakos") (Fig. 3-20) that often has a central umbilication. Microscopically, masses of large eosinophilic histiocytes (von Hansemann histiocytes) are present, many of which contain basophilic inclusions (Michaelis-Gutmann bodies). Periodic acid–Schiff (PAS) stain and special stains for calcium and iron enhance the targetoid appearance of these cytoplasmic inclusions and indicate their mineralized nature. Malakoplakia is discussed in detail in Chapter 4.

RETROPERITONEAL FIBROSIS

Retroperitoneal fibrosis is a proliferative process of inflammation and fibrosis of middle and old age.[59-61] Retroperitoneal structures may be encased, with the ureters frequently exhibiting medial deviation on intravenous pyelography. Retroperitoneal fibrosis may be primary and idiopathic, although a variety of secondary causes have been identified, including iatrogenic (drugs, surgery, irradiation), inflammatory (vasculitis, aneurysms, diverticulitis, inflammatory bowel disease), and neoplastic (sclerosing lymphoma and urothelial carcinoma) disorders.[59-61] Regardless of the etiology, the typical histology is a prominent mixed inflammatory cell infiltrate with fibroplasia and edema. The major challenge is to identify those secondary causes that may merit different therapy.

NEOPLASMS

Neoplasms of the ureter and pelvis represent 20% to 25% of upper tract tumors in adults, and renal cell carcinoma comprises most of the remaining cases.[62] Ureteral and pelvic neoplasms occur with approximately equal frequency but collectively are only one tenth as common as their bladder counterpart.[63,64] Ninety-five percent are epithelial and 80% are malignant, with urothelial carcinoma accounting for 90% of these.[62]

BENIGN EPITHELIAL NEOPLASMS

Inverted papilloma

Inverted papilloma is a benign urothelial tumor that occurs less commonly in the renal pelvis and ureter than in the urinary bladder.[65,66] It is almost twice as common in the ureter as in the renal pelvis.[67] Men predominate and the mean age of presentation is about 65 years.[67] In the upper tract it is found incidentally by intravenous pyelography[66] or may cause hematuria.[68,69] Inverted papilloma may be multiple and associated with urothelial carcinoma at other sites.[70] Grossly, it may form a mass mimicking carcinoma (Fig. 3-21). The tumor consists of trabeculae of histologically typical urothelium, which often forms small glandular structures lined by metaplastic mucinous epithelium.[71] The histologic features of these tumors are discussed in more detail in Chapter 5. Rarely, urothelial carcinoma may arise within an inverted papilloma of the ureter.[72,73]

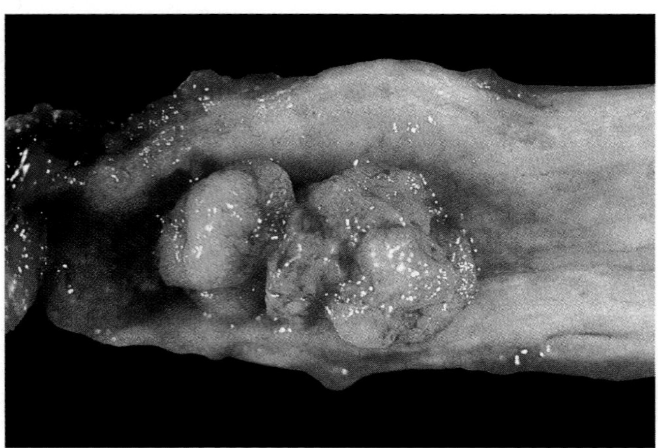

3-21. Inverted papilloma of the ureter.

Urothelial papilloma

Urothelial papilloma is rare. It is usually a small (several millimeters or less), delicate papillary structure most often found incidentally and only rarely biopsied. The latter has been attributed to the tendency for urologists to fulgurate this small, clinically innocent appearing lesion. Microscopically, papilloma consists of thin delicate fibrovascular fronds invested by epithelium of normal thickness that lacks atypia. By definition, there is no extension into the lamina propria.

MALIGNANT NEOPLASMS

Urothelial dysplasia and carcinoma in situ

In keeping with the concept of the urothelium of the renal pelvis, ureter, and bladder as a single anatomic unit affected by similar neoplastic influences, the same relationships between dysplasia and cancer shown for bladder cancer have also been established in the upper tract. The mucosa adjacent to invasive pelvic and ureteral tumors is abnormal (dysplasia or carcinoma in situ) in

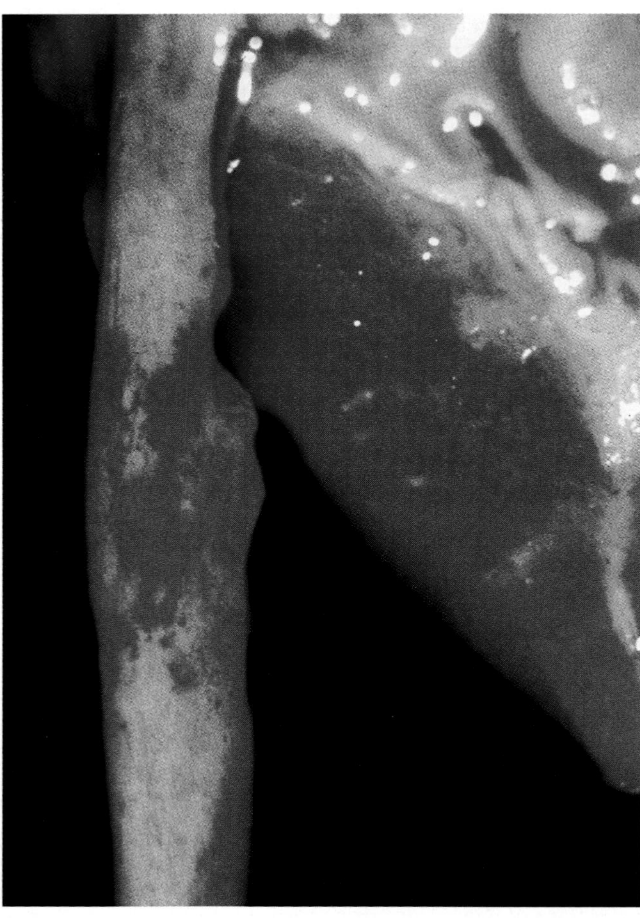

3-22. Red patches of urothelial carcinoma in situ of the ureter. *(Courtesy of Robert H. Young, M.D.)*

95% of specimens. The severity of the mucosal dysplasia correlates with the grade of the adjacent carcinoma and identifies patients at risk for metachronous tumors of other sites.[74-76] Furthermore, ureteral or pelvic muscle invasion occurs in 86% to 90% of cases of flat urothelial carcinoma but only 30% to 36% of cases of papillary urothelial carcinoma.[75,76] Grossly, the mucosa appears erythematous (Fig. 3-22) or normal.

Urothelial carcinoma

Urothelial carcinoma of the upper tract is epidemiologically similar to that of the bladder[77]: There is male predominance,[78] it is most common in older individuals, and tobacco[79] and industrial carcinogens are risk factors. Phenacetin abuse[80,81] is the most important etiologic factor in some populations, accounting for nearly one quarter of renal pelvic tumors and more than 10% of ureteral tumors. Balkan nephropathy and exposure to thorium-containing radiologic contrast material[82,83] are risk factors for upper tract carcinoma but not for urinary bladder tumors. Tumors of the renal pelvis and calyces are approximately twice as common as tumors of the ureters.[78] Hematuria is the principal symptom but flank pain also is frequent.[84] Multifocality is a significant problem for patients with upper tract tumors.[78,85] Nearly 50% of patients have a history of urothelial carcinoma of the bladder or ureters or later develop urothelial carcinoma.[86] In the ureter the most common location is the distal segment.[87] Grade and stage are the most important prognostic factors in urothelial carcinoma of the upper tract, while multiplicity of tumors also has an effect.[85] Approximately 75% of cases are low grade and low stage.[88] The grading scheme is identical to that applied in the bladder, and the staging system is generally similar to that used in the bladder. There is no international standard on staging. The TNM of the Jewett system for staging bladder carcinomas has been used extensively and is shown in the box on this page. Carcinoma, which is grade 1 and stage 1 at the time of resection, has little or no effect on survival.[89] Muscle invasion is a critical point in the progression of these tumors and survival decreases markedly when it is present. The lung is the most common site of metastasis.[90] Due to the high rate of recurrence (more than 15%) in the ureter distal to the resected tumor, nephroureterectomy with resection of a cuff of urinary bladder is the operation of choice.[76]

Gross pathology. The gross appearance of the tumors is similar to that seen in the bladder (Fig. 3-23) except that large papillary tumors frequently fill the ureters and cause obstruction, resulting in hydronephrosis (Fig. 3-24). Large tumors of the pelvis may extensively invade the renal parenchyma in an ill-defined infiltrative manner (Fig. 3-25), even extending into the paracortical fat with a scirrhous response. In some such tumors little evidence remains of a mucosal origin in the pelvis and extensive histologic sampling is necessary to demonstrate it.

Microscopic pathology. The histopathology of urothelial carcinoma of the renal pelvis and ureter (Fig. 3-26) has the same spectrum as urothelial carcinoma of the

STAGING CARCINOMA OF THE RENAL PELVIS AND URETER

Ta	Noninvasive papillary carcinoma
Tis	Carcinoma in situ
T1	Invasion of subepithelial connective tissue
T2	Invasion of muscularis propria
T3	Invasion of peripelvic fat or renal parenchyma (renal pelvic tumors only) Invasion of periureteric fat (ureteral tumors only)
T4	Invasion of adjacent organs or through kidney into perirenal fat
N1	Metastasis to a single lymph node less than or equal to 2 cm in maximum diameter
N2	Metastasis to a single lymph node between 2 cm and 5 cm in maximum diameter or metastasis to multiple lymph nodes none larger than 5 cm in maximum diameter
N3	Metastasis to a lymph node larger than 5 cm in maximum diameter

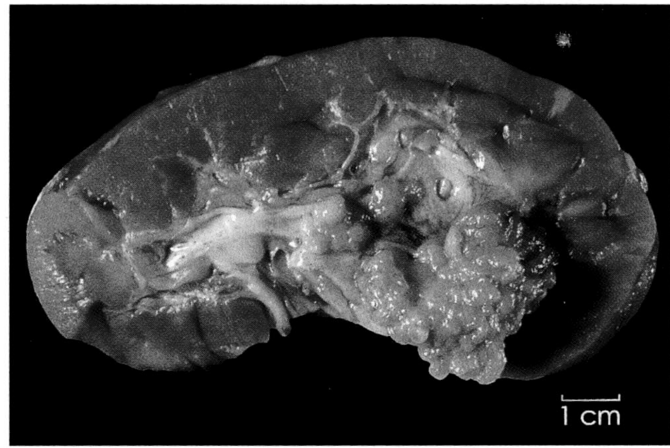

3-23. Papillary urothelial carcinoma of the renal pelvis.

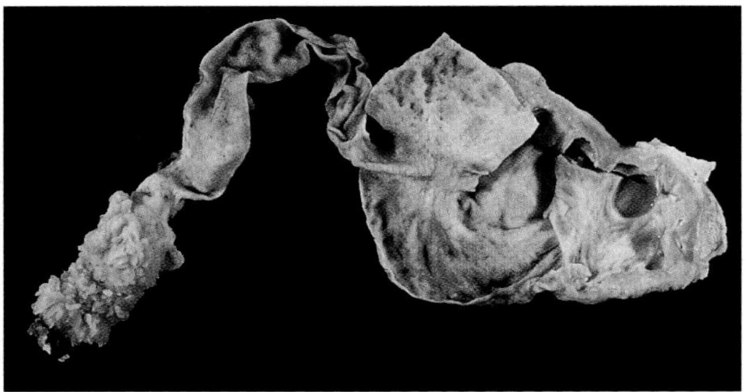

3-24. Papillary urothelial carcinoma of the ureter causing hydronephrosis.

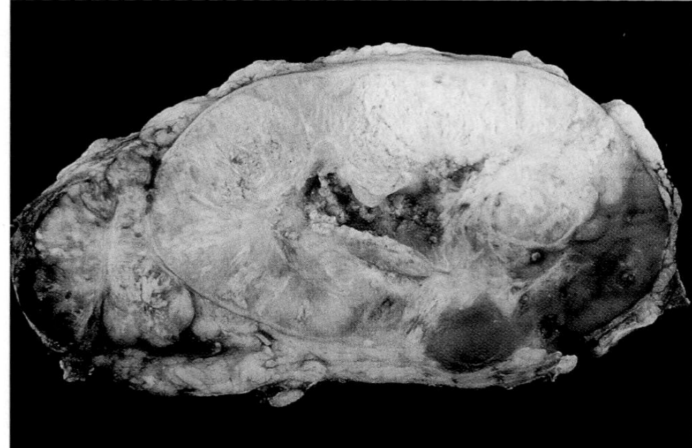

3-25. Infiltrative urothelial carcinoma of the pelvis, replacing most of the kidney.

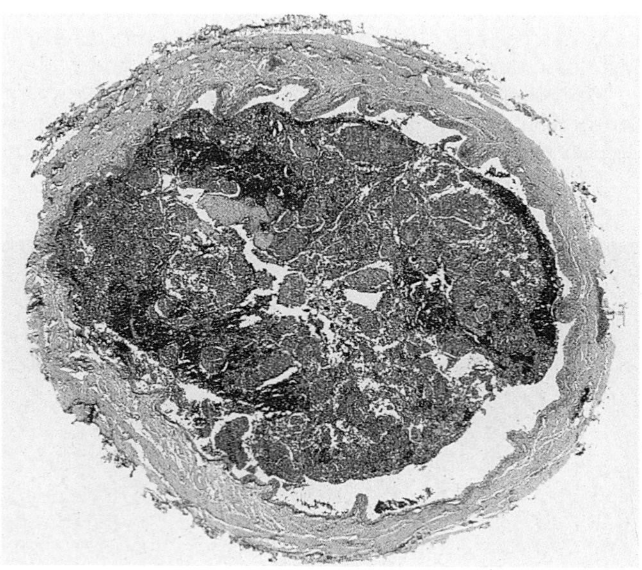

3-26. Papillary urothelial carcinoma filling the lumen of the ureter.

urinary bladder, including squamous and glandular[91] differentiation and the sarcomatoid[92-94] and small cell[95] variants. A complete discussion of the microscopic pathology of urothelial carcinoma appears in Chapter 5. Rare variants, including those with trophoblastic differentiation and osteoclast-type giant cells[96,97] have been reported. When the sarcomatoid elements obscure the clearly carcinomatous elements, immunohistochemical studies[92,94] or ultrastructural examination[91] may be of diagnostic help. Mapping studies have shown that virtually all cases of urothelial carcinoma of the renal pelvis and ureter are associated with changes ranging from hyperplasia to carcinoma in situ in the mucosa elsewhere in the specimen.[98] Thickening of basement membranes around capillaries in the lamina propria of the renal pelvis and ureter has recently been found to be a histologic marker for analgesic abuse and termed *capillarosclerosis*.[80]

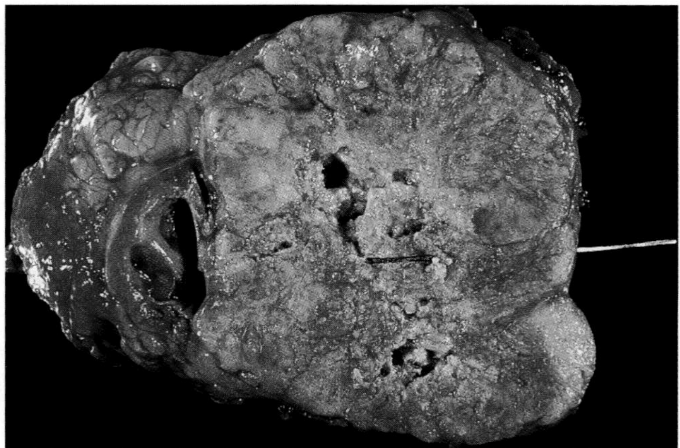

3-27. Squamous cell carcinoma of the renal pelvis. The probe indicates the course of the ureter.

Squamous cell carcinoma

Approximately 10% of renal pelvic tumors are squamous cell carcinoma[99] and the percentage of cases of ureteral carcinoma is even smaller. Calculi and chronic infection often are associated with squamous cell carcinoma. The relationship with squamous metaplasia is more controversial, with some studies of squamous cell carcinoma reporting a strong association[100,101] while some studies of squamous metaplasia have reported little association.[44] The disagreement may be the result of the rarity of squamous cell carcinoma of the upper urinary tract. Most squamous cell carcinomas of the renal pelvis and ureters are high stage[102]; extensive infiltration of the renal parenchyma is common (Fig. 3-27) and survival for 5 years is rare.[101] The histopathology of this tumor is similar to squamous cell carcinoma in the urinary bladder. This tumor should be distinguished from metastatic squamous cell carcinoma, which usually is straightforward when clinical and pathological features are considered. An exceptional case of adenosquamous carcinoma of the renal pelvis without urothelial carcinoma was described in association with staghorn calculi.[103]

Adenocarcinoma

Primary adenocarcinoma of the upper tract is rare and the reports consist of single cases or small series of cases.[104-109] Most occur in adults but rare pediatric cases have been described.[110] Calculi, chronic inflammation, and infection appear to be predisposing conditions. Most patients present with advanced cancer, similar to those with squamous cell carcinoma, and have a poor prognosis. Glandular metaplasia[42,47] may be a precursor lesion, and noninvasive carcinoma is sometimes found in the adjacent mucosa (Fig. 3-28). Papillary architecture and resemblance to mucinous adenocarcinoma of the colon (Fig. 3-29) are common. One tumor had hepatoid areas and contained bile pigment.[108]

Metastases

Neoplastic involvement of ureters may occur by direct local extension or metastasis.[111,112] Contiguous ureteral involvement is more frequent and is usually caused by

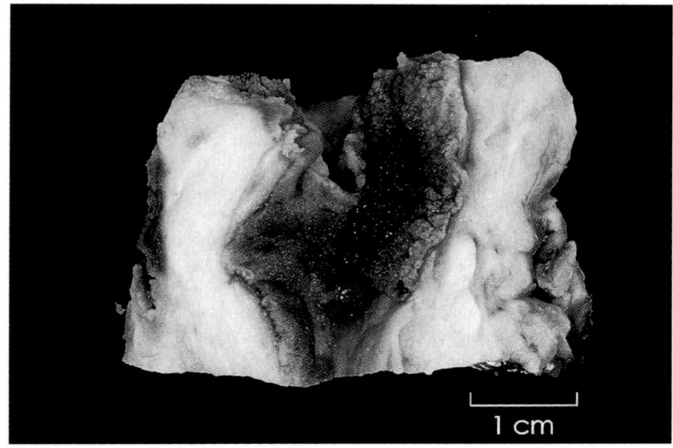

3-28. Mucinous adenocarcinoma of the renal pelvis.

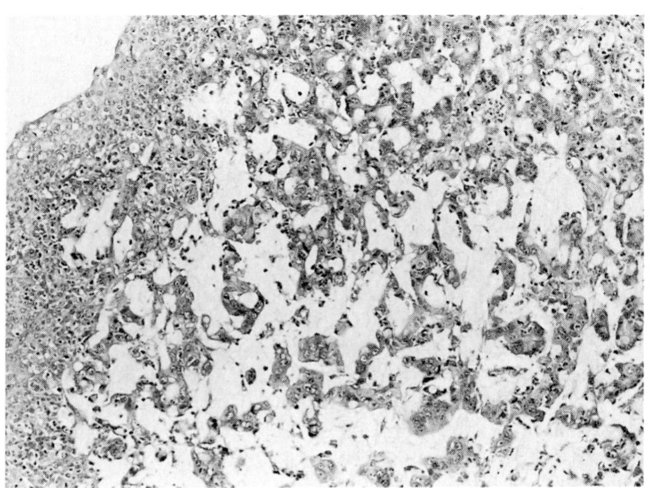

3-29. Mucinous adenocarcinoma of the ureter infiltrating the lamina propria.

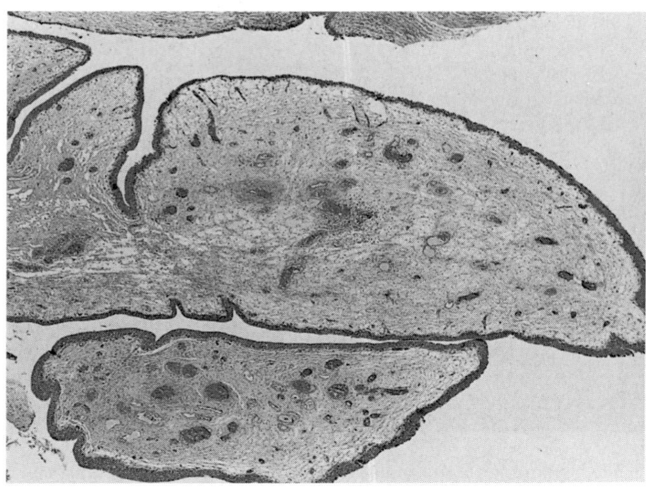

3-30. Fibroepithelial polyp consisting of a fibrovascular core with scattered inflammatory cells and a covering of normal urothelium.

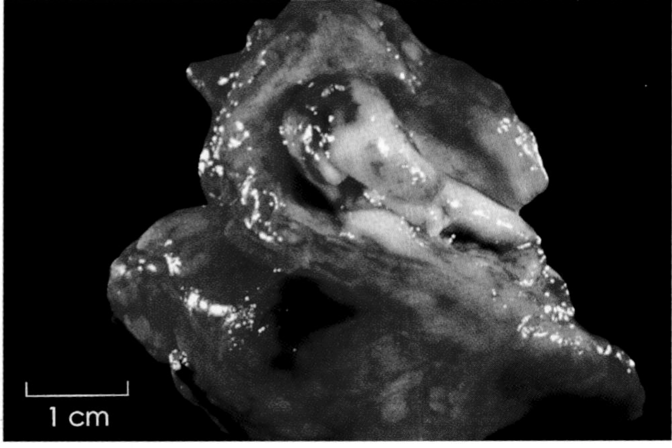

3-31. Leiomyosarcoma of ureter. *(Courtesy of Robert H. Young, M.D.)*

carcinoma of the cervix, prostate, or bladder.[111] Metastatic involvement is less common, and breast and colon are the most common sites of primaries.[112] Ureteral involvement is rarely the initial manifestation of the neoplasm.

MESENCHYMAL NEOPLASMS

Mesenchymal neoplasms are uncommon in the ureter and pelvis. Fibroepithelial polyp is most common, followed by benign and malignant smooth muscle tumors. A variety of additional tumors have been reported as single cases, including hemangioma, neurofibroma, and malignant schwannoma.

Fibroepithelial polyp

Fibroepithelial polyp is more common in the ureters and renal pelvis than in the bladder. It is an uncommon benign mesenchymal tumor of the renal pelvis[113] and ureter.[114] Approximately 70% of patients with fibroepithelial polyp are male.[115] Fibroepithelial polyp occurs at all ages, from infancy to old age (the mean is approximately 40 years).[116-118] Fibroepithelial polyp is the most common benign polypoid lesion of the ureters in children.[117] Colicky flank pain and hematuria are the most common symptoms. The etiology is uncertain.[119]

Grossly, fibroepithelial polyp consists of single or multiple slender smooth-surfaced vermiform polyps that usually arise from a common base. The ureteropelvic junction is a common site and the polyp may cause obstruction at that narrow point. Rarely, fibroepithelial polyp is bilateral. Microscopically, the polyp is covered by normal urothelium which may be focally eroded. The core of the polyp is composed of a loose edematous and vascular stroma with few inflammatory cells (Fig. 3-30).

Leiomyoma and leiomyosarcoma

Smooth muscle tumors of the ureter and pelvis are much rarer than those of the kidney, and patients have an approximately equal frequency of benign and malignant tumors.[120-125] Patients present with hematuria, pain, or mass findings indistinguishable from the presentation of urothelial neoplasms. Grossly, small tumors may form polypoid masses (Fig. 3-31) while larger tumors

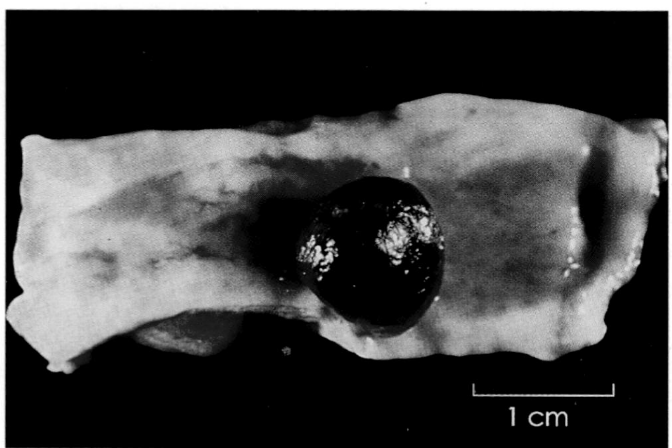

3-32. Hemangioma of the ureter. *(Courtesy of Robert H. Young, M.D.)*

are often infiltrative. Histologically, they resemble their counterparts elsewhere.

Hemangioma

Hemangioma of the ureter and renal pelvis is an uncommon polypoid tumor (Fig. 3-32) consisting of hypervascular fibrous stroma covered by normal urothelium.[126,127] Occurring in children and adults, this lesion may be multiple and frequently causes obstruction.

Other tumors

Other sarcomas, such as osteogenic sarcoma[128] and malignant schwannoma[129] are extremely rare. Malignant melanoma may arise in the mucosa of the renal pelvis.[130] Carcinosarcoma, combining squamous or urothelial carcinoma with heterologous sarcoma such as osteogenic sarcoma, chondrosarcoma, or rhabdomyosarcoma, is extremely rare.[131,132] A pure choriocarcinoma of the renal pelvis has been reported.[133] Obstruction caused by secondary infiltration by malignant lymphoma occurs in approximately 16% of cases of disseminated lymphoma.[134]

References

1. Mackie GG: Abnormalities of the ureteral bud, Urol Clin North Am 5:161-174, 1978.
2. Ruano-Gil D, Coca-Payeras A, Tejedo-Mateu A: Obstruction and normal recanalization of the ureter in the human embryo. Its relation to congenital ureteric obstruction, Eur Urol 1:287-293, 1975.
3. Matsuno T, Tokunaka S, Koyanagi T: Muscular development in the urinary tract, J Urol 132:148-152, 1984.
4. Itatani H, Koide T, Okuyama A et al: Development of the calyceal system in the human fetus, Invest Urol 16:388-394, 1979.
5. Itatani H, Koide T, Okuyama A et al: Development of the ureterovesical junction in human fetus: in consideration of the vesicoureteral reflux, Invest Urol 15:232-238, 1977.
6. Elbadawi A: Anatomy and function of the ureteral sheath, J Urol 102:224-229, 1972.
7. Notley RG: Electron microscopy of the upper ureter and the pelvi-ureteric junction, Br J Urol 40:37-52, 1968.
8. Rizzo M, Faussone Pellegrini MS, Arbi Riccardi R et al: Ultrastructure of the urinary tract muscle coat in man: calices, renal pelvis, pelvi-ureteric junction and ureter, Eur Urol 7:171-177, 1981.
9. Vaughan ED Jr, Middleton GW: Pertinent genitourinary embryology, review for practicing urologists, Urology 6:139-149, 1975.
10. Lenaghan D: Bifid ureters in children: an anatomical, physiological and clinical study, J Urol 87:808-817, 1962.
11. Barry JE, Auldist AW: The VATER association, one end of a spectrum of anomalies, Am J Dis Child 128:769-771, 1974.
12. Straub E, Spranger J: Etiology and pathogenesis of the prune belly syndrome, Kidney Int 20:695-699, 1981.
13. Egli F, Stalder G: Malformations of kidney and urinary tract in common chromosomal aberrations. I. Clinical studies, Humangenetik 18:1-15, 1973.
14. Atwell JD, Cook PL, Howell CJ et al: Familial incidence of bifid and double ureters, Arch Dis Child 49:390-393, 1974.
15. Atwell JD: Familial pelviureteric junction hydronephrosis and its association with a duplex pelvicaliceal system and vesicoureteric reflux. A family study, Br J Urol 57:365-369, 1985.
16. Roodhooft AM, Birnholz JC, Holmes LB: Familial nature of congenital absence and severe dysgenesis of both kidneys, N Engl J Med 310:1341-1345, 1984.
17. Jerkins GR, Noe HN: Familial vesicoureteral reflux: a prospective study, J Urol 128:774-778, 1982.
18. Belman AB: Megaureter, classification, etiology, and management, Urol Clin North Am 1:497-513, 1974.
19. Emanuel B, Nachman R, Aronson N et al: Congenital solitary kidney: a review of 74 cases, J Urol 111:394-397, 1974.
20. Caldamone AA: Duplication anomalies of the upper tract in infants and children, Urol Clin North Am 12:75-91, 1985.
21. Mackie GG, Stephens FD: Duplex kidneys: a correlation of renal dysplasia with position of the ureteral orifice, J Urol 114:274-280, 1975.
22. Tanagho EA, Guthrie TH, Lyon RP: The intravesical ureter in primary reflux, J Urol 101:824-832, 1969.
23. Hawtrey CE, Culp DA, Loening S et al: Ureterovesical reflux in an adolescent and adult population, J Urol 130:1067-1069, 1983.
24. Johnston JH, Evans JP, Glassberg KI et al: Pelvic hydronephrosis in children: a review of 219 personal cases, J Urol 117:97-101, 1977.
25. Foote JW, Blennerhassett JB, Wiglesworth FW et al: Observations on the ureteropelvic junction, J Urol 104:252-257, 1970.
26. Hanna MK, Jeffs RD, Sturgess JM et al: Ureteral structure and ultrastructure. Part II. Congenital ureteropelvic junction obstruction and primary obstructive megaureter, J Urol 116:725-730, 1976.
27. Maizels M, Stephens FD: Valves of the ureter as a cause of primary obstruction of the ureter: anatomic, embryologic and clinical aspects, J Urol 123:742-747, 1980.
28. Stephens FD: Ureterovascular hydronephrosis and the "aberrant" renal vessels, J Urol 128:984-987, 1982.
29. Tanagho EA, Smith DR, Guthrie TH: Pathophysiology of functional ureteral obstruction, J Urol 104:73-88, 1970.

30. Tokunaka S, Koyanagi T: Morphologic study of primary nonreflux megaureters with particular emphasis on the role of ureteral sheath and ureteral dysplasia, J Urol 128:399-402, 1982.
31. Hanna MK: Ureteral structure and ultrastructure. Part V. The dysplastic ureter, J Urol 122:796-798, 1979.
32. Tokunaka S, Gotoh T, Koyanagi T et al: Muscle dysplasia in megaureters, J Urol 131:383-390, 1984.
33. Tanagho EA: Anatomy and management of ureteroceles, J Urol 107:729-736, 1972.
34. Tokunaka S, Gotoh T, Koyanagi T et al: Morphological study of the ureterocele: a possible clue to its embryogenesis as evidenced by a locally arrested myogenesis, J Urol 126:726-729, 1981.
35. Mandell J, Colodny AH, Lebowitz R et al: Ureteroceles in infants and children, J Urol 123:921-926, 1980.
36. Wickramasinghe SF, Stephens FD: Paraureteral diverticula: associated renal morphology and embryogenesis, Invest Urol 14:381-385, 1977.
37. Tokunaka S, Koyanagi T, Matsuno T et al: Paraureteral diverticula: clinical experience with 17 cases with associated renal dysmorphism, J Urol 124:791-796, 1980.
38. Mostofi FK: Potentialities of bladder epithelium, J Urol 71:705-714, 1954.
39. Wiener DP, Koss LG, Sablay B et al: The prevalence and significance of Brunn's nests, cystitis cystica and squamous metaplasia in normal bladders, J Urol 122:317-321, 1979.
40. Morse HD: The etiology and pathology of pyelitis cystica, ureteritis cystica and cystitis cystica, Am J Pathol 4:33-49, 1928.
41. Askari A, Herrera HH: Pyeloureteritis cystica, Urology 16:398-399, 1980.
42. Bullock PS, Thoni DE, Murphy WM: The significance of colonic mucosa (intestinal metaplasia) involving the urinary tract, Cancer 59:2086-2090, 1987.
43. Reece RW, Koontz WW Jr: Leukoplakia of the urinary tract: a review, J Urol 114:165-171, 1975.
44. Hertle L, Androulakakis P: Keratinizing desquamative squamous metaplasia of the upper urinary tract: leukoplakia-cholesteatoma, J Urol 127:631-635, 1982.
45. Kinn A-C: Squamous cell carcinoma of the renal pelvis, Scand J Urol Nephrol 14:77-80, 1979.
46. Li MK, Cheung WL: Squamous cell carcinoma of the renal pelvis, J Urol 138:269-271, 1987.
47. Gordon A: Intestinal metaplasia of the urinary tract epithelium, J Pathol Bacteriol 85:441-444, 1963.
48. Ward AM: Glandular neoplasia within the urinary tract. The aetiology of adenocarcinoma of the urothelium with a review of the literature I. Introduction: the origin of glandular epithelium in the renal pelvis, ureter and bladder, Virchows Arch [A] 352:296-311, 1971.
49. Krag DO, Alcott DL: Glandular metaplasia of the renal pelvis, report of a case, Am J Clin Pathol 27:672-680, 1957.
50. Satodate R, Koike H, Sasou S et al: Nephrogenic adenoma of the ureter, J Urol 131:332-334, 1984.
51. Lugo M, Petersen RO, Elfenbein IB et al: Nephrogenic metaplasia of the ureter, Am J Clin Pathol 80:92-97, 1983.
52. Murphy WM, Soloway MS, Finebaum PJ: Pathological changes associated with topical chemotherapy for superficial bladder cancer, J Urol 126:461-464, 1981.
53. Mukamel E, Glanz I, Nissenkorn I et al: Unanticipated vesicoureteral reflux: a possible sequela of long-term thio-tepa instillations to the bladder, J Urol 127:245-246, 1982.
54. Michaelis L, Gutmann C: Ueber Einschlüsse in Blasentumoren, Z Klin Med 47:208-215, 1902.
55. Von Hansemann D: Über Malakoplakie der Harnblase, Virchows Arch Pathol Anat Physiol Klin Med 173:302-308, 1903.
56. Stanton MJ, Maxted W: Malacoplakia: a study of the literature and current concepts of pathogenesis, diagnosis and treatment, J Urol 125:139-146, 1981.
57. McClure J: Malakoplakia of the urinary tract, Br J Urol 54:181-185, 1982.
58. McClure J: Malakoplakia, J Pathol 140:275-330, 1983.
59. Mitchinson MJ: The pathology of idiopathic retroperitoneal fibrosis, J Clin Pathol 23:681-689, 1970.
60. Lepor H, Walsh PC: Idiopathic retroperitoneal fibrosis, J Urol 122:1-6, 1979.
61. Mitchinson MJ: Retroperitoneal fibrosis revisited, Arch Pathol Lab Med 110:784-786, 1986.
62. Bennington JL, Beckwith JB: Atlas of tumor pathology, second series, fasicle 12, tumors of the kidney, renal pelvis, and ureter. Bethesda, 1975, Armed Forces Institute of Pathology.
63. Booth CM, Cameron KM, Pugh RCB: Urothelial carcinoma of the kidney and ureter, Br J Urol 52:430-435, 1980.
64. McCarron JP, Mills C, Vaughan ED Jr: Tumors of the renal pelvis and ureter: current concepts and management, Semin Urol 1:75-81, 1983.
65. Naito S, Minoda M, Hirata H: Inverted papilloma of ureter, Urology 22:290-291, 1983.
66. Lausten GS, Anagnostaki L, Thomsen OF: Inverted papilloma of the upper urinary tract, Eur Urol 10:67-70, 1984.
67. Kyriakos M, Royce RK: Multiple simultaneous inverted papillomas of the upper urinary tract. A case report with a review of ureteral and renal pelvic inverted papillomas, Cancer 63:368-380, 1989.
68. Embon OM, Saghi N, Bechar L: Inverted papilloma of ureter, Eur Urol 10:139-140, 1984.
69. Arrufat JM, Vera-Román JM, Casas V et al: Papiloma invertido de uréter, Actas Urol Esp 7:225-228, 1983.
70. Palvio DHB: Inverted papillomas of the urinary tract, a case of multiple, recurring inverted papillomas of the renal pelvis, ureter and bladder associated with malignant change, Scand J Urol Nephrol 19:299-302, 1985.
71. Kunze E, Schauer A, Schmitt M: Histology and histogenesis of two different types of inverted urothelial papillomas, Cancer 51:348-358, 1983.
72. Kimura G, Tsuboi N, Nakajima H et al: Inverted papilloma of the ureter with malignant transformation: a case report and review of the literature, Urol Int 42:30-36, 1987.
73. Grainger R, Gikas PW, Grossman HB: Urothelial carcinoma occurring within an inverted papilloma of the ureter, J Urol 143:802-804, 1990.
74. McCarron JP Jr, Chasko SB, Gray GF Jr: Systematic mapping of nephroureterectomy specimens removed for urothelial cancer: pathological findings and clinical correlations, J Urol 128:243-246, 1982.
75. Heney NM, Nocks BN, Daly JJ et al: Prognostic factors in carcinoma of the ureter, J Urol 125:632-636, 1981.

76. Nocks BN, Heney NM, Daly JJ et al: Transitional cell carcinoma of renal pelvis, Urology 19:472-477, 1982.
77. Kvist E, Lauritzen AF, Bredesen J et al: A comparative study of transitional cell tumors of the bladder and upper urinary tract, Cancer 61:2109-2112, 1988.
78. Mazeman E: Tumours of the upper urinary tract calyces, renal pelvis and ureter, Eur Urol 2:120-128, 1976.
79. McLaughlin JK, Blot WJ, Mandel JS et al: Etiology of cancer of the renal pelvis, J Natl Cancer Inst 71:287-291, 1983.
80. Palvio DHB, Andersen JC, Falk E: Transitional cell tumors of the renal pelvis and ureter associated with capillarosclerosis indicating analgesic abuse, Cancer 59:972-976, 1987.
81. Steffens J, Nagel R: Tumours of the renal pelvis and ureter, observations in 170 patients, Br J Urol 61:277-283, 1988.
82. Christensen P, Rørbæk Madsen M, Myhre Jensen O: Latency of thorotrast-induced renal tumors, Scand J Urol Nephrol 17:127-130, 1983.
83. Verhaak RLOM, Harmsen AE, van Unnik AJM: On the frequency of tumor induction in a thorotrast kidney, Cancer 34:2061-2068, 1974.
84. Nielsen K, Ostri P: Primary tumors of the renal pelvis: evaluation of clinical and pathological features in a consecutive series of 10 years, J Urol 140:19-21, 1988.
85. Corrado F, Ferri C, Mannini D et al: Transitional cell carcinoma of the upper urinary tract: evaluation of prognostic factors by histopathology and flow cytometric analysis, J Urol 145:1159-1163, 1991.
86. Bonsib SM: Pathology of the renal pelvis and ureter. In Eble JN, ed: Tumors and tumor-like conditions of the kidneys and ureters, New York, 1990, Churchill Livingstone.
87. Anderström C, Johansson SL, Pettersson S et al: Carcinoma of the ureter: a clinicopathologic study of 49 cases, J Urol 142:280-283, 1989.
88. Blute ML, Tsushima K, Farrow GM et al: Transitional cell carcinoma of the renal pelvis: nuclear deoxyribonucleic acid ploidy studied by flow cytometry, J Urol 140:944-949, 1988.
89. Murphy DM, Zincke H, Furlow WL: Primary grade 1 transitional cell carcinoma of the renal pelvis and ureter, J Urol 123:629-631, 1980.
90. Huben RP, Mounzer AM, Murphy GP: Tumor grade and stage as prognostic variables in upper tract urothelial tumors, Cancer 62:2016-2020, 1988.
91. Tajima Y, Aizawa M: Unusual renal pelvic tumor containing transitional cell carcinoma, adenocarcinoma and sarcomatoid elements (so-called sarcomatoid carcinoma of the renal pelvis), a case report and review of the literature, Acta Pathol Jpn 38:805-814, 1988.
92. Piscioli F, Bondi A, Scappini P et al: 'True' sarcomatoid carcinoma of the renal pelvis, Eur Urol 10:350-355, 1984.
93. Rao SS, Rao NN, Venkataratnam G: Carcino-sarcoma of renal pelvis in a child, a case report, Indian J Pathol Microbiol 29:313-316, 1986.
94. Wick MR, Perrone TL, Burke BA: Sarcomatoid transitional cell carcinoma of the renal pelvis, an ultrastructural and immunohistochemical study, Arch Pathol Lab Med 109:55-58, 1985.
95. Essenfeld H, Manivel JC, Benedetto P et al: Small cell carcinoma of the renal pelvis: a clinicopathological, morphological and immunohistochemical study of 2 cases, J Urol 144:344-347, 1990.
96. Kenney RM, Prat J, Tabernero M: Giant-cell tumor-like proliferation associated with a papillary transitional cell carcinoma of the renal pelvis, Am J Surg Pathol 8:139-144, 1984.
97. Tarry WF, Morabito RA, Belis JA: Carcinosarcoma of the renal pelvis with extension into the renal vein and vena cava, J Urol 128:582-585, 1982.
98. Mahadevia PS, Karwa GL, Koss LG: Mapping of urothelium in carcinomas of the renal pelvis and ureter, Cancer 51:890-897, 1983.
99. Utz DC, McDonald JR: Squamous cell carcinoma of the kidney, J Urol 78:540-552, 1957.
100. Vyas MCR, Joshi KR, Mathur DR et al: Primary squamous cell carcinoma of the renal pelvis, a report of four cases with review of literature, Indian J Pathol Microbiol 25:151-155, 1982.
101. Blacher EJ, Johnson DE, Abdul-Karim FW et al: Squamous cell carcinoma of renal pelvis, Urology 25:124-125, 1985.
102. Strobel SL, Jasper WS, Gogate SA et al: Primary carcinoma of the renal pelvis and ureter, evaluation of clinical and pathologic features, Arch Pathol Lab Med 108:697-700, 1984.
103. Howat AJ, Scott E, Mackie B et al: Adenosquamous carcinoma of the renal pelvis, Am J Clin Pathol 79:731-733, 1983.
104. Martínez García R, Boronat Tormo F, Domínguez Hinarejos C et al: Adenocarcinoma de pelvis renal, Actas Urol Esp 13:470-472, 1989.
105. Takezawa Y, Saruki K, Jinbo S et al: A case of adenocarcinoma of the renal pelvis, Acta Urol Jpn 36:841-845, 1990.
106. Stein A, Sova Y, Lurie M et al: Adenocarcinoma of the renal pelvis, report of two cases, one with simultaneous transitional cell carcinoma of the bladder, Urol Int 43:299-301, 1988.
107. Kim YI, Yoon DH, Lee SW et al: Multicentric papillary adenocarcinoma of the renal pelvis and ureter: report of a case with ultrastructural study, Cancer 62:2402-2407, 1988.
108. Ishikura H, Ishiguro T, Enatsu C et al: Hepatoid adenocarcinoma of the renal pelvis producing alpha-fetoprotein of hepatic type and bile pigment, Cancer 67:3051-3056, 1991.
109. Brawer MK, Waisman J: Papillary adenocarcinoma of ureter, Urology 19:205-209, 1982.
110. Moncino MD, Friedman HS, Kurtzberg J et al: Papillary adenocarcinoma of the renal pelvis in a child: case report and brief review of the literature, Med Pediatr Oncol 18:81-86, 1990.
111. Richie JP, Withers G, Ehrlich RM: Ureteral obstruction secondary to metastatic tumors, Surg Gynecol Obstet 148:355-357, 1979.
112. Cohen WM, Freed SZ, Hasson J: Metastatic cancer to the ureter: a review of the literature and case presentations, J Urol 112:188-189, 1974.
113. Wolgel CD, Parris AC, Mitty HA et al: Fibroepithelial polyp of renal pelvis, Urology 19:436-439, 1982.
114. Goldman SM, Bohlman ME, Gatewood OMB: Neoplasms of the renal collecting system, Semin Roentgenol 22:284-291, 1987.
115. Williams PR, Feggeter J, Miller RA et al: The diagnosis and management of benign fibrous ureteric polyps, Br J Urol 52:253-256, 1980.
116. Bartone FF, Johansson SL, Markin RJ et al: Bilateral fibroepithelial polyps of ureter in a child, Urology 35:519-522, 1990.

117. Macksood MJ, Roth DR, Chang C-H et al: Benign fibroepithelial polyps as a cause of intermittent ureteropelvic junction obstruction in a child: a case report and review of the literature, J Urol 134:951-952, 1985.
118. van Poppel H, Nuttin B, Oyen R et al: Fibroepithelial polyps of the ureter, etiology, diagnosis, treatment and pathology, Eur Urol 12:174-179, 1986.
119. Stuppler SA, Kandzari SJ: Fibroepithelial polyps of ureter, a benign ureteral tumor, Urology 5:553-558, 1975.
120. Kao VCT, Graff PW, Rappaport H: Leiomyoma of the ureter, a histologically problematic rare tumor confirmed by immunohistochemical studies, Cancer 24:535-542, 1969.
121. Zaitoon MM: Leiomyoma of ureter, Urology 28:50-51, 1986.
122. Fitko R, Gallagher L, Gonzalez-Crussi F et al: Urothelial leiomyomatous hamartoma of the kidney, Am J Clin Pathol 95:481-483, 1991.
123. Gislason T, Arnarson OO: Primary ureteral leiomyosarcoma, Scand J Urol Nephrol 18:253-254, 1984.
124. Tolia BM, Hajdu SI, Whitmore WF Jr: Leiomyosarcoma of the renal pelvis, J Urol 109:974-976, 1973.
125. Rushton HG, Sens MA, Garvin AJ et al: Primary leiomyosarcoma of the ureter: a case report with electron microscopy, J Urol 129:1045-1046, 1983.
126. Uhlíř K: Hemangioma of the ureter, J Urol 110:647-649, 1973.
127. Jansen TTH, van deWeyer FPH, deVries HR: Angiomatous ureteral polyp, Urology 20:426-427, 1982.
128. Eble JN, Young RH, Störkel S et al: Primary osteosarcoma of the kidney: a report of three cases, J Urogenital Pathol 1:83-88, 1991.
129. Fein RL, Hamm FC: Malignant schwannoma of the renal pelvis: a review of the literature and a case report, J Urol 94:356-361, 1965.
130. Frasier BL, Wachs BH, Watson LR et al: Malignant melanoma of the renal pelvis presenting as a primary tumor, J Urol 140:812-813, 1988.
131. Chen KTK, Workman RD, Flam MS et al: Carcinosarcoma of renal pelvis, Urology 22:429-431, 1983.
132. Yano S, Arita M, Ueno F et al: Carcinosarcoma of the ureter, Eur Urol 10:71, 1984.
133. Vahlensieck W, Riede U, Wimmer B et al: Beta-human chorionic gonadotropin-positive extragonadal germ cell neoplasia of the renal pelvis, Cancer 67:3051-3056, 1991.
134. Scharifker D, Chalasani A: Ureteral involvement by malignant lymphoma, ten years' experience, Arch Pathol Lab Med 102:541-542, 1978.

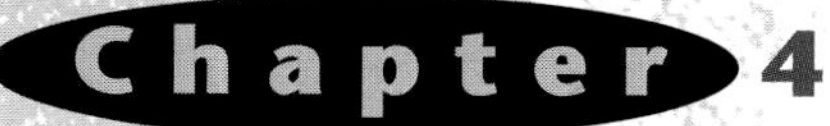

NON-NEOPLASTIC DISORDERS OF THE URINARY BLADDER

ROBERT H. YOUNG, M.D.
JOHN N. EBLE, M.D.

EMBRYOLOGY AND ANATOMY

EMBRYOLOGY

The common excretory ducts (the dilated segments of the mesonephric ducts distal to the ureteral buds) become absorbed into the urogenital sinus after the fourth week of gestation. Their epithelium merges toward the midline and forms a triangular patch that will become the trigone of the urinary bladder. The ends of the developing ureters implant there. The anterior abdominal wall closes with the caudal migration of the cloacal membrane and in this process mesenchyme is induced to form the anterior wall of the bladder. During the seventh week of gestation, the urorectal septum of the cloaca fuses with the proctodeum, separating the rectum from the parts of the urogenital sinus, which will form the dome and posterior wall of the bladder. Thus, most of the bladder is derived from the rostral part of the urogenital sinus.

In early embryogenesis, the allantois projects outward from the yolk sac into the body stalk, which later forms the umbilical cord. The allantois originates from the part of the yolk sac that gives rise to the cloaca. As the urinary bladder forms, the allantois remains connected to its apex. The urachus (from the Greek ὁ οὐραχύς, plural urachi) is the intraabdominal structure that connects the apex of the bladder to the umbilicus and contains the allantois. The urachus grows with the embryo to maintain its bridge between the dome of the bladder and the body stalk. By the sixth month of gestation, the urachus has become a cord-like structure little more than 1 mm in diameter between the umbilicus and the dome of the bladder. At birth, the dome of the bladder is near the umbilicus, the urachus is 2 to 3 mm long, the adjacent umbilical arteries are 5 to 7 mm in diameter, and the umbilical vein is 10 mm in diameter. Superiorly, the urachus usually divides into three bands of fibrous tissue. The middle band passes through the abdominal wall into the umbilical cord where it disperses into fine strands. The other two bands attach to the adventitia of the umbilical arteries.

GROSS ANATOMY

The bladder is located within the pelvis minor, beneath the peritoneum. When it fills, it expands into the abdomen and may reach the level of the umbilicus. In children younger than 6 years, the empty bladder is partially in the abdomen. Between age 6 and puberty, the bladder descends to its adult position. At the bladder neck, the bladder is fixed in place by the pubovesical ligaments in the female and the puboprostatic ligaments in the male. The rest of the bladder is loosely contained by the pelvic fat and fibrous tissue and is free to expand as the need arises. The empty bladder has roughly the shape of an inverted pyramid. The superior surface, the dome, is covered by peritoneum. The most anterior and superior point, the apex, is the usual point of insertion of the median umbilical ligament and the urachus. The posterior surface faces posteriorly and inferiorly, forming the base of the bladder. Between it and the rectum are the uterine cervix and superior end of the vagina in females and the lower vasa deferentia and seminal vesicles in the male. On either side, the lateral surfaces are in contact with the fascia of the levator ani muscles.

The trigone lies at the base of the bladder and borders the posterior side of the bladder neck.[1] At the lateral points of the trigone, the ureters empty into the bladder cavity through the ureteral orifices.[2] The muscle of the trigone is derived from the detrusor muscle of the bladder and the muscle of the ureters.[3] Within the wall of the bladder, the ureters are surrounded by sheaths of muscle and fibrous tissue known as Waldeyer's sheath.[4] The ureters pass obliquely through the wall of the bladder in such a way that when the bladder fills, the pressure compresses and closes the ureters, preventing reflux.[5,6] The region where the walls of the bladder converge and connect with the urethra is the neck of the bladder.[7] In this area, muscle fibers from the detrusor muscle, the muscle of the trigone, and the muscle of the urethra merge.[3] The internal sphincter is in the bladder neck and consists principally of fibers from the detrusor muscle.[8]

The urachus lies in Retzius' space anterior to the peritoneum and surrounded anteriorly and posteriorly by the umbilicovesical fascia. On either side, it lies between the umbilical arteries, which are enveloped in the umbilicovesical fascia. Caudally, the layers of the umbilicovesical fascia spread over the dome of the bladder. This space is pyramidal and separated from the peritoneum and other structures by fascial planes. After birth, the apex of the bladder descends and draws the urachus with it, bringing along the obliterated umbilical arteries. Within the umbilical fascial tunnel, the adventitia of the umbilical arteries is teased out into fibrous strands referred to as the *plexus of Luschka*.

Hammond et al[9] recognized four anatomic variants of the urachus (Fig. 4-1). Type I consists of a well-formed urachus that extends from the bladder to the umbilicus, distinct from the umbilical arteries. In type II, the urachus is joined with one of the umbilical arteries and these continue jointly to the umbilicus. In type III, the urachus and both umbilical arteries join and continue to the umbilicus as the ligamentum commune. Type IV consists of a short tubular urachus that terminates before fusing with either of the umbilical arteries. Hammond et al[9] found urachi of type I in almost 33% of adults, type II in 20%, type III in 20%, and type IV in 25%. Blichert-Toft et al[10] found a different distribution of the types in a study of 81 specimens: 9% type I, 12% type II, 25% type 3, and 54% type IV. In adults, the urachus outside the bladder wall is usually 5 to 5.5 cm long and at its junction with the bladder is 4 to 8 mm broad and tapers to approximately 2 mm at the umbilical end. Pathologically and clinically, it is convenient to divide the urachus into supravesical, intramural, and intramucosal segments (Fig. 4-2).

The urinary bladder is supplied by two pairs of vessels, the superior and inferior vesical arteries.[11,12] The lymphatics of the anterior and posterior bladder walls drain through the internal and middle chains of the external iliac lymph nodes, while those of the trigone drain both to the external iliac nodes and the hypogastric nodes.[13]

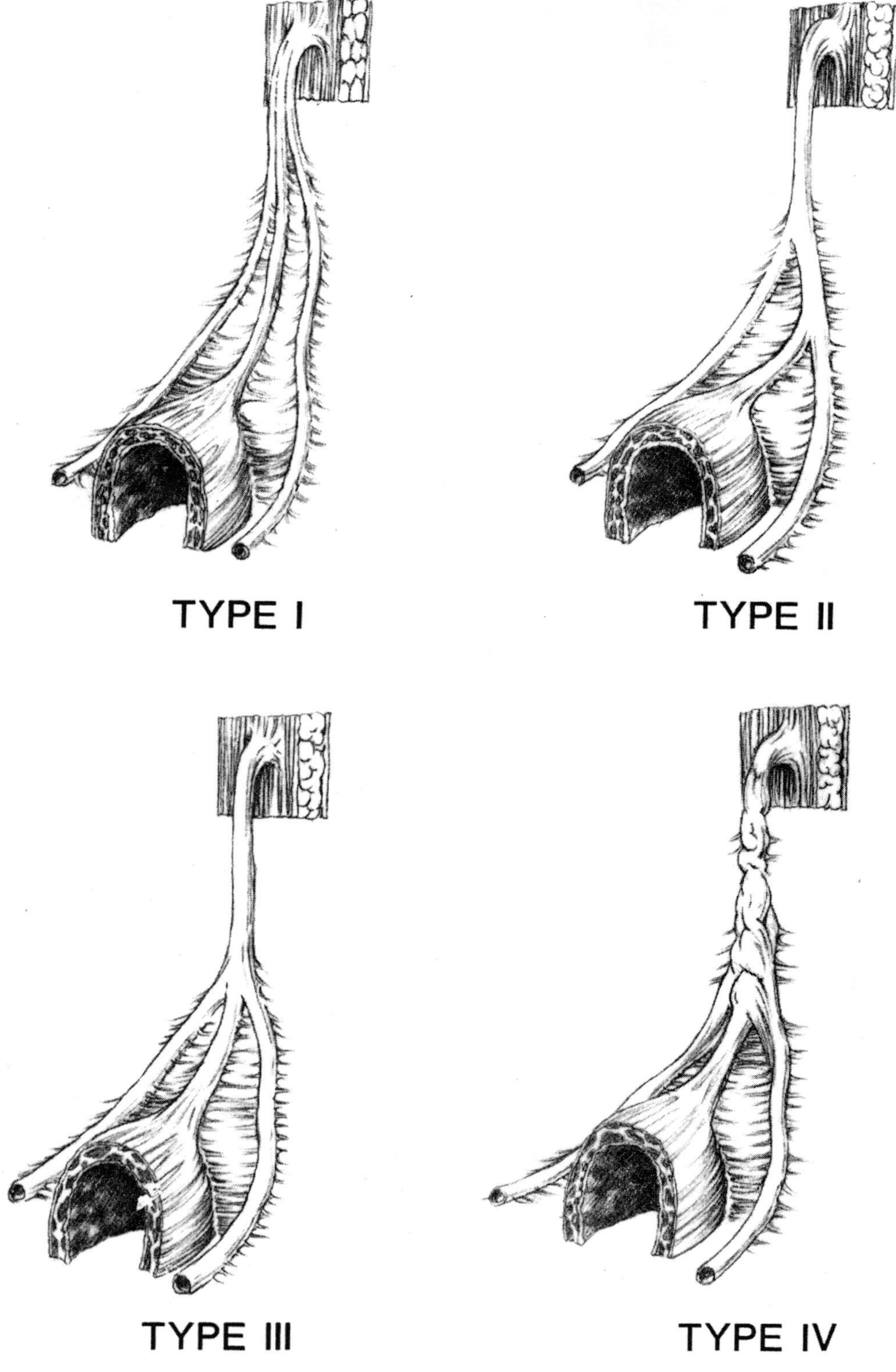

4-1. The four common variants of urachal anatomy. Type I: The urachus extends to the umbilicus (fetal type). Type II: The urachus joins one of the umbilical arteries. Type III: The urachus and umbilical arteries merge and continue to the umbilicus. Type IV: The urachus and umbilical arteries form a complex of fine strands, the plexus of Luschka.

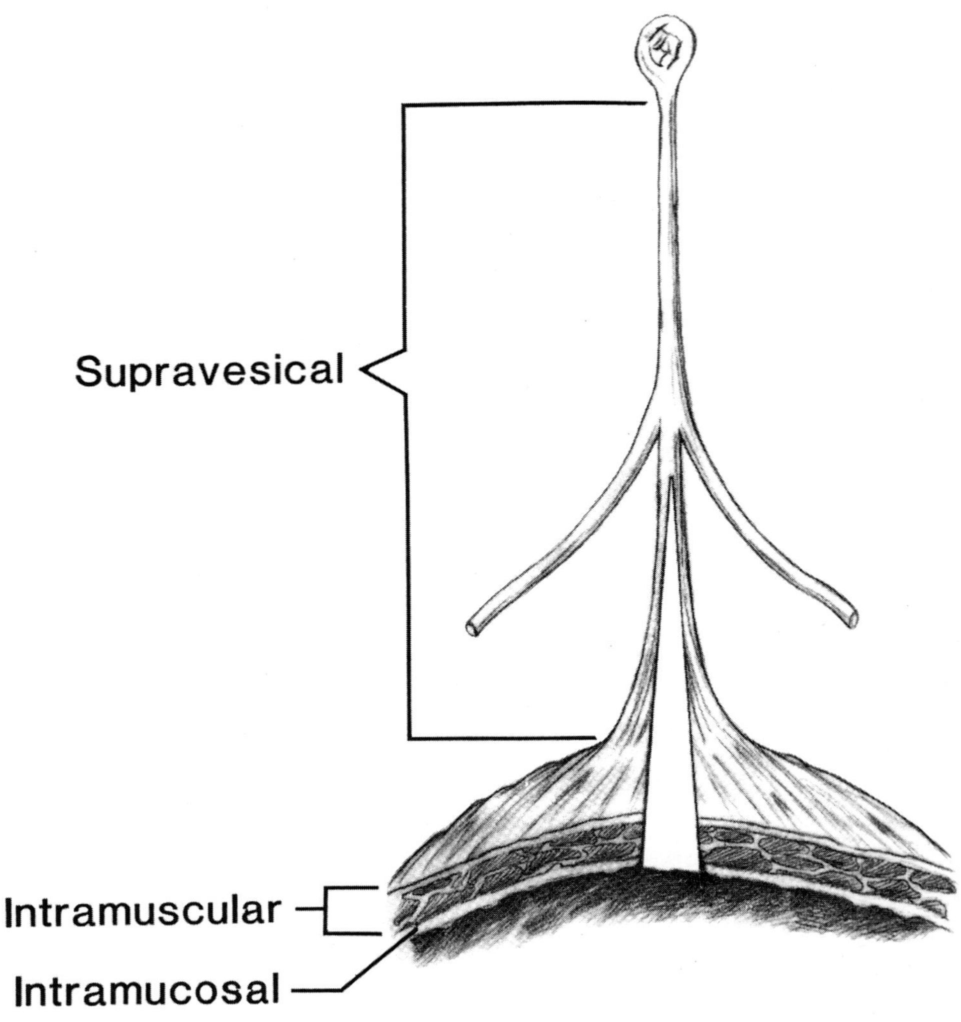

4-2. The urachus is composed of the intramucosal, intramuscular, and supravesical segments.

HISTOLOGY

The bladder is lined by a specialized epithelium variously referred to as *urothelium* for its adaptation to the urinary environment or *transitional cells* after the anal transition zone, a vestige of the cloaca, or because of its morphology, which early microscopists perceived as transitional between squamous and glandular. The designation *urothelium* is preferred here for its reflection of the function of these cells. The urothelial lining of the human urinary tract is composed of three to six layers of cells. The apparent number of layers varies with the degree of distention or stretching at the time of fixation. There are two subtypes of urothelial cells: the umbrella cells, which cover the surface and are in direct contact with urine, and the underlying cells, which comprise the other layers.

The umbrella cells are the largest cells of the urothelium (Fig. 4-3), with eosinophilic cytoplasm, which may contain small amounts of mucin. Their nuclei are large and often somewhat irregular with condensed hyperchromatic chromatin and inconspicuous nucleoli. Ultrastructurally, umbrella cells have asymmetrical cell membranes with a thick outer layer,[14] an irregular angular surface resulting from insertion of stiff segments of membrane, and a variety of intercellular connections.[15] These specializations enable the umbrella cells to cope with the rigors of the urinary environment and maintain the blood-urine barrier as the bladder expands and contracts.[14]

The urothelial cells of the other layers are smaller and more uniform than the umbrella cells,[16] with pale cytoplasm. The nuclei are central, predominantly oval, and, in the deeper layers, oriented perpendicular to the basement membrane. Often, there is a noticeable nuclear groove. The chromatin is very fine and evenly dispersed, and nucleoli are small and inconspicuous. Mitotic figures are uncommon and DNA replication studies reveal that the urothelium is renewed approximately once a year. The basal layer of urothelium rests on a basement membrane.[17] Beneath the basement membrane is the lamina propria, a zone of loose connective tissue that contains delicate vessels and thin, delicate bundles of smooth muscle fibers referred to as the *muscularis mucosae* (Fig. 4-4). The muscularis mucosae of the bladder is variable, ranging from an essentially complete layer analogous to

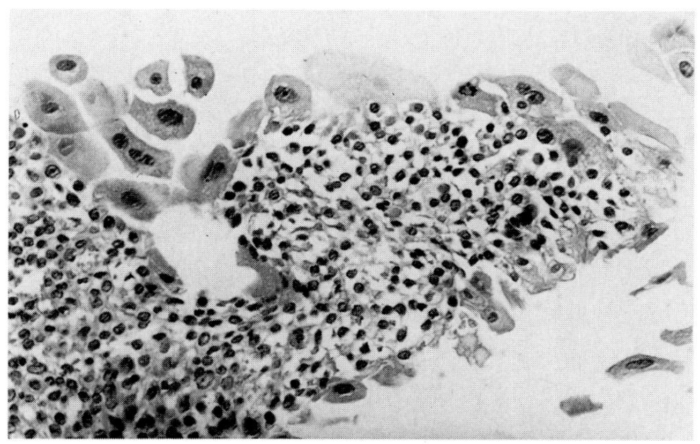

4-3. Umbrella cells have voluminous cytoplasm and large nuclei with inconspicuous nucleoli.

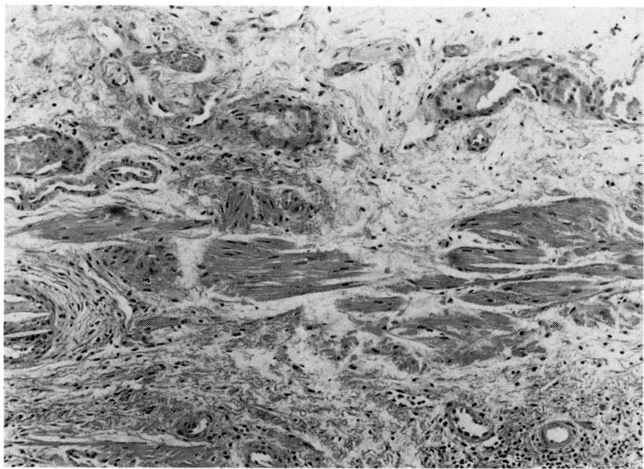

4-4. Smooth muscle in lamina propria is arranged in small irregular bundles.

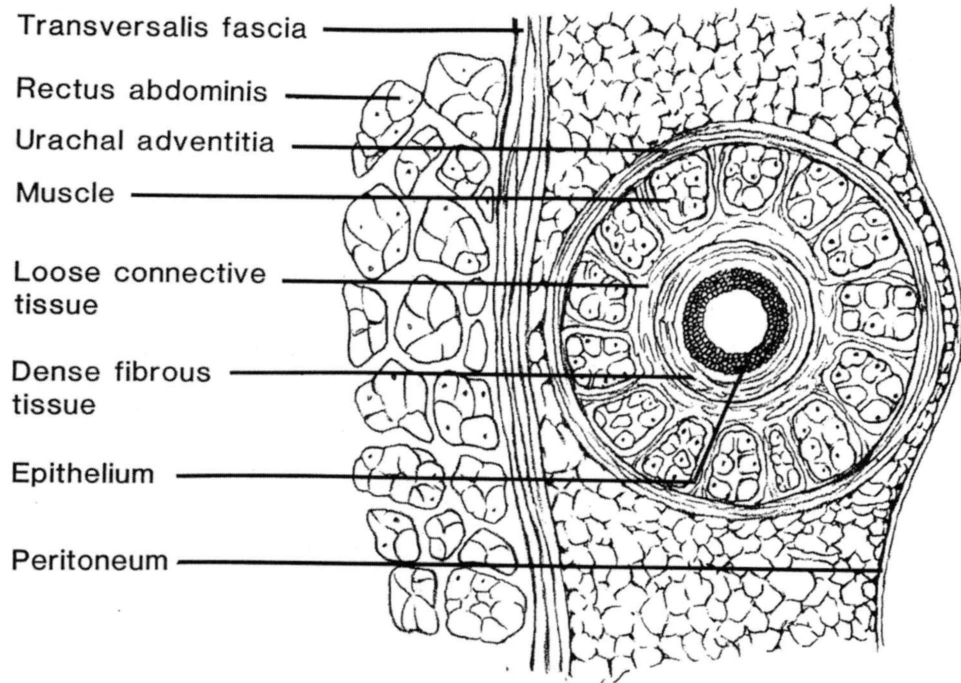

4-5. The structure of the urachus in cross-section.

that seen in the colon to a sparse and incomplete array of smooth muscle fibers.[18-22] The connective tissue beneath the muscularis mucosae contains an arcade of larger vessels. Beneath this is the *muscularis propria* composed of large bundles of muscle fibers with a scant amount of loose connective tissue. The arrangement of muscle bundles varies in pattern and thickness at different locations in the bladder. Distinct layers, analogous to those of the bowel, are seen only in the area of the internal sphincter. In the bladder neck and superior urethral regions, the muscle bundles are more uniform and densely packed than elsewhere.

Histologically, urachal remnants typically consist of a central lumen lined by epithelium and surrounded by a narrow zone of dense connective tissue, then bundles of smooth muscle fibers, and finally a connective tissue adventitia (Fig. 4-5).[23] Such tubular remnants are present in about 33% of adults.[24] Schubert et al[24] classified intramural urachal remnants into three groups, ranging from simple tubular structures to more complex canals (Fig. 4-6, Fig. 4-7). The mucosal segment of the urachus may consist of a papilla, a small opening flush with the surface, a wide diverticular opening, or may be absent (Fig. 4-8, Fig. 4-9). Hammond et al[9] found a mucosal opening

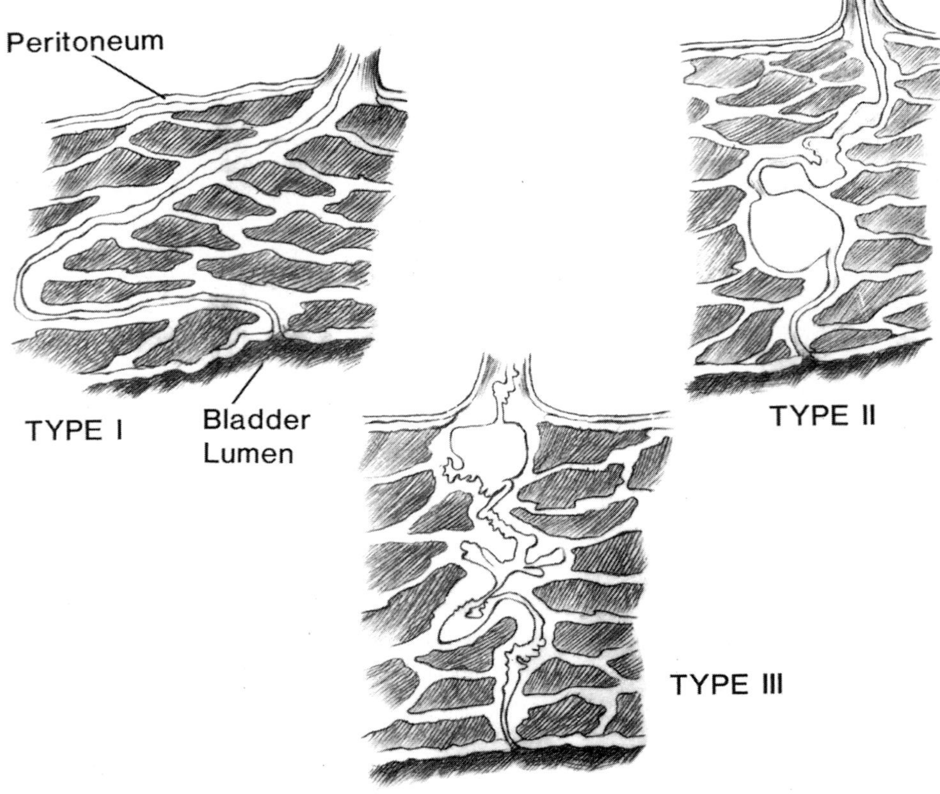

4-6. Variation in the course and structure of the urachus. Type I is a simple canal with a smooth course. Type II has saccular dilations. Type III is more complex with dilations, outpouchings, and an irregular course.

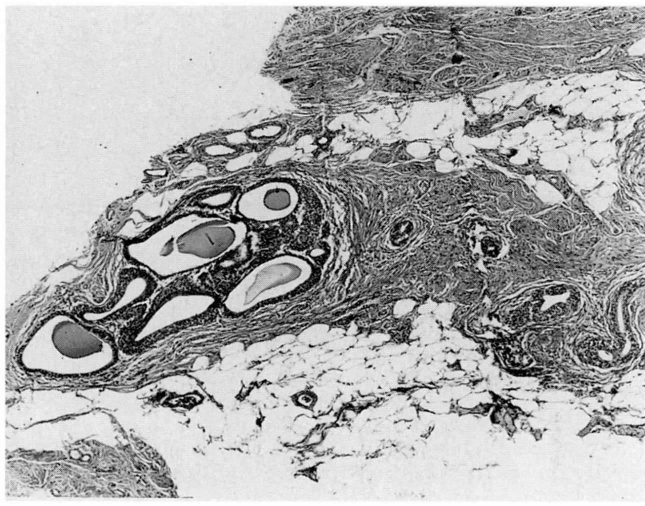

4-7. A complex of urachal channels with focal dilation in the supravesical segment.

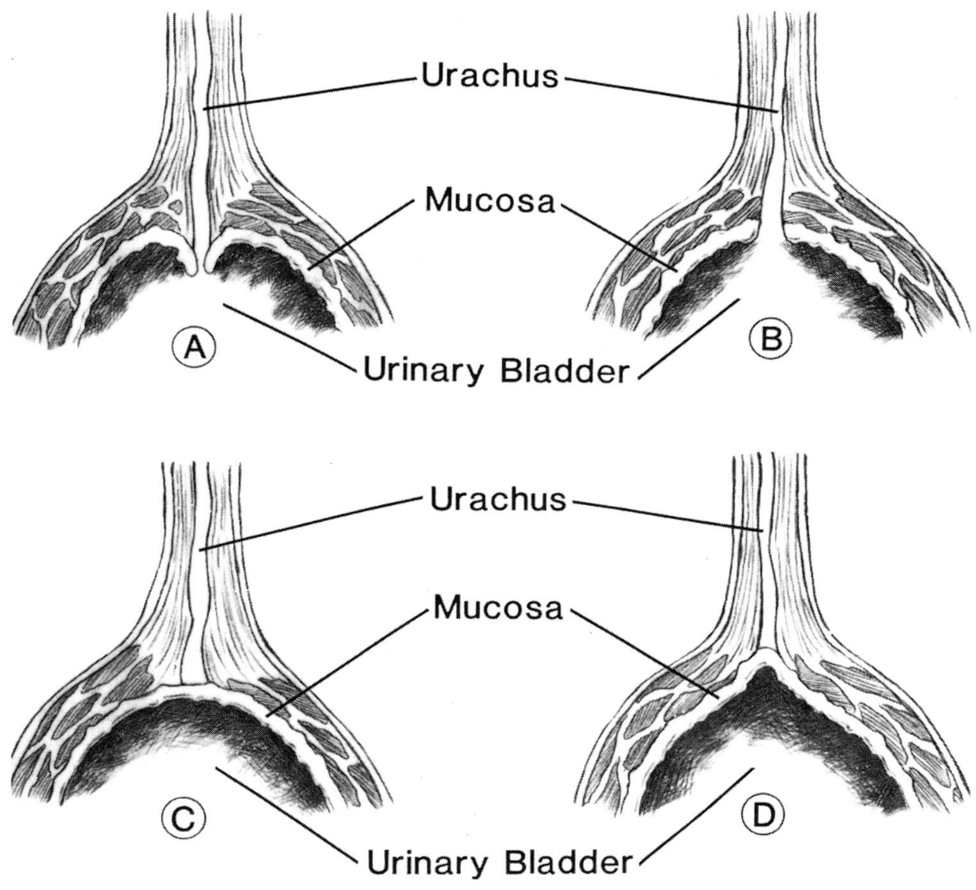

4-8. The intramucosal urachus varies from a lumen terminating in a papilla (**A**), a patent lumen smoothly continuous with bladder mucosa (**B**), smooth bladder mucosa closing the urachal lumen (**C**), to dimpled bladder mucosa covering the urachal lumen (**D**).

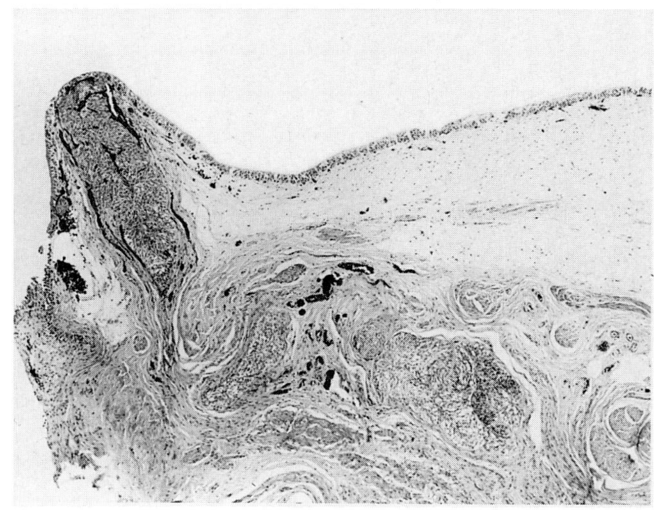

4-9. Type A intramucosal urachus ending in a papilla.

in 10% of specimens. Blichert-Toft et al[10] found that the epithelial component was present in more than 50% of supravesical segments of the type I variant but was often absent or limited to the segment immediately above the bladder in the type IV variant. Urothelium is the most common lining, present in more than 66% of intramural remnants.[24] The remaining intramural remnants are lined by columnar cells that occasionally may be mucus-secreting.[25] The urachus is not always a straight tube; Begg[26] and Schubert et al[24] showed that the urachus often has saccular dilations, outpouchings, and a tortuous course through the bladder wall.

EPITHELIAL ABNORMALITIES

VON BRUNN'S NESTS

Well-circumscribed nests of urothelial cells in the lamina propria, von Brunn's nests,[27-31] arise by a process of budding from the overlying epithelium or by migration[32] and may or may not be attached to the epithelium. Autopsy studies find von Brunn's nests in 85% to 95% of bladders, more commonly in the trigone than elsewhere.[28,30,31,33] Previously, some considered these nests to be related to inflammation or a precursor of carcinoma, but neither view is currently accepted. Today they are viewed as normal features of the bladder mucosa.

Histologically, von Brunn's nests are rounded, well-circumscribed groups of urothelial cells in the lamina propria, usually close to the urothelium but occasionally appreciably deep (Fig. 4-10). Their regular shape and orderly spatial arrangement contrast with the features of rare carcinomas with a nested pattern that are occasionally confused with von Brunn's nests (see Fig. 5-35 in Chapter 5). The nuclei of the cells in von Brunn's nests lack significant atypia. Reactive and metaplastic changes in the surface urothelium may also occur in von Brunn's nests. Urothelial carcinoma in situ may extend into von Brunn's nests and should not be mistaken for invasion of the lamina propria. When von Brunn's nests are numerous, closely packed, and hyperplastic, the distinction from inverted papilloma may be difficult and arbitrary.

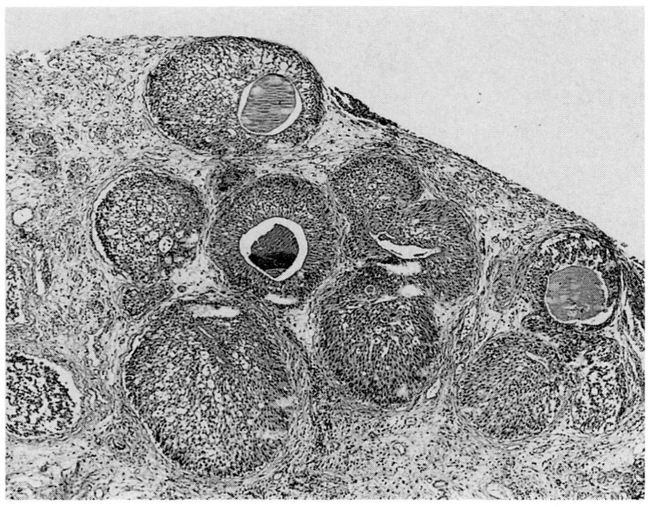

4-10. von Brunn's nests at the mucosal surface and deeper in the lamina propria. Note smooth round contours of the nests.

CYSTITIS GLANDULARIS AND CYSTITIS CYSTICA

The term *cystitis glandularis* refers to a lesion that evolves from and merges imperceptibly with von Brunn's nests.[34-41] Cystitis glandularis is so common that it may be considered a normal feature of the vesical mucosa. Autopsy studies reveal its presence in up to 71% of bladders, most commonly in the trigone.[33] Most foci of cystitis glandularis are microscopic. However, it occasionally forms irregular, rounded, or nodular elevations of the mucosa.[42] Exceptionally, it forms larger polypoid lesions that may be mistaken for a neoplasm prior to microscopic examination.[43-46] Microscopically, cystitis glandularis is composed of glands in the lamina propria, which are lined by cuboidal to columnar cells surrounded by one or more layers of urothelial cells (Fig. 4-11). Similar epithelium may also be present on the mucosal surface. The glands of cystitis glandularis may be dilated. Although the lining cells are sometimes characterized as mucinous, they usually do not appear overtly mucinous in sections stained with

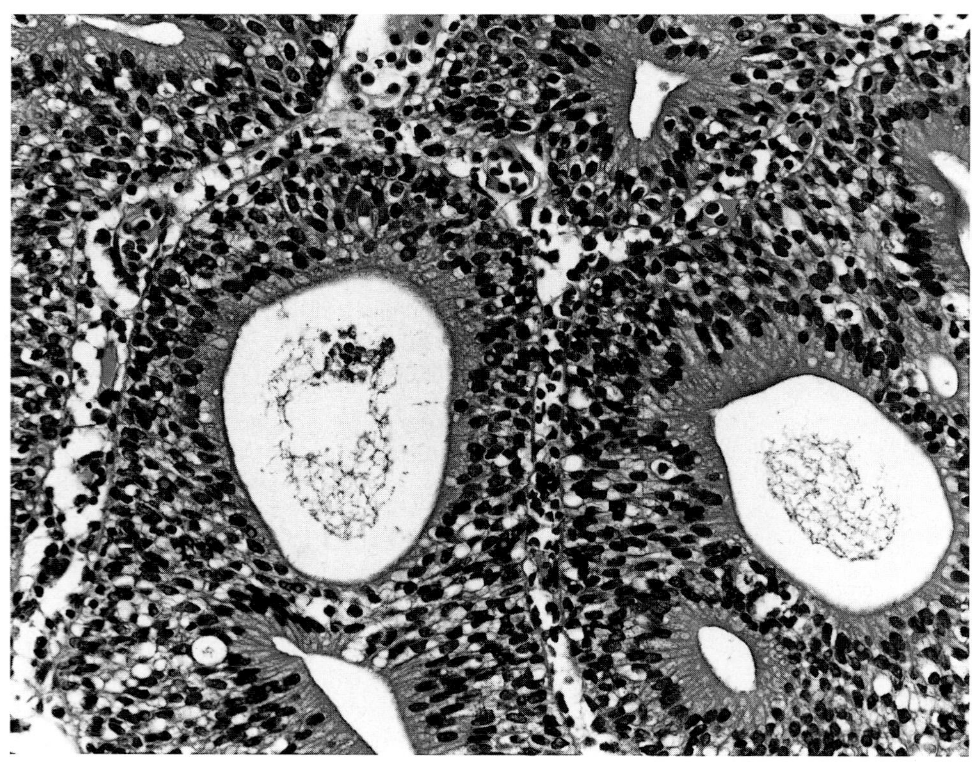

4-11. Cystitis glandularis of the typical type. The lining cells are columnar, goblet cells are not present, and mucus is absent or inconspicuous.

hematoxylin and eosin,[34] and mucin stains are often negative or weakly positive. Less frequently, the lining cells are tall and columnar with obvious mucin production. In such cases, goblet cells often are present and the glands closely resemble colonic glands. Rarely, Paneth cells and argentaffin or argyrophil cells are present.[36,41,47,48] The distinction between nonmucinous and mucinous cystitis glandularis has been recognized for many years but is not always made. The more common form can be referred to as the *typical type* of cystitis glandularis and the second form as the *intestinal type*.[34] The two may coexist, or one may predominate or be present exclusively.

Cystitis glandularis of the intestinal type may be extensive, affecting both the lamina propria and the mucosa.[34,46,48,49] Biopsies from such areas closely resemble colonic mucosa, with tubular glands and numerous goblet cells (Fig. 4-12). The mucin produced by these cells is of the colonic type.[50,51] In some cases, the cells also stain immunohistochemically with antibodies to prostate-specific antigen and prostatic acid phosphatase.[52,53] Rarely, colonic epithelium may be present in the bladder as a developmental abnormality.[54]

Diffuse cystitis glandularis of the intestinal type is termed *intestinal metaplasia* and usually occurs in chronically irritated bladders such as those of paraplegics or in patients with stones or long-term catheterization (Fig. 4-13). Unlike focal cystitis glandularis of the intestinal type, persistent extensive or diffuse intestinal metaplasia is associated with an increased risk of bladder carcinoma.[41,47,55] This risk probably exceeds that of patients with World Health Organization grade 1 noninvasive papillary urothelial carcinoma.[56] It is only the intestinal type of cystitis glandularis that is associated with adenocarcinoma.[57-64]

Cystitis glandularis usually poses no diagnostic problem, but occasional cases are difficult to distinguish from adenocarcinoma.[57,65] This is particularly true of the intestinal type, especially when mucin extravasates into the stroma. An irregular haphazard arrangement of glands in the deeper lamina propria and cytologic atypia should raise the suspicion of adenocarcinoma.

Cystitis cystica consists of von Brunn's nests in which the central cells have degenerated to form small cystic cavities.[30,58,66-68] While somewhat less common than von Brunn's nests and cystitis glandularis, cystitis cystica is present in up to 60% of bladders.[31] It is most common in adults but also occurs in children.[68] At cystoscopy, its cystic nature is usually apparent. Grossly, the lesions appear as translucent, submucosal cysts that are pearly-white to yellow-brown (Fig. 4-14).[42] Most are less than 5 mm in diameter[67] but rare examples of a few centimeters in diameter have been reported. The cysts contain clear yellow fluid. Microscopically, the cysts are lined by urothelium or cuboidal epithelium (Fig. 4-15) and filled by eosinophilic fluid in which a few inflammatory cells often are present.

SQUAMOUS METAPLASIA

Metaplastic squamous epithelium is common in patients with severe chronic cystitis,[69-74] such as those with nonfunctioning bladders[75,76] or schistosomiasis.[77] It is about four times more common in women than men. Squamous metaplasia may occur anywhere in the bladder but is most frequent on the anterior wall. Areas of metaplasia often are white or gray-white (Fig. 4-16) and may blend into the surrounding mucosa[69] or be sharply demarcated.[71] Abundantly keratinizing lesions may have a bulky irregular appearance similar to carcinoma.[78,79] Histologically, the lesions show squamous epithelium of variable thickness, often covered by a layer of keratin (Fig. 4-17). In most cases, there is no nuclear atypia, but changes as severe as those of carcinoma in situ are occasionally seen (Fig. 4-18) and should raise the possibility of invasive carcinoma elsewhere in the specimen or in nearby mucosa.

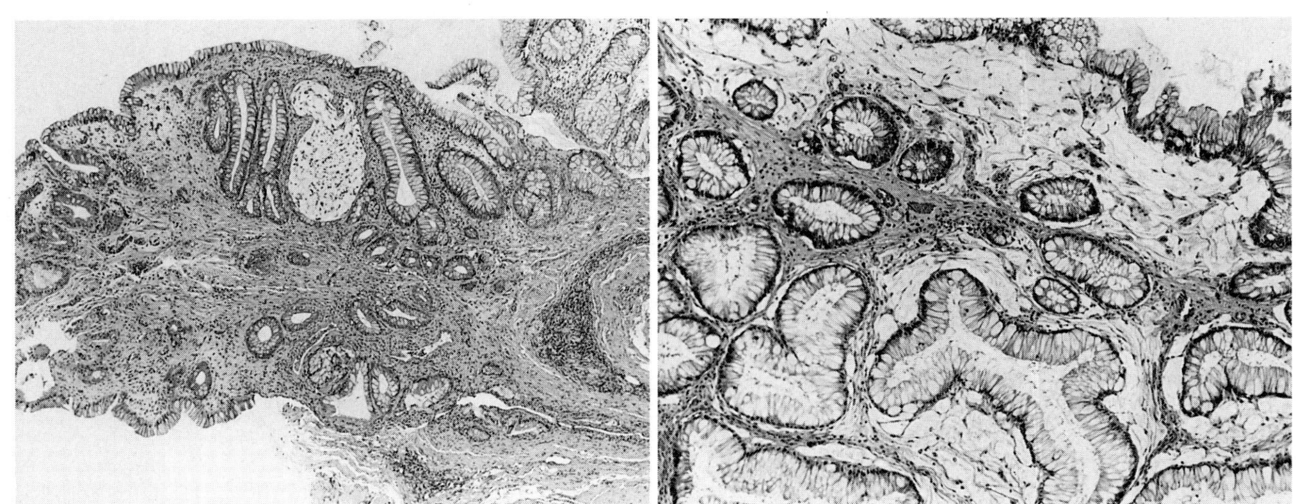

4-12. **A**, Cystitis glandularis, intestinal type. There are irregularly spaced tubular glands lined by goblet cells. The surface epithelium also is mucinous. **B**, Cystitis glandularis, intestinal type. The glands closely resemble colonic glands.

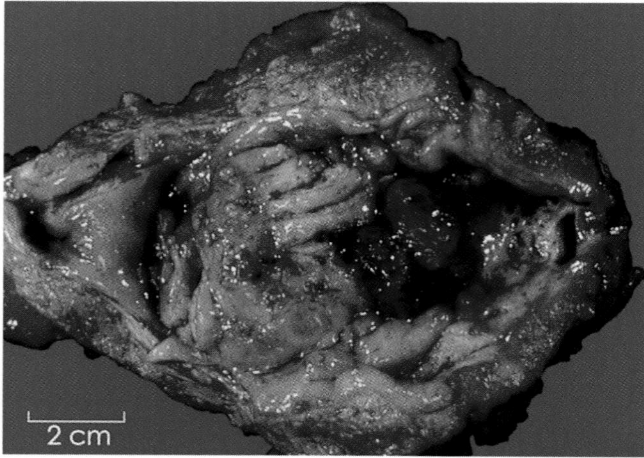

4-13. Extensive cystitis glandularis, intestinal type (intestinal metaplasia). Large and small foci of glistening red mucosa mimic a bladder tumor. Cystitis cystica also is present in the upper left quadrant.

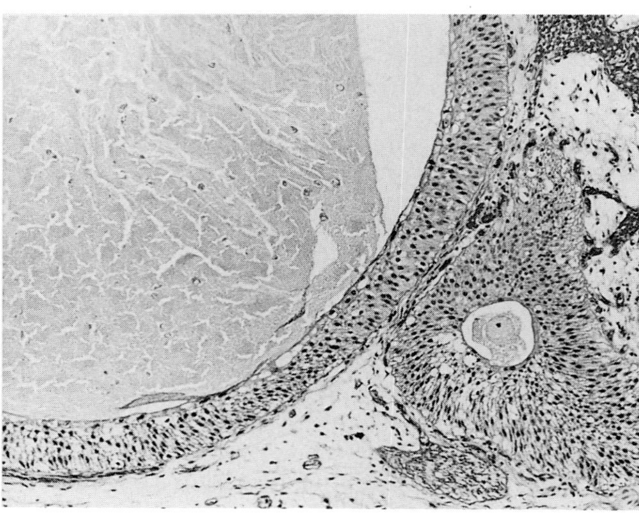

4-15. Cystitis cystica. The cysts are lined by urothelium and the lumen contains proteinaceous fluid.

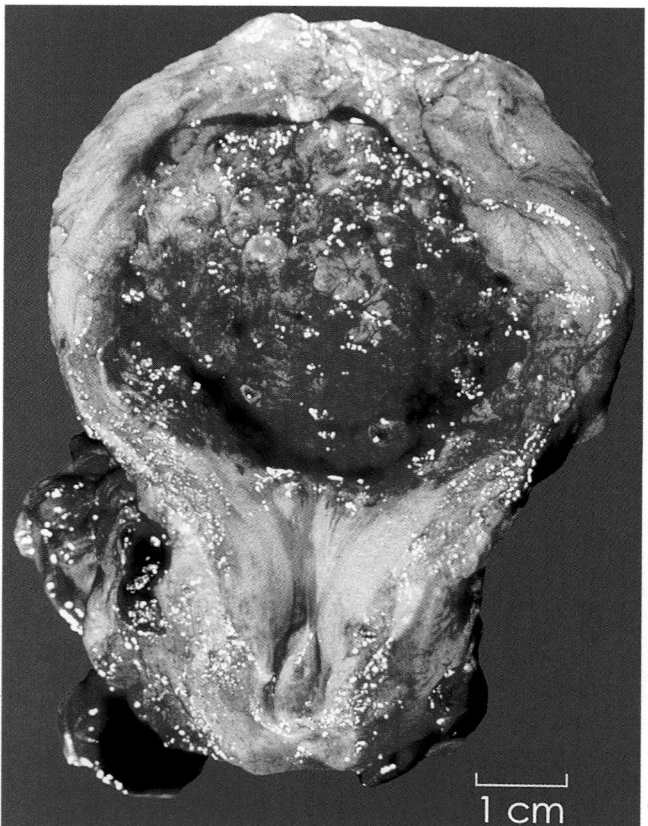

4-14. Cystitis cystica appears as thin-walled domed mucosal cysts or blebs.

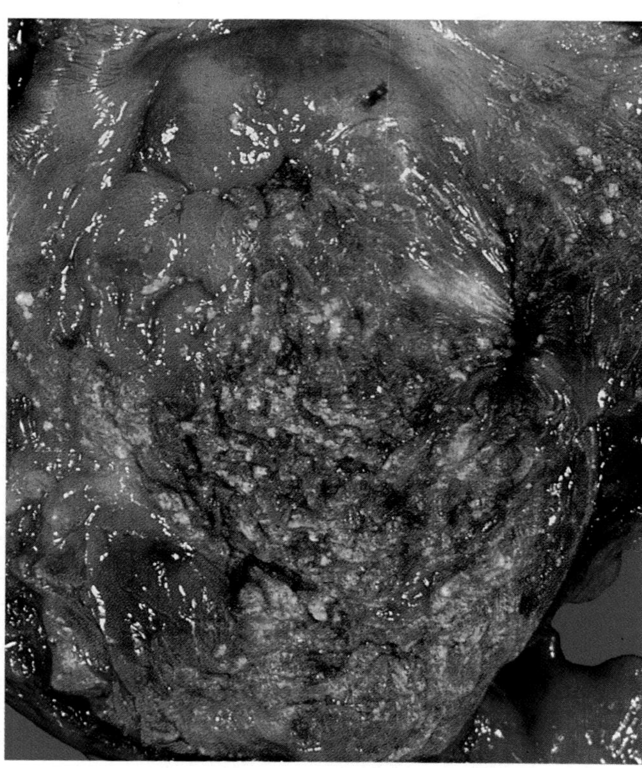

4-16. Keratinizing squamous metaplasia is gray with flecks of light-colored keratin.

Keratinizing squamous metaplasia (leukoplakia) appears to be a significant risk factor for the development of carcinoma of the urinary mucosa.[80-82] A study of 78 patients with keratinizing squamous metaplasia from the Mayo Clinic found that 22% had synchronous carcinoma and another 20% later developed carcinoma (the mean interval was 11 years).[83] Most were squamous cell carcinoma. Where schistosomiasis is endemic, squamous metaplasia commonly precedes squamous cell carcinoma.[84,85]

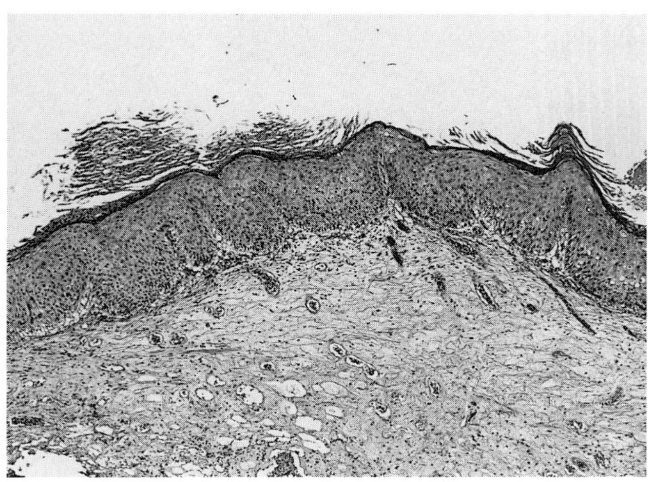

4-17. Keratinizing squamous metaplasia replacing the urothelium.

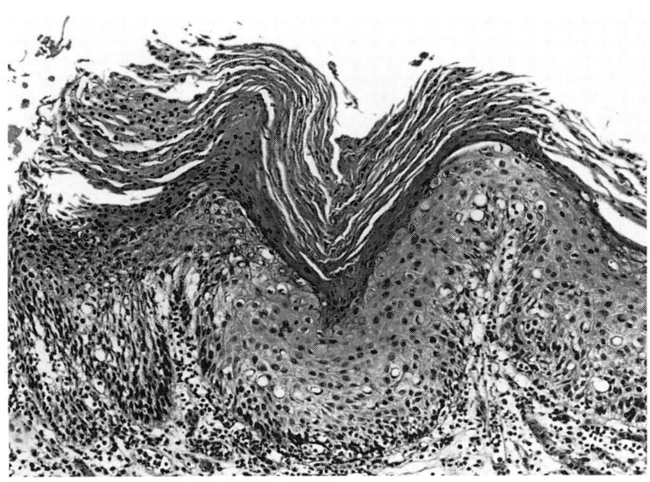

4-18. Keratinizing squamous metaplasia with nuclear atypia and parakeratosis.

Nonkeratinizing glycogenated squamous epithelium, resembling vaginal epithelium (Fig. 4-19), is present in the trigone and bladder neck in up to 86% of women of reproductive age and in almost 75% of postmenopausal women.[86-91] This normal finding should not be diagnosed as squamous metaplasia. Cystoscopically, these areas are pale gray-white with irregular borders, often with a surrounding zone of erythema. The clinical association of this cystoscopic finding with symptoms of urgency and frequency has been called *pseudomembranous trigonitis*. This type of squamous epithelium is very rare in men, but has been reported in patients receiving estrogen therapy for adenocarcinoma of the prostate.[88,92]

NEPHROGENIC ADENOMA

First described as a hamartoma in 1949 by Davis,[93] the name *nephrogenic adenoma* was given a year later by Friedman and Kuhlenbeck[94] in a report of eight cases.

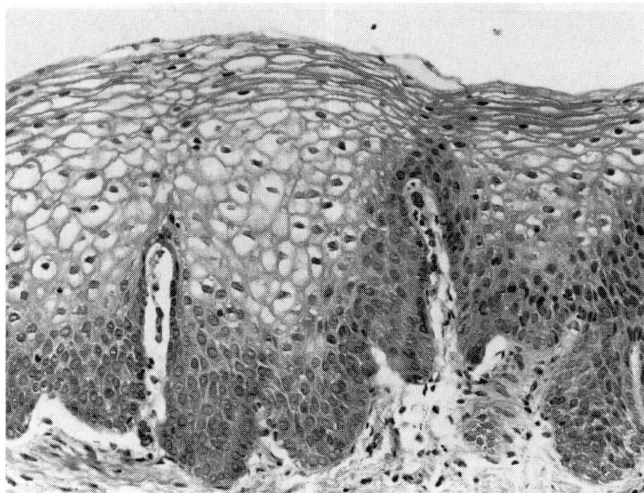

4-19. Nonkeratinizing glycogenated squamous epithelium from the trigone of a woman of reproductive age.

They chose this name because in its most common form it is composed of small tubules resembling renal tubules. Today it is recognized as a metaplastic process[95-101] and the terms *nephrogenic metaplasia*[102,103] and *adenomatous metaplasia*[98] are preferred by some authors. More than 75% of reported cases have involved the bladder, but lesions in the urethra, ureter, and rarely the renal pelvis have also been reported.[99]

Approximately 90% of patients with nephrogenic adenoma are adults and there is a male predominance of 2:1. In children, it is more common in girls than in boys.[104,105] Nephrogenic adenoma is frequently found following genitourinary surgery (61% of cases) or associated with calculi (14% of cases), trauma (9% of cases), and cystitis.[99] Renal transplant recipients make up about 8% of patients.[99,106] Complaints of hematuria, dysuria, and frequency are common, but the association with other lesions makes it difficult to attribute any of these to the nephrogenic adenoma.

Approximately 56% are papillary, 34% sessile, and 10% polypoid. It is rare on the anterior wall of the bladder,[99] but nearly evenly distributed over the rest of the mucosa. About two thirds are smaller than 1 cm in diameter, ranging down to incidentally discovered microscopic lesions. Approximately 25% are from 1 to 4 cm in diameter and only 10% are larger. In less than 20% of cases, there are multiple lesions, which rarely include diffuse involvement of the bladder.

Microscopically, nephrogenic adenoma displays tubular, cystic, polypoid, papillary, and diffuse patterns.[107] The most common architecture is tubular (present in 96% of cases). The tubules are typically small round structures lined by cuboidal epithelium (Fig. 4-20), but occasionally are elongate and solid. Sometimes, they are surrounded by a prominent basement membrane. Cystic dilatation of the tubules is common (Fig. 4-21) (present in 72% of cases) and may predominate. Tubules and cysts often contain eosinophilic or basophilic secretions, which may react with mucicarmine (present in 25% of

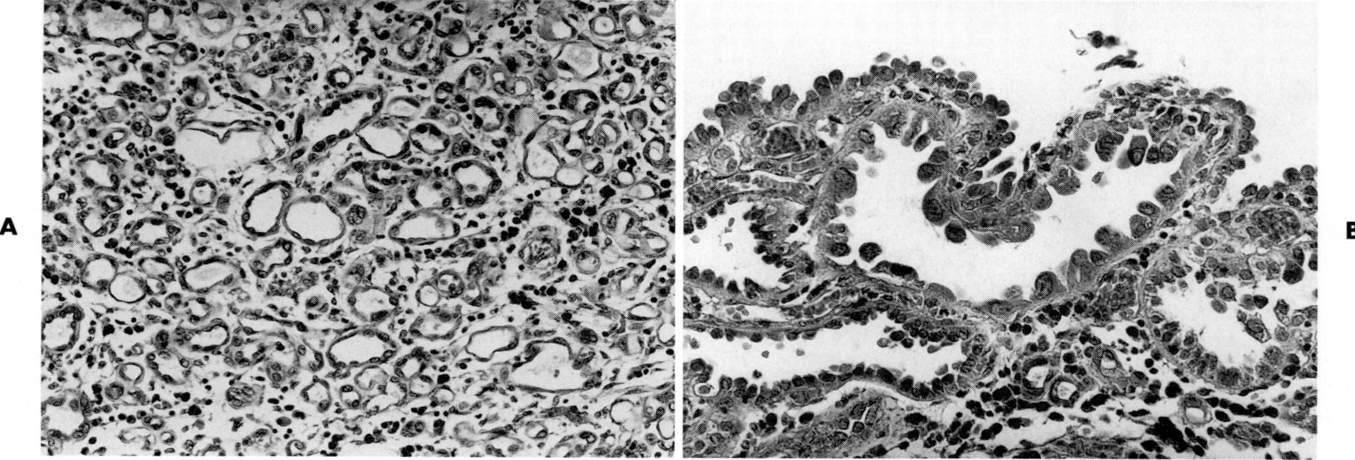

4-20. **A**, Tubules of nephrogenic adenoma lined by cuboidal epithelium resembling renal medullary tubules. **B**, Tubules of nephrogenic adenoma lined by hobnail cells.

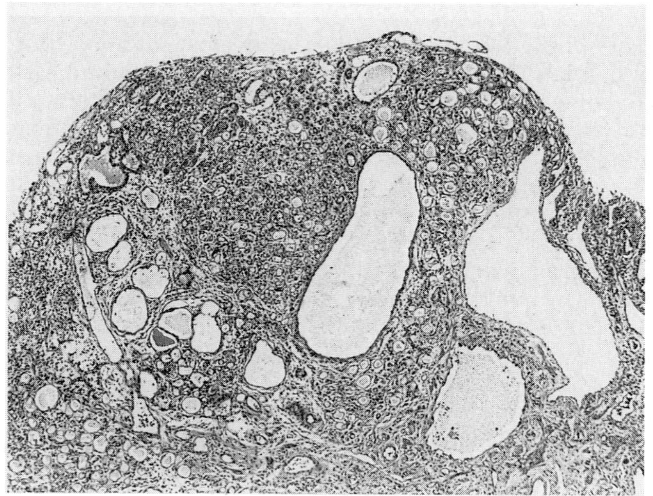

4-21. Cystic dilation of tubules in nephrogenic adenoma.

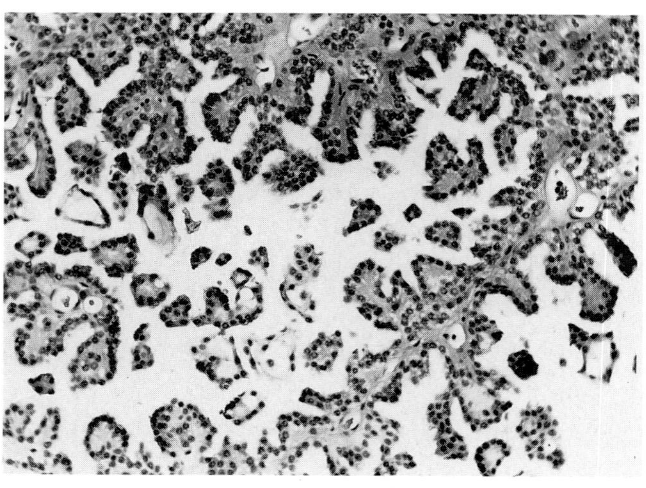

4-22. Papillary nephrogenic adenoma. The papillae are covered by a single layer of cuboidal cells.

cases). Polypoid and papillary structures (Fig. 4-22) are present in 65% of cases. Edematous polyps are more common than delicate papillae, which are present in only 10% of cases. Focal solid growth (Fig. 4-23) is uncommon.

Most tubules, cysts, and papillae have cuboidal to low columnar epithelium with scant cytoplasm, but epithelium with abundant clear cytoplasm is seen in 40% of cases.[108] While hobnail cells (Fig. 4-20*B*) focally line the tubules and cysts in 70% of cases, they rarely are predominant.[107] Larger cysts may be lined by flat epithelium and a small amount of mucin may be found in the epithelial cells. Glycogen is present in some cells in 10% to 15% of cases.[108] The nuclei are regular and round, and atypia is rare, usually appearing degenerative. Mitotic figures are absent or rare.[107,109] Nephrogenic adenoma is often associated with chronic cystitis, which may obscure it. Rarely, it is associated with stromal calcification,[95,110] squamous metaplasia, or cystitis glandularis.

Nephrogenic adenoma has a number of features that may cause confusion with bladder carcinoma. Tiny mucin-filled tubules apparently lined by a single cell with a compressed nucleus may resemble signet ring cells. The irregular disposition of the tubules may simulate invasive adenocarcinoma, especially when the tubules are among the fibers of the muscularis mucosae. Hobnail cells may bring to mind clear cell adenocarcinoma, which shares architectural features of tubular, cystic, and papillary structures with nephrogenic adenoma (see Chapter 5). Clinical and pathologic features that help to distinguish nephrogenic adenoma from clear cell adenocarcinoma are shown in Table 4-1.

In a few cases of nephrogenic adenoma, papillae are the predominant feature (Fig. 4-24) and may cause confusion with other papillary lesions, such as urothelial carcinoma and papillary cystitis. Recognition of the cuboidal epithelium covering the papillae of nephro-

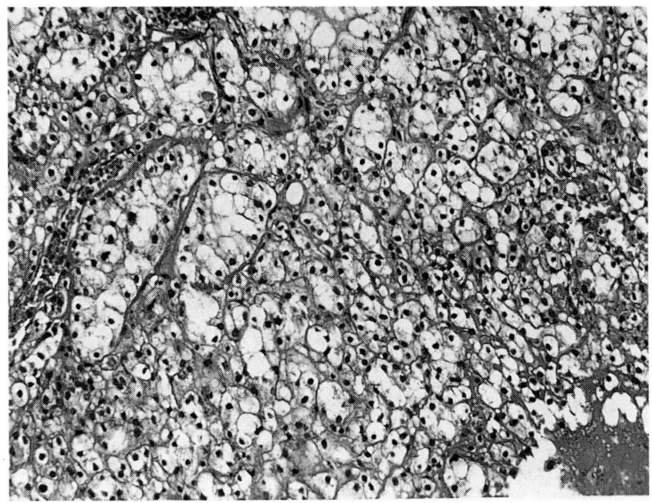

4-23. The diffuse or solid pattern of nephrogenic adenoma. The cells have abundant clear cytoplasm.

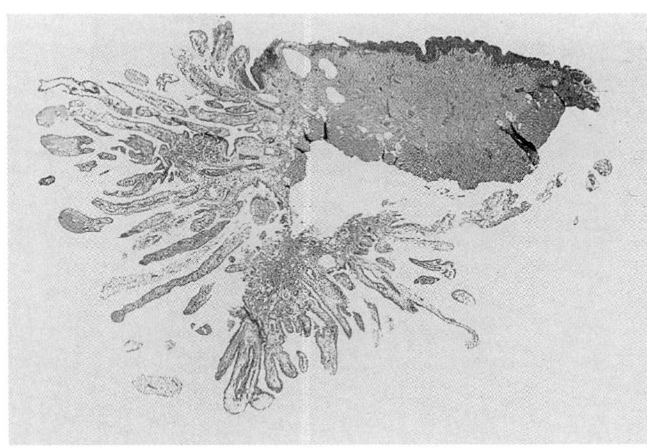

4-24. Nephrogenic adenoma with predominance of the papillary component.

TABLE 4-1.
FEATURES DISTINGUISHING NEPHROGENIC ADENOMA FROM CLEAR CELL ADENOCARCINOMA

Feature	Nephrogenic Adenoma	Clear Cell Adenocarcinoma
Gender predominance	Male	Female
Age	33% < 30 years	All > 43 years
Associated genitourinary conditions	Very common	Absent
Size	Usually small	Often large
Solid growth pattern	Rare	Common
Clear cells	Uncommon	Common
Glycogen in cytoplasm	Rare	Common and abundant
Nuclear atypia and mitotic figures	Rare	Common

genic adenoma differentiates it from these lesions, which are covered by urothelium.

PAPILLARY HYPERPLASIA

The urothelial mucosa overlying inflammatory or neoplastic processes may occasionally have a papillary appearance on microscopic examination. In some cases, discovery of the bladder lesion precedes identification of the underlying condition and in these cases the bladder lesion is referred to as a *herald lesion*.[111] The term *papillary hyperplasia* is used when papillae are not seen grossly or at cystoscopy.[42] Most often, the underlying lesion originates in the prostate, female genital tract, or colon.[111,112] When associated with prostatic disease, the papillary lesions are found in the trigone in the midline; those associated with uterine disease are found in the midline above the trigone. When associated with intestinal disease, the bladder lesions are often on the left and posterior.[42] Non-specific papillary hyperplasia should be distinguished from the papillary hyperplasia that is seen at the earliest manifestation of papillary carcinoma.

INFLAMMATION AND INFECTION

NONSPECIFIC CYSTITIS

Polypoid and papillary cystitis

Polypoid and papillary cystitis result from inflammation and edema in the lamina propria leading to papillary and polypoid mucosal lesions.[113-117] The term *papillary cystitis* is used for finger-like papillae (Fig. 4-25) and *polypoid cystitis* for broad-based edematous lesions (Fig. 4-26). The latter are more common. Chronic inflammation in the lamina propria and dilated blood vessels are prominent and diagnostically helpful features of both papillary and polypoid cystitis. Depending on the degree of edema of the lamina propria, there is a continuous morphological spectrum from papillary cystitis to polypoid cystitis to *bullous cystitis* (Fig. 4-27). In papillary and polypoid cystitis the lesion is taller than it is wide, while in bullous cystitis the opposite applies. There may be associated metaplastic changes in the epithelium covering or adjacent to the lesion.

In the clinical settings of indwelling catheter and vesical fistula, the surgical pathologist should be alert to the

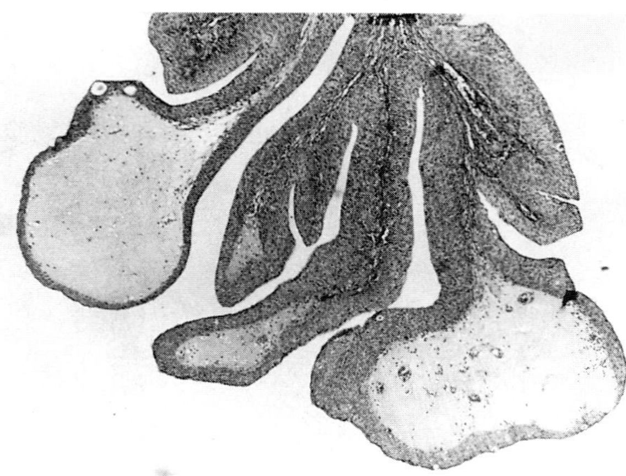

4-25. Papillary cystitis with finger-like fronds covered by a few layers of urothelium.

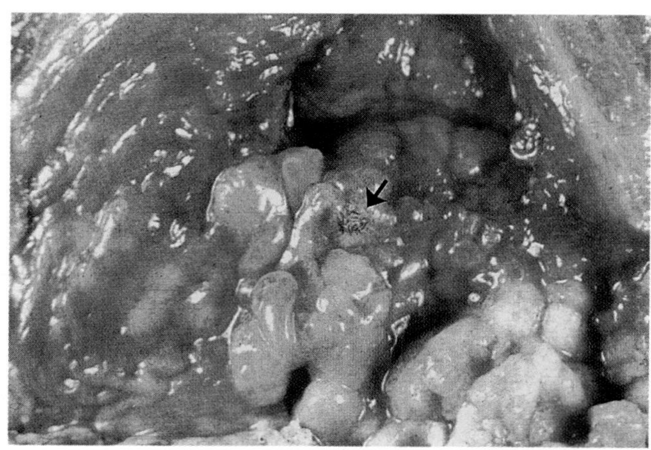

4-26. Polypoid cystitis. Arrow shows biopsy site. *(Courtesy of Dr. M. El-Bolkainy.)*

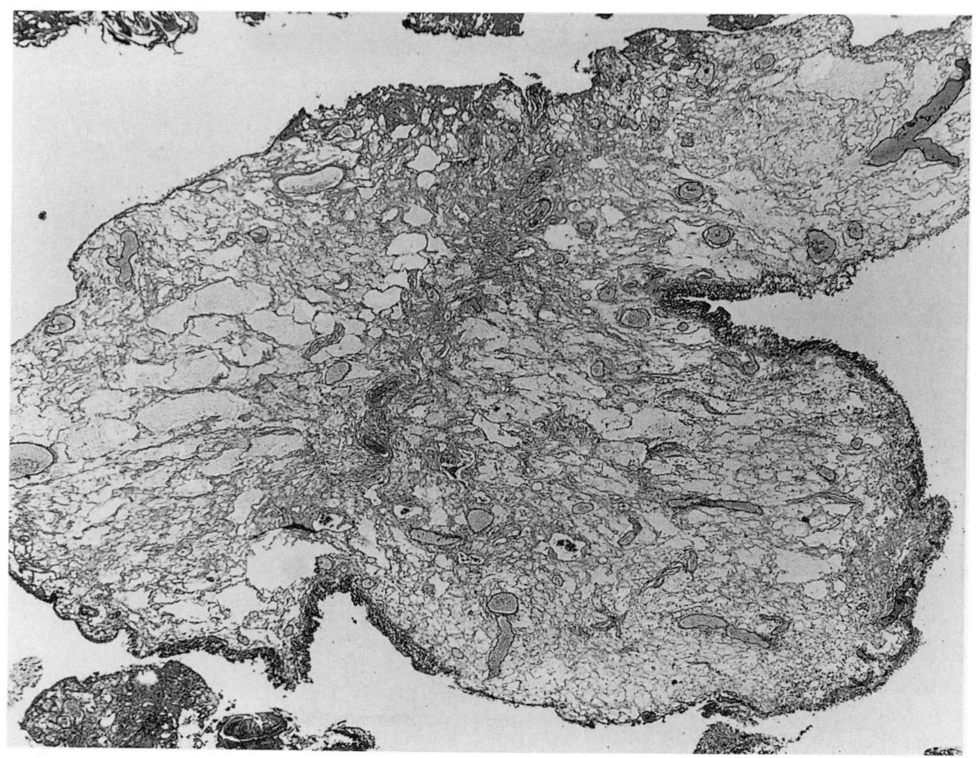

4-27. Bullous cystitis.

possibility that an exophytic bladder lesion may be inflammatory.[118] Polypoid cystitis is present in up to 80% of patients with indwelling catheters.[116] While most lesions are of microscopic size, polypoid or bullous lesions up to 5 mm in diameter (mostly in the dome or on the posterior wall) are found in about 33% of cases. Prolonged catheterization may induce widespread polypoid and bullous cystitis. Most lesions disappear within 6 months of removal of the irritant.[115]

Vesical fistulae, whether resulting from intestinal diverticulitis,[119] Crohn's disease, colorectal cancer (Fig. 4-28),[119] or appendicitis, often are associated with polypoid cystitis, and, less commonly, with papillary cystitis.[120-125] Fistulae between the urinary bladder and the alimentary tract are about three times more common in men than in women.[121,126] Pneumaturia and fecaluria are typical symptoms.[121] In about 50% of cases, indications of extravesical disease are initially absent, making the diagnosis more difficult. Patients may present with frequency, urgency, and dysuria. Cystoscopically, the appearance often suggests bladder carcinoma.[114]

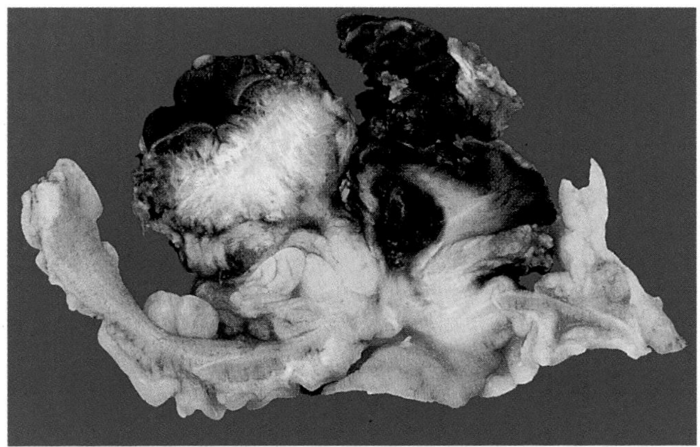

4-28. Colovesical fistula secondary to adenocarcinoma of colon. The dimpled outlet in the bladder mucosa (*above*) connects with the colon (*below*).

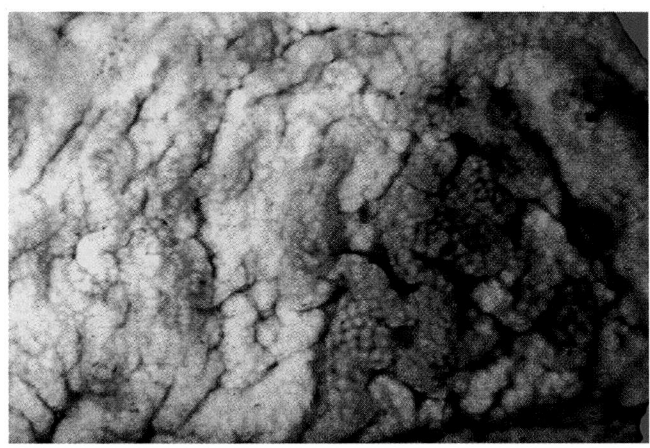

4-29. Follicular cystitis. The lymphoid aggregates are visible as small domed lesions on the mucosal surface.

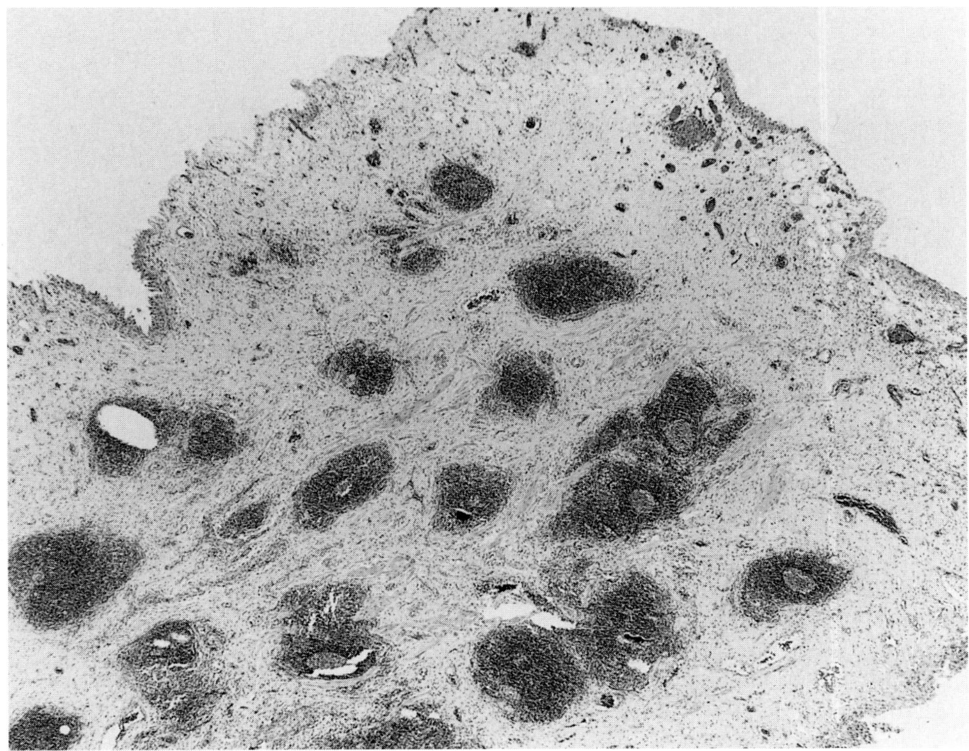

4-30. Follicular cystitis. The lamina propria contains numerous lymphoid follicles.

Papillary and polypoid cystitis must be distinguished from papillary urothelial carcinoma. Grossly and microscopically, the fronds of polypoid cystitis are much broader than those of most papillary carcinomas. The delicate papillae of papillary cystitis more closely resemble those of carcinoma. Branching is much less prominent in papillary cystitis than in papillary carcinoma. In papillary cystitis, the epithelium may be hyperplastic, but usually not to the degree seen in carcinoma. Umbrella cells are more often present in papillary cystitis than in carcinoma.

Follicular cystitis

Follicular cystitis occurs in up to 40% of patients with bladder cancer[127] and 35% of patients with urinary tract infection.[128] Grossly, the mucosa is erythematous with pink, white, or gray nodules (Fig. 4-29).[129-132] Microscopically, the nodules consist of lymphoid follicles in the lamina propria, usually with germinal centers (Fig. 4-30). Malignant lymphoma is the most important differential diagnostic consideration, particularly in biopsies. The criteria used to distinguish lymphoma from chronic inflammation at other sites apply here.

Giant cell cystitis

Atypical mesenchymal cells with enlarged, hyperchromatic, or multiple nuclei are frequently seen in the lamina propria of the bladder. Wells[133] found them in 33% of cases of cystitis at autopsy and coined the term *giant cell cystitis*. Such cells are common in bladder biopsies, including those without other evidence of cystitis. Histologically, the cells often have bipolar or multipolar tapering eosinophilic cytoplasmic processes (Fig. 4-31). The nuclei are often irregular in size and shape and hyperchromatic. Mitotic figures are absent or rare. If present in large numbers, these cells may bring to mind pseudoneoplastic lesions such as postoperative spindle cell nodule and neoplasms like sarcomatoid urothelial carcinoma or sarcoma. Similar cells may be seen in the lamina propria after radiation therapy and anticancer chemotherapy.[134-137]

Hemorrhagic cystitis

Cystitis with a predominantly hemorrhagic clinical presentation (Fig. 4-32) may be caused by chemical toxins, radiation, viral infection, or may be idiopathic.[138]

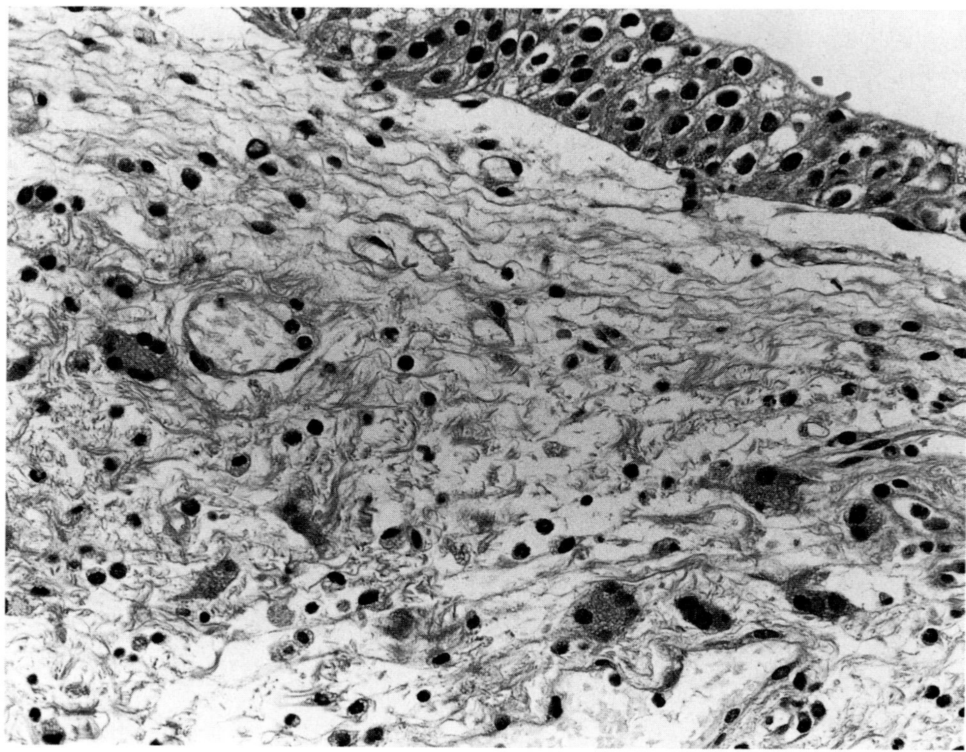

4-31. Giant cell cystitis. The lamina propria contains large stromal cells, some with elongate cytoplasmic processes and some that are multinucleated.

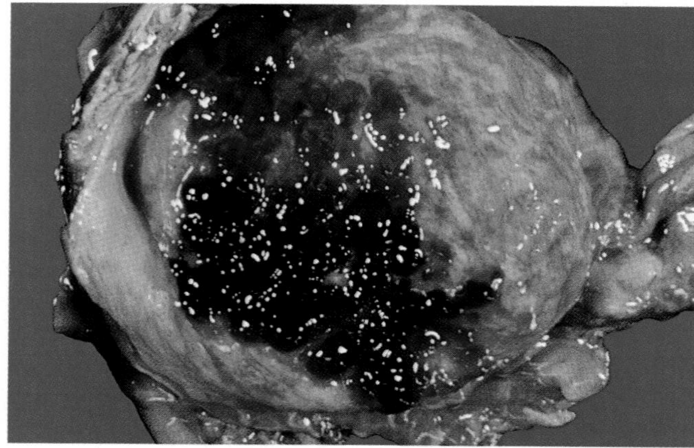

4-32. Hemorrhagic cystitis. *(Courtesy of Dr. I. Damjanov.)*

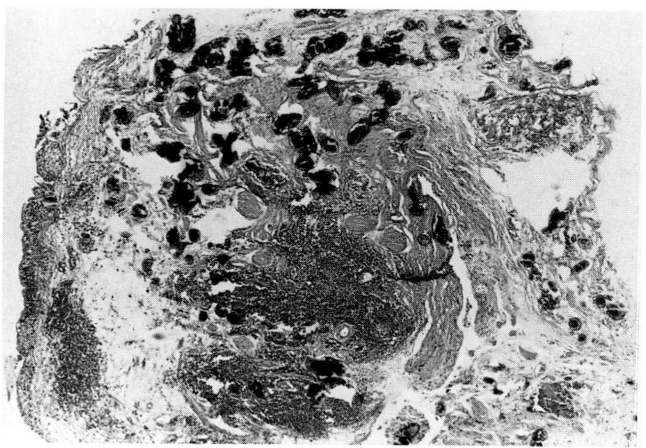

4-33. Hemorrhagic cystitis. The vasculature is congested and there is hemorrhage in the lamina propria.

Chemical causes include drugs (such as cyclophosphamide, busulfan, and thiotepa), derivatives of aniline and toluidine (such as dyes and insecticides), and a host of other compounds.[138,139] Radiation and chemotherapy for cancer account for most cases.

Since its introduction in the late 1950s, cyclophosphamide has been recognized as a potent bladder toxin associated with hemorrhagic cystitis.[136,140,141] Hemorrhage may be severe[142] and early experience reported mortality of nearly 4%.[141] Hemorrhage usually begins during or shortly after treatment. Within 4 hours, the mucosa is edematous and congested (Fig. 4-33) and the epithelium shows changes similar to those seen in the irradiated bladder, including nuclear pleomorphism and variable cell size. As the bladder heals, the urothelium becomes hyperplastic and may form papillae. High doses of cyclophosphamide and repeated exposure may lead to irreversible fibrosis and a small contracted bladder.[134] Epithelial and mesenchymal neoplasms have arisen in the bladder following cyclophosphamide therapy.[143-145]

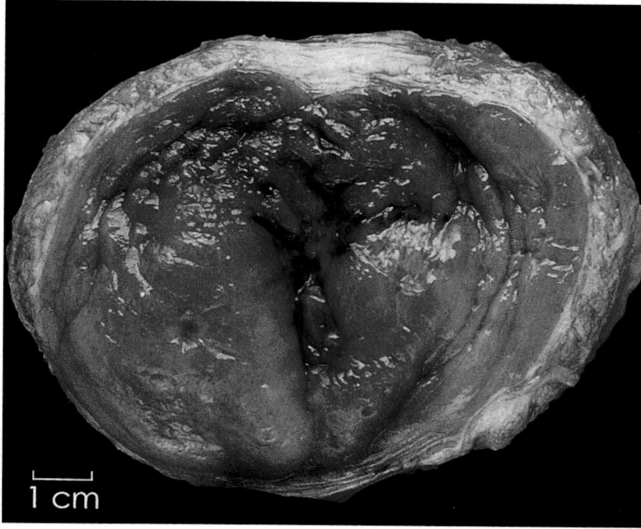

4-34. Chronic interstitial cystitis. The mucosa is punctuated by depressed scars and the wall is thick and rigid.

SPECIAL TYPES OF CYSTITIS

Interstitial cystitis

Interstitial cystitis has also been referred to as *Hunner's ulcer*, but that name is used less frequently today as it has been recognized that ulcers are not always present. The term *interstitial cystitis* was introduced by Skene[146] in 1887, and Nitze[147] described most of the characteristic features prior to the work by Hunner in 1914.[148] Interstitial cystitis poses diagnostic problems for both pathologists and urologists. The pathologic features are not specific, and the pathologist must correlate them with the clinical and cystoscopic features.

At least 90% of patients with interstitial cystitis are women and it is seen most often in middle age and old age.[149-154] Patients complain of marked frequency,

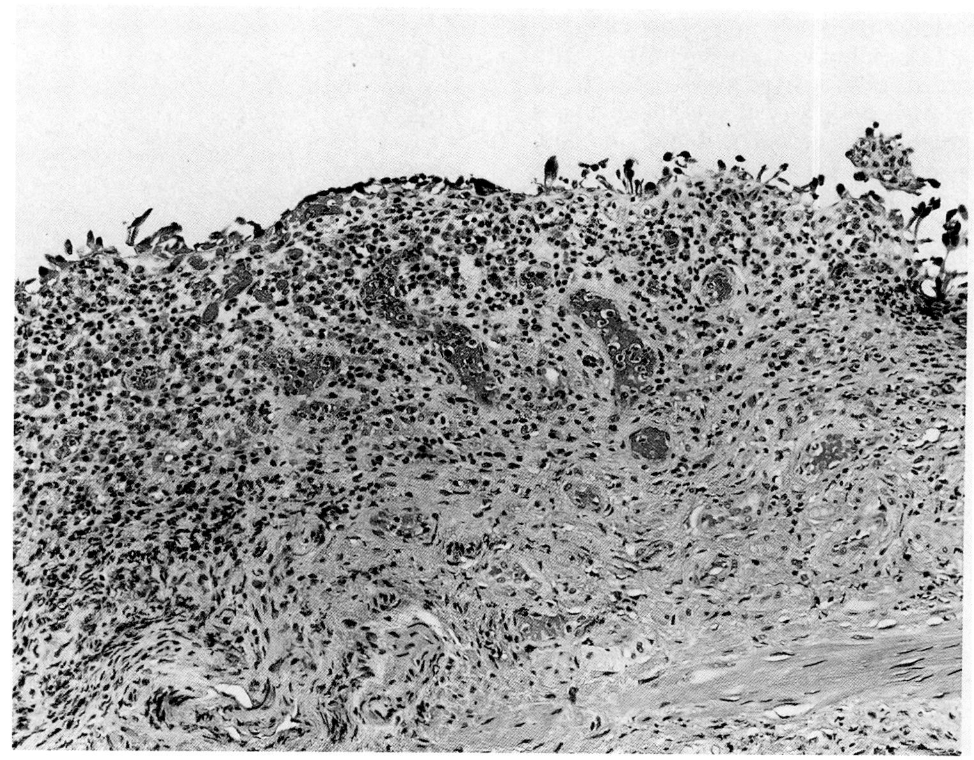

4-35. The mucosa is denuded and the lamina propria inflamed in interstitial cystitis.

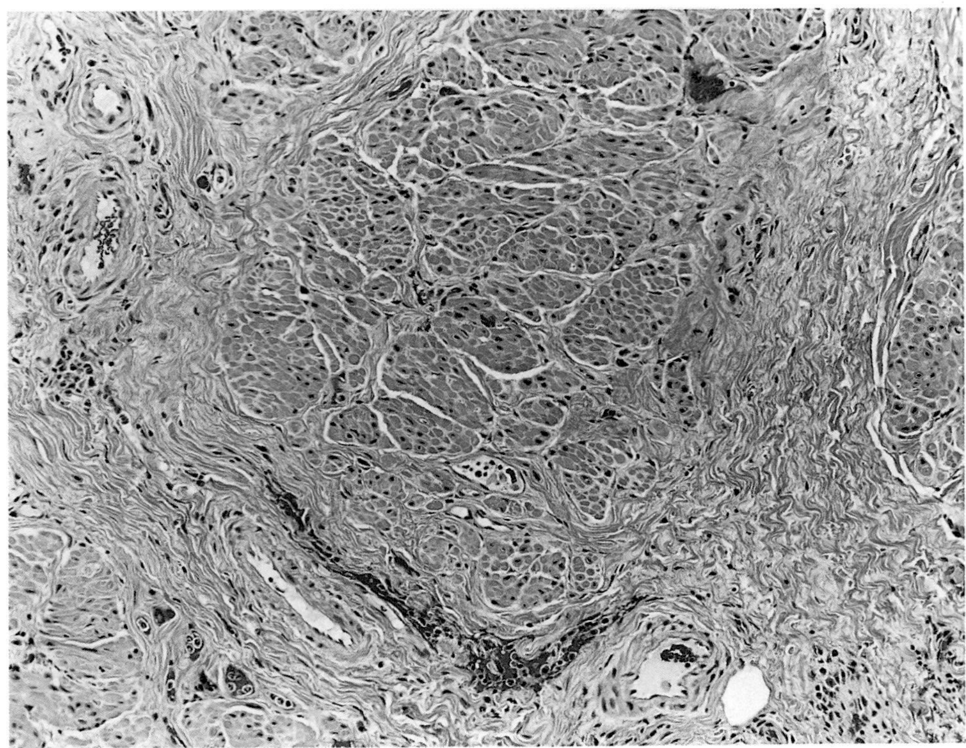

4-36. Interfascicular and intrafascicular fibrosis in interstitial cystitis.

urgency, and pain when the bladder becomes full and when it is emptied.[155] The urine is sterile. Cystoscopy may reveal small foci of hemorrhage (glomerulations), hemorrhagic spots that ooze blood, and linear cracks in the mucosa.[155,156] Occasionally, there are ulcers with radiating scars. Ulcers and scars are more frequent in older patients with long-standing cystitis.[157] In advanced cases, the wall of the bladder becomes fibrotic and contracted, resulting in very low bladder capacity (Fig. 4-34). Interstitial cystitis most often affects the dome and posterior and lateral walls.

Biopsy specimens from patients with interstitial cystitis have a variety of appearances. When present, ulcers are often wedge-shaped, and the urothelium is either absent or mixed with a surface exudate of fibrin, erythrocytes, and inflammatory cells (Fig. 4-35). The ulcers usually extend deep into the lamina propria, which is edematous and congested. The muscularis propria may also be edematous or fibrotic (Fig. 4-36). Generally, there is a dense infiltrate of lymphocytes and plasma cells. When ulcers are not present, the changes are less striking. Small mucosal ruptures, edema of the lamina propria, and foci of hemorrhage in the lamina propria are usually present and correspond to the glomerulations seen at cystoscopy.

Mast cells are often seen in the mucosa, lamina propria, and muscularis propria (Fig. 4-37) in interstitial cystitis. Their significance has been debated for the last 4 decades. Simmons and Bunce[158] first described an increase in mast cells in interstitial cystitis in 1958. Kastrup et al[159] concluded that more than 20 mast cells per mm^2 in the muscularis propria was strongly suggestive of interstitial cystitis, while Larsen et al[160] found that 28 mast cells per mm^2 was the upper limit for normal bladders. Johansson and Fall[157] found an average of 164 mast cells per mm^2 in the lamina propria of patients with ulcers, 93 per mm^2 in those without, and 88 per mm^2 in a control group. The difficulty of counting mast cells and the lack of consensus on what is "normal" are evident. Conditions of tissue fixation also affect the counts. Thus, the histologic features of interstitial cystitis are not pathognomonic.

4-37. Mast cells in the muscularis propria in interstitial cystitis (Giemsa stain).

The extensive mucosal denudation that often occurs with carcinoma in situ may result in an appearance of ulceration, inflammation, and vascular congestion closely resembling that seen in interstitial cystitis. When urothelium is absent or scant in a biopsy, multiple sections should be obtained to look for foci of atypical cells.

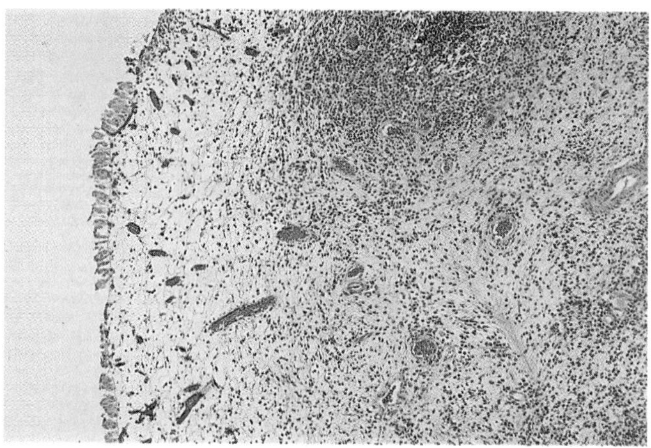

4-38. In eosinophilic cystitis the lamina propria contains sheets of eosinophils.

When other conditions are excluded, often the pathologist can only report that the pathologic findings are consistent with interstitial cystitis.

Eosinophilic cystitis

Bladder inflammation with a striking infiltrate of eosinophils occurs in two settings: in association with allergic diseases or without allergic association but usually in association with transurethral resection or invasive urothelial carcinoma.[161] In some cases, there is no associated condition.[162] Eosinophilic cystitis associated with allergic diseases is rare and most cases have involved patients with asthma or eosinophilic gastroenteritis.[163,164] Very rarely, eosinophilic cystitis is associated with parasitic infection.[165,166] Patients range in age from newborn to elderly, and more than 33% are children. The ratio of females to males is 2:1. The usual symptoms are dysuria, frequency, and hematuria.[161] At cystoscopy, there often are polypoid lesions resembling those of polypoid cystitis and in children sarcoma botryoides may come to mind. Nodular and sessile lesions and ulcers also are seen. Occasionally, the lesions mimic carcinoma.[167,168] Histologically, the lamina propria is edematous, containing a mixed inflammatory infiltrate in which eosinophils are prominent (Fig. 4-38). Occasionally, edema causes ureteral obstruction and upper tract complications, but most patients respond to

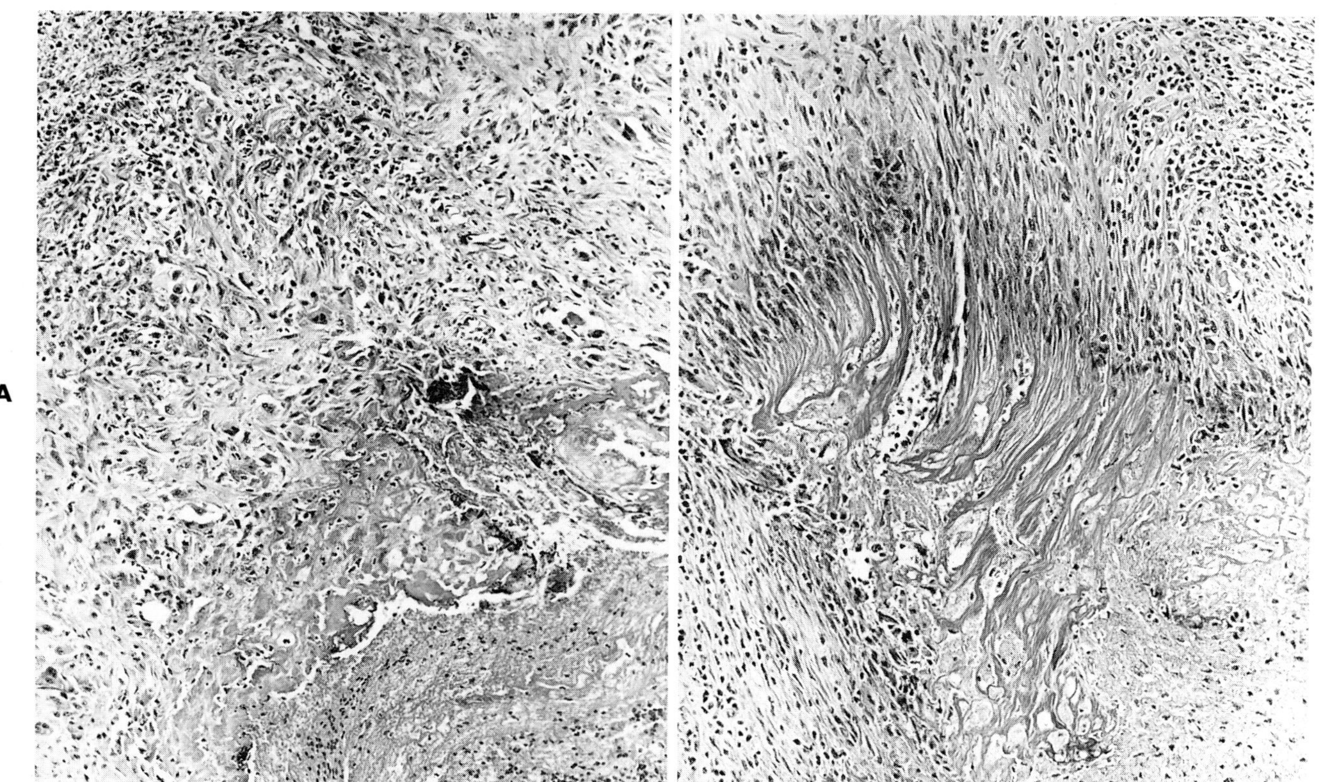

4-39. **A,** Postsurgical granuloma with amorphous debris in the center of the lesions (*lower right*) and fragments of brown cauterized material in the adjacent layer (*very dark foci*). **B,** Postsurgical granuloma with strands of coagulated tissue in the center and a palisade of histiocytes surrounding the necrotic material.

medical treatment including antihistamines, steroids, and antibiotics. However, the disease tends to be persistent.[162]

Patients with no history of allergy are typically older men with various urologic diseases, such as prostatic hyperplasia and carcinoma of the bladder.[169] Many patients give histories of transurethral resection or biopsy, and eosinophilic cystitis may be a reaction to bladder injury. Inflammation with prominent eosinophils also is commonly seen at the periphery of invasive carcinoma in cystectomy specimens.

Postsurgical necrobiotic granulomas

After transurethral surgery with diathermic cauterization, the bladder may contain necrotizing palisading granulomas.[170-172] Similar lesions have been reported subsequent to laser surgery.[173] Postsurgical granulomas are found in approximately 10% of cases, and the frequency increases with the number of operations. Typically, these granulomas have elongate linear or serpiginous outlines. Their centers contain acellular, finely granular eosinophilic material in which flecks of brown debris often are present (Fig. 4-39). Around the necrotic areas is a band of histiocytes arranged radially like the stakes of a palisade fence. Epithelioid histiocytes and foreign body giant cells also are commonly present. Surrounding this layer is a layer of dense chronic inflammation in which eosinophils may be numerous. Eventually the granulomas are replaced by fibrous scars, sometimes with dystrophic calcification.

Bacillus Calmette-Guérin granulomas

Since 1976, urothelial carcinoma in situ has been treated with intravesical instillation of the mycobacterium *bacillus Calmette-Guérin*.[174] This therapy often produces remissions but usually is not curative.[175,176] A profound inflammatory reaction ensues following instillation[177] with the result that the urothelium is lost and the lamina propria develops dense chronic inflammatory infiltrates among which are interspersed small granulomas composed of epithelioid histiocytes and multinucleated giant cells (Fig. 4-40).[178-182] These granulomas are usually round or ovoid lesions in the superficial lamina propria and lack necrosis. Acid-fast stains only rarely demonstrate organisms.[179] Granulomatous inflammatory changes may also be seen in urine cytology specimens.[183,184] Rarely, nephrogenic adenoma may arise following therapy with bacillus Calmette-Guérin.[185]

Other noninfectious granulomas

Suture granuloma may produce an inflammatory mass in or near the bladder following herniorrhaphy.[186-192] Usually the herniorrhaphy wound has been infected. Because of the long interval between herniorrhaphy and bladder symptoms (up to 11 years), the clinical diagnosis is often of bladder neoplasm. Microscopic examination shows a predominantly inflammatory process with foreign body giant cells and fibrosis around fragments of suture.

Rarely, diffuse infiltrates of histiocytes without the features specific for malakoplakia may form nodules in the

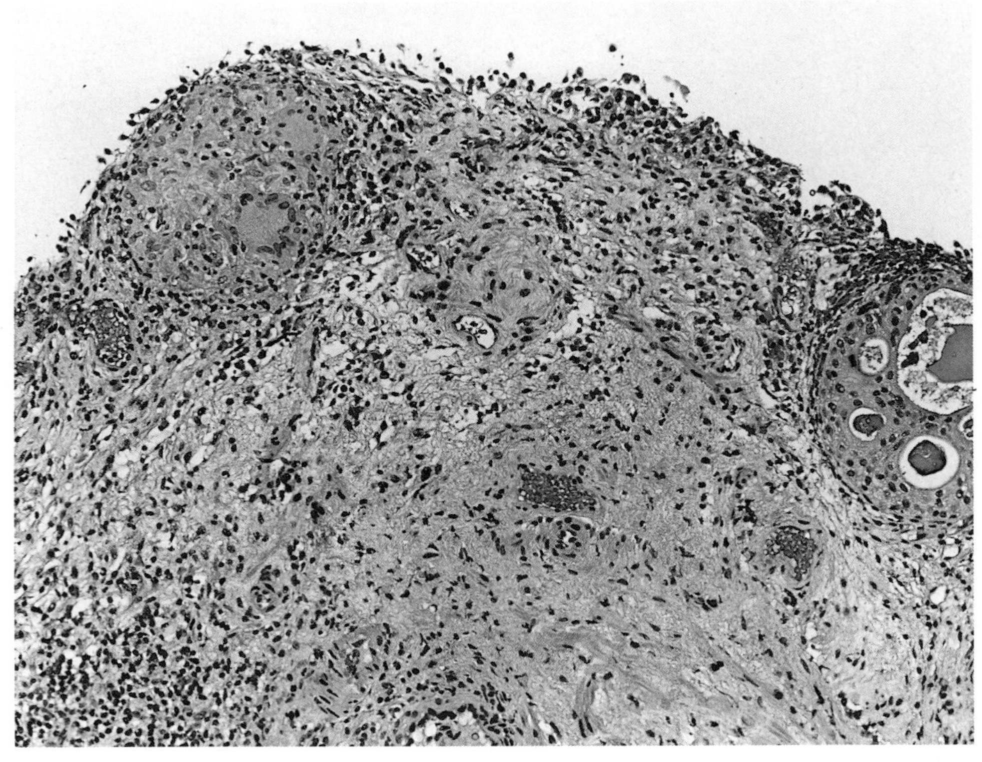

4-40. Granuloma of bacillus Calmette-Guérin associated with denudation of the mucosa.

bladder, and this has been termed *xanthogranulomatous cystitis*.[193] Collections of foamy histiocytes may also be found in the lamina propria in patients with disorders of lipid metabolism and have been called *xanthoma of the bladder*.[194] Granulomatous inflammation of the bladder has also been reported in association with granulomatous disease of childhood,[195] rheumatoid arthritis,[196] and fistulae of Crohn's disease.[197] Sarcoidosis rarely affects the bladder.[198]

Radiation cystitis

Radiation frequently induces a variety of abnormalities in the bladder.[199,200] Three to six weeks after treatment, there is acute cystitis with loss of the urothelium and congestion and edema in the lamina propria.[201] The remaining urothelial cells show varying degrees of nuclear atypicality. Features of radiation injury in the urothelium include vacuoles in the cytoplasm and nuclei, karyorrhexis, and normal nuclear/cytoplasmic ratio. In the stroma, marked edema and telangiectasis are common. Blood vessels also undergo hyalinization and thrombosis. The lamina propria usually contains atypical spindle cells similar to those of giant cell cystitis (Fig. 4-41). Later, ulcers and fibrosis and contraction of the bladder wall and stricture of the ureters may occur.[201,202]

Reaction to topical chemotherapy

Urothelial carcinoma in situ is commonly treated with intravesical topical chemotherapy. The most frequently used agents are the alkylating agents triethylenethiophosphoramide (thiotepa) and mitomycin C. These drugs induce denudation of the bladder mucosa in 37% of biopsies.[137] The remaining epithelium often shows nuclear changes such as pleomorphism and hyperchromasia which may be mistaken for residual carcinoma in situ (Fig. 4-42).[203]

INFECTIOUS CYSTITIS

Bacterial cystitis

Bacterial infection is the most common cause of cystitis and is usually caused by coliform organisms such as *Escherichia coli*, *Klebsiella pneumoniae*, and *Streptococcus faecalis*. Less commonly, *Proteus vulgaris*, *Pseudomonas pyocyanea*, *Neisseria gonorrhoea*, *Salmonella typhi*, and diphtheroids are implicated. Predisposition to bacterial cystitis is associated with structural factors including exstrophy, urethral malformations, fistulae with other pelvic organs, diverticula, calculi, and foreign bodies. Urine stasis and alkalinity also promote infection. Systemic illnesses such as diabetes mellitus, chronic renal disease, and immunosuppression are predisposing conditions. Most pathogens gain access to the bladder by ascending the urethra. Mycobacteria are an exception and usually descend from the upper tract in the urine.

Early in bacterial infection, the appearance of the mucosa ranges from moderately erythematous to deeply hemorrhagic; these changes may be diffuse or focal. In addition to the classic symptoms of dysuria, urgency, and frequency, hematuria may result from leakage of erythrocytes through the mucosa. Later, a gray fibrinous membrane may cover the mucosal surface. With progression, a thin purulent exudate may adhere to the surface, creating a suppurative or exudative cystitis. Edema may thicken the vesical wall and in chronic infections fibrosis may thicken and stiffen the wall and the mucosa may be ulcerated (Fig. 4-43).

Microscopically, the urothelium may be hyperplastic or metaplastic. Ulceration may be extensive and the surface of the ulcer may be covered by a fibrinous exudate in which neutrophils are mixed with bacterial colonies. Early in the infection edema is often the predominant

4-41. Radiation cystitis with atypical stromal cells and vascular thickening.

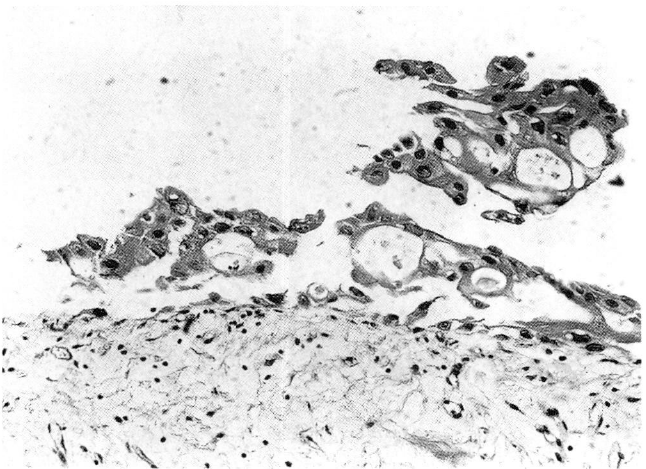

4-42. Epithelial atypia and sloughing associated with intravesical therapy with thiotepa.

finding. Initially leukocytes are not numerous, but as the infection progresses they become prominent in the lamina propria. In severe cases, suppuration is followed by abscess formation, which may involve the entire thickness of the bladder wall. When the inflammatory reaction is less intense and more indolent, the process may be characterized as subacute. In such cases the mucosa is usually denuded, the lamina propria is edematous, and eosinophils may be prominent.

In chronic cystitis the mucosa may be ulcerated and the urothelium thin or hyperplastic. The urothelium may display reactive atypia. Granulation tissue may replace

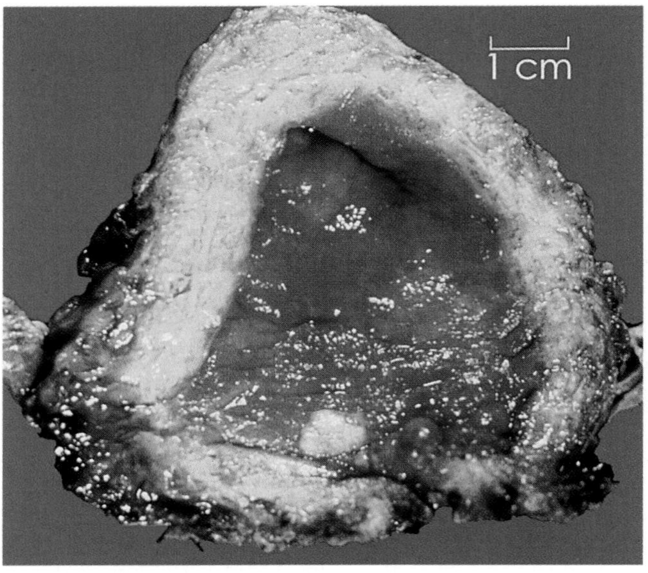

4-43. Bladder of spinal cord injury patient with chronic and acute cystitis.

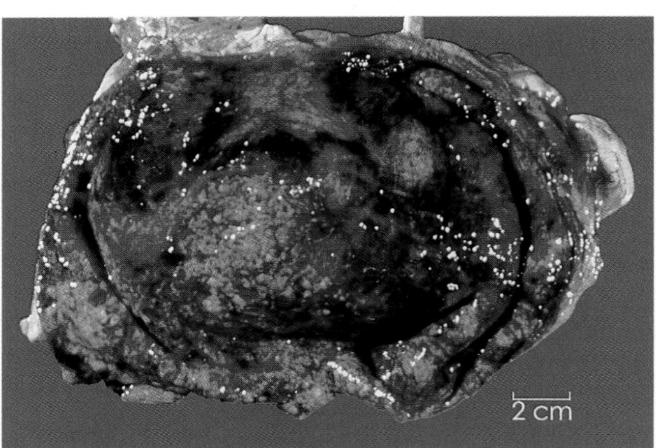

4-44. Gangrenous cystitis from a patient dying with *Klebsiella* sepsis. The mucosa is diffusely necrotic.

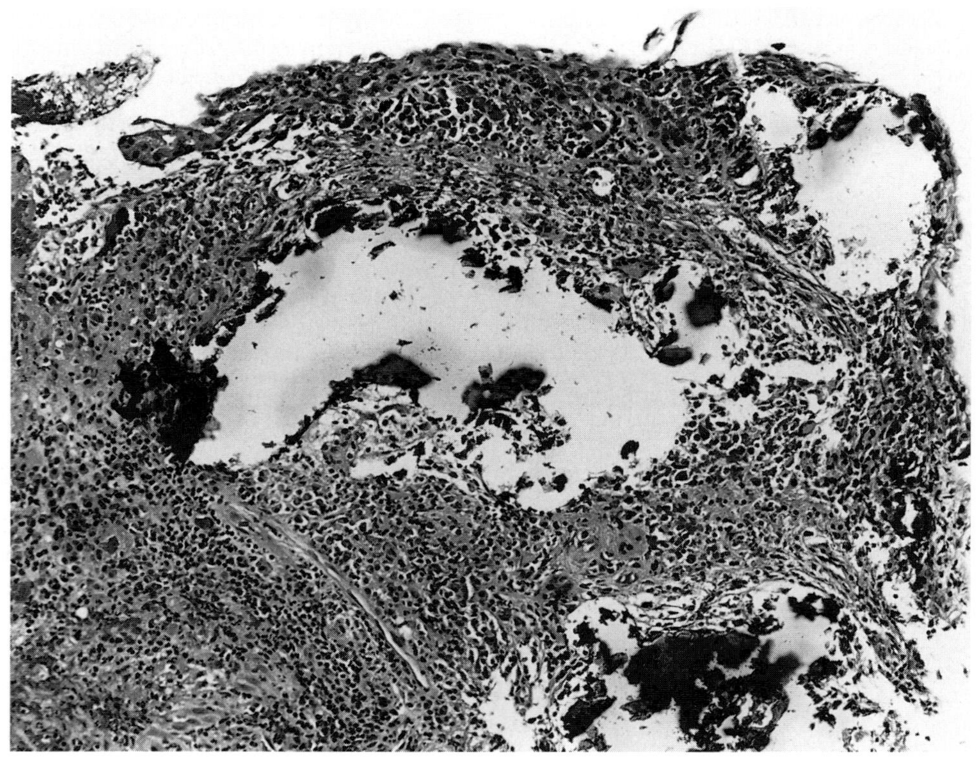

4-45. Encrusted cystitis with deposits of calcium salts in the lamina propria.

parts of the lamina propria and muscularis propria, eventually becoming densely fibrotic.

Gangrene

Gangrene is a dangerous complication of vesical infection and may arise as a consequence of circulatory compromise, debilitating systemic illness (such as uncontrolled diabetes mellitus or carcinoma), vascular insufficiency, or instillation of corrosive chemicals.[204-207] Gangrene usually begins in the mucosa and the necrotic tissue is sloughed to expose deeper structures (Fig. 4-44). Occasionally, the muscularis propria is deeply penetrated and gangrene extends to the serosa. Deposition of mineral salts from the urine may give the sloughed material a gritty texture.

Encrusted cystitis. When urea-splitting bacteria alkalinize the urine and inorganic salts are deposited in a damaged mucosa (Fig. 4-45), the term *encrusted cystitis* is applied.[208-214] Encrusted cystitis is most common in women and may occur in association with conditions in which inflammation or trauma damages the mucosa. Patients complain of long-standing dysuria, frequency, and sometimes hematuria. The urine contains gritty material, blood, mucus, and pus. When the salts are rich in calcium, the deposits may be visible in radiographs.[214,215] Cystoscopically, the lesions are usually multiple and have a gritty appearance. Rarely, the entire mucosa is involved. Histologically, the lesions are covered with a shaggy coat of fibrin mixed with calcified necrotic debris and inflammatory cells. The underlying tissue may be quite inflamed early in the course of the disease, but later inflammatory cells become scant and the lamina propria becomes fibrotic. Mineral salts may also be deposited on the surface of urothelial carcinoma, particularly in areas of necrosis or fulguration.[215]

Emphysematous cystitis. In some cases of cystitis, gas-filled blebs are seen by cystoscopy or at gross examination, a condition termed *emphysematous cystitis*.[216-225] Emphysematous cystitis is more common in women than men. Approximately half the patients are diabetic, usually with bacterial infections with *Escherichia coli* or *Aerobacter aerogenes*.[226] Less frequently, the infection is fungal.[221,225] Other predisposing conditions include cystoscopy, trauma, fistula, and urinary stasis. The blebs range from 0.5 to 3 mm in diameter and may be present throughout the mucosa. Histologically, the blebs are cavities lined by flattened cells and surrounded by thin septa in the lamina propria. Occasionally they extend into the muscularis propria.

Urachal abscess

Most bacterial infections of the urachus are associated with a urachal malformation or cyst.[227-229] Many of these develop into abscesses (Fig. 4-46) that may drain into the bladder or through the umbilicus. Rupture through the peritoneum can cause severe peritonitis, a serious complication. When the abscess is large and associated with much inflammation and fibrosis in surrounding tissues, it may be difficult or impossible to precisely determine the nature of the underlying urachal abnormality. The combination of antibiotic therapy with surgical excision of the urachal malformation and abscess is usually curative.[230] On rare occasions, urachal abscess may be caused by tuberculous, echinococcal, or actinomycotic infections.[23]

Malakoplakia

First described in 1902 and 1903 by Michaelis and Gutmann[231] and by von Hansemann,[232] malakoplakia occurs most frequently in the urinary bladder where it is visible as yellow-white soft raised plaques on the mucosal surface.[233] It was this appearance, combined with a reluctance to speculate on the pathogenesis of the disorder, which prompted von Hansemann to combine the Greek roots for plaque (*plakos*) and soft (*malakos*) to coin the term

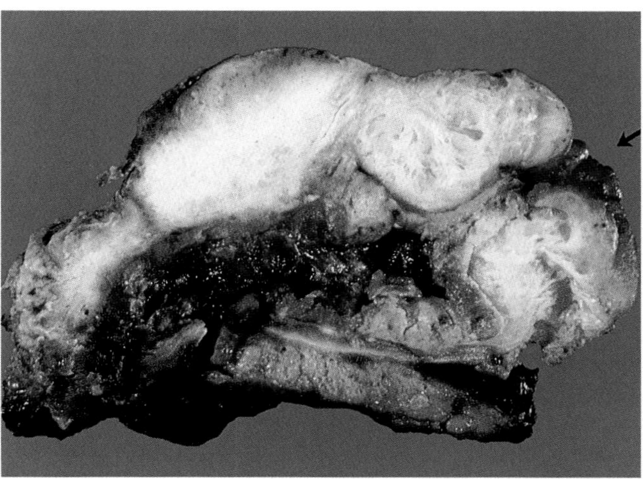

4-46. Urachal abscess. Arrow indicates outlet of urachus in mucosa of bladder.

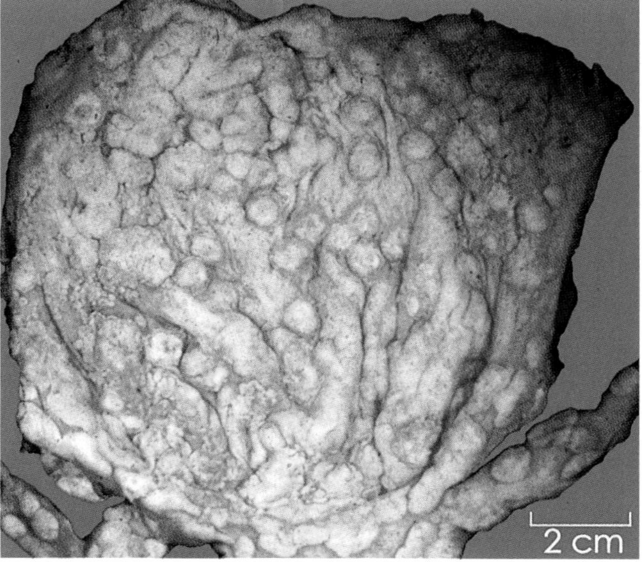

4-47. Malakoplakia of the bladder and ureters.

malakoplakia for the condition.[234] Urinary tract malakoplakia primarily affects women (more than 75% of cases) and has a peak incidence in the fifth decade.[234] It occasionally occurs in children.[235] Malakoplakia is an uncommon granulomatous process that results from impairment of the capacity of mononuclear cells to kill phagocytosed bacteria.[236,237] It is usually associated with infection by coliform organisms. Most patients present with the usual symptoms of urinary tract infection, including hematuria. *Escherichia coli* is most frequently cultured from the urine but *Proteus vulgaris, Aerobacter aerogenes, Klebsiella pneumoniae,* and alpha-hemolytic streptococci have also been isolated. Despite this, bacteria have rarely been identified within the lesions of malakoplakia without the use of transmission electron microscopy.[238,239]

Grossly, the lesions are usually multiple, soft yellow or yellow-brown plaques (Fig. 4-47). Often there is a central dimple and a rim of congestion about the plaque. Lesions larger than 2 cm are unusual. In some cases the lesions are nodular, but rarely large and polypoid.

Microscopically, there is an accumulation of histiocytes with granular eosinophilic cytoplasm (von Hansemann histiocytes) in the superficial lamina propria beneath the urothelium, which usually is intact (Fig. 4-48). The histiocytes contain the characteristic intracytoplasmic inclusions known as Michaelis-Gutmann bodies. These are typically spherical, 5 to 8 micron, concentrically laminated bodies with a bull's-eye appearance (Fig. 4-49). Often they are basophilic but also may be pale and difficult to see. They always contain calcium and some-

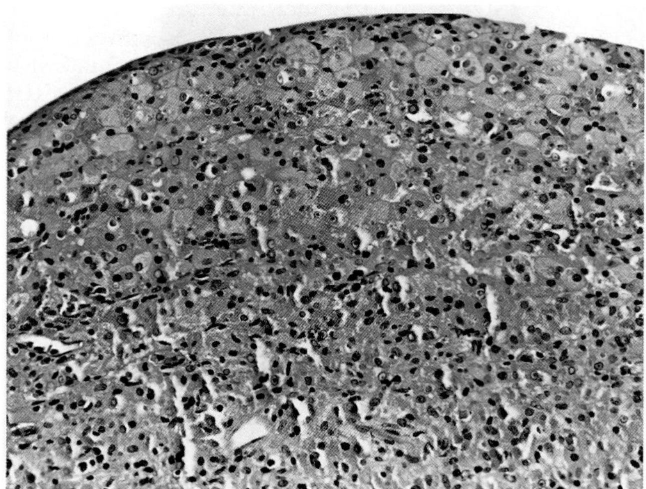

4-48. Malakoplakia. The lamina propria is filled with von Hansemann histiocytes.

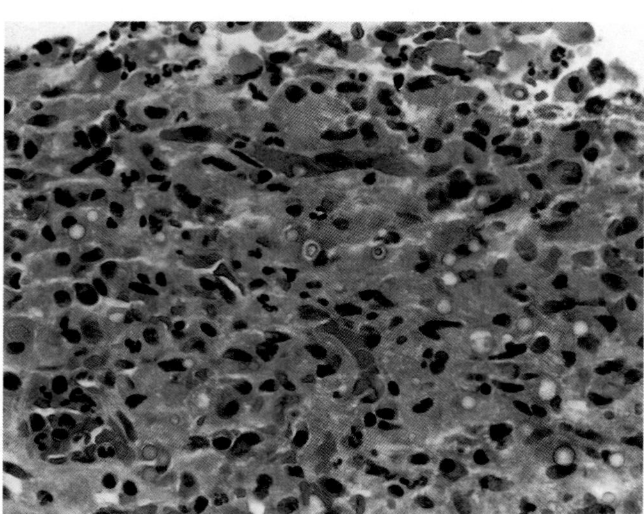

4-49. Malakoplakia. Michaelis-Gutmann bodies in the lamina propria.

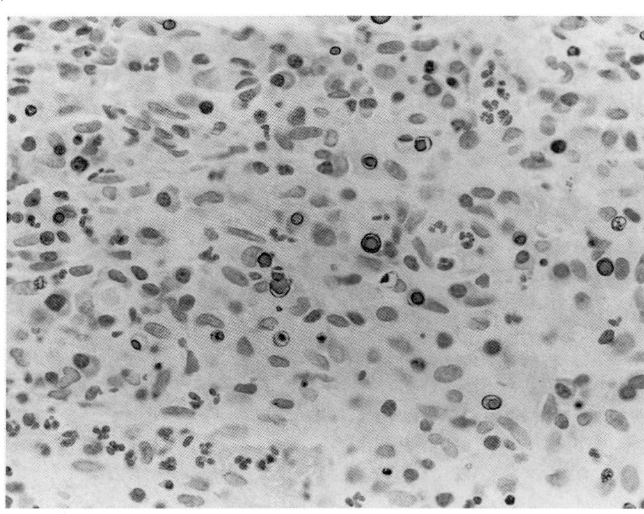

4-50. Malakoplakia. The von Kossa stain for calcium highlights the Michaelis-Gutmann bodies.

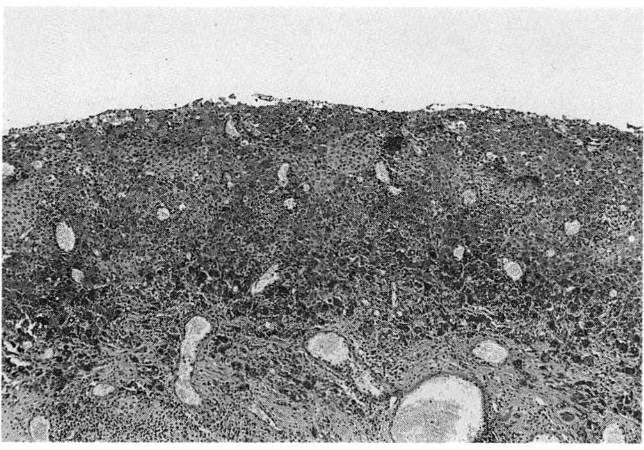

4-51. Malakoplakia. The von Hansemann histiocytes react strongly with the periodic acid-Schiff stain.

times iron salts so the von Kossa (Fig. 4-50) and Perl's Prussian blue stains highlight them. They also react with the periodic acid-Schiff stain but so does the cytoplasm of the von Hansemann histiocytes (Fig. 4-51), so this technique is less helpful than staining for calcium. Early in the disease, Michaelis-Gutmann bodies may be scant and very difficult to appreciate in sections stained with hematoxylin and eosin. Thus, when there is an infiltrate of histiocytes in the bladder, a section should be stained for calcium to find inapparent Michaelis-Gutmann bodies. Michaelis-Gutmann bodies are required for the diagnosis so it is possible that there is an early prediagnostic phase of the disease in which there is insufficient calcification to make the bodies detectable. In some cases, there is abundant granulation tissue, extensive fibrosis, or a dense infiltrate of acute and chronic inflammatory cells that may obscure the von Hansemann histiocytes and Michaelis-Gutmann bodies. Late in the disease, there may be extensive fibrosis and few Michaelis-Gutmann bodies.

Ultrastructural and immunohistochemical studies have shown that the cytoplasm of von Hansemann histiocytes contains many phagolysosomes in which there are fragments of bacterial cell walls.[240] It appears that Michaelis-Gutmann bodies form when the phagolysosomes fuse and calcium is transported across the phagolysosomal membranes and forms hydroxyapatite crystals with phosphate from the bacterial cell walls. The bodies enlarge over time, producing the typical laminated structure. Ultrastructurally, Michaelis-Gutmann bodies range from 5 to 10 microns in diameter (Fig. 4-52).[241] At the center is a dense crystalline core that is surrounded by a homogeneous zone that is not crystalline but rather is granular or composed of myelin figures.

Tuberculous cystitis

Tuberculous cystitis is almost always caused by *Mycobacterium tuberculosis*;[242,243] *Mycobacterium bovis* accounts for only about 3% of cases.[244] Tuberculous cystitis is almost always secondary to renal tuberculosis from which organisms in infected urine implant in the bladder. In one study 66% of patients with surgically treated renal tuberculosis had vesical tuberculosis.[245] Some cases in men appear to be secondary to genital infection, in which case spread of the infection is directly along the mucosa. Frequency, urgency, hematuria, and dysuria are common symptoms.

Early in the infection, the lesions are in the region of the ureteral orifices and consist of marked mucosal congestion, sometimes with edema. These lesions may progress to form 1 to 3 mm tubercles or may ulcerate and become covered by friable necrotic material. Initially the tubercles are sharply circumscribed, firm, and solid. As they enlarge they coalesce and ulcerate.

The tuberculous granuloma in which central caseous necrosis is surrounded by multinucleated giant cells, plasma cells, and lymphocytes is the characteristic histological lesion. Acid-fast or auramine-rhodamine–stained sections usually will disclose mycobacteria.

Chronic tuberculous cystitis may result in a small scarred bladder of low capacity. The ureteral orifices may be distorted and obstructed, causing hydronephrosis and hydroureter. Rarely, the infection penetrates the wall of the bladder causing peritonitis or a fistula.

Fungal and actinomycotic cystitis

Fungal cystitis is uncommon and most often is caused by *Candida albicans*.[246-248] Infection may ascend the urethra or may be hematogenous. Ascending infection usually is limited to the trigone. Most candidal cystitis occurs

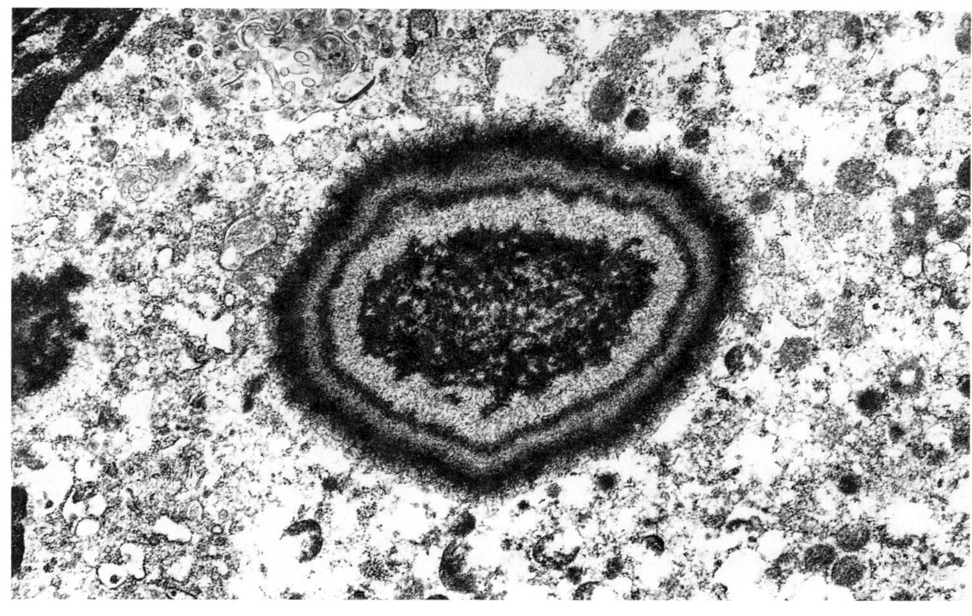

4-52. Ultrastructural appearance of a Michaelis-Gutmann body. *(Courtesy of Dr. A. Billis.)*

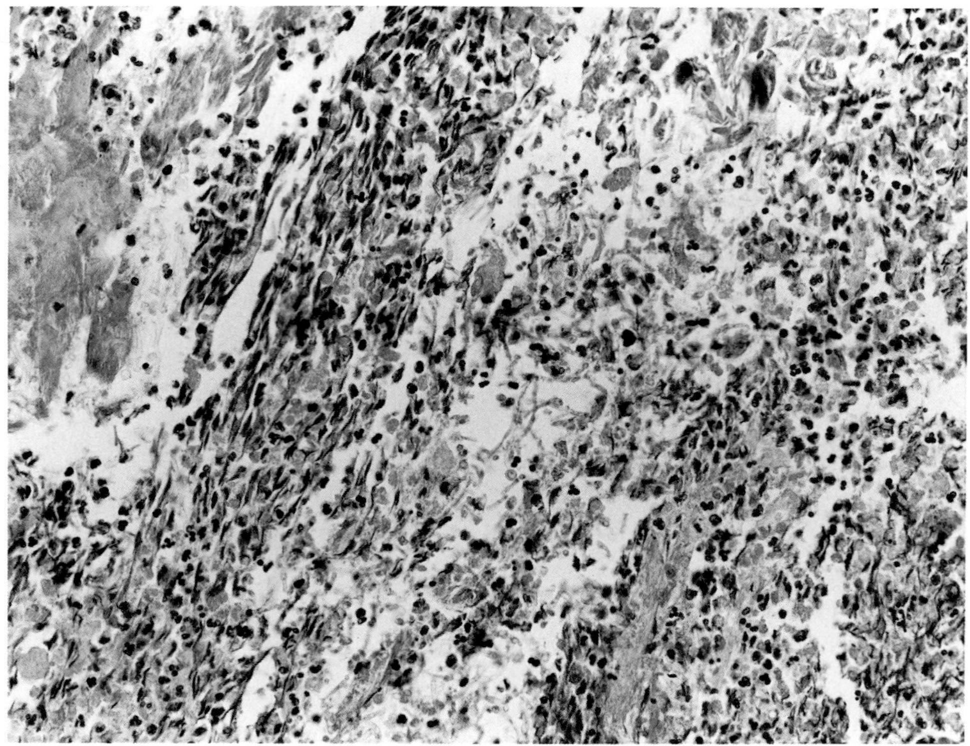

4-53. Candidal cystitis. Fungus is present in the inflammatory exudate and debris.

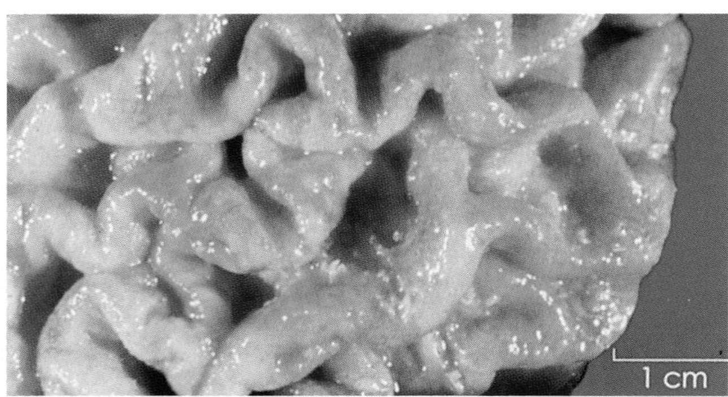

4-54. Condyloma of the bladder with prominent folds.

in debilitated patients or patients on antibiotic therapy. Many are diabetic and most are women. Nocturia, constant pain, and marked frequency are typical symptoms. The urine is usually turbid and bloody.

The lesions are typically slightly raised and sharply demarcated white plaques with irregular shapes. Occasionally, a fungus ball may form in the lumen of the bladder. Microscopically, there is ulceration and inflammation of the lamina propria. The typical hyphae and budding yeast forms may be seen in routine sections (Fig. 4-53) or with periodic acid-Schiff or Gomori's methenamine silver stains.

Rare cases of fungal cystitis caused by *Aspergillus* species[249] and other fungi have been reported.[247]

Vesical actinomycosis is rare in the general population but complicates actinomycosis of the ovary or fallopian tube in about 10% of cases.[250] Symptoms are nonspecific. Microscopically, the bladder wall is focally or diffusely thickened and there is often continuity with the lesions in adjacent organs. The infection may form a mass simulating a neoplasm. The mucosa may be edematous or ulcerated and, if the infection is transmural, a fistula may form. Microscopically, there is abundant granulation tissue within which are small abscesses containing colonies of *Actinomyces* (sulfur granules).

Viral cystitis

Human papillomavirus. A few dozen cases of condyloma acuminatum of the bladder have been reported.[251-257] There is a predominance of females to males of approximately 2:1. Patients range in age from early adulthood to old age, but most have been younger than 50 years. Most patients, many of whom are immunocompromised, have had condylomata of the urethra, vulva, vagina, anus, or perineum, but some have had condylomata only in the bladder. In some immunocompromised patients, the lesions have been particularly difficult to eradicate.

Cystoscopy usually shows a solitary lesion in the bladder neck or trigone. These appear papillary and the clinical differential diagnosis includes papillary carcinoma and other papillary lesions of the vesical mucosa. Alternately, the mucosa may have prominent folds and scattered white flecks (Fig. 4-54).[253]

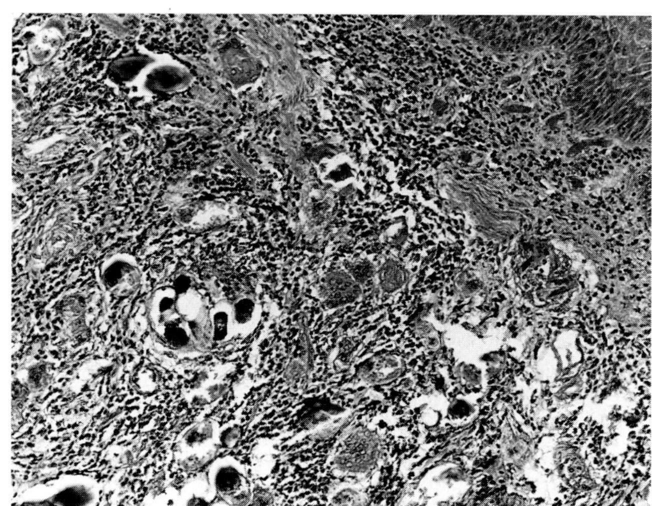

4-55. Schistosomiasis, active form with numerous ova and marked granulomatous inflammation.

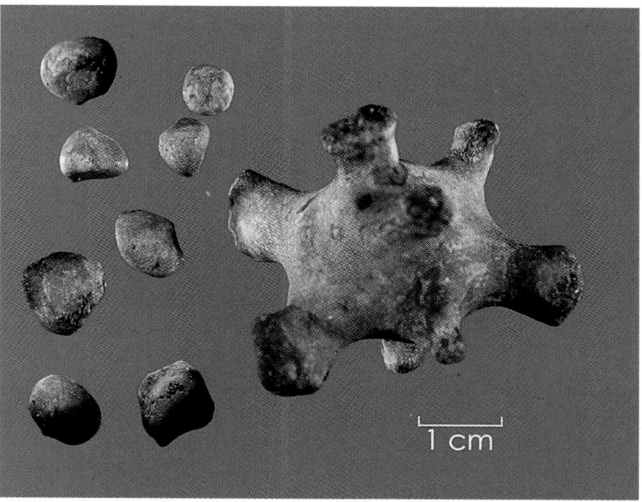

4-56. Bladder calculi from a man with obstructive prostatic hyperplasia.

Microscopically, the lesions show the characteristic features of condylomata, including koilocytotic cells with abundant clear cytoplasm and wrinkled hyperchromatic nuclei. These features distinguish the lesions from the rare squamous papilloma and papillary squamous cell carcinoma of the bladder.

Other viruses. Adenovirus is recognized as an important cause of hemorrhagic cystitis, especially in children.[258] Otherwise healthy children may be affected, as well as children after bone marrow transplantation. Adenovirus types 11 and 21 are most frequently identified.[259-263] Papovavirus also causes hemorrhagic cystitis in children and adults.[264] Herpes simplex type 2 has caused hemorrhagic cystitis in a few patients[265] and herpes zoster has also caused cystitis.[266] Cytomegalovirus also is sometimes seen in the bladder, particularly in immunosuppressed patients.[267]

Schistosomiasis

Schistosomiasis is the fourth most prevalent disease in the world and the world's leading cause of hematuria.[268] In humans, the trematode *Schistosoma hematobium* commonly resides in the paravesical veins and causes urinary schistosomiasis, which also is known as *bilharziasis*.[269] The adult forms of these flat worms are dioecious, living as pairs in veins, with the male surrounding the female. Estimates of adults' life spans vary from 2 to 20 years, and each pair is capable of producing up to 200 eggs per day. In endemic areas, children have the highest incidence of infection, but it is adults who suffer the severe effects of chronic infection.

Schistosomiasis has varied clinical manifestations but the underlying process begins with the deposition of eggs in small veins and venules. Subsequently, the eggs may pass into the lumens of hollow organs, such as the bladder, or become trapped in the walls of viscera where they produce a granulomatous response and may be destroyed or calcified. Alternately, they may enter the circulation from the small veins and embolize other sites. For unknown reasons, the predominant site for oviposition by *S. hematobium* is the venous systems of the lower urinary tract. *S. hematobium* deposits eggs in clusters, causing a patchy distribution of lesions.[270] The eggs of *S. hematobium* are not acid-fast in histologic sections whereas those of other common human schistosomes, *S. mansoni*, *S. intercalatum*, and *S. japonicum* are acid-fast. *S. mattheei*, which usually infects animals but may cause urinary schistosomiasis in humans, also is not acid-fast. In humans, the eggs of *S. hematobium* are intermediate in size between those of *S. mansoni* and *S. japonicum*.

Schistosomiasis may be categorized as active or inactive. The active form is characterized by the presence of active pairs of flatworms depositing eggs, which elicit a strong granulomatous response (Fig. 4-55). Polypoid inflammatory masses may obstruct the ureters or the bladder outlet.[271] The number of ova in the urine correlates with the burden of eggs in the bladder wall and the active stage is most readily diagnosed by examination of the urine. The inactive form occurs after the worms have died and there are no viable eggs in urine or tissue. However, eggs remain in the tissue, and high concentrations of calcified eggs may be detected radiographically. Evaluation of the quantity of ova in tissue requires special digestion techniques.[272-275] In the inactive phase, the patient is not infectious.

The principal nonneoplastic manifestations of schistosomiasis in the bladder are polyps and ulcers. In most cases, the trigone and ureteral orifices are the sites of the lesions,[276] which may lead to bladder neck obstruction.[277] The deposits of ova are heaviest in the submucosa.[77] During active disease, heavy burdens of eggs produce multiple large inflammatory polyps, which may obstruct the ureteral orifices and may bleed sufficiently to cause anemia or clot retention.[271,278,279] Obstruction may lead to stone formation in the kidneys, ureters, and bladder.[280,281] In inactive schistosomiasis, the polyps are fibrocalcific. In a small percentage of cases, the polyps are composed of hyperplastic epithelium that appears more villous than polypoid. The inflammation in the bladder also gives rise to polypoid cystitis, biopsy specimens of which may not contain any eggs. In the early active stage, ulcers rarely form when a necrotic polyp detaches. Ulcers are more common in the chronic stage, when large numbers of eggs (greater than 250,000/g of bladder tissue) are present. These constantly painful ulcers are often in the posterior bladder wall of young adults and have stellate or ovoid contours.[282] Metaplastic changes, including keratinizing squamous metaplasia and intestinal metaplasia also are common.[268] The bladder mucosa may also contain raised granules known as *bilharzial tubercles*.[276] These may calcify to form the classic sandy patches. Neoplastic complications of schistosomiasis are discussed in Chapter 5.

CALCULI

Bladder stones are most common in men with bladder outlet obstruction (Fig. 4-56) and in children in underdeveloped countries. Most are free in the bladder, but occasionally calculi form about a suture after surgery. The symptoms are similar to those of bladder outlet obstruction, including hesitancy, frequency, and nocturia. Other symptoms include hematuria, dysuria, and suprapubic pain radiating down the penis. Radiography or cystoscopy are usually diagnostic of bladder calculus. Because bladder stones may be composed of radiolucent uric acid, cystoscopy is the most definitive diagnostic procedure.

Bladder calculi were common in children in Europe before 1800 and remain relatively common in some parts of Asia and the Middle East. Most patients are boys younger than 10 years and the stones are composed of calcium oxalate and ammonium acid urate. Patients usually do not have renal stones. Diet low in protein and minerals, along with low fluid intake, seem to be factors promoting stone formation in these children. In North America and Europe, only 2% to 3% of patients with bladder calculi are children. Most of these also have renal or ureteral calculi and their stones are composed of calcium oxalate, calcium phosphate, or mixtures of the two. While most of these children have bacterial infections, the causative organisms do not often produce urease. Children with histories of multiple urologic procedures are more likely to have struvite stones and infections with *Proteus* species.

POLYPS AND OTHER MASS LESIONS

ECTOPIC PROSTATE

Polyps composed of prostatic epithelium resembling those more commonly seen in the prostatic urethra rarely occur in the bladder.[283-286] Reported cases have occurred in men from 20 to 67 years old and hematuria has been the most consistent symptom. About two thirds of the lesions arise in the trigone and the architecture varies from papillary to polypoid. The stroma contains prostatic glands and the surface is covered by columnar epithelium or urothelium. Immunohistochemistry confirms the prostatic character of the glands and columnar cells. Prostatic hyperplasia may also expand into the bladder lumen as a polypoid mass.[287-289]

OTHER POLYPS

Fibroepithelial polyps of the bladder are rare and resemble the more common counterpart in the ureter.[290-292] They are distinguished from polypoid cystitis by being solitary, with a more fibrous core and a paucity of inflammatory cells.

HAMARTOMA

Hamartoma of the bladder is a rare polypoid mass (Fig. 4-57) composed of epithelial elements resembling von Brunn's nests, cystitis glandularis, or cystitis cystica distributed irregularly in a stroma that may be muscular, fibrous, or edematous.[293-295] Occasional cases have intestinal metaplasia of the glands, small tubules resembling renal tubules, or markedly cellular stroma.[295]

4-57. Bladder hamartoma consisting of polypoid fronds of cellular stroma containing small tubular structures lined by epithelium.

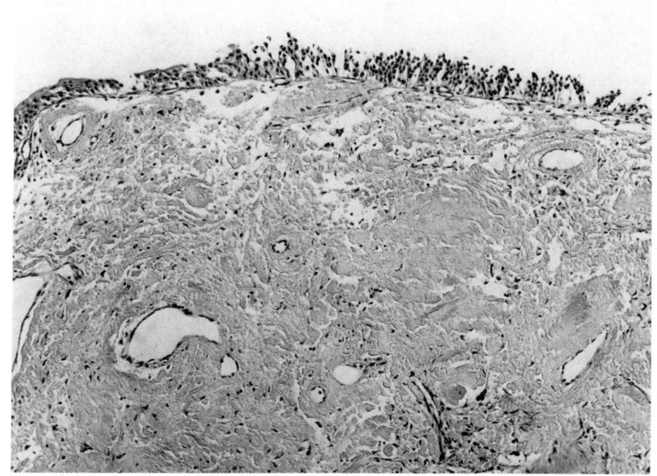

4-58. Amyloid fills the lamina propria in this biopsy specimen.

AMYLOIDOSIS

More than 50 cases of primary amyloidosis of the bladder have been reported.[296-304] The lesions appear throughout adulthood and are equally common in both sexes. In most cases, the deposits are limited to the bladder, but the ureters and urethra have also been involved in some cases. Hematuria is almost always the presenting symptom.[305] By cystoscopy, the lesions range from sessile and ulcerated to nodular or polypoid, and often are mistaken for carcinoma.[101] In about 25% of cases, there are multiple lesions. Histologically, the amyloid deposits are predominantly in the lamina propria and muscularis propria (Fig. 4-58). Vascular involvement is less prominent. A foreign body giant cell reaction may be present adjacent to the deposits, and rarely the deposits become calcified.

Secondary involvement of the bladder is rare in systemic amyloidosis.[306] Reported cases are associated with rheumatoid arthritis, Crohn's disease, ankylosing spondylitis, myeloma, and familial Mediterranean fever. Hematuria is universal and often very severe.[305,306] While primary localized amyloidosis often presents with hematuria, it is generally much less severe than that associated with secondary amyloidosis. By cystoscopy there is diffuse erythema, sometimes with petechiae or necrosis. Histologically, the amyloid is mainly in the blood vessels; occasionally there are lesser deposits in the lamina propria.

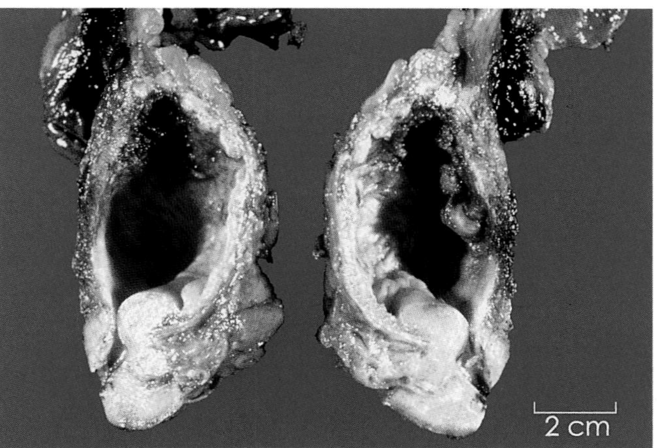

4-59. Postoperative spindle cell nodule in bladder neck.

POSTOPERATIVE SPINDLE CELL NODULE

The term *postoperative spindle cell nodule* was coined by Proppe et al[307] in 1984 for a proliferative spindle cell lesion occurring in the lower urinary tract and female genital tract within 120 days of surgery at the site where the lesions arise. Subsequently, others have reported identical lesions.[308,309] At cystoscopy, the bladder lesions are nodular (Fig. 4-59) and described as "heaped up tumor" and a "friable vegetant mass." The possibility of confusion with malignancy is heightened by the microscopic examination that shows interlacing fascicles (Fig. 4-60) of mitotically active spindle cells (Fig. 4-61) resembling leiomyosarcoma or some other spindle cell sarcoma. Other histologic features include delicate vasculature, scattered inflammatory cells, small foci of hemorrhage, edema, and focal myxoid change. Although there may be many mitotic figures, the nuclei usually show little pleomorphism or hyperchromasia.

The original and subsequent reports have shown that postoperative spindle cell nodules are benign reactive proliferations that resolve spontaneously or with medical therapy and must be distinguished from sarcoma. Well-differentiated leiomyosarcoma is the most important consideration in this differential diagnosis. This distinction may be very difficult because both postoperative spindle cell nodule and well-differentiated leiomyosarcoma have similarly bland nuclei, may infiltrate the muscularis propria, and have similar numbers of mitotic figures. The prominent array of delicate blood vessels seen in many postoperative spindle cell nodules is not a common feature of leiomyosarcoma. Myxoid change may be

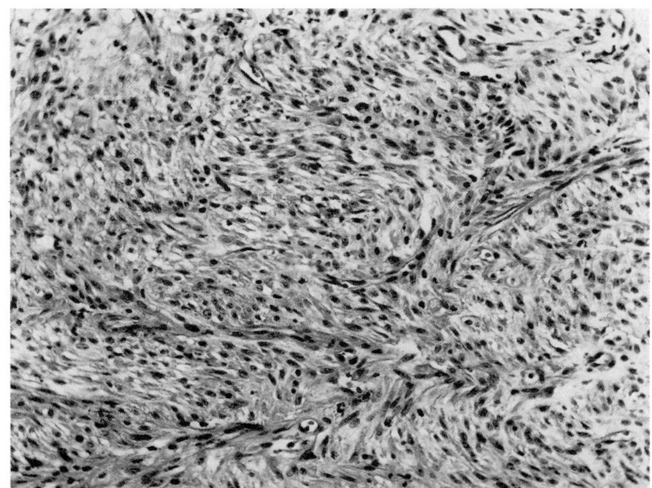

4-60. Postoperative spindle cell nodule composed of cellular bundles of spindle cells.

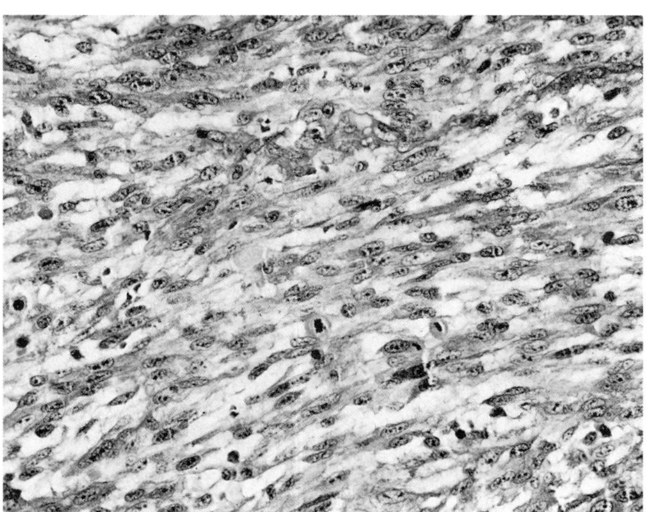

4-61. Postoperative spindle cell nodule with mitotic figure.

seen in both and is not helpful unless extensive, a finding more common in leiomyosarcoma. The clinical history of recent surgery at the site powerfully suggests postoperative spindle cell nodule. In these cases, follow up with cystoscopy and additional biopsies is warranted.

INFLAMMATORY PSEUDOTUMOR

Patients without histories of recent surgery may also have benign proliferative spindle cell lesions that mimic sarcoma.[310] A variety of terms have been applied to these, but *inflammatory pseudotumor* is preferred because it is in wide use for similar lesions at other sites.[311-317] Most patients range in age from 20 to 50 years and there appears to be a slight predominance of women.[316] Gross hematuria is the most common presenting symptom.

Grossly, the lesions have ranged from pedunculated masses protruding into the bladder cavity (Fig. 4-62) to small nodules or ulcers in the mucosa. Usually, the lesions are solitary, 2 to 5 cm polyps with broad bases. Some lesions are sessile and deeply infiltrate the muscularis propria (Fig. 4-63). The cut surface may be gelatinous or mucoid.

Histologically, inflammatory pseudotumor is typically composed of spindle cells arranged in a widely spaced haphazard pattern in a myxoid matrix containing a prominent network of small blood vessels (Fig. 4-64).[316] A second pattern that is sometimes seen is more cellular with spindle cells arranged in fascicles with variable amounts of collagen between them (Fig. 4-65). In both patterns, the spindle cells are similar with long bipolar eosinophilic or amphophilic cytoplasmic processes. In the myxoid pattern, stellate and polygonal cells also are present. The nuclei are large and occasionally multiple. In most cases there are fewer than two mitotic figures per 10 high-power fields, but occasional cases have more (Fig. 4-66).[316] The myxoid pattern usually contains a sparse inflammatory infiltrate whereas in the second pattern lymphocytes and plasma cells may be prominent. An example of the second pattern has been reported as a plasma cell granuloma.[318] Eosinophils often are common in both patterns. Infiltration of the muscularis propria is common and the process may extend into perivesical fat.

The main differential diagnostic consideration for inflammatory pseudotumor is malignancy, particularly myxoid sarcomatoid carcinoma and myxoid leiomyosarcoma. Inflammation and vascularity are more prominent in inflammatory pseudotumor than in leiomyosarcoma, and the cellularity is more variable. Immunohistochemical evidence of smooth muscle differentiation favors leiomyosarcoma, but this is not absolutely reliable. Although a destructively infiltrative margin favors leiomyosarcoma, inflammatory pseudotumor also may invade the muscularis propria.

MÜLLERIAN LESIONS

ENDOMETRIOSIS

The bladder is the most common site of urinary tract involvement in endometriosis,[319-324] but only about 1% of women with endometriosis have bladder involvement.[325] As many as 50% of these patients have a history of pelvic surgery, and approximately 12% lack evidence of endometriosis at any other site. The average age is approximately 35 years. Frequency, dysuria, and hematuria are the most common symptoms, but more than 50% of patients have no vesical symptoms. Endo-

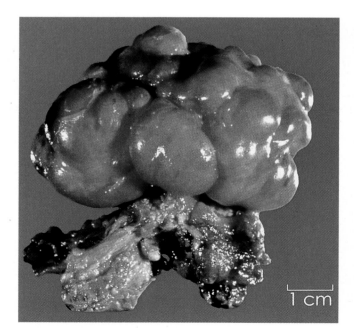

4-62. Inflammatory pseudotumor. A polypoid mass projects into the bladder lumen.

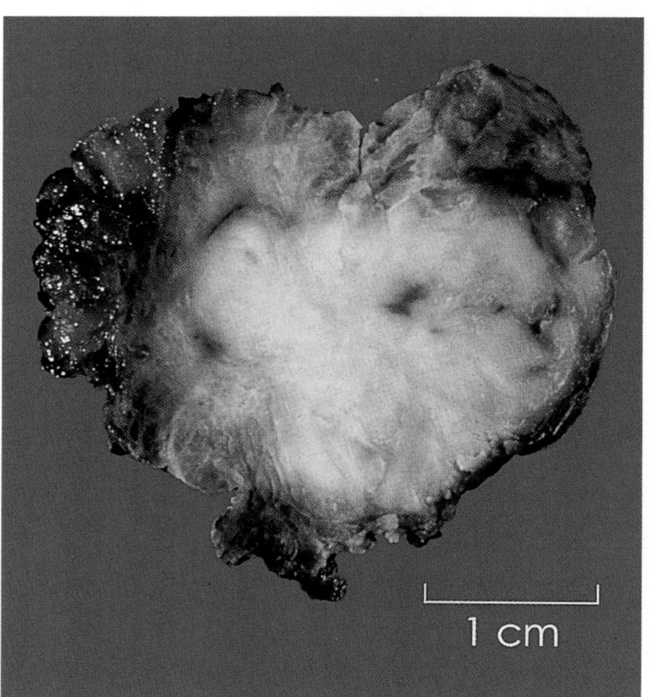

4-63. Inflammatory pseudotumor. The cut surface shows involvement of the full thickness of the bladder wall.

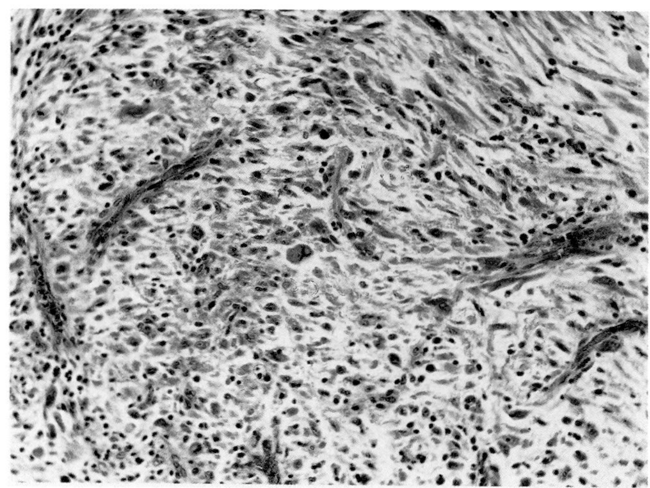

4-64. Inflammatory pseudotumor showing delicate blood vessels in a background of spindle cells.

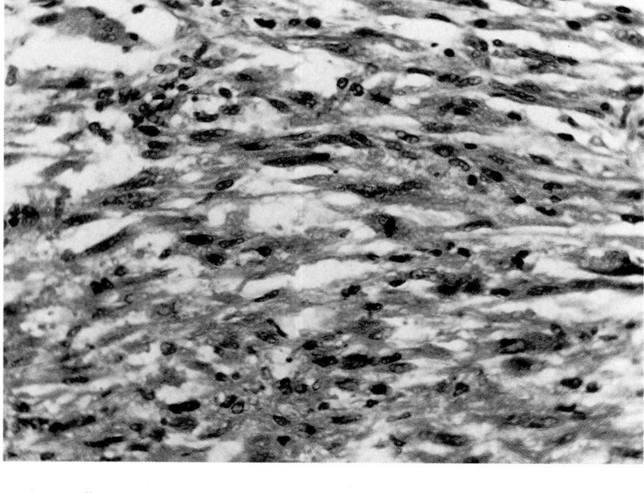

4-66. Inflammatory pseudotumor with pleomorphic nuclei and a mitotic figure.

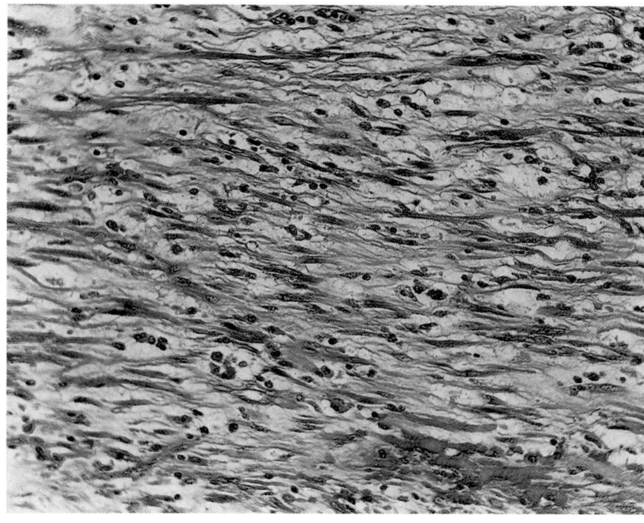

4-65. Inflammatory pseudotumor composed of fascicles of spindle cells.

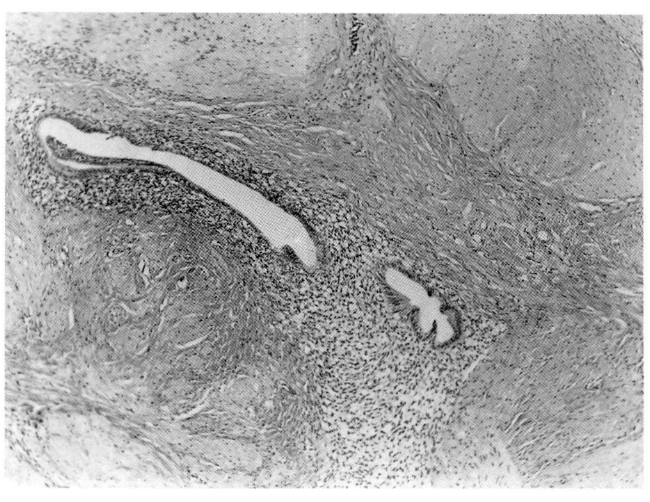

4-67. Endometriosis. Endometrial glands surrounded by endometrial stroma.

metriosis of the muscularis propria may give symptoms similar to those of interstitial cystitis.[326] There is a palpable suprapubic mass in almost 50% of cases and this may undergo catamenial enlargement. Rarely, endometriosis has been reported in post-menopausal women treated with estrogen[327-329] and in men treated with estrogen for prostate cancer.[330-332] At cystoscopy, the lesions usually appear as congested, edematous mucosal elevations overlying blue, blue-black, or red-brown cysts. The overlying urothelium may be intact or eroded. If the lesions are limited to the muscularis propria (Fig. 4-67, 4-68) or serosa, the mucosa may be normal. Fibrosis and hyperplastic muscle around the lesions may thicken the bladder wall. Microscopically, the lesions resemble endometriosis as seen elsewhere. In some cases, not all of the glands are surrounded by endometrial stroma and in some foci stroma is absent.[320]

ENDOCERVICOSIS

Endocervicosis of the bladder is less common than endometriosis.[333,334] Patients typically present in their fourth and fifth decades with symptoms such as suprapubic pain, dysuria, frequency, or hematuria and may have catamenial exacerbation of symptoms. They often have a history of caesarean section. Most lesions are in the muscularis propria, but the mucosa (Fig. 4-69*A*) and adventitia also may be involved. In endocervicosis, there is a haphazard proliferation of irregularly shaped mucinous glands in the bladder wall (Fig. 4-69*B*). The epithelium lining the glands consists of a single layer of columnar cells with abundant pale cytoplasm that reacts with periodic acid-Schiff and mucicarmine stains. Ciliated cells often are interspersed among the mucinous cells. When the glands are dilated, the epithelium is cuboidal or flattened. The glandular lumens usually contain mucus.

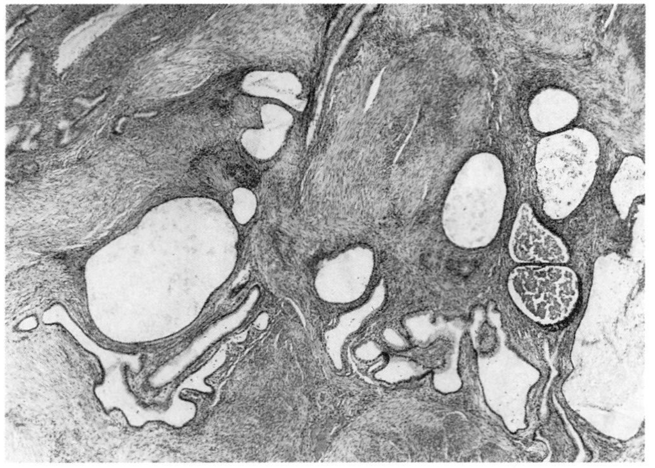

4-68. Endometriosis deep in the muscularis propria.

Ruptured glands with extravasated mucus and a stromal reaction may be seen. The most common of the benign müllerian glandular lesions in women, endosalpingiosis, is, enigmatically, the one least often seen in the bladder. Indeed, it has only recently been described.[334a] Vesical endosalpingiosis consists of numerous tubal-type glands (Fig. 4-70*A*) lined at least focally by ciliated cells (Fig. 4-70*B*). The müllerian epithelium may replace the urothelium of the mucosa and cover polypoid intraluminal projections (Fig. 4-71). In some cases, a mixture of several different types of müllerian epithelium is present and the term *müllerianosis* may be appropriate.[334a]

MÜLLERIAN CYST

Müllerian duct cyst in men usually lies between the bladder and rectum and may involve the posterior wall of the bladder.[335,336] Patients usually present with irritative bladder symptoms and clinical evaluation reveals a mid-

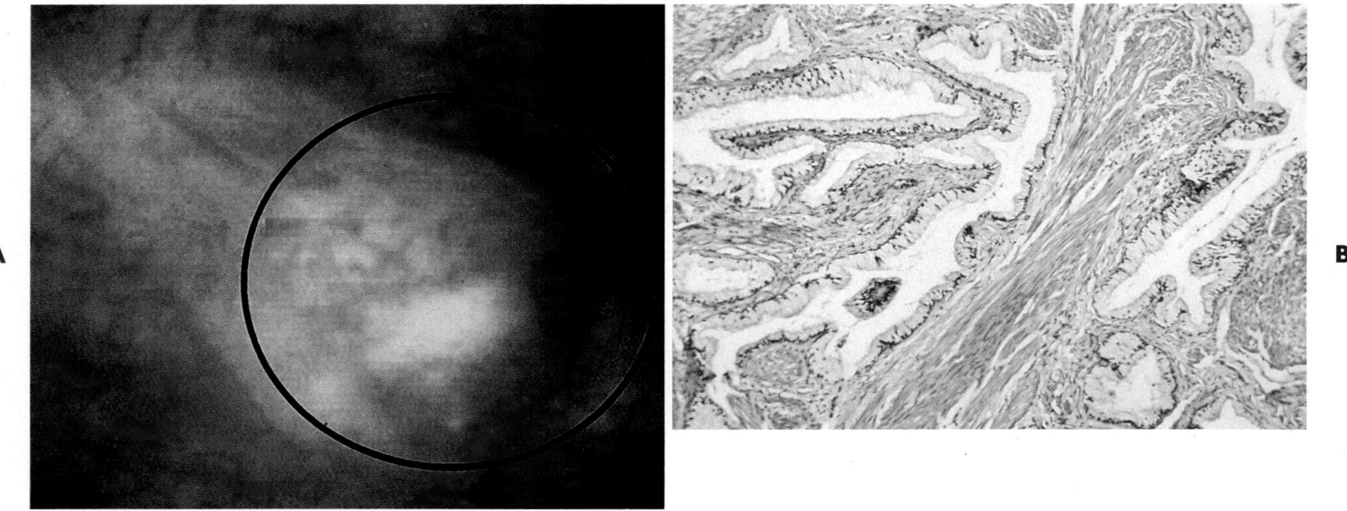

4-69. Endocervicosis. **A**, Cystoscopy shows vesical endocervicosis as a submucosal nodule. **B**, Glands lined by benign columnar epithelium are present in the muscularis propria.

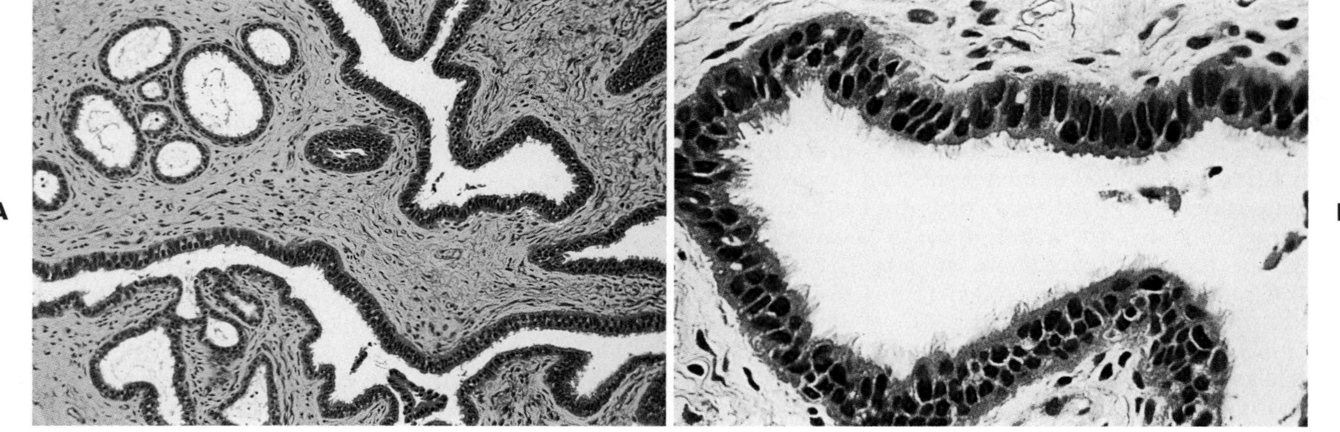

4-70. Endosalpingiosis. **A**, Glands, some of them branching, are lined by tubal-type epithelium. **B**, Higher magnification demonstrates cilia on the surfaces of the epithelial cells.

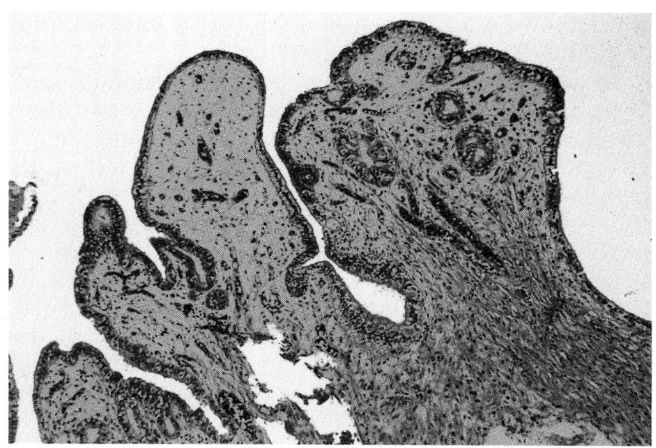

4-71. Müllerianosis. Polyps lined by müllerian epithelium protrude into the bladder lumen. Epithelia of endocervical, endometrial, and tubal types are present in this case.

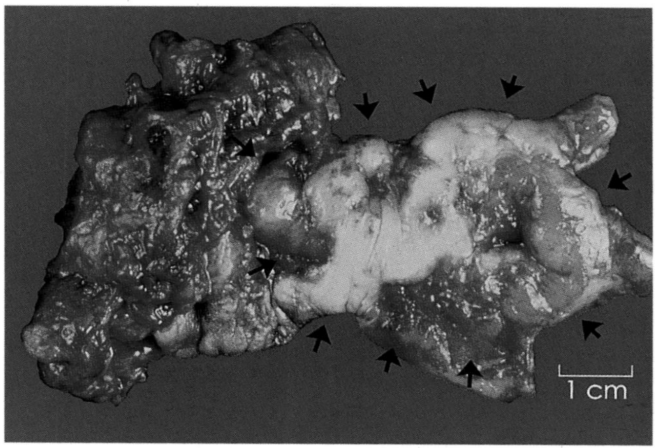

4-72. Exstrophy of the bladder. The mucosa (*arrows*) shows congestion, edema, and fibrosis.

line supraprostatic mass. Grossly, the cyst is unilocular or multilocular and filled with clear or hemorrhagic fluid. Microscopically, the cyst lining is often lost throughout much of its area but a layer of müllerian epithelium can usually be found at least focally. In contrast to seminal vesicle cyst, spermatozoa are absent from müllerian duct cyst.

Müllerian sinus lined by mucus-secreting epithelium connecting the posterolateral wall of the bladder with the broad ligament is a rare lesion.[337]

MALFORMATIONS

AGENESIS

Agenesis of the bladder is rare[338] and only a few dozen cases have been recorded, almost all of them in girls.[339-343] Agenesis results from failure of separation of the ureters from the wolffian ducts. In this situation, the ureters enter the müllerian tract or posterior urethra. Alternately, the urorectal septum fails to form and the cloaca remains. Usually there is ureteral obstruction with megaureter and hydronephrosis. When development of the distal ureters fails, the trigone of the bladder does not develop. Vesical agenesis is strongly associated with sirenomelia, a syndrome characterized by fusion of the lower extremities and other anomalies. Most such cases have no ureters, lending support to the concept that vesical agenesis is related to failure of ureteral development.

EXSTROPHY

Exstrophy (incomplete closure) of the bladder and its associated malformations has long been recognized and the 1855 description and review by Duncan[344] can hardly be improved upon today. Exstrophy is more common than agenesis and occurs in approximately 1 of 10,000 to 40,000 live births.[345] While there is little risk (1%) to siblings of patients with exstrophy,[346] among offspring of parents with exstrophy the rate is 1 in 70 live births.[347] Exstrophy occurs in two variants: bladder exstrophy and cloacal exstrophy. The latter is much less common than the former (1 in 200,000 live births).[348]

Exstrophy results from perforation of an abnormally developed cloacal membrane. In normal development, the ingrowth of mesenchyme between the ectodermal and endodermal layers of the cloacal membrane permits fusion of the midline structures below the umbilicus and closure of the abdominal wall. Downward growth of the urorectal septum divides the cloaca into the bladder anteriorly and the rectum posteriorly. The urorectal septum joins the cloacal membrane in the perineum before perforating it to produce the anal and urogenital openings. Before perforation, the genital tubercles migrate medially and fuse in the midline. Defective development of the cloacal membrane with premature perforation results in a variety of abnormalities, including superior vesical fissure, bladder exstrophy, and cloacal exstrophy.[349]

Bladder exstrophy is five to seven times more common in boys than in girls.[350] It often is accompanied by other malformations such as epispadias, intestinal malformations, and defects of spinal closure. Genital malformations are the rule, with epispadias in 86% of boys and unfused labia in 71% of girls.[351] Epispadias is so often associated with exstrophy that the two are sometimes called the exstrophy-epispadias complex.[347] Spina bifida is present in 18% of cases.[351]

Bladder exstrophy is a true malformation rather than an arrest of development.[352] In exstrophy, the urinary tract is open to the body wall from the urethral meatus to the umbilicus.[349] The mucosa of the bladder and urethra is fused to the adjacent skin, and the urethra and bladder are foreshortened. The ureters end in a widened trigone and are prone to reflux after surgical closure. The pubic symphysis is widely open (3 to 10 cm).[349] The rectus muscles are widely separated, and umbilical and inguinal hernias are common. At birth, the exstrophic bladder mucosa is usually smooth and has a normal appearance. This condition is short-lived, and trauma and infection quickly produce ulcers and inflammation (Fig. 4-72). The anus is often anteriorly displaced, and there may be rectal prolapse. In girls, the müllerian system shows variable duplication and failure of closure.[353] In boys, the penis is short, with a dorsal chordee. Incomplete variants of this constellation of anatomical lesions are rare.[354]

Histologically, the mucosa often shows acute and chronic inflammation with ulceration and metaplastic changes at the time of surgical closure.[355] Squamous and intestinal metaplasia are absent or slight at birth and become extensive and profound with time.[356] After closure, the mucosa often remains inflamed and squamous metaplasia is common, although changes such as cystitis cystica and glandularis diminish.[355]

Without surgery, more than 66% of patients with bladder exstrophy die by age 20.[350] Early surgical intervention, with or without urinary diversion, is successful in many cases, allowing preservation of renal function, urinary continence, and eliminating urinary infections in more than 50% of patients.[357,358] The chronic inflammation and metaplasia of untreated exstrophy predispose the patient to carcinoma, particularly adenocarcinoma.[350] Surgical reconstruction prevents this, and exstrophy-associated carcinoma has become rare.[359]

Cloacal exstrophy is a complex malformation that also is known as *exstrophia splanchnia*, which conveys the extensiveness of the defects.[360] Typically, the lower abdominal wall consists of a large area of exposed mucosa, above which is usually an omphalocele. At the center of the area of mucosa is a patch of intestinal mucosa with one to four orifices. The most superior orifice connects to the ileum, while the lowest orifice connects to a short segment of colon that ends blindly. The other orifices are appendices. The anus is imperforate. Lateral to the intestinal mucosa is exstrophic bladder mucosa containing the ureteral orifices and occasionally the vasa deferentia and vagina. Patches of bladder mucosa may join above or below the intestinal mucosa or may encircle it. The testes are undescended and the external genitalia are absent or malformed. Double penis is common in boys.[361] The pubic symphysis is diastatic and vertebral abnormalities are common. Abnormalities of other organ systems are rare. Cloacal exstrophy was invariably fatal 4 decades ago, but modern surgical techniques have greatly improved patient outcome and survival is now near 50%.[348]

DUPLICATION AND SEPTATION OF THE BLADDER

The complete form of duplication is very rare and consists of two fully formed urinary bladders with complete mucosal and muscular elements.[362,363] Each unit receives the ureter from its side and drains into a duplicate urethra.[364] In the great majority of cases, this anomaly is accompanied by either diphallus or duplication of the uterus and vagina. In nearly 50% of cases, the hindgut is duplicated and the lumbar vertebrae may also be duplicated.[365]

In partial duplication, the bladder is divided either sagittally or coronally by a complete wall, and each side is connected to the ureter from the kidney on its side.[362,363,366] Partial duplication differs from complete duplication in that the two units usually communicate and drain into a common urethra. Partial duplication is even rarer than complete duplication.

In septation of the urinary bladder, a septum composed of mucosa with or without muscularis partitions the bladder in either the sagittal or coronal planes.[362,366] The partition may be complete or incomplete. When the septum is in the sagittal plane, the ureter from each side connects with its respective chamber. Because there is a single bladder neck and urethra, complete septation is associated with dysplasia and obstruction of one side.[367] If the partition is incomplete, drainage may be normal. Hourglass bladder is an allied condition in which the bladder narrows near its middle, giving it the shape of an hourglass.[368,369]

URACHAL CYSTS AND PERSISTENCE

Completely patent urachus is a dramatic lesion in which urine flows from the umbilicus or stump of the umbilical cord. This abnormality is uncommon, with fewer than 300 reported cases.[23,370] The ratio of males to females is approximately 2:1. Most patients with patent urachus have no other developmental abnormality, although Lattimer[371] found that 50% of patients with prune-belly syndrome (congenital deficiency of the abdominal musculature) had patent urachus. In most cases, patent urachus does not appear to result from increased intravesical pressure. Schreck and Campbell[372] found that only two of eight children with patent urachus had urinary outlet obstruction. Embryologically, the sequence of development indicates that the urachus is normally already closed before the development of other structures could lead to increased pressure, which might keep it open. The concept that increased pressure later in development might lead to the reopening of the urachus after normal closure was refuted by Begg's[26] anatomical studies.

Incompletely patent urachus is classified by Vaughan[373] as umbilico-urachal sinus, vesico-urachal sinus or diverticulum, and the blind variant in which the urachus is closed at both ends but remains open centrally (Fig. 4-73). Later, Hinman[374] added alternating urachal sinus to the classification to account for individuals without histories of umbilical urinary drainage in whom urachal infections drained both into the bladder and from the umbilicus. Alternating urachal sinus should be distinguished from completely patent urachus in which the lumen is patent from bladder to umbilicus at birth. Hinman[374] concluded that, in patients with alternating urachal sinus, the lumen is a potential space in which accumulating epithelial cellular debris becomes a focus for infection. Rarely, stones form within urachal malformations. These may be of urinary origin, similar in composition to other urinary calculi, or may be of different origin in which case they are usually small and yellow-brown or brown.

Urachal cysts are found at any point in the urachus (Fig. 4-74) and range from small lesions found incidentally (Fig. 4-75, 4-76) to immense masses containing as much as 50 liters of fluid.[375] Small cysts are usually lined by urothelium or cuboidal epithelium (Fig. 4-77), but columnar epithelium may be present. The lining of large cysts is usually flattened.

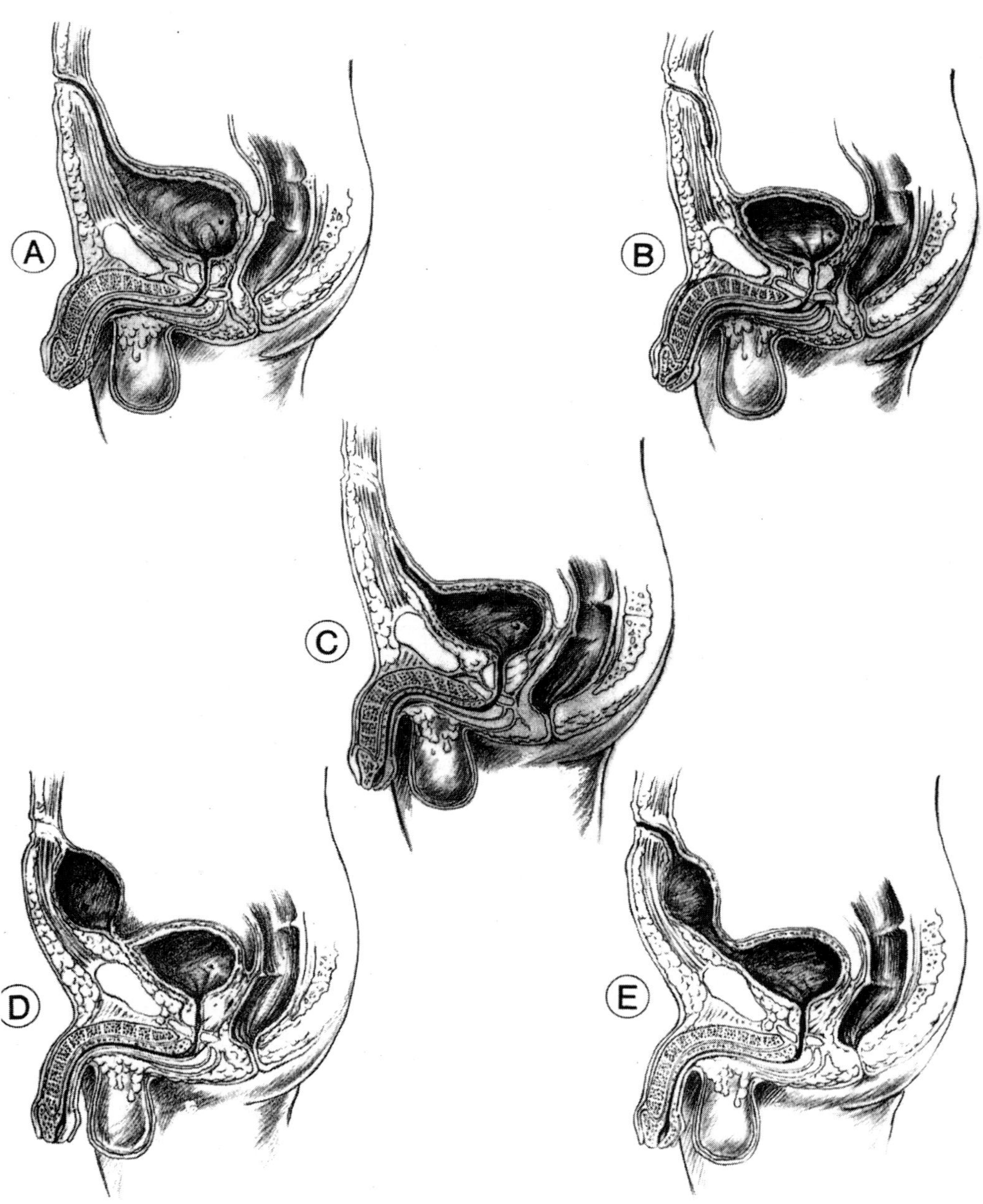

4-73. Types of persistent or patent urachus. Complete patency (**A**). Umbilicourachal sinus (**B**). Vesicourachal sinus (**C**). Blindly patent urachus (**D**). Alternating urachal sinus (**E**).

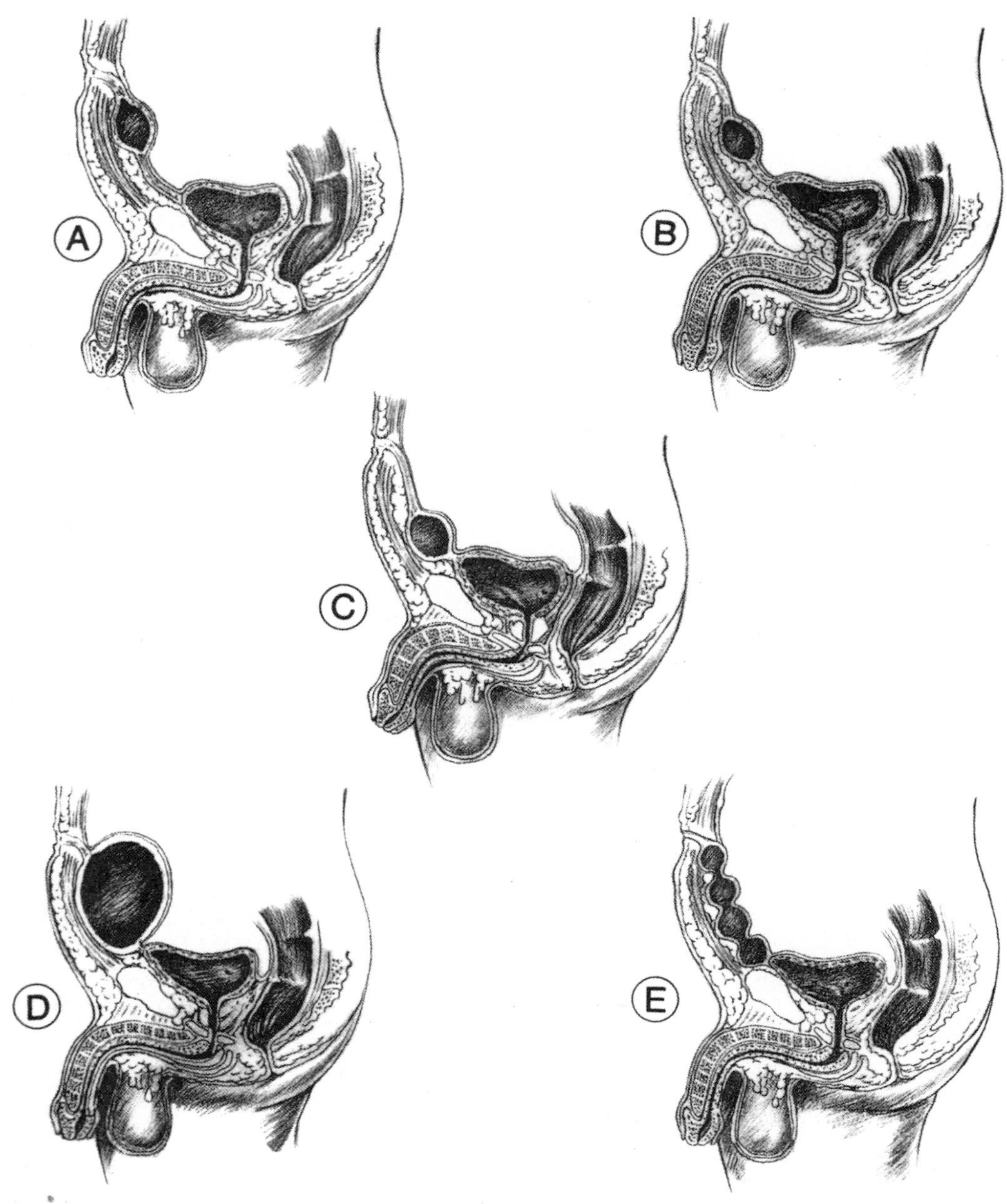

4-74. Classification of urachal cysts. Juxta-umbilical (**A**). Intermediate (**B**). Juxtavesical (**C**). Giant cyst (**D**). Multiple cysts (**E**).

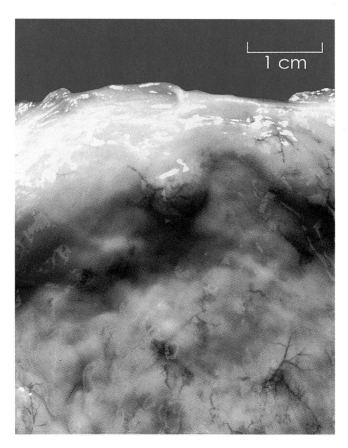

4-75. Small urachal cyst found as a submucosal nodule in the bladder dome.

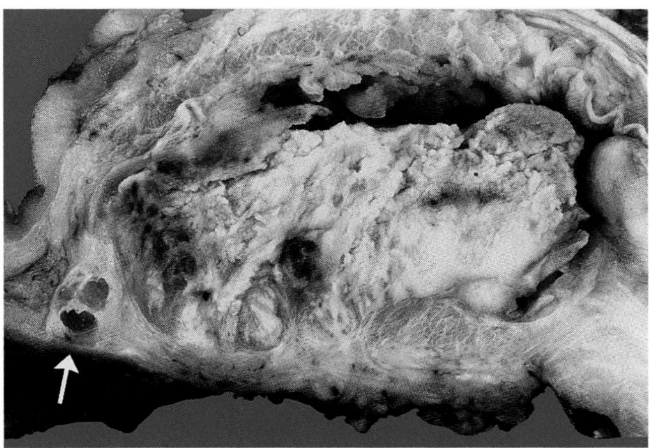

4-76. Urachal cyst. An incidental finding in a radical cystoprostatectomy specimen.

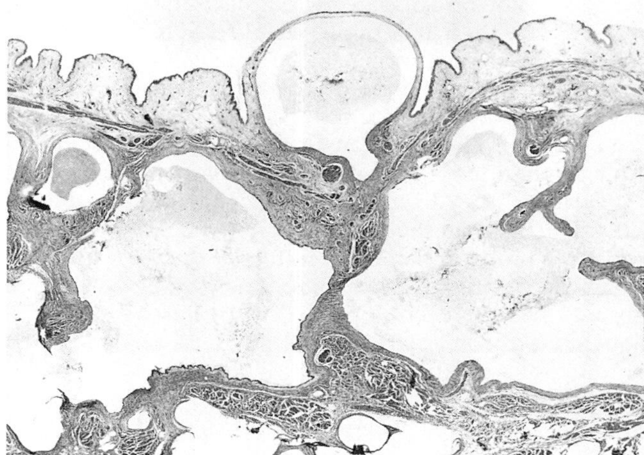

4-77. Multilocular urachal cyst lined by cuboidal and atrophic epithelium.

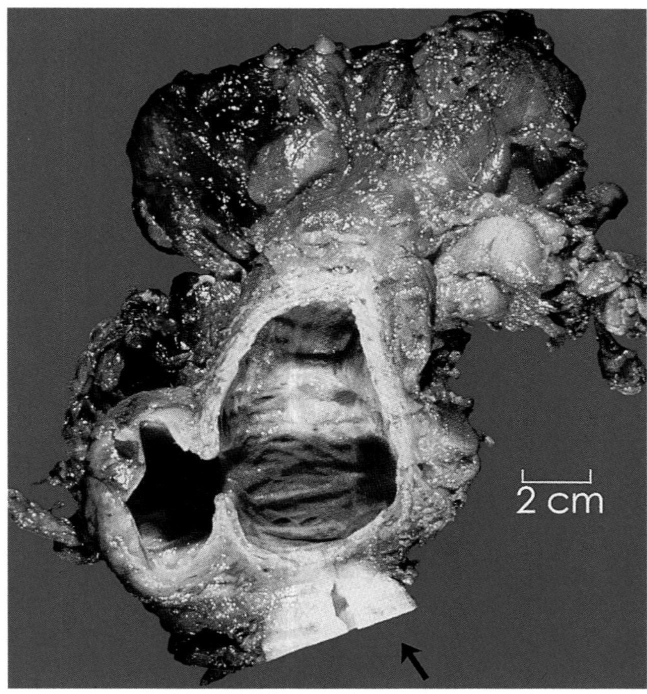

4-78. Bladder diverticulum (*arrow indicates hyperplastic prostate*).

DIVERTICULUM

Diverticulum of the bladder (Fig. 4-78) is a common clinical problem that infrequently requires surgical treatment. The etiology of bladder diverticulum is generally attributed to increased lumenal pressure,[376] although some lesions in children are attributable to localized deficiency of the muscularis propria[377-381] and others to syndromes such as Ehlers-Danlos syndrome.[382] Diverticula are common in children with Menkes' syndrome (kinky hair syndrome).[383] Diverticula are found in patients of all ages,[384] but most often in men older than 50 years[376] with outflow obstruction caused by prostatic hyperplasia, suggesting that they are caused by increased pressure.[385] Diverticula are most common in the vicinity of the ureteral orifices. At this site, diverticula can cause ureteral obstruction or reflux and predispose the patient to infection. While most diverticula are small and asymptomatic, large ones may rival or exceed the volume of the bladder[376] and be associated with infection and stone formation. Less than 10% of diverticula develop neoplasms, most of which are urothelial carcinoma.[386-389]

The excised specimen usually includes a small orifice connecting the bladder and the diverticulum.[385] The passage between the two consists of a narrow intramural neck in the inner layer of the muscularis propria, while the wall of the diverticulum may contain attenuated muscle fibers from the outer layer in patients without histories of chronic inflammation. In patients with histories of chronic inflammation the muscle fibers often are absent, having been replaced with fibrous tissue.[390] Squamous metaplasia also is seen in association with chronic inflammation.[390]

References

1. Tanagho EA, Smith DR, Meyers FH: The trigone: anatomical and physiological considerations. 2. In relation to the bladder neck, J Urol 100:633-639, 1968.
2. Tanagho EA, Meyers FH, Smith DR: The trigone: anatomical and physiological considerations. 1. In relation to the ureterovesical junction, J Urol 100:623-632, 1968.
3. Woodburne RT: Anatomy of the bladder and bladder outlet, J Urol 100:474-487, 1968.
4. Elbadawi A: Anatomy and function of the ureteral sheath, J Urol 107:224-229, 1972.
5. Gosling J: The structure of the bladder and urethra in relation to function, Urol Clin North Am 6:31-38, 1979.
6. Tanagho EA, Pugh RCB: The anatomy and function of the ureterovesical junction, Br J Urol 35:151-165, 1963.
7. Tanagho EA, Smith DR: The anatomy and function of the bladder neck, Br J Urol 38:54-71, 1966.
8. Hutch JA, Rambo ON, Jr: A study of the anatomy of the prostate, prostatic urethra and the urinary sphincter system, J Urol 104:443-452, 1970.
9. Hammond G, Yglesias L, Davis JE: The urachus, its anatomy and associated fasciae, Anat Rec 80:271-287, 1941.
10. Blichert-Toft M, Koch F, Nielsen OV: Anatomic variants of the urachus related to clinical appearance and surgical treatment, Surg Gynecol Obstet 137:51-54, 1973.
11. Shehata R: The arterial supply of the urinary bladder, Acta Anat 96:128-134, 1976.
12. Braithwaite JL: The arterial supply of the male urinary bladder, Br J Urol 24:64-71, 1952.
13. Parker AE: The lymph collectors from the urinary bladder and their connections with the main posterior lymph channels of the abdomen, Anat Rec 65:443-460, 1936.
14. Koss LG: The asymmetric unit membranes of the epithelium of the urinary bladder of the rat, an electron microscopic study of a mechanism of epithelial maturation and function, Lab Invest 21:154-168, 1969.
15. Battifora H, Eisenstein R, McDonald JH: The human urinary bladder mucosa, an electron microscopic study, Invest Urol 1:354-361, 1964.
16. Newman J, Antonakopoulos GN: The fine structure of the human fetal urinary bladder. Development and maturation. A light, transmission and scanning electron microscopic study, J Anat 166:135-150, 1989.
17. Alroy J, Gould VE: Epithelial-stromal interface in normal and neoplastic human bladder epithelium, Ultrastruct Pathol 1:201-210, 1980.
18. Ro JY, Ayala AG, El-Naggar A: Muscularis mucosa of urinary bladder, importance for staging and treatment, Am J Surg Pathol 11:668-673, 1987.
19. Keep JC, Piehl M, Miller A et al: Invasive carcinomas of the urinary bladder, evaluation of tunica muscularis mucosae involvement, Am J Clin Pathol 91:575-579, 1989.
20. Younes M, Sussman J, True LD: The usefulness of the level of the muscularis mucosae in the staging of invasive transitional cell carcinoma of the urinary bladder, Cancer 66:543-548, 1990.
21. Weaver MG, Abdul-Karim FW: The prevalence and character of the muscularis mucosae of the human urinary bladder, Histopathology 17:563-566, 1990.
22. Hasui Y, Kitada S, Nishi S: Significance of invasion to the muscularis mucosae on the progression of superficial bladder cancer, Urology 43:782-786, 1994.
23. Eble JN: Abnormalities of the urachus. In Young RH, ed: Pathology of the urinary bladder, New York, 1989, Churchill Livingstone.
24. Schubert GE, Pavkovic MB, Bethke-Bedürftig BA: Tubular urachal remnants in adult bladders, J Urol 127:40-42, 1982.
25. Tyler DE: Epithelium of intestinal type in the normal urachus: a new theory of vesical embryology, J Urol 92:505-507, 1964.
26. Begg RC: The urachus: its anatomy, histology and development, J Anat 64:170-182, 1930.
27. von Brunn A: Ueber drüsenähnliche Bildungen in der Schleimhaut des Nierenbeckens, des Ureters und der Harnblase beim Menschen, Archiv fur mikroscopische Anatomie 41:294-302, 1893.
28. Morse HD: The etiology and pathology of pyelitis cystica, ureteritis cystica and cystitis cystica, Am J Pathol 4:33-49, 1928.
29. Patch FS, Rhea LJ: The genesis and development of von Brunn's nests and their relation to cystitis cystica, cystitis glandularis and primary adeno-carcinoma of the bladder, Can Med Assoc J 33:597-606, 1935.
30. Andersen JA, Hansen BF: The incidence of cell nests, cystitis cystica and cystitis glandularis in the lower urinary tract revealed by autopsies, J Urol 108:421-424, 1972.
31. Wiener DP, Koss LG, Sablay B et al: The prevalence and significance of von Brunn's nests, cystitis cystica and squamous metaplasia in normal bladders, J Urol 122:317-321, 1979.
32. Goldstein AMB, Fauer RB, Chinn M et al: New concepts on formation of von Brunn's nests and cysts in urinary tract mucosa, Urology 11:513-517, 1978.
33. Ito N, Hirose H, Shirai T et al: Lesions of the urinary bladder epithelium in 125 autopsy cases, Acta Pathol Jpn 31:545-557, 1981.
34. Emmett JL, McDonald JR: Proliferation of glands of the urinary bladder simulating malignant neoplasm, J Urol 48:257-265, 1942.
35. Lowry EC, Hamm FC, Beard DE: Extensive glandular proliferation of the urinary bladder resembling malignant neoplasm, J Urol 52:133-138, 1944.
36. Foot NC: Glandular metaplasia of the epithelium of the urinary tract, South Med J 37:137-142, 1944.

37. Sauer HR, Blick MS: Cystitis glandularis: a consideration of symptoms, diagnosis and clinical course of the disease, J Urol 61:446-458, 1948.
38. Lane TJD: An uncommon bladder condition simulating carcinoma. Glandular proliferation in the epithelium of the urinary tract, with special reference to cystitis cystica and cystitis glandularis, Br J Urol 20:175-179, 1948.
39. Kittredge WE, Brannan W: Cystitis glandularis, J Urol 81:419-430, 1959.
40. Gingell JC, Burn JI: Cystitis glandularis—case report, Br J Urol 42:446-449, 1970.
41. Ward AM: Glandular neoplasia within the urinary tract. The aetiology of adenocarcinoma of the urothelium with a review of the literature I. Introduction: the origin of glandular epithelium in the renal pelvis, ureter and bladder, Virchows Arch A Pathol Anat Histopathol 352:296-311, 1971.
42. Stirling WC, Ash JE: Chronic proliferative lesions of the urinary tract, J Urol 45:342-360, 1941.
43. Dann RH, Arger PH, Enterline HT: Benign proliferation processes presenting as mass lesions in the urinary bladder, AJR Am J Roentgenol 116:822-829, 1972.
44. Imray TJ, Kaplan P: Lower urinary tract infections and calculi in the adult, Semin Roentgenol 18:276-287, 1983.
45. Davies G, Castro JE: Cystitis glandularis, Urology 10:128-129, 1977.
46. Edelman L: Muciparous glands in the mucosa of the urinary bladder, report of two cases, J Urol 20:211-224, 1928.
47. Young RH, Parkhurst EC: Mucinous adenocarcinoma of bladder. Case associated with extensive intestinal metaplasia of urothelium in patient with nonfunctioning bladder for twelve years, Urology 24:192-195, 1984.
48. Bullock PS, Thoni DE, Murphy WM: The significance of colonic mucosa (intestinal metaplasia) involving the urinary tract, Cancer 59:2086-2090, 1987.
49. Gordon A: Intestinal metaplasia of the urinary tract epithelium, J Pathol Bacteriol 85:441-444, 1963.
50. Wells M, Anderson K: Mucin histochemistry of cystitis glandularis and primary adenocarcinoma of the urinary bladder, Arch Pathol Lab Med 109:59-61, 1985.
51. Hasegawa R, Fukushima S, Hirose M et al: Histochemical demonstration of colonic type mucin in glandular metaplasia and adenocarcinoma of the human urinary bladder, Acta Pathol Jpn 37:1097-1103, 1987.
52. Nowels K, Kent E, Rinsho K et al: Prostate specific antigen and acid phosphatase-reactive cells in cystitis cystica and glandularis, Arch Pathol Lab Med 112:734-737, 1988.
53. Golz R, Schubert GE: Prostatic specific antigen: immunoreactivity in urachal remnants, J Urol 141:1480-1482, 1989.
54. Hasegawa R, Fukushima S, Furukawa F et al: Abberant colonic epithelium in the bladder: report of a case, J Urol 136:901-902, 1986.
55. Elem B, Alam SZ: Total intestinal metaplasia with focal adenocarcinoma in a schistosoma-infested defunctioned urinary bladder, Br J Urol 56:331-343, 1984.
56. Eble JN, Young RH: Benign and low-grade papillary lesions of the urinary bladder: a review of the papilloma-papillary carcinoma controversy, and a report of five typical papillomas, Semin Diagn Pathol 6:351-371, 1989.
57. Bell TE, Wendel RG: Cystitis glandularis: benign or malignant? J Urol 100:462, 1968.
58. Parker C: Cystitis cystica and glandularis: a study of 40 cases, Proc R Soc Med 63:239-242, 1970.
59. Shaw JL, Gislason GJ, Imbriglia JE: Transition of cystitis glandularis to primary adenocarcinoma of the bladder, J Urol 79:815, 1958.
60. Lin JI, Tseng CH, Choy C et al: Diffuse cystitis glandularis associated with adenocarcinomatous change, Urology 15:411-415, 1980.
61. Kittredge WE, Collett AJ, Morgan C: Adenocarcinoma of the bladder associated with cystitis glandularis: a case report, J Urol 91:145, 1964.
62. Salm R: Neoplasia of the bladder and cystitis cystica, Br J Urol 39:67-72, 1967.
63. Susmano D, Rubenstein AB, Dakin AR et al: Cystitis glandularis and adenocarcinoma of the bladder, J Urol 105:671, 1971.
64. Edwards PD, Hurm RA, Jaeschke WH: Conversion of cystitis glandularis to adenocarcinoma, J Urol 108:568, 1972.
65. Talbert ML, Young RH: Carcinomas of the urinary bladder with deceptively benign-appearing foci, a report of three cases, Am J Surg Pathol 13:374-381, 1989.
66. Kretschmer HL: The pathology and cystoscopy of cystitis cystica, Surg Gynecol Obstet 7:274-279, 1908.
67. Warrick WD: Cystitis cystica: bacteriological studies in a series of 28 cases, J Urol 45:835-843, 1941.
68. Kaplan GW, King LR: Cystitis cystica in childhood, J Urol 103:657-659, 1970.
69. Thompson GJ, Stein JJ: Leukoplakia of the urinary bladder: a report of 34 clinical cases, J Urol 44:639-649, 1940.
70. Rabson SM: Leukoplakia and carcinoma of the urinary bladder, report of a case with a review of the literature, J Urol 35:321-341, 1936.
71. O'Flynn JD, Mullaney J: Leukoplakia of the bladder, a report on 20 cases, including 2 cases progressing to squamous cell carcinoma, Br J Urol 39:461-471, 1967.
72. Scholl AJ: Squamous cell changes and infection in the urinary tract, J Urol 44:759-767, 1940.
73. Reece RW, Koontz WW, Jr: Leukoplakia of the urinary tract: a review, J Urol 114:165-171, 1975.
74. Widran J, Sanchez R, Gruhn J: Squamous metaplasia of the bladder: a study of 450 patients, J Urol 112:479-482, 1974.
75. Polsky MS, Weber CH, Jr, Williams JE, III et al: Chronically infected and postdiversionary bladders, cytologic and histopathologic study, Urology 7:531-535, 1976.
76. Kaufman JM, Fam B, Jacobs SC et al: Bladder cancer and squamous metaplasia in spinal cord injury patients, J Urol 118:967-971, 1977.
77. Zahran MM, Kamel M, Mooro H et al: Bilharziasis of urinary bladder and ureter, comparative histopathologic study, Urology 8:73-79, 1976.
78. Witherington R: Leukoplakia of the bladder: an 8-year follow up, J Urol 112:600-602, 1974.
79. Thomas SD, Sanders PW, III, Sanders PW, Jr: Cholesteatoma of the bladder, J Urol 112:598-599, 1974.
80. Connery DB: Leukoplakia of the urinary bladder and its association with carcinoma, J Urol 69:121-127, 1953.
81. O'Flynn JD, Mullaney J: Vesical leukoplakia progressing to carcinoma, Br J Urol 46:31-37, 1974.
82. DeKock MLS, Anderson CK, Clark PB: Vesical leukoplakia progressing to squamous cell carcinoma in women, Br J Urol 53:316-317, 1981.

83. Benson RC, Jr, Swanson SK, Farrow GM: Relationship of leukoplakia to urothelial malignancy, J Urol 131:507-511, 1984.
84. El Bolkainy MN, Mokhtar NM, Ghoneim MA et al: The impact of schistosomiasis on the pathology of bladder carcinoma, Cancer 48:2643-2648, 1981.
85. Khafagy MM, El Bolkainy MN, Mansour MA: Carcinoma of the bilharzial urinary bladder, a study of the associated mucosal lesions in 86 cases, Cancer 30:150-159, 1972.
86. Cifuentes L: Epithelium of vaginal type in the female trigone: the clinical problem of trigonitis, J Urol 57:1028-1037, 1947.
87. Packham DA: The epithelial lining of the female trigone and urethra, Br J Urol 43:201-205, 1971.
88. Tyler DE: Stratified squamous epithelium in the vesical trigone and urethra: findings correlated with the menstrual cycle and age, Am J Anat 111:319-335, 1962.
89. Long ED, Shepherd RT: The incidence and significance of vaginal metaplasia of the bladder trigone in adult women, Br J Urol 55:189-194, 1983.
90. Ney C, Ehrlich JC: Squamous epithelium in the trigone of the human female urinary bladder, with a note on cystoscopic observations during estrogen therapy, J Urol 73:809-819, 1955.
91. Stephenson TJ, Henry L, Harris SC et al: Pseudomembranous trigonitis of the bladder: hormonal aetiology, J Clin Pathol 42:922-926, 1989.
92. Henry L, Fox M: Histological findings in pseudomembranous trigonitis, J Clin Pathol 24:605-608, 1971.
93. Davis TA: Hamartoma of the urinary bladder, Northwest Med 48:182-185, 1949.
94. Friedman NB, Kuhlenbeck H: Adenomatoid tumors of the bladder reproducing renal structures (nephrogenic adenomas), J Urol 64:657-670, 1950.
95. O'Shea PA, Callaghan JF, Lawlor JB et al: "Nephrogenic adenoma": an unusual metaplastic change of urothelium, J Urol 125:249-252, 1981.
96. Navarre RJ, Jr, Loening SA, Platz C et al: Nephrogenic adenoma: a report of 9 cases and review of the literature, J Urol 127:775-779, 1982.
97. Devine P, Ucci AA, Krain H et al: Nephrogenic adenoma and embryonic kidney tubules share PNA receptor sites, Am J Clin Pathol 81:728-732, 1984.
98. Ford TF, Watson GM, Cameron KM: Adenomatous metaplasia (nephrogenic adenoma) of urothelium, an analysis of 70 cases, Br J Urol 57:427-433, 1985.
99. Young RH, Scully RE: Nephrogenic adenoma: a report of 15 cases, review of the literature, and comparison with clear cell carcinoma of the urinary tract, Am J Surg Pathol 10:268-275, 1986.
100. Sørensen FB, Jacobsen F, Nielsen JB et al: Nephroid metaplasia of the urinary tract, a survey of the literature, with the contribution of 5 new immunohistochemically studied cases, including one case examined by electron microscopy, Acta Pathol Microbiol Scand [A] 95:67-81, 1987.
101. Young RH: Pseudoneoplastic lesions of the urinary bladder, Pathol Annu 23:67-104, 1988.
102. Lugo M, Petersen RO, Elfenbein IB et al: Nephrogenic metaplasia of the ureter, Am J Clin Pathol 80:92-97, 1983.
103. Billerey C, Khamlu K, Regin JP et al: La métaplasie néphrogénique de la muqueuse urothéliale, à propos de onze observations, Ann Urol 17:340-346, 1983.
104. de Jong EAJM, Scholtmeijer RJ: Nephrogenic adenoma of the bladder in children, Eur Urol 10:187-190, 1984.
105. Kay R, Lattanzi C: Nephrogenic adenoma in children, J Urol 133:99-101, 1985.
106. Gonzalez JA, Watts JC, Alderson TP: Nephrogenic adenoma of the bladder: report of 10 cases, J Urol 139:45-47, 1988.
107. Oliva E, Young RH: Nephrogenic adenoma of the urinary tract: a review of the microscopic appearances of 80 cases with emphasis on unusual features, Mod Pathol 8:722-730, 1995.
108. Alsanjari N, Lynch MJ, Fisher C et al: Vesical clear cell adenocarcinoma versus nephrogenic adenoma: a diagnostic problem, Histopathology 27:43-49, 1995.
109. McIntire TL, Soloway MS, Conway S: Nephrogenic adenoma, Urology 29:237-241, 1987.
110. Patel PS, Wilbur AC: Nephrogenic adenoma presenting as a calcified mass, AJR Am J Roentgenol 150:1071-1072, 1988.
111. Melicow MM, Uson AC: The "herald" lesion of the bladder: a lesion which portends the approach of cancer or inflammation from outside the bladder, J Urol 85:543-551, 1961.
112. Melicow MM, Uson AC, Stams U: Herald lesion of urinary bladder, a nonspecific but significant process, Urology 3:140-147, 1974.
113. Mostofi FK: Potentialities of bladder epithelium, J Urol 71:705-714, 1954.
114. Buck EG: Polypoid cystitis mimicking transitional cell carcinoma, J Urol 131:963, 1984.
115. Ekelund P, Johansson S: Polypoid cystitis, a catheter associated lesion of the human bladder, Acta Pathol Microbiol Scand [A] 87:179-184, 1979.
116. Ekelund P, Anderström C, Johansson SL et al: The reversibility of catheter-associated polypoid cystitis, J Urol 130:456-459, 1983.
117. Young RH: Papillary and polypoid cystitis, a report of eight cases, Am J Surg Pathol 12:542-546, 1988.
118. Milles G: Catheter-induced hemorrhagic pseudopolyps of the urinary bladder, JAMA 193:968-969, 1965.
119. Slade N, Gaches C: Vesico-intestinal fistulae, Br J Surg 59:593-597, 1972.
120. Goldstein MJ, Bragg D, Sherlock P: Granulomatous bowel disease presenting as a bladder tumor, report of a case, Dig Dis 16:337-341, 1971.
121. Pugh JI: On the pathology and behaviour of acquired nontraumatic vesico-intestinal fistula, Br J Surg 51:644-657, 1964.
122. Joffe N: Roentgenologic abnormalities of the urinary bladder secondary to Crohn's disease, AJR Am J Roentgenol 127:297-302, 1976.
123. Lazarus JA, Marks MS: Vesico-intestinal fistula: actual and incipient. Early diagnosis and treatment, Am J Surg 59:526-535, 1943.
124. Demos TC, Moncada R: Inflammatory gastrointestinal disease presenting as genitourinary disease, Urology 13:115-121, 1979.
125. Gray FW, Newman HR: Granuloma of the bladder associated with regional enteritis: case report, J Urol 78:393-397, 1957.

126. Carson CC, Malek RS, ReMine WH: Urologic aspects of vesicoenteric fistulas, J Urol 119:744-746, 1978.
127. Sarma KP: On the nature of cystitis follicularis, J Urol 104:709-714, 1970.
128. Marsh FP, Banerjee R, Panchamia P: The relationship between urinary infection, cystoscopic appearance and pathology of the bladder in man, J Clin Pathol 27:297-307, 1974.
129. Hinman F, Cordonnier J: Cystitis follicularis, J Urol 34:302-308, 1935.
130. Stirling WC: Cystitis follicularis, with a discussion of the other proliferative lesions of the bladder and report of four cases, JAMA 112:1326-1331, 1939.
131. Alexander S: Some observations respecting the pathology and pathological anatomy of nodular cystitis, Journal of Cutaneous and Genito-urinary Diseases 11:245-262, 1893.
132. Kretschmer HL: On the occurrence of lymphoid tissue in the urinary organs, J Urol 68:252-260, 1952.
133. Wells HG: Giant cells in cystitis, Arch Pathol Lab Med 26:32-43, 1938.
134. Johnson WW, Meadows DC: Urinary-bladder fibrosis and telangiectasia associated with long-term cyclophosphamide therapy, N Engl J Med 284:290-294, 1971.
135. Beyer-Boon ME, De Voogt HJ, Schaberg A: The effects of cyclophosphamide treatment on the epithelium and stroma of the urinary bladder, Eur J Cancer 14:1029-1035, 1978.
136. Millard RJ: Busulfan-induced hemorrhagic cystitis. Urology 18:143-144, 1981.
137. Murphy WM, Soloway MS, Finebaum PJ: Pathological changes associated with topical chemotherapy for superficial bladder cancer, J Urol 126:461-464, 1981.
138. deVries CR, Freiha FS: Hemorrhagic cystitis: a review, J Urol 143:1-9, 1990.
139. Treible DP, Skinner D, Kasimain D et al: Intractable bladder hemorrhage requiring cystectomy after use of intravesical thiotepa, Urology 30:568-570, 1987.
140. Rubin JS, Rubin RT: Cyclophosphamide hemorrhagic cystitis, J Urol 96:313-316, 1966.
141. Lawrence HJ, Simone J, Aur RJA: Cyclophosphamide-induced hemorrhagic cystitis in children with leukemia, Cancer 36:1572-1576, 1975.
142. Stillwell TJ, Benson RC, Jr: Cyclophosphamide-induced hemorrhagic cystitis, a review of 100 patients, Cancer 61:451-457, 1988.
143. Rowland RG, Eble JN: Bladder leiomyosarcoma and pelvic fibroblastic tumor following cyclophosphamide therapy, J Urol 130:344-346, 1983.
144. Pedersen-Bjergaard J, Ersbøll J, Hansen VL et al: Carcinoma of the urinary bladder after treatment with cyclophosphamide for non-Hodgkin's lymphoma, N Engl J Med 318:1028-1032, 1988.
145. Fairchild WV, Spence CR, Solomon HD et al: The incidence of bladder cancer after cyclophosphamide therapy, J Urol 122:163-164, 1979.
146. Skene AJC. Treatise on diseases of the bladder and urethra in women, New York, 1887, William and Wood.
147. Nitze M: Lehrbuch der kystoscopie, ed 2, Berlin, 1907.
148. Hunner GL: A rare type of bladder ulcer in women: report of cases, Transactions of Southern Surgeons and Gynecologists 27:247-292, 1914.
149. Kretschmer HL: Elusive ulcer of the bladder, J Urol 42:385-395, 1939.
150. Higgins CC: Hunner ulcer of the bladder (review of 100 cases), Ann Intern Med 15:708-715, 1941.
151. Hand JR: Interstitial cystitis: report of 223 cases (204 women and 19 men), J Urol 61:291-310, 1949.
152. Burford EH, Burford CE: Hunner ulcer of the bladder: a report of 187 cases, J Urol 79:952-955, 1958.
153. de Juana CP, Everett JC, Jr: Interstitial cystitis: experience and review of recent literature, Urology 10:325-329, 1977.
154. Koziol JA, Clark DC, Gittes RF et al: The natural history of interstitial cystitis: a survey of 374 patients, J Urol 149:465-469, 1993.
155. Messing EM, Stamey TA: Interstitial cystitis: early diagnosis, pathology and treatment, Urology 12:381-392, 1978.
156. Meares EM, Jr: Guest editorial: interstitial cystitis—1987, Urology 29:46-48, 1987.
157. Johansson SL, Fall M: Clinical features and spectrum of light microscopic changes in interstitial cystitis, J Urol 143:1118-1124, 1990.
158. Simmons JL, Bunce PL: On the use of an antihistamine in the treatment of interstitial cystitis, Am Surg 24:664-667, 1958.
159. Kastrup J, Hald T, Larsen S et al: Histamine content and mast cell count of detrusor muscle in patients with interstitial cystitis and other types of chronic cystitis, Br J Urol 55:495-500, 1983.
160. Larsen S, Thompson SA, Hald T et al: Mast cells in interstitial cystitis, Br J Urol 54:283-286, 1982.
161. Hellstrom HR, Davis BK, Shonnard JW: Eosinophilic cystitis, a study of 16 cases, Am J Clin Pathol 72:777-784, 1979.
162. Castillo J, Jr, Cartagena R, Montes M: Eosinophilic cystitis: a therapeutic challenge, Urology 32:535-537, 1988.
163. Rubin L, Pincus MB: Eosinophilic cystitis: the relationship of allergy in the urinary tract to eosinophilic cystitis and the pathophysiology of eosinophilia, J Urol 112:457-460, 1974.
164. Gregg JA, Utz DC: Eosinophilic cystitis associated with eosinophilic gastroenteritis, Mayo Clin Proc 49:185-187, 1974.
165. Perlmutter AD, Edlow JB, Kevy SV: Toxocara antibodies in eosinophilic cystitis, J Pediatr 73:340-344, 1968.
166. Oh SJ, Chi JG, Lee SE: Eosinophilic cystitis caused by vesical sparganosis: a case report, J Urol 149:581-583, 1993.
167. Thijssen A, Gerridzen RG: Eosinophilic cystitis presenting as invasive bladder cancer: comments on pathogenesis and management, J Urol 144:977-979, 1990.
168. Hansen MV, Kristensen PB: Eosinophilic cystitis simulating invasive bladder carcinoma. Case report, Scand J Urol Nephrol 27:275-277, 1993.
169. Lowe D, Jorizzo J, Hutt MSR: Tumour-associated eosinophilia: a review, J Clin Pathol 34:1343-1348, 1981.
170. Eble JN, Banks ER: Post-surgical necrobiotic granulomas of urinary bladder, Urology 35:454-457, 1990.
171. Spagnolo DV, Waring PM: Bladder granulomata after bladder surgery, Am J Clin Pathol 86:430-437, 1986.
172. Sørensen FB, Marcussen N: Iatrogenic granulomas of the prostate and the urinary bladder, Pathol Res Pract 182:822-830, 1987.
173. Washida H, Watanabe H, Noguchi Y et al: Tissue effects in the bladder wall after contact Nd: YAG laser irradiation for bladder tumors, World J Urol 10:115-119, 1992.

174. Witjes JA, van der Meijden APM, Debruyne FMJ: Use of intravesical bacillus Calmette-Guérin in the treatment of superficial transitional cell carcinoma of the bladder: an overview, Urol Int 45:129-136, 1990.
175. Harland SJ, Charig CR, Highman W et al: Outcome in carcinoma in situ of bladder treated with intravesical bacille Calmette-Guérin, Br J Urol 70:271-275, 1992.
176. Akaza H, Hinotsu S, Aso Y et al: Bacillus Calmette-Guérin treatment of existing papillary bladder cancer and carcinoma in situ of the bladder, Cancer 75:552-559, 1995.
177. Patard JJ, Chopin DK, Boccon-Gibod L: Mechanisms of action of bacillus Calmette-Guérin in the treatment of superficial bladder cancer, World J Urol 11:165-168, 1993.
178. Adolphs HD, Schwabe HW, Helpap B et al: Cytomorphological and histological studies on the urothelium during and after chemoimmune prophylaxis, Urol Res 12:129-133, 1984.
179. Lage JM, Bauer WC, Kelley DR et al: Histological parameters and pitfalls in the interpretation of bladder biopsies in bacillus Calmette-Guérin treatment of superficial bladder cancer, J Urol 135:916-919, 1986.
180. Shapiro A, Lijovetzky G, Pode D: Changes of the mucosal architecture and of urine cytology during BCG treatment, World J Urol 6:61-64, 1988.
181. Pagano F, Bassi P, Milani C et al: Pathologic and structural changes in the bladder after BCG intravesical therapy in men, Prog Clin Biol Res 310:81-91, 1989.
182. Rigatti P, Colombo R, Montorsi F et al: Local bacillus Calmette-Guérin therapy for superficial bladder cancer: clinical, histological and ultrastructural patterns, Scand J Urol Nephrol 24:191-198, 1990.
183. Badalament RA, Gay H, Cibas ES et al: Monitoring intravesical bacillus Calmette-Guérin treatment of superficial bladder carcinoma by postoperative urinary cytology, J Urol 138:763-765, 1987.
184. Betz SA, See WA, Cohen MB: Granulomatous inflammation in bladder wash specimens after intravesical bacillus Calmette-Guérin therapy for transitional cell carcinoma of the bladder, Am J Clin Pathol 99:244-248, 1993.
185. Stilmant MM, Siroky MB: Nephrogenic adenoma associated with intravesical bacillus Calmette-Guérin treatment: a report of 2 cases, J Urol 135:359-361, 1986.
186. Brandt WE: Unusual complications of hernia repairs: large symptomatic granulomas, Am J Surg 92:640-643, 1956.
187. Stearns DB, Gordon SK: Granuloma of the bladder following inguinal herniorrhaphy: report of a case with gross hematuria, Boston Med Q 10:52-53, 1959.
188. Daniel WJ, Aarons BJ, Hamilton NT et al: Paravesical granuloma presenting as a late complication of herniorrhaphy, Aust N Z J Surg 43:38-40, 1973.
189. Helms CA, Clark RE: Post-herniorrhaphy suture granuloma simulating a bladder neoplasm, Radiology 124:56, 1977.
190. Pearl GS, Someren A: Suture granuloma simulating bladder neoplasm, Urology 15:304-306, 1980.
191. Katz PG, Crawford JP, Hackler RH: Infected suture granuloma simulating mass of urachal origin: case report, J Urol 135:782-783, 1986.
192. Flood HD, Beard RC: Post-herniorrhaphy paravesical granuloma, Br J Urol 61:266-268, 1988.
193. Walther M, Glenn JF, Vellios F: Xanthogranulomatous cystitis, J Urol 134:745-746, 1985.
194. Nishimura K, Nozawa M, Hara T et al: Xanthoma of the bladder, J Urol 153:1912-1913, 1995.
195. Cyr WL, Johnson H, Balfour J: Granulomatous cystitis as a manifestation of chronic granulomatous disease of childhood, J Urol 110:357-359, 1973.
196. Berman HH, Wilets AJ: Rheumatoid pseudotumor of urinary bladder simulating carcinoma, Urology 9:83-85, 1977.
197. Greenstein AJ, Janowitz HD, Sachar DB: The extra-intestinal complications of Crohn's disease and ulcerative colitis: a study of 700 patients, Medicine 55:401-412, 1976.
198. Tammela T, Kallioinen M, Kontturi M et al: Sarcoidosis of the bladder: a case report and literature review, J Urol 141:608-609, 1989.
199. Gowing NFC: III. Pathological changes in the bladder following irradiation, a contribution to a symposium on "Treatment of carcinoma of the bladder" at the British Institute of Radiology on January 14, 1960, Br J Radiol 33:484-487, 1960.
200. Fajardo LF, Berthrong M: Radiation injury in surgical pathology. Part I, Am J Surg Pathol 2:159-199, 1978.
201. Warren S: Effects of radiation on tissues. VII. Effects of radiation on the urinary system, the kidneys and ureters, Arch Pathol 34:1079-1084, 1942.
202. Suresh UR, Smith VJ, Lupton EW et al: Radiation disease of the urinary tract: histological features of 18 cases, J Clin Pathol 46:228-231, 1993.
203. Murphy WM, Soloway MS, Lin CJ: Morphologic effects of thio-TEPA on mammalian urothelium, changes in abnormal cells, Acta Cytol 22:550-554, 1978.
204. Stirling WC, Hopkins GA: Gangrene of the bladder, review of two hundred seven cases; report of two personal cases, J Urol 31:517-525, 1934.
205. Cristol DS, Greene LF: Gangrenous cystitis, etiologic classification and treatment, Surgery 18:343-346, 1945.
206. Maggio AJ, Jr, Lupu A: Gangrene of bladder, Urology 18:390-391, 1981.
207. Devitt AT, Sethia KK: Gangrenous cystitis: case report and review of the literature, J Urol 149:1544-1545, 1993.
208. Hager BH, Magath TB: The etiology of incrusted cystitis with alkaline urine, JAMA 85:1352-1355, 1925.
209. Hager BH: Clinical data on alkaline incrusted cystitis, J Urol 16:447-457, 1926.
210. Letcher HG, Matheson NM: Encrustation of the bladder as a result of alkaline cystitis, Br J Surg 23:716-720, 1935.
211. Randall A, Campbell EW: Alkaline incrusted cystitis, J Urol 37:284-299, 1937.
212. Jameson RM: The treatment of phosphatic encrusted cystitis (alkaline cystitis) with nalidixic acid, Br J Urol 38:89-92, 1966.
213. Jameson RM: Phosphatic encrusted cystis, Br J Clin Pract 21:463-465, 1967.
214. Harrison RB, Stier FM, Cochrane JA: Alkaline encrusting cystitis, AJR Am J Roentgenol 130:575-577, 1978.
215. Pollack HM, Banner MP, Martinez LO et al: Diagnostic considerations in urinary bladder wall calcification, AJR Am J Roentgenol 136:791-797, 1981.
216. Mills RG: Cystitis emphysematosa, I. Report of cases in men, J Urol 23:289-306, 1930.
217. Mills RG: Cystitis emphysematosa, II. Report of a series of cases in women, JAMA 94:321-332, 1930.
218. Redewill FH: Cystitis cystica emphysematosa, Urol Cutan Rev 38:537-543, 1934.

219. Levin HA: Gas cysts of urinary bladder, J Urol 39:45-52, 1938.
220. Bailey H: Cystitis emphysematosa, 19 cases with intraluminal and interstitial collections of gas, AJR Am J Roentgenol 86:850-862, 1961.
221. Singh CR, Lytle WF, Jr: Cystitis emphysematosa caused by *Candida albicans*, J Urol 130:1171-1173, 1983.
222. Rocca JM, McClure J: Cystitis emphysematosa, Br J Urol 57:585, 1985.
223. Hawtrey CE, Williams JJ, Schmidt JD: Cystitis emphysematosa, Urology 3:612-614, 1974.
224. Maliwan N: Emphysematous cystitis associated with *Clostridium perfringens* bacteremia, J Urol 121:819-820, 1979.
225. Bartkowski DP, Lanesky JR: Emphysematous prostatitis and cystitis secondary to *Candida albicans*, J Urol 139:1063-1065, 1988.
226. Quint HJ, Drach GW, Rappaport WD et al: Emphysematous cystitis: a review of the spectrum of disease, J Urol 147:134-137, 1992.
227. Brodie N: Infected urachal cysts, Am J Surg 69:243-248, 1945.
228. MacMillan RW, Schullinger JN, Santulli TV: Pyourachus: an unusual surgical problem, J Pediatr Surg 8:387-389, 1973.
229. Hinman F, Jr: Surgical disorders of the bladder and umbilicus of urachal origin, Surg Gynecol Obstet 113:605-614, 1961.
230. Newman BM, Karp MP, Jewett TC et al: Advances in the management of infected urachal cysts, J Pediatr Surg 21:1051-1054, 1986.
231. Michaelis L, Gutmann C: Ueber Einschlüsse in Blasentumoren, Z Klin Med 47:208-215, 1902.
232. von Hansemann D: Über Malakoplakie der Harnblase, Virchows Arch Pathol Anat Physiol Klin Med 173:302-308, 1903.
233. Damjanov I, Katz SM: Malakoplakia, Pathol Annu 16:103-128, 1981.
234. McClure J: Malakoplakia, J Pathol 140:275-330, 1983.
235. Sinclair-Smith C, Kahn LB, Cywes S: Malacoplakia in childhood, case report with ultrastructural observations and review of the literature, Arch Pathol 99:198-203, 1975.
236. Lou TY, Teplitz C: Malakoplakia: pathogenesis and ultrastructural features, Hum Pathol 5:191-207, 1974.
237. Abdou NI, NaPombejara C, Sagawa A et al: Malakoplakia: evidence for monocyte lysosomal abnormality correctable by cholinergic agonist in vitro and in vivo, N Engl J Med 297:1413-1419, 1977.
238. McClurg FV, D'Agostino AN, Martin JH et al: Ultrastructural demonstration of intracellular bacteria in three cases of malakoplakia of the bladder, Am J Clin Pathol 60:780-788, 1973.
239. Qualman SJ, Gupta PK, Mendelsohn G: Intracellular *Escherichia coli* in urinary malakoplakia: a reservoir of infection and its therapeutic implications, Am J Clin Pathol 81:35-42, 1984.
240. Steven S, McClure J: The histochemical features of the Michaelis-Gutmann body and a consideration of the pathophysiological mechanisms of its formation, J Pathol 137:119-127, 1982.
241. McClure J, Cameron CHS, Garrett R: The ultrastructural features of malakoplakia, J Pathol 134:13-25, 1981.
242. Auerbach O: The pathology of urogenital tuberculosis, New International Clinics 3:21-61, 1940.
243. Christensen WI: Genitourinary tuberculosis: review of 102 cases, Medicine 53:377-390, 1974.
244. Stoller JK: Late recurrence of *Mycobacterium bovis* genitourinary tuberculosis: case report and review of literature, J Urol 134:565-566, 1985.
245. Lazarus JA: Prevention and treatment of delayed wound healing and ulcerative cystitis following surgery for tuberculosis of the urinary tract, J Urol 55:160-163, 1946.
246. Michigan S: Genitourinary fungal infections, J Urol 116:390-397, 1976.
247. Wise GJ, Silver DA: Fungal infections of the genitourinary system, J Urol 149:1377-1388, 1993.
248. Rohner TJ, Tuliszewski RM: Fungal cystitis: awareness, diagnosis and treatment, J Urol 124:142-144, 1980.
249. Sakamoto S, Ogato J, Sakazaki Y et al: Fungus ball formation of Aspergillus in the bladder, an unusual case report, Eur Urol 4:388-389, 1978.
250. McClure J, Young RH: Infectious disease of the urinary bladder, including malacoplakia. In Young RH, ed: Pathology of the urinary bladder, New York, 1989, Churchill Livingstone.
251. Kleiman H, Lancaster Y: Condyloma acuminata of the bladder, J Urol 88:52-55, 1962.
252. Pompeius R, Ekroth R: A successfully treated case of condyloma acuminatum of the urethra and urinary bladder, Eur Urol 2:298-299, 1976.
253. Keating MA, Young RH, Carr CP et al: Condyloma acuminatum of the bladder and ureter: case report and review of the literature, J Urol 133:465-467, 1985.
254. van Poppel H, Stessens R, de Vos R et al: Isolated condyloma acuminatum of the bladder in a patient with multiple sclerosis: etiological and pathological considerations, J Urol 136:1071-1073, 1986.
255. Walther M, O'Brien DP, Birch HW: Condyloma acuminata and verrucous carcinoma of the bladder: case report and literature review, J Urol 135:362-365, 1986.
256. Del Mistro A, Koss LG, Braunstein J et al: Condyloma acuminata of the urinary bladder, natural history, viral content, and DNA content, Am J Surg Pathol 12:205-215, 1988.
257. Shirai T, Yamamoto K, Adachi T et al: Condyloma acuminatum of the bladder in two autopsy cases, Acta Pathol Jpn 38:399-405, 1988.
258. Mufson MA, Belshe RB: A review of adenoviruses in the etiology of acute hemorrhagic cystitis, J Urol 115:191-194, 1976.
259. Numazaki Y, Shigeta S, Kumasaka T et al: Acute hemorrhagic cystitis in children, isolation of adenovirus type 11, N Engl J Med 278:700-704, 1968.
260. Hanash KA, Pool TL: Interstitial and hemorrhagic cystitis: viral, bacterial and fungal studies, J Urol 104:705-706, 1970.
261. Shindo K, Kitayama T, Ura T et al: Acute hemorrhagic cystitis caused by adenovirus type 11 after renal transplantation, Urol Int 41:152-155, 1986.
262. Mufson MA, Belshe RB, Horrigan TJ et al: Cause of acute hemorrhagic cystitis in children, Am J Dis Child 126:605-609, 1973.

263. Ambinder RF, Burns W, Forman M et al: Hemorrhagic cystitis associated with adenovirus infection in bone marrow transplantation, Arch Intern Med 146:1400-1401, 1986.
264. Apperley JF, Rice SJ, Bishop JA et al: Late-onset hemorrhagic cystitis associated with urinary excretion of polymaviruses after bone marrow transplantation, Transplantation 43:108-112, 1987.
265. DeHertogh DA, Brettman LR: Hemorrhagic cystitis due to herpes simplex virus as a marker of disseminated herpes infection, Am J Med 84:632-635, 1988.
266. Richmond W: The genito-urinary manifestations of herpes zoster, three case reports and a review of the literature, Br J Urol 46:193-200, 1974.
267. Wong T-W, Warner NE: Cytomegalic inclusion disease in adults, report of 14 cases with review of literature, Arch Pathol 74:403-422, 1962.
268. Smith JH, Christie JD: The pathobiology of *Schistosoma haematobium* infection in humans, Hum Pathol 17:333-345, 1986.
269. Bilharz T: Distomum Haematobium und sein Verhältniss zu gewissen pathologischen Veränderungen der menschlichen Harnorgane, Wiener Medizinische Wochenschrift 6:49-52, 1856.
270. von Lichtenberg F, Erickson DG, Sadun EH: Comparative histopathology of schistosome granulomas in the hamster, Am J Pathol 72:149-178, 1973.
271. Smith JH, Kelada AS, Khalil A et al: Surgical pathology of schistosomal obstructive uropathy: a clinicopathologic correlation, Am J Trop Med Hyg 26:96-108, 1977.
272. Kamel IA, Cheever AW, Elwi AM et al: *Schistosoma mansoni* and *S. haematobium* infections in Egypt. I. Evaluation of techniques for recovery of worms and eggs at necropsy, Am J Trop Med Hyg 26:696-701, 1977.
273. Cheever AW, Kamel IA, Elwi AM et al: *Schistosoma mansoni* and *S. haematobium* infections in Egypt. II. Quantitative parasitological findings at necropsy, Am J Trop Med Hyg 26:702-716, 1977.
274. Christie JD, Crouse D, Pineda J et al: Patterns of *Schistosoma haematobium* egg distribution in the human lower urinary tract. I. Noncancerous lower urinary tracts, Am J Trop Med Hyg 35:743-751, 1986.
275. Gelfand M, Ross CMD, Blair DM et al: Schistosomiasis of the male pelvic organs, severity of infection as determined by digestion of tissue and histologic methods in 300 cadavers, Am J Trop Med Hyg 19:779-784, 1970.
276. Makar N: Cystoscopic appearances of bilharziosis of the bladder, Br J Urol 4:209-216, 1932.
277. Fam A, Le Golvan PC: Bilharzial bladder-neck obstruction, Br J Urol 32:165-177, 1960.
278. Smith JH, Torky H, Kelada AS et al: Schistosomal polyposis of the urinary bladder, Am J Trop Med Hyg 26:85-88, 1977.
279. El-Badawi AA: Bilharzial polypi of the urinary bladder, Br J Urol 38:24-35, 1966.
280. Ibrahim A: The relationship between urinary bilharziasis and urolithiasis in the Sudan, Br J Urol 50:294-297, 1978.
281. Cutajar CL: The role of schistosomiasis in urolithiasis, Br J Urol 55:349-352, 1983.
282. Smith JH, Kelada AS, Khalil A: Schistosomal ulceration of the urinary bladder, Am J Trop Med Hyg 26:89-95, 1977.
283. Gutierrez J, Nesbit RM: Ectopic prostatic tissue in bladder, J Urol 98:474-478, 1967.
284. Rubin J, Khanna OP, Damjanov I: Adenomatous polyp of the bladder: a rare cause of hematuria in young men, J Urol 126:549-550, 1981.
285. Klein HZ, Rosenberg ML: Ectopic prostatic tissue in bladder trigone, distinctive cause of hematuria, Urology 23:81-82, 1984.
286. Remick DG, Jr, Kumar NB: Benign polyps with prostatic-type epithelium of the urethra and the urinary bladder, a suggestion of histogenesis based on histologic and immunohistochemical studies, Am J Surg Pathol 8:833-839, 1984.
287. Bernstein RG, Siegelman SS, Tein AB et al: Huge filling defect in the bladder caused by intravesical enlargement of the prostate, Radiology 92:1447-1452, 1969.
288. Korsower JM, Reeder MM: Filling defect in the urinary bladder, JAMA 231:408-409, 1975.
289. Faber RB, Kirchner FK, Jr, Braren V: Benign prostatic hyperplasia presenting as a massive bladder filling defect in a young man, J Urol 118:347-348, 1977.
290. Musselman P, Kay R: The spectrum of urinary tract fibroepithelial polyps in children, J Urol 136:476-477, 1986.
291. Ganem EJ, Ainsworth LB: Benign neoplasms of the urinary bladder in children: review of the literature and report of a case, J Urol 73:1032-1038, 1955.
292. Young RH: Fibroepithelial polyp of the bladder with atypical stromal cells, Arch Pathol Lab Med 110:241-242, 1986.
293. Moose LT, Garvey FK: Hamartoma of the bladder, J Urol 89:185-187, 1963.
294. Borski AA: Hamartoma of the bladder, J Urol 104:718-719, 1970.
295. Keating MA, Young RH, Lillehei CW et al: Hamartoma of the bladder in a 4-year-old girl with hamartomatous polyps of the gastrointestinal tract, J Urol 138:366-369, 1987.
296. Kinzel RC, Harrison EG, Jr, Utz DC: Primary localized amyloidosis of the bladder, J Urol 85:785-799, 1961.
297. Tripathi VNP, Desautels RE: Primary amyloidosis of the urogenital system: a study of 16 cases and brief review, J Urol 102:96-101, 1969.
298. Malek RS, Greene LF, Farrow GM: Amyloidosis of the urinary bladder, Br J Urol 43:189-200, 1971.
299. Akhtar M, Valencia M, Thomas AM: Solitary primary amyloidosis of urinary bladder, light and electron microscopic study, Urology 12:721-724, 1978.
300. Nakajima K, Hisazumi H, Okasyo A et al: Primary localized amyloidosis of bladder, Urology 15:302-303, 1980.
301. Caldamone AA, Elbadawi A, Moshtagi A et al: Primary localized amyloidosis of urinary bladder, Urology 15:174-181, 1980.
302. Khan SM, Birch PJ, Bass PS et al: Localized amyloidosis of the lower genitourinary tract: a clinicopathological and immunohistochemical study of nine cases, Histopathology 21:143-147, 1992.
303. Ehara H, Deguchi T, Yanagihara M et al: Primary localized amyloidosis of the bladder: an immunohistochemical study of a case, J Urol 147:458-460, 1992.
304. Grainger R, O'Riordan B, Cullen A et al: Primary amyloidosis of lower urinary tract, Urology 31:14-16, 1988.
305. Missen GAK, Tribe CR: Catastrophic haemorrhage from the bladder due to unrecognised secondary amyloidosis, Br J Urol 42:43-49, 1970.
306. Nurmi MJ, Ekfors TO, Puntala PV: Secondary amyloidosis of the bladder: a cause of massive hematuria, J Urol 138:44-45, 1987.

307. Proppe KH, Scully RE, Rosai J: Postoperative spindle cell nodules of the genitourinary tract resembling sarcomas, a report of eight cases, Am J Surg Pathol 8:101-108, 1984.
308. Huang W-L, Ro JY, Grignon DJ et al: Postoperative spindle cell nodule of the prostate and bladder, J Urol 143:824-826, 1990.
309. Vekemans K, Vanneste A, Van Oyen P et al: Postoperative spindle cell nodule of bladder, Urology 35:342-344, 1990.
310. Roth JA: Reactive pseudosarcomatous response in urinary bladder, Urology 16:635-637, 1980.
311. Nochomovitz LE, Orensteim JM: Inflammatory pseudotumor of the urinary bladder—possible relationship to nodular fasciitis, two case reports, cytologic observations, and ultrastructural observations, Am J Surg Pathol 9:366-373, 1985.
312. Ro JY, Ayala AG, Ordóñez NG et al: Pseudosarcomatous fibromyxoid tumor of the urinary bladder, Am J Clin Pathol 86:583-590, 1986.
313. Young RH, Scully RE: Pseudosarcomatous lesions of the urinary bladder, prostate gland, and urethra, Arch Pathol Lab Med 111:354-358, 1987.
314. Stark GL, Feddersen R, Lowe BA et al: Inflammatory pseudotumor (pseudosarcoma) of the bladder, J Urol 141:610-612, 1989.
315. Dietrick DD, Kabalin JN, Daniels GF, Jr et al: Inflammatory pseudotumor of the bladder, J Urol 148:141-144, 1992.
316. Jones EC, Clement PB, Young RH: Inflammatory pseudotumor of the urinary bladder: a clinicopathological, immunohistochemical, ultrastructural and flow cytometric study of 13 cases, Am J Surg Pathol 17:264-274, 1993.
317. August CZ, Khazoum SG, Mutchnik DL: Inflammatory pseudotumor of the bladder: a case report with DNA content analysis, J Urol Pathol 1:211-217, 1993.
318. Jufe R, Molinolo AA, Fefer SA et al: Plasma cell granuloma of the bladder: a case report, J Urol 131:1175-1176, 1984.
319. Lichtenheld FR, McCauley RT, Staples PP: Endometriosis involving the urinary tract, a collective review, Obstet Gynecol 17:762-768, 1961.
320. O'Conor VJ, Greenhill JP: Endometriosis of the bladder and ureter, Surg Gynecol Obstet 80:113-119, 1945.
321. Beecham CT, McCrea LE: Endometriosis of the urinary tract, Urol Surv 7:2-24, 1957.
322. Arap Neto W, Lopes RN, Cury M et al: Vesical endometriosis, Urology 24:271-274, 1984.
323. Aldridge KW, Burns JR, Singh B: Vesical endometriosis: a review and 2 case reports, J Urol 134:539-541, 1985.
324. Stanley KE, Jr, Utz DC, Dockerty MB: Clinically significant endometriosis of the urinary tract, Surg Gynecol Obstet 120:491-498, 1965.
325. Abeshouse BS, Abeshouse G: Endometriosis of the urinary tract: a review of the literature and a report of four cases of vesical endometriosis, J Int Coll Surg 34:43-63, 1960.
326. Sircus SI, Sant GR, Ucci AA, Jr: Bladder detrusor endometriosis mimicking interstitial cystitis, Urology 32:339-342, 1988.
327. Stewart WW, Ireland GW: Vesical endometriosis in a postmenopausal woman: a case report, J Urol 118:480-481, 1977.
328. Skor AB, Warren MM, Mueller EO, Jr: Endometriosis of bladder, Urology 9:689-692, 1977.
329. Vorstman B, Lynne C, Politano VA: Postmenopausal vesical endometriosis, Urology 22:540-542, 1983.
330. Pinkert TC, Catlow CE, Straus R: Endometriosis of the urinary bladder in a man with prostatic cancer, Cancer 43:1562-1567, 1979.
331. Oliker AJ, Harris AE: Endometriosis of the bladder in a male patient, J Urol 106:858-859, 1971.
332. Schrodt GR, Alcorn MO, Ibanez J: Endometriosis of the male urinary system: a case report, J Urol 124:722-723, 1980.
333. Clement PB, Young RH: Endocervicosis of the urinary bladder, a report of six cases of a benign müllerian lesion that may mimic adenocarcinoma, Am J Surg Pathol 16:533-542, 1992.
334. Parivar F, Bolton DM, Stoller ML: Endocervicosis of the bladder, J Urol 153:1218-1219, 1995.
334a. Young RH, Clement PB: Müllerianosis of the urinary bladder, Mod Pathol, 1996 (in press).
335. Ritchey ML, Benson RC, Jr, Kramer SA et al: Management of Müllerian duct remnants in the male patient, J Urol 140:795-799, 1988.
336. Felderman T, Schellhammer PF, Devine CJ, Jr et al: Müllerian duct cysts: conservative management, Urology 29:31-34, 1987.
337. Steele AA, Byrne AJ: Paramesonephric (müllerian) sinus of urinary bladder, Am J Surg Pathol 6:173-176, 1982.
338. Glenn JF: Agenesis of the bladder, JAMA 169:2016-2018, 1959.
339. Graham SD: Agenesis of bladder, J Urol 107:660-661, 1972.
340. Vakili BF: Agenesis of the bladder: a case report, J Urol 109:510-511, 1973.
341. Metoki R, Orikasa S, Ohta S et al: A case of bladder agenesis, J Urol 136:662-664, 1986.
342. Krull CL, Heyns CF, de Klerk DP: Agenesis of the bladder and urethra: a case report, J Urol 140:793-794, 1988.
343. Palmer JM, Russi MF: Persistent urogenital sinus with absence of the bladder and urethra, J Urol 102:590-594, 1969.
344. Duncan A: An attempt towards a systematic account of the appearances connected with that malconformation of the urinary organs in which the ureters, instead of terminating in a perfect bladder, open externally on the surface of the abdomen, Edinburgh Medical and Surgical Journal 1805-82:43-60, 1855.
345. Rickham PP: The incidence and treatment of ectopia vesicae, Proc R Soc Med 54:389-392, 1961.
346. Ives E, Coffey R, Carter CO: A family study of bladder exstrophy, J Med Genet 17:139-141, 1980.
347. Shapiro E, Lepor H, Jeffs RD: The inheritance of the exstrophy-epispadias complex, J Urol 132:308-310, 1984.
348. Hurwitz RS, Manzoni GAM, Ransley PG et al: Cloacal exstrophy: a report of 34 cases, J Urol 138:1060-1064, 1987.
349. Jeffs RD: Exstrophy and cloacal exstrophy, Urol Clin North Am 5:127-140, 1978.
350. McIntosh JF, Worley G, Jr: Adenocarcinoma arising in exstrophy of the bladder: report of two cases and review of the literature, J Urol 73:820-829, 1955.
351. Engel RM, Wilkinson HA: Bladder exstrophy, J Urol 104:699-704, 1970.
352. Marshall VF, Muecke EC: Variations in exstrophy of the bladder, J Urol 88:766-796, 1962.
353. Blakeley CR, Mills WG: The obstetric and gynaecological complications of bladder exstrophy and epispadias, Br J Obstet Gynaecol 88:167-173, 1981.

354. Hamdy MH, El-Kholi NA, El-Zayat S: Incomplete exstrophy of the bladder, Br J Urol 62:484-485, 1988.
355. Rudin L, Tannenbaum M, Lattimer JK: Histologic analysis of the exstrophied bladder after anatomical closure, J Urol 108:802-807, 1972.
356. Culp DA: The histology of the exstrophied bladder, J Urol 91:538-548, 1964.
357. Mesrobian H-GJ, Kelalis PP, Kramer SA: Long-term follow up of 103 patients with bladder exstrophy, J Urol 139:719-722, 1988.
358. Oesterling JE, Jeffs RD: The importance of a successful initial bladder closure in the surgical management of classical bladder exstrophy: analysis of 144 patients treated at The Johns Hopkins Hospital between 1975 and 1985, J Urol 137:258-262, 1987.
359. Nielsen K, Nielsen KK: Adenocarcinoma in exstrophy of the bladder—the last case in Scandinavia? A case report and review of the literature, J Urol 130:1180-1182, 1983.
360. Spencer R: Exstrophia splanchnia (exstrophy of the cloaca), Surgery 57:751-766, 1965.
361. Johnston JH: The genital aspects of exstrophy, J Urol 113:701-705, 1975.
362. Senger FL, Santare VJ: Congenital multilocular bladder: a case report, Trans Am Assoc Genitourinary Surg 43:114-119, 1951.
363. Abrahamson J: Double bladder and related anomalies: clinical and embryological aspects and a case report, Br J Urol 33:195-214, 1961.
364. Satter EJ, Mossman HW: A case report of a double bladder and double urethra in the female child, J Urol 79:274-278, 1958.
365. Ravitch MM, Scott WW: Duplication of the entire colon, bladder, and urethra, Surgery 34:843-858, 1953.
366. Burns E, Cummins H, Hyman J: Incomplete reduplication of the bladder with congenital solitary kidney: report of a case, J Urol 57:257-269, 1947.
367. Tacciuoli M, Laurenti C, Racheli T: Double bladder with complete sagittal septum: diagnosis and treatment, Br J Urol 47:645-649, 1975.
368. Ockerblad NF, Carlson HE: Congenital hourglass bladder, Surgery 8:665-671, 1940.
369. Uhlíř K: Rare malformations of the bladder, J Urol 99:53-58, 1968.
370. Sterling JA, Goldsmith R: Lesions of urachus which appear in the adult, Ann Surg 137:120-128, 1953.
371. Lattimer JK: Congenital deficiency of the abdominal musculature and associated genitourinary anomalies: a report of 22 cases, J Urol 79:343-352, 1958.
372. Schreck WR, Campbell WA, III: The relation of bladder outlet obstruction to urinary-umbilical fistula, J Urol 108:641-643, 1972.
373. Vaughan GT: Patent urachus. Review of the cases reported. Operation on a case complicated with stones in the kidneys. A note on tumors and cysts of the urachus, Trans Am Surg Assoc 23:273-294, 1905.
374. Hinman F, Jr: Urologic aspects of the alternating urachal sinus, Am J Surg 102:339-342, 1961.
375. Cullen TS: Embryology, anatomy, and diseases of the umbilicus together with diseases of the urachus, Philadelphia, 1916, W. B. Saunders.
376. Fox M, Power RF, Bruce AW: Diverticulum of the bladder—presentation and evaluation of treatment of 115 cases, Br J Urol 34:286-298, 1962.
377. Barrett DM, Malek RS, Kelalis PP: Observations on vesical diverticulum in childhood, J Urol 116:234-236, 1976.
378. Kretschmer HL: Diverticula of the urinary bladder, a clinical study of 236 cases, Surg Gynecol Obstet 71:491-503, 1940.
379. Hernanz-Schulman M, Lebowitz RL: The elusiveness and importance of bladder diverticula in children, Pediatr Radiol 15:399-402, 1985.
380. Livne PM, Gonzales ET, Jr: Congenital bladder diverticula causing ureteral obstruction, Urology 15:273-276, 1985.
381. Verghese M, Belman AB: Urinary retention secondary to congenital bladder diverticula in infants, J Urol 132:1186-1188, 1984.
382. Breivik N, Refsum S, Jr, Oppedal BR et al: Ehlers-Danlos syndrome and diverticula of the bladder, Z Kinderchir 40:243-246, 1985.
383. Harcke HT, Capitanio MA, Grover WD et al: Bladder diverticula and Menkes' syndrome, Radiology 124:459-461, 1977.
384. Schiff M, Jr, Lytton B: Congenital diverticulum of the bladder, J Urol 104:111-115, 1970.
385. Miller A: The aetiology and treatment of diverticulum of the bladder, Br J Urol 30:43-56, 1958.
386. Abeshouse BS, Goldstein AE: Primary carcinoma in a diverticulum of the bladder; a report of four cases and a review of the literature, J Urol 49:534-557, 1943.
387. Knappenberger ST, Uson AC, Melicow MM: Primary neoplasms occurring in vesical diverticula: a report of 18 cases, J Urol 83:153-159, 1960.
388. Faysal MH, Freiha FS: Primary neoplasm in vesical diverticula, a report of 12 cases, Br J Urol 53:141-143, 1981.
389. Montague DK, Boltuch RL: Primary neoplasms in vesical diverticula: report of 10 cases, J Urol 116:41-42, 1976.
390. Peterson LJ, Paulson DF, Glenn JF: The histopathology of vesical diverticula, J Urol 110:62-64, 1973.

Benign Epithelial Neoplasms
- Urothelial papilloma
- Inverted urothelial papilloma
- Villous adenoma

Malignant Epithelial Neoplasms
- Urothelial carcinoma
- Squamous cell carcinoma
- Adenocarcinoma
- Small cell carcinoma

Malignant Melanoma

Paraganglioma (Pheochromocytoma)

Germ Cell Neoplasms
- Choriocarcinoma
- Dermoid cyst
- Yolk Sac tumor

Benign Mesenchymal Neoplasms
- Leiomyoma
- Hemangioma
- Neurofibroma
- Granular cell tumor

Malignant Soft Tissue Neoplasms
- Rhabdomyosarcoma
- Leiomyosarcoma
- Malignant fibrous histiocytoma
- Osteosarcoma
- Fibrosarcoma
- Malignant mesenchymoma
- Angiosarcoma
- Hemangiopericytoma
- Liposarcoma
- Rhabdoid tumor

Lymphoreticular and Hematopoietic Neoplasms
- Malignant lymphoma
- Plasmacytoma
- Leukemia

Metastases

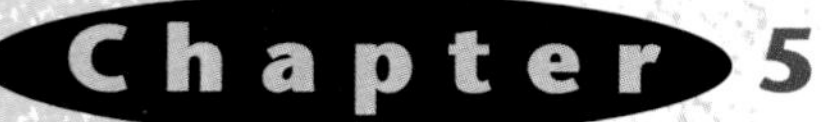

NEOPLASMS OF THE URINARY BLADDER

DAVID J. GRIGNON, M.D.

Tumors of the urinary bladder include neoplasms of virtually all types of tissue derivation, and the World Health Organization (WHO) classification reflects this diversity (see box on this page).[1] This chapter deals with conditions encompassed by Groups I through V (tumors); entities in Groups VI and VII (tumorlike lesions) are presented in chapter 4.

> **WORLD HEALTH ORGANIZATION: HISTOLOGICAL CLASSIFICATION OF URINARY BLADDER TUMORS**
>
> I. Epithelial Tumors
>   A. Transitional cell papilloma
>   B. Transitional cell papilloma, inverted type
>   C. Squamous cell papilloma
>   D. Transitional cell carcinoma
>   E. Variants of transitional cell carcinoma
>   1. With squamous metaplasia
>   2. With glandular metaplasia
>   3. With squamous and glandular metaplasia
>   F. Squamous cell carcinoma
>   G. Adenocarcinoma
>   H. Undifferentiated carcinoma
> II. Nonepithelial Tumors
>   A. Benign
>   B. Malignant
>   1. Rhabdomyosarcoma
>   2. Others
> III. Miscellaneous Tumors
>   A. Pheochromocytoma
>   B. Lymphoma
>   C. Carcinosarcoma
>   D. Malignant melanoma
>   E. Others
> IV. Metastatic Tumors and Secondary Extensions
> V. Unclassified Tumors
> VI. Epithelial Abnormalities
>   A. Papillary (polypoid) "cystitis"
>   B. von Brunn's nests
>   C. "Cystitis" cystica
>   D. Glandular metaplasia
>   E. "Nephrogenic" adenoma
>   F. Squamous metaplasia
> VII. Tumorlike Lesions
>   A. Follicular cystitis
>   B. Malakoplakia
>   C. Amyloidosis
>   D. Fibrous (fibroepithelial) polyp
>   E. Endometriosis
>   F. Hamartoma
>   G. Cysts

BENIGN EPITHELIAL NEOPLASMS

UROTHELIAL PAPILLOMA

Perhaps no topic in bladder pathology has sparked as much debate as the existence of and diagnostic criteria for urothelial papilloma of the urinary bladder. This controversy was reviewed in detail by Eble and Young.[2] Although most authorities currently accept the infrequent occurrence of such lesions based on restricted diagnostic criteria, the debate has now moved on to one of extending the diagnosis to a larger number of papillary tumors.

Historically the diagnosis of papilloma was limited to a small number of cases amounting to no more than 2% to 3% of papillary urothelial tumors.[3-5] These lesions are small, usually unifocal, and consist of delicate fibrovascular stalks covered by cytologically and architecturally normal urothelium (Fig. 5-1, 5-2).[5] Utilizing these criteria, papilloma occurs in a younger age group (usually younger than age 50 years) than most urothelial cancers. Development of new additional papillary tumors (often called *recurrences*) is common (73% in one series of 100 patients followed for a minimum of 180 months[6]) and later development of invasive urothelial carcinoma elsewhere in the urinary mucosa has been reported in up to 10% of patients.[3,6,7]

Jordan et al[8] and Murphy[9] have advocated extension of the diagnosis of papilloma to include all WHO grade 1 urothelial carcinomas. Reuter and Melamed[10] have also supported this extension of the definition of papilloma, and in the 1994 Armed Forces Institute of Pathology Fascicle, Murphy et al[11] recommend this approach. Arguments supporting this position maintain that these tumors are not malignant and do not have the capacity to invade or metastasize. Rather, these lesions are considered to be neoplastic based on their propensity to recur and an association with the subsequent development of carcinoma in a proportion of cases.[11] Using this approach, WHO grades 2 and 3 papillary urothelial carcinomas would be termed low- and high-grade urothelial carcinoma respectively. Urothelial papilloma as defined above made up 25% of newly diagnosed cases in the study of Jordan et al.[8] Of these patients, 3.3% later developed higher grade lesions and 4.4% died of bladder cancer.[8]

Many authorities,[6,12] including the National Bladder Cancer Study Group,[7] have not supported this position and see clinical value and prudence in continuing with current terminology. Although grade 1 papillary urothelial carcinoma rarely invades, patients with these tumors often later develop new, more aggressive, urothelial tumors;[7] in the National Bladder Cancer Study Group series, 61% of patients with noninvasive grade 1 tumor subsequently developed additional tumors, and 4.5% progressed to invasive disease.[7] In 16%, the new tumors were of higher histologic grade.

A major problem with adopting this suggestion relates to the lack of uniformity in the histological grading of tumors. Several authors have studied the interobserver and intraobserver variability in the grading of papillary urothelial neoplasms.[13-15] In the study of Ooms et al,[13] correlation coefficients for interobserver variability ranged from 0.46 to 0.67 and intraobserver variability from 0.50 to 0.67. These data suggest that up to 50% of patients with WHO grade 2 tumors would be misclassified as grade 1 (papilloma) with death from bladder cancer occurring in 12% of cases with WHO grade 2 tumor.[7]

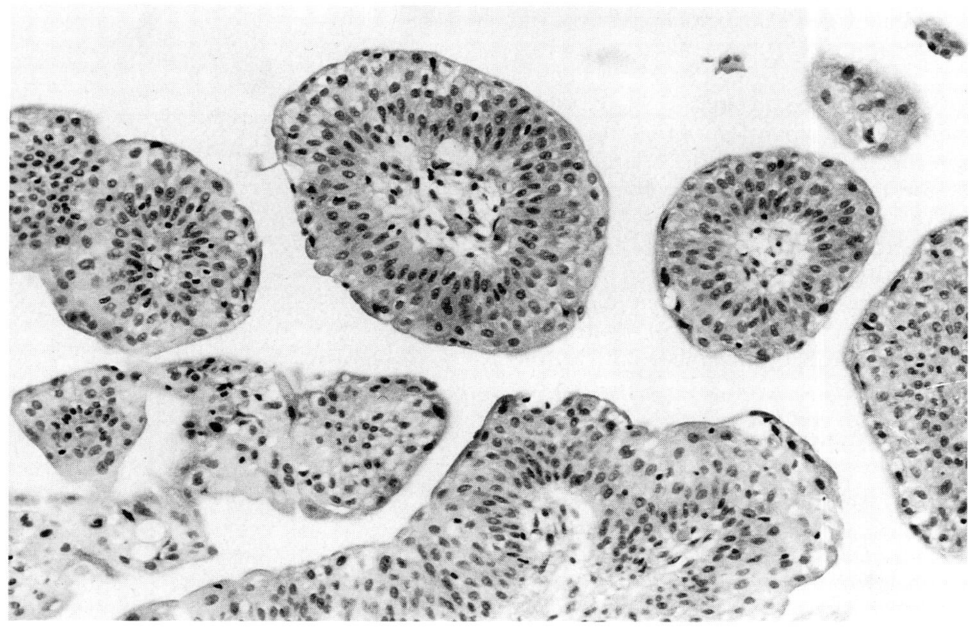

5-1. Urothelial papilloma with small fibrovascular cores covered by architecturally and cytologically normal urothelium.

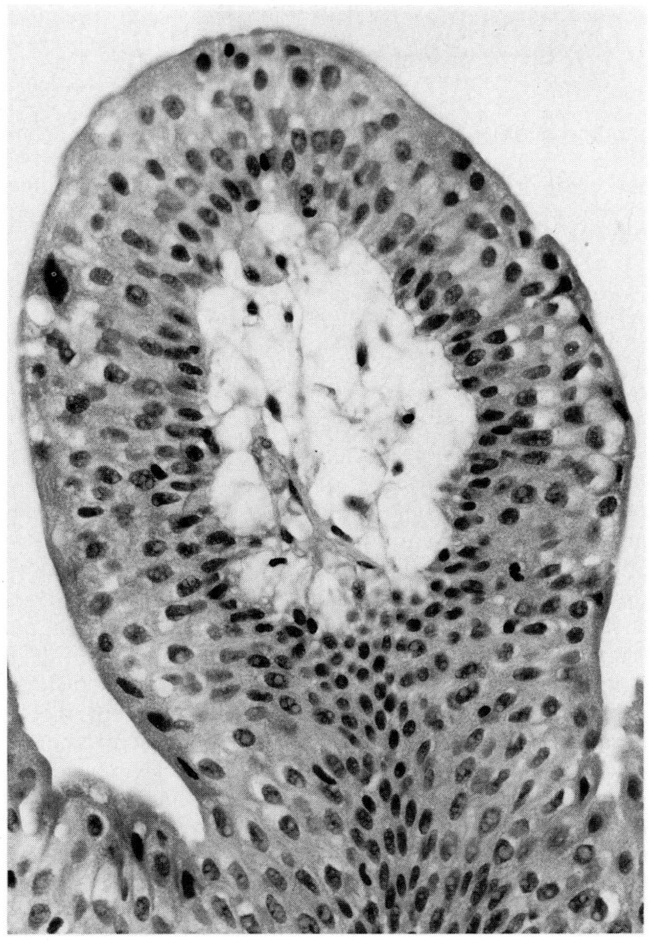

5-2. Urothelial papilloma highlighting the normal appearance of the surface urothelium.

The net effect would be a higher than anticipated rate of progression and death among patients diagnosed with urothelial papilloma.[8]

This limitation is highlighted in studies of invasive carcinoma. Proponents of the expansion of the urothelial papilloma category consider WHO grade 1 tumors to have no potential for invasion.[11] Reports from many groups have, however, considered a proportion, albeit a small one, of invasive carcinomas to actually be grade 1.[16-18] Until histologic criteria are better defined and it is demonstrated that they can be consistently applied, we recommend restriction of the diagnosis of urothelial papilloma to those tumors meeting the WHO criteria for papilloma.

INVERTED UROTHELIAL PAPILLOMA

Etiology and pathogenesis

This distinctive lesion was described by Paschkis in 1927,[19] and the term *inverted papilloma* was introduced by Potts and Hirst in 1963.[20] Other terms that have been applied to this lesion include *adenoma* and *Brunnian adenoma*.[21] The etiology of inverted papilloma of the urinary tract remains unknown. Some authors have viewed it as a neoplasm[22,23] but others consider it to be reactive, similar to proliferative urothelial lesions like cystitis glandularis and cystitis cystica.[24] Ultrastructural studies indicate similarity to normal urothelium and low-grade papillary urothelial tumors.[25,26]

Clinical features

Inverted papilloma accounts for 1% or less of urothelial tumors of the urinary bladder.[9] It occurs at all ages, with the youngest reported case occurring in a 14-year-old boy;[27] most patients are middle-aged, with a median age of 55 years.[28] It is more common in males (ratio 6.9:1) and usually presents with hematuria or irritative symptoms, but infrequently may produce obstructive symptoms.[28] Most cases are located in the trigone. The tumors are characteristically sessile or pedunculated with a smooth surface. Most are small (<3cm) and single, but lesions up to 8 cm in diameter have been reported[29] and multifocal lesions have been described.[30,31] Urine cytology may show atypical cells.[28]

Gross pathology

Inverted papilloma is usually removed by transurethral resection, and the surgical pathologist rarely has the opportunity to appreciate the gross characteristics of this lesion.[32] Cystoscopically, it often appears as a smooth, domed mass in the trigone.

Microscopic pathology

Inverted papilloma is characterized by anastomosing islands and trabeculae of urothelium originating from the overlying mucosa and growing downward into the stroma (Fig. 5-3). The surface urothelium may be normal or attenuated but should not have an exophytic papillary component.

Kunze et al[24] divided inverted papilloma into trabecular and glandular subtypes. The trabecular type is composed of anastomosing cords or sheets of urothelium, which are arranged at various angles to the mucosal surface (Fig. 5-4). These cords arise from the overlying urothelium. In some cases, cystic spaces lined by attenuated urothelium may be present within the islands. These spaces sometimes contain eosinophilic secretions that stain with periodic acid–Schiff reaction but not with mucicarmine.[23] The glandular subtype is composed of nests of urothelium with pseudoglandular or glandular differentiation. In pseudoglandular spaces, the lining remains urothelial in type, while in true glandular differentiation there is a layer of mucus-secreting cells lining the lumen (Fig. 5-5). The secretions stain with mucicarmine.[24] Intestinal metaplasia with goblet cells may be present. The epithelial elements are surrounded by basement membrane and separated by a delicate fibrovascular stroma.

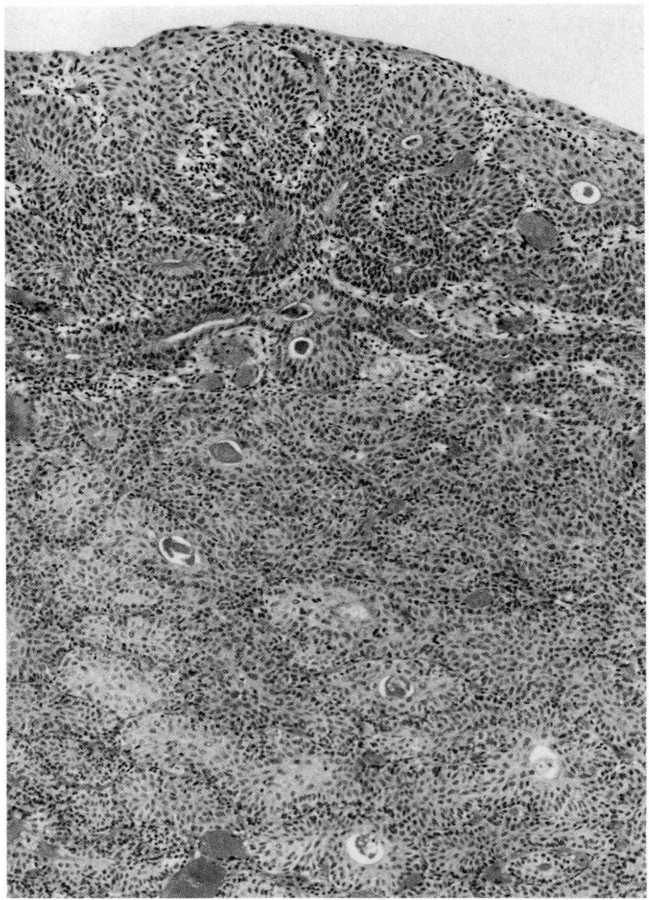

5-3. Inverted urothelial papilloma with normal urothelium at the surface and anastomosing trabeculae of urothelium extending downward into the lamina propria.

Nonkeratinizing squamous metaplasia is common. Although keratinization can occur, its presence is an indication of possible carcinoma. A single case was reported that contained cells with brightly eosinophilic granular cytoplasm indicating neuroendocrine differentiation;[33] chromogranin positive cells were subsequently identified immunohistochemically in three of eight other examples of inverted papilloma.[33]

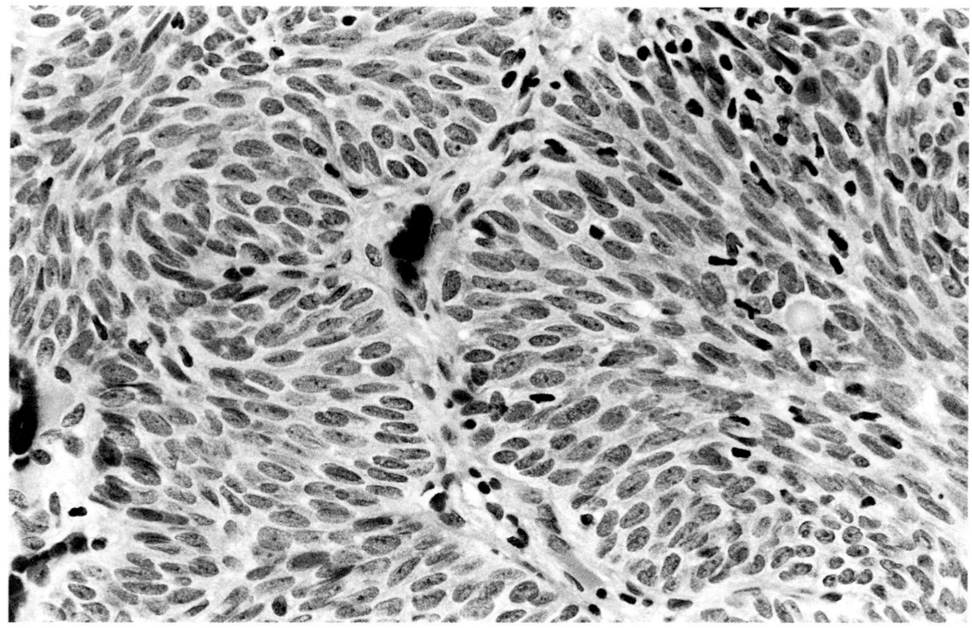

5-4. Inverted urothelial papilloma, trabecular type with anastomosing trabeculae of urothelium showing minimal atypia.

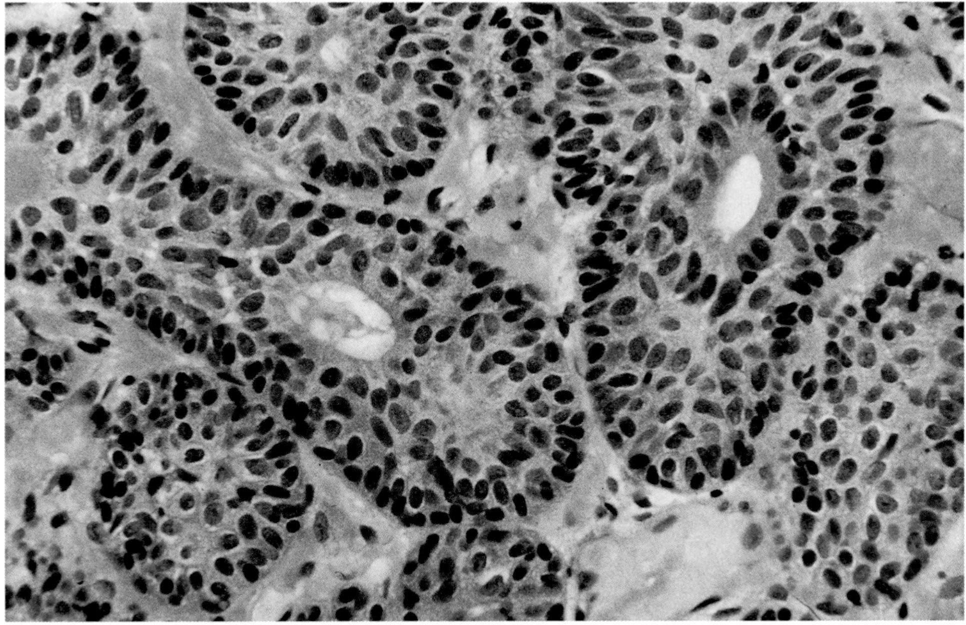

5-5. Inverted urothelial papilloma, glandular type with glandular spaces lined by columnar mucin-secreting cells within the trabeculae.

There is usually little or no cytologic atypia in inverted papilloma, but minor focal cytologic atypia is acceptable according to most authors.[9,22,24] Mitotic figures should be rare or absent.[22,24] Uyama et al[32] described a case with a medullary component containing spindle cell areas within the urothelial nests; scattered mitotic figures were present within these areas. The lesion was considered to be questionably malignant and the patient received adjuvant chemotherapy, but there was no evidence of recurrence at 4 months.

Relationship to urothelial carcinoma

The relationship between inverted papilloma and papillary urothelial lesions remains unresolved. The natural history of inverted papilloma is benign, and only rare cases have recurred.[28] Caro and Tessler[28] reported a recurrence rate of less than 1% based on a review of 104 cases, a rate much lower than would be expected with even low grade papillary urothelial neoplasms.[7] An increasing number of cases of inverted papilloma with recurrences[23,34-36] and coexistent urothelial carcinoma have been reported in the last few years.[23,31,34-40] In some of these cases, foci of papillary urothelial carcinoma appear to be arising from otherwise typical examples of inverted papilloma.* Some probably are urothelial carcinoma with an inverted growth pattern.[22,35,41,42] In a study of DNA content in inverted papilloma, Kunimi et al[43] found five inverted papillomas to be diploid and one of three inverted papillomas with associated urothelial carcinoma to be aneuploid.

Differential diagnosis

The major differential diagnostic consideration is urothelial carcinoma. The presence of an exophytic papillary component is incompatible with the diagnosis of inverted papilloma. When inverted papilloma becomes fragmented during transurethral resection, a pseudoexophytic pattern can result. The stromal cores in this instance will be wider and more variable than the fibrovascular cores of true papillary neoplasms. In those rare cases of typical inverted papilloma associated with an exophytic papillary lesion, both diagnoses should be rendered. Recognition that invasive urothelial carcinoma may have an inverted architecture mimicking inverted papilloma is important,[22,41] but this lesion is distinguished by significant cytologic atypia and mitotic activity and may focally have an invasive, infiltrative pattern typical of urothelial carcinoma.

Treatment and outcome

The treatment of choice for inverted papilloma is complete transurethral resection. In view of the rarity of local recurrence, additional therapy is not indicated. Follow-up with urine cytology and cystoscopic evaluations has been recommended by most authors.[35,36,44]

VILLOUS ADENOMA

There have been four documented examples of tumors occurring in the urinary bladder that are histologically identical to villous adenoma of the colon.[45-48] Similar lesions are more frequently described in the urachus.[49] Villous adenoma in the urinary bladder occurred in three men (73, 79, and 52 years old) and one woman (58 years old). All tumors appeared cystoscopically as exophytic papillary masses. Histologically, papillary fronds were covered by columnar mucus-secreting epithelium with goblet cells (Fig. 5-6, 5-7). In two tumors there was crowding and pseudostratification of the epithelium corresponding to mild dysplasia.[47,48] Argyrophilic neuroendocrine cells were demonstrated in one case.[47] In two cases, loss of normal ABO blood group expression was found in both the villous adenoma and associated cystitis glandularis.[46,48] In one case, lakes of extravasated mucin were present in the stroma, raising the possibility of invasion. Three patients were treated by transurethral resection and one by cystoprostatectomy; follow-up in three cases treated by transurethral resection showed no recurrence after 14, 18, and 60 months.

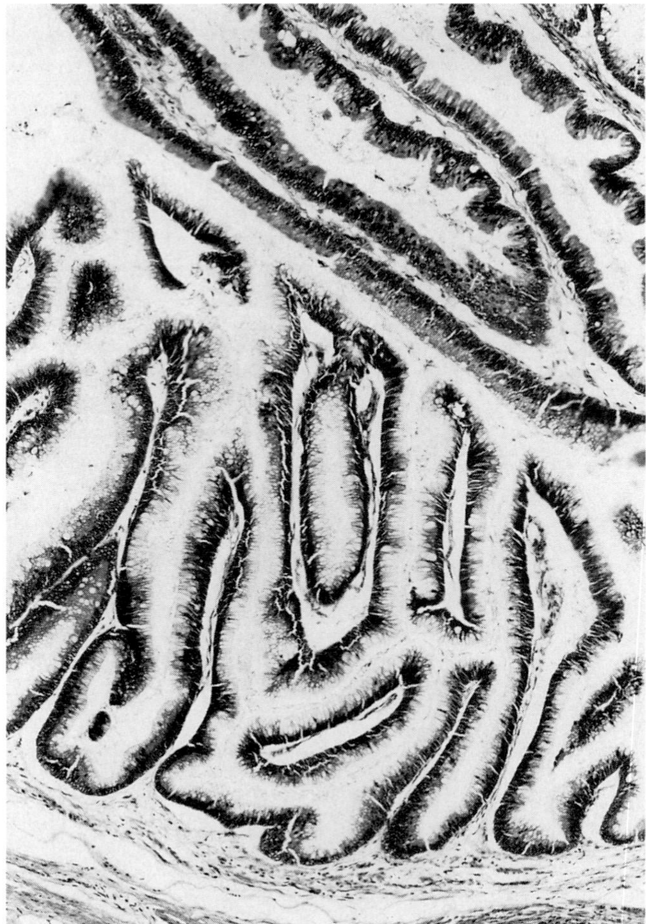

5-6. Villous adenoma of bladder with complex branching papillary structures lined by a pseudostratified epithelium containing goblet cells. There is no invasion into the underlying bladder wall.

The differential diagnosis of villous adenoma includes florid cystitis glandularis (polypoid cystitis glandularis) and well differentiated adenocarcinoma. The former does not have the well formed villous structures that are typi-

*References 31, 34, 36, 37, 39, 40.

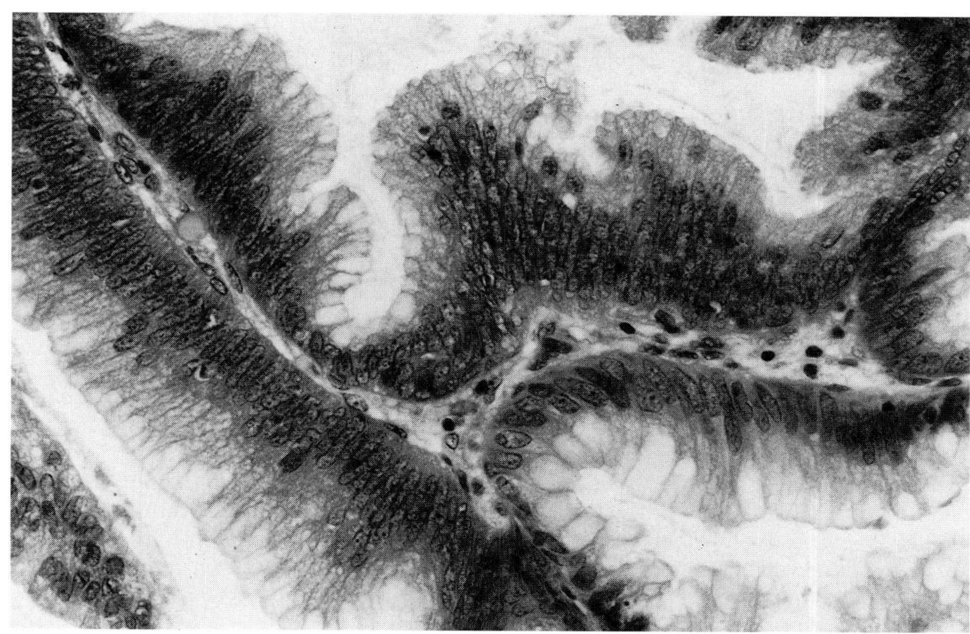

5-7. Epithelium of villous adenoma with pseudostratification, nuclear hyperchromasia and crowding, and goblet cells.

cal of villous adenoma. Adenocarcinoma with villous architecture occurs in the urinary bladder,[50] usually with severe atypia of the epithelium and invasion of the underlying stroma. In well differentiated villous adenocarcinoma, the epithelium is pseudostratified, and the nuclei are enlarged, crowded, and hyperchromatic,[50] features not present in cystitis glandularis.

MALIGNANT EPITHELIAL NEOPLASMS

UROTHELIAL CARCINOMA

Epidemiology

The incidence of bladder cancer varies throughout the world, with the highest rates in North America and Western Europe and the lowest in Japan.[51] In the United States, bladder cancer is approximately twice as common in whites as in African-Americans.[52] Bladder cancer also has a distinctive gender distribution, with a 2.7-fold higher incidence in men than women.[52] This difference is reflected in a nearly double death rate in men.[52]

Most bladder cancers develop in late adulthood, with the median age at diagnosis over 65 years of age.[52] Although uncommon, bladder cancer can develop in young patients and rarely in children.[53-58] The vast majority of the latter are low-grade papillary lesions, but rare examples of aggressive epithelial tumors have been described in the urinary bladder.

Etiology and pathogenesis

Many models of carcinogenesis have been based on the urinary bladder, highlighting this organ's importance in the development of our understanding of the neoplastic process. In part, this resulted from the recognition of carcinogenic agents and their relationship to bladder cancer in the nineteenth century (see box on this page). The exact mechanism of carcinogenesis remains uncertain in most cases; as in other tumor systems, new data regarding the role of cytogenetics, oncogenes, and suppressor genes are opening up new understanding of possible mechanisms. A comprehensive review of bladder carcinogenesis is beyond the scope of this discussion. In the next few paragraphs specific agents of general interest are discussed and overviews of current knowledge regarding cytogenetics, oncogenes, and suppressor genes are provided.

UROTHELIAL CARCINOMA: CARCINOGENIC AGENTS

Tobacco (smoking)
- Nitrosamines
- 2-naphthylamine

Occupational
- Benzidine
- 2-naphthylamine
- Chlorinated aliphatic hydrocarbons
- Arylamines
- Nitrosamines
- Other

Drugs
- Phenacetin
- Cyclophosphamide

Infections
- *S. haematobium*

Other

Tobacco smoke. It is estimated that 33% of bladder cancer cases are related to tobacco smoke.[59] Cigarette smokers have a 2- to 4-fold increase in risk of bladder cancer compared to nonsmokers.[60-62] The increased risk is similar in men and women and in different parts of the world.[60] The risk increases with increasing amounts smoked, increased duration of smoking, and inhalation practices.[60] Smoking filter-tipped cigarettes slightly reduces the risk.[63,64] Ex-smokers have a reduced risk, but the level of reduction and the length of time needed for the risk to return to that of nonsmokers is unknown.[60,65,66] There is a much lower increase in risk with cigar and pipe smoking.[61,67] Smokeless tobacco is not associated with an increased risk.[67]

Nitrosamines and 2-naphthylamine are known bladder carcinogens that are present in cigarette smoke, but whether they contribute to the increased risk in tobacco smokers remains unknown.[68] Histologic study of bladders of smokers reveals an increased number of atypical cells and thickening of the basal cell layer compared with nonsmokers.[69] The degree of change correlates strongly with the number of cigarettes smoked.[69]

Occupational exposure. It is estimated that occupational exposure accounts for up to 33% of bladder cancer cases in North America.[70] As early as 1895, it was recognized that workers in the dye industry had an increased risk of bladder cancer,[71] and subsequent studies demonstrated that these workers had death rates from bladder cancer that were 10 to 50 times higher than the general population.[72] The increased risk depends on the intensity and duration of the exposure; the chemicals most often implicated are benzidine (4,4-diaminodiphenyl) and 2-naphthylamine (aromatic amines).

Other industries have been linked to bladder cancer by case-control studies, but the association has been weaker than that for the dye industry.[60] Combustion gases, soot from coal, and chlorinated aliphatic hydrocarbons have been implicated.[73] Occupations reported to have an increased risk of bladder cancer include autoworkers, railway workers, machinists, drill press operators, electrical and electronic workers, plumbers, painters, truck drivers, leather workers, shoemakers and repairers, apparel manufacturers, rope and twine makers, dry cleaners, paper manufacturers, rubber workers (including shipping and warehousing), hairdressers, dental technicians, and physicians.[60,74-77]

Artificial sweeteners. The development of bladder tumors in male rats exposed to high levels of saccharin in utero or in the early prenatal period led to tremendous controversy concerning the risk for humans during the 1970s.[78] The animal results were initially supported by a case-control study that reported a 1.6-fold increased risk for men who used artificial sweeteners,[79] but subsequent studies failed to confirm these findings.[60,80] Histologic studies on human bladders revealed no difference in the urothelium of users of artificial sweeteners and controls.[69] The current opinion is that use of artificial sweeteners confers little or no risk of bladder cancer.[60]

Phenacetin. The data linking analgesic use to urothelial carcinoma in the bladder are not as strong as in the renal pelvis.[60] Case-control studies show a weak association between phenacetin use and bladder cancer.[81-83] The risk was significant only when high cumulative doses (in the range of 2 kg) were reached.[82] Other analgesics have no association with bladder cancer.[81,84]

Cyclophosphamide. Since the first report associating bladder carcinoma with cyclophosphamide in 1971,[85] a number of similar cases have been documented.[86-96] A cumulative risk of 10.7% at 12 years has been reported, with a latency period of 65 to 141 months.[95] In one study, 7 of 9 patients eventually died of bladder carcinoma.[95] The development of bladder cancer is believed to be the effect of the accumulation of acrolein, a degradation product of cyclophosphamide. Although the majority of reported tumors have been urothelial carcinoma, other histologic types of bladder cancer such as squamous cell carcinoma,[92] adenocarcinoma,[92] and leiomyosarcoma[97] have been described. Leiomyosarcoma occurred in a patient with hereditary retinoblastoma, a condition also known to be associated with the development of other malignancies including sarcomas.[98] In addition, a fibroblastic tumor of uncertain malignant potential has been described.[93]

Radiation. The development of bladder carcinoma has been reported in patients treated with radiation therapy.[99-101] The risk of urothelial carcinoma is increased 2- to 4-fold in women treated with radiation for cervical carcinoma.[99,101] In one study, the average interval between radiation exposure and development of bladder cancer was 20.5 years.[101] All nine patients in this report presented with advanced urothelial cancer without prior superficial disease.[101] The high grade and stage of radiation-associated bladder cancer have been recognized by other investigators.[100] In addition to urothelial carcinoma, adenocarcinoma[101] and sarcoma have also been described in patients with histories of radiation exposure.[102]

Coffee and tea. Some but not all studies have suggested an increased risk of bladder cancer in coffee and tea drinkers.[60,64,103-105] Morrison[60] concluded that the cumulative evidence linking coffee to bladder cancer indicates that the relationship, if any exists, must be weak. The confounding effect of coincidental cigarette smoking makes conclusions difficult.

Human papilloma virus. Human papilloma virus infection has been implicated as a causative factor in cancers of the anogenital region and upper respiratory tract. To date, there have been only limited studies of the association of human papilloma virus with bladder cancer, and these have had conflicting results.[106-109] Using in situ DNA hybridization and polymerase chain reaction, Kerley et al[106] found human papilloma virus DNA in only one of twenty-seven bladder cancers (a keratinizing squamous cell carcinoma in an immunocompromised 61-year-old woman). Similarly, Knowles[108] and Chang et al[109] found no evidence of human papilloma virus in over 200 cases studied by in situ hybridization and polymerase chain reaction. In contrast, Anwar et al[107] also used in situ hybridization and polymerase chain reaction, and identified human papilloma virus DNA in 81% of carcinomas studied (39 of 48). In the latter study, normal bladder mucosa from the same patients was positive for human papilloma virus in one third, raising the question of contamination. Taken in sum, current evidence indicates little if any role for human papilloma virus in the development of urothelial carcinoma.

Cytogenetics. Bladder cancer has been extensively studied cytogenetically during the past decade by karyotyping and a variety of molecular cytogenetic techniques. A review of the cytogenetics of bladder cancer was recently published by Sandberg and Berger.[110]

Numerical alterations in chromosome number were among the earliest cytogenetic changes reported in urothelial carcinoma. Increased modal chromosomal number has been associated with increased grade, stage, and adverse outcome.[111-113] Commonly reported numerical abnormalities include loss of chromosome 9, trisomy of chromosome 7,[110] and loss of the Y chromosome. In men, loss of the Y chromosome has correlated with an unfavorable outcome.[110]

One of the most frequent structural alterations is a deletion on the long arm of chromosome 9 (9q-).[110] This abnormality has been reported in up to 50% of urothelial carcinomas and is independent of stage and grade.[114] In one report,[114] loss of heterozygosity for chromosome 9q was found in 14 of 25 (56%) grade 1 urothelial carcinomas and in 19 of 40 (48%) stage pTa/pT1 tumors. These results suggest that a critical tumor suppressor gene is located at this site. It has been suggested that this loss is an early event, and may be the first detected cytogenetic event in urothelial carcinogenesis.[110] Other frequently reported structural alterations involve chromosomes 1 and 5.[110]

Fluorescent in situ hybridization studies are valuable in studying bladder cancer.[115-118] This technique has been applied to surgical specimens and urine cytology preparations, and these have most often demonstrated abnormalities of chromosomes 1, 7, 9, 11, 15, and 17.[116-119] Loss of chromosome 9 (-9) has been the most frequently observed abnormality in low grade papillary tumors.[120]

There are other potential tumor suppressor genes involved in bladder cancer. Loss of heterozygosity has been observed on chromosomes 1p, 1q, 3p, 5q, 6q, 9q, 11p, 13q, 17p, and 18q.[110,114,121] Involvement of 13q and 17p implicates the retinoblastoma and p53 tumor suppressor genes in bladder cancer; these appear to be involved at a later stage than the suppressor gene on 9q.[122-124] The prognostic importance of these suppressor gene lesions is discussed below in the section titled Other Prognostic Markers.

Heredity. The development of bladder cancer is not strongly related to heredity. Several studies have reported familial clusters of cases indicating that there may be a small percentage of cases associated with autosomal dominant inheritance,[125-127] although such occurrences may also reflect common environmental exposure.[128] Urothelial carcinoma has been reported in association with cancer family syndromes such as the Muir-Torre syndrome.[129,130]

Clinical features

The most common presenting symptom of bladder cancer is painless hematuria, present in up to 90% of patients.[131-134] Irritative symptoms, including frequency, urgency, and dysuria, may be seen in up to 20% of cases.[131-134] Less frequently, patients complain of flank pain resulting from ureteral obstruction, lower extremity edema caused by lymphatic obstruction, or symptoms related to a pelvic mass. Rarely, patients may present with metastases prior to detection of the bladder primary.[135-138] Leukemoid reaction[139,140] and rare paraneoplastic syndromes such as thrombocytosis, hypercalcemia, and encephalomyelitis may also occur.[139,141]

Diagnosis

Urine cytology. Urine cytology (voided, catheterized, and washes) is an indispensable tool in the management of bladder cancer patients. The major contribution of urine cytology is in follow-up and monitoring of the therapeutic response. Urine cytology is also a valuable diagnostic tool in screening high risk patients,[142,143] but it is not recommended for other populations. It also has a role in the clinical work up of patients suspected of having bladder cancer. The diagnostic accuracy of urine cytology has been a subject of considerable debate over the years. These controversies have focused on the ability to diagnose low-grade and intermediate-grade papillary tumors on voided urine and bladder wash specimens. Sensitivity for these tumors has ranged from 22% to more than 60%.[144,145] In high-grade tumors, including carcinoma in situ and invasive cancer, urine cytology is highly sensitive and specific.[146]

Cystoscopy and biopsy. Cystoscopy is the primary diagnostic tool in patients suspected of having a bladder tumor, allowing direct visualization of the bladder mucosa, biopsy of suspicious lesions, and random biopsies of normal mucosa in selected patients. Bladder washings obtained at the time of cystoscopic evaluation also provide useful cytologic material.[147]

The role of random biopsies has changed in recent years. In an effort to identify dysplasia and carcinoma in situ in patients with papillary tumors, some groups have recommended random mucosal biopsies. However, enthusiasm for this has decreased because of the low yield in patients with low-grade tumors, and many now suggest restricting random biopsies to patients with non-invasive grade 2 and 3 papillary urothelial carcinoma, patients with stage T1 cancer, patients with low-grade papillary tumors but positive urine cytology, and those considered for partial cystectomy.[148]

Cystograms and excretory urography. All patients evaluated for bladder tumors require assessment of the upper tracts.[128] It is important to screen for the presence of upper tract disease as the cause of the presenting symptom (hematuria) and to exclude synchronous upper tract cancer in patients with urinary bladder carcinoma. Voiding cystograms may demonstrate a bladder filling defect in larger tumors and aid in localization.

Staging of bladder cancer

Clinical and pathologic staging of bladder cancer is critical in stratifying patients for therapy. Bladder cancer has long been divided clinically into superficial and invasive cancer. Superficial cancer includes tumors that have not invaded the muscularis propria of the bladder (stages Ta, TIS, and T1), and invasive cancer includes tumors that extend into the muscularis propria or beyond (stages T2, T3, and T4). Unfortunately, this terminology classifies T1 tumors as superficial (noninvasive) despite invasion through the basal lamina into the lamina propria. It is, therefore, crucial that the pathology report clearly indicate the depth of invasion seen; if invasion is present, a statement regarding involvement of the muscularis propria must be made. If muscularis propria is not included in the submitted material, this should be explicitly indicated.

The most important task of local staging is to determine whether the muscularis propria has been invaded. This is the single most crucial piece of information for therapeutic decisionmaking. The most useful means to determine this is transurethral resection of the bladder tumor with histological examination for muscle invasion. Bimanual physical examination performed at the time of cystoscopy is also helpful because palpable tumors are almost always muscle invasive. Imaging modalities such as computed tomography, magnetic resonance imaging, and ultrasound may be of value as adjuncts, but are not adequately sensitive to detect early muscle invasion.[128]

For patients with muscle-invasive cancer, the extent of the carcinoma greatly influences therapy. Local extension beyond the urinary bladder may result in unresectability, and imaging studies are often used to look for local extension into perivesical soft tissues or adjacent organs. The sensitivity and specificity of the various modalities are debated and reviewed in the clinical literature.[128]

Of importance to pathologists is the use of biopsies and transurethral resections of the prostate to evaluate the degree of involvement, if any, of this organ.[149,150] Several studies have documented relatively high rates of involvement of the prostate gland by urothelial carcinoma in selected subgroups of patients. In patients with muscle-invasive bladder cancer, the frequency of involvement of the prostate gland approaches 50%.[151,152] The frequency is even greater in patients who have multifocal carcinoma in situ associated with the invasive tumor. In the current staging systems, involvement of the prostate indicates advanced cancer (stages D1 or T4) regardless of the extent of involvement. Recently, some authors have suggested that the degree of involvement should be considered in staging such patients. Hardeman and Soloway[153] recommended classifying prostatic involvement (when present) into three groups: carcinoma confined to the prostatic urethral mucosa, carcinoma extending into ducts and acini but confined by the basement membrane, and carcinoma invading the prostatic stroma. Several studies have indicated that prostatic involvement necessitates aggressive therapy (radical cystoprostatectomy),[154-157] while others consider conservative treatment an option.[152] However, all agree that the presence of prostatic stromal invasion indicates a need for aggressive therapy; consequently, this feature needs to be documented pathologically in all such specimens.

Wishnow et al[156] reported the development of metastatic cancer in 100% (5 of 5) of patients with stromal invasion in the prostate compared to 11% (2 of 11) when the prostatic involvement remained in situ (all patients had urothelial carcinoma in situ in the urinary bladder and were treated by cystoprostatectomy). In another study of patients treated by radical cystectomy, the presence of prostatic ductal involvement, without stromal invasion, did not adversely affect outcome; however, the presence of prostatic stromal invasion was an unfavorable prognostic factor.[158] The presence of prostatic urethral carcinoma in situ also indicates a high risk for urethral recurrence (see Chapter 9).[159]

Regional and distant metastases also are important in guiding therapy. A variety of imaging modalities are available for assessing regional lymph nodes, including computed tomography, magnetic resonance imaging, ultrasound, and lymphangiography, but pelvic lymphadenectomy with pathologic examination remains the most accurate.[128] Computed tomography is the most widely used imaging tool for this purpose, and in patients with gross (incurable) nodal involvement, fine needle aspiration is useful in confirming the diagnosis.[160] In most cases, however, staging lymph node dissection is performed at the time of cystectomy. The

TABLE 5-1.
PATHOLOGICAL STAGING OF BLADDER CARCINOMA

Depth of Invasion	AJCC/UICC	Marshall
Noninvasive, papillary	Ta	0
Noninvasive, flat	TIS	0
Lamina propria	T1	A
Superficial muscularis propria	T2	B1
Deep muscularis propria	T3a	B2
Perivesicle fat	T3b	C
Adjacent structures	T4	D1
Lymph node metastases	N1-3*	D1
Distant metastases	M1	D2

N1, regional lymph node, < 2 cm; N2, regional lymph nodes, 2 to 5 cm; N3, regional lymph nodes, > 5 cm or other lymph nodes.

clinical urology literature maintains that some patients with limited nodal involvement may be cured by cystectomy and lymph node dissection.[161,162] LaPlante and Brice[161] reported a 5 year survival rate of 12.8% for patients with positive lymph nodes at or below the iliac bifurcation compared with 0% if higher level nodes contained carcinoma in patients treated by radical cystectomy and lymph node dissection. Pathologists should be aware of this, recognizing that a surgeon may proceed with radical surgery despite the diagnosis of lymph node metastasis at frozen section. Many urologists do not request frozen sections on lymph nodes at the time of cystectomy unless grossly involved nodes are found.

Clinical and pathologic staging of bladder cancer remains the single most important determinant of prognosis and therapy. Currently, the Marshall modification of the Jewett-Strong system[163] and the American Joint Commission for Cancer–Union Internationale Contre le Cancer (AJCC-UICC) classifications[164] are the two main systems in clinical use. They are summarized and compared in Table 5-1 and important features are discussed below.

Both staging systems are based on the depth of invasion into the bladder wall and the pattern of regional and distant spread. Although TIS and Ta tumors are noninvasive, they differ in clinical outcome, which makes separation important, a feature lacking in the Marshall protocol. The other significant difference between these two systems is the classification of invasion of contiguous organs and regional lymph node metastases; these are combined in a single stage (D1) in the Marshall system. Although such patterns of spread are unfavorable prognostic features, from a biologic perspective it is logical to place these in separate categories. In both systems, invasion of the muscularis propria is a major staging determinant (B or T2).

Traditionally, tumors without muscle invasion have been treated by transurethral resection (with or without intravesical therapy) and muscle-invasive tumors have been treated with radical surgery or radiation therapy. The fundamental importance of muscle invasion creates a dichotomous branch in the therapeutic approach; recent advances in the treatment of bladder cancer have resulted in several treatment alternatives in the nonmuscle–invasive group, which are influenced by the tumor stage (Ta versus TIS versus T1). The simplistic terminology of *superficial* and *invasive* should be avoided and the pathology report should indicate the specific AJCC-UICC stage. The histological issues regarding these distinctions are discussed below in the section titled Diagnosis of Invasion and Pathologic Staging.

Clinical staging of localized urothelial carcinoma correlates poorly with pathologic staging at radical cystectomy.[132,163,165,166] Nonetheless, clinical stage remains a powerful predictor of tumor behavior in clinical studies.

Urothelial carcinoma in situ

In 1952, Melicow[167] first described highly atypical epithelium in the mucosa adjacent to bladder cancer. Since that early description, urothelial carcinoma in situ has become extremely important in the study of histogenesis, pathology, and treatment of urothelial carcinoma.

Clinical features. Carcinoma in situ can occur in the absence of other urothelial tumors, so-called primary carcinoma in situ. This is rare, accounting for 1% or less of bladder cancers,[168] and occurs almost exclusively in men over the age of 50 years.[168-174] Symptoms typically include dysuria, pain (perineal, penile, and suprapubic), frequency, hematuria, and sterile pyuria. Occasionally, carcinoma in situ may be asymptomatic. The clinical presentation may closely mimic interstitial cystitis. This is a significant pitfall; in a study of 486 patients from the Mayo Clinic who were initially considered to have interstitial cystitis, 23% of men were found to have carcinoma in situ (in contrast to 1.3% of women).[175] In most cases, carcinoma in situ is multifocal, appearing cystoscopically as red, velvety patches (Fig. 5-8), although it may appear normal and be invisible to the cystoscopist.

The association of carcinoma in situ with prior or synchronous urothelial tumors is much more common. The frequency of carcinoma in situ increases with increasing grade and stage of the associated tumor.[167,176] Random biopsies in patients with superficial (Ta/T1) carcinomas show epithelial abnormalities (dysplasia or carcinoma in situ) in up to 24% of patients.[177,178] Such biopsies are routine in the management of these patients, particularly those with high-grade lesions. Mapping studies in

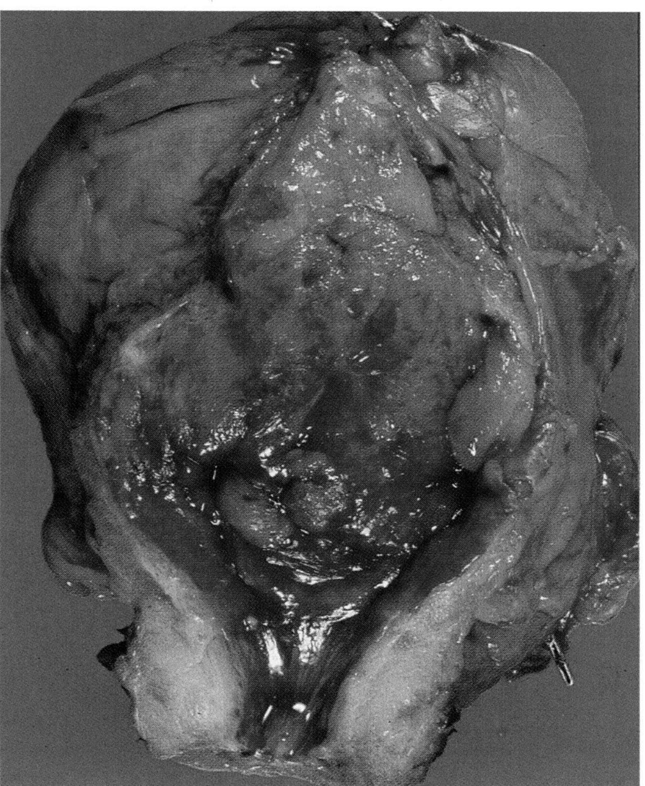

5-8. Diffuse urothelial carcinoma in situ with red mucosal surface.

cystectomy specimens have shown that carcinoma in situ may be extensive.[168,179] In addition, patients with carcinoma in situ in the bladder often have involvement of the prostatic urethra (up to 67%),[159,168,172,180] prostate gland (up to 40%),[168,181-184] and ureters (up to 57%).[168,185-188] In rare cases, urothelial carcinoma in situ can extend in a pagetoid fashion to involve the skin of the external genitalia[189,190] and seminal vesicles.[191] This can occur with or without the presence of invasive urothelial carcinoma.

Pathology. Many studies have used the original criteria for carcinoma in situ of Melicow,[167] limiting the diagnosis to lesions with full thickness replacement of the epithelium by cytologically malignant cells.[179,192] Currently, most authors agree that the diagnosis of carcinoma in situ is based more on the presence of severe cytologic atypia, and the presence of a full thickness change is not necessary.[10,11,193,194]

The usual type of carcinoma in situ is characterized by full thickness replacement of the urothelium by large pleomorphic cells with moderate to abundant cytoplasm (Fig. 5-9). Occasionally, the cells may be small with a high nuclear to cytoplasmic ratio (Fig. 5-10). The number of cell layers is not important to the diagnosis as it can be normal, increased, or decreased. The pattern with small cells particularly may be associated with an increased number of cell layers. The nuclei are enlarged and hyperchromatic, with coarse unevenly distributed chromatin and scattered prominent nucleoli, which are often irregular in shape and angulated. Mitotic figures are frequently present, often with abnormal forms. The cells are randomly oriented producing a disorganized appearance. There is often striking cellular discohesion, which, in some cases, results in few or no recognizable epithelial cells on the surface—so-called *denuding cystitis* (Fig. 5-11).[174] Ultrastructural studies have demonstrated focal discontinuity of the basement membrane in areas of carcinoma in situ.[195,196] In some cases, there is intense chronic inflammation in the superficial

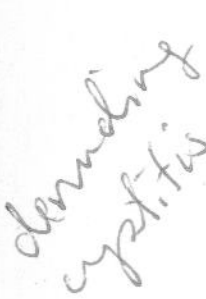

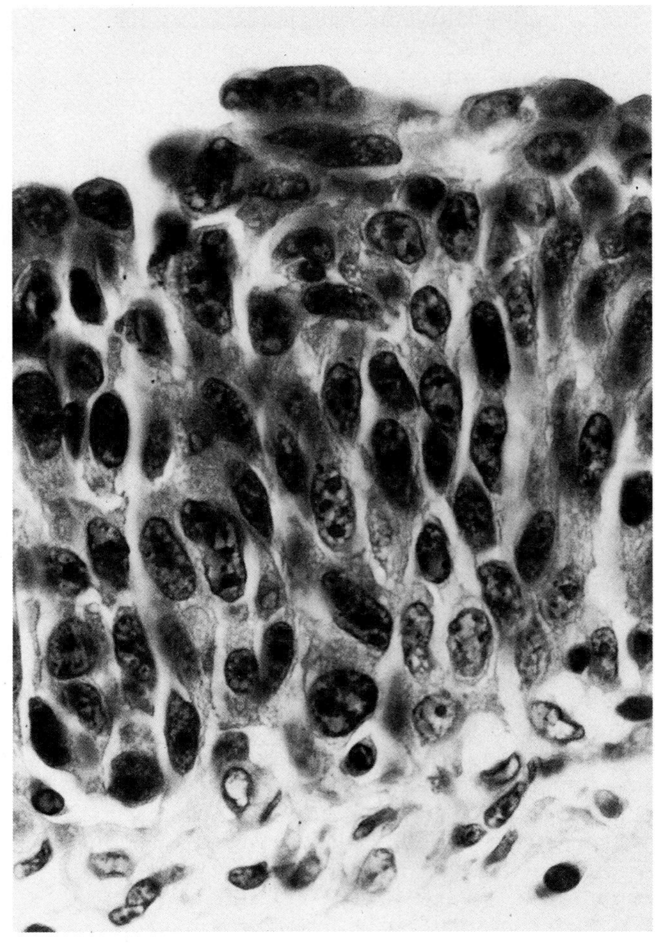

5-9. Typical urothelial carcinoma in situ with full thickness replacement of the urothelium by large pleomorphic cells that have open nuclei and a coarse chromatin pattern.

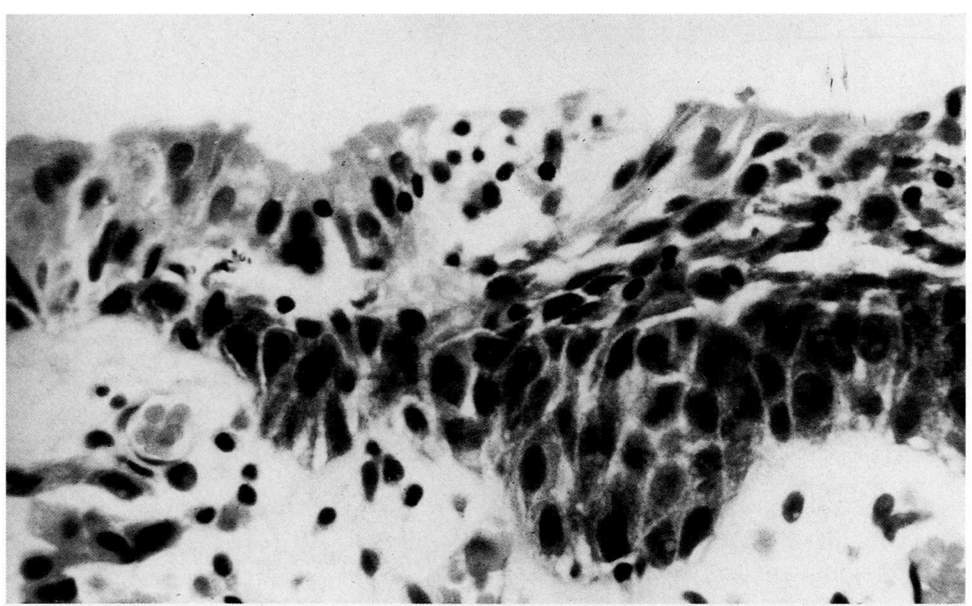

5-10. Small cell pattern of urothelial carcinoma in situ with cells that have dense hyperchromatic nuclei and a moderate amount of cytoplasm. Note the undermining of the normal urothelium in the left half of the photomicrograph.

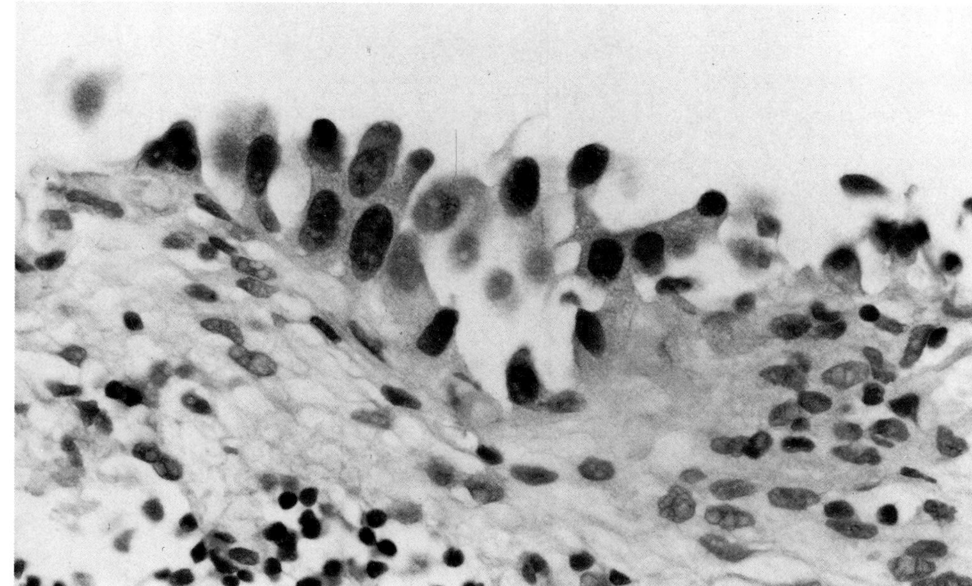

5-11. Urothelial carcinoma in situ with loss of intercellular cohesion resulting in a denuding pattern. The severe cytologic atypia warrants the diagnosis of carcinoma in situ in cases such as this.

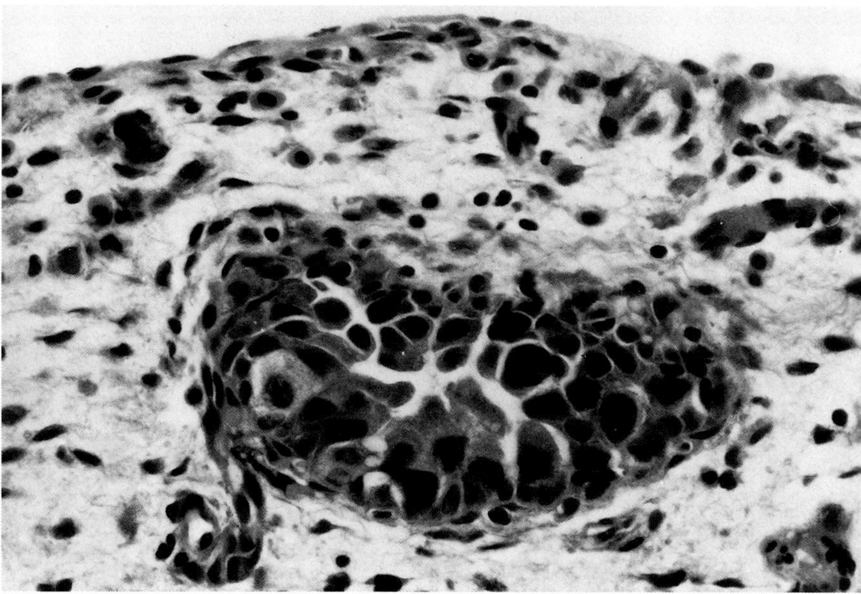

5-12. Urothelial carcinoma in situ within a von Brunn's nest. Note the completely denuded mucosal surface in this case.

lamina propria. Vascular ectasia and proliferation of small capillaries are frequent.

Recognition of the denuded pattern is crucial in random bladder biopsies from patients with synchronous bladder tumors or those taken during the follow-up of bladder cancer. It is insufficient to simply report such a biopsy as negative without obtaining deeper sections of the biopsy and indicating in the report that the surface epithelium is partially or completely absent. Recuts may demonstrate carcinoma in situ in von Brunn's nests or foci of preserved surface carcinoma in situ in such cases (Fig. 5-12). Correlation with urine cytology often is helpful, because most cases with these biopsy findings have positive urine cytology.

In rare cases, urothelial carcinoma in situ has a pagetoid pattern of growth,[197,198] characterized by large, single, or clustered cells within an otherwise normal urothelium (Fig 5-13). The carcinoma cells have large nuclei with coarse chromatin, single or multiple nucleoli, and abundant pale to eosinophilic cytoplasm that does not react with stains for mucin.[198] In one study, this pattern was never identified in a pure form but was invariably associated with a more typical pattern of carcinoma in situ.[198]

Cytology. Urine cytology is quite useful in the diagnosis of carcinoma in situ. The cells in this lesion are typically discohesive, and large numbers are shed into the urine. The cells show marked variability in size.[5,173,199,200] The urine often contains numerous single cells with few small cohesive clusters (Fig 5-14). Nuclei tend to be markedly hyperchromatic and irregular with coarse chromatin, and the cytoplasm tends to

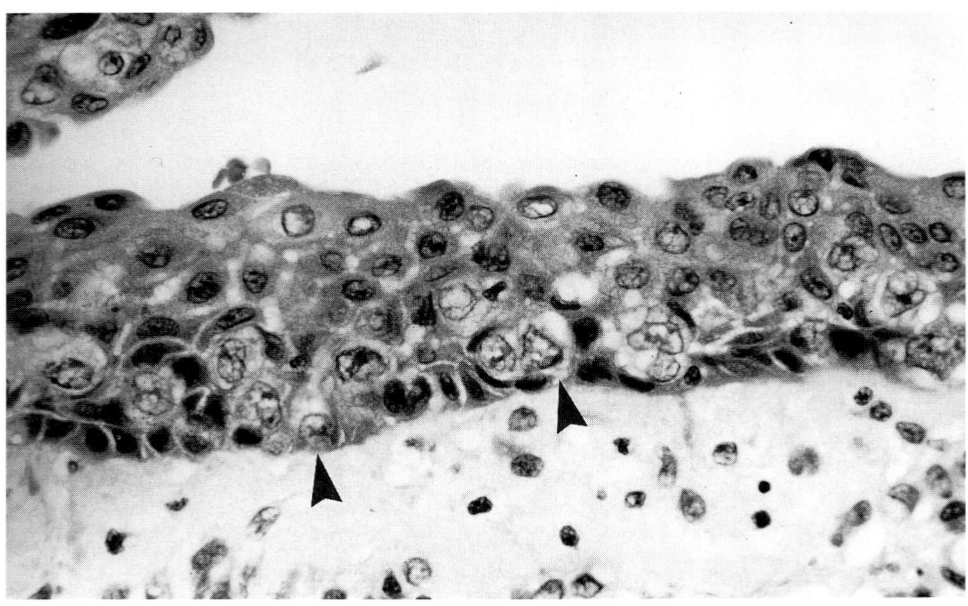

5-13. Urothelial carcinoma in situ with pagetoid spread of large pleomorphic cells (*arrows*) into adjacent epithelium.

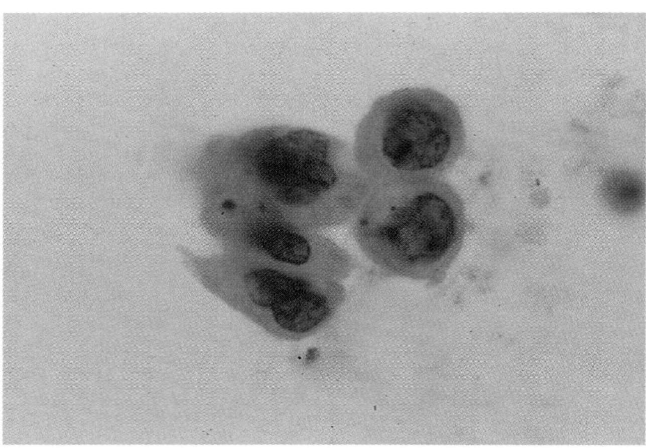

5-14. Urine cytology specimen from a patient with urothelial carcinoma in situ. This example shows poorly cohesive cells with large nuclei and irregular chromatin.

be scant. It is difficult to distinguish high grade urothelial carcinoma, with or without invasion, from carcinoma in situ in cytology specimens.[200,201]

Special studies. There is typically loss of normal A, B, and H blood group antigens in carcinoma in situ.[202-205] Carcinoembryonic antigen is frequently found in carcinoma in situ, whereas it is absent from normal urothelium.[204] Morphometry has shown increases in nuclear area, nuclear perimeter, and maximum nuclear diameter in carcinoma in situ.[204] DNA ploidy studies by both image analysis and flow cytometry have demonstrated a high frequency of aneuploidy in carcinoma in situ.[206,207]

Urothelial dysplasia and atypia. For epithelial changes that have some but not all features of carcinoma in situ, other terms such as dysplasia, atypia, or atypical hyperplasia are used.[11,179,192,208,209] Mostofi et al,[210] and Nagy and Friedell[211] have argued in favor of using a grading system similar to that applied to papillary transitional cell neoplasms, with epithelial abnormalities reported as low, moderate, and high grade dysplasia. Mostofi et al[210] suggested the term *carcinoma in situ, grades 1, 2, and 3* for these abnormalities, a terminology we discourage. Several studies have documented the lack of reproducibility in grading dysplasia.[15,212,213] Many authors continue to advocate attempting to grade these atypical lesions[192,193,211] whereas others, recognizing the lack of reproducible criteria, would combine high-grade dysplasia with carcinoma in situ, acknowledging this as a clinically significant lesion that requires the same treatment.[10,194,209,214] Reuter and Melamed have pushed this argument to the point of recommending that "even the earliest carcinomatous transformation, if so recognized, should be classified as carcinoma in situ,"[10] and discourage the use of *dysplasia*, resulting in essentially a two-tiered diagnostic system. Murphy et al[11] recommend including moderate dysplasia with carcinoma in situ, but recognize a dysplastic lesion distinguishable from other atypias, maintaining three levels of diagnosis (atypia, dysplasia, and carcinoma in situ). We also favor a three-tiered system, and would restrict the diagnosis of carcinoma in situ to lesions falling into the groups of carcinoma in situ and severe (high-grade) dysplasia (see above). Lesser lesions that are believed to be dysplastic and not reactive in nature are included under the term *moderate dysplasia*, although some argue that moderate dysplasia should not be considered neoplastic.[209] Lesions that fit into the spectrum of low-grade dysplasia are not distinguishable from a variety of reactive atypias and are left in the non-neoplastic group. Interested readers are referred to more detailed discussions of this controversy elsewhere.[192,210,212]

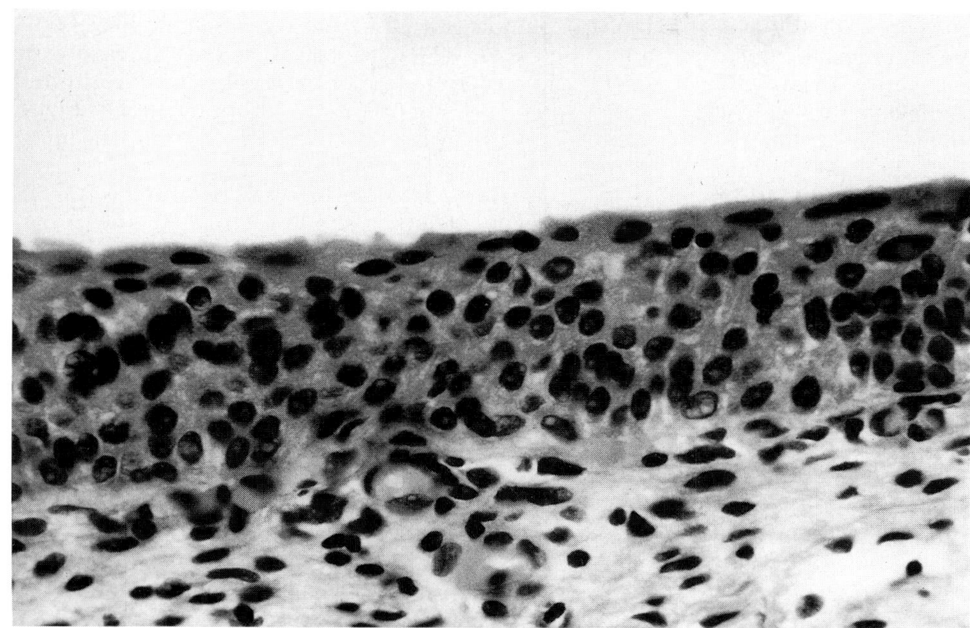

5-15. Urothelial dysplasia with some haphazardly arranged cells that have hyperchromatic nuclei but retain some architectural organization and an umbrella cell layer.

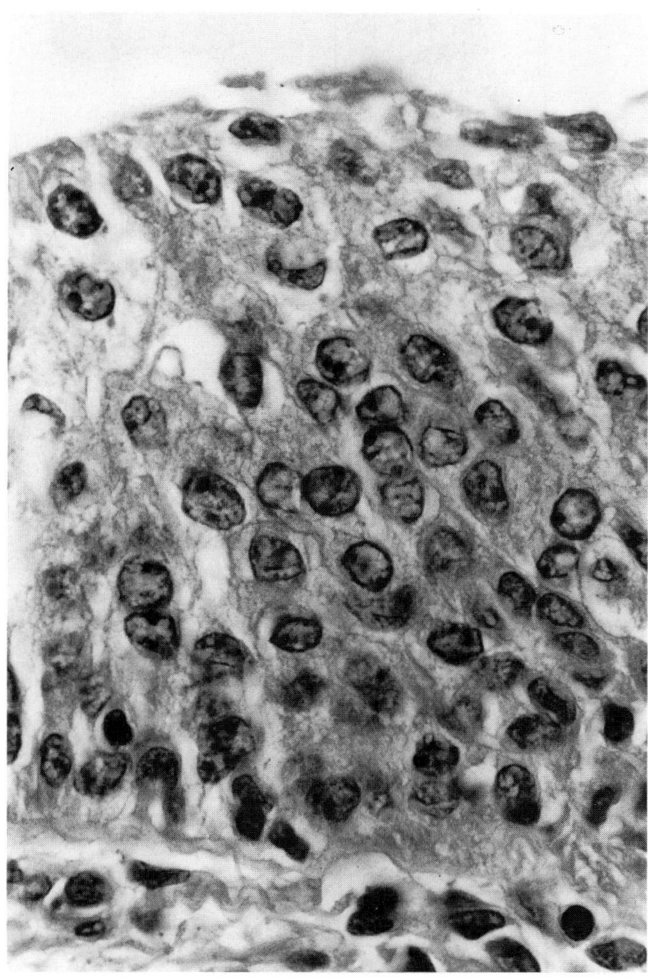

5-16. Urothelial dysplasia showing open nuclei with irregular clumped chromatin; there is general preservation of the architecture and the umbrella cell layer.

In moderate dysplasia, the cytologic abnormalities are less severe than carcinoma in situ and restricted to the basal and intermediate layers. Abnormalities include nuclear enlargement, coarse chromatin, and variation in nuclear shape, with notching of the nuclear membrane. Nucleoli are small and inconspicuous. Mitotic figures are usually absent. An intact umbrella cell layer is present (Fig. 5-15). Murphy et al[11] stress the nuclear (and architectural) features in distinguishing dysplasia from atypia (Fig 5-16).

The significance of dysplasia remains unresolved. Studies of blood group antigen expression, morphometry, and DNA ploidy suggest that dysplasia is an intermediate lesion between normal urothelium and carcinoma in situ.[204,206] However, there is little clinical data available concerning whether dysplasia remains the same, progresses, or regresses. The presence of dysplasia in the mucosa adjacent to papillary urothelial carcinoma is associated with an increased risk of subsequent recurrence[212,215] and progression.[216,217] Smith et al[215] found that 73% of patients with dysplasia developed recurrences, compared with 43% of those without dysplasia.

Natural history and treatment. Initial studies showed the development of invasive cancer in 32% of untreated patients with carcinoma in situ.[169] Subsequent studies have confirmed the high risk of progression for this lesion and the development of invasive cancer in up to 83% of cases.[170,171,218-220] These observations led some to treat carcinoma in situ with radical cystectomy. Examination of these cystectomy specimens has revealed foci of microinvasion in 34% of bladders[175] and muscle-invasive cancer in up to 9%.[221] Five-year cause-specific survival for patients with carcinoma in situ treated by radical surgery ranges from 85% to 100%.[221,222] Recently, carcinoma in situ has been treated with a variety of intravesical agents including bacillus Calmette-Guérin (BCG), thiotepa, mitomycin, and others.[173,223-226] Because of the high frequency and adverse implications of prostatic involvement, biopsy of the prostatic urethra and prostatic ducts is usually performed prior to conservative therapy.[227] Failure rates for intravesical therapy have varied widely, but significant numbers of patients do ultimately progress, indicating the need for close clinical follow-up with repeated urine cytologies and biopsy specimens. In some instances, the separation of residual or recurrent carcinoma in situ from reactive atypia caused by therapy may be difficult or impossible. The morphologic changes associated with various topical therapies, and the distinction of reactive atypia from residual carcinoma in situ is covered in detail in Chapter 4.

Gross pathology

Papillary urothelial carcinoma. Grossly, papillary tumors are exophytic, appearing as single or multiple and small fingerlike or larger complex lesions that are nearly solid in appearance. In most series, approximately 66% of papillary tumors are single at the time of presentation.[217,228,229] Clinically, the documentation of single versus multiple tumors is significant, as patients with multiple tumors have a higher risk of recurrence[7,230,231] and progression.[230,231] Tumors occur most often on the lateral and posterior walls of the bladder, and least often at the dome.[232,233] In one study, location correlated with prognosis, with tumors at the dome having the most aggressive behavior.[232]

Nonpapillary urothelial carcinoma. Nonpapillary urothelial carcinoma shows a range of growth patterns, including polypoid, sessile, and ulcerated and infiltrative (Fig. 5-17). In some cases, the polypoid pattern can be associated with a stalk. A polypoid pattern is characteristic of the sarcomatoid variant of urothelial carcinoma.[234] On sectioning, such tumors tend to be solid, gray-white, and infiltrative.

Microscopic pathology

Papillary urothelial carcinoma. Papillary urothelial carcinoma is exophytic, with papillae containing well-defined thin fibrovascular cores (Fig. 5-18). The cores are covered by urothelium, which may vary from nearly normal to anaplastic. There may be foci of squamous differentiation, a feature more often seen in high-grade

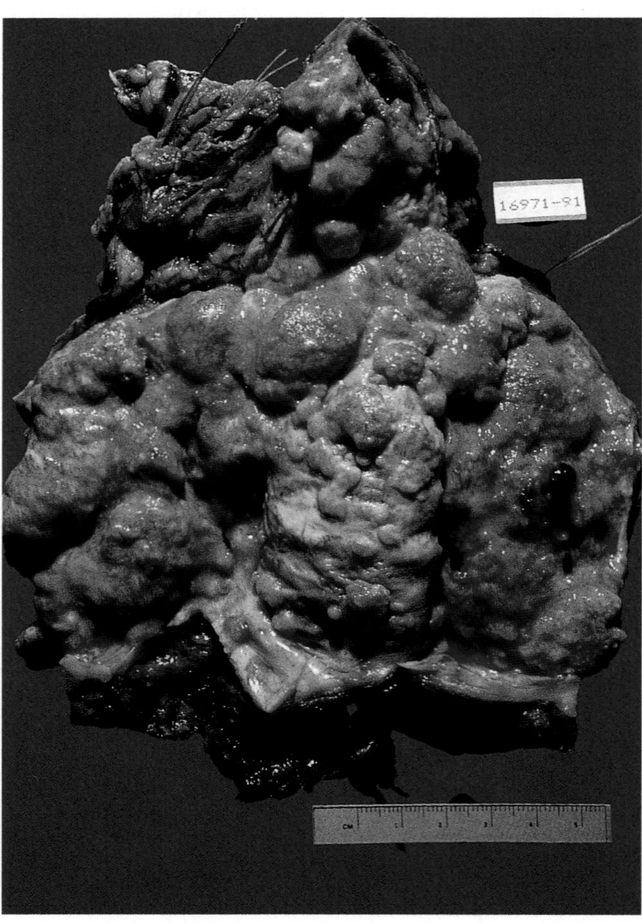

5-17. Gross photograph of multifocal sessile urothelial carcinoma in a cystoprostatectomy specimen. *(Photograph courtesy of Dr. D. Ian Turnbull.)*

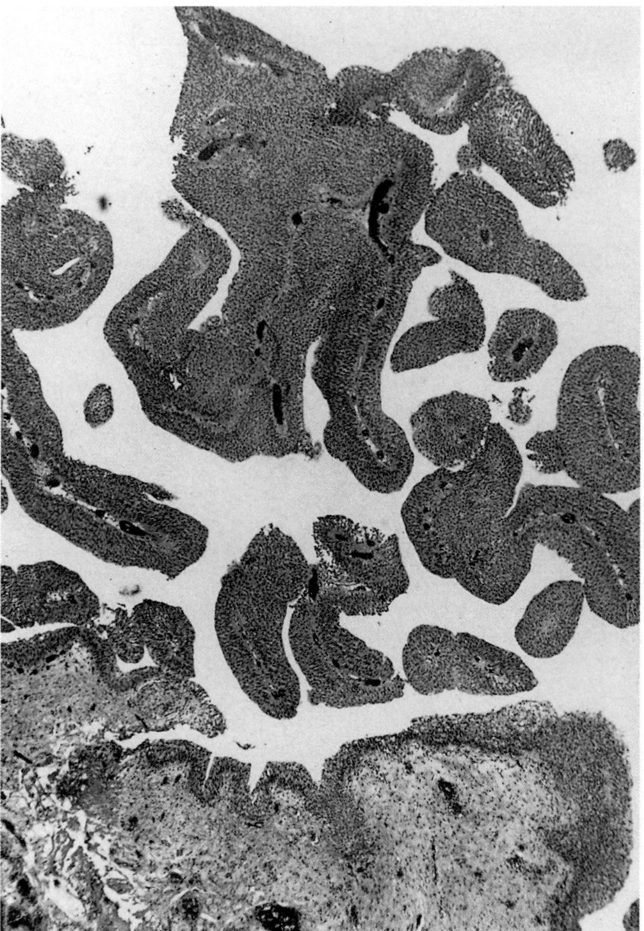

5-18. Papillary urothelial carcinoma. Numerous papillary fronds appear to float in space above the mucosal surface in this photomicrograph.

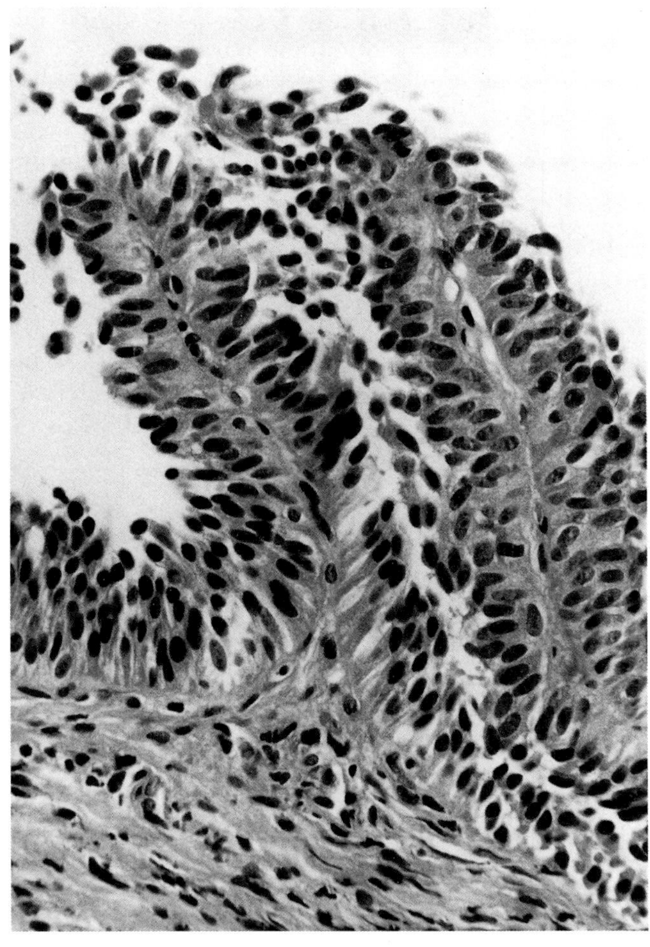

5-19. Micropapillary urothelial carcinoma. Note the thin fibrovascular cores within the centers of the two papillae.

tumors. Mucinous cells may also be present, occasionally in large numbers. Oncocytic change is rarely encountered, with the cells having abundant, finely granular eosinophilic cytoplasm. These morphologic variations have no apparent clinical significance.

Occasionally, papillary tumors contain only small, short papillae, resulting in a micropapillary appearance (Fig. 5-19). In these cases, the cores are typically very fine, with scant stroma and only one or two thin vascular channels in the center. Such papillae may be complex or branching, features not seen in normal infoldings of the bladder mucosa or in papillary hyperplasia. Cytologic atypia encompasses the full range of grades discussed below.

The differential diagnosis of papillary urothelial carcinoma includes all entities that produce papillae or papillary structures. The urinary bladder mucosa is elastic, allowing it to stretch and contract; in the contracted state, normal folds may mimic papillae. In folds, the stroma appears normal and lacks the fine vascular channels extending the length of the papillae typical of urothelial carcinoma. Papillary cystitis has wider papillary structures with more stromal tissue and vascular structures than papillary carcinoma. In papillary cystitis, the surface epithelium may show reactive atypia, but more severe cytologic atypia and disturbances of the normal epithelial architecture are absent.[235] Polypoid cystitis, a condition associated with indwelling catheters, also mimics papillary neoplasia.[236,237] Typically, it consists of an exophytic lesion with edematous lamina propria covered by attenuated, normal, or hyperplastic urothelium. The stroma may be less edematous in some cases, but always is wider and contains more inflammatory cells and more capillaries than the cores of papillary carcinoma. Nephrogenic adenoma often has small papillary projections covered by cuboidal cells with tubular structures in the underlying lamina propria.[238-240] Clinically, it can mimic papillary urothelial carcinoma.

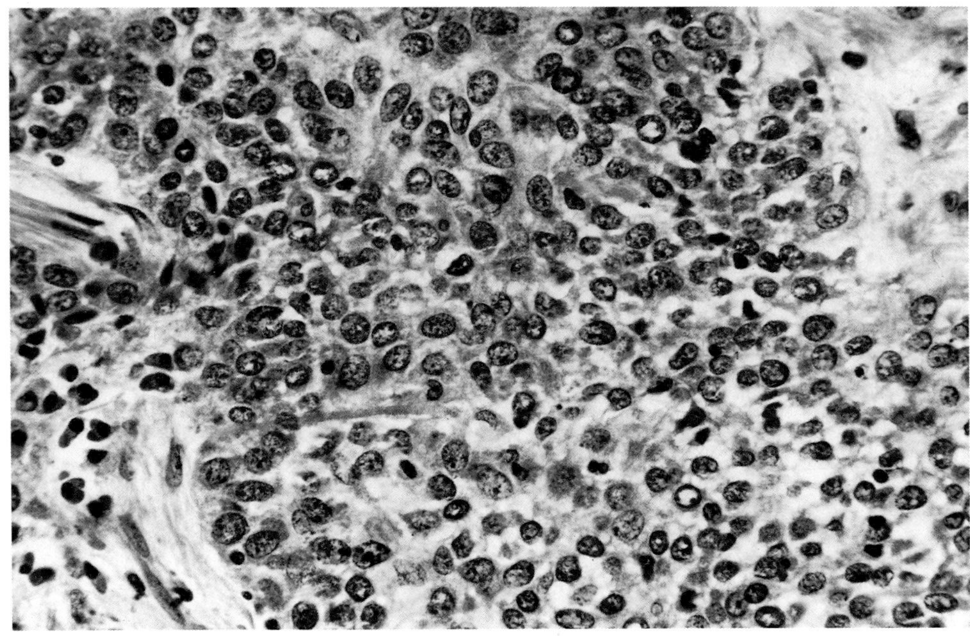

5-20. Invasive high-grade (WHO grade 3) urothelial carcinoma growing in large solid islands.

Nonpapillary urothelial carcinoma. The histology of invasive nonpapillary urothelial carcinoma is highly varied, with numerous variants described. Some of the specialized histologic types are described in specific sections later in this chapter; others are highlighted in the following discussion.

Typical urothelial carcinoma. The great majority of invasive urothelial carcinomas are high grade, corresponding to World Health Organization grade 3 lesions. These consist of cohesive nests or islands of cells with moderate to abundant amphophilic cytoplasm and large hyperchromatic nuclei (Fig 5-20). In a minority of invasive tumors, remnants of papillary architecture persist. In larger nests, palisading of nuclei is seen at the edges of the nests, with apparent stratification towards the center, a helpful finding in diagnosis (Fig. 5-21). This feature has recently been used to subclassify the high-grade tumors.[16] Frequently, carcinoma cells are arranged in small clusters or single cells (Fig. 5-22). Less often, the tumor invades as solid sheets with little intervening stroma (Fig 5-23).

The nuclei are typically pleomorphic and often have irregular contours with angular profiles (Fig. 5-24). Nuclear grooves, characteristic of low-grade urothelial cancer, may be identified in some cells. Nucleoli are highly variable in number and appearance, with some

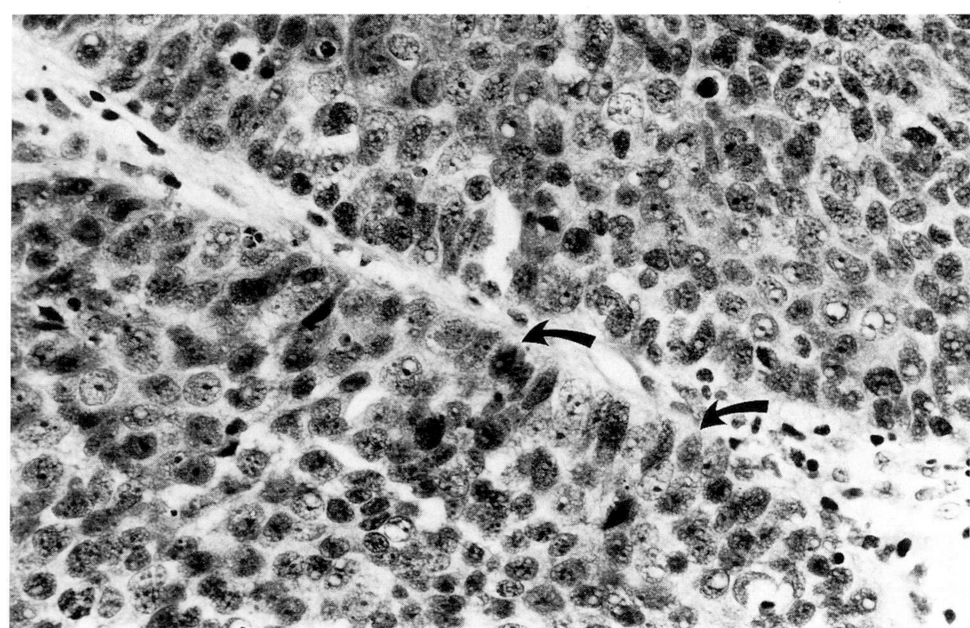

5-21. Invasive urothelial carcinoma growing in solid nests; there is focal palisading of the nuclei at the periphery of the nests (*arrows*).

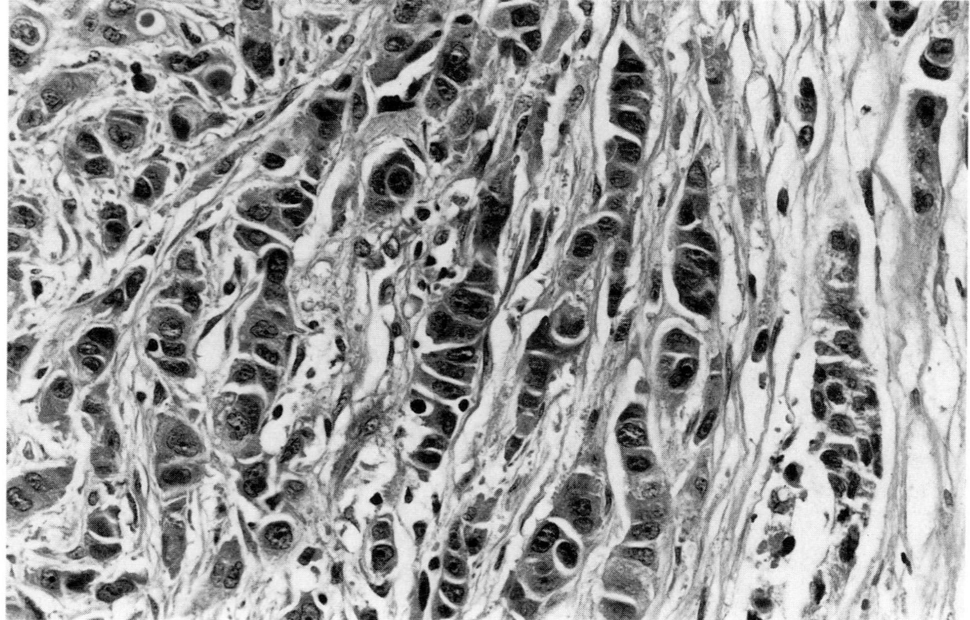

5-22. Invasive urothelial carcinoma growing in solid cords and small nests.

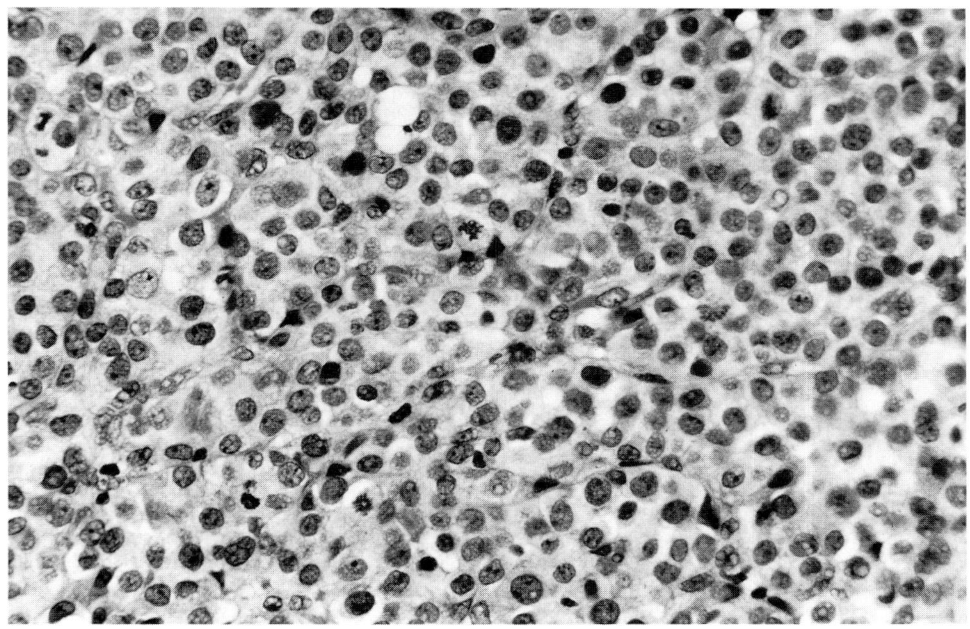

5-23. Invasive urothelial carcinoma composed of small nests of pleomorphic cells separated by scant compressed stroma.

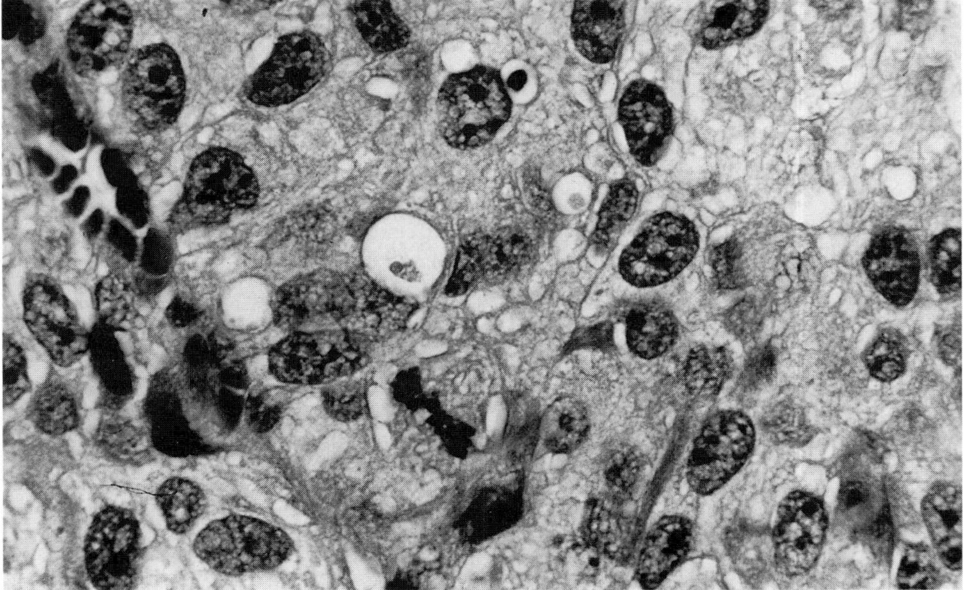

5-24. High power photomicrograph of invasive urothelial carcinoma illustrating the variability in nuclear size and shape, coarse chromatin, and single or multiple nucleoli.

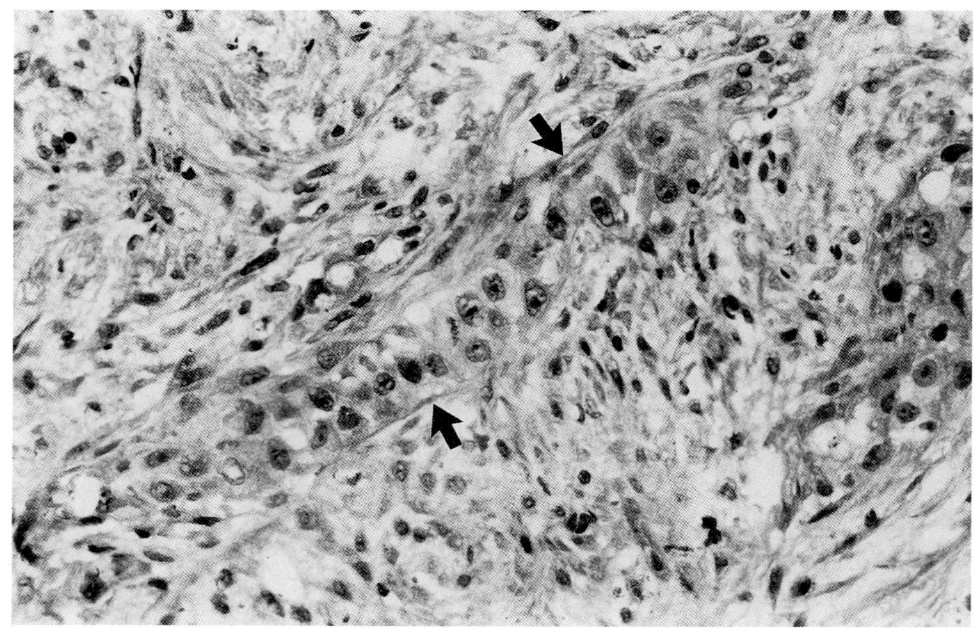

5-25. Invasive urothelial carcinoma with pseudosarcomatous stroma. The epithelial component can be recognized as a cohesive cord of cells (*arrows*).

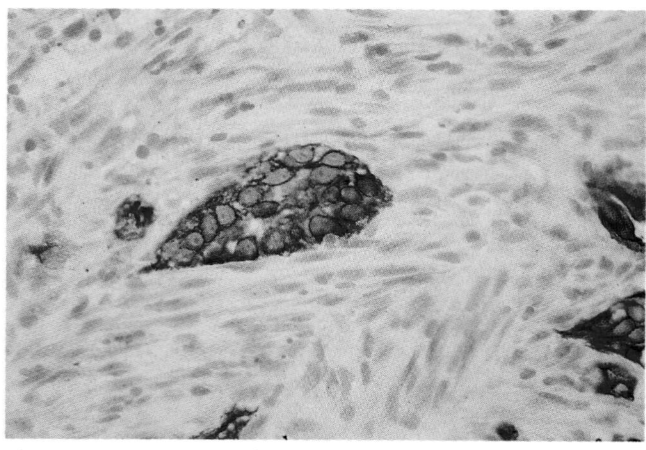

5-26. Invasive urothelial carcinoma with pseudosarcomatous stroma immunohistochemically stained for cytokeratin; the stromal cells are nonreactive.

cells containing single or multiple small nucleoli and others having large eosinophilic nucleoli. Foci of marked pleomorphism may be seen, with bizarre and multinuclear tumor cells in solid areas. Mitotic figures are common, with numerous abnormal forms. Some authors have stressed the mitotic rate as a prognostic indicator.[241]

The invasive nests usually induce a striking desmoplastic stromal reaction, a feature that is helpful in diagnosing invasion in early lesions. The desmoplastic reaction is occasionally very great and can mimic a malignant spindle cell component (Fig. 5-25, 5-26).[175,242] In formalin-fixed paraffin-embedded specimens, artifactual clefts are often present around the nests of carcinoma cells, mimicking vascular invasion (Fig. 5-27, 5-28). It is important to be aware of this feature to avoid overdiagnosis of vascular invasion.

Squamous differentiation occurs in up to 20% of cases of invasive urothelial carcinoma, and is an important feature that should be reported (see the next section).[243,244] However, it is common to see areas of urothelial carcinoma that have a squamoid appearance. These consist of cells with more abundant eosinophilic or clear glycogenated cytoplasm near the centers of tumor nests (Fig. 5-29). These foci should not be classified as squamous differentiation unless there is definite keratinization or intercellular bridges.

Urothelial carcinoma with squamous or glandular differentiation. Urothelial tumors have a great capacity for divergent differentiation.[245] Russell et al[246] found ultrastructural evidence of squamous and glandular differentiation in xenografted urothelial carcinoma cells. High-grade urothelial carcinoma often shows foci of squamous, glandular, or small cell differentiation. Unusual tumors demonstrating multiple lines of differentiation have been described.[92]

Squamous differentiation, defined by the presence of intercellular bridges or keratinization, occurs in up to 20% of urothelial carcinomas (Fig. 5-30).[243,244] Sakamoto et al[243] recently described detailed histologic maps of 28 cases of urothelial carcinoma with squamous differentiation. The proportion of the squamous component was shown to vary considerably, with some cases having urothelial carcinoma in situ as the only urothelial component. Sakamoto et al suggested that pure squamous cell carcinoma can arise in association with squamous metaplasia of the urothelium or may represent urothelial carcinoma with extensive squamous differentiation. The

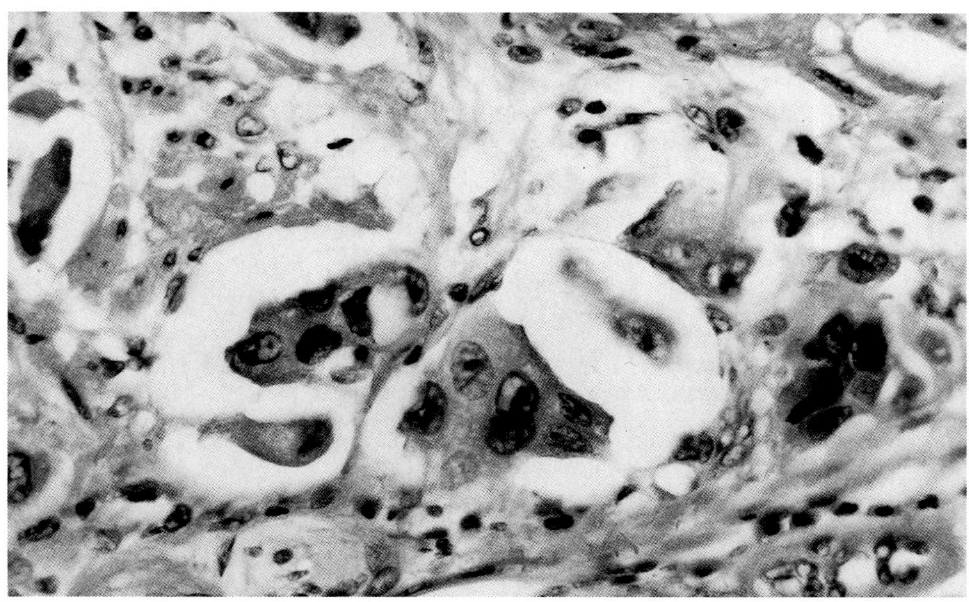

5-27. Invasive urothelial carcinoma with retraction artifact around nests of carcinoma cells, simulating vascular invasion.

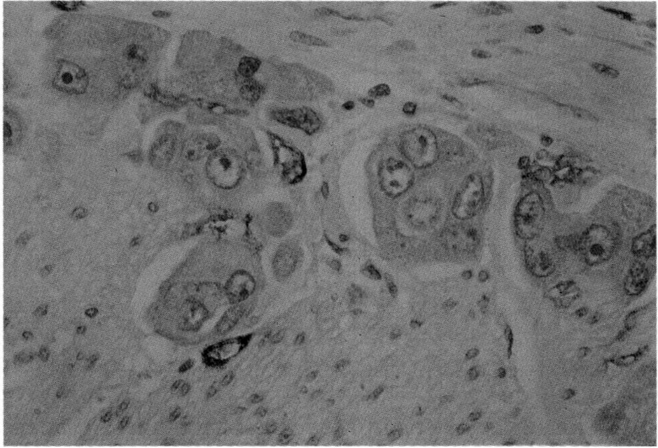

5-28. Invasive urothelial carcinoma (same focus as Fig. 5-27) stained immunohistochemically for Factor VIII–related antigen demonstrating the absence of endothelial cells around the nests of carcinoma.

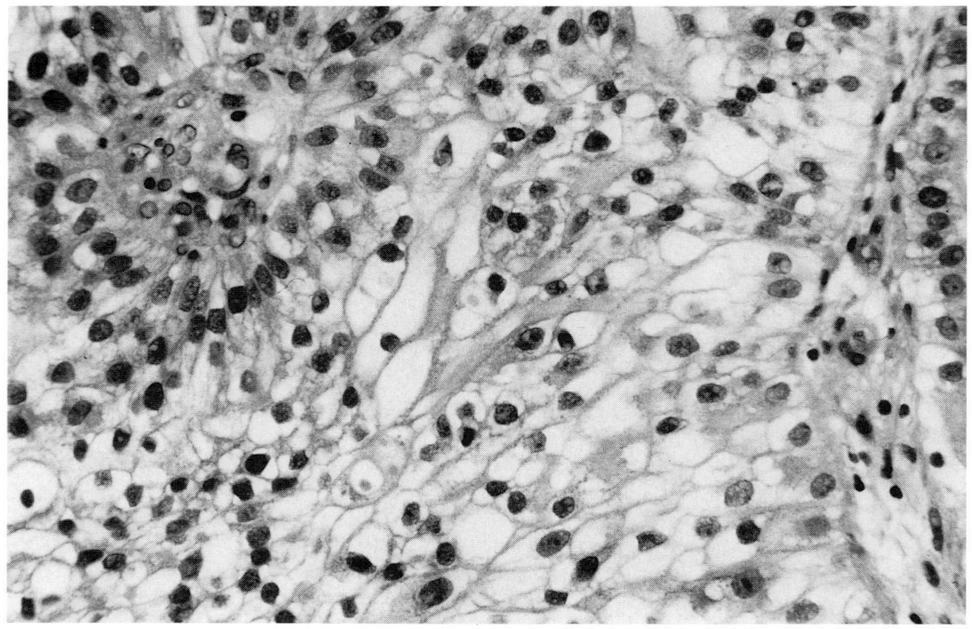

5-29. Invasive urothelial carcinoma with stratified architecture and clear cells resembling a glycogenated squamous epithelium; this is not considered to be squamous differentiation.

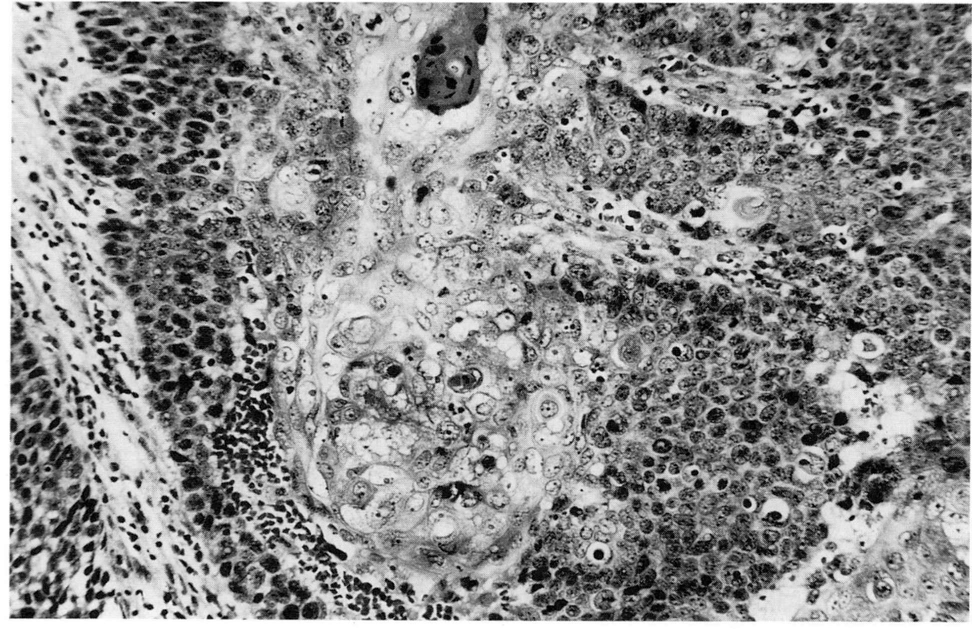

5-30. Invasive urothelial carcinoma with squamous differentiation; keratinization and intercellular bridges are present.

diagnosis of squamous cell carcinoma is reserved for pure lesions without any associated urothelial component, including urothelial carcinoma in situ. Tumors with any identifiable urothelial element are classified as urothelial carcinoma with squamous differentiation.

The clinical significance of squamous differentiation remains uncertain; it is an unfavorable prognostic feature in patients undergoing radical cystectomy, according to Frazier et al,[158] possibly because of its association with high-grade urothelial carcinoma. Martin et al[244] and Akdas and Turkeri[247] reported that squamous differentiation was predictive of a poor response to radiation therapy. In another report, squamous differentiation was associated with a poor response to systemic chemotherapy.[248]

Glandular differentiation is less common than squamous differentiation.[249,250] Glandular differentiation is

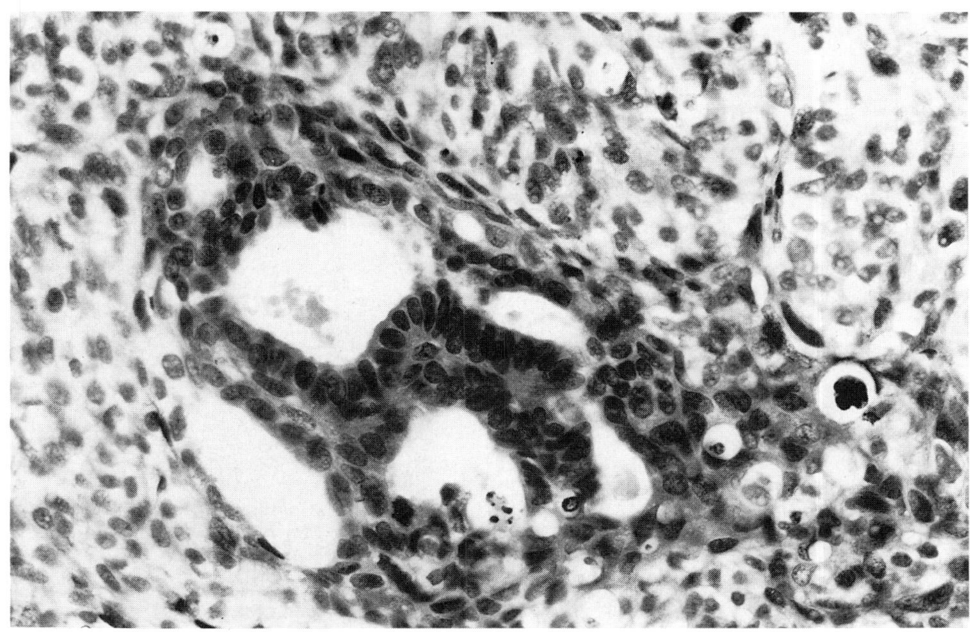

5-31. Invasive urothelial carcinoma with glandular differentiation.

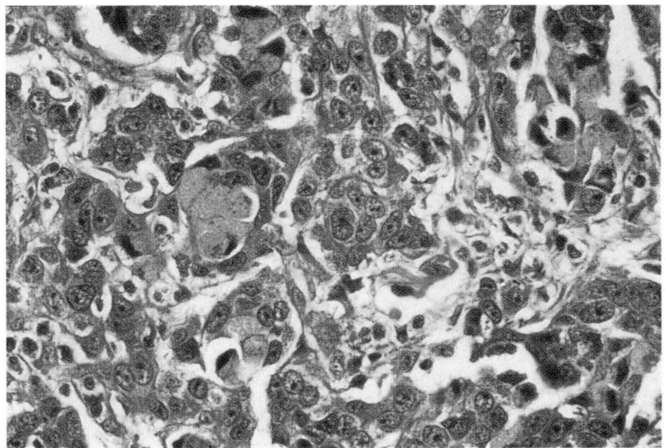

5-32. Invasive urothelial carcinoma containing numerous mucin-containing alcian blue–positive cells; this is not classified as glandular differentiation.

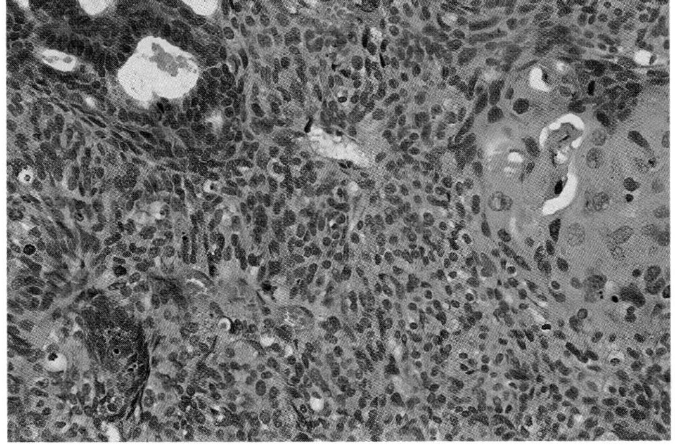

5-33. Invasive urothelial carcinoma with squamous, glandular, and small cell differentiation.

defined as the presence of true glandular spaces within the tumor (Fig. 5-31).[1,251] Pseudoglandular spaces caused by necrosis or artifact should not be considered evidence of glandular differentiation. Mucin-containing cells are common in high-grade urothelial carcinoma (Fig. 5-32). Donhuijsen et al[252] found mucin-positive cells in 14% of grade 1, 49% of grade 2, and 63% of grade 3 urothelial carcinomas. The diagnosis of adenocarcinoma is reserved for pure tumors, although some authors disagree,[253] and a tumor with mixed glandular and urothelial differentiation is classified as urothelial carcinoma with glandular differentiation regardless of the extent of the glandular differentiation (Fig. 5-33).[254] Rare cases of coexistent adenocarcinoma and a geographically separate urothelial carcinoma have been described.[255]

The clinical significance of glandular differentiation and mucin positivity in urothelial carcinoma remains uncertain. In one study, the presence of glandular differentiation was associated with a poorer response to systemic chemotherapy.[248]

Nested variant. In 1992, Murphy and Deana[256] described four cases of invasive urothelial carcinoma with a distinctive growth pattern of small nests of benign-appearing urothelial cells, closely resembling von Brunn's nests, infiltrating the lamina propria (Fig. 5-34). Some nests have small tubular lumens. Nuclei generally show little or no atypia, but invariably the tumor contains foci of unequivocal cancer with enlarged nucleoli and a coarse chromatin pattern (Fig. 5-35). This feature tends to be most apparent in the deeper parts of the lesion. This

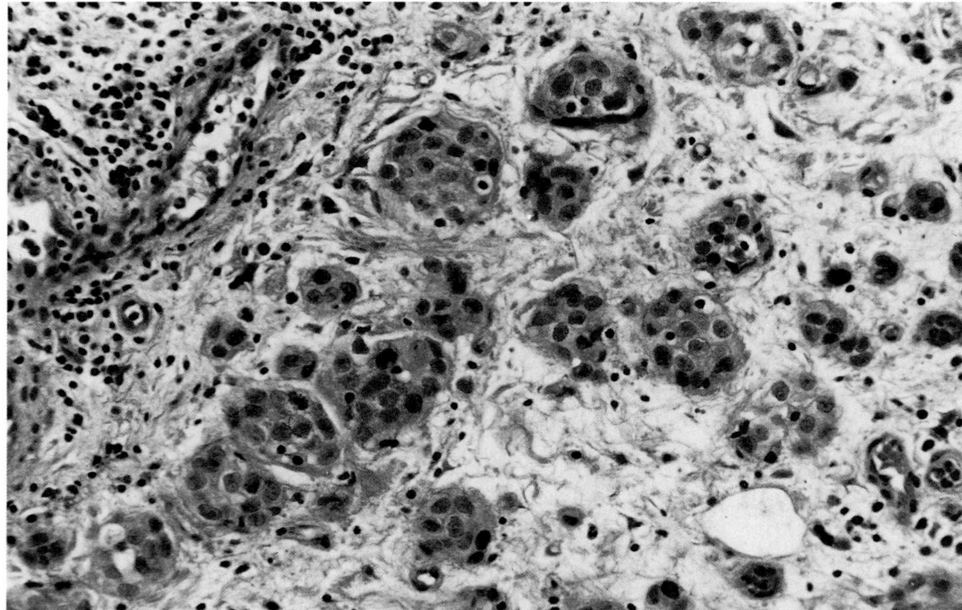

5-34. Nested variant of urothelial carcinoma; the tumor is growing as relatively uniform round nests.

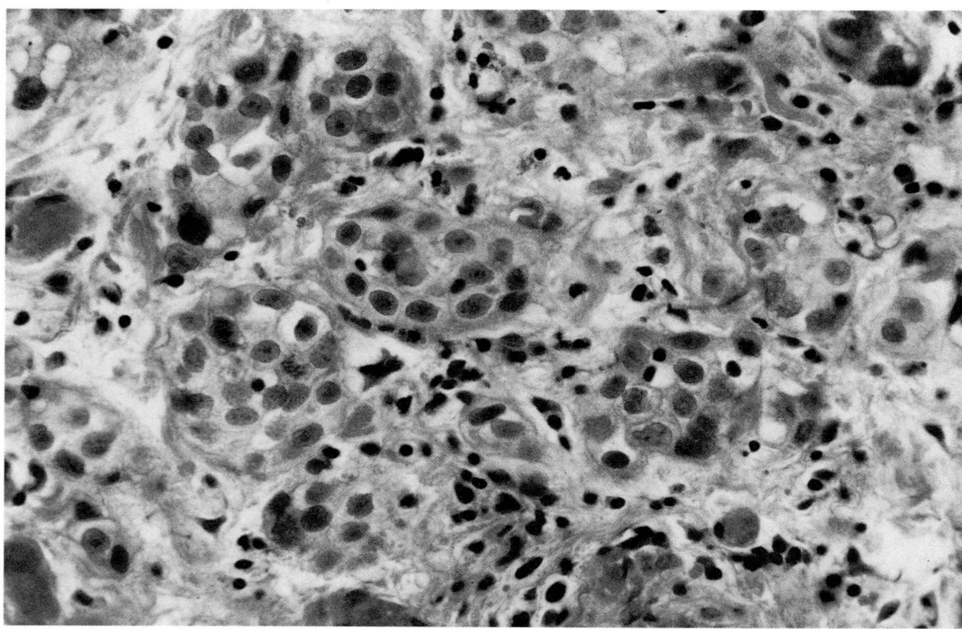

5-35. Nested variant of urothelial carcinoma demonstrating uniform nuclei with dispersed chromatin and small nucleoli. In other areas the tumor showed greater atypia and muscle invasion.

rare pattern of urothelial carcinoma had previously been described by Talbert and Young[257] in a paper describing a group of tumors having deceptively benign appearances. Useful features in recognizing this lesion as malignant are the tendency for increasing cellular anaplasia in the deeper portions of the lesion, the infiltrative nature, and the presence of muscle invasion.

The differential diagnosis of the nested variant of urothelial carcinoma includes prominent von Brunn's nests, cystitis cystica and glandularis, inverted papilloma, nephrogenic adenoma, and paraganglionic tissue and paraganglioma. The presence of deep invasion is most useful in distinguishing carcinoma from benign proliferations; nuclear atypia is of secondary value.[256,257] Closely packed small nests and irregularly distributed nests would also favor carcinoma.[257] Inverted papilloma lacks a nested architecture and consists of anastomosing trabeculae of urothelium with minimal nuclear atypia.[22,24] Nephrogenic adenoma typically has a papillary component and prominent tubular growth pattern.[240,258] The nested variant of carcinoma may mimic paraganglioma, but the prominent vascular network of paraganglioma that surrounds individual nests is different from carcinoma; immunohistochemistry may be useful in distinguishing carcinoma from paraganglioma in difficult cases.[259] Paraganglioma

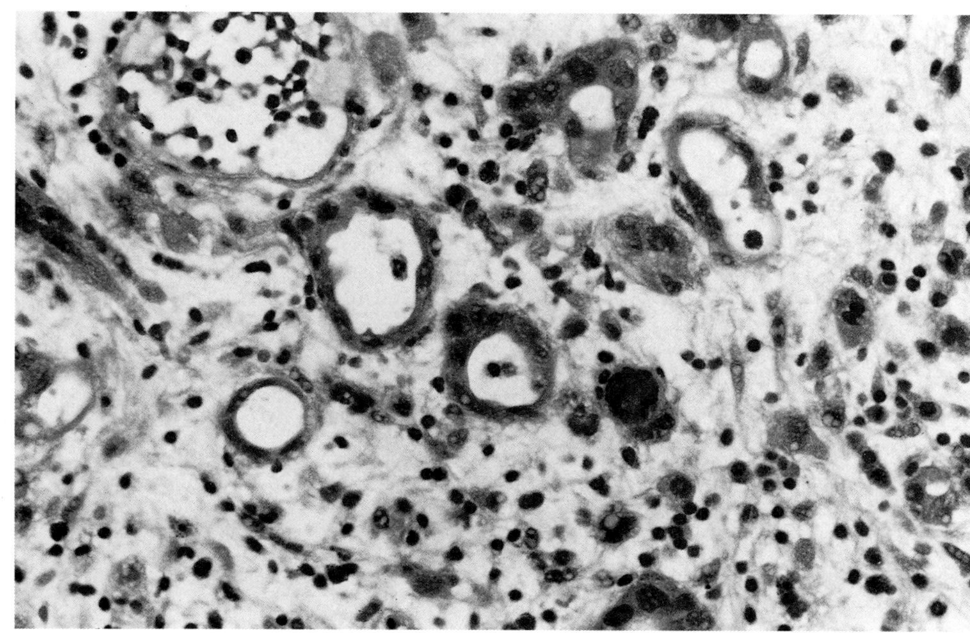

5-36. Microcystic variant of urothelial carcinoma with nests of tumor cells having central lumens.

consistently expresses neuroendocrine markers (neuron specific enolase, chromogranin, and others) and is nonreactive for cytokeratin.[259] Urothelial carcinoma expresses cytokeratin and other epithelial markers.[260,261]

Microcystic pattern. In 1991, Zukerberg and Young [262] described four cases of invasive urothelial carcinoma characterized by the formation of microcysts (Fig. 5-36). The pattern was similar to some foci of tubular differentiation included in the nested variant of Murphy and Deana[256] and deceptively benign appearing bladder cancer of Talbert and Young.[257] The reported cases included lesions with intermediate- to high-grade urothelial carcinoma having areas of microcystic or macrocystic change or tubular (glandular) differentiation. The cysts and tubules may be empty or may contain necrotic debris or mucin.

It is important to distinguish cystic change in urothelial carcinoma from benign and malignant mimics. It may be confused with benign proliferations such as cystitis cystica and glandularis and nephrogenic adenoma. The presence of significant nuclear atypia, at least focally, and areas of typical invasive urothelial carcinoma allow accurate separation. More problematic is the separation of the microcystic pattern of urothelial carcinoma and adenocarcinoma of the bladder. The diagnosis of adenocarcinoma should be restricted to pure tumors with true gland formation.[254] In microcystic urothelial cancer, the lining cells are urothelial.

Inverted growth pattern. In 1976, Cameron and Lupton[22] described two cases of urothelial carcinoma that mimicked inverted papilloma architecturally, but possessed high-grade cytologic abnormalities (Fig. 5-37). The potential for misinterpretation of such cases as inverted papilloma has been confirmed by other authors.[148,257] By definition, this variant of urothelial carcinoma has significant nuclear pleomorphism, mitotic

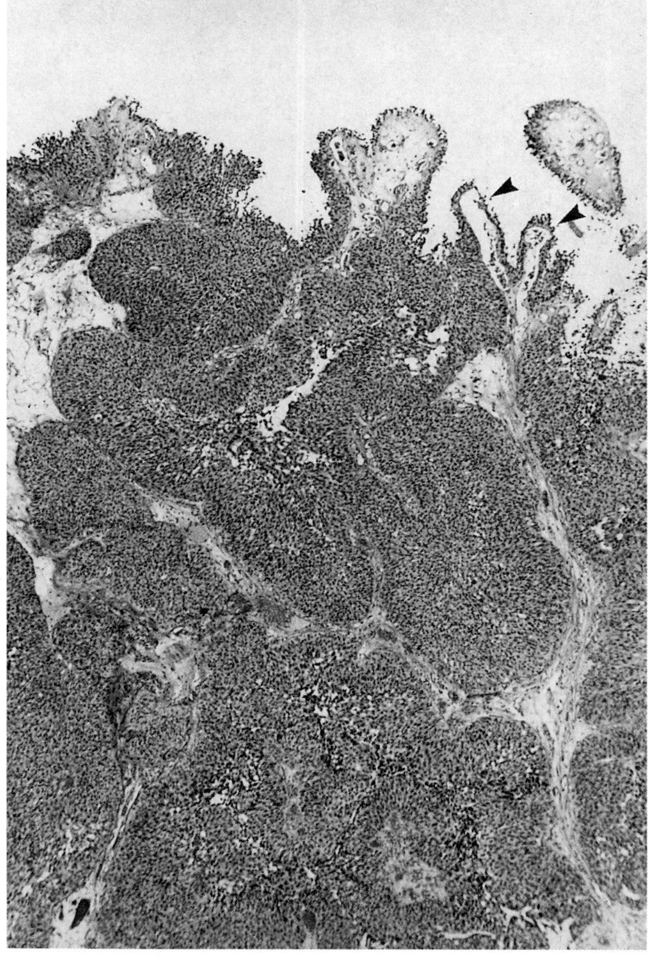

5-37. Invasive urothelial carcinoma with a predominantly inverted architecture mimicking inverted papilloma. Note the presence of a minor exophytic papillary component (*arrows*).

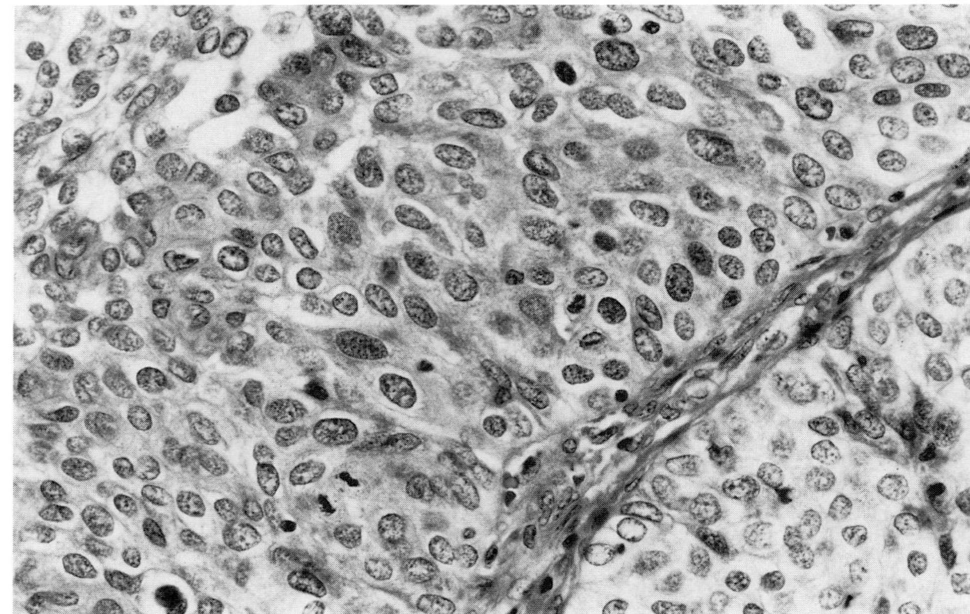

5-38. Invasive urothelial carcinoma with inverted pattern demonstrating architectural and cytologic pleomorphism incompatible with inverted papilloma.

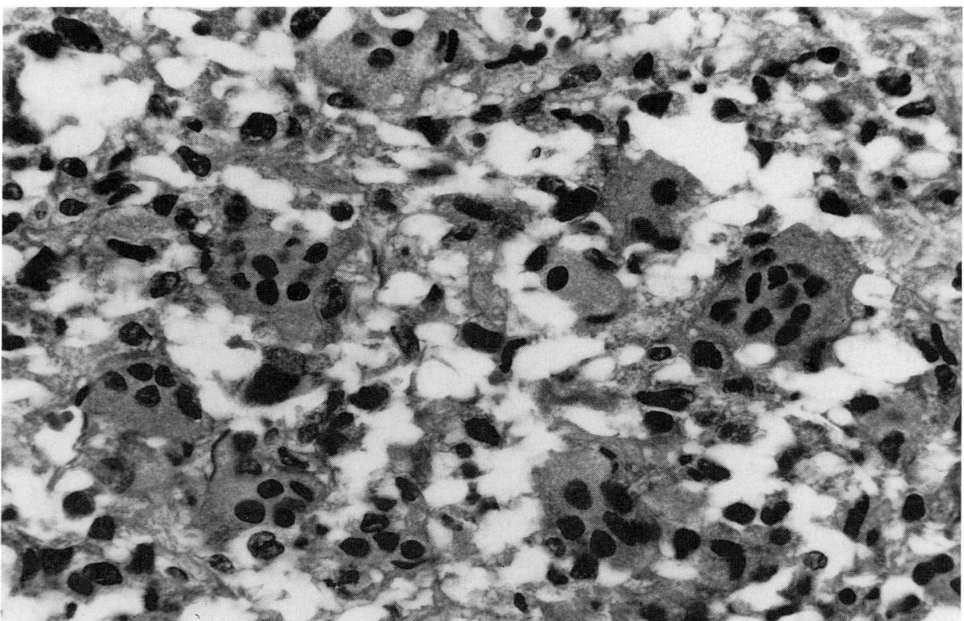

5-39. Urothelial carcinoma with numerous osteoclast-like giant cells.

figures, and architectural disruption consistent with WHO grades 2 or 3 (Fig. 5-38). In most, the overlying epithelium has similar abnormalities. An exophytic papillary or invasive component is often associated with the inverted element.

Giant cell variant. Giant cells have been reported in bladder tumors in a variety of different contexts. Giant cell carcinoma with malignant epithelial giant cells has been described,[5,263,264] and the giant cells stain positively for cytokeratin.[264] This tumor has a very poor prognosis.

Giant cells may also be found in urothelial carcinoma associated with human chorionic gonadotropin production, and are indicative of syncytiotrophoblastic differentiation (discussed in detail in the section titled Choriocarcinoma).[265]

Zukerberg et al[264] described the presence of osteoclast-like giant cells in two cases of invasive high-grade urothelial carcinoma, both of which had a sarcomatoid spindle cell component. The giant cells had abundant eosinophilic cytoplasm and numerous small, round, regular nuclei, and they stained positively for vimentin and tartrate-resistant acid phosphatase but not for epithelial markers (Fig. 5-39). Similar tumors have been described by other authors[266-268] as giant cell reparative granuloma and giant cell tumor. The giant cells probably reflect a stromal response to the tumor. There is no evidence to

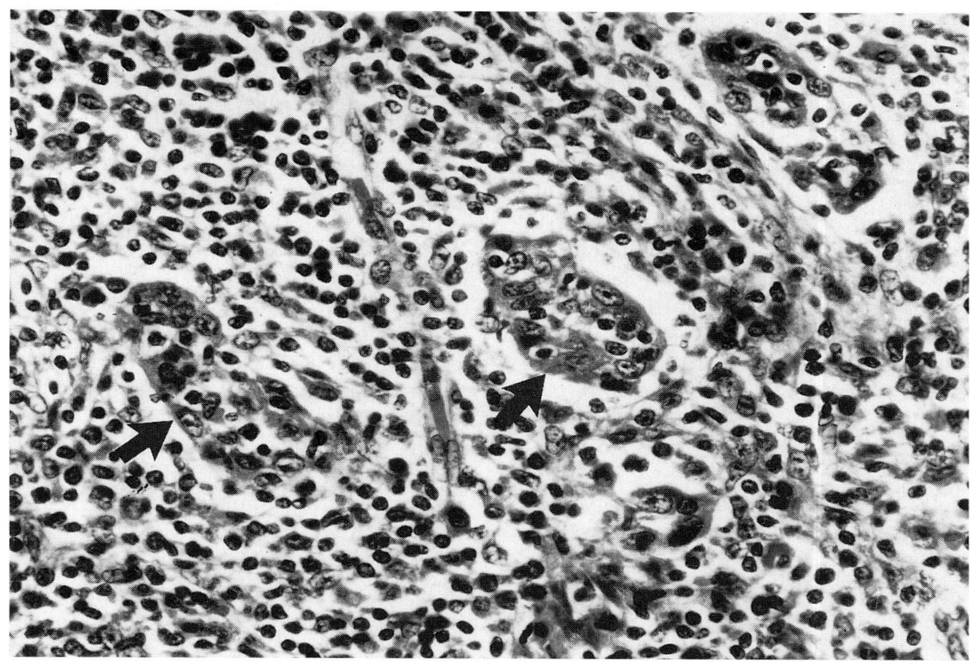

5-40. Lymphoepithelioma-like carcinoma of bladder with syncytial islands of tumor cells (*arrows*) in a cellular inflammatory background.

indicate that osteoclast-like giant cells indicate increased aggressiveness.

Giant cells are also seen in association with urothelial carcinoma in two other situations. In patients who have received bacillus Calmette-Guérin therapy, a granulomatous response that includes Langhans giant cells can be seen. Also, in patients who have undergone prior resection or biopsy, foreign body–type giant cells may be seen.

Lymphoepithelioma-like variant. Carcinoma that histologically resembles lymphoepithelioma of the nasopharynx[269,270] has recently been described in the urinary bladder, with 13 cases reported to date.[251,271-273] Histologically, similar tumors have been described in other sites[273] and some are related to Epstein-Barr virus infection.[274,275] Cases in the urinary bladder are more common in men than in women (10:3 ratio) and occur in late adulthood (range, 52 to 81 years; mean, 69 years). Most patients present with hematuria.

The tumor usually involves the dome, posterior wall, or trigone with a sessile growth pattern. Histologically, it may be pure or mixed with typical urothelial carcinoma, the latter being focal and inconspicuous in some instances. Glandular and squamous differentiation can be seen.[273] The tumor is composed of nests, sheets, and cords of undifferentiated cells with large pleomorphic nuclei and prominent nucleoli. The cytoplasmic borders are poorly defined, giving a syncytial appearance. The background consists of a prominent lymphoid stroma that includes lymphocytes, plasma cells, histiocytes, and occasional neutrophils or eosinophils (Fig. 5-40).

The major differential diagnostic considerations are poorly differentiated urothelial carcinoma, squamous cell carcinoma, and lymphoma, the last being most important. The presence of a recognizable urothelial or squamous cell carcinoma component does not exclude the diagnosis; rather, the diagnosis is based on finding areas typical of lymphoepithelioma reminiscent of that in the nasopharynx. Differentiation from lymphoma may be difficult,[271] but the presence of a syncytial pattern of large malignant cells with a dense polymorphous lymphoid background are important clues. Immunohistochemistry shows cytokeratin in the malignant cells, confirming their epithelial nature (Fig. 5-41).[273] It is possible to overlook the malignant cells in the background of inflamed bladder mucosa and misdiagnose the condition as florid chronic cystitis.[271,273] Cases submitted as tumors or masses should be carefully evaluated for the presence

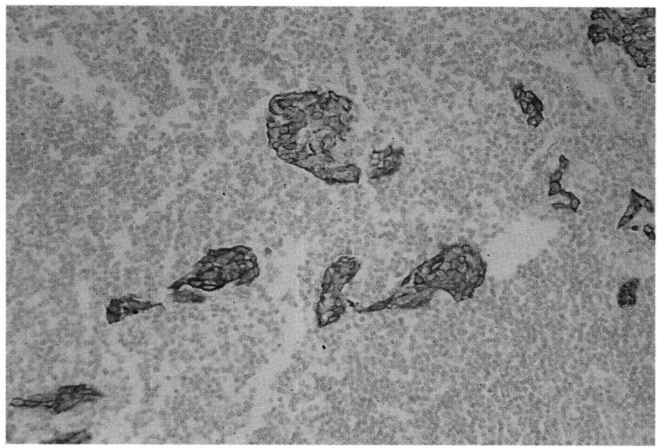

5-41. Lymphoepithelioma-like carcinoma stained immunohistochemically for cytokeratin highlighting the carcinoma cells in the inflammatory infiltrate.

of malignant cells; in difficult cases, immunohistochemistry should be employed as an adjunct to define an epithelial component within the inflammation.

The clinical significance of lymphoepithelioma-like carcinoma rests with its apparent responsiveness to chemotherapy.[273,276] In four cases reported from The M.D. Anderson Cancer Center,[273] there was complete response to transurethral resection combined with chemotherapy, allowing preservation of the bladder.

Lymphoma-like variant. Rare carcinomas of the urinary bladder can mimic malignant lymphoma. The following discussion does not include small cell carcinoma or lymphoepithelioma-like carcinoma, which are discussed in detail later in this chapter and above.

Zukerberg et al[271] described two cases of bladder carcinoma that diffusely permeated the bladder wall and were composed of cells with a monotonous appearance mimicking lymphoma. In both cases, the tumor cells were medium-sized, with eosinophilic cytoplasm and eccentric nuclei producing a plasmacytoid appearance. Typical urothelial carcinoma was found in one case. The diagnosis of carcinoma was confirmed by immunoreactivity for cytokeratin and carcinoembryonic antigen, and negative staining for lymphoid markers. A similar tumor, presenting as a scalp metastasis mimicking multiple myeloma, was reported by Sahin et al.[277] The author has also seen such a case (Fig. 5-42, 5-43).

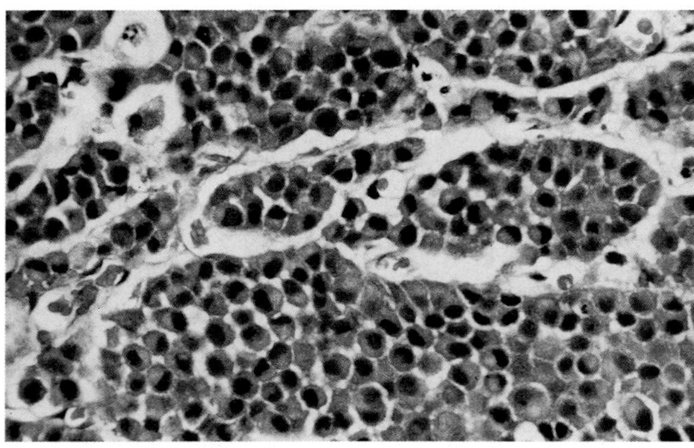

5-42. Invasive urothelial carcinoma composed of cells having a distinctive plasmacytoid morphology.

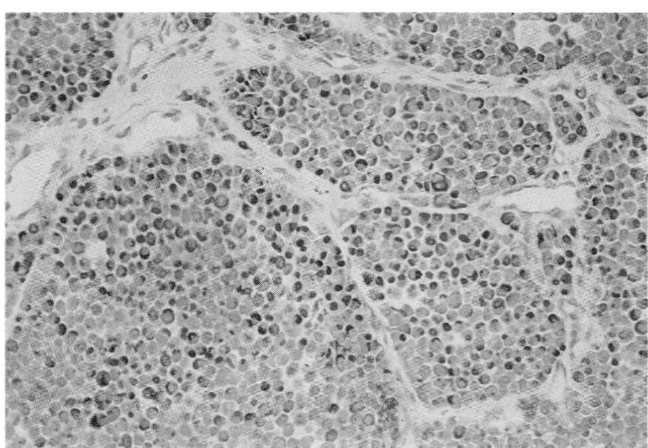

5-43. Plasmacytoid urothelial carcinoma (same case as Fig. 5-42) stained immunohistochemically for cytokeratin, confirming the epithelial nature of the tumor.

The differential diagnostic considerations are plasmacytosis, lymphoma, and multiple myeloma. Identification of an epithelial component confirms the diagnosis, but immunohistochemistry may be necessary to confirm the histologic impression.

Sarcomatoid urothelial carcinoma (carcinosarcoma). Rare cancers of the urinary bladder contain both malignant epithelial and malignant spindle cell components.[278,279] As in other organs, various terms have been used for these neoplasms, including carcinosarcoma,[280-284] sarcomatoid carcinoma,[285,286] pseudosarcomatous transitional cell carcinoma,[287] malignant mesodermal mixed tumor,[288,289] spindle cell and giant cell carcinoma,[263] and malignant teratoma.[278] There is considerable debate concerning the appropriate nomenclature for these tumors. Some authors include all such tumors under the term *sarcomatoid carcinoma*[286,288] or *carcinosarcoma*,[284] while others advocate using *sarcomatoid carcinoma* for those cases without heterologous elements in the spindle cell element and *carcinosarcoma* for cases with heterologous elements in the spindle cell component.[251,253,285,290-292] The two poten-

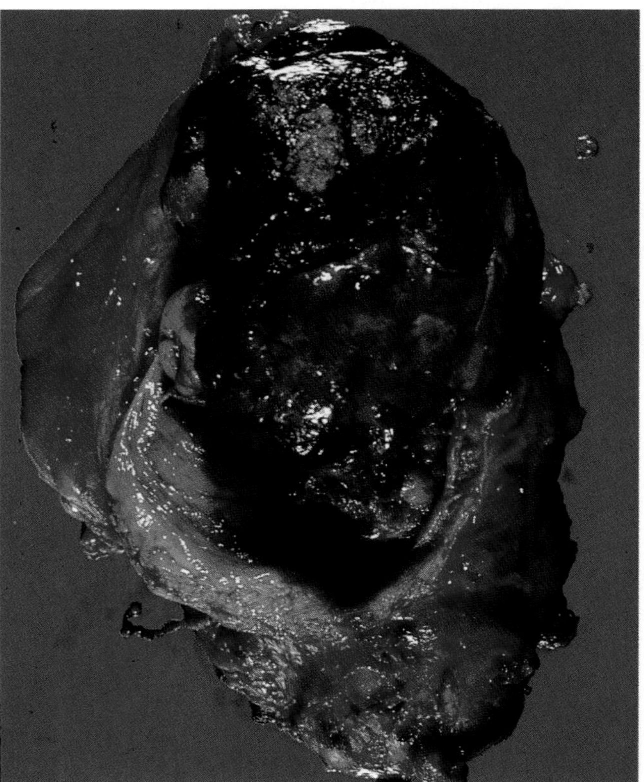

5-44. Sarcomatoid urothelial carcinoma having the characteristic exophytic polypoid gross appearance. *(Photograph courtesy of Dr. Alberto Ayala.)*

tial categories have similar clinical characteristics (patient age, sex, presentation, and outcome) and there is no compelling evidence to date which favors one or the other term. It is appropriate to report the presence of heterologous elements when present. The term *sarcomatoid carcinoma* is used in the remainder of this section for both types.

Clinical features. Sarcomatoid carcinoma affects males more frequently than females (2-3:1) and tends to occur in older patients (seventh and eighth decades), with only rare cases in patients under the age of 50 years. The most frequent presenting sign is hematuria, although irritative and obstructive symptoms can occur.

Pathology. Grossly, sarcomatoid carcinoma is usually exophytic, often with a polypoid or pedunculated growth pattern (Fig. 5-44); rarely, it is a sessile mass. Most are large, up to 12 cm in diameter.[234]

Histologically, the tumors contain a mixture of carcinoma and malignant spindle cells. The epithelial component is most often urothelial with squamous being next most frequent; adenocarcinoma[285,292] and small cell carcinoma[251,284,285,292] can also occur. In some cases, the epithelial component consists only of carcinoma in situ, while in others the epithelial component cannot be recognized histologically, and special studies are required to prove the epithelial nature of the spindle cells.[286,292]

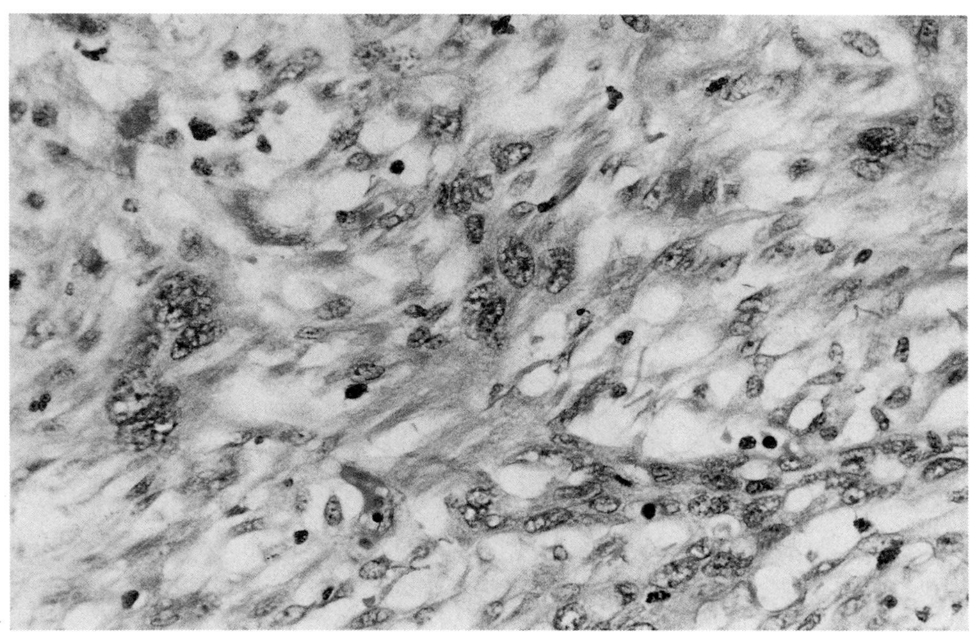

5-45. Sarcomatoid urothelial carcinoma composed of spindle shaped cells in a myxoid stroma.

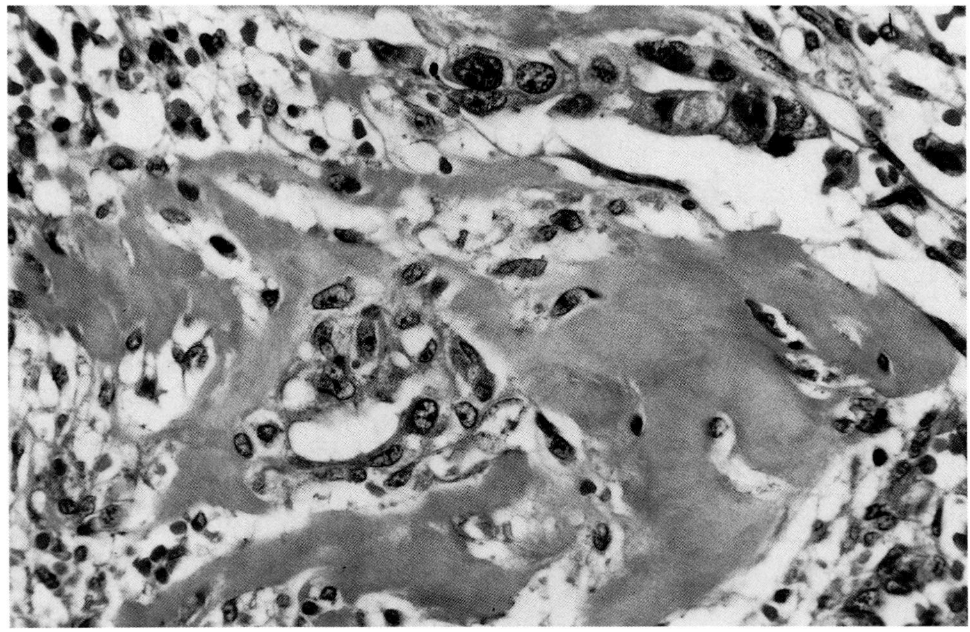

5-46. Sarcomatoid urothelial carcinoma with osteoid production.

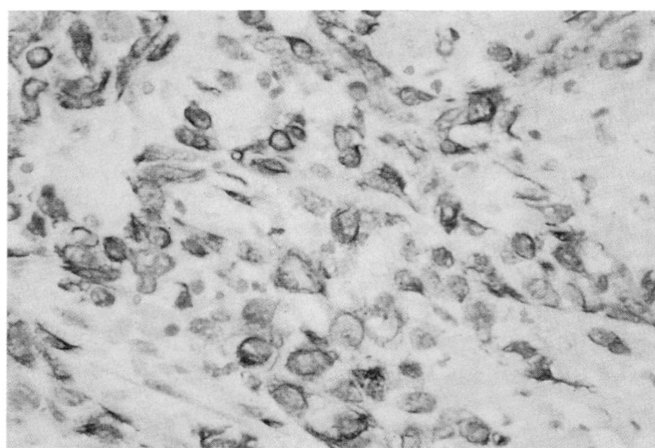

5-47. Sarcomatoid urothelial carcinoma stained immunohistochemically for cytokeratin showing strong cytoplasmic reactivity in the spindle cells.

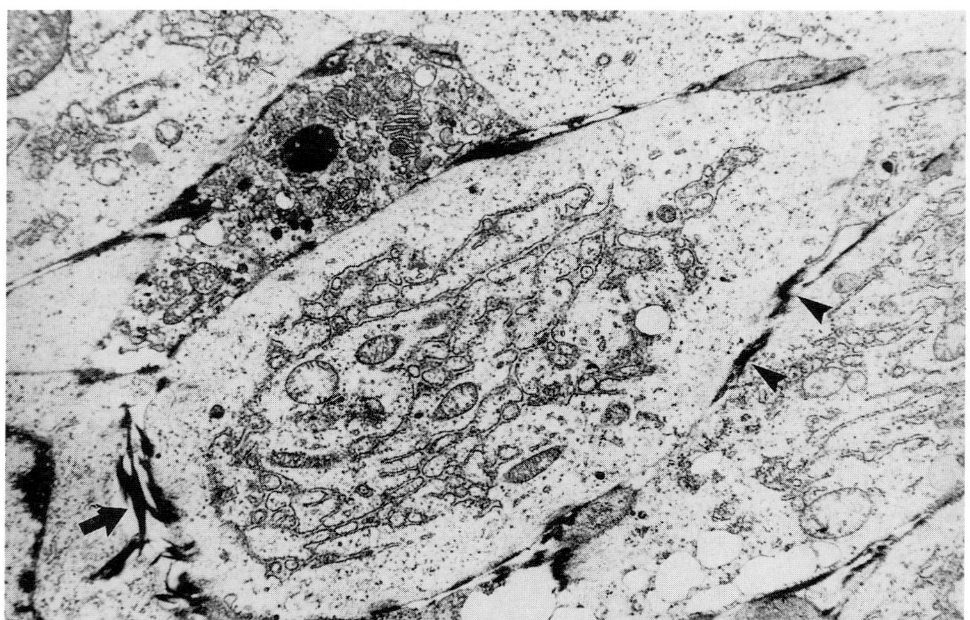

5-48. Electron micrograph of a sarcomatoid urothelial carcinoma demonstrating the presence of desmosomes (*arrowheads*) and tonofilaments (*arrow*).

In most cases, the spindle cell component consists of pleomorphic cells in poorly formed fascicles without a specific pattern of differentiation (Fig. 5-45).[286] The merging of the epithelial and spindle cell components is helpful in the diagnosis. In some cases the epithelial element appears as discrete nests in a background of malignant spindle cells. Heterologous differentiation, when present, usually consists of chondrosarcoma (47%), osteosarcoma (31%) (Fig. 5-46), or rhabdomyosarcoma (24%).[293]

Special studies. Several immunohistochemical studies of sarcomatoid carcinoma have been reported.* In most reports, the spindle cell element has been found to express cytokeratin at least focally (Fig. 5-47),[242,285,287,294] although in some cases cytokeratin has not been demonstrable.[242,281,292] Other epithelial markers such as epithelial membrane antigen may also be expressed although even less consistently.[242,292] Coexpression of vimentin in the spindle cell component is usual.[242,285,292] Occasionally, the spindle cells express muscle-specific actin, but are negative for desmin.[242] Heterologous elements express markers appropriate to the type of differentiation.[290]

Ultrastructural studies[290,295,296] indicate that the spindle cells in some cases do not have epithelial features[295,296] whereas in others there are desmosomes and tonofilament insertions (Fig. 5-48),[292] similar to sarcomatoid carcinomas in other organs.[297] Appropriate features have been described in the heterologous elements.[290,296]

Differential diagnosis. In cases with carcinoma and a malignant spindle cell component, the major differential diagnostic consideration is urothelial carcinoma with a pseudosarcomatous stroma,[242,298,299] a rare entity with reactive stroma that shows sufficient cellularity and atypia to raise a serious concern of sarcomatoid carcinoma (see Fig. 5-25). The stroma varies from myxoid with stellate or multinucleated cells to cellular and spindled

*References 242, 281, 285, 287, 290, 292, 294.

with fascicle formation. Immunohistochemically the stromal cells of pseudosarcoma show fibroblastic and myofibroblastic differentiation and invariably lack cytokeratin (see Fig. 5-26).[242]

Osseous metaplasia is present in some cases of urothelial carcinoma and should be differentiated from an osteosarcoma component.[300-303] This finding has also been described in metastatic urothelial carcinoma.[304-306] The metaplastic bone is histologically benign, with a normal lamellar pattern; it is usually found adjacent to areas of hemorrhage.[303] The cells in the adjacent stroma are cytologically benign.

The giant cells of giant cell cystitis should not be confused with sarcomatoid carcinoma. These cells typically have several small, round uniform nuclei and scant cytoplasm.[307-310]

In cases without obvious carcinoma, the main differential diagnostic consideration is sarcoma. Because of the rarity of primary bladder sarcoma, a malignant spindle cell tumor in the urinary bladder of an adult should be considered sarcomatoid carcinoma until proven otherwise. Extensive sectioning of the tumor and surrounding mucosa may reveal an in situ or invasive epithelial component. Immunohistochemical studies with antibodies to low– molecular weight cytokeratin may give evidence of epithelial differentiation; ultrastructural studies may also be helpful.

Treatment and outcome. Sarcomatoid urothelial carcinoma is highly malignant, with crude 1- and 2-year sur-

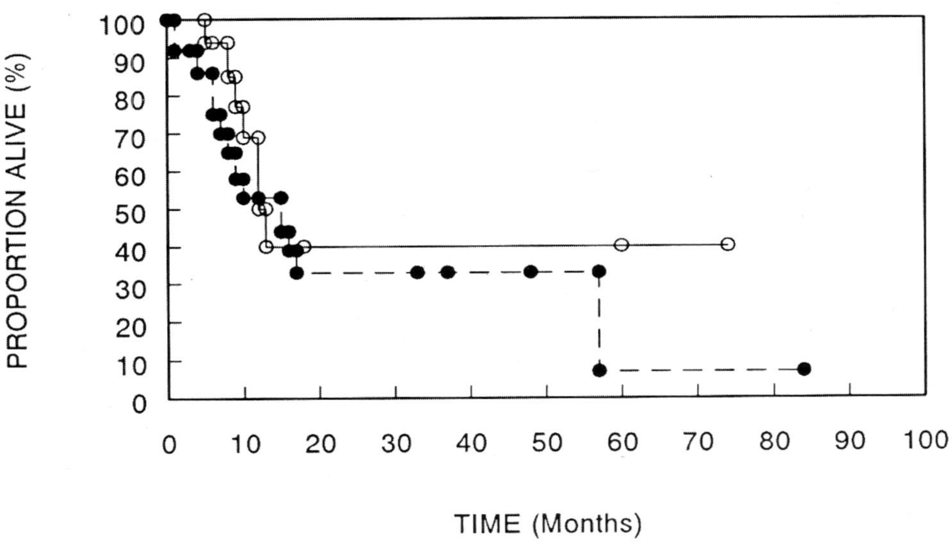

5-49. Kaplan-Meier survival curves for sarcomatoid urothelial carcinoma with (*dark circles*) and without (*open circles*) heterologous elements; there is no significant difference between the two (p>0.1, Log-rank test).

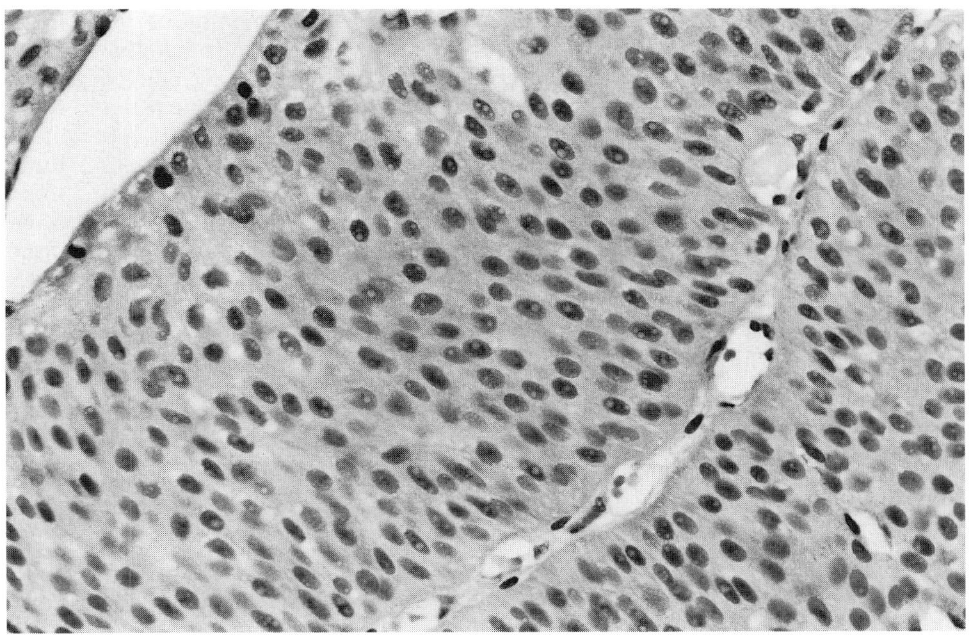

5-50. Papillary urothelial carcinoma, WHO grade 1. Note the thickened epithelium, mild nuclear atypia, preservation of architecture, and intact umbrella cell layer.

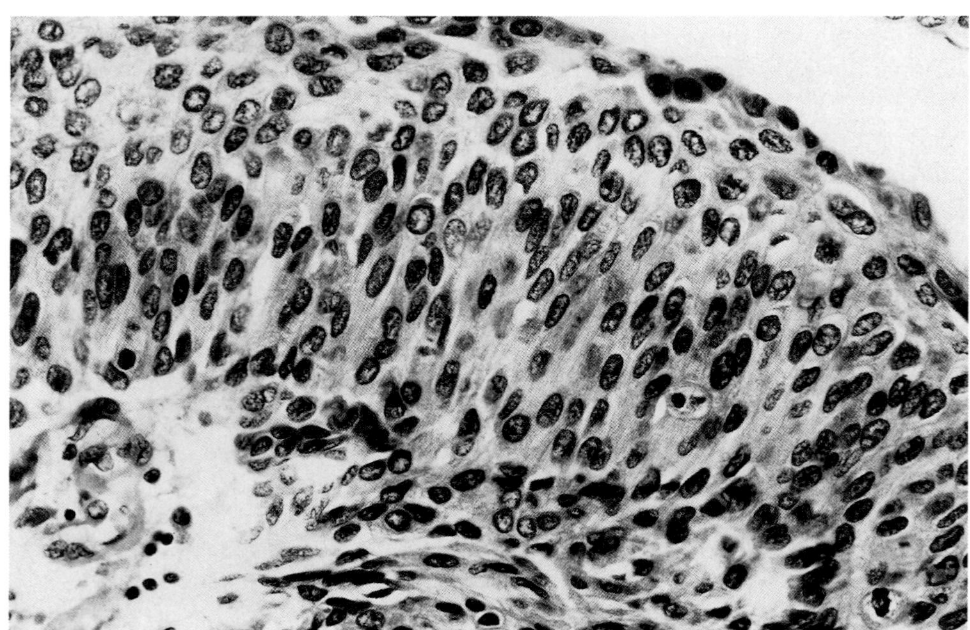

5-51. Papillary urothelial carcinoma, WHO grade 2. Note the variability in nuclear size, coarse chromatin pattern, focal crowding of cells with disturbance in architecture, and intact umbrella cell layer.

TABLE 5-2
HISTOLOGICAL GRADING CATEGORIES FOR PAPILLARY UROTHELIAL TUMORS

WHO	Murphy	Bergkvist	Pauwels
Papilloma	Papilloma	Papilloma	Papilloma
Grade 1	Papilloma	Grade 1	Grade 1
Grade 2	Low grade	Grade 2	Grade 2a
Grade 3	High grade	Grade 3	Grade 2b
		Grade 4	Grade 3

vivals of about 50% and 25%, respectively. Survival curves for 32 cases without heterologous elements* and 24 cases with heterologous elements† are shown in Figure 5-49; no significant differences are found between the two groups ($p>0.1$, log-rank test). Presently these tumors are treated the same as high-grade urothelial carcinoma.

Grading of urothelial carcinoma

The first grading scheme for urothelial carcinoma was proposed by Broders at the Mayo Clinic in 1922,[320] and was based on an estimate of the percentage of tumor cells that were differentiated; that is, the proportion of cells resembling normal urothelial cells. Since that time, a number of other grading systems have been proposed for urothelial carcinoma.[1,8,321,322] These have focused on papillary neoplasms and have had 4 (including papilloma) or 5 grades. The most widely applied grading system is that adopted by WHO.[1] In Table 5-2, the WHO system is compared with other commonly applied systems.[321,322] Grade 1 carcinoma has thickened epithelium, defined as more than seven cell layers. The cells show slight nuclear enlargement, maintain normal architecture, and contain rare or absent mitotic figures (Fig. 5-50). In grade 2 carcinoma, there is a greater degree of nuclear pleomorphism, with coarse chromatin and some disruption of the normal architecture. The number of cell layers may be increased, normal, or decreased. Mitotic figures remain infrequent (Fig. 5-51). Grade 3 carcinoma has severe nuclear atypia, similar to that seen in carcinoma in situ. There is loss of normal architecture and the cells become discohesive. Mitotic figures are usually frequent (Fig. 5-52). Lack of detailed histologic criteria has been a weakness of the WHO system and many recent attempts at modifying it have provided more detailed histologic criteria.[17,241,323]

One of the inevitable results of the inexact criteria for histological grading of urothelial carcinoma has been poor reproducibility.[13-15] Ooms et al[13] had six pathologists grade 57 cases of urothelial carcinoma and found only fair interobserver and intraobserver correlation. Strikingly, the percentage of cases called grade 3 (high grade) ranged from 18% to 44%. This finding has considerable significance because of the prognostic

*References 263, 285, 287, 292, 311, 312.

†References 266, 280-282, 288, 289, 291, 293, 296, 313-319.

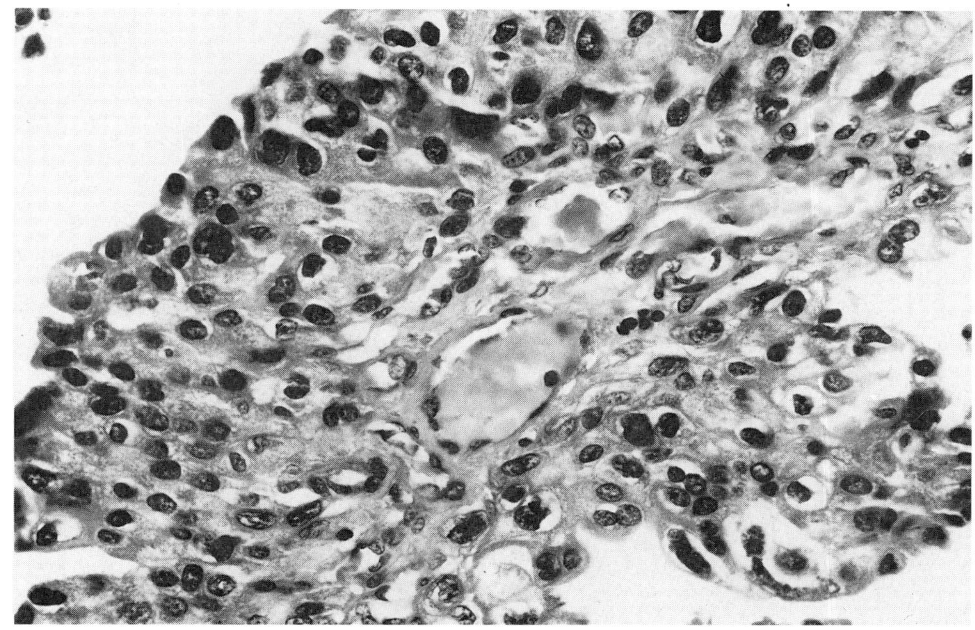

5-52. Papillary urothelial carcinoma, WHO grade 3. Note the nuclear pleomorphism and hyperchromasia, loss of architecture, and presence of pleomorphic cells at the surface.

importance of histological grade and the influence of grade on therapeutic decisionmaking. In a similar study with eight participating pathologists, Robertson et al[15] found an overall "poor" to "fair" degree of interobserver concordance and a "poor" degree of intraobserver agreement. The importance of this problem is readily apparent when comparing various clinicopathologic studies of urothelial carcinoma. Jordan et al[8] studied 407 consecutive unselected cases of urothelial carcinoma and found a WHO distribution of 25% grade 1, 13% grade 2, and 63% grade 3. In their hands, 96.5% of invasive cancers (stage T1 or greater) were grade 3, and no grade 1 cancers were invasive. In contrast, in a study of 168 consecutive carcinomas by Pauwels et al,[17] the WHO distribution was 8% grade 1, 69% grade 2, and 23% grade 3. Of the invasive cancers, only 43.5% were grade 3. A study of 103 invasive urothelial carcinomas by Lipponen et al[18] found that 14% were grade 1, 58% grade 2, and 28% grade 3. Despite this wide variation in histologic grading, these[8,17,18] and other studies have convincingly demonstrated the powerful prognostic importance of grading urothelial carcinoma.[324,325]

In most investigators' hands, a large proportion of cases fall into the intermediate (WHO grade 2) group. Pauwels et al[17] stressed the degree of nuclear deviation and polarity of cells as a way of subdividing this large intermediate grade group. Grade 2a tumors showed slight cellular deviation and some variation in nuclear size and retained the normal polarity of the cells. In contrast, grade 2b tumors had obvious variability in nuclear size and shape with some loss of normal polarity. Tumor progression occurred in 4% (2 of 54) grade 2a, pTa/pT1 carcinomas, compared to 33% (7 of 21) grade 2b, pTa/pT1 urothelial carcinomas.[17] The application of these criteria to muscle invasive cancer has also been found to significantly predict outcome.[16] Lipponen et al,[241] with a similar goal in mind, found the mitotic index to be most useful. Other groups have applied nuclear morphometry to separate the low- and high-grade groups.[326-330]

Jordan et al[8] did not find heterogeneity within individual cases to be a significant problem in grading bladder cancer, but other authors have noted a high degree of heterogeneity.[323] Grade is assigned based on the worst grade present.[322,323,331]

Histological grading is important and should be reported for all cases of urothelial carcinoma. No one system seems to be superior to another, although the criteria used in the WHO system[1] and by Bergkvist et al[322] are most widely used. The College of American Pathologists recommends use of the WHO grading system (Dr. E. Hammond, personal communication, 1995). In reporting grade, the denominator should be indicated so as to avoid possible confusion, and the grade assigned should represent the highest grade present.

Immunohistochemistry

Several groups have evaluated the expression of cytokeratins in urothelial carcinoma.[260,332,333] The normal urothelium expresses simple cytokeratins and cytokeratins associated with stratified epithelia.[332] Higher grade urothelial carcinoma tends to lose the high molecular weight cytokeratins associated with stratified epithelia.[332] Urothelial carcinoma has also been shown to express other epithelial markers including epithelial membrane antigen,[261] Leu-M1,[334] and carcinoembryonic antigen.[335]

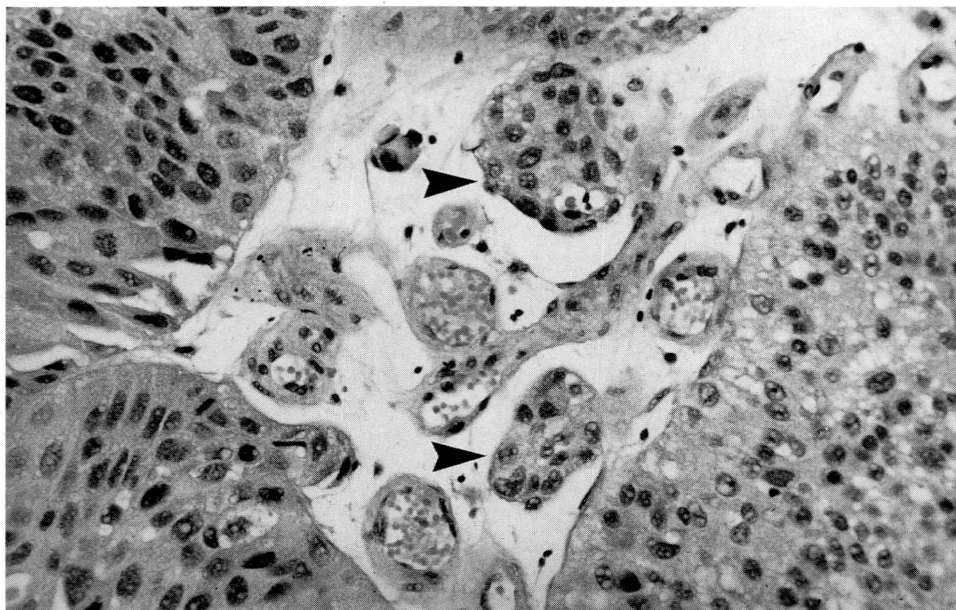

5-53. Papillary urothelial carcinoma, WHO grade 2, with early stromal invasion at the base of the papillae (*arrows*).

Electron microscopy

Ultrastructural studies of urothelial carcinoma reveal typical features of epithelial differentiation, including desmosomes and tonofilaments.[336,337] In one report, increased tumor grade was associated with a decrease in the number of desmosomes per unit area.[336] Scanning electron microscopy has demonstrated the presence of microvilli on the surface of urothelial carcinoma.[196,337]

Diagnosis of invasion and pathologic staging

Up to 80% of cases of urothelial carcinoma are noninvasive at the time of presentation. The presence of early invasion (stage T1) has therapeutic and prognostic significance,[229,338] and should be carefully looked for in both papillary and flat lesions. Farrow and Utz[338] found that microinvasion (in this study defined as invasion of 5 mm or less into lamina propria) was associated with a significantly increased risk of metastatic cancer. Once invasion is identified, it is critical to determine microscopically the depth of invasion. Assessment of involvement of the muscularis propria is perhaps the single most important role the pathologist plays in the management of bladder cancer.

Papillary tumors are often difficult to evaluate for invasion. They have pushing borders and may encroach on the muscularis propria without showing a truly infiltrative pattern of invasion,[192] although an infiltrative component can be found at the base of the papillae (Fig. 5-53). Invasive urothelial carcinoma typically appears as small nests or cords of cells with a prominent desmoplastic tissue response. The cells in the nests are often of higher grade than the papillary component above. Although invasion can occur with grade 1 papillary carcinoma, the majority are grade 2 or 3.

Significance of muscularis mucosae. In 1985, Dixon and Gosling[339] described the muscularis mucosae of the human urinary bladder. Subsequently this struc-

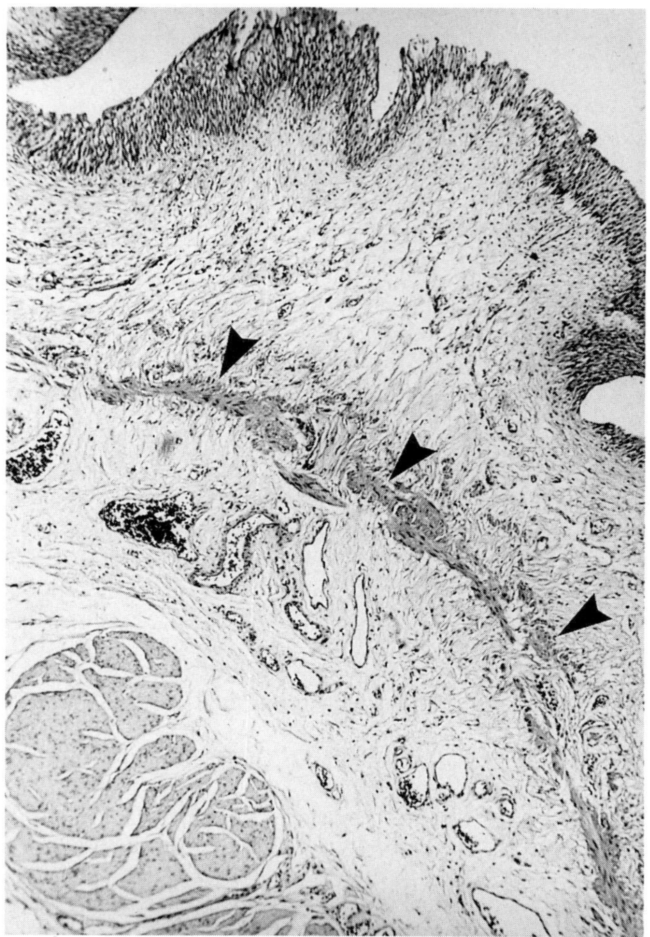

5-54. Normal urinary bladder wall with a well-developed muscularis mucosae (*arrows*). Note also the layer of vascular channels immediately beneath the muscularis mucosae.

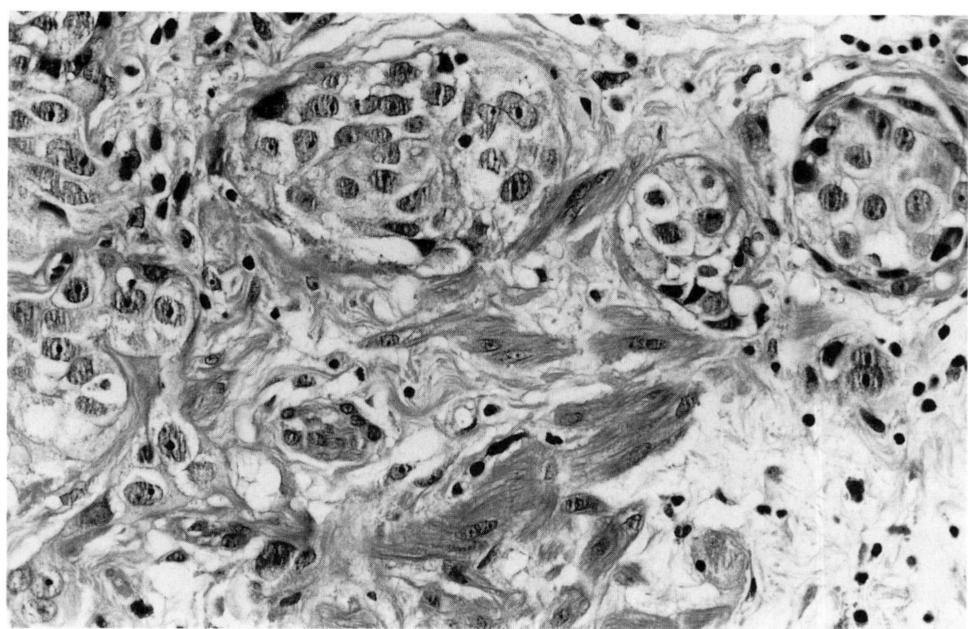

5-55. Invasive urothelial carcinoma involving the muscularis mucosae, characterized by thin wispy smooth muscle fibers (compare with Fig. 5-56).

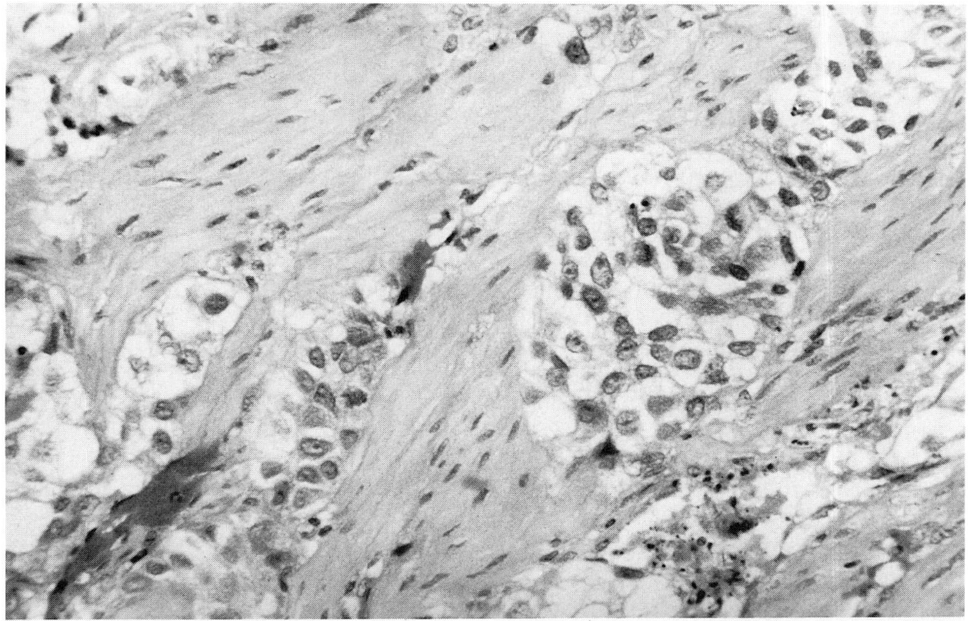

5-56. Invasive urothelial carcinoma involving the muscularis propria, characterized by thick, dense bundles of smooth muscle cells.

ture was studied by other groups.[340,341] A complete or nearly complete muscularis mucosae was found in 23% to 60% of bladders, with at least scattered muscle fibers present in the lamina propria in up to 100% of bladders (Fig. 5-54).[340,341] The muscle fibers of the muscularis mucosae are small and typically form small wispy groups, unlike the thick bundles of the muscularis propria. In the trigone, the muscle fibers have a loose interwoven architecture, and, in this region, separation of the muscularis mucosae and muscularis propria is difficult. Another feature defining the muscularis mucosae is its association with a layer of medium-sized arterial and venous vessels.

Ro et al[340] cautioned against overstaging patients with stage T1 disease by misinterpreting extension into the muscularis mucosae as invasion of the muscularis propria (Fig. 5-55, 5-56). Abel et al[14] documented this problem, noting that 6 of 29 patients were erroneously diagnosed with muscle-invasive cancer; one actually had stage pTa carcinoma and five had pT1 carcinoma. The latter was misdiagnosed because of over interpretation of muscularis mucosae fiber involvement in biopsies.

The potential for substaging patients with stage T1 bladder cancer using the muscularis mucosae as an anatomic level has been studied. Younes et al[342] reported that survival of patients with stage T1 cancer with invasion beyond the muscularis mucosae is similar to survival of those with invasion of the muscularis propria, and significantly worse than the survival of those with invasion of the lamina propria superficial to the muscularis mucosae. Hasui et al[343] studied 88 patients with stage T1 disease and classified them into T1a (60 patients with invasion superficial to muscularis mucosae) and T1b (28 patients with invasion deep to muscularis mucosae). The progression rate was 53.5% in patients with T1b tumors compared to 6.7% in those with T1a tumors. Another study reported similar results,[344] indicating that substaging of T1 carcinoma may be recommended in the future.

Other prognostic markers

Increased understanding of the natural history of bladder cancer combined with therapeutic advances indicate a need for more accurate prediction of the behavior of a bladder cancer in individual patients. In the following sections, less studied histologic features and more recent tumor markers are discussed.

Invasion of blood vessels and lymphatics. Invasion of blood and lymphatic channels has been considered an important prognostic factor in urothelial carcinoma.[229,345-349] Bell et al[345] reported 5-year survivals of 29% and 51% for patients with and without vascular invasion, respectively. However, two recent studies of stage T1 tumors failed to demonstrate prognostic value for blood or lymphatic vessel invasion when endothelial markers were used to confirm this feature.[345,350]

Identification of vascular invasion may be difficult.[350,351] Artifactual clefting around nests of invasive carcinoma mimics vascular invasion (see Fig. 5-27, 5-28). Endothelial cell markers such as *Ulex europaeus* and factor VIII–related antigen have been utilized to confirm vascular involvement (Fig. 5-57).[350,351] That overdiagnosis is a problem is underscored by the study of Larsen et al,[351] in which the lectin *Ulex europaeus* agglutinin I confirmed the presence of vascular invasion in only 5 of 36 cases (14%) initially considered to have this feature. In a similar study, Ramani et al[350] used several endothelial markers, but confirmed the presence of vascular/lymphatic invasion in only 2 of 5 stage T1 bladder cancers (40%) considered to have this feature by routine light microscopy.

DNA content (ploidy). DNA content has been extensively studied in urothelial carcinoma, and the review of Wheeless et al[352] has covered this in depth. There is a strong correlation between aneuploidy and high grade and high stage.[353-360] One exception to the latter is urothelial carcinoma in situ, which is almost always aneuploid. In papillary carcinoma, Blomjous et al[354] detected aneuploidy in 0% of grade 1, 61% of grade 2, and 100% of grade 3 tumors; they also found the frequency of aneuploidy increased from 14% in stage Ta tumors to 83% in muscle-invasive (stages T2-T4) carcinoma.

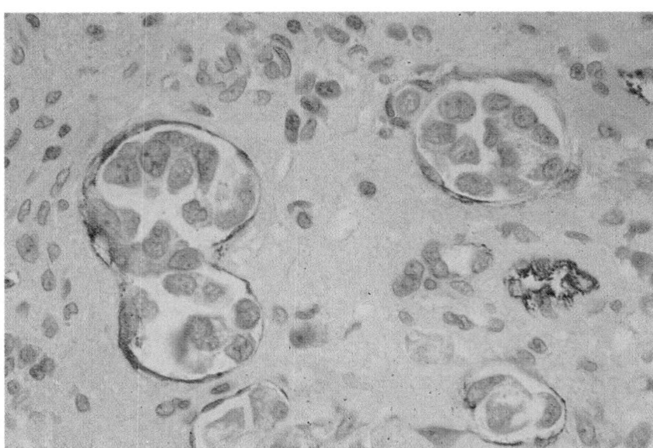

5-57. Urothelial carcinoma with vascular invasion; the endothelial cells are highlighted by immunohistochemical staining for Factor VIII–related antigen.

DNA ploidy has repeatedly been shown to be a significant prognostic indicator for urothelial carcinoma.[353,354,357] For noninvasive (Ta) and invasive tumors limited to the submucosa (T1), which are treated conservatively, DNA content is a powerful indicator of the potential for recurrence and progression.[329,354,360-363] Blomjous et al[329] reported recurrences in 87% of patients with DNA aneuploid pTa/pT1 tumors and in 66% of diploid cases. Progression occurred in 60% of patients with DNA aneuploid pTa/pT1 urothelial carcinomas, but only in 2% of patients with DNA diploid tumors. Between 73% and 97% of muscle-invasive tumors are DNA aneuploid,[355,356] so DNA content is of less value as a prognostic marker for these tumors.[352,361]

Recent studies indicate that the presence of an aneuploid population predicts a better response to radiation therapy[358,364] or to combined radiation therapy and chemotherapy[365] although these have not been uniformly found.[366]

Cellular proliferation. Cellular proliferation in urothelial carcinoma has been assessed by different methods, including mitotic figure counting,[367] flow cytometry (S-phase fraction),[353,355,358,359] immunohistochemistry for proliferating cell nuclear antigen (PCNA)[368,369] and Ki-67,[370,371] and bromodeoxyuridine incorporation.[370,372,373] Most studies have shown a positive correlation between increased proliferation and higher grade and stage.* In studies with outcome data, a positive correlation with prognosis has also been demonstrated.[353,363] Lipponen et al[363,367,374,375] have reported in several studies that mitotic rate is a powerful prognostic indicator independent of grade and stage.

Morphometry. Morphometric analysis of nuclear size, nuclear area, and other features can assist in grading urothelial carcinoma.[376] The prognostic significance of

*References 353,355,358,359,367,370,371,373.

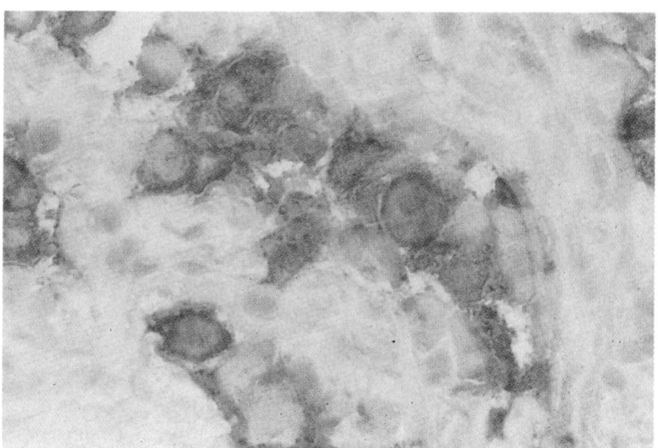

5-58. Invasive urothelial carcinoma: immunohistochemical reaction showing expression of epidermal growth factor receptor (EGFR).

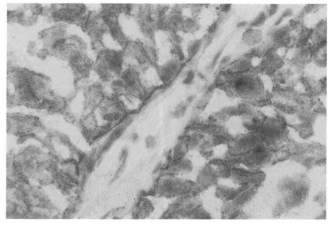

5-59. Invasive urothelial carcinoma: immunohistochemical demonstration of excessive expression of the c-erbß-2 oncogene.

these indices has also been studied.[367,377] In a large series reported by Lipponen et al,[367] the mean nuclear area, standard deviation of the mean nuclear area, and mean nuclear area of the 10 largest nuclei correlated significantly with prognosis. In Cox regression analysis, mean nuclear area added power to the prediction of outcome.

Basement membrane integrity. Several studies, based on immunohistochemistry for collagen and laminin, have evaluated the importance of basement membranes in bladder cancer.[378-381] These have shown an intact basement membrane surrounding some invasive tumor nests while in others there is complete absence of a basement membrane. The pattern of basement membrane staining (degree of completeness) correlates with survival.[378,379,381] Schapers et al[381] showed that the 5-year survival for patients with tumors with intact basement membranes was 61%, compared to 32% for those with patchy or absent basement membrane staining.

Blood group antigens. There has been considerable interest in the blood group antigens expressed by urothelial tumors. Depending on the individual, normal urothelium expresses A, B, and precursor H antigens, as well as the related M, N, T, and Lewis antigens. Loss of blood group antigens correlates with histological grade, and, in some studies, indicates an increased risk of progression in patients with noninvasive papillary urothelial carcinoma.[382-385] Interpretation of staining in patient material has been difficult because of the heterogeneity within individual cases[383,386] as well as the occurrence of loss of expression in non-neoplastic inflammatory conditions.[387] For these and other reasons, this technique has never gained widespread acceptance in clinical practice.

Other antigens. Class I and class II HLA antigens are expressed by some invasive urothelial carcinomas.[368,388,389] Levin et al[368] found that patients with HLA class I antigen-positive tumors had a 5-year survival of 74% compared with 36% for patients with antigen-negative tumors.

Tissue polypeptide antigen (TPA) is a metabolic product of cytokeratin that can be detected in urine and serum. Elevated levels in the serum and urine of patients with urothelial carcinoma are associated with higher grade, higher stage, and an increased risk of progression and death from cancer.[390-392] The practical use of this marker is limited by its lack of specificity, and because elevated levels can appear in patients with inflammatory conditions and in some normal individuals.[393]

Growth factors. Expression of epidermal growth factor receptor correlates with histologic grade[394-396] and stage[394,395] of urothelial carcinoma of the urinary bladder (Fig. 5-58). In lower stage tumors (Ta and T1) expression correlates with recurrence and progression, and, in higher stage tumors with death.[395] The mechanism by which epidermal growth factor receptor is expressed appears to be related to mRNA over expression and not DNA amplification.[397]

Oncogenes. The *ras* oncogene was discovered in human bladder and lung carcinoma cells and has received considerable attention in bladder cancer.[398-401] Increased *ras* oncogene expression is seen in dysplastic and malignant urothelium.[398-400,402] Recently, *H-ras* mutations in cells from urine specimens have been examined as a diagnostic test for bladder cancer with some success;[403] no defined role as a prognostic marker has been demonstrated.

The HER-2\neu oncogene (c-erbß-2) is expressed in a significant number of urothelial carcinomas (Fig. 5-59).[401,404-409] This oncogene codes for a membrane receptor protein related to the epidermal growth factor receptor. Most studies show a positive correlation between c-erbß-2 expression and histologic grade, stage, and, in some reports, prognosis. However, a recent study found an inverse relationship between c-erbß-2 expression and survival.[410] Increased c-erbß-2 expression is probably caused by increased mRNA expression, although not all cases with increased mRNA expression show increased protein expression.[406]

Suppressor genes. There is presently great interest in two suppressor genes as prognostic indicators in bladder cancer. Mutations of the p53 suppressor gene have been found in urothelial carcinoma,[411-419] and are associated with allelic deletion on chromosome 17p, the site of the p53 suppressor gene (Fig. 5-60).[122,124] Abnormalities in the p53 gene are also present in dysplastic epithelium

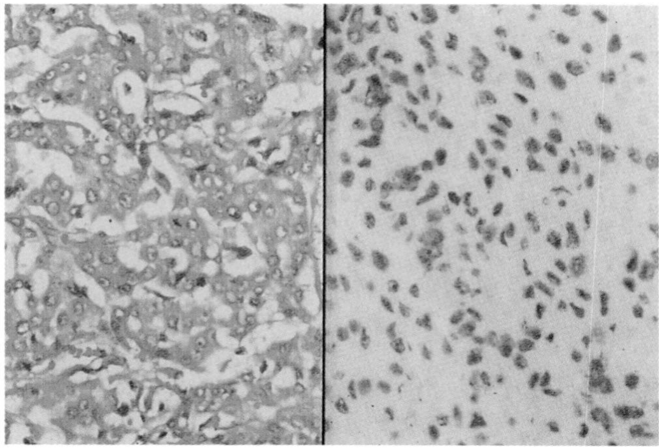

5-60. Urothelial carcinoma with excessive expression of the p53 tumor suppressor gene as detected by immunohistochemistry (DO7 antibody, right photo).

adjacent to tumors.[417] Several studies have demonstrated a positive correlation between p53 abnormalities and higher tumor stage.[411,417-419] Sarkis et al[415] reported a much higher risk of progression in patients with pT1 tumors with abnormal p53 protein expression than in those without. In a study of 212 patients, Lipponen[420] confirmed the prognostic significance of p53 protein status, but did not find it to be a predictor of survival independent of stage and mitotic index. Esrig et al[421] studied 243 patients with urothelial carcinoma treated by cystectomy using immunohistochemistry for p53 protein accumulation. Over expression correlated significantly with recurrence and crude survival, and, on multivariate regression analysis, was independent of pathologic stage and histologic grade. For muscle invasive tumors (pT2 and pT3a), the 5-year survivals were 79% and 64% for p53 negative cases, and 30% and 22% for p53 positive cases, respectively. The specific type and site of p53 gene mutations have also been related to the presumed mechanism of carcinogenesis.[416,422]

The retinoblastoma suppressor gene product is also lost in high-grade bladder cancer.[423-425] Two reports have shown a significant correlation between loss of retinoblastoma suppressor gene protein expression and decreased survival in patients with urothelial carcinoma.[426,427]

Treatment and natural history

One of the greatest problems in assessing the treatment of bladder cancer has been the tendency to group patients with different stages (Ta, TIS, and T1) into a single group. The lack of stratification makes interpretation of many studies difficult and results of different treatment trials are often not comparable. For this reason, these three stage groupings are discussed separately.

Stage Ta. The mainstay of treatment for noninvasive papillary urothelial carcinoma is transurethral resection and fulguration of the visible tumors (TURBT). With this treatment, the crude 5-year survival ranges from 80% to 90%.[229,428] For these patients, the rate of recurrence and progression is particularly important. *Recurrence* refers to the subsequent development of new tumors following initial therapy, although some studies restrict this term to new tumors of a similar grade and stage. *Progression* refers to the development of new tumors of higher grade and of higher stage. The most important predictors of new tumor development are the original number of tumors,[6,7,217,231] tumor size,[6,7,217] histologic grade,[216,217] history of previous recurrences, and associated dysplasia and carcinoma in situ in the adjacent urothelium.[216,217] Predictors of progression to invasive carcinoma are the number of tumors,[231] tumor size,[217] histologic grade,[216,217,231,429] and associated dysplasia and carcinoma in situ.[216,217] The relationship of these factors to the risk of recurrence and progression are not the same in all studies.[430] Kiemeney et al[231] developed a prognostic index for the risk of recurrence and progression based on a cohort of 1745 patients with pTa and pT1 tumors. The 3-year risk of recurrence was 55%, with stage, tumor extent, and multicentricity being most significant. Histologic grade and the status of the adjacent epithelium were not significant predictors of recurrence. The risk of progression was 10%, and was most strongly predicted by multicentricity, histologic grade, and stage.

In patients at high risk for recurrence and progression, a variety of adjuvant therapies have been applied, including intravesical chemotherapy (triethylenethiophosphoramide [Thiotepa], mitomycin-C, and doxorubicin [Adriamycin]), intravesical immunotherapy (bacillus Calmette-Guérin and interferon), photoradiation, laser, and vitamin therapy. Currently, bacillus Calmette-Guérin and intravesical chemotherapy with Thiotepa and mitomycin-C are widely used.[431-437] Accurate pathologic assessment of histologic grade of the tumor and the status of the adjacent mucosa are important in guiding the selection of adjuvant therapy based on the relative risk of tumor recurrence and progression.[438] These features should be carefully documented in all specimens.

Follow-up in these patients depends on the characteristics of the tumor, but most are followed with repeat cystoscopy (with urine and bladder wash cytologies and biopsy as indicated) every 3 months for 2 years, every 6 months for the next 2 years, and once a year thereafter.[128] Up to 5% of patients develop upper tract tumors,[431] indicating the need for annual upper tract studies.

Rarely, extensive superficial papillary carcinomas are cystoscopically unresectable, requiring cystectomy. Metastases rarely develop from papillary tumors in the absence of demonstrable invasion.[439]

Stage TIS (urothelial carcinoma in situ). Carcinoma in situ occurs most often in association with bladder tumors of other types. Whether de novo carcinoma in situ is more aggressive than carcinoma in situ associated with other tumors is unknown, and treatment depends on the extent of carcinoma. Transurethral resection may be adequate in localized cases, but adjuvant intravesical therapy is usually required. Bacillus Calmette-Guérin and intravesical chemotherapy remain the standard treatments.[433,436,437]

Patients with carcinoma in situ require close follow-up. In those with extensive carcinoma in situ, the risk of progression to invasive disease is up to 80% at 5 years.[440]

In one study, 34% of patients undergoing cystectomy for carcinoma in situ had microinvasion when the cystectomy specimen was evaluated pathologically.[175] Follow-up biopsies are frequently performed in this group irrespective of the cystoscopic findings as areas of carcinoma in situ may not be grossly recognizable. Interpretation of biopsy and cytology specimens from these patients often is complicated by treatment-induced alterations in benign epithelium. Pathologists must be aware of the treatment given to these patients and the morphological changes induced by these agents. Patients who fail to respond to topical therapy may require radical surgery (cystectomy or cystoprostatectomy).[441]

Stage T1. Invasion of the lamina propria without extension into the muscularis propria does not require radical surgery.[128,442] These patients are usually treated by transurethral resection with or without adjuvant intravesical therapy. The presence of invasion does increase the risk of progression compared with stages Ta and TIS carcinoma,[217,231,429,442,443] and most patients receive adjuvant intravesical therapy.[436-438,444] Crude 3- and 5-year survival for patients with pT1 tumors is about 80% and 70%, respectively.[228] For patients with grade 3 carcinoma, 3- and 5-year survival decreases to about 75% and 60%, respectively.[228,229] Some urologists consider cystectomy the treatment of choice for patients with grade 3 pT1 tumors because of this risk.[445]

Stages T2, T3, and T4. In North America, the standard treatment for muscle-invasive bladder cancer is total cystectomy or cystoprostatectomy. Conservative treatment by transurethral resection or partial cystectomy may yield comparable results in selected patients,[446,447] but most restrict this approach to small tumors in the bladder dome or posterior wall without associated urothelial carcinoma in situ.[448] In contrast, radiation therapy is the most frequent treatment for muscle invasive bladder cancer in other parts of the world.

Survival rates following total cystectomy vary widely and depend on stage. Survival rates following radiation therapy also vary widely.[449-451]

Recently, there has been enthusiasm for bladder preservation, utilizing chemotherapy and radiation therapy, reserving cystectomy for patients failing initial therapy. Up to 40% of these patients retain their bladders 2 years after treatment[452] but long-term follow-up is not available on significant numbers of patients.

The role of chemotherapy for patients at high risk for metastatic urothelial carcinoma is under investigation, especially with the discovery of chemotherapeutic combinations active against urothelial carcinoma.[248,453] One popular combination is methotrexate, vinblastine, Adriamycin (doxorubicin), and cisplatin (M-VAC).[454,455]

SQUAMOUS CELL CARCINOMA

Clinical features

The prevalence of squamous cell carcinoma varies in different parts of the world. In areas where schistosomiasis is endemic, squamous cell carcinoma accounts for up to 73% of bladder cancers.[456] In England and the United States, it comprises only 3% to 6% of bladder malignancies.[457,458]

In the past 25 years, there have been 10 large series aggregating 541 patients with pure squamous cell carcinoma of the urinary bladder from England[457,459] and the United States.[458,460-466] This group included 337 males and 204 females (M:F ratio of 1.7:1), ranging in age from 30 to 90 years (mean, 65.5 years). Most patients presented with hematuria or irritative symptoms. Rarely, there is associated hypercalcemia.[467,468] A high proportion of patients have advanced cancer at the time of diagnosis.[457,465]

Etiology and pathogenesis

Many patients with squamous cell carcinoma have a long history of bladder irritation caused by infections,[460,461,464] stones,[461,464] indwelling catheters,[464] intermittent self-catheterization,[469] or urinary retention.[461] Keratinizing squamous metaplasia (leukoplakia) is an important risk factor for the development of squamous cell carcinoma (Fig. 5-61).[470-478] In one series, 33 of 78 patients with keratinizing squamous metaplasia had simultaneous or subsequent carcinoma. In those who subsequently developed cancer, the tumor arose between 3 months and 30 years after the diagnosis of metaplasia (mean, 12 years). Many tumors arising in bladder diverticula are squamous cell carcinoma.[479-485] In one case, squamous cell carcinoma arose 17 months after treatment of urothelial carcinoma in situ with bacillus Calmette-Guérin.[486] Rarely, cancers arising in bladder exstrophy and in the urachus are squamous cell carcinomas.[487-492]

Schistosomiasis. Schistosome infection is a worldwide medical problem,[493,494] and its role in the pathogenesis of bladder cancer in endemic areas is of considerable importance. There are three major species pathogenic in humans: *S. mansoni*, *S. japonicum*, and *S. haematobium*. Only *S. haematobium* causes bladder cancer.[494] In Egypt, squamous cell carcinoma of the urinary bladder has been called the "foremost oncologic problem."[456] In a series of 1095 cases of bladder cancer, schistosome eggs were identified in the bladder wall in 902 cases (82%).[456]

The life cycle of *S. haematobium* begins with adult trematodes in the urogenital system of mammals. Eggs are produced, excreted in urine, and hatch in fresh water. The larvae infect snails and undergo asexual reproduction, producing cercaria, which are excreted back into the water. The cercaria are able to penetrate the skin of mammals (including humans) that they come into contact with in the water, and migrate to the pelvic and mesenteric venous plexuses where they mature, reproduce, and lay eggs, completing the life cycle.

The eggs incite a severe inflammatory and fibrotic reaction, and many are trapped within the muscularis and lamina propria of the bladder wall (Fig. 5-62). The eggs are destroyed or become calcified. The calcified eggs create the characteristic granular, yellow tan lesion known as a sandy patch. Bladder infection by *S. haematobium* may result in polyposis, ulceration, urothelial hyperplasia and metaplasia, dysplasia, or carcinoma.[495] Although squamous cell carcinoma is the most frequent type of cancer, a relatively high prevalence of adenocarcinoma (5.8%) is also seen.[456] Urinary schistosomiasis probably acts as a co-carcinogen or promoter for bladder cancer.[495]

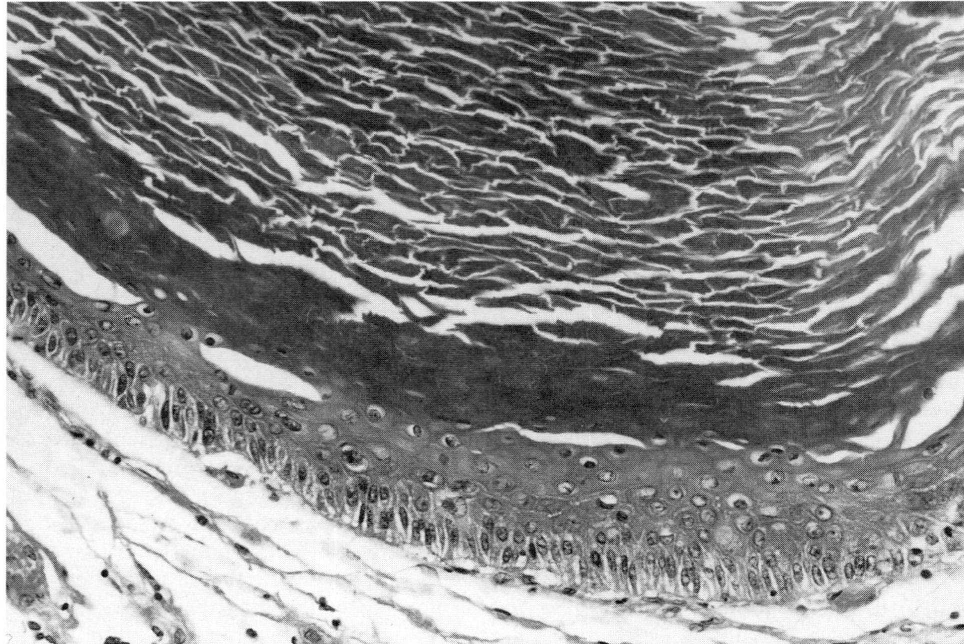

5-61. Keratinizing squamous metaplasia in the urinary bladder.

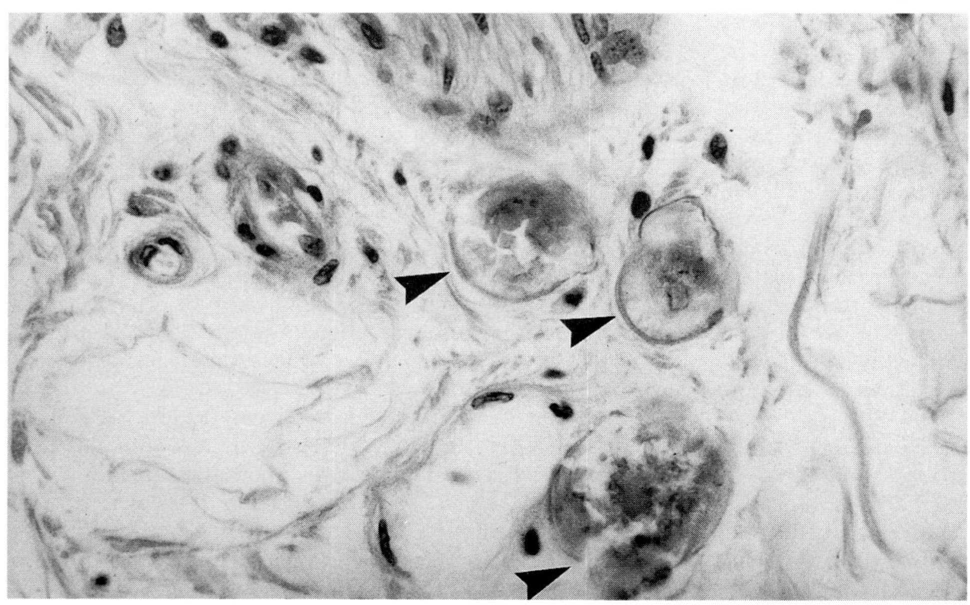

5-62. Schistosome ova (*arrows*) in the wall of the urinary bladder.

Gross pathology

Most squamous cell carcinomas are bulky, polypoid, solid, necrotic masses, often filling the bladder lumen,[457,461] although some are predominantly flat and irregularly bordered[460] or ulcerated and infiltrating (Fig. 5-63).[462] The presence of necrotic material and keratin debris on the surface is relatively constant. There is an apparent propensity for the lateral wall and trigone.[459,462]

Microscopic pathology

The diagnosis of squamous cell carcinoma is restricted to pure tumors without identifiable urothelial carcinoma (see section on urothelial carcinoma with squamous or glandular differentiation).[457-459,461-466] The tumor may be well differentiated, consisting of well defined islands of squamous cells with keratinization, prominent intercellular bridges, and minimal nuclear pleomorphism, or poorly differentiated, with marked nuclear pleomorphism and only focal squamous differentiation (Fig. 5-64). Squamous metaplasia is present in the adjacent epithelium in 17% to 60% of cases from Europe and North America.[459,461,462]

Verrucous carcinoma. Rare cases of verrucous carcinoma of the bladder have been described.[496-498] Another case reported as verrucous carcinoma invaded in

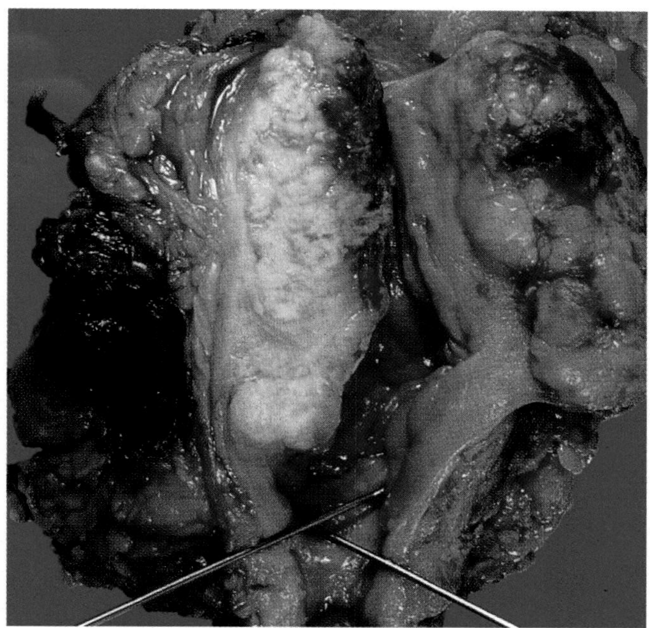

5-63. Squamous cell carcinoma of the urinary bladder.

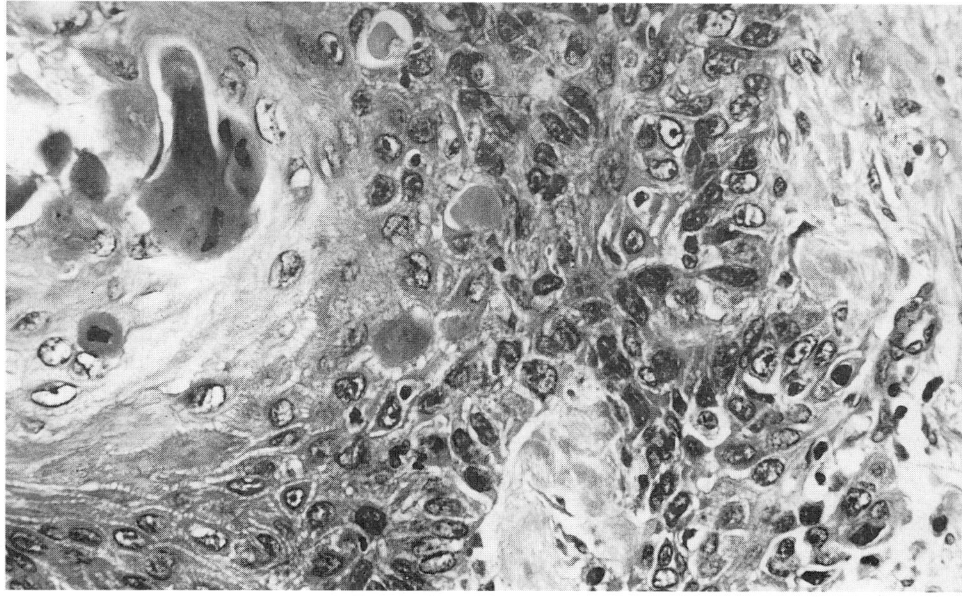

5-64. Invasive squamous cell carcinoma with intercellular bridges and keratin formation.

nests with areas of perineural invasion, and probably represented typical well differentiated squamous cell carcinoma.[499] Verrucous carcinoma is more common in patients with schistosomiasis, accounting for 3% of bladder cancers in one series.[456] This cancer appears as an exophytic, papillary, or warty mass with epithelial acanthosis and papillomatosis, minimal nuclear and architectural atypia and rounded, pushing, deep borders (Fig. 5-65, 5-66). In other organs, verrucous carcinoma has a good prognosis, but data on its behavior in the bladder are meager. Three cases were free of recurrence and progression after 3, 24, and 36 months.[496-498]

Verrucous carcinoma at other sites has been linked to human papilloma virus infection. One case in the urinary bladder developed in a patient with longstanding anogenital condyloma acuminata, suggesting a possible link with the bladder tumor.[498] Condyloma acuminata occur in the bladder[498,500-502] and have been shown to contain human papilloma virus.[500] Cases reported as locally aggressive condylomata in the bladder may represent verrucous carcinoma.[498]

Grading

Squamous cell carcinoma of the bladder is graded according to the amount of keratinization and the degree of nuclear pleomorphism.[460,463-465] Histologic grade may correlate with stage and outcome[463,464] although results have not been uniform.[460] Winkler et al[465] found that

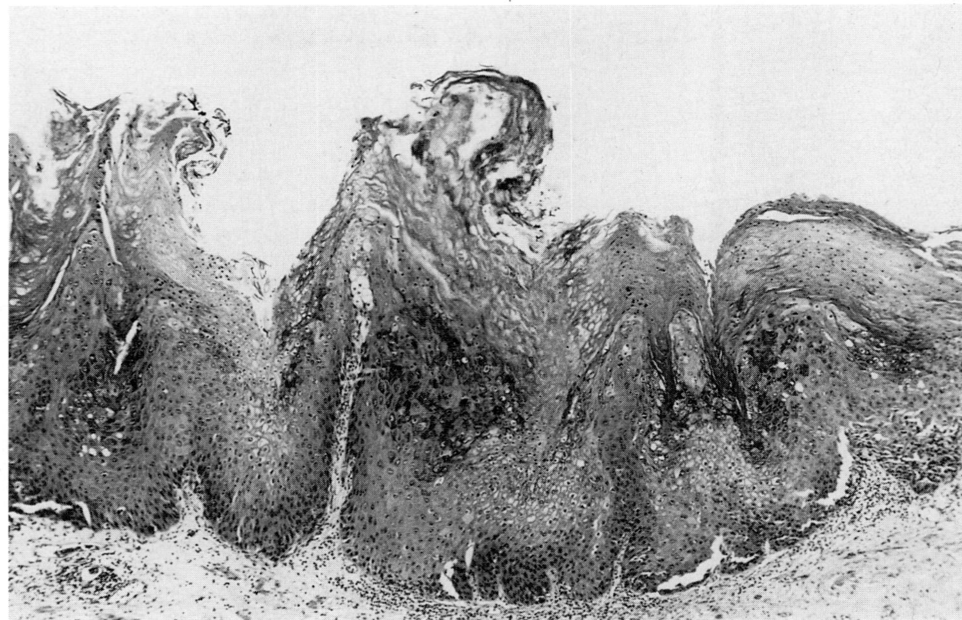

5-65. Verrucous carcinoma of the bladder. Note the blunt pushing architecture at the base.

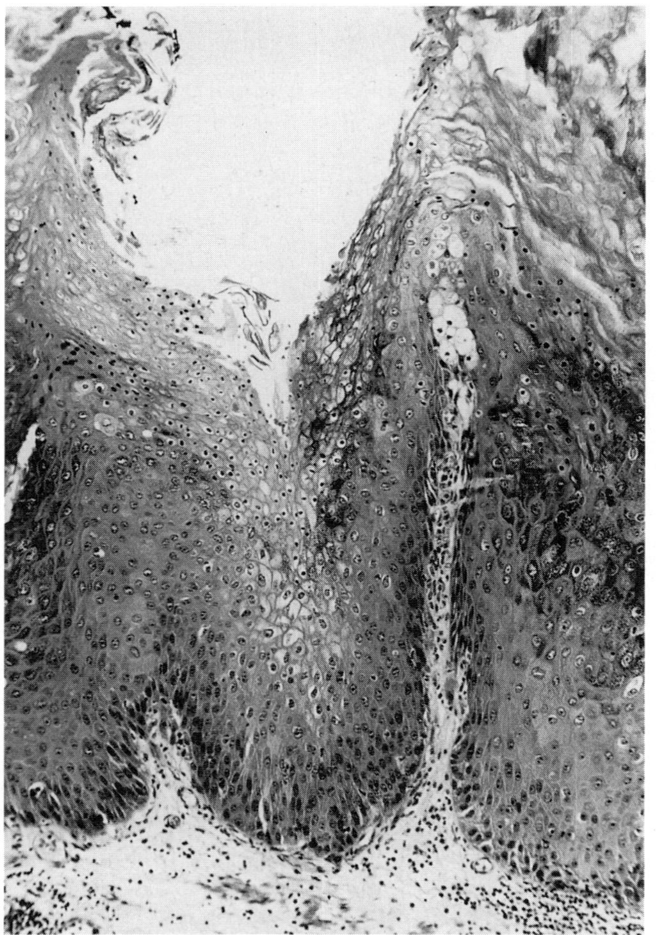

5-66. Verrucous carcinoma showing koilocytic atypia, minimal nuclear pleomorphism, and pushing deep margin.

tumor grade correlated with DNA content but not with survival.

DNA ploidy

Winkler et al[465] studied 76 cases of pure squamous cell carcinoma by DNA flow cytometry using paraffin embedded material, and found 37% of cases were diploid, 23% tetraploid, and 40% aneuploid. DNA ploidy was a powerful predictor of progression, with progression in 35%, 45%, and 92% of patients with diploid, tetraploid, and aneuploid tumors, respectively. Shaaban et al[503] studied 100 cases and found a strong correlation of DNA aneuploidy and high S-phase fraction with high grade tumors. In a subsequent study, they found that DNA content was a significant predictor of outcome, with 5-year survival of 54% and 21% for patients with diploid and aneuploid tumors, respectively.[504]

The karyotype of a single case of squamous cell carcinoma showed changes similar to those frequently seen in urothelial carcinoma, including -9 and del(11p).[505]

Differential diagnosis

The major differential diagnostic consideration for squamous cell carcinoma is urothelial carcinoma with squamous differentiation, which occurs in up to 20% of high-grade urothelial carcinomas.[243,244] In North America, Europe, and other regions where primary squamous cell carcinoma is uncommon, such tumors should be carefully studied for a urothelial component. If an identifiable urothelial element (including urothelial carcinoma in situ) is found, the tumor should be classified as urothelial carcinoma with squamous differentiation.[243] The presence of keratinizing squamous metaplasia, especially if associated with dysplasia, favors the diagnosis of squamous cell carcinoma. Secondary invasion of the bladder by an adjacent primary such as squamous cell carcinoma of the cervix or vagina should always be considered and excluded clinically.

Staging

Tumor stage, by either the AJCC-TNM or Jewett (or Marshall modification of Jewett) staging system, is the most important prognostic indicator for squamous cell carcinoma.[457,459,460,462,464] These systems are presented in detail in the section on urothelial carcinoma.

Treatment and natural history. The treatment of choice for pure squamous cell carcinoma of the bladder has been radical cystectomy or cystoprostatectomy. Radiation therapy alone is not effective.[506] Recent reports suggest that preoperative radiation therapy with[507] or without[466] adjuvant chemotherapy may be useful. Chemotherapy presently is ineffective in dealing with metastatic squamous cell carcinoma of the bladder.

The prognosis is poor for patients with squamous cell carcinoma. In the M.D. Anderson series, survival at 5 and 10 years was only 13.5% and 5.3%, respectively.[462] Other studies have reported 5-year survival ranging from 7.4%[461] to 50%;[466] the latter was seen in a small series of patients treated with preoperative radiation and radical cystectomy.[466] The biological behavior of squamous cell carcinoma is different from that of urothelial carcinoma. In most patients, death is caused by local recurrence rather than metastasis.[459,461,466] Metastases show a striking predilection for bone.[457,459,461]

ADENOCARCINOMA

Primary adenocarcinoma accounts for less than 1% of malignant bladder tumors.[508,509] Petersen[253] reviewed the literature in 1985 and found 321 cases. There are 14 institutional series with a minimum of 10 patients each;[254,508-520] the largest, with 72 cases, was reported by Grignon et al.[254] Adenocarcinoma of the bladder is divided into two principal categories: those occurring in the urachus and those developing in the bladder proper.

Urachal adenocarcinoma

Diagnostic criteria. The separation of urachal from nonurachal adenocarcinoma requires correlation of clinical and pathologic findings. Criteria that establish urachal origin include location in the bladder dome, primary involvement of muscle or deeper structures, presence of a suprapelvic mass, tumor growth in the bladder wall extending into the space of Retzius, sharp demarcation between tumor and normal surface epithelium, an intact or ulcerated epithelium, absence of cystitis cystica and glandularis elsewhere in the bladder, and the presence of urachal remnants (see box on this page).[513,516,517] Wheeler and Hill[521] suggested that "from a clinical standpoint, it is justifiable to consider all adenocarcinomas of the dome as urachal unless a transition from nonneoplastic bladder epithelium to adenocarcinoma is demonstrated." The criteria of Johnson et al[515] are perhaps most practical: the tumor should be located anteriorly or in the dome, there should be a sharp demarcation between tumor and normal epithelium, and a primary tumor elsewhere must be excluded.

CRITERIA TO DISTINGUISH URACHAL FROM NONURACHAL ADENOCARCINOMA

- Location in bladder dome
- Epicenter in bladder wall (not mucosa)
- Absence of cystitis glandularis or intestinal metaplasia in urothelium
- Other primary sites excluded

There are no specific histologic features that distinguish urachal from nonurachal tumors. A higher proportion of urachal tumors are mucinous (colloid), but there is too much overlap with nonurachal tumors to allow the histologic subtype to be helpful.[254] Studies of mucin histochemistry[254,522] and immunohistochemistry[254] have shown no difference between the two types.

Clinical features. Adenocarcinoma of the urachus occurs throughout adulthood, and the youngest case was in a 15-year-old girl.[523] The majority of cases occur in the fifth and sixth decades, with a mean age of 50.6 years,* approximately 10 years younger than the mean for adenocarcinoma elsewhere in the bladder.† There is a predominance of men over women (1.8:1),* lower than the 2.6 to 1 ratio for nonurachal adenocarcinoma.† The most frequent presenting symptoms are hematuria (71%), pain (42%), irritative symptoms (40%), mucusuria (25%), and umbilical discharge (2%).[492]

Etiology and pathogenesis. Intestinal metaplasia of the urachal epithelium is the favored mechanism accounting for the preponderance of adenocarcinomas of the urachus (Fig. 5-67).[526] Cases arising from villous adenoma of the urachus have been described.[527]

Gross pathology. Most urachal adenocarcinomas form discrete masses in the dome of the bladder and often appear centered in the wall of the bladder, rather than in the mucosa as is typical for nonurachal tumors (Fig. 5-68). The bladder mucosa may be intact or ulcerated. The cut surface of the tumor may be solid, but often has a glistening gelatinous appearance caused by abundant mucus production. Sometimes the tumor extends along the urachal tract, and the tumor may be found within the abdominal wall.

Microscopic pathology. Urachal adenocarcinoma has a variety of histologic appearances. The most frequent is mucinous (colloid) carcinoma with nests and single cells appearing to float in pools of extracellular mucin (Fig. 5-69). The cells may have signet ring cell or columnar cell morphology. The next most frequent pattern is enteric adenocarcinoma, which resembles colorectal adenocarcinoma, and may include Paneth cells and argyrophilic neuroendocrine cells.[528,529] An uncommon pattern is linitis plastica-like signet ring cell carcinoma.[530] Histochemical stains reveal neutral and acid (sulfated and nonsulfated) mucin in these tumors.[254]

Immunohistochemistry. Urachal adenocarcinoma expresses cytokeratin,[516] carcinoembryonic antigen,[254,516]

*References 254, 492, 510, 511, 517, 520, 524, 525.
†References 254, 508, 510, 511, 513, 514, 517, 520.

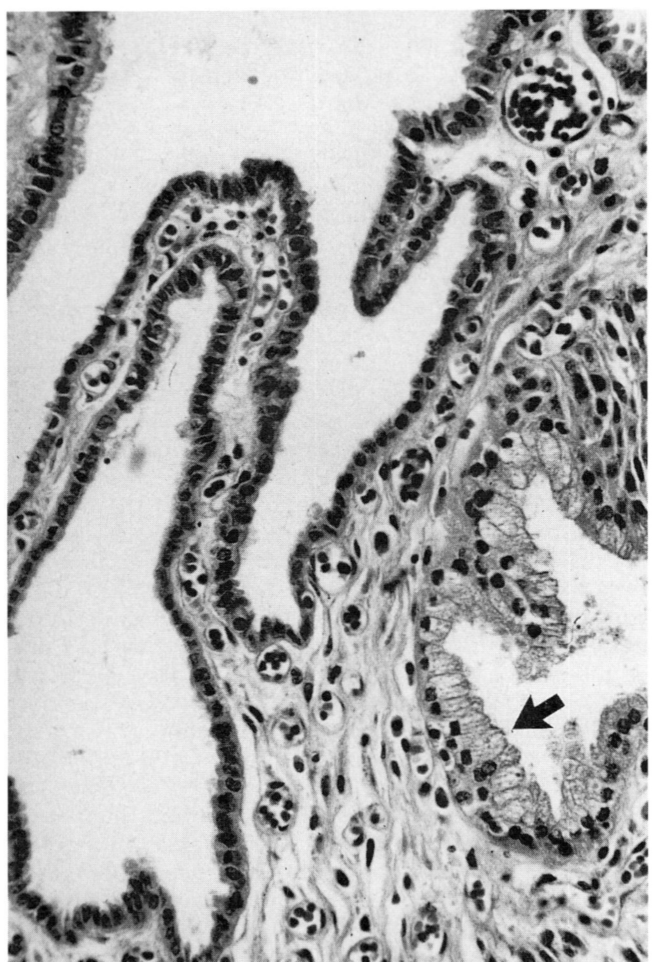

5-67. Urachal remnant in the dome of the bladder having focal mucinous metaplasia (*arrow*).

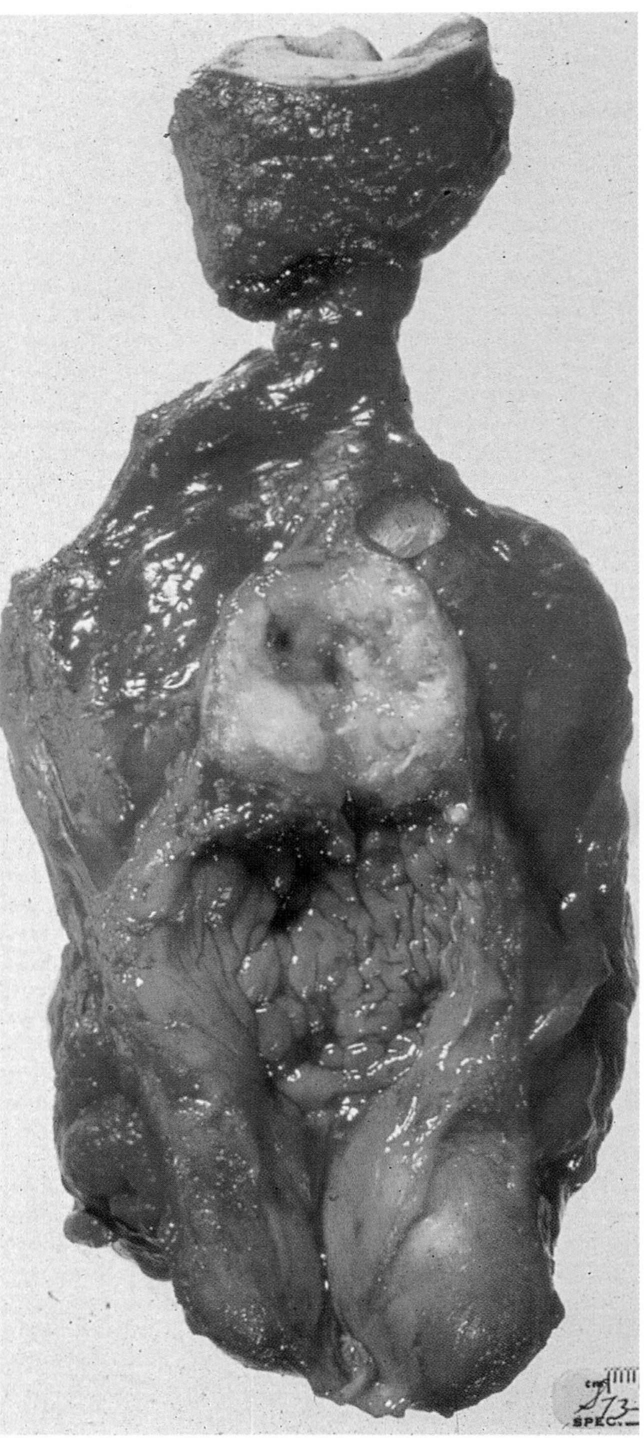

5-68. Urachal adenocarcinoma resected en bloc with the urachal tract and umbilicus. The tumor has its epicenter in the wall of the bladder at the dome, and has a glistening mucoid cut surface. *(Photograph courtesy of Dr. Alberto Ayala.)*

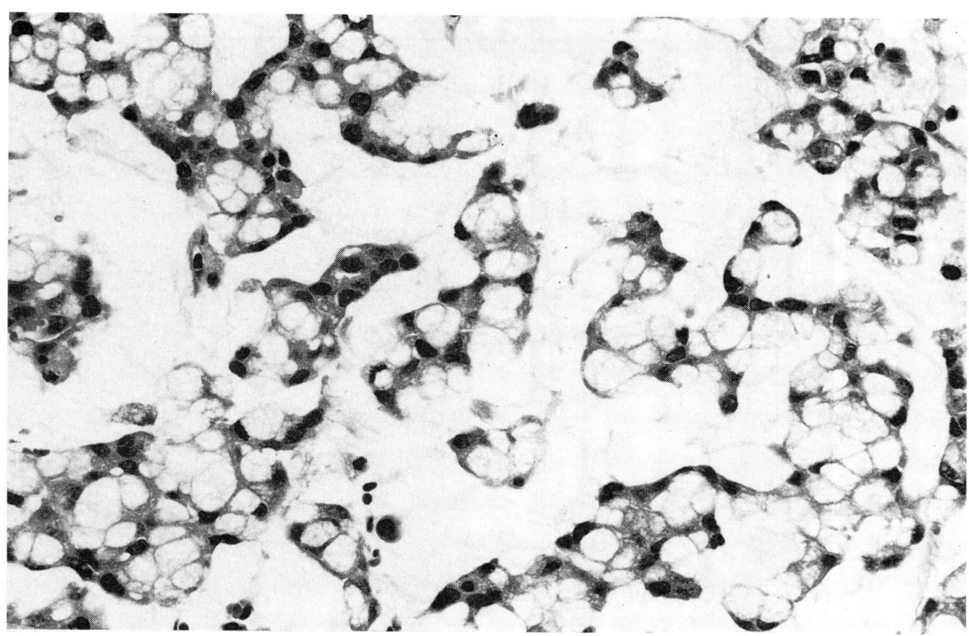

5-69. Urachal adenocarcinoma with a mucinous pattern characterized by small nests of cells appearing to float in extracellular mucin.

Leu-M1,[254,516] and epithelial membrane antigen.[516] There have been conflicting reports concerning immunoreactivity for prostate specific antigen and prostatic acid phosphatase. Urachal remnants were positive for prostate specific antigen in 4 of 25 cases using a polyclonal antibody,[531] and in 1 of 7 cases of urachal adenocarcinoma with a polyclonal prostate specific antigen antibody but not with a monoclonal antibody.[254] None of the cases studied by Abenoza et al[516] stained for prostate specific antigen. Epstein et al[532] studied 15 bladder adenocarcinomas, one or two of which appear to have been urachal; these tumors were negative for prostate specific antigen and focally positive for prostatic acid phosphatase in one.

Differential diagnosis. The major differential diagnostic consideration is nonurachal bladder adenocarcinoma. As discussed above, this distinction requires clinicopathologic correlation. Urachal adenocarcinoma should be distinguished from urachal villous adenoma;[49] this rare lesion is histologically identical to those found in the gastrointestinal tract. The presence of invasion indicates malignancy. Secondary invasion of the bladder by adenocarcinoma arising elsewhere, particularly the colon, must always be excluded clinically.

Staging. Urachal adenocarcinoma is staged with the same systems used for urothelial bladder cancer.* Application of these systems is problematic in urachal carcinoma because, by virtue of their anatomic origin, almost all are muscle invasive. Recognizing this, Sheldon et al[492] proposed a system specific for urachal tumors. Stage I cancer is confined to the urachal mucosa; Stage II cancer is invasive but confined to the urachus; Stage III includes local extension to the bladder (IIIA), abdominal wall (IIIB), peritoneum (IIIC), or viscera other than the bladder (IIID); and Stage IV includes metastases to regional lymph nodes (IVA) or distant sites (IVB). The applicability and utility of this system have not been tested.

Treatment and natural history. The treatment of urachal adenocarcinoma remains unsettled. In 1971, Whitehead et al[533] advocated segmental resection of the tumor with en bloc resection of the urachus and umbilicus, an approach supported by others.[511,534,535] In contrast, Sheldon et al[492] and others[518,536] advocated en bloc cystectomy with pelvic lymphadenectomy and umbilectomy. Whether partial or radical cystectomy is performed, the inclusion of the entire urachal tract is of critical importance. Urachal adenocarcinoma appears resistant to radiation therapy.[492]

Some authors report a better prognosis for urachal than for nonurachal adenocarcinoma,[254,509,519] while others have found no difference[512,518] or a worse prognosis.[517,525] In a study of 72 cases, Grignon et al[254] reported 5-year crude survival of 61% and 31% for urachal and nonurachal adenocarcinoma, respectively ($p=0.07$, Log-rank test). The 10-year survival for urachal cases was 46%.[254] Two other large series reported 5-year survivals of 67%[509] and 27%.[519] Survival curves, based on 71 patients reported in the literature, combined with raw data obtained from Grignon et al,[254] reveal 5- and 10-year survival of 37% and 17%, respectively (Fig. 5-70). In this analysis, there was no significant difference in crude survival between adenocarcinoma of urachal and nonurachal origin ($0.05<p<0.1$, Log-rank test). In a study of signet ring cell adenocarcinoma of the bladder, Grignon et al[530] reported a significantly better survival for those originating in the urachus.

*References 254, 510, 512, 513, 516, 518, 519.

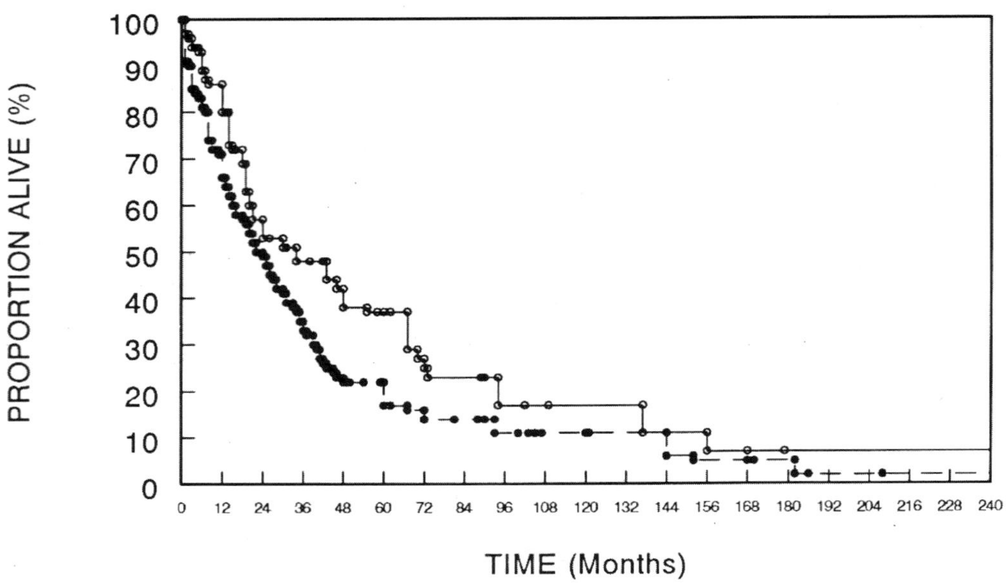

5-70. Kaplan-Meier survival curves comparing urachal (*open circles*) with nonurachal (*dark circles*) bladder adenocarcinoma; the difference in the curves is not statistically significant ($0.05<p<0.1$, Log-rank test).

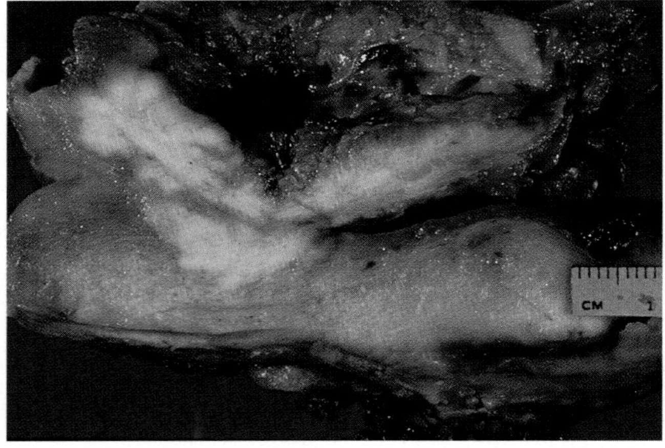

5-71. Nonurachal adenocarcinoma arising in the posterior wall of the bladder and invading into the wall of the lower uterine segment. *(Photograph courtesy of Dr. D. Ian Turnbull.)*

Nonurachal adenocarcinoma

Clinical features. Nonurachal adenocarcinoma accounts for 61% to 80% of primary bladder adenocarcinomas.[517] This tumor occurs over a wide age range, with a mean of 59.4 years, and is more common in males than females (2.6:1).* Hematuria is the most common presentation (88%), followed by irritative symptoms (48%) and, rarely, mucusuria (2%).[254] The tumors are often advanced, with metastatic cancer in up to 40% of patients at the time of presentation.[254]

Etiology and pathogenesis. Most cases of primary nonurachal adenocarcinoma arise from metaplasia of the urothelium. Support for this mechanism comes from cases arising in patients with longstanding diffuse intestinalization of the bladder mucosa associated with a nonfunctioning bladder,[537-540] chronic irritation,[541,542] obstruction,[543] and cystocele.[544] Cystitis glandularis is present in 14% to 67% of patients with nonurachal adenocarcinoma.[509,516] Origin from metaplasia is also considered to be the mechanism in patients with exstrophy.[545-553] Most cancers arising in association with exstrophy are adenocarcinoma, although occasional examples of squamous cell carcinoma[487,488] and urothelial carcinoma have been described.[554] The risk of adenocarcinoma in patients with exstrophy is in the range of 4.1% to 7.1%.[551,552] There also appears to be an increased risk of adenocarcinoma in patients with pelvic lipomatosis, which is attributed to its association with cystitis glandularis.[555,556] Adenocarcinoma also occurs in patients with *S. haematobium* infection.[456,557,558] Rare cases of adenocarcinoma[559,560] and adenosarcoma[561] have occurred in association with endometriosis involving the bladder.

Gross pathology. Primary nonurachal adenocarcinoma can appear as an exophytic, papillary, solid, sessile, ulcerating, or infiltrative mass (Fig. 5-71). The signet ring cell variant frequently shows diffuse thickening of the bladder wall, producing a linitis plastica-like appearance, and urothelial mucosal biopsies may be negative.

Microscopic pathology. There has been some variability in defining adenocarcinoma in the literature. Some reports excluded any case containing a recognizable urothelial carcinoma component, preferring to classify these as urothelial carcinoma with glandular differentiation.[254,509,516] Although other studies included such cases as adenocarcinoma if the adenocarcinoma-

*References 254, 508, 510, 511, 513, 514, 517, 520

tous elements predominated,[253,517,519] the former definition is recommended. Grignon et al[254] recognized six histologic variants of adenocarcinoma of the urinary bladder:

1. Adenocarcinoma of no specific type—the tumor did not resemble another recognized pattern (Fig. 5-72)
2. Enteric—the cancer was composed of pseudostratified columnar cells forming glands, often with central necrosis, resembling colonic adenocarcinoma (Fig. 5-73)
3. Mucinous (colloid)—the tumor cells were single or in nests appearing to float in extracellular mucin (see Fig. 5-69)
4. Signet ring cell—the tumor consisted of signet ring cells diffusely infiltrating the bladder wall (Fig. 5-74, 5-75)
5. Clear cell—the tumor was composed of papillary and tubular structures with cytologic features similar to mesonephric adenocarcinoma of the female genital system (Fig. 5-76, 5-77)
6. Mixed—two or more of the described patterns were found.

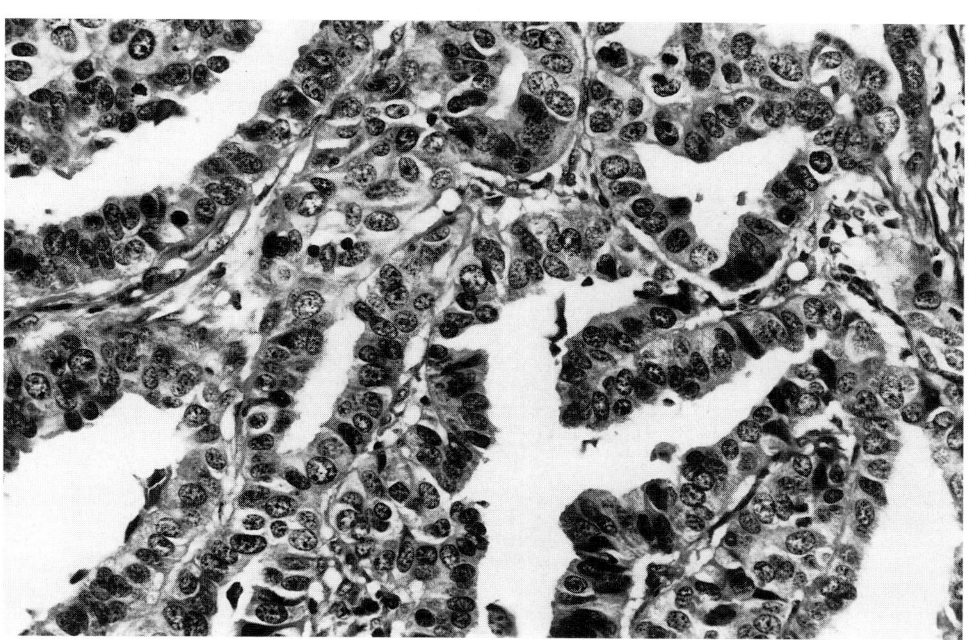

5-72. Bladder adenocarcinoma classified as adenocarcinoma of no specific type; the tumor forms glands but does not resemble any of the specific patterns of adenocarcinoma.

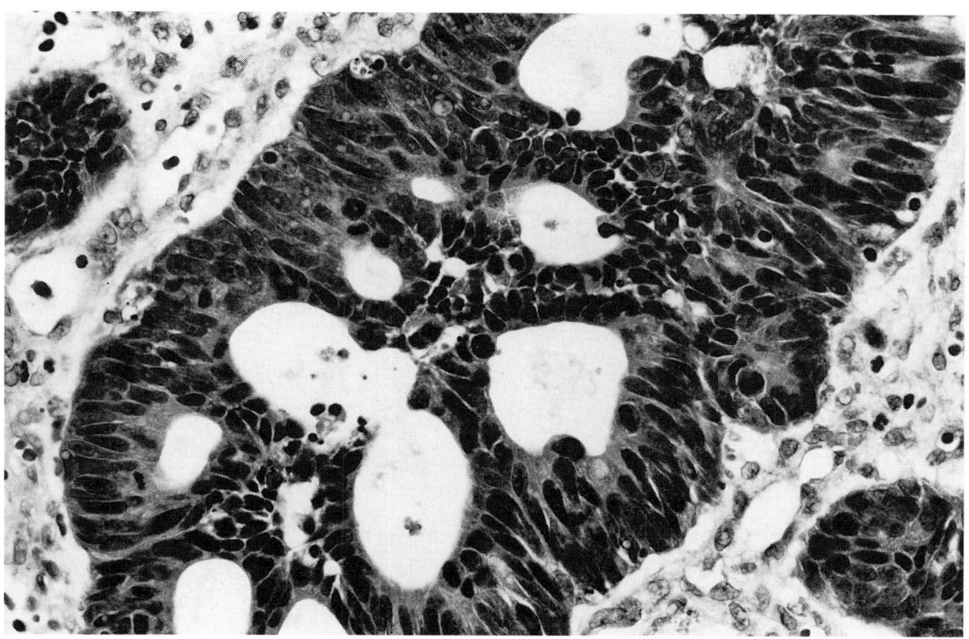

5-73. Bladder adenocarcinoma classified as enteric-type; the cells are columnar with pseudostratification and a cribriform architecture.

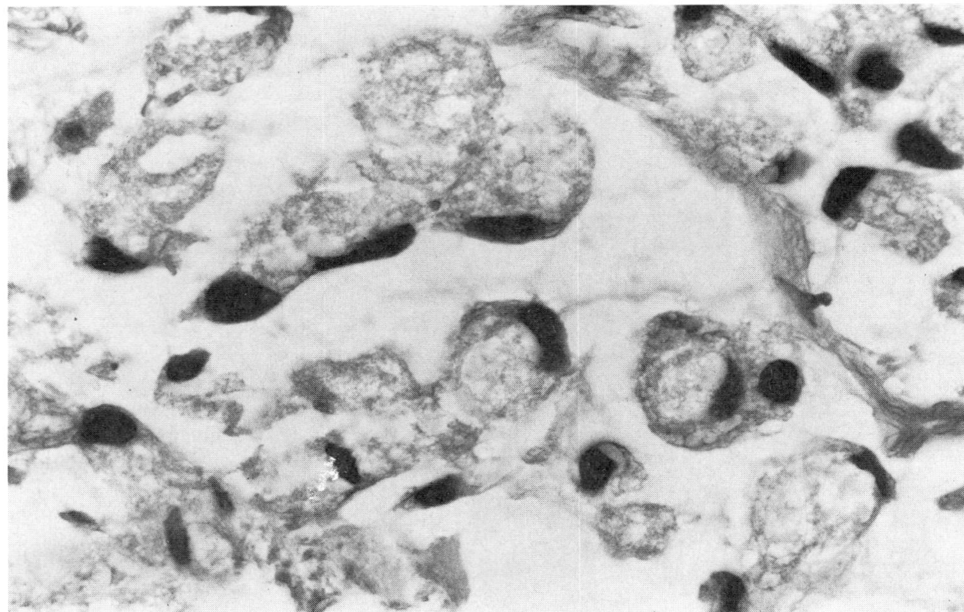

5-74. Signet ring cell adenocarcinoma of the bladder with cells having abundant finely vacuolated bubbly cytoplasm.

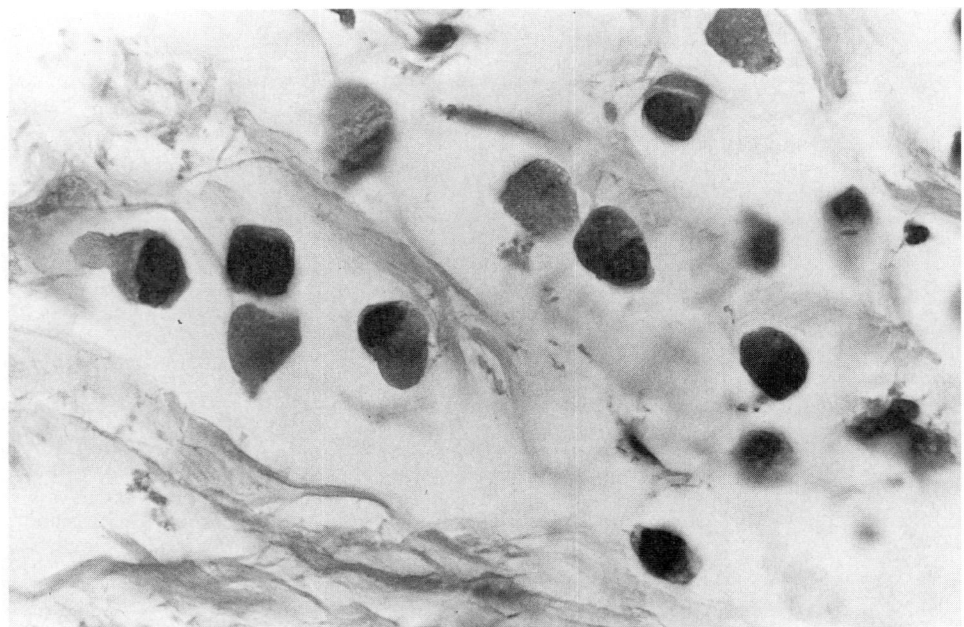

5-75. Signet ring cell adenocarcinoma of the bladder which consists of cells with eccentric nuclei and pale staining cytoplasm, a morphology that has been termed *monocytoid*.

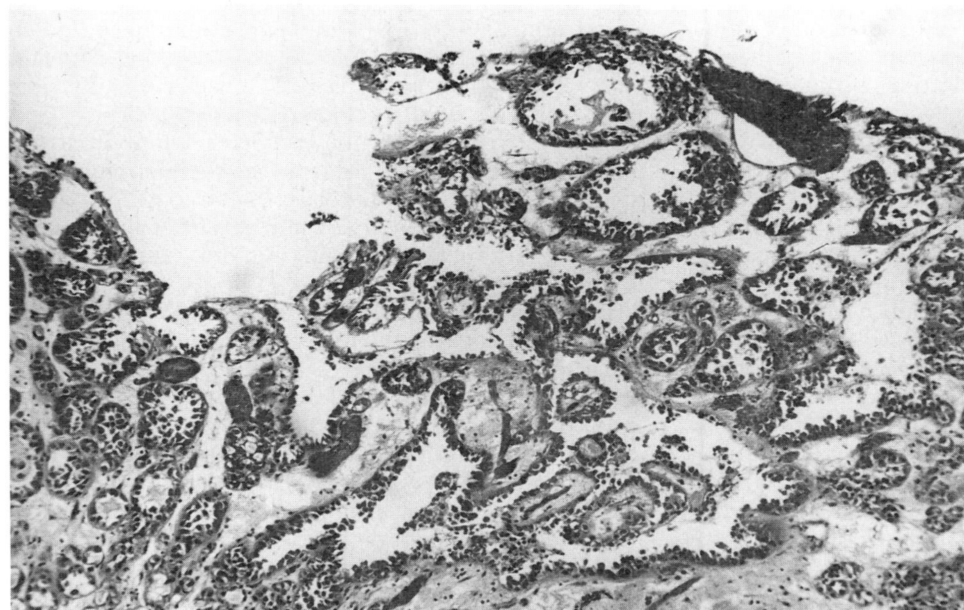

5-76. Clear cell adenocarcinoma of the bladder with papillary and tubular architecture. Many of the spaces are dilated, producing a microcystic pattern.

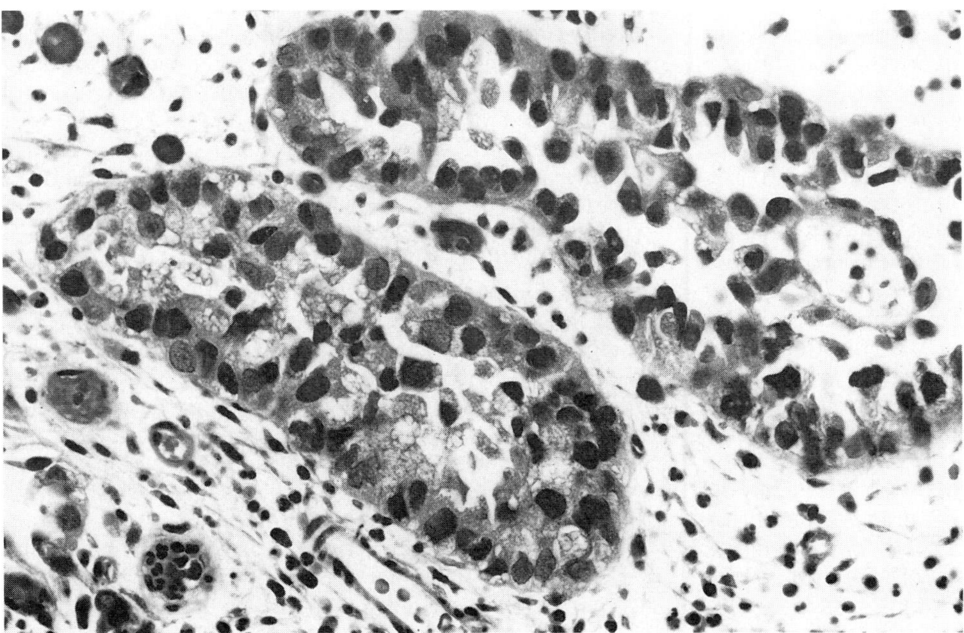

5-77. Clear cell adenocarcinoma showing nuclear atypia and hobnail cells.

For nonurachal tumors, the nonspecific and enteric types were most common. Paneth cells and argentaffin cells may be present in the enteric-type tumors.[528] One case of endometrioid adenocarcinoma arising from endometriosis has been reported[559] and a case of adenocarcinoma occurring synchronously with lymphomatous involvement of the bladder has been described.[562] Ultrastructural findings in primary adenocarcinoma reveal typical features of glandular differentiation.[522,563]

Grading. A uniform grading system has not been applied to adenocarcinoma of the bladder.[509,519] Anderström et al[519] found grade to be a significant prognostic indicator, while Thomas et al[509] did not find a correlation between grade and outcome. In the former system, grade was assessed based on the degree of gland formation, with two specific histologic subtypes (pure colloid and signet ring cell) considered to be poorly differentiated. The histologic pattern did not correlate with outcome in the M.D. Anderson series, although the poor prognosis of the signet ring cell variant was noted.[254]

Immunohistochemistry. There have been few studies of the immunohistochemistry of primary bladder adenocarcinoma.[254,516,532] Results in urachal and nonurachal adenocarcinoma were identical. Both groups consistently express carcinoembryonic antigen and Leu-M1.[254] Epstein et al[532] reported focal reactivity for prostate specific antigen and prostatic acid phosphatase in some nonurachal tumors, although results varied with antibodies tested.

DNA flow cytometry. Badalament et al[564] evaluated urine specimens from four patients and obtained DNA aneuploid histograms in three. Grignon et al[565] retrospectively performed DNA analysis on 36 cases and found 12 diploid, 19 aneuploid, and 3 tetraploid tumors; DNA content did not correlate with outcome. In contrast, Song et al[566] studied DNA ploidy in 38 cases and found it to be a significant predictor of outcome. The crude 5- and 10-year survival for patients with diploid tumors was 80% and 70%, respectively, but for nondiploid cancers the corresponding survival was 20% and 12%, respectively.

Differential diagnosis. The differential diagnosis of adenocarcinoma is extensive. First, benign mimics of adenocarcinoma must be excluded. In some cases, cystitis cystica and cystitis glandularis may be florid, producing pseudopapillary or polypoid lesions that may mimic a tumor.[9,567] The benign cytology of the lining cells and lack of invasion are important features. In unusual cases, extracellular mucin is present, and careful evaluation for malignant cells is necessary. Patients with longstanding intestinal metaplasia are at risk for the development of adenocarcinoma, and biopsies from such cases should be carefully evaluated for early evidence of neoplastic transformation.[540,544] Villous adenoma rarely occurs in the urinary bladder,[45,47] and shows cytologic and architectural abnormalities of adenomatous epithelium without stromal invasion. Nephrogenic adenoma must be distinguished from adenocarcinoma, particularly the clear cell variant (see below). Endometriosis often involves the bladder, and should be considered in women of child-bearing age to distinguish it from adenocarcinoma.[253,568,569] The histology is similar to endometriosis elsewhere, with variable proportions of endometrial glands and stroma, often associated with hemosiderin-laden macrophages.

Staging. Nonurachal adenocarcinoma, in contrast with urachal adenocarcinoma, is staged using the standard AJCC-TNM or Marshall modification of the Jewett staging system. Although stage is generally thought to be the most significant prognostic indicator in bladder adenocarcinoma,[512,513,515,516] only two studies have statistically confirmed this.[254,519] Both found few long-term survivors in patients with transmural invasion.[254,519]

Treatment and natural history. Radical cystectomy or cystoprostatectomy with pelvic lymph node dissection is the preferred therapy for adenocarcinoma of the bladder.[254,509,518] The roles of radiation therapy and chemotherapy remain uncertain,[519] although a recent report found bladder adenocarcinoma responsive to chemotherapy.[570]

Prognosis for this tumor is poor. The overall 5- and 10-year survival for the 48 cases of nonurachal adenocarcinoma reported by Grignon et al[254] were 31% and 28%, respectively. These data indicate that most patients dying of this tumor do so in the first 5 years, with uncommon late recurrence and death. The 5-year survival for patients with Stage B (T2 and T3a) cancer was 76%, indicating the potential curability of earlier stages.[254] Survival curves, based on 171 cases from the world literature and raw data obtained from Grignon et al,[254] show 5- and 10-year crude survival rates of 17% and 11%, respectively (see Fig. 5-71). As previously indicated, there is no significant difference between adenocarcinoma of urachal and nonurachal origin.

Signet ring cell adenocarcinoma

The first report of the signet ring cell variant of bladder adenocarcinoma as a distinct clinicopathologic entity is attributed to Saphir in 1955.[571] In 1991, Grignon et al[530] reported 12 cases and reviewed 56 cases from the literature. They provided a detailed analysis of their 12 cases and 37 of the cases from the literature for which their criteria for diagnosis were met and sufficient clinical details were available.[509,517,571-593] They required at least a focal component of diffuse linitis plastica-like signet ring cell adenocarcinoma and there could not be an element of urothelial carcinoma. Seven other cases fulfilling these criteria have subsequently been reported.[535,594-596] In 47% of cases, cystoscopy did not show a mucosal or mass lesion, with the mucosa most often described as *edematous* or *bullous*. Biopsies revealed diffuse permeation by single signet ring cells, some with single cytoplasmic vacuoles and others with bubbly cytoplasm (see Fig. 5-74). In some cases, the cytoplasm was pale and eosinophilic, with the nucleus pushed to one end, a pattern referred to as monocytoid (see Fig. 5-75).[530,571]

The significance of this subtype of adenocarcinoma is its extremely poor prognosis. The 5-year survival for patients with a pure signet ring cell pattern was 13%, compared with 33% in tumors with a mixed pattern.[530]

Clear cell adenocarcinoma

Primary clear cell adenocarcinoma of the urinary bladder is rare, with only six well-documented cases in the

English language literature.[560,597-601] Only a single case of clear cell carcinoma was described[519] in the four largest published series of bladder adenocarcinoma, totalling 232 cases.[254,509,517,519]

Grossly, the tumors are typically solid or papillary, and located in the trigone or posterior wall. Histologically, all have a tubular component, some of which is cystically dilated (see Fig. 5-76). The lining cells are flattened, cuboidal, or columnar, with clear cytoplasm and at least focally, the characteristic hobnail cells (Fig. 5-77). The cells have significant nuclear pleomorphism with frequent mitotic figures. Special stains demonstrate abundant cytoplasmic glycogen, and, in most, focal cytoplasmic and lumenal mucin.

The major differential diagnostic considerations are nephrogenic adenoma and metastatic clear cell carcinoma. Nephrogenic adenoma is typically small, has papillary and tubular components, lacks solid areas, and shows minimal cytologic atypia.[240,258] Nephrogenic adenoma can infiltrate the muscularis propria, and this feature should not be used alone as a diagnostic criterion for malignancy.[239,240,258] A history of trauma or instrumentation may be helpful. Metastatic clear cell carcinoma should be excluded in all female patients and requires clinical correlation. Renal cell carcinoma can metastasize to the bladder.[602] Recognition of the typical vascular pattern, lack of tubular differentiation, absence of mucin, and clinical features should resolve this diagnosis.

The pathogenesis of clear cell adenocarcinoma in the bladder remains unresolved. Origin from embryonic rests of mesoderm from the mesonephric ducts was generally accepted in early reports;[597-599] this has been challenged, and a metaplastic origin from urothelium suggested.[601] There has also been a recent case reported in association with endometriosis, suggesting müllerian origin for at least some cases.[560]

SMALL CELL CARCINOMA

Clinical features

Small cell carcinoma in the bladder, histologically resembling that occurring in the lung,[603] is being reported with increasing frequency, with over 100 cases now described.[604-626] Angulo et al[627] summarized 106 cases from the world literature, including 2 of their own. The tumor has been estimated to represent 0.5% of bladder malignancies,[619] but this is probably an underestimate. It develops much more frequently in men than women (ratio, 4:1) and is usually a tumor of older patients (range, 20 to 85 years; mean, 66 years).[627] Hematuria is the most frequent presentation (90% of cases), with symptoms of bladder irritability or obstruction occurring less frequently. The patients often present with locally advanced or metastatic cancer. Paraneoplastic syndromes have been rarely reported, including ectopic adrenocorticotropic hormone production,[611] hypercalcemia[613,619] and hypophosphatemia.[614] At least four cases have arisen in bladder diverticula,[609,614,616,619] and one case in a patient following augmentation cystoplasty.[621]

Etiology and pathogenesis

At least three theories have been proposed to account for these tumors in the bladder. The most often cited and currently favored theory is origin from multipotential undifferentiated or stem cells present in the urothelium.[609,610,616,619] The frequent association of this tumor with other histologic variants such as urothelial carcinoma and adenocarcinoma supports this theory.[617] A second theory is origin from neuroendocrine cells within normal[283] or metaplastic urothelium.[614] A third theory is origin from an undefined population of submucosal neuroendocrine cells.[607]

Gross pathology

There are no specific gross features separating small cell carcinoma from other carcinomas of the bladder. This tumor ranges in size from 2 cm polypoid lesions[613] to 10 cm solid masses (Fig. 5-78).[619] It can develop at any location, including the dome and within diverticula. The overlying mucosa may be ulcerated.

Microscopic pathology

The tumor fulfills the light microscopic criteria used for small cell carcinoma of the lung.[603] It can show either an oat cell or intermediate cell pattern, and both may be present in the same tumor. The oat cell type consists of a relatively uniform population of cells with scant cytoplasm, hyperchromatic nuclei with dispersed chromatin, and absent or inconspicuous nucleoli. The intermediate cell type has more abundant cytoplasm, larger nuclei with less hyperchromasia, and a similar chromatin pattern and nucleolar features. In some cases, the intermediate type of small cell carcinoma contains elongate or spindled cells. Both types have extensive necrosis, prominent nuclear molding, frequent mitotic figures, and may have DNA encrustation of blood vessel walls (Azzopardi phenomenon) (Fig. 5-79, 5-80). A single case with a large cell neuroendocrine carcinoma phenotype has been described,[605] and the presence of scattered cells with monstrous nuclei has also been reported.[628]

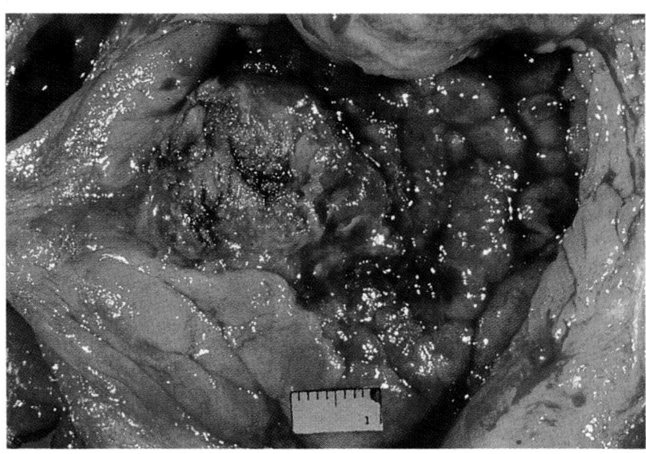

5-78. Small cell carcinoma of the bladder.

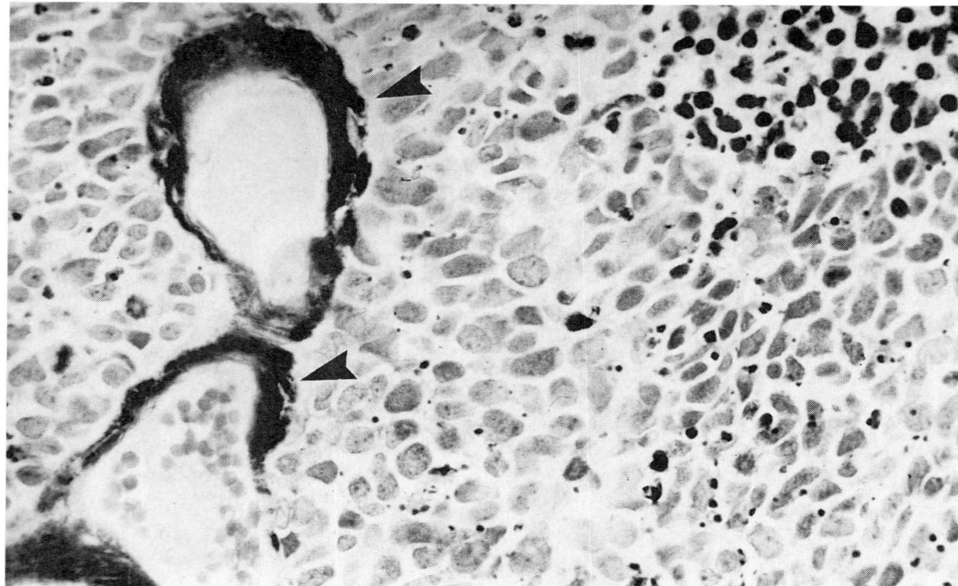

5-79. Small cell carcinoma of the bladder with areas of necrosis and DNA deposition in blood vessel walls (Azzopardi phenomenon, *arrows*).

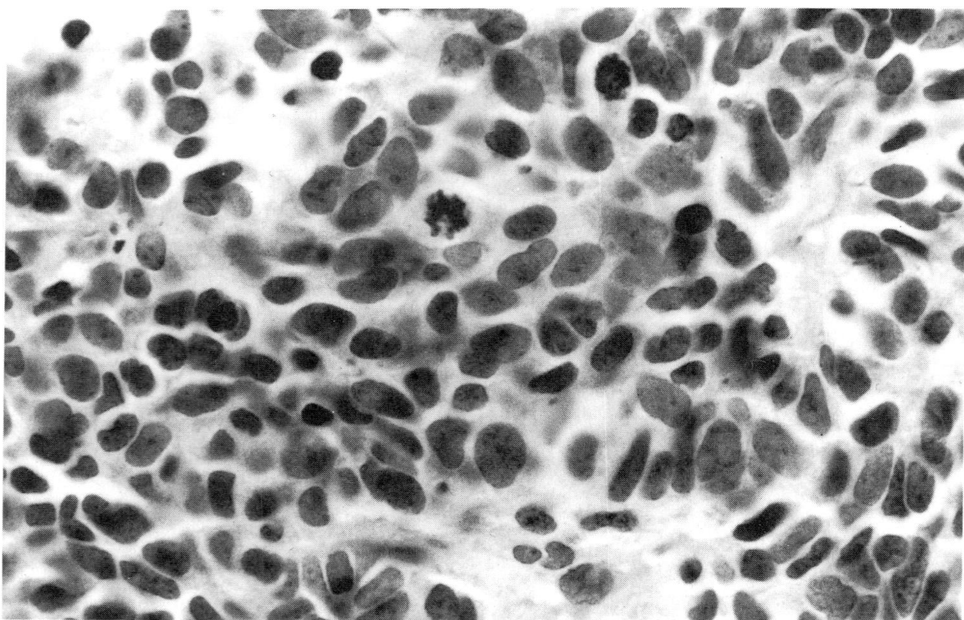

5-80. Small cell carcinoma of the bladder composed of cells with nuclei having fine, evenly distributed chromatin and inconspicuous nucleoli.

Between 23%[628] and 67%[617] of cases are mixed with other histologic patterns (Fig. 5-81). A urothelial carcinoma component (papillary or nonpapillary) is most common, but glandular and squamous differentiation have been observed. One case of small cell carcinoma arose in association with urachal adenocarcinoma.[580] In at least 11 cases, the adjacent urothelium had severe dysplasia or urothelial carcinoma in situ.[607,613,615,618–620,628] Unlike urothelial carcinoma with squamous or glandular differentiation, mixed tumors are reported as small cell carcinoma with other histologic patterns. This difference in terminology is related to therapy (see the section titled Treatment and Natural History below).

Rare examples of well differentiated neuroendocrine neoplasms showing histologic features of carcinoid tumor, without associated urothelial carcinoma, have been described.[629,630] In these cases, an organoid growth pattern was present and the cells had more abundant cytoplasm. Too few cases, with limited follow-up, have been reported to allow conclusions regarding treatment or clinical behavior.

Special studies

Dense core neurosecretory granules have been found in most reported cases studied by electron microscopy.*

*References 605, 607, 609, 613-615, 617, 618, 620, 628.

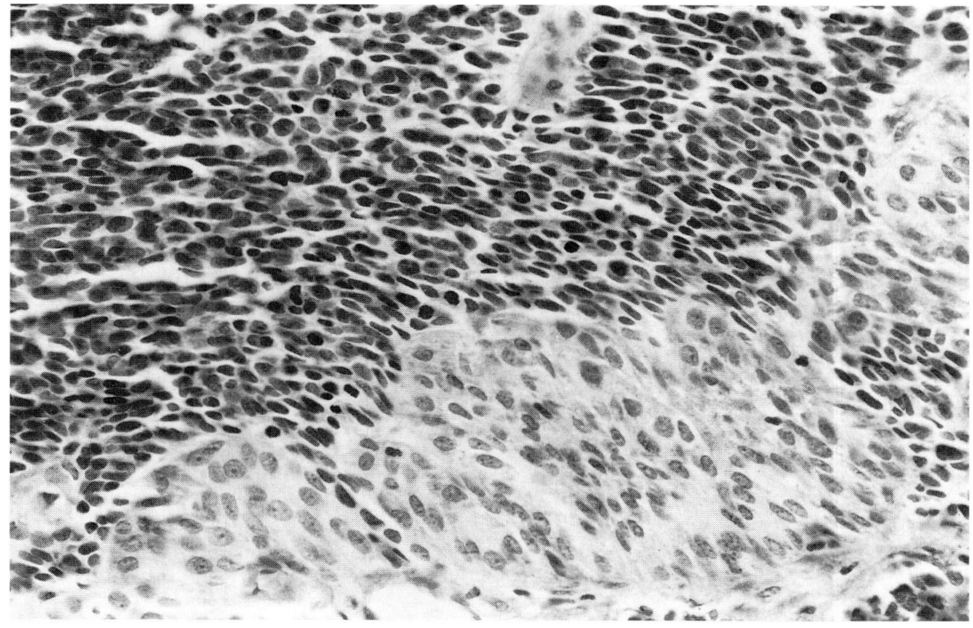

5-81. Small cell carcinoma of the bladder mixed with urothelial carcinoma.

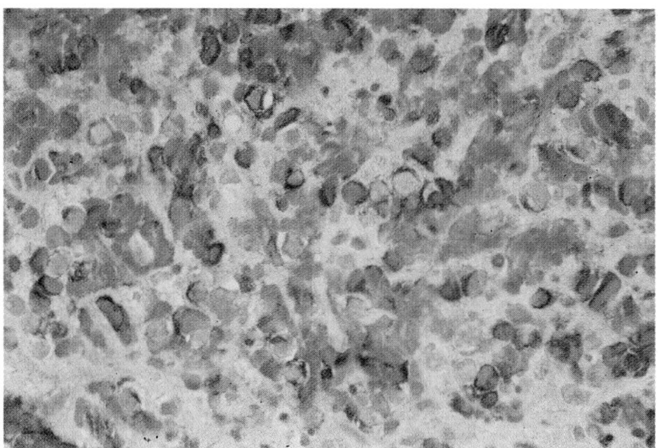

5-82. Small cell carcinoma immunohistochemically stained for chromogranin and showing intense cytoplasmic reactivity.

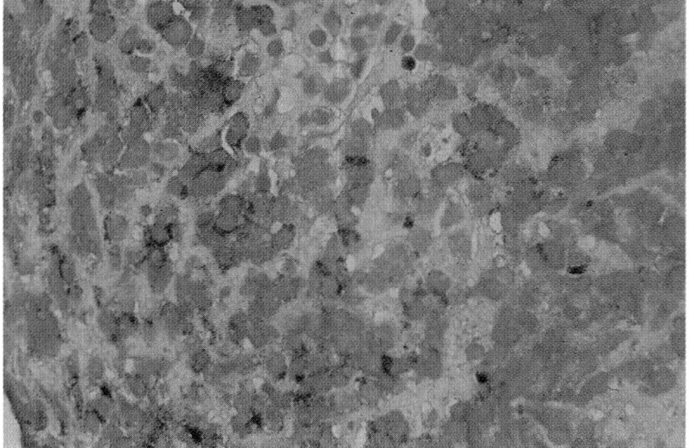

5-83. Small cell carcinoma immunohistochemically stained for cytokeratin, demonstrating cytoplasmic reactivity, which in some cells has a dotlike pattern.

In the majority of cases, immunohistochemical evidence of neuroendocrine differentiation can be found, with neuron specific enolase immunoreactivity being most frequent; other neuroendocrine markers are less often positive (Fig. 5-82). Although cytokeratin is present in most tumors, some are nonreactive; and this is significant in differential diagnosis. The presence of a dotlike pattern for cytokeratin has been noted in some cases (Fig. 5-83).[628]

Differential diagnosis

The major differential diagnostic considerations are small cell carcinoma from another site and malignant lymphoma. Small cell carcinoma may arise in the prostate, and, in about 50% of cases, there is coexistent adenocarcinoma; positive staining of this element for prostate specific antigen and prostatic acid phosphatase indicates prostatic origin. The small cell component usually is negative for prostate specific antigen and prostatic acid phosphatase,[631] so, in pure cases, clinical correlation may be essential to distinguish prostate and bladder primaries. Metastases from other sites also must be considered; interestingly, symptomatic bladder metastasis from bronchogenic small cell carcinoma is rare,[632] but clinical correlation is necessary to exclude this possibility. The identification of a urothelial component, including urothelial carcinoma in situ, would strongly support primary bladder origin.[617,628] Malignant lymphoma should be distinguishable in most cases on histologic grounds, but immunohistochemical staining for cytokeratin and leukocyte common antigen in difficult cases should readily distinguish the two.[617,628]

Treatment and natural history

The aggressive behavior of this tumor has been repeatedly noted, and overall survival is poor. Recent reports suggest that patients may respond to combination therapy if it is given early enough.[607,619,628] In a series from the M.D. Anderson Cancer Center,[628] six patients treated with cystectomy or cystoprostatectomy combined with adjuvant multiagent chemotherapy, were alive at the time of the report, 10 to 77 months after treatment, including three patients who had metastases at the time of diagnosis. In the review of Angulo et al,[627] tumor stage and method of treatment were the most important predictors of outcome. Patients receiving chemotherapy had a 5-year survival of 46%, while patients whose treatment did not include systemic therapy had a 5-year survival of 20%, despite having an overall lower stage. This report and others underscore the importance of recognizing this distinct form of bladder cancer, which may respond to multimodal therapy.[606,607,619,627,628]

MALIGNANT MELANOMA

Malignant melanoma is rarely primary in the bladder, with only 11 reported cases.[633-641] It occurs more frequently in women than men (8:3), appearing in the sixth to seventh decades (range, 46 to 81 years; median, 57 years). Most patients present with gross hematuria (64%) or metastases (27%). In three cases, the bladder primary was detected only at autopsy.[638,639,641]

Grossly, melanoma is dark brown to black, polypoid or fungating, and solid or infiltrating. Some cases have had a flat or macular appearance. It has been reported throughout the bladder, and ranges from 5 mm to 8 cm in diameter. Histologically, these resemble other melanoma and consist of large malignant cells arranged in nests with variable amounts of pigment (Fig. 5-84). In some cases, melanocytes have been found in the adjacent epithelium, occasionally in association with squamous metaplasia.[635-637,641] All cases studied by immunohistochemistry have shown immunoreactivity for S100 protein[638,640,641] and HMB45.[641] Ultrastructural studies revealed typical melanosomes in six cases.[635,637-639]

The major diagnostic concern is excluding metastasis to the bladder from another site. Metastatic melanoma is much more common in the bladder than primary melanoma.[602] In a review of malignant melanoma of the genitourinary tract, Stein and Kendall[642] noted that between 14% and 22% of patients dying of metastatic melanoma have bladder metastases. Strict criteria for the diagnosis of primary bladder melanoma were first proposed by Ainsworth et al[635] and refined by Stein and Kendall.[642] These criteria are:

1. There should be no history of cutaneous melanoma
2. Careful examination of the entire skin surface (including use of a Woods light to exclude a depigmented area which may represent a regressed melanoma) must be negative
3. Comprehensive clinical studies that exclude an ophthalmic or other visceral primary site must be negative
4. The pattern of metastases or recurrence should be consistent with a primary bladder tumor rather than disseminated metastatic melanoma
5. Atypical melanocytes should be present in the mucosa adjacent to the tumor nodule

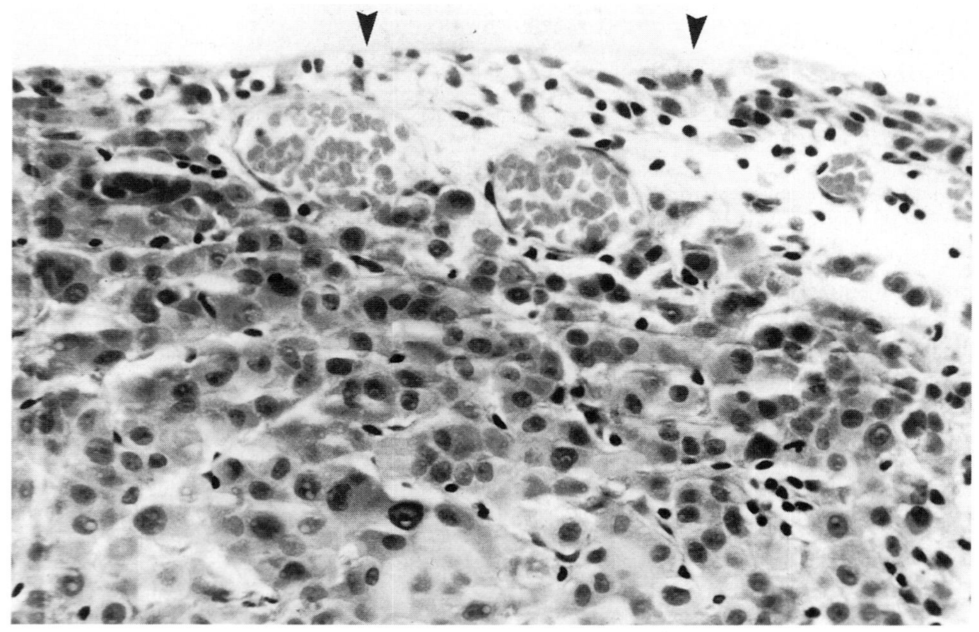

5-84. Malignant melanoma (metastatic) involving the lamina propria of the bladder (*arrows indicate mucosal surface*).

The histogenesis of this tumor remains unknown, and three theories have been proposed: (1) origin from ectopic or dysembryoplastic remnants containing melanocytes;[635] (2) development from argyrophilic cells found in normal urothelium;[637] and (3) origin from metaplastic change in the urothelium.[637]

There are too few reported cases to draw conclusions about treatment. Melanoma has an aggressive clinical course and most patients die of disseminated metastases.

PARAGANGLIOMA (PHEOCHROMOCYTOMA)

Clinical features

The first case of paraganglioma (pheochromocytoma) of the urinary bladder was reported by Zimmerman et al[643] in 1953; since that report, almost 200 cases have been described.[259,644-648] Paraganglioma probably arises from paraganglionic tissue within the bladder wall.[649,650] It occurs from childhood to old age, and is found equally in males and females.[259,648] Rare examples have been reported in association with neurofibromatosis,[651] intestinal carcinoid,[652] and long-term dialysis.[653]

Patients characteristically present with symptoms of catecholamine excess, including tachycardia, hypertension, headaches, fainting, and dizziness. Hematuria is common, and paroxysmal hypertension with painless hematuria at the time of micturition is pathognomonic. Diagnosis is usually confirmed by measurement of catecholamines and their metabolites in urine and serum. Localization of the lesion in the urinary bladder may be confirmed with ^{131}I-MIBG scintigraphy.[654,655]

Pathology

Grossly, paraganglioma is intramural, with a predilection for the trigone, anterior wall, and dome.[648] The overlying mucosa may be intact or ulcerated. It is usually circumscribed, lobulated, and pink to yellow-brown,[652] ranging from 0.2 to 15 cm in greatest dimension, with 66% being less than 4 cm.[645]

Histologically, paraganglioma of the bladder is identical to those occurring elsewhere. The tumor is composed of cells arranged in discrete nests ("Zellballen") separated by a prominent sinusoidal vascular network (Fig. 5-85). Individual cells have abundant pale eosinophilic or clear cytoplasm with central nuclei. Nuclei usually have finely dispersed chromatin, but may show considerable variation in size with some nuclear atypia (Fig. 5-86). Mitotic figures are usually infrequent, and necrosis is not prominent. In some cases, flattened sustentacular cells can be recognized around the cell nests. A single case contained foci of ganglioneuroma.[656]

Pathologic predictors of behavior for these tumors are not well defined.[259,645,646] Features associated with aggressive behavior in other paragangliomas, such as mitotic figures, necrosis, and vascular invasion, have not been studied in urinary bladder tumors.[657] Grignon et al[259] reported a case with multiple recurrences in which the development of overt malignant behavior was associated with an increase in the numbers of mitotic figures.

Special studies

At least 13 tumors have been studied immunohistochemically.[259,652,658-661] Most diagnostically useful are the lack of immunoreactivity for cytokeratin, epithelial membrane antigen, and carcinoembryonic antigen, and positive reaction with antibodies to neuroendocrine

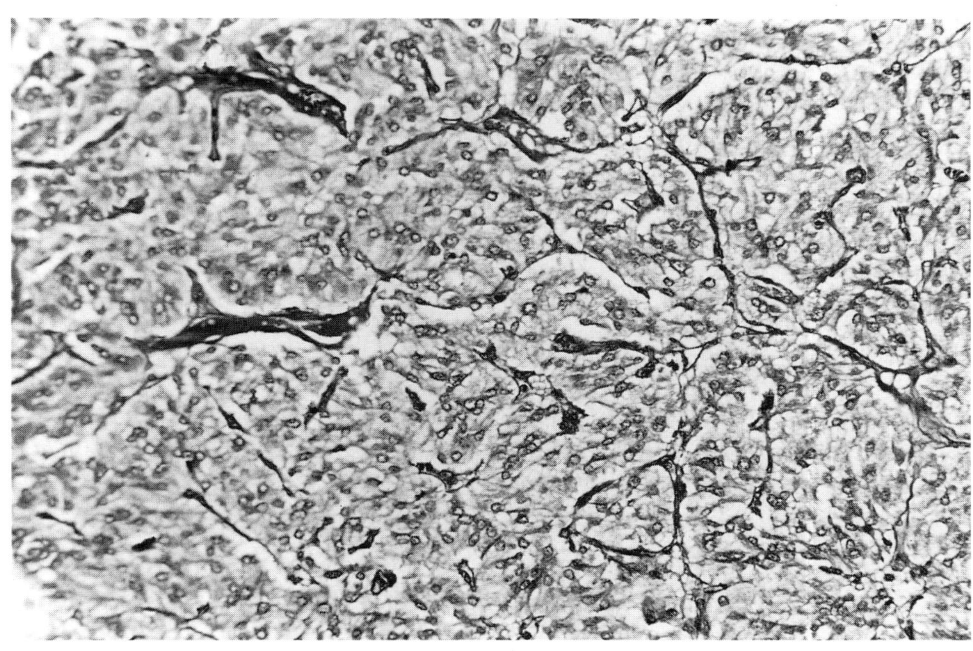

5-85. Paraganglioma of the bladder; the cells are arranged in nests (Zellballen).

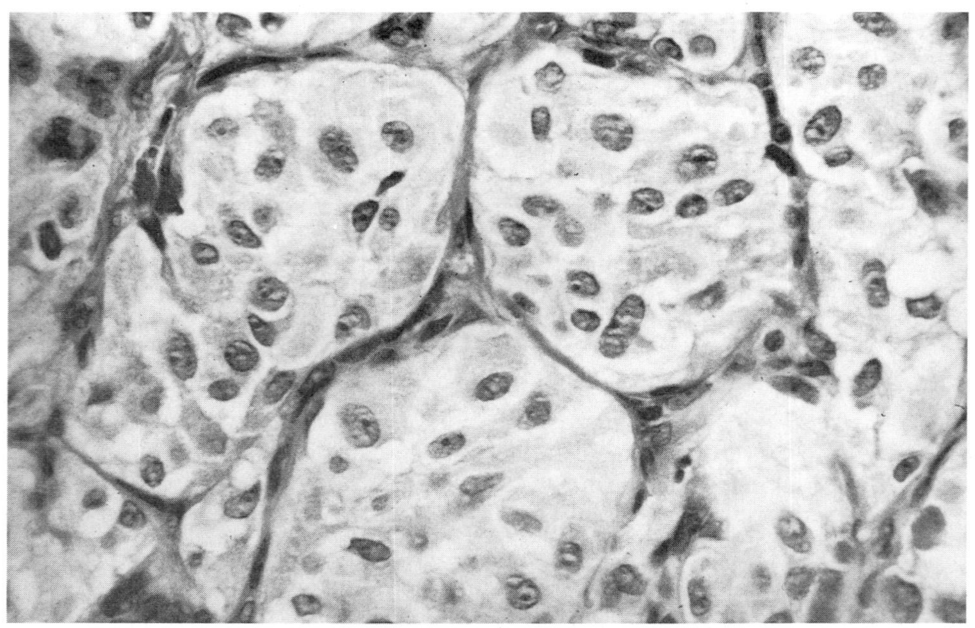

5-86. Paraganglioma of the bladder with cells having abundant cytoplasm and uniform nuclei.

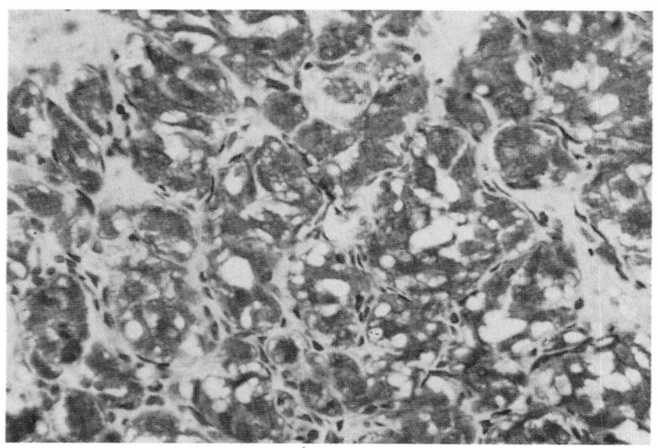

5-87. Paraganglioma of the bladder with intense cytoplasmic immunoreactivity for chromogranin.

markers, including neuron specific enolase, chromogranin, serotonin, somatostatin, and others (Fig. 5-87). Sustentacular cells stain positively for S-100 protein.

Eight tumors have been studied by electron microscopy.[259,645,659,660,662] All contained dense core neurosecretory granules, seven had the typical morphology of catecholamine-secreting tumors with eccentric dense cores. In one tumor, the granules were pleomorphic and the tumor metastasized.[259] Intercellular junctions are usually present, but well formed desmosomes are not.

DNA flow cytometry in three cases was reported by Grignon et al.[259] Two cases were aneuploid and both were cured by surgery. A third case was diploid through two recurrences, but tetraploid when it metastasized.

Differential diagnosis

The main differential diagnostic consideration is invasive urothelial carcinoma, although the possibility of metastasis from another site might be considered. Urothelial carcinoma shows a wide range of morphologic patterns, including rare cases with a discrete nesting pattern.[256] In such cases, the prominent sinusoidal vascular pattern of paraganglioma is a useful diagnostic clue. Immunohistochemistry may be necessary to confirm the histologic impression and exclude urothelial carcinoma, with cytokeratin and neuroendocrine markers being most helpful.

Treatment and natural history

Urinary bladder paraganglioma is treated by complete surgical resection. With small tumors, transurethral resection may be adequate, although partial cystectomy is usually recommended. There is a significant risk of local recurrence if the tumor is not completely resected. Some researchers advocate pelvic lymph node dissection for staging purposes.[648] Metastasis occurs in less than 15% of cases. Davaris et al[645] found lymph node metastases in 12 of 86 well documented cases (13.8%) and distant metastases in only 2 cases (2.3%). An additional patient reported by Grignon et al[259] developed lymph node and peritoneal metastases 24 years after the initial diagnosis following multiple local recurrences. This tendency for late recurrence has been noted by others.[663,664]

GERM CELL NEOPLASMS

CHORIOCARCINOMA

Since the first report, by Djewitzki in 1904,[665] of choriocarcinoma arising in the bladder, 22 cases have been described,[251,666,667] and other cases have been reported elsewhere in the urinary tract.[265,668] Young and Eble[251] found that no cases of pure choriocarcinoma of the bladder have appeared in the recent literature; this may indicate that a urothelial carcinoma component is present in these cases, supporting a metaplastic origin.

The histogenesis of this tumor is uncertain. Grammatico et al[265] proposed a metaplastic theory, suggesting that typical urothelial carcinoma develops the ability to produce human chorionic gonadotropin and subsequently displays tumor giant cells and then syncytiotrophoblastic giant cells before complete evolution of choriocarcinoma.

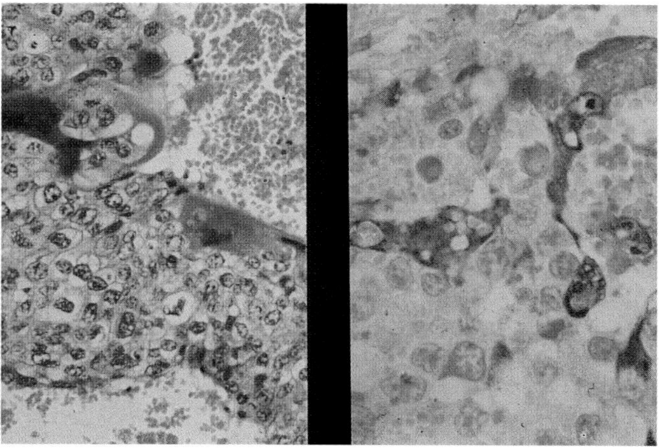

5-88. Choriocarcinoma showing both syncytiotrophoblastic giant cells and cytotrophoblast (*left*) and immunoreactivity for human chorionic gonadotropin in the syncytiotrophoblast (*right*). This tumor also contained areas of high-grade urothelial carcinoma.

Clinical features

Most patients have symptoms typical of other bladder cancers, including hematuria, dysuria, and frequency. Gynecomastia has been reported in some men, and increased levels of serum or urinary gonadotropins may be present.[666,667,669-673]

The significance of human chorionic gonadotropin production by urothelial carcinoma with or without trophoblastic differentiation remains uncertain. In most cases with human chorionic gonadotropin immunoreactivity, there is elevation of the serum chorionic gonadotropin level. Dexeus et al[674] reported elevated serum chorionic gonadotropin in 17% of 69 patients with metastatic urothelial carcinoma. The level of serum chorionic gonadotropin did not correlate with tumor response to chemotherapy; however, decreasing levels during chemotherapy correlated with a positive response, and increasing levels following an initial decrease indicated failure.

Pathology

Grossly, choriocarcinoma is large, exophytic, or fungating, with hemorrhage and necrosis.

Histologically, typical features of choriocarcinoma are present, including a mixture of syncytiotrophoblastic and cytotrophoblastic elements (Fig 5-88). In more than two thirds of cases, and all reported since 1967, urothelial carcinoma is also present. Tumor giant cells and syncytiotrophoblastic giant cells may be seen without cytotrophoblasts;[265] in these cases, there is often intermingling and transition from urothelial carcinoma to giant cells (Fig. 5-89). Such cases should be classified as urothelial carcinoma with syncytiotrophoblastic differentiation rather than choriocarcinoma. Some cases of urothelial carcinoma display chorionic gonadotropin immunoreactivity in mononuclear cells without evidence of trophoblastic differentiation (Fig. 5-90).

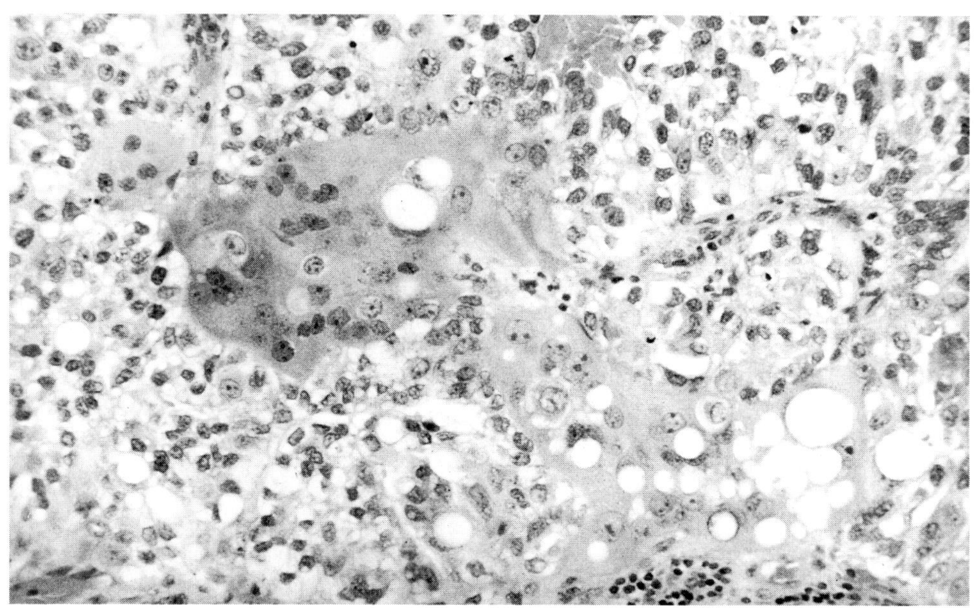

5-89. Urothelial carcinoma containing syncytiotrophoblastic giant cells.

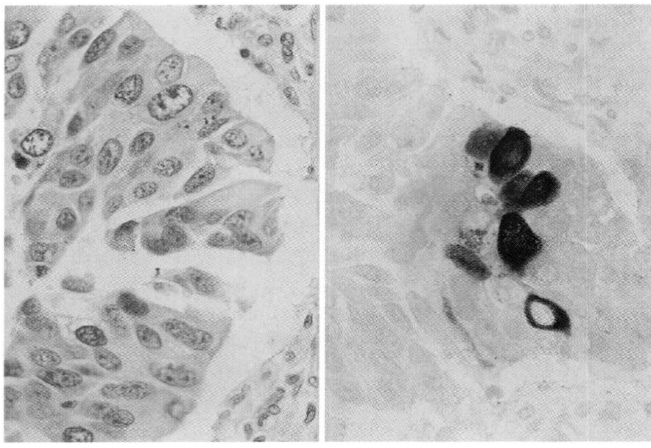

5-90. Invasive urothelial carcinoma without giant cells (*left*) which shows immunoreactivity for human chorionic gonadotropin (*right*).

Special studies

In cases of typical choriocarcinoma or urothelial carcinoma with syncytiotrophoblastic differentiation, the syncytiotrophoblasts express human chorionic gonadotropin. Immunohistochemical studies of urothelial carcinoma reveal chorionic gonadotropin expression in 12% to 46% of cases.[265,668,675-679] The frequency of positivity correlates with grade; Shah et al[677] found positivity in 0 of 41 grade 1 and 2 tumors, compared with 12 of 56 grade 3 and 4 carcinomas; Campo et al[668] reported positivity in 0 of 16 low-grade tumors, compared with 9 of 47 high-grade cancers. Similarly, Seidal et al[679] showed a significant association between chorionic gonadotropin positivity and increased histologic grade. In the series reported by Martin et al,[678] the presence of chorionic gonadotropin immunoreactivity correlated significantly with the presence of squamous metaplasia. Chorionic gonadotropin immunoreactivity has also been found in squamous cell carcinoma of the bladder associated with schistosomiasis.[680]

Grammatico et al[265] performed immunogold ultrastructural studies of urothelial carcinoma with syncytiotrophoblastic cells and urothelial carcinoma with chorionic gonadotropin immunoreactivity but without morphologic evidence of trophoblastic differentiation. They localized human chorionic gonadotropin within cytoplasmic granules and larger flocculent bodies.

Treatment and natural history

Too few cases are available to make treatment recommendations for choriocarcinoma. Cases with morphologic evidence of trophoblastic differentiation are highly aggressive neoplasms with early metastases and death.[251] The value of chemotherapy in managing these patients is unknown. Martin et al[678] reported that tumors with human chorionic gonadotropin immunoreactivity were less responsive to radiation therapy than those without human chorionic gonadotropin immunoreactivity. Seidal et al[679] found that human chorionic gonadotropin positivity indicated a worse outcome in patients of all stages and grades. Dexeus et al[674] reported that elevated serum human chorionic gonadotropin in patients with metastatic bladder cancer did not predict chemoresponsiveness.

DERMOID CYST

At least four cases of dermoid cyst arising in the bladder have been described,[681,682] all in women between 30 and 49 years of age. Complaints were nonspecific, although the passing of hair in the urine was occasionally seen.

Pathologically, dermoid cyst of the bladder has features typical of dermoid cyst in the ovary. Hair, teeth, and calcifications may be present. In one case, a connection was found between the bladder dermoid cyst and an apparently normal ovary. The possibility of direct extension from an ovarian primary or metastatic teratoma should be considered prior to accepting a case as originating in the bladder.

YOLK SAC TUMOR

A single case of yolk sac tumor developing in the urinary bladder has been reported.[683] The tumor arose in the bladder of a 1-year-old boy who presented with gross hematuria. The lesion was grossly polypoid, with a hemorrhagic, gelatinous, and necrotic cut surface. Histologically, it consisted of solid and cystic areas with cuboidal to columnar cells displaying eosinophilic to clear cytoplasm. Schiller-Duval bodies and hyaline globules were present. The patient was treated with partial cystectomy, pelvic lymph node dissection, and chemotherapy; follow-up at 4 months showed no evidence of recurrence.

BENIGN MESENCHYMAL NEOPLASMS

Benign mesenchymal neoplasms are uncommon in the bladder and the majority are leiomyoma (estimated 35%[684]), hemangioma, or neurofibroma. In the review by Melicow,[4] benign soft tissue tumors accounted for only 0.9% of primary bladder lesions. Rare examples of other benign soft tissue tumors have been reported including granular cell tumor,[685] lymphangioma,[686] benign fibrous histiocytoma,[687,688] and ganglioneuroma.[689]

LEIOMYOMA

In 1986, Knoll et al[690] reported 5 examples of leiomyoma of the bladder, and found approximately 155 further cases in the literature. Subsequently, 10 more cases have been reported.[684,691-697] Leiomyoma is more common in women (male:female ratio, 1:2) and the majority occur in adults, although rare examples in children are reported.[698] Obstructive symptoms are most common, because of a ball-valve effect of the pedunculated tumor.[697,699-702] Less often the tumor produces pelvic pain[693] or ureteral obstruction with hydronephrosis.[694] Bladder leiomyoma may be associated with paraurethral leiomyoma.[703]

Grossly, leiomyoma is submucosal (endovesical) in two thirds of cases, producing a polypoid or pedunculated mass. Less commonly it arises within the wall or subserosally. The overlying epithelium is usually intact.

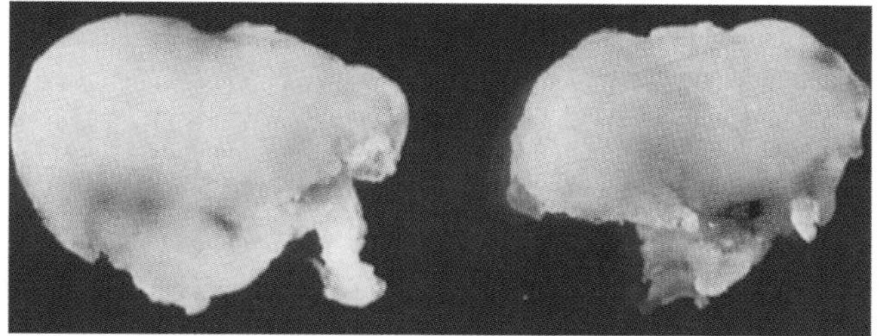

5-91. Leiomyoma of the bladder, which shelled out at the time of transurethral resection.

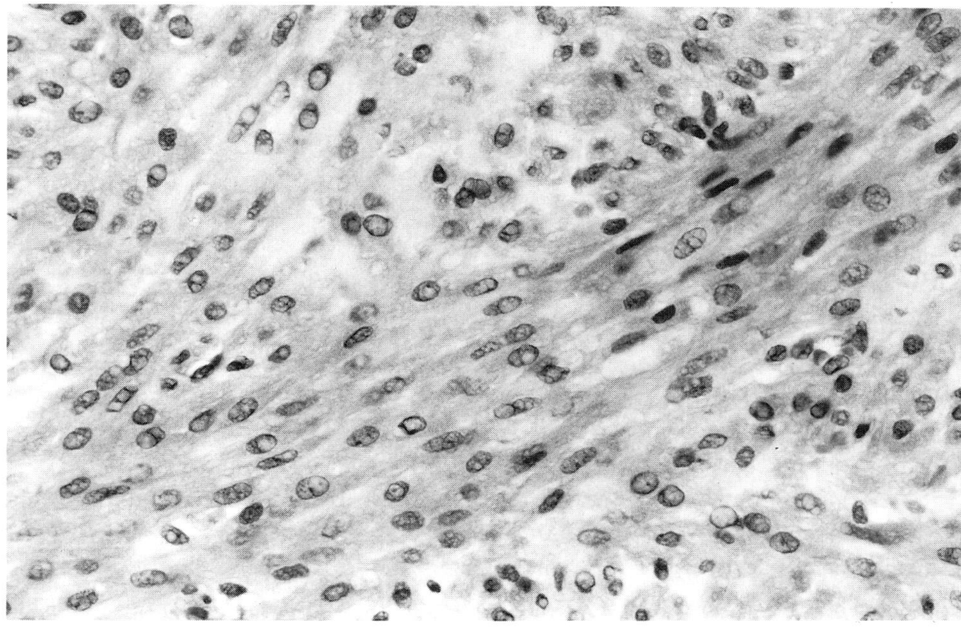

5-92. Leiomyoma of the bladder with fascicles of spindle-shaped cells showing minimal nuclear atypia and no mitotic figures.

Most are small, 1 to 4 cm in diameter, although tumors as large as 25 cm have been described (Fig. 5-91).[696] One patient had multiple leiomyomata.[704] The cut surface is typically circumscribed and bulging, with a whorled gray-white appearance. Histologically, the typical features of leiomyoma are present, including fascicles of spindle-shaped cells with fusiform, blunt-ended nuclei, and eosinophilic cytoplasm. There is minimal atypia and few mitotic figures (Fig. 5-92). In tumors with atypical features (nuclear pleomorphism, frequent mitotic figures, or necrosis), no criteria allow precise separation of benign and malignant lesions. Mills et al[705] recommended that a smooth muscle tumor with rare or absent mitotic figures and an infiltrative pattern be considered low-grade leiomyosarcoma. The presence of an infiltrative pattern argues against a benign diagnosis. Focal myxoid change can occur in leiomyoma, but a prominent myxoid character is more likely in leiomyosarcoma.[706] One case that was studied ultrastructurally demonstrated typical features of smooth muscle.[695]

Treatment of leiomyoma is conservative. Depending on tumor size, transurethral resection or segmental resection is indicated. In cases with atypical features, resection with frozen sections to ensure negative margins may be appropriate.[706] In most cases, treatment is curative, although leiomyoma can recur if incompletely resected.[697] No cases of sarcoma developing from a leiomyoma have been reported.

HEMANGIOMA

In 1991, Jahn and Nissen[707] reviewed the literature on hemangioma of the urinary tract and identified 106 cases in the bladder. In Melicow's series,[4] hemangioma accounted for 40% of benign soft tissue tumors, and 0.6% of primary tumors. It occurs at any age, with the majority presenting prior to age 30; there is a slight male preponderance. Most patients present with hematuria, but irritation, pain, and obstructive symptoms may occur. Up to 30% of patients have cutaneous hemangiomas.[708] Bladder hemangioma occurs in 3% to 6% of patients with Klippel-Trenaunay syndrome,[708-710] and has also been reported in patients with Sturge-Weber syndrome.[710,711] Cystoscopically, hemangioma appears purple, multilobulated, and sessile, and may be mistaken for endometriosis, melanoma, or sarcoma.[707] Arteriography and ultrasonography may be useful in diagnosis and assessment of the extent of the lesion.[711,712]

Grossly, hemangioma may be single (66%[713]) or multiple, and be superficial or extend through the full thickness of the bladder wall. The majority are small (1 to 2 cm), although lesions up to 10 cm in diameter have been

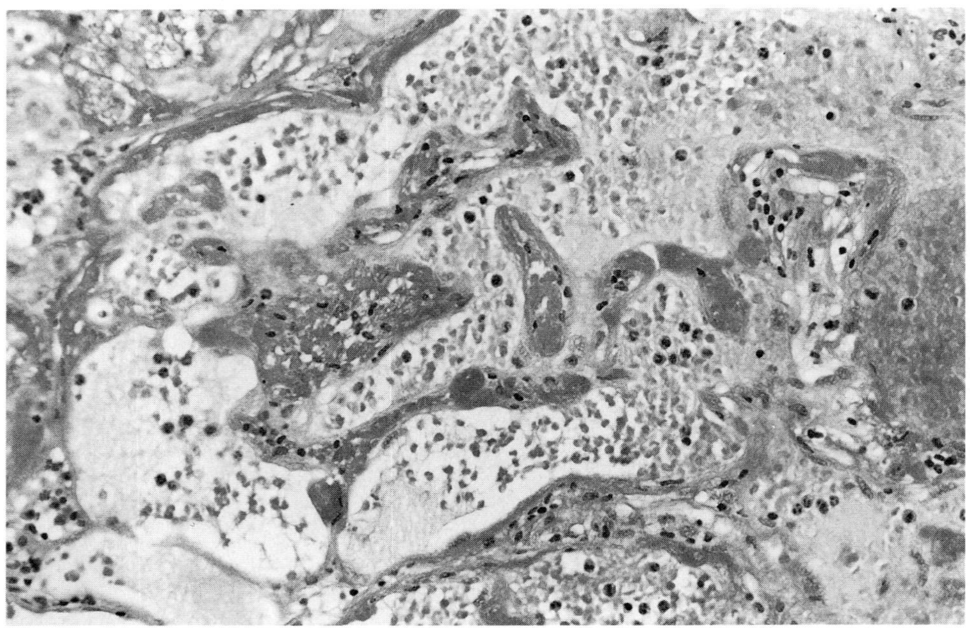

5-93. Cavernous hemangioma of the bladder with dilated vascular channels filled with red blood cells.

described. It is soft, spongy, and hemorrhagic. Histologically, it consists of vascular spaces containing blood and thrombi. Depending on the pattern, hemangioma is classified as cavernous, capillary, venous, or racemose, with cavernous being most common (Fig. 5-93).[707] The major differential diagnostic consideration is angiosarcoma, although these typically have nuclear pleomorphism and numerous mitotic figures.[714] Involvement of the bladder by Kaposi's sarcoma in AIDS patients has also been described.[715] Rarely hemangiopericytoma arises in the bladder;[716,717] this tumor is more cellular than hemangioma and has a characteristic vascular pattern.

Treatment depends on the size and location of the hemangioma. Most investigators recommend partial cystectomy or local excision.[707,713,718,719] Biopsy and transurethral resection risk massive hemorrhage.[707,720,721] Recently, obliteration with the Nd:YAG laser has been successful.[708] There is a risk of local recurrence if resection is incomplete.[707]

NEUROFIBROMA

In 1986, Ogawa and Watanabe[722] described a case of neurofibroma in the bladder, and reviewed approximately 50 other reported cases. The majority occur in patients with von Recklinghausen's disease, although rare cases occur in the absence of this syndrome.[723,724] In von Recklinghausen's disease, the urinary bladder is the most frequent site of involvement in the genitourinary tract. Neurofibroma can appear at any age, including infancy, and is slightly more common in males.[253] The majority of patients complain of hematuria, dysuria, or irritative symptoms.[725] In some cases, there is concomitant involvement of other genitourinary sites, including the ureter, spermatic cord, penis, and scrotum.[722,726-728]

Grossly, neurofibroma may be single or multiple, consisting of discrete variably sized nodules within the bladder wall or submucosa, which may be polypoid or pedunculated. Most are small, but may be up to several centimeters in diameter. Neurofibroma may also appear as diffuse thickening of the bladder wall without discrete margins; this pattern corresponds to the plexiform variant characteristically associated with von Recklinghausen's disease. In these patients, neurofibroma may extensively involve the muscularis propria, ureters, and adjacent soft tissues.

Histologically, neurofibroma of the bladder is identical to neurofibroma occurring elsewhere, composed of fascicles of elongated spindle-shaped cells with thin wavy nuclei in a collagenized and fibrillar background (Fig. 5-94). Small nerve fibers are usually present within the mass, and myxoid areas may also be present. Immunohistochemical results are similar to other neurofibromas; the case reported by Winfield and Catalona[724] was S-100 protein positive.

The differential diagnostic considerations with neurofibroma include other benign spindle cell lesions such as leiomyoma[690,694,697] and inflammatory (fibromyxoid) pseudotumor.[729,730] The majority of leiomyomata in the bladder show typical features, and separation should be straightforward. In problem cases, immunohistochemistry reveals evidence of muscle differentiation. Inflammatory pseudotumor is characterized by cytologically benign spindle or stellate cells in a loose myxoid background mixed with inflammatory cells.[729,730] The spindle cells contain vimentin and actin, reflecting their fibroblastic and myofibroblastic nature.[731] Because most bladder neurofibromata occur in patients with von Recklinghausen's disease, clinical history should be obtained when this diagnosis is entertained. Malignant change in neurofibroma in the bladder has been reported only once.[732]

Treatment of neurofibroma remains controversial. Most investigators recommend radical resection with uri-

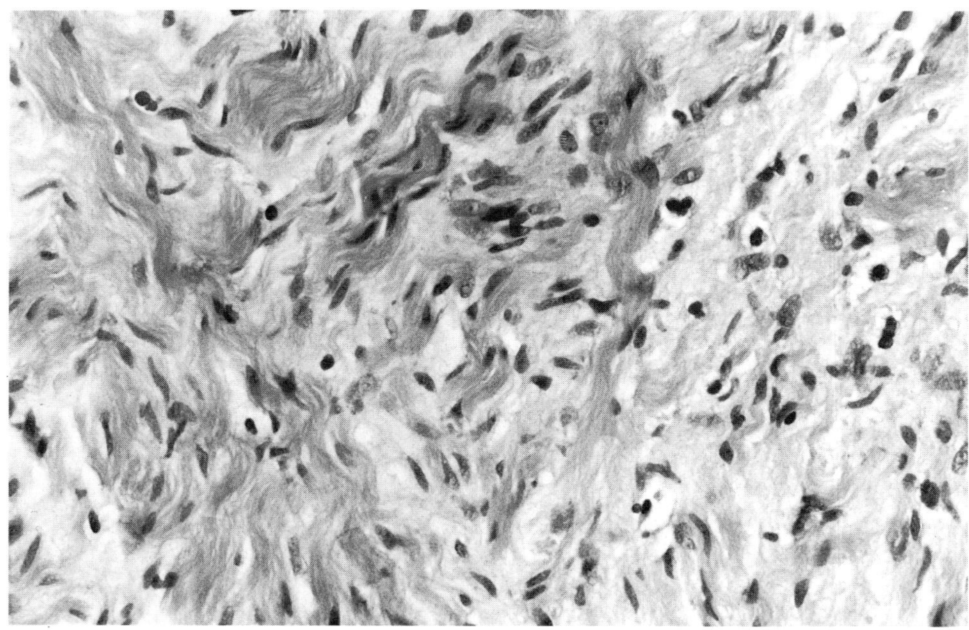

5-94. Neurofibroma of the bladder with wavy spindle cells arranged in loose, poorly formed fascicles.

nary diversion because of the high rate of recurrence with partial resection.[723,728] Urinary diversion alone may be useful in cases with extensive involvement,[727,733] although conservative management has been advocated by some until the tumor becomes too extensive for transurethral resection or until ureteral obstruction develops.[734,735] Neurofibroma frequently recurs and can cause death by urinary obstruction and renal failure.[735]

GRANULAR CELL TUMOR

Granular cell tumor is rare in the urinary bladder, with 10 cases found in the literature.[685,736-744] All have arisen in adults, with equal sex distribution. All patients presented with hematuria.

Grossly, granular cell tumor is circumscribed or encapsulated, appearing as a yellow-white nodule up to 12 cm in diameter;[736] in one case, multiple nodules were found.[743] Histologically, the tumor is composed of spindle to polygonal shaped cells with abundant coarsely granular eosinophilic cytoplasm. The granules are PAS-positive and diastase resistant. Although this tumor is considered to be neurogenic (Schwann cell) in origin,[745] the only bladder lesion studied ultrastructurally had myogenic features.[741] The tumor is S-100 protein positive, similar to granular cell tumor elsewhere.[746]

All cases have been benign except for the one reported by Ravich et al.[736] The latter case showed benign histologic features in the bladder lesion but subsequently recurred and metastasized. Recent authors suggest conservative treatment given the benign course in all cases but one.[744]

MALIGNANT SOFT TISSUE NEOPLASMS

Sarcoma of the urinary bladder is uncommon, and there is a distinctive age distribution according to histologic type. Rhabdomyosarcoma is the most frequent tumor of the bladder in childhood, whereas leiomyosarcoma is the most frequent sarcoma in adults. In the review by Melicow,[4] sarcoma accounted for 2.7% of all primary bladder neoplasms. It is difficult to accurately assess the old literature regarding sarcoma because of the inclusion of lymphosarcoma and cases of carcinoma mimicking soft tissue tumors. The following discussion is limited to cases reported in the last 20 to 30 years.

BLADDER TUMORS IN CHILDHOOD (IN APPROXIMATE ORDER OF FREQUENCY)

- Rhabdomyosarcoma (>75%)
- Hemangioma
- Neurofibroma
- Urothelial carcinoma
- Leiomyoma
- Leukemia/lymphoma
- Others

RHABDOMYOSARCOMA

Rhabdomyosarcoma of all sites accounts for between 4% and 8% of all malignant tumors in children under the age of 15 years.[747] However, not all malignant neoplasms of the bladder in children are rhabdomyosarcoma; other types of sarcoma and a variety of epithelial tumors have also been described (see box on this page).[748] Rhabdomyosarcoma of the bladder is rare in adults.[749-751] In children, it occurs more frequently in boys (ratio, 3:2), and most develop before age 5 years. It most often presents with hematuria and bladder neck obstruction. Cystoscopically, the characteristic finding is a polypoid mass filling the bladder lumen.

Grossly, rhabdomyosarcoma forms polypoid masses that may be single or multiple, producing a sarcoma

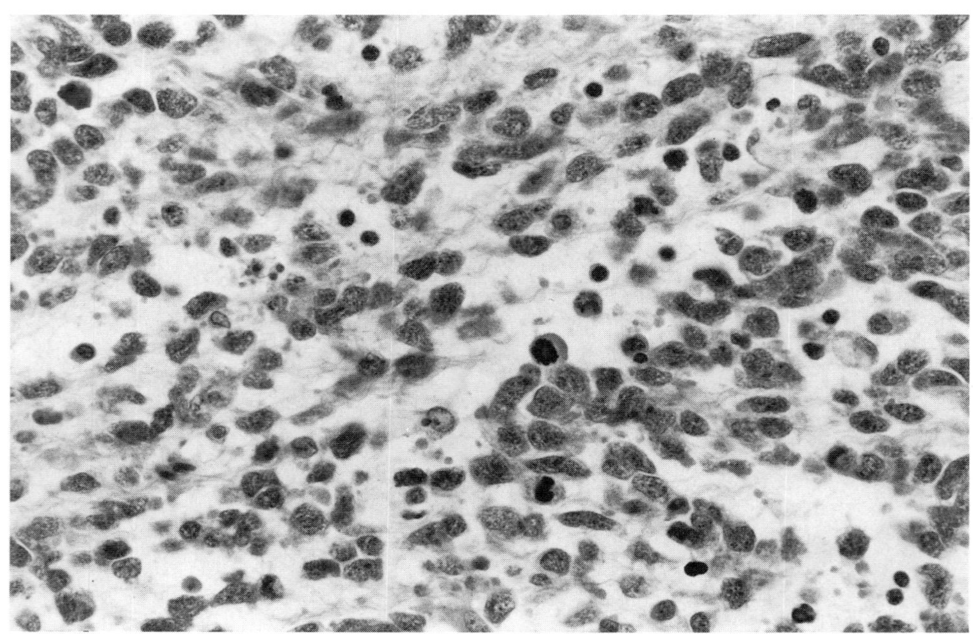

5-95. Embryonal rhabdomyosarcoma of the bladder composed of small blue round cells.

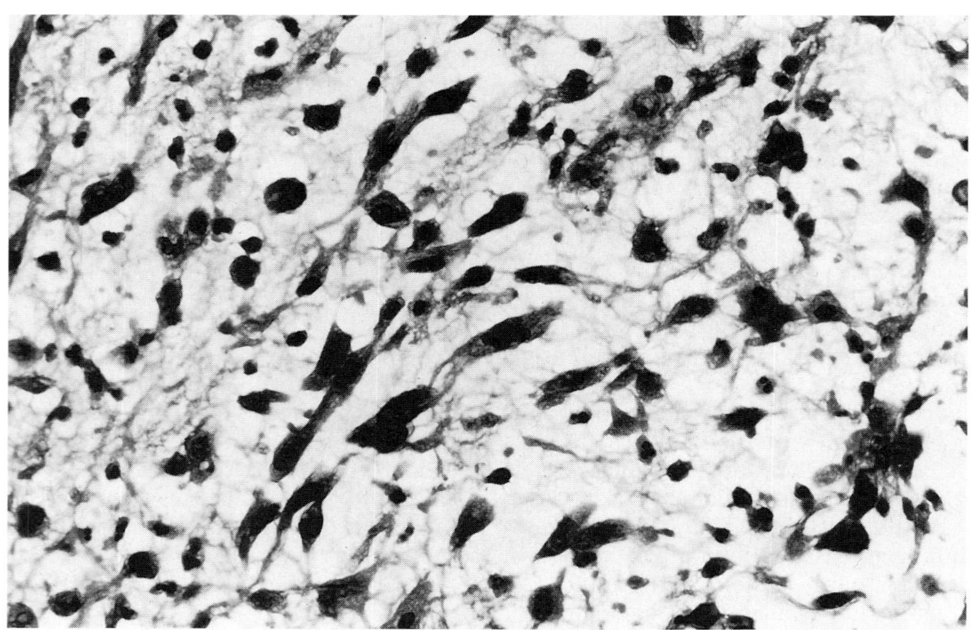

5-96. Rhabdomyosarcoma of the bladder with strap cells in a myxoid stroma.

botryoides (grapelike) appearance. The trigone is the most common location. Histologically, most are embryonal rhabdomyosarcoma, with diffuse infiltration of small round blue cells with scant cytoplasm (Fig. 5-95). In the sarcoma botryoides type, the cells are scattered in a loose myxoid stroma, with condensation of rhabdomyoblasts beneath the surface epithelium in a cambium layer. Although rare rhabdoid or strap cells containing cross striations may be found (Fig. 5-96), this is not necessary for diagnosis and most cases require immunohistochemistry or electron microscopic examination to prove rhabdomyoblastic differentiation.

Until recently, rhabdomyosarcoma had a dismal prognosis; however, combinations of surgery, radiation therapy, and chemotherapy have markedly improved survival.[747,752,753] In the first Intergroup Rhabdomyosarcoma Study, 28% of children (11 of 31) with primary bladder rhabdomyosarcoma died of tumor following combined therapy.[753]

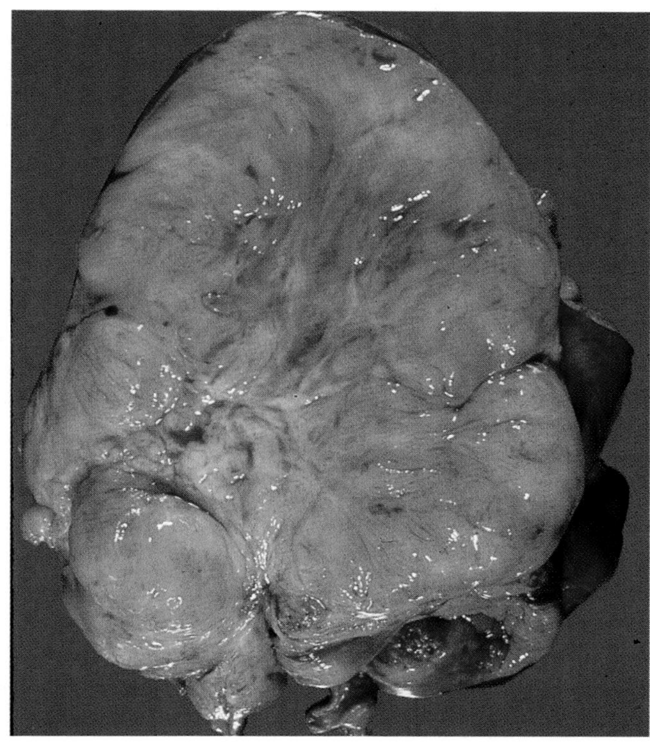

5-97. Primary leiomyosarcoma of the bladder. The tumor is 12x16 cm. *(Photograph courtesy of Dr. Alberto Ayala.)*

LEIOMYOSARCOMA

Clinical features

Leiomyosarcoma is the most common sarcoma of the bladder in adults. Since 1960, more than 64 cases have been reported.[53,97,705,706,754-775] There is a wide age range (7 to 81 years) with a mean age of 52 years; nine cases occurred in patients under the age of 21 years.* Several cases have developed following cyclophosphamide therapy for other conditions.[97,768,770,773] Two of these reports concern the same case.[768,770] One case was associated with a family history of bone abnormalities,[769] and one patient had bilateral retinoblastoma as an infant.[97] The most common presentation is hematuria and obstructive symptoms.

Pathology

Grossly, leiomyosarcoma is most often lobulated or polypoid, and may be ulcerated. A mushroom shape at cystoscopy is typical.[776] Most tumors are 2 to 5 cm in diameter, occasional examples range up to 13 cm (Fig. 5-97).[757]

Histologically, the majority have the typical appearance of leiomyosarcoma, composed of interwoven fascicles of spindle shaped cells with long blunt-ended nuclei and eosinophilic cytoplasm (Fig. 5-98). Nuclear pleomorphism is variable, as is the mitotic rate. Necrosis may be present. In a few cases, the tumor has been myxoid,[705,706] and epithelioid leiomyosarcoma has also been described.[253]

Ultrastructural studies show features typical of smooth muscle cells, including thin filaments with dense bodies and pinocytotic vesicles.[769] Tumors evaluated by immunohistochemistry have been uniformly cytokeratin negative and vimentin and muscle-specific actin positive; desmin shows variable reactivity.[705]

Leiomyosarcoma has occurred with urothelial carcinoma in situ,[774] noninvasive papillary carcinoma,[771] and invasive urothelial carcinoma.[754]

Differential diagnosis

The differential diagnosis of spindle cell lesions in the bladder is extensive.[777] If the tumor is clearly malignant, the major considerations are other types of sarcoma and sarcomatoid carcinoma. Other sarcomas are distinguished by histologic features and immunohistochemical findings. Sarcomatoid carcinoma (discussed above in the section titled Sarcomatoid Urothelial Carcinoma) may mimic high-grade leiomyosarcoma. In most cases, extensive sampling reveals a recognizable epithelial component; however, there are cases of sarcomatoid carcinoma without identifiable foci of carcinoma,[286] and immunohistochemistry is invaluable in such instances. The majority of cases of sarcomatoid carcinoma express cytokeratin at least focally in the spindle cell component and do not stain with muscle markers such as actin and desmin.[242,285,286,292] This distinction is not merely academic; sarcomatoid carcinoma has a much poorer prognosis than leiomyosarcoma.[286,705]

Distinction from leiomyoma may be difficult because of the lack of well-established criteria. The presence of more than slight nuclear pleomorphism, high mitotic rate, infiltrative growth, and necrosis suggest malignancy. Mills et al[705] suggested that any tumor with 5 or more

*References 53, 97, 705, 706, 759, 762, 768-770.

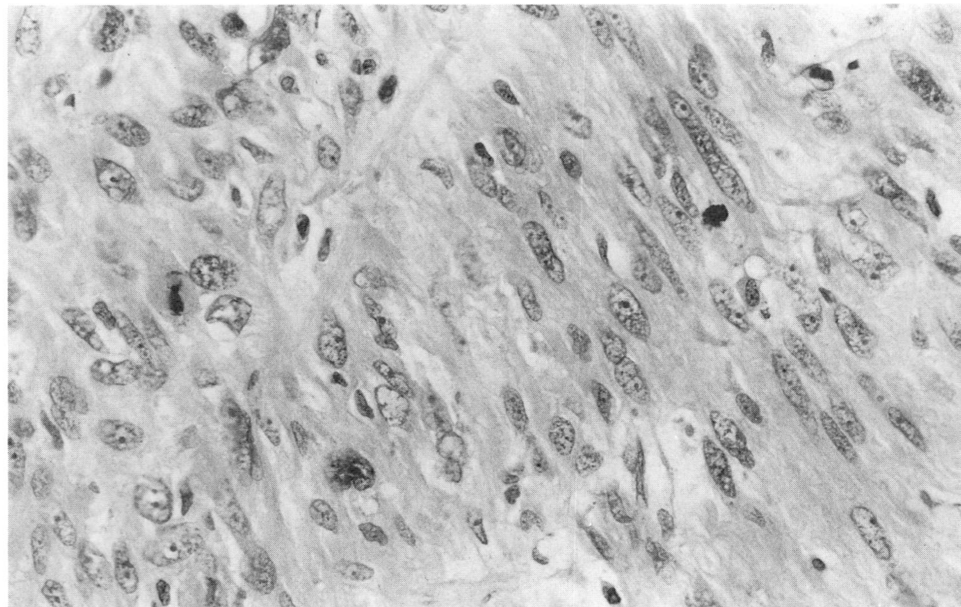

5-98. Leiomyosarcoma of bladder with fascicles of spindle cells showing nuclear pleomorphism and mitotic figures.

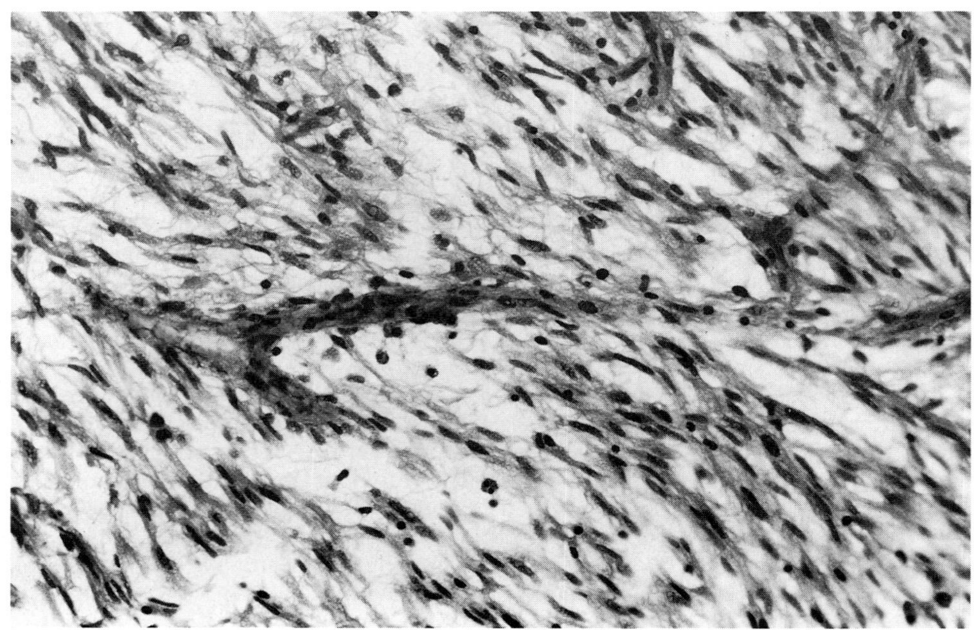

5-99. Inflammatory (fibromyxoid) pseudotumor with spindle and stellate cells in a myxoid stroma with numerous inflammatory cells in the background.

mitotic figures per 10 high power fields was leiomyosarcoma, and cautioned that tumors with even 0 or 1 mitotic figures should be considered malignant if there is an infiltrative growth pattern. Caution is indicated in calling any mitotically active smooth muscle tumor of the bladder benign.

In any spindle cell lesion of the bladder, the possibility of a benign process should be considered. Several entities produce spindle cell proliferations, which can be quite alarming in their histologic appearance. Pseudosarcomatous fibromyxoid tumor,[729,731] or inflammatory pseudotumor,[730,778] is typically polypoid and can be quite large. Histologically, it has a loose myxoid appearance with numerous slitlike blood vessels and a background of acute and chronic inflammatory cells (Fig. 5-99). Individual cells are spindle-shaped or stellate with little nuclear pleomorphism, although occasional bizarre nuclei may be seen; mitotic figures are infrequent and morphologically normal. The process is infiltrative and can involve the muscularis propria,[730] a feature that makes distinction from myxoid leiomyosarcoma difficult and, in small samples, often impossible.[705] With adequate sampling, the latter should show features diagnostic of leiomyosarcoma. The results of immunohistochemistry have been variable; inflammatory pseudotumor is usually vimentin

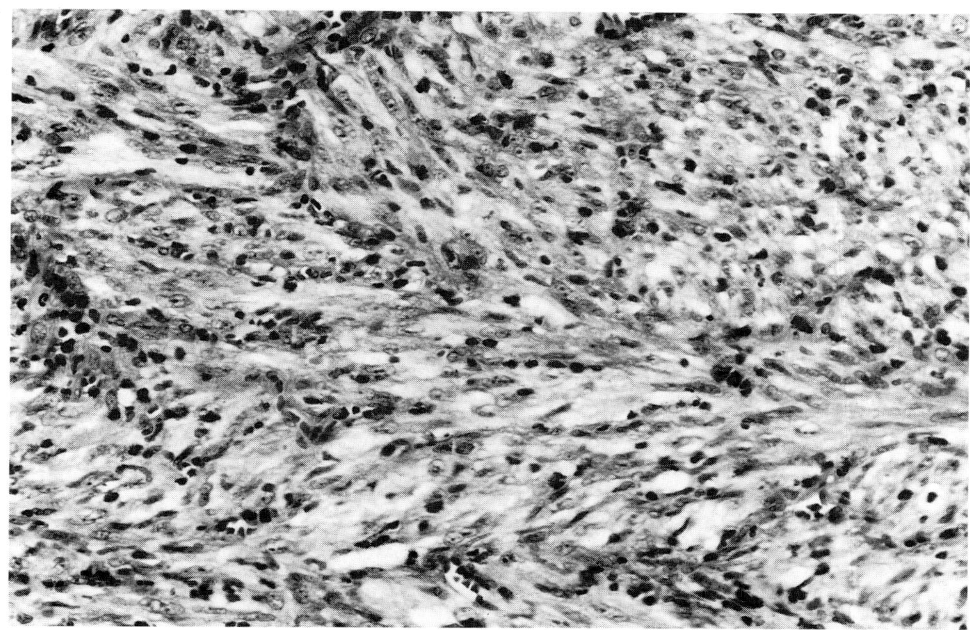

5-100. Postoperative spindle cell nodule having moderate cellularity with admixed inflammatory cells.

and actin positive and desmin negative, reflecting the myofibroblastic nature of the cells.[729,731,778] However, desmin positivity has been reported,[730,779] making immunohistochemistry of little value.

Postoperative spindle cell nodule can also be confused with leiomyosarcoma. It is most often an incidental finding and develops following surgery or trauma.[779-782] Histologically, it resembles inflammatory pseudotumor with spindle-shaped cells arranged in short haphazard fascicles reminiscent of granulation tissue (Fig. 5-100). Although mitotic activity can be brisk, abnormal mitotic figures and nuclear pleomorphism are not found. Immunohistochemical and ultrastructural studies show features of fibroblasts and myofibroblasts, although cytokeratin positivity has been reported.[779,782]

Treatment and natural history

Leiomyosarcoma is treated by partial cystectomy if localized or radical cystectomy if more extensive.[769,772] The use of combination chemotherapy has been advocated.[772] Many investigators have commented on the aggressive nature of these tumors,[756,757] but review of 62 cases with outcome data reported since 1960* reveals crude 2- and 5-year survival of 81% and 67%, respectively (Fig. 5-101). None of eight patients under the age of 21 years with follow-up available died of leiomyosarcoma.†

MALIGNANT FIBROUS HISTIOCYTOMA

Only nine examples of malignant fibrous histiocytoma arising in the bladder have been described since 1970.[688,783-790] In four of these, the pathologic description is sketchy and it is difficult to know if sarcomatoid carcinoma was adequately excluded.[790] There were five men and four women, with ages ranging from 20 to 84 years. Hematuria and lower abdominal pain were the most common presentations, and all tumors were locally advanced.

Grossly, the tumors are large and necrotic; one case was polypoid.[790] Histologically, four cases were considered inflammatory malignant fibrous histiocytoma,[688,783,784,786] two cases storiform,[785,791] and one case each myxoid[789] and pleomorphic (Fig. 5-102).[790] Ultrastructural[688,784,789,790] and immunohistochemical[688,789,790] studies, when reported, have been consistent with malignant fibrous histiocytoma arising elsewhere in the body.

The major differential diagnostic consideration is sarcomatoid carcinoma, which also is usually large and polypoid. Histologically, sarcomatoid carcinoma frequently shows a malignant fibrous histiocytoma-like growth pattern.[286] Prior to accepting a diagnosis of primary malignant fibrous histiocytoma, this possibility must be excluded by extensive sampling to identify a recognizable epithelial element. If no epithelial component is found, immunohistochemical or ultrastructural studies should be employed to look for evidence of epithelial differentiation.

Too few cases are reported to draw any conclusions concerning treatment. Of seven patients with follow up, three died of their tumor at 5, 7, and 11 months,[4,785,791] and the remaining four were alive and well at 18, 24, and 36 months,[786,788,789] or dead of unrelated causes without evidence of progression.[784]

OSTEOSARCOMA

In 1987, Young and Rosenberg[792] reported an osteosarcoma primary in the bladder and reviewed 21 cases from the world literature. Counting the Young and Rosenberg

*References 53, 97,705, 706, 755-764, 766, 767, 769-775.
†References 53, 97, 705, 706, 759, 762, 769, 770.

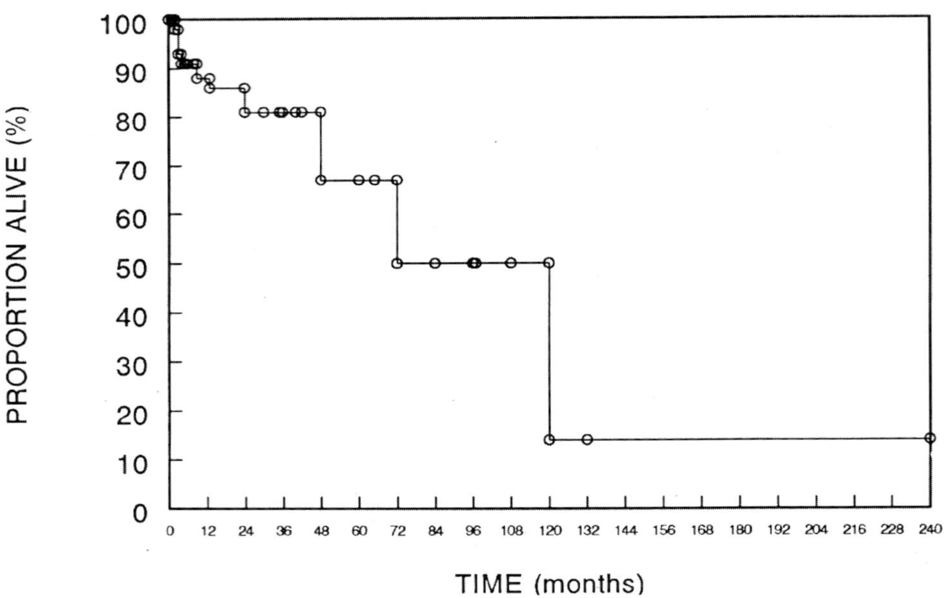

5-101. Kaplan-Meier survival curve of reported cases of bladder leiomyosarcoma.

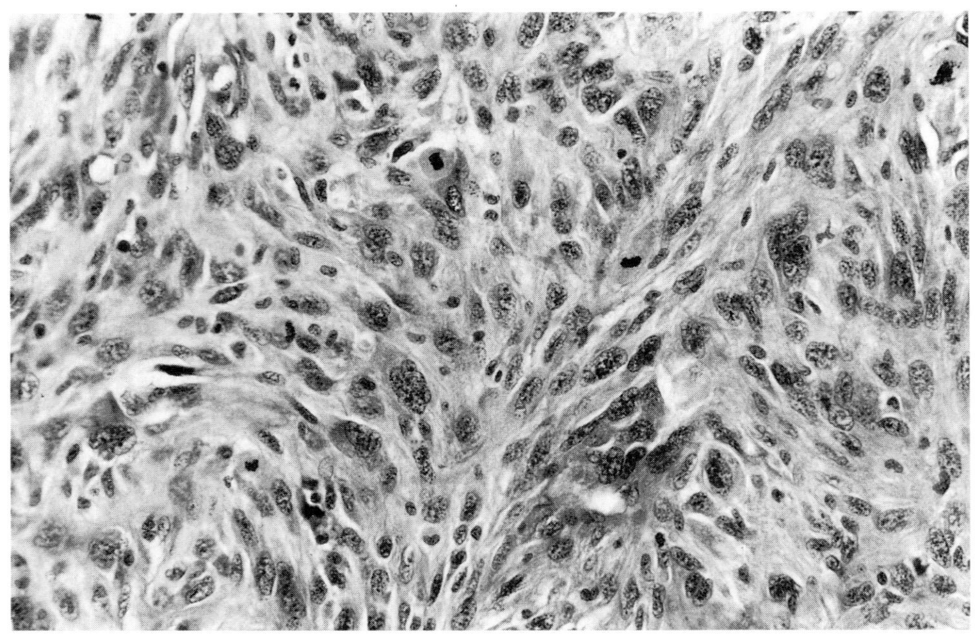

5-102. Primary malignant fibrous histiocytoma of the bladder.

case, only seven cases have been reported since 1970.[102,761,792-796] The majority occur in men (4.5:1 male to female ratio), with an average age of 62 years.[792] Presentation includes hematuria, irritative symptoms, and abdominal mass. In one patient, the tumor developed 27 years after radiation therapy for urothelial carcinoma.[102]

Grossly, osteosarcoma is large, polypoid, and deeply infiltrative. Histologically, the tumor is high-grade sarcoma with osteoid production. Sarcomatoid urothelial carcinoma and urothelial carcinoma with osseous metaplasia must be considered in the differential diagnosis. Osteoid formation can be seen in sarcomatoid carcinoma (carcinosarcoma).[281,285,286] This tumor is differentiated by the presence of an identifiable epithelial component within the tumor, which may require immunohistochemical or ultrastructural studies. Areas of osseous metaplasia have been described in urothelial carcinoma without a sarcomatous component.[303] The bone in these cases is mature with a lamellar architecture and no cytologic atypia. Bone has been seen in malignant mesenchymoma of the bladder.[797,798]

The prognosis of patients with osteosarcoma is poor. In the review of Young and Rosenberg,[792] 18 of 21 patients with follow up were dead of tumor within 6 months.

FIBROSARCOMA

Primary fibrosarcoma of the bladder is exceedingly rare; since 1970, only three cases have been published under this name.[761,765,799] The only case with detailed pathologic findings contained extensive areas of chondroid differentiation, raising questions about the appropriateness of the classification.[799] To qualify for this diagnosis, a tumor should meet the criteria utilized for fibrosarcoma elsewhere in the body.[800] In two cases with gross descriptions, the tumor was large, with one extensively involving the retroperitoneum and the bladder.[765] Follow-up was available in two cases; one patient died of other causes at 12 months[799] and the other had recurrence at 2 months.[761]

MALIGNANT MESENCHYMOMA

In 1948, Stout[801] defined malignant mesenchymoma as "a malignant tumor showing two or more unrelated, differentiated tissue types in addition to the fibrosarcomatous element." To date, there have been two acceptable examples of this entity in the bladder. One of these cases included leiomyosarcoma and osteosarcoma as the differentiated components,[798] and the other contained leiomyosarcoma, chondrosarcoma, and osteosarcoma.[797] Both were pedunculated and polypoid, measuring 3 and 18 cm in greatest dimension, respectively. One patient died of progressive tumor 21 months after diagnosis,[797] and the other was alive and well at 18 months.[798]

ANGIOSARCOMA

Rare examples of primary angiosarcoma of the bladder have been reported. Stroup and Chang[714] described a case in a 68-year-old man and identified three reported cases since 1907. In 1983, Schwartz et al[715] reported a case in a homosexual male resembling Kaposi's sarcoma, which involved the skin and bladder. In retrospect, this case probably was disseminated Kaposi's sarcoma in association with HIV infection. The major differential diagnostic consideration is hemangioma, which is much more common. Most hemangiomas of the bladder are cavernous, and all types lack significant cytologic atypia.

HEMANGIOPERICYTOMA

At least five examples of hemangiopericytoma arising in the bladder have been described,[716,717,802-804] including three apparently originating in the urachus.[716,802,804] All have occurred in adults (four women and one man; age range, 29 to 50 years) with one case developing in a patient exposed to polyvinyl alcohol.[716] Grossly, the tumor is solid, ovoid, and well circumscribed. Histologically, the typical features of hemangiopericytoma are present.[800] Hemangiopericytoma-like areas can be found in sarcomatoid carcinoma of the bladder and this entity must be considered in the differential diagnosis. This change is usually only focal, and the sarcomatous component of such tumors is usually high grade; in addition, an epithelial element is often found. Follow-up was available in three cases; two patients were alive and well at 6 and 48 months,[717,804] and one had pulmonary metastases 9 years after resection of the primary tumor.[716]

LIPOSARCOMA

In 1983, Rosi et al[805] reported a case of myxoid liposarcoma developing in the bladder of a 36-year-old man. Following partial cystectomy, the patient was alive and tumor free after 30 months.

RHABDOID TUMOR

Three rhabdoid tumors arising in the bladder have been reported.[806-808] The first case, described in a 46-year-old woman, contained a mixture of urothelial carcinoma, high-grade sarcoma, and rhabdoid tumor. Rhabdoid cells can be found in other sarcomas and in sarcomatoid carcinoma,[809,810] and this case is considered to be an example of the latter. The other cases developed in 6- and 14-year-old girls, and showed histologic, immunohistochemical, and ultrastructural features typical of rhabdoid tumor.[807,808] Key features for the diagnosis are (1) the characteristic rhabdoid morphology, (2) constant expression of vimentin with variable coexpression of cytokeratin, (3) young age, and (4) whorled cytoplasmic intermediate filaments on electron microscopy.[808]

LYMPHORETICULAR AND HEMATOPOIETIC NEOPLASMS

MALIGNANT LYMPHOMA

Clinical features

Involvement of the bladder by malignant lymphoma is usually secondary to systemic lymphoma. In autopsy series of patients dying with non-Hodgkin's lymphoma, bladder involvement has been present in up to 13% of cases.[811,812] The majority of patients are asymptomatic.[812] Much less frequent is the development of primary malignant lymphoma in the bladder in the absence of systemic lymphoma. Such cases account for only 0.2% of all cases of extranodal malignant lymphoma.[813] Ohsawa et al[814] recently reported three cases and critically reviewed the world literature, identifying 27 additional examples. Two other cases have recently been described.[815,816]

The majority of patients with primary lymphoma of the bladder are women (male to female ratio, 1:6.5), usually in the seventh and eighth decades (median age, 64 years).[814] A single case of primary malignant lymphoma in a child was described.[817] Most patients present with gross hematuria, but may complain of dysuria or irritative symptoms. Cystoscopically, the tumor is single or multiple, and sessile or polypoid. In a few cases, there may be diffuse involvement without formation of a discrete mass.[818,819] The presence of intact mucosa overlying the mass is a useful clue to the diagnosis.[820] One case was diagnosed initially on a urine cytology specimen.[821]

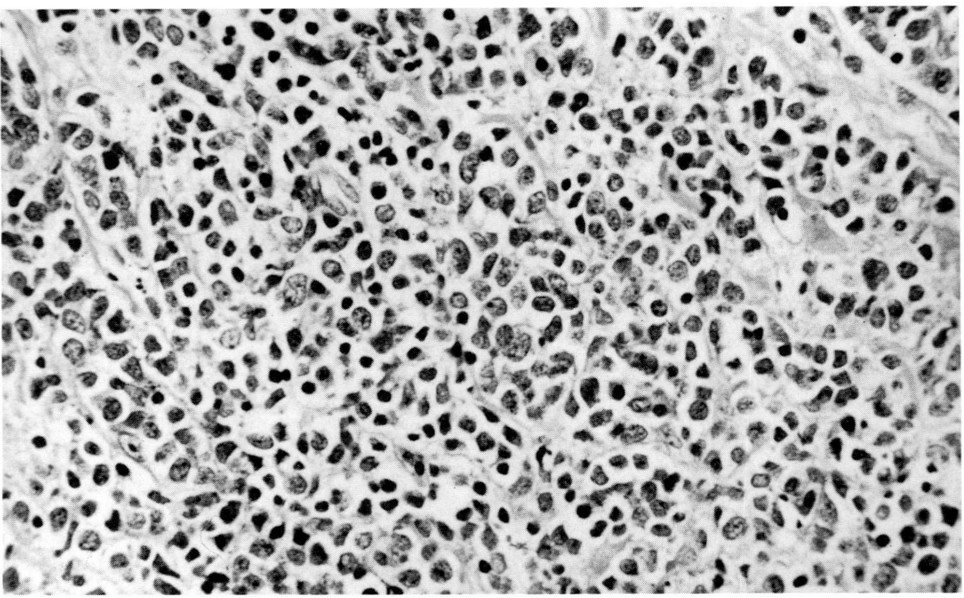

5-103. Large cell lymphoma diffusely infiltrating the bladder with haphazardly arranged noncohesive cells.

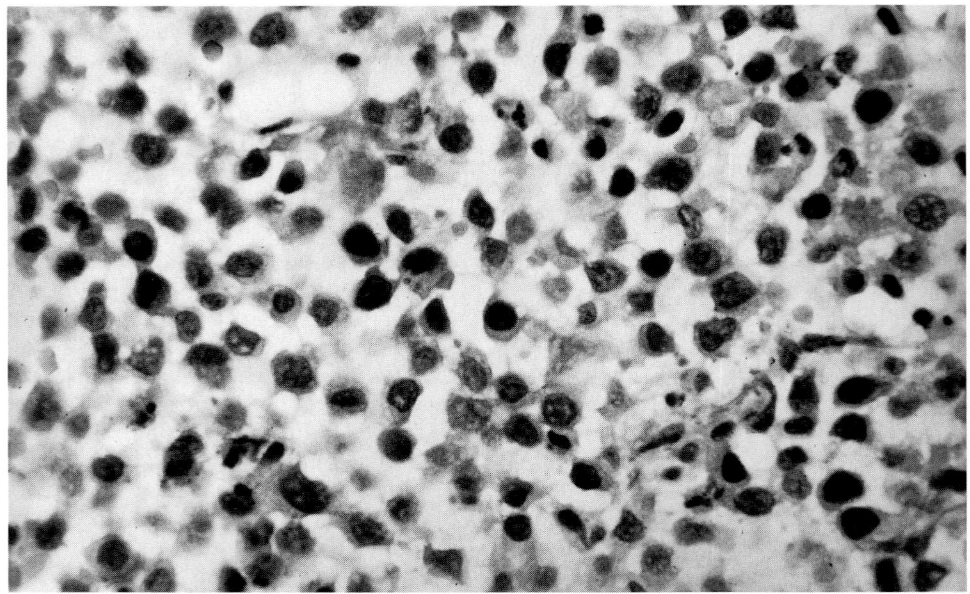

5-104. Malignant lymphoma with plasmacytoid features in the urinary bladder.

Pathology

Lymphoma appears as a solid mass, forming sessile or polypoid lesions. Treatment is surgical, and pathologic material is usually a biopsy or transurethral resection specimen. Histologically, the tumor consists of a diffuse, infiltrative proliferation of lymphoid cells surrounding and permeating normal structures rather than replacing them (Fig. 5-103). The most common types are diffuse large cell and small lymphocytic lymphoma; less frequent are follicular, plasmacytoid, mantle zone, and monocytoid lymphoma (Fig. 5-104). One case of lymphoma arising synchronously with adenocarcinoma in the bladder was described by Stitt and Colapinto.[562] Cases studied immunohistochemically have all been of B-cell origin and display monoclonality.[814,816,817,822-824] Hodgkin's disease primary in the bladder is extremely rare.[814,825,826]

Differential diagnosis

The major differential diagnostic considerations of malignant lymphoma are a florid chronic inflammatory process, small cell carcinoma, and lymphoma-like carcinoma. Inflammatory processes should not be a significant

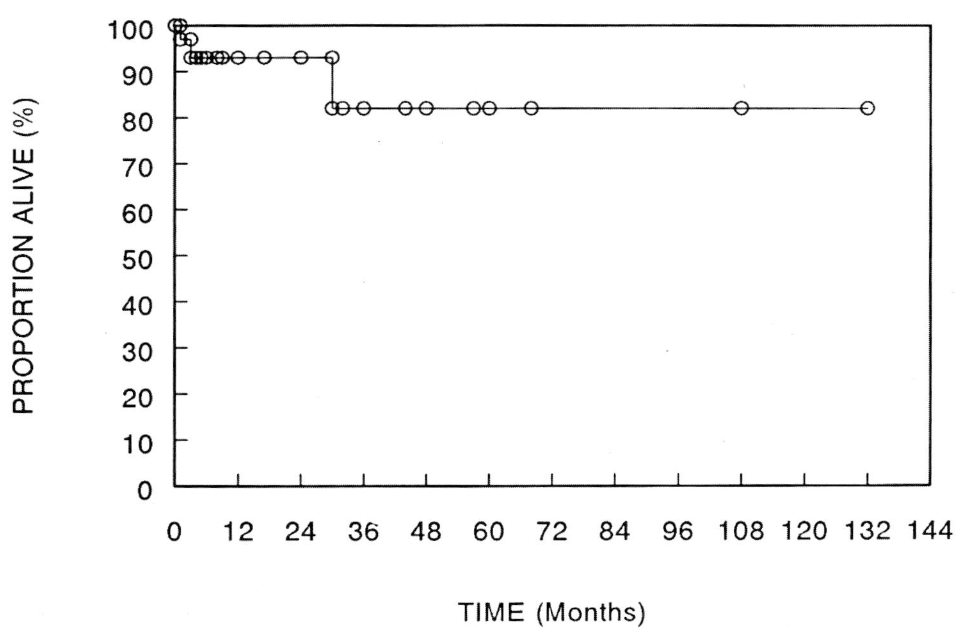

5-105. Kaplan-Meier survival curve of reported cases of malignant lymphoma primarily involving the bladder.

problem; these lesions contain a polymorphous infiltrate without formation of a mass, and immunohistochemistry documenting polyclonality may be helpful. Small cell carcinoma is increasingly reported in the bladder.[628] It has histologic features identical to small cell carcinoma elsewhere in the body. A cohesive growth pattern, prominent nuclear molding, and, in up to 50% of cases, an identifiable urothelial or other epithelial component should allow its diagnosis. In biopsies, the use of immunohistochemistry can be helpful; lymphoma should be cytokeratin negative and leukocyte common antigen positive. Most cases of small cell carcinoma are cytokeratin positive and all should be leukocyte common antigen negative. Several examples of carcinoma other than the small cell type resembling malignant lymphoma have been described.[271] Examples of lymphoepithelioma-like carcinoma resembling nasopharyngeal carcinoma have been described.[271,273] This tumor (described above in the section titled Lymphoepithelioma-like Variant) consists of syncytial groups of cytokeratin-positive carcinoma cells in a polymorphous inflammatory background. Awareness of the entity, combined with immunohistochemical results should prevent misdiagnosis.

Treatment and natural history

The treatment of choice for these tumors is radiotherapy. Systemic therapy may be indicated in cases with the tumor outside the bladder. Although the prognosis for these patients has historically been poor, it is now clear that patients presenting with disease limited to the bladder have a good outcome following radiotherapy. In 27 cases summarized by Ohsawa et al,[814] only 3 died of tumor, and the 5-year survival was 82% (Fig. 5-105).

PLASMACYTOMA

The bladder may contain neoplastic plasma cells in disseminated multiple myeloma[827] or solitary plasmacytoma.[823,828-832] One reported case of plasmacytoma probably was a benign pseudotumor with polyclonality of the plasma cell population documented by immunohistochemistry.[830] The few reported cases showed no sex predilection and occurred over a wide age range (28 to 89 years).[832] Most patients presented with hematuria; in one case, urine cytology revealed malignant plasma cells.[829]

Grossly, the tumors form solid masses, which may be polypoid or pedunculated. The surface mucosa is typically intact. Histologically, the tumor is composed of sheets of plasma cells with varying degrees of atypia.

The major differential diagnostic consideration is plasmacytoid urothelial carcinoma.[271,277] In this case, the epithelial nature of the tumor is indicated by a cohesive growth pattern or the presence of carcinoma in situ, and immunohistochemical staining for cytokeratin and light chains should distinguish the two.

Treatment for solitary plasmacytoma of the urinary bladder is radiation therapy.[832] Of the nine patients summarized by Ho et al,[832] all were alive and tumor free up to 12 years after diagnosis; no patients had synchronous or subsequent development of multiple myeloma.

LEUKEMIA

Infiltration of the bladder in patients with leukemia rarely presents clinically.[823,833] In patients dying of chronic lymphocytic leukemia and chronic myelogenous leukemia, autopsy studies reveal bladder involvement in 15.5% and 17.7%, respectively.[811] The frequency is somewhat higher with acute leukemia (25.8%

in one study).[811] Only 6 of 349 autopsied patients with acute and chronic leukemia reported by Givler[811] had gross evidence of bladder involvement. In these cases, involvement was described as mucosal nodules or hemorrhagic mucosal thickening; none of these patients had significant clinical symptoms. One case of granulocytic sarcoma involving the bladder has been described (Fig 5-106).[823]

METASTASES

In the compilation by Melicow,[4] secondary tumors accounted for 148 of 1102 (13.4%) bladder neoplasms. The majority (106) were direct invasion from malignancies arising in adjacent organs (71.6%). There were 17 cases of lymphoma and leukemia (11.5%), and 25 cases of metastases from distant organs (16.9%). Overall, distant metastases accounted for 2.3% of cases. This is similar to other autopsy studies, which have identified bladder metastases in up to 3.6% of patients dying with cancer.[834,835] In 1967, Goldstein[602] published a comprehensive review of the literature and found that malignant melanoma (38%) and carcinomas of the stomach (23%), breast (11%), kidney (10%), and lung (8%) were the most common primaries.

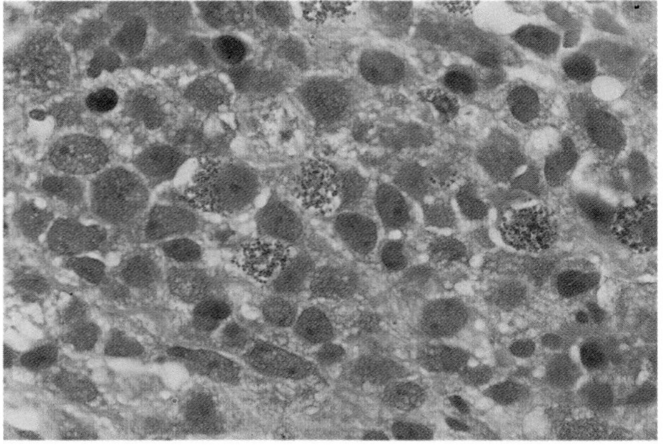

5-106. Granulocytic sarcoma involving the urinary bladder. *(Case courtesy of Dr. P. Engbers.)*

In most cases, bladder metastases are discovered incidentally at autopsy,[834,835] or bladder symptoms develop late in the course of known cancer.[834,836-839] Rare cases presenting primarily in the bladder from gastric adenocarcinoma,[840,841] breast carcinoma,[842] and malignant melanoma[843,844] have occurred. In one case of breast cancer, the urinary bladder was the only site of metastasis (Fig. 5-107).[842] Young and Johnston[845] recently described a case of serous adenocarcinoma from the uterus metastatic to the bladder, which was detected during follow-up cystoscopy for papillary urothelial carcinoma. In rare cases of malignant melanoma metastatic to the bladder, sufficient melanoma pigment may be released to darken the urine.[602,837]

Metastasis should be suspected in any bladder tumor with unusual histology. In cases of pure adenocarcinoma or squamous cell carcinoma, clinical correlation is necessary to exclude the possibility of secondary involvement. In squamous carcinoma, the finding of keratinizing squamous metaplasia in the adjacent epithelium would support bladder origin. Most cases of secondary involvement by prostatic adenocarcinoma are readily recognized by the distinctive histology of the tumor and the immunohistochemical results.[254] Bladder melanoma is almost always secondary.[641]

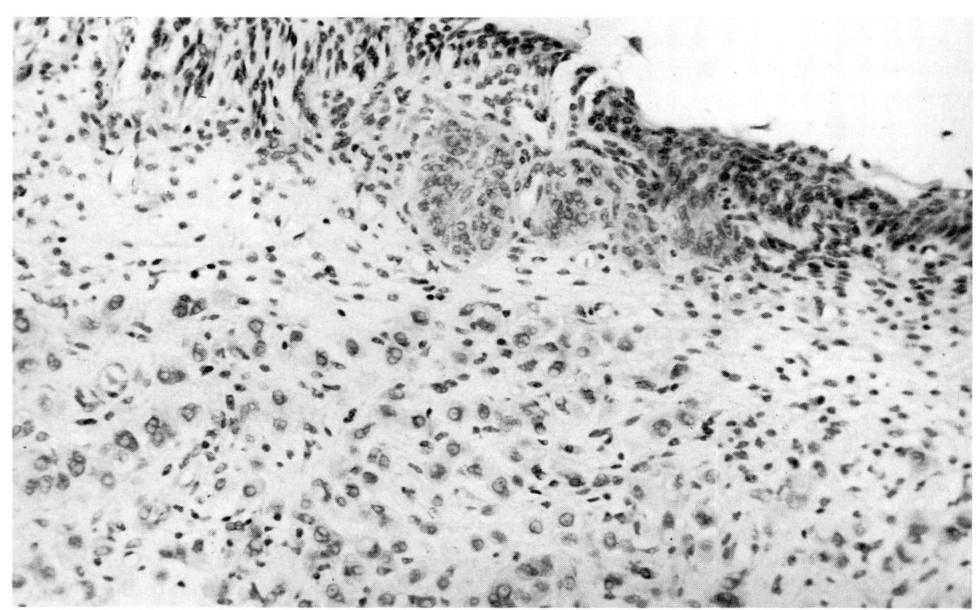

5-107. Metastatic lobular carcinoma of the breast involving the lamina propria of the bladder.

REFERENCES

1. Mostofi FK, Sobin HL, Torlini H: Histologic typing of urinary bladder tumors, Geneva, 1973, World Health Organization.
2. Eble JN, Young RH: Benign and low-grade papillary lesions of the urinary bladder: a review of the papilloma-papillary carcinoma controversy and a report of 5 typical papillomas, Semin Diagn Pathol 6:351-371, 1989.
3. Deming CL: The biological behavior of transitional cell papilloma of the bladder, J Urol 63:815-820, 1950.
4. Melicow MM: Tumors of the urinary bladder: a clinicopathological analysis of over 2500 specimens and biopsies, J Urol 74:498-521, 1955.
5. Koss LG: Tumors of the urinary bladder, second series, Washington, DC, 1974, Armed Forces Institute of Pathology.
6. Greene LF, Hanash KA, Farrow GM: Benign papilloma or papillary carcinoma of the bladder? J Urol 110:205-207, 1973.
7. Prout GR Jr, Barton BA, Griffin PP et al: Treated history of noninvasive grade 1 transitional cell carcinoma, J Urol 148:1413-1419, 1992.
8. Jordan AM, Weingarten J, Murphy WM: Transitional cell neoplasms of the urinary bladder: can biologic potential be predicted from histologic grading? Cancer 60:2766-2774, 1987.
9. Murphy WM (ed): Urologic pathology, Philadelphia, 1989, W.B. Saunders.
10. Reuter VE, Melamed MR: The lower urinary tract. In Sternberg SS (ed): Diagnostic surgical pathology, ed 2, New York, 1994, Raven Press.
11. Murphy WM, Beckwith JB, Farrow GM: Tumors of the kidney, bladder, and related structures, third series, Washington, DC, 1994, Armed Forces Institute of Pathology.
12. Friedell GH, Parija GC, Nagy GK et al: The pathology of human bladder cancer, Cancer 45:1823-1831, 1980.
13. Ooms ECM, Anderson WAD, Alons CL et al: Analysis of the performance of pathologists in the grading of bladder tumors, Hum Pathol 14:140-143, 1983.
14. Abel PD, Henderson D, Bennett MK et al: Differing interpretations by pathologists of the pT category and grade of transitional cell cancer of the bladder, Br J Urol 62:339-342, 1988.
15. Robertson AJ, Swanson Beck J, Burnett RA et al: Observer variability in histopathological reporting of transitional cell carcinoma and epithelial dysplasia in bladders, J Clin Pathol 43:17-21, 1990.
16. Angulo JC, Lopez JL, Flores N et al: The value of tumour spread, grading and growth pattern as morphological predictive parameters in bladder carcinoma: a critical revision of the 1987 TNM classification, J Cancer Res Clin Oncol 119:578-593, 1993.
17. Pauwels RPE, Schapers RFM, Smeets AWGB et al: Grading in superficial bladder cancer: (1) morphological criteria, Br J Urol 61:129-134, 1988.
18. Lipponen PK: Histological and quantitative prognostic factors in transitional cell bladder cancer treated by cystectomy, Anticancer Res 12:1527-1532, 1992.
19. Paschkis R: Über Adenoma der Harnblase, Z Urol Nephrol 21:313-327, 1927.
20. Potts IF, Hirst E: Inverted papilloma of the bladder, J Urol 90:175-179, 1963.
21. Kim YH, Reiner L: Brunnian adenoma (inverted papilloma) of the urinary bladder: report of a case, Hum Pathol 9:229-231, 1978.
22. Cameron KM, Lupton CH: Inverted papilloma of the lower urinary tract, Br J Urol 48:567-577, 1976.
23. Sullivan JJ, Watson JG, Kingston CW et al: Inverted papilloma of the urinary bladder: a report of two cases, Aust N Z J Surg 41:60-62, 1971.
24. Kunze E, Schauer A, Schmitt M: Histology and histogenesis of two different types of inverted urothelial papillomas, Cancer 51:348-358, 1983.
25. Iwata H, Yokoyama M, Morita M et al: Inverted papilloma of the urinary bladder: scanninng and electron microscopic observations, Urology 19:322-324, 1982.
26. Alroy J, Miller AW III, John S et al: Inverted papilloma of the urinary bladder, Cancer 46:64-70, 1980.
27. Francis RR: Inverted papilloma in a 14-year-old male, Br J Urol 51:327, 1979.
28. Caro DJ, Tessler A: Inverted papilloma of the bladder: a distinct urologic lesion, Cancer 42:708-713, 1978.
29. Tannenbaum M: Inverted papilloma: urothelial tumor of benign biological potential, Urology 7:76-79, 1976.
30. Henderson DW, Allen PW, Bourne AJ: Inverted urinary papilloma: report of five cases and review of the literature, Virchows Arch [A] 366:177-186, 1975.
31. Khoury JM, Stutzman RE, Sepulveda RA: Inverted papilloma of the bladder with focal transitional cell carcinoma: a case report, Milit Med 150:562-563, 1985.
32. Uyama T, Nakamura S, Moriwaki S: Inverted papilloma of bladder, Urology 16:152-154, 1980.
33. Summers DE, Rushin JM, Frazier HA et al: Inverted papilloma of the urinary bladder with granular eosinophilic cells, Arch Pathol Lab Med 115:802-806, 1991.
34. Palvio DHB: Inverted papillomas of the urinary tract: a case of multiple recurring inverted papilloma of the renal pelvis, ureter and bladder associated with malignant change, Scand J Urol Nephrol 19:299-302, 1985.
35. Risio M, Coverlizza S, Lasaponara F et al: Inverted urothelial papilloma: a lesion with malignant potential, Eur Urol 14:333-338, 1988.
36. Renfer LG, Kelley L, Belville WD: Inverted papilloma of the urinary tract: histogenesis, recurrence and associated malignancy, J Urol 140:832-834, 1988.
37. Stein DS, Rosen S, Kendall AR: The association of inverted papilloma and transitional cell carcinoma of the urothelium, J Urol 131:751-752, 1984.
38. Anderström C, Johansson S, Petersson S: Inverted papilloma of the urinary tract, J Urol 127:1132-1134, 1982.
39. Whitesel JA: Inverted papilloma of the urinary tract: malignant potential, J Urol 127:539-540, 1982.
40. Lazarevic B, Garret R: Inverted papilloma and papillary transitional cell carcinoma of urinary bladder, Cancer 42:1904-1911, 1978.
41. Schürch W, Seemayer TA, Lagace R: Stromal myofibroblasts in primary invasive and metastatic carcinomas, Virchows Arch [A] 391:125-139, 1981.
42. Tsujimura A, Nishimura K, Yasunaga Y et al: Transitional cell carcinoma of the ureter with inverted proliferation: a case report, Acta Urol Jpn 38:941-944, 1992.

43. Kunimi K, Uchibayashi T, Lee S-W et al: Nuclear deoxyribonucleic acid content in inverted papilloma of the urothelium, Eur Urol 26:149-152, 1994.
44. Berkhoff WBC, Jobsis AC, Bruijnes E et al: The inverted urothelial papilloma, Urol Int 40:93-96, 1985.
45. Assor D: A villous tumor of the bladder, J Urol 119:287-288, 1978.
46. Miller DC, Gang DG, Gavris VE et al: Villous adenoma of the urinary bladder: a morphologic or biologic entity? Am J Clin Pathol 79:728-731, 1983.
47. Channer JL, Williams JL, Henry L: Villous adenoma of the bladder, J Clin Pathol 46:450-452, 1993.
48. Soli M, Bercovich E, Botteghi B et al: A rare case of mucous-secreting villous adenoma of the bladder, It J Surg Sci 3:261-264, 1987.
49. Eble JN, Hull MT, Rowland RG et al: Villous adenoma of the urachus with mucusuria: a light and electron microscopic study, J Urol 135:1240-1244, 1986.
50. Daroca PJ Jr, Mackenzie F, Reed RJ et al: Primary adenovillous carcinoma of the bladder, J Urol 115:41-45, 1976.
51. Morrison AS, Cole P: Epidemiology of urologic cancer. In Javadpour N (ed): Principles and management of urologic cancer, Baltimore, 1979, Williams and Wilkins.
52. Boring CC, Squires TS, Tong T et al: Cancer statistics 1994, CA-A 44:7-26, 1994.
53. Ray B, Grabstald H, Exelby PR et al: Bladder tumors in children, Urology 2:426-435, 1973.
54. McCarthy JP, Gavrell GJ, LeBlanc GA: Transitional cell carcinoma of bladder in patients under thirty years of age, Urology 13:487-489, 1979.
55. Paduano L, Chiella E: Primary epithelial tumors of the bladder in children, J Urol 139:794-795, 1988.
56. Khasidy LR, Khashu B, Mallett EC et al: Transitional cell carcinoma of bladder in children, Urology 35:142-144, 1990.
57. Yanase M, Tsukamoto T, Yoshiaki K et al: Transitional cell carcinoma of the bladder or renal pelvis in children, Eur Urol 19:312-314, 1991.
58. Keetch DW, Manley CB, Catalona WJ: Transitional cell carcinoma of bladder in children and adolescents, Urology 42:447-449, 1993.
59. Howe GR, Burch JD, Miller AB et al: Tobacco use, occupation, coffee, various nutrients, and bladder cancer, J Natl Cancer Inst 64:701-703, 1980.
60. Morrison AS: Advances in the etiology of urothelial cancer, Urol Clin North Am 11:557-566, 1984.
61. Burch JD, Rohan TE, Howe GR et al: Risk of bladder cancer by source and type of tobacco exposure: a case-control study, Int J Cancer 44:622-628, 1989.
62. Clavel J, Cordier S, Boccon-Gibod L et al: Tobacco and bladder cancer in males: increased risk for inhalers and smokers of black tobacco, Int J Cancer 44:605-610, 1989.
63. Wynder EL, Augustine A, Kabat GC: Effect of the type of cigarette smoked on bladder cancer risk, Cancer 61:622-627, 1988.
64. Miller AB: The etiology of bladder cancer from the epidemiological viewpoint, Cancer Res 37:2939-2942, 1977.
65. Slattery ML, Schumacher MC, West DW et al: Smoking and bladder cancer, Cancer 61:402-408, 1988.
66. Augustine A, Hebert JR, Kabat GC et al: Bladder cancer in relation to cigarette smoking, Cancer Res 48:4405-4408, 1988.
67. Hartge P, Hoover R, Kantor A: Bladder cancer risk and pipes, cigars, and smokeless tobacco, Cancer 55:901-906, 1985.
68. Lower GM Jr: Concepts in causality: chemically induced human urinary bladder cancer, Cancer 49:1056-1066, 1982.
69. Auerbach O, Garfinkel L: Histologic changes in the urinary bladder in relation to cigarette smoking and use of artificial sweeteners, Cancer 64:983-987, 1989.
70. Cole P, Hoover R, Friedell GH: Occupation and cancer of the lower urinary tract, Cancer 29:1250-1260, 1972.
71. Rehn L: Ueber Blasentumoren bei Fuchsinarbeitern, Arch Kind Chir 50:588-600, 1895.
72. Case RAM, Hosker ME, McDonald DB et al: Tumours of the urinary bladder in workmen engaged in the manufacture and use of certain dyestuff intermediates in the British chemical industry, Br J Ind Med 11:75-104, 1954.
73. Steineck G, Plato N, Norell SE et al: Urothelial cancer and some industrial-related chemicals: an evaluation of the epidemiologic literature, Am J Ind Med 17:371-391, 1990.
74. Malker HS, McLaughlin JK, Silverman DT et al: Occupational risks for bladder cancer among men in Sweden, Cancer Res 47:6763-6766, 1987.
75. Silverman DT, Levin LI, Hoover RN et al: Occupational risks of bladder cancer in the United States. I. White men, J Natl Cancer Inst 81:1472-1480, 1989.
76. Silverman DT, Levin LI, Hoover RN et al: Occupational risks of bladder cancer in the United States. II. Nonwhite men, J Natl Cancer Inst 81:1480-1483, 1989.
77. Dolin PJ, Cook-Mozaffari P: Occupation and bladder cancer: a death-certificate study, Br J Cancer 66:568-578, 1992.
78. Hoover R: Saccharin—bitter aftertaste, N Engl J Med 302:573-575, 1980 (editorial).
79. Miller AB, Morrison B: Artificial sweeteners and human bladder cancer, Lancet 2:578-581, 1977.
80. Morrison AS, Buring JE: Artificial sweeteners and cancer of the lower urinary tract, N Engl J Med 302:537-541, 1980.
81. McCredie M, Stewart JH, Ford JM et al: Phenacetin-containing analgesics and cancer of the bladder or renal pelvis in women, Br J Urol 55:220-224, 1983.
82. Fokkens W: Phenacetin abuse related to bladder cancer, Environ Res 20:192-198, 1979.
83. Piper JM, Tonascia J, Matanoski GM: Heavy phenacetin use and bladder cancer in women aged 20 to 49 years, N Engl J Med 313:292-295, 1985.
84. Wahlqvist L: Chemical carcinogenesis—a review and personal observations with special reference to the role of tobacco and phenacetin in the production of urothelial tumors. In Pavone-Maculoso M (ed): Bladder tumors and other topics in urologic oncology, New York, 1980, Plenum Press.
85. Worth PHL: Cyclophosphamide and the bladder, Br Med J 3:182, 1971.
86. Dale GL, Smith RB: Transitional cell carcinoma of the bladder associated with cyclophosphamide, J Urol 112:603-604, 1974.
87. Ansell ID, Castro JE: Carcinoma of the bladder complicating cyclophosphamide therapy, Br J Urol 47:413-418, 1975.

88. Fairchild WV, Spence CR, Solomon HD et al: The incidence of bladder cancer after cyclophosphamide therapy, J Urol 122:163-164, 1979.
89. Ershler WB, Gilchrist KW, Citrin DL: Adriamycin enhancement of cyclophosphamide induced bladder injury, J Urol 123:121-122, 1980.
90. Glucksman MA: Bladder cancer after cyclophosphamide therapy, Urology 16:553, 1980.
91. Hoover R, Fraumeni JF Jr: Drug-induced cancer, Cancer 47:1071-1080, 1981.
92. Chodak GW, Straus FW II, Schoenberg HW: Simultaneous occurrence of transitional, squamous, and adenocarcinoma of the bladder after 15 years of cyclophosphamide ingestion, J Urol 125:424-426, 1981.
93. Carney CN, Stevens PS, Fried FA et al: Fibroblastic tumor of the urinary bladder after cyclophosphamide therapy, Arch Pathol Lab Med 106:247-249, 1982.
94. Tuttle TM, Williams GM, Marshall FF: Evidence for cyclophosphamide induced transitional cell carcinoma in a renal transplant patient, J Urol 140:1009-1011, 1988.
95. Pedersen-Bjergaard J, Ersbøll J, Hansen VL et al: Carcinoma of the urinary bladder after treatment with cyclophosphamide for non-Hodgkin's lymphoma, N Engl J Med 318:1028-1032, 1988.
96. Levine LA, Richie JP: Urological complications of cyclophosphamide, J Urol 141:1063-1069, 1989.
97. Kawamura J, Sakurai M, Tsukamoto K et al: Leiomyosarcoma of the bladder eighteen years after cyclophosphamide therapy for retinoblastoma, Urol Int 51:49-53, 1993.
98. Friend SH, Horowitz JM, Gerber MR et al: Deletions of a DNA sequence in retinoblastomas and mesenchymal tumors: organisation of the sequence and its encoded protein, Proc Natl Acad Sci USA 84:9059-9063, 1987.
99. Duncan RE, Bennett DW, Evans AT et al: Radiation induced bladder tumors, J Urol 118:43-45, 1977.
100. Quilty PM, Kerr GR: Bladder cancer following low- or high-dose pelvic irradiation, Clin Radiol 38:583-585, 1987.
101. Sella A, Dexeus FH, Chong C et al: Radiation therapy–associated invasive bladder tumors, Urology 33:185-188, 1989.
102. Ferrie BG, Imrie JEA, Paterson PJ: Osteosarcoma of bladder 27 years after local radiotherapy, J Royal Soc Med 77:962-963, 1984.
103. Weinberg DM, Ross RK, Mack TM et al: Bladder cancer etiology, Cancer 51:675-680, 1983.
104. Ciccone G, Vineis P: Coffee drinking and bladder cancer, Cancer Lett 41:45-52, 1988.
105. Slattery ML, West DW, Robinson LM: Fluid intake and bladder cancer in Utah, Int J Cancer 42:17-22, 1988.
106. Kerley SW, Persons DL, Fishback JL: Human papillomavirus and carcinoma of the urinary bladder, Mod Pathol 4:316-319, 1991.
107. Anwar K, Naiki H, Nakakuki K et al: High frequency of human papillomavirus infection in carcinoma of the urinary bladder, Cancer 70:1967-1973, 1992.
108. Knowles MA: Human papillomavirus sequences are not detectable by Southern blotting or general primer-mediated polymerase chain reaction in transitional cell tumors of the bladder, Eur Urol 20:297-301, 1992.
109. Chang F, Lipponen P, Tervahauta A et al: Transitional cell carcinoma of the bladder: failure to demonstrate human papillomavirus deoxyribonucleic acid by in situ hybridization and polymerase chain reaction, J Urol 152:1429-1433, 1994.
110. Sandberg AA, Berger CS: Review of chromosome studies in urological tumors. II. Cytogenetics and molecular genetics of bladder cancer, J Urol 151:545-560, 1994.
111. Sandberg AA: Chromosome changes in bladder cancer: clinical and other correlations, Cancer Genet Cytogenet 19:163-175, 1986.
112. Falor WH, Ward-Skinner RM: The importance of marker chromosomes in superficial transitional cell carcinoma of the bladder: 50 patients followed up to 17 years, J Urol 139:929-932, 1988.
113. Micic S, Micic M, Milasin J: Chromosome analysis in patients with bladder tumor, Urol Int 43:201-204, 1988.
114. Knowles MA, Elder PA, Williamson M et al: Allelotype of human bladder cancer, Cancer Res 54:531-538, 1994.
115. Hopman AHN, Ramaekers FCS, Raap AK et al: In situ hybridization as a tool to study numerical chromosome aberrations in solid bladder tumors, Histochemistry 89:307-316, 1988.
116. Hopman AHN, Poddighe PJ, Smeets AWGB et al: Detection of numerical chromosome aberrations in bladder cancer by in situ hybridization, Am J Pathol 135:1105-1117, 1989.
117. Hopman AHN, van Hooren E, van de Kaa CA et al: Detection of numerical chromosome aberrations using in situ hybridization in paraffin sections of routinely processed bladder cancers, Mod Pathol 4:503-513, 1991.
118. Hopman AHN, Moesker O, Smeets AWGB et al: Numerical chromosome 1,7,9, and 11 aberrations in bladder cancer detected by in situ hybridization, Cancer Res 51:644-651, 1991.
119. Poddighe PJ, Ramaekers FCS, Smeets AWGB et al: Structural chromosome 1 aberrations in transitional cell carcinoma of the bladder: interphase cytogenetics combining a centromeric telomeric, and library DNA probe. Cancer Res 52:4929-4934, 1992.
120. Miyao N, Tsai YC, Lerner SP et al: Role of chromosome 9 in bladder cancer, Cancer Res 53:4066-4070, 1993.
121. Wu S-Q, Storer BE, Bookland EA et al: Nonrandom chromosome losses in stepwise neoplastic transformation in vitro of human uroepithelial cells, Cancer Res 51:3323-3326, 1991.
122. Habuchi T, Ogawa O, Kakehi Y et al: Allelic loss of chromosome 17p in urothelial cancer: strong association with invasive phenotype, J Urol 148:1595-1599, 1992.
123. Tsai YC, Nichols PW, Hiti AL et al: Allelic losses of chromosomes 9, 11 and 17 in human bladder cancer, Cancer Res 50:44-47, 1990.
124. Olumi AF, Tsai YC, Nichols PW et al: Allelic loss of chromosome 17p distinguishes high grade from low grade transitional cell carcinoma of the bladder, Cancer Res 50:7081-7083, 1990.
125. Aherne G: Retinoblastoma associated with other primary malignant tumors, Trans Ophthalmol Soc U K 94:938, 1974.
126. Fraumeni JF Jr, Thomas LB: Malignant bladder tumors in a man and his three sons, JAMA 201:507-509, 1967.

127. McCullough DL, Lamm DL, McLaughlin AP III et al: Familial transitional cell carcinoma of the bladder, J Urol 113:629-635, 1975.
128. Catalona WJ: Urothelial tumors of the urinary tract. In Walsh PC, Retik AB, Stamey TA et al (eds): Campbell's Urology, ed 6, Philadelphia, 1994, W B Saunders.
129. Orphali SLJ, Shols GW, Hagewood J et al: Familial transitional cell carcinoma of renal pelvis and upper ureter, Urology 27:394-396, 1986.
130. Grignon DJ, Shum DT, Bruckschwaiger O: Transitional cell carcinoma in the Muir-Torre syndrome, J Urol 138:406-408, 1987.
131. Francis RR: Carcinoma of the bladder, J Urol 85:552-555, 1961.
132. Richie JP, Skinner DG, Kaufman JJ: Radical cystectomy for carcinoma of the bladder: 16 years of experience, J Urol 113:186-189, 1975.
133. Kaye KW, Lange PH: Mode of presentation of invasive bladder cancer: reassessment of the problem, J Urol 128:31-33, 1982.
134. Hopkins SC, Ford KS, Soloway MS: Invasive bladder cancer: support for screening, J Urol 130:61-64, 1983.
135. Feggeter JGW: An osteolytic lesion as a presentation of bladder carcinoma, Br J Urol 48:254, 1976.
136. Schwartz RA, Fleishman JS: Transitional cell carcinoma of the urinary tract presenting with a cutaneous metastasis, Arch Dermatol 117:513-515, 1981.
137. Cieplinski W, Ciesielski TE, Hainne C et al: Choroid metastases from transitional cell carcinoma of the bladder, Cancer 50:1596-1600, 1982.
138. Mughal TI, Phillips RH, Robinson WA: Bladder carcinoma presenting as a solitary bony metastasis, J Urol 130:973, 1983.
139. Block NL, Whitmore WF Jr: Leukemoid reaction, thrombocytosis and hypercalcemia associated with bladder cancer, J Urol 110:660-663, 1973.
140. Sires C, Neely S, Skinner D: Leukemoid reaction in a patient with bladder and prostatic cancer, J Urol 135:366-367, 1986.
141. Richardson EP Jr, Hedley-White ET: Case records of the Massachusetts General Hospital, N Engl J Med 313:249-257, 1985.
142. Crabbe JG, Cresdee WD, Scott TS et al: The cytologic diagnosis of bladder tumors amongst dyestuff workers, Br J Ind Med 13:270-276, 1956.
143. Melamed MR, Koss LG, Ricci A et al: Cytohistological observations on developing carcinoma of the urinary bladder in man, Cancer 13:67-74, 1960.
144. Murphy WM, Soloway MS, Jukkola AF et al: Urinary cytology and bladder cancer, Cancer 53:1555-1565, 1984.
145. Farrow GM: Urine cytology of transitional cell carcinoma. In Wied GL, Keebler CM, Koss LG (eds): Compendium of diagnostic cytology, ed 6, Chicago, 1988, International Academy of Cytology.
146. Flanagan MJ, Miller A: Evaluation of bladder washing cytology for bladder cancer surveillance, J Urol 119:42-43, 1978.
147. Matzkin H, Moinuddin S, Soloway MS: Value of urine cytology versus bladder washing in bladder cancer, Urology 39:201-203, 1992.
148. Paulson J, Metwalli N, Wu B et al: Transitional cell carcinoma of bladder with features of inverted papilloma, Lab Invest 58:71A, 1988 (Abstract).
149. Rikken CHM, van Helsdingen PJRO, Kazzaz BA: Are biopsies from the prostatic urethra useful in patients with superficial bladder carcinoma? Br J Urol 59:145-147, 1987.
150. Bryan RL, Newman J, Suarez V et al: The significance of prostatic urothelial dysplasia, Histopathology 22:501-503, 1993.
151. Mahadevia PS, Koss LG, Tar IJ: Prostatic involvement in bladder cancer: prostate mapping in 20 cystoprostatectomy specimens, Cancer 58:2096-2102, 1986.
152. Wood DP Jr, Montie JE, Pontes JE et al: Transitional cell carcinoma of the prostate in cystoprostatectomy specimens removed for bladder cancer, J Urol 141:346-349, 1989.
153. Hardeman SW, Soloway MS: Transitional cell carcinoma of the prostate: diagnosis, staging and management, World J Urol 6:170-174, 1988.
154. Matzkin H, Soloway MS, Hardeman S: Transitional cell carcinoma of the prostate, J Urol 146:1207-1212, 1991.
155. Hardeman SW, Perry A, Soloway MS: Transitional cell carcinoma of the prostate following intravesical therapy for transitional cell carcinoma of the bladder, J Urol 140:289-292, 1988.
156. Wishnow KI, Ro JY: Importance of early treatment of transitional cell carcinoma of prostatic ducts, Urology 32:11-12, 1988.
157. Orihuela E, Herr HW, Whitmore WF Jr: Conservative treatment of superficial transitional cell carcinoma of prostatic urethra with intravesical BCG, Urology 34:231-237, 1989.
158. Frazier HA, Robertson JE, Dodge RK et al: The value of pathologic factors in predicting cancer-specific survival among patients treated with radical cystectomy for transitional cell carcinoma of the bladder and prostate, Cancer 71:3993-4001, 1993.
159. Richie JP, Skinner DG: Carcinoma in situ of the urethra associated with bladder carcinoma: the role of urethrectomy, J Urol 119:80-81, 1978.
160. Piscioli F, Pusiol T, Leonardi E et al: Role of percutaneous pelvic node aspiration cytology in the management of bladder carcinoma, Acta Cytol 29:37-43, 1985.
161. LaPlante M, Brice M: The upper limits of hopeful application of radical cystectomy for vesical carcinoma: does nodal metastasis always indicate incurability? J Urol 109:261-264, 1973.
162. Skinner DG: Management of invasive bladder cancer: a meticulous pelvic node dissection can make a difference, J Urol 128:34-36, 1982.
163. Marshall VF: The relation of the preoperative estimate to the pathologic demonstration of the extent of vesical neoplasms, J Urol 68:714-723, 1952.
164. International Union Against Cancer: TNM Classification of Malignant Tumours, ed 4, Geneva, 1987, Springer-Verlag.
165. Wajsman Z, Merrin C, Moore R et al: Current results from treatment of bladder tumors with total cystectomy at Roswell Park Memorial Institute, J Urol 113:806-810, 1975.
166. Whitmore WF Jr, Batata MA, Ghoneim MA et al: Radical cystectomy with or without prior irradiation in the treatment of bladder cancer, J Urol 118:184-187, 1977.

167. Melicow MM: Histological study of vesical urothelium intervening between gross neoplasms in total cystectomy, J Urol 68:261-279, 1952.
168. Farrow GM, Utz DC, Rife CC: Morphological and clinical observations of patients with early bladder cancer treated with total cystectomy, Cancer Res 36:2495-2501, 1976.
169. Melamed MR, Voutsa NG, Grabstald H: Natural history and clinical behavior of in situ carcinoma of the human urinary bladder, Cancer 17:1533-1545, 1964.
170. Utz DC, Hanash KA, Farrow GM: The plight of the patient with carcinoma in situ of the bladder, J Urol 103:160-164, 1970.
171. Yates-Bell AJ: Carcinoma in situ of the bladder, Br J Surg 58:359-364, 1971.
172. Barlebo H, Sørensen BL, Søeborg Ohlsen A: Carcinoma in situ of the urinary bladder, Scand J Urol Nephrol 6:213-223, 1972.
173. Farrow GM, Utz DC, Rife CC et al: Clinical observations on sixty-nine cases of in situ carcinoma of the urinary bladder, Cancer Res 37:2794-2798, 1977.
174. Elliot GB, Moloney PJ, Anderson GH: "Denuding cystitis" and in situ urothelial carcinoma, Arch Pathol 96:91-94, 1973.
175. Zincke H, Utz DC, Farrow GM: Review of Mayo Clinic experience with carcinoma in situ, Urology Suppl 26:39-46, 1985.
176. Wolf H, Rosenkilde Olsen P, Fischer A et al: Urothelial atypia concomitant with primary bladder tumour, Scand J Urol Nephrol 21:33-38, 1987.
177. Dona ST, Flamm J: The significance of bladder quadrant biopsies in patients with primary superficial bladder carcinoma, Eur Urol 16:81-85, 1989.
178. Mufti GR, Singh M: Value of random mucosal biopsies in the management of superficial bladder cancer, Eur Urol 22:288-293, 1992.
179. Koss LG: Mapping of the urinary bladder: its impact on the concepts of bladder cancer, Hum Pathol 10:533-548, 1979.
180. Schellhammer PF, Whitmore WF Jr: Transitional cell carcinoma of the urethra in men having cystectomy for bladder cancer, J Urol 115:56-60, 1976.
181. Franks LM, Chesterman FC: Intra-epithelial carcinoma of prostatic urethra, peri-urethral glands and prostatic ducts ("Bowen's disease of urinary epithelium"), Br J Cancer 10:223-225, 1956.
182. Thelmo WL, Seemayer TA, Madarnas P et al: Carcinoma in situ of the bladder with associated prostatic involvement, J Urol 111:491-494, 1974.
183. Seemayer TA, Knaack J, Thelmo WL et al: Further observations on carcinoma in situ of the urinary bladder: silent but extensive intraprostatic involvement, Cancer 36:514-520, 1975.
184. Grabstald H: Prostatic biopsy in selected patients with carcinoma in situ of the bladder: preliminary report, J Urol 132:1117-1118, 1984.
185. Culp OS, Utz DC, Harrison EG Jr: Experiences with ureteral carcinomas in situ detected during operations for vesical neoplasm, J Urol 97:679-682, 1967.
186. Sharma TC, Melamed MR, Whitmore WF Jr: Carcinoma in-situ of the ureter in patients with bladder carcinoma treated by cystectomy, Cancer 26:583-587, 1970.
187. Schade ROK, Tubingen MD, Serck-Hanssen A et al: Morphological changes in the ureter in cases of bladder carcinoma, Cancer 27:1267-1272, 1971.
188. Skinner DG, Richie JP, Cooper PH et al: The clinical significance of carcinoma in situ of the bladder and its association with overt carcinoma, J Urol 112:68-71, 1974.
189. Fukutani K, Kawabe K, Niijima T et al: Transitional cell carcinoma of the urinary tract associated with vulvar Paget's disease: a report of two cases, Urol Int 42:71-73, 1987.
190. Bégin LR, Deschenes J, Mitmaker B: Pagetoid carcinomatous involvement of the penile urethra in association with high-grade transitional cell carcinoma of the urinary bladder, Arch Pathol Lab Med 115:632-635, 1991.
191. Jakse G, Putz A, Hofstädter F: Carcinoma in situ of the bladder extending into the seminal vesicles, J Urol 137:44-45, 1987.
192. Ayala AG, Ro JY: Premalignant lesions of the urothelium and transitional cell tumors. In Young RH (ed): Pathology of the urinary bladder, New York, 1989, Churchill Livingstone.
193. Nochomovitz LE, Manyak MJ, Kahn LB: Bladder biopsy interpretation, New York, 1992, Raven Press.
194. Epstein JI: Differential diagnosis in pathology: urologic disorders, New York, 1992, Igaku-Shoin Medical Publishers.
195. Tannenbaum M, Tannenbaum S, Carter HW: SEM, BEI, and TEM ultrastructural characteristics of normal, preneoplastic, and neoplastic human transitional epithelia, Electron Microsc 2:949-958, 1978.
196. Jacobs JB, Cohen SM: Scanning electron microscopic features of human urinary bladder cancer, Cancer 48:1399-1409, 1981.
197. Farrow GM: Pathology of carcinoma in situ of the urinary bladder and related lesions, J Cell Biochem Suppl 161:39-43, 1992.
198. Orozco RE, Vander Zwaag R, Murphy WM: The pagetoid variant of urothelial carcinoma in situ, Hum Pathol 24:1199-1202, 1993.
199. Voutsa NG, Melamed MR: Cytology of in situ carcinoma of the urinary bladder, Cancer 16:1307-1316, 1963.
200. Boon ME, Blomjous CEM, Zwartendijk J et al: Carcinoma in situ of the urinary bladder: clinical presentation, cytologic pattern and stromal changes, Acta Cytol 30:360-366, 1986.
201. Esposti PL, Zajicek J: Grading of transitional cell neoplasms of the urinary bladder from smears of bladder washings: a critical review of 326 tumors, Acta Cytol 16:529-537, 1972.
202. Coon JS, McCall A, Miller AW III et al: Expression of blood-group-related antigens in carcinoma in situ of the urinary bladder, Cancer 56:797-804, 1985.
203. Coon JS, Weinstein RS: Detection of ABH tissue isoantigens by immunoperoxidase methods in normal and neoplastic urothelium, Am J Clin Pathol 76:163-171, 1981.
204. Sanchez-Fernandez de Sevilla C, Morell-Quadreny L, Gil-Salom M et al: Morphometric and immunohistochemical characterization of bladder carcinoma in situ and its preneoplastic lesions, Eur Urol 21:5-9, 1992.
205. Nakanishi K, Kawai T, Suzuki M: Lectin binding and expression of blood group–related antigens in carcinoma in situ and invasive carcinoma of urinary bladder, Histopathology 23:153-158, 1993.

206. Hofstädter F, Delgado R, Jakse G et al: Urothelial dysplasia and carcinoma in situ of the bladder, Cancer 57:356-361, 1986.
207. Norming U, Tribukait B, Gustafson H et al: Deoxyribonucleic acid profile and tumor progression in primary carcinoma in situ of the bladder: a study of 63 patients with grade 3 lesions, J Urol 147:11-15, 1992.
208. Boon ME, Ooms ECM: Carcinoma in situ of transitional cell epithelium: clinical and pathological considerations, Prog Surg Pathol 8:153-168, 1988.
209. Murphy WM, Soloway MS: Urothelial dysplasia, J Urol 127:849-854, 1982.
210. Mostofi FK, Sesterhenn IA, Davis CJ Jr: Dysplasia versus atypia versus carcinoma in situ of bladder. In McCullough DL (ed): Difficult diagnoses in urology, New York, 1988, Churchill Livingstone.
211. Nagy GK, Friedell GHY: Urinary bladder. In Henson DE, Albores-Saavedra J (eds): Pathology of incipient neoplasia, ed 2, Philadelphia, 1993, W B Saunders.
212. Friedell GH, Soloway MS, Hilgar AG et al: Summary of workshop on carcinoma in situ of the bladder, J Urol 136:1047-1048, 1986.
213. Droller MJ: A rose is a rose is a rose, or is it? J Urol 136:1057-1058, 1986.
214. Brodsky GL: Pathology of bladder carcinoma, Hematol Oncol Clin North Am 6:59-80, 1992.
215. Smith G, Elton RA, Beynon LL et al: Prognostic significance of biopsy results of normal-looking mucosa in cases of superficial bladder cancer, Br J Urol 55:665-669, 1983.
216. Rübben H, Lutzeyer W, Fischer N et al: Natural history and treatment of low and high risk superficial bladder tumors, J Urol 139:283-285, 1988.
217. Heney NM, Ahmed S, Flanagan MJ et al: Superficial bladder cancer: progression and recurrence, J Urol 130:1083-1086, 1983.
218. Moloney PJ, Elliott GB, Mclaughlin M et al: In situ transitional carcinoma and the non-specifically inflamed contracting bladder, J Urol 111:162-164, 1974.
219. Althausen AF, Prout GR Jr, Daly JJ: Non-invasive papillary carcinoma of the bladder associated with carcinoma in situ, J Urol 116:575-580, 1976.
220. Jacobsen F, Møller-Nielsen C, Mommsen S: Flat intraepithelial carcinoma in situ of the urinary bladder, Scand J Urol Nephrol 29:253-255, 1985.
221. Amling CL, Thrasher JB, Dodge RK et al: Radical cystectomy for stages TA, TIS and T1 transitional cell carcinoma of the bladder, J Urol 151:31-36, 1994.
222. Malkowicz SB, Nichols P, Lieskovsky G et al: The role of cystectomy in the management of high grade superficial bladder cancer (PA, P1, PIS and P2), J Urol 144:641-645, 1990.
223. Prout GR Jr, Griffin PP, Daly JJ: The outcome of conservative treatment of carcinoma in situ of the bladder, J Urol 138:766-770, 1987.
224. Stanisic TH, Donovan JM, Lebouton J et al: 5-year experience with intravesical therapy of carcinoma in situ: an inquiry into the risks of "conservative" management, J Urol 138:1158-1161, 1987.
225. Mukamel E, Dekernion JB: Conservative treatment of diffuse carcinoma in situ of the bladder with repeated courses of intravesical therapy, Br J Urol 64:143-146, 1989.
226. Bretton PR, Herr HW, Whitmore WF Jr et al: Intravesical bacillus Calmette-Guerin therapy for in situ transitional cell carcinoma involving the prostatic urethra, J Urol 141:853-856, 1989.
227. Sakamoto N, Tsuneyoshi M, Naito S et al: An adequate sampling of the prostate to identify prostatic involvement by urothelial carcinoma in bladder cancer patients, J Urol 149:318-321, 1993.
228. Williams JL, Hammonds JC, Saunders N: T1 bladder tumours, Br J Urol 49:663-668, 1977.
229. Anderström C, Johansson S, Nilsson S: The significance of lamina propria invasion on the prognosis of patients with bladder tumors, J Urol 124:23-26, 1980.
230. Parmar MKB, Freedman LS, Hargreave TB et al: Prognostic factors for recurrence and follow up policies in the treatment of superficial bladder cancer: report from the British Medical Research Council subgroup on superficial bladder cancer (Urological Cancer Working Party), J Urol 142:284-288, 1989.
231. Kiemeney LALM, Witjes JA, Heijbroek RP et al: Predictability of recurrent and progressive disease in individual patients with primary superficial bladder cancer, J Urol 150:60-64, 1993.
232. Stephenson WT, Holmes FF, Noble MJ et al: Analysis of bladder carcinoma by subsite, Cancer 66:1630-1635, 1990.
233. Utz DC, Schmitz SE, Fugelso PD et al: A clinicopathologic evaluation of partial cystectomy for carcinoma of the urinary bladder, Cancer 32:1075-1077, 1973.
234. Shivde AV, Kherdekar MS: Carcinosarcoma of the urinary bladder: a case report and review of literature, Ind J Med Sc 27:932-934, 1973.
235. Young RH: Papillary and polypoid cystitis, Am J Surg Pathol 12:542-546, 1988.
236. Ekelund P, Anderström C, Johansson SL et al: The reversibility of catheter associated polypoid cystitis, J Urol 130:456-459, 1983.
237. Buck EG: Polypoid cystitis mimicking transitional cell carcinoma, J Urol 131:963-965, 1984.
238. Davis TA: Hamartoma of the urinary bladder, Northwest Med 48:182-187, 1949.
239. Bhagavan BS, Tiamson EM, Wenk RE et al: Nephrogenic adenoma of the urinary bladder and urethra, Hum Pathol 12:907-916, 1981.
240. Ford TF, Watson GM, Cameron KM: Adenomatous metaplasia (nephrogenic adenoma) of urothelium: an analysis of 70 cases, Br J Urol 57:427-433, 1985.
241. Lipponen PK, Eskelinen MJ, Jauhiainen K et al: Prognostic factors in WHO grade 2 transitional-cell bladder cancers (TCC): a novel two-grade classification system for TCC based on mitotic index, J Cancer Res Clin Oncol 118:615-620, 1992.
242. Bannach B, Grignon DJ, Shum DT: Sarcomatoid transitional cell carcinoma vs pseudosarcomatous stromal reaction in bladder carcinoma, J Urol Pathol 1:105-119, 1993.
243. Sakamoto N, Tsuneyoshi M, Enjoji M: Urinary bladder carcinoma with neoplastic squamous component: a mapping study of 31 cases, Histopathology 21:135-141, 1992.
244. Martin JE, Jenkins BJ, Zuk RJ et al: Clinical importance of squamous metaplasia in invasive transitional cell carcinoma of the bladder, J Clin Pathol 42:250-253, 1989.

245. Mostofi FK: Potentialities of bladder epithelium, J Urol 71:705-714, 1954.
246. Russell PJ, Wills EJ, Philips J et al: Features of squamous and adenocarcinoma in the same cell in a xenografted human transitional cell carcinoma: evidence of a common histogenesis, Urol Res 16:79-84, 1988.
247. Akdas A, Turkeri L: The impact of squamous metaplasia in transitional cell carcinoma of the bladder, Int J Urol Nephrol 23:333-336, 1990.
248. Logothetis CJ, Dexeus FH, Chong C et al: Cisplatin, cyclophosphamide and doxorubicin chemotherapy for unresectable urothelial tumors: the MD Anderson experience, J Urol 141:33-37, 1989.
249. Grace DA, Winter CC: Mixed differentiation of primary carcinoma of the urinary bladder, Cancer 21:1239-1243, 1968.
250. Fegen JP, Albert DJ, Persky L: Adenocarcinoma and transitional cell carcinoma occurring simultaneously in the urinary bladder (mixed tumor), J Surg Oncol 3:387-392, 1971.
251. Young RH, Eble JN: Unusual forms of carcinoma of the urinary bladder, Hum Pathol 22:948-965, 1991.
252. Donhuijsen K, Schmidt U, Richter HJ et al: Mucoid cytoplasmic inclusions in urothelial carcinomas, Hum Pathol 23:860-864, 1992.
253. Petersen RO: Urologic pathology, ed 2, Philadelphia, 1992, JB Lippincott.
254. Grignon DJ, Ro JY, Ayala AG et al: Primary adenocarcinoma of the urinary bladder: a clinicopathologic analysis of 72 cases, Cancer 67:2165-2172, 1991.
255. Wiener M, Sarma DP, Weilbaecher TG: Simultaneous occurrence of adenocarcinoma and transitional cell carcinoma as two separate primary tumors in the bladder, J Surg Oncol 25:48-49, 1984.
256. Murphy WM, Deana DG: The nested variant of transitional cell carcinoma: a neoplasm resembling proliferation of Brunn's nests, Mod Pathol 5:240-243, 1992.
257. Talbert ML, Young RH: Carcinomas of the urinary bladder with deceptively benign-appearing foci, Am J Surg Pathol 13:374-381, 1989.
258. Young RH, Scully RE: Nephrogenic adenoma, Am J Surg Pathol 10:268-275, 1986.
259. Grignon DJ, Ro JY, Mackay B et al: Paraganglioma of the urinary bladder: immunohistochemical, ultrastructural, and DNA flow cytometric studies, Hum Pathol 22:1162-1169, 1991.
260. Cintorino M, Del Vecchio MT, Bugnoli M et al: Cytokeratin pattern in normal and pathological bladder urothelium: Immunohistochemical investigation using monoclonal antibodies, J Urol 139:428-432, 1988.
261. Asamoto M, Fukushima S, Oosumi H et al: Immunohistochemical distribution of epithelial membrane antigen in bladder carcinomas as detected with a monoclonal antibody, Urol Res 17:273-277, 1989.
262. Zukerberg LR, Young RH: Microcystic transitional cell carcinomas of the urinary bladder, Am J Clin Pathol 96:635-639, 1991.
263. Komatsu H, Kinoshita K, Mikata N et al: Spindle and giant cell carcinoma of the bladder, Eur Urol 11:141-144, 1985.
264. Zukerberg LR, Armin A-R, Pisharodi L et al: Transitional cell carcinoma of the urinary bladder with osteoclast-type giant cells: a report of two cases and review of the literature, Histopathology 17:407-411, 1990.
265. Grammatico D, Grignon DJ, Eberwein P et al: Transitional cell carcinoma of the renal pelvis with choriocarcinomatous differentiation: immunohistochemical and immunoelectron microscopic assessment of human chorionic gonadotropin production by transitional cell carcinoma of the urinary bladder, Cancer 71:1835-1841, 1993.
266. Holtz F, Fox JE, Abell MR: Carcinosarcoma of the urinary bladder, Cancer 29:294-304, 1972.
267. Kitazawa M, Kobayashi H, Ohnishi Y et al: Giant cell tumor of the bladder associated with transitional cell carcinoma, J Urol 133:472-475, 1985.
268. Lidgi S, Embon OM, Turani H et al: Giant cell reparative granuloma of the bladder associated with transitional cell carcinoma, J Urol 142:120-122, 1989.
269. Pao WJ, Hustu HO, Douglass EC et al: Pediatric nasopharyngeal carcinoma: long term follow-up of 29 patients, Int J Rad Oncol Biol Phys 17:299-305, 1989.
270. Rahima M, Rakowsky E, Barzilay J et al: Carcinoma of the nasopharynx: an analysis of 91 cases and a comparison of differing treatment approaches, Cancer 58:843-849, 1986.
271. Zukerberg LR, Harris NL, Young RH: Carcinomas of the urinary bladder simulating malignant lymphoma, Am J Surg Pathol 15:569-576, 1991.
272. Young RH, Eble JN: Lymphoepithelioma-like carcinoma of the urinary bladder, J Urol Pathol 1:63-67, 1994.
273. Amin MB, Ro JY, Lee KM et al: Lymphoepithelioma-like carcinoma of the urinary bladder, Am J Surg Pathol 18:466-473, 1994.
274. Burke AP, Yen TSB, Shekitka KM et al: Lymphoepithelial carcinoma of the stomach with Epstein-Barr virus demonastrated by polymerase chain reaction, Mod Pathol 3:377-380, 1990.
275. Pittaluga S, Wong MP, Chung LP et al: Clonal Epstein-Barr virus in lymphoepithelioma-like carcinoma of the lung, Am J Surg Pathol 17:678-682, 1993.
276. Dinney CPN, Ro JY, Babaian RJ et al: Lymphoepithelioma of the bladder: a clinicopathological study of 3 cases, J Urol 149:840-842, 1993.
277. Sahin AA, Myhre M, Ro JY et al: Plasmacytoid transitional cell carcinoma: report of a case with initial presentation mimicking multiple myeloma, Acta Cytol 35:277-280, 1991.
278. Pollack AD: Malignant teratoma of the urinary bladder, Am J Pathol 12:561-568, 1936.
279. Hirsch EF, Gasser GW: Cancerous mixed tumor of the urinary bladder, Arch Pathol 37:24-26, 1944.
280. Orsatti G, Corgan FJ, Goldberg SA: Carcinosarcoma of urothelial organs: sequential involvement of urinary bladder, ureter, and renal pelvis, Urology 41:289-291, 1993.
281. Bloxham CA, Bennett MK, Robinson MC: Bladder carcinosarcomas: three cases with diverse histogenesis, Histopathology 16:63-67, 1990.
282. Signal SH, Tomaszewski JE, Brooks JJ et al: Carcinosarcoma of bladder following long-term cyclophosphamide therapy, Arch Pathol Lab Med 115:1049-1051, 1991.
283. Sen SE, Malek RS, Farrow GM et al: Sarcoma and carcinosarcoma of the bladder in adults, J Urol 133:29-30, 1985.
284. Mazzucchelli L, Kraft R, Gerber H et al: Carcinosarcoma of the urinary bladder: a distinct variant characterized by small cell undifferentiated carcinoma with neuroendocrine features, Virchows Arch [A] 421:477-483, 1992.

285. Young RH, Wick MR, Mills SE: Sarcomatoid carcinoma of the urinary bladder. A clinicopathological analysis of 12 cases and review of the literature, Am J Clin Pathol 90:653-661, 1988.
286. Ro JY, Ayala AG, Wishnow KI et al: Sarcomatoid bladder carcinoma: clinical, pathologic and immunohistochemical study on 44 cases, Surg Pathol 1:359-374, 1988.
287. Pearson JM, Banerjee SS, Haboubi NY: Two cases of pseudosarcomatous invasive transitional cell carcinoma of the urinary bladder mimicking malignant fibrous histiocytoma, Histopathology 15:93-99, 1989.
288. Fromowitz FB, Bard RH, Koss LG: The epithelial origin of a malignant mesodermal mixed tumor of the bladder: report of a case with long-term survival, J Urol 132:978-981, 1984.
289. Babaian RJ, Johnson DE, Manning J et al: Mixed mesodermal tumors of urinary bladder, Urology 15:261-264, 1980.
290. Grossman HB, Sonda LB, Lloyd RV et al: Carcinosarcoma of bladder, Urology 24:387-389, 1984.
291. Kusaba Y, Yushita Y, Suzu H et al: Carcinosarcoma of the bladder, J Urol 131:118-119, 1984.
292. Torenbeek R, Blomjous CEM, de Bruin PC et al: Sarcomatoid carcinoma of the urinary bladder: clinicopathologic analysis of 18 cases with immunohistochemical and electron microscopic findings, Am J Surg Pathol 18:241-249, 1994.
293. Young RH: Carcinosarcoma of the bladder, Cancer 59:1333-1339, 1987.
294. Rodenburg CJ, Kruseman ACN, de Maaker HA et al: Immunohistochemical localization and chromatographic characterization of human chorionic gonadotropin in a bladder carcinoma, Arch Pathol Lab Med 109:1046-1048, 1985.
295. Duong HD, Jackson AG, Kovi J et al: Mixed mesodermal tumor of urinary bladder, Urology 17:377-380, 1981.
296. Murao T, Tanahashi T: Carcinosarcoma of the urinary bladder, Acta Pathol Jpn 35:981-988, 1985.
297. Bonsib SM, Fischer J, Plattner S et al: Sarcomatoid renal tumors: Clinicopathologic correlation of three cases, Cancer 59:527-532, 1987.
298. Young RH, Wick MR: Transitional cell carcinoma of the urinary bladder with pseudosarcomatous stroma, Am J Clin Pathol 89:216-219, 1988.
299. Jao W, Soto JM, Gould VE: Squamous carcinoma of bladder with pseudosarcomatous stroma, Arch Pathol 99:461-464, 1975.
300. Yushita Y, Suzu H, Imamura A et al: A case of primary vesical undifferentiated carcinoma with heterotopic ossification, Acta Urol Jpn 28:1419-1426, 1982.
301. Toma H, Yamashita N, Nakazawa H et al: Transitional cell carcinoma with osteoid metaplasia, Urology 27:174-176, 1986.
302. Nakachi K, Miyamoto I, Kuroda J et al: A case of transitional cell carcinoma of the bladder with heterotopic bone formation, Acta Urol Jpn 34:1651-1655, 1988.
303. Eble JN, Young RH: Stromal osseous metaplasia in carcinoma of the bladder, J Urol 145:823-825, 1991.
304. Cornes JS, Sussman T, Dawson IMP: Bone formation in metastasis from carcinoma of urinary bladder: report of a case with review of the literature, Br J Urol 32:290-294, 1960.
305. Chinn D, Genant HK, Quivey JM et al: Heterotopic-bone formation in metastatic tumor from transitional-cell carcinoma of the urinary bladder: a case report, J Bone Joint Surg 58-A:881-883, 1976.
306. Evison G, Pizey N, Roylance J: Bone formation associated with osseous metastases from bladder cancer, Clin Radiol 32:303-309, 1981.
307. Wells HG: Giant cells in cystitis, Arch Pathol 26:32-43, 1938.
308. Gowing NFC: Pathological changes in the bladder following irradiation, Br J Radiol 33:484-487, 1960.
309. Beyer-Boon ME, De Voogt HJ, Schaberg A: The effects of cyclophosphamide treatment on the epithelium and stroma of the urinary bladder, Eur J Cancer 14:1029-1035, 1978.
310. Young RH: Pathology of the urinary bladder, New York, 1989, Churchill Livingstone.
311. Uyama T, Moriwaki S: Carcinosarcoma of urinary bladder, Urology 18:191-194, 1981.
312. Brinton JA, Ito Y, Olsen BS: Carcinosarcoma of the urinary bladder, Cancer 1183-1186, 1970.
313. Guirguis AB, Milam JH, Richardson DH: Carcinosarcoma, Urology 22:553-555, 1983.
314. Smith JA Jr, Herr HW, Middleton RG: Bladder carcinosarcoma: histologic variation in metastatic lesions, J Urol 129:829-831, 1983.
315. Schoborg TW, Saffos RO, Rodriquez AP et al: Carcinosarcoma of the bladder, J Urol 124:724-727, 1980.
316. Johansen SE, Stenwig AE, Tveter KJ: Carcinosarcoma of the urinary bladder in an adult male, Scand J Urol Nephrol 13:117-122, 1979.
317. Patterson TH, Dale GA: Carcinosarcoma of the bladder: case report and review of the literature, J Urol 115:753-755, 1976.
318. McCarthy LJ, Wahle WM, Moosey NA: Carcinosarcoma of the urinary bladder—a case report, J Indiana State Med Assoc 68:722-724, 1975.
319. Delides GS: Bone and cartilage in malignant tumours of the urinary bladder, Br J Urol 44:571-581, 1972.
320. Broders AC: Epithelioma of the genitourinary organs, Ann Surg 75:574-604, 1922.
321. Ash JE: Epithelial tumors of the bladder, J Urol 44:135-145, 1940.
322. Bergkvist A, Ljungqvist A, Moberger G: Classification of bladder tumours based on the cellular pattern, Acta Chir Scand 130:371-378, 1965.
323. Colpaert C, Goovaerts G, Buyssens N: Factors influencing the subjective grading of bladder cancer, Virchows Arch [A] 411:479-484, 1987.
324. Takashi M, Murase T, Mizuno S et al: Multivariate evaluation of prognostic determinants in bladder cancer patients, Urol Int 42:368-374, 1987.
325. Torti FM, Lum BL, Aston D et al: Superficial bladder cancer: the primacy of grade in the development of invasive disease, J Clin Oncol 5:125-130, 1987.
326. Ooms ECM, Kurver PHJ, Veldhuizen RW et al: Morphometric grading of bladder tumors in comparison with histologic grading by pathologists, Hum Pathol 14:144-150, 1983.
327. Nielsen K: Need for morphometric analysis in grading bladder tumours, Anal Cell Pathol 3:183-185, 1991.

328. Sowter C, Slavin G, Sowter G et al: Morphometry of bladder carcinoma: morphometry and grading complement each other, Anal Cell Pathol 3:1-9, 1991.
329. Blomjous CEM, Schipper NW, Baak JPA et al: The value of morphometry and DNA flow cytometry in addition to classic prognosticators in superficial urinary bladder carcinoma, Am J Clin Pathol 91:243-248, 1989.
330. Nielsen K, Ørntoft T, Wolf H: Stereologic estimates of nuclear volume in noninvasive bladder tumors (Ta) correlated with the recurrence pattern, Cancer 64:2269-2274, 1989.
331. Carbin B-E, Ekman P, Gustafson H et al: Grading of human urothelial carcinoma based on nuclear atypia and mitotic frequency. I. Histological description, J Urol 145:968-971, 1991.
332. Moll R, Achtstatter T, Becht E et al: Cytokeratins in normal and malignant transitional epithelium, Am J Pathol 132:123-144, 1988.
333. Ramaekers FCS, Beck JLM, Feitz WFJ et al: Keratin expression during neoplastic progression of bladder cancer, Eur Urol 14(suppl 1):7-8, 1988.
334. Hoshi S, Orikasa S, Numata I et al: Expression of Leu-M1 antigens in carcinoma of the urinary bladder, J Urol 135:1075-1077, 1986.
335. Shevchuk MM, Fenoglio CM, Richart RM: Carcinoembryonic antigen localization in benign and malignant transitional epithelium, Cancer 47:899-905, 1981.
336. Alroy J, Pauli BU, Weinstein RS: Correlation between numbers of desmosomes and the aggressiveness of transitional cell carcinoma in human urinary bladder, Cancer 47:104-112, 1981.
337. Hopkins DM, Morris JA, Oates K et al: Low-temperature and conventional scanning electron microscopy of human urothelial neoplasms, J Pathol 158:45-51, 1989.
338. Farrow GM, Utz DC: Observations on microinvasive transitional cell carcinoma of the urinary bladder, Clin Oncol 1:609-614, 1982.
339. Dixon JS, Gosling JA: Histology and fine structure of the muscularis mucosae of the human urinary bladder, J Anat 136:265-271, 1983.
340. Ro JY, Ayala AG, El-Naggar AK: Muscularis mucosa of urinary bladder: importance for staging and treatment, Am J Surg Pathol 11:668-673, 1987.
341. Keep JC, Piehl M, Miller A et al: Invasive carcinomas of the urinary bladder: evaluation of tunica muscularis mucosae involvement, Am J Clin Pathol 91:575-579, 1989.
342. Younes M, Sussman J, True LD: The usefulness of the level of the muscularis mucosae in the staging of invasive transitional cell carcinoma of the urinary bladder, Cancer 66:543-548, 1990.
343. Hasui Y, Osada Y, Kitada S et al: Significance of invasion to the muscularis mucosae on the progression of superficial bladder cancer, Urology 43:782-786, 1994.
344. Angulo JC, Lopez JI, Grignon DJ et al: The muscularis mucosae distinguishes two populations with different prognosis in stage T1 bladder cancer, Urology 45:47-53, 1995.
345. Bell JT, Burney SW, Friedell GH: Blood vessel invasion in human bladder cancer, J Urol 105:675-678, 1971.
346. Heney NM, Proppe K, Prout GR Jr et al: Invasive bladder cancer: tumor configuration, lymphatic invasion and survival, J Urol 130:895-897, 1983.
347. Jewett HJ, King LR, Shelley WM: A Study of 365 cases of infiltrating bladder cancer: relation of certain pathological characteristics to prognosis after extirpation, J Urol 92:668-678, 1964.
348. McDonald JR, Thompson GJ: Carcinoma of the urinary bladder: a pathologic study with a special reference to invasiveness and vascular invasion, J Urol 60:435-445, 1948.
349. Slack NH, Prout GR Jr: The heterogeneity of invasive bladder carcinoma and different responses to treatment, J Urol 123:644-652, 1980.
350. Ramani P, Birch BRP, Harland SJ et al: Evaluation of endothelial markers in detecting blood and lymphatic channel invasion in pT1 transitional carcinoma of bladder, Histopathology 19:551-554, 1991.
351. Larsen MP, Steinberg GD, Brendler CB et al: Use of *Ulex europaeus* agglutinin I (UEAI) to distinguish vascular and pseudovascular invasion in transitional cell carcinoma of bladder with lamina propria invasion, Mod Pathol 3:83-88, 1990.
352. Wheeless LL, Badalament RA, deVere White RW et al: Consensus review of the clinical utility of DNA cytometry in bladder cancer, Cytometry 14:478-481, 1993.
353. Lipponen PK, Collan Y, Eskelinen MJ et al: Comparison of morphometry and DNA flow cytometry with standard prognostic factors in bladder cancer, Br J Urol 65:589-597, 1990.
354. Blomjous CEM, Schipper NW, Baak JPA et al: Retrospective study of prognostic importance of DNA flow cytometry of urinary bladder carcinoma, J Clin Pathol 41:21-25, 1988.
355. Tribukait B, Gustafson H, Esposti PL: The significance of ploidy and proliferation in the clinical and biological evaluation of bladder tumours: a study of 100 untreated cases, Br J Urol 54:130-135, 1982.
356. Chin JL, Huben RP, Nava E et al: Flow cytometric analysis of DNA content in human bladder tumors and irrigation fluids, Cancer 56:1677-1681, 1985.
357. Masters JRW, Camplejohn RS, Constance Parkinson M et al: DNA ploidy and the prognosis of stage T1 bladder cancer, Br J Urol 64:403-408, 1989.
358. Jacobsen A, Pettersen EO, Åmellem Ø et al: The prognostic significance of deoxyribonucleic acid flow cytometry in muscle invasive bladder carcinoma treated with preoperative irradiation and cystectomy, J Urol 147:34-37, 1992.
359. Farsund T, Hoestmark JG, Laerum OD: Relation between flow cytometric DNA distribution and pathology in human bladder cancer, Cancer 54:1771-1777, 1984.
360. Shaaban AA, Tribukait B, Abdel-Fattah A et al: Prediction of lymph node metastases in bladder carcinoma with deoxyribonucleic acid flow cytometry, J Urol 144:884-887, 1990.
361. Gustafson H, Tribukait B: Characterization of bladder carcinomas by flow DNA analysis, Eur Urol 11:410-417, 1985.
362. deVere White RW, Deitch AD, West B et al: The predictive value of flow cytometric information in the clinical management of stage 0 (Ta) bladder cancer, J Urol 139:279-282, 1988.

363. Lipponen PK, Nordling S, Eskelinen MJ et al: Flow cytometry in comparison with mitotic index in predicting disease outcome in transitional cell bladder cancer, Int J Cancer 53:42-47, 1993.
364. Wijkstrom H, Tribukait B: Deoxyribonucleic acid flow cytometry in predicting response to radical radiotherapy of bladder cancer, J Urol 144:646-651, 1990.
365. Hug EB, Donnelly SM, Shipley WU et al: Deoxyribonucleic acid flow cytometry in invasive bladder carcinoma: a possible predictor for successful bladder preservation following transurethral surgery and chemotherapy-radiotherapy, J Urol 148:47-51, 1992.
366. Sandlow J, Cohen MB, Robinson RA et al: DNA ploidy and p-glycoprotein expression as predictive factors of response to neoadjuvant chemotherapy for invasive bladder cancer, Urology 43:787-791, 1994.
367. Lipponen PK, Eskelinen MJ, Kiviranta J et al: Prognosis of transitional cell bladder cancer: a multivariate prognostic score for improved prediction, J Urol 146:1535-1540, 1991.
368. Levin I, Klein T, Goldstein J et al: Expression of class I histocompatibility antigens in transitional cell carcinoma of the urinary bladder in relation to survival, Cancer 68:2591-2594, 1991.
369. Malmstrom PU, Wester K, Vasko J et al: Expression of proliferative cell nuclear antigen (PCNA) in urinary bladder carcinoma. Evaluation of antigen retrieval methods, APMIS 100:988-992, 1992.
370. Tsujihashi H, Nakanishi A, Matsuda H et al: Cell proliferation of human bladder tumors determined by BRDURD and Ki-67 immunostaining, J Urol 145:846-849, 1991.
371. Okamura K, Miyake K, Koshikawa T et al: Growth fractions of transitional cell carcinomas of the bladder defined by the monoclonal antibody Ki-67, J Urol 144:875-878, 1990.
372. Tachibana M, Deguchi N, Jitsukawa S et al: Quantification of cell kinetic characteristics using flow cytometric measurements of deoxyribonucleic acid and bromodeoxyuridine for bladder cancer, J Urol 145:963-967, 1991.
373. Nemoto R, Uchida K, Hattori K et al: S phase fraction of human bladder tumor measured in situ with bromodeoxyuridine labeling, J Urol 139:286-289, 1988.
374. Lipponen PK, Eskelinen MJ: Volume-corrected mitotic index and mitotic activity index in transitional cell bladder cancer, Eur Urol 18:258-262, 1990.
375. Lipponen PK, Eskelinen MJ, Kivaranta J et al: Classic prognostic factors, flow cytometric data, nuclear morphometric variables and mitotic indexes as predictors in transitional cell bladder cancer, Anticancer Res 11:911-916, 1991.
376. DeSanctis PN, Tannenbaum M, Tannenbaum S et al: Morphologic quantitation of nuclear size in various grades of transitional cell carcinoma of urinary bladder, Urology 20:196-199, 1982.
377. Blomjous CEM, Vos W, Schipper NW et al: The prognostic significance of selective nuclear morphometry in urinary bladder carcinoma, Hum Pathol 21:409-413, 1990.
378. Conn IG, Crocker J, Wallace DMA et al: Basement membranes in urothelial carcinoma, Br J Urol 60:536-542, 1987.
379. Daher N, Abourachid H, Bove N et al: Collagen IV staining pattern in bladder carcinomas: relationship to prognosis, Br J Cancer 55:665-671, 1987.
380. Zuk RJ, Baithun SI, Martin JE et al: The immunocytochemical demonstration of basement membrane deposition in transitional cell carcinoma of bladder, Virchows Arch [A] 414:447-452, 1989.
381. Schapers RFM, Pauwels RPE, Havenith MG et al: Prognostic significance of type IV collagen and laminin immunoreactivity in urothelial carcinomas of the bladder, Cancer 66:2583-2588, 1990.
382. Limas C: Blood group antigen expression in urothelial neoplasia, Eur Urol Suppl 14:9-10, 1988.
383. Coon JS, Schwartz D, Weinstein RS: Markers in the analysis of human urinary bladder carcinoma, Adv Pathol 1:201-228, 1988.
384. Pauwels RPE, Schapers RFM, Smeets AWGB et al: Blood group isoantigen deletion and chromosomal abnormalities in bladder cancer, J Urol 140:959-963, 1988.
385. Abel PD, Thorpe SJ, Williams G: Blood group antigen expression in frozen sections of presenting bladder cancer: 3-year prospective follow-up of prognostic value, Br J Urol 63:171-175, 1989.
386. Cordon-Cardo C, Lloyd KO, Finstad CL et al: Immunoanatomic distribution of blood group antigens in the human urinary tract, Lab Invest 55:444-454, 1986.
387. Ørntoft TF, Nielsen MJS, Wolf H et al: Blood group ABO and Lewis antigen expression during neoplastic progression of human urothelium, Cancer 60:2641-2648, 1987.
388. Meyers FJ, Gumerlock PH, Kawasaki ES et al: Human leukocyte antigen II, interleukin-6, and interleukin-6 receptor expression determined by the polymerase chain reaction, Cancer 67:2087-2095, 1991.
389. Stefanini GF, Bercovich E, Mazzeo V et al: Class I and class II HLA antigen expression by transitional cell carcinoma of the bladder: correlation with T-cell infiltration and BCG treatment, J Urol 141:1449-1453, 1989.
390. Costello CB, Kumar S: Prognostic value of tissue polypeptide antigen in urological neoplasia, J Royal Soc Med 78:207-210, 1985.
391. Khanna OP, Wu B: Tissue polypeptide antigen (TPA) as a predictor for genitourinary cancers and their metastases, Urology 30:106-110, 1987.
392. Carbin B-E, Ekman P, Eneroth P et al: Urine-TPA (tissue polypeptide antigen), flow cytometry and cytology as markers for tumor invasiveness in urinary bladder carcinoma, Urol Res 17:269-272, 1989.
393. Tizzanil A, Cassetta G, Cicigoil A et al: Tumor markers (CEA, TPA and CA 19-9) in urine of bladder cancer patients, Ant J Biol Markers 2:121-124, 1987.
394. Neal DE, Smith K, Fennelly JA et al: Epidermal growth factor receptor in human bladder cancer: a comparison of immunohistochemistry and ligand binding, J Urol 141:517-521, 1989.
395. Neal DE, Sharples L, Smith K et al: The epidermal growth factor receptor and the prognosis of bladder cancer, Cancer 65:1619-1625, 1990.
396. Messing EM: Clinical implications of the expression of epidermal growth factor receptors in human transitional cell carcinoma, Cancer Res 50:2530-2537, 1990.
397. Wood DP Jr, Fair WR, Chaganti RSK: Evaluation of epidermal growth factor receptor DNA amplification and mRNA expression in bladder cancer, J Urol 147:274-277, 1992.

398. Meyers FJ, Gumerlock PH, Kokoris SP et al: Human bladder and colon carcinomas contain activated *ras* p21, Cancer 63:2177-2181, 1989.
399. Agnantis NJ, Constantinidou A, Poulios C et al: Immunohistochemical study of the *ras* oncogene expression in human bladder endoscopy specimens, Eur J Surg Oncol 16:153-160, 1990.
400. Stock LM, Brosman SA, Fahey JL et al: *ras* related oncogene protein as a tumor marker in transitional cell carcinoma of the bladder, J Urol 137:789-792, 1987.
401. Ye D-W, Zheng J-F, Qian S-X et al: Correlation between the expression of oncogenes *ras* and C-erb-2 and the biological behavior of bladder tumors, Urol Res 21:39-43, 1993.
402. Dunn TL, Seymour GJ, Gardiner RA et al: Immunocytochemical demonstration of $p21^{ras}$ in normal and transitional cell carcinoma urothelium, J Pathol 156:59-65, 1988.
403. Levesque P, Ramchurren N, Saini K et al: Screening of human bladder tumors and urine sediments for the presence of H-*ras* mutation, Int J Cancer 55:785-790, 1993.
404. Swanson PE, Frierson HF Jr, Wick MR: c-erb-2 (HER-2/neu) oncopeptide immunoreactivity in localized, high grade transitional cell carcinoma of the bladder, Mod Pathol 5:531-536, 1992.
405. McCann A, Dervan PA, Johnston PA et al: c-erbB-2 oncoprotein expression in primary human tumors, Cancer 65:88-92, 1990.
406. Wood DP Jr, Wartinger DD, Reuter V et al: DNA, RNA and immunohistochemical characterization of the HER-2/neu oncogene in transitional cell carcinoma of the bladder, J Urol 146:1398-1401, 1991.
407. Asamoto M, Hasegawa R, Masuko T et al: Immunohistochemical analysis of c-erbB-2 oncogene product and epidermal growth factor receptor expression in human urinary bladder carcinomas, Acta Pathol Jpn 40:322-326, 1990.
408. Moriyama M, Akiyama T, Yamamoto T et al: Expression of c-erB-2 gene product in urinary bladder cancer, J Urol 145:423-427, 1991.
409. Lipponen P: Expression of c-erbB-2 oncoprotein in transitional cell bladder cancer, Eur J Cancer 29:749-753, 1993.
410. Nguyen PL, Swanson PE, Jaszcz W et al: Expression of epidermal growth factor receptor in invasive transitional cell carcinoma of the urinary bladder: a multivariate survival analysis, Am J Clin Pathol 101:166-176, 1994.
411. Wright C, Mellon K, Johnston P et al: Expression of mutant p53, C-erbB-2 and the epidermal growth factor receptor in transitional cell carcinoma of the human urinary bladder, Br J Cancer 63:967-970, 1991.
412. Bartek J, Bartkova J, Vojtesek B et al: Aberrant expression of the p53 oncoprotein is a common feature of a wide spectrum of human malignancies, Oncogene 6:1699-1703, 1991.
413. Oka K, Ishikawa J, Bruner JM et al: Detection of loss of heterozygosity in the p53 gene in renal cell carcinoma and bladder cancer using the polymerase chain reaction, Mol Carcin 4:10-13, 1991.
414. Sidransky D, von Eschenbach A, Tsai YC et al: Identification of p53 mutations in bladder cancers and urine samples, Science 25:705-709, 1991.
415. Sarkis AS, Dalbagni G, Cordon-Cardo C et al: Nuclear overexpression of p53 protein in transitional cell bladder carcinoma: a marker for disease progression, J Natl Cancer Inst 85:53-59, 1993.
416. Habuchi T, Takahashi R, Yamada H et al: Influence of cigarette smoking and schistosomiasis on p53 gene mutation in urothelial cancer, Cancer Res 53:3795-3799, 1993.
417. Soini Y, Turpeenniemi-Hujanen T, Kamel D et al: p53 immunohistochemistry in transitional cell carcinoma and dysplasia of the urinary bladder correlates with disease progression, Br J Cancer 68:1029-1035, 1993.
418. Esrig D, Spruck CH III, Nichols PW et al: P53 nuclear protein accumulation correlates with mutations in the p53 gene, tumor grade, and stage in bladder cancer, Am J Pathol 143:1389-1397, 1993.
419. Furihata M, Inoue K, Ohtsuki Y et al: High-risk human papilloma virus infections and overexpression of p53 protein as prognostic indicators in transitional cell carcinoma of the urinary bladder, Cancer Res 53:4823-4827, 1993.
420. Lipponen PK: Over-expression of p53 nuclear oncoprotein in transitional-cell bladder cancer and its prognostic value, Int J Cancer 53:365-370, 1993.
421. Esrig D, Elmajian D, Groshen S et al: Accumulation of nuclear p53 and tumor progression in bladder cancer, N Engl J Med 331:1259-1264, 1994.
422. Spruck CH III, Rideout WM III, Olumi AF et al: Distinct pattern of p53 mutations in bladder cancer: relationship to tobacco usage, Cancer Res 53:1162-1166, 1993.
423. Ishikawa J, Xu H-J, Hu S-X et al: Inactivation of the retinoblastoma gene in human bladder and renal cell carcinomas, Cancer Res 51:5736-5743, 1991.
424. Presti JC Jr, Reuter VE, Galan T et al: Molecular genetic alterations in superficial and locally advanced human bladder cancer, Cancer Res 51:5405-5409, 1991.
425. Takahashi R, Hashimoto T, Xu H et al: The retinoblastoma gene functions as a growth and tumor suppressor in human bladder carcinoma cells, Proc Natl Acad Sci USA 88:5257-5261, 1991.
426. Cordon-Cardo C, Wartinger D, Petrylak D et al: Altered expression of the retinoblastoma gene product: prognostic indicator in bladder cancer, J Natl Cancer Inst 84:1251-1256, 1992.
427. Logothetis CJ, Xu H-J, Ro JY et al: Altered expression of retinoblastoma protein and known prognostic variables in locally advanced bladder cancer, J Natl Cancer Inst 84:1256-1261, 1992.
428. Kiemeney LALM, Witjes JA, Verbeek ALM et al: The clinical epidemiology of superficial bladder cancer, Br J Cancer 67:806-812, 1993.
429. Gilbert HA, Loga JL, Kagan AR et al: The natural history of papillary transitional cell carcinoma of the bladder and its treatment in an unselected population on the basis of histologic grading, J Urol 119:488-492, 1978.
430. Loening S, Narayana A, Yoder L et al: Factors influencing the recurrence of bladder cancer, J Urol 123:29-31, 1980.
431. Koontz WW, Prout GR, Jr, Smith W et al: The use of intravesical thiotepa in the management of non-invasive carcinoma of the bladder, J Urol 125:307-312, 1981.

432. Zincke H, Utz DC, Taylor WF et al: Influence of thiotepa and doxorubicin instillation at the time of transurethral surgical treatment of bladder cancer on tumor recurrence: a prospective, randomized, double-blind, controlled trial, J Urol 129:505-509, 1983.
433. Issell BF, Prout GR, Jr, Soloway MS et al: Mitomycin C intravesical therapy in noninvasive bladder cancer after failure on thiotepa, Cancer 53:1025-1028, 1984.
434. Stricker CN, Grant AB, Hosken BM et al: Topical mitomycin C therapy for carcinoma of the bladder, J Urol 138:1164-1166, 1987.
435. Soloway MS: Intravesical and systemic chemotherapy in the management of superficial bladder cancer, Urol Clin North Am 11:623-635, 1984.
436. Catalona WJ, Ratliff TL: Bacillus Calmette-Guérin and superficial bladder cancer: clinical experience and mechanism of action, Surg Annu 22:363-378, 1990.
437. Martinez-Pineiro JA, Muntanola P: Nonspecific immunotherapy with BCG vaccine in bladder tumors: a preliminary report, Eur Urol 3:11-22, 1977.
438. Rubben H, Lutzeyer W, Fischer N et al: Natural history and treatment of low and high risk superficial bladder tumors, J Urol 139:283-285, 1988.
439. Matthews PN, Madden M, Bidgood KA et al: The clinicopathological features of metastatic superficial papillary bladder cancer, J Urol 132:904-906, 1984.
440. Utz DC, Farrow GM: Carcinoma in situ of the urinary tract, Urol Clin North Am 11:735-740, 1984.
441. Herr HW, Laudone VP, Badalament RA et al: Bacillus Calmette-Guérin therapy alters the progression of superficial bladder cancer, J Clin Oncol 6:1450-1455, 1988.
442. Soloway MS, Murphy WM, Johnson DE et al: Initial evaluation and response criteria for patients with superficial bladder cancer, Br J Urol 66:380-385, 1990.
443. Kaubisch S, Lum BL, Reese J et al: Stage T1 bladder cancer: grade is the primary determinant for risk of muscle invasion, J Urol 146:28-31, 1991.
444. Huland H, Otto U, Droese M et al: Long-term mitomycin C instillation after transurethral resection of superficial bladder carcinoma: influence on recurrence, progression, and survival, J Urol 132:27-29, 1984.
445. Birch BRP, Harland SJ: The pT1 G3 bladder tumour, Br J Urol 64:109-116, 1989.
446. Resnick MI, O'Connor VJ: Segmental resection for carcinoma of the bladder: review of 102 cases, J Urol 109:1007-1010, 1973.
447. Herr HW: Conservative management of muscle-infiltrating bladder cancer: prospective experience, J Urol 138:1162-1163, 1987.
448. Fair ER, Fuks ZY, Scher HI: Cancer of the bladder. In DeVita VT Jr, Hellman S, Rosenberg SA (eds): Cancer: principles and practice of oncology, ed 4, Philadelphia, 1993, J. B. Lippincott.
449. Gospodarowicz MK, Hawkins NV, Rawlings GA et al: Radical radiotherapy for muscle invasive transitional cell carcinoma of the bladder: failure analysis, J Urol 142:1448-1454, 1989.
450. Greven KM, Solin LJ, Hanks GE: Prognostic factors in patients with bladder carcinoma treated with definitive irradiation, Cancer 65:908-912, 1990.
451. Jenkins BL, Martin JE, Baithun SI et al: Prediction of response to radiotherapy in invasive bladder cancer, Br J Urol 65:345-348, 1990.
452. Kaufman DS, Shipley WU, Griffin PP et al: Selective bladder preservation by combination treatment of invasive bladder cancer, N Engl J Med 329:1377-1382, 1993.
453. Logothetis CJ, Johnson DE, Chong C et al: Adjuvant cyclophosphamide, doxorubicin, and cisplatin chemotherapy for bladder cancer: an update, J Clin Oncol 6:1590-1596, 1988.
454. Sternberg CN, Arena MG, Calabresi F et al: Neoadjuvant M-VAC (methotrexate, vinblastine, doxorubicin, and cisplatin) for infiltrating transitional cell carcinoma of the bladder, Cancer 72:1975-1982, 1993.
455. Scher HI, Yagoda A, Herr HW et al: Neoadjuvant M-VAC (methotrexate, vinblastine, doxorubicin and cisplatin) effect on the primary bladder lesion, J Urol 139:470-474, 1988.
456. El-Bolkainy MN, Mokhtar NM, Ghoneim MA et al: The impact of schistosomiasis on the pathology of bladder carcinoma, Cancer 48:2643-2648, 1981.
457. Sarma KP: Squamous cell carcinoma of the bladder, Int Surg 53:313-318, 1970.
458. Rous SN: Squamous cell carcinoma of the bladder, J Urol 120:561-562, 1978.
459. Sakkas JL: Clinical pattern and treatment of squamous cell carcinoma of the bladder, Int Surg 45:71-76, 1966.
460. Newman DM, Brown JR, Jay AC et al: Squamous cell carcinoma of the bladder, J Urol 100:470-473, 1968.
461. Bessette PL, Abell MR, Herwig KR: A clinicopathologic study of squamous cell carcinoma of the bladder, J Urol 112:66-67, 1974.
462. Johnson DE, Schoenwald MB, Ayala AG et al: Squamous cell carcinoma of the bladder, J Urol 115:542-544, 1976.
463. Richie JP, Waisman J, Skinner DG et al: Squamous carcinoma of the bladder: treatment by radical cystectomy, J Urol 115:670-672, 1976.
464. Faysal MH: Squamous cell carcinoma of the bladder, J Urol 126:598-599, 1981.
465. Winkler HZ, Nativ O, Hosaka Y et al: Nuclear deoxyribonucleic acid ploidy in squamous cell bladder cancer, J Urol 141:297-302, 1989.
466. Swanson DA, Liles A, Zagars GK: Preoperative irradiation and radical cystectomy for stages T2 and T3 squamous cell carcinoma of the bladder, J Urol 143:37-40, 1990.
467. Boissonnas A, Dallot JY, Caquet R et al: Bladder carcinoma with paraneoplastic hypercalcemia, Br J Urol 54:320, 1982.
468. Desai PG, Ali Khan S, Jayachandran S et al: Paraneoplastic syndrome in squamous cell carcinoma of urinary bladder, Urology 30:262-264, 1987.
469. Kaye MC, Levin HS, Montague DK et al: Squamous cell carcinoma of the bladder in a patient on intermittent self-catheterization, Cleveland Clin Q 59:645-646, 1992.
470. Connery DB: Leukoplakia of the urinary bladder and its association with carcinoma, J Urol 69:121-127, 1953.
471. Holley PS, Mellinger GT: Leukoplakia of the bladder and carcinoma, J Urol 48:235-241, 1961.
472. O'Flynn JD, Mullaney J: Leukoplakia of the bladder: a report on 20 cases, including 2 cases progressing to squamous cell carcinoma, Br J Urol 39:461-471, 1967.

473. Witherington R: Leukoplakia of the bladder: an 8-year followup, J Urol 112:600-602, 1974.
474. Widran J, Sanchez R, Gruhn J: Squamous metaplasia of the bladder: a study of 450 patients, J Urol 112:479-482, 1974.
475. Reece RW, Koontz WW, Jr: Leukoplakia of the urinary tract: a review, J Urol 114:165-171, 1975.
476. Morgan RJ, Cameron KM: Vesical leukoplakia, Br J Urol 52:96-100, 1980.
477. Benson RC, Jr, Swanson SK, Farrow GM: Relationship of leukoplakia to urothelial malignancy, J Urol 131:507-511, 1984.
478. Roehrborn CG, Teigland CM, Spence HM: Progression of leukoplakia of the bladder to squamous cell carcinoma 19 years after complete urinary diversion, J Urol 140:603-604, 1988.
479. Pearlman CK, Bobbitt RM: Carcinoma within a diverticulum of the bladder, J Urol 59:1127-1129, 1948.
480. Knappenberger ST, Uson AC, Melicow MM: Primary neoplasms occurring in vesical diverticula: a report of 18 cases, J Urol 83:153-158, 1960.
481. Fox M, Power RF, Bruce AW: Diverticulum of the bladder—presentation and evaluation of treatment of 115 cases, Br J Urol 34:286-298, 1962.
482. Montague DK, Boltuch RL: Primary neoplasms in vesical diverticula: report of 10 cases, J Urol 116:41-42, 1976.
483. Faysal MH, Freiha FS: Primary neoplasms in vesical diverticula: a report of 12 cases, Br J Urol 53:141-143, 1981.
484. Shirai T, Arai M, Sakata T et al: Primary carcinomas of urinary bladder diverticula, Acta Pathol Jpn 34:417-424, 1984.
485. Bjerklund Johansen TE: Primary neoplasms in vesical diverticula: report of two cases, Scand J Urol Nephrol 22:347-348, 1988.
486. Brenner DW, Yore LM, Schellhammer PF: Squamous cell carcinoma of bladder after successful intravesical therapy with bacillus Calmette-Guérin, Urology 34:93-95, 1989.
487. Stuart WT: Carcinoma of the bladder associated with exstrophy: report of a case and review of the literature, Va Med Mon 89:39-42, 1962.
488. Gupta S, Gupta IM: Ectopia vesicae complicated by squamous cell carcinoma: short case report, Br J Urol 48:244, 1976.
489. Shaw RE: Squamous cell carcinoma in a cyst of the urachus, Br J Urol 30:87-89, 1958.
490. Rankin FW, Parker B: Tumors of the urachus: with a report of seven cases, Surg Gynecol Obstet 42:19-27, 1926.
491. Lin R-Y, Rappoport AE, Deppisch LM et al: Squamous cell carcinoma of the urachus, J Urol 118:1066-1067, 1977.
492. Sheldon CA, Clayman RV, Gonzalez R et al: Malignant urachal lesions, J Urol 131:1-8, 1984.
493. Warren KS: The relevance of schistosomiasis, N Engl J Med 303:203-206, 1980.
494. Nash TE, Cheever AW, Ottesen EA et al: Schistosome infections in humans: perspectives and recent findings, Ann Int Med 97:740-754, 1982.
495. Smith JH, Christie JD: The pathobiology of *Schistosoma haematobium* infection in humans, Hum Pathol 17:333-345, 1986.
496. Wyatt JK, Craig I: Verrucous carcinoma of urinary bladder, Urology 16:97-99, 1980.
497. Holck S, Jorgensen L: Verrucous carcinoma of urinary bladder, Urology 22:435-437, 1983.
498. Walther M, O'Brien DP III, Birch HW: Condylomata acuminata and verrucous carcinoma of the bladder: case report and literature review, J Urol 135:362-365, 1986.
499. Boileau MA, Hui KKS, Cowan DF: Invasive verrucous carcinoma of urinary bladder treated by irradiation, Urology 27:56-59, 1986.
500. Del Mistro A, Koss LG, Braunstein J et al: Condylomata acuminata of the urinary bladder, Am J Surg Pathol 12:205-215, 1988.
501. Pettersson S, Hansson G, Blohme I: Condyloma acuminatum of the bladder, J Urol 115:535-536, 1976.
502. Keating MA, Young RH, Carr CP et al: Condyloma acuminatum of the bladder and ureter: case report and review of the literature, J Urol 133:465-467, 1985.
503. Shaaban AA, Tribukait B, Abdel-Fattah A et al: Characterization of squamous cell bladder tumors by flow cytometric deoxyribonucleic acid analysis: a report of 100 cases, J Urol 144:879-883, 1990.
504. Shaaban AA, Javadpour N, Tribukait B et al: Prognostic significance of flow-DNA analysis and cell surface isoantigens in carcinoma of bilharzial bladder, Urology 39:207-210, 1992.
505. Lundgren R, Elfving P, Heim S et al: A squamous cell bladder carcinoma with karyotypic abnormalities reminiscent of transitional cell carcinoma, J Urol 142:374-376, 1989.
506. Rundle JSH, Hart AJL, McGeorge A et al: Squamous cell carcinoma of bladder: a review of 114 patients, Br J Urol 54:522-526, 1982.
507. Patterson JM, Ray EH Jr, Mendiondo OA et al: A new treatment for invasive squamous cell bladder cancer: the NIGRO regimen: preoperative chemotherapy and radiation therapy, J Urol 140:379-380, 1988.
508. Jacobo E, Loening S, Schmidt JD et al: Primary adenocarcinoma of the bladder: a retrospective study of 20 patients, J Urol 117:54-56, 1977.
509. Thomas DG, Ward AM, Williams JL: A study of 52 cases of adenocarcinoma of the bladder, Br J Urol 43:4-15, 1971.
510. Wilson TG, Pritchett TR, Lieskovsky G et al: Primary adenocarcinoma of bladder, Urology 38:223-226, 1991.
511. Kamat MR, Kulkarni JN, Tongaonkar HB: Adenocarcinoma of the bladder: study of 14 cases and review of the literature, Br J Urol 68:254-257, 1991.
512. Nocks BN, Heney NM, Daly JJ: Primary adenocarcinoma of the urinary bladder, Urology 21:26-29, 1983.
513. Jones WA, Gibbons RP, Correa RJ Jr et al: Primary adenocarcinoma of bladder, Urology 15:119-122, 1980.
514. Kramer SA, Bredael JJ, Croker BP et al: Primary non-urachal adenocarcinoma of the bladder, J Urol 121:278-281, 1979.
515. Johnson DE, Hogan JM, Ayala AG: Primary adenocarcinoma of the urinary bladder, South Med J 65:527-530, 1972.
516. Abenoza P, Manivel C, Fraley EE: Primary adenocarcinoma of urinary bladder: clinicopathologic study of 16 cases, Urology 29:9-14, 1987.
517. Mostofi FK, Thomson RV, Dean AL Jr: Mucous adenocarcinoma of the urinary bladder, Cancer 8:741-758, 1955.
518. Fuselier HA Jr, Brannan W, Ochsner MG et al: Adenocarcinoma of the bladder as seen at Ochsner Medical Institutions, South Med J 71:804-806, 1978.

519. Anderström C, Johansson SL, von Schultz L: Primary adenocarcinoma of the urinary bladder: a clinicopathologic and prognostic study, Cancer 52:1273-1280, 1983.
520. Gill HS, Dhillon HK, Woodhouse CRJ: Adenocarcinoma of the urinary bladder, Br J Urol 64:138-142, 1989.
521. Wheeler JD, Hill WT: Adenocarcinoma involving the urinary bladder, Cancer 7:119-135, 1954.
522. Alroy J, Roganovic D, Banner BF et al: Primary adenocarcinomas of the human urinary bladder: histochemical, immunological and ultrastructural studies, Virchows Arch [A] 393:165-181, 1981.
523. Cornil C, Reynolds CT, Kickham CJE: Carcinoma of the urachus, J Urol 98:93-95, 1967.
524. Loening SA, Jacobo E, Hawtrey CE et al: Adenocarcinoma of the urachus, J Urol 119:68-71, 1978.
525. Kakizoe T, Matsumoto K, Andoh M et al: Adenocarcinoma of urachus: report of 7 cases and review of the literature, Urology 21:360-366, 1983.
526. Begg RC: The colloid adenocarcinomata of the bladder vault arising from the epithelium of the urachal canal: with a critical survey of the tumours of the urachus, Br J Surg 18:422-464, 1931.
527. Lucas DR, Lawrence WD, McDevitt WJ et al: Mucinous papillary adenocarcinoma of the bladder arising within a villous adenoma of urachal remnants: an immunohistochemical and ultrastructural study, J Urol Pathol 2:173-182, 1994.
528. Pallesen G: Neoplastic Paneth cells in adenocarcinoma of the urinary bladder: a first case report, Cancer 47:1834-1837, 1981.
529. Satake T, Matsuyama M: Neoplastic nature of argyrophil cells in urachal adenocarcinoma, Acta Pathol Jpn 36:1587-1592, 1986.
530. Grignon DJ, Ro JY, Ayala AG et al: Primary signet-ring cell carcinoma of the urinary bladder, Am J Clin Pathol 95:13-20, 1991.
531. Golz R, Schubert GE: Prostatic specific antigen: immunoreactivity in urachal remnants, J Urol 141:1480-1482, 1989.
532. Epstein JI, Kuhajda FP, Lieberman PH: Prostate-specific acid phosphatase immunoreactivity in adenocarcinomas of the urinary bladder, Hum Pathol 17:939-942, 1986.
533. Whitehead ED, Tessler AN: Carcinoma of the urachus, Br J Urol 43:468-476, 1971.
534. Johnson DE, Hodge GB, Abdul-Karim FW et al: Urachal carcinoma, Urology 26:218-221, 1985.
535. Ravi R, Shrivastava BR, Chandrasekhar GM et al: Adenocarcinoma of the urachus, J Surg Oncol 50:201-203, 1992.
536. Ohman U, von Garrelts B, Moberg A: Carcinoma of the urachus: review of the literature and report of two cases, Scand J Urol Nephrol 5:91-95, 1971.
537. Bullock PS, Thoni DE, Murphy WM: The significance of colonic mucosa (intestinal metaplasia) involving the urinary tract, Cancer 59:2086-2090, 1987.
538. Young RH, Parkhurst EC: Mucinous adenocarcinoma of bladder: case associated with extensive intestinal metaplasia of urothelium in patient with nonfunctioning bladder for twelve years, Urology 24:192-195, 1984.
539. Lin JI, Tseng CH, Choy C et al: Diffuse cystitis glandularis associated with adenocarcinomatous change, Urology 15:411-415, 1980.
540. Kittredge WE, Collett AJ, Morgan C Jr: Adenocarcinoma of the bladder associated with cystitis glandularis: a case report, J Urol 91:145-150, 1964.
541. Edwards PD, Hurm RA, Jaeschke WH: Conversion of cystitis glandularis to adenocarcinoma, J Urol 108:568-570, 1972.
542. Susmano D, Rubenstein AB, Dakin AR et al: Cystitis glandularis and adenocarcinoma of the bladder, J Urol 105:671-674, 1971.
543. Shaw JL, Gislason GJ, Imbriglia JE: Transition of cystitis glandularis to primary adenocarcinoma of the bladder, J Urol 79:815-822, 1958.
544. O'Kane HOJ, Megaw JMcI: Carcinoma in the exstrophic bladder, Br J Surg 55:631-635, 1968.
545. Sayegh ES, Ishak KG: Adenocarcinoma associated with schistosomiasis in an ectopia vesicae: report of a case, Br J Surg 44:426-429, 1957.
546. Davidson JA: Report of three cases of carcinoma occuring in exstrophy of the bladder, Urol Cutan Rev 54:206-208, 1950.
547. Staubitz WJ, Oberkircher OJ, Lent MH: Carcinoma in exstrophy of the bladder, N Y State J Med 56:386-390, 1956.
548. McCown PE: Carcinoma in exstrophy of the bladder, J Urol 43:533-542, 1940.
549. Scott LS, Sorbie C: The development of carcinoma in an ectopic bladder, Br J Urol 28:264-267, 1956.
550. Engel RM, Wilkinson HA: Bladder exstrophy, J Urol 104:699-704, 1970.
551. Goyanna R, Emmett JL, McDonald JR: Exstrophy of the bladder complicated by adenocarcinoma, J Urol 65:391-400, 1951.
552. McIntosh JF, Worley G Jr: Adenocarcinoma arising in exstrophy of the bladder: report of two cases and review of the literature, J Urol 73:820-829, 1955.
553. Wattenberg CA, Beare JB, Tormey AR, Jr: Exstrophy of the urinary bladder complicated by adenocarcinoma, J Urol 76:583-594, 1956.
554. Cordonnier JJ, Spjut HJ: Vesical exstrophy and transitional cell carcinoma: unusual longevity after ureterosigmoidostomy, J Urol 78:242-249, 1957.
555. Heyns CF, De Kock MLS, Kirsten PH et al: Pelvic lipomatosis associated with cystitis glandularis and adenocarcinoma of the bladder, J Urol 145:364-366, 1991.
556. Yalla SV, Ivker M, Burros HM et al: Cystitis glandularis with perivesical lipomatosis: frequent association of two unusual proliferative conditions, Urology 5:383-386, 1975.
557. Elem B, Alam SZ: Total intestinal metaplasia with focal adenocarcinoma in a Schistosoma-infested defunctioned urinary bladder, Br J Urol 56:331-343, 1984.
558. Khafagy MM, El-Bolkainy MN, Mansour MA: Carcinoma of the bilharzial urinary bladder, Cancer 30:150-159, 1972.
559. Yoshimura S, Ito Y: Malignant transformation of endometriosis of the urinary bladder: case report, Gann 42:2, 1951.
560. Chor PJ, Gaum LD, Young RH: Clear cell adenocarcinoma of the urinary bladder: report of a case of probable mullerian origin, Mod Pathol 6:225-228, 1993.
561. Vara AR, Ruzics EP, Moussabeck O et al: Endometrioid adenosarcoma of the bladder arising from endometriosis, J Urol 143:813-815, 1990.

562. Stitt RB, Colapinto V: Multiple simultaneous bladder malignancies: primary lymphosarcoma and adenocarcinoma, J Urol 96:733-736, 1966.
563. Trillo AA, Kuchler LL, Wood AC et al: Adenocarcinoma of the urinary bladder: histologic, cytologic and ultrastructural features in a case, Acta Cytol 25:285-290, 1981.
564. Badalament RA, Cibas ES, Reuter VE et al: Flow cytometric analysis of primary adenocarcinoma of the bladder, J Urol 137:1159-1162, 1987.
565. Grignon DJ, El-Naggar A, Ro JY et al: Deoxyribonucleic acid flow cytometry on primary adenocarcinoma of the bladder: an analysis of 36 cases, J Urol 142:1206-1210, 1989.
566. Song J, Farrow GM, Lieber MM: Primary adenocarcinoma of the bladder: favorable prognostic significance of deoxyribonucleic acid diploidy measured by flow cytometry, J Urol 144:1115-1118, 1990.
567. Davies G, Castro JE: Cystitis glandularis, Urology 10:128-129, 1977.
568. Aldridge KW, Burns JR, Singh B: Vesical endometriosis: a review and 2 case reports, J Urol 134:539-541, 1985.
569. Arap Neto W, Lopes RN, Cury M et al: Vesical endometriosis, Urology 24:271-274, 1984.
570. Bavendam TG, Kramolowsky EV, Mitros FA: Invasive adenocarcinoma of bladder response to cisplatinum, methotrexate, and vinblastine chemotherapy, Urology 33:53-56, 1989.
571. Saphir O: Signet-ring cell carcinoma of the urinary bladder, Am J Pathol 31:223-231, 1955.
572. Blute ML, Engen DE, Travis WD et al: Primary signet ring cell adenocarcinoma of the bladder, J Urol 141:17-21, 1989.
573. Choi H, Lamb S, Pintar K et al: Primary signet-ring cell carcinoma of the urinary bladder, Cancer 53:1985-1990, 1984.
574. DeFillipo N, Blute R, Klein LA: Signet-ring cell carcinoma of bladder: evaluation of three cases with review of literature, Urology 29:479-483, 1987.
575. Rosas-Uribe A, Luna MA: Primary signet ring cell carcinoma of the urinary bladder: report of two cases, Arch Pathol 88:294-297, 1969.
576. Bowlby LS, Smith ML: Signet-ring cell carcinoma of the urinary bladder: primary presentation as a Krukenberg tumor, Gynecol Oncol 25:376-381, 1986.
577. Braun EV, Majid A, Fayemi AO et al: Primary signet-ring cell carcinoma of the urinary bladder: review of the literature and report of a case, Cancer 47:1430-1435, 1981.
578. Corwin SH, Tassy F, Malament M et al: Rare signet ring cell variant of mucinous adenocarcinoma of the bladder, J Urol 106:697-700, 1971.
579. DeMay RM, Grathwohl MA: Signet-ring-cell (colloid) carcinoma of the urinary bladder: cytologic, histologic and ultrastructural findings in one case, Acta Cytol 29:132-136, 1985.
580. Deture FA, Dein R, Hackett RL et al: Primary signet ring cell carcinoma of bladder exemplifying vesical epithelium multipotentiality, Urology 6:240-244, 1975.
581. Hirasawa S, Oki M, Abe H et al: A case of signet ring cell carcinoma of the urinary bladder, Acta Urologica Jponica 31:2049-2053, 1985.
582. Jakse G, Schneider H-M, Jacobi GH: Urachal signet-ring cell carcinoma, a rare variant of vesical adenocarcinoma: incidence and pathological criteria, J Urol 120:764-766, 1978.
583. Kitamura H, Sumikawa T, Fukuoka H et al: Primary signet-ring cell carcinoma of the urinary bladder: report of two cases with histochemical studies, Acta Pathol Jpn 35:675-686, 1985.
584. Kondo A, Ogisu B, Mitsuya H: Signet-ring cell carcinoma involving the urinary bladder: report of a case and review of 21 cases, Urol Int 36:373-379, 1981.
585. Kums JJM, van Helsdingen PJRO: Signet-ring cell carcinoma of the bladder and prostate: report of 4 cases, Urol Int 40:116-119, 1985.
586. Ponz M, Luzuriaga J, Robles JE et al: Primary signet-ring cell carcinoma of the urinary bladder (linitis plastica), Eur Urol 11:212-214, 1985.
587. Poore E, Egbert B, Jahnke R et al: Signet ring cell adenocarcinoma of the bladder, Arch Pathol Lab Med 105:203-204, 1981.
588. Sagalowsky A, Donohue JP: Sixteen year survival with metastatic signet ring cell carcinoma, Urology 15:501-504, 1980.
589. Tanaka T, Kanai N, Sugie S et al: Primary signet-ring cell carcinoma of the urinary bladder, Pathol Res Pract 182:130-132, 1987.
590. Townsend GH, Sarma DP: Signet-ring cell carcinoma of the urinary bladder, J La State Med Soc 139:47-48, 1987.
591. Yoshida H, Iwata H, Ochi K et al: Primary signet-ring cell carcinoma of urinary bladder, Urology 17:481-483, 1981.
592. Young RH, Scully RE: Urothelial and ovarian carcinomas of identical cell types: problems in interpretation: a report of three cases and review of literature, Int J Gynecol Pathol 7:197-211, 1988.
593. Alonso-Correa M, Mompo-Sanchis JA, Jorda-Cuevas M et al: Signet ring cell adenocarcinoma of the urachus, Eur Urol 11:282-284, 1985.
594. Horne DW, Fauver HE: Primary signet-ring cell carcinoma of bladder, Urology 30:574-578, 1987.
595. Azadeh B, Vijayan P, Chejfec G: Linitis plastica-like carcinoma of the urinary bladder, Br J Urol 63:479-482, 1989.
596. Kumar PVN, Youssefi A, Ahmad A: Primary signet ring cell adenocarcinoma of the urinary bladder with calculi, Br J Urol 58:342-343, 1986.
597. Kanokogi M, Uematsu K, Kakudo K et al: Mesonephric adenocarcinoma of the urinary bladder: an autopsy case, J Surg Oncol 22:118-120, 1983.
598. Dow JA, Young JD Jr: Mesonephric adenocarcinoma of the bladder, J Urol 100:466-469, 1968.
599. Skor AB, Warren MM: Mesonephric adenocarcinoma of bladder, Urology 10:64-65, 1977.
600. Schultz RE, Bloch MJ, Tomaszewski JE et al: Mesonephric adenocarcinoma of the bladder, J Urol 132:263-265, 1984.
601. Young RH, Scully RE: Clear cell adenocarcinoma of the bladder and urethra: a report of three cases and review of the literature, Am J Surg Pathol 9:816-826, 1985.
602. Goldstein AG: Metastatic carcinoma to the bladder, J Urol 98:209-215, 1967.
603. World Health Organization: The World Health Organization histological typing of lung tumours, ed 2, Am J Clin Pathol 77:123-136, 1982.
604. Aoyama H, Yoshida K, Kondo T et al: Primary carcinoid tumor of the urinary bladder (report of a case), Jpn J Urol 69:124-133, 1978.

605. Abenoza P, Manivel C, Sibley RK: Adenocarcinoma with neuroendocrine differentiation of the urinary bladder: clinicopathologic, immunohistochemical and ultrastructural study, Arch Pathol Lab Med 110:1062-1066, 1986.
606. Davis MP, Murthy MSN, Simon J et al: Successful management of small cell carcinoma of the bladder with cisplatin and etoposide, J Urol 142:817, 1989.
607. Oesterling JE, Brendler CB, Burgers JK et al: Advanced small cell carcinoma of the bladder: successful treatment with combined radical cystoprostatectomy and adjuvant methotrexate, vinblastine, doxorubicin and cisplatin chemotherapy, Cancer 65:1928-1936, 1990.
608. Ibrahim NBN, Briggs JC, Corbishley CM: Extrapulmonary oat cell carcinoma, Cancer 54:1645-1661, 1984.
609. Davis BH, Ludwig ME, Cole SR et al: Small cell neuroendocrine carcinoma of the urinary bladder: report of three cases with ultrastructural analysis, Ultrastruct Pathol 4:197-204, 1983.
610. Kim CK, Lin JI, Tseng CH: Small cell carcinoma of urinary bladder: ultrastructural study, Urology 24:384-386, 1984.
611. Partanen S, Asikainen U: Oat cell carcinoma of the urinary bladder with ectopic adrenocorticotropic hormone production, Hum Pathol 16:313-315, 1985.
612. Blomjous CEM, Vos W, Schipper NW et al: Morphometric and flow cytometric analysis of small cell undifferentiated carcinoma of the bladder, J Clin Pathol 42:1032-1039, 1989.
613. Reyes CV, Soneru I: Small cell carcinoma of the urinary bladder with hypercalcemia, Cancer 56:2530-2533, 1985.
614. Cramer SF, Aikawa M, Cebelin M: Neurosecretory granules in small cell invasive carcinoma of the urinary bladder, Cancer 47:724-730, 1981.
615. Williams MR, Dunn M, Ansell ID: Primary oat cell carcinoma of the urinary bladder, Br J Urol 58:225, 1986.
616. Podesta AH, True LD: Small cell carcinoma of the bladder: report of five cases with immunohistochemistry and review of the literature with evaluation of prognosis according to stage, Cancer 64:710-714, 1989.
617. Mills SE, Wolfe JT III, Weiss MA et al: Small cell undifferentiated carcinoma of the urinary bladder: a light-microscopic, immunocytochemical, and ultrastructural study of 12 cases, Am J Surg Pathol 11:606-617, 1987.
618. Ordóñez NG, Khorsand J, Ayala AG et al: Oat cell carcinoma of the urinary tract: an immunohistochemical and electron microscopic study, Cancer 58:2519-2530, 1986.
619. Blomjous CEM, Vos W, De Voogt HJ et al: Small cell carcinoma of the urinary bladder: a clinicopathologic, morphometric, immunohistochemical, and ultrastructural study of 18 cases, Cancer 64:1347-1357, 1989.
620. Swanson PE, Brooks R, Pearse H et al: Small cell carcinoma of urinary bladder, Urology 32:558-563, 1988.
621. Golomb J, Klutke CG, Lewin KJ et al: Bladder neoplasms associated with augmentation cystoplasty: report of 2 cases and literature review, J Urol 142:377-380, 1989.
622. Yu DS, Chang SY, Wang J et al: Small cell carcinoma of the urinary tract, Br J Urol 66:590-595, 1990.
623. Hobarth K, Wrba F, Hofbauer J: Primary small cell carcinoma of the urinary bladder, Urol Int 48:95-98, 1992.
624. Cheng C, Nicholson A, Lowe DG et al: Oat cell carinoma of urinary bladder, Urology 34:504-507, 1992.
625. Lertprasertsuke N, Tsutsumi Y: Neuroendocrine carcinoma of the urinary bladder: case report and review of the literature, Jpn J Clin Oncol 21:203-210, 1991.
626. Cassidy J, Kaye SB: An unusual case of haematuria, Eur J Cancer 29A:906-907, 1993.
627. Angulo JC, Lopez JI, Sanchez-Chapado M et al: Small cell carcinoma of the urinary bladder: a report of two cases with complete remission and a comprehensive literature review with emphasis on therapeutic decisions, J Urol Pathol, 1996 (in press).
628. Grignon DJ, Ro JY, Ayala AG et al: Small cell carcinoma of the urinary bladder: a clinicopathologic analysis of 22 cases, Cancer 69:527-536, 1992.
629. Colby TV: Carcinoid tumor of the bladder, Arch Pathol Lab Med 104:199-200, 1980.
630. Walker BF, Someren A, Kennedy JC et al: Primary carcinoid tumor of the urinary bladder, Arch Pathol Lab Med 116:1217-1220, 1992.
631. Têtu B, Ro JY, Ayala AG et al: Small cell carcinoma of the prostate. Part I: a clinicopathologic study of 20 cases, Cancer 59:1803-1809, 1987.
632. Coltart RS, Stewart S, Brown CH: Small cell carcinoma of the bronchus: a rare cause of haematuria from a metastasis in the urinary bladder, J Royal Soc Med 78:1053-1054, 1985.
633. Wheelock MC: Sarcoma of the urinary bladder, J Urol 48:628-634, 1942.
634. Su C-T, Prince CL: Melanoma of the bladder, J Urol 87:365-367, 1962.
635. Ainsworth AM, Clark WH Jr, Mastrangelo M et al: Primary malignant melanoma of the urinary bladder, Cancer 37:1928-1936, 1976.
636. Willis AJ, Huang AH, Carroll P: Primary melanoma of the bladder: a case report and review, J Urol 123:278-281, 1980.
637. Anichkov NM, Nikonov AA: Primary malignant melanomas of the bladder, J Urol 128:813-815, 1982.
638. Ironside JW, Timperley WR, Madden JW et al: Primary melanoma of the urinary bladder presenting with intracerebral metastases, Br J Urol 57:593-594, 1985.
639. Goldschmidt SJ, Py JM, Kostakopoulos A et al: Primary malignant melanomas of the urinary bladder, Br J Urol 61:359-366, 1988.
640. Van Ahlen H, Nicolas V, Lenz W et al: Primary melanoma of urinary bladder, Urology 40:550-554, 1992.
641. Kojima T, Tanaka T, Yoshimi N et al: Primary malignant melanoma of the urinary bladder, Arch Pathol Lab Med 116:1213-1216, 1992.
642. Stein DS, Kendall AR: Malignant melanoma of the genitourinary tract, J Urol 132:859-868, 1984.
643. Zimmerman IJ, Biron RE, MacMahon HE: Pheochromocytoma of the urinary bladder, N Engl J Med 249:25-26, 1953.
644. Schutz W, Vogel E: Pheochromocytoma of the urinary bladder—a case report and review of the literature, Urol Int 39:250-255, 1984.
645. Davaris P, Petraki K, Arvantis D et al: Urinary bladder paraganglioma (U.B.P), Pathol Res Pract 181:101-105, 1986.
646. Kliewer KE, Cochran AJ: A review of the histology, ultrastructure, immunohistology, and molecular biology of extra-adrenal paragangliomas, Arch Pathol Lab Med 113:1209-1218, 1989.

647. Heyman J, Cheung Y, Ghali V et al: Bladder pheochromocytoma: evaluation with magnetic resonance imaging, J Urol 141:1424-1426, 1989.
648. Thrasher JB, Rajan RR, Perez LM et al: Pheochromocytoma of urinary bladder: contemporary methods of diagnosis and treatment options, Urology 41:435-439, 1993.
649. Leestma JE, Price EB Jr: Paraganglioma of the urinary bladder, Cancer 28:1063-1073, 1971.
650. Rode J, Bentley A, Parkinson C: Paraganglion cells of urinary bladder and prostate: potential diagnostic problem, J Clin Pathol 43:13-16, 1990.
651. Burton EM, Schellhammer PF, Weaver DL et al: Paraganglioma of urinary bladder in a patient with neurofibromatosis, Urology 27:550-552, 1986.
652. Lam KY, Chan ACL: Paraganglioma of the urinary bladder: an immunohistochemical study and report of an unusual association with intestinal carcinoid, Aust N Z J Surg 63:740-745, 1993.
653. Misawa T, Shibasaki Y, Toshima S et al: A case of pheochromocytoma of the urinary bladder in a long-term hemodialysis patient, Nephron 64:443-446, 1993.
654. Whalen RK, Althausen AF, Daniels GH: Extra-adrenal pheochromocytoma, J Urol 147:1-10, 1992.
655. Nomura S, Kinoshita Y, Takeda M et al: A case of vesical paraganglioma behind the symphysis pubis, J Urol 146:830-832, 1991.
656. Hurwitz R, Fitzpatrick T, Ackerman I et al: A neuro-ectodermal tumor in the bladder, J Urol 124:417-421, 1980.
657. Kliewer KE, Wen D-R, Cancilla PA et al: Paragangliomas: assessment of prognosis by histologic, immunohistochemical, and ultrastructural techniques, Hum Pathol 20:29-39, 1989.
658. Hamid Q, Varndell IM, Ibrahim NB et al: Extraadrenal paragangliomas: an immunocytochemical and ultrastructural report, Cancer 60:1776-1781, 1987.
659. Moyana TN, Kontozoglou T: Urinary bladder paragangliomas: an immunohistochemical study, Arch Pathol Lab Med 112:70-72, 1988.
660. Lunde S, Nesland JM, Holm R et al: A urinary bladder tumor in a 65-year old man, Ultrastruct Pathol 11:79-82, 1987.
661. Schmid KW, Schroder S, Dockhorn-Dworniczak B et al: Immunohistochemical demonstration of chromogranin A, chromogranin B, and secretogranin II in extra-adrenal paragangliomas, Mod Pathol 7:347-353, 1994.
662. Brown WJ, Barajas L, Waisman J et al: Ultrastructural and biochemical correlates of adrenal and extra-adrenal pheochromocytoma, Cancer 29:744-759, 1972.
663. Yoffa DE, Withycombe JFR: Bladder—phaeochromocytoma metastases, Lancet 2:422, 1967.
664. Maddocks RA, Fagan WT: Paraganglioma of bladder with recurrence ten years later, Urology 7:430-432, 1976.
665. Djewitzki WS: Primary chorionepithelioma of the urinary bladder in a male: report of a case, Virchows Archiv 178:451-464, 1904.
666. Yokoyama S, Hayashida Y, Nagahama J et al: Primary and metaplastic choriocarcinoma of the bladder: a report of two cases, Acta Cytol 36:176-182, 1992.
667. Cho JH, Yu E, Kim KH et al: Primary choriocarcinoma of the urinary bladder, J Korean Med Sci 7:369-372, 1992.
668. Campo E, Algaba F, Palacin A et al: Placental proteins in high-grade urothelial neoplasms: an immunohistochemical study of human chorionic gonadotropin, human placental lactogen, and pregnancy specific beta-1-glycoprotein, Cancer 63:2497-2504, 1989.
669. Hyman A, Leiter HE: Extratesticular chorioepithelioma in a male, probably primary in the urinary bladder, J Mt Sinai Hosp 10:212, 1943.
670. Ainsworth RW, Gresham GA: Primary choriocarcinoma of the urinary bladder in a male, J Path Bacteriol 79:185-192, 1960.
671. Kawamura J, Machida S, Yoshida O et al: Bladder carcinoma associated with ectopic production of gonadotropin, Cancer 42:2773-2780, 1978.
672. Hattori M, Yoshimoto Y, Matsukura S et al: Qualitative and quantitative analyses of human chorionic gonadotropin and its subunits produced by malignant tumors, Cancer 46:355-361, 1980.
673. Turner AG, Dennis PM: Primary choriocarcinoma of the bladder evolving from a transitional cell carcinoma, J Clin Pathol 37:503-505, 1984.
674. Dexeus FH, Logothetis C, Hossan E et al: Carcinoembryonic antigen and beta-human chorionic gonadotropin as serum markers for advanced urothelial malignancies, J Urol 136:403-407, 1986.
675. Yamase HT, Wurzel RS, Nieh PT et al: Immunohistochemical demonstration of human chorionic gonadotropin in tumors of the urinary bladder, Ann Clin Lab Sci 15:414-417, 1985.
676. Wurzel RS, Yamase HT, Nieh PT: Ectopic production of human chorionic gonadotropin by poorly differentiated transitional cell tumors of the urinary tract, J Urol 137:502-504, 1987.
677. Shah VM, Newman J, Crocker J et al: Ectopic ß-human chorionic gonadotropin production by bladder urothelial neoplasia, Arch Pathol Lab Med 110:107-111, 1986.
678. Martin JE, Jenkins BJ, Zuk RJ et al: Human chorionic gonadotropin expression and histological findings as predictors of response to radiotherapy in carcinoma of the bladder, Virchows Arch [A] 414:273-277, 1989.
679. Seidal T, Breborowicz J, Malmstrom PU et al: Immunoreactivity to human chorionic gonadotropin in urothelial carcinoma: correlation with tumor grade, stage, and progression, J Urol Pathol 1:397-410, 1993.
680. Tungekar MF, Abdul-Sattar S, Al Adnani MS: Expression of chorionic gonadotropin by Schistosomiasis-associated squamous carcinoma of bladder, Eur Urol 14:30-33, 1988.
681. Cauffield EW: Dermoid cysts of the bladder, J Urol 75:801-804, 1956.
682. Lazebnik J, Kamhi D: A case of vesical teratoma associated with vesical stones and diverticulum, J Urol 85:796-799, 1961.
683. Taylor G, Jordan M, Churchill B et al: Yolk sac tumor of the bladder, J Urol 129:591-594, 1983.
684. Jacobs MA, Bavendam TG, Leach GE: Bladder leiomyoma, Urology 34:56-57, 1989.
685. Mintz ER: Pedunculated neurofibroma of the bladder, J Urol 43:268-274, 1940.
686. Bolkier M, Ginesin Y, Lichtig C et al: Lymphangioma of bladder, J Urol 129:1049, 1983.

687. Karol JB, Eason AA, Tanagho EA: Fibrous histiocytoma of bladder, Urology 10:593-595, 1977.
688. Egawa S, Uchida T, Koshiba K et al: Malignant fibrous histiocytoma of the bladder with focal rhabdoid tumor differentiation, J Urol 151:154-156, 1994.
689. Wyman HE, Chappell BS, Jones WR Jr: Ganglioneuroma of bladder: report of a case, J Urol 63:526-532, 1950.
690. Knoll LD, Segura JW, Scheithauer BW: Leiomyoma of the bladder, J Urol 136:906-908, 1986.
691. Van Regemorter G, Germeau F: Leiomyoma of the bladder, Eur Urol 10:210-211, 1984.
692. Bollinger B, Mikkelsen AL: Leiomyoma of the urinary bladder, Urol Int 40:43-44, 1985.
693. McLucas B, Stein JJ: Bladder leiomyoma: a rare cause of pelvic pain, Am J Obstet Gynecol 153:896, 1985.
694. Bazeed MA, Aboulenien H: Leiomyoma of the bladder causing urethral and unilateral ureteral obstruction: a case report, J Urol 140:143-144, 1988.
695. Aneiros J, Camara M, O'Valle F et al: An ultrastructural analysis of vascular leiomyoma of the bladder, Urol Int 43:185-187, 1988.
696. Bramwell SP, Pitts J, Goudie SE et al: Giant leiomyoma of the bladder, Br J Urol 60:178-184, 1987.
697. Kabalin JN, Freiha FS, Neibel JD: Leiomyoma of bladder, Urology 35:210-212, 1990.
698. Mutchler RW, Gorder JL: Leiomyoma of the bladder in a child, Br J Radiol 45:538-540, 1972.
699. Thompson IM, Coppridge AJ: Bladder sarcoma, J Urol 82:329-332, 1959.
700. O'Connell K, Edson M: Leiomyoma of bladder, Urology 6:114-115, 1975.
701. Katz RB, Waldbaum RS: Benign mesothelial tumor of bladder, Urology 5:236-238, 1975.
702. Belis JA, Post GJ, Rochman SC et al: Genitourinary leiomyomas, Urology 13:424-429, 1979.
703. Lake MH, Kossow AS, Bokinsky G: Leiomyoma of the bladder and urethra, J Urol 125:742-743, 1981.
704. Chavez CA, Neto M: Multiple leiomyomata of the urinary bladder, J Kans Med Soc 85:298-299, 1984.
705. Mills SE, Bova SG, Wick MR et al: Leiomyosarcoma of the urinary bladder, Am J Surg Pathol 13:480-489, 1989.
706. Young RH, Proppe KH, Dikersin GR et al: Myxoid leiomyosarcoma of the urinary bladder, Arch Pathol Lab Med 111:359-362, 1987.
707. Jahn H, Nissen HM: Haemangioma of the urinary tract: review of the literature, Br J Urol 68:113-117, 1991.
708. Hockley NM, Bihrle R, Bennett RM III et al: Congenital genitourinary hemangiomas in a patient with the Klippel-Trenaunay syndrome: management with the neodymium: YAG laser, J Urol 141:940-941, 1989.
709. Klein TW, Kaplan GW: Klippel-Trenaunay syndrome associated with urinary tract hemangiomas, J Urol 114:596-600, 1975.
710. Hall BD: Bladder hemangiomas in Klippel-Trenaunay-Weber syndrome, N Engl J Med 2885:1032-1033, 1971.
711. Esguerra A, Carvajal A, Mouton H: Pelvic arteriography in the diagnosis of hemangioma of the bladder, J Urol 109:609-611, 1973.
712. Pakter R, Nussbaum A, Fishman EK: Hemangioma of the bladder: sonographic and computerized tomography findings, J Urol 140:601-602, 1988.
713. Hendry WF, Vinnicombe J: Hemangioma of bladder in children and young adults, Br J Urol 43:309-316, 1971.
714. Stroup RM, Chang YC: Angiosarcoma of the bladder: a case report, J Urol 137:984-985, 1987.
715. Schwartz RA, Kardashian JF, McNutt NS et al: Cutaneous angiosarcoma resembling anaplastic Kaposi's sarcoma in a homosexual man, Cancer 51:721-726, 1983.
716. Prout MN, Davis HL Jr: Hemangiopericytomas of the bladder after polyvinyl alcohol exposure, Cancer 39:1328-1330, 1977.
717. Sutton R, Hopper IP, Munson KW: Haemangiopericytoma of the bladder, Br J Urol 63:548-554, 1989.
718. Fuleihan FM, Cordonnier JJ: Hemangioma of the bladder: report of a case and review of the literature, J Urol 102:581-585, 1969.
719. Susset J, Korzinstone C, Masse S: Cavernous hemangioma of vesical neck, Urology 17:75-76, 1981.
720. Leonard MP, Nickel JC, Morales A: Cavernous hemangiomas of the bladder in the pediatric age group, J Urol 140:1503-1504, 1988.
721. Gottesman JE, Seale RH: Cavernous haemangioma of the bladder, Br J Urol 55:450-451, 1983.
722. Ogawa A, Watanabe K: Genitourinary neurofibromatosis in a child presenting with an enlarged penis and scrotum, J Urol 135:755-757, 1986.
723. Kramer SA, Barrett DM, Utz DC: Neurofibromatosis of the bladder in children, J Urol 126:693-694, 1981.
724. Winfield HN, Catalona WJ: An isolated plexiform neurofibroma of the bladder, J Urol 134:542-543, 1985.
725. Cameron KM: Neurofibromatosis of the bladder, Br J Urol 36:77-81, 1964.
726. Gonzalez-Angulo A, Reyes HA: Neurofibromatosis involving the lower urinary tract, J Urol 89:804-811, 1963.
727. Daneman A, Grattan-Smith P: Neurofibromatosis involving the lower urinary tract in children: a report of three cases and review of the literature, Pediatr Radiol 4:161-166, 1976.
728. Rink RC, Mitchell ME: Genitourinary neurofibromatosis in childhood, J Urol 130:1176-1179, 1983.
729. Ro JY, Ayala AG, Ordóñez NG et al: Pseudosarcomatous fibromyxoid tumor of the urinary bladder, Am J Clin Pathol 86:583-590, 1986.
730. Jones EC, Clement PB, Young RH: Inflammatory pseudotumor of the urinary bladder, Am J Surg Pathol 17:264-274, 1994.
731. Ro JY, El-Naggar AK, Amin MB et al: Pseudosarcomatous fibromyxoid tumor of the urinary bladder and prostate, Hum Pathol 24:1203-1210, 1993.
732. Ross JA: A case of sarcoma of the urinary bladder in von Recklinghausen's disease, Br J Urol 29:121-126, 1957.
733. Borden TA, Shrader AD: Neurofibromatosis of bladder in a child: unusual cause of enuresis, Urology 15:155-158, 1980.
734. Torres H, Bennett MJ: Neurofibromatosis of the bladder: case report and review of the literature, J Urol 96:910-912, 1966.
735. Clark SS, Marlett MM, Prudencio RF et al: Neurofibromatosis of the bladder in children: case report and literature review, J Urol 118:654-656, 1977.
736. Ravich A, Stout AP, Ravich RA: Malignant granular cell myoblastoma involving the urinary bladder, Ann Surg 121:361-372, 1945.

737. Andersen R, Hoeg K: Myoblastoma of the bladder neck: report of a case, Br J Urol 33:76-126, 1961.
738. Marsh RJ, Ceccarelli FE: Ten-year analysis of primary bladder tumors at Brooke General Hospital, J Urol 91:530-532, 1964.
739. Seery WH: Granular cell myoblastoma of the bladder: report of a case, J Urol 100:735-737, 1968.
740. Okuda N, Ohkawa T, Nakamura T et al: Granular cell myoblastoma of the urinary bladder: report of a case, Jpn J Urol 15:505-513, 1969.
741. Christ ML, Ozzello L: Myogenous origin of a granular cell tumor of the urinary bladder, Am J Clin Pathol 56:736-749, 1971.
742. Mizutani S, Okuda N, Sonoda T: Granular cell myoblastoma of the bladder: report of an additional case, J Urol 110:403-405, 1973.
743. Mouradian JA, Coleman JW, McGovern JH et al: Granular cell tumor (myoblastoma) of the bladder, J Urol 112:343-345, 1974.
744. Fletcher MS, Aker M, Hill JT et al: Granular cell myoblastoma of the bladder, Br J Urol 57:109-110, 1985.
745. Fisher ER, Wechsler H: Granular cell myoblastoma—a misnomer: electron microscopic and histochemical evidence concerning its Schwann cell derivation and nature (granular cell schwannoma), Cancer 15:936-957, 1962.
746. Stefansson K, Wollmann RL: S-100 protein in granular cell tumors (granular cell myoblastomas), Cancer 49:1834-1838, 1982.
747. Kaplan WE, Firlit CF, Berger RM: Genitourinary rhabdomyosarcoma, J Urol 130:116-119, 1983.
748. Dehner LP: Pathology of the urinary bladder in children. In Young RH (ed): Pathology of the urinary bladder, New York, 1989, Churchill Livingstone.
749. Hellstrom HR, Fisher ER: Embryonal rhabdomyosarcoma of the bladder in the aged, J Urol 86:336-339, 1961.
750. Evans AT, Bell TE: Rhabdomyosarcoma of the bladder in adult patients: report of three cases, J Urol 94:573-575, 1965.
751. Bhansali SK: Sarcoma botryoides of the bladder in infancy and childhood, J Urol 87:871-875, 1962.
752. McDougal WS, Persky L: Rhabdomyosarcoma of the bladder and prostate in children, J Urol 124:882-885, 1980.
753. Hays DM, Raney RB Jr, Lawrence W Jr et al: Bladder and prostatic tumors in the Intergroup Rhabdomyosarcoma Study (IRS-1): results of therapy, Cancer 50:1472-1482, 1982.
754. Hejtmancik JH, Klatt WW: Co-existing carcinoma and sarcoma of the bladder, J Urol 84:320-321, 1960.
755. Bohne AW, Urwiller RD, Pantos TG: Leiomyosarcoma of the urinary bladder with review of the literature, Henry Ford Hosp Med Bull 10:445-448, 1962.
756. Uehling D, Frable WJ: Myosarcoma of the bladder: report of two cases, J Urol 91:354-356, 1964.
757. Reeves JF Jr, Powell EB, Powell NB: Leiomyosarcoma of the bladder: case report with autopsy, J Urol 97:486-489, 1967.
758. Mackenzie AR, Whitmore WF Jr, Melamed MR: Myosarcomas of the bladder and prostate, Cancer 22:833-844, 1968.
759. Mackenzie AR, Sharma TC, Whitmore WF Jr et al: Nonextirpative treatment of myosarcomas of the bladder and prostate, Cancer 28:329-334, 1971.
760. Tara HH, Mentus NL: Leiomyosarcoma of urinary bladder, Urology 2:460-462, 1973.
761. Narayana AS, Loening S, Weimar GW et al: Sarcoma of the bladder and prostate, J Urol 119:72-76, 1978.
762. Weitzner S: Leiomyosarcoma of urinary bladder in children, Urology 12:450-452, 1978.
763. Papacharalambous AN, Pavlakis AJ: Leiomyosarcoma of the bladder, Br J Urol 51:321, 1979.
764. Wilson TM, Fauver HE, Weigel JW: Leiomyosarcoma of urinary bladder, Urology 13:565-567, 1979.
765. Savir A, Meiraz D: Malignant mesodermal (mesenchymal) tumors of bladder, Urology 16:307-309, 1980.
766. Holmquist ND: Detection of urinary cancer with urinalysis sediment, J Urol 123:188-189, 1980.
767. Patterson DE, Barrett DM: Leiomyosarcoma of urinary bladder, Urology 21:367-369, 1983.
768. Rowland RG, Eble JN: Bladder leiomyosarcoma and pelvic fibroblastic tumor folowing cyclophosphamide therapy, J Urol 130:344-346, 1983.
769. Swartz DA, Johnson DE, Ayala AG et al: Bladder leiomyosarcoma: a review of 10 cases with 5-year followup, J Urol 133:200-202, 1985.
770. Seo IS, Clark SA, McGovern FD et al: Leimyosarcoma of the urinary bladder 13 years after cyclophosphamide therapy for Hodgkin's disease, Cancer 55:1597-1603, 1985.
771. Chen KT: Coexisting leiomyosarcoma and transitional cell carcinoma of the urinary bladder, J Surg Oncol 33:36-37, 1986.
772. Ahlering TE, Weintraub P, Skinner DG: Management of adult sarcomas of the bladder and prostate, J Urol 140:1397-1399, 1988.
773. Thrasher JB, Miller GJ, Wettlaufer JN: Bladder leiomyosarcoma following cyclophosphamide therapy for lupus nephritis, J Urol 143:119-121, 1990.
774. Ozteke O, Demirel A, Aydin NE et al: Bladder leiomyosarcoma: report of three cases, Int Urol Nephrol 24:393-396, 1992.
775. Brown HE: Leiomyosarcoma of the bladder: followup report of two cases with 4 and 10 years' survival, J Urol 94:247-251, 1965.
776. Tripathi VN, Dick VS: Primary sarcoma of the urogenital system in adults, J Urol 101:898-904, 1969.
777. Jones EC, Young RH: Nonneoplastic and neoplastic spindle cell proliferations and mixed tumors of the urinary bladder, J Urol Pathol 2:105-134, 1994.
778. Nochomovitz LE, Orenstein JM: Inflammatory pseudotumor of the urinary bladder—possible relationship to nodular fasciitis, Am J Surg Pathol 9:366-373, 1985.
779. Wick MR, Brown BA, Young RH et al: Spindle cell proliferations of the urinary tract, Am J Surg Pathol 12:379-389, 1988.
780. Proppe KH, Scully RE, Rosai J: Postoperative spindle cell nodules of genitourinary tract resembling sarcomas, Am J Surg Pathol 8:101-108, 1984.
781. Vekemans K, Vanneste A, Van Oyen P et al: Postoperative spindle cell nodule of bladder, Urology 35:342-344, 1990.
782. Huang W-L, Ro JY, Grignon DJ et al: Postoperative spindle cell nodule of the prostate and bladder, J Urol 143:824-826, 1990.

783. Anderson JD, Scardino P, Smith RB: Inflammatory fibrous histiocytoma presenting as a renal pelvic and bladder mass, J Urol 118:470-471, 1977.
784. Henriksen OB, Mogensen P, Engelholm AJ: Inflammatory fibrous histiocytoma of the urinary bladder: clinicopathological report of a case, Acta Pathol Microbiol Immunol Scand 90:333-337, 1982.
785. McCormick SR, Dodds PR, Kraus PA et al: Nonepithelial neoplasms arising within vesical diverticula, Urology 25:405-408, 1985.
786. Turner AG: Malignant fibrous histiocytoma involving the bladder, Br J Urol 57:237-247, 1985.
787. Goodman AJ, Greany MG: Malignant fibrous histiocytoma of the bladder, Br J Urol 57:106-107, 1985.
788. Harrison GSM: Malignant fibrous histiocytoma of the bladder, Br J Urol 58:457-458, 1986.
789. Oesterling JE, Epstein JI, Brendler CB: Myxoid malignant fibrous histiocytoma of the bladder, Cancer 66:1836-1842, 1990.
790. Song T, Grignon DJ, Sakr W et al: Primary malignant fibrous histiocytoma of the urinary bladder: a case report and review of the literature, J Urol Pathol 1996 (in press).
791. Kaczmarek A: Unusual complication of foreign body in the bladder, Br J Urol 57:106-115, 1985.
792. Young RH, Rosenberg AE: Osteosarcoma of the urinary bladder: report of a case and review of the literature, Cancer 59:174-178, 1987.
793. Beltrami CA, Fabris G, Siciliano C et al: Osteocondrosarcoma vescicale primitivo, Riv Pathol Clin Sper 11:213-221, 1972.
794. Chitiyo ME: Primary osteogenic sarcoma of the urinary bladder, J Pathol 111:53-56, 1973.
795. Murat J, Huten N, Crassas Y: Sarcome osteogénique de la vessie, J Chir (Paris) 109:327-332, 1975.
796. Berenson RJ, Flynn S, Freiha FS et al: Primary osteogenic sarcoma of the bladder: case report and review of the literature, Cancer 57:350-355, 1986.
797. Terada Y, Saito I, Morohoshi T et al: Malignant mesenchymoma of the bladder, Cancer 60:858-863, 1987.
798. Jones HM, Ross CF: Osteogenic leiomyosarcoma of the bladder, Br J Surg 38:242-245, 1950.
799. Suster S, Huszar M, Bubis JJ et al: Fibrosarcoma of the urinary bladder: study of a case showing extensive chondroid differentiation, Arch Pathol Lab Med 111:767-770, 1987.
800. Enzinger FM, Weiss SW: Soft tissue tumors, ed 3, St. Louis, 1995, Mosby–Year Book.
801. Stout AP: Mesenchymoma, the mixed tumor of mesenchymal derivatives, Ann Surg 127:278-290, 1948.
802. Baglio CM, Crowson CN: Hemangiopericytoma of urachus: report of a case, J Urol 91:660-662, 1964.
803. Baumgartner G, Gaeta J, Wajsman Z et al: Hemangiopericytoma of the urinary bladder: a case report and review of the literature, J Surg Oncol 8:281-286, 1976.
804. Burgess NA, Hudd C, Matthews PN: Two cases of haemangiopericytoma, Br J Urol 71:238-239, 1993.
805. Rosi P, Selli C, Carini M et al: Myxoid liposarcoma of the bladder, J Urol 130:560-561, 1983.
806. Harris M, Eyden BP, Joglekar VM: Rhabdoid tumour of the bladder: a histological, ultrastructural and immunohistochemical study, Histopathology 11:1083-1092, 1987.
807. Carter RL, McCarthy KP, Al-Sam SZ et al: Malignant rhabdoid tumor of the bladder with immunohistochemical and ultrastructural evidence suggesting histiocytic origin, Histopathology 14:179-190, 1989.
808. McBride JA, Ro JY, Hicks J et al: Malignant rhabdoid tumor of the bladder in an adolescent: case report and discussion of extrarenal rhabdoid tumor, J Urol Pathol 2:255-263, 1994.
809. Sotelo-Avila C, Gonzalez-Crussi F, deMello DE et al: Renal and extrarenal rhabdoid tumors in children: a clinicopathologic study of 14 patients, Semin Diagn Pathol 3:151-163, 1986.
810. Tsuneyoshi M, Daimaru Y, Hashimoto H et al: The existence of rhabdoid cells in specified soft tissue sarcoma, Virchows Arch [A] 411:509-514, 1987.
811. Givler RL: Involvement of the bladder in leukemia and lymphoma, J Urol 105:667-670, 1971.
812. Sufrin G, Keogh B, Moore RH et al: Secondary involvement of the bladder in malignant lymphoma, J Urol 118:251-253, 1977.
813. Freeman C, Berg JW, Cutler ST: Occurrence and prognosis of extranodal lymphomas, Cancer 29:252-260, 1972.
814. Ohsawa M, Aozasa K, Horiuchi K et al: Malignant lymphoma of bladder: report of three cases and review of the literature, Cancer 72:1969-1974, 1993.
815. Aigen AB, Phillips M: Primary malignant lymphoma of urinary bladder, Urology 28:235-237, 1986.
816. Abraham NZ Jr, Maher TJ, Hutchison RE: Extra-nodal monocytoid B-cell lymphoma of the urinary bladder, Mod Pathol 6:145-149, 1993.
817. Salem YH, Rushton HG: A case of primary malignant lymphoma of the bladder in childhood, J Urol 150:1469-1471, 1993.
818. Borski AA: Lymphosarcoma of the bladder, J Urol 48:551-554, 1960.
819. Makinen J, Alfthan O, Vuori J: Malignant lymphoma of the urinary bladder: a report of 2 cases, Eur Urol 5:45-47, 1979.
820. Bhansali SK, Cameron KM: Primary malignant lymphoma of the bladder, Br J Urol 32:440-454, 1960.
821. Mincione GP: Primary malignant lymphoma of the urinary bladder with a positive cytologic report, Acta Cytol 26:69-72, 1982.
822. Forrest JB, Saypol DC, Mills SE et al: Immunoblastic sarcoma of the bladder, J Urol 130:350-351, 1983.
823. Chaitin BA, Manning JT, Ordóñez NG: Hematologic neoplasms with initial manifestations in lower urinary tract, Urology 23:35-42, 1984.
824. De Bruyne R, Peters O, Goossens A et al: Primary IgG-lambda immunocytoma of the urinary bladder, Eur J Surg Oncol 13:361-364, 1987.
825. Marconis JT: Primary Hodgkin's (paragranulomatous type) disease of the bladder, J Urol 81:275-281, 1959.
826. Jones MW: Primary Hodgkin's disease of the urinary bladder, Br J Urol 63:438, 1989.
827. Weide R, Pflüger KH, Görg C et al: Multiple myeloma of the bladder and vagina, Cancer 66:989-991, 1990.
828. Gorfain AD: Extramedullary plasmacytoma of the bladder with local metastasis, Calif Med 71:147-148, 1949.
829. Yang C, Motteram R, Sandeman TF: Extramedullary plasmacytoma of the bladder: a case report and review of literature, Cancer 50:146-149, 1982.

830. Jufe R, Molinolo AA, Fefer SA et al: Plasma cell granuloma of the bladder: a case report, J Urol 131:1175-1176, 1984.
831. Thornhill JA, Dervan P, Otridge BW et al: Symptomatic plasmacytoma (myeloma) involving the bladder, Br J Urol 65:542-543, 1990.
832. Ho DS, Patterson AL, Orozco RE et al: Extramedullary plasmacytoma of the bladder: case report and review of the literature, J Urol 150:473-474, 1993.
833. Pentecost CL, Pizzolato P: Involvement of the genito-urinary tract in leukemia: with the report of a case of involvement of the urinary bladder, J Urol 53:725-731, 1945.
834. Sheehan EE, Greenberg SD, Scott R Jr: Metastatic neoplasms of the bladder, J Urol 90:281-284, 1963.
835. Abrams HL, Spiro R, Goldstein N: Metastases in carcinoma: analysis of 1000 autopsied cases, Cancer 3:74-81, 1950.
836. Ganem EJ, Batal JT: Secondary malignant tumors of the urinary bladder metastatic from primary foci in distant organs, J Urol 75:965-972, 1956.
837. Bartone FF: Metastatic melanoma of the bladder, J Urol 91:151-155, 1964.
838. Haid M, Ignatoff J, Khandekar JD et al: Urinary bladder metastases from breast carcinoma, Cancer 46:229-232, 1980.
839. Berger Y, Nissenblatt M, Salwitz J et al: Bladder involvement in metastatic breast carcinoma, J Urol 147:137-139, 1992.
840. Van Driel MF, Ypma AFGVM, Van Gelder B: Gastric carcinoma metastatic to the bladder, Br J Urol 59:193-194, 1987.
841. Leddy FF, Peterson NE, Ning TC: Urogenital linitis plastica metastatic from stomach, Urology 39:464-467, 1992.
842. Silverstein LI, Plaine L, Davis JE et al: Breast carcinoma metastatic to bladder, Urology 29:544-547, 1987.
843. Meyer JE: Metastatic melanoma of the urinary bladder, Cancer 34:1822-1824, 1974.
844. Chin JL, Sales JL, Silver MM et al: Melanoma metastatic to the bladder and bowel: an unusual case, J Urol 127:541-542, 1982.
845. Young RH, Johnston WH: Serous adenocarcinoma of the uterus metastatic to the urinary bladder mimicking primary bladder neoplasia: report of a case, Am J Surg Pathol 14:877-880, 1990.

Embryology and Fetal-Prepubertal History

Anatomy

- Zones
- Capsule
- Neurovascular bundles
- Cowper's glands

Histology

Function

Prostatic Hyperplasia

- Relation to age
- Clinical symptoms
- Etiology
- Pathogenesis of symptoms
- Location
- Treatment
- Pathology
- Infarcts
- Atypical stromal hyperplasia

Prostatitis

- Abscess
- Granulomatous prostatitis
- Mycotic prostatitis
- Mycobacterial prostatitis
- Malakoplakia
- Nonspecific granulomatous prostatitis
- Postbiopsy granulomas
- Systemic granulomatous prostatitis
- Viral infections
- Miscellaneous infections

Atypical Adenomatous Hyperplasia

Sclerosing Adenosis

Basal Cell Hyperplasia

Clear Cell Cribriform Hyperplasia

Benign Non-neoplastic Conditions

- Amyloid
- Corpora amylacea
- Calculi and calcification
- Cysts
- Multilocular cysts (multilocular prostatic cystadenoma)
- Melanotic lesions
- Antiandrogen therapy
- Atrophy
- Metaplasia

Miscellaneous Conditions

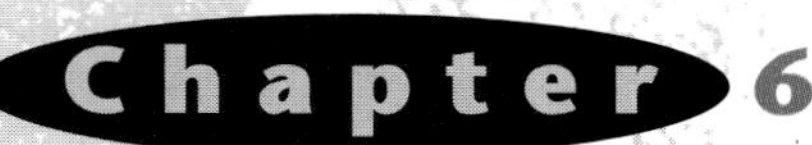

6

NON-NEOPLASTIC DISEASES OF THE PROSTATE

JONATHAN I. EPSTEIN

EMBRYOLOGY AND FETAL-PREPUBERTAL HISTOLOGY

The prostate begins development from the mesenchyme surrounding the urogenital sinus in the third month of gestation.[1] Its development depends on dihydrotestosterone (DHT), which is produced from fetal testosterone, by the enzyme 5 alpha-reductase within the urogenital sinus.[2] Epithelial buds invaginate from the posterior urogenital sinus on either side of the verumontanum. The mesenchymal stroma does not appear to be a passive substrate into which the tubules grow; the type of epithelium that develops in this region depends on stromal influences. Concurrently, wolffian ducts develop into seminal vesicles, epididymis, vas deferens, and ejaculatory ducts, which are stimulated by fetal testosterone rather than dihydrotestosterone. By the fourth month of gestation the basic structure of the prostate is complete.

In the fetal prostate, glandular buds begin as solid outgrowths of cells. Small lumina develop lined by cuboidal or columnar cells.[3] In the perinatal period, active secretion may be seen in the peripheral portion of the prostate along with squamous metaplasia of the urethral epithelium, utricle, and central portion of the prostate; these are the effects of maternal estrogens and regress several months after birth.[4] Prostatic acini in the term infant and young male resemble those seen in basal cell hyperplasia, hence its synonyms *embryonal hyperplasia* and *fetalization of the prostate*.[5] The glands are simple tubular structures without significant branching, and are lined by multiple layers of immature cells with round nuclei and scant cytoplasm.

ANATOMY

By age 20 the prostate weighs approximately 20 g and has the shape of an inverted cone with the base at the bladder neck and the apex at the urogenital diaphragm.[6] The prostatic urethra does not follow a straight line as it runs through the center of the gland but rather is bent anteriorly approximately 35 degrees at the verumontanum.[7] Posteriorly, the prostate and seminal vesicles are separated from the rectum by a thin, filmy layer of connective tissue known as Denonvilliers' fascia. At its apex the skeletal muscle of the urogenital diaphragm extends into the prostate (Fig. 6-1). Striated muscle continues predominantly in the anterior and anterolateral regions of the gland to form a sleeve around the prostate.[8,9] Though mostly exterior to the gland, these skeletal muscle fibers extend into the peripheral portion of the prostate gland, especially apically and anteriorly. Consequently, the finding of a few benign-appearing prostatic glands admixed with skeletal muscle fibers does not indicate that the glands are neoplastic. The finding of skeletal muscle fibers on transurethral resection is not associated with an increase in postsurgical incontinence.[10]

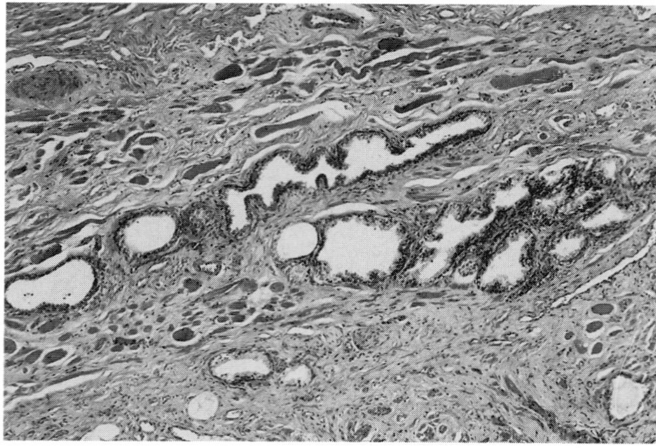

6-1. Prostatic apex containing benign prostate glands admixed with skeletal muscle fibers.

ZONES

Initially, the prostate was thought to be composed of distinct anatomical lobes.[11] Today's anatomical theories divide the prostate into inner and outer regions, the inner being that affected predominantly by nodular hyperplasia and the outer having a predilection for carcinoma, although carcinomas occur centrally as well. McNeal has taken this generalized concept of the prostate and has refined it with the addition of other anatomical zones.[7] In McNeal's model the prostate is divided into four zones: anterior fibromuscular stroma; central zone; peripheral zone; and preprostatic region, which encompasses the periurethral ducts and the larger transition zone (Fig. 6-2).

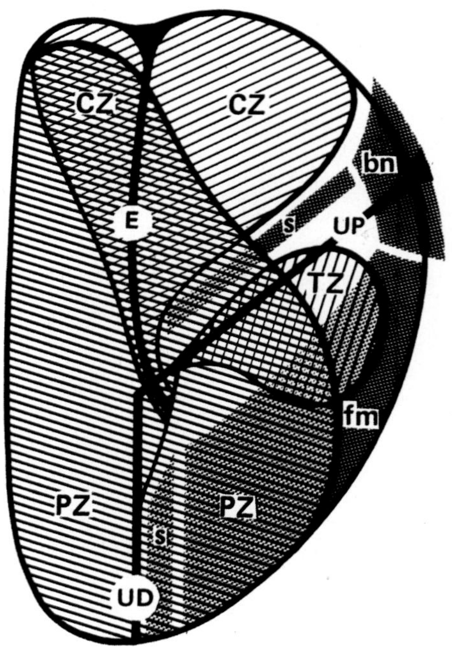

6-2. Diagram of prostate and urethra in sagittal section. Distal prostatic urethral segment (*UD*), proximal urethral segment (*UP*), and ejaculatory ducts (*E*) in relation to sagittally cut anteromedial nonglandular tissues (bladder neck, *bn*; anterior fibromuscular stroma, *fm*; preprostatic sphincter, *S*). These structures are shown in relation to a three-dimensional representation of the glandular prostate tissue (central zone, *CZ*; peripheral zone, *PZ*; transition zone, *TZ*). *(From McNeal JE: Normal histology of the prostate, Am J Surg Pathol 12:619, 1988, with permission).*

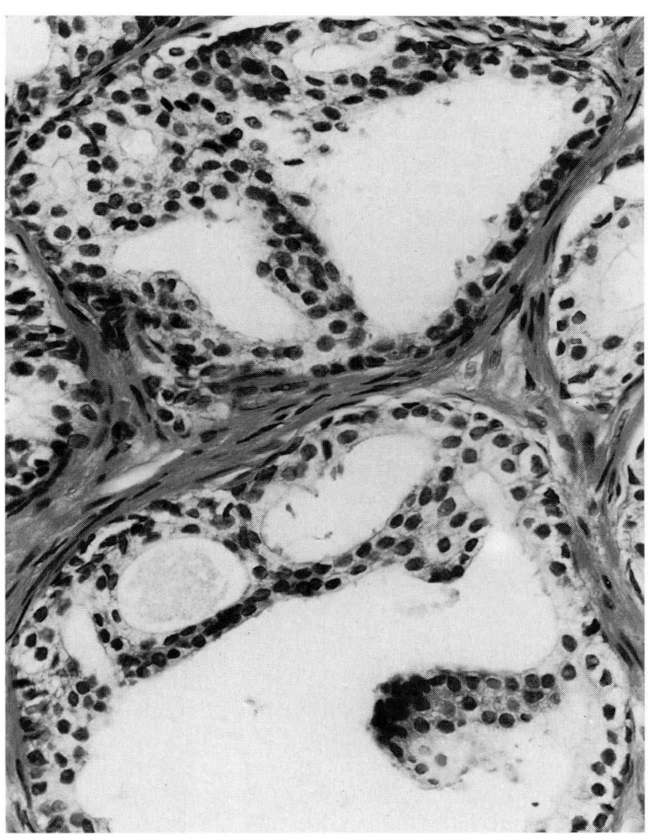

6-3. Benign Roman bridge and cribriform formations at the base of the prostate.

The anterior fibromuscular stroma, which occupies approximately one third of the prostate, contains very few glands and consists of smooth muscle tissue and dense fibrous tissue. The anterior fibromuscular stroma merges with the internal sphincter of the bladder neck proximally and with the striated muscle of the external sphincter at the apex.

The central zone forms a cone-shaped volume surrounding the ejaculatory ducts with its apex at the verumontanum and its base at the bladder neck. Glands within the central zone are complex and large with numerous papillary infoldings and often are lined by pseudostratified epithelium. In these glands one can see Roman bridge and cribriform patterns where the nuclei stream parallel to the glandular bridges (Fig. 6-3). These benign epithelial proliferations may be confused with prostatic intraepithelial neoplasia but are distinguished by their lack of cytologic atypia. It is thought by McNeal that the central zone may be derived from the wolffian duct similar to the seminal vesicle.

The peripheral zone is the largest zone and contains 75% of the glandular tissue of the prostate. The peripheral zone is distal to the central zone and corresponds to a horseshoe-shaped structure extending posteriorly, posterolaterally, and laterally around the inner aspect of the prostate (Fig. 6-4). It is a flat disk of tissue whose ducts branch out laterally and anteriorly from either side of the distal urethra. In contrast to the central zone, the glands of the peripheral zone are composed of smaller rounder acini with small, dark, basally located nuclei. Glands within the peripheral zone also tend to have smoother and straighter luminal borders than those in the central zone.

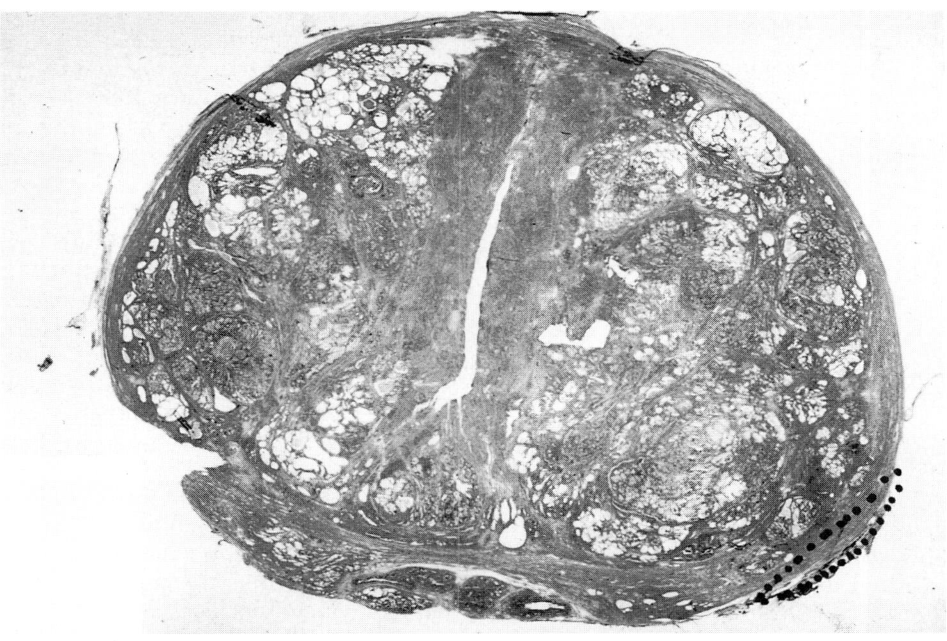

6-4. Whole mount of the prostate showing massive enlargement of the transition zone by nodular hyperplasia, with a compressed horseshoe-shaped peripheral zone. A small focus of adenocarcinoma is outlined with black dots in the posterolateral peripheral zone.

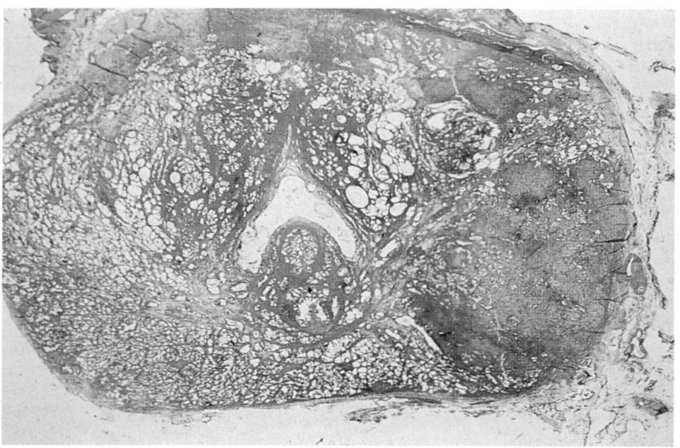

6-5. Whole mount of the prostate showing neurovascular bundles (*bottom right*). Contrast with contralateral region (*bottom left*) where the bundle has been spared and left within the patient.

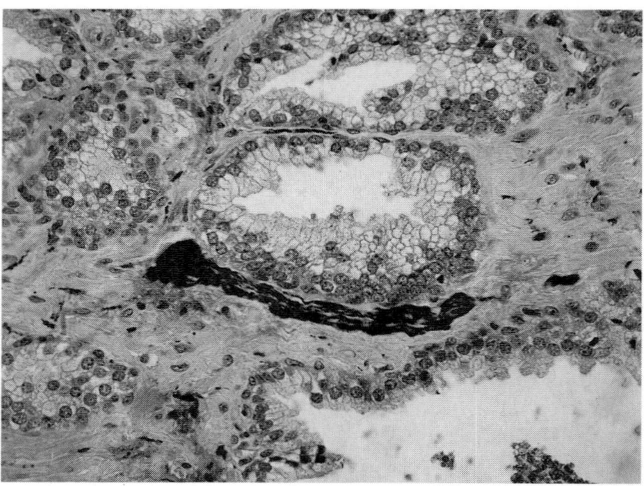

6-6. Perineural abutment by benign gland. Immunostain for S-100 protein accentuates nerve.

The preprostatic region is most affected by hyperplasia. It is subdivided into two regions. The first is a cylindrical smooth muscle sphincter surrounding the entire urethral submucosa from the verumontanum to the bladder neck. This area contains tiny periurethral glands, the development of which is restrained by the sphincter. Thus only small hyperplastic nodules develop there. At the distal end of the preprostatic region, ducts escape from the sphincter laterally at the verumontanum to form the transition zone. Although the transition zone comprises only 5% of the glandular prostate, it may grow significantly with the development of glandular-stromal hyperplasia. These larger mixed glandular-stromal hyperplasia nodules are more laterally situated and originate more distally along the urethra closer to the proximal end of the verumontanum.

The central and peripheral zones taken together encompass what others had previously referred to as the outer aspect of the prostate, in contrast to the inner area affected by hyperplasia. The rationale for separating the outer aspect of the prostate into central and peripheral zones is in part based on both histological differences and differences in the diseases affecting these two areas. The peripheral zone is much more frequently affected by carcinoma. The central zone is an uncommon site for origin of carcinoma, although it may be secondarily invaded by large peripheral zone tumors. Furthermore, McNeal has identified cytochemical differences between the peripheral and central zones.[12] Despite these differences, experts in the field still find difficulties in distinguishing between the central and peripheral zones and often combine them into one zone when investigating various aspects of prostatic disease. From this standpoint, McNeal's more complicated scheme is often simplified into a two-zone concept, corresponding to the inner (transition zone) and outer (peripheral and central zones) sections of the prostate.

CAPSULE

The prostate, although well defined grossly, lacks a discrete capsule around much of the gland.[13,14] In some areas there may be the appearance of a fibromuscular band surrounding the prostate; in others, however, glands extend right up to its edge. At the base and apex of the prostate its edge is particularly ill defined, and prostatic glands on occasion appear almost to extend out of the prostate. At the apex of the prostate skeletal muscle fibers are admixed with benign prostate glands and the prostatic boundary is often obscure. This vagueness as to what constitutes the edge of the prostate, especially in these regions, has important implications for assessing capsular penetration by carcinoma and whether the prostate has been cut into (capsular incision) as a source of positive margins.

NEUROVASCULAR BUNDLES

One area that has received growing attention in the study of normal prostate anatomy is that of its neurovascular supply. In the early 1980s Walsh described paired posterolateral neurovascular bundles running exterior to the prostate from the base to the apex[15,16] (Fig. 6-5). It was demonstrated that these bundles play an important role in potency. Consequently, modified techniques for performing radical prostatectomy were developed that selectively spared or resected the neurovascular bundle(s) depending on the likelihood of carcinoma invading these structures. When pathologists describe the location of extracapsular spread and positive margins, their relationship to the neurovascular bundles should be stated; in certain cases positive margins may be avoided by more liberally sacrificing part or all of the neurovascular bundle(s).

The neurovascular bundles often contain ganglion cells. Although more common exterior to the prostate, ganglion cells and nerves are also present within the prostate. Consequently, perineural or ganglion cell invasion by carcinoma does not equate with extracapsular spread of tumor. Occasionally, benign glands may be seen in close proximity to nerves, mimicking perineural invasion by cancer (Fig. 6-6). These benign glands indent the nerves on one side rather than circumferentially involv-

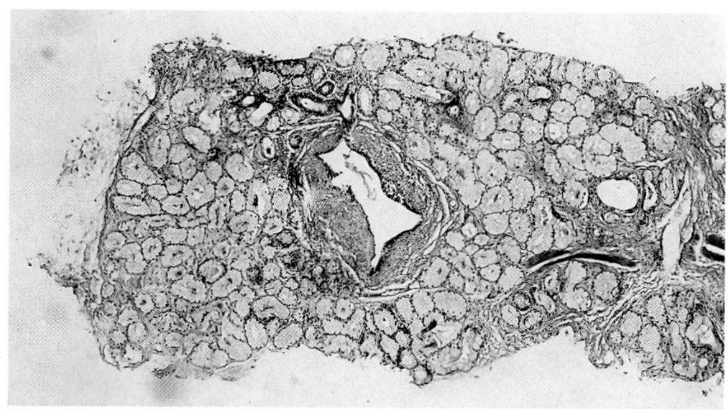

6-7. Cowper's gland in a needle biopsy specimen.

ing the nerve as seen in carcinoma.[17,18] The bland cytology of benign prostate glands with perineural indentation further distinguishes them from carcinoma.

COWPER'S GLANDS

Although not within the prostate gland proper, Cowper's glands are often considered in the discussion of the prostate because they may be sampled in the biopsy of the prostate and may be confused with adenocarcinoma of the prostate. Cowper's glands (bulbourethral glands) are paired pea-sized compound tubular glands located directly distal to the prostate. The distinction of Cowper's glands from carcinoma of the prostate is based on several features. Cowper's glands have a lobular configuration with central ducts lined by cuboidal cells which often have amphophilic cytoplasm (Fig. 6-7). These ducts give Cowper's glands a bimorphic appearance lacking in adenocarcinoma. The other cell type in Cowper's glands are goblet cells, which are distended with mucin to the extent that the lumina are almost occluded. In contrast, glands of adenocarcinoma of the prostate lack such abundant mucin-filled cytoplasm and narrowing of their lumina. Cowper's glands are situated within skeletal muscle fibers, which further mimics the infiltrative pattern of adenocarcinoma. Mucin stains may help to definitively identify Cowper's glands by demonstrating their abundant mucin-filled cytoplasm.

HISTOLOGY

From puberty to middle age the prostate becomes more complex with ducts and branching glands arranged in lobules and surrounded by stroma. The distinction between prostatic ducts and acini is primarily based on their architectural pattern at low magnification. The ducts consist of elongated branching tubular structures as opposed to the more rounded acini. Ducts cut on cross section are indistinguishable from acini. In benign prostatic glands the luminal surface has an undulating and ruffled contour whereas in many carcinomas the glandular lumina have a straight, even border. Although rarely carcinomas may have papillary infoldings and branching,[19] these features are more typically seen in benign prostate glands where papillary processes lined by fibrovascular cores project into the lumen. Corpora amylacea are seen in approximately 25% of men aged 20 to 40 years, whereas they are rare in carcinomas.[20,21]

The prostate consists of stromal and epithelial cells. The stromal cells are smooth muscle cells, fibroblasts, and endothelial cells. The epithelial cells of the prostate are secretory cells, basal cells, and neuroendocrine cells.

The columnar secretory epithelial cells are tall with pale to clear cytoplasm, in contrast to some adenocarcinomas which have amphophilic cytoplasm. Secretory cells are connected to adjacent cells by adhesion molecules and to the basement membrane through integrin receptors, laminin, and fibronectin. These cells are terminally differentiated and stain positively with prostate-specific antigen, prostatic acid phosphatase, and other enzymes. In general, benign prostate glands stain more intensely with antisera to prostate-specific antigen and prostatic acid phosphatase than do malignant glands.[22-24] Why benign prostate glands, which stain more intensely with prostate-specific antigen and prostatic acid phosphatase than carcinoma, are associated with lower serum prostate-specific antigen and prostatic acid phosphatase levels is unclear. Possible explanations include the excretion of prostate-specific antigen and prostatic acid phosphatase into the urethra by benign glands. In addition, benign prostate glands are invested by basal cells and have more complete basal lamina than do neoplastic glands, which may prevent leakage of prostate-specific antigen into the surrounding stroma and vasculature.

It has been claimed that secretory cells lack acid mucin.[25-29] This belief has been used in the past to support the use of acid mucin stains in differentiating adenocarcinoma from its mimics. However, recently it has been demonstrated that non-neoplastic prostate glands may contain acid mucin.[30] In particular, atypical adenomatous hyperplasia, atrophic glands, and transitional cell metaplasia can show acid mucin positivity. Mucin may also be seen in the prostate in the form of goblet cells, as discussed in the mucous gland metaplasia section of this chapter. Secretory cells may also contain a scant amount of neutral mucin.[31,32]

Although classically the finding of lipofuscin was thought to be diagnostic of seminal vesicle epithelium, this concept has recently been questioned. Several investigators have noted that the cytoplasm of prostatic secretory epithelial cells frequently contains pigment granules.[33] On hematoxylin-eosin-stained sections, these granules may be either yellow-brown or pale gray-brown with a dark blue rim (Fig. 6-8). The granules are coarse and have been shown to be lipofuscin by histochemical and ultrastructural methods. This pigment is autofluorescent and is positive with the following stains: Fontana-Masson, periodic acid-Schiff with diastase, Congo red, alcian blue, Giemsa, and oil red-O, all reactions typical of lipofuscin. This pigment may also be seen within stromal macrophages. While visible in approximately 50% of cases in hematoxylin-eosin-stained sections, when studied by special stains such as Fontana-Masson, lipofuscin may be seen in almost all cases. Recognition that lipofuscin may be present within non-neoplastic prostatic glands is of great clinical importance. Carcinoma adjacent to pigmented prostate glands on needle biopsy could

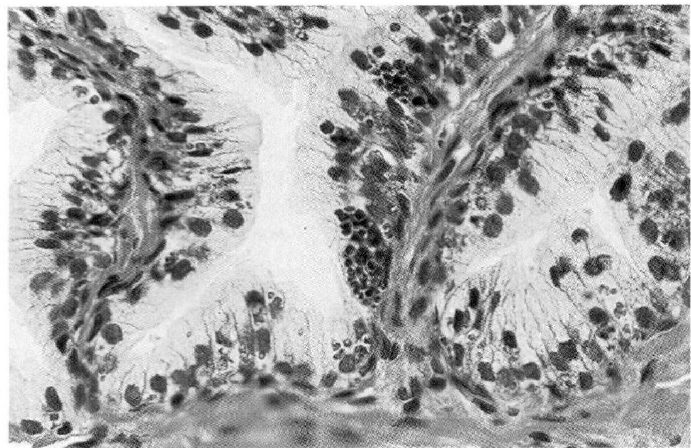

6-8. Lipofuscin pigment within prostatic epithelium.

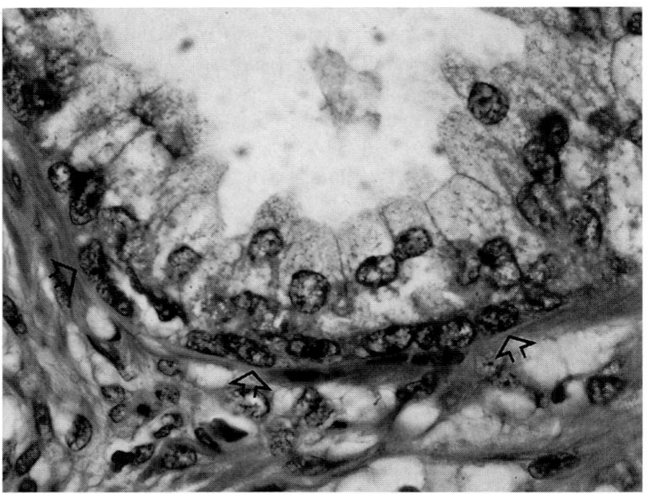

6-9. Flattened basal cells within benign prostate glands (*arrows*).

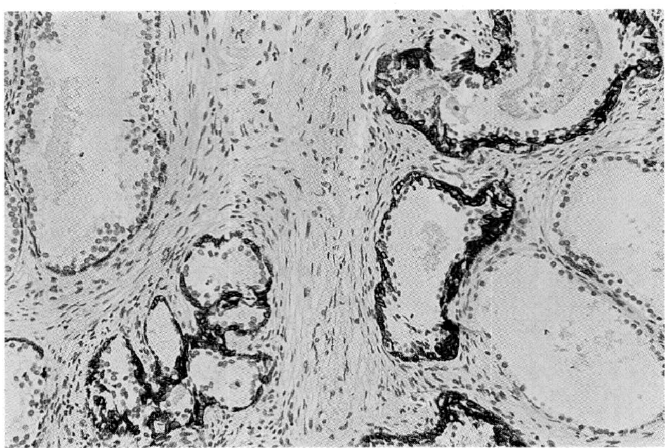

6-10. Immunohistochemical demonstration of basal cells using antibodies to cytokeratin 34ßE12.

be misinterpreted as cancer invading the seminal vesicle, implying a stage where the patient would have been denied potentially curative surgery. Further distinction between seminal vesicle tissue and benign prostatic epithelium is based on the architectural and nuclear features of seminal vesicle epithelium (see chapter 8).

Less commonly, melanin occurs in prostatic secretory cells and stromal cells. This pigment has been verified as melanin by immunohistochemistry and electron microscopy.[34-39] The terms *melanosis* and *blue nevus* have been used to refer to melanin containing glands and stroma, respectively.

The basal cells lie beneath the secretory cells. They are cigar-shaped or fibroblastic in shape and are oriented parallel to the basement membrane (Fig. 6-9). The cells may be inconspicuous in benign glands and difficult to distinguish from the surrounding fibroblasts. It is important to recognize basal cells and distinguish them from surrounding fibroblasts or an artifactual two-cell layer in cancer, because basal cells are absent in adenocarcinoma of the prostate and may be identified in conditions that mimic prostate cancer.[40,41] Whereas fibroblasts have extremely hyperchromatic and pointed nuclei, often basal cells are recognizable by their more ovoid nuclei with lighter chromatin resembling those of smooth muscle cells. Basal cells also may be identified by their immunohistochemical reaction with antibodies to basal cell–specific high molecular weight cytokeratin[42-47] (Fig. 6-10). Basal cells in hyperplastic glands usually are uniformly labeled with these antisera, although an occasional gland stains discontinuously or even not at all. The staining patterns of basal cells in other benign processes are discussed in their respective sections.

Basal cells are less differentiated than secretory cells and are almost devoid of secretory products such as prostate-specific antigen and prostatic acid phosphatase.[48] They rest on the basement membrane and appear wedged between the bases of adjacent tall columnar epithelial cells. It is believed, though not proved, that these undifferentiated basal cells give rise to secretory epithelial cells and function as stem cells. Basal cells are not myoepithelial cells and do not react with antibodies to muscle-specific actin or S-100, and ultrastructural studies reveal a lack of contractile elements.[49,50]

The third group of prostatic epithelial cells are those with neuroendocrine differentiation. The prostate contains the largest number of endocrine-paracrine cells of any genitourinary organ.[51] These cells are irregularly distributed throughout ducts and acini, with a greater population in ducts. Di Sant'Agnese et al[51] have shown that these cells are of two types: open and closed. Open cells have long apical cytoplasmic processes extending to the lumen with long specialized microvilli on the apical surface protruding into the luminal secretion. The morphology of the open cell type suggests that the long apical microvilli contain receptors that monitor the luminal contents and regulate their secretions. Closed cells lack such extension to the lumen. Most endocrine-paracrine cells of the prostate contain serotonin. Other peptides include calcitonin, gene-related peptides, katacalcin, bombesin-like substance, somatostatin, alpha-human chorionic gonadotropin, and thyroid-stimulating hormonelike substance. Neuroendocrine cells co-express prostate-specific antigen and prostatic acid phosphatase and hence arise from differentiation of secretory epithelium rather than migration from the neural crest. Little is known of their function, but it is speculated that these cells play a role in the regulation of the prostate gland by paracrine release of peptides to regulate adjacent cells or by endocrine or neurocrine mechanisms.

FUNCTION

At present the functional role of the prostate is incompletely understood.[2] The prostate provides the bulk of the volume of the ejaculate. The ejaculate includes high concentrations of prostaglandins, spermine, potassium, fructose, phosphorylcholine, free amino acids, citric acid, and zinc. In addition, there are enzymes such as proteases, esterases, and phosphatase. The function of these secretory products in the seminal plasma is unclear. The seminal plasma does not contain factors that are essential for fertilization, although they may optimize conditions for fertilization. It has been suggested that high concentrations of sugars within the seminal plasma provide nutrients to the sperm. One potential role of zinc is as a prostatic antibacterial factor. Prostate specific antigen (also termed *gamma-seminal protein*) is a glycoprotein of 33,000 molecular weight and is detected only in the epithelial cells of the prostate.[52] Prostate-specific antigen is a serine protease with chymotrypsin-like and trypsin-like activity. The sequence of the protein is similar to the kallikreins which are important proteolytic enzymes. One of the possible roles of prostate-specific antigen is lysis of the ejaculate clot, yet it is unknown why this clotting and lysing mechanism is important for reproduction. Another important enzyme is prostatic acid phosphatase. Acid phosphatase activity in the prostate is more than 200 times greater than in any other tissue.[2] Phosphatase enzymes hydrolyze organic monophosphate esters to yield inorganic phosphate ions and alcohol. The biologic functions of this enzyme are also not known. Other products found within the prostate are prostate-specific protein-94 (beta-inhibin, beta microseminoprotein) and leucine amino-petidase.

PROSTATIC HYPERPLASIA

Prostatic hyperplasia, also referred to as nodular hyperplasia, is the most common urologic disease of men. It has been estimated that in the United States the probability of a 40-year-old man undergoing a prostatectomy for hyperplasia is 30% to 40% if he lives to 80 years of age.[53] In recent years there has been a renewed interest in the study of prostatic hyperplasia with the development of new pharmacologic and nonoperative approaches to its management. There is potential in the future for the pathologist also to have a greater role in selection of therapy based on the histological components of the disease.

RELATION TO AGE

The prostate slowly enlarges from birth to puberty. Thereafter the prostate rapidly increases in size until the age of 21 to 30, at which point it weighs, on average, 20 g.[54] Hyperplasia is first seen in a small percentage of prostates around the mid-20s and its incidence rises rapidly after age 40. Pathological evidence of hyperplasia is present in 50% of men 50 to 60 years of age and 90% of men in their 80s. Approximately 4% of the prostates in men older than 70 years of age weigh over 100 g.[54]

McNeal considers that the progression of hyperplasia in men less than 70 years of age occurs predominantly by an increase in the number of nodules. Nevertheless, nodules account for approximately 14% of the mass of the transition zone in men 50 to 70 years of age.[55] In some elderly men a second phase of evolution occurs where there is enlargement and gland proliferation within preexisting nodules.

CLINICAL SYMPTOMS

Hyperplasia results in a smooth firm enlargement of the prostate. However, the size of the prostate does not correlate closely with the degree of urinary tract obstruction or symptoms. Early symptoms of urinary tract obstruction include decrease in the caliber and force of the urinary stream, hesitancy in initiating urination, inability to abruptly terminate micturition without dribbling, sensations of incomplete emptying of the bladder, and occasionally urinary retention. As symptoms progress and bladder compliance decreases, bladder instability develops with frequency, nocturia, urgency, and urgency incontinence.

Other obstructive conditions may simulate hyperplasia. These include urethral stricture, bladder neck contracture, bladder calculi, and carcinoma of the prostate. Irritative symptoms mimicking those of hyperplasia may also occur with urinary tract infections, neurogenic bladder, and diffuse carcinoma in situ of the bladder.

ETIOLOGY

Little is known about the pathogenesis of hyperplasia. In a recent study the risk of surgery for hyperplasia was elevated in Jewish men and in blacks to 1.6 times that seen in men of other religions and races, respectively.[56] Nationality, diet, and other factors have not been shown to be significantly associated with hyperplasia.

Both estrogens and androgens appear to play a role in the control of hyperplasia.[57] There are multiple ways in which estrogen may influence the proliferation of prostatic cells. Estrogen has been shown to induce the androgen receptors. Estrogen can also alter steroid metabolism to favor an increase in the formation of dihydrotestosterone within the prostate, which is the potent androgen within the prostate. When given with androgens, estrogens can also inhibit cell death. Another role of estrogen may be in stimulating stromal collagen synthesis.

The importance of androgens in established hyperplasia has been demonstrated by observing changes in the disease following androgen withdrawal. When treated with LH-RH agonists, which inhibit the hypothalamic-pituitary axis, prostates regress in size with a corresponding regression of glandular epithelial height.[58] Furthermore, the majority of men show improvement in urologic symptoms and some experience improvements of urinary flow rates. These changes are reversible following cessation of treatment. More recently, the use of 5 alpha-reductase inhibitors, which inhibit the conversion of testosterone to dihydrotestosterone, has been shown to decrease prostatic weight significantly in approximately one third of treated men.[59,60] However, dihydrotestosterone accumulation does not appear to be the cause of hyperplasia since hyperplasia occurs in the presence of normal levels of dihydrotestosterone.[61]

In summary, persistent androgen stimulation, possibly with estrogen synergism, is involved in growth of hyperplasia with age. In aging men, patients with more prominent hyperplasia have higher serum androgen and estrogen levels. The finding of increased nuclear androgen receptor in men with hyperplasia supports the possibility that estrogen induction of the androgen receptor may be responsible for the increase in hyperplasia volume seen with age. However, it has not been possible to demonstrate increased estrogen receptors in human hyperplasia.

Both stromal and epithelial cells are thought to contribute to hyperplasia. Basic fibroblastic growth factor is mitogenic for stromal and epithelial cells.[2] Transforming growth factor beta-2 inhibits epithelial growth but continues to support stromal growth.

Histological observations of hyperplasia have also resulted in various concepts of its evolution. McNeal has asserted that in normal embryonic development epithelium provides the inductive stimulus for primitive stroma to mature into adult smooth muscle.[55] He hypothesizes that the initial abnormality in hyperplasia is spontaneous reversion of a clone of stromal cells to the embryonic state, possibly under the influence of hormones. This concept notes that the majority of periurethral nodules are purely stromal, consisting of what he considers to be embryonic mesenchyme with a myxoid matrix. Furthermore, as the stroma of embryonic glandular organs has limited capacity for self-stimulation, these pure stromal nodules tend to be small. Only with the interaction of epithelium and stroma do most embryonic organs grow; similarly, only when prostatic epithelium and stroma grow in concert do more sizable nodules form.

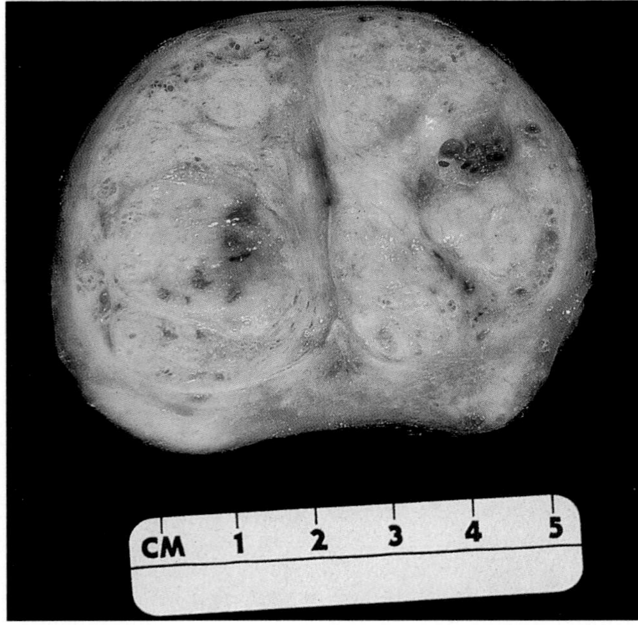

6-11. Prostatic hyperplasia with numerous central nodules and compression of the urethra and peripheral zone. A small focus of carcinoma is present in the peripheral zone in the lower right of the photograph (*patient's right*).

PATHOGENESIS OF SYMPTOMS

Urinary obstructive symptoms have both an anatomic component of obstruction produced by the enlarging hyperplastic tissue and a dynamic component related to smooth muscle tone.

Clinically, hyperplasia is classified into lateral enlargement, middle lobe enlargement, and posterior lobe hyperplasia. Typical hyperplasia of tissue lateral to the urethra is designated as lateral lobe enlargement (Fig. 6-11). Middle lobe enlargement refers to a nodule arising at the bladder neck, which may then project into the bladder, creating a ball valve obstruction (Fig. 6-12). In posterior lobe hyperplasia there is a bar of tissue, termed the *median bar*, which arises posterior to the urethra. Because of the strategic location of middle or posterior lobe enlargement, relatively small prostates may be associated with marked urinary obstructive symptoms. Consequently, there may be little correlation between the size of the prostate and the degree of obstruction.[62]

In addition to mechanical obstruction, dynamic obstruction results from increased smooth muscle tone. This has been demonstrated by improvements in urinary flow rates and symptom scores in men after treatment with alpha$_1$-adrenergic blockers.[63]

The third factor in the pathophysiology of the symptoms of hyperplasia is the response of the bladder detrusor muscle. The obstructed detrusor muscle develops hyperplasia, hypertrophy, and fibrosis. This leads to detrusor muscle instability and loss of the normal control which gives rise to irritative symptoms. Bladder capacity

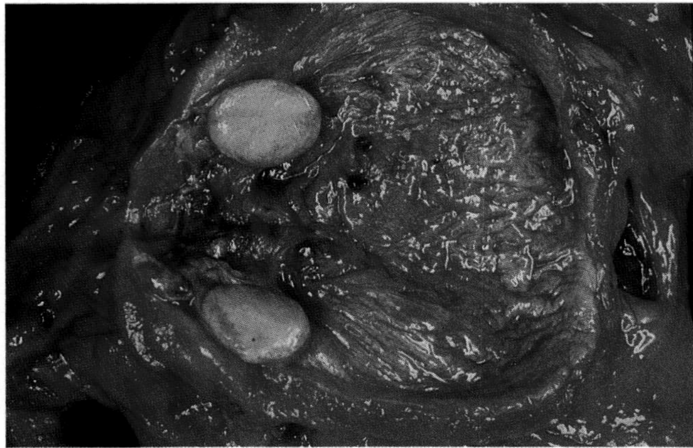

6-12. Middle lobe hyperplasia with ball-valve obstruction. The bladder is opened and a nodular mass is present at the base (the mass is bisected).

is reduced, giving rise to frequency, urgency, nocturia, and urgency incontinence. Muscle wall trabeculation, thickening of the detrusor musculature, and herniation with formation of diverticula occurs with progressive obstruction. Finally, bladder decompensation may result with dilation of the bladder, increased residual urine, and secondary hydronephrosis and hydroureter formation.

LOCATION

McNeal has described four zones within the prostate (see Anatomy) and asserts that the preprostatic tissue is the exclusive site of origin of hyperplasia.[7,55] The preprostatic tissue surrounds the proximal segment of the urethra from the base of the verumontanum to the bladder neck. Consequently, hyperplasia never involves the tissue surrounding the distal urethral segment.

One component of the preprostatic zone is a cylindrical smooth muscle sphincter that surrounds the urethra. This sphincter prevents reflux of semen into the bladder at the time of ejaculation. Inside this cylinder of smooth muscle are tiny periurethral glands. These glands lie entirely confined within the preprostatic sphincter and are the site of origin of periurethral stromal nodules. Because of their confinement by the preprostatic sphincter, these periurethral stromal nodules tend to be limited in size.

A larger component of the preprostatic region is the transition zone. The transition zone consists of bilateral lobules of tissue that are immediately external to the sphincter. These nodules arise at the most distal rings of the preprostatic sphincter at the junction of the proximal and distal urethral segments. Nodules within the transition zone tend to be glandular from their inception and later in life form the main mass of hyperplasia tissue.

Hyperplastic nodules may on occasion be seen in the peripheral zone, which can mimic carcinoma on digital rectal exam and on ultrasound. There are several theories to explain this phenomenon. These include ectopic transition zone tissue in the peripheral zone and an abnormal response of the peripheral zone to embryonic mesenchymal signals. Less likely, these peripheral hyperplastic nodules represent herniation of transition zone nodules, because many of the prostates with peripheral hyperplastic nodules have not had prominent hyperplasia in the transition zone.

TREATMENT

The major form of treatment for hyperplasia is simple prostatectomy, which encompasses transurethral resection of the prostate for low volumes of tissue and enucleation of the prostate for larger volumes. New pharmacological therapies include finasteride (a 5 alpha-reductase inhibitor preventing testosterone's conversion to dihydrotestosterone—the most potent prostatic androgen) and alpha$_1$-adrenergic blockers, which relax smooth muscle. Other recent techniques to treat hyperplasia include transurethral incision of the prostate,[64] balloon dilation of the prostate,[65] and hyperthermia.[66]

PATHOLOGY

Franks described five histologic subtypes of prostatic hyperplasia based on their differing epithelial and stromal components (Fig. 6-13).[67] The smallest nodules are predominantly stromal, often composed of loose mesenchyme containing prominent small round vessels[68] (Fig. 6-14). In a needle biopsy specimen, these vessels help in differentiating between a mesenchymal tumor and a stromal nodule. These nodules are located in the periurethral submucosa and seldom reach large size except near the bladder neck, where they may protrude into the bladder lumen as a solitary midline mass creating a ball-valve type of obstruction. More commonly, enlargements of midline nodules are confined by the internal urethral sphincter, and are termed *median* or *posterior lobes*.

Occasionally, one can see pure stromal nodules composed almost entirely of smooth muscle.[68] Several reports of leiomyomas of the prostate probably are descriptions of these sorts of nodules. The diagnosis of prostatic leiomyoma should be restricted to large symptomatic masses of smooth muscle.

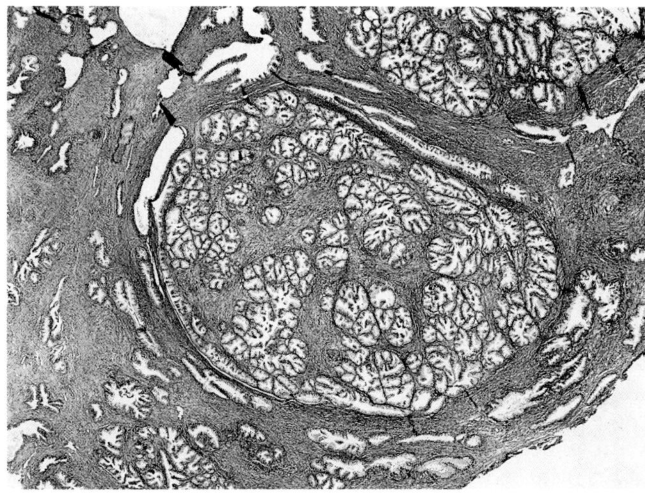

6-13. Mixed epithelial and stromal nodule of prostatic hyperplasia.

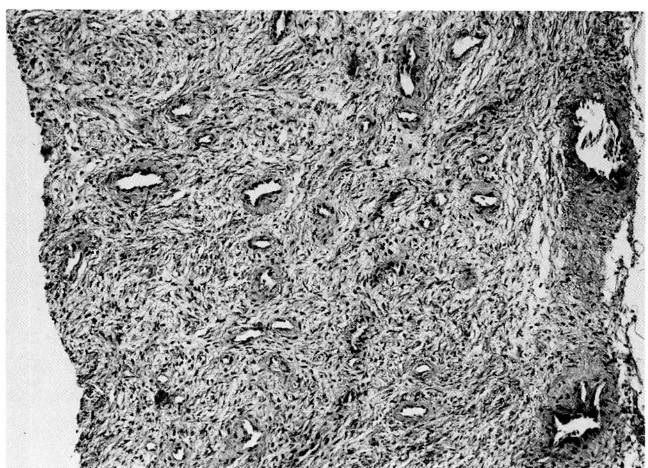

6-14. Stromal hyperplasia with myxoid appearance on needle biopsy.

Fibroadenoma-like foci are another variant of stromal hyperplasia.[69,70] These resemble intracanalicular fibroadenomas of the breast where cytologically benign stroma compresses prostatic glands into slitlike spaces. They are usually microscopic, involving only a few glands, and are uncommon, seen in less than 1% of prostatic specimens.[70]

The largest and most numerous hyperplastic nodules are almost always laterally situated and tend to occur in the periurethral zone near the proximal end of the verumontanum.[7] These nodules are predominantly glandular from inception and are the cause of most clinically evident hyperplasia. The glandular component is made up of small and large acini, some showing papillary infoldings and projections containing central fibrovascular cores. The luminal secretory epithelium consists of tall columnar cells with pale-staining granular cytoplasm. Within hyperplastic areas there often is an infiltrate of lymphocytes and plasma cells around the glands. Usually these are not associated with any infection or with symptoms of prostatitis.[71,72]

More limited hyperplasia is characterized by less nodule formation. Tissue removed by transurethral resection in these cases contains fairly unremarkable prostatic tissue with the exception of greater frequency of focal atrophy and chronic inflammation.[55] These small transurethral resection specimens contain a higher percentage component of bladder neck and anterior fibromuscular tissue. Specimens of intermediate size, weighing up to 50 g also have mainly an increase in non-nodular transition zone tissue. In larger specimens, usually obtained by enucleation, the nodules become a more dominant feature. These nodules frequently show a prominence of the epithelial component. As a result of ductal obstruction, the glands are often cystically dilated.

In many cases the diagnosis of nodular hyperplasia does not relate to specific histological findings but rather to clinical findings of an enlarged prostate resulting in obstructive symptoms. Only in some cases are there distinct nodules that are specific for hyperplasia. The presence of papillary infoldings, although more prominent in hyperplasia, is not specific. By definition, transurethral resection specimens may be diagnosed as hyperplasia since surgery has been performed for urinary obstructive symptoms. Needle biopsy specimens should not be diagnosed as showing hyperplasia. First, many needle biopsy specimens do not even sample the transition zone. Second, because the presence of papillary infolding is not specific for hyperplasia and nodules are rarely seen on needle biopsy, one can only rarely identify hyperplasia on needle biopsy.

INFARCTS

In 20% to 25% of specimens removed for hyperplasia, there are small infarcts ranging in size from a few millimeters to 5 cm.[68,73] Grossly, these are yellow or mottled with a hemorrhagic margin and are somewhat firmer than the surrounding tissue. Prostate glands with acute infarcts are twice as large as those without infarcts.[73] Patients with infarcts are more prone to acute urinary retention and gross hematuria than patients without

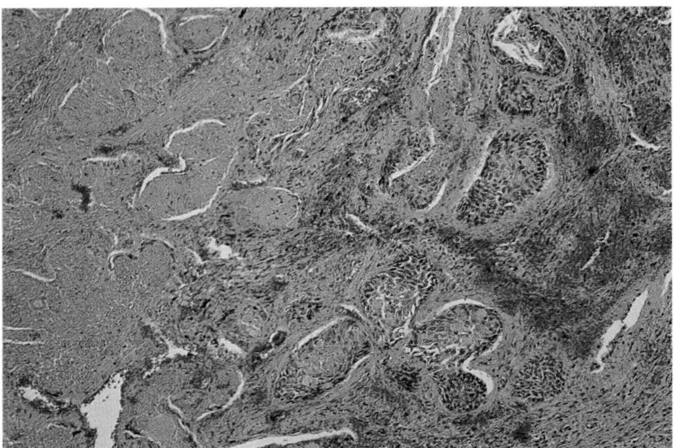

6-15. Acute prostatic infarct with acute coagulative necrosis (*left*) and adjacent squamous metaplasia (*right*).

infarcts. These symptoms, however, may not be due to the infarcts but may result from the larger size of the gland containing them, since the infarcts are often small and not close to the urethra.

Histologically, acute prostatic infarcts have a characteristic zonation. Acute coagulative necrosis and recent hemorrhage are found in the center of the infarct (Fig. 6-15). Immediately adjacent to the infarct there may be reactive epithelial nests with prominent nucleoli and mitotic figures. Farther away there is more mature squamous metaplasia that may also show some reactive nuclear features.[74] These squamous islands may be cystic with intraluminal cellular debris but rarely show keratinization. Recognizing that the reactive squamous epithelium is immediately adjacent to an infarct should prevent a misdiagnosis of squamous cell carcinoma. Furthermore, the squamous epithelium adjacent to infarcts shows changes typical of reactive nuclei; the nuclei are vesicular and enlarged with prominent nucleoli but without pleomorphism. Remote infarcts are recognized by areas of dense fibrotic stroma admixed with small glands containing immature squamous metaplasia. Infarction of the prostatic urethra and surrounding prostate has also been described at autopsy in men with marked hypotension who had urethral catheters.[75]

ATYPICAL STROMAL HYPERPLASIA

In this uncommon condition there are stromal cells with marked yet degenerative-appearing cytologic atypia[76,77] (Fig. 6-16). These cells have hyperchromatic, enlarged, and pleomorphic nuclei. However, the nuclei appear smudgy with indistinct chromatin and nuclear vacuolation, lacking the prominent nucleoli seen in neoplastic atypia. Mitotic figures are either rare or absent and usually the lesions are sparsely cellular. For lesions where these atypical stromal cells are interspersed between prostatic glands and the lesion focus is small, the diagnosis of atypical stromal hyperplasia is appropriate. For cases with similar cytology where there is also a mass or the lesion is extensive, a more appropriate diagnosis would

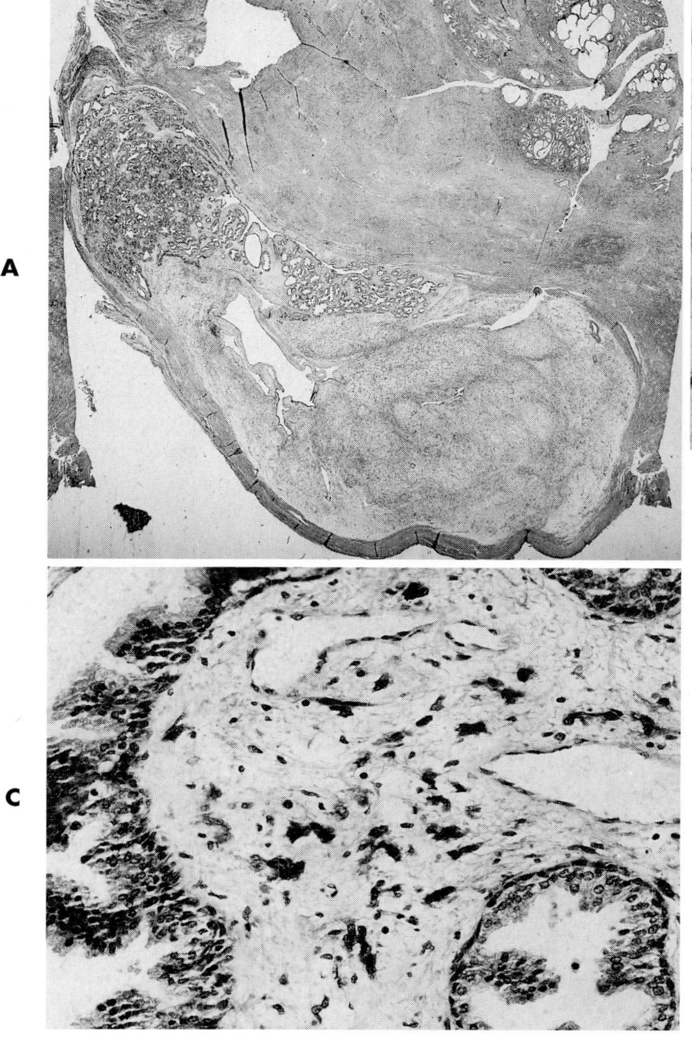
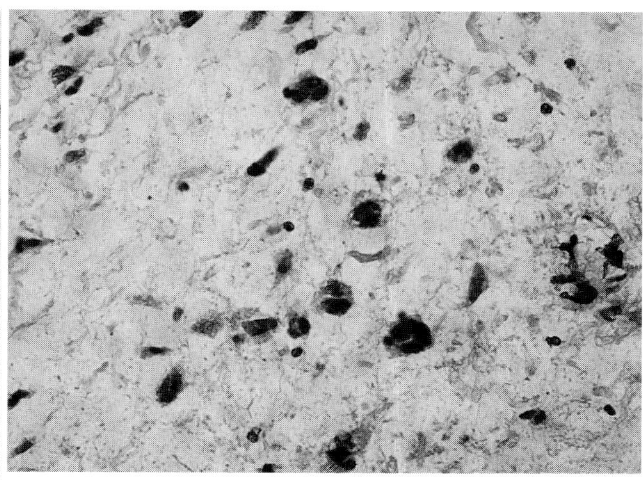

A B C

6-16. **A**, Low magnification view of stromal nodule with atypia. **B**, Stromal area of nodule, with myxoid background and scattered atypical cells. **C**, Mixed glandular and stromal area with atypical degenerate stromal cells between benign prostate glands.

be benign phyllodes tumor (see Chapter 7). Although the histologic appearances of benign phyllodes tumor and atypical stromal hyperplasia are virtually identical, there have been rare reports of lesions with the morphology of benign phyllodes tumor that recurred showing the histology of phyllodes sarcoma.[78,79] Only when the findings of atypical stromal hyperplasia are limited and appear to be an alteration of usual hyperplastic stroma rather than a neoplasm can one can be confident of its benignity and diagnose it as atypical stromal hyperplasia. The glands in areas of atypical stromal hyperplasia may be normal or cystically dilated.

Similarly, when a small nodule of smooth muscle contains degenerative atypical stromal changes, the diagnosis of atypical stromal nodule is more appropriate than atypical leiomyoma.[80] Although most patients with larger atypical smooth muscle tumors (atypical leiomyomas) have remained without evidence of disease, a few have experienced recurrences. Ultrastructural studies of atypical stromal hyperplasia have in some cases shown smooth muscle differentiation[77] but some have more fibroblastic features.

PROSTATITIS

Clinically, prostatitis is classified into acute and chronic bacterial prostatitis, and nonbacterial prostatitis. Bacterial prostatitis is associated with urinary tract infections, increased number of inflammatory cells in prostatic secretions, and growth of bacterial organisms from prostatic secretions. The organisms causing bacterial prostatitis are similar in type and incidence to those resulting in urinary tract infections.[81] Chronic bacterial prostatitis is characterized by recurrent urinary tract infections caused by the same pathogens. Patients with HIV infections and AIDS have an increased incidence of bacterial prostatitis. The majority of these infections also are caused by Gram-negative organisms.[82] Nonbacterial prostatitis is an inflammatory condition of unknown cause and the most common prostatitis syndrome. Nonbacterial prostatitis is clinically similar to chronic bacterial prostatitis except that both cultures and history of urinary tract infections are negative. Mycoplasma and Ureaplasma do not appear to be causative agents of nonbacterial prostatitis.[83] Despite conflicting reports, chlamydia and *Trichomonas vaginalis* have yet to be shown to play a major role in the etiology of prostatitis.[83]

Although acute and chronic prostatitis are common diseases in urologic practice, they are usually diagnosed clinically and treated with antibiotics so the histologic examination of specimens removed for symptomatic prostatitis is uncommon. Acute bacterial prostatitis is characterized by sheets of neutrophils within and around acini, intraductal desquamated cellular debris, and stromal edema and hyperemia. Histologically, symptomatic chronic prostatitis is identical to the chronic inflammation commonly seen in specimens removed for hyperplasia. Several studies have shown that in many prostatic specimens with prominent chronic inflammation, no organisms can be cultured.[71,72] Also, in specimens with positive cultures there often is not prominent inflammation within the tissue.[84] Consequently, it is preferable to diagnose inflamed prostate specimens as showing acute or chronic inflammation as opposed to acute or chronic prostatitis.

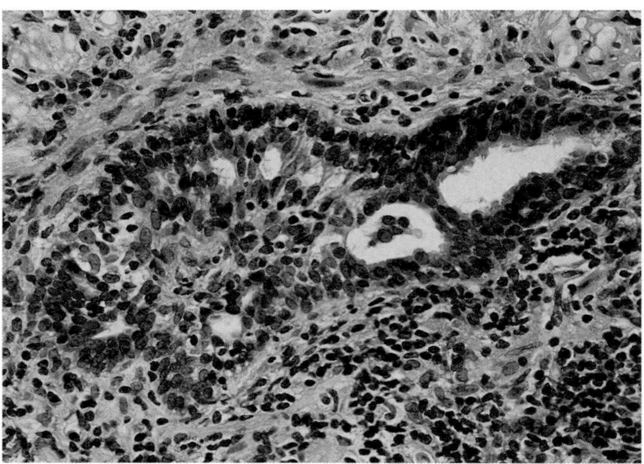

6-17. Reactive cribriform glandular architecture in an area of chronic inflammation.

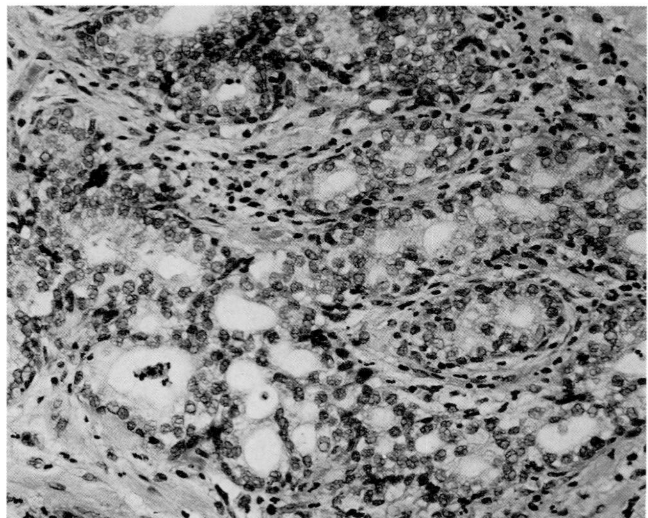

6-18. Inflamed cribriform glands with reactive vesicular nuclei.

In men with bacterial prostatitis, prostatic calculi may become infected and serve as sources for persistent urinary tract infections.[85] In these cases surgical means may be used to attempt removal of infected calculi whereby pathologists may have tissue for examination. In order to remove infected calculi, a "radical" transurethral prostatectomy must be performed because the peripheral zone of the prostate is the greatest source of infected stones.

Acute and chronic inflammation within the prostate may cause both architectural and cytologic abnormalities that may be confused with carcinoma. The glands often appear atrophic at low magnification, occasionally with budding off of little glands in a pseudocribriform architecture (Fig. 6-17, 6-18). At higher magnification the epithelium may show typical features of atrophy or there may be streaming of basophilic epithelium resembling urothelial metaplasia. Occasional large nucleoli are not uncommon in areas of chronic or acute inflammation (Fig. 6-19). The inflammatory infiltrate in these areas may be mild and composed predominantly of lymphocytes. The distinction of inflammatory atypia from carcinoma rests first on the recognition that the atypical glands are in an area of inflammation and that they are atrophic. Consequently, caution must be exercised in diagnosing adenocarcinoma of the prostate in the setting of chronic or acute inflammation. In the uncommon case of carcinoma associated with acute or chronic inflammation, an unequivocal malignant diagnosis can be rendered only when atypical glands also are found in areas away from inflammation or when the pattern of small crowded glands is so characteristic of adenocarcinoma that their appearance cannot be attributed to the inflammation.[86]

ABSCESS

The availability of antibiotics has made symptomatic prostatic abscess a rarity. The most common type of prostatic abscess occurs in patients with bladder outlet

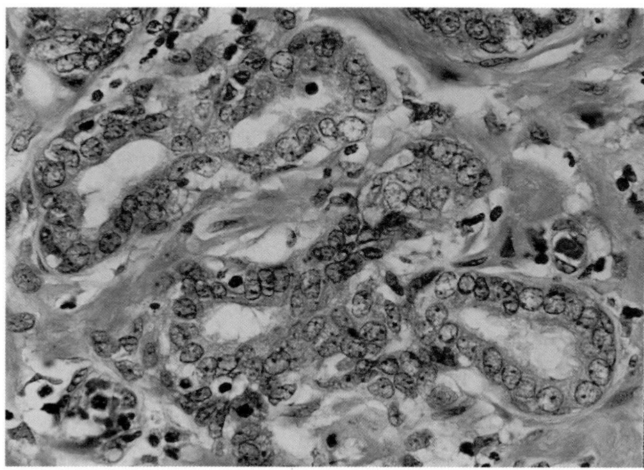

6-19. Inflamed atrophic glands with visible nucleoli.

obstruction and is a complication of their lower urinary tract infection, usually caused by coliform organisms.[87] Much less frequently, prostatic abscesses result by dissemination from an extraurinary source of infection, the most common being staphylococcal infections of the skin. Prostatic abscess may also arise as a complication of biopsy or instrumentation.[88] Other risk factors include immunosuppression, diabetes, internal prosthesis, chronic renal failure, indwelling catheters, and chronic prostatitis.[83,87,88,89] Patients present with voiding symptoms, fever, and rectal tenesmus and may have acute urinary retention. Urine cultures may be negative, which is why culture of the prostatic fragments removed by transurethral resection is important. The treatment includes either transurethral resection or incisional drainage with antibiotic therapy. Complications include chronic prostatitis, infertility, sepsis, and spontaneous rupture into the urethra, perineum, bladder, or rectum.

GRANULOMATOUS PROSTATITIS

Granulomatous prostatitis is subclassified into infectious granulomas, nonspecific granulomatous prostatitis, biopsy granulomas, and allergic granulomatous prostatitis.[90,91] Stillwell et al have also proposed that instead of *allergic granulomatous prostatitis*, a more general designation such as *systemic granulomatous prostatitis* should be utilized.[91] In a series of 200 cases of granulomatous prostatitis, nonspecific granulomatous prostatitis (138 cases) and postbiopsy granulomas (49 cases) were the most common.[91] Infectious granulomatous prostatitis occurred in only seven cases with the remaining six being those due to systemic granulomatous disorders.

MYCOTIC PROSTATITIS

Fungal infections of the prostate usually occur in immunocompromised hosts with disseminated mycoses.[92] Of the deep mycoses, the largest number of prostatic infections are observed with blastomycosis, coccidioidomycosis, and cryptococcosis. In AIDS patients, the prostate may be a sequestered reservoir for cryptococcosis from which systemic relapses may occur.[93] Cases have also been reported of histoplasmosis, paracoccidioidomycosis, aspergillosis, and candidiasis of the prostate; a case of *Aspergillus flavus* confined to the prostate in an otherwise healthy 50-year-old man has also been described.[92] The histology in these cases is identical to that seen in nonprostatic sites.

MYCOBACTERIAL PROSTATITIS

Mycobacterial prostatitis may occur in patients with systemic tuberculosis but today is more commonly a complication of bacillus Calmette-Guérin immunotherapy for superficial bladder carcinoma. The incidence of prostatic involvement in systemic tuberculosis ranges from 3% to 12% with over 90% of these cases also having pulmonary tuberculosis.[94,95] The prostate is involved in 75% to 95% of patients with urogenital tuberculosis. However, in only 7% to 13% of these cases is the prostate the sole organ involved. Most cases of tuberculous prostatitis appear to arise from hematogenous dissemination rather than contact with infected urine. Evidence supports hematogenous dissemination: the largest tuberculous foci are usually found peripherally, the earliest tuberculous infiltrate is in the periglandular stroma and only extends into the acinus when the lesion enlarges, and only 18% of the cases of advanced prostatic tuberculosis show extension into the prostatic urethra. Even in cases with prominent prostatic urethral tuberculosis, only one third have renal tuberculosis. Atypical mycobacterial infections of the prostate are exceedingly rare. *Mycobacterium avium intracellulare* infection of the prostate has been described in an immunocompromised host.[96] There has also been one report of granulomatous prostatitis with isolation of *Mycobacterium kansasii* and *Mycobacterium fortuitum* in an otherwise healthy man.[97]

Following bacillus Calmette-Guérin therapy for superficial bladder carcinoma, patients present with fever, mild hematuria, and urinary frequency. Approximately 40% of men will have an abnormal rectal exam and 55% will have ultrasonographic abnormalities.[98-100] These lesions may further mimic carcinoma by elevating serum prostate-specific antigen levels. Following bacillus Calmette-Guérin therapy, biopsies show caseating or noncaseating granulomas in 22% of cases and acid-fast stains are positive in approximately 50% of these cases.

Histologically, the findings in bacillus Calmette-Guérin prostatitis are indistinguishable from those of tuberculous prostatitis occurring as a result of systemic infection. Small noncaseating granulomas are found in the periglandular stroma, as seen in early hematogenous dissemination of systemic tuberculosis (Fig. 6-20). There also may be large caseating granulomas that are well demarcated from the surrounding prostatic stroma. Characteristically, the necrosis within tuberculous prostatitis is caseous and consists of grummous fine granular debris (Fig. 6-21). This differs from the coagulative necrosis seen in postbiopsy granulomas. Caseating larger granulomas predominate within the peripheral zone of the prostate although the transition zone or central zone may be involved as well. In addition to the more peripherally located caseating and noncaseating granulomas, there are

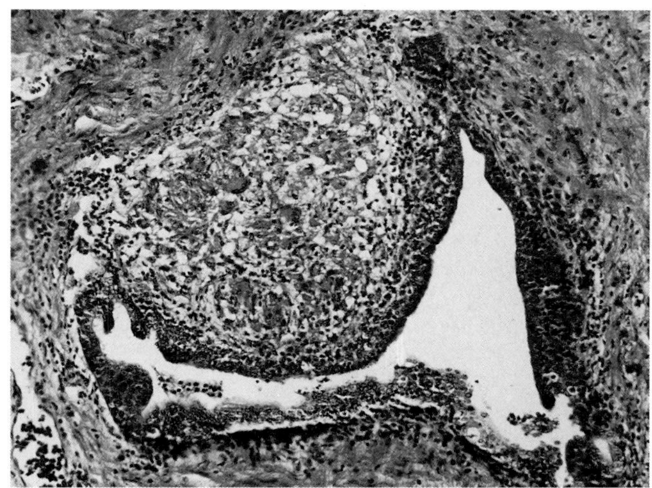

6-20. Small periglandular noncaseating granuloma resulting from bacillus Calmette-Guérin therapy for bladder cancer.

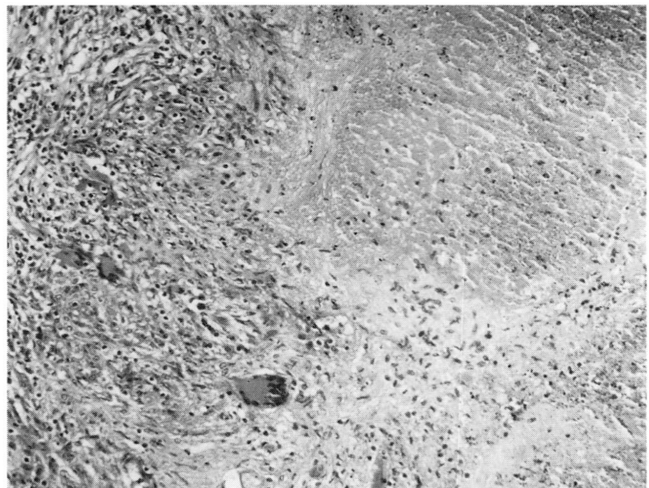

6-21. Tuberculous prostatitis with multinucleated giant cells and caseous necrosis.

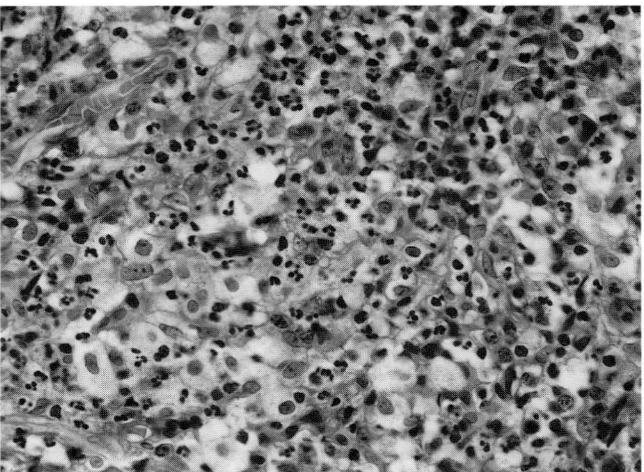

6-22. Nonspecific granulomatous prostatitis with acute and chronic inflammation and pale-staining histiocytes.

almost always small suburethral granulomas. In some instances the suburethral granulomas are well formed and discrete and in other areas more ill-defined granulomatous inflammation is seen.

Bacillus Calmette-Guérin granulomatous prostatitis is localized and self-limited and need not be treated with antibiotics.[98,99] Regardless of the histologic pattern of bacillus Calmette-Guérin–related granulomatous prostatitis or the presence or absence of acid-fast bacilli on special stains, patients usually remain asymptomatic and require no specific therapy. Consequently, it is not necessary to perform stains for acid-fast organisms in these cases; stains for fungi should be done for completeness. Patients are followed for systemic signs and symptoms because on rare occasions disseminated infection with bacillus Calmette-Guérin has occurred.

MALAKOPLAKIA

Twenty-nine cases of malakoplakia have been reported in the prostate.[101-103] As in the bladder, its most frequent site, the majority of men with prostatic malakoplakia have urinary tract infections, most commonly with *E. coli*. The ages of patients with prostatic malakoplakia range from 47 to 85. Symptoms include urinary retention, dysuria, urinary frequency, hematuria, and fever. Clinically, malakoplakia may mimic cancer by giving rise to an indurated prostate on rectal examination as well as appearing as a hypoechoic lesion on transrectal ultrasound. Histologically, the lesions are indistinguishable from those occurring in other sites. Just as nonspecific granulomatous prostatitis may be histologically misdiagnosed as prostate cancer, malakoplakia may similarly be misdiagnosed.

NONSPECIFIC GRANULOMATOUS PROSTATITIS

The most commonly diagnosed noninfectious granulomatous process within the prostate is nonspecific granulomatous prostatitis.[91] In a study of 25,387 benign prostate specimens, the incidence of nonspecific granulomatous prostatitis was 0.5%. Lesions occurred over broad ages ranging from 18 to 86 years of age with a mean and median age of 62 years. Common symptoms included irritative voiding symptoms (50%), fever (46%), chills (44%), and obstructive voiding symptoms (32%). In 82% of men there was pyuria and in 46% there was hematuria. Seventy-one percent of men experienced urinary tract infection at an average of 4 weeks prior to diagnosis. In 59% of men the rectal exam revealed an indurated prostate suggestive of adenocarcinoma. The process appeared to be diffuse throughout the prostate in 80% of men. Five of the 138 cases of nonspecific granulomatous prostatitis contained large numbers of eosinophils yet no hypereosinophilia was noted within the blood. However, in another report a patient with nonspecific granulomatous prostatitis containing eosinophils had over 30% eosinophils within the blood.[104] None of these men experienced allergic symptoms, suggesting that the eosinophils reflect a subacute inflammatory reaction rather than an allergic disorder.

The etiology of this lesion is thought to be a reaction to bacterial toxins, cell debris, and secretions spilling into the stroma from blocked ducts. Its major significance for pathologists is that it mimics prostate carcinoma on rectal exam and on ultrasound, and can result in an elevated serum prostate-specific antigen level. At the same time as being presented with this clinical scenario of prostate cancer, the pathologist is confronted with a biopsy where the histology closely mimics carcinoma.

The earliest lesion in nonspecific granulomatous prostatitis consists of dilated ducts and acini filled with neutrophils, debris, foamy histiocytes, and desquamated epithelial cells. Rupture of these ducts and acini results in a localized granulomatous and chronic inflammatory reaction. Surrounding the ruptured acini are multinucleated giant cells, epithelioid histiocytes, lymphocytes, plasma cells, and some eosinophils. Extension of the infiltrate into surrounding ductal and acinar units results in the characteristic lobular dense infiltrate of lymphocytes, plasma cells, and histiocytes typical of more advanced nonspecific granulomatous prostatitis (Fig. 6-22). Often

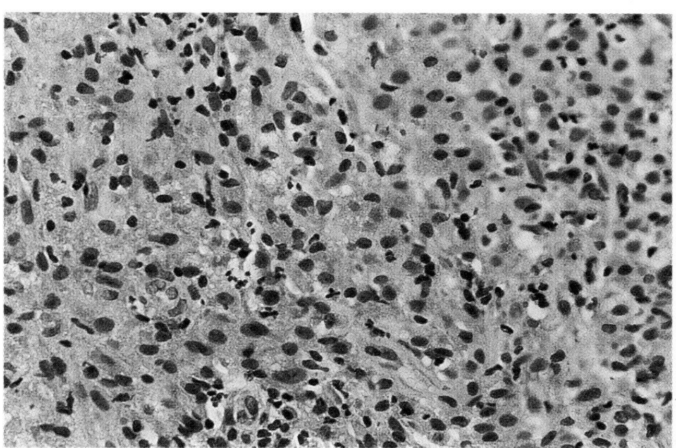

6-23. Nonspecific granulomatous prostatitis on needle biopsy with abundant epithelioid pale-staining histiocytes resembling poorly differentiated adenocarcinoma.

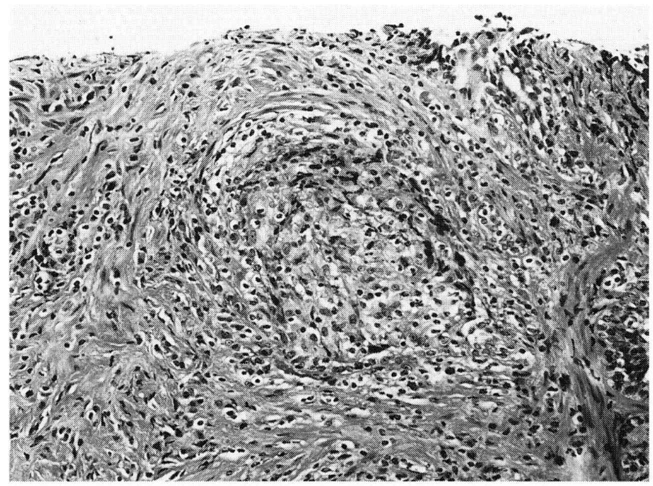

6-24. Nonspecific granulomatous prostatitis on needle biopsy showing clusters of epithelioid histiocytes surrounding ruptured ducts.

within the center of these large inflammatory nodules there are dilated and partially effaced acini. Many of the histiocytes have foamy cytoplasm and some are multinucleated. Neutrophils and eosinophils make up a smaller component of the inflammatory infiltrate.

In most cases, there is little histologic similarity between nonspecific granulomatous prostatitis and infectious granulomatous inflammation of the prostate. In general, the lesions of nonspecific granulomatous prostatitis are not as granulomatous as those due to infection and are composed of a more mixed inflammatory infiltrate. Though discrete small granulomas can be seen in nonspecific granulomatous prostatitis, they are invariably seen with the early lesion surrounding a ruptured dilated duct or acinus. In contrast, infectious early noncaseating granulomas surround intact acini. Nonspecific granulomatous prostatitis also lacks caseous necrosis, although there may be small abscesses at the centers of nodules of nonspecific granulomatous prostatitis. In some instances nonspecific granulomatous prostatitis has a prominent epithelioid histiocytic component that can be difficult to distinguish from an infectious granulomatous process. In such cases, where the light microscopic diagnosis of nonspecific granulomatous prostatitis is unclear, special stains for organisms are necessary to exclude an infection. Recognition that nonspecific granulomatous prostatitis may contain abundant eosinophils should prevent a misdiagnosis of allergic granulomatous prostatitis. Older lesions of nonspecific granulomatous prostatitis show a more prominent fibrous component.

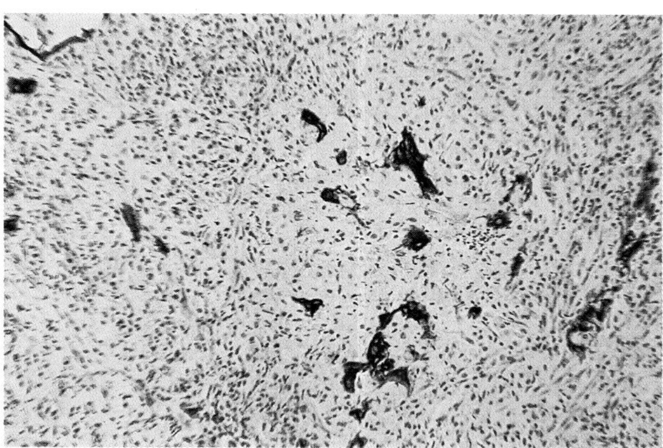

6-25. Nonspecific granulomatous prostatitis. Immunostaining with antibodies to keratin shows ruptured glands and ducts.

Nonspecific granulomatous prostatitis with prominent epithelioid histiocytes may be misdiagnosed as adenocarcinoma of the prostate on needle biopsy (Fig. 6-23). It should be borne in mind that the clinical findings, while suggestive of carcinoma, are nonspecific. The histologic finding of plasma cells, neutrophils, and eosinophils helps to identify the lesion as prostatitis. High-grade prostate cancer rarely is associated with a prominent inflammatory infiltrate. The clustering of the epithelioid histiocytes around partially ruptured acini, which may sometimes be appreciated on needle biopsy, contrasts with the diffuse pattern of high-grade prostate cancer (Fig. 6-24). Immunohistochemical stains for histiocytic markers and epithelial markers can help to differentiate between the two.[105] Epithelial markers in nonspecific granulomatous prostatitis must be interpreted cautiously because disrupted acini may result in isolated cords and individual keratin-positive cells; these epithelial fragments are distinguished from carcinoma by their localized nature and the fact that the vast majority of epithelioid cells (histiocytes) are keratin-negative (Fig. 6-25). As with chronic prostatitis, there may sometimes be seen reactive epithelial changes that could be confused with carcinoma, especially in needle biopsies.

The lesion is treated with warm sitz baths, fluids, and antibiotics if a urinary tract infection is documented. Most patients' symptoms will resolve within a few months although slightly over 50% of men will have a persistent abnormal rectal exam 2 to 8 years following diagnosis. If new nodules or increased firmness develops, then another biopsy should be performed to rule out concurrent carcinoma.

POSTBIOPSY GRANULOMAS

Granulomas with characteristic morphology may be seen in the prostate from 9 days to 52 months following transurethral resection.[90,106] The post–transurethral resection granuloma appears to be a reaction to altered epithelium and stroma from the trauma of diathermic cautery. Although the centers of most post–transurethral resection granulomas contain only amorphous fibrinoid material, in some cases there may be necrotic epithelial and stromal components. The recognition of similar granulomas following cautery in other sites argues against the process resulting solely from altered epithelium or secretions unique to the prostate. Although it is much more common to have a granulomatous reaction following transurethral resection, similar linear granulomas may develop after needle biopsy.[91] More commonly following needle biopsy, there is an irregular stellate defect surrounded by laminar fibrosis.[107] Near these defects at the edge of the prostate there is capsular fibrosis with hemosiderin deposition tracking away from the needle biopsy site.

Post–transurethral resection granulomas are composed of a central region of fibrinoid necrosis surrounded by palisading epithelioid histiocytes[90,106] (Fig. 6-26). The number of granulomas in a case is variable. Though lesions may be round, ovoid, triangular, or rectangular, characteristically some are elongated and tortuous. In the tissue surrounding the necrobiotic granulomas, multinucleated giant cells and granulomas without central necrosis are common. Inflammation surrounding the granulomas is usually minimal, consisting predominantly of lymphocytes and plasma cells with scattered eosinophils.

In cases where the interval between transurethral resections is approximately 1 month or less, eosinophils are often abundant. Prior to the recognition of this disorder, post–transurethral resection granulomas with numerous eosinophils had been reported in the literature as allergic granulomatous prostatitis. In contrast to allergic granulomatous prostatitis, the eosinophils are localized around post–transurethral resection granulomas rather than diffusely infiltrating the stroma. Also, the postbiopsy granulomas tend be more variable in size and shape.

Postbiopsy granulomas must also be distinguished from infectious granulomas. In contrast to the amorphous granular necrosis seen in caseous infectious granulomas, the necrosis in postbiopsy granulomas contains ghostlike structures of vessels, acini, and stroma seen with coagulative necrosis. The lesion is so characteristic and histologically distinct from infectious granulomas that stains for organisms are usually not necessary.

Postbiopsy granulomas are incidental findings and are commonly seen in radical prostatectomy specimens removed for carcinoma after a prior transurethral resection.

SYSTEMIC GRANULOMATOUS PROSTATITIS

This category encompasses cases with tissue eosinophilia such as allergic granulomatous prostatitis and Churg-Strauss syndrome,[91] as well as those without eosinophilia such as Wegener's granulomatosis.[108] Allergic granulomatous prostatitis as a reflection of a generalized allergic reaction is an exceedingly uncommon condition.[90,109] Of the 12 patients with allergic granulomatous prostatitis reported in the literature, all have had either asthma or evidence of systemic allergic reactions at the time of diagnosis of their prostatic lesions, and the majority of affected individuals have had increased blood eosinophil counts. In some instances the severity of the asthmatic symptoms fluctuated synchronously with the severity of the urinary obstructive symptoms. In a few cases the condition has been systemic with granulomas in other organs, and in one individual the systemic granulomatous process was a contributing factor in his death. Because allergic granulomatous prostatitis may be associated with systemic illness requiring prompt and aggressive treatment with steroids, it is important to distinguish the rare allergic granulomatous prostatitis from other granulomatous prostatic lesions with eosinophils.

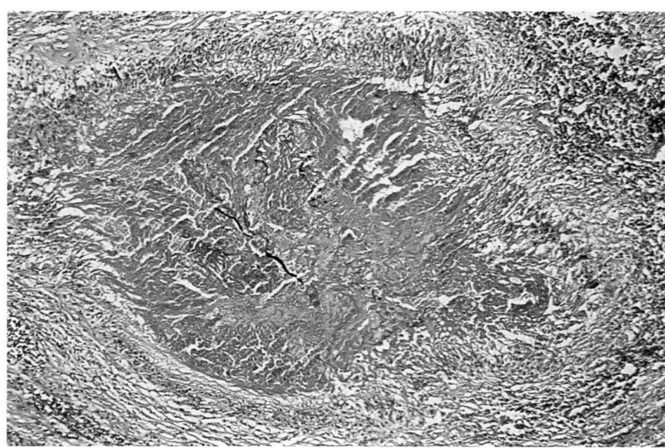

6-26. Post–transurethral resection granuloma.

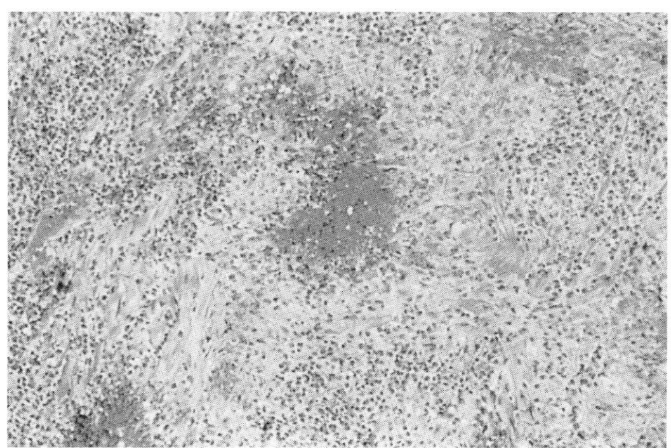

6-27. Allergic granulomatous prostatitis with necrosis and numerous eosinophils.

Histologically, allergic granulomatous prostatitis consists of multiple small, ovoid necrobiotic granulomas surrounded by numerous eosinophils (Fig. 6-27). Usually the granulomas of allergic granulomatous prostatitis are more eosinophilic and more regular in size and shape than postbiopsy granulomas. However, some postbiopsy granulomas may resemble these. In these instances, the history of a transurethral resection and the localization of eosinophils around the granuloma distinguish postbiopsy granulomas from allergic granulomatous prostatitis. Nonspecific granulomatous prostatitis with numerous eosinophils must also be distinguished from allergic granulomatous prostatitis.

VIRAL INFECTIONS

A case of disseminated cytomegalovirus with numerous inclusions within the prostatic epithelial cells has been described at autopsy in one patient.[110] One report described two cases of sacral herpes zoster where there was granulomatous prostatitis with necrosis.[111] However, no inclusions were identified.

MISCELLANEOUS INFECTIONS

Other prostatic infections, some of which are more commonly seen in developing countries, are exceedingly rare in North America and Europe. These include: schistosomiasis,[112] amoebic prostatitis,[113] syphilis,[114] actinomycosis,[115] echinococcosis,[116] and brucellosis.[117]

ATYPICAL ADENOMATOUS HYPERPLASIA

One of the most common lesions that may be confused with carcinoma is atypical adenomatous hyperplasia.[118,119] Other terms for atypical adenomatous hyperplasia include *adenosis*,[118] *small gland hyperplasia*,[120] *atypical adenosis*,[121] and *small acinar atypical hyperplasia*.[122] Although recently a group of urologic pathologists came out in support of the term *atypical adenomatous hyperplasia*, I prefer the term *adenosis*.[123] Prefacing *adenomatous hyperplasia* with *atypical* has the potential for adverse consequences both in terms of practical patient management and in the theoretical framework for this entity. There is very little data in support of a relation between atypical adenomatous hyperplasia and carcinoma. By designating these lesions *atypical*, patients may be subjected to unnecessary repeated biopsies. Conceptually, as has happened in the past, use of the term *atypical adenomatous hyperplasia* may result in this entity being combined with prostatic intraepithelial neoplasia as precursors to carcinoma of the prostate. Whereas there is strong evidence that prostatic intraepithelial neoplasia is a precursor to some prostate cancers, this evidence is lacking for atypical adenomatous hyperplasia. Notwithstanding these points, in deference to common usage, the term *atypical adenomatous hyperplasia* will be used in this chapter for this entity.

Atypical adenomatous hyperplasia is a common (found at Johns Hopkins Hospital in 1.6% of benign transurethral resections and 0.8% of all needle biopsies) benign glandular lesion with histologic features that may be confused with carcinoma.[118,119,125] In general, atypical adenomatous hyperplasia consists of a crowded focus of small glands that mimics low-grade adenocarcinoma. In the spectrum of architectural atypia, which ranges from obviously benign glands that are somewhat crowded to areas that are difficult to distinguish from carcinoma, the diagnosis of atypical adenomatous hyperplasia should be restricted to cases that are sufficiently atypical in their growth pattern that one must seriously consider the diagnosis of low-grade cancer.

The distinction of atypical adenomatous hyperplasia from low-grade adenocarcinoma is based on architectural and cytologic features[118,125] (Table 6-1). In order to minimize misdiagnoses, the constellation of histologic

TABLE 6-1.
DIAGNOSTIC CRITERIA FOR ATYPICAL ADENOMATOUS HYPERPLASIA

Atypical Adenomatous Hyperplasia	Low Grade Carcinoma
FEATURES SEEN AT LOW MAGNIFICATION	
Lobular growth	Infiltrative/haphazard
Small crowded glands admixed with larger glands	May be pure population of small crowded glands
FEATURES SEEN AT HIGH MAGNIFICATION	
Huge (≥3 μm) nucleoli absent	Occasionally huge nucleoli present
Small glands share cytoplasmic and nuclear features with admixed larger benign glands	Small glands differ from surrounding benign glands in cytoplasmic and/or nuclear features
Pale to clear cytoplasm	May have amphophilic cytoplasm
Blue-tinged mucinous secretions rare	Blue-tinged mucinous secretions common
Corpora amylacea common	Corpora amylacea rare
Occasional glands with basal cells	Basal cells absent
Basal cell–specific antikeratin antibodies stain basal cells in some small glands	Small glands are not immunoreactive with basal cell–specific antikeratin antibodies

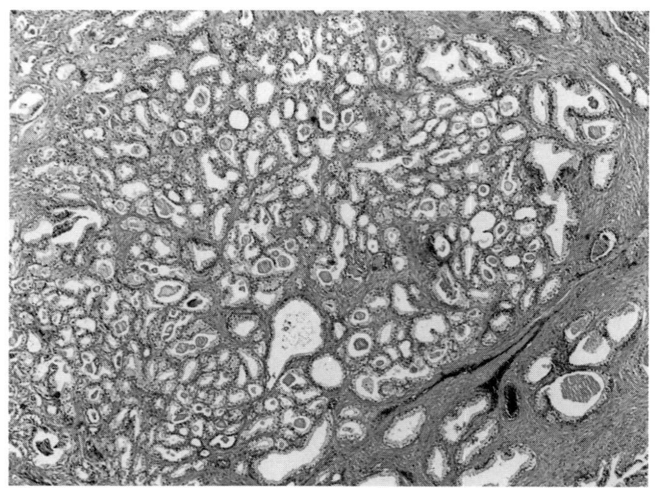

6-28. Low-power view of atypical adenomatous hyperplasia.

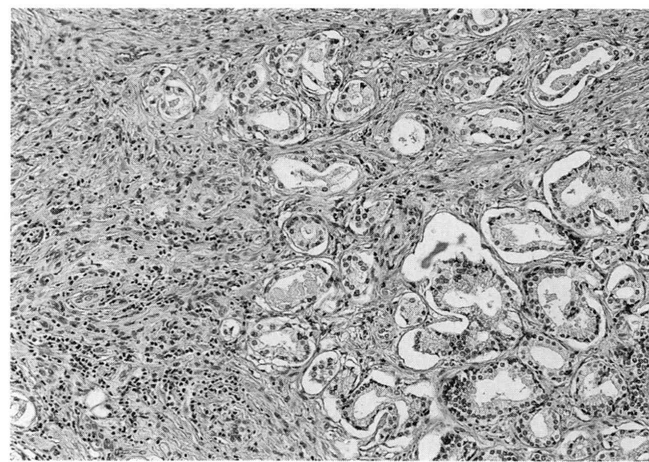

6-29. Irregular border at the edge of a nodule of atypical adenomatous hyperplasia.

NONDIAGNOSTIC FEATURES IN ATYPICAL ADENOMATOUS HYPERPLASIA AND CARCINOMA

Features shared in AAH and cancer

- Crowded (back-to-back glands)
- Intraluminal crystalloids
- Medium-sized (≤1.5 μm) nucleoli
- Scattered poorly formed glands and single cells
- Minimal infiltration at periphery of nodule

features seen in a lesion should outweigh the significance of any one diagnostic feature. That atypical adenomatous hyperplasia and low-grade adenocarcinoma have overlapping features is clear (see box on this page). At scanning magnification, atypical adenomatous hyperplasia is characterized by a lobulated proliferation of small glands (Fig. 6-28). In contrast, low-grade carcinomas have a haphazard, irregular, infiltrative growth pattern. Despite the overall lobular pattern seen in atypical adenomatous hyperplasia, in 19% of cases there may be some infiltration into the surrounding stroma[118] (Fig. 6-29).

Within a nodule of atypical adenomatous hyperplasia there are elongated glands with papillary infolding and branching lumens typical of more benign glands, but in their cytoplasmic features they look similar to the adjacent small glands suggestive of carcinoma (Fig. 6-30). Another common feature is the budding off of glands of atypical adenomatous hyperplasia from obviously benign glands. In contrast, there is an abrupt interface between the small glands of adenocarcinoma and the larger architecturally benign surrounding glands.

At higher power, atypical adenomatous hyperplasia typically is composed of small glands with pale to clear cytoplasm, as opposed to some carcinomas that have more amphophilic cytoplasm (Fig. 6-31). In order for this feature to be diagnostically useful, the cytoplasm of benign prostate glands should appear pale or clear on

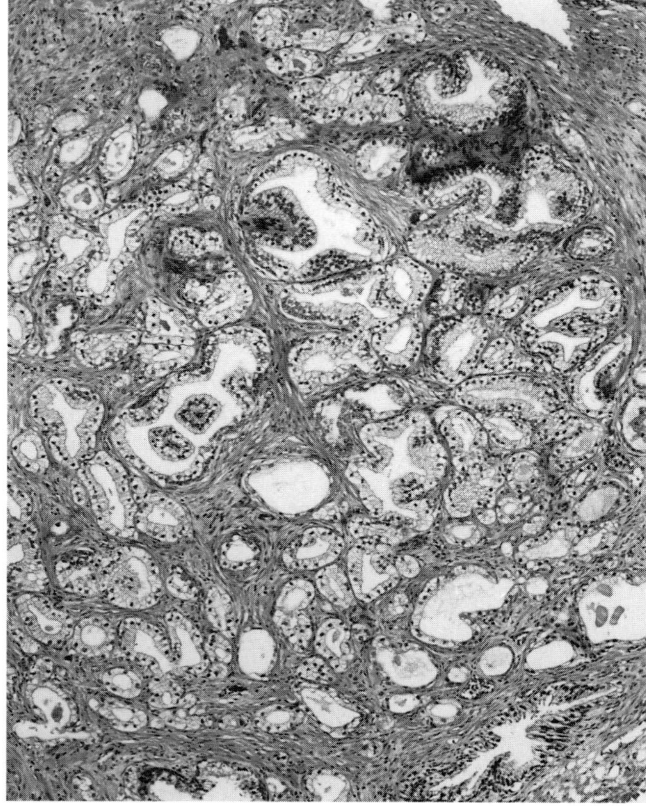

6-30. Nodule of atypical adenomatous hyperplasia.

routinely stained slides. A diagnosis of carcinoma should not be reached based on a few individual cells or poorly formed glands within a nodule of what otherwise is typical of atypical adenomatous hyperplasia (Fig. 6-32). These mimics of carcinoma are tangential sections of the small crowded glands of atypical adenomatous hyperplasia and are seen in 16% of cases found on transurethral resection.[118] Usually, atypical adenomatous hyperplasia has

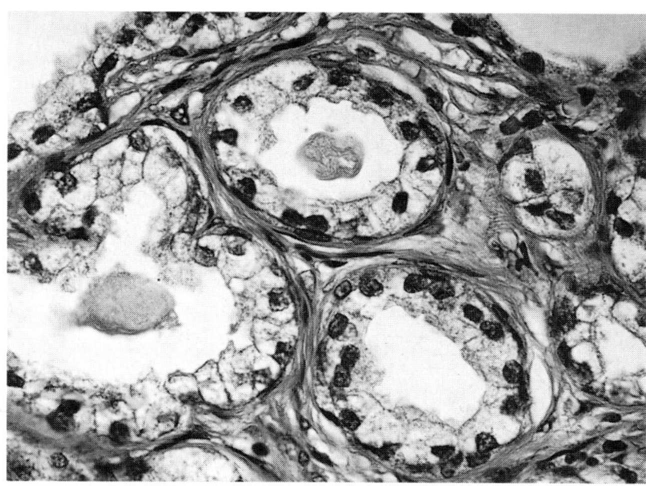

6-31. Atypical adenomatous hyperplasia with pale-staining glands, corpora amylacea, and inconspicuous basal cells.

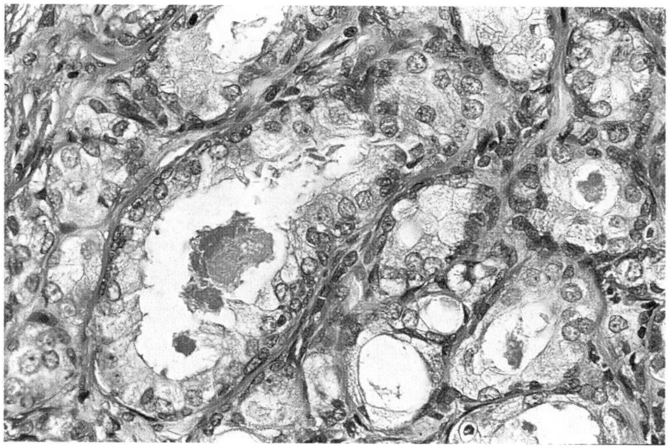

6-32. Atypical adenomatous hyperplasia with visible nucleoli. Note scattered flattened basal cells, luminal proteinaceous material, and small crystalloids.

been described as having completely bland nuclei without nucleoli. This is generally valid; 60% of the lesions contain no, or at most rare, visible nucleoli. In the other 40% small nucleoli are present, which should not lead to the diagnosis of carcinoma[126] (Fig. 6-32). In one study of 38 lesions, 18% contained nucleoli larger than 1 μm.[119] Only huge nucleoli (>3 μm) are incompatible with a diagnosis of atypical adenomatous hyperplasia. In contrast, the majority (70%) of foci of low grade adenocarcinoma have occasional or frequent large nucleoli.[126] These findings emphasize that, although nucleoli are generally helpful in differentiating atypical adenomatous hyperplasia from adenocarcinoma, there is overlap at both ends of the spectrum of visible nucleoli. In this differential diagnosis, the presence of nucleoli should not necessarily be given any more diagnostic weight than the many other light microscopic features to be evaluated. In most cases a constellation of features must be evaluated to differentiate the two entities.

The luminal contents also may be useful in this differential diagnosis. Corpora amylacea are commonly seen in atypical adenomatous hyperplasia and are rare in carcinoma. Carcinomas, on the other hand, may contain amorphous pink homogeneous secretions or intraluminal blue mucinous secretions visible in hematoxylin-eosin-stained sections. Only 2% of cases of atypical adenomatous hyperplasia contain blue intraluminal secretions.[118] In contrast to the diagnostic value of the mucinous secretions visible on hematoxylin-eosin-stained sections, it is not helpful to perform special stains for mucin. Several early studies claimed that the presence of acid mucin was diagnostic of carcinoma, although examples of atypical adenomatous hyperplasia were never analyzed. A later study found that 54% of foci of atypical adenomatous hyperplasia contained acid mucin secretions, evidenced by high-iron diamine alcian-blue positivity.[30] Crystalloids are another intraluminal structure that has been touted as distinguishing atypical adenomatous hyperplasia from carcinoma.[127-130] However, 18% to 39% of foci of atypical adenomatous hyperplasia contain crystalloids,[118,119] and they may be numerous (Fig. 6-32). Thus the presence of crystalloids should not be used to differentiate atypical adenomatous hyperplasia from carcinoma. If crystalloids, single cells, and minimal infiltration are considered characteristic of atypical adenomatous hyperplasia, and mitotic figures, blue mucin, and nucleoli are uncharacteristic, 76% of foci of atypical adenomatous hyperplasia have no uncharacteristic features, 20% have one, and only 4% have two.

Basal cells are the one feature seen in atypical adenomatous hyperplasia that is never seen in carcinoma. Although basal cells may be difficult to identify within many of the glands, a flattened basal cell layer can be seen in at least some of the glands. As long as the glands with a basal cell layer are otherwise identical to the glands where a basal cell layer can not be identified, the entire lesion is benign. It is important to distinguish the basal cell layer from adjacent fibroblasts. While fibroblasts have elongated pointed hyperchromatic nuclei, those basal cells that are recognizable in routine sections have a more cigar-shaped ovoid contour with chromatin similar to that of the overlying secretory cells (see Fig. 6-31). In foci of glandular crowding where all of the features are characteristic of atypical adenomatous hyperplasia and there is no cytologic atypia, one can make the diagnosis without immnohistochemical stains even if basal cells are not visible on routine sections. In cases where the architectural pattern favors atypical adenomatous hyperplasia but there are large nucleoli, the diagnosis can be clarified using immunohistochemistry for basal cells. The use of a basal cell–specific antibody to high molecular weight keratin, such as 34ßE12, is helpful because some glands will show a thin rim of keratin immunoreactivity underneath the cuboidal or columnar secretory cells.[42] The attenuated appearance of this immunoreactivity shows why the basal cell layer is often so difficult to see in routine sections. Corresponding to the discontinuous patchy distribution of basal cells seen in routine sections, as few as 10% of the glands in a nodule of atypical adenomatous hyperplasia may be labeled with antibodies to high molecular keratin, although usually more than half of the glands will show some staining. In an entire nodule, at least some of the glands show basal cell staining, thereby excluding adenocarcinoma. If some glands suggestive of atypical adenomatous hyperplasia lack keratin 34ßE12 immunoreactivity, but are otherwise indistinguishable from adjacent glands that demonstrate basal cell keratin immunoreactivity, the absence of a basal cell layer in some glands should not be the basis of a diagnosis of carcinoma. Some of the variability in basal cell immunoreactivity within atypical adenomatous hyperplasia and other lesions may be caused by tissue processing since more uniform immunoreactivity has been observed in frozen tissue. To date more than 200 cases of adenocarcinoma of the prostate have been studied with antibodies to high molecular weight cytokeratin, and in only one example was there rare positive staining.[42-47]

Atypical adenomatous hyperplasia occurs most frequently within the central region of the prostate and is often seen in transurethral resection specimens where one can appreciate its typical architectural pattern at low magnification as well as evaluate a substantial number of glands for the presence of a basal cell layer. Recently the number of cases of atypical adenomatous hyperplasia seen on needle biopsy has increased. These are more likely to be misdiagnosed as carcinoma, because it is difficult to appreciate the architectural pattern. In order to minimize the potential for misdiagnosing atypical adenomatous hyperplasia on needle biopsy, one should always question whether a lesion may be atypical adenomatous hyperplasia when considering the diagnosis of low-grade carcinoma. If the crowded glands merge with surrounding more recognizable glands, then the focus may be atypical adenomatous hyperplasia. In contrast, glands of carcinoma differ from surrounding benign glands by their darker cytoplasm, enlarged nuclei, prominent nucleoli, and intraluminal contents.

Basal cell–specific antibodies must be interpreted with caution in needle biopsies. Because basal cell staining may be patchy in atypical adenomatous hyperplasia, negative staining in a small focus of glands is not necessarily indicative of malignancy. However, if some of the glands within a crowded glandular focus in a needle biopsy demonstrate a basal cell layer, then atypical adenomatous hyperplasia can be diagnosed. Because of the difficulty in diagnosing atypical adenomatous hyperplasia on needle biopsy, it is useful to verify the diagnosis with high molecular weight cytokeratin antibodies (Fig. 6-33). Similar to the results with transurethral resection specimens, a study of 77 foci of atypical adenomatous hyperplasia in needle biopsies found that mitotic figures and blue mucin were uncommon.[131] Some single cells and a minimally infiltrative pattern were seen in about 12% of lesions and crystalloids were present in 24% of cases. Some nucleoli were present in 13% of atypical adenomatous hyperplasia foci in needle biopsy specimens.

Atypical adenomatous hyperplasia often appears to be multifocal. In a study of 44 cases of atypical adenomatous hyperplasia in transurethral resection specimens, 30 had two or more foci (mean 3.3 foci per case).[118] In a few cases the foci were so numerous that had they been misdiagnosed as carcinoma, they would have been classified as stage T_1b, possibly leading to unwarranted radical therapy. The distinction between atypical adenomatous hyperplasia and low-grade adenocarcinoma in even a single focus may be critical, because diagnosis of even a single focus of carcinoma on transurethral resection may lead to aggressive surgery.[132,133]

Although atypical adenomatous hyperplasia mimics carcinoma, there is no conclusive evidence that these patients have an increased risk of synchronous or metachronous adenocarcinoma of the prostate. In one study, only 6 of 44 patients with atypical adenomatous hyperplasia on transurethral resection had foci of carcinoma.[118] Prior reports of transitions between atypical adenomatous hyperplasia and carcinoma were not verified with the use of basal cell–specific antibodies and may have been atypical adenomatous hyperplasia with foci of individual cells, minimal infiltration, or visible nucleoli. Another argument that has been raised to suggest that atypical adenomatous hyperplasia is a precursor to prostate cancer is that the two entities share certain morphologic features. Several studies have shown that atypical adenomatous hyperplasia may contain acid mucin, crystalloids, nucleoli, and have a patchy basal cell layer. Rather than proving a relation between atypical adenomatous hyperplasia and carcinoma, these findings demonstrate that any one of these features, by itself, is not specific for carcinoma. For example, acid mucin may be seen in atrophy,[30] and a patchy basal cell layer is seen in clear cell cribriform hyperplasia,[134] while nucleoli can be seen in basal cell hyperplasia.[135] None of these lesions is a precursor to prostate cancer. The interpretation of these features must be made in the context of the totality of a lesion's architectural and cytologic features.

A study from the M.D. Anderson Cancer Center[136] analyzed 60 prostates from men who underwent cystoprostatectomy for bladder cancer. Forty-one were found to have incidental prostate cancer and 12 were found to have atypical adenomatous hyperplasia, which the

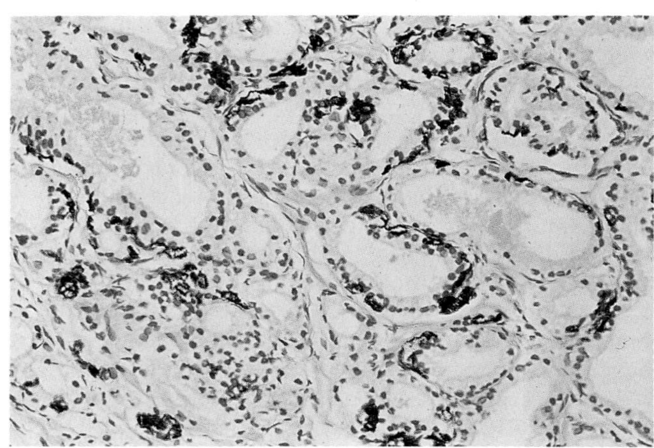

6-33. Atypical adenomatous hyperplasia labeled with antibodies to high molecular weight cytokeratin, demonstrating the basal cells.

authors termed *atypical small glandular proliferations*. They subcategorized the cases of atypical adenomatous hyperplasia into those with and without architectural or cytologic atypia. The overall prevalence of atypical adenomatous hyperplasia in prostates with and without carcinoma was not significantly different. The distribution of atypical adenomatous hyperplasia with and without atypical features also did not differ significantly between cases with and without carcinoma. There was no topographic association between either form of atypical adenomatous hyperplasia and carcinoma. This reinforces the conclusion that atypical adenomatous hyperplasia is not related to carcinoma.

Those studies suggesting a higher risk of carcinoma in men with atypical adenomatous hyperplasia have defined it differently, including many examples of what most authorities would call carcinoma. Whether cases of atypical adenomatous hyperplasia with more prominent nucleoli differ from more ordinary cases in their association with adenocarcinoma remains unknown. Until long-term follow-up studies are performed to assess the risk of developing adenocarcinoma, atypical adenomatous hyperplasia should not be classified as a premalignant lesion. In reporting atypical adenomatous hyperplasia, it may be helpful to add the following note: "Atypical adenomatous hyperplasia, although mimicking adenocarcinoma of the prostate, has not been shown to be associated with either an increased risk of concurrent or subsequent carcinoma."

SCLEROSING ADENOSIS

A lesion with the morphology of sclerosing adenosis was first reported in 1983 as an adenomatoid prostatic tumor.[137] The lesion has also been referred to as *pseudoadenomatoid tumor*. More recently, the term *sclerosing adenosis* has been preferred. In one series, sclerosing adenosis was found in approximately 2% of prostatic specimens.[138] Most lesions are discovered incidentally in routine transurethral resection specimens. Although as many as 10 prostatic chips have been involved in one case, usually only one or two small foci of sclerosing adenosis are present.

Histologically, sclerosing adenosis has a biphasic appearance consisting of well-formed small glands admixed with a densely cellular spindle cell stroma.[138-140] In some lesions glands predominate, while in others the stroma is dominant. The glands are relatively small with pale to lightly acidophilic cytoplasm. In general the nuclei are small and uniform, although occasional nucleoli may be prominent. These glands merge with clusters, cords, and individual epithelial cells with similar nuclear and cytoplasmic features, and react with antibodies to prostate-specific antigen and prostatic acid phosphatase. A thick rim of hyalinized connective tissue invests at least some of the glands within a focus of sclerosing adenosis. Mitotic figures are rare or absent. Although cellular, the spindle cell component lacks pleomorphism or mitotic figures. The transition between the epithelial and spindle cell components is often gradual with the two components seeming to merge together.

Several features should prevent the misdiagnosis of adenocarcinoma in these cases:

1. Sclerosing adenosis, if it was prostate cancer, would be assigned a high Gleason score (7 or 8) because it comprises an admixture of glands, poorly formed glandular structures, and single cells. Prostatic adenocarcinomas with these scores are only rarely seen as limited foci within a transurethral resection specimen. Consequently, the finding of only one or several small foci of a cellular lesion when one is entertaining a diagnosis of high-grade carcinoma should prompt a consideration of sclerosing adenosis (Fig. 6-34). Furthermore, although sclerosing adenosis may be minimally infiltrative at its perimeter, it is still relatively circumscribed compared with high-grade prostate adenocarcinoma.

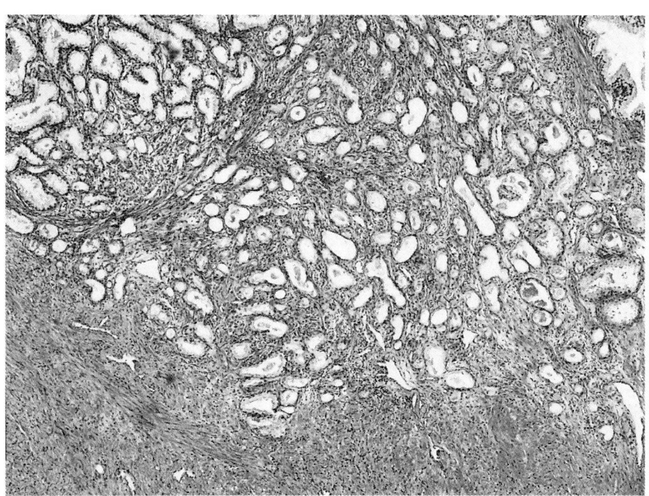

6-34. Sclerosing adenosis at low magnification.

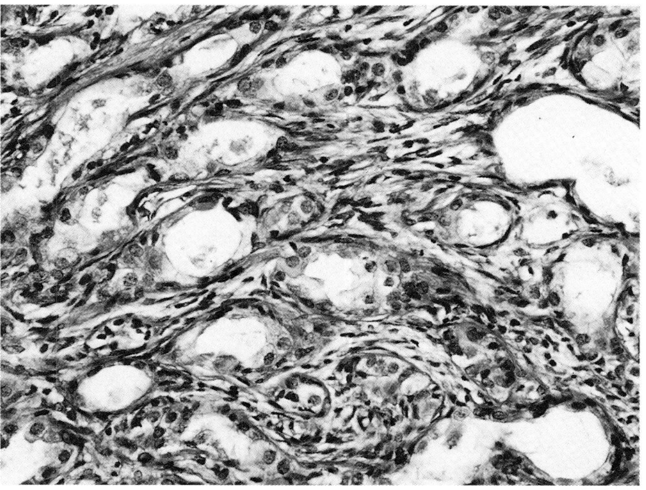

6-35. Sclerosing adenosis with glands resembling atypical adenomatous hyperplasia embedded in spindle-cell stroma.

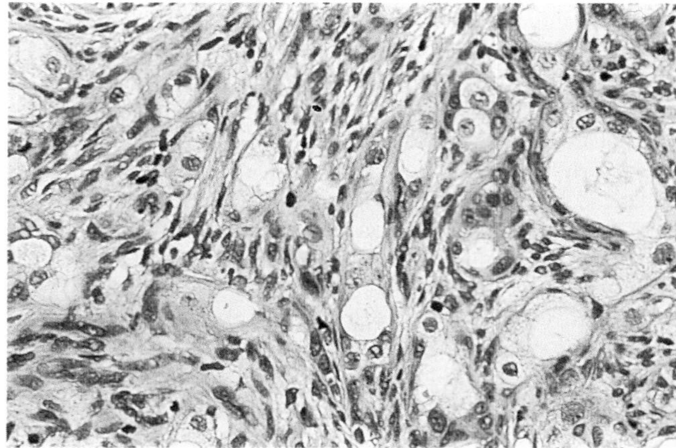

6-36. Stroma of sclerosing adenosis. Note epithelial cells, some with visible nucleoli.

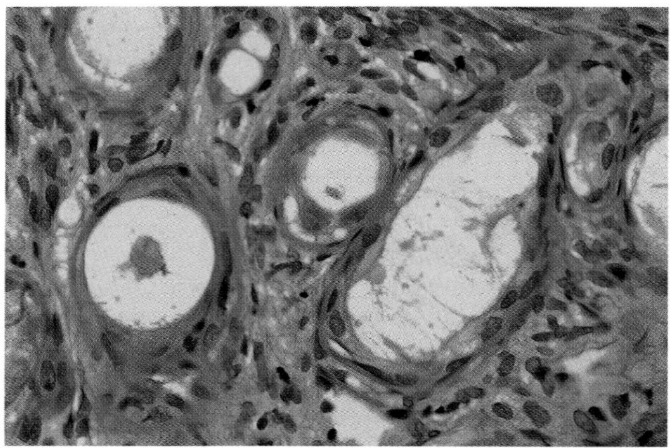

6-37. Eosinophilic hyaline connective tissue sheath surrounding some of the glands within sclerosing adenosis.

2. The glandular structures in sclerosing adenosis resemble those seen in atypical adenomatous hyperplasia (Fig. 6-35). They are composed of cells with pale to clear cytoplasm and bland-appearing nuclei. In many of them a basal cell layer is visible on routine sections. This contrasts with carcinoma, where basal cells are absent.
3. Sclerosing adenosis contains a densely cellular spindle cell (Fig. 6-36). Usually, adenocarcinomas of the prostate either show no apparent stromal response or at most a hypocellular fibrotic reaction.
4. A distinctive feature of sclerosing adenosis is a hyaline sheathlike structure around some of the glands (Fig. 6-37). The glands in ordinary adenocarcinoma lack such a collarette and have a "naked" appearance as they infiltrate the stroma.
5. The relatively bland cytology is also useful for distinguishing sclerosing adenosis from adenocarcinoma, although some nuclei within sclerosing adenosis may be moderately enlarged and contain nucleoli (see Fig. 6-36). The absence of mitotic figures in sclerosing adenosis is not particularly useful in the differential diagnosis because most adenocarcinomas of the prostate, even relatively high-grade ones, lack prominent mitotic activity.

These light microscopic features are diagnostic for sclerosing adenosis, which can usually be diagnosed on routine sections. However, immunohistochemistry is very helpful in difficult cases. Ordinary adenocarcinomas of the prostate of all grades lack basal cells and do not react with antibodies to high molecular weight cytokeratin. In contrast, sclerosing adenosis contains a basal cell layer around most of the glandular structures as well as among the individual cells and cords of cells.[138,139] Ordinary basal cells of the prostate show no myoepithelial cell differentiation. They lack muscle-specific actin and ultrastructurally do not show contractile elements.[49] In sclerosing adenosis, the basal cells react with antibodies to muscle-specific actin and, to a lesser extent, S-100 protein consistent with myoepithelial cell differentiation (Fig. 6-38).[138,139] The dense spindle cell component in sclerosing adenosis reacts to a lesser extent with antibodies to keratin and muscle-specific actin, consistent with myoepithelial cell differentiation. The presence of cells that do not react with these antibodies suggests that there is a fibroblastic component. Ultrastructural studies have confirmed the myoepithelial differentiation in sclerosing adenosis.[141] There has been no association between sclerosing adenosis and adenocarcinoma of the prostate.

BASAL CELL HYPERPLASIA

A spectrum of basaloid lesions ranging from hyperplasia to carcinoma exists in the prostate. Ordinary basal cell hyperplasia resembles the fetal prostate and has been referred to as *fetalization of the prostate* or *embryonal hyperplasia*.[5,142,143] It may occur in association with nodular hyperplasia and grow as well-circumscribed nodules. Alternatively, it can mimic cancer with diffuse infiltration of the prostate. The glands appear basophilic at low power due to multilayering of the basal cells which have scant cytoplasm (Fig. 6-39). Hyperplasia of the basal cells ranges from glands with a few layers of basal cells to solid nests. The cells often palisade around the edge of the nests and the nests may have central lumens. Basal cell hyperplasia is one of the few entities in the prostate that occasionally contains calcified laminated structures resembling psammoma bodies (Fig. 6-40). These structures may be diagnostically useful because they are exceedingly rare in prostate cancer. Basal cell hyperplasia may occasionally contain focal cribriform glands. These glands occur in association with more ordinary basal cell hyperplasia and appear to be the result of fusion of glands of basal cell hyperplasia (Fig. 6-41).

Usually basal cell hyperplasia has been described as having bland nuclear features without nucleoli or pleomorphism[5,142,143,144] (see Fig. 6-39). Recent reports have described cases that would otherwise be considered ordinary basal cell hyperplasia, except for the presence of atypical cytologic features[135,145] (Fig. 6-42).

Ordinary and atypical basal cell hyperplasia are characterized by multilayering of basal cells, as contrasted with the single cell layer and the lack of basal cells in

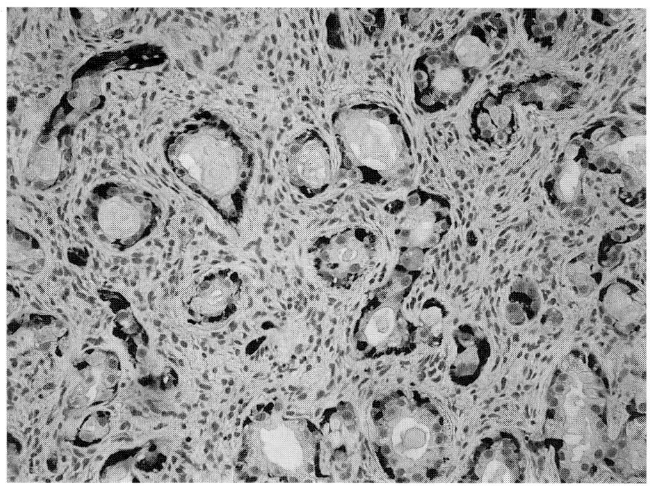

6-38. Sclerosing adenosis with intense S-100 protein immunoreactivity in the basal cells.

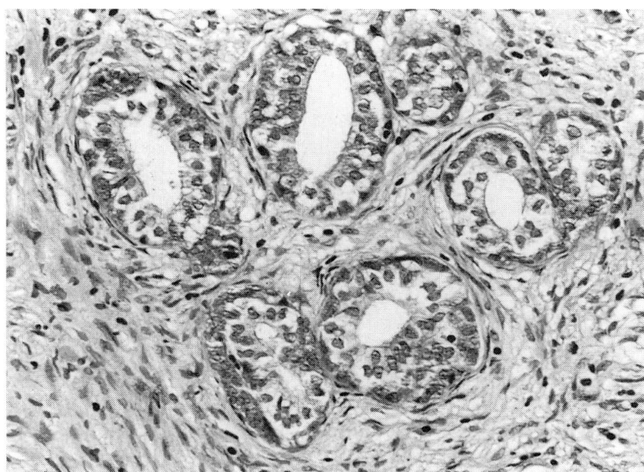

6-39. Basal cell hyperplasia with multilayering of bland nuclei and scant cytoplasm.

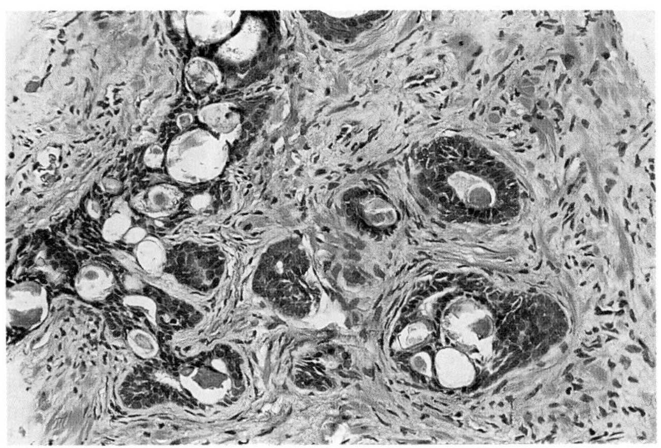

6-40. Basal cell hyperplasia on needle biopsy with numerous calcifications.

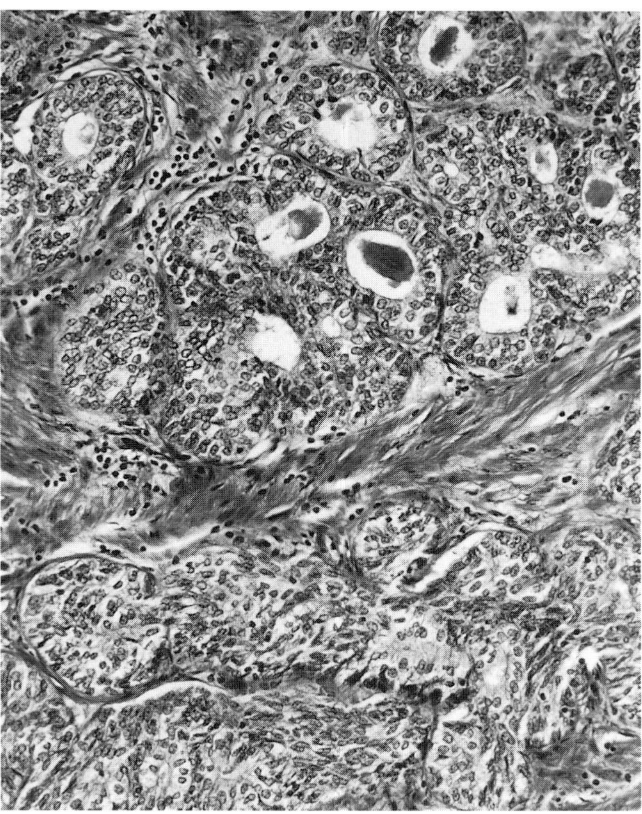

6-41. Focal cribriform architecture within basal cell hyperplasia. Note surrounding zone of typical basal cell hyperplasia composed of individual open multilayered glands and solid basaloid nests.

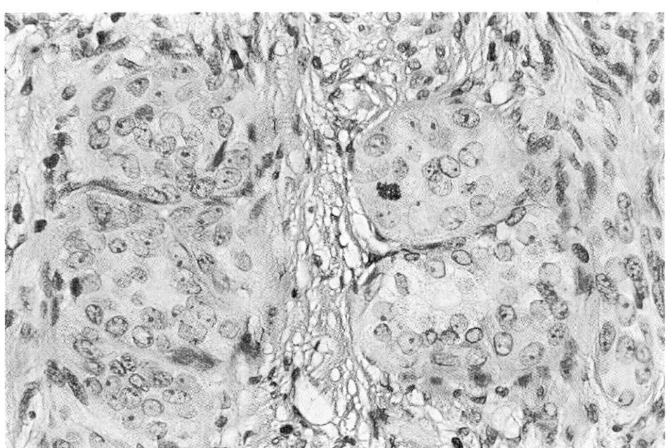

6-42. Atypical basal cell hyperplasia consisting of solid nests of cells with prominent nucleoli. Note mitotic figure.

adenocarcinoma of the prostate. Verification of the presence or absence of basal cells can be accomplished with basal cell specific antibodies, such as keratin 34ßE12.[42,44,45,47,143] Distinguishing atypical basal cell hyperplasia from prostatic intraepithelial neoplasia is more difficult. In most cases the glands of atypical basal cell hyperplasia are small and round. In contrast, glands of prostatic intraepithelial neoplasia tend to be larger with branching and papillary infoldings. Whereas areas of basal cell hyperplasia often consist of crowded glands, prostatic intraepithelial neoplasia glands are separated by a greater amount of stroma, similar to normal glands. At higher magnification, the cells in atypical basal cell hyperplasia have round nuclei, whereas in prostatic intraepithelial neoplasia the nuclei are elongated and pseudostratified. Within areas of atypical basal cell hyperplasia one can occasionally see the atypical basal cells undermining the overlying secretory cells, which have benign nuclei. The basal cells in these foci tend to have a streaming morphology parallel to the basement membrane. On the other hand, prostatic intraepithelial neoplasia has full thickness cytologic atypia with the nuclei oriented perpendicular to the basement membrane. The finding of solid epithelial nests in atypical basal cell hyperplasia further distinguishes it from prostatic intraepithelial neoplasia. An additional difference between prostatic intraepithelial neoplasia and atypical basal cell hyperplasia is that most cases of atypical basal cell hyperplasia are found in transurethral resection specimens, indicating growth in the central part of the prostate. This central distribution parallels that seen with ordinary basal cell hyperplasia and contrasts with prostatic intraepithelial neoplasia which is preferentially located in the periphery of the prostate.[146]

The use of antibodies to cytokeratin 34ßE12 may help in differentiating prostatic intraepithelial neoplasia from atypical basal cell hyperplasia. Within some of the glands of atypical basal cell hyperplasia, cytokeratin 34ßE12 immunohistochemistry will demonstrate multilayered staining of the atypical basal cells, identical to ordinary basal cell hyperplasia. These immunohistochemical results must be interpreted with caution because high molecular weight keratin antibodies may label the periphery of the glands of atypical basal cell hyperplasia more intensely, mimicking the staining seen with prostatic intraepithelial neoplasia.[135] However, the cells that are 34ßE12 reactive in atypical basal cell hyperplasia are cytologically atypical and identical to cells that are not staining within the center of the lumen. High molecular weight keratin staining of prostatic intraepithelial neoplasia shows only a single immunoreactive cell layer confined to cytologically benign appearing flattened basal cells beneath the unreactive atypical columnar cells of prostatic intraepithelial neoplasia.[42,44,45]

When a well-formed distinct nodule of basaloid nests is formed, the term *basal cell adenoma* is sometimes employed, though others prefer to consider these lesions as more pronounced examples of basal cell hyperplasia.[147] In these nodules there may be cribriform structures as well as solid nests.

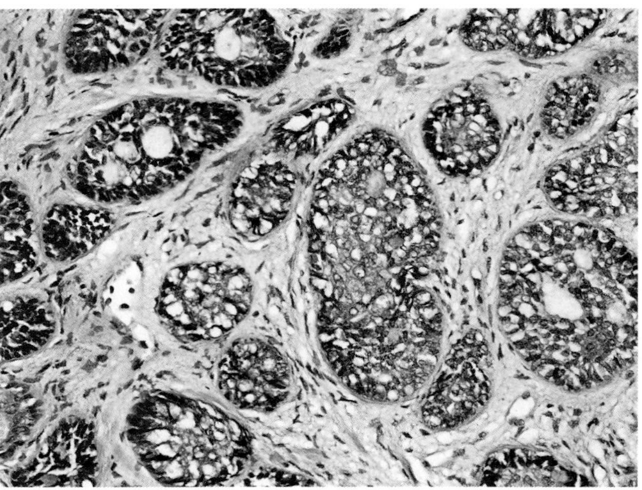

6-43. Adenoid basal cell pattern of basal cell hyperplasia.

A more controversial form of basal cell hyperplasia is the adenoid basal cell pattern, where there are basaloid nests with peripheral palisading and cribriform architecture[140,143,145,148] (Fig. 6-43). These lesions resemble salivary gland neoplasms such as basal cell adenoma or adenoid cystic carcinoma. When present as a focal lesion within the prostate, some authorities regard this as a variant of basal cell hyperplasia.[140] However, in extensive cases the distinction of the adenoid basal form of basal cell hyperplasia from basaloid carcinoma is problematic (see Chapter 7). The distinction of basal cell hyperplasia, adenoid basal cell tumor, and basaloid carcinoma of the prostate cannot be made using basal cell antibodies because all three of these entities show similar immunoreactivity.

Ordinary and atypical basal cell hyperplasia have not been associated with either adenocarcinoma of the prostate or basaloid carcinomas. Whether atypical basal cell hyperplasia carries an increased risk of progression to malignant basaloid tumors is unknown, although the rarity of basaloid carcinomas as compared with atypical basal cell hyperplasia argues against this association. Because of the uncertain nature of atypical basal cell hyperplasia careful follow-up of these patients is recommended.

CLEAR CELL CRIBRIFORM HYPERPLASIA

Clear cell cribriform hyperplasia is a recently described benign lesion that may be confused with either prostatic intraepithelial neoplasia or adenocarcinoma of the prostate.[134] It typically occurs within the central region of the prostate and is seen in specimens removed for urinary obstructive symptoms.

In its most readily recognized form, clear cell cribriform hyperplasia is composed of numerous cribriform glands separated from one another by a modest amount of stroma in a pattern of nodular hyperplasia. In florid cases the glands infiltrate the stroma more diffusely (Fig. 6-44). The epithelial cells have distinctive clear cytoplasm and small bland nuclei with inconspicuous or small nucleoli (Fig. 6-

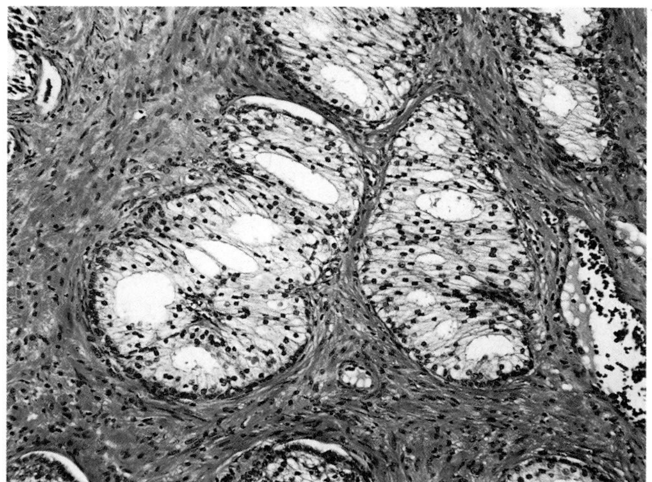
6-44. Clear cell cribriform hyperplasia with glands containing pale to clear cytoplasm.

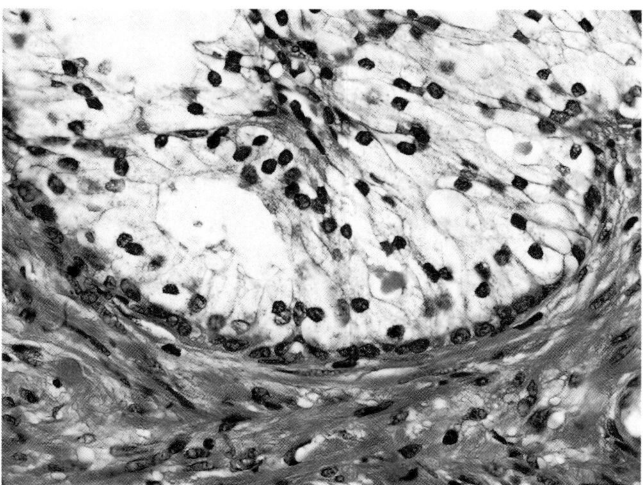
6-45. Clear cell cribriform hyperplasia showing bland cytology and basal cell layer around the gland.

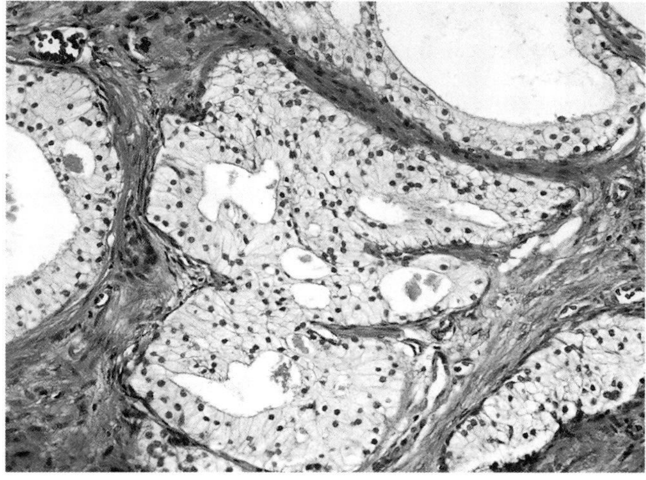
6-46. Glands of clear cell cribriform hyperplasia with inconspicuous basal cell layer.

45). Around many of the glands of clear cell cribriform hyperplasia is a strikingly prominent basal cell layer, consisting of a row of cuboidal darkly staining cells beneath the clear cells (see Fig. 6-45). The basal cells may form small knots at the periphery of some of the glands. Occasionally the basal cells may have small nucleoli. The basal cell layer may be incomplete and in some glands may be invisible in routine sections (Fig. 6-46). Tangential sections can also result in the appearance of nests of clear cells without cribriform architecture or basal cells. Although usually unnecessary, immunostains for high molecular weight cytokeratin can highlight the basal cell layer.[149]

Cribriform prostatic intraepithelial neoplasia also contains large cribriform glands that fit within the normal architectural pattern of the prostate. Architecturally, the cribriform bridges in clear cell cribriform hyperplasia are more tenuous and have more streaming of the nuclei (comparable to the epithelial bridges seen within papillomatosis of the breast). Within cribriform prostatic intraepithelial neoplasia the bridges appear more sturdy (similar to intraductal carcinoma of the breast). Cribriform prostatic intraepithelial neoplasia also is seen only infrequently in transurethral resection specimens, because prostatic intraepithelial neoplasia usually occurs in the periphery of the prostate.

Additional differences between prostatic intraepithelial neoplasia and clear cell cribriform hyperplasia are seen at higher magnification. In prostatic intraepithelial neoplasia the secretory cells have enlarged nuclei with prominent nucleoli. There is often a gradation of nuclear atypia with enlarged nuclei with prominent nucleoli at the periphery of the gland and smaller more bland nuclei toward the center. In clear cell cribriform hyperplasia the clear cells lack nuclear atypia. The very prominent basal cell layer around some of the glands also distinguishes this entity from prostatic intraepithelial neoplasia, where the basal cell layer is inapparent. One cannot use immunostaining with high molecular weight cytokeratin antibodies to differentiate between these two entities because their staining patterns are identical.

The distinction between clear cell cribriform hyperplasia and infiltrating cribriform carcinoma is easier. First, the presence of basal cells around some of the glands in clear cell cribriform hyperplasia rules out carcinoma. Second, the glands in clear cell cribriform hyperplasia lack cytologic atypia in contrast to infiltrating cribriform carcinoma, which almost always shows nuclear atypia. Also it is uncommon to see carcinoma when cribriform glands are unaccompanied by small infiltrating glands.

Clear cell cribriform hyperplasia is uncommon and its natural history is unknown. Although 3 of 25 cases were associated with adenocarcinoma of the prostate, there were no areas of transition from clear cell cribriform hyperplasia to carcinoma of the prostate.[134,149] With prostate cancer's high incidence in elderly men, caution must be exercised before assuming a causal association between it and another entity.

BENIGN NON-NEOPLASTIC CONDITIONS

AMYLOID

Vascular amyloid can be identified in 2% to 10% of prostates removed for hyperplasia or carcinoma.[150-152] Patients with multiple myeloma, primary amyloidosis of the kidney, or chronic debilitating diseases have a higher incidence of prostatic amyloidosis. In these cases amyloid is located in subepithelial areas as well as in vessels. Usually amyloid within the prostate is an incidental finding, although rarely it may mimic carcinoma on rectal examination and give rise to slightly elevated serum acid phosphatase levels.[152] Corpora amylacea often stain nonspecifically for amyloid.[153]

CORPORA AMYLACEA

Corpora amylacea are round laminated hyaline structures found within benign prostatic glands. It is thought that these structures result from growth around a central nidus. Based on the finding of lipid and phospholipid within the central portions of the corpora amylacea, as well as one study that located a keratin dot within the center of the structures, the nidus is thought to originate from degenerated prostatic epithelial cells.[154-157] Ultrastructurally, corpora amylacea are composed of concentric branching fibrils that differ from those seen in amyloid; interspersed are fine particles and granules. Corpora amylacea are Congo red positive and it is thought that the amyloid is derived from beta$_2$-microglobulin coming from urinary reflux into the prostate. Occasionally sperm may also be seen within corpora amylacea.[158]

CALCULI AND CALCIFICATION

Prostatic calculi are found within the tissues or acini of the gland, in contrast to urinary calculi which are found within the prostatic urethra.[159,160] Prostatic calculi are present in 70% to 100% of the glands studied at autopsy, most commonly in men over 50 years of age. Generally, prostatic calculi are multiple and small with an average diameter of less than 5 mm. Occasionally, larger ones up to 4 cm in diameter have occurred. They are brownish-gray, round to ovoid, and usually have smooth surfaces. They are most common within large central prostatic ducts and, when peripherally located, may sometimes be found in cystic cavities. Histologically, the calculi are composed of concentric layers resembling calcified corpora amylacea. They form by the consolidation and calcification of corpora amylacea or by calcification of precipitated prostatic secretions. Although prostatic calculi are common, they are usually asymptomatic and are discovered incidentally. Abscesses may occur in patients who have urinary tract infections resistant to antimicrobial therapy in which the prostatic calculi are infected and provide a continual source of infection. Prostatic calculi are also significant in that they may be confused on clinical examination with carcinoma of the prostate.

Laminated calcifications resembling psammoma bodies may occasionally be seen in benign prostatic conditions. Basal cell hyperplasia is the most common lesion (see Fig. 6-40). This finding may be a diagnostic aid, because only rarely do carcinomas contain laminated calcifications. Calcifications that are seen in prostate cancers tend to be small stippled granular calcifications in areas of central necrosis, most commonly seen in high-grade carcinomas and ductal adenocarcinomas.

CYSTS

Prostatic cysts can be subdivided into utricle cysts and retention cysts.[161,162] The utricle is a small potential space at the apex of the verumontanum posterior to the urethra. Most utricle cysts (müllerian duct cysts) are midline and lie outside the prostate between the bladder and rectum. In the approximately 25% of utricle cysts that are congenital there are also abnormalities of the external genitalia, and in about 10% of all utricle cysts there is unilateral renal dysgenesis or agenesis. Utricle cysts may also arise secondarily due to inflammation. The cysts often are asymptomatic but when large cause bladder obstruction. The patients range in age from 2 months to 75 years, with a median age of 26 years. Histologically, the cyst walls may lack an epithelial lining or may be composed of columnar, cuboidal, transitional, or, less frequently, squamous epithelium. In approximately 10% of cases there are calculi within the cyst. Other associations include four cases of cystadenoma and isolated cases of squamous-cell carcinoma and adenocarcinoma arising in the cysts.

Retention cysts arise when prostatic acini become distended with clear fluid. Clusters of dilated prostatic glands may appear hypoechoic on transrectal ultrasound, mimicking carcinoma.[163] Since small asymptomatic dilated acini are common, the term *retention cyst* should be reserved only for those that are symptomatic. Defined accordingly, the cysts range from 1 to 2 cm, are usually unilocular, and are found adjacent to the urethra. Histologically, the cysts are lined by flattened prostatic glandular epithelium or transitional epithelium.

MULTILOCULAR CYSTS (MULTILOCULAR PROSTATIC CYSTADENOMA)

Several reports have described large multilocular cystic lesions composed of prostatic glands between the bladder and the rectum[164-169] (Fig. 6-47). They may be either separate from the prostate or attached to the prostate by a pedicle. These masses have weighed up to 6,500 g, ranging from 7.5 to 20 cm in diameter. On cross section they are well circumscribed and resemble nodular hyperplasia with multiple cysts, ranging from microscopic to several centimeters in diameter. Cyst contents include serous, mucinous, serosanguineous, or purulent fluid. Atrophic prostatic epithelium, reactive with antibodies to prostate-specific antigen and prostatic acid phosphatase, lines the cysts. Some multilocular cysts are more solid with less intervening stroma and prominent arborization of prostatic glands. The epithelial lining in these cases may be cuboidal, low columnar, or show squamous metaplasia. The stroma may be either collagenous or fibromuscular. There also have been several reports of similar lesions within the prostate.

The distinction of intraprostatic multilocular cysts from cystic nodular hyperplasia may be difficult. The

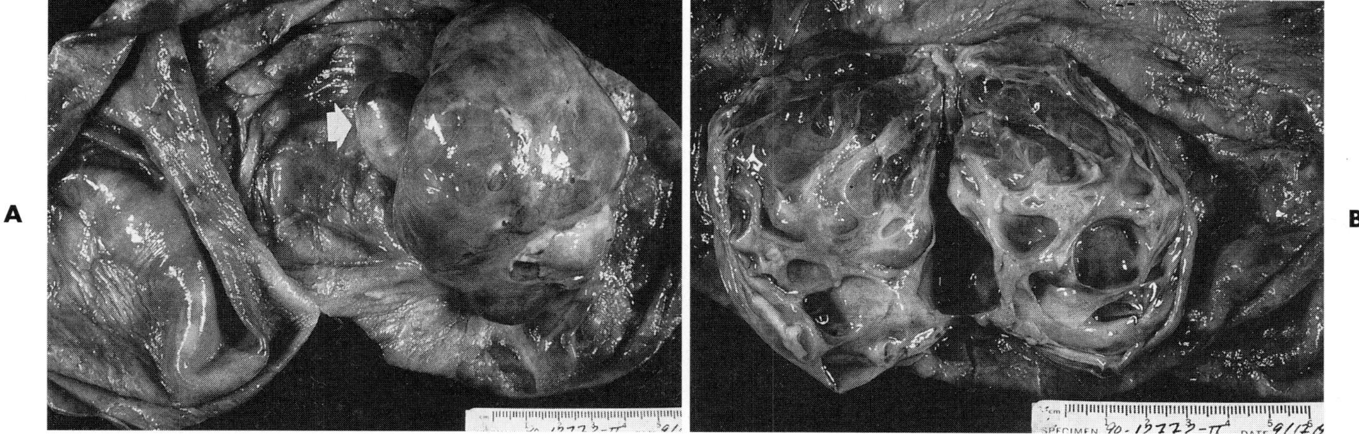

6-47. A, Opened multilocular cyst containing a large round projection and smaller sausage-shaped projection (*arrow*) that proved to be a seminal vesicle. B, Sectioned large projection showing multilocular cyst of the prostate. *(From Lim DJ, Hayden RT, Murad T et al: Multilocular prostatic cystadenoma presenting as a large complex pelvic cystic mass, J Urol 149:856-859,1993; with permission.)*

diagnosis of intraprostatic cystadenoma should be restricted to cases where one half of the prostate resembles normal prostate tissue and the remaining prostate is enlarged by a solitary encapsulated nodule composed of epithelium, cysts, or both.[168,169] Extraprostatic cystadenomas may represent ectopic prostatic tissue resulting from abnormal embryogenesis. In support of this concept the lesions often are found in men in their 20s and 30s. Also, there are other examples of ectopic prostate tissue in the region such as in the anus and bladder. Another alternative is that in cases with severe prostatic hyperplasia, nodules may herniate into surrounding soft tissue, attached only by a thin pedicle or separate from the prostate. Prostatic cystadenomas may recur if incompletely excised and may require extensive surgery because of their large size and impingement on surrounding structures.

MELANOTIC LESIONS

Melanin may be found within the stroma, glands, or both stroma and glands.[34-39] The term *melanosis*, if not otherwise specified, usually refers to melanin found in any location within the prostate. Blue nevus is used to describe stromal melanin deposition, and glandular melanosis denotes the presence of melanin within epithelial cells. In about 50% of the cases of prostatic blue nevi, pigment is grossly evident. The areas of pigment deposition may be extensive, in some cases up to 2 cm in diameter. Microscopically, blue nevi consist of deeply pigmented melanin-filled spindle cells within the fibromuscular stroma. Ultrastructurally, the cells are melanocytes with melanosomes in different stages of differentiation. When melanin is present in prostatic epithelium, it is most prominent along the basement membrane. Nonneoplastic and neoplastic prostatic epithelial cells with melanin contain only mature melanosomes, suggesting that epithelial melanin results from a transfer of pigment from the stromal melanocytes. In addition to glandular and stromal melanosis, melanin may rarely be seen in glands of adenocarcinoma of the prostate. The incidence of microscopic prostatic blue nevi and glandular melanosis is about 4% each. Cases with more prominent melanosis, such as those with grossly visible pigment, are much less common and have been published as isolated case reports.

ANTIANDROGEN THERAPY

Antiandrogen therapy results in squamous metaplasia in both the overlying urethra as well as diffusely throughout the prostate.[170-172] Another situation associated with urethral squamous metaplasia within urethra is transurethral resection. The diffuse nature of squamous metaplasia with antiandrogen therapy is characteristic since the only other situation in which squamous metaplasia occurs within the prostate is localized to the immediate vicinity of prostatic infarcts. Other changes with antiandrogen therapy include atrophy of the glandular epithelium with piling up of the nuclei resembling basal cell hyperplasia and some stromal fibrosis.[172]

ATROPHY

Atrophy, although typically considered to be a process affecting the elderly, was recently demonstrated by Gardner and Culberson to be present in at least 70% of men between the ages of 19 and 29.[173] Atrophic prostate glands may be firm at digital rectal examination and may give rise to hypoechoic lesions on transrectal ultrasound; such areas may be biopsied as lesions suggestive of cancer.[174] There are several different patterns of atrophy. Regardless of the pattern all forms of atrophy can be recognized at medium power magnification. The presence of well-formed open glands with a very basophilic appearance is characteristic of atrophy (Fig. 6-48). The basophilia results from scant cytoplasm rather than nuclear enlargement, such that at low power one is virtually seeing the nuclear outline of the gland. In contrast, gland-forming adenocarcinomas of the prostate have abundant cytoplasm. Even those carcinomas with amphophilic

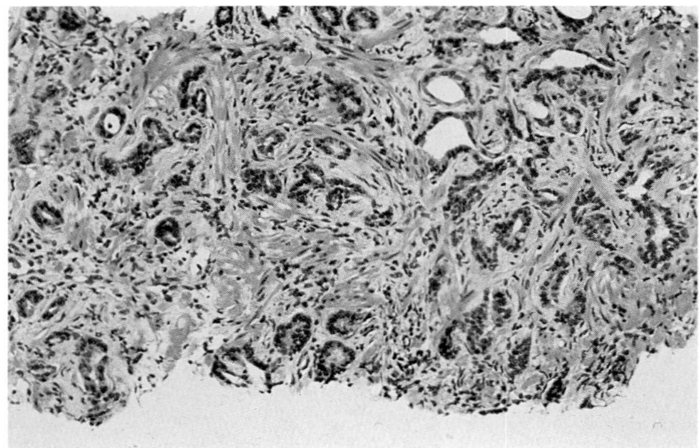

6-48. Glandular atrophy.

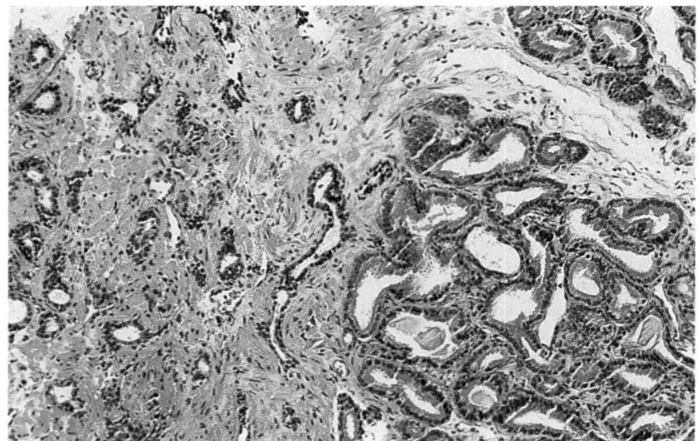

6-49. Atrophy (*left*) adjacent to carcinoma with amphophilic cytoplasm (*right*).

cytoplasm do not appear as dark, open glands at low power (Fig. 6-49).

Atrophy is most readily diagnosed when the glands are arranged in a lobular configuration. On occasion, atrophic glands appear more infiltrative and may be misdiagnosed as cancer. This invasive appearance is an artifact of the limited sampling of needle biopsy material. In contrast with prostate cancer, individual atrophic glands are not seen infiltrating between benign prostate glands. A particularly invasive pattern occurs with sclerotic atrophy where benign atrophic glands are set in a fibrotic stroma. The diagnosis of sclerotic atrophy should be made at low-medium power. In general once one makes the diagnosis of atrophy based on the low-power appearance, one need not examine the focus at higher power. Although atrophic glands generally have bland cytologic features, a few have nuclear enlargement and occasional large nucleoli (Fig. 6-50). The low-power appearance of basophilic open glands is so characteristic of atrophy that, except for rare cases (see Chapter 7, section on atrophic cancers), one should not let the occasional high

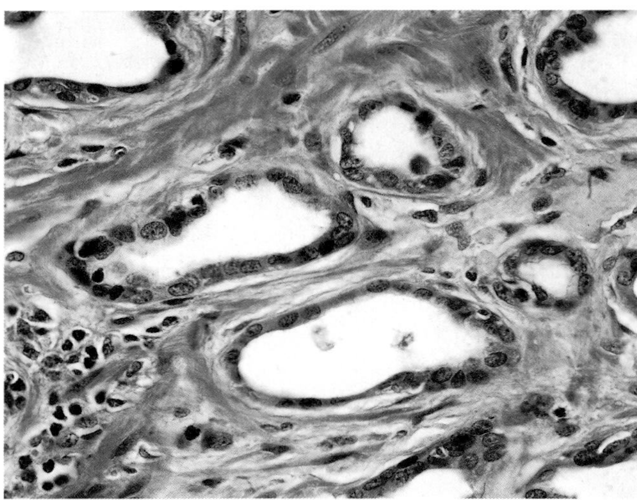

6-50. Atrophic glands with scant cytoplasm and some nuclei showing prominent nucleoli.

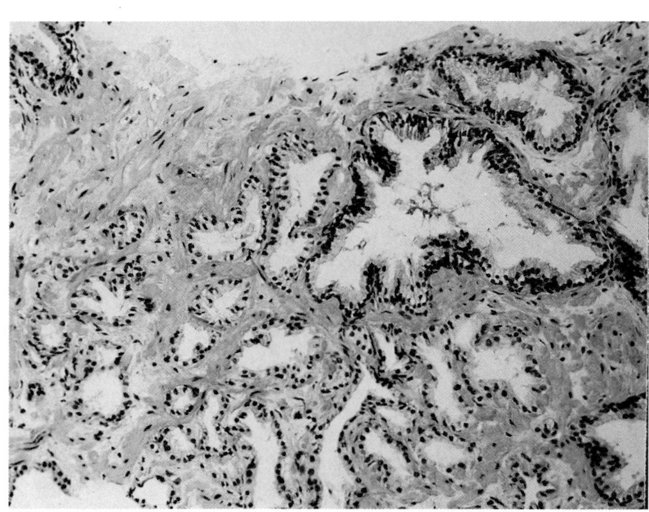

6-51. Pale-staining atrophic glands adjacent to larger glands.

magnification finding of nuclei with atypia dissuade one from a benign diagnosis. Although atrophic glands with more pronounced atypia are usually associated with inflammation, the degree of inflammation leading to these changes may be mild and predominantly composed of lymphocytes. Furthermore, atrophy-associated atypia need not be accompanied by an inflammatory infiltrate.

Another pattern, which has been termed *partial atrophy*, may be misdiagnosed as carcinoma of the prostate.[175] The lesion can have a lobular appearance in which pale-staining glands cluster around more recognizably benign large glands (Fig. 6-51). In more pronounced examples, the pale glands are distributed diffusely throughout the needle biopsy and have a disorganized infiltrative appearance. These glands have attenuated cytoplasm and the nuclei almost reach the luminal surface. Because of the scant but visible cytoplasm, the

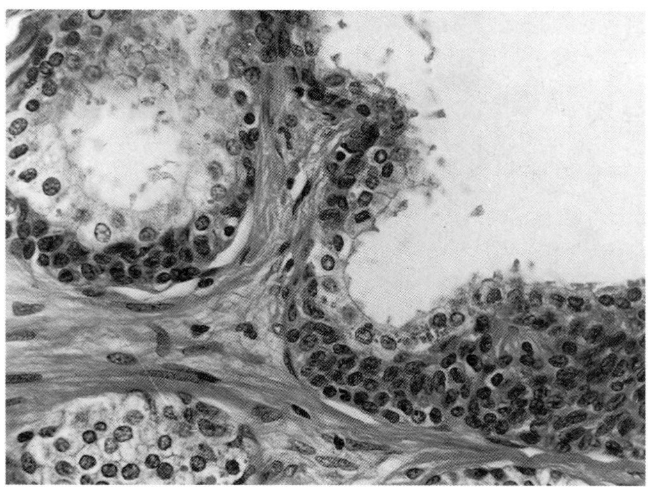

6-52. Metaplastic urothelium beneath prostatic glandular epithelium.

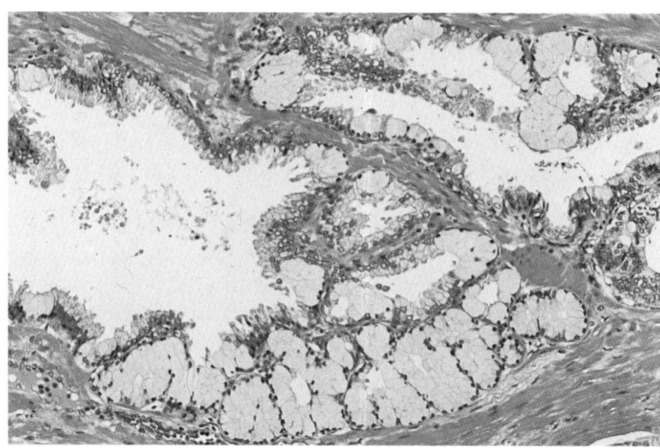

6-53. Mucinous metaplasia.

glands are not as basophilic at low power as are those of fully developed atrophy. The pale to clear attenuated cytoplasm in partially atrophic glands differs from gland-forming cancers which have more abundant cytoplasm. The nuclei in partially atrophic glands are small, somewhat crinkly, and without nucleoli, in contrast with spherical nuclei of carcinoma in which nucleoli often are visible. Although the routine histological appearance of atrophy is usually diagnostic, the diagnosis can be verified with basal cell–specific keratin antibodies, which label atrophic glands uniformly and intensely.

METAPLASIA

Urothelial

The central segments of the prostatic ducts are lined by urothelium similar to that of the urethra. In the peripheral segments of the prostatic ducts, as well as in scattered prostatic acini, there may be alternating areas of cuboidal and columnar epithelium admixed with urothelium. When urothelium is present in the more peripheral prostatic ducts and acini, it is referred to as *urothelial metaplasia*. Urothelial metaplasia may be a misnomer in that there is no evidence that this process results from metaplasia of a different epithelial cell type. Urothelial metaplasia may be seen throughout the prostate in infants and neonates. It is composed of spindle-shaped epithelial cells that are often oriented with their long axes perpendicular to the lumen. The urothelium contains ovoid nuclei that often overlap in a streaming manner (Fig. 6-52). These areas differ from ordinary urothelium in that they lack umbrella cells and often are lined by eosinophilic secretory cells. In areas of intense chronic inflammation, morphologic alterations occur consisting of streaming of basophilic epithelium resembling urothelial metaplasia.

Paneth cell

A form of metaplasia designated *Paneth cell-like metaplasia* or *Paneth cell-like change* has been described in a few cases.[176-178] Histologically, it is characterized by bright eosinophilic granules filling the apical cytoplasm. Usually this is found in only a few groups or scattered individual cells within glands that otherwise appear unremarkable. The granules stain with periodic acid-Schiff and are diastase resistant. They show no reaction with Fontana-Masson and Grimelius stains and do not react with antibodies to neuroendocrine markers. Prostate-specific antigen and prostatic acid phosphatase are present in these cells. In one case electron microscopy revealed electron-dense variably sized lysosome-like or exocrine-like granules. Unlike normal Paneth cells, the granules of Paneth cell-like metaplasia are lysosyme and IgA-negative. These granules do not appear to be degenerative in nature, in contrast to lipofuscin which stains positive with Fontana-Masson. Despite the above findings, a recent study has questioned whether Paneth cell-like metaplasia is a distinct entity or merely represents cells with prominent neuroendocrine differentiation.[179]

Mucous gland

Mucous gland metaplasia is found in approximately 1% of prostates.[180,181] The lesion consists of tall mucin-filled goblet cells (Fig. 6-53). The cells are positive for periodic acid-Schiff, mucicarmine, and alcian blue, and are diastase resistant. The cells are negative for prostate-specific antigen and prostatic acid phosphatase. These may occur as randomly scattered individual cells or in groups of 5 to 10 cells. Most foci are small, very rarely measuring over 1 square mm. The nuclei are tiny, dark, and basal. Mucinous gland metaplasia may be found in normal and hyperplastic prostate and in areas of urothelial metaplasia, basal cell hyperplasia, or atrophy. It does not appear to be related to cancer or inflammation.

Squamous

Squamous metaplasia is common adjacent to infarcts,[74] following antiandrogen therapy,[170-172] and in neonates,[4] as described earlier in this chapter. In general the cells of squamous metaplasia lack immunoreactivity for prostatic markers, although one study demonstrated some cells to contain prostatic acid phosphatase.[182]

Mesenchymal

One case of cartilaginous metaplasia in the prostate has been reported.[183]

MISCELLANEOUS CONDITIONS

In a study of prostates from a medical examiner's office, 9% of prostates contained sperm.[158] Rare cases of prostatic endometriosis[184] and polyarteritis nodosa[185] have been reported with prostatic symptoms and diagnosed on biopsy material. Extramedullary hematopoiesis and ectopic salivary gland tissue have been described in the prostate.[186,187]

One case of paraganglion cells in the prostate has been reported.[188] This occurred in a transurethral resection specimen where clusters of clear cells with fine cytoplasmic granules were present between muscle fibers. Their nuclei had moderate pleomorphism. These cells were intimately related to nerves and blood vessels and were highly vascularized. Verification of their nature was accomplished with immunostaining, demonstrating them to be positive for neuroendocrine markers and negative for keratin. This lesion closely mimicked adenocarcinoma of the prostate. The highly vascular setting along with the neuroendocrine type of atypia are clues to prevent a misdiagnosis.

References

1. Aumuller G: Prostate gland and seminal vesicles, Berlin, 1979, Springer-Verlag.
2. Coffey DS: The molecular biology, endocrinology, and physiology of the prostate and seminal vesicles. In Walsh PC, Retik AB, Stamey TA et al, eds: Campbell's urology, ed 6, Philadelphia, 1992, WB Saunders.
3. Glenister TW: The development of the utricle and the so-called "middle" or "median" lobe of the prostate, J Anat 96:443-455, 1962.
4. Zondek T, Zondek LH: The fetal and neonatal prostate. In Goland M, ed: Normal and abnormal growth of the prostate. Springfield, Ill, 1975, Charles C Thomas.
5. Bennett ED, Gardner WA Jr: Embryonal hyperplasia of the prostate, Prostate 7:411-417, 1985.
6. Berry SW, Coffey DS, Walsh PC et al: The development of human benign prostate hyperplasia with age, J Urol 132:474-479, 1984.
7. McNeal JE: Normal and pathologic anatomy of prostate, Urology 17(suppl):11-16, 1981.
8. Kost LV, Evans GW: Occurrence and significance of striated muscle within the prostate, J Urol 92:703-704, 1964.
9. Manley CB Jr: The striated muscle of the prostate, J Urol 95:234-240, 1966.
10. Graversen PH, England DM, Madsen PO et al: Significance of striated muscle in curettings of the prostate, J Urol 139:751-753, 1988.
11. Lowsley OS: The development of the human prostate gland with reference to the development of other structures at the neck of the urinary bladder, Am J Anat 13:299-349, 1912.
12. Reese JH, McNeal JE, Redwine EA et al: Differential distribution of pepsinogen II between zones of the human prostate and the seminal vesicle, J Urol 136:1148-1152, 1986.
13. Ayala AG, Ro JY, Babaian R et al: The prostate capsule: does it exist? Its importance in the staging and treatment of prostatic carcinoma, Am J Surg Pathol 13:21-27, 1989.
14. Epstein JI: The prostate and seminal vesicles. In Sternberg SS, ed: Diagnostic surgical pathology, New York, 1989, Raven Press.
15. Walsh PC, Lepor H, Eggleston JC: Radical prostatectomy with preservation of sexual function: anatomical and pathological considerations, Prostate 4:473-485, 1983.
16. Lepor H, Gregerman M, Crosby R et al: Precise localization of the autonomic nerves from the pelvic plexus to the corpora cavernosa: a detailed anatomical study of the adult male pelvis, J Urol 133:207-212, 1985.
17. Carstens PHB: Perineural glands in normal and hyperplastic prostate, J Urol 123:686-688, 1980.
18. McIntyre TL, Franzini DA: The presence of benign prostatic glands in perineural spaces, J Urol 135:507-509, 1986.
19. Epstein JI: Differential diagnosis in pathology: urologic disorders, New York, 1992, Igaku-Shoin.
20. Moore RA: The evolution and involution of the prostate gland, J Urol 60:599-603, 1948.
21. Andrews GS: The histology of the human foetal and prepubertal prostates, J Anat 85:44-54, 1951.
22. Jobsis AC, DeVries DP, Anholt RRH: Demonstration of the prostatic origin of metastases: an immunohistochemical method for formalin-fixed embedded tissue, Cancer 41:1788-1793, 1978.
23. Shevchuk MM, Romas NA, Ng PY et al: Acid phosphatase localization in prostatic carcinoma, Cancer 52:1642-1646, 1983.
24. Yam LT, Janckila AJ, Lam KW et al: Immunohistochemistry of prostatic acid phosphatase, Prostate 2:97-107, 1981.
25. Franks LM, O'Shea JD, Thomson AER: Mucin in the prostate: an immunohistochemical study in normal glands, latent, clinical and colloid cancers, Cancer 17:983-991, 1964.
26. Hukill PB, Vidone RA: Histochemistry of mucous and other polysacchyrides in tumors: carcinoma of the prostate, Lab Invest 16:395-406, 1967.
27. Pinder SE, McMahon RFT: Mucins in prostatic carcinoma, Histopathology 16:433-446, 1990.
28. Ro JY, Grignon DJ, Troncoso P et al: Mucin in prostatic adenocarcinoma, Semin Diagn Pathol 5:273-283, 1988.
29. Taylor NS: Histochemistry in the diagnosis of early prostatic carcinoma, Hum Pathol 10:513-520, 1979.
30. Epstein JI, Fynheer J: Acidic mucin in the prostate: can it differentiate adenosis from adenocarcinoma? Hum Pathol 23:1321-1325, 1992.
31. Foster EA, Levine AG: Mucin production in metastatic carcinomas, Cancer 16:506-509, 1963.
32. Levine AJ, Foster EA: Relation of mucicarmine-staining properties of carcinomas of the prostate to differentiation, metastasis, and prognosis, Cancer 17:21-25, 1964.

33. Brennick JB, O'Connell JS, Dickersin GR et al: Lipofuscin pigmentation (so-called "melanosis") of the prostate, Am J Surg Pathol 18:446-454, 1994.
34. Aguilar M, Gaffney EF, Finnerty DP: Prostatic melanosis with involvement of benign and malignant epithelium, J Urol 128:825-827, 1982.
35. Botticelli AR, DiGregorio C, Losi L et al: Melanosis (pigmented melanocytosis) of the prostate gland, Eur Urol 16:229-232, 1989.
36. Jao W, Fretzin DF, Christ NL et al: Blue nevus of the prostate gland, Arch Pathol 91:187-191, 1971.
37. Ro JY, Grignon DJ, Ayala AG et al: Blue nevus and melanosis of the prostate. Electron-microscopic and immunohistochemical studies, Am J Clin Pathol 90:530-535, 1988.
38. Ryan J, Crow J: Melanin in the prostate gland, Br J Urol 61:455-456, 1988.
39. Martinez MCJ, Garcia GR, Castaneda CAL: Blue nevus of the prostate: Report of two new cases with immunohistochemical and electron microscopic studies, Eur Urol 22:339-342, 1992.
40. Totten RS, Heinemann NW, Hudson PB et al: Microscopic differential diagnosis of latent carcinoma of prostate, Arch Pathol 55:131-141, 1953.
41. Brandes D, Kirchein D, Scott WW: Ultrastructure of the human prostate. Normal and neoplastic, Lab Invest 13:1541-1560, 1964.
42. Hedrick L, Epstein JI: Use of keratin 903 as an adjunct in the diagnosis of prostate carcinoma, Am J Surg Pathol 13:389-396, 1989.
43. Nagle RB, Ahmann FR, McDaniel KM et al: Cytokeratin characterization of human prostatic carcinoma and its derived cell lines, Cancer Res 47:281-286, 1987.
44. Shah IA, Schlageter M, Stinnett P et al: Cytokeratin immunohistochemistry as a diagnostic tool for distinguishing malignant from benign epithelial lesions of the prostate, Mod Pathol 4:220-224, 1991.
45. Brawer MK, Peehl DM, Stamey TA et al: Keratin immunoreactivity in the benign and neoplastic human prostate, Cancer Res 45:3663-3667, 1985.
46. Brawer MK, Nagle RB, Pitts W et al: Keratin immunoreactivity as an aid to the diagnosis of persistent adenocarcinoma in irradiated human prostate, Cancer 63:454-460, 1989.
47. O'Malley FP, Grignon DJ, Shum DT: Usefulness of immunoperoxidase staining with high-molecular-weight cytokeratin in the differential diagnosis of small-acinar lesions of the prostate gland, Virchows Arch A Pathol Anat Histopathol 417:191-196, 1990.
48. Warhol MJ, Longtine JA: The ultrastructural localization of prostatic specific antigen and prostatic acid phosphatase in hyperplastic and neoplastic human prostates, J Urol 134:607-613, 1985
49. Srigley JR, Dardick I, Hartwick RWJ et al: Basal epithelial cells of human prostate gland are not myoepithelial cells: a comparative immunohistochemical and ultrastructural study with the human salivary gland, Am J Pathol 126:957-966, 1990.
50. Howat AJ, Mills PM, Lyons TJ et al: Absence of S-100 protein in prostatic glands, Histopathology 13:468-470, 1988.
51. Di Sant'Agnese PA: Neuroendocrine differentiation in human prostatic carcinoma, Hum Pathol 23:287-296, 1992.
52. Oesterling JE: Prostate specific antigen: A critical assessment of the most useful tumor marker for adenocarcinoma of the prostate, J Urol 145:907-923, 1991.
53. Glynn RJ, Campion EW, Bouchard GR et al: The development of benign prostatic hyperplasia among volunteers in the normative aging studies, Am J Epidemiol 121:78-90, 1985.
54. Berry SJ, Coffey DS, Walsh PC et al: The development of human benign prostatic hyperplasia with age, J Urol 132:474-479, 1984.
55. McNeal J: Pathology of benign prostatic hyperplasia: insight into etiology, Urol Clin N Am 17:477-486, 1990.
56. Morrison AS: Risk factors for surgery for prostatic hypertrophy, Am J Epidemiol 135:974-980, 1992.
57. Walsh PC: Benign prostatic hyperplasia. In Walsh PC, Retik AB, Stamey TA et al, eds: Campbell's urology, ed 6, Philadelphia, 1992, WB Saunders.
58. Peters CA, Walsh PC: The effect of Nafarelin acetate, a luteinizing hormone-releasing hormone agonist on benign prostatic hyperplasia, N Eng J Med 217:599-604, 1987.
59. Stoner E, Finasteride Study Group: Clinical effects of 5 alpha-reductase inhibitor, Finasteride on benign prostatic hyperplasia, J Urol 147:1298-1302, 1992.
60. Gormley GJ, Stoner E, Bruskewitz RC et al: The effect of Finasteride on men with benign prostatic hyperplasia, N Engl J Med 327:1185-1191, 1992.
61. Walsh PC, Hutchins GM, Ewing LL: Tissue content of dihydrotestosterone in human prostatic hyperplasia is not supranormal, J Clin Invest 72:1772-1777, 1983.
62. Bartsch G, Muller HR, Oberholzer M et al: Light microscopic stereological analysis of the normal human prostate and of benign prostatic hyperplasia, J Urol 122:487-491, 1979.
63. Lepor H, Auerbach S, Puras-Baez A et al: A randomized placebo-controlled multicentric study of the efficacy and safety of terazosin in the treatment of benign prostatic hyperplasia, J Urol 148:1467-1474, 1992.
64. Bruskewitz RT, Christensen MM: Critical evaluation of transurethral resection and incision of the prostate, Prostate 3(suppl):27-38, 1990.
65. Dowd JE, Smith JJ: Balloon dilatation of the prostate, Urol Clin North Am 17:671-677, 1990.
66. Sapozink MD, Boyd SD, Astrahan MA et al: Transurethral hyperthermia for benign prostatic hyperplasia: preliminary clinical results, J Urol 143:944-950, 1990.
67. Franks LM: Benign nodular hyperplasia of the prostate: a review, Ann R Coll Surg Engl 14:92-106, 1954.
68. Moore RA: Benign hypertrophy of the prostate: a morphologic study, J Urol 50:680-710, 1943.
69. Attah EB, Powell NEA: Atypical stromal hyperplasia of the prostate gland, Am J Clin Pathol 67:324-327, 1977.
70. Kafandarif PM, Polyzonis MD: Fibroadenoma-like foci in human prostatic nodular hyperplasia, Prostate 4:33-36, 1983.
71. Kohnen PW, Drach GW: Patterns of imflammation in prostatic hyperplasia: a histologic and bacteriologic study, J Urol 121:755-760, 1979.

72. Nielsen ML, Asnaes S, Hattel T: Inflammatory changes in the noninfected prostate gland. A clinical, microbiological and histological investigation, J Urol 110:423-426, 1973.
73. Baird HH, McKay HW, Kimmelstiel P: Ischemic infarction of the prostate gland, South Med J 43:234-240, 1950.
74. Mostofi FK, Morse WH: Epithelial metaplasia in "prostatic infarction," Arch Pathol 51:340-345, 1951.
75. Jones TJ, Howie AJ: Necropsy study of infarcts of prostate and prostatic urethra, J Clin Pathol 39:1221-1223, 1986.
76. Eble JN, Tejada E: Prostatic stromal hyperplasia with bizarre nuclei, Arch Pathol Lab Med 115:87-89, 1991.
77. Leong SS, Vogt PF, Yu GM: Atypical stroma with muscle hyperplasia of prostate, Urology 31:163-167, 1988.
78. Young JF, Jensen TE, Wiley EA: Malignant phyllodes tumor of the prostate: a case report with immunohistochemistry clinical and ultrastructural studies, Arch Pathol Lab Med 116:296-299, 1992.
79. Yum M, Miller JC, Agrawal DL: Leiomyosarcoma arising in atypical fibromuscular hyperplasia (phyllodes tumor) of the prostate with distant metastasis, Cancer 68:910-915, 1991.
80. Rosen Y, Ambiadagar PC, Vuletin JC: Atypical leiomyoma of prostate, Urology 15:183-185, 1980.
81. Meares EM Jr: Acute and chronic prostatitis: diagnosis and treatment, Infect Dis Clin North Am 1:855-873:, 1987.
82. Leport C, Rousseau F, Perronne C et al: Bacterial prostatitis in patients infected with the human immunodeficiency virus, J Urol 141:334-336, 1989.
83. Meares EM Jr: Prostatitis and related disorders. In Walsh PC, Retik AB, Stamey TA et al, eds: Campbell's urology, ed 6, Philadelphia, 1992, WB Saunders.
84. Gorlick JI, Senterfit LB, Vaughan ED Jr: Quantitative bacterial tissue cultures from 209 prostatectomy specimens: findings and implications, J Urol 139:57-60, 1988.
85. Meares EM Jr: Infection stones of the prostate gland: laboratory diagnosis and clinical management, Urology 4:560-566, 1974.
86. Epstein JI: Differential diagnosis in pathology: urologic disorders. New York, 1992, Igaku-Shoin.
87. Granados EA, Riley G, Salvador J et al: Prostatic abscess: diagnosis and treatment, J Urol 148:80-82, 1992.
88. Sohlberg OE, Chetner M, Ploch N et al: Prostatic abscess after transrectal ultrasound guided biopsy, J Urol 146:420-422, 1991.
89. Mamo GJ, Rivero MA, Jacobs SC: Cryptococcal prostatic abscess associated with the acquired immunodeficiency syndrome, J Urol 148:889-890, 1192.
90. Epstein JI, Hutchins GM: Granulomatous prostatitis. Distinction among allergic, non-specific, and post-transurethral resection lesions, Hum Pathol 15:818-825, 1984.
91. Stillwell TJ, Engen DE, Farrow GM: The clinical spectrum of granulomatous prostatitis: a report of 200 cases, J Urol 138:320-323, 1987.
92. Wise GJ, Silver DA: Fungal infections of the genitourinary system, J Urol 149:1377-1388, 1993.
93. Adams JR Jr, Mata JA, Culkin TJ et al: Acquired immuodeficiency syndrome manifesting as prostate nodules secondary to cryptococcal infection, Urology 39:289-291, 1992.
94. Auerbach O: Tuberculosis of the genital system, Q Bull Sea View Hosp 7:188-207, 1942.
95. Moore RA: Tuberculosis of the prostate gland, J Urol 37:372-384, 1937.
96. Mikolich DJ, Metes SM: Granulomatous prostatitis due to *Mycobacterium avium* complex, Clin Infect Dis 14:589-591, 1992.
97. Lee LW, Burgher LW, Price EB et al: Granulomatous prostatitis: Association with isolation of *Mycobacterium kansasii* and *Mycobacterium fortuitum*, JAMA 237:2408-2409, 1987.
98. Oates RD, Stilmant MM, Freedlund MC et al: Granulomatous prostatitis following bacillus Calmette-Guérin immunotherapy of bladder cancer, J Urol 140:751-754, 1988.
99. Mukamel E, Konichezky M, Engelstein D et al: Clinical and pathological findings in prostates following intravesicle bacillus Calmette-Guérin installation, J Urol 144:1399-1400, 1990.
100. Miyashita H, Troncoso P, Babaian RJ: BCG-induced granulomatous prostatitis: a comparative ultrasound and pathologic study, Urology 39:364-367, 1992.
101. Koga S, Arakaki Y, Matsuoka M et al: Malakoplakia of prostate, Urology 37:160-161, 1986.
102. Sujka SK, Nalin BT, Asirwatham JE: Prostatic malakoplakia associated with prostatic adenocarcinoma and multiple prostatic abscesses, Urology 34:159-161, 1989.
103. Thrasher JB, Sutherland RS, Limoge JP et al: Transrectal ultrasound and biopsy in diagnosis of malakoplakia of prostate, Urology 39:262-265, 1992.
104. Sugiura H, Hayashi M, Shimamura M: Nonspecific simple eosinophilic granulomatous prostatitis with eosinophilia in peripheral blood: a case report, Acta Pathol Jpn 37:1973-1977, 1987.
105. Presti B, Weidner N: Granulomatous prostatitis and poorly differentiated prostate carcinoma: the distinction with the use of immunohistochemical methods, Am J Clin Pathol 95:330-334, 1991.
106. Mies C, Balogh K, Stadecker M: Palisading prostate granulomas following surgery, Am J Surg Pathol 8:217-221, 1984.
107. Bastacky SI, Walsh PC, Epstein JI: Relationship between perineural tuomor invasion on needle biopsy and radical prostatectomy capsular penetration in clinical stage B adenocarcinoma of the prostate, Am J Surg Pathol 17:336-341, 1993.
108. Bray VJ, Hasbergen JA: Prostatic involvement in Wegener's granulomatosis, Am J Kidney Dis 17:578-580, 1991.
109. Kelalis PP, Harrison EG Jr, Greene LF: Allergic granulomas of the prostate in asthmatics, JAMA 180:963-967, 1964.
110. Benson PJ, Smith CS: Cytomegaloprostatitis, Urology 30:165-167, 1992.
111. Clason AE, McGeorge A, Garland C et al: Urinary retention and granulomatous prostatitis following herpes zoster infection: a report of 2 cases with a review of the literature, Br J Urol 54:166-169, 1982.
112. Zaher MF, El-Deeb A: Bilharziasis of the prostate: its relation to bladder neck obstruction and its management, J Urol 106:257-261, 1971.
113. Goff DA, Davidson RA: Amebic prostatitis, South Med J 77: 1053-1054, 1984.
114. Thompson L: Syphilis of the prostate, Am J Syphilol 4:323-341, 1920.

115. DeSouza E, Katz DA, Dwarzack DL et al: Actinomycosis of the prostate, J Urol 133:290-291, 1985.
116. Houston W: Primary hydatid cyst of the prostate gland, J Urol 113:732-733, 1975.
117. Kelalis PP, Greene LF, Weed LA: Brucellosis of the urogenital tract: a mimic of tuberculosis, J Urol 88:347-353, 1962.
118. Gaudin P, Epstein JI: Adenosis of the prostate: histologic features in transurethral resection specimens, Am J Surg Pathol 18:863-870, 1994.
119. Bostwick DG, Srigley J, Grignon D et al: Atypical adenomatous hyperplasia of the prostate: morphologic criteria for its distinction from well-differentiated carcinoma, Hum Pathol 24:819-832, 1993.
120. Ayala AG, Troncoso P, Ro JY: Prostate gland. In Henson DE, Albores-Saavedra J, eds: Pathology of incipient neoplasia, Philadelphia, 1993, WB Saunders.
121. Epstein JI: Disorders of the prostate gland. In Sternberg SS, ed: Diagnosis in surgical pathology, New York, 1989, Raven Press.
122. Petersen RO: Urologic pathology, Philadelphia, 1992, JB Lippincott.
123. Bostwick DG, Algaba F, Amin MB et al: Consensus on terminology: recommendation to use atypical adenomatous hyperplasia in place of adenosis of the prostate, Am J Surg Pathol 18:1069-1072, 1994.
124. Kovi J: Microscopic differential diagnosis of small acinar adenocarcinoma of the prostate, Pathol Annu 20 (pt. 1):157-196, 1985.
125. Epstein JI: Differential diagnosis in pathology, Urologic disorders, New York, 1992, Igaku-Shoin.
126. Kramer CE, Epstein JI: Nucleoli in low-grade prostate adenocarcinoma and adenosis, Hum Pathol 24:618-623, 1993.
127. Bennett B, Gardner WA Jr: Crystalloids in prostatic hyperplasia, Prostate 1:31-35, 1980.
128. Ro JY, Ayala AG, Ordonez NG et al: Intraluminal crystalloids in prostatic adenocarcinoma: immunohistochemical, electron microscopic and X-ray microanalytic studies, Cancer 57:2397-2407, 1986.
129. Ro JY, Grignon DJ, Troncoso P: Intraluminal crystalloids and whole-organ sections of prostate, Prostate 13:233-239, 1988.
130. Furusato M, Kato H, Takahashi H et al: Crystalloids in latent prostatic carcinoma, Prostate 15:259-262, 1989.
131. Gaudin P, Epstein JI: Adenosis of the prostate: histologic features in needle biopsy specimens, Am J Pathol 19:737-747, 1995.
132. Epstein JI, Paul G, Eggleston JC et al: Prognosis of untreated stage A1 prostatic carcinoma: a study of 94 cases with extended follow-up, J Urol 136:837-839, 1986.
133. Larsen MP, Carter HB, Epstein JI: Can stage A1 tumor extent be predicted by transurethral resection tumor volume, percent, or grade? A study of 64 stage A1 radical prostatectomies with comparison to prostates removed for stage A2 and B disease, J Urol 146:1059-1063, 1991.
134. Ayala AG, Srigley JR, Ro JY et al: Clear cell cribriform hyperplasia of prostate: report of ten cases, Am J Surg Pathol 10:665-671, 1986.
135. Epstein JI, Armas OA: Atypical basal cell hyperplasia of the prostate, Am J Surg Pathol 16:1205-1214, 1992.
136. Troncoso P, Ayala AG: Atypical small glandular proliferations of the transition zone in cystoprostatectomy specimens, Mod Pathol 7:85A, 1994.
137. Chen KTK, Schiff JJ: Adenomatoid prostatic tumor, Urology 21:88-89, 1983.
138. Sakamoto N, Tsuneyoshi M, Enjoji M: Sclerosing adenosis of the prostate: histopathologic and immunohistochemical analysis, Am J Surg Pathol 15:660-667, 1991.
139. Jones EC, Clement PB, Young RH: Sclerosing adenosis of the prostate gland: a clinicopathological and immunohistochemical study of 11 cases, Am J Surg Pathol 15:1171-1180, 1991.
140. Ronnett BM, Epstein JI: A case showing sclerosing adenosis and an unusual form of basal cell hyperplasia of the prostate, Am J Surg Pathol 13:866-872, 1989.
141. Grignon DJ, Ro JY, Srigley JR et al: Sclerosing adenosis of the prostate gland: a lesion showing myoepithelial differentiation, Am J Surg Pathol 16:383-391, 1992.
142. Cleary KR, Choi HY, Ayala AG: Basal cell hyperplasia of the prostate, Am J Clin Pathol 80:850-854, 1983.
143. Grignon DJ, Ro JY, Ordonez NG et al: Basal cell hyperplasia, adenoid basal cell tumor, and adenoid cystic carcinoma of the prostate: an immunohistochemical study, Hum Pathol 19:1425-1433, 1988.
144. Young RH: Pseudoneoplastic lesions of the prostate gland, Pathol Annu 23:105-128, 1988.
145. Devaraj LT, Bostwick DG: Atypical basal cell hyperplasia of the prostate: immunophenotypic profile and proposed classification of basal cell proliferations, Am J Surg Pathol 17:645-659, 1993.
146. Quinn BD, Cho KR, Epstein JI: Relationship of severe dysplasia to stage B adenocarcinoma of the prostate, Cancer 65:2328-2337, 1990.
147. Lin JI, Cohen EL, Villacin AB et al: Basal cell adenoma of prostate, Urology 11:409-410, 1978.
148. Young RH, Frierson HL, Mills SE et al: Adenoid cystic-like tumor of the prostate gland: report of 2 cases and review of the literature on "adenoid cystic carcinoma" of the prostate, Am J Clin Pathol 89:49-56, 1988.
149. Frauenhoffer EE, Ro JY, El-Naggar AK et al: Clear cell cribriform hyperplasia of the prostate: immunohistochemical and flow cytometric study, Am J Clin Pathol 95:446-453, 1991.
150. Lupovitch A: The prostate and amyloidosis, J Urol 108:301-302, 1972.
151. Wilson SK, Buchanan RD, Stone WJ et al: Amyloid deposition in the prostate, J Urol 110:322-323, 1973.
152. Carris CK, McLaughlin AP III, Gittes RF: Amyloidosis of the lower genitourinary tract, J Urol 115:423-426, 1976.
153. Cross PA, Bartley CJ, McClure J: Amyloid in prostatic corpora amylacea, J Clin Pathol 45:894-897, 1992.
154. Battagia S, Barbolini G, Botticelli AR et al: Apoptotic amyloid: a study on prostatic amyloidosis with particular reference to corpora amylacea, Appl Pathol 3:105-114, 1985.
155. Marx AJ, Gueft B, Moskal JF: Prostatic corpora amylacea, Arch Pathol 80:487-494, 1965.
156. Schrodt GR, Murray M: The keratin structure of corpora amylacea, Arch Pathol 82:518-525, 1966.
157. Seaman AR: Cytochemical observations on the corpora amylacea of the human prostate gland, J Urol 76:99-106, 1956.
158. Nelson G, Delberson DE, Gardner WA Jr: Intraprostatic spermatozoa, Hum Pathol 19:541-544, 1988.

159. Hassler O: Calcifications in the prostate gland and adjacent tissues: a combined biophysical and histologic study, Pathol Microbiol (Basel) 31:97-107, 1968.
160. Drach GW: Urinary lithiasis: etiology, diagnosis and medical management. In Walsh PC, Reti Ab, Stamey TA et al, eds: Campbell's urology, ed 6, Philadelphia, 1992, WB Saunders.
161. Magri J: Cysts of the prostate gland, Br J Urol 32:295-301, 1960.
162. Schuhrke TD, Kaplan GW: Prostatic utricle cysts (müllerian duct cysts), J Urol 119:765-767, 1978.
163. Hamper UM, Epstein JI, Scheff S et al: Cystic lesions of the prostate gland: a sonographic-pathologic correlation, J Ultrasound Med 9:395-402, 1990.
164. Lim DJ, Hayden RT, Murad T et al: Multilocular prostatic cystadenoma presenting as a large complex pelvic cystic mass, J Urol 149:856-859, 1993.
165. Yasukawa S, Aoshi H, Pakamatsu M: Ectopic adenoma in retrovesicle space, J Urol 137:998-999, 1987.
166. Maluf HM, King ME, DeLuca FR et al: Giant multilocular prostatic cystadenoma. A distinctive lesion of the retroperitoneum in men: a report of 2 cases, Am J Surg Pathol 15:131-135, 1991.
167. Eyrah LN: Retrovesicle tumours: a report of 3 cases, Br J Urol 26:75-83, 1954.
168. Kirkland JL, Bale PM: A cystic adenoma of the prostate, J Urol 97:324-327, 1967.
169. Melen DR: Multilocular cysts of the prostate, J Urol 27:343-349, 1932.
170. Bainborough AR: Squamous metaplasia of prostate following estrogen therapy, J Urol 68:329-336, 1952.
171. Levine AC, Kirschenbaum A, Droller M et al: Effect of the addition of estrogen to medical castration on prostatic size, symptoms, histology and serum prostate specific antigen in 4 men with benign prostatic hypertrophy, J Urol 146:790-793, 1991.
172. Têtu D, Srigley JR, Boivin J et al: Effect of combination endocrine therapy (LHRH agonist and flutamide) on normal prostate and prostatic adenocarcinoma: a histopathologic and immunohistochemical study, Am J Surg Pathol 15:111-120, 1991.
173. Gardner WA Jr, Culberson DE: Atrophy and proliferation in the young adult prostate, J Urol 137:53-56, 1987.
174. Hamper UM, Scheff S, Walsh PC et al: Stage B adenocarcinoma of the prostate: transrectal US and pathologic correlation of non-malignant hypoechoic peripheral lesions, Radiology 180:101-104, 1991.
175. Epstein JI: Differential diagnoses in pathology: urologic disorders, New York, 1992, Igaku-Shoin.
176. Frydman CP, Bleiweiss IJ, Unger PD et al: Paneth cell-like metaplasia of the prostate gland, Arch Pathol Lab Med 116:274-276, 1992.
177. Weaver MG, Abdul-Karim FW, Srigley J et al: Paneth cell-like changes of the prostate gland: a histological, immunohistochemical, and electron microscopic study, Am J Surg Pathol 16:62-68, 1992.
178. Weaver MG, Abdul-Karim FW: Paneth cell-like change of the prostate, Arch Pathol Lab Med 116:1101-1102, 1992.
179. Adlakha H, Bostwick DG: Paneth cell-like change in prostatic adenocarcinoma represents neuroendocrine differentiation: report of 30 cases, Hum Pathol 25:135-139,1994.
180. Shiraishi T, Kusano I, Watanabe M et al: Mucous gland metaplasia of the prostate, Am J Surg Pathol 17:618-622, 1993.
181. Grignon DJ, O'Malley FP: Mucinous metaplasia in the prostate gland, Am J Surg Pathol 17:287-290, 1993.
182. Lager DJ, Goeken JA, Kemp JD et al: Squamous metaplasia of the prostate: an immunohistochemical study, Am J Clin Pathol 90:597-601, 1988.
183. Bedrosian SA: Heterotopic cartilage in prostate, Urology 21:536-537, 1983.
184. Beckman EN, Leonard GL, Pintado SO et al: Endometriosis of the prostate, Am J Surg Pathol 9:374-379, 1985.
185. Cheatam DE, Sowell DS, Dulaney RB: Hepatitis B antigen-associated periarteritis nodosa with prostatic vasculitis, Arch Intern Med 141:107-108, 1981.
186. Humphrey PA, Vollmer RT: Extramedullary hematopoiesis in the prostate, Am J Surg Pathol 15:486-490, 1991.
187. Dickman SH, Toker C: Seromucinous gland ectopia within the prostatic stroma, J Urol 109:852-854, 1973.
188. Rode J, Bentley A, Parkinson C: Paraganglial cells of the urinary bladder and prostate: potential diagnostic problem, J Clin Pathol 43:13-16, 1990.

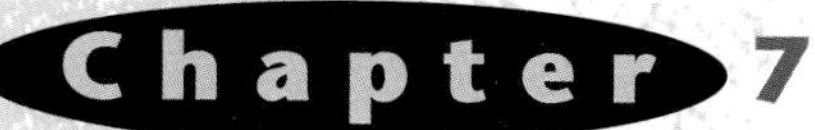

7

NEOPLASMS OF THE PROSTATE

DAVID G. BOSTWICK

Prostate cancer is the most common cancer of men in the United States and is second only to lung cancer as a cause of cancer death. In 1996 41,400 Americans died of prostate cancer and 317,000 new cases were diagnosed.[1] The probability of developing prostate cancer rose from 1 in 78 (1.28) in men between 40 and 59 years of age to 1 in 6 (15.60) for men between 60 and 79 years; for all men, the overall probability was 1 in 5 (18.54).[1] Despite prevalence at autopsy of up to 80% by age 80 years, the clinical incidence is much lower, indicating that most men die *with* prostate carcinoma rather than *of* prostate carcinoma.[2-6] Little is known about the causes of prostate cancer despite its high incidence and prevalence. This chapter reviews the pathology of adenocarcinoma of the prostate and other prostatic tumors. Issues of grading and staging are addressed, and diagnostic and prognostic markers are discussed.

EPITHELIAL NEOPLASMS

PROSTATIC INTRAEPITHELIAL NEOPLASIA

Two histopathologic lesions have been proposed as premalignant in the prostate. The first, prostatic intraepithelial neoplasia, consists of severe cytologic changes in the epithelium within preexisting ducts and acini. The second, atypical adenomatous hyperplasia, is characterized by architectural changes with proliferation of small acini but lacking significant cytologic atypia. The evidence for premalignancy is greatest for prostatic intraepithelial neoplasia; atypical adenomatous hyperplasia was discussed in Chapter 6 in the section on prostatic hyperplasia and is chiefly in the transition zone.

Prostatic intraepithelial neoplasia refers to the precancerous end of the morphologic continuum of cellular proliferations within prostatic ducts, ductules, and acini.[7,8] Two grades of prostatic intraepithelial neoplasia are recognized (low grade and high grade), and high-grade prostatic intraepithelial neoplasia is considered an immediate precursor of invasive adenocarcinoma. The continuum from low-grade prostatic intraepithelial neoplasia to high-grade prostatic intraepithelial neoplasia and early invasive cancer is characterized by basal cell layer disruption, progressive loss of markers of secretory differentiation, increasing nuclear and nucleolar abnormalities, increasing proliferative activity, neovascularization, genetic instability, and increasing variation in DNA content. Clinical studies suggest that prostatic intraepithelial neoplasia precedes carcinoma by 10 years or more, with low-grade prostatic intraepithelial neoplasia first emerging in men in the third decade of life.[9,10] The clinical importance of recognizing prostatic intraepithelial neoplasia is based on its strong association with carcinoma; its identification in biopsy specimens warrants further search for invasive carcinoma.

The term *prostatic intraepithelial neoplasia* was proposed in 1987[8] and endorsed by consensus at a 1989 international conference[11] to replace other synonymous terms used in the literature, including *intraductal dysplasia*,[7] *large acinar atypical hyperplasia*,[9] *atypical primary hyperplasia, hyperplasia with malignant change, marked atypia*, and *duct-acinar dysplasia*.[12,13] The conference participants also agreed that prostatic intraepithelial neoplasia should be divided into two grades (low grade and high grade) to replace the previous three-grade system (prostatic intra-

TABLE 7-1.
PROSTATIC INTRAEPITHELIAL NEOPLASIA (PIN): DIAGNOSTIC CRITERIA

	Low-grade PIN (Formerly PIN 1)	High-grade PIN (Formerly PIN 2 and 3)
Architecture	Epithelial cell crowding and stratification, with irregular spacing	Similar to low-grade PIN; more crowding and stratification; 4 patterns: tufting, micropapillary, cribriform, and flat
Cytology		
Nuclei	Enlarged, with marked size variation	Enlarged; some size and shape variation
Chromatin	Normal	Increased density and clumping
Nucleoli	Rarely prominent	Occasionally to frequently large and prominent, similar to invasive carcinoma; sometimes multiple
Basal Cell Layer	Intact	May show some disruption
Basement Membrane	Intact	Intact

Modified from Bostwick DG, Brawer MK: Prostatic intra-epithelial neoplasia and early invasion in prostate cancer, Cancer 59:788-794, 1987; with permission.

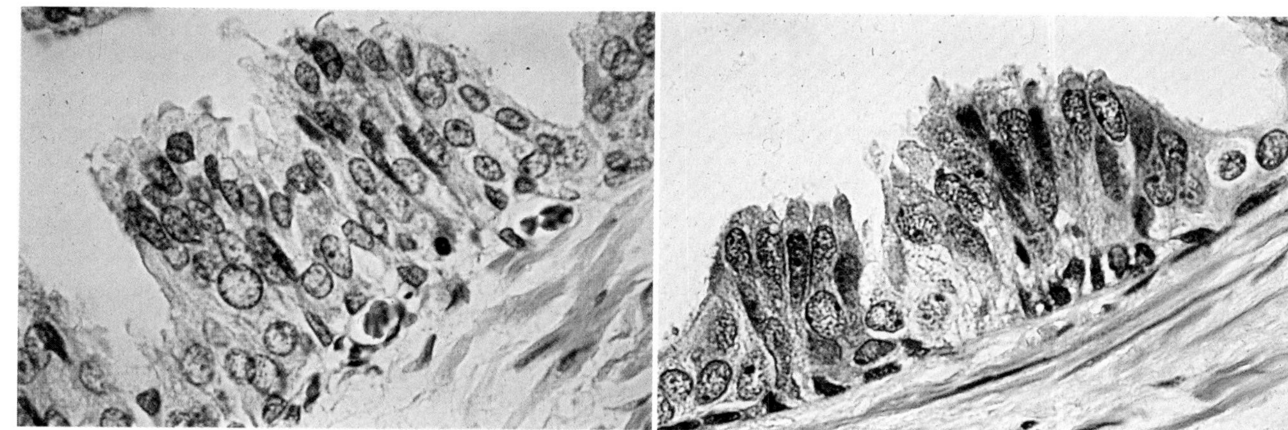

7-1. Prostatic intraepithelial neoplasia. **A**, Low grade. **B**, High grade.

epithelial neoplasia 1 is considered low grade, and prostatic intraepithelial neoplasia 2 and 3 are considered high grade). A subsequent consensus conference sponsored by the American Cancer Society concluded that prostatic intraepithelial neoplasia is the most likely precursor of prostate adenocarcinoma.[14]

Microscopic pathology

In low-grade prostatic intraepithelial neoplasia, the epithelium lining ducts and acini are heaped up, crowded, and irregularly spaced, with marked variation in nuclear size (Table 7-1). Elongate hyperchromatic nuclei and small nucleoli are also present, but usually are not prominent. The diagnosis of prostatic intraepithelial neoplasia requires a combination of cytologic and architectural features, and lesions displaying some but not all features are considered atypical but not neoplastic. High-grade prostatic intraepithelial neoplasia resembles low-grade prostatic intraepithelial neoplasia, but cell crowding and stratification are more pronounced, and nuclear size is less variable because the majority of nuclei are enlarged (Fig. 7-1). The presence of prominent nucleoli, often multiple, is typical of high-grade prostatic intraepithelial neoplasia and of great diagnostic utility.[15]

There are four main architectural patterns of high-grade prostatic intraepithelial neoplasia: tufting, micropapillary, cribriform, and flat (Fig. 7-2).[16] The patterns often merge with each other, although fields with only a single pattern may be present. Familiarity with these patterns aids in recognition of prostatic intraepithelial neoplasia and avoids potential diagnostic pitfalls. Other than diagnostic utility, there is no known clinical significance to the different patterns.

Prostatic intraepithelial neoplasia spreads through prostatic ducts in three different patterns, similar to prostatic adenocarcinoma.[17] In the first pattern neoplastic cells replace the normal luminal secretory epithelium, with preservation of the basal cell layer and basement membrane. Foci of high-grade prostatic intraepithelial neoplasia are usually indistinguishable from ductal spread of carcinoma by routine light microscopy. In the second pattern there is direct invasion through the ductal or acinar wall. In the third pattern neoplastic cells grow between the basal cell layer and columnar secretory cell layer ("pagetoid spread"), a rare finding.

The peripheral zone of the prostate, in which 70% of prostatic carcinomas occur, is also the most common location for prostatic intraepithelial neoplasia. Cancer and prostatic intraepithelial neoplasia are frequently multifocal in the peripheral zone, indicating a "field" effect similar to the multifocality of urothelial carcinoma of the bladder.

PROSTATIC INTRAEPITHELIAL NEOPLASIA: DIFFERENTIAL DIAGNOSIS

- Normal anatomic structures and embryonic rests
  - Seminal vesicles and ejaculatory ducts
  - Cowper's glands
  - Paraganglionic tissue
  - Mesonephric remnants
  - Ectopic prostatic tissue of the urethra
- Hyperplasia
  - Benign epithelial hyperplasia
  - Cribriform hyperplasia (including clear cell hyperplasia)
  - Atypical basal cell hyperplasia
  - Postatrophic hyperplasia
  - Simple lobular atrophy
  - Sclerosing adenosis
- Metaplasia and reactive changes
  - Urothelial metaplasia
  - Infarction-induced atypia
  - Inflammation-induced atypia
  - Radiation-induced atypia
  - Nephrogenic metaplasia of the prostatic urethra
- Carcinoma
  - Acinar adenocarcinoma
  - Urothelial dysplasia and carcinoma
  - Cribriform pattern of prostatic adenocarcinoma
  - Ductal (endometrioid) prostatic adenocarcinoma

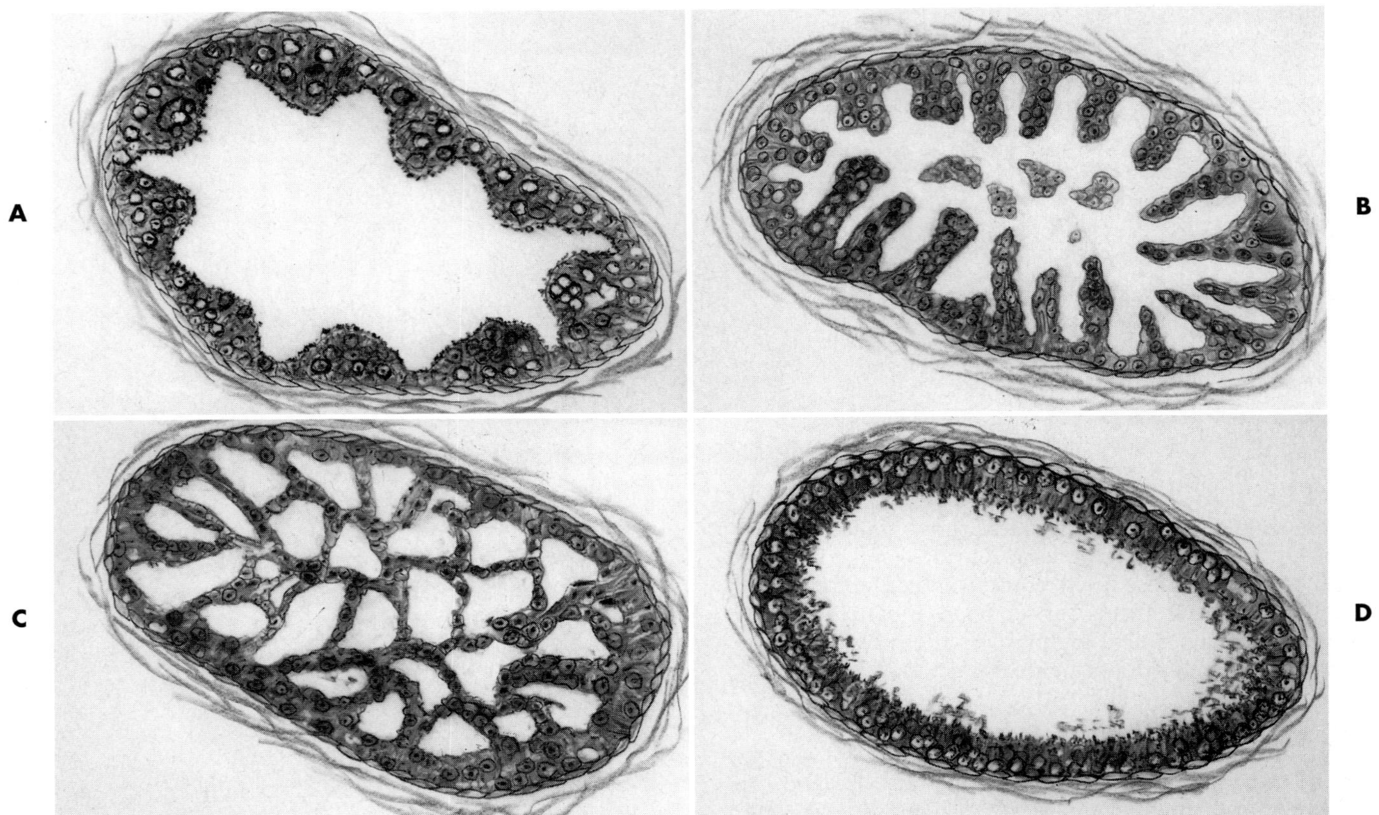

7-2. Architectural patterns of high-grade prostatic intraepithelial neoplasia. **A**, Tufting pattern. **B**, Micropapillary pattern. **C**, Cribriform Pattern. **D**, Flat pattern. *(From Bostwick DG, Amin MB, Dundore P et al: Architectural patterns of high grade prostatic intraepithelial neoplasia, Hum Pathol 24:298-310, 1993; with permission.)*

The transition zone and periurethral area, the anatomic areas in which nodular hyperplasia occurs, account for about 25% of cases of prostate carcinoma and harbor foci of prostatic intraepithelial neoplasia in only 8% of such cases.[18-26] By contrast, atypical adenomatous hyperplasia is found in up to 24% of transurethral resection specimens.[27]

Differential diagnosis

The histologic differential diagnosis of prostatic intraepithelial neoplasia includes lobular atrophy, postatrophic hyperplasia, atypical basal cell hyperplasia, cribriform hyperplasia, and metaplastic changes associated with radiation, infarction, and prostatitis (see box on page 347). Many of these display architectural and cytologic atypia, including enlarged nucleoli, and small specimens, cauterized or distorted specimens, and specimens submitted with incomplete patient history should be interpreted with caution. Cribriform adenocarcinoma, ductal carcinoma, and urothelial carcinoma involving prostatic ducts and acini may also be confused with prostatic intraepithelial neoplasia.

Evidence linking prostatic intraepithelial neoplasia and cancer

High-grade prostatic intraepithelial neoplasia is strongly associated with prostatic adenocarcinoma (see box on page 347).

Frequency and extent of prostatic intraepithelial neoplasia. The frequency of prostatic intraepithelial neoplasia in prostates with adenocarcinoma is much greater than in prostates without cancer.[7,18-25] Prostatic intraepithelial neoplasia was present in 82% of step-sectioned prostates with adenocarcinoma but in only 43% of age-matched controls.[7] Prostatic intraepithelial neoplasia was more extensive in prostates with lower stage tumors, probably due to "overgrowth" or obliteration of prostatic intraepithelial neoplasia by larger high-stage tumors.[20] The grade of prostatic intraepithelial neoplasia was greater in prostates with adenocarcinoma than in controls.[18]

Relationship of prostatic intraepithelial neoplasia and patient age. Prostatic intraepithelial neoplasia increases in incidence with patient age, according to most studies, but the correlation is weak. Sakr et al[10] described the onset of prostatic intraepithelial neoplasia in men in their 20s and 30s in an autopsy study of step-sectioned whole prostates (9% and 22% frequency, respectively); most foci of prostatic intraepithelial neoplasia in young males were low grade, with increasing frequency of high-grade prostatic intraepithelial neoplasia with advancing age (Fig. 7-3). The prevalence of prostatic intraepithelial neoplasia was similar in men of African ancestry and men of European ancestry. Qian et

EVIDENCE FOR THE ASSOCIATION OF HIGH-GRADE PROSTATIC INTRAEPITHELIAL NEOPLASIA (PIN) AND PROSTATIC CARCINOMA

- Histology
  - Similar architectural and cytologic features.
- Location
  - Both are located chiefly in the peripheral zone and are multicentric.
  - Close spatial association of PIN and cancer.
- Correlation with cell proliferation and death (apoptosis)
  - Growth fraction of PIN is similar to cancer.
  - Number of apoptotic bodies in PIN is similar to cancer.
  - Apoptosis-suppressing oncoprotein bcl-2 expression is increased in PIN and cancer.
- Loss of basal cell layer
  - The highest grade of PIN has loss of basal cell layer, similar to cancer.
- Increased frequency of PIN in the presence of cancer
- Increased extent of PIN in the presence of cancer
- Increased severity of PIN in the presence of cancer
- Immunophenotype
  - PIN is more closely related to cancer than benign epithelium.
  - For some biomarkers there is progressive loss of expression with increasing grades of PIN and cancer, including prostate-specific antigen, neuroendocrine cells, cytoskeletal proteins, and secretory proteins.
- Immunophenotype, cont'd
  - For some biomarkers there is progressive increase in expression with increasing grades of PIN and cancer, including type IV collagenase, TGF-alpha, EGF, EGFR, Lewis Y antigen, and c-erbB-2 oncogene.
- Morphometry
  - High-grade PIN and cancer have similar nuclear area, chromatin content and distribution, nuclear perimeter, nuclear diameter, and nuclear roundness.
  - High-grade PIN and cancer have similar nucleolar number, size, and location.
- DNA content
  - High-grade PIN and cancer have similar frequency of aneuploidy.
- Genetic instability
  - High-grade PIN and cancer have similar frequency of allelic loss.
  - High-grade PIN and cancer have similar foci of allelic loss.
- Microvessel density
  - Progressive increase in microvessel density from PIN to cancer.
- Origin
  - Cancer found to arise in foci of PIN.
- Age
  - Age incidence peak of PIN precedes cancer.
- Predictive value of high-grade PIN
  - PIN on biopsy has high predictive value for cancer on subsequent biopsy.

al[18] found a positive but weak correlation of volume of high-grade prostatic intraepithelial neoplasia with patient age between 44 and 77 years. Lee et al[26] studied 256 ultrasound-guided biopsies of hypoechoic lesions and identified 103 cancers and 27 cases of prostatic intraepithelial neoplasia; those with prostatic intraepithelial neoplasia had a mean age of 65 years, whereas those with cancer had a mean age of 70 years. Conversely, Humphrey et al[20] found no relationship between estimated extent of prostatic intraepithelial neoplasia and patient age in a series of 81 patients treated by radical prostatectomy, and McNeal and Bostwick[7] did not find a significant difference in the frequency of prostatic intraepithelial neoplasia in cancer patients with advancing age. Also, Kovi et al[9] studied 429 step-sectioned whole prostates and found that the prevalence of prostatic intraepithelial neoplasia in prostates with cancer decreased with age but predated the onset of carcinoma by more than 5 years.

Basal cell layer disruption. Increasing grades of prostatic intraepithelial neoplasia are associated with progressive disruption of the basal cell layer.[8] Basal cell–specific monoclonal antibodies directed against high molecular weight keratin (e.g., clone 34ß-E12) selectively label the prostatic basal cell layer.[27-29] Carcinoma cells consistently fail to react with this antibody, whereas normal prostatic epithelium invariably reacts, with a continuous circumferential basal cell layer observed in most instances. Basal cell layer disruption is present in 56% of cases of high-grade prostatic intraepithelial neoplasia and more commonly in acini adjacent to invasive carcinoma than in distant acini (Fig. 7-4).[8] Also, the amount of disruption increases with increasing grades of prostatic intraepithelial neoplasia, with loss of more than one third of the basal cell layer in 52% of foci of high-grade prostatic intraepithelial neoplasia. Early invasive carcinoma occurs at sites of acinar outpouching and basal cell disruption.[8,12] A model of prostatic carcinogenesis has been proposed based on the morphologic continuum of prostatic intraepithelial neoplasia and the multistep theory of transformation (Fig. 7-5).[8]

Morphometric studies. Virtually all measures of nuclear abnormality by image analysis show the similarity of prostatic intraepithelial neoplasia to adenocarcinoma, in contrast with normal and hyperplastic epithelium.[30-32] The changes include increased nuclear

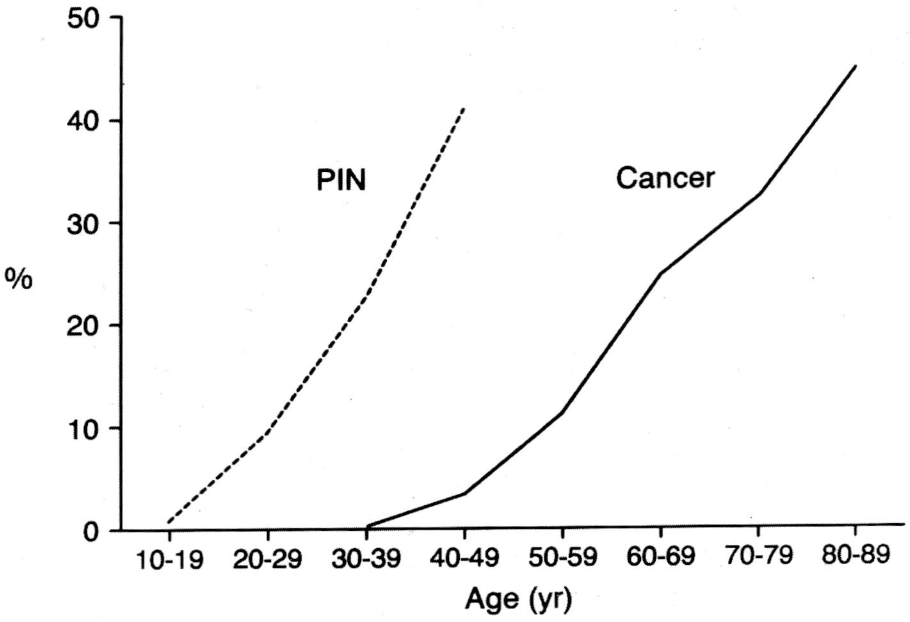

7-3. Frequency of prostatic intraepithelial neoplasia and cancer with increasing age. There is a parallel increase in the frequency of prostatic intraepithelial neoplasia and cancer, according to serially sectioned autopsy prostates, although prostatic intraepithelial neoplasia appears to precede cancer by more than 10 years. *(From Sakr WA, Haas GP, Cassin BJ et al: The frequency of carcinoma and intraepithelial neoplasia of the prostate in young male patients, J Urol 150: 379-385, 1993; Bostwick DG, Cooner WH, Denis L et al: The association of benign prostatic hyperplasia and cancer of the prostate, Cancer 70: 291-301, 1992; with permission.)*

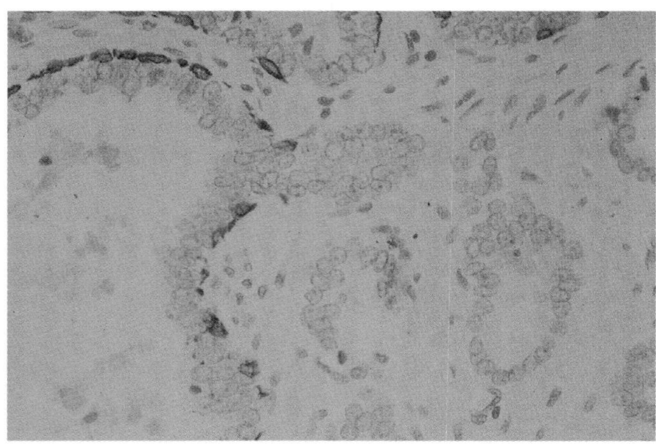

7-4. Basal cell layer disruption in high-grade prostatic intraepithelial neoplasia (*left*) and absent basal cell layer in cancer (*right*). The tongue of cells (*center*) protruding from the large acinar structure with prostatic intraepithelial neoplasia is thought to represent early invasion (basal cells stained immunohistochemically with antikeratin 34ß-E12).

area, chromatin content and distribution, nuclear perimeter, nuclear diameter, and nuclear roundness. Also, most morphometric measures of nucleoli show the similarity of prostatic intraepithelial neoplasia and cancer.[30,33-37] These data indicate that the continuum from prostatic intraepithelial neoplasia to adenocarcinoma is characterized by progressive abnormalities of nuclei and nucleoli.

Phenotypic and genotypic abnormalities. Prostatic intraepithelial neoplasia is associated with abnormalities of phenotype and genotype, which are intermediate between normal prostatic epithelium and adenocarcinoma, indicating impairment of cell differentiation and regulatory control with advancing stages of prostatic carcinogenesis. There is progressive loss of some markers of secretory differentiation, including prostate-specific antigen,[13] secretory proteins,[13,38,39] cytoskeletal proteins,[39] and glycoproteins.[40] Changes in cytoskeletal proteins in prostatic intraepithelial neoplasia probably affect transport of cell products, accounting for the differences in secretory protein distribution.[39] Reduction of cytoplasmic differentiation markers during the preinvasive phase may be followed by abrupt reexpression at the site of microinvasion.[12,13,41] There also is progressive decrease in the number of neuroendocrine cells in normal epithelium, high-grade prostatic intraepithelial neoplasia, and carcinoma.[42]

Other markers show progressive increase, including including c-erbB-2 oncoproteins,[43] bcl-2 oncoprotein,[44] epidermal growth factor and epidermal growth factor receptor,[45] type IV collagenase,[46] Lewis Y antigen,[40] transforming growth factor–alpha, apoptotic bodies,[47] mitotic figures,[48] proliferating cell nuclear antigen expression,[49] aneuploidy and genetic abnormalities,[32,50-55] and microvessel density.[56] Montironi et al[30] suggested that two successive phases of genetic instability occur: The first occurs in hyperplastic epithelium and low-grade prostatic intraepithelial neoplasia and is characterized by DNA duplication without nuclear division, resulting in euploidy

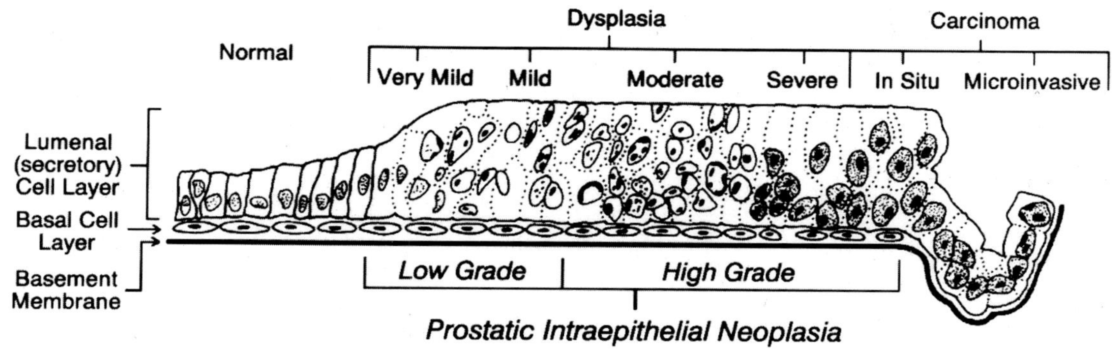

7-5. Morphologic continuum from normal prostatic epithelium through increasing grades of prostatic intraepithelial neoplasia to early invasive carcinoma, according to the disease-continuum concept. Low-grade prostatic intraepithelial neoplasia (grade 1) corresponds to very mild to mild dysplasia. High-grade prostatic intraepithelial neoplasia (grades 2 and 3) corresponds to moderate to severe dysplasia and carcinoma in situ. The precursor state ends when malignant cells invade the stroma; this invasion occurs where the basal cell layer is disrupted. Dysplastic changes occur in the superficial (luminal) secretory cell layer, perhaps in response to lumenal carcinogens. Disruption of the basal cell layer accompanies the architectural and cytologic features of high-grade prostatic intraepithelial neoplasia, and appears to be a necessary prerequisite for stromal invasion. Basement membrane is retained with high-grade prostatic intraepithelial neoplasia and early invasive carcinoma. *(Modified from Bostwick DG, Brawer MK: Prostatic intra-epithelial neoplasia and early invasion in prostate cancer, Cancer 59:788-794, 1987; with permission.)*

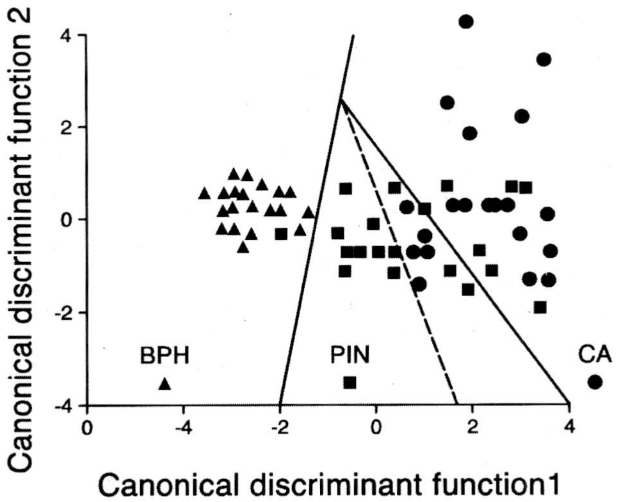

7-6. Scatterplot of the spatial distribution of benign prostatic hyperplasia (*BPH*), prostatic intraepithelial neoplasia (*PIN*), and cancer (*CA*). The cases appear as continuous categories, with overlap mainly between PIN and cancer. The two lines divide the scatterplot into three parts, corresponding to three categories. The part corresponding to PIN is subdivided into two parts (*interrupted line*), separating low-grade PIN (*close to BPH*) and high-grade PIN (*close to cancer*). *(Modified from Montironi R, Scarpelli M, Sisti S et al: Quantitative analysis of prostatic intra-epithelial neoplasia on tissue sections, Anal Quant Cytol Histol 12:366-372, 1990; with permission.)*

(diploidy [2n] or tetraploidy [4n]) (Fig. 7-6). The second phase occurs only in high-grade prostatic intraepithelial neoplasia and cancer and includes aneuploid elements.

Animal studies. Evidence supporting the hypothesis of progression from prostatic intraepithelial neoplasia to adenocarcinoma have been obtained in animal models.[57-65] Leav et al[57] reported induction of prostatic hyperplasia, "dysplasia," and carcinoma in the Noble rat by administration of testosterone and 17ß-estradiol. This report suggested that dysplasia may progress to carcinoma and that long-term hormonal stimulation plays a significant role in the genesis of these lesions. Histopathologic studies indicate a sequence of changes that culminate in prostatic adenocarcinoma, indicating a multistep process.[61] Substantial alteration of the serum ratio of testosterone to estrogen with malignancy supports the role of steroid hormones as promotors of carcinogenesis.[61,62] Estrogenization of neonatal mice resulted in dysplasia within 12 to 18 months, accompanied by increased expression of c-*myc* oncogene.[63]

The Lobund-Wistar rat has a 10% incidence of prostatic carcinoma with metastases when raised in a germ-free environment. Pollard et al demonstrated prevention of the development of primary and metastatic tumors in this rat model by administration of synthetic retinoids (N-[4-hydroxyphenyl] retinamide).[62] These results were confirmed by Slayter et al,[64] although the inhibitory effect was smaller, and they also described a grading system for carcinogen-induced prostate and seminal vesicle carcinoma in rats.[64]

Effect of androgen deprivation therapy on prostatic intraepithelial neoplasia

There is a marked decrease in the prevalence and extent of high-grade prostatic intraepithelial neoplasia after androgen deprivation therapy when compared with untreated cases (Fig. 7-7).[65] These findings indicate that the dysplastic prostatic epithelium is hormone dependent. The loss of normal, hyperplastic, and dysplastic epithelial cells with androgen deprivation is probably due to acceleration of programmed single-cell death (apoptosis) with subsequent exfoliation into acinar lumens.[65]

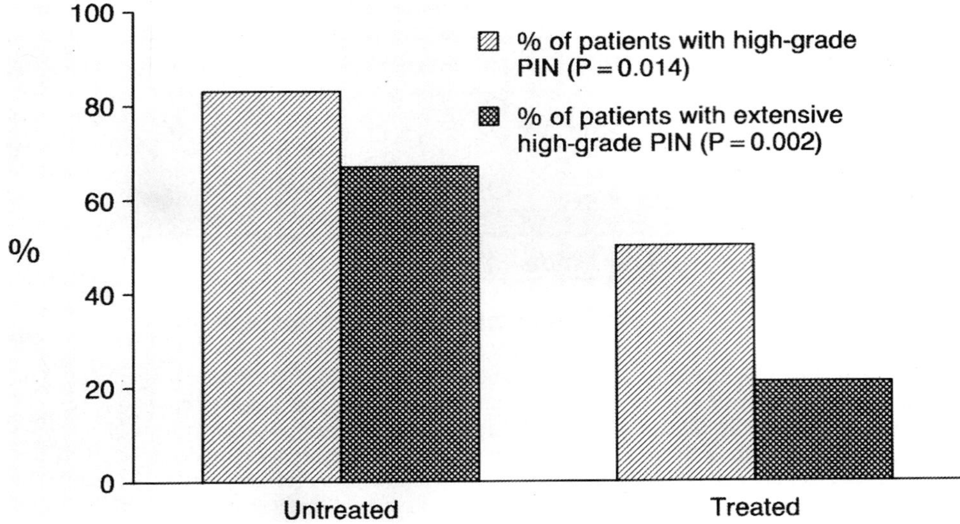

7-7. Histogram comparing the prevalence and extent of high-grade prostatic intraepithelial neoplasia following androgen deprivation in 24 treated and 24 untreated patients. Light bars indicate prevalence; dark bars indicate extent in high-power microscopic fields. *(From Ferguson J, Zincke H, Ellison E et al: Decrease of prostatic intraepithelial neoplasia (PIN) following androgen deprivation therapy in patients with stage T3 carcinoma treated by radical prostatectomy, Urology 44:91-95, 1994; with permission.)*

Clinical importance of high-grade prostatic intraepithelial neoplasia

The clinical importance of recognizing high-grade prostatic intraepithelial neoplasia is based on its strong association with prostatic carcinoma. Because prostatic intraepithelial neoplasia has a high predictive value as a marker for adenocarcinoma, its identification in biopsy specimens warrants further search for concurrent invasive carcinoma.[66]

The predictive value of high-grade prostatic intraepithelial neoplasia was evaluated in a retrospective case control study of 100 patients with needle biopsies with high-grade prostatic intraepithelial neoplasia and 112 biopsies without prostatic intraepithelial neoplasia matched for clinical stage, patient age, and serum prostate-specific antigen.[67] Adenocarcinoma was identified in 35% of subsequent biopsies from cases with prostatic intraepithelial neoplasia, compared with 13% in the control group. The likelihood of finding cancer increased as the time interval from first biopsy increased (32% incidence of cancer within 1 year, compared with 38% incidence in follow-up biopsies obtained after more than 1 year) (Fig. 7-8). High-grade prostatic intraepithelial neoplasia, patient age, and serum prostate-specific antigen level were jointly highly significant predictors of cancer, with prostatic intraepithelial neoplasia providing the highest risk ratio (14:9). Prostatic intraepithelial neoplasia was more predictive of cancer in older patients and those with serum prostate-specific antigen level over 4 ng/mL; within 2 years of first biopsy, 90% of patients with elevated serum prostate-specific antigen were found to have cancer. Other smaller series have also found a high predictive value of prostatic intraepithelial neoplasia for cancer.[66-72] These data underscore the strong association of prostatic intraepithelial neoplasia and adenocarcinoma and indicate that vigorous diagnostic follow-up is needed.

High-grade prostatic intraepithelial neoplasia is encountered in prostatic specimens in 10% to 16% of contemporary 18-gauge needle biopsies.[73] In such cases all tissue should be examined and serial sections of suspicious foci prepared. Antibodies to high molecular weight cytokeratin may be used to look for the presence of basal cells, recognizing that prostatic intraepithelial neoplasia retains an intact or fragmented basal cell layer whereas adenocarcinoma does not.[8] Unfortunately, needle biopsy specimens often fail to show the suspicious focus on deeper levels.

Biopsy remains the definitive method for detecting prostatic intraepithelial neoplasia and early invasive cancer, but noninvasive methods are being evaluated. By transrectal ultrasound, prostatic intraepithelial neoplasia has been reported as being hypoechoic, indistinguishable from carcinoma, but this is not widely accepted.[26,74] Transrectal ultrasound–directed biopsy allows localization of the needle and tissue being sampled. Repeat biopsy is suggested if the first attempt is unrevealing. Serum prostate-specific antigen levels may be elevated in patients with prostatic intraepithelial neoplasia, according to one author,[75] although these findings have been disputed.[76] If all diagnostic procedures fail to identify coexistent carcinoma, follow-up appears to be indicated. Follow-up with repeat digital rectal examination, prostate-specific antigen, and biopsy is suggested at 6-month intervals for 2 years, and thereafter at 12-month intervals for life.[15] It is generally agreed that prostatic intraepithelial neoplasia alone is not a justification for radical prostatectomy or radiation therapy.[15, 66-72] Prostatic intraepithelial neoplasia also offers promise as an

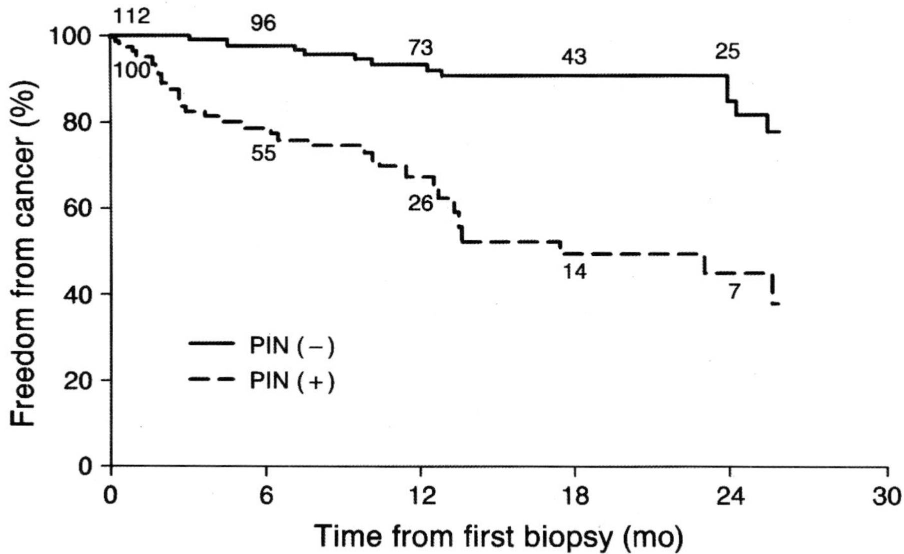

7-8. Freedom from cancer from time of first biopsy according to the presence or absence of high-grade prostatic intraepithelial neoplasia *(From Davidson D, Bostwick DG, Qian J et al: Prostatic intraepithelial neoplasia is a risk factor for adenocarcinoma: predictive accuracy in needle biopsies, J Urol 154:1295-1299, 1995; with permission.)*

intermediate end-point biomarker in studies of chemoprevention of prostatic carcinoma.[77]

ADENOCARCINOMA

Adenocarcinoma accounts for about 95% of prostatic malignancies.

Clinical aspects

Epidemiology. The incidence of prostatic adenocarcinoma has risen dramatically in the past decade, probably owing to early detection programs which employ digital rectal examination, serum prostate-specific antigen, and transrectal ultrasonography. As competing causes of mortality, such as lung cancer and heart disease, decline, men are living longer and increasing their risk of developing clinically apparent prostatic adenocarcinoma. The probability of developing clinically apparent prostatic adenocarcinoma in the United States has risen from 6.1% in 1985 to 8.7% in 1986 for men of European ancestry, and the lifetime risk of dying of prostatic adenocarcinoma is 2.6% for men of European ancestry and 4.3% for men of African ancestry.[3,78,79]

Prostatic adenocarcinoma is rare before 40 years of age, but the incidence rises quickly thereafter. Autopsy studies of thoroughly evaluated prostates from men without clinical evidence of cancer have shown a very high level of latent cancer, increasing from about 10% at 50 years of age to 80% by age 80.[2] The incidence of prostatic adenocarcinoma is much higher in men of African ancestry (100 per 100,000) than in men of European ancestry (70.1 per 100,000), and men of African ancestry in the United States have the world's highest mortality rate from prostatic adenocarcinoma.[3,6,45] The prevalence of clinically occult cancer is similar in different geographic and ethnic groups despite wide variation in the prevalence of clinically apparent adenocarcinoma.[2,4,80] The incidence is low in American Indians, Hispanics, and Orientals, but high in American men of African and European ancestry.

PROPOSED RISK FACTORS FOR PROSTATE CANCER

- Family history
- Diet
- Fat
- Cadmium
- Zinc
- Obesity
- Alcohol
- Hormones
- Smoking
- Sexual activity
- Early sexual activity
- Multiple sexual partners
- Occupational exposure
- Agricultural fertilizers and pesticides
- Rubber
- Ionizing radiation
- Venereal diseases
- Herpesvirus type 2
- Cytomegalovirus
- Vasectomy
- Benign prostatic hyperplasia
- Prostatic intraepithelial neoplasia

Etiology and pathogenesis. Normal prostatic epithelium and stroma require stimulation by testosterone and dihydrotestosterone for growth and development; these androgens are also essential for maintenance and growth of adenocarcinoma cells.

A large number of risk factors of prostatic adenocarcinoma have been proposed (see box on this page). Familial association, with early onset of prostatic adenocarcinoma, probably accounts for about 9% of cases, with risk increasing as the number of affected relatives increases.[81-85] A man's risk is twofold higher if a first-degree relative such as a father or brother has prostatic adenocarcinoma, and the risk is fivefold to elevenfold higher if two or three first-degree relatives have cancer. Heredity appears to be one of the most consistent and strongest risk factors for the development of prostatic adenocarcinoma.

Dietary fat may also be related to prostatic adenocarcinoma, according to cross-cultural comparisons, but the relationship is complex and ill defined, perhaps due in part to the influence of diet on the production of sex hormones.[86] Obesity and alcohol abuse may also be risk factors. The data linking smoking, sexual activity, and occupational exposure with prostatic adenocarcinoma are inconclusive, and early studies that implicated venereal diseases such as gonorrhea have been refuted. Viruses such as herpesvirus type 2 and cytomegalovirus may be involved, but the data are not conclusive.

Surgical sterilization with segmental removal of the vas deferens (vasectomy) has been proposed as a risk factor for prostatic adenocarcinoma, but reports to date have been affected by patient selection bias.[87,88] Further studies are needed to determine the validity of these findings; the level of risk, if confirmed, appears to be low.

Prostatic hyperplasia is frequently seen in association with prostatic adenocarcinoma and there are a number of compelling similarities, including increasing incidence and prevalence with age, concordant natural history, and hormonal requirements for growth and development, but no causal relationship has been established or seriously suggested.[2] Patients with prostatic intraepithelial neoplasia are at increased risk for prostatic adenocarcinoma and many are found to have cancer on repeat biopsy.[67-72]

Signs and symptoms. Prostatic adenocarcinoma has no specific presenting symptoms, and is usually clinically silent, although it may cause urinary obstructive symptoms mimicking nodular hyperplasia. As a consequence, cancer is often initially manifest in metastatic sites such as cervical lymph nodes and bone. The diagnosis may be made in the following clinical instances: (1) if, in routine surveillance for prostatic adenocarcinoma in men over 40 years of age, digital rectal examination shows a nodular or diffusely enlarged prostate (clinical stage T_2, T_3, or T_4); serum prostate-specific antigen level is greater than 4 ng/mL (clinical stage T_1c); or transrectal ultrasound and biopsies are positive for malignancy (lesion-directed, random, or systematic sextant needle biopsies); (2) incidental carcinoma in transurethral resection specimens (clinical stage T_1a and T_1b carcinoma); (3) metastatic adenocarcinoma of unknown primary; (4) carcinoma of the prostate presenting as a rectal mass (prostate carcinoma very rarely produces an eccentric or circumferential rectal and perirectal mass with or without mucosal involvement of the rectum).

Adenocarcinoma in children and young adults. Prostatic adenocarcinoma is rare in patients under age 40. In the literature fewer than 10 cases of adenocarcinoma have been found in each of the following groups: children less than 12 years old, adolescents, and young adults between 20 and 25 years old.[89,90] In all cases the tumors were poorly differentiated, clinically aggressive, and unresponsive to hormonal therapy and radiation therapy.

Tissue methods of detection

Needle core biopsy. The introduction of the automatic spring-driven 18-gauge core biopsy gun in the late 1980s began a new era in the sampling of the prostate for histologic diagnosis. The 18-gauge needle offered important advantages over the previously used 14-gauge needle. The rate of postbiopsy infection declined from 7%–39% to 0.81%, and hemorrhage with urinary clot retention fell from 3.2% to less than 1%.[91] The false negative rate declined from 11%–25% to 11%, and there was an improvement in the quality of the tissue sample obtained, usually with little or no compression artifact at the lateral edges of the specimens. Also, the 18-gauge needle allows sextant biopsies of the prostate with minimal discomfort.[92-94] The main disadvantage of the 18-gauge needle is that it provides less than half as much tissue per needle core for pathologic examination as the traditional 14-gauge biopsy.[91]

Fine needle aspiration. Fine needle aspiration remains popular for cytologic examination of the prostate in parts of Europe, but interest in this method in the United States has dropped precipitously because of the ease of acquisition and interpretation of the 18-gauge needle core biopsy. Both techniques have similar sensitivity in the diagnosis of prostatic adenocarcinoma, and both are limited by small sample size; they are best considered as complementary techniques.[95,96] Complications of fine needle aspiration occur in less than 2% of cases and are similar to those with needle core biopsy, including epididymitis, transient hematuria, hemospermia, fever, and sepsis.

Fine needle aspiration produces clusters and small sheets of epithelial cells without stroma.[95,96] This enrichment for epithelium allows evaluation of single-cell morphology and the relationship between cells. Benign and hyperplastic prostatic epithelium consist of orderly sheets of cells with distinct margins creating a honeycomb-like pattern. Benign nuclei are uniform with finely granular chromatin and indistinct nucleoli; basal cells are often present at the edge. Prostatic carcinoma is distinguished from benign epithelium by increased cellularity, loss of cell adhesion, variation in nuclear size and shape, and nucleolar enlargement (Fig. 7-9).

Transurethral resection. The region of the prostate sampled by transurethral resection and needle biopsy tend to be different.[97] Transurethral resection specimens usually consist of tissue from the transition zone, urethra, periurethral area, bladder neck, and anterior fibromuscular stroma. Studies of radical prostatectomies performed after transurethral resection show that the resection does not usually include tissue from the central or peripheral zones, and not all of the transition zone is removed. Most needle biopsy specimens consist only of tissue from the peripheral zone, seldom including the central or transition zones.

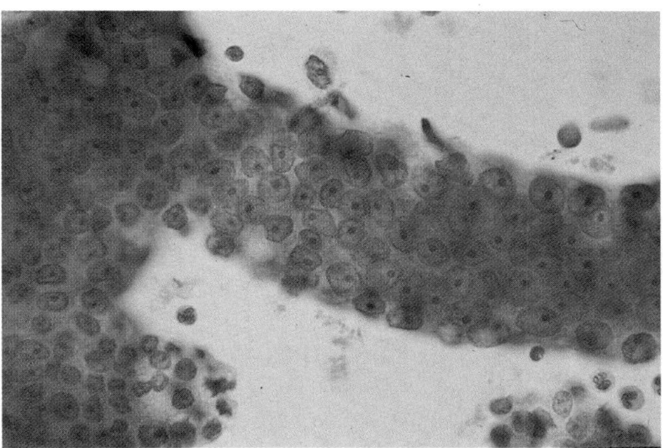

7-9. Moderately differentiated prostatic adenocarcinoma on fine needle aspiration. *(Courtesy Dr. John Maksem.)*

Well-differentiated adenocarcinoma found incidentally in transurethral resection chips usually has arisen in the transition zone.[98] These tumors are frequently small and may be completely resected by transurethral resection. Poorly differentiated adenocarcinoma in transurethral resection chips usually represents part of a larger tumor that has invaded the transition zone after arising in the peripheral zone.

The optimal number of chips to submit for histologic evaluation from a transurethral resection specimen remains controversial, with some experts advocating complete submission even with large specimens that would require many cassettes.[99-102] The Cancer Committee of the College of American Pathologists recommends a minimum of 6 cassettes for the first 30 g of tissue and 1 cassette for every 10 g thereafter.[103]

Prostatic enucleation (suprapubic prostatectomy; adenectomy). In patients with massive benign prostatic hyperplasia, open surgical enucleation may be preferred to transurethral resection. The specimen usually consists exclusively of transition zone tissue and periurethral tissue with grossly visible nodules.

Radical prostatectomy. There are two main surgical approaches to radical prostatectomy. The first, retropubic prostatectomy, is the most popular approach in the United States, allowing staging lymph node biopsies with frozen section evaluation prior to removal of the prostate. The second surgical approach, perineal prostatectomy, does not allow lymph node biopsy during the same operation due to the anatomic approach employed.

The completeness of the pathologic examination of prostatectomy specimens affects the determination of pathologic stage.[104-109] Haggman and colleagues compared the results of limited sectioning (sections of palpable tumor and two random sections of apex and base) with complete sectioning and found a significant increase in positive surgical margins (12% versus 59%, respectively) and pathologic stage with complete sectioning.[109] Also, the presence and extent of extraprostatic extension in clinical stage T2 (B) adenocarcinoma (and hence clinical staging error) is related to the number of blocks processed.[106] The Cancer Committee of the College of American Pathologists has issued guidelines for the examination of radical prostatectomy specimens.[103] A variety of methods for partial and complete sampling of prostatectomy specimens has been described.[102-107]

The Mayo Clinic protocols for preparing and reporting radical prostatectomy specimens are shown in Figure 7-10 and the box above. Complete and careful submission of tissue for histologic evaluation allows the following: unequivocal orientation of specimen and tumor (left, right; transition zone, peripheral zone; anterior, mid, posterior; apex, base, etc.); evaluation of the extent and location of positive surgical margins; assessment and quantitation of the extent and location of extra-prostatic extension and seminal vesicle invasion; quality control data for the surgeon, particularly in regard to surgical margins in nerve-sparing prostatectomy; postoperative

SAMPLE SURGICAL PATHOLOGY REPORT

Tissue description

Prostate (5.5 x 3.8 x 3.5 cm) and seminal vesicles (4 x 3.2 x 1 cm) are submitted and weigh 40g and 15g, respectively. Tumor is identified grossly involving both sides of the prostate extensively, chiefly on the right. Pelvic lymphadenectomy tissue (right, 5.5 x 3 x 1 cm and 3 x 1 x 1 cm; left 4.5 x 2 x 1 cm and 3 x 0.5 x 0.5 cm) submitted separately.

Diagnosis

Radical Retropubic Prostatoseminovesiculectomy—Adenocarcinoma (Gleason Grade 4 + 5 = 9)
Size: about 27.72 cc
Location: bilateral peripheral zone and transition zone
Resection margins: negative
Perineural invasion: extensive
Involvement of capsule: bilateral invasion and extensive multifocal right-sided perforation (extra-prostatic extension)
Premalignant change: patchy high-grade prostatic intraepithelial neoplasia
Pelvic lymph nodes: metastases to 2 of 9 right and 1 of 6 left pelvic lymph nodes
Apex: involvement of the right anterior and posterior and left posterior quadrants without extension to the margin
Bladder base: negative
Gleason grade 4 pattern: 80%
Gleason grade 5 pattern: 10%
Vascular/lymphatic invasion: extensive
Clear cell change: 20%
Other: nodular hyperplasia
focal papillary growth in the peripheral zone cancer
DNA content (flow cytometry): tetraploid (block C8; 60% cancer)
TNM (1992 revision) stage (pathologic): T3cN2Mx ("M" best determined by review of clinical chart)

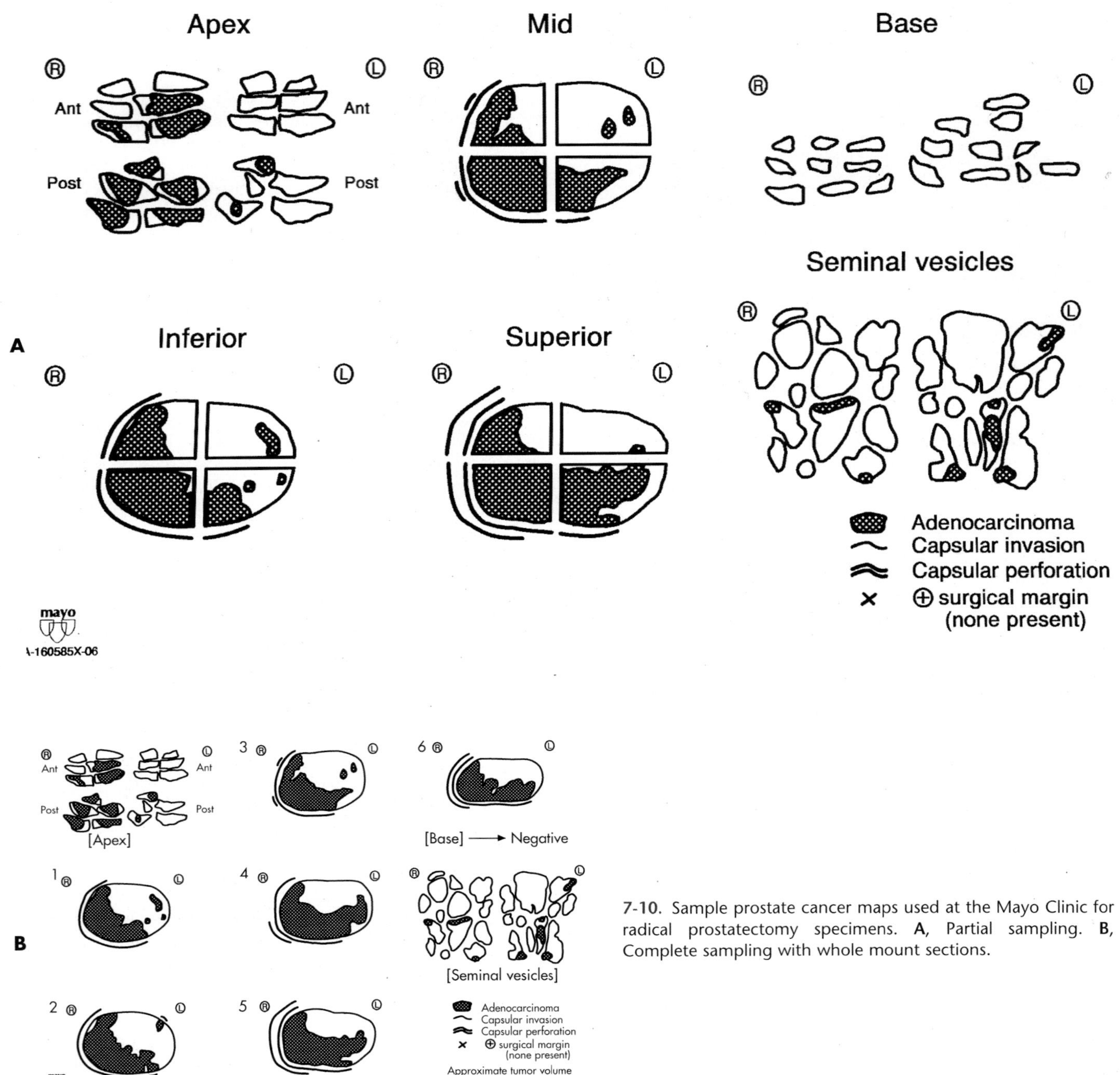

7-10. Sample prostate cancer maps used at the Mayo Clinic for radical prostatectomy specimens. **A**, Partial sampling. **B**, Complete sampling with whole mount sections.

measurement of tumor volume for correlation with imaging studies, as desired; evaluation of tumor grade (percentage of poorly differentiated adenocarcinoma); fulfillment of all recommendations by the Cancer Committee of the College of American Pathologists[103]; and comparison of results with published studies. Standard protocols are useful because of the frequent multifocality of prostatic adenocarcinoma, the inability to fully identify the location and extent of tumor by examining tissue slices, and the inability to grossly identify positive surgical margins and capsular perforation. Partial submission is practical for most cases, does not require special processing, and provides all necessary clinical information.

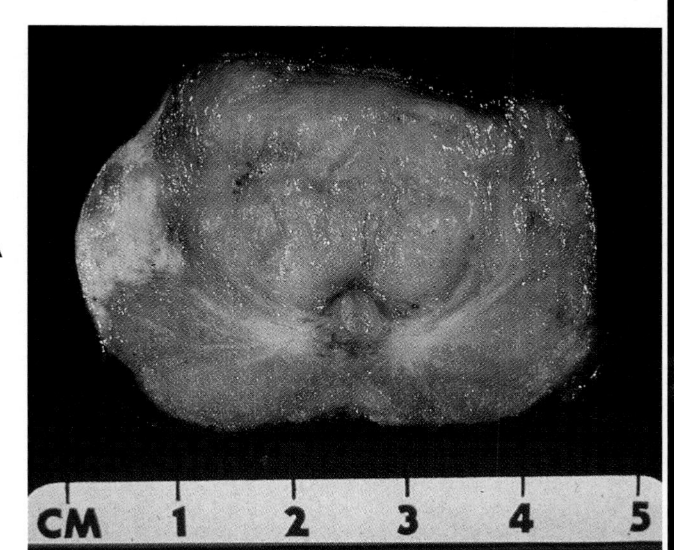

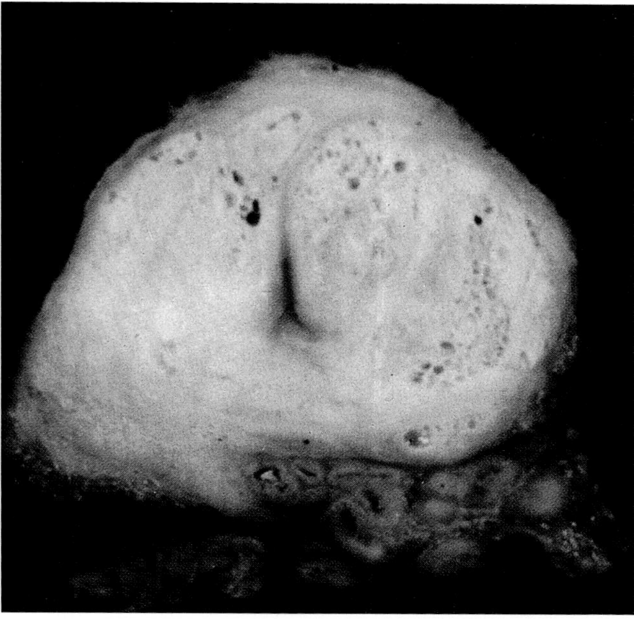

7-11. Gross appearance of prostatic adenocarcinoma. **A**, Large firm yellow tumor mass is grossly visible on one side, but microscopic foci were present throughout the peripheral zone bilaterally. The yellow color is due to abundant cytoplasmic lipid in tumor cells, which was confirmed histochemically. **B**, Large unilateral cancer extending into the seminal vesicles, confirming the clinical impression based on palpability.

Gross pathology

Gross identification of prostatic adenocarcinoma is often difficult or impossible, and definitive diagnosis requires microscopic examination. In transurethral resection specimens, adenocarcinoma is rarely grossly identified unless extensive due to the confounding macroscopic features of nodular hyperplasia. In prostatectomies, adenocarcinoma tends to be multifocal, with a predilection for the peripheral zone.[98] Grossly apparent tumor foci are at least 5 mm in greatest dimension and appear yellow-white with a firm consistency due to stromal desmoplasia (Fig. 7-11). Some tumors appear as yellow granular masses, which contrast sharply with the normal spongy prostatic parenchyma. Similar gross findings may be caused by tuberculosis, granulomatous prostatitis, and acute and chronic prostatitis.

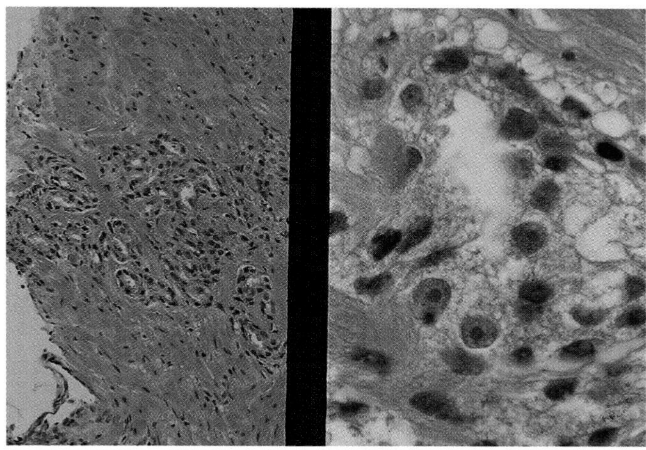

7-12. Prostatic adenocarcinoma on needle biopsy. This solitary focus, occupying less than 5% of the linear extent of the needle core biopsy specimen, displays architectural and cytologic findings diagnostic of adenocarcinoma (Gleason 3 + 3 = 6). Subsequent radical prostatectomy revealed extensive carcinoma of similar grade.

Microscopic pathology

Microscopically, most prostatic adenocarcinomas are composed of small acini arranged in one or more patterns. Diagnosis relies on a combination of architectural and cytologic findings and may be aided by ancillary studies such as immunohistochemistry.

Architectural features can be assessed at low-power to medium-power magnification. The acini in suspicious foci are usually small or medium sized, with irregular contours that contrast with the smooth contours of normal prostatic acini. The arrangement of the acini is diagnostically useful; carcinomatous acini often have an irregular haphazard arrangement, sometimes splitting or distorting muscle fibers in the stroma, and the spacing between acini often varies widely. Variation in acinar size can also be of value, particularly when there are small irregular abortive acini with primitive lumens at the periphery. Comparison with the adjacent benign prostatic acini is always of value (Fig. 7-12). The stroma frequently contains young collagen that appears lightly eosinophilic, and desmoplasia may be prominent. An understanding of the Gleason grading system[110] is of value in interpretation of small foci because of its reliance on architectural patterns (see the section on grading discussed in this chapter).

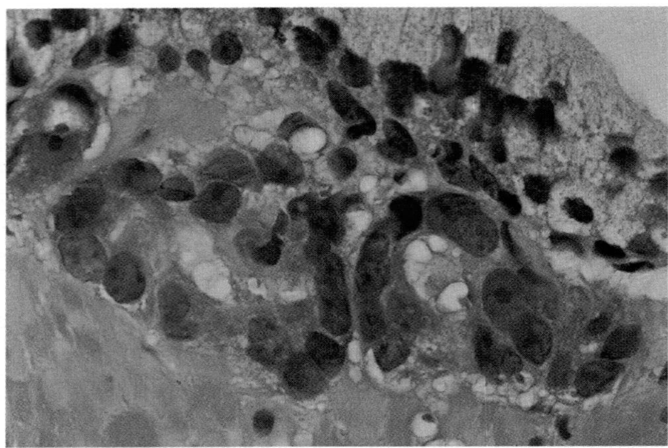

7-13. Nuclear and nucleolar enlargement in prostate cancer.

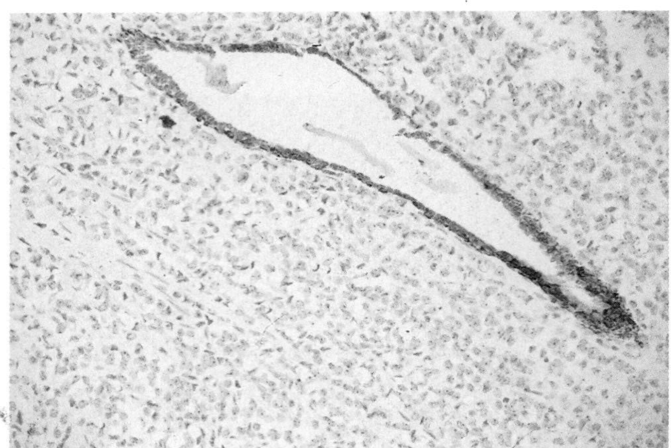

7-14. Lack of basal cell immunoreactivity (antikeratin 34ß-E12) in high-grade prostate cancer (signet ring cell pattern). Note intact layer surrounding benign duct.

Cytologic features of adenocarcinoma include nuclear and nucleolar enlargement, and these features are important for the diagnosis of malignancy. Enlarged nuclei are usually present in the majority of adenocarcinoma cells, and enlarged nucleoli are present in many (Fig. 7-13). Every cell has a nucleolus, so one searches for "prominent" nucleoli, which are at least 1.25 µm to 1.50 µm in diameter or larger.[111] The identification of two or more nucleoli is virtually diagnostic of malignancy, according to Helpap,[34] particularly when the nucleoli are eccentrically located in the nucleus. Overstaining of nuclei and other artifacts may obscure the nucleoli.

The basal cell layer is absent in adenocarcinoma, an important feature which may be difficult to evaluate in sections stained with hematoxylin-eosin.[8] Compressed stromal fibroblasts can mimic basal cells but are usually only seen focally at the periphery of acini. An intact basal cell layer is present at the periphery of benign acini, whereas carcinoma entirely lacks a basal cell layer. Sometimes, small foci of adenocarcinoma cluster around larger acini that have intact basal cell layers, compounding the difficulty. In problematic cases it may be useful to employ monoclonal antibodies directed against high molecular weight cytokeratin (e.g., clone 34ß-E12) to evaluate the basal cell layer (Fig. 7-14).

Other histologic features aid in the diagnosis of adenocarcinoma (Fig. 7-15). Perineural invasion is common in adenocarcinoma (Fig. 7-15*A*) and is strong evidence of malignancy, but it is not pathognomonic because it has been reported rarely with benign acini.[112-114] However, circumferential growth or intraneural invasion is found only with malignancy. Perineural invasion often indicates tumor spread along paths of least resistance which accompany intraprostatic nerves but does not represent lymphatic invasion as originally suggested. Acidic sulfated and nonsulfated mucin is often seen in acini of adenocarcinoma (Fig. 7-15*B*), appearing as wispy, faintly basophilic secretions in hematoxylin-eosin-stained sections. This mucin stains with Alcian blue and is best demonstrated at pH 2.5, whereas the normal prostatic epithelium contains periodic acid-Schiff reactive neutral mucin. Acidic mucin is not specific for carcinoma, and may be found in prostatic intraepithelial neoplasia, atypical adenomatous hyperplasia, sclerosing adenosis, and rarely in nodular hyperplasia.[115-118] Crystalloids are needlelike eosinophilic structures that are often seen in the lumens of well-differentiated and moderately differentiated carcinoma (Fig. 7-15*C*).[119,120] Ultrastructurally, they are composed of electron-dense material that lacks the periodicity of crystals; thus, the term *crystalloids* is appropriate. X-ray microanalysis has demonstrated uniformly high sulfur peaks with small sodium peaks.[120] Their pathogenesis is uncertain, but they probably result from abnormal protein and mineral metabolism by malignant acini. Crystalloids are not specific for carcinoma, and can be found infrequently in prostatic intraepithelial neoplasia, atypical adenomatous hyperplasia, nodular hyperplasia, and normal prostatic epithelium. Collagenous micronodules are an incidental finding in mucin-producing prostatic adenocarcinoma, consisting of microscopic nodular masses of paucicellular eosinophilic fibrillar stroma which impinge on acinar lumens (Fig. 7-15*D*). They probably result from extravasation of acidic mucin into the stroma.[121,122] Collagenous micronodules are present in about 13% of cases of adenocarcinoma and are not observed in benign epithelium, nodular hyperplasia, or prostatic intraepithelial neoplasia. Collagenous micronodules are an infrequent finding, present in 0.6% of needle biopsies and 12.7% of prostatectomies; they are a useful but infrequent diagnostic clue in prostatic adenocarcinoma and may be particularly valuable in challenging needle biopsy specimens. Microvascular invasion is a strong indicator of malignancy (Fig. 7-15*E*) and its presence correlates with histologic grade, although it is sometimes difficult to distinguish from fixation-associated retraction artifact of acini.[123,124] Tumor within adipose tissue is indicative of extra-prostatic extension (Fig. 7-15*F*), although this is a rare finding in biopsy specimens.

Inflammation is diagnostically useful in the evaluation of small acinar proliferations, particularly when the architectural features are equivocal and one is relying on the cytologic findings of enlarged nuclei and nucleoli for the

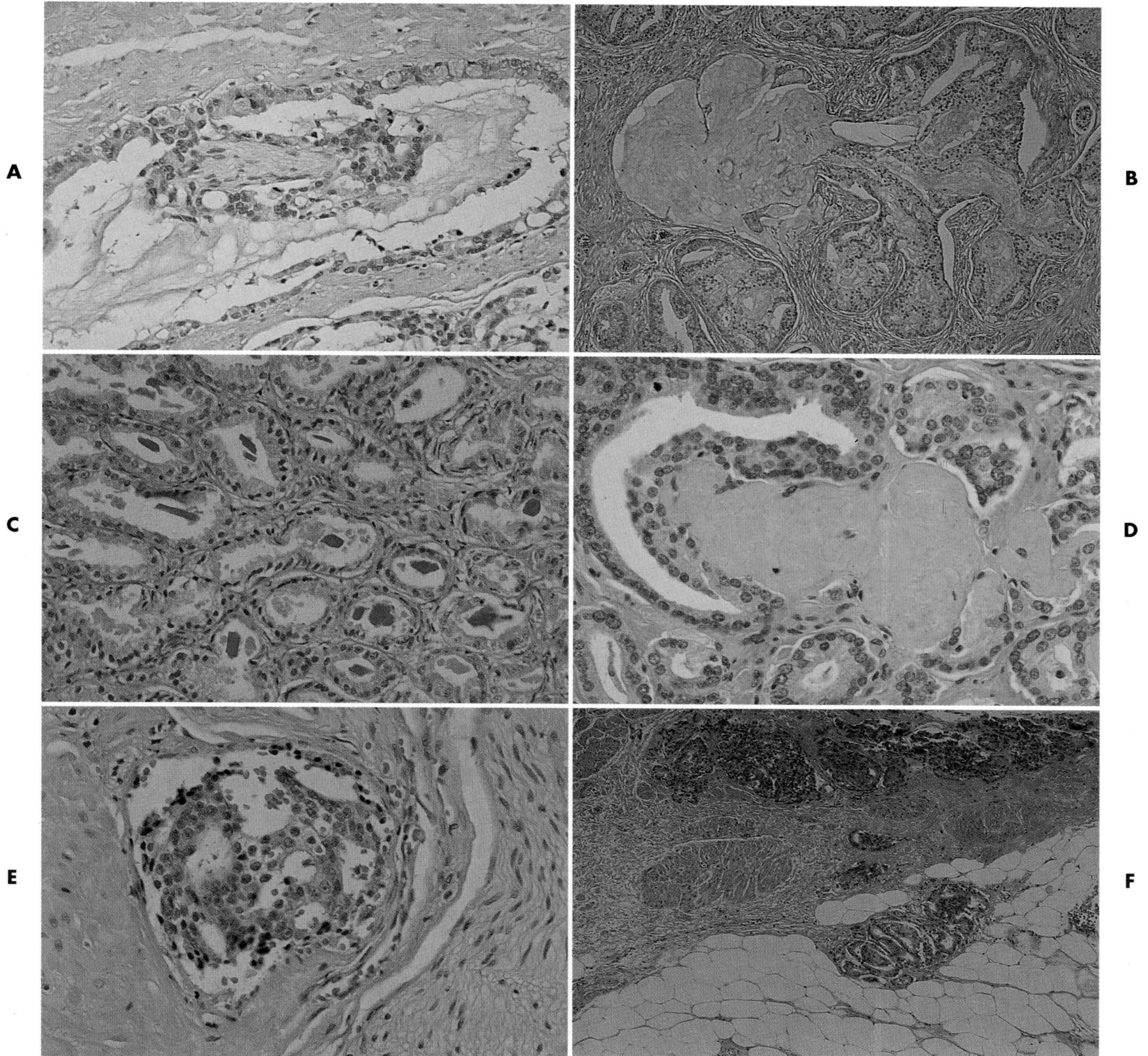

7-15. Ancillary histologic features of prostate cancer. **A**, Perineural invasion. **B**, Mucin production. **C**, Crystalloids. **D**, Collagenous micronodule. **E**, Microvascular invasion. **F**, Extra-prostatic extension.

diagnosis of carcinoma. Inflammation and other stimuli, such as radiation and infarction, may cause reactive atypia.

Common problems in needle biopsy interpretation

Suspicious small acinar proliferations. In some needle biopsies, a proliferation of small acini is found that is highly suggestive of carcinoma but falls below the diagnostic threshold for adenocarcinoma. This is often caused by the small size of the focus, distorted acini with architectural features of malignancy that lack convincing cytologic features, and acinar atrophy or prominent inflammation in which the adjacent benign acini show distortion and reactive atypia with nuclear and nucleolar enlargement. In such cases, it may be appropriate to describe the case as "small acinar proliferation suspicious for but not diagnostic of malignancy" and to suggest rebiopsy. Such lesions are found in up to 3% of needle biopsy specimens.[73] In view of the serious consequences of the diagnosis of adenocarcinoma, it is prudent to diagnose adenocarcinoma only when one has absolute confidence in the histologic findings. A wide variety of small acinar proliferations may mimic adenocarcinoma, particularly in small specimens[73] (see box on page 358).

Atypical adenomatous hyperplasia versus adenocarcinoma. Small acinar proliferations in the prostate form a morphologic continuum ranging from benign proliferations with minimal architectural and cytologic atypia to well differentiated adenocarcinoma.[111] Lesions with a degree of atypia that raise the possibility of carcinoma have recently been the subject of much interest, and those which arise in the transition zone with nodular hyperplasia are referred to as atypical adenomatous hyperplasia. Atypical adenomatous hyperplasia is rarely observed in the peripheral zone or in needle biopsies. It is distinguished from well-differentiated carcinoma primarily by inconspicuous nucleoli, infrequent crystalloids, lack of basophilic mucin, and fragmented basal cell layer seen with basal cell–specific antikeratin antibodies (Fig. 7-16).

DIFFERENTIAL DIAGNOSIS OF SMALL ACINAR PROLIFERATION IN THE PROSTATE

- Atypical adenomatous hyperplasia
- Basal cell hyperplasia (typical and atypical)
- Adenoid basal cell tumor
- Sclerosing adenosis
- Nephrogenic adenoma of the prostatic urethra
- Atrophy
    - Simple lobular atrophy
    - Cystic atrophy
    - Sclerotic atrophy
- Postatrophic hyperplasia
- Seminal vesicles
- Paraganglia
- Cowper's glands
- Florid hyperplasia of mesonephric remnants
- Xanthoma
- Verumontanum mucosal gland hyperplasia

Prostatic intraepithelial neoplasia versus large acinar variant of Gleason grade 3 carcinoma. Prostatic intraepithelial neoplasia encompasses the spectrum of dysplastic cytologic abnormalities within preexisting structures in the prostate that are invested with an intact basal cell layer. In contrast, the large acinar variant of Gleason grade 3 carcinoma, including the cribriform variant, does not have a circumferential basal cell layer and is usually associated with areas of small acinar adenocarcinoma.[126] In equivocal cases diagnosis may be aided by staining with basal cell–specific antibodies to high molecular weight cytokeratin 34ß-E12. Small-sized to medium-sized acini indicate invasive carcinoma rather than prostatic intraepithelial neoplasia.

Clear cell pattern of carcinoma versus benign acini. Numerous forms of adenocarcinoma contain clear cytoplasm. Adenocarcinoma arising in the transition zone characteristically contains clear cells and is well or moderately differentiated.[2,15,16] In contrast, Gleason grade 4 carcinoma may contain cells with clear cytoplasm, referred

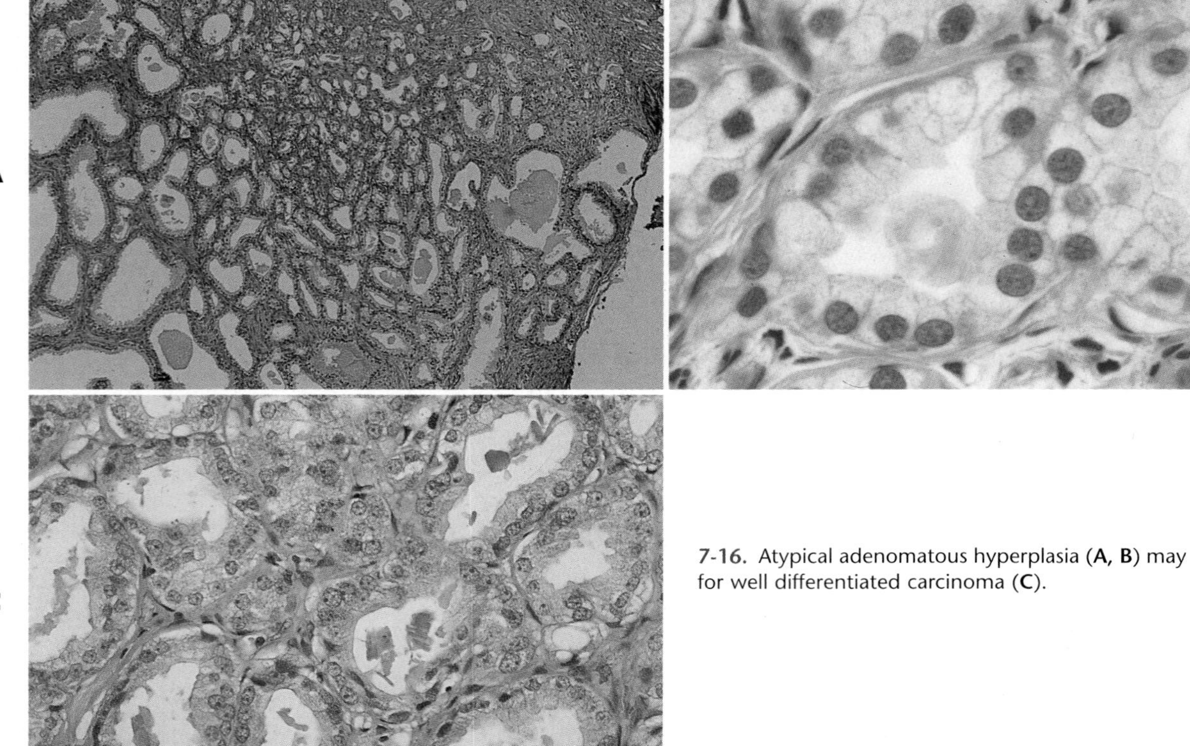

7-16. Atypical adenomatous hyperplasia (**A, B**) may be mistaken for well differentiated carcinoma (**C**).

TABLE 7-2.
GRADING SYSTEMS FOR PROSTATE ADENOCARCINOMA: BRIEF SUMMARIES

Gleason[129-132]	Mostofi (World Health Organization)[135]	Broders[127] and M.D. Anderson Cancer Center[139]	Böcking[138]	Gaeta[128]	Helpap[143]
Pattern 1: Lobular cluster of closely packed single, separate, round uniform glands	Grade 1:Well differentiated, with slight nuclear anaplasia	Grade 1: 75% to 100% of tumor composed of glands	Grade 1: Uniform glands with or without nuclear and nucleolar variation	Grade 1: Single, separate glands; small nuclei with inconspicuous nucleoli	Grade 1a: Well-differentiated glands
Pattern 2: Same as pattern 1, except for less uniformity of gland spacing and shape, and tumor margin not well defined	Grade 2: Moderately to poorly differentiated, with moderate nuclear anaplasia	Grade 2: 50% to 75% of tumor composed of glands	Grade 2: Cribriform, without nuclear anaplasia, or pleomorphic glands and small glands with variable nuclear and nucleolar size	Grade 2: Small or medium glands; pleomorphic nuclei with nucleomegaly	Grade 1b: Moderately differentiated glands
Pattern 3: Single separate, irregular glands, including cribriform and papillary patterns	Grade 3: Poorly differentiated, with marked nuclear anaplasia, or undifferentiated carcinoma	Grade 3: 25% to 50% of tumor composed of glands	Grade 3: Cribriform, with enlarged nuclei and nucleoli, or sheets of cells without glands and variable nuclear and nucleolar size	Grade 3: Small glands, including cribriform and scirrhous patterns; pleomorphic nuclei with nucleomegaly	Grade 2a: Poorly differentiated, with moderate nuclear and nucleolar atypia, or mixed pattern with minor cribriform component
Pattern 4: Coalescing and fused glands form cords, including solid and cribriform patterns; may have hypernephroid appearance (clear cells)		Grade 4: 0% to 25% of tumor composed of glands		Grade 4: Sheets of cells without glands; nuclei and nucleoli of any size; mitotic figures >3 per high-power field	Grade 2b: Poorly differentiated, with marked nuclear and nucleolar atypia, or mixed pattern, with chiefly cribriform pattern
Pattern 5: Few or no glands; tumor in sheets or comedo pattern					Grade 3: Solid trabecular pattern with marked atypia, with or without cribriform pattern

to as the *hypernephroid* pattern. In addition, therapy such as androgen deprivation induces abundant clear cell change in benign and carcinomatous acini, and the diagnosis of adenocarcinoma in such cases may be difficult (see discussion later in this chapter). The clear cell pattern of carcinoma may be confused with histiocytes, vacuolated stromal smooth muscle cells, and metaplastic cells.

Grading

Histologic grade is a strong prognostic factor in prostatic adenocarcinoma and is valuable, even in 18-gauge needle biopsies. Numerous grading systems have been proposed since the pioneering work of Broders more than 60 years ago,[110,127-143] and all successfully identify well-differentiated adenocarcinoma, which progresses slowly, and poorly differentiated adenocarcinoma, which progresses rapidly. However, grading systems are less successful in subdividing the majority of moderately differentiated adenocarcinomas which have intermediate clinical and biologic potential. Some of the popular grading systems are compared in Table 7-2.

Problems with grading include interobserver and intraobserver variability, imprecise predictive value, and lack of a single universal system. In biopsies these problems are compounded by small sample size, tumor heterogeneity, and undergrading of biopsy samples. Also, significant histologic changes in adenocarcinoma occur as a result of radiation and androgen deprivation therapy. The sections that follow on grading describe the current role of grading in prostatic adenocarcinoma, including possible improvements in grading, correlation of biopsy grade with prostatectomy grade, the influence of treatment on adenocarcinoma grade, and correlation of grade with anatomic and

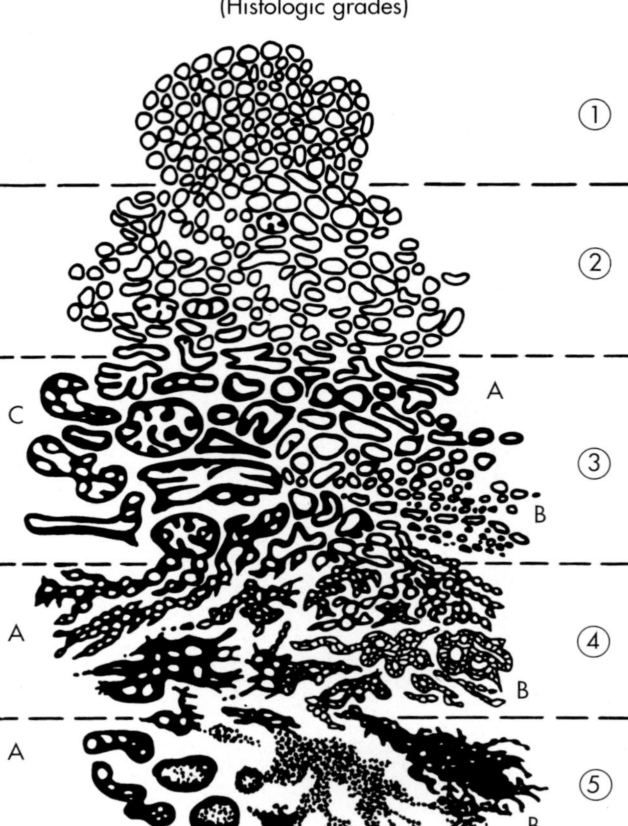

7-17. Standardized drawing for grading prostate cancer (Gleason grading system). See Table 7-3 for a description of the patterns.

TABLE 7-3.
GLEASON GRADING SYSTEM FOR PROSTATIC ADENOCARCINOMA: HISTOLOGIC PATTERNS

Pattern	Peripheral Borders	Stromal Invasion	Appearance of Glands	Size of Glands	Architecture of Glands	Cytoplasm
1	Circumscribed pushing, expansile	Minimal	Simple, round, monotonously replicated	Medium, regular	Closely packed rounded masses	Similar to benign epithelium
2	Less circumscribed; early infiltration	Mild, with definite separation of glands by stroma	Simple, round, some variability in shape	Medium, less regular	Loosely packed rounded masses	Similar to benign epithelium
3A	Infiltration	Marked	Angular, with variation in shape	Medium to large	Variable packed irregular masses	More basophilic than patterns 1 and 2
3B	Infiltration	Marked	Angular, with variation in shape	Small	Variable packed irregular masses	More basophilic than patterns 1 and 2
3C	Smooth, rounded	Marked	Papillary and cribriform	Irregular	Round to elongate masses	More basophilic than patterns 1 and 2
4A	Ragged infiltration	Marked	Microacinar, papillary, and cribriform	Irregular	Fused, with chains and cords	Dark
4B	Ragged infiltration	Marked	Microacinar, papillary, and cribriform	Irregular	Fused, with chains and cords	Clear (hypernephroid)
5A	Smooth, rounded	Marked	Comedocarcinoma	Irregular	Round to elongate masses	Variable
5B	Ragged infiltration	Marked	Difficulty to identify gland lumens	Irregular	Fused sheets and masses	Variable

biochemical markers of progression. Emphasis is placed on the commonly used Gleason grading system.

Gleason grading system. The Gleason grading system, based on the Veterans Administration Cooperative Urological Research Group study of more than 4000 patients between 1960 and 1975, is the de facto grading standard in the United States and other parts of the world.[110,129-134,144] Other systems in use internationally are the Mostofi (World Health Organization)[135] and Böcking systems.[138] These systems are clinically useful, showing a positive correlation with tumor volume, preoperative serum prostate-specific antigen level, and the likelihood of pelvic lymph node metastases and tumor recurrence after surgical and radiation therapy.

The Gleason system is based on the degree of architectural differentiation (Table 7-3; Fig. 7-17, 7-18). Tumor heterogeneity is accounted for by assigning a primary pattern for the dominant grade and a secondary pattern

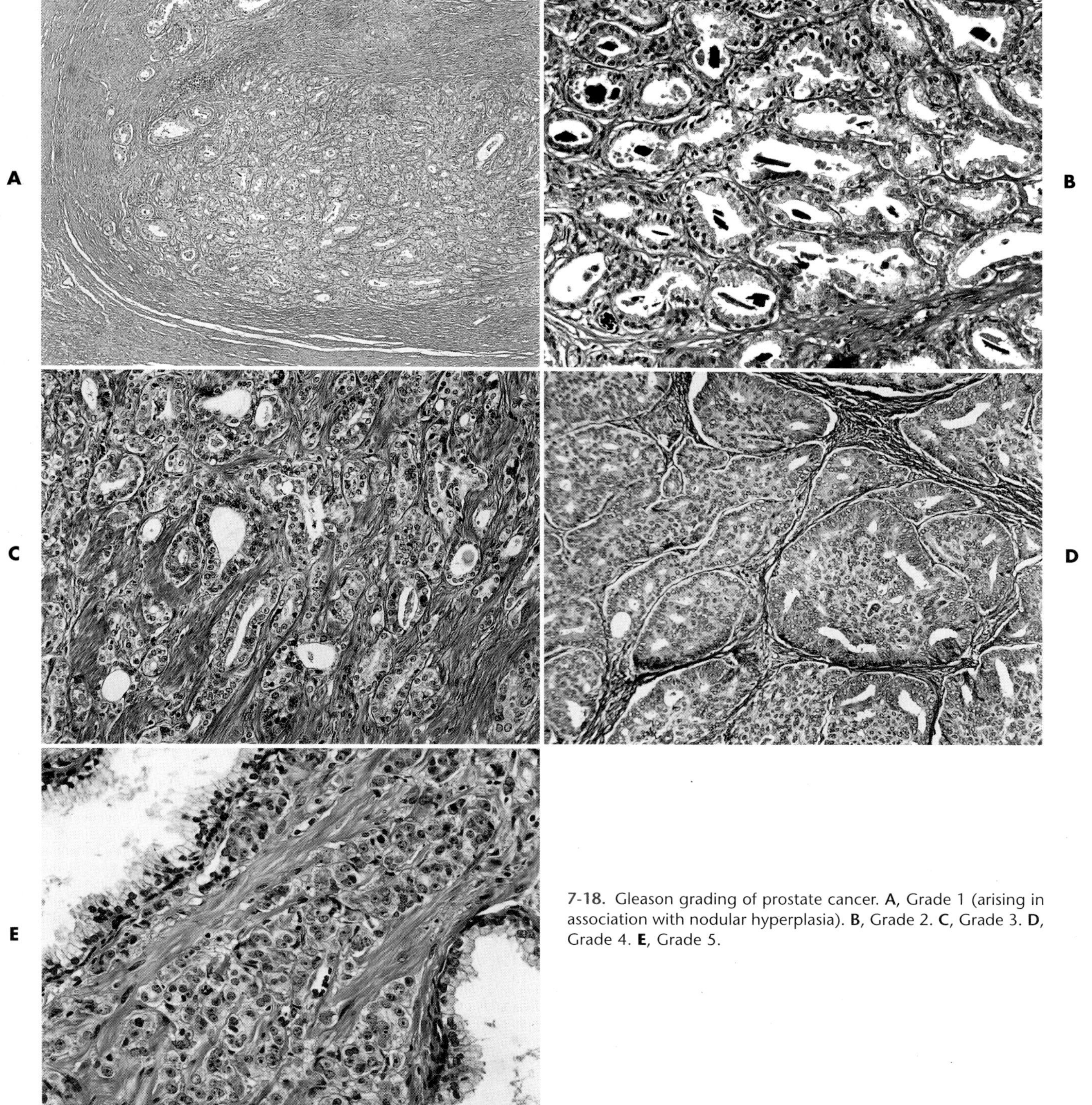

7-18. Gleason grading of prostate cancer. **A**, Grade 1 (arising in association with nodular hyperplasia). **B**, Grade 2. **C**, Grade 3. **D**, Grade 4. **E**, Grade 5.

for the nondominant grade; the histologic score is derived by adding these two patterns together. Early studies described the addition of the clinical stage (1–4 scale) to create the Gleason "sum," but this did not achieve widespread use.[131,134]

The success of the Gleason grading system is due to four factors: (1) histologic patterns are identified by the degree of acinar differentiation without relying on morphogenetic or histogenetic models; (2) a simplified and standardized drawing is available; (3) the Veterans Administration study provided abundant prospective information that allowed objective development of this self-defining grading system; and, (4) unlike any other grading system in the body, the Gleason system provided for tumor heterogeneity by identifying primary and secondary patterns.

Gleason noted that more than 50% of adenocarcinomas in his series contained two or more patterns.[134] Similarly, Aihara et al[145] found an average of 2.7 different Gleason grades per case (range, 1–5) in a series of 101 totally embedded prostatectomies, and more than 50% of adenocarcinomas contained at least 3 different grades. Also, the number of grades increased with greater cancer volume, and the most common finding was high-grade adenocarcinoma within a larger well-differentiated or moderately differentiated adenocarcinoma (53% of cases).[145] In addition to this morphologic heterogeneity, prostatic adenocarcinoma shows heterogeneity for nuclear DNA ploidy.[146-151]

The Gleason score is a scalar measurement that combines discrete primary and secondary groups into a total of nine discrete groups (scores 2–10). Bibbo et al[152,153] noted that optimal grading creates a continuum that incorporates the findings of a variety of diagnostic clues, including acinar formation, lumen area, acinar fusion, type of acinus fusion, acinar packing, acinar size, acinar uniformity, thickness of acinar epithelial layer, nuclear size, nuclear variability, nuclear shape, chromatin pattern, and nucleolar size. Using these architectural and nuclear features, Bibbo et al[153] developed and tested a Bayesian belief network for grading prostatic adenocarcinoma and attained agreement with Gleason grading in 241 of 256 microscopic fields. They noted that four diagnostic clues allowed unique mapping of Gleason primary patterns, and additional clues offered redundancy and robustness to the network.

Proposed modifications to Gleason grading. Numerous modifications or additions have been proposed for Gleason grading to improve its discriminative capabilities, including nuclear grading and morphometric grading, grade compression, measuring the amount of high-grade adenocarcinoma, and considering the extent of the cribriform pattern.

Nuclear grading and morphometric grading. Nuclear and nucleolar enlargement are important diagnostic clues for the diagnosis of malignancy. Morphometric methods allow objective evaluation of nuclear size, roundness, shape, chromatin texture, and other features. In an effort to create an objective method of grading prostatic adenocarcinoma, Blom et al[154] employed morphometric estimates of variation in nuclear size, separating patients undergoing prostatectomy into two groups with differing survival rates. Other investigators have utilized morphometry to improve the predictive value of Gleason grading, but these methods are not used routinely.[155-167]

Nuclear roundness has been the subject of considerable interest since the first report by Diamond et al in 1982.[159-167] Average nuclear roundness accurately predicted prognosis in patients with untreated stage T1b (A2) prostatic adenocarcinoma and other clinical stage adenocarcinomas. However, many of these reports were limited by small sample size (less than 30 patients), use of the same patient cohort in multiple publications, failure to describe the morphologic variations and nuclear roundness extremes, and bias in patient selection. Further, significant problems of reproducibility have been encountered, and the results with different digitizing instruments are not comparable. Nuclear roundness failed to identify patients with tumor recurrence following radiation therapy except in those with well-differentiated adenocarcinoma.[167] The good correlation of morphologic nuclear grade in biopsies and prostatectomies is probably due to the large number of cases that fall into the grade 2 (of 3) category.[91]

Tannenbaum et al[168] compared nucleolar surface area in 40 biopsies and matched prostatectomies with adenocarcinoma, reporting no significant difference in 70% of cases. Nucleolar grading of prostatic adenocarcinoma has also been proposed, but has not been adopted (grade 1: large and prominent nucleoli in virtually every cell; grade 2: intermediate; grade 3: tiny nucleoli that are difficult to find).[169]

Grade compression. Many authors have simplified the Gleason grading system by compressing the scores into groups, usually creating three groups: 2-3-4, 5-6-7, and 8-9-10.[170] Unfortunately, grade compression diminishes the statistical strength of grading.[134] Further, the choice of grouping is often problematic; the most important "cut point" is between Gleason score 6 and 7 due to the emergence of poorly differentiated adenocarcinoma (pattern 4) in score 7, yet many studies combine these scores. Gleason argued against grade compression except in studies with a small number of patients in which grouping is unavoidable; in such cases, a cut point between scores 6 and 7 is preferred.[134,171] The probability of lymph node metastases is significantly greater in patients with score 7 adenocarcinoma than in those with score 6.[172,173]

Amount of high-grade adenocarcinoma. The volume of high-grade adenocarcinoma appears to be an important prognostic factor; as tumor volume increases, the frequency and volume of high-grade tumor increases.[14,173-176] McNeal et al[173] suggested that the Gleason grade stratifies adenocarcinomas into three subgroups with different levels of aggressiveness. Gleason pattern 1 and 2 adenocarcinomas are almost always small, usually less than 1 cm^3, and are indolent, localized, and frequently located in the transition zone. Grade 3 adenocarcinomas are variable in size and very common. Grades 4 and 5 adenocarcinomas are usually larger and more aggressive than lower grade tumors, and are likely to extend beyond the prostate or metastasize. In a study of 209 radical prostatectomies from patients with clinical stage T1 and T2 adenocarcinomas, McNeal et al[173,174] found that the volume of high-grade adenocarcinoma (Gleason grades 4 and 5) had the highest predictive value for lymph node metastases, greater even than tumor volume. Twenty-two of 38 patients (58%) with more than 3.2 cm^3 of high-grade adenocarcinoma had pelvic lymph node metastases, compared with only 1 of 171 patients (0.6%) with smaller volumes of high-grade adenocarcinoma. Gaffney et al[177] studied the extent of solid undifferentiated carcinoma in 24 cases and found a strong correlation with tumor progression. Bostwick et al[176] also found that Gleason score and percent of patterns 4 and 5 adenocarcinoma showed a positive correlation with tumor volume. Egawa et al[178] showed that poorly differentiated adenocarcinoma was the strongest predictor of tumor progression and cancer-specific survival in a series of 107 patients with clinically localized prostatic adenocarcinoma. The cumulative data suggest that the volume of high-grade adenocarcinoma is of prognostic significance, refuting Gleason's contention that prostatic carcinoma behaves according to the average of histologic grades. However, many of these studies grouped the Gleason scores, raising questions of grade compression (as discussed in the previous section).

Histologic dedifferentiation of prostatic adenocarcinoma has been reported by numerous investigators, but these studies included only cases with more than one resection, probably selecting for adenocarcinomas which are more aggressive and thus more likely to require repeat operation.[173,179,180] Brawn[179] reported dedifferentiation in 65% of repeat transurethral resections. Cumming et al[180] described 74 patients with repeated transurethral resections with a mean interval of 2.4 years; Gleason score remained constant in 12, increased in 49, and decreased in 7, and dedifferentiation occurred in untreated adenocarcinomas and in those subjected to expectant management. Whittemore et al[181] suggested that dedifferentiation to high-grade adenocarcinoma is unusual in low-grade (Gleason patterns 1-3), small-volume (1 cm^3) adenocarcinomas, occurring in only 2.4% of patients in 7 years. Their hypothesis explains the large discrepancy in the incidence of clinical cancer among populations with similar prevalences of occult cancer, and indicates that volume of occult cancer is an important marker of aggressive adenocarcinoma.

Reproducibility of Gleason grading and comparison with other grading systems. Interobserver and intraobserver variability have been studied with the Gleason grading system and other grading systems.[134,170,182-186] The subjective nature of grading precludes absolute precision, no matter how carefully the system is defined, but the significant correlation of prostatic adenocarcinoma grade with virtually every outcome measure attests to the predictive strength and utility of grading in the hands of most investigators. Gleason himself noted exact reproducibility of score in 50% of needle biopsies and ± 1 score in 85%, similar to the findings of Bain et al.[134,183]

Some investigators have expressed concerns with Gleason grading because of the significant incidence of interobserver variability in their studies.[170,183,184] Di Loreto et al[184] found a high level of disagreement in grading among 3 pathologists evaluating 41 cases of well-differentiated to moderately differentiated adenocarcinoma. De Las Morenas[170] and colleagues compared the level of interobserver agreement with 4 grading systems in a consecutive series of 100 prostatic adenocarcinomas and found the Gleason grading system to be the least reproducible, with complete agreement of score in only 66% of cases. To perform the analysis, the authors compressed the Gleason scores into three grade groups: 2–5, 6–7 and 8–10. Gallee et al[185] compared the prognostic accuracy of 5 grading systems (Broders, Gleason, M.D. Anderson Cancer Center, Mostofi, and Mostofi-Schröder) in 50 prostatectomy specimens, and averaged the results from 5 participating pathologists to reduce the impact of interobserver variation. Using time-to-recurrence and time-to-death as outcome variables, they found the Gleason system had the lowest predictive ability, whereas the Broders and Mostofi-Schröder systems had reasonable ability, although there was a high level of interobserver variation with the Mostofi-Schröder system. Conversely, Cintra and Billis[186] compared the level of intraobserver agreement with the Gleason, Mostofi, and Böcking systems, and found no significant differences; further, the level of variability was unaffected by type of specimen or amount of tissue examined. Despite questions of exact reproducibility, the collective experience supports the clinical utility of grading prostatic adenocarcinoma.

Grading needle biopsies. Needle core biopsy underestimates tumor grade in 33% to 45% of cases and overestimates grade in 4% to 32% (Table 7-4).[81,187-192] Grading errors are common in biopsies with small amounts of tumor and low-grade tumor, and are probably due to tissue sampling error, tumor heterogeneity, and undergrading of needle biopsies.[91] Biopsy grading error did not correlate with amount of adenocarcinoma on the biopsy or with clinical staging error.[91,193] In one study, the accuracy of biopsy was highest for the primary Gleason pattern, but the secondary pattern on biopsy appeared to be sufficiently accurate in predicting prostatectomy grade to provide useful predictive information, particularly when combined with primary pattern to create the Gleason score (Fig. 7-19). Based on these results, Gleason grading is recommended for all needle biopsies, even those with small amounts of tumor, similar to the original recommendations of Gleason.[91]

Kramer et al[194,195] compared the Gleason score in 14-gauge needle biopsies with matched lymph node metastases and found exact correlation in 17 of 42 cases (40%), ± 1 in 32 of 42 cases (76%), and ± 2 in 40 of 42 cases (95%). The lack of a more anaplastic pattern in the metastatic deposits implied that factors other than loss of differentiation were responsible for the cells' ability to metastasize.[196]

Grading after therapy

Grading after radiation therapy. Grading of specimens after radiation therapy has yielded conflicting results, with some observers noting no difference from

TABLE 7-4.
CORRELATION OF BIOPSY GRADE AND PROSTATECTOMY GRADE: REVIEW OF THE LITERATURE

	Number of Patients	Biopsy Specimens	Grading System	Correlation of Biopsy and Prostatectomy Grade (Gleason Score)				Other
				Exact	± 1 unit	Needle Higher	Needle Lower	
14-GAUGE BIOPSIES								
Kastendieck, 1980[191]	120	Needle biopsies: 120	Glandular differentiation	63%	-	-	-	
Catalona et al, 1982[187]	66	Needle biopsies: 66	Well, moderately, poorly	59%	-	8%	33%	*No correlation of grading error and clinical understaging
Lange and Narayan, 1982[189]	72	Needle biopsies: 66 TURP: 6	Gleason score	74%	-	14%	39%	*Grading error greatest with low-grade tumors
Garnett et al, 1984[188]	115	Needle biopsies: 111 TURP: 4	Gleason score	30%	72%	32%	38%	*Grading error greatest with low-grade tumors
Mills and Fowler, 1986[190]	53	Needle biopsies: 38 TURP:15	Gleason score	51%	74%	4%	45%	*Grading error greatest with low-grade tumors and small amounts of tumor *No correlation of grading error and clinical understaging
18-GAUGE BIOPSIES								
Spires et al, 1994[192]	67	Needle biopsies: 67	Gleason score	58%	94%	-	-	*No correlation of grading error and clinical understaging
Bostwick, 1994[91]	316	Needle biopsies: 316	Gleason score	35%	74%	25%	40%	*Grading error greatest with low-grade tumors and small amounts of tumor *No correlation of grading error and clinical understaging

TURP = transurethral resection of the prostate.

From Bostwick DG: Gleason grading of prostatic needle biopsies: correlation with grade in 316 matched prostatectomies, Am J Surg Pathol 18:796-803, 1994; with permission.

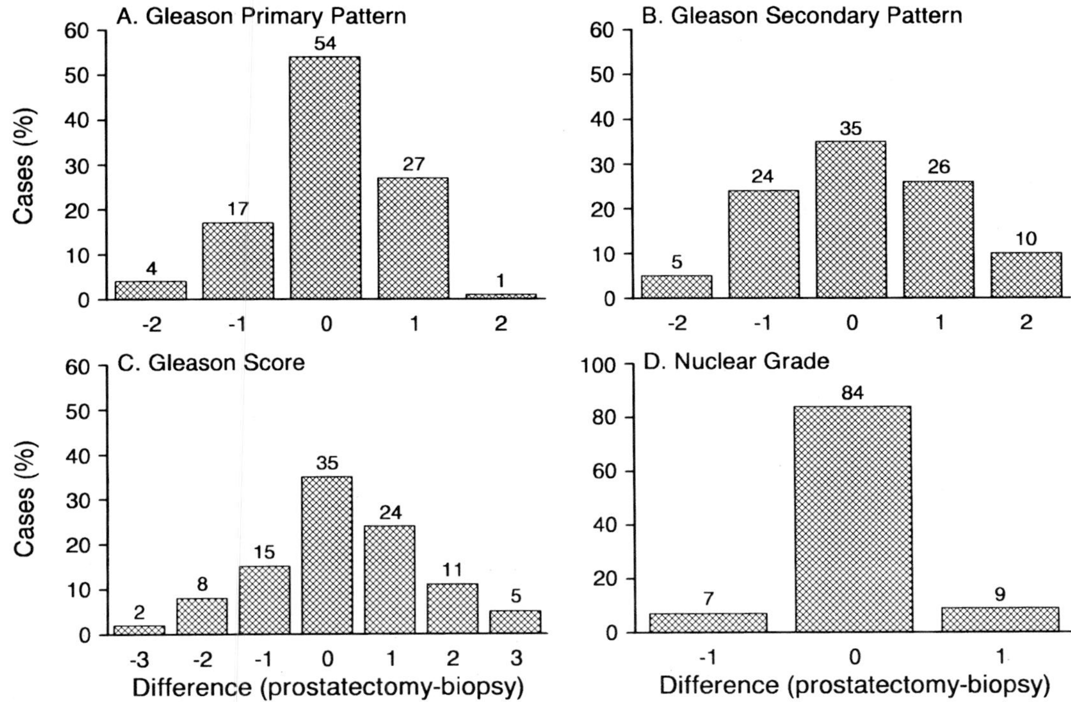

7-19. Distribution of grading differences between prostatectomy and biopsy in 316 matched cases. **A**, Gleason primary pattern. **B**, Gleason secondary pattern. **C**, Gleason score (sum of primary and secondary patterns). **D**, Nuclear grade. *(From Bostwick DG: Gleason grading of prostatic needle biopsies: correlation with grade in 316 matched prostatectomies, Am J Surg Pathol 18:796-803, 1994; with permission.)*

pretherapy grade and others finding a substantial increase in grade.[196-204] Bostwick et al found no apparent difference in grade before and after external beam therapy in 40 patients.[197] Conversely, Wheeler et al[199] found an increase in tumor grade following treatment which they attributed to time-dependent tumor progression. Similarly, Siders and Lee[202] evaluated matched tissue specimens from 58 men before therapy and more than 18 months after therapy, and found a significant increase in Gleason score; there were 24% more poorly differentiated adenocarcinomas (scores 8–10) and an associated shift toward aneuploid DNA content in 31% of pretreatment diploid tumors, indicating increasing histologic and biologic tumor aggressiveness; no outcome data were provided to support this assertion. Despite conflicting results, most investigators recommend grading of specimens after therapy, recognizing that the biologic significance of grade may be different than in untreated cancer.

Grading systems have been proposed for therapy-induced adenocarcinoma regression, chiefly by German investigators, but have not been adopted by others.[205,206] These systems are considered useful following androgen deprivation therapy and radiation therapy because the effects on adenocarcinoma cells may be similar. Böcking[205] suggested that reversible cell damage in prostate cancer is characterized by cytoplasmic vacuolization, nuclear shrinkage, and reduction in the number and size of nucleoli, whereas irreversible cell damage is characterized by rupture of the cytoplasm, nuclear pyknosis, and loss of nucleoli.

Grading after androgen deprivation therapy. Following androgen deprivation therapy (e.g., leuprolide, flutamide), there is an increase in the Gleason grade of the tumor which is accompanied by a marked reduction in nuclear and nucleolar size and prominent cytoplasmic clearing.[50,207-212] Ellison et al[209] found a significant increase in Gleason grade, a decrease in nuclear grade, and a decrease in extent of high-grade prostatic intraepithelial neoplasia in a control study of cases treated with androgen deprivation therapy; the "uncoupling" of the architectural and cytologic pattern was considered vexing due to the identification of small shrunken nuclei within malignant acini. Despite an apparent increase in grade, adenocarcinoma following androgen deprivation therapy and perhaps radiation therapy is probably not more clinically aggressive than when untreated; however, outcome data are not available to confirm this assertion. (This issue is discussed later in this chapter under Carcinoma after androgen deprivation therapy.)

Clinical significance of grading. Grade is one of the strongest predictors of biologic behavior in prostatic adenocarcinoma, including invasiveness and metastatic potential, but is not reliable when used alone in predicting pathologic stage or patient outcome for individual patients.[171] Grade is included among other prognostic factors in therapeutic decisionmaking, including patient age and health, clinical stage, and serum prostate-specific antigen level.

Correlation of grade with recurrence and survival. Virtually every measure of recurrence and survival is strongly correlated with adenocarcinoma grade, including crude survival, tumor-free survival following treatment, metastasis-free survival, and cause-specific survival.[196,213-232] Humphrey et al[232] found that the Gleason score was the strongest predictor of time to recurrence after radical prostatectomy.

Schroeder et al[140-142] quantitated the impact on cancer-specific survival of 12 histopathologic characteristics used in grading prostatic adenocarcinoma. In their analysis of 346 patients treated by perineal prostatectomy, they found that four characteristics provided independent predictive value: acinar arrangement (architecture), nuclear size, nuclear shape, and the presence of mitotic figures.

Correlation of grade and tumor volume. The strong correlation between the Gleason grade and cancer volume has been shown in specimens from transurethral resections and radical prostatectomies.[173,174,176,179,233] McNeal et al[54] showed that low-grade adenocarcinoma (Gleason patterns 1 and 2) was rarely larger than 1 cm^3, whereas high-grade adenocarcinoma (patterns 4 and 5) was almost always larger than 1 cm^3. The probability of tumor progression is best indicated by grade and volume[216,234,235]; when tumor volume was held constant, grade had residual prognostic value, indicating that it provided additional independent information, although these two prognostic factors are closely linked.[216]

Correlation of grade and prostate-specific antigen. Adenocarcinoma associated with elevated serum prostate-specific antigen is more likely to be of higher grade, larger volume, and more advanced pathologic stage than adenocarcinoma associated with a normal serum prostate-specific antigen level.[236-238] Blackwell et al[236] found a significant positive correlation between serum prostate-specific antigen and primary Gleason grade, the percentage of Gleason patterns 4 and 5, nuclear grade, and DNA content in a large series of totally embedded prostatectomies. Adenocarcinoma with Gleason scores ≥7 had a significantly higher median serum prostate-specific antigen and median cancer volume than cancer with lower (<7) Gleason scores. Also, patients with adenocarcinoma consisting of >30% Gleason patterns 4 and 5 had a significantly higher median serum prostate-specific antigen and cancer volume than patients with ≤30% Gleason patterns 4 and 5. Further, the median serum prostate-specific antigen level was greater in tumors with Gleason pattern >3 than in those with Gleason pattern <3 after controlling for tumor volume in 5 cm^3 increments.

Partin et al[237] found that serum prostate-specific antigen was of limited usefulness for staging localized prostatic adenocarcinoma because of the influence of tumor grade; by controlling for cancer volume but not gland volume (prostate-specific antigen/cancer volume), they found a negative correlation with the Gleason score, suggesting that serum prostate-specific antigen concentration was determined by multiple confounding factors. However, Blackwell et al[236] found that combining prostate-specific antigen with gland volume and cancer volume (prostate-specific antigen cancer density) increased the reliability and predictive value for pathologic stage and tumor grade. Although individual cells in poorly differentiated adenocarcinoma produce less prostate-specific antigen than cells in well-differentiated and moderately differentiated adenocarcinoma, they are usually present in such large numbers (greater tumor volume) and replace more of the prostate that serum prostate-specific antigen level is higher.

Serial measurements of prostate-specific antigen suggest that prostatic adenocarcinoma has a constant log-linear growth rate, with mean prostate-specific antigen doubling times of 2.4 years for localized adenocarcinoma and 1.8 years for metastatic adenocarcinoma.[213,214] Higher Gleason grades are associated with faster doubling times.

Correlation of grade and pathologic stage. Grade is one of the strongest and most useful predictors of pathologic stage and other clinical and pathologic features, according to numerous univariate and multivariate studies.* This predictive ability applies to virtually every measure of pathologic stage, including extraprostatic extension, seminal vesicle invasion, lymph node metastases, and bone metastases. Some investigators claim that a Gleason score of 8 or higher on biopsy is strongly predictive of lymph node metastases and suggest dispensing with staging lymph node dissections in these cases.[134,194,239-241] Despite the optimism for grading to predict clinical stage, the predictive value is not high enough to permit its application for individual patients, particularly in those with moderately differentiated adenocarcinoma.

Correlation of grade and tumor location. Grade may be related to the site of origin of adenocarcinoma within the prostate.[2,98,242-244] Adenocarcinoma arising in the transition zone of the prostate appears to be lower grade and less aggressive clinically than the more common adenocarcinoma arising in the peripheral zone (discussed later in this chapter). The majority of transition zone adenocarcinomas arise in foci adjacent to nodular hyperplasia, with one third actually originating within nodules. These adenocarcinomas are better differentiated than those in the peripheral zone, accounting for the majority of Gleason pattern 1 and 2 tumors.

Variants of prostatic adenocarcinoma

A number of histologic variants of prostatic carcinoma have been identified in recent years (Table 7-5). The biologic behavior of many of these variants may differ from typical acinar adenocarcinoma, and proper clinical management depends on accurate diagnosis and separation from tumors arising in other sites. Unusual tumors arising in the prostate also raise questions of histogenesis.[244-248] These variants represent the spectrum of changes that can occur in adenocarcinoma and may not represent separate clinicopathologic entities, although data remain limited for many.

Ductal carcinoma (papillary carcinoma; endometrioid carcinoma). Ductal carcinoma arises as a polypoid or papillary mass within the prostatic urethra and large periurethral prostatic ducts, and histologically

*References 147-151,171,173,176,216,232,236,237.

TABLE 7-5.
VARIANTS OF PROSTATIC CARCINOMA

Adenocarcinoma and Associated Tumors	Gleason Primary Pattern
Ductal carcinoma (endometrioid carcinoma)	3 (no necrosis); 5 (necrosis)
Mucinous carcinoma	4
Signet ring cell carcinoma	5
Sarcomatoid carcinoma	5
Adenocarcinoma with neuroendocrine cells	Variable
Neuroendocrine carcinoma	5 (small cell carcinoma)
Squamous and adenosquamous carcinoma	Variable; usually high grade
Adenocarcinoma with oncocytic features	Variable
Lymphoepithelioma-like carcinoma	5

resembles endometrial adenocarcinoma of the female uterus.[249-281] In the initial description, Melicow and Pachter[249] suggested that the morphologic appearance and consistent location of this tumor near the prostatic verumontanum indicated origin from the müllerian (female) remnant of the utriculus masculinus, implying that these tumors are estrogen dependent. The therapeutic importance of estrogen-dependent prostatic carcinoma would be considerable, because hormonal (estrogen) therapy would be contraindicated. The hypothesis of true uterine ("endometrial") carcinoma arising in the male is intriguing, but all studies have shown that endometrioid carcinoma is merely a histopathologic variant of prostatic adenocarcinoma. Most refer to this tumor as *adenocarcinoma with endometrioid features* or simply *ductal carcinoma*. The term *endometrial* should not be used in the prostate.

Clinical features. Ductal carcinoma accounts for about 0.2% to 0.8% of prostatic adenocarcinomas, with less than 100 cases reported to date.[251,262,280] It occurs exclusively in older men who have symptoms of hematuria, urinary urgency, and frequency, and rarely with acute retention. The clinical symptoms of pure ductal carcinoma and mixed ductal-acinar carcinoma are identical to typical acinar carcinoma.[281] In some cases the adenocarcinoma is detected by digital rectal examination in asymptomatic patients, usually in association with peripherally located acinar adenocarcinoma. Cystoscopically, ductal carcinoma consists of multiple friable polypoid wormlike white masses protruding from ducts at or near the mouth of the prostatic utricle of the verumontanum. The prostate is usually enlarged, with palpable induration or nodularity in up to 54% of cases. At the time of symptom presentation the majority of patients have tumors confined to the prostate or urethra, with concurrent invasive acinar prostatic adenocarcinoma in at least 77% of cases.[251] Ro et al[268] noted that 9 of 35 patients had clinical stage T3 (C) tumors, and 11 others had stage N+ (D) tumors. Hoang and associates[279] described a papillary ductal carcinoma at the urinary bladder neck that displayed prostate-specific antigen and prostatic acid phosphatase immunoreactivity. Aydin[281] described a patient with urinary obstructive symptoms from an anterior penile urethral implant from ductal carcinoma.

Serum levels of prostate-specific antigen and prostatic acid phosphatase may be normal at the time of diagnosis except in patients with bone metastases.[251] This is in contrast with the typical acinar prostatic adenocarcinoma, which has elevated serum prostatic acid phosphatase levels in 64% of cases and often has elevated prostate-specific antigen. This discrepancy in levels of serum prostatic acid phosphatase might be due to early onset of obstructive symptoms and rapid diagnosis of centrally located (periurethral or intraurethral) ductal carcinoma as compared with the typical peripheral prostatic carcinoma. It is also possible that ductal carcinoma has a smaller tumor volume at the time of diagnosis.

Pathology. Ductal carcinoma usually involves the large periurethral prostatic ducts and verumontanum, with direct spread through the ductal and ductular system. The tumor is at least focally indistinguishable from uterine carcinoma, consisting of masses of complex papillae or glands lined by variably stratified columnar epithelium. It may be found in association with a urethral adenomatous polyp at the verumontanum, suggesting origin at that site. Two architectural patterns have been observed: papillary and cribriform (Fig. 7-20).[268] These patterns coexist in about half of cases, and both display nuclear anaplasia and frequent mitotic figures. The characteristic appearance of ductal carcinoma may result from exophytic growth into luminal spaces such as large ducts or the urethra, in a manner similar to endometrial tumors expanding into the uterine cavity or ovarian tumors growing into cystic spaces or the peritoneal cavity.[251] The limited space and stromal influences in the peripheral zone of the prostate usually cannot accommodate formation of papillae or complex acini, accounting for the infrequent occurrence of tumors with endometrioid pattern at that location. However, papillary and cribriform carcinoma can occur in the peripheral zone of the prostate without ductal involvement, so the histologic findings alone on needle biopsy cannot be considered sufficient for the diagnosis of ductal carcinoma. Clinical and pathologic evidence of involvement of the large periurethral prostatic ducts or urethra is required for definitive diagnosis.

Ductal carcinoma invariably displays intense cytoplasmic immunoreactivity for prostatic acid phosphatase

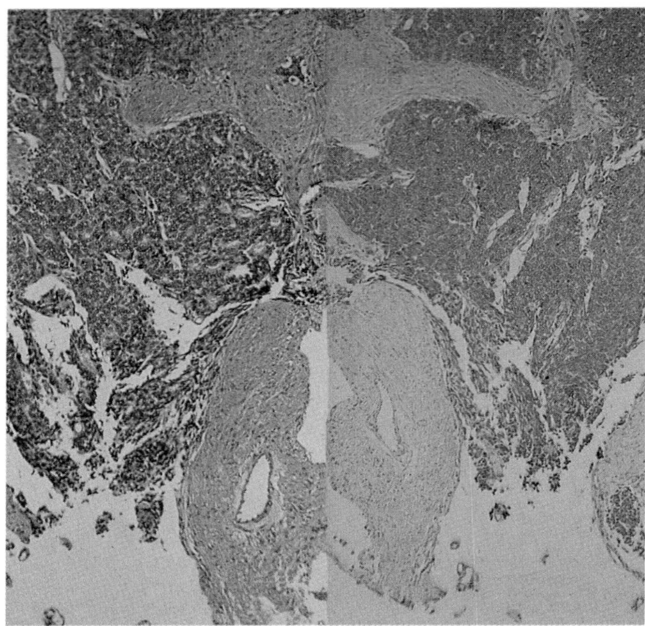

7-20. Ductal carcinoma in large periurethral prostatic ducts. Tumor cells displayed cytoplasmic immunoreactivity for prostatic acid phosphatase (*right*).

and prostate-specific antigen. Focal carcinoembryonic antigen immunoreactivity has also been observed in a minority of cases. Lee et al[280] described focal patchy immunoreactivity for estrogen-regulated protein and estrogen-receptor-related protein, indicating prostatic origin. Ultrastructural findings include well-developed acini with distinct basal lamina, luminal microvilli, large nuclei with prominent nucleoli, desmosomes, secretory droplets, lysosomes, and abundant rough endoplasmic reticulum. Two types of tumor cells are distinguished on the basis of cytoplasmic differentiation: light cells are most common, containing secretory droplets, lipid-filled vacuoles, and pinocytotic vesicles; dark cells contain electron-dense cytoplasm with abundant endoplasmic reticulum and free ribosomes. Transitional forms of each of these cell types are present. Although Carney and Kelalis[256] described tumor cell cilia, subsequent studies indicate that these are microvilli, similar to typical prostatic carcinoma.[251,268,270,279]

Treatment and prognosis. Ductal carcinoma appears to have the same prognosis as typical acinar adenocarcinoma, although conflicting results have been found. Between 25% and 36% of cases have metastases at the time of diagnosis, similar to acinar carcinoma. Bostwick et al[251] reported 13 patients, 7 of whom died of metastases within 6 years of diagnosis. Epstein and Woodruff[270] reported a series of 10 patients, three of whom were alive with metastases at 24, 41, and 44 months, and 2 of whom were dead with metastases in less than 4 years. Ro et al[268] noted that 7 of 8 patients followed for more than eight years died of metastases. The 5-year survival rates range from 15% to 43%. The pattern of metastases is identical to that of the typical acinar prostatic adenocarcinoma. Metastases usually reveal a tumor histologically similar to ductal carcinoma, even when coexistent acinar carcinoma is present in the prostate, suggesting that the endometrioid pattern is more aggressive. Androgen deprivation therapy provides palliative relief in many cases but does not appear to influence survival. In the study by Ro et al[268] 7 patients showed a clinical response to orchiectomy or estrogen therapy, with decreased serum levels of prostatic acid phosphatase and marked symptomatic improvement. Radiation therapy has been used to palliate voiding difficulty and hematuria, as well as to control bone pain, and these tumors appear to be sensitive to treatment with radiation. Nonetheless, the prognosis is poor.

Differential diagnosis. Ductal carcinoma must be distinguished from urothelial carcinoma of the prostate, ectopic prostatic tissue,[282] benign polyp,[283,284] nephrogenic metaplasia,[285] proliferative papillary urethritis,[286] inverted papilloma, and accentuated mucosal folds. There is usually morphologic evidence of glandular differentiation in ductal carcinoma, allowing separation from urothelial carcinoma; in difficult cases or those with small samples, immunohistochemical stains for prostate-specific antigen and prostatic acid phosphatase are useful (positive in ductal carcinoma and negative in urothelial carcinoma). Benign mimics are distinguished from ductal carcinoma by the absence of dysplasia. Primary duct (large duct) and secondary duct prostatic adenocarcinoma[258,259] are histologically indistinguishable from endometrioid carcinoma, and most authors consider these as a single entity. There are no clinical or pathological criteria for separation of ductal carcinoma into utricular and nonutricular types.

Mucinous carcinoma. About 50 cases of mucinous carcinoma of the prostate have been reported.[117,121,287-315] Typical acinar adenocarcinoma may produce mucin following high-dose estrogen therapy.

Clinical features. The signs and symptoms of mucinous carcinoma are similar to typical acinar carcinoma. There are no apparent differences in patient age, stage at presentation, cancer volume, or serum prostate-specific antigen level.[117,121,300] In one case, mucinous carcinoma presented as a 10-cm diameter retrovesical cyst.[289]

Pathology. Focal mucinous differentiation is observed in at least one third of cases of prostatic carcinoma, but the diagnosis of mucinous carcinoma requires that at least 25% of the tumor consist of pools of extracellular mucin, according to Elbadawi et al.[294] Mucinous carcinoma consists of tumor cell nests and clusters floating in mucin, similar to mucinous carcinoma of the breast. In small specimens such as needle biopsies, rare cases consist only of mucin pools, without identifiable tumor cells, although serial sectioning usually reveals carcinoma cells on deeper levels. Three patterns of mucinous carcinoma have been described: acinar carcinoma with luminal distension, cribriform carcinoma with luminal distension, and "colloid carcinoma" with cell nests embedded in mucinous lakes (Fig. 7-21).[121] Other histologic patterns of adenocarcinoma are typically present in association with mucinous carcinoma, including cribriform and comedocarcinoma patterns. The cells of mucinous carcinoma usually have enlarged nuclei and display

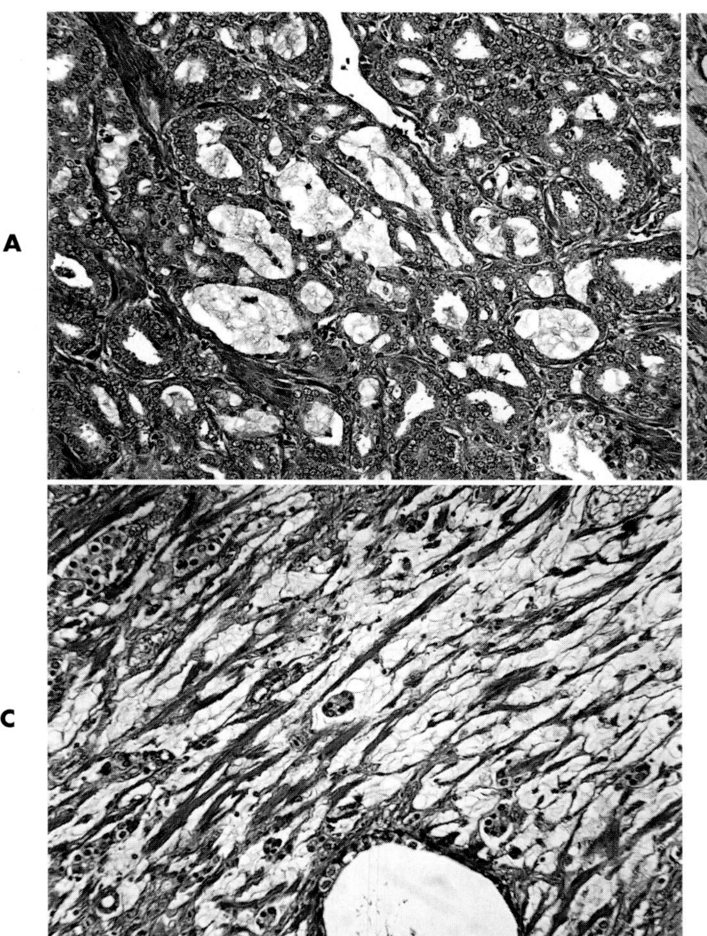
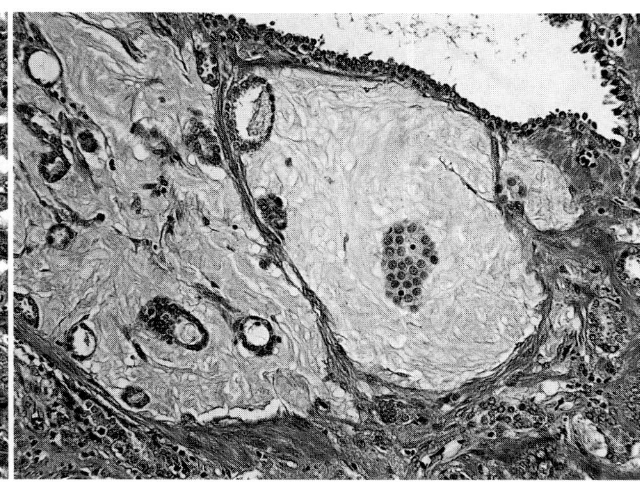

7-21. Mucinous carcinoma. **A**, Luminal mucin. **B**, Mucin lakes. **C**, Extraacinar mucin dissects between the stromal muscle fibers.

the entire spectrum of cytologic abnormalities observed in typical adenocarcinoma. In some cases the nuclei have low-grade cytologic findings, with uniform finely granular chromatin and inconspicuous nucleoli, but their presence within mucin pools is diagnostic of malignancy. Signet ring cells are usually not seen in mucinous carcinoma, although Alfthan and Koivuniemi[297] illustrated a case in which such cells were abundant. Another case of mucinous carcinoma arose in the transition zone in association with large numbers of neuroendocrine cells with large eosinophilic granules.[302] McNeal et al[121] considered "colloid" carcinoma a variant of Gleason grade 4 carcinoma.

Prostatic mucin stains with periodic acid-Schiff, Alcian blue, and mucicarmine. Most studies have found neutral mucin in benign acini and acidic mucin in malignant acini, although benign acini rarely produce small quantities of acidic mucin.[115-117,304,306,311] Based on these findings, some have suggested that acidic mucin is a useful supportive feature in the diagnosis of adenocarcinoma, present in about 60% of cases, but this has been refuted.* Acidic mucin has also been described in atypical adenomatous hyperplasia, mucinous metaplasia, prostatic intraepithelial neoplasia, sclerosing adenosis, and basal cell hyperplasia.[115,116,118]

The cells of mucinous carcinoma contain prostate-specific antigen and prostatic acid phosphatase, but usually do not produce carcinoembryonic antigen. In one case, neuron-specific enolase immunoreactivity was observed, confirming histochemical results with the Grimelius stain.[302] Proia and associates[296] identified estrogen receptors in one case of mucinous carcinoma. Ultrastructurally, the tumor cells are joined by zonula adherens junctions and set in an amorphous background. Microvilli and cytoplasmic projections are prominent. Nuclei are compressed to one side of the cells, with cytoplasmic organelles and mucinogen granules filling the remainder of the cells.

Collagenous micronodules are an incidental finding in mucin-producing carcinoma that probably result from extracellular acid mucin (see Fig. 7-15*D*).[121,122] The amount of collagenous micronodules is correlated with mucin production by the tumor, including luminal mucin and extraacinar mucin; there is a weak negative correlation of collagenous micronodules with the percent of tumor composed of signet ring cells. Collagenous micronodules in prostatic adenocarcinoma are not prognostically significant, although they indicate the likelihood of mucin production by the tumor.[122]

*References 115-118,305,306,309,311,312.

Treatment and prognosis. The pattern of metastases of mucinous carcinoma of the prostate is similar to typical prostatic adenocarcinoma. Early reports suggested that these tumors were less aggressive and of lower stage than other forms of prostatic adenocarcinoma, with no tendency for bone metastasis, but in a recent study of eight patients, osteoblastic bone metastases frequently occurred, and six of eight patients showed symptoms of stage T3 (C) or N+ (D) tumors.[301]

Patients have been treated with radiation therapy, hormonal therapy, or both. Five of eight patients reported by Ro et al[301] died from tumor within 7 years, and the remaining three patients are alive with tumor up to 15 months. The aggregate data are limited and uncontrolled but suggest that these tumors do not respond well to endocrine therapy[300,315] or radiation therapy and are highly aggressive; rare cases respond to androgen deprivation therapy.[313,314]

Differential diagnosis. Mucinous carcinoma of the rectum and urinary bladder may invade the prostate, mimicking mucinous carcinoma of the prostate. Similarly, Cowper's gland carcinoma displays prominent mucinous differentiation. These distinctions are important because of significant differences in treatment and prognosis. Immunohistochemical stains for prostate-specific antigen and prostatic acid phosphatase are positive in mucinous carcinoma of the prostate and confirm prostatic origin.

Signet ring cell carcinoma. Signet ring cell carcinoma of the prostate is rare, with fewer than 20 reported cases.[316-326] The characteristic cytoplasmic clearing is rarely mucicarminophilic, in contrast with mucicarmine-positive signet ring cell carcinoma of the bladder, urachus, stomach, and other sites.

Clinical features. The presenting signs and symptoms of signet ring cell carcinoma are similar to typical acinar adenocarcinoma. Catton et al[323] described a unique case of signet ring cell carcinoma presenting with malignant ascites, one of only three reported cases of prostatic adenocarcinoma with this clinical manifestation. Rectal examination of the prostate with signet ring cell carcinoma may reveal stony-hard induration.

Pathology. The diagnosis of signet ring cell carcinoma requires that 25% or more of the tumor is composed of signet ring cells, although some authors require 50%. Tumor cells show distinctive nuclear displacement by clear cytoplasm (Fig. 7-22). Signet ring cells are present in 2.5% of cases of acinar adenocarcinoma, but rarely in sufficient numbers to be considered signet ring cell carcinoma.[325] Almost all reported cases are associated with other forms of poorly differentiated prostatic adenocarcinoma, including cribriform carcinoma, comedocarcinoma, and solid (Gleason grade 5) carcinoma. Tumor cells diffusely infiltrate through the stroma, invading perineural and vascular spaces and often perforating the prostatic capsule.

Histochemical and immunohistochemical stains for mucin, lipid, prostate-specific antigen, prostatic acid phosphatase, and carcinoembryonic antigen have provided variable results, suggesting variants of signet ring cell carcinoma (Table 7-6). Giltman[321] reported a case of pure signet ring cell carcinoma that was periodic acid-Schiff–positive and diastase-resistant but negative for acid mucin and fat (mucicarmine, Alcian blue, and oil red O). In another case, tumor cells were shown to stain with sudan black, indicating the presence of intracellular lipid. Mucin stains are variably positive.[324] Ro et al[316] reported eight cases in which the tumor cells did not stain for Alcian blue, mucicarmine, or periodic acid-Schiff with or without diastase. Prostate-specific antigen, prostatic acid phosphatase, and keratin immunoreactivity was observed within signet ring cells and the non–signet ring cell component, but no carcinoembryonic antigen staining was detected, similar to the findings of Catton et al.[323] Conversely, Remmele et al[319] reported one case with carcinoembryonic antigen immunoreactivity that was negative for prostate-specific antigen and prostatic acid phosphatase, and others have reported carcinoembryonic antigen staining with prostate-specific antigen and prostatic acid phosphatase staining.[322] The signet ring cell appearance results from different factors in different cases, including cytoplasmic lumens, mucin granules, and fat vacuoles, thus accounting for the contradictory histochemical and immunohistochemical results.

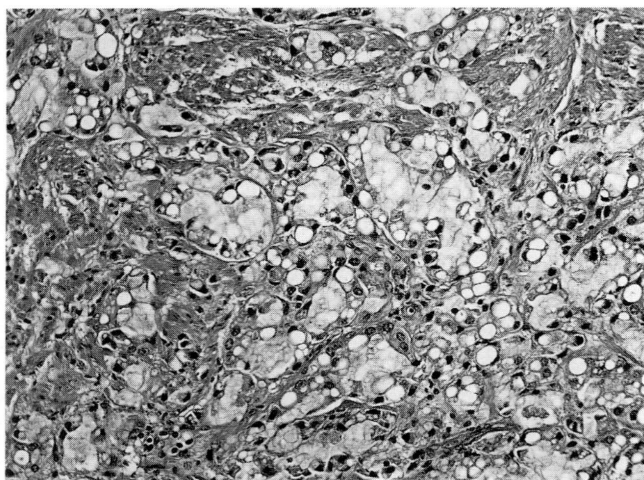

7-22. Signet ring cell carcinoma of the prostate.

Ultrastructurally, signet ring cells contain cytoplasmic vacuoles and intracytoplasmic lumens, sometimes lined by microvilli, sometimes with no demonstrable mucin or lipid vacuoles. Occasional rod-shaped intraluminal crystalloids are observed in metastatic sites, similar to crystalloids observed in typical acinar adenocarcinoma.

Treatment and prognosis. All reported patients have clinical stage T3 (C) or N+ (D) adenocarcinoma. Treatment is variable, including hormonal therapy, radiation therapy, or both. Five of eight patients reported by Ro et al[316] died between 32 and 60 months after diagnosis, and two patients were alive with less than 12 months of follow-up.

Differential diagnosis. Signet ring cell carcinoma of the prostate should be distinguished from similar tumors arising in other sites, particularly the gastrointestinal tract and stomach. Prostatic origin should be

TABLE 7-6.
SIGNET RING CELL CARCINOMA OF THE PROSTATE: LABORATORY FINDINGS

	Number of Cases	Preoperative Serum PAP	Preoperative Serum PSA	PAS	Lipid Stain	Alcian Blue	Muci-carmine	PSA	PAP	CEA	Other Findings
Lipid-Rich											
Kums and van Helsdingen, 1985[320]	2			—	1/2	—	—	—	—	—	
Glycogen or Mucin-Rich											
Giltman, 1981[321]	1			1/1	0/1	0/1	0/1	—	—	—	
Remmele et al, 1988[319]	1			1/1	—	1/1	1/1	0/1	0/1	1/1	
Uchijima et al, 1990[318]	1			0/1	—	1/1	—	1/1	—	—	
Alline and Cohen, 1992[322]	1	Normal	5.2	0/1	—	1/1	1/1	0/1	0/1	1/1	
Catton et al, 1992[323]	1	33.6	—	—	—	0/1	0/1	1/1	1/1	0/1	
Segawa and Kakehi, 1993[324]	1	Normal	<4.0*	1/1	—	—	1/1	0/1	0/1	1/1	CA19-9 positive
Guerin et al, 1993[325]	5	2.4/1.5/21.9		5/5	0/1	5/5	—	5/5	5/5	1/2	
Smith et al, 1994[326]	1	1.7	4.6*	1/1	—	—	1/1	1/1	1/1	1/1	Diploid primary; aneuploid metastases; loss of Y chromosome
Lipid, Glycogen, and Mucin-Poor											
Ro et al, 1988[316]	8			0/8	—	0/8	0/8	4/4	4/4	0/4	

*Normal Postoperative (never rose above normal despite death from metastases)
Number positive cases/Number cases studied
PAS: periodic acid-Schiff; PSA: prostate-specific antigen; PAP: prostatic acid phosphatase; CEA: carcinoembryonic antigen

considered in metastatic signet ring cell carcinoma of supraclavicular lymph nodes that exhibit negative mucin staining; prostate-specific antigen and prostatic acid phosphatase immunostaining may be useful. There have been no reported cases of signet ring cell lymphoma involving the prostate.

Artifactual changes mimicking signet ring cell carcinoma have been described in transurethral resection specimens, with lymphocytes and vacuolated smooth muscle cells causing diagnostic difficulty.[327] In these cases, prostate-specific antigen and prostatic acid phosphatase staining of the suspicious cells is negative, although leukocyte common antigen immunoreactivity is observed within the inflammatory cells.

Sarcomatoid carcinoma (carcinosarcoma; metaplastic carcinoma). Sarcomatoid carcinoma is considered by many to be synonymous with carcinosarcoma.[328-331] Authors who separate these tumors define sarcomatoid carcinoma as an epithelial tumor showing spindle cell (mesenchymal) differentiation; carcinosarcoma is defined as adenocarcinoma intimately admixed with malignant soft tissue elements (Fig. 7-23). Tumors containing areas of bone, cartilage, or striated muscle differentiation are sometimes referred to as sarcomatoid carcinoma with heterologous elements. Regardless of terminology, these tumors are rare and have a poor prognosis.

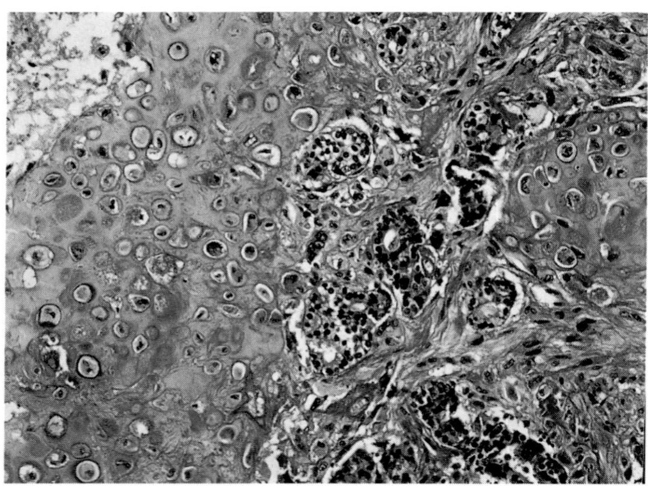

7-23. Sarcomatoid carcinoma (carcinosarcoma). There is an intimate admixture of adenocarcinoma and chondrosarcoma.

Clinical features. Patients tend to be older men who have symptoms of urinary outlet obstruction, similar to typical adenocarcinoma. Serum prostate-specific antigen level may be normal at the time of diagnosis.[331] About half of the patients have a prior history of typical acinar adenocarcinoma treated by radiation therapy or androgen deprivation therapy.

Pathology. The distinction between sarcomatoid carcinoma and carcinosarcoma is often difficult and of no apparent clinical significance; many authors consider these tumors to be the same entity. In the five cases studied by Shannon and associates,[329] three displayed an intimate mixture of sarcomatoid carcinoma and typical acinar adenocarcinoma, with transitions between them. Coexistent adenocarcinoma is almost always high grade (Gleason score 9 or 10). According to Dundore et al,[331] the most common soft tissue elements are osteosarcoma and leiomyosarcoma.

The epithelial component displays cytoplasmic immunoreactivity for keratin, prostate-specific antigen, and prostatic acid phosphatase, similar to typical prostatic adenocarcinoma. The soft tissue component usually displays immunoreactivity for vimentin, with variable staining for desmin, actin, and S-100 protein. Ultrastructurally, tumor cells within the sarcomatoid areas occasionally display desmosomes and filaments which apparently are cytokeratin. In two cases of Shannon et al,[329] there was no ultrastructural evidence of epithelial differentiation.

Treatment and prognosis. Treatment is variable and has no apparent influence on the poor prognosis. Dundore et al[331] found a 41% 5-year cancer-specific survival and 12% 7-year cancer-specific survival in a series of 21 patients from the Mayo Clinic, similar to survival in Gleason score 9 and 10 adenocarcinomas without sarco-

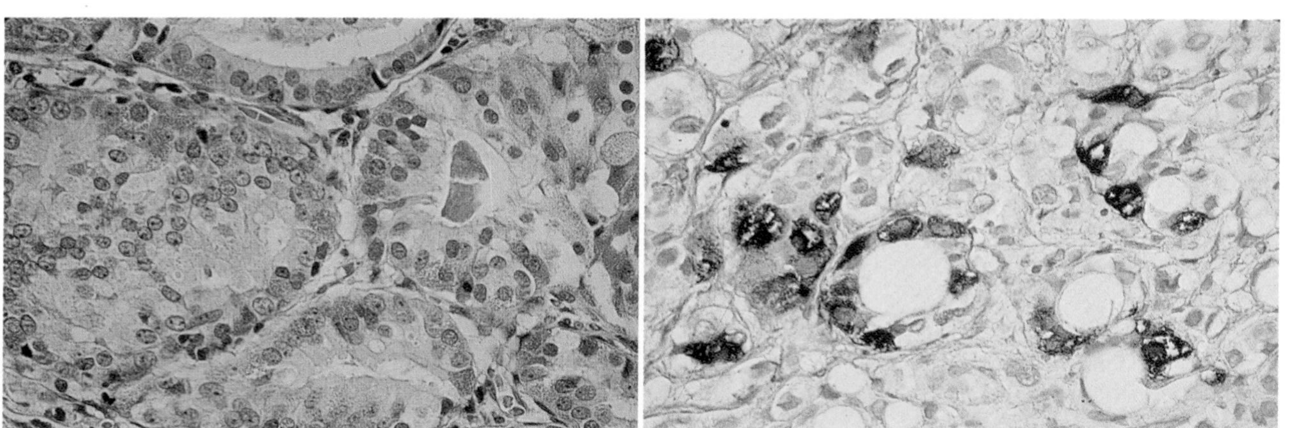

7-24. A, Adenocarcinoma with large eosinophilic granules. B, Another case, with serotonin-immunoreactive cells corresponding to cells with granules.

matoid features. Of five patients reported by Shannon et al.,[329] three died of tumor within 46 months of diagnosis, one was alive with tumor at 48 months, and one was lost to follow-up after 1 month.

Differential diagnosis. The separation of sarcomatoid carcinoma from sarcoma and carcinosarcoma may be difficult and clinically unimportant, although immunohistochemical stains and electron microscopy are helpful. Keratin immunoreactivity has been identified in some cases of leiomyosarcoma, so this finding alone may not be sufficient to determine epithelial differentiation.

Adenocarcinoma with neuroendocrine cells, including those with large eosinophilic granules (Paneth cell-like change). Virtually all prostatic adenocarcinomas contain at least a small number of neuroendocrine cells, but special studies such as histochemistry and immunohistochemistry are necessary to identify them.[42,332-372] About 10% of adenocarcinomas contain cells with large eosinophilic granules (formerly called *adenocarcinoma with Paneth cell-like change*), but these usually consist of only rare foci of scattered cells and small clusters that may be overlooked (Fig. 7-24).[347,367-371] Although cells with large eosinophilic granules in the normal epithelium and adenocarcinoma resemble Paneth cells of the intestine and other sites by light microscopy, they differ from Paneth cells by their neuroendocrine differentiation (producing chromogranin, neuron-specific enolase, and serotonin expression) and their lack of lysozyme.[347,367-371]

Clinical features. The clinical features of adenocarcinoma with neuroendocrine cells are apparently the same as typical acinar adenocarcinoma.

Pathology. The number of neuroendocrine cells is greater than the number of cells with large eosinophilic granules in the benign prostatic epithelium and adenocarcinoma, suggesting that there are neuroendocrine cells with granules that are not apparent on hematoxylin-eosin-stained sections. Neuroendocrine differentiation in the benign and malignant prostatic epithelium typically consists of scattered cells that are not apparent by light microscopy but revealed by stains positive for neuroendocrine markers.

Prostate-specific antigen and prostatic acid phosphatase immunoreactivity are present in cells with large eosinophilic granules.[42,345,372,332] Recently Abrahamsson et al[346] showed androgen receptor immunoreactivity in cells with neuroendocrine differentiation.

Treatment and prognosis. Neuroendocrine differentiation in prostatic adenocarcinoma may indicate a poor prognosis,[343,366] although this has been disputed.[42,332,344] Cohen et al[343] suggested that neuroendocrine differentiation is an independent prognostic variable in prostatic adenocarcinoma, but they examined only a small number of cases and did not control for tumor grade, clinical and pathologic stage, and DNA content. Other authors were unable to identify prognostic significance for neuroendocrine differentiation, and there was no correlation between the number of neuroendocrine cells and pathologic stage, metastases, and a variety of clinical and pathologic factors.[42,332,344]

There is evidence that the neuroendocrine component of prostatic carcinoma is resistant to hormonal therapy. Stratton et al[351] noted that typical acinar carcinoma with focal neuroendocrine differentiation recurred as neuroendocrine carcinoma following hormonal therapy. Di Sant'Agnese[334] suggested an autocrine mechanism for stimulation of growth of tumor cells with epithelial and neuroendocrine differentiation.

Differential diagnosis. The differential diagnosis of adenocarcinoma with neuroendocrine cells is the same as typical acinar adenocarcinoma. Areas with neuroendocrine differentiation may be misinterpreted as poorly differentiated adenocarcinoma.

Neuroendocrine carcinoma (small cell carcinoma and carcinoid). Neuroendocrine differentiation in typical prostatic adenocarcinoma was first observed by Azzopardi and Evans[348] in 1971. Subsequent studies have confirmed these findings, observing argentaffin-positive and argyrophil-positive cells in up to 33% of tumors. Using the argyrophil stain and immunohistochemical neuroendocrine markers, Di Sant'Agnese and de Mesy Jensen[356] found neuroendocrine differentiation in 47% of cases of prostatic adenocarcinoma. Abrahamsson et al[339] found neuroendocrine differentiation in 100% of cases of prostatic carcinoma evaluated histochemically and immunohistochemically when using a special fixative.

The biologic significance of neuroendocrine cells in the benign and neoplastic prostate is unknown. These cells are thought to have an endocrine-paracrine regulatory role in growth and development, similar to neuroendocrine cells in other organs, and contain multiple neuropeptides that can modulate cell growth and proliferation. Somatostatin analogues inhibit the growth of androgen-dependent human prostatic adenocarcinoma xenograft PC-82 and the Dunning rat prostatic adenocarcinoma.[373-375] Bombesin (gastrin-releasing peptide) is mitogenic for the androgen-independent human prostatic adenocarcinoma cell line PC-3 in vitro,[376] and bombesin antagonists suppress growth of the xenograft PC-82.[374] Neuroendocrine cells in the benign epithelium are probably postmitotic, whereas adjacent cells are frequently proliferative, according to studies with Ki-67 immunoreactivity in the benign epithelium.[335] Androgen deprivation therapy does not appear to influence the number or distribution of neuroendocrine cells in the normal or neoplastic prostate.[332] Neuroendocrine cells coexpress prostate-specific antigen[332,375] and androgen receptors,[346] suggesting a common cell of origin for epithelial cells and neuroendocrine cells in the prostate. However, pure small cell carcinoma of the prostate does not usually display immunoreactivity for prostate-specific antigen.

Tissue fixation is critical in preservation of neuroendocrine cell immunoreactivity, according to Abrahamsson et al,[339] and routine formalin fixation is not optimal for all markers.

Clinical features. Most cases of neuroendocrine carcinoma have typical signs and symptoms of prostatic adenocarcinoma, and serum prostate-specific antigen levels vary according to tumor volume and stage.[377-387] In addition, paraneoplastic syndromes are frequent in patients with small cell carcinoma and carcinoid of the prostate. Cushing's syndrome is most common, invariably in association with adrenocorticotropic hormone immunoreactivity in tumor cells.[379] Other clinical conditions include malignant hypercalemia,[383,384] the syndrome of inappropriate antidiuretic hormone secretion,[385] and myasthenic (Eaton-Lambert) syndrome.[378]

Pathology. A spectrum of neuroendocrine differentiation can be seen in prostatic adenocarcinoma, varying from a carcinoidlike pattern (low-grade neuroendocrine carcinoma) to small cell undifferentiated (oat cell) carcinoma (high-grade neuroendocrine carcinoma) (Fig. 7-25). These tumors are morphologically identical to carcinoid tumor and small cell carcinoma of the lung and other sites. Typical acinar adenocarcinoma is present, at least focally, in about 25% of cases, and transition patterns may be seen. In cases with a solid Gleason 5 pattern suggestive of neuroendocrine carcinoma, immunohistochemical stains are recommended.

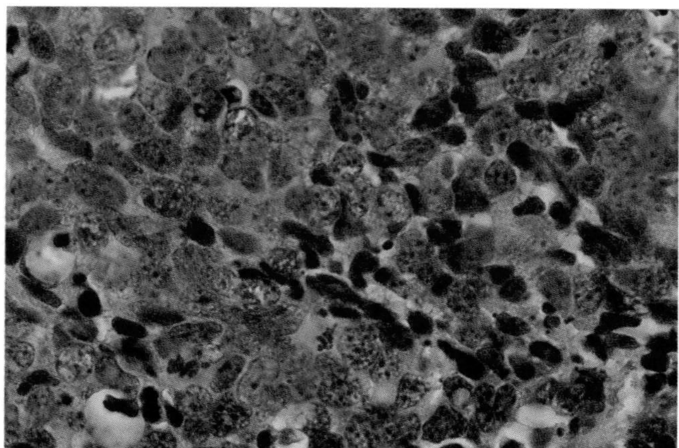

7-25. Small cell undifferentiated adenocarcinoma.

Immunohistochemically, a wide variety of secretory products may be detected within the carcinoma cells, including serotonin, calcitonin, adrenocorticotropic hormone, human chorionic gonadotropin, thyroid-stimulating hormone, bombesin, calcitonin gene-related peptide, atachalcin, and inhibin.[381,387] The same cells may express peptide hormones and prostate-specific antigen and prostatic acid phosphatase. Azumi et al[345] and others identified concomitant prostate-specific antigen and neuroendocrine marker immunoreactivity in prostatic carcinoid and other prostatic tumors.

Serotonin and chromogranin are the most often identified markers of neuroendocrine cells in formalin-fixed sections of prostate.[42,334,339] Aprikian and associates[332] found neuroendocrine cells in 77% of untreated prostatic

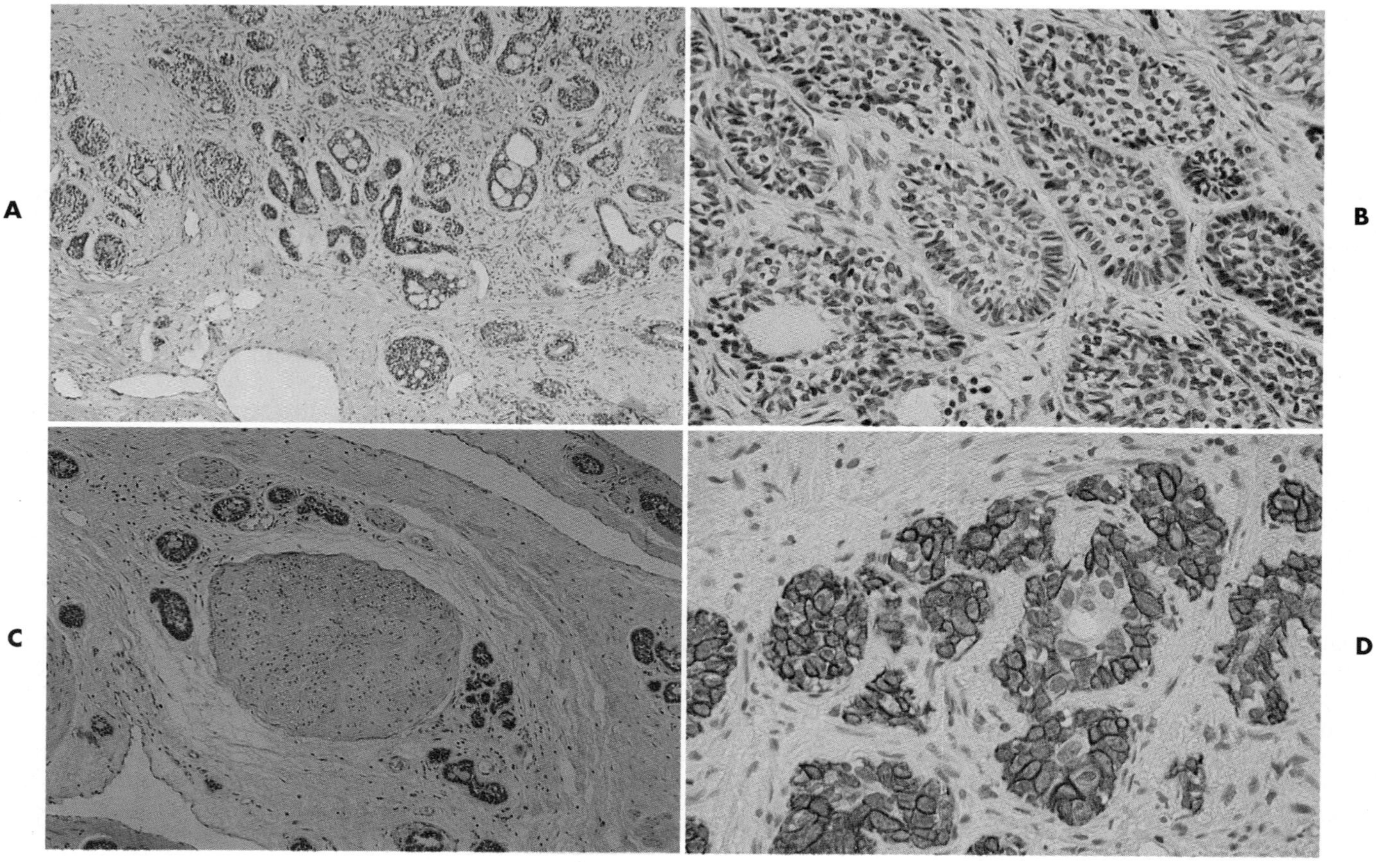

7-26. Adenoid basal cell tumor of the prostate. **A**, Adenoid cystic carcinoma-like pattern. **B**, Basal cell carcinoma-like pattern. **C**, Prominent perineural invasion. **D**, Intense immunoreactivity for antikeratin 34ß-E12.

adenocarcinomas, 60% of hormone-refractory adenocarcinomas, and 52% of metastases, with a small number of dispersed positive cells in each of these cases. Berner et al[333] found no difference in neuron-specific enolase expression in pretreatment and posttreatment specimens from 47 cases of hormone-resistant prostatic adenocarcinoma.

Ultrastructurally, small cell carcinoma and carcinoid tumors display features similar to their counterparts in the lung. The characteristic finding is variable numbers of round, regular 100 to 400 nm membrane-bound neurosecretory granules. Well-defined cytoplasmic processes are usually present, with approximately 8 to 15 granules per process. The cells are small, with dispersed chromatin and small inconspicuous nucleoli. Acinar formation is lacking in the neuroendocrine component and no tonofilaments are present.

Treatment and prognosis. Small cell carcinoma is aggressive and rapidly fatal[381,386,387] and is a variant of Gleason pattern 5 adenocarcinoma. Ferguson et al[388] found that androgen receptor expression in small cell carcinoma was predictive of a poorer outcome (median survival, 10 months) than in cases without expression (median survival, more than 30 months), regardless of treatment.

Differential diagnosis. Although unusual, metastases to the prostate from other sites may mimic carcinoid and small cell carcinoma of the prostate. High-grade carcinoma from the bladder that invades the prostate may be mistaken for neuroendocrine carcinoma. Other rare tumors, such as peripheral neuroectodermal tumor, desmoplastic small round cell tumor, and malignant lymphoma, may be mistaken for prostatic neuroendocrine carcinoma, particularly in extraprostatic sites.

Adenoid basal cell tumor (basal cell carcinoma; adenoid cysticlike tumor). Neoplastic basal cell proliferations in the prostate exhibit a morphologic continuum ranging from basal cell adenoma in the setting of nodular hyperplasia to florid adenoid basal cell tumor.[389-413] These diverse proliferations have been referred to by a variety of terms, including basal cell tumor,[395] basal cell adenoma,[397] basaloid carcinoma,[390] adenoid basal cell tumor,[393,400] prostatic adenoma of ductal origin,[398] adenoid cysticlike tumor,[406] and adenoid cystic carcinoma.[393,397,400,413] Benign and neoplastic basal cell proliferations (including basal cell hyperplasia) are uncommon lesions, comprising 22 of 247 (8.9%) cases in one study[407] and 10 of 172 (5.8%) cases in another series[399]; the rarest of these are basal cell carcinoma and adenoid cysticlike tumor. Grignon et al[393] suggested that there was a continuum of basal cell hyperplasia, basal cell adenoma, adenoid basal cell tumor, and adenoid cystic carcinoma, and this was confirmed by Deveraj and Bostwick.[407]

Clinical features. The age, presenting symptoms, and clinical findings of adenoid basal cell tumor are similar to typical acinar adenocarcinoma. All reported cases have been confined to the prostate at presentation and follow-up as long as 6 years after diagnosis. Serum prostate-specific antigen and prostatic acid phosphatase levels are not apparently elevated.

Pathology. Adenoid basal cell tumor of the prostate is histologically similar to adenoid cystic carcinoma in the salivary glands and other sites (Fig. 7-26). The criteria for distinguishing these lesions have recently been refined (Table 7-7), and the malignant nature of cases previously reported as adenoid cystic carcinoma has been questioned. Young et al[406] reclassified four previously reported cases of adenoid cystic carcinoma as adenoid cysticlike tumor following review of the histologic slides and added two cases from their files. Published cases illustrated in the World Health Organization Monograph and 1973 Armed Forces Institute of Pathology Fascicle have been reclassified as variants of adenoid basal cell tumor.[245,246] Young et al[406] stated that virtually all cases of adenoid cystic carcinoma of the prostate in the literature resemble basal cell hyperplasia and should not be considered malignant.

Adenoid basal cell tumor is histologically similar to basal cell hyperplasia and basal cell adenoma, but the tumor usually involves large areas of the prostate with little or no circumscription.[407] It can form two distinct architectural patterns: adenoid cystic[400,406] and basaloid.[390] The first of these consists of irregular clusters of crowded basaloid cells punctuated by round spaces, many of which contain mucinous material resembling salivary gland adenoid cystic carcinoma. The basaloid pattern consists of variably sized round basaloid cell nests with prominent peripheral palisading. These patterns frequently coexist in the same lesion,[406] although pure forms have been described.[390]

In adenoid basal cell tumor, the basal cell nests are large and irregular in outline, separated by benign myxoid stroma, and the tumor cells are predominantly elongate, with narrow tapering nuclei and peripheral palisading. Cell crowding is prominent, and the basal cell masses frequently display multiple lumens, some of which are sharply circumscribed and rounded ("punched-out"). Nucleoli are inconspicuous, similar to basal cell hyperplasia. In limited samples, such as transurethral resection specimens, it may be difficult to separate basal cell adenoma and adenoid basal cell tumor. Squamous differentiation with keratin production is frequent in these prostatic tumors but is rare in adenoid cystic carcinoma arising at other sites. Perineural invasion has been reported but is rare. Grignon and associates[393] described an adenoid basal cell tumor with extensive perineural invasion, which was interpreted as adenoid cystic carcinoma; however, that case lacked significant cytologic atypia and no capsular perforation or follow-up was reported.

In some areas the tumor nests are punctuated by small cystic spaces, imparting a prominent adenoid pattern. These spaces are filled with hyaline material, mucin, or eosinophilic deposits. Two cell types are present: basaloid cells with delicate stippled chromatin and scant cytoplasm, and an inner lining of cuboidal to columnar ductal cells with moderate amounts of pale eosinophilic cytoplasm. Rarely, mitotic figures and mild cytologic atypia are present. In some areas prominent keratinization of the secretory luminal cells is observed; foci of basal cell hyperplasia are invariably present. These tumors are expansive, extending into the stroma of the

TABLE 7-7.
BASAL CELL PROLIFERATIONS OF THE PROSTATE: DIAGNOSTIC CRITERIA AND IMMUNOHISTOCHEMICAL PROFILE

	Normal Basal Cell Layer	Basal Cell Hyperplasia (BCH)	Atypical Basal Cell Hyperplasia	Basal Cell Adenoma	Adenoid Basal Cell Tumor
Architecture	Near-continuous single cell layer	Small cell nests (solid or cystic), usually in nodular hyperplasia, 2-cell-layer minimum	Same as BCH	Round circumscribed nodule of BCH	Infiltrating "adenoid cystic" pattern or basaloid pattern,myxoid stroma
Cytology	Small elongate cells, ovoid nuclei, scant cytoplasm	Large ovoid nuclei indistinct nucleoli, scant cytoplasm, may have clear cytoplasm	Same as BCH, but with nucleolomegaly	Same as BCH, may have nucleolomegaly	Basaloid cells with large nuclei
Immunohistochemical findings					
Basal cell–specific keratin 34ß-E12	+	+	+	+	+ (patchy)
Prostate-specific antigen	-	+ (patchy)	+ (patchy)	+ (focal)	±
Prostatic acid phosphatase	-	+ (patchy)	+ (patchy)	+ (focal)	±
Chromogranin	-	±	±	±	±
S-100 protein	-	±	±	±	-
Neuron-specific enolase	-	±	±	-	-

±, <5% of cells were positive.

From Deveraj LT, Bostwick DG: Atypical basal cell hyperplasia of the prostate. Immunophenotypic profile and proposed classification of basal cell proliferations, Am J Surg Pathol 17:645-659, 1993; with permission.

prostate without entrapping acinar elements and are accompanied by a myxoid matrix. Adenocarcinoma may be present in adjacent foci, but is never in direct contact with the adenoid basal cell tumor.

The watery basophilic material within the cystic spaces stains with Alcian blue at pH 2.5, but staining is eliminated by hyaluronidase digestion. Periodic acid-Schiff stain after diastase digestion is positive, as is the mucicarmine stain. The myxoid stroma surrounding the tumor nests stains strongly with Alcian blue at pH 2.5, weakly with periodic acid-Schiff, and is unstained with mucicarmine.

Adenoid basal cell tumor shows variable immunoreactivity with basal cell–specific high molecular weight antikeratin 34ß-E12. Also, rare scattered cells may show prostate-specific antigen and prostatic acid phosphatase immunoreactivity, and rare cells display chromogranin staining. S-100 protein and neuron-specific enolase stains are negative.[407]

Ultrastructurally, the basaloid cells form cohesive nests surrounded by prominent basal laminae. Well-formed desmosomes are present, and intercellular spaces are occasionally lined by microvilli or rare cilia. In nests with true lumens, the cells exhibit superficial microvilli and have nuclei with conspicuous heterochromatin. The lumens are filled with abundant vesicles, granular material, and cellular debris. In solid nests the tumor cells have round nuclei with uniform chromatinic rims and prominent euchromatin. There is no evidence of myoepithelial differentiation.

Treatment and prognosis. Most patients with adenoid basal cell tumor have been treated by transurethral resection, although other forms of therapy have been employed, including radical prostatectomy and radiation therapy. The malignant potential of adenoid basal cell tumor remains uncertain due to the small number of reported cases. These tumors are best classified as adenoid basal cell tumors, as suggested by Young et al[406]; they differ from adenoid cystic carcinoma by the absence of cytoplasmic myofilaments, the absence of consistent basal lamina proliferation around cell nests, and the absence of documented malignant behavior. A recent case reported as basal cell carcinoma was considered malignant by the identification of tumor on a perineal biopsy; however, there was no definite evidence of extraprostatic extension, and the tumor followed a benign clinical course.[413] One of the cases reported by Deveraj and Bostwick[407] exhibited prominent perineural invasion and focal extraprostatic spread suggestive of malignancy; however, follow-up at 5 months indicated no evidence of recurrence or metastasis, and pelvic lymph nodes were uninvolved at the time of radical prostatectomy. At present adenoid basal cell tumor is probably best considered as a tumor of low malignant potential pending long-term follow-up study of other cases.

Differential diagnosis. The differential diagnosis of adenoid basal cell tumor and other basal cell proliferations includes a wide variety of benign and malignant lesions. Atypical adenomatous hyperplasia may be confused with basal cell hyerplasia and adenoid basal cell tumor but does not usually have a prominent basal cell layer and displays a fragmented keratin 34ß-E12–immunoreactive basal cell layer. Sclerosing adenosis may be difficult to separate from sclerosing basal cell hyperplasia, and these lesions may coexist; however, sclerosing adenosis is distinguished by the absence of smooth muscle in the sclerotic stroma and the presence of myoepithelial differentiation (intense cytoplasmic immunoreactivity with keratin 34ß-E12, S-100 protein, and muscle-specific actin, as well as ultrastructural evidence of cytoplasmic myofilaments).

Well-differentiated adenocarcinoma is distinguished from basal cell hyperplasia and adenoid basal cell tumor by the presence of prostate-specific antigen and prostatic acid phosphatase–immunoreactive luminal secretory cells with enlarged nucleoli, frequent luminal crystalloids, and absence of a keratin 34ß-E12–immunoreactive basal cell layer. Similar criteria allow separation of the cribriform variant of adenocarcinoma, adenoid basal cell tumor, basal cell hyperplasia with or without clear cell change, and clear cell cribriform hyperplasia. There has been no report of adenoid cystic carcinoma from another organ metastasizing to the prostate.

Adenocarcinoma with oncocytic features. Rare cases of prostatic adenocarcinoma with diffuse oncocytic change have been reported, characterized by tumor cells with abundant eosinophilic granular cytoplasm reflecting the presence of abundant mitochondria.[414-416] Tumor cells displayed prostate-specific antigen immunoreactivity. The clinical behavior appears to be the same as typical acinar adenocarcinoma.[416] Differential diagnosis includes prostatic nodular hyperplasia with oncocytic change (oncocytoma),[414] neuroendocrine carcinoma, and rhabdoid tumor.

Lymphoepithelioma-like carcinoma. Carcinoma accompanied by a dense lymphocytic infiltrate is termed *lymphoepithelioma*, *lymphoepithelioma-like carcinoma*, and *medullary carcinoma*. This histologically distinctive tumor is most common in the head and neck but has rarely arisen in the breast, bladder, and other sites. A single case has been reported in the prostate (Fig. 7-27).[417] Although prostatic adenocarcinoma may be associated with granulomatous prostatitis or patchy acute and chronic inflammation, it rarely appears as solid islands of epithelial cells

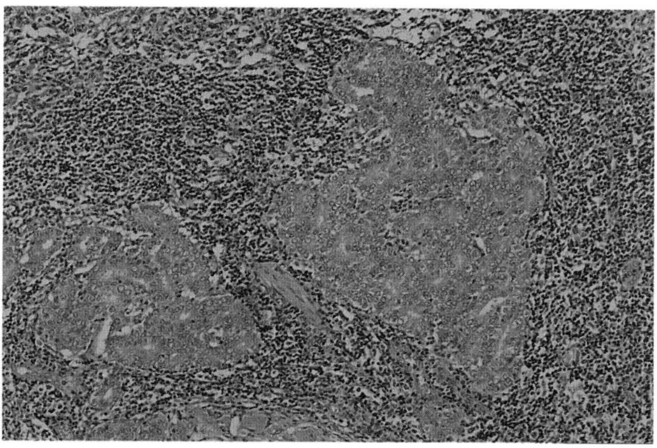

7-27. Lymphoepithelioma-like carcinoma of the prostate.

punctating a sheetlike infiltrate of lymphocytes characteristic of lymphoepithelioma-like carcinoma at other sites. The tumor had large areas of typical adenocarcinoma, but the different patterns were not intermingled.

Immunohistochemistry revealed that the lymphocytic infiltrate was composed chiefly of T cells, similar to the lymphocytic response in lymphoepithelioma-like carcinomas at other sites. No atypical lymphocytes were observed, and these were not the features of malignant lymphoma or leukemia involving the prostate. Flow cytometry revealed that the tumor was aneuploid. In situ hybridization was negative for Epstein-Barr virus.[417]

Cribriform carcinoma. The cribriform pattern is a histologically distinct variant of Gleason grade 3 carcinoma, characterized by large epithelial cell masses punctuated by multiple small lumens. Unlike cribriform prostatic intraepithelial neoplasia, cribriform carcinoma does not have a basal cell layer at the periphery of acini (Fig. 7-28*A*, *B*).[16,126,418,419] Amin et al[126] studied 23 prostatectomies with adenocarcinoma which contained cribriform acini, and found that 55% of these acini were cribriform prostatic intraepithelial neoplasia rather than cribriform adenocarcinoma. These results are similar to those of McNeal et al,[419] who found that up to 70% of cribriform masses were intraductal; however, they described this as "cribriform carcinoma" and suggested that the cribriform pattern has the same biologic behavior as Gleason pattern 4 adenocarcinoma. No follow-up information was provided to support their claim, and the number of cases studied (21 cases) was too small to draw conclusions regarding biologic behavior. The association of cribriform prostatic intraepithelial neoplasia and Gleason pattern 4 carcinoma was not confirmed in another study of 60 totally sectioned prostatectomies.[16] The term *cribriform carcinoma*, if used at all, is most commonly employed only as a descriptive term and does not refer to a specific histogenetic category of prostatic adenocarcinoma. The cribriform pattern is invariably found in association with other patterns of adenocarcinoma.

Comedocarcinoma. Comedocarcinoma is characterized by luminal necrosis within round masses of malignant cells, similar to comedocarcinoma of the breast (Fig. 7-28*C*). This morphologic variant of adenocarcinoma is included in the Gleason grading system as poorly differentiated (grade 5) carcinoma based on the degree of acinar differentiation. Currin et al[420] studied the biologic potential of prostatic comedocarcinoma by flow cytometry and found a high frequency of aneuploidy, suggesting aggressiveness. Prostatic acid phosphatase and prostate-

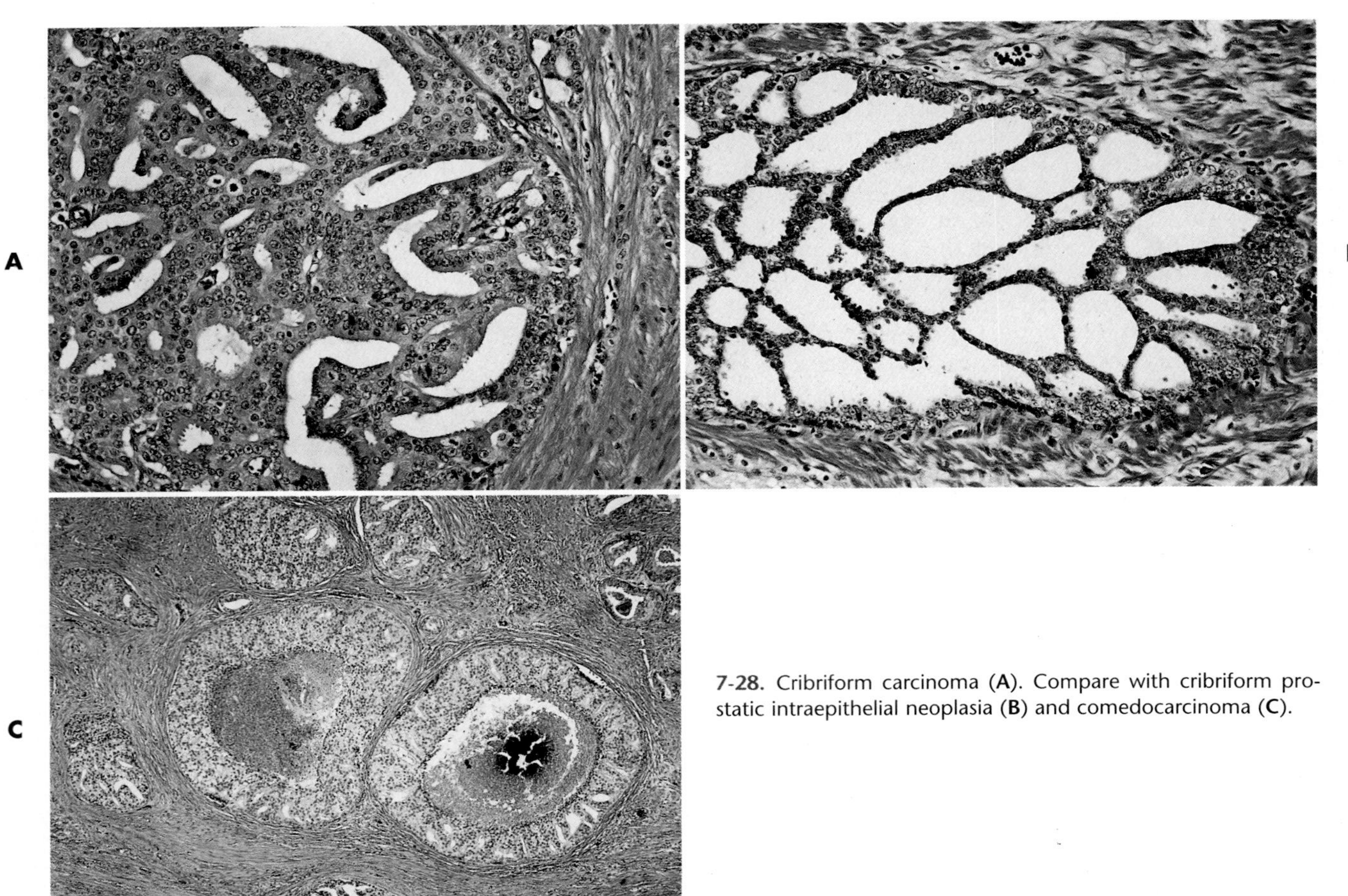

7-28. Cribriform carcinoma (**A**). Compare with cribriform prostatic intraepithelial neoplasia (**B**) and comedocarcinoma (**C**).

specific antigen were present in the majority of tumor cells. Comedocarcinoma is invariably found in association with other patterns of adenocarcinoma and does not warrant separation as a clinicopathologic entity.

Squamous and adenosquamous carcinoma. Squamous cell carcinoma is very rare in the prostate, with only about 50 published cases.[421-435] Adenosquamous carcinoma refers to the combination of squamous cell carcinoma and typical acinar carcinoma,[432] and appears to be even more rare than pure squamous cell carcinoma, with fewer than 10 reported cases.

Clinical features. Presenting signs and symptoms are similar to those of the typical prostatic adenocarcinoma, although there is often a history of hormonal therapy or radiation therapy. Patients are more than 50 years of age, with a mean in the seventh decade. Prostate-specific antigen and prostatic acid phosphatase levels are usually normal, even with metastases, and bone metastases are typically osteolytic rather than osteoblastic.[424,427,428] Squamous cell carcinoma of the prostate may arise in patients infected with *Schistosoma haematobium*.[434]

Pathology. Squamous cell carcinoma of the prostate is histologically similar to its counterpart in other organs, consisting of irregular nests and cords of malignant cells with keratinization and squamous differentiation, rarely with squamous pearls (Fig. 7-29). Keratinizing squamous cell carcinoma of the prostate usually arises in the periurethral ducts and is very rare; otherwise, the site of origin of squamous cell carcinoma is unknown.[428] Mott[424] required an absence of acinar differentiation for the diagnosis of squamous cell carcinoma, as well as a lack of bladder involvement; mixed tumors are best classified simply as adenosquamous carcinoma. Mott also required no prior estrogen therapy, but we consider this exclusion unnecessary. Metastases may consist of adenosquamous carcinoma in cases without a squamous component in the primary tumor, perhaps due to sampling error.[433]

Saito et al[430] identified prostatic acid phosphatase immunoreactivity in the acinar and squamous components of their case of adenosquamous carcinoma. Conversely, Gattuso et al[432] found staining only in the acinar component of their case; interestingly, they noted immunoreactivity in the squamous component for high molecular weight keratin AE-3, but not in the acinar component. The adenosquamous carcinoma reported by Devaney et al[435] showed prostate-specific antigen and prostatic acid phosphatase immunoreactivity in the acinar component but not in the squamous component; both components were diploid. Prostate-specific antigen immunoreactivity was identified by Al Adani[434] in two Iraqi patients with squamous cell carcinoma arising in intimate association with calcified schistosomal ova; prostatic acid phosphatase was negative.

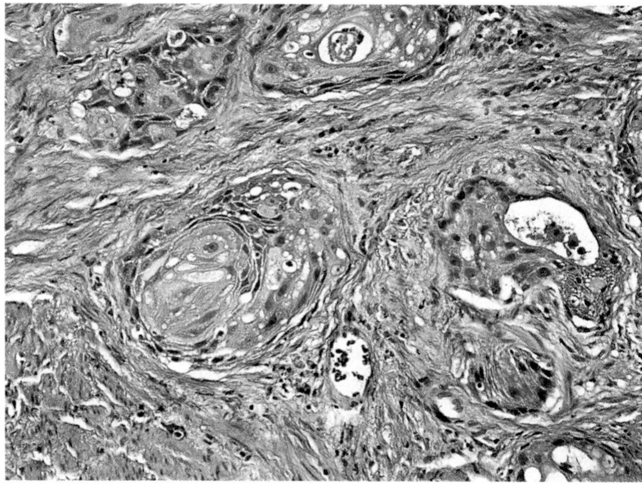

7-29. Squamous cell carcinoma of the prostate.

The histogenesis of squamous and adenosquamous carcinoma is unknown, but proposed origins include multipotential stem cells,[431] basal cells or reserve cells,[422,426] columnar secretory cells,[424] prostatic urethral or periurethral urothelial cells,[423] cells of adenocarcinoma,[430] and metaplastic squamous cells.[429,434]

Treatment and prognosis. Squamous cell carcinoma of the prostate is aggressive, with a mean survival of about 14 months regardless of therapy.[424] These tumors appear to be unresponsive to androgen deprivation therapy.

Differential diagnosis. Squamous cell carcinoma of the prostate may be confused with squamous metaplasia due to infarction, radiation therapy, and hormonal therapy. Rarely, adenocarcinoma may exhibit benign squamous metaplasia. Squamous cell carcinoma of the bladder may invade the prostate and must be excluded.

Changes due to therapy

The histologic changes in adenocarcinoma following therapy, such as androgen deprivation or radiation therapy, often present a significant diagnostic challenge.

Carcinoma after androgen deprivation therapy. In 1942 Schenken et al[436] reported that estrogen therapy for prostatic adenocarcinoma caused nuclear size reduction in up to 56% of cases compared with untreated controls, and loss of recognizable nucleoli, chromatin condensation, nuclear pyknosis, and cytoplasmic vacuolation. Similar findings have been reported in prostatic epithelium in animal models, normal human prostate, and prostatic adenocarcinoma, underscoring the androgen sensitivity of these tissues.[205-213]

There is an increase in the Gleason grade and a substantial reduction in nuclear and nucleolar size in prostatic adenocarcinoma following androgen deprivation therapy, accompanied by prominent cytoplasmic clearing (Fig. 7-30).[205-213] While these changes are rarely seen in untreated adenocarcinoma, the combination of features following therapy is sufficiently distinctive to warrant recognition of this entity. It is important for pathologists to be aware of these changes because of the reliance placed on nuclear and nucleolar size in the diagnosis of prostatic adenocarcinoma, particularly in small specimens and lymph nodes metastases.

Tetu et al[207] also found changes in benign acini, including marked lobular and acinar atrophy, epithelial vacuolation, basal cell hyperplasia, squamous metaplasia,

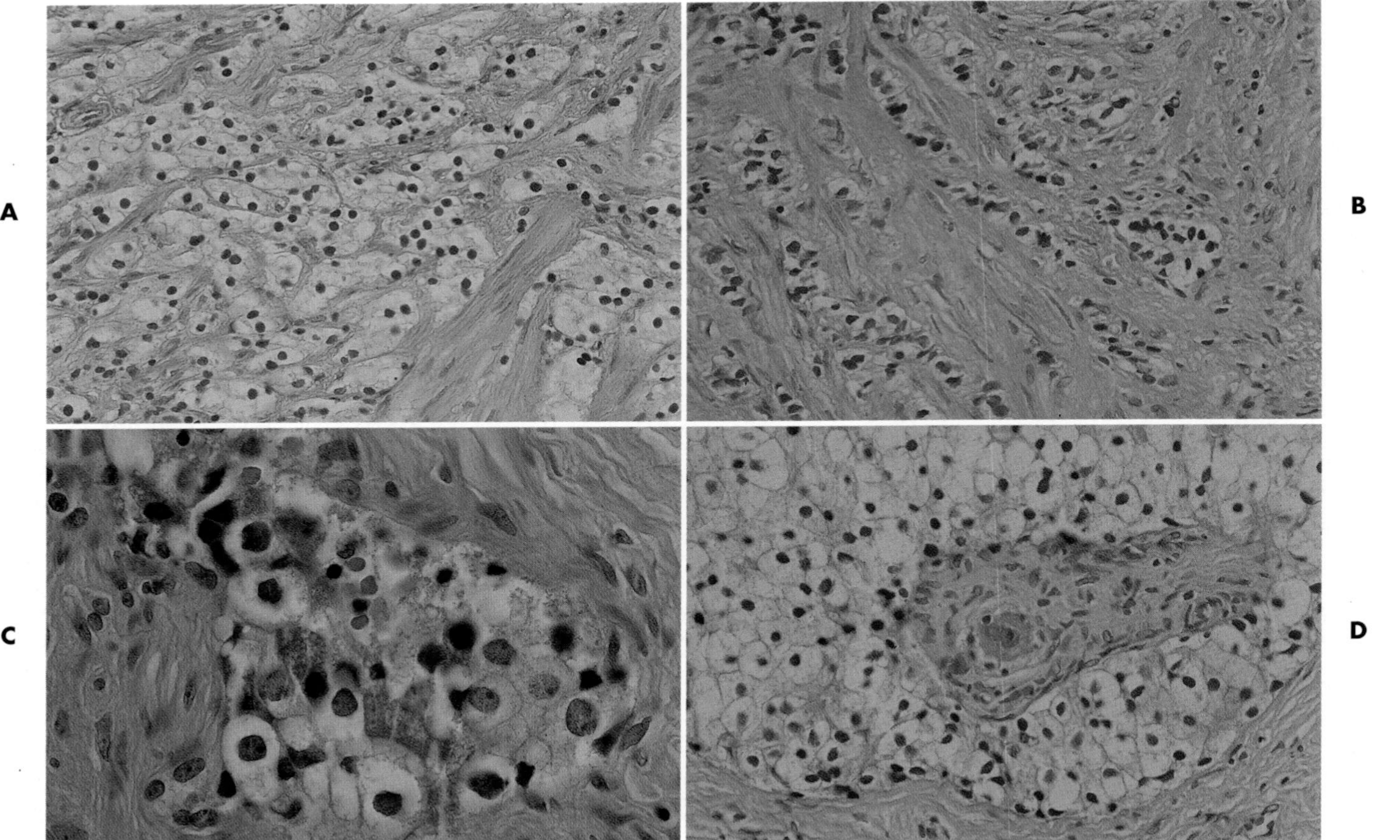

7-30. Prostate cancer following androgen deprivation therapy. **A**, Tumor cells contain abundant clear cytoplasm with shrunken hyperchromatic nuclei. **B**, The infiltrative pattern often consists of ribbons and nests of cells. **C**, Tumor nuclei are often hyperchromatic and "nucleolus-poor." **D**, Extraprostatic ganglion surrounded by cancer showing treatment effect.

transitional metaplasia, and acinar rupture with extravasation of secretions. In treated adenocarcinoma they described atypical microacini characterized by a single cell lining with large nucleoli, cytoplasmic vacuolation, and a "hemangiopericytoma-like" arrangement. Ellison et al[209] confirmed many of these findings and noted decreased nucleolar size. In another study Murphy et al[208] compared paired prostatic specimens before and after androgen deprivation, noting the presence after therapy of infiltrative small acini as well as a significant reduction in benign acinar size and density.[212] These studies indicate that consistent and characteristic changes occur in the benign and neoplastic prostate after therapy.

What is the the biologic potential of treated prostatic adenocarcinoma? Does the consistent high-grade pattern reflect aggressive androgen-insensitive clones or, conversely, collapsed carcinoma of low viability? DNA ploidy analysis in 27 cases by Ellison et al[209] revealed a trend toward aneuploidy after treatment; also, there was no correlation of ploidy and stage. Despite an apparent increase in grade, adenocarcinoma following therapy is probably not more clinically aggressive than when untreated; however, outcome data are not available to confirm this assertion.

Androgen deprivation stimulates expression of a variety of genes, including transforming growth factor ß, testosterone-repressed prostate message, c-myc, glutathione S-transferase Xb1, Mr 70,000 heat shock, and c-fos.[436-439] Androgen ablation of normal, hyperplastic, and dysplastic epithelial cells causes acceleration of programmed cell death of single cells (apoptosis), characterized by fragmentation of tumor DNA, appearance of apoptotic bodies, and inhibition of cell growth.[437-439]

The main differential diagnostic considerations of carcinoma following androgen deprivation therapy include a variety of atrophic and hyperplastic changes in benign acini, such as clear cell cribriform hyperplasia, sclerosing adenosis, acinar atrophy, atypical adenomatous hyperplasia, and atypical basal cell hyperplasia (see box on page 383). Significant difficulty may also be encountered in separating minute clusters and single file ribbons of tumor cells after androgen deprivation from lymphocytes, myocytes, and fibroblasts, particularly on a cell-by-cell basis in some foci. Low-power scanning may fail to identify tumor because of the deceptively benign appearance of the cytoplasm and nuclei after therapy. Untreated prostatic adenocarcinoma may have a clear cell pattern, particularly when arising in the transition zone in associ-

CLEAR CELL PROLIFERATIONS IN THE PROSTATE: DIFFERENTIAL DIAGNOSIS

- Benign
  - Paraganglioma with clear cell pattern
  - Mucinous metaplasia
  - Storage disease
  - Cowper's glands
  - Basal cell hyperplasia with clear cell change
  - Atypical adenomatous hyperplasia with clear cell change
  - Mesonephric remnants
  - Xanthoma
- Malignant
  - Clear cell adenocarcinoma of the prostrate
  - Transition zone cancer with clear cell pattern
  - Cancer following androgen deprivation
  - Mucinous and signet ring cell carcinoma
  - Epithelioid leiomyoma and leiomyosarcoma
  - Secondary malignancies
  - Clear cell carcinoma of the bladder
  - Metastatic renal cell carcinoma, clear cell pattern
  - Signet ring cell lymphoma

ation with nodular hyperplasia, but it is usually well differentiated (Gleason patterns 1, 2, 3), has prominent nucleoli, and is not associated with atrophic acini with abundant clear cell change.

Immunohistochemical studies for prostate-specific antigen, prostatic acid phosphatase, and basal cell–specific keratin 34ß-E12 are of value in separating carcinoma following therapy and some of its mimics. Prostate-specific antigen and prostatic acid phosphatase are retained in tumor cells after therapy, and keratin 34ß-E12 remains negative, indicating an absent basal cell layer. No differences are found in expression of neuroendocrine differentiation markers such as chromogranin, neuron-specific enolase, ß-hCG, and serotonin.

The use of androgen deprivation therapy is expected to increase with the introduction of new agents such as the recently approved 5 alpha-reductase inhibitor, finasteride (Proscar). Androgen deprivation has been used for preoperative tumor shrinkage and treatment of prostatic hyperplasia and may be effective for cancer prophylaxis, although this remains speculative. Ferguson et al[65] recently showed that androgen deprivation therapy causes a marked reduction in the presence and extent of high-grade prostatic intraepithelial neoplasia. Because the mechanism of action varies among the different androgen deprivation agents, further study is needed to assess subtle differences beyond those noted here and to define the possible biologic significance of these changes.

Carcinoma after radiation therapy. As a result of the delayed manifestation of tumor cell death, needle biopsy is usually of little value for 12 months after irradiation.[197] After this period, however, biopsy is the best method for assessing local tumor control (Fig. 7-31), with a low level of sampling error that is minimized by taking serial specimens.[197-204,440]

No definitive method exists for assessment of tumor viability after irradiation. Musselman and associates[441] demonstrated monolayer growth from explants of prostatic carcinoma two years or more after definitive radiation. Conversely, Mollenkamp et al[442] were unable to culture any of 19 irradiated tumors, but their success rate for in vitro cultivation of untreated carcinoma was poor (less than 7%). Mahan et al[440] identified intense cytoplasmic immunoreactivity for prostatic acid phosphatase in 23 of 27 irradiated cases of adenocarcinoma, leading them to suggest that tumor cells capable of protein production probably retain the potential for cell division and consequent metastatic spread. Other reports have claimed that if prostatic carcinoma is not histologically ablated by radiotherapy after 12 months, it is probably biologically active.[197,201,202] Keisling et al[204] noted that the ultrastructural features of prostatic adenocarcinoma after irradiation were indistinguishable from those of untreated carcinoma, suggesting that residual tumor is viable.

Ancillary studies

Immunohistochemistry

Prostate-specific antigen. Prostate-specific antigen is the most important, accurate, and clinically useful biochemical marker in the prostate because it is so specific for prostatic tissue.[443-445] This 34 kilodalton serine protease is manufactured by the epithelial cells and secreted into the prostatic ductal system, where it catalyzes the liquefaction of the seminal coagulum after ejaculation. Serum levels are normally below about 4.0 ng/mL, but vary with patient age (Table 7-8)[445]; any process that disrupts the normal architecture of the prostate allows diffusion of prostate-specific antigen into the stroma, where it gains access to the blood through the microvasculature. Elevated serum prostate-specific antigen levels are seen with prostatitis, hyperplasia, and transiently following biopsy, but the most important elevations are seen with prostatic adenocarcinoma. Although adenocarcinoma produces less prostate-specific antigen *per cell* than benign epithelium, the greater number of malignant cells and the associated stromal disruption accounts for the elevated serum prostate-specific antigen levels.[236,237] The clinical utility of prostate-specific antigen is generally recognized.[446-448]

The major form of measurable prostate-specific antigen in the serum is a complex between the prostate-specific antigen molecule and alpha 1-antichymotrypsin; there is a higher proportion of complex prostate-specific antigen in the serum of patients with adenocarcinoma than in other patients, and this serum fractionation may be diagnostically useful.[449] New assays for prostate-specific antigen allow detection of blood concentrations as low as 0.1 ng/mL.[450]

Immunohistochemical detection of prostate-specific antigen is useful for the pathologist in distinguishing high-grade prostatic adenocarcinoma from urothelial carcinoma, colonic carcinoma, granulomatous prostatitis, lymphoma, and other histologic mimics.[448,451-460] It also

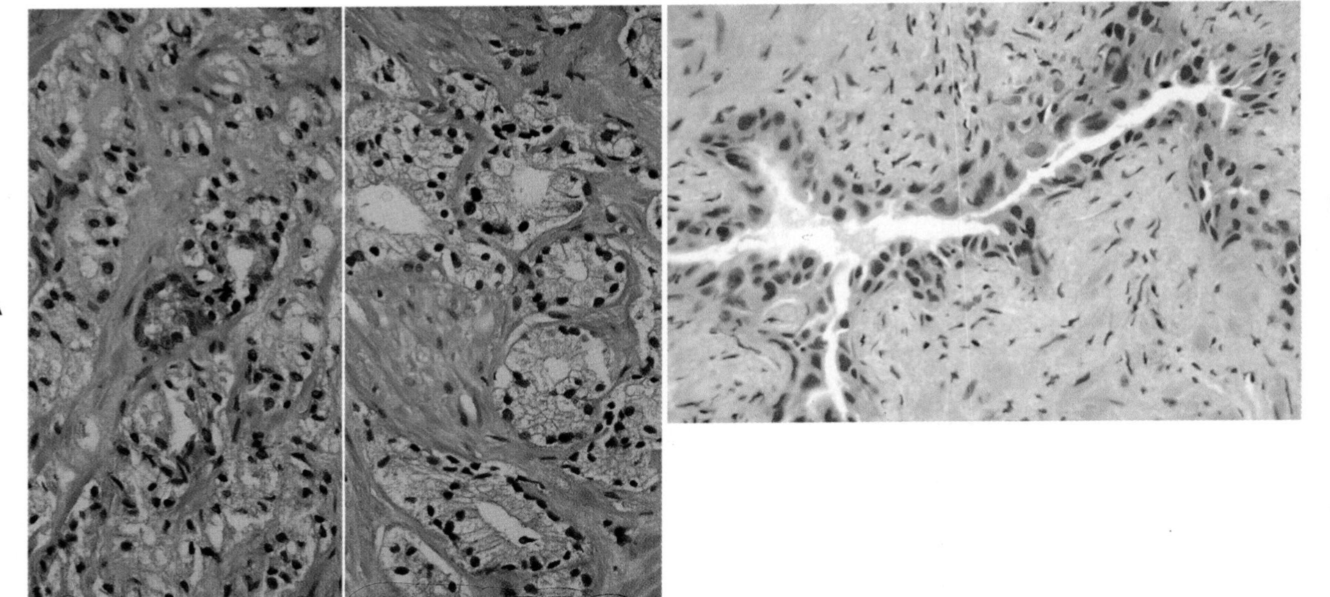

7-31. Changes following radiation therapy. **A**, Prostatic adenocarcinoma before (*left*) and 24 months after (*right*) external beam radiation therapy. In this case recurrence is histologically similar to the initial cancer. Compare with **B**, showing acinar atrophy, severe cytologic atypia, and stromal fibrosis without evidence of residual cancer.

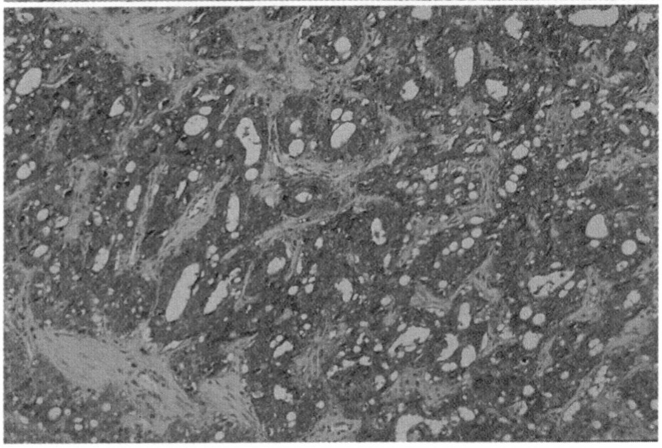

7-32. Prostate-specific antigen immunoreactivity. Prostate-specific antigen expression in the cytoplasm of poorly differentiated prostatic adenocarcinoma (**A**), metastic prostatic adenocarcinoma in cervical lymph nodes (**B**), and Skene's gland adenocarcinoma of the female urethra (**C**.)

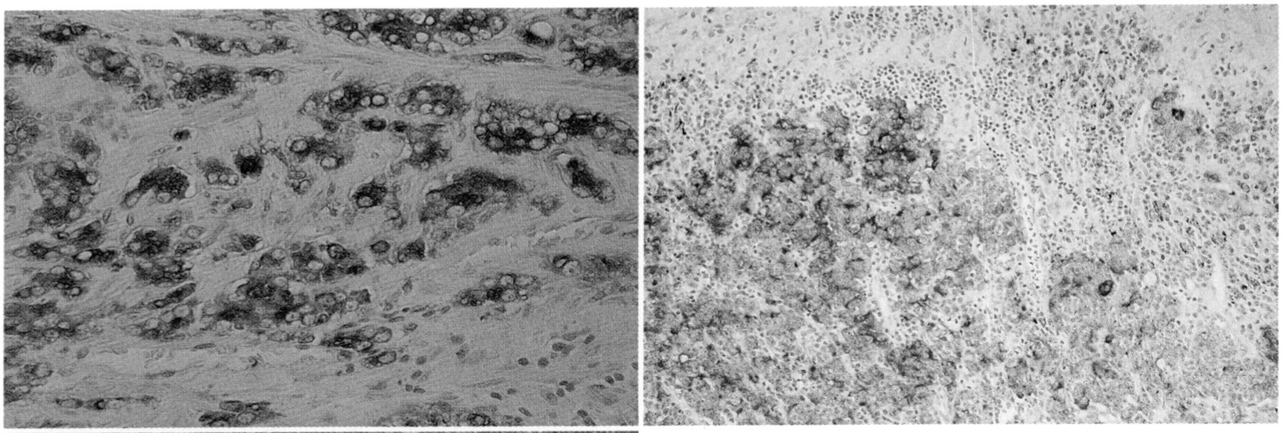

TABLE 7-8.
AGE-SPECIFIC REFERENCE RANGE FOR SERUM PROSTATE-SPECIFIC ANTIGEN (PSA)

Age (year)	PSA Range (ng/mL)	Age (year)	PSA Range (ng/mL)*
40	2.0	60	3.8
41	2.1	61	4.0
42	2.2	62	4.1
43	2.3	63	4.2
44	2.3	64	4.4
45	2.4	65	4.5
46	2.5	66	4.6
47	2.6	67	4.7
48	2.6	68	4.9
49	2.7	69	5.1
50	2.8	70	3.3
51	2.9	71	3.4
52	3.0	72	3.6
53	3.1	73	3.8
54	3.2	74	6.0
55	3.3	75	6.2
56	3.4	76	6.4
57	3.5	77	6.6
58	3.6	78	6.8
59	3.7	79	7.0

*From 0.0 to the specified value

From Oesterling JE, Jacobsen SJ, Chute CG et al: Serum prostate-specific antigen in a community-based population of healthy men: establishment of age-specific reference ranges, JAMA 270:860-866, 1993; with permission.

allows identification of the site of origin in metastatic adenocarcinoma (Fig. 7-32). Prostate-specific antigen expression is generally greater in low-grade tumors than in high-grade tumors, but there is significant heterogeneity from cell to cell. The box on this page lists extraprostatic tissues and tumors that have been reported to show prostate-specific antigen immunoreactivity.[458, 461-467]

Prostate-specific antigen can be detected in frozen sections, paraffin-embedded sections, cell smears, and cytologic preparations of normal and neoplastic prostatic epithelium. Microwave antigen retrieval is usually not necessary, even in tissues that have been immersed in formalin for years. Sinha et al[460] found that formalin fixation was optimal for localization of prostate-specific antigen, and variations in staining intensity were not due to fixation and embedding effects. Immunoreactivity is preserved in decalcified specimens.

Prostate-specific antigen in carcinoma. The intensity of prostate-specific antigen immunoreactivity often varies from field to field within a tumor, and the correlation of staining intensity with tumor differentiation is inconsistent. Up to 1.6% of poorly differentiated adenocarcinomas will be negative for both prostate-specific antigen and prostatic acid phosphatase.[457,468,469]

IMMUNOREACTIVITY OF PROSTATE-SPECIFIC ANTIGEN (PSA) IN EXTRAPROSTATIC TISSUES AND TUMORS

- Extraprostatic tissues
  - Urethra, periurethral glands (male and female)
  - Bladder, cystitis cystica and glandularis
  - Urachal remnants
  - Neutrophils
  - Anus, anal glands (male only)
- Extraprostatic tumors
  - Mature teratoma
  - Urethra, periurethral gland adenocarcinoma (female)
  - Bladder, villous adenoma and adenocarcinoma
  - Penis, extramammary Paget's disease
  - Salivary gland, pleomorphic adenoma (male only)
  - Salivary gland, carcinoma (male only)

Caveat: In many of these tissues and tumors, staining may be patchy, weak, or equivocal. Many of these reports have not been confirmed or validated. Also, contemporary antibodies to PSA may have different specificity and sensitivity than those used in some of these studies.

Neuroendocrine cells coexpress prostate-specific antigen[332,381,387] and androgen receptors,[346,387] suggesting a common cell of origin for epithelial cells and neuroendocrine cells in the prostate. High-grade neuroendocrine carcinoma (small cell carcinoma) of the prostate usually does not express prostate-specific antigen or prostatic acid phosphatase.[381,387]

Prostate-specific antigen in prostatic intraepithelial neoplasia. Prostatic intraepithelial neoplasia has little or no influence on serum prostate-specific antigen level.[76] Some studies have found a positive correlation of prostate-specific antigen and prostatic intraepithelial neoplasia, but this is probably the result of the confounding influence of associated adenocarcinoma.[75] There is decreased expression of prostate-specific antigen in prostatic intraepithelial neoplasia when compared with normal epithelium and adenocarcinoma.[13] Because prostatic intraepithelial neoplasia occurs in preexisting ducts and acini, secretory products such as prostate-specific antigen would be expected to empty into the lumen rather than the stroma and blood vessels, so a strong correlation of serum prostate-specific antigen and prostatic intraepithelial neoplasia would be surprising.

Prostate-specific antigen in adenocarcinoma after treatment. Prostate-specific antigen expression is usually retained after androgen deprivation therapy and radiation therapy.[198,470] Immunohistochemical studies for prostate-specific antigen, prostatic acid phosphatase, and basal cell–specific keratin 34ß-E12 are of value in separating treated adenocarcinoma and some of its mimics: Prostate-specific antigen and prostatic acid phosphatase are retained in tumor cells and keratin 34ß-E12 remains negative, indicating an absent basal cell layer.[198]

Prostate-specific antigen expression: primary versus metastases. The histologic appearance of metastatic prostatic adenocarcinoma does not always mirror the primary tumor. Metastases are frequently composed of only one of the patterns seen in the primary tumor and are usually moderately or poorly differentiated.[195,196] In 1993 Bovenberg et al[471] evaluated the immunoreactivity of three monoclonal antibodies against different epitopes of prostate-specific antigen in metastatic prostatic adenocarcinoma and found that the expression of prostate-specific antigen was similar but not identical to the primary tumor. Fidler[472] suggested that prostatic adenocarcinoma, like other heterogeneous tumors, is composed of populations of cells with differing immunologic properties and metastatic potential. These findings show that when adenocarcinoma metastasizes, it often retains expression of prostate-specific antigen antigenicity. The cascade theory of metastases predicts that generalized metastases do not usually occur directly from the primary tumor but from prior metastases, allowing for additional heterogeneity. The conservation of prostate-specific antigen expression in metastases has important implications for the use of radiopharmaceuticals for in vivo imaging and therapy of adenocarcinoma utilizing prostate-specific antigen.

Prostatic acid phosphatase. Prostatic acid phosphatase as a serum marker was useful for identifying the presence and extent of prostatic adenocarcinoma prior to widespread use of prostate-specific antigen, but has fallen into disfavor in recent years because of inherent problems in accuracy of measurement, including the requirement for special handling due to enzyme instability, diurnal fluctuation, variation resulting from prostatic digital examination and biopsy, and cross-reactivity with nonprostatic serum acid phosphatases produced by liver, bone, kidney, and blood cells. At present serum prostatic acid phosphatase has little or no clinical utility, but this marker is valuable for immunohistochemical staining when used in combination with stains for prostate-specific antigen.[473] Hammond et al[474] found that the intensity of prostatic acid phosphatase immunoreactivity correlated with patient survival, probably due to greater androgen responsiveness in the immunoreactive group. A list of extraprostatic tissues and tumors that may display prostatic acid phosphatase immunoreactivity is shown in the box above.[345,456,458,463,475-488]

Androgen receptors. Androgen receptors are present within androgen-responsive and androgen-unresponsive cells in prostatic adenocarcinoma (Fig. 7-32*D*). These receptors are widely distributed in the nuclei of the basal cell layer of the normal prostate and in hyperplasia[489] and can be identified in localized and metastatic prostatic carcinoma.[490] The percentage of adenocarcinoma cells with androgen receptors is not predictive of time to progression after androgen deprivation therapy[491]; however, greater heterogeneity of androgen receptor immunoreactivity is seen in adenocarcinomas that responded poorly to therapy.[490] Androgen receptor expression in small cell carcinoma appears to be predictive of a poorer outcome (see the section on neuroendocrine carcinoma in this chapter).[387]

IMMUNOREACTIVITY OF PROSTATIC ACID PHOSPHATASE (PAP) IN EXTRAPROSTATIC TISSUES AND TUMORS

- Extraprostatic cells and tissues
  - Urethra, periurethral glands (male and female)
  - Bladder, cystitis cystica and glandularis
  - Pancreas, islet cells
  - Kidney, renal tubules
  - Neutrophils
  - Colon, neuroendocrine cells
  - Anus, anal glands (male only)
  - Stomach, parietal cells
  - Liver, hepatocytes
  - Breast, ductal epithelial cells
- Extraprostatic tumors
  - Bladder, adenocarcinoma
  - Anus, cloacogenic carcinoma
  - Rectum, carcinoid
  - Other gastrointestinal carcinoids
  - Pancreas, islet cell tumor
  - Mature teratoma
  - Breasts, ductal epithelial cells
  - Salivary gland, pleomorphic adenoma (male only)
  - Salivary gland, carcinoma (male only)

Caveat: In many of these tissues and tumors, staining may be patchy, weak, or equivocal. Many of these reports have not been confirmed or validated. Also, contemporary antibodies to PAP may have different specificity and sensitivity than those used in some of these studies.

Neuroendocrine cells. Neuroendocrine cells may be present in large numbers in adenocarcinoma (see the section on adenocarcinoma with neuroendocrine cells in this chapter). The claim that this indicates a poor prognosis, perhaps due to insensitivity to hormonal growth regulation,[343] has been refuted.[42,332,333,344] The progressive loss of markers of neuroendocrine differentiation with increasing grades of prostatic intraepithelial neoplasia and adenocarcinoma indicates that there is progressive impairment of cell differentiation and regulatory control with advancing stages of prostatic carcinogenesis.[42] Early reports indicated that neuroendocrine differentiation was present in only a minority of cases of adenocarcinoma, but recent studies identified at least focal staining in most if not all cases, with variable results due to use of different fixatives, variable number of sections stained, and smaller number of antibodies employed.[339] Further studies are needed to evaluate the function and prognostic utility of neuroendocrine cells in the normal and neoplastic prostate. At present there is no practical value for determining neuroendocrine immunoreactivity in prostatic adenocarcinoma.

Peptide growth factors. Peptide growth factors appear to control development of normal and neoplastic prostatic epithelium by acting as paracrine mediators of epithelial-stromal interaction and growth.[492-498] The epidermal growth factor family of peptides includes epidermal growth factor, transforming growth factor alpha, and other factors that act through the same transmembrane glycoprotein receptor and a tyrosine kinase. Prostatic adenocarcinoma cells favor synthesis of transforming growth factor alpha, and this stimulates epithelial and fibroblastic proliferation. The transforming growth factor beta family of peptides, including transforming growth factor beta1 and transforming growth factor beta2, appear to be regulators of cell differentiation and proliferation.[493,496-498] Expression of the transforming growth factor beta receptor appears to be under negative androgenic regulation, suggesting that transforming growth factor beta plays a role in cell death following androgen deprivation. The transforming growth factor beta binding protein is produced in benign and hyperplastic tissue but not in malignant tissue.[498] Growth factors in prostatic adenocarcinoma have recently been reviewed.[492]

Other prostatic biomarkers. There are many other investigational tumor markers in prostatic adenocarcinoma.[499,500] Prostate-associated glycoprotein complex, a sialic acid–based group of glycoproteins identified by monoclonal antibody TURP-27, appears to be a differentiation antigen, expressed in only 10% of normal prostatic epithelial cells but in up to 100% of nodular hyperplasia and malignant cells, including metastastic adenocarcinoma.[499] Prostate mucin antigen, a high molecular weight non–sialic acid glycoprotein identified by monoclonal antibody PD41, is expressed only in prostatic intraepithelial neoplasia and prostatic adenocarcinoma cells but not in benign or hyperplastic epithelial cells; maximal expression is seen in poorly differentiated adenocarcinoma and metastases.[499] The antigen recognized by monoclonal antibody 7E11-C5 is a mixture of glycoproteins expressed on normal and neoplastic prostatic tissues, with greatest intensity in carcinoma and metastases. This antigen is not affected by androgen deprivation therapy; currently, clinical trials are evaluating the utility of this marker for radioimmunodetection and radioimmunotherapy of prostatic adenocarcinoma.[499] Other markers are described in recent reviews.[500]

DNA ploidy analysis. DNA content analysis of prostatic adenocarcinoma by flow cytometry,[501-506] static image analysis,[507] and fluorescence in situ hybridization[508] may provide independent prognostic information that supplements histopathologic examination (Fig. 7-33). Patients with diploid tumors have a more favorable outcome than those with aneuploid tumors; for example, among patients with lymph node metastases treated with radical prostatectomy and androgen deprivation therapy, those with diploid tumors may survive 20 years or more, whereas those with aneuploid tumors die within 5 years.[501] However, the ploidy pattern of prostatic adenocarcinoma is often heterogeneous, creating potential problems with sampling error. An international DNA Cytometry Consensus Conference reviewed the literature and concluded that the clinical significance was uncertain of DNA ploidy analysis and did not warrant routine clinical use.[505]

The minimum amount of needle core tissue necessary to yield satisfactory results with flow cytometry is a 0.2 cm length of malignant acini, which corresponds to approximately 2,500 to 5,000 nuclei.[506] Fluorescence in situ hybridization requires even less tissue but is labor intensive and expensive.[508] Concordance of static image analysis on needle biopsy and flow cytometry from radical prostatectomy specimens was 82%.[507]

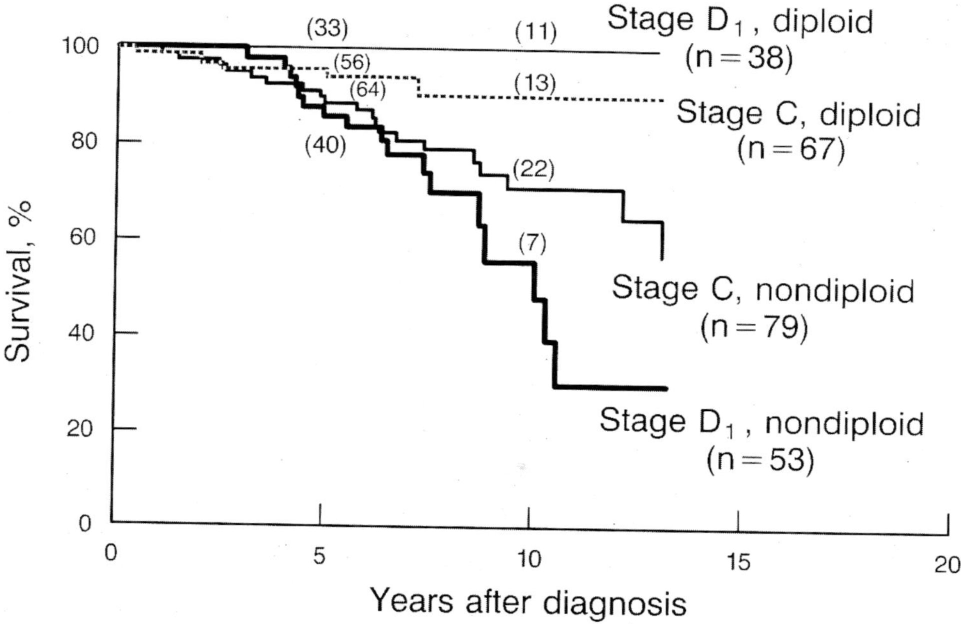

7-33. Postoperative probability of survival of pathologic stage T3 (C) and N+(D1) prostatic carcinoma according to DNA ploidy pattern. *(From Nativ O, Winkler HZ, Raz Y et al: Stage C prostatic adenocarcinoma. Flow cytometric nuclear DNA ploidy analysis, Mayo Clin Proc 64:911-919, 1989; with permission.)*

Cytogenetics and allelic loss. Allelic loss is a common finding in prostatic adenocarcinoma, present in more than 50% of cases on chromosomes 8p, 10q, and 16q.[509-513] One or more tumor suppressor genes appear to be present on 8p, which may be involved in carcinogenesis (Fig. 7-34).[510,511] Allelic loss appears to be more common in high-grade tumors.[510] Fluorescence in situ hybridization studies with centromere-specific probes for chromosomes 7, 8, 11, and 12 reveal that gains of chromosomes 7 and 8 are consistent numerical alterations and may be markers of tumor aggressiveness and prognosis.[508]

Inactivation of p53, a tumor suppressor gene on chromosome 17p, is present in up to 25% of advanced prostatic adenocarcinomas but is rare in early adenocarcinomas, suggesting that it may play a role in late progression.[514-517] Another tumor suppressor gene, DCC, shows allelic deletion and loss of expression in 45% of cases, indicating that it is a frequent feature of prostatic adenocarcinoma.[518] Loss of expression of the retinoblastoma gene on chromosome 13q is seen in a minority of prostatic adenocarcinomas, usually in advanced stages.[519]

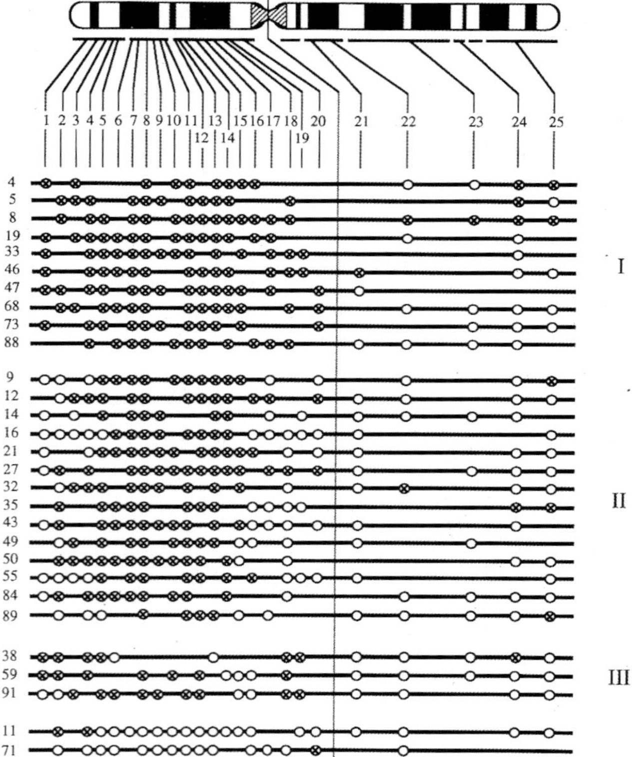

7-34. Map of allelic imbalances at 25 microsatellite repeat loci. Numbered loci (*top*) are illustrated at their approximate position on chromosome 8 (*left to right*, 8p to 8q). Twenty-nine prostate cancers (cases numbered at left) with any loss of microsatellite repeat alleles are diagrammed in four groups based on the pattern of loss; 34 others had no loss. Empty circle indicates allele retained; X within circle indicates allele lost. *(From MacGrogan D, Levy A, Bostwick D et al: Loss of chromosome arm 8p loci in prostate cancer: mapping by quantitative allelic balance, Genes Chromosom Cancer 10:151-159, 1994; with permission.)*

Activated oncogenes such as *ras* appear to be infrequent in early prostatic adenocarcinomas.[520]

c-erbB-2 (HER2-neu) and c-erbB-3. The role of the c-erbB-2 and c-erbB-3 oncogenes in prostatic growth and differentiation is uncertain. Transfection of the rat HER2-neu–activated gene into the rat ventral prostatic epithelial cells line NbE-1.4 resulted in acquisition of a tumorigenic phenotype,[521] indicating that this oncogene is involved in tumor growth. The expression of c-erbB-2 is upregulated by androgens in vitro and in vivo, paralleling expression of prostate-specific antigen.[522]

The expression of c-erbB-2 may be a potentially useful prognostic factor in the clinical management of prostatic adenocarcinoma.[517,523-531] However, the predictive value of this and other molecular markers in management of prostatic adenocarcinoma has not been validated, and results with c-erbB-2 have been contradictory. Overexpression of c-erbB-2 was found to be an independent predictive marker of poor prognosis in two recent studies,[529,530] but not in other reports.[517,523,528,531] Veltri et al[530] undertook a large multivariate analysis, and found that c-erbB-2 expression provided significant predictive information for adenocarcinoma recurrence and progression. Ross et al[531] described a positive correlation of c-erbB-2 expression with grade, aneuploid DNA content, and metastases in a series of 100 cases of prostatic adenocarcinoma, but found that it offered no independent value. Other reports have not identified a correlation of c-erbB-2 with prostatic tumor grade,[517,523,528] stage,[517,528] progression,[528] or p53 expression.[517] Studies of c-erbB-2 oncoprotein expression have found inconsistent patterns of immunoreactivity, probably resulting from differences in tissue preparation and fixation, immunohistochemical techniques, antibody specificity, and interpretation of results[525-527]; these results demonstrate the pitfall of interpreting negative immunohistochemical results without independent confirmation from other tests.[527,532]

The expression of c-erbB-2 and c-erbB-3 in high-grade prostatic intraepithelial neoplasia is intermediate between that in normal prostatic epithelium and prostatic adenocarcinoma.[533] Also, a recent consensus conference concluded that c-erbB-2 expression was one of seven promising surrogate endpoint biomarkers for screening candidate chemopreventive compounds for prostatic adenocarcinoma in short-term phase II clinical trials.[77]

Other prognostic factors in prostatic adenocarcinoma

Numerous pathologic, biochemical, and genetic markers have been described in prostatic adenocarcinoma but comparative analysis of most of these factors has not been performed. It is possible that a combination of factors would be useful as an adjunct to current staging or as a surrogate endpoint biomarker in clinical trials.

Zonal origin of adenocarcinoma. The site of origin appears to be a significant prognostic factor.[2,97,98,233,242-244] Adenocarcinoma arising in the transition zone of the prostate appears to be less aggressive than typical acinar adenocarcinoma arising in the peripheral zone (Table 7-9). The majority of transition zone adenocarcinomas arise adjacent to nodules of hyperplasia, with one-third actually originating within nodules. These adenocarcinomas are better differentiated than those in the peripheral zone, accounting for the majority of Gleason primary grade 1 and 2 tumors (Fig. 7-35). The volume of these low-grade tumors tends to be smaller than those arising in the peripheral zone, although frequent exceptions are seen. The confinement of transition zone adenocarcinomas to their anatomic site of origin may account in part for the favorable prognosis of clinical stage T1 (A) tumors. The transition zone boundary may act as a relative barrier to tumor extension, as malignant acini appear to frequently fan out along this boundary before invasion into the peripheral and central zones.

Volume of adenocarcinoma in needle biopsy. The ability of needle biopsy to predict volume of tumor in the prostate is uncertain. Some investigators have found a strong correlation between tumor burden in sextant core biopsies and lymph node metastases.[92-94] Hammerer et al[93] found lymph node metastases in 52 of 57 patients (91% specificity) and 10 of 14 patients (71% sensitivity) when adenocarcinoma replaced two core biopsies and 80% of a third from the sextant sample. They noted that the addition of grade to tumor volume improved the sensitivity and specificity. Stamey et al[94] developed algorithms to increase accuracy of preoperative volume estimates by combining serum prostate-specific antigen level with ultrasonographic assessment of prostatic volume as measured by 2-mm axial step sections, biopsy Gleason grade, and amount of adenocarcinoma in sextant biopsies; they found an excellent correlation (r = 0.76) for organ-confined adenocarcinoma and noted that digital rectal examination added no additional information to the multiple regression analysis.[92] Conversely, a retrospective study of 162 patients with prostatic adenocarcinoma treated at the Mayo Clinic compared the tumor burden on needle biopsy with that of matched, step-sectioned, whole-mount radical prostatectomies. Linear regression analysis revealed a weak correlation of the amount of tumor in the needle biopsy and radical prostatectomy specimens (r = 0.39).[534] Low tumor burden on needle biopsy did not appear predictive of low-volume prostatic adenocarcinoma, whether measured as percentage of biopsy cores involved, percentage of adenocarcinoma area in biopsy cores, millimeters of adenocarcinoma in the entire biopsy, or millimeters of adenocarcinoma per core. Patients with less than 30% of cores involved had a mean volume of 6.06 cm^3 (range,

TABLE 7-9.
COMPARISON OF TRANSITION ZONE AND PERIPHERAL ZONE CARCINOMA*

	Transition Zone Cancer	Peripheral Zone Cancer
Incidence		
Stage T1a	75%	—
Stage T1b	79%	—
All Stage T1	78%	—
All Stages	24%	70%
Origin		
In or near BPH	Yes	No
Near apex	Yes	Yes
Detection rate by TURP	78%	—
Pathologic features		
Tumor volume	Usually small	Small to large
Tumor pattern	Alveolar-medullary	Tubular-scirrhous
Tumor grade (Gleason)	Usually 1 or 2	Usually 2, 3, or 4
Clear cell pattern	Most cases	Rare
Stromal fibrosis	Uncommon	Common
Associated putative premalignant changes	AAH or PIN	PIN
Aneuploidy	6%	31%
Clinical behavior		
Extracapsular extension	11%	44%
Site of extracapsular extension	Anterolateral and apical	Lateral
Average tumor size with extracapsular extension	4.98 cc	3.86 cc
Risk of seminal vesicle invasion	0%	19%
Risk of lymph node metastases	Low	High

BPH: benign prostatic hyperplasia; TURP: transurethral resection of the prostate; AAH: atypical adenomatous hyperplasia; PIN: prostatic intraepithelial neoplasia.

*Central zone cancers (5% to 10% of total) were excluded.

From Bostwick DG, Cooner WH, Denis L et al: The association of benign prostatic hyperplasia and cancer of the prostate, Cancer 70:291-301, 1992; with permission.

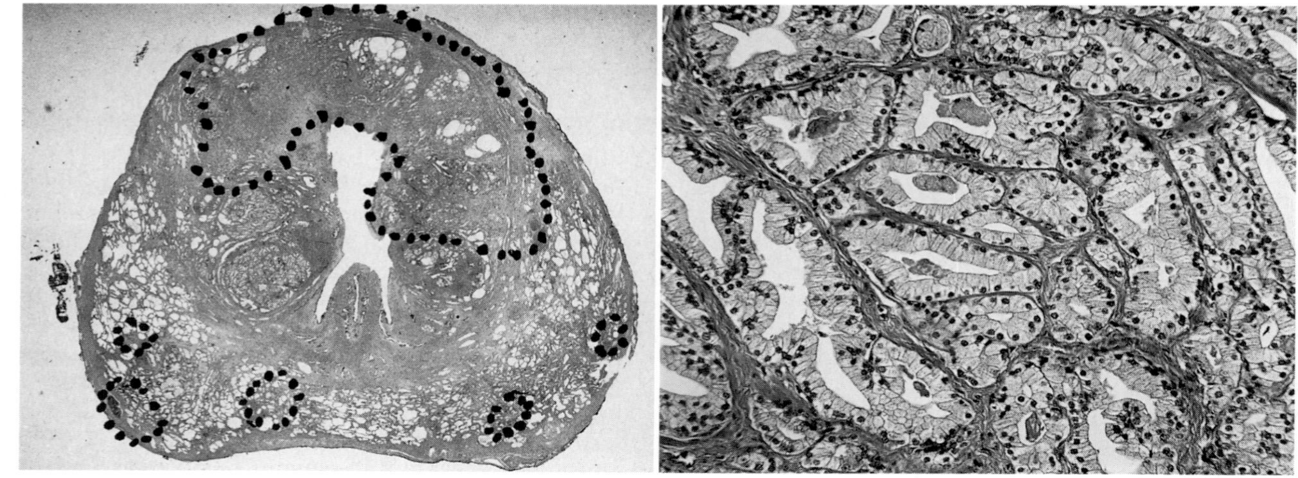

7-35. Transition zone cancer. **A**, Whole mount section, showing large transition zone cancer (*top*) and smaller foci in the peripheral zone (*bottom*). **B**, Tumor is well differentiated, with clear cytoplasm and uniform nuclei.

0.19–16.8 cm^3), indicating that the amount of tumor on transrectal needle biopsy was not a good predictor of tumor volume and should not influence therapeutic decisions. This study was limited by the variability in needle biopsy sampling, with the number of cores ranging from 4–10 (mean, 5.7 cores).[534] The combined results from these studies indicate that biopsy extent of tumor provides some predictive value for extent in radical prostatectomy specimens and should be reported. Cupp et al[534] provides an estimate of the percentage of the biopsy specimen involved with cancer based on the results of a comparative study with millimeters per core and number of cores involved.

Tumor volume. Tumor volume has been proposed as an adjunct to digital rectal examination–based staging of prostatic adenocarcinoma because of its powerful prognostic ability[14,174,535,536]; this approach may be feasible with improvements in imaging techniques such as transrectal ultrasonography. A tumor volume-based prognostic index has been proposed as an adjunct for staging based on the evidence linking adenocarcinoma volume with patterns of progression (capsular perforation, seminal vesicle invasion, and lymph node metastases).[14,536] For organ-confined tumors, three main categories were recognized: V1: cancer less than 1 cm^3; V2a: cancer 1–5 cm^3; and V2b: tumor more than 5 cm^3. The goal of the prognostic index was to achieve greater precision in predicting outcome for individual patients. The index was considered preliminary, pending standardization of methods of volume quantitation and definitions of capsular invasion and perforation, as well as field testing with both pathologic specimens and imaging techniques. As such, it represents a proposed "telescopic ramification" of the 1992 revision of the TNM staging (see TNM Staging System in this chapter).[104,537]

Several studies have found a positive correlation between serum prostate-specific antigen level and tumor volume (Fig. 7-36).[162,236,237,538] However, the additive and confounding effect of nodular hyperplasia limits the usefulness of prostate-specific antigen in estimating preoperative tumor size and extent.[237] As adenocarcinoma enlarges, it usually becomes less differentiated and loses some of its capacity for prostate-specific antigen production. Partin and associates[237] showed that prostate-specific antigen levels increased with increasing Gleason grade, but when tumor volume was held constant prostate-specific antigen levels actually decreased (prostate-specific antigen levels declined as Gleason grade increased). This finding was probably due to less production of prostate-specific antigen *per cell* in more poorly differentiated tumors. In a series of 311 radical prostatectomy specimens, Blackwell et al[236] observed a positive and significant correlation of cancer volume and serum prostate-specific antigen level (R= 0.58, linear regression), similar to the findings of Stamey and colleagues.[538] There is no accepted standard for reporting tumor volume in prostatectomy specimens; the easiest and most practical approach is an estimate of the percentage of cancer in the entire specimen.

Multiple prognostic index. A prognostic index that combines multiple variables would probably be more precise in predicting outcome for individual patients than current clinical staging, which relies on only a few variables and is being investigated by the American Joint Committee on Cancer.[539] A multiple prognostic index for prostatic adenocarcinoma would probably include such variables as clinical stage, ultrasonographic findings, tumor volume, serum prostate-specific antigen level, Gleason grade, percentage of Gleason grades 4 and 5, tumor origin, and DNA content.[104,162,540]

Spread of prostatic adenocarcinoma

Staging. Current clinical and pathologic staging of early prostatic adenocarcinoma separates patients into two groups: those with palpable tumors and those with nonpalpable tumors.[104,537] This reliance on palpability of the tumor as determined by digital rectal examination is unique among organ staging systems and is hampered by

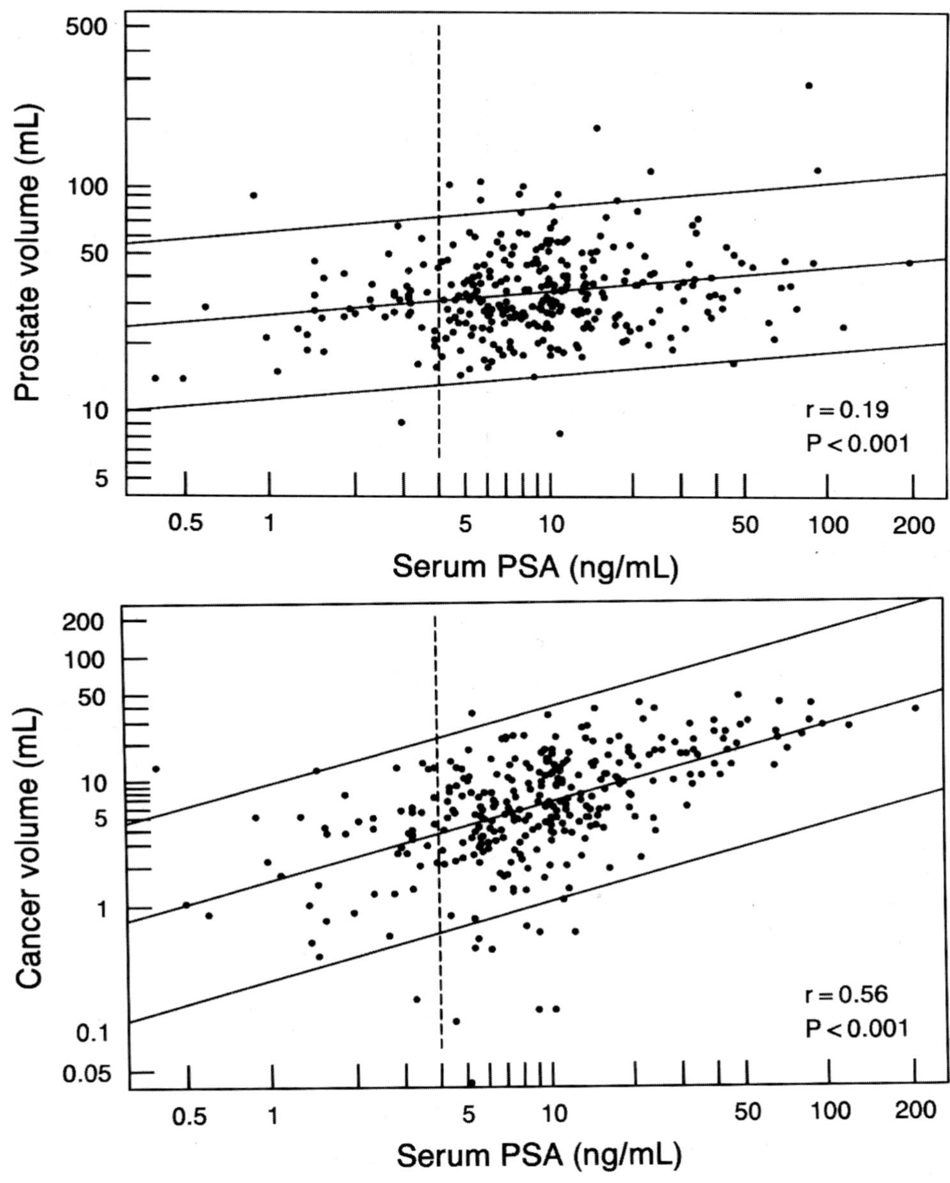

7-36. Preoperative serum prostate-specific antigen and its relationship with prostate volume (**A**) and cancer volume (**B**) in 311 patients treated with radical prostatectomy. Parallel lines indicate 95% confidence intervals for prediction according to preoperative serum prostate-specific antigen level. Vertical line indicates upper limit of normal serum prostate-specific antigen value. *(From Blackwell KL, Bostwick DG, Zincke H et al: Combining prostate specific antigen with cancer and gland volume to predict more reliably pathologic stage: the influence of prostate specific antigen cancer density, J Urol 151:1565-1570, 1994; with permission.)*

the low sensitivity, low specificity, and low positive predictive value of digital rectal examination.[541] Recent refinements in staging have led to the introduction of a new stage of nonpalpable adenocarcinoma detected by elevated serum prostate-specific antigen level, referred to as stage T1c or B0; however, this new stage was introduced without supportive clinical evidence and recent studies show that it does not identify a distinct group of patients.[542-545] The question remains whether those patients who will benefit from early detection and intervention can be separated from those who will not.

The 1992 revision of the TNM system is now considered the international standard for prostatic adenocarcinoma staging.[104,537] It is possible that future staging of early prostatic adenocarcinoma will rely on objective measures such as image-based determination of tumor volume rather than on palpability by digital rectal examination or number of involved chips in a transurethral resection specimen. Preoperative assessment of volume may also alert the urologist to an increased probability of positive surgical margins. Improvements in staging will allow more precise stratification of patients into

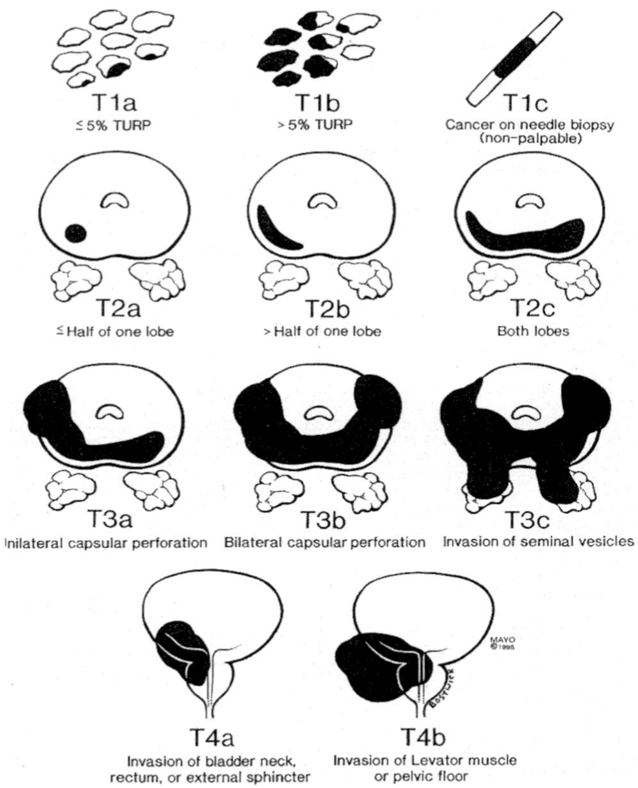

7-37. Prostate cancer staging using the TNM system, 1992 revision, for the T (tumor) category. Black indicates extent of cancer.

prognostically distinct groups. However, at present there is no reliable system to predict tumor volume preoperatively or extent of the tumor. Further efforts directed toward standardization of staging, including guidelines for pathologic evaluation of specimens, will allow comparison of results from different centers (Fig. 7-37).[103]

Current staging systems. The two principal clinical staging systems currently in widespread use are the TNM system and American system (modified Whitmore-Jewett)[104,537]; they are presented in Table 7-10. Although these two systems are similar, the TNM system contains a greater number of subdivisions for most stages. Also, the TNM system includes stage groupings that consist of combined clinical stage and tumor grade.

The TNM staging system. The TNM classification for prostatic adenocarcinoma was first published by the American Joint Committee on Cancer and the Union Internationale Contre le Cancer in 1978, but their definitions at that time contained significant differences.[537] By 1987 these differences were resolved, but the resulting classification was criticized by the European Organization for Research on Treatment of Cancer Genitourinary Group and others, particularly for the T (primary tumor) category and the proposed stage groupings. A consensus conference was held to resolve discrepancies and included representatives from the American Joint Committee on Cancer, Union Internationale Contre le Cancer, European Organization for Research on Treatment of Cancer Genitourinary Group, and the American Urological Association. From this meeting a revised and uniform TNM classification was published in 1992, which is now considered the international standard for prostatic adenocarcinoma staging.[537]

The 1992 revision of the TNM system included four significant changes from the 1987 version.[537] First, a new category (T1c) was introduced to recognize nonpalpable nonvisible adenocarcinomas identified by random biopsy following detection of elevated serum prostate-specific antigen level (see discussion later in this chapter). Second, palpable adenocarcinomas confined to the prostate (T2) were subdivided into three groups rather than two based on relative involvement of the prostate (involvement of half a lobe or less, more than half a lobe but not both lobes, and both lobes) instead of absolute tumor size by digital rectal examination. Third, adenocarcinomas with local extraprostatic extension (T3) were subdivided into three groups rather than two based on laterality and seminal vesicle invasion (unilateral, bilateral, and seminal vesicle invasion). Finally, the concept of *telescopic ramification* was introduced to allow for additional prognostic factors without altering existing categories.

American (modified Whitmore-Jewett) staging system. The American staging system, introduced by Whitmore in 1956, consists of letters A through D, which denote stages. It was modified by Jewett to allow the substaging of stage B; he and others noted that patients with a palpably discrete nodule (B1 nodule; "Jewett nodule") had increased cancer-free survival. Recently, the American system was modified to accommodate prostate-specific antigen–detected adenocarcinomas (stage B0).[537] The current stage divisions are similar to the TNM system (Table 7-10) but do not include tumor grade except in the separation of stages A1 and A2 (see discussion later in this chapter).

Limitations of current staging systems. Current staging systems are limited by a number of factors, including: clinical understaging with transurethral resection, clinical understaging with digital rectal examination, limited ability of imaging studies to evaluate the presence and extent of prostatic adenocarcinoma, heterogeneity of stage T1c (B0) adenocarcinomas, variability in pathologic staging of stage T1 (A) adenocarcinomas, and variability in examination of radical prostatectomy specimens.

Clinical understaging of transition zone adenocarcinomas with transurethral resection. Clinical understaging with transurethral resection of the prostate is a recognized problem in early prostatic adenocarcinoma. The sensitivity of transurethral resection in detecting stage T1 (A) carcinoma is only 28%, and up to 60% of patients with stage T1a (A1) tumors who undergo repeat transurethral resection have residual adenocarcinoma, with 26% of these being upstaged.[176,242,546-548] Parfitt and colleagues[549] identified residual carcinoma in 12 of 31 partially sampled prostates (40%) removed for stage T1a (A1) adenocarcinoma. Similarily, Epstein and coworkers[550] identified residual adenocarcinoma in 37 of 40 thoroughly sampled prostates (92%), noting that the location of residual adenocarcinoma at the apex and periphery made it inaccessible to transurethral resection. They also noted that the presence and amount of residual tumor could not be predicted from the transurethral resection specimen. Christenson and associates[551] found

TABLE 7-10.
STAGING OF PROSTATIC ADENOCARCINOMA

	American	TNM*†
Nonpalpable cancer		
≤ 5% of TURP tissue‡	A1	T1a
> 5% of TURP tissue‡	A2	T1b
Cancer detected by biopsy (e.g., elevated prostate-specific antigen)	B0	T1c
Palpable or visible cancer clinically confined within the capsule		
≤ Half of one lobe	B1	T2a
> Half of one lobe, but not both lobes	B1	T2b
Both lobes	B2	T2c
Cancer with local extracapsular extension		
Unilateral	C1	T3a
Bilateral	C1	T3b
Seminal vesicle invasion	C2	T3c
Invasion of bladder neck, rectum, or external sphincter	C2	T4a
Invasion of levator muscle or pelvic wall	C2	T4b
Metastatic cancer		
Single regional lymph node, ≤ 2 cm in greatest dimension	D1	N1§
Single regional lymph node, 2-5 cm, or multiple regional lymph nodes, ≤ 5 cm	D1	N2
Single regional lymph node, > 5 cm	D1	N3
Distant metastasis	D2	M1
Nonregional lymph node(s)	D2	M1a
Bone(s)	D2	M1b
Other sites	D2	M1c

*N_O or N_XM_O for T1-T4

†STAGE GROUPINGS FOR TNM STAGING SYSTEMS (G = GRADE ON 1–4 SCALE)

Stage 0	T1a	N0	M0	G1
Stage I	T1a	N0	M0	G2,3,4
	T1b	N0	M0	Any G
	T1c	N0	M0	Any G
	T1	N0	M0	Any G
Stage II	T2	N0	M0	Any G
Stage III	T3	N0	M0	Any G
Stage IV	T4	N0	M0	Any G
	Any T	N1,2,3	M0	Any G
	Any T	Any N	M1	Any G

‡Different definitions exist for substaging A1 and A2 cancers.

§N_X: regional lymph nodes not assessable; M_X: distant metastasis not assessable

that 10 of 39 men (26%) with clinical stage T1b (A2) carcinoma had higher final pathologic stage (8 were stage T3 [C], 2 were stage T1-4N+ [D]), and all had residual adenocarcinoma. They found that final pathologic stage correlated with tumor volume and Gleason grade in both transurethral resection and radical prostatectomy specimens. Despite the limitations of examining transurethral resection specimens to stage some prostatic adenocarcinomas, this remains the standard of care.

Clinical understaging with digital rectal examination. Current staging of palpable organ-confined adenocarcinoma relies on digital rectal examination to separate unilateral from bilateral tumors or small from large tumors (less than half of one lobe, between one half and one lobe, and more than one lobe). However, there is a high level of inaccuracy and interobserver variability of digital rectal examination in determining tumor size and pathologic stage.[541] Prostatic adenocarcinoma staging is unique among organ staging systems by relying on the presence or absence of palpability and by substaging T2 (B) adenocarcinomas based upon the proportion of organ induration identified.

Bostwick[176] identified clinical understaging in 59% and clinical overstaging in 5% of cases in a series of 311 serially sectioned radical retropubic prostatectomies removed for clinically localized prostatic adenocarcinoma excluding stages T1a (A1), T1b (A2), and T1c (B0); note that there is no equivalent pathologic stage for clinical stage T1c (B0), so this group will always be restaged pathologically (see below). These results are similar to those reported by others who have also undertaken careful pathologic sectioning of prostatectomy specimens. This substantial error rate must be accounted for when evaluating recurrence and survival rates, especially when comparing studies of clinically staged patients followed with active surveillance (watchful waiting) and surgically (pathologically) staged patients. There was considerable overlap in the volume of adenocarcinoma in clinical stages T2a+b (B1) and T2c (B2), with tumors measuring up to 41 and 43 cm^3, respectively. These data indicate that digital rectal examination is inaccurate for preoperative assessment of tumor volume.

Limitations of imaging studies. Imaging studies to assess tumor volume and extent would be invaluable in clinical staging. However, the present level of accuracy attained by such methods limits the utility of these methods. The accuracy of correctly identifying extraprostatic extension is 63% with transrectal ultrasonography,[552] 71% with body coil magnetic resonance imaging,[552] and 83% with endorectal and surface coil magnetic resonance imaging.[553]

Pathology of prostate-specific antigen–detected adenocarcinomas (clinical stage T1c). Prior to widespread clinical use of prostate-specific antigen, most organ-confined adenocarcinomas were discovered by digital rectal examination (clinical stage T2 [B]) or at the time of transurethral resection (clinical stage T1 [A]). Routine use of serum prostate-specific antigen increases the detection rate of prostatic adenocarcinoma and discovers some adenocarcinomas that cannot be detected by digital rectal examination.[554-558] There was a seven-fold increase in prostate-specific antigen–detected adenocarcinomas at the Mayo Clinic in the 3-year period from 1988 to 1991 (14 versus 118 cases, respectively).[542] These adenocarcinomas were designated clinical stage T1c in the 1992 revision of the TNM classification and clinical stage B0 in the modified American classification.[542]

There is no pathologic stage equivalent for clinical stage T1c, and such tumors are invariably upstaged at surgery, usually to pathologic stage T2 (B) or T3 (C) (Table 7-11).[542] Oesterling et al[542] found that clinical stage T1c

TABLE 7-11.
PATHOLOGIC CHARACTERISTICS OF 416 CLINICAL STAGES T1c, T2a, AND T2b PROSTATE CANCERS

Parameter	Stage T1c	Stages T2a and T2b	P Value
Tumor volume (cc)*	6.4 (range: 0.03–56)	5.2 (range: 0.01–98)	0.03
Maximum diameter (cm)*	2.1 (range: 0.1–5.0)	2.0 (range: 0.3–6.8)	0.17
Focality			0.63
Unifocal	152 (73%)	162 (78%)	
Multifocal	56 (27%)	46 (22%)	
Gleason score			0.37
2–4	48 (23%)	42 (20%)	
5–6	124 (60%)	128 (62%)	
7–10	36 (17%)	38 (18%)	
DNA ploidy			0.61
Diploid	153 (74%)	153 (74%)	
Tetraploid	27 (13%)	30 (14%)	
Aneuploid	11 (5%)	9 (4%)	
Not interpretable	17 (8%)	16 (8%)	
Pathologic stage			0.86
Organ confined	110 (53%)	115 (55%)	
Capsular perforation	74 (35%)	75 (36%)	
Seminal vesicle invasion	18 (9%)	14 (7%)	
Pelvic lymph node involvement	6 (3%)	4 (2%)	
Surgical margins			0.05
Negative	138 (66%)	156 (75%)	
Microscopic involvement	66 (32%)	51 (24.5%)	
Macroscopic involvement	4 (2%)	1 (0.5%)	
Prostate gland size (cc)*	57 (range: 20–290)	47 (range: 20–110)	0.001
Predominant tumor location			0.44
Peripheral zone	179 (86%)	199 (96%)	
Transition and/or central zone	19 (9%)	6 (3%)	

* Mean value

From Oesterling JE, Suman VJ, Zincke H et al: PSA-detected (clinical stage T1c or B0) prostate cancer: pathologically significant tumors, Urol Clin N Am 20:687-693, 1993; with permission.

(B0) adenocarcinoma and clinical stage T2a+b (B1) adenocarcinoma had similar maximum tumor diameters, frequencies of multifocality, tumor grades, DNA content results, pathologic stages, and tumor locations; interestingly, they had different serum prostate-specific antigen values, tumor volumes, positive surgical margins, and prostate gland sizes, with the T1c (B0) tumors having higher values for each feature. These findings indicate that prostate-specific antigen detects adenocarcinoma, which is clinically important and potentially curable. Also, prostate-specific antigen–detected tumors that are visible on transrectal ultrasonography have pathologic features similar to those that are not visible.[545]

Further long-term follow-up of prostate-specific antigen–detected prostatic adenocarcinomas is necessary to establish the prognosis of these tumors and determine whether a separate staging category is warranted for them.

Pathologic staging of stage T1 (A) adenocarcinomas. Staging of adenocarcinoma in transurethral resection specimens is not standardized, and numerous methods have been developed to objectively measure tumor volume and define substages T1a (A1) and T1b (A2) (Table 7-12).[559] The pathologist's "eyeball" estimate of tumor volume correlated well with morphometrically determined measures, and the predictive ability was similar to that of other methods of tumor quantitation.[560-561] Also, percent tumor was slightly more predictive of tumor progression than absolute tumor volume for both stage T1 and stage T2 tumors.[551,562] Some methods employ additional factors such as tumor grade in an effort to stratify patients more precisely, but this "blending of stage and grade seems somewhat incongruous," according to Weems and Morris.[563] Nevertheless, the distinction between the two substages of stage T1 (A) is critically important in clinical practice.

Radical prostatectomy specimens. Methods of examining radical prostatectomy specimens were discussed above. Four practical problems have been described for pathologic staging using the TNM system in radical prostatectomy specimens.[104] First, separation of substages T2a (less than half of one lobe) and T2b (more than half of one lobe) is difficult, particularly in specimens that are partially sampled rather than whole-mounted; this problem is resolved by reporting such cases as T2a+b, an

TABLE 7-12.
METHODS OF DEFINING SUBSTAGES A1 AND A2 OF PROSTATIC CARCINOMA

Method	Description	Advantages	Disadvantages
TURP chip counting	Stage A1: Fewer than 3 or 5 chips involved Stage A2: More than 3 or 5 chips involved	Simple to use; popular	Few supporting studies for 3 to 5 chip threshold; cannot apply to enucleation specimens
Area ratio estimation	Stage A1: 5% or less of specimen area	Simple to use; strong empirical support; used in 1992 revision of TNM system	Incompatible with current concepts of cancer risk factors; supporting studies only from one institution (Johns Hopkins)
Volume estimate	Stage A1: 1 cm^3 or less Stage A2: Greater than 1 cm^3 cancer volume	Theoretically sound; modest empirical support	Requires measurement and calculation; based on volume
TURP chip ratio	Ratio of benign to malignant chips in TURP specimens	Simple to use; low interobserver variability; correlates with prognosis	Does not lend itself to two-tier A1-A2 substaging; cannot apply to enucleation specimens
TURP chip grid ratio	Ratio of malignant to total "grids" in TURP specimens	Simple to use; slightly better than area ratio estimation method	Requires grid or ruler; only recently introduced; does not lend itself to two-tier A1-A2 substaging
Cancer foci counting	Stage A1 (T1a): 3 or fewer microscopic foci Stage A2 (T1b): More than 3 foci of cancer	Simple to use; formerly used in TNM system (prior to 1992)	"Foci" not defined; same problems as area ratio estimation method; addition of grade T1a and T1b to obtain final stage in TNM system is awkward (T1a and low grade = stage 0; T1a and higher grade = stage I; T1b with any grade is stage II)

TURP = transurethral resection of prostate.
From Bostwick DG, Choi C: Prognostic factors in early prostate cancer, Urol Annu 6:129-146, 1992; with permission.

approach that necessarily compresses data. Second, the pathologist rarely if ever has access to clinical information pertaining to distant metastases at the time of histologic evaluation of the prostatectomy specimen, and thus cannot accurately report the "M" of TNM; this problem is resolved by reporting all cases as "Mx" with a brief qualification that refers to the clinical record. The third problem is the pathologic "upstaging" of adenocarcinoma which usually occurs with prostatectomy following transurethral resection; as already noted, transurethral resection–detected adenocarcinomas are T1 (a or b), but additional adenocarcinoma identified on prostatectomy frequently results in upstaging to T2 and T3. This problem is resolved by reporting both TNM stages (transurethral resection and prostatectomy) with a brief note describing this issue. The fourth problem in pathologic staging is encountered in cases without extraprostatic tissue and tumor extending to the surgical margin; these foci should be considered Tx or T2+ rather than T3, although many pathologists express confusion with this guideline.

Metastases. The usual sites of metastases for prostatic adenocarcinoma are pelvic lymph nodes, bone (chiefly osteoblastic metastases), and lungs (Fig. 7-38).[564-566] However, many unusual sites of metastases have been described, including kidney, breast, and brain. No important differences are seen in the pattern of metastases at autopsy in Japan and the United States.[565,566] De La Monte[565] found a similar number of metastatic sites in patients who received estrogen therapy and those who did not, although patients who received estrogen had more frequent metastases to the central nervous system. Cluster analysis of metastases revealed a subset of men of African ancestry who developed distant metastases with minimal local spread of tumor.

Staging pelvic lymph node biopsy is usually performed prior to prostatectomy, and most urologists discontinue surgery if metastases are identified. Lymph node dissection may be an open or laparoscopic procedure. Radical perineal prostatectomy and lymph node dissection are performed as separate procedures because the surgical approaches are different, whereas radical retropubic prostatectomy and lymphadenectomy are often performed as a single procedure. The pathologist should carefully evaluate the fibroadipose tissue obtained by lymphadenectomy and submit all lymph nodes for pathologic examination. It may not be necessary to submit obvious adipose tissue, although it is my policy to do so. Sampling error by frozen section accounts for a false negative rate of lymph node metastases of 2% to 3% in my experience (D. Bostwick, unpublished observations). Surgeons at Wayne State University do not undertake frozen section evaluation of pelvic lymph nodes that are not palpably enlarged due to the potential for histopathologic sampling error (D. Grignon, personal communication).

There is a low incidence of micrometastatic occult prostatic carcinoma in serum and pelvic lymph nodes that cannot be detected by routine hematoxylin-eosin staining (Table 7-13).[567] Using immunohistochemical studies directed against cytokeratin, Moul et al[567] found lymph node micrometastases in 3% of patients with clinically localized prostatic adenocarcinoma, similar to the results of Gomella et al.[568] In another study, circulating prostate-specific antigen–immunoreactive cells in the blood were identified by flow cytometry in all cases of adenocarcinoma with distant metastases and 47% of lower stage adenocarcinomas.[569] Reverse transcriptase polymerase chain reaction studies to detect prostate-specific antigen mRNA revealed prostate-specific antigen–positive cells

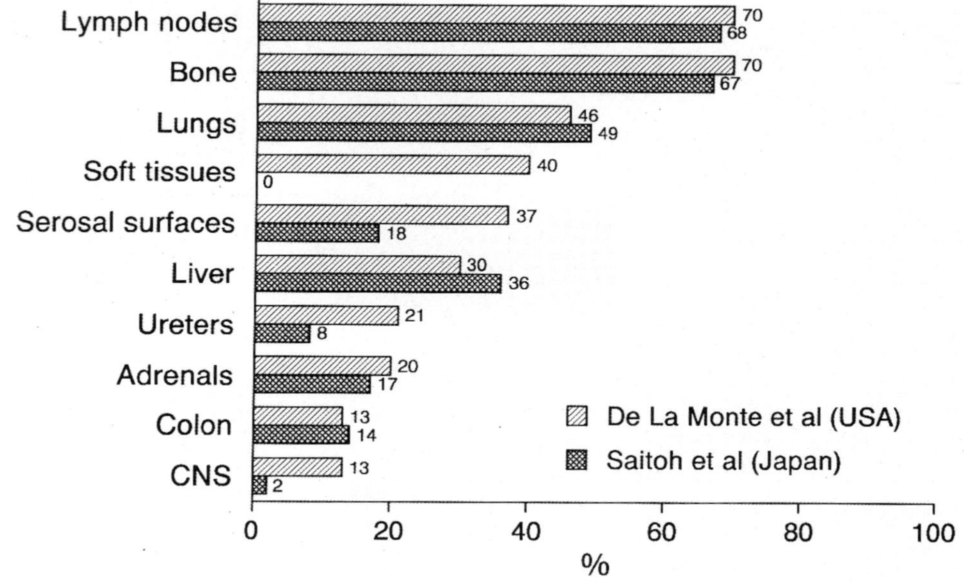

7-38. Ten most common sites of prostate cancer metastases at autopsy in the United States and Japan. *(From Bostwick DG, Eble JN: Prostatic adenocarcinoma metastatic to inguinal hernia sac, J Urol Pathol 1: 193-199, 1993; with permission.)*

TABLE 7-13.
MICROMETASTASES IN PATIENTS WITH PROSTATE CANCER

Site	Author and Year	Number of Cancer Patients	Method of Detection	Results
Lymph Nodes	Deguchi et al, 1993[682]	22	RTPCR and immunohistochemistry (anti–PSA)	Micrometastases by RTPCR in 6 patients (27.3%), including 4 with both histologic and immunohistochemical confirmation
	Gomella et al, 1993[568]	32	Immunohistochemistry (anti–PSA, PAP, and cytokeratin)	Micrometastases in 1 of 32 patients (3%)
	Moul et al, 1994[567]	32	Immunohistochemistry (anti–PSA and cytokeratin)	Micrometastases in 1 of 32 patients (3%)
Bone Marrow	Mansi et al, 1988[683]	40	Immunohistochemistry (anti–PSA)	Micrometastases in 73% of patients with clinically metastatic cancer and 13% with clinically organ-confined cancer
	Wood et al, 1994[684]	55	RTPCR and immunohistochemistry (anti–PSA)	Micrometastases in 65% of patients with extraprostatic cancer, immunohistochemistry confirmed micrometastases in 79% of those with positive RTPCR
Serum	Hamdy et al, 1992[569]	40	Flow cytometry and immunohistochemistry (anti–PSA)	PSA–positive cells in 47% patients with stage non-D2 cancers and 100% with stage D2 cancer
	Moreno et al, 1992[685]	12	RTPCR (anti–PSA)	PSA–positive cells in 4 of 12 patients with stage N+ cancer (33%)
	Katz et al, 1994[571]	83	RTPCR (anti–PSA)	PSA–positive cells in 77.8% of patients with stage N+ cancers, and 38.5% with clinically organ-confined cancer

RTPCR = reverse transcriptase polymerase chain reaction for PSA mRNA sequences
PSA: prostate-specific antigen
PAP: prostatic acid phosphatase

circulating in the peripheral blood of 4 of 12 patients with adenocarcinoma with pelvic lymph node metastases.[570] Katz et al[571] demonstrated the clinical utility of this test in predicting stage and referred to it as "molecular staging."

Treatment and patient outcome

Treatment of prostatic adenocarcinoma remains controversial, consisting of one or more of four major options: radical prostatectomy, radiation therapy, androgen deprivation therapy, and active surveillance (deferred treatment). At present there is no role for chemotherapy. The choice of treatment is based on patient age and health, life expectancy, clinical stage of the adenocarcinoma, serum prostate-specific antigen level, and tumor grade. Clinical management of prostatic adenocarcinoma is addressed in a number of recent reviews.[572]

It is difficult to compare precisely the efficacy of different treatments and outcomes in prostatic adenocarcinoma because of the significant clinical staging error, the paucity of rigorous prospective and randomized clinical trials, and the lengthy follow-up needed to obtain results with a relatively slow-growing tumor such as prostatic adenocarcinoma.[6] Fleming et al[573] evaluated the impact of various therapies on quality-adjusted life expectancy using decision analysis in men between 60 and 75 years of age with clinically localized prostatic adenocarcinoma. They concluded that radical prostatectomy and radiation therapy offered only a slight marginal benefit for selected patients when compared with no therapy. In an accompanying editorial, Whitmore[574] noted that optimal management of prostatic adenocarcinoma "may be more a matter of opinion than a matter of fact."

The 10-year cancer-specific survival for all stages of adenocarcinoma is about 51%, with an estimated "cure" rate of 32% (Table 7-14).[6] Clinically localized adenocarcinoma had the most favorable outcome. Long-term progression for untreated stage T1a (A1) adenocarcinoma varied from 8% to 37%, with the risk of progression increasing with additional years of follow-up (Table

TABLE 7-14.
PROSTATE CANCER: DIAGNOSIS, RISK OF DEATH, AND CURE RATE BY CLINICAL STAGE

Patients (%)	Stage	Prognosis	10-year Cancer-Specific Survival Rate (%)	Estimated Cure Rate (%)
10	T1a (A1)	Treatment "unnecessary"	95	85
30	T1b-T2 (A2-B2)	Often curable	80	65
10	T3-4 (C1-2)	Occasionally curable	60	25
20	N+ (D1)	Rarely curable	40	<5
30	M+ (D2)	Incurable	10	<1
100	All stages		51	32
	Excluding T1a (stage A1)		45	25

Modified from Scardino PT, Weaver R, Hudson MA: Early detection of prostate cancer, Hum Pathol 23:211-222, 1992, with permission.

TABLE 7-15.
LONG-TERM FOLLOW-UP OF PATIENTS WITH UNTREATED CLINICAL STAGE T1A (A1) ADENOCARCINOMA

	Method of Defining Stage T1a (A1)	Mean Age in Years (range)	Mean Follow-up in Years (range)	Progression (%)	Mean Time to Progression in Years (range)
Thompson and Zeidman[575]	Cancer foci counting	NA	7.5 (1-20)	3/37 (8%)	8.7 (2-19)
Zhang et al[576]	Area ratio estimation	NA	8.2 (5-23)	12/132 (10%)	7 (0.5-20)
Lowe and Listrom[235]	Area ratio estimation	NA (46-99)	NA	12/80 (15%)	13.5 (1-26.5)
Orestano[577]	Cancer foci counting	72 (59-87)	9	11/30 (37%)	7
Epstein et al[546]	Area ratio estimation	65 (50-87)	10 (8-18)	8/50 (16%)	7 (3.5-8)
Blute et al[547]	Volume estimation	55 (48-59)	12.2 (10-25)	4/15 (27%)	10.2 (9-19)

NA: Data not given

7-15)[235,546,547,575-577]; survival at 10 years was 95%, similar to the age-specific survival, suggesting to some authors that treatment for this stage may be unnecessary.[6] Larger organ-confined adenocarcinomas (T1b and T2) and those with local extraprostatic extension (T3 and T4) showed progressively lower survival and "cure" rates, but the worst outcomes were observed with adenocarcinomas metastatic to regional lymph nodes (T1-4 N+M0)(40% survival at 10 years) and distant organs (M+)(10% survival). For stage T1c (B0) there are insufficient data available to determine outcome because it was only recently defined.

OTHER EPITHELIAL NEOPLASMS

Urothelial carcinoma

Urothelial carcinoma of the prostate is rarely primary, accounting for less than 4% of tumors originating in the prostate, and usually represents synchronous or metachronous spread from carcinoma in the bladder and urethra (Fig. 7-39).[578-596] It involves the prostate in about 40% of radical cystoprostatectomy specimens for bladder carcinoma.[578,579,582,587]

Clinical features. Patients usually have symptoms of hematuria, urinary obstruction, or prostatitis. Serum prostate-specific antigen and prostatic acid phosphatase levels are not elevated. Clinically, urothelial carcinoma may be mistaken for prostatitis or nodular hyperplasia. Most clinical findings are due to tumor arising elsewhere in the urothelium.

Pathology. Urothelial carcinoma of the prostate involves the periurethral prostatic ducts and acini. Diagnostic criteria are identical to those for urothelial cancer of the bladder; most cancers are moderately differentiated and usually associated with prominent chronic inflammation. Squamous metaplasia is infrequent.

Treatment and outcome. Radical cystoprostatectomy is the treatment of choice for urothelial carcinoma of the prostate.[578-580,595,596] In a study of 21 patients by Hardeman and Soloway,[580] radical surgery was found to be the most useful therapy. These authors also noted that bladder cancer extending into the prostate can easily be missed cystoscopically and recommended random biopsies of the prostate.

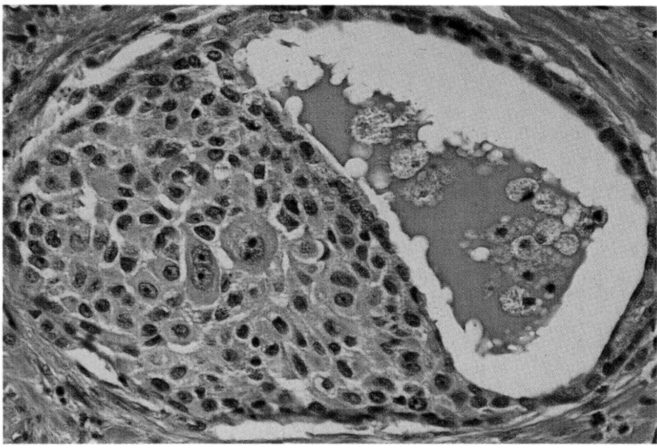

7-39. Urothelial carcinoma involving prostatic ducts.

Differential diagnosis. Distinguishing urothelial carcinoma from adenocarcinoma is clinically important because of the estrogen unresponsiveness of the former; these tumors often coincidentally coexist. By light microscopy adenocarcinoma usually displays some evidence of acinar differentiation, although this may be difficult to identify in high grade cancers or cases of urothelial carcinoma with pseudoglandular pattern. Immunohistochemical stains for prostate-specific antigen and prostatic acid phosphatase will distinguish these tumors, with immunoreactivity exclusively in adenocarcinoma.

Mixed tumors

Phyllodes tumor. Phyllodes tumor of the prostate (also known as Cystic epithelial-stromal tumor, phyllodes type of atypical hyperplasia, cystadenoleiomyofibroma, and cystosarcoma phyllodes) is a rare lesion that should be considered a neoplasm rather than atypical hyperplasia because of its frequent early recurrences, infiltrative growth, and potential for extraprostatic spread in some cases.[597-616] Dedifferentiation with multiple recurrences in some cases is further evidence of the potentially aggressive nature of this tumor.[610,615,616] Although a benign clinical course has been emphasized in some reports,[611] the cumulative evidence in the literature indicates that some patients develop local recurrences.[610,616]

Clinical features. Patients with prostatic phyllodes tumor typically display such symptoms as urinary obstruction, hematuria, and dysuria. There may be severe urinary obstruction, often occurring at a younger age than expected for typical symptomatic prostatic hyperplasia. The youngest reported patient was 22-years-old with a 20-cm diameter retrovesicular mass.[599] Most tumors range in size from 4 to 25 cm, with one report of a 58 cm tumor weighing 11.2 kg.[604,608] Phyllodes tumor can arise centrally near the verumontanum or involve the lateral part of the peripheral zone unilaterally. At the time of transurethral resection, the cystoscopist may note an unusual spongy or cystic texture of the involved prostate.

Pathology. The diagnosis of phyllodes tumor is usually made on resected tissue, and it may be overlooked on needle biopsy in which it is difficult to appreciate the pattern of the tumor. Important diagnostic clues include the diffuse infiltration, variably cellular stroma surrounding cysts, and compressed elongated channels that often have a leaflike configuration.

Prostatic phyllodes tumor exhibits a spectrum of histologic features, similar to its counterpart in the breast. It may be subdivided into low-grade, intermediate-grade, and high-grade groups, but even low-grade tumors may recur.[616] High-grade prostatic phyllodes tumor has a high stromal-epithelial ratio, prominent stromal cellularity and overgrowth, marked cytologic atypia, and increased mitotic activity (Fig. 7-40). A sarcomatous component may arise within a low-grade tumor over time, invariably after multiple recurrences over many years.[615,616] One reported case consisted of a phyllodes tumor containing an incidental focus of well-differentiated adenocarcinoma.[604] Rarely, tumors with overtly malignant stroma

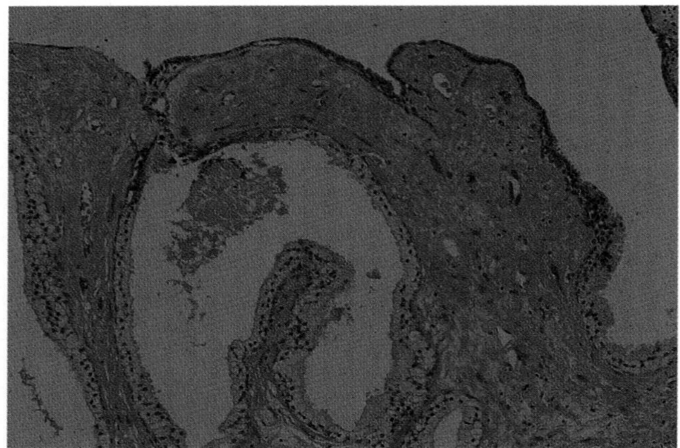

7-40. Low-grade phyllodes tumor of the prostate.

have given rise to lung, bone, and abdominal wall metastases of sarcoma. Lymph node metastases have not been observed.

The histogenesis is uncertain but is not considered müllerian for the following reasons: (1) no müllerian remnants exist in the adult prostate; the müllerian epithelium in the prostatic utricle is replaced by the urogenital sinus early in life; (2) prostate-specific antigen and prostatic acid phosphatase have been demonstrated in the epithelium of the adult utricle, indicating the endodermal (prostatelike) nature of this tissue; and (3) prostate-specific antigen has been demonstrated in the epithelium of prostate phyllodes tumors.[609,610,614,616]

Treatment and outcome. Phyllodes tumor must be considered potentially aggressive and an individualized approach to complete excision of the tumor is needed. Low-grade tumors may be treated conservatively, recognizing that recurrences may be higher grade and require complete excision.[616]

Differential diagnosis. The differential diagnosis of prostatic phyllodes tumor includes stromal hyperplasia with bizarre nuclei, giant multilocular prostatic cystadenoma, hyperplasia with cystic acini, and cysts such as müllerian duct cysts and congenital and acquired seminal vesicle cysts. Phyllodes tumor may also arise in the seminal vesicle as a supraprostatic retrovesicular mass, but it is separated from its prostatic counterpart by the absence of prostate-specific antigen and prostatic acid phosphatase immunoreactivity in the epithelial component. Stromal hyperplasia with bizarre nuclei is a hypocellular lesion with enlarged hyperchromatic degenerative-appearing nuclei occurring in the stroma adjacent to typical hyperplastic acini or within nodules of nodular hyperplasia. Giant multilocular cystadenoma of the prostate is a solitary tumor with cysts lined by prostatic epithelium surrounded by dense fibrous stroma. Cystic adenoma of the prostate has also been described, consisting of complex inward growth of papillary epithelial fronds with scant stroma. Nodular hyperplasia commonly contains small cystic acini within hyperplastic nodules, and infrequently small fibroadenoma-like foci may be misinterpreted as phyllodes tumor. Müllerian duct cysts (typically midline) and seminal vesicle cysts (typically lateral) are usually unilocular, lacking the prostatic epithelial lining and stromal cellularity of phyllodes tumor. Primary sarcoma of the prostate such as leiomyosarcoma is also a diagnostic consideration, but this tumor consists of a monophasic densely cellular proliferation of spindle cells that lacks the epithelial component of phyllodes tumor. Sarcomatoid carcinoma is a concern when an overtly malignant spindle cell component is present, but it is distinguished by the presence of a malignant epithelial component or evidence of epithelial differentiation within the neoplastic spindle cells.

Wilms' tumor. A single case of primary Wilms' tumor of the prostate was reported, arising in a 32-year-old man with hemospermia and obstructive symptoms.[617] The characteristic triphasic pattern was observed, including blastema, epithelial tubules, and spindled stroma. The patient developed pulmonary metastases 1 year after presentation. Extrarenal Wilms' tumor is thought to arise from embryonic rests of metanephric blastema, explaining the occurrence of this tumor in other urogenital areas such as the scrotum, spermatic cord, and in an ovotestis. The differential diagnosis includes sarcoma such as rhabdomyosarcoma, sarcomatoid carcinoma, and teratoma.

Carcinoma metastatic to prostate

Tumors arising in other organs occasionally involve the prostate, usually due to contiguous spread, but metastases are extremely rare, with involvement at autopsy in 0.5% to 2.2% of men dying of malignancies.[618,619] The most common tumor metastasizing to the prostate is squamous cell carcinoma of the bronchus, accounting for almost half of all metastases.[618,619] Malignant melanoma accounts for approximately 27% of prostatic metastases, with an incidence of prostatic involvement of 1.1% of patients with malignant melanoma at autopsy.[618-626] Grignon et al[620] described an unusual case of tumor-to-tumor metastasis of malignant melanoma to prostatic adenocarcinoma. The remaining 25% of metastases to prostate arise from a variety of sites,[624,625] including pancreatic carcinoma[626] and a recent case of goblet cell carcinoid of the appendix involving the prostate 21 years after appendectomy.[622]

SOFT TISSUE NEOPLASMS

BENIGN

Leiomyoma and fibroma

These benign soft tissue tumors are often confused with nodular hyperplasia. Leiomyoma is defined as a circumscribed solitary smooth muscle nodule greater than 1 cm in diameter.[627-630] It is identical to leiomyoma occurring in the uterus and other sites, consisting of a proliferation of benign smooth muscle cells with variable amounts of collagen. Fibroma is a similar nodule composed of collagen with few fibroblasts; fibroma may be indistinguishable from a pure stromal nodule of nodular hyperplasia. Some authors have questioned the existence of these tumors, preferring to consider them within the spectrum of nodular hyperplasia.

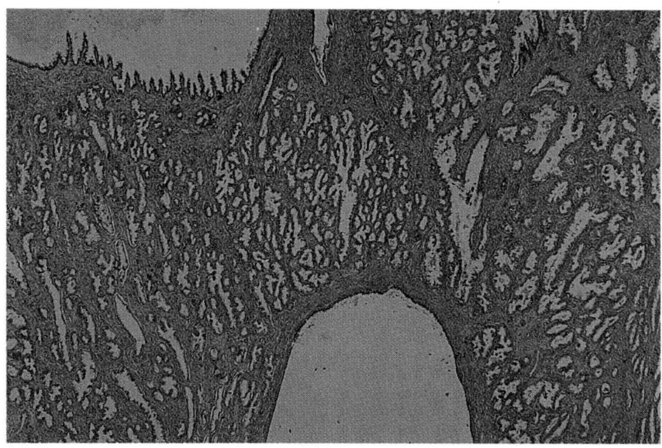

7-41. Giant multilocular cystic hyperplasia of the prostate in a 20-year-old patient with urinary obstructive symptoms. The patient was treated by radical prostatectomy owing to the failure of conservative management.

Variants of leiomyoma include cellular leiomyoma, atypical leiomyoma,[630] and leiomyoblastoma. The cellular variant is distinguished by increased density of cells. Although some cases have been reported as having occasional mitotic figures, these are usually absent. The atypical (symplastic; bizarre) variant contains multinucleated giant cells with smudged nuclear detail, probably representing degenerative changes. Mitotic figures are rare or absent.

The differential diagnostic considerations are leiomyosarcoma and stromal hyperplasia with atypia. The small number of published cases limits conclusions regarding behavior of the variants of leiomyoma, but they appear to be benign. No strict morphologic criteria separate atypical leiomyoma from stromal hyperplasia with atypia.

Hemangiopericytoma

Fewer than 10 cases of hemangiopericytoma have been reported.[631-633] The diagnostic features are similar to those at other sites. Of three cases with follow-up, one is free of tumor 3 years after diagnosis, and two have had recurrences, including one with metastases to the bone and skin.

Other benign tumors

Pheochromocytoma (paraganglioma) of the prostate is rare. The patients usually have hypertension.[634] Extra-adrenal pheochromocytomas have been decribed in the retroperitoneum, mediastinum, bladder, and prostate, and are likely to secrete norepinephrine alone. Surgical manipulation of the tumor may precipitate hypertensive crisis, and precautions must be taken to avoid this.

Giant multilocular prostatic cystadenoma is a large tumor composed of acini and cysts lined by prostatic-type epithelium lying in a hypocellular fibrous stroma (Fig. 7-41).[635-638] This tumor arises in men between ages 28 and 80 years as a large midline prostatic or extraprostatic mass causing urinary obstruction. The epithelial lining displays intense prostate-specific antigen immunoreactivity, indicating prostatic derivation. Surgical excision is usually curative, although it may recur if incompletely excised. The differential diagnosis includes phyllodes tumor, multilocular peritoneal inclusion cyst, müllerian duct cyst, seminal vesicle cyst, lymphangioma, and hemangiopericytoma; the nature of the cyst lining is useful in separating these lesions.

Other benign tumors arise in the prostate, including hemangioma, lymphangioma, neurofibroma, neurilemoma, and others.

SARCOMA

Sarcoma of the prostate is rare and accounts for less than 0.1% of the primary prostatic neoplasms. One third occur in children under 10 years of age and most of these are rhabdomyosarcoma; leiomyosarcoma is most common in adults. Symptoms include prostatism and pelvic pain, which is usually refractory to medical management. Tumors measure up to 15 cm or more in diameter and are usually soft with areas of necrosis. The lung is the most common site of metastases, although rhabdomyosarcoma often involves regional lymph nodes.[639]

Rhabdomyosarcoma

Rhabdomyosarcoma of the prostate has a peak incidence between birth and 6 years of age, although sporadic cases have been reported in men as old as 80 years.[640] The prostate accounts for 21% of cases in children, second only to head and neck origin. Serum prostate-specific antigen and prostatic acid phosphatase levels are normal. Three adults had hypercalcemia due to bone metastases.[639]

The tumor is usually extensive, with a mean diameter of 5 to 9 cm, and involves the prostate, bladder, and periurethral, perirectal, and perivesicular soft tissues. It may be difficult to determine the precise site of origin in large tumors. Urethral involvement may not be apparent cytoscopically.[641] Symptoms include urethral obstruction, often acute, as well as bladder displacement and rectal compression. The prostate may be palpably normal, although large tumors often fill the pelvis and can be palpated suprapubically.

Most are embryonal rhabdomyosarcoma (Fig. 7-42), and the remainder are alveolar, botryoid, and spindle cell subtypes.[642] Tumor cells are arranged in sheets of immature round to spindle cells set in a myxoid stroma. Polypoid tumor fragments ("botryoid pattern") may fill the urethral lumen, covered by intact urothelium with condensed underlying tumor cells creating a distinctive cambium layer. Nuclei are usually pleomorphic and darkly staining. Scattered rhabdomyoblasts may be present with eosinophilic cytoplasmic processes containing cross striations.

Tumor cells may display immunoreactivity for myoglobin, desmin, and vimentin but are negative for prostate-specific antigen and prostatic acid phosphatase. Ultrastructural study reveals two cell types, similar to rhabdomyosarcoma at other sites; large oval or elongate tumor cells contain segments of sarcomere with abundant glycogen, and smaller round cells contain abundant cytoplasmic organelles but lack myofibrils. All tumors appear to be aneuploid by flow cytometry.[643]

Combination chemotherapy in conjunction with surgery and radiotherapy has improved patient outcome in the past 2 decades, with 3-year survival rates of over 70% reported for pelvic sites in the Intergroup Rhabdomyosarcoma Study[644]; long-term survival has been reported.[645] The outcome is similar for the embryonal and alveolar subtypes.

The differential diagnosis includes other small cell neoplasms, including lymphoma, acute leukemia, neuroblastoma, neuroendocrine carcinoma, poorly differentiated carcinoma, primitive neuroectodermal tumor, and other high-grade sarcomas. The botryoid pattern may be mistaken for a benign fibroepithelial polyp.

Leiomyosarcoma

Leiomyosarcoma of the prostate presents as a large bulky mass that replaces most of the prostate and periprostatic tissues. It is the most common sarcoma in adults and accounts for 26% of all prostate sarcomas. Patients range in age from 40 to 71 years (mean, 59 years), with sporadic reports in younger patients.[646,647] The histologic findings are typical of leiomyosarcoma at other sites (Fig. 7-43). Although the criteria separating leiomyoma from low-grade leiomyosarcoma have not been precisely defined in the prostate, they are probably similar to those in other organs, including degree of cellularity and cytologic anaplasia, mitotic activity, necrosis, vascular invasion, and size.

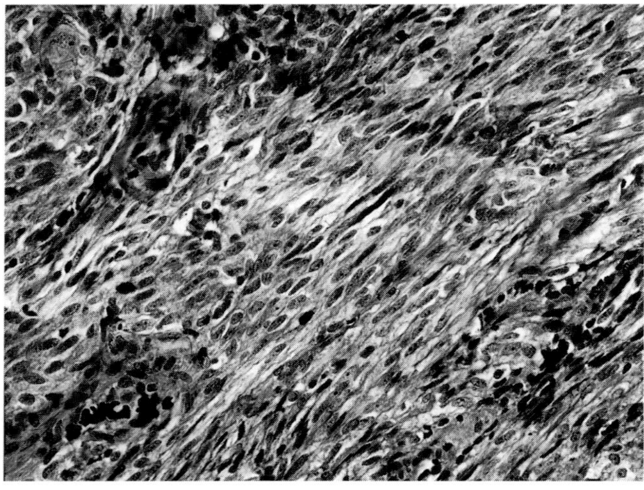

7-42. Rhabdomyosarcoma in a 2-year-old.

Tumor cells usually display intense cytoplasmic immunoreactivity for smooth muscle specific actin and vimentin and weak desmin immunoreactivity. Some cases may be unreactive to any antibody due to prolonged fixation. Most are negative for cytokeratin (AE1/AE3) and S-100 protein, but exceptions have been described.[646-648]

Local recurrence and distant metastasis are frequent with these tumors and the prognosis is poor. Treatment includes radical surgery with postoperative radiation or radiation therapy alone. Mean survival after diagnosis was less than 3 years in one series (range, 0.2 to 6.5 years), and most patients died from tumor.[647] Rare long-term survivors have been reported. All reports indicate that prostatic leiomyosarcoma has a poor prognosis and that radical surgery is the preferred treatment, although limited data are available.[646-648]

Other sarcomas

Other rare sarcomas reported in the prostate include malignant phyllodes tumors, fibrosarcoma, osteosarcoma, malignant fibrous histiocytoma,[649,650] angiosarcoma,[651] chondrosarcoma, neurofibrosarcoma, liposarcoma, and undifferentiated sarcoma. Sarcomatoid carcinoma, although not truly mesenchymal, must be included in the differential diagnoses of pleomorphic spindle cell neoplasms with necrosis and significant mitotic activity. Recognition of transition of carcinoma to sarcomatous differentiation and immunostaining with cytokeratin, prostate-specific antigen, and prostatic acid phosphatase may be helpful. Sarcoma of the prostate frequently resists efforts at subclassification, and I refer to this as undifferentiated sarcoma. Regardless of classification, the prognosis of prostatic sarcoma is poor.

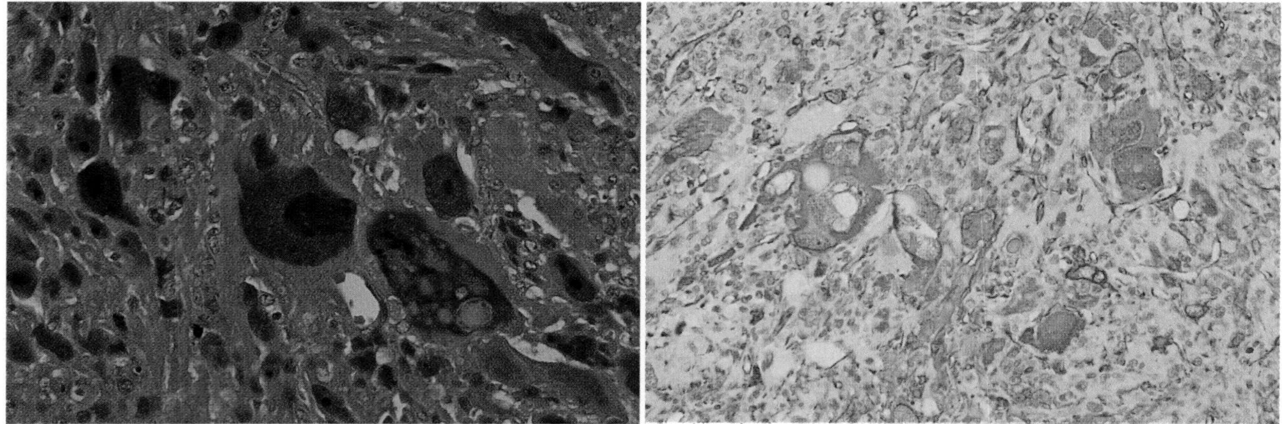

7-43. Leiomyosarcoma of the prostate. **A,** Light microscopy reveals bizarre giant cells in some areas. **B,** Intense cytoplasmic immunoreactivity for actin in the majority of tumor cells.

Rhabdoid tumor

Rhabdoid tumor is a poorly differentiated malignant neoplasm with light microscopic features of rhabdomyosarcoma that displays epithelial differentiation, including intense cytoplasmic immunoreactivity for keratin proteins and epithelial membrane antigen, rare cell junctions, occasional intracytoplasmic lumens, and distinctive paranuclear aggregates of intermediate filaments. Most cases occur in the kidney but rare extrarenal tumors have been identified, including rare cases in the prostate.[652]

OTHER NEOPLASMS AND TUMORLIKE PROLIFERATIONS

TUMORLIKE PROLIFERATIONS

Postoperative spindle cell nodule

Postoperative spindle cell nodule is a rare benign reparative response that occurs within months of surgery, and consists of nodules of spindle cells arranged in fascicles with occasional or numerous mitotic figures (up to 25 mitotic figures per 10 high-power fields).[653,654] The cells have central elongate to ovoid nuclei, small prominent nucleoli, and abundant cytoplasm. Necrosis may be present but is usually not a prominent feature. The main differential diagnostic consideration is sarcoma, but postoperative spindle cell nodule is distinguished by the small size of the nodules, the presence of chronic inflammation, the plexiform pattern of blood vessels, the lack of signficant nuclear pleomorphism and atypical mitotic figures, and the lack of recurrence after conservative excision.

Spindle cell proliferations with no prior operation

The appearance of spindle cell proliferations in a patient without a history of prior surgery (inflammatory pseudotumor, pseudosarcoma, nodular fasciitis, pseudosarcomatous fibromyxoid tumor) is a rare benign pathologic occurrence of unknown etiology in the bladder, prostate, and urethra.[655-659] Patients range in age from 16 to 73 years (mean, 41 years), with a slight female predilection in the bladder. Mean tumor size is 3.6 cm but can measure up to 8 cm in diameter. Histologically, spindle cell proliferation with no prior operation is similar to postoperative spindle cell nodule, although the tumor nodules tend to be larger. The stroma is loose, edematous, and myxoid, with abundant small slitlike blood vessels resembling granulation tissue (Fig. 7-44). Mitotic figures are infrequent, with less than 3 per 10 high-power fields; none is atypical. Ulceration and focal necrosis is present in most cases but is not prominent.

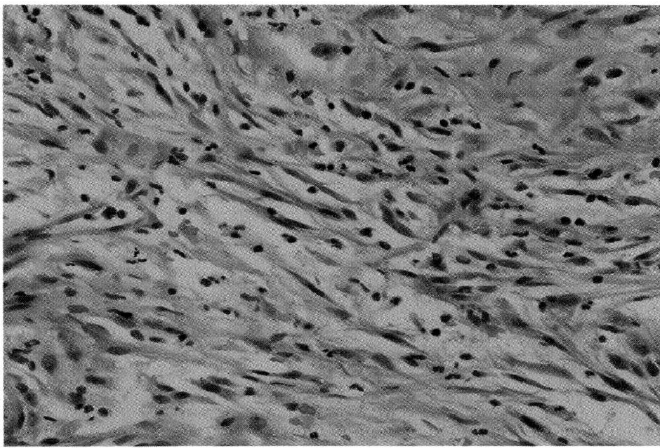

7-44. Inflammatory pseudotumor of the prostate.

The myxoid stroma contains abundant nonsulfated acid mucopolysaccharides, with strong staining for alcian blue at pH 2.7 but not at pH 0.9. The spindle cells display vimentin immunoreactivity and rarely stain for smooth muscle actin, desmin, and keratin; S-100 protein and myoglobin are negative. Ultrastructural studies show some cells with myofibroblastic differentiation, including cytoplasmic microfilaments and dense bodies; no epithelial differentiation is evident. Tumors are usually diploid, with a low S-phase fraction.

The differential diagnosis is the same as postoperative spindle cell nodule, with leiomyosarcoma, other myxoid sarcomas, and sarcomatoid carcinoma representing the greatest pitfalls (Table 7-16). Other mimics include leiomyoma, aggressive angiomyxoma, and phyllodes tumor. In addition, pseudosarcomatous stromal reaction can be seen in association with urothelial carcinoma which may mimic spindle cell tumor with no prior operation. Ro et al[655] urge extreme caution when making this diagnosis in small biopsy specimens.

Follow-up for as long as 13 years indicates that this is a benign tumor even with conservative excision or biopsy, with no cases of metastasis or death from tumor; some bulky tumors require wide excision.

HEMATOLOGIC MALIGNANCIES

Hematologic maligancies are rare in the prostate, with primary involvement or secondary spread from systemic lymphoma, leukemia, or myeloma.

Malignant lymphoma

Patients with malignant lymphoma involving the prostate are usually older men (mean, 61 years), who have urinary obstructive symptoms, including urinary urgency, urinary frequency, acute urinary retention, urinary tract infections, and hematuria.[660-666] Systemic symptoms, including fever, chills, night sweats, and weight loss, are infrequent and are found only in patients with widespread lymphoma. Two reported patients had a history of urinary tract infections, and two others had a history of gonorrhea.[660-666] Grossly, the prostate gland with malignant lymphoma is diffusely enlarged, nontender, and firm or rubbery. Serum prostate-specific antigen level is usually not elevated.

Primary lymphoma is much less frequent than secondary involvement. Ewing[662] and others challenged the existence of primary extranodal lymphoma due to the paucity of lymphoid tissue in the prostate. However, identification of rudimentary lymphoid nodules in the prostate by Fukase,[663] the recognition of malignant

TABLE 7-16.
DIFFERENTIAL DIAGNOSIS OF MYXOID LESIONS OF THE PROSTATE

	Inflammatory Pseudotumor*	Postoperative Spindle Cell Nodule	Sarcomatoid Carcinoma	Myxoid Leiomyo-sarcoma	Myxoid Rhabdomyo-sarcoma	Myxoid Malignant Fibrous Histiocytoma
Light Microscopic Findings						
Cellularity	Variable, often low	Variable, often low	High	Variable	Variable	Variable
Growth pattern	Tissue culture–like	Tissue culture–like	Biphasic	Intersecting fasicles	Subepithelial condensation	Storiform
Pleomorphism	+	-	+++	±	++	+++
Vessels	Slitlike	Unremarkable	Unremarkable	Unremarkable	Unremarkable	Unremarkable
Necrosis	±	±	++	++	+	++
Mitotic figures	+	++	++	+ (variable)	++	+++
Atypical mitotic figures	-	-	+	+	+	+
Ultrastructural Findings	Fibroblasts and myofibroblasts	Fibroblasts and myofibroblasts	Epithelial ± mesenchymal	Smooth muscle	Striated muscle	Fibroblasts and myofibroblasts
Immunohistochemical Findings						
Cytokeratin	- (rarely +)	- (rarely +)	+	- (rarely +)	- (rarely +)	- (rarely +)
Vimentin	+	+	+	+	+	+
Epithelial membrane antigen	-	-	±	-	-	-
Desmin	±	±	±	+	+	- (rarely +)
Smooth muscle actin	+	+	±	+	-	-
Muscle-specific actin	+	+	±	+	+	- (rarely +)
S-100 protein	-	-	±	-	-	-
Clinical Course	Benign	Benign	Malignant	Malignant	Malignant	Malignant

*Also referred to as spindle cell proliferation with no prior operation.

±:Variably positive; +: positive; -: negative.

Note: Myxoid rhabdomyosarcoma is a subset of embryonal rhabdomyosarcoma.

lymphoma arising in extranodal sites, and histologic documentation of cases with involvement limited to the prostate confirmed the existence of lymphoma arising in the prostate. The prevalence of primary prostatic lymphoma at autopsy is 0.2% of extranodal lymphoma.[664] Diagnostic criteria that have been proposed for primary lymphoma include symptoms attributable to prostatic enlargement; lymphoma chiefly involving the prostate with or without involvement of adjacent tissues; and lack of liver, spleen, lymph nodes, and peripheral blood involvement within 1 month of diagnosis.[660]

Microscopically, the infiltrate may be diffuse or patchy within the stroma, with characteristic preservation of the prostatic acini (Fig. 7-45); by contrast, granulomatous prostatitis causes acinar destruction. The lymphomatous infiltrate is usually extensive but may be irregular and patchy, often extending into the extraprostatic soft tissues. Tumor cell infiltration into the acinar epithelium is uncommon and rarely includes aggregates in the lumens. The most frequent lymphoma involving the prostate is diffuse non-Hodgkin's lymphoma, including small cleaved-cell, large cell, and mixed-cell types; Hodgkin's disease is very rare, with fewer than five documented cases.[660] Angiotropic lymphomas have also been described, including one case with spurious immunoreactivity for prostatic acid phosphatase (prostate-specific antigen was negative) presumably due to tumor cell absorption from the phosphatase-rich vessel contents.[665,666] Rare cases have coincidental adenocarcinoma.

The prognosis of lymphoma involving the prostate is usually poor regardless of patient age, stage of the tumor, histologic classification, type of involvement (primary or secondary), or type of therapeutic regimen employed. Twelve of 13 patients reported by Bostwick and Mann[660] died within 2 years after diagnosis. More than 60% of patients die of lymphoma, although survival of up to 10 years is possible with combination chemotherapy. Surgery is used chiefly for symptomatic relief of urinary obstruction.

The differential diagnosis of lymphoma includes leukemia, granulomatous prostatitis, chronic prostatitis with follicular hyperplasia, and neuroendocrine carcinoma. A 68-year-old man with prostatic pseudolymphoma was described by Peison et al.[667] The patient had no prior history of lymphoma and showed symptoms of acute urinary obstruction and normal blood count. Histologically, there was prominent lymphoid hyperplasia in the transurethral resection specimen without evidence of malignancy. Long-term follow-up was not available. Humphrey and Vollmer[668] described the first case of extramedullary hematopoiesis of the prostate appearing in a 75-year-old man with a history of myelofibrosis and progressive outlet obstruction. The transurethral resection specimen revealed a diffuse stromal infiltrate of atypical megakaryocytes, immature myeloid elements, and normoblasts; the epithelium was preserved. Chloroacetate esterase stain was useful in confirming the myeloid nature of the infiltrate.

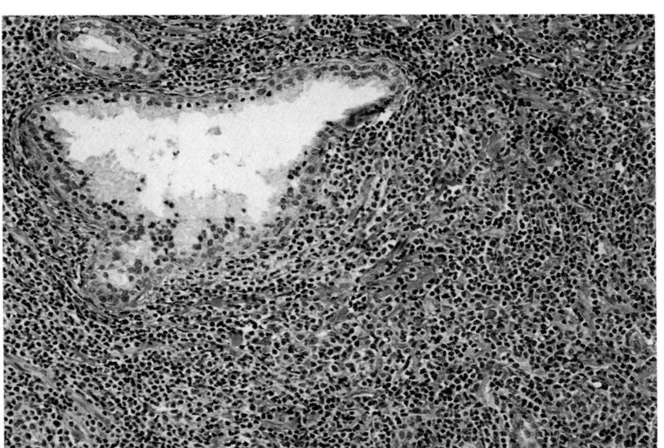

7-45. Malignant lymphoma of the prostate, diffuse large cell type.

Leukemia

Chronic lymphocytic leukemia is the most common leukemia involving the prostate, with more than 100 reported cases.[669-671] The autopsy prevalence of prostatic involvement is about 20% of cases of leukemia.[669] Cachia et al[670] followed 46 men with chronic lymphocytic leukemia, and all 6 who underwent transurethral resection for urinary obstructive symptoms had prostatic involvement. The clinical symptoms and histologic pattern in the prostate are similar to malignant lymphoma, and leukemia is distinguished chiefly from lymphoma by the presence of blood involvement. Thalhammer and colleagues[672] reported an unusual case of late relapse of granulocytic sarcoma (chloroma) detected by urinary obstructive symptoms due to prostatic enlargement after 9 years of remission; diagnosis was made by transurethral resection. Bladder neck obstruction in patients with leukemia may respond to surgery if chemotherapy is ineffective, although Frame et al[673] recommended radiation therapy.

Multiple myeloma

Multiple myeloma involving the prostate is rare, with less than 10 cases reported.[674] Most are diagnosed at autopsy, usually after systemic diagnosis. IgD and IgA myelomas have been described and rarely may cause urinary obstructive symptoms. The incidence of prostatic involvement by myeloma is uncertain.[674]

GERM CELL TUMORS

Rare cases of germ cell tumor arising in the prostate have been reported, invariably with metastases and massive prostatic involvement. These tumors probably arise from sequestration of germ cells during migration, usually occurring in the midline; this theory also accounts for germ cell tumors in the vagina, mediastinum, liver, retroperitoneum, and liver.

Two patients with yolk sac tumor, aged 29 and 51 years, died 10 months after diagnosis despite radical surgery and chemotherapy.[675,676] A patient with retroperitoneal seminoma and simultaneous occurrence in the prostate was described by Arai et al.[677] Michel et al[678] reported a 40-year-old with mixed germ cell tumor (embryonal carcinoma and teratoma) who was alive 2 years after treatment. Choriocarcinoma of the prostate has also been described in older reports.[679,680]

The main differential diagnostic considerations include sarcomatoid carcinoma (carcinosarcoma), mucinous carcinoma, typical acinar adenocarcinoma, ductal carcinoma, and metastases from testicular or retroperitoneal primary. The diagnosis of primary germ cell tumor of the prostate should only be considered after all other possibilities are excluded. The usual histologic features of germ cell tumor at other sites are present. For yolk sac tumor, these include Schiller-Duval bodies, hyaline periodic acid-Schiff–positive globules, and elevated serum alpha-fetoprotein levels; prostate-specific antigen and prostatic acid phosphatase are normal.[676]

OTHER TUMORLIKE CONDITIONS

A case of endometriosis of the prostate was documented by Beckman et al.[681] It arose as a small red-tan raised mass proximal to the internal urethral orifice, which extended into the prostate in a 78-year-old man with a long history of estrogen therapy (chlorotrianisene) for prostatic carcinoma. This case and similar cases reported in the male bladder were invariably associated with hematuria and chlorotrianisene therapy for prostatic adenocarcinoma.

MISCELLANEOUS NEOPLASMS

A single case of neuroblastoma has been reported in the prostate.[246]

REFERENCES

1. Parker SL, Tong T, Bolden S: Cancer statistics, 1996, CA Cancer J Clin 65:5-27, 1996.
2. Bostwick DG, Cooner WH, Denis L et al: The association of benign prostatic hyperplasia and cancer of the prostate, Cancer 70:291-301, 1992.
3. Seidman H, Mushinski MH, Gelb SK et al: Probabilities of eventually developing or dying of cancer—United States, 1985, CA Cancer J Clin 35:36-56, 1985.
4. Morra MN, Das S: Prostate cancer. Epidemiology and etiology. In Das S, Crawford ED, eds: Cancer of the prostate, New York, 1993, Marcel Dekker.
5. Nomura AMY, Kolonel LN: Prostate cancer: a current perspective, Am J Epidemiol 13:200-227, 1991.
6. Scardino PT: Early detection of prostate cancer, Urol Clin North Am 16:635-655, 1989.
7. McNeal JE, Bostwick DG: Intraductal dysplasia: a premalignant lesion of the prostate, Hum Pathol 17:64-71, 1986.
8. Bostwick DG, Brawer MK: Prostatic intra-epithelial neoplasia and early invasion in prostate cancer, Cancer 59:788-794, 1987.
9. Kovi J, Mostofi FK, Heshmat MY et al: Large acinar atypical hyperplasia and carcinoma of the prostate, Cancer 61:555-561, 1988.
10. Sakr WA, Haas GP, Cassin BJ et al: The frequency of carcinoma and intraepithelial neoplasia of the prostate in young male patients, J Urol 150:379-385, 1993.
11. Drago JR, Mostofi FK, Lee F: Introductory remarks and workshop summary, Urology 34(suppl):2-3, 1989.
12. McNeal JE, Villers A, Redwine EA et al: Microcarcinoma in the prostate: its association with duct-acinar dysplasia, Hum Pathol 22:644-652, 1991.
13. McNeal JE, Alroy J, Leav I et al: Immunohistochemical evidence for impaired cell differentiation in the premalignant phase of prostate carcinogenesis, Am J Clin Pathol 90:23-32, 1988.
14. Graham SD Jr, Bostwick DG, Hoisaeter A et al: Report of the committee on staging and pathology, Cancer 70(suppl):359-361, 1992.
15. Bostwick DG: High-grade prostatic intraepithelial neoplasia: the most likely precursor of prostate cancer, Cancer 75:1823-1836, 1995.
16. Bostwick DG, Amin MB, Dundore P et al: Architectural patterns of high-grade prostatic intraepithelial neoplasia, Hum Pathol 24:298-310, 1993.
17. Kovi J, Jackson MA, Heshmat MY: Ductal spread in prostatic carcinoma, Cancer 56:1566-1573, 1985.
18. Qian J, Wollan P, Bostwick DG: The extent and multicentricity of high-grade prostatic intraepithelial neoplasia in clinically localized prostatic adenocarcinoma, Hum Pathol, 1996 (in press).
19. De La Torre, Haggman M, Brandstedt S et al: Prostatic intraepithelial neoplasia and invasive carcinoma in total prostatectomy specimens: distribution, volume and DNA ploidy, Br J Urol 72:207-213, 1993.
20. Humphrey PA, Frazier HA, Paulson DF et al: Extent of severe dysplasia in the prostate is inversely related to pathologic stage, Mod Pathol 5:54A, 1992.
21. Troncosco P, Babaian RJ, Ro JY et al: Prostatic intraepithelial neoplasia and invasive prostatic adenocarcinoma in cystoprostatectomy specimens, Urology 24(suppl):52-56, 1989.
22. Tsukamoto T, Kumamoto Y, Masumori N et al: Studies on incidental carcinoma of the prostate, Nippon Hinyokika Gakkai Zasshi 81:1343-1350, 1990.
23. Sentinelli S, Rondanelli E: La neoplasia intraepiteliale prostatica: una nuova lesione displastica della prostata, Pathologica 81:127-137, 1989.
24. Kastendieck H, Helpap B: Prostatic "dysplasia/atypical hyperplasia," Urology 24(suppl):28-42, 1989.
25. Quinn BD, Cho KR, Epstein JI: Relationship of severe dysplasia to stage B adenocarcinoma of the prostate, Cancer 65:2328-2337, 1990.
26. Lee F, Torp-Pedersen ST, Carroll JT et al: Use of transrectal ultrasound and prostate-specific antigen in diagnosis of prostatic intraepithelial neoplasia, Urology 24(suppl):4-8, 1989.
27. Brawer MK, Peehl DM, Stamey TA et al: Keratin immunoreactivity in benign and neoplastic human prostate, Cancer Res 45:3665-3669, 1985.
28. O'Malley FP, Grignon DJ, Shum DT: Usefulness of immunoperoxidase staining with high-molecular-weight cytokeratin in the differential diagnosis of small-acinar lesions of the prostate gland, Virchows Arch A Pathol Anat Histopathol 417:191-196, 1990.
29. Hedrick L, Epstein JI: Use of keratin 903 as an adjunct in the diagnosis of prostate carcinoma, Am J Surg Pathol 13:389-396, 1989.
30. Montironi R, Scarpelli M, Sisti S et al: Quantitative analysis of prostatic intra-epithelial neoplasia on tissue sections, Anal Quant Cytol Histol 12:366-372, 1990.

31. Montironi R, Bracciſchi A, Matera G et al: Quantitation of prostatic intra-epithelial neoplasia. Analysis of the nuclear size, number and location, Pathol Res Pract 187:307-314, 1990.
32. Petein M, Michel P, Van Velthoven R et al: Morphonuclear relationship between prostatic intraepithelial neoplasia and cancers as assessed by digital cell image analysis, Am J Clin Pathol 96:628-634, 1991.
33. Sesterhenn IA, Becker RL, Avallone FA et al: Image analysis of nucleoli and nucleolar organizer regions in prostatic hyperplasia, intraepithelial neoplasia, and prostatic carcinoma, J Urogen Pathol 1:61-74, 1991.
34. Helpap B: Observations on the number, size and location of nucleoli in hyperplastic and neoplastic prostatic disease, Histopathology 13:203-211, 1988.
35. Min KW, Jin J-K, Blank J et al: AgNOR in the human prostatic gland, Am J Clin Pathol 95:508, 1990.
36. Layfield LJ, Goldstein NS: Morphometric analysis of borderline atypia in prostatic aspiration biopsy specimen, Anal Quant Cytol Histol 13:288-292, 1991.
37. Deschenes J, Weidner N: Nucleolar organizer regions (NOR) in hyperplastic and neoplastic prostate disease, Am J Surg Pathol 14:1148-1155, 1990.
38. Humphrey PA: Mucin in severe dysplasia in the prostate, Surg Pathol 4:137-143, 1991.
39. Nagle RB, Brawer MK, Kittelson J et al: Phenotypic relationships of prostatic intraepithelial neoplasia to invasive prostatic carcinoma, Am J Pathol 138:119-128, 1991.
40. Perlman EJ, Epstein JI: Blood group antigen expression in dysplasia and adenocarcinoma of the prostate, Am J Surg Pathol 14:810-818, 1990.
41. McNeal JE, Leav I, Alroy J et al: Differential lectin staining of central and peripheral zones of the prostate and alterations in dysplasia, Am J Clin Pathol 89:41-48, 1988.
42. Bostwick DG, Dousa MK, Crawford BG et al: Neuroendocrine differentiation in prostatic intraepithelial neoplasia and adenocarcinoma, Am J Surg Path 18:1240-1246, 1994.
43. Myers RB, Srivastava S, Oelschlager DK et al: Expression of p160erbB-3 and p185erbB-2 in prostatic intraepithelial neoplasia and prostatic adenocarcinoma, J Natl Cancer Inst 86:1140-1144, 1994.
44. Colombel M, Symmans F, Gil S et al: Detection of the apoptosis-suppressing oncoprotein bcl-2 in hormone-refractory human prostate cancers, Am J Pathol 143:390-400, 1993.
45. Maygarden SJ, Strom S, Ware JL: Localization of epidermal growth factor receptor by immunohistochemical methods in human prostatic carcinoma, prostatic intraepithelial neoplasia, and benign hyperplasia, Arch Pathol Lab Med 116:269-273, 1992.
46. Boag AH, Young ID: Immunohistochemical analysis of type IV collagenase expression in prostatic hyperplasia and adenocarcinoma, Mod Pathol 6:65-68, 1993.
47. Montironi R, Magi Galluzzi C, Scarpelli M et al: Occurrence of cell death (apoptosis) in prostatic intra-epithelial neoplasia, Virchows Arch A Pathol Anat Histopathol 423:351-357, 1993.
48. Gainnulis I, Montironi R, Galluzzi CM et al: Frequency and location of mitoses in prostatic intraepithelial neoplasia (PIN), Anticancer Res 13:2447-2452, 1993.
49. Montironi R, Magi Galluzzi C, Diamanti L et al: Prostatic intra-epithelial neoplasia. Expression and location of proliferating cell nuclear antigen (PCNA) in epithelial, endothelial and stromal nuclei, Virchows Arch A Pathol Anat Histopathol 422:185-192, 1993.
50. Baretton GB, Vogt T, Blasenbreu S et al: Comparison of DNA ploidy in prostatic intraepithelial neoplasia and invasive carcinoma of the prostate: an image cytometric study, Hum Pathol 25:506-513, 1994.
51. Sakr WA, Haas GP, Drozdowicz SM et al: Nuclear DNA content of prostatic carcinoma and intraepithelial neoplasia (PIN) in young males. An image analysis study, Mod Pathol 5:58A, 1992.
52. Amin MB, Schultz DS, Zarbo RJ et al: Computerized static DNA ploidy analysis of prostatic intraepithelial neoplasia, Arch Pathol Lab Med 117:794-798, 1993.
53. Weinberg DS, Weidner N: Concordance of DNA content between prostatic intraepithelial neoplasia and concomitant carcinoma. Evidence that prostatic intraepithelial neoplasia is a precursor of invasive prostatic carcinoma, Arch Pathol Lab Med 117:1132-1137, 1993.
54. Crissman JD, Sakr WA, Hussein ME et al: DNA quantitation of intraepithelial neoplasia and invasive carcinoma of the prostate, Prostate 22:155-162, 1993.
55. O'Malley F, Grignon D, Keeney M et al: DNA flow cytometric studies of prostatic intraepithelial neoplasia, Mod Pathol 4:50A, 1991.
56. Montironi R, Magi Galluzzi C, Diamanti L et al: Prostatic intra-epithelial neoplasia. Qualitative and quantitative analyses of the blood capillary architecture on thin tissue sections, Pathol Res Pract 189:542-548, 1993.
57. Leav I, Ho SM, Ofner P et al: Biochemical alterations in sex hormone-induced hyperplasia and dysplasia of the dorsolateral prostates of Noble rats, J Natl Cancer Inst 80:1045-1053, 1988.
58. Pollard M: Spontaneous prostate adenocarcinoma in aged germ-free Wistar rats, J Natl Cancer Inst 51:1235, 1973.
59. Isaacs JT: The aging ACI/Seg versus male Copenhagen rat as a model system for the study of prostatic carcinogenesis, Cancer Res 44:1, 1984.
60. Ward JM, Reznick G, Stinson SF et al: Histogenesis and morphology of a naturally occurring prostatic carcinoma in the ACI/Seg HAP BR rat, Lab Invest 43:517, 1980.
61. Shain SA, McCullough B, Nutchuck M et al: Prostate carcinogenesis in the AXC rat, Oncology 34:114, 1977.
62. Pollard M, Luckert PH, Sporn MB: Prevention of primary prostate cancer in Lobund-Wistar rats by N-(4-hydroxyphenyl) retinamide, Cancer Res 51:3610-3611, 1991.
63. Pylkkanen L, Makela S, Valve E et al: Prostatic dysplasia associated with increased expression of c-myc in neonatally estrogenized mice, J Urol 149:1593-1601, 1993.
64. Slayter MV, Anzano MA, Kadomatsu K et al: Histogenesis of induced prostate and seminal vesicle carcinoma in Lobund-Wistar rats: a system for histological scoring and grading, Cancer Res 54:1440-1445, 1994.
65. Ferguson J, Zincke H, Ellison E et al: Decrease of prostatic intraepithelial neoplasia (prostatic intraepithelial neoplasia) following androgen deprivation therapy in patients with stage T3 carcinoma treated by radical prostatectomy, Urology 44:91-95, 1994.

66. Bostwick DG: The pathology of early prostate cancer, CA Cancer J Clin 39:376-393, 1989.
67. Davidson D, Bostwick DG, Qian J et al. Prostatic intraepithelial neoplasia is a risk factor for adenocarcinoma: predictive accuracy in needle biopsies, J Urol 154:1295-1299, 1995.
68. Brawer MK, Bigler SA, Sohlberg OE et al: Significance of prostatic intraepithelial neoplasia on prostate needle biopsy, Urology 38:103-107, 1991.
69. Weinstein MH, Epstein JI: Significance of high-grade prostatic intraepithelial neoplasia on needle biopsy, Hum Pathol 24:624-629, 1993.
70. Park C, Galang C, Johennig P et al: Follow-up aspiration biopsies for dysplasia of the prostate, Lab Invest 60:70A, 1989.
71. Markham CW: Prostatic intraepithelial neoplasia. Detection and correlation with invasive cancer in fine-needle biopsy, Urology 24(suppl):57-61, 1989.
72. Berner A, Danielsen HE, Pettersen EO et al: DNA distribution in the prostate. Normal gland, benign and premalignant lesions, and subsequent adenocarcinomas, Anal Quant Cytol Histol 15:247-252, 1993.
73. Bostwick DG, Qian J, Frankel K: The incidence of high-grade prostatic intraepithelial neoplasia in needle biopsies, J Urol 154:1791-1794, 1995.
74. Shinohara K, Scardino PT, Carter SSC et al: Pathologic basis of the sonographic appearance of the normal and malignant prostate, Urol Clin N Am 16:675-691, 1989.
75. Brawer MK, Lange PH: Prostate-specific antigen and premalignant change. Implications for early detection. CA Cancer J Clin 39:361-375, 1989.
76. Ronnett BM, Carmichael MJ, Carter HB et al: Does high-grade prostatic intraepithelial neoplasia result in elevated serum prostate specific antigen levels? J Urol 150:386-389, 1993.
77. Bostwick DG, Burke HB, Wheeler TM et al: The most promising surrogate endpoint biomarkers for screening candidate chemopreventive compounds for prostatic adenocarcinoma in short-term phase II clinical trials, J Cell Biochem 19(suppl):283-289, 1994.
78. Miller BA, Ries LAG, Hankey BF et al: Cancer statistics review: 1973–1989, NIH publication 92-2789, Bethesda, 1992, National Cancer Institute.
79. Silverberg E: Statistical and epidemiologic data on urologic cancer, Cancer 60:692-717, 1987.
80. Doll R: Geographic variation in cancer incidence: a clue to causation, World J Surg 2:595-602, 1978.
81. Carter BS, Bova GS, Beaty TH et al: Hereditary prostate cancer: epidemiologic and clinical features, J Urol 150:797-802, 1993.
82. Cannon L, Bishop D, Skolnick M et al: Genetic epidemiology of prostate cancer in the Utah Mormon genealogy, Cancer Surv 1:47-69, 1982.
83. Steinberg G, Carter B, Beaty T et al: Family history and the risk of prostate cancer, Prostate 17:337-347, 1990.
84. Keetch D, Catalona W: Familial aspects of prostate cancer: a case-control review, J Urol 145:250A, 1991.
85. Spitz M, Currier R, Fueger J et al: Familial patterns of prostate cancer: a case-control analysis, J Urol 146:1305-1307, 1991.
86. Pienta KJ, Esper PS: Is dietary fat a risk factor for prostate cancer? J Natl Cancer Instit 85:1538-1540, 1993.
87. Giovannucci E, Ascherio A, Rimm E et al: A prospective cohort study of vasectomy and prostate cancer in U.S. men, JAMA 269:873-877, 1993.
88. Giovannucci E, Tosteson TD, Speizer FE et al: A retrospective cohort study of vasectomy and prostate cancer in U.S. men, JAMA 269:878-882, 1993.
89. Culkin DJ, Wheeler JS Jr, Castelli M et al: Carcinoma of the prostate in a 25-year-old man: a case report and review of the literature, J Urol 136:684-686, 1986.
90. Shimada H, Misugi K, Sasaki Y et al: Carcinoma of the prostate in childhood and adolescence: report of a case and review of the literature, Cancer 46:2534-2538, 1980.
91. Bostwick DG: Gleason grading of prostatic needle biopsies: correlation with grade in 316 matched prostatectomies, Am J Surg Pathol 18:796-803, 1994.
92. Terris MK, McNeal JE, Stamey TA: Detection of clinically significant prostate cancer by transrectal ultrasound-guided systematic biopsies, J Urol 148:829-832, 1992.
93. Hammerer P, Huland H, Sparenberg S: Digital rectal examination, imaging, and systematic-sextant biopsy in identifying operable lymph node–negative prostatic carcinoma, Eur Urol 22:281-287, 1992.
94. Stamey TA, Freiha FS, McNeal JE et al: Localized prostate cancer. Relationship of tumor volume to clinical significance for treatment of prostate cancer, Cancer 71:933-938, 1993.
95. Maksem JA, Galang CF, Johenning PW et al: Aspiration biopsy cytology of the prostate. In Bostwick DG, ed: Pathology of the prostate, New York, 1990, Churchill Livingstone.
96. Stilmant MM, Freedlund MC, De La Morenas A et al: Expanded role for fine needle aspiration of the prostate. A study of 335 specimens, Cancer 63:583-589, 1989.
97. McNeal JE, Price H, Redwine EA et al: Stage A versus stage B adenocarcinoma of the prostate: morphologic comparison and biologic significance, J Urol 139:61-68, 1988.
98. McNeal JE, Redwine EA, Freiha FS et al: Zonal distribution of prostatic adenocarcinoma. Correlation with histologic pattern and direction of spread, Am J Surg Pathol 12:897-906, 1988.
99. Rohr LR: Incidental adenocarcinoma in transurethral resection of the prostate. Partial versus complete microscopic examination, Am J Surg Pathol 11:53-58, 1987.
100. Murphy WM, Dean PJ, Brasfield JA et al: Incidental carcinoma of the prostate. How much sampling is adequate? Am J Surg Pathol 10:170-176, 1986.
101. Eble JN, Tejada E: Cost implications of sampling strategies for prostatic transurethral resection specimens: analysis of 549 cases, Am J Clin Pathol 85:382, 1986.
102. Vollmer RT: Prostate cancer and chip specimens: complete versus partial sampling, Hum Pathol 17:285-290, 1986.
103. Henson DE, Hutter RVP, Farrow GM: Practice protocol for the examination of specimens removed from patients with carcinoma of the prostate gland, Arch Pathol Lab Med 118:779-783, 1994.
104. Bostwick DG, Myers RP, Oesterling JE: Staging of prostate cancer, Semin Surg Oncol 10:60-73, 1994.
105. Hall GS, Kramer CE, Epstein JI: Evaluation of radical prostatectomy specimens: a comparative analysis of sampling methods, Am J Surg Pathol. 16:315-324, 1992.

106. Schmid H-P, McNeal JE: An abbreviated standard procedure for accurate tumor volume estimation in prostate cancer, Am J Surg Pathol 16:184-191, 1992.
107. Haggman M, Norberg M, de la Torre M et al: Characterization of localized prostatic cancer: distribution, grading and pT-staging in radical prostatectomy specimens, Scand J Urol Nephrol 27:7-13, 1993.
108. Humphrey PA, Vollmer RT: Intraglandular tumor extent and prognosis in prostatic carcinoma: application of a grid method to prostatectomy specimens, Hum Pathol 21:799-804, 1990.
109. Wheeler TM: Anatomic considerations in carcinoma of the prostate, Urol Clin N Am 16:623-634, 1989.
110. Gleason DF: Histologic Grading of Prostatic Carcinoma. In Bostwick DG, ed: Pathology of the Prostate, New York, 1990, Churchill Livingstone.
111. Bostwick DG, Srigley J, Grignon D et al: Atypical adenomatous hyperplasia of the prostate: morphologic criteria for its distinction from well-differentiated carcinoma, Hum Pathol 24:819-832, 1993.
112. Bastacky SI, Walsh PC, Epstein JI: Relationship between perineural tumor invasion on needle biopsy and radical prostatectomy capsular penetration in clinical stage B adenocarcinoma of the prostate, Am J Surg Pathol 17:336-341, 1993.
113. Hasson MO, Maksem J: The prostatic perineural space and its relation to tumor spread. An ultrastructural study, Am J Surg Pathol 4:143-148, 1980.
114. McIntire TL, Franzina DA: The presence of benign prostate glands in perineural spaces, J Urol 135:507-509, 1986.
115. Epstein JI, Fynheer J: Acid mucin in the prostate: can it differentiate adenosis from adenocarcinoma? Hum Pathol 23:1321-1325, 1992.
116. Goldstein, N, Qian J, Bostwick DG: Mucin expression in atypical adenomatous hyperplasia of the prostate, Hum Pathol 26:887-891, 1995.
117. Ro JY, Grignon DJ, Troncoso P et al: Mucin in prostatic adenocarcinoma, Semin Diagn Pathol 5:273-283, 1988.
118. Humphrey PA: Mucin in severe dysplasia in the prostate, Surg Pathol 4:137-143, 1991.
119. Holmes EJ: Crystalloids of prostatic carcinoma: relationship to Bence-Jones crystals, Cancer 29:2073-2080, 1977.
120. Del Rosario AD, Bui HX, Abdulla M et al: Sulfur-rich prostatic intraluminal crystalloids: a surgical pathologic and electron probe x-ray microanalytic study, Hum Pathol 24:1159-1167, 1993.
121. McNeal JE, Alroy J, Villers A et al: Mucinous differentiation in prostatic adenocarcinoma, Hum Pathol 22:979-988, 1991.
122. Bostwick DG, Wollan P, Adlakha K: Collagenous micronodules in prostate cancer: a specific but infrequent diagnostic finding, Arch Pathol Lab Med 119:444-447, 1995.
123. Bahnson RR, Dresner SM, Gooding W et al: Incidence and prognostic significance of lymphatic and vascular invasion in radical prostatectomy specimens, Prostate 15:149-155, 1989.
124. Napalkov P, Watts L, Gansler T et al: Microvascular invasion of the seminal vesicles in adenocarcinoma of the prostate: prognostic value, Prostate, 1996 (in press).
125. Bostwick DG, Dundore PA: Biopsy Pathology of the Prostate, London, 1996, Chapman-Hall (in press).
126. Amin MB, Schultz DS, Zarbo RJ: Analysis of cribriform morphology in prostate neoplasia using antibody to high molecular weight cytokeratins, Arch Pathol Lab Med 118:260-264, 1994.
127. Broders AC: Carcinoma grading and practical application, Arch Pathol Lab Med 2:376-381, 1926.
128. Gaeta JF, Asirwatham JE, Miller G et al: Histologic grading of primary prostatic cancer: a new approach to an old problem, J Urol 123:689-693, 1980.
129. Gleason DF: Classification of prostatic carcinomas, Cancer Chemother Rep 50:125-128, 1966.
130. Mellinger GT, Gleason D, Bailar J III: The histology and prognosis of prostatic Cancer, J Urol 97:331-333, 1967.
131. Gleason D, Mellinger G, Veterans Administration Cooperative Urological Research Group: Prediction of prognosis for prostatic adenocarcinoma by combined histological grading and clinical staging, J Urol 111:58-64, 1974.
132. Gleason D: Histologic grading and clinical staging of carcinoma of the prostate. In Tannenbaum M, ed: Urologic Pathology: The Prostate, Philadelphia, 1977, Lea & Febiger.
133. Gleason DF: Atypical hyperplasia, benign hyperplasia, and well-differentiated adenocarcinoma of the prostate, Am J Surg Pathol 9:53-67, 1985.
134. Gleason DF: Histologic grading of prostate cancer: a perspective, Hum Pathol 23:273-279, 1992.
135. Mostofi FK: Grading of prostatic carcinoma, Cancer Chemotherapy Reports Part I. 59:111-117, 1975.
136. Utz DC, Farrow GM: Pathologic differentiation and prognosis of prostatic carcinoma, JAMA 209:1701-1705, 1969.
137. Murphy GP, Whitmore WF: A report of the workshop on the current status of the histologic grading of prostate cancer, Cancer 44:1490-1494, 1979.
138. Böcking A, Kiehn J, Heinzel-Wach M: Combined histologic grading of prostatic carcinoma, Cancer 50:288-294, 1982.
139. Brawn PN, Ayala AG, von Eschenbach AC et al: Histologic grading study of a new system and comparison with other methods. A preliminary study, Cancer 49:525-532, 1982.
140. Schroeder FH, Blom JHM, Hop WCJ et al: Grading of prostatic cancer: I. An analysis of the prognostic significance of single characteristics, Prostate 6:81-100, 1985.
141. Schroeder FH, Blom JHM, Hop WCJ et al: Grading of prostatic cancer: II. The prognostic significance of the presence of multiple architectural patterns, Prostate 6:403-415, 1985.
142. Schroeder FH, Hop WCJ, Blom JHM et al: Grading of prostate cancer: III. Multivariate analysis of prognostic parameters, Prostate 7:13-20, 1985.
143. Helpap B: Review of the morphology of prostatic carcinoma with special emphasis on subgrading and prognosis, J Urol Pathol 1:3-19, 1993.
144. Gardner WA Jr, Coffey D, Karr JP et al: A uniform histopathologic grading system for prostate cancer, Hum Pathol 19:119-120, 1988.
145. Aihara M, Wheeler TM, Ohori M et al: Heterogeneity of prostate cancer in radical prostatectomy specimens, Urology 43:60-66, 1994.
146. O'Malley FP, Grignon DJ, Keeney M et al: DNA heterogeneity in prostatic adenocarcinoma. A DNA flow cytometric mapping study with whole organ sections of prostate, Cancer 71:2797-2802, 1993.

147. Kucuk O, Demirer T, Gilman-Sachs A et al: Intratumor heterogeneity of DNA ploidy and correlations with clinical stage and histologic grade in prostate cancer, J Surg Oncol 54:171-174, 1993.
148. Jones EC, McNeal J, Bruchovsky N et al: DNA content in prostatic adenocarcinoma. A flow cytometry study of the predictive value of aneuploidy for tumor volume, percentage gleason grade 4 and 5, and lymph node metastases, Cancer 66:752-757, 1990.
149. Konchuba AM, Schellhammer PF, Kolm P et al: Deoxyribonucleic acid cytometric analysis of prostate core biopsy specimens—relationship to serum prostate specific antigen and prostatic acid phosphatase, clinical stage and histopathology, J Urol 150:115-119, 1993.
150. Wu WJ, Huang MS, Wang HJ et al: Flow cytometric DNA analysis of advanced prostatic adenocarcinoma, Kaohsiung J Med Sci 9:122-130, 1993.
151. Al-Abadi H, Nagel R: Nuclear DNA analysis: DNA heterogeneity in the monitoring of patients with locally advanced prostatic carcinoma, Eur Urol 22:303-310, 1992.
152. Bibbo M, Kim DH, Galera-Davidson G et al: Architectural, morphometric and photometric features and their relationship to the main subjective diagnostic clues in the grading of prostatic cancer, Anal Quant Cytol Histol 12:85-90, 1990.
153. Bibbo M, Bartels PH, Pfeifer T et al: Belief network for grading prostate lesions, Anal Quant Cytol Histol 15:124-135, 1993.
154. Blom JH, Ten Kate FJ, Schroeder FH et al: Morphometrically estimated variation in nuclear size. A useful tool in grading prostatic cancer, Urol Res 18:93-99, 1990.
155. Robutti F, Pilato FP, Betta P-G: A new method of grading malignancy of prostate carcinoma using quantitative microscopic nuclear features, Pathol Res Pract 185:701-703, 1989.
156. Schultz DS, Harry T, Wong KL et al: Computer-assisted grading of adenocarcinoma in prostatic aspirates, Anal Quant Cytol Histol 12:91-97, 1990.
157. Irinopoulou T, Rigaut JP, Benson MC: Toward objective prognostic grading of prostatic carcinoma using image analysis, Anal Quant Cytol Histol 15:341-344, 1993.
158. Aragona F, Franco V, Rodolico V et al: Interactive computerized morphometric analysis of the differential diagnosis between dysplasia and well differentiated adenocarcinoma of the prostate, Urol Res 17:35-40, 1989.
159. Diamond DA, Berry SJ, Jewett HJ et al: A new method to assess metastatic potential of human prostate cancer: relative nuclear roundness, J Urol 128:729-734, 1982.
160. Epstein JI, Berry SJ, Eggleston JC: Nuclear roundness factor. A predictor of progression in untreated stage A2 prostate cancer, Cancer 54:1666-1671, 1984.
161. Mohler JL, Partin AW, Coffey DS: Correlation of prognosis to nuclear roundness and to flow cytometric light scatter, Anal Quant Cytol Histol 9:156-164, 1987.
162. Mohler JL, Partin AW, Lohr WD et al: Nuclear roundness factor measurement for assessment of prognosis of patients with prostatic carcinoma. I. Testing of a digitization system, J Urol 139:1080-1084, 1988.
163. Mohler JL, Partin AW, Epstein JI et al: Nuclear roundness factor measurement for assessment of prognosis of patients with prostatic carcinoma. II. Standardization of methodology for histologic sections, J Urol 139:1085-1090, 1988.
164. Partin AW, Walsh AC, Pitcock RV et al: A comparison of nuclear morphometry and Gleason grade as a predictor of prognosis in stage A2 prostate cancer: a critical analysis, J Urol 142:1254-1258, 1989.
165. Partin AW, Steinberg GD, Pitcock RV et al: Use of nuclear morphometry, gleason histologic scoring, clinical stage, and age to predict disease-free survival among patients with prostate cancer, Cancer 70:161-168, 1992.
166. Armas OA, Pizov G, Pitcock RV et al: Nuclear morphology of prostatic carcinoma: comparison of computerized image analysis (CAS 200) versus video planimetry (DynaCELL), Mod Pathol 4:763-767, 1991.
167. Shaeffer J, Tegeler JA, Kuban DA et al: Nuclear roundness factor and local failure from definitive radiation therapy for prostatic carcinoma, Int J Radiat Biol Phys 24:431-434, 1992.
168. Tannenbaum M, Tannenbaum S, DeSnactis PN et al: Prognostic significance of nucleolar surface area in prostate cancer, Urology 19:546-551, 1982.
169. Myers RP, Neves RJ, Farrow GM et al: Nucleolar grading of prostatic adenocarcinoma: light microscopic correlation with disease progression, Prostate 3:423-432, 1982.
170. De Las Morenas A, Siroky MB, Merriam J et al: Prostatic adenocarcinoma: reproducibility and correlation with clinical stages of four grading systems, Hum Pathol 19:595-597, 1988.
171. Oesterling JE, Brendler CB, Epstein JI et al: Correlation of clinical stage, serum prostatic acid phosphatase and preoperative Gleason grade with final pathological stage in 275 patients with clinically localized adenocarcinoma of the prostate, J Urol 138:92-98, 1987.
172. Thomas R, Lewis R, Sarma D et al: Aid to accurate clinical staging—histopathologic grading in prostatic cancer, J Urol 128:726-728, 1982.
173. McNeal JE, Villers AA, Redwine EA et al: Histologic differentiation, cancer volume, and pelvic lymph node metastasis in adenocarcinoma of the prostate, Cancer 52:246-251, 1990.
174. McNeal JE, Bostwick DG, Kindrachuk RA et al: Patterns of progression in prostate cancer, Lancet 1:60-63, 1986.
175. Bostwick DG, Graham SD Jr, Napalkov P et al: Staging of early prostate cancer: a proposed tumor volume-based prognostic index, Urology 41:403-411, 1993
176. Bostwick DG: The significance of tumor volume in prostate cancer, Urol Ann 8:1-22, 1994.
177. Gaffney EF, O'Sullivan SN, O'Brien A: A major solid undifferentiated carcinoma pattern correlates with tumor progression in locally advanced prostatic carcinoma, Histopathology 21:249-255, 1992.
178. Egawa S, Go M, Kuwao S et al: Long-term impact of conservative management on localized prostate cancer. A twenty-year experience in Japan, Urology 42:520-526, 1993.
179. Brawn PN: The dedifferentiation of prostatic carcinoma, Cancer 52:246-251, 1983.
180. Cumming JA, Ritchie AW, Goodman CM et al: Dedifferentiation with time in prostate cancer and the influence of treatment on the course of the disease, Br J Urol 65:271-274, 1990.
181. Whittemore AS, Keller JB, Betensky R: Low-grade, latent prostate cancer volume: predictor of clinical cancer incidence? J Natl Cancer Inst 83:1231-1235, 1991.

182. Ten Kate FJW, Gallee MPW, Schmitz PIM et al: Problems in grading of prostatic carcinoma. Interobserver reproducibility of five different grading systems, World J Urol 4:147-152, 1986.
183. Bain G, Koch M, Hanson J: Feasibility of grading prostatic carcinomas, Arch Pathol Lab Med 106:265-267, 1982.
184. Di Loreto C, Fitzpatrick B, Underhill S et al: Correlation between visual clues, objective architectural features and interobserver agreement in prostate cancer, Am J Clin Pathol 96:70-75, 1991.
185. Gallee MP, Ten Kate FJ, Mulder PG et al: Histological grading of prostatic carcinoma in prostatectomy specimens. Comparison of prognostic accuracy of five grading systems, Br J Urol 65:368-375, 1990.
186. Cintra ML, Billis A: Histologic grading of prostatic adenocarcinoma: intraobserver reproducibility of the Mostofi, Gleason and Böcking grading systems, Int Urol Nephrol 23:449-454, 1991.
187. Catalona WJ, Stein AJ, Fair WR: Grading errors in prostatic needle biopsies: relation to the accuracy of tumor grade in predicting pelvic lymph node metastases, J Urol 127:919-922, 1982.
188. Garnett JE, Oyasu R, Grayhack JT: The accuracy of diagnostic biopsy specimens in predicting tumor grades by Gleason's classification of radical prostatectomy specimens, J Urol 131:690-693, 1984.
189. Lange PH, Narayan P: Understaging and undergrading of prostate cancer, Urology 21:113-118, 1983.
190. Mills SE, Fowler JE: Gleason histologic grading of prostatic carcinoma. Correlations between biopsy and prostatectomy specimens, Cancer 57:346-349, 1986.
191. Kastendieck H: Morphologie des Prostatacarcinoms in Stanzbiopsien und totalen Prostatektomien. Untersuchungen zur Frage der Relevanz bioptischer Befundaussagen, Pathologe 2:31-43, 1980.
192. Spires SE, Cibull ML, Wood DP Jr et al: Gleason histologic grading in prostatic carcinoma: correlation of 18-gauge core biopsy with prostatectomy, Arch Pathol Lab Med 118:705-708, 1994.
193. Epstein JI, Steinberg GD: The significance of low-grade prostate cancer on needle biopsy. A radical prostatectomy study of tumor grade, volume, and stage of the biopsied and multifocal tumor, Cancer 66:1927-1932, 1990.
194. Kramer SA, Spahr J, Brendler CB et al: Experience with Gleason's histopathologic grading in prostatic cancer, J Urol 124:223-225, 1980.
195. Kramer SA, Farnham R, Glenn JF et al: Comparative morphology of primary and secondary deposits of prostatic adenocarcinoma, Cancer 48:271-273, 1981.
196. Brawn P, Kuhl D, Johnson C et al: Stage D1 prostate carcinoma. The histologic appearance of nodal metastases and its relationship to survival, Cancer 65:538-543, 1990.
197. Bostwick DG, Egbert BM, Fajardo LF: Radiation injury of the normal and neoplastic prostate, Am J Surg Pathol 6:541-548, 1982.
198. Brawer MK, Bostwick DG: Interpretation of postradiation prostate biopsies. In: Bostwick DG, ed: Pathology of the Prostate, New York, 1990, Churchill Livingstone.
199. Wheeler JA, Zagars GK, Ayala AG: Dedifferentiation of locally recurrent prostate cancer after radiation therapy, Cancer 71:3783-3787, 1993.
200. Dugan TC, Shipley WU, Young RH et al: Biopsy after external beam radiation therapy for adenocarcinoma of the prostate: correlation with original histological grade and current prostate specific antigens levels, J Urol 146:1313-1316, 1991.
201. Helpap B, Koch V: Histological and immunohistochemical findings of prostatic carcinoma after external or interstitial radiotherapy, J Cancer Res Clin Oncol 117:608-614, 1991.
202. Siders DB, Lee F: Histologic changes of irradiated prostatic carcinoma diagnosed by transrectal ultrasound, Hum Pathol 23:344-351, 1992.
203. Kabalin JN: Biopsy after external beam radiation therapy for adenocarcinoma of the prostate: correlation with original histological grade and current prostate specific antigen levels, J Urol 148:1565-1566, 1992 (letter).
204. Kiesling VJ, Friedman HI, McAninch JW et al: The ultrastructural changes of prostatic adenocarcinoma following external beam radiation therapy, J Urol 122:633-636, 1979.
205. Böcking A, Auffermann W: Cytological grading of therapy-induced tumor regression in prostatic carcinoma: proposal of a new system, Diagn Cytopathol 3:108-111, 1987.
206. Schmeller NT, Jocham D, Staehler G et al: Cytologic regression grading of hormone-treated prostatic cancer, Prostate 9:1-7, 1986.
207. Tetu B, Srigley JR, Boivin J et al:. Effect of combination endocrine therapy (LHRH agonist and flutamide) on normal prostate and prostatic adenocarcinoma, Am J Surg Pathol 15:111-120, 1991.
208. Murphy WM, Soloway MS, Barrows GH: Pathologic changes associated with androgen deprivation therapy for prostate cancer, Cancer 68:821-828, 1991.
209. Ellison E, Chuang S-S, Zincke H et al: Prostate adenocarcinoma following androgen deprivation therapy. A comparative study of morphology, morphometry, immunohistochemistry, and DNA ploidy, Pathol Case Studies 1996 (in press).
210. Hellström M, Häggman M, Brändstedt S et al: Histopathological changes in androgen-deprived localized prostatic cancer. A study in total prostatectomy specimens, Eur Urol 24:461-465, 1993.
211. Smith DM, Murphy WM: Histologic changes in prostate carcinomas treated with leuprolide (luteinizing hormone-releasing hormone effect). Distinction from poor tumor differentiation, Cancer 73:1472-1744, 1994.
212. Civantos F, Marcial MA, Banks ER et al: Pathology of androgen deprivation therapy in prostatic carcinoma. A comparative study of 173 patients, Cancer 75:1634-1641, 1995.
213. Hanks GE, D'Amico A, Epstein BE et al: Prostatic-specific antigen doubling times in patients with prostate cancer: a potentially useful reflection of tumor doubling time, Int J Radiat Oncol Biol Phys 27:125-127, 1993.
214. Schmid HP, McNeal JE, Starney TA: Observations on the doubling time of prostate cancer. The use of serial prostate-specific antigen in patients with untreated disease as a measure of increasing cancer volume, Cancer 71:2031-2040, 1993.
215. Nielsen K, Overgaard J, Bentzen SM et al: Histological grade, DNA ploidy and mean nuclear volume as prognostic factors in prostatic cancer, APMIS 101:614-620, 1993.
216. Humphrey PA, Walther PJ, Currin SM et al: Histologic grade, DNA ploidy, and intraglandular tumor extent as indicators of tumor progression of clinical stage B prostatic carcinoma, Am J Surg Pathol 15:1165-1170, 1991.

217. Anscher MS, Prosnitz LR: Multivariate analysis of factors predicting local relapse after radical prostatectomy—possible indications for postoperative radiotherapy, Int J Radiat Oncol 21:941-947, 1991.
218. Wirth MP, Muller HA, Manseck A et al: Value of nuclear DNA ploidy patterns in patients with prostate cancer after radical prostatectomy, Eur Urol 20:248-252, 1991.
219. Voges GE, Eigner EB, Ross W et al: Pathologic parameters and flow cytometric ploidy analysis in predicting recurrence in carcinoma of the prostate, Eur Urol 24:132-139, 1993.
220. Epstein JI, Pizov G, Walsh PC: Correlation of pathologic findings with progression after radical retropubic prostatectomy, Cancer 71:3582-3593, 1993.
221. Cheng WS, Frydenberg M, Bergstralh EJ et al: Radical prostatectomy for pathologic stage C prostate cancer: influence of pathologic variables and adjuvant treatment on disease outcome, Urology 42:283-291, 1993.
222. Pisansky TM, Cha SS, Earle JD et al: Prostate-specific antigen as a pretherapy prognostic factor in patients treated with radiation therapy for clinically localized prostate cancer, J Clin Oncol 11:2158-2166, 1993.
223. Zagars GK, von Eschenbach AC, Ayala AG: Prognostic factors in prostate cancer. Analysis of 874 patients treated with radiation therapy, Cancer 72:1709-1725, 1993.
224. Van den Ouden D, Tribukait B, Blom JH et al: Deoxyribonucleic acid ploidy of core biopsies and metastatic lymph nodes of prostate cancer patients: impact on time to progression, J Urol 150:400-406, 1993.
225. Chodak GW, Thisted RA, Gerber GS et al: Results of conservative management of clinically localized prostate cancer, New Engl J Med 330:242-248, 1994.
226. Forsslund G, Esposti PL, Nilsson B et al: The prognostic significance of nuclear DNA content in prostatic carcinoma, Cancer 69:1432-1439, 1992.
227. Visakorpi T, Kallioniemi OP, Heikkinen A et al: Small subgroup of aggressive, highly proliferative prostatic carcinomas defined by p53 accumulation, J Natl Cancer Inst 84:883-887, 1992.
228. Ritter MA, Messing EM, Shanahan TG et al: Prostate-specific antigen as a predictor of radiotherapy response and patterns of failure in localized prostate cancer, J Clin Oncol 10:1208-1217, 1992.
229. Bagshaw MA, Kaplan ID, Cox RC: Prostate cancer. Radiation therapy for localized disease, Cancer 71:939-952, 1993.
230. Tribukait B: Nuclear deoxyribonucleic acid determination in patients with prostate carcinomas: clinical research and application, Eur Urol 23:64-76, 1993.
231. Cadeddu JA, Pearson JD, Partin AW et al: Relationship between changes in prostate-specific antigen and prognosis of prostate cancer, Urology 42:383-389, 1993.
232. Humphrey PA, Frazier HA, Vollmer RT et al: Stratification of pathologic features in radical prostatectomy specimens that are predictive of elevated initial postoperative serum prostate-specific antigen levels, Cancer 71:1821-1827, 1993.
233. McNeal JE: Prostatic microcarcinomas in relation to cancer origin and the evolution to clinical cancer, Cancer 71:984-991, 1993.
234. Cantrell BB, DeKlerk DP, Eggleston JC et al: Pathological factors that influence prognosis in stage A prostatic cancer: the influence of extent versus grade, J Urol 125:516-520, 1981.
235. Lowe BA, Listrom MB: Incidental carcinoma of the prostate: an analysis of the predictors of progression, J Urol 140:1340-1344, 1988.
236. Blackwell KL, Bostwick DG, Zincke H et al: Combining prostate specific antigen with cancer and gland volume to predict more reliably pathologic stage: the influence of prostate specific antigen cancer density, J Urol 151:1565-1570, 1994.
237. Partin AW, Carter HB, Chan DW et al: Prostate specific antigen in the staging of localized prostate cancer: influence of tumor differentiation, tumor volume, and benign hyperplasia, J Urol 143:747-752, 1990.
238. Tomita T, Dalton T, Kwok S et al: Profile of prostatic-specific antigen in prostatic carcinomas, Mod Pathol 6:259-264, 1993.
239. Barzel W, Bean M, Hilaris B et al: Prostatic adenocarcinoma: relationship of grade and local extent to pattern of metastases, J Urol 118:278-282, 1977.
240. Paulson D, Piserchia P, Garner W: Predictors of lymphatic spread in prostatic carcinoma: uro-oncology Research Group study, J Urol 123:697-699, 1980.
241. Fournier GR Jr, Narayan P: Re-evaluation of the need for pelvic lymphadenectomy in low grade prostate cancer, Br J Urol 72:484-488, 1993.
242. Greene DR, Wheeler TM, Egawa S et al: Relationship between clinical stage and histological zone of origin in early prostate cancer: morphometric analysis, Br J Urol 68:499-509, 1991.
243. McNeal JE: Cancer volume and site of origin of adenocarcinoma in the prostate: relationship to local and distant spread, Hum Pathol 23:258-266, 1992.
244. Lee F, Siders DB, Torp-Pedersen ST et al: Prostate cancer: transrectal ultrasound and pathology comparison. A preliminary study of outer gland (peripheral and central zones) and inner gland (transition zone) cancer, Cancer 67:1132-1142, 1991.
245. Mostofi FK, Sesterhenn I, Sobin LH: Histological typing of prostate tumors. Internation histologic classification of tumours, no. 22. Geneva, 1980, World Health Organization.
246. Mostofi FK, Price EB Jr: Tumors of the Male Genital System, Fascicle 8, second series, Atlas of Tumor Pathology. Washington, DC, 1973, Armed Forces Institute of Pathology.
247. Amin MB, Ro JY, Ayala AG: The clinical relevance of histologic variants of prostate cancer, Cancer Bull 45:403-410, 1993.
248. Dhom G: Unusual prostatic carcinomas, Pathol Res Pract 186:28-36, 1990.
249. Melicow MM, Pachter MR: Endometrial carcinoma of prostatic utricle (uterus masculinus), Cancer 20:1715-1721, 1967.
250. Melicow MM, Tannenbaum M: Endometrial carcinoma of uterus masculinus (prostatic utricle). Report of 6 cases, J Urol 106:892-902, 1971.
251. Bostwick DG, Kindrachuk RW, Rouse RV: Prostatic adenocarcinoma with endometrioid features, Am J Surg Pathol 9:595-609, 1985.
252. August CZ, Oyasu R: Adenocarcinoma of the prostate gland. A spectrum of differentiation, Arch Pathol Lab Med 107:501-502, 1983.

253. Bates, HR Jr, Thornton JL: Adenocarcinoma of primary prostatic ducts and utricle, Arch Pathol Lab Med 96:207, 1973.
254. Belter LF, Dodson AI Jr: Papillomatosis and papillary adenocarcinoma of prostatic ducts. A case report, J Urol 104:880-883, 1970.
255. Cantrell BB, Leifer G, DeKlerk DP et al: Papillary adenocarcinoma of the prostatic urethra with clear-cell appearance, Cancer 48:2661-2667, 1981.
256. Carney JA, Kelalis PP: Endometrial carcinoma of the prostatic utricle, Am J Clin Pathol 60:565-573, 1973.
257. Drake WM, Burrows S: Papillary carcinoma of prostatic ducts, Urology 3:621-623, 1974.
258. Dube VE, Farrow GM, Greene LF: Prostatic adenocarcinoma of ductal origin, Cancer 32:402-409, 1973.
259. Greene LF, Farrow GM, Ravits JM et al: Prostatic adenocarcinoma of ductal origin, J Urol 121:303-305, 1979.
260. Merchant RF, Grahm AR, Bucher WC Jr et al: Endometrial carcinoma of prostatic utricle with osseous metastases, Urology 8:169-173, 1976.
261. Satter EJ, Blumenfeld CM: Endometrial carcinoma of the prostatic utricle, J Urol 112:505-506, 1974.
262. Tannenbaum M: Endometrial tumors and or associated carcinomas of prostate, Urology 6:372-375, 1975.
263. Walter AN, Mills SE, Fechner RE et al: "Endometrial" adenocarcinoma of the prostatic urethra arising in a villous polyp. A light microscopic and immunoperoxidase study, Arch Pathol Lab Med 106:624-627,1982.
264. Young BW, Lagios MD: Endometrial (papillary) carcinoma of the prostatic utricle-response to orchiectomy, Cancer 32:1293-1300, 1973.
265. Zaloudek C, Williams JW, Kempson RL: "Endometrial" adenocarcinoma of the prostate. A distinctive tumor of probable prostatic duct origin, Cancer 37:2255-2262, 1976.
266. Kuhajda FP, Gipson T, Mendelsohn G: Papillary adenocarcinomas of the prostate: an immunohistochemical study, Cancer 54:1328-1332, 1984.
267. Cueva C, Urdiales J, Nogales F et al: Papillary endometrioid carcinoma of the prostate, Br J Urol 61:1988.
268. Ro JY, Ayala AG, Wishow KI et al: Prostatic duct adenocarcinoma with endometrioid features: immunohistochemical and electron microscopic study, Semin Diagn Pathol 5:301-311, 1988.
269. Walther MM, Massar V, Harruff HC et al: Endometrial carcinoma of the prostatic utricle: a tumor of prostatic origin, J Urol 134:769-773, 1985.
270. Epstein JI, Woodruff JM: Adenocarcinoma of the prostate with endometrioid features: a light microscopic and immunohistochemical study of ten cases, Cancer 57:111-119, 1986.
271. Christenson WN, Steinberg C, Walsh PC et al: Prostatic duct adenocarcinoma: findings at radical prostatectomy, Cancer 67:2118-2124, 1991.
272. Keith RL, Flegel G: Endometrial carcinoma of the prostatic utricle: report of a case, J Am Osteopath Assoc 82:551-553, 1983.
273. Sufrin G, Gaeta J, Staubitz WJ et al: Endometrial carcinoma of prostate, Urology 27:18-23, 1986.
274. Rotterdam HZ, Melicow MM: Double primary prostatic adenocarcinoma, Urology 6:245-248, 1975.
275. Scott MB, Goldstein AM, Onofri RC et al: Papillary adenocarcinoma of the prostate, Urology 8:227-230, 1976.
276. Walther MM: Endometrial carcinoma of prostate, Urology 27:574, 1986 (letter).
277. Wernert N, Luchtrath H, Seeliger H et al: Papillary carcinoma of the prostate, location, morphology, and immunohistochemistry: the histogenesis and entity of so-called endometrioid carcinoma, Prostate 10:123-132, 1987.
278. Witters S, Moerman P, Bussche LV et al: Papillary adenocarcinoma of the prostatic urethra, Eur Urol 12:143-146, 1986.
279. Hoang C, Wasse M, Cortesse A et al: Adenocarcinome papillaire "endometrioide" du col vesical: microscopie optique et electronique et immunohistochimie, Ann Pathol 5:125-129, 1985.
280. Lee SS: Endometrioid adenocarcinoma of the prostate. A clinicopathologic and immunohistochemical study, J Surg Oncol 55:235-238, 1994.
281. Aydin F: Endometrioid adenocarcinoma of prostatic urethra presenting with anterior urethral implantation, Urology 41:91-95, 1993.
282. Butterick JD, Schnitzer B, Abell MR: Ectopic prostatic tissue in urethra: a clinicopathological entity and a significant cause of hematuria, J Urol 105:97-104, 1971.
283. Craig JR, Hart WR: Benign polyps with prostatic-type epithelium of the urethra, Am J Clin Pathol 63:343-347, 1975.
284. Eglen DE, Pontius EE: Benign prostatic epithelial polyp of the urethra, J Urol 1312:120-122, 1984.
285. Bhagavan BS, Tiamso EM, Wenk RE et al: Nephrogenic adenoma of the urinary bladder and urethra, Hum Pathol 12:907-916, 1981.
286. Schinella R, Thurm J, Feiner H: Papillary pseudotumor of the prostatic urethra: proliferative papillary urethritis, J Urol 11:38-40, 1974.
287. Dickmen SH, Toker C: Seromucinous gland ectopia within the prostatic stroma, J Urol 109:852-855, 1973.
288. Ro JY, Grignon DJ, Ayala AG et al: Mucinous adenocarcinoma of the prostate gland, J Urol 141:1447-1451, 1989.
289. Krogh J, Lund PG: Mucinous adenocarcinoma of the prostate presenting as a retrovesical cyst, Scand J Urol Nephrol 22:235-236, 1988.
290. Odom DG, Donatucci CF, Dedshon GE: Mucinous adenocarcinoma of the prostate, Hum Pathol 17:863-868, 1986.
291. Chica G, Johnson DE, Ayala AG: Mucinous adenocarcinoma of the prostate, J Urol 118:124-127, 1977.
292. Hsueh Y, Tsung SH: Prostatic mucinous adenocarcinoma, Urology 24:626-628, 1984.
293. Patel RS, Dias R, Fernandes M et al: Adenocarcinoma of the prostate—mucin secreting, NY State J Med 18:936-937, 1981.
294. Elbadawi A, Graig W, Linke CA et al: Prostatic mucinous carcinoma, Urology 13:658-659, 1979.
295. Uyama T, Moriwaki S: Papillary and mucus-forming adenocarcinomas of prostate, Urology 13:432-434, 1979.
296. Proia, AD, McCarty S, Woodard, BH: Prostatic mucinous adenocarcinoma, Am J Surg Pathol 5:701-706, 1981.
297. Alfthan O, Koivuniemi A: Mucinous carcinoma of the prostate, Scand J Urol Nephrol 4:78-80, 1970.
298. Sika JV, Bugkley JJ: Mucus-forming adenocarcinoma of prostate, Cancer 17:949-952, 1964.
299. Bhargava S, Trivedi, Agarwal VK et al: Mucinous adenocarcinoma of prostate, Indian J Cancer 17:64-66, 1980.

300. Epstein JI, Lieberman PH: Mucinous adenocarcinoma of the prostate gland, Am J Surg Pathol 9:299-308, 1985.
301. Ro JY, Grignon DJ, Ayala AG et al: Mucinous adenocarcinoma of the prostate: histochemical and immunohistochemical studies, Hum Pathol 21:593-600, 1990.
302. Van de Voorde W, Poppel HV, Haustermans K et al: Mucin-secreting adenocarcinoma of the prostate with neuroendocrine differentiation and Paneth-like cells, Am J Surg Pathol 18:200-207, 1994.
303. Levine AJ, Foster JD: The relation of mucicarmine staining properties of carcinomas of the prostate to differentiation, metastasis, and prognosis, Cancer 17:21-25, 1964.
304. Franks LM, O'Shea DD, Thompson AER: Mucin in the prostate. A histochemical study in normal glands, latent, clinical, and colloid carcinoma, Cancer 17:983-991, 1964.
305. Hukill PB, Vidone RA: Histochemistry of mucus and other polysaccharides in tumors II. Carcinoma of the prostate, Lab Invest 16:395-406, 1967.
306. Taylor NS: Histochemistry in the diagnosis of early prostatic carcinoma, Hum Pathol 10:513-520, 1979.
307. Dobrogorski OJ, Braunstein H: Histochemical study of staining lipid, glycogen, and mucin in human neoplasms, Am J Clin Pathol 40:435-443, 1963.
308. Foster EA, Levine AJ: Mucin production in metastatic carcinomas, Cancer 16:506-509, 1963.
309. Pinder SE, McMahon RFT: Mucins in prostatic carcinoma, Histopathology 16:43-46, 1990.
310. Tannenbaum M: Mucin-secreting carcinoma of prostate, Urology 5:543-544, 1975.
311. Grignon DJ, O'Malley FP: Mucinous metaplasia in the prostate gland, Am J Surg Pathol 17:287-290, 1993.
312. Ro JY, Ayala AG, Ordonez NG: Intraluminal crystalloids in prostatic adenocarcinoma. Immunohistochemical, electron microscopic, and x-ray microanalytic studies, Cancer 57:2397-2407, 1986.
313. Teichman JMH, Shabaik A, Demby AM: Mucinous adenocarcinoma of the prostate and hormone sensitivity, J Urol 151:701-702, 1994.
314. Ishizu K, Yoshihiro S, Joko K et al: Mucinous adenocarcinoma of the prostate with good response to hormonal therapy: a case report, Acta Urol Jpn 37:1057-1059, 1991.
315. Efros MD, Fischer J, Mallouh C et al: Unusual primary prostatic malignancies, Urology 39:407-411, 1992.
316. Ro JY, El-Naggar A, Ayala AG et al: Signet-ring-cell carcinoma of the prostate, Am J Surg Pathol 12:453-460, 1988.
317. Hejka AG, England DM: Signet ring cell carcinoma of prostate: immunohistochemical and ultrastructural study of a case, Urology 24:155-158, 1989.
318. Uchijima Y, Ito H, Takahashi M et al: Prostate mucinous adenocarcinoma with signet ring cell, Urology 36:267-268, 1990.
319. Remmele W, Weber A, Harding P: Primary signet-ring cell carcinoma of the prostate, Hum Pathol 19:478-480,1988.
320. Kums JJ, van Helsdingen PJ: Signet-ring cell carcinoma of the bladder and the prostate. Report of 4 cases, Urol Int 40:116-121, 1985.
321. Giltman, LI: Signet ring cell adenocarcinoma of the prostate, J Urol 126:134-135, 1981.
322. Alline KM, Cohen MB: Signet-ring cell carcinoma of the prostate, Arch Pathol Lab Med 116:99-102, 1992.
323. Catton PA, Hartwick RWJ, Srigley JR: Prostate cancer presenting with malignant ascites. Signet-ring cell variant of prostatic adenocarcinoma, Urology 39:495-497, 1992.
324. Segawa T, Kakehi Y: Primary signet ring cell adenocarcinoma of the prostate: a case report and literature review, Acta Urol Jpn 39:565-568, 1993.
325. Geurin D, Hasan N, Keen CE: Signet ring cell differentiation in adenocarcinoma of the prostate: a study of five cases, Histopathology 22:367-371, 1993.
326. Smith C, Feddersen RM, Dressler L et al: Signet ring cell adenocarcinoma of prostate, Urology 43:397-400, 1994.
327. Alguacil-Garcia A: Artifactual changes mimicking signet ring cell carcinoma in transurethral prostatectomy specimens, Am J Surg Pathol 10:795-800, 1986.
328. Wick MR, Young RH, Malvesta R et al: Prostatic carcinosarcomas: clinical, histologic, and immunohistochemical data on two cases, with a review of the literature, Am J Clin Pathol 92:131-139, 1989.
329. Shannon RL, Ro JY, Grignon DJ et al: Sarcomatoid carcinoma of the prostate. A clinicopathologic study of 12 cases, Cancer 69:2676-2682, 1992.
330. Lauwers GY, Schevchuk M, Armenakas N et al: Carcinosarcoma of the prostate, Am J Surg Pathol 17:342-349, 1993.
331. Dundore PA, Cheville JC, Nascimento AG et al: Carcinosarcoma of the prostate. Report of 21 cases, Cancer 76:1035-1042, 1995.
332. Aprikian AG, Cordon-Cardo C, Fair WR et al: Characterization of neuroendocrine differentiation in human benign prostate and prostatic adenocarcinoma, Cancer 71:3952-3965, 1993.
333. Berner A, Nesland JM, Waehre H et al: Hormone resistant prostatic adenocarcinoma. An evaluation of prognostic factors in pre- and post-treatment specimens, Br J Cancer 68:380-384, 1993.
334. Di Sant'Agnese PA: Neuroendocrine differentiation in carcinoma of the prostate. Diagnostic, prognostic, and therapeutic implications, Cancer 70:254-268, 1992.
335. Bonkhoff H, Wernert N, Dhom G et al: Relation of endocrine-paracrine cells to cell proliferation in normal, hyperplastic and neoplastic human prostate, Prostate 19:91-98, 1991.
336. Helpap B, Oehler U, Bollmann R: Das endokrin differenzierte Prostatakarzinom. Histologie and Immunohistochemie, Pathologe 11:18-24, 1990.
337. Wernert N, Kern L, Heitz P et al: Morphological and immunohistochemical investigations of the utriculus prostaticus from the fetal period up to adulthood, Prostate 17:19-30, 1990.
338. Davis NS, di Sant'Agnese PA, Ewing JF et al: The neuroendocrine prostate: characterization and quantitation of calcitonin in the human gland, J Urol 142:884-888, 1989.
339. Abrahamsson PA, Wadstrom LB, Alumets J et al: Peptide-hormone- and serotonin-immunoreactive tumour cells in carcinoma of the prostate, Pathol Res Pract 182:298-307, 1987.
340. Abrahamsson PA, Wadstrom LB, Alumets J et al: Peptide-hormone- and serotonin-immunoreactive cells in normal and hyperplastic prostate glands, Pathol Res Pract 181:675-683, 1986.

341. Di Sant'Agnese PA, de Mesy Jensen KL: Human prostatic endocrine-paracrine (APUD) cells: distributional analysis with a comparison of serotonin and neuron-specific enolase immunoreactivity and silver stains, Arch Pathol Lab Med 109:607-612, 1985.
342. Di Sant'Agnese PA, de Mesy Jensen KL: Endocrine-paracrine cells of the prostate and prostatic urethra: an ultrastructural study, Hum Pathol 15:1034-1041, 1984.
343. Cohen RJ, Glezerson G, Haffejee Z et al: Prostatic carcinoma: histological and immunohistological factors affecting prognosis, Br J Urol 66:405-410, 1990.
344. Wright C, Grignon D, Shum D et al: Neuroendocrine differentiation in prostatic adenocarcinoma is not an independent prognostic indicator, Mod Pathol 5:61A, 1992 (abstract).
345. Azumi N, Shibuya H, Ishikura M: Primary prostatic carcinoid tumor with intracytoplasmic prostatic acid phosphatase and prostate-specific antigen, Am J Surg Pathol 8:545-551, 1984.
346. Abrahamsson P-A, Ptak A, Nakada SY et al: Immunohistochemical localization of the androgen receptor in neuroendocrine cells in human prostatic tissue and prostatic carcinoma, Mod Pathol 6:54A, 1993 (abstract).
347. Adlakha H, Bostwick DG: Paneth cell-like change in prostatic adenocarcinoma represents neuroendocrine differentiation: report of 30 cases, Hum Pathol 25:135-139, 1994.
348. Azzopardi JG, Evans DJ: Argentaffin cells in prostatic carcinoma: differentiation from lipofuscin and melanin in prostatic epithelium, Pathology 104:247-251, 1971.
349. Di Sant'Agnese PA: Neuroendocrine differentiation and prostatic carcinoma: the concept "comes of age," Arch Pathol Lab Med 112:1097-1099, 1988.
350. Turbat-Herrera EA, Herrera GA, Gore I et al: Neuroendocrine differentiation in prostatic carcinomas: a retrospective autopsy study, Arch Pathol Lab Med 112:1100-1106, 1988.
351. Stratton M, Evans DJ, Lampert IA: Prostatic adenocarcinoma evolving into carcinoid: selective effect of hormonal treatment? J Clin Pathol 39:750-756, 1986.
352. Ghali VS, Gargia RL: Prostatic adenocarcinoma with carcinoidal features producing adrenocorticotropic syndrome, Cancer 54:1042-1048, 1984.
353. Fetissof F, Bruandet P, Arbeille B et al: Calcitonin-secreting carcinomas of the prostate: an immunohistochemical and ultrastructural analysis, Am J Surg Pathol 10:702-710, 1986.
354. Schron DS, Gipson T, Mendelsohn G: The histogenesis of small cell carcinoma of the prostate, Cancer 53:2478-2480, 1984.
355. Fetissof F, Dubois MP, Arbeille-Brassart B et al: Endocrine cells in the prostate gland, urothelium and Brenner tumors, Virchows Arch B Cell Pathol 42:53-64, 1983.
356. Di Sant'Agnese PA, de Mesy Jensen KL: Endocrine-paracrine cells of the prostate and prostatic urethra: an ultrastructural study, Hum Pathol 15:1034-1041, 1984.
357. Di Sant'Agnese PA, de Mesy Jensen KL, Churukian CG et al: Human prostatic endocrine paracrine (APUD) cells, Arch Pathol Lab Med 109:607-612, 1985.
358. Di Sant'Agnese PA: Calcitoninlike immunoreactive and bombesin like immunoreactive endocrine-paracrine cells of the human prostate, Arch Pathol Lab Med 110:412-415, 1986.
359. Di Sant'Agnese PA, de Mesy Jensen KL: Neuroendocrine differentiation in prostatic carcinoma, Hum Pathol 18:849-856, 1987.
360. Kazzaz BA: Argentaffin and argyrophil cells in the prostate, J Pathol 112:189-193, 1974.
361. Capella C, Usellini L, Buffa R et al: The endocrine component of prostatic carcinomas, mixed adenocarcinoma-carcinoid tumours and on-tumour prostate: histochemical and ultrastructural identification of the endocrine cells, Histopathology 5:175-192, 1981.
362. Ro JY, Tetu B, Ayala AG et al: Small cell carcinoma of the prostate: II. Immunohistochemical and electron microscopic studies of 18 cases, Cancer 59:977-982, 1987.
363. Ansari MA, Pintozzi RL, Choi YS et al: Diagnosis of carcinoid-like metastatic prostatic carcinoma by an immunoperoxidase method, Am J Clin Pathol 76:94-99, 1981.
364. Almagro UA, Tieu TM, Remeniuk E et al: Argyrophilic "carcinoid-like" prostatic carcinoma, Arch Pathol Lab Med 110:916-919, 1986.
365. Dauge MC, Delmas V: APUD type endocrine tumour of the prostate: incidence and prognosis in association with adenocarcinoma. In Murphy GP, Kuss R, Khoury S et al, eds. Progress in clinical and biological medicine. Prostate cancer Part A: research, endocrine treatment, and histopathology, New York, 1987, Alan R Liss.
366. Cohen RJ, Glezerson G, Haffejee Z: Neuroendocrine cells. A new prognostic parameter in prostate cancer, Br J Urol 68:258-262, 1991.
367. Weaver MG, Abdul-Karim FW, Srigley J et al: Paneth cell-like change of the prostate gland: a histological immunohistochemical and electron microscopic study, Am J Surg Pathol 16:62-68, 1992.
368. Weaver MG, Abdul-Karim FW, Srigley JR et al: Paneth cell-like change and small cell carcinoma of the prostate. Two divergent forms of prostatic neuroendocrine differentiation, Am J Surg Pathol 16:1013-1016, 1992.
369. Frydman CP, Bleiweiss IJ, Unger PD et al: Paneth cell-like metaplasia of the prostate gland, Arch Pathol Lab Med 116:274-276, 1992.
370. Weaver MG, Abdul-Karim FW, Srigley JR et al: Paneth cell-like change of the prostate, Arch Pathol Lab Med 116:1101-1102, 1992 (letter).
371. Haratake J, Akio H, Kenji I: Argyrophilic adenocarcinoma of the prostate with Paneth cell-like granules, Acta Pathol Jpn 37:831-836, 1987.
372. Cohen RJ, Glezerson G, Haffejee Z: Prostate specific antigen and prostate specific acid phosphatase in neuroendocrine cells of prostate cancer, Arch Pathol Lab Med 116:65-66, 1992.
373. Bogden AE, Taylor JE, Moreau JP et al: Treatment of R-3327 prostate tumors with a somatostatin analogue (somatuline) as adjuvant therapy following surgical castration, Cancer Res 50:2646-2650, 1990.
374. Milovanovic SR, Radulovic S, Groot K et al: Inhibition of growth of PC-82 human prostate cancer cell line xenografts in nude mice by bombesin antagonist RC-3095 or combination of agonist [D-Trp^6]-LH-RH and somatostatin analog RC-160, Prostate 20:269-280, 1992.

375. Schally AV, Redding TW: Somatostatin analogues as adjuncts to agonists of luteinizing hormone-releasing hormone in the treatment of experimental prostate cancer, Proc Natl Acad Sci U S A 84:7275-7279, 1987.
376. Bologna M, Festuccia C, Muzi P et al: Bombesin stimulates growth of human prostatic cancer cells in vitro, Cancer 63:1714-1720, 1989.
377. Wasserstein PW, Goldman RL: Primary carcinoid of prostate, Urology 18:407-409, 1981.
378. Tetu B, Ro JY, Ayala AG et al: Small cell carcinoma of prostate associated with myasthenic (Eaton-Lambert) syndrome, Urology 33:148-152, 1989.
379. Tetu B, Ro JY, Ayala AG et al: Small cell carcinoma of the prostate. I. A clinicopathologic study of 20 cases, Cancer 59:1803-1809, 1987.
380. Hindson DA, Knight LL, Ocker JM: Small cell cancer of prostate: transient complete remission with chemotherapy, Urology 26:182-184, 1985.
381. Ro JY, Tetu B, Ayala AG et al: Small cell carcinoma of the prostate: immunohistochemical and electron microscopic studies of 18 cases, Cancer 59:977-984, 1987.
382. Wenk RE, Bhagavan BS, Levy R et al: Ectopic ACTH, prostatic oat cell carcinoma, and marked hypernatremia, Cancer 40:773-778, 1977.
383. Mahadevia PS, Ramaswamy A, Greenwald ES et al: Hypercalcemia in prostatic carcinoma. Report of eight cases, Arch Intern Med 143:1339-1342,1983.
384. Barkin J, Crassweller PO, Roncari DAK et al: Hypercalcemia associated with cancer of prostate without any metastases, Urology 24:368-379, 1984.
385. Ghandur-Mnaynmah L, Satterfield S, Block NL: Small cell carcinoma of the prostate gland with inappropriate antidiuretic hormone secretion: morphological, immunohistochemical, and clinical expressions, J Urol 135:1263-1266, 1986.
386. Moore SR, Reinberg Y, Zhang G: Small cell carcinoma of prostate: effectiveness of hormonal versus chemotherapy, Urology 39:411-416, 1992.
387. Oesterling JE, Hauzear CG, Farrow GM: Small cell anaplastic carcinoma of the prostate: a clinical, pathological and immunohistological study of 27 patients, J Urol 147:804-809, 1992.
388. Ferguson JK, Sebo TA, Husmann DA et al: Androgen receptor expression predicts survival in small cell carcinoma of the prostate (submitted).
389. Cleary KR, Choi HY, Ayala AG: Basal cell hyperplasia of the prostate, Am J Clin Pathol 80:850-854, 1983.
390. Denholm SW, Webb JN, Howard GCW et al: Basaloid carcinoma of the prostate gland: histogenesis and review of the literature, Histopathology 20:151-155, 1992.
391. Dermer GB: Basal cell proliferation in benign prostatic hyperplasia, Cancer 41:1857-1862, 1978.
392. Elbadawi A: Benign proliferative lesions of the prostate gland. In Spring-Mills E, Hafez ESE, eds: Male Accessory Sex Glands, The Netherlands, 1980, Elsevier/North Holland Biomedical Press.
393. Grignon DJ, Ro JY, Ordonez NG et al: Basal cell hyperplasia, adenoid basal cell tumor, and adenoid cystic carcinoma of the prostate gland: an immunohistochemical study, Hum Pathol 19:1425-1433, 1988.
394. Kirkland KL, Bale PM: A cystic adenoma of the prostate, J Urol 97:324-327, 1967.
395. Krompecher E: Uber Basalzellenhyperplasien und Basalzellenkrebse der Prostata, Eingegangen 284-293, 1925.
396. Lawrence JB, Mazur MT: Adenoid cystic carcinoma. A comparative pathologic study of tumors in salivary gland, breast, lung, and cervix, Hum Pathol 13:916-924, 1982.
397. Lin JI, Cohen EL, Villacin AB et al: Basal cell adenoma of prostate, Urology 11:409-410, 1978.
398. Min KW, Gyorkey F: Prostatic adenoma of ductal origin, Urology 16:95-96, 1980.
399. Mittal BV, Amin MB, Kinare SG: Spectrum of histological lesions in 185 consecutive prostatic specimens, J Postgrad Med 35:157-161, 1989.
400. Reed RJ: Consultation case, Am J Surg Pathol 8:699-704, 1984.
401. Ronnett BM, Epstein JI: A case showing sclerosing adenosis and an unusual form of basal cell hyperplasia of the prostate, Am J Surg Pathol 13:866-872, 1989.
402. Sarma DP, Guileyardo JM: Basal cell hyperplasia of the prostate, J La State Med Soc 134:23-27, 1982.
403. Srigley JR, Dardick I, Hartwick RWJ et al: Basal epithelial cells of human prostate gland are not myoepithelial cells. A comparative immunohistochemical and ultrastructural study with the human salivary gland, Am J Pathol 136:957-966, 1990.
404. Tannenbaum M: Adenoid cystic or "salivary gland" carcinomas of prostate, Urology 6:2338, 1975.
405. Wernert N, Seitz G: Immunohistochemical investigation of different cytokeratins and vimentin in the prostate from the fetal period up to adulthood and in prostate carcinoma, Pathol Res Pract 182:617-626, 1987.
406. Young RH, Frierson HF, Mills SE et al: Adenoid cystic-like tumor of the prostate gland. A report of two cases and review of the literature on "adenoid cystic carcinoma" of the prostate, Am J Clin Pathol 89:49-56, 1988.
407. Devaraj LT, Bostwick DG: Atypical basal cell hyperplasia of the prostate. Immunophenotypic profile and proposed classification of basal cell proliferations, Am J Surg Pathol 17:645-659, 1993.
408. Shond-San C, Walters MNI: Adenoid cystic carcinoma of prostate. Report of a case, Pathology 16:337-338, 1984.
409. Frankel KC Jr: Adenoid cystic carcinoma of the prostate. Report of a case, Am J Clin Pathol 62:639-645, 1974.
410. Gilmour AM, Bell TJ: Adenoid cystic carcinoma of the prostate, Br J Urol 58:105-106, 1986.
411. Kramer SA, Bredael JJ, Krueger RP: Adenoid cystic carcinoma of the prostate: report of a case, J Urol 120:383-384, 1978.
412. Kuhajda FP, Mann RG: Adenoid cystic carcinoma of the prostate. A case report with immunoperoxidase staining for prostate-specific acid phosphatase and prostate-specific antigen, Am J Clin Pathol 81:257-260, 1984.
413. Cohen RJ, Goldberg RD, Verhaart MJ et al: Adenoid cyst-like carcinoma of the prostate, Arch Pathol Lab Med 117:799-801, 1993.
414. Beer M, Occhionero F, Welsch U: Oncocytoma of the prostate: a case report with ultrastructural and immunohistochemical evaluation, Histopathology 17:370-372, 1990.
415. Ordóñez NG, Ro JY, Ayala AG: Metastatic prostatic carcinoma presenting as an oncocytic tumor, Am J Surg Pathol 16:1007-1012, 1992.

416. Pinto JA, Gonzalez JE, Granadillo MA: Primary carcinoma of the prostate with diffuse oncocytic changes, Histopathology 25:286-288, 1994.
417. Bostwick DG, Adlakha K: Lymphoepithelioma-like carcinoma of the prostate, J Urol Pathol 2:319-325, 1994.
418. Montironi R, Santinelli A, Galluzzi CM et al: Proliferating cell nuclear antigen (PCNA) evaluation in the diagnostic quantitative pathology of cribriform adenocarcinoma of the prostate, In Vivo 7:343-346, 1993.
419. McNeal JE, Reese JH, Redwine EA et al: Cribriform adenocarcinoma of the prostate, Cancer 58:1714-1719, 1986.
420. Currin SM, Lee SE, Walther PJ: Flow cytometric analysis of comedocarcinoma of the prostate: an uncommon histopathological variant of prostatic adenocarcinoma, J Urol 140:96-100, 1988.
421. Kahler JE: Carcinoma of the prostate gland: a pathologic study, J Urol 41:447-562, 1939.
422. Sieracki JC: Epidermoid carcinoma of the human prostate. Report of three cases, Lab Invest 4:232-235, 1955.
423. Gray GF Jr, Marshall VF: Squamous carcinoma of the prostate, J Urol 113:736-738, 1975.
424. Mott LJM: Squamous cell carcinoma of the prostate. Report of 2 cases and review of the literature, J Urol 121:833-836, 1979.
425. Sharma SK, Malik KAK, Bapna BC: Squamous cell carcinoma of prostate, Indian J Cancer 17:134-135, 1980.
426. Wernert N, Goebbels R, Bonkhoff H et al: Squamous cell carcinoma of the prostate, Histopathology 17:339-344, 1990.
427. Sarma DP, Weilbaecher TG, Moon TD: Squamous cell carcinoma of prostate, Urology 37:260-262, 1991.
428. Moskovitz N, Munichor M, Bolkier M et al: Squamous cell carcinoma of the prostate, Urol Int 51:181-183, 1993.
429. Bennett RS, Edgerton EO: Mixed prostatic carcinoma, J Urol 110:561-563, 1973.
430. Saito R, Davis BK, Ollipally EP: Adenosquamous carcinoma of the prostate, Hum Pathol 15:87-89, 1984.
431. Moyana TN: Adenosquamous carcinoma of the prostate, Am J Surg Pathol 11:402-407, 1987.
432. Gattuso P, Carson HJ, Candel A et al: Adenosquamous carcinoma of the prostate, Hum Pathol 26:123-126, 1995.
433. Acceta PA, Gardner WA Jr: Squamous metastases from prostatic adenocarcinoma, Lab Invest 46:2A, 1982.
434. Al Adani MS: Schistosomiasis, metaplasia and squamous cell carcinoma of the prostate: histogenesis of the squamous cells determined by localization of specific markers, Neoplasma 32:613-622, 1985.
435. Devaney DM, Dorman A, Leader M: Adenosquamous carcinoma of the prostate: a case report, Hum Pathol 22:1046-1050, 1991.
436. Schenken JR, Burns EL, Kahle PJ: The effect of diethylstilbestrol and diethylstilbestrol dipropionate on carcinoma of the prostate gland. II. Cytologic changes following treatment, J Urol 48:99-112, 1942.
437. English HF, Kyprianou N, Isaacs JT: Relationship between DNA fragmentation and apoptosis in the programmed cell death in the rat prostate following castration, Prostate 15:233-250, 1989.
438. Kyprianou N, Isaacs JT: Expression of transforming growth factor-ß in the rat ventral prostate during castration-induced programmed cell death, Mol Endocrinol 3:1515-1522, 1989.
439. Kyprianou N, English H, Isaacs JT: Programmed cell death during regression of PC-82 human prostate cancer following androgen ablation, Cancer Res 50:3748-3753, 1990.
440. Mahan DE, Bruce AW, Manley PN et al: Immunohistochemical evaluation of prostatic carcinoma before and after radiotherapy, J Urol 124:488-492, 1980.
441. Musselman PW, Tubbs R, Connelly RW et al: Biological significance of prostatic carcinoma after definitive radiation therapy, J Urol 137:114A, 1987.
442. Mollenkamp JS, Cooper JF, Kagan AR: Clinical experience with supervoltage radiotherapy in carcinoma of the prostate: a preliminary report, J Urol 113:374-377, 1975.
443. Kuriyama J, Wang MC, Lee CL et al: Multiple marker evaluation in human prostate cancer with use of tissue-specific antigens, J Natl Cancer Inst 68:99-105, 1982.
444. Nadji J, Tabei SZ, Castro A et al: Prostatic origin of tumors. An immunohistochemical study, Am J Clin Pathol 73:735-739, 1980.
445. Oesterling JE, Jacobsen SJ, Chute CG et al: Serum prostate-specific antigen in a community-based population of healthy men: establishment of age-specific reference ranges, JAMA 270:860-866, 1993.
446. Ruckle HC, Klee GG, Oesterling JE: Prostate-specific antigen: critical issues for the practicing physician, Mayo Clin Proc 69:59-68, 1994.
447. Ruckle HC, Klee GG, Oesterling JE: Prostate-specific antigen: concepts for staging prostate cancer and monitoring response to therapy, Mayo Clin Proc 69:69-79, 1994.
448. Bostwick DG: Prostate-specific antigen. Current role in diagnostic pathology of prostate cancer, Am J Clin Pathol 102(suppl 1):S31-S37, 1994.
449. Lilja H: Significance of different molecular forms of serum prostate-specific antigen: the free, noncomplexed form of prostate-specific antigen versus that complexed to alpha-1-antichymotrypsin, Urol Clin N Am 20:681-686, 1993.
450. Vessella RL, Lange PH: Issues in the assessment of prostate-specific antigen immunoassays, Urol Clin N Am 20:607-620, 1993.
451. Brawn P, Johnson EH, Foster DM et al: Characteristics of prostatic infarcts and their effects on serum prostate-specific antigen and prostatic acid phosphatase, Urology 44:71-75, 1994.
452. Ordonez NG, Ro JY, Ayala AG: Application of immunocytochemistry in pathology. In Bostwick DG, ed: Pathology of the prostate, New York, 1990, Churchill Livingstone.
453. Vernon SE, Williams WD: Pre-treatment and post-treatment evaluation of prostatic adenocarcinoma for prostatic specific acid phosphatase and prostatic specific antigen by immunohistochemistry, J Urol 130:95-98, 1983.
454. Nadji M, Tabei SZ, Castro A et al: Prostatic-specific antigen. An immunohistologic marker for prostatic neoplasms, Cancer 48:1229-1232, 1981.
455. Stein BS, Vangore S, Petersen RO et al: Immunoperoxidase localization of prostate-specific antigen, Am J Surg Pathol 6:553-558, 1982.
456. Fishleder A, Tubbs RR, Levin HS: An immunoperoxidase technique to aid in differential diagnosis of prostatic carcinoma, Cleve Clin Q 48:331-334, 1981.

457. Keillor JS, Aterman K: The response of poorly differentiated prostatic tumors to staining for prostate specific antigen and prostatic acid phosphatase: a comparative study, J Urol 137:894-898, 1987.
458. Cote RJ, Taylor CR: Prostate, bladder, and kidney. In Taylor CR, Cote RJ, eds: Immunomicroscopy: a diagnostic tool for the surgical pathologist, ed 2, Philadelphia, 1994, WB Saunders.
459. Epstein JI, Eggleston JC: Immunohistochemical localization of prostate-specific acid phosphatase and prostate-specific antigen in stage A_2 adenocarcinoma of the prostate: prognostic implications, Hum Pathol 15:853-859, 1984.
460. Sinha AA, Hagen KA, Sibley RK et al: Analysis of fixation effects on immunohistochemical localization of prostatic specific antigen in human prostate, J Urol 136:722-727, 1986.
461. Frazier HA, Humphrey PA, Burchette JL et al: Immunoreactive prostate specific antigen in male periurethral glands, J Urol 147:246-250, 1992.
462. Elgamal A, van de Voorde W, van Poppel et al: Immunohistochemical localization of prostate-specific markers within the accessory male sex glands of Cowper, Littre, and Morgagni, Urology 434:84-90, 1994.
463. Nowels K, Kent E, Rinsho K: Prostate specific antigen and acid phosphastase-reactive cells in cystitis cystica and glandularis, Arch Pathol Lab Med 112:734-738, 1988.
464. Golz R, Schubert GE: Prostate specific antigen. Immunoreactivity in urachal remnants, J Urol 141:1480-1484, 1989.
465. Kamoshida S, Tsutsumi Y: Extraprostatic localization of prostatic acid phosphatase and prostate specific antigen: distribution in cloacogenic glandular epithelium and sex-dependent expression in human anal gland, Hum Pathol 21:1108-1115, 1990.
466. Spencer JR, Brodin AG, Ignatoff JM: Clear cell adenocarcinoma of the urethra: evidence for origin within paraurethral ducts, J Urol 143:122-125, 1990.
467. Minkowitz G, Peterson P, Godwin TA: A histochemical and immunohistochemical study of adenocarcinomas involving urinary bladder, Mod Pathol 3:68A, 1990 (abstract).
468. Ellis DW, Leffers S, Davies JS et al: Multiple immunoperoxidase markers in benign hyperplasia and adenocarcinoma of the prostate, Am J Clin Pathol 81:279-283, 1984.
469. Svanholm H: Evaluation of commercial immunoperoxidase kits for prostate specific antigen and prostatic specific acid phosphatase, Acta Pathol Microbiol Immunol Scand [A] 94:7-15, 1986.
470. Grignon D, Troster M: Changes in immunohistochemical staining in prostatic adenocarcinoma following diethylstilbesterol therapy, Prostate 7:195-202, 1985.
471. Bovenberg SA, van der Zwet CJJ, van der Kwast TH et al: Prostate-specific antigen expression in prostate cancer and its metastases, J Urol Pathol 1:55-62, 1993.
472. Fidler IJ: Tumor heterogeneity and the biology of cancer invasion and metastasis, Cancer Res 38:2651-2657, 1978.
473. Lowe FC, Trauzzi SJ: Prostatic acid phosphatase in 1993. Its limited clinical utility, Urol Clin N Am 20:589-596, 1993.
474. Hammond ME, Sause WT, Martz KL et al: Correlation of prostatespecific acid phosphatase and prostate-specific antigen immunocytochemistry with survival in prostate carcinoma, Cancer 63:461-466, 1989.
475. Tepper SL, Jagirdar J, Heath D et al: Homology between the female paraurethral (Skene's glands) and the prostate, Arch Pathol Lab Med 108:423-427, 1984.
476. Pollen JJ, Dreiling A: Immunohistochemical identification of prostatic acid phosphatase and prostate specific antigen in female periurethral glands, Urology 23:303-307, 1984.
477. Van Krieken JHJM: Prostate marker immunoreactivity in salivary gland neoplasms. A rare pitfall in immunohistochemistry, Am J Surg Pathol 17:410-414, 1993.
478. Bentz MS, Cohen C, Budgeon LR et al: Evaluation of commercial immunoperoxidase kits in diagnosis of prostate carcinoma, Urology 23:75-81, 1984.
479. Shaw LM, Yang N, Brooks JJ et al: Immunochemical evaluation of the organ specificity of prostatic acid phosphatase, Clin Chem 27:1505-1510, 1981.
480. Epstein JI, Kuhajda FP, Lieberman PH: Prostate-specific acid phosphastase immunoreactivity in adenocarcinomas of the urinary bladder, Hum Pathol 17:939-945, 1986.
481. Sobin LH, Hjermstad BM, Sesterhenn IA et al: Prostatic acid phosphatase activity in carcinoid tumors, Cancer 58:136-143, 1986.
482. Choe BK, Pontes EJ, Rose NR et al: Expression of human prostatic acid phosphatase in a pancreatic islet cell carcinoma, Invest Urol 15:312-316, 1978.
483. Li C-Y, Lam WKW, Yam LT: Immunohistochemical diagnosis of prostatic carcinoma with metastasis, Cancer 46:706-710, 1980.
484. Fernandez PL, Gomez M, Caballero T et al: Prostatic acid phosphatase in cloacogenic carcinoma, Am J Surg Pathol 16:526-531, 1992.
485. Kimura N, Sasano N: Prostate-specific acid phosphatase in carcinoid tumors, Virchows Arch A Pathol Anat Histol 410:247-252, 1986.
486. Yam LT, Janckila AJ, Lam KW et al: Immunohistochemistry of prostatic acid phosphatase, Prostate 2:97-107, 1981.
487. Sleater JP, Ford MJ, Beers BB: Extramammary Paget's disease associated with prostate adenocarcinoma, Hum Pathol 25:615-617, 1994.
488. Lam KW, Li CY, Yam LT et al: Improved immunohistochemical detection of prostatic acid phosphatase by a monoclonal antibody, Prostate 15:13-18, 1989.
489. Bonkhoff H, Remberger K: Widespread distribution of nuclear androgen receptors in the basal cell layer of the normal and hyperplastic human prostate, Virchows Arch A Pathol Anat Histol 422:35-38, 1993.
490. Sadi MV, Barrack ER: Image analysis of androgen receptor immunostaining in metastatic prostate cancer, Cancer 71:2574-2580, 1993.
491. Sadi MV, Walsh PC, Barrack ER: Immunohistochemical study of androgen receptors in metastatic prostate cancer. Comparison of receptor content and response to hormonal therapy, Cancer 67:3057-3064, 1991.
492. Steiner MS: Role of peptide growth factors in the prostate: a review, Urology 42:99-110, 1993.
493. Myers RB, Kudlow JE, Grizzle WE: Expression of transforming growth factor-alpha, epidermal growth factor and the epidermal growth factor receptor in adenocarcinoma of the prostate and benign prostatic hyperplasia, Mod Pathol 6:733-737, 1993.

494. Harper ME, Goddard L, Glynne-Jones E et al: An immunocytochemical analysis of transforming growth factor alpha expression in benign and malignant prostatic tumors, Prostate 23:9-23, 1993.
495. Maygarden SJ, Strom S, Ware JL: Localization of epidermal growth factor receptor by immunohistochemical methods in human prostatic carcinoma, prostatic intraepithelial neoplasia, and benign hyperplasia, Arch Pathol Lab Med 116:269-273, 1992.
496. Kyprianou N, Isaacs JT: Identification of a cellular receptor for transforming growth factor-beta in rat ventral prostate and its negative regulation by androgens, Endocrinology 27:2124-2131, 1988.
497. Thompson TC, Truong LD, Timme TL et al: Transforming growth factor beta-1 as a biomarker for prostate cancer, J Cell Biochem suppl 16H:54-61, 1992.
498. Eklov S, Funa K, Nordgren H et al: Lack of the latent transforming growth factor beta binding protein in malignant, but not benign prostatic tissue, Cancer Res 53:3193-3197, 1993.
499. Schellhammer PF, Wright GL Jr: Biomolecular and clinical characteristics of prostate-specific antigen and other candidate tumor markers, Urol Clin N Am 20:597-606, 1993.
500. Bostwick DG, Qian J: Current and proposed biologic markers in prostate cancer: 1994, J Cell Biochem Suppl 19:197-201, 1994.
501. Zincke H, Bergstrahl EJ, Larson-Keller JJ et al: Stage D1 prostate cancer treated by radical prostatectomy and adjuvant hormonal treatment. Evidence for favorable survival in patients with DNA diploid tumors, Cancer 70(suppl 1):311-323, 1992.
502. Nativ O, Winkler HZ, Raz Y et al: Stage C prostatic adenocarcinoma. Flow cytometric nuclear DNA ploidy analysis, Mayo Clin Proc 64:911-919, 1989.
503. Montgomery BT, Nativ O, Blute ML et al: Stage B prostate adenocarcinoma. Flow cytometric nuclear DNA ploidy analysis, Arch Surg 125:327-331, 1990.
504. DeVere White RW, Deitch AD, Meyer-Haass GM et al: Deoxyribonucleic acid ploidy in the irradiated prostate, World J Urol 10:173-178, 1992.
505. Shankey TV, Kallioniemi O-P, Koslowski JM et al: Consensus review of the clinical utility of DNA content cytometry in prostate cancer, Cytometry 14:497-500, 1993.
506. Takai K, Goellner JR, Katzmann JA et al: Static image and flow DNA cytometry of prostatic adenocarcinoma: studies of needle biopsy and radical prostatectomy specimens, J Urol Pathol 2:39-48, 1994.
507. Warzynski MJ, Soechtig CE, Maatman TJ et al: DNA analysis by flow cytometry of paraffin embedded core biopsies of the prostate, Prostate 24:313-319, 1994.
508. Takahashi S, Qian J, Brown JA et al: Potential markers of prostate cancer aggressiveness detected by fluorescence in situ hybridization in needle biopsies, Cancer Res 54:3574-3579, 1994.
509. Sandberg AA: Chromosomal abnormalities and related events in prostate cancer, Hum Pathol 23:368-380, 1992.
510. MacGrogan D, Levy A, Bostwick D et al: Loss of chromosome arm 8p loci in prostate cancer: mapping by quantitative allelic balance, Genes Chromosom Cancer 10:151-159, 1994.
511. Bova GS, Carter BS, Bussemakers MJG et al: Homozygous deletion and frequent allelic loss of chromosome 8p22 loci in human prostate cancer, Cancer Res 53:3869-3873, 1993.
512. Bergerheim USR, Kunimi K, Collins VP et al: Deletion mapping of chromosomes 8, 10, and 16 in human prostatic carcinoma, Genes Chromosom Cancer 3:215-220, 1991.
513. Carter BS, Ewing CM, Ward WS et al: Allelic loss of chromosomes 16q and 10q in human prostate cancer, Proc Natl Acad Sci U S A 87:8751-8755, 1990.
514. Bookstein R, MacGrogan D, Hilsenbeck SG et al: p53 is mutated in a subset of advanced-stage prostate cancers, Cancer Res 53:3369-3373, 1993.
515. Effert PJ, McCoy RH, Walther PJ et al: p53 gene alterations in human prostate carcinoma, J Urol 150:257-261, 1993.
516. Van Veldhuizen PJ, Sadasivan R, Garcia F et al: Mutant p53 expression in prostate carcinoma, Prostate 22:23-30, 1993.
517. Mellon K, Thompson S, Charlton RG et al: p53, c-erbB-2 and the epidermal growth factor receptor in the benign and maligant prostate, J Urol 147:496-499, 1992.
518. Gao X, Honn KV, Grignon D et al: Frequent loss of expression and loss of heterozygosity of the putative tumor suppressor gene DCC in prostatic carcinomas, Cancer Res 53:2723-2727, 1993.
519. Bookstein R, Rio P, Madreperla S et al: Promoter deletion and loss of retinoblastoma gene expression in human prostate carcinoma, Proc Natl Acad Sci U S A 87:7762-7766, 1990.
520. Moul JW, Friedrichs PA, Lance RS et al: Infrequent RAS oncogene mutations in human prostate cancer, Prostate 20:327-333, 1992.
521. Sikes RA, Chung LWK: Acquistion of a tumorigenic phenotype by a rat ventral prostate epithelial cell line expressing a transfected activated neu oncogene, Cancer Res 52:3174-3178, 1992.
522. Zhau HE, Wan DS, Zhou J et al: Expression c-erbB-2/neu proto-oncogene in human prostatic cancer tissues and cell lines, Mol Carcinog 5:320-327, 1992.
523. Ibrahim GK, MacDonald JA, Kerns BJM et al: Differential immunoreactivity of her-2/neu oncoprotein in prostatic tissues, Surg Oncol 1:151-155, 1992.
524. Giri DK, Wadhwa SN, Upadhaya SN et al: Expression of neu/her-2 oncoprotein ($p185^{neu}$) in prostate tumors: an immunohistochemical study, Prostate 23:329-336, 1993.
525. Visakorpi T, Kallioniemi O-P, Koivula T et al: Expression of epidermal growth factor receptor and ERBB2 (her-2/neu) oncoprotein in prostatic carcinomas, Mod Pathol 5:643-648, 1992.
526. McCann A, Dervan PA, Johnston PA et al: c-erbB-2 oncoprotein expression in primary human tumors, Cancer 65:88-94, 1990.
527. Ware JL, Maygarden SJ, Koontz WW Jr et al: Immunohistochemical detection of c-erbB-2 protein in human benign and neoplastic prostate, Hum Pathol 22:254-259, 1991.
528. Kuhn EJ, Kurnot RA, Sesterhenn IA et al: Expression of the c-erbB-2 (HER2/neu) oncoprotein in human prostatic carcinoma, J Urol 150:1427-1433, 1993.
529. Sadasivan R, Morgan R, Jennings S et al: Overexpression of HER2/neu may be an indicator of poor prognosis in prostate cancer, J Urol 150:126-131, 1993.

530. Veltri RW, Partin AW, Epstein JI et al: Quantitative nuclear morphometry, Markovian texture descriptors, and DNA content captured on a CAS-200 image analysis system, combined with PCNA and HER-2/neu immunohistochemistry for prediction of prostate cancer progression, J Cell Biochem Suppl 19:249-258, 1994.
531. Ross JS, Nazeer T, Church K et al: Contribution of HER-2/neu oncogene expression to tumor grade and DNA content analysis in the prediction of prostatic carcinoma metastasis, Cancer 72:3020-3028, 1993.
532. Grizzle WE, Myers RB, Arnold MM et al: Biomarkers in breast and prostate cancer: effects of tissue processing and other variables, J Cell Biochem Suppl 19:259-266, 1994.
533. Myers RB, Srivastava S, Oelschlager DK et al: Expression of $p160^{erbB-3}$ and $p185^{erbB-2}$ in prostatic intraepithelial neoplasia and prostatic adenocarcinoma, J Natl Cancer Inst 86:1140-1145, 1994.
534. Cupp MR, Bostwick DG, Meyrs RP et al: The volume of prostate cancer in the biopsy specimen cannot reliably predict the quantity of cancer in the radical prostatectomy specimen on an individual basis, J Urol 153:1543-1548, 1995.
535. Graham SD Jr: Critical assessment of prostate cancer staging, Cancer 70:269-274, 1992.
536. Bostwick DG, Graham SD Jr, Napalkov P et al: Staging of early prostate cancer: a proposed tumor volume-based prognostic index, Urology 41:403-411, 1993.
537. Shroder FH, Hermanek P, Denis L et al: The TNM classification of prostate carcinoma, Prostate 4(suppl):129-138, 1992.
538. Stamey TA, Yang N, Hay AR et al: Prostate-specific antigen as a serum marker for adenocarcinoma of the prostate, N Engl J Med 317:909-916, 1987.
539. Fielding LP, Fenoglio-Preiser CM, Freedman LS: The future of prognostic factors in outcome prediction for patients with cancer, Cancer 70:2367-2377, 1992.
540. Lee F, Littrup PJ, Loft-Christensen L et al: Predicted prostate specific antigen results using transrectal ultrasound gland volume, Cancer 70(suppl):211-220, 1992.
541. Friedman GD, Hiatt RA, Quesenberry CP et al: Case-control study of screening for prostate cancer by digital rectal examinations, Lancet 337:1526-1529, 1991.
542. Oesterling JE, Suman VJ, Zincke H et al: PSA-detected (Clinical stage T1c or B0) prostate cancer: pathologically significant tumors, Urol Clin N Am 20:687-693, 1993.
543. Epstein JI, Walsh PC, Carmichael M et al: Pathologic and clinical findings to predict tumor extent of nonpalpable (stage T1c) prostate cancer, JAMA 271:368-374, 1994.
544. Scaletscky R, Koch MO, Eckstein CW et al: Tumor volume and stage in carcinoma of the prostate detected by elevations in prostate specific antigen, J Urol 152:129-131, 1994.
545. Ferguson JK, Bostwick DG, Suman V et al: Prostate-specific antigen detected prostate cancer. Pathological characteristics of ultrasound visible versus ultrasound invisible tumors, Eur Urol 27:8-12, 1995.
546. Epstein JI, Paull G, Eggleston JC et al: Prognosis of untreated stage A1 prostatic carcinoma: a study of 94 cases with extended followup, J Urol 136:837-839, 1986.
547. Blute ML, Zincke H, Farrow GM: Long-term followup of young patients with Stage A adenocarcinoma of the prostate, J Urol 136:840-843, 1986.
548. Greene DR, Egawa S, Neerhut G et al: The distribution of residual cancer in radical prostatectomy specimens in stage A prostate cancer, J Urol 145:324-329, 1991.
549. Parfitt HE, Smith JA, Gliedman JB et al: Accuracy of staging in A1 carcinoma of the prostate, Cancer 51:2346-2350, 1983.
550. Epstein JI, Oesterling JE, Walsh PC: The volume and anatomical location of residual tumor in radical prostatectomy specimens removed for stage A1 prostate cancer, J Urol 139:975-979, 1988.
551. Christenson WN, Parfitt AW, Walsh PC et al: Pathologic findings in clinical stage A2 prostate cancer. Relation of tumor volume, grade, and relation to pathologic stage, Cancer 65:1021-1027, 1990.
552. Rifkin MD, Zerhouni EA, Garsonis CA et al: Comparison of magnetic resonance imaging and ultrasonography in staging early prostate cancer: results of a multi-institutional cooperative trial, N Engl J Med 323:621-627, 1990.
553. Ramchandani P, Schnall MD: Magnetic resonance imaging of the prostate, Semin Roentgenol 28:74-82, 1993.
554. Brawer MK, Chetner MP, Beatie J et al: Screening for prostatic carcinoma with prostate-specific antigen, J Urol 147:841-844, 1992.
555. Catalona WJ, Smith DS, Ratliff TL et al: Measurement of prostate-specific antigen in serum as a screening test for prostate cancer, N Engl J Med 324:1156-1161, 1991.
556. Cooner WH, Mosley BR, Rutherford CL Jr et al: Prostate cancer detection in a clinical urological practice by ultrasonography, digital rectal examination and prostate-specific antigen, J Urol 143:1146-1151, 1990.
557. Labrie F, Dupont A, Suburu R et al: Serum prostate-specific antigen as pre-sceening test for prostate cancer, J Urol 147:846-850, 1992.
558. Mettlin C, Lee F, Drago J et al:. Findings on the detection of early prostate cancer in 2425 men, Cancer 67:2949-2957, 1991.
559. Bostwick DG, Choi C: Prognostic factors in early prostate cancer, Urol Annu 6:63-101, 1992.
560. Cantrell BB, DeKlerk DP, Eggleston JC et al: Pathological factors that influence prognosis in stage A prostatic cancer: the influence of extent versus grade, J Urol 125:516-519, 1981.
561. Foucar E, Haake G, Dalton L et al: The area of cancer in transurethral resection specimens as a prognostic indicator in carcinoma of the prostate: a computer-assisted morphometric study, Hum Pathol 21:586-592, 1990.
562. Partin AW, Epstein JI, Cho R et al: Morphometric measurement of tumor volume and per cent of gland involvement as predictors of pathological stage in clinical stage B prostate cancer, J Urol 141:341-346, 1989.
563. Weems WL, Morris JS: The limits of resectability of prostate cancer, Urol Annu 6:129-146, 1992.
564. Bostwick DG, Eble JN: Prostatic adenocarcinoma metastatic to inguinal hernia sac, J Urol Pathol 1:193-199, 1993.
565. De La Monte SM, Moore GW, Hutchins GM: Metastatic behavior of prostate cancer. Cluster analysis of pattern with respect to estrogen treatment, Cancer 58:985-993, 1986.
566. Saitoh H, Hida M, Shimbo T et al: Metastatic patterns of prostatic cancer. Correlation between sites and number of organs involved, Cancer 54:3078-3084, 1984.

567. Moul JW, Kahn DG, Lewis DJ et al: Immunohistologic detection of prostate cancer pelvic lymph node micrometastases: correlation to preoperative serum prostate-specific antigen, Urology 43:68-73, 1994.
568. Gomella LG, White JL, McCue PA et al: Screening for occult nodal metastases in localized carcinoma of the prostate, J Urol 149:776-778, 1993.
569. Hamdy FC, Lawry J, Anderson JB et al: Circulating prostate specific antigen–positive cells correlate with metastatic prostate cancer, Br J Urol 69:392-396, 1992.
570. Moreno JG, Croce CM, Fischer R et al: Detection of hematogenous micrometastasis in patients with prostate cancer, Cancer Res 52:6110-6112, 1992.
571. Katz AE, Olsson CA, Raffo AJ et al: Molecular staging of prostate cancer with the use of an enhanced reverse transcriptase-PCR assay, Urology 43:765-775, 1994.
572. See WA, Williams RD: Management of prostate cancer: stage by stage. In Das S, Crawford ED, eds: Cancer of the prostate, New York, 1993, Marcel Dekker.
573. Fleming C, Wasson J, Albertson PC et al: A decision analysis of alternative treatment strategies for clinically localized prostate cancer, JAMA 269:2650-2658, 1993.
574. Whitmore WF Jr: Management of clinically localized prostatic cancer. An unresolved problem, JAMA 269:2676-2677, 1993 (editorial).
575. Thompson IM, Zeidman EJ: Extended followup of stage A1 carcinoma of the prostate, Urology 33:455-458, 1989.
576. Zhang G, Wasserman NF, Sidi AM et al: Long-term follow-up results after expectant management of stage A1 prostatic cancer, J Urol 146:99-103, 1991.
577. Orestano F: Problems of wait-and-see policy in incidental carcinoma of the prostate. In Altwein JE, Faul P, Schneider W, eds: Incidental carcinoma of the prostate, Berlin, 1991, Springer Verlag.
578. Babaian RJ, Troncoso P, Ayala AG et al: Involvement of prostatic urethra and prostatic ducts by transitional cell carcinoma in patients with bladder cancer, J Urol 141:1415, 1989.
579. Wood DP Jr, Montie JE, Pontes JE et al: Transitional cell carcinoma of the prostate in cystoprostatectomy specimens removed for bladder cancer, J Urol 141:346-349, 1989.
580. Handeman SW, Soloway MS: Transitional cell carcinoma of the prostate: diagnosis, staging and management, Urology 6:170-174, 1988.
581. Wendelken JR, Schellhammer PF, Ladaga LE et al: Transitional cell carcinoma: cause of refractory cancer of the prostate, Urology 13:557-560, 1979.
582. Mahadevia PS, Koss LG, Tar IJ: Prostatic involvement in bladder cancer, Cancer 58:2096-2102, 1986.
583. Taylor HG, Blom J: Transitional cell carcinoma of the prostate, Cancer 51:1800-1802, 1983.
584. Schujman E, Mukamel E, Slutzker D et al: Prostatic transitional cell carcinoma. Concept of its pathogenesis and classification, Isr J Med Sci 19:794-800, 1983.
585. Kopelson G, Harisiadis L, Romas NA et al: Periurethral prostatic duct carcinoma, Cancer 42:2894-2902, 1978.
586. Schellhammer PF, Bean MA, Whitmore WF Jr: Prostatic involvement by transitional cell carcinoma: pathogenesis, patterns and prognosis, J Urol 118:399-403,1977.
587. Seemayer TA, Knaack J, Thelmo WL et al: Further observations on carcinoma in situ of the urinary bladder. Silent but extensive intraprostatic involvement, Cancer 36:514-520, 1975.
588. Johnson DE, Hogan JM, Ayala AG: Transitional cell carcinoma of the prostate, Cancer 29:287-293,1972.
589. Rhamy RK, Buchanan RD, Spalding MJ: Intraductal carcinoma of the prostate gland, J Urol 109:457-460, 1973.
590. Rubenstein ARB, Rubnitz ME: Transitional cell carcinoma of the prostate, Cancer 3:543-546, 1969.
591. Ullmann AS, Ross OA: Hyperplasia, atypism, and carcinoma in situ in prostatic periurethral glands, Am J Clin Pathol 47:497-504, 1967.
592. Ende N, Woods LP, Shelly HS: Carcinoma originating in ducts surrounding the prostatic urethra, Am J Clin Pathol 40:183-189, 1963.
593. Frank LM, Chesterman FC: Intra-epithelial carcinoma of prostatic urethra, peri-urethral glands and prostatic ducts (Bowen's disease of urinary epithelium), Br J Cancer 10:223-225, 1956.
594. Wishnow KI, Ro JY: Importance of early treatment of transitional cell carcinoma of prostatic ducts, Urology 32:11-12, 1988.
595. Frazier HA, Robertson JE, Dodge RK et al: The value of pathologic factors in predicting cancer-specific survival among patients treated with radical cystectomy for transitional cell carcinoma of the bladder and prostate, Cancer 71:3993-4001, 1993.
596. Takashi M, Sakata T, Nagai T et al: Primary transitional cell carcinoma of prostate: case with lymph node metastasis eradicated by neoadjuvant methotrexate, vinblastine, doxorubicin, and cisplatin (M-VAC) therapy, Urology 36:96-99, 1990.
597. Attah EB, Nkposong EO: Phyllodes type of atypical prostatic hyperplasia, J Urol 115:762-764, 1976.
598. Cox R, Dawson IMP: A curious prostatic tumor: probably a true mixed tumor, Br J Urol 32:306-311, 1960.
599. Cummine HG, Johnson AS: Report of a case of retrovesical polycystic tumor of probable prostatic origin, Aust N Z J Surg 19:91-92, 1950.
600. Gueft B, Walsh MA: Malignant prostatic cystosarcoma phyllodes, N Y State J Med 75:2226-2228, 1975.
601. Ito H, Ito M, Nitsuhata N et al: Phyllodes tumor of the prostate. A case report, Jpn J Clin Oncol 19:299-304, 1989.
602. Kafandaris PM, Polyyzonis MB: Fibroadenoma-like foci in human prostatic nodular hyperplasia, Prostate 4:33-36, 1983.
603. Kendall AR, Stein BS, Shea FJ et al: Cystic pelvic mass, J Urol 135:550-553, 1986.
604. Kerley SW, Pierce P, Thomas J: Giant cystosarcoma phyllodes of the prostate associated with adenocarcinoma, Arch Pathol Lab Med 116:195-197, 1992.
605. Kevwitch MK, Walloch JL, Waters WB et al: Prostatic cystic epithelial-stromal tumors: a report of 2 new cases, J Urol 149:860-864, 1993.
606. Kirkland KL, Bale PM: A cystic adenoma of the prostate, J Urol 97:324-327, 1967.
607. Lopez-Beltran A, Gaeta JF, Huben R et al: Malignant phyllodes tumor of the prostate, Urology 35:164-167, 1990.
608. Maluf HM, King ME, DeLuca FR et al: Giant multilocular prostatic cystadenoma: a distinctive lesion of the retroperitoneum in men, Am J Surg Pathol 15:131-135, 1991.

609. Manivel C, Shenoy BV, Wick MR et al: Cystosarcoma phyllodes of the prostate: a pathologic and immunohistochemical study, Arch Pathol Lab Med 110:534-538, 1986.
610. Mishina T, Shimada N, Toki J et al: A case report of phyllodes tumor of the prostate: review of the literature and analysis of bizarre giant cell origin, Acta Urol Jpn 36:1185-1188, 1990.
611. Reese JH, Lombard CM, Krone K et al: Phyllodes type of atypical prostatic hyperplasia: a report of 3 new cases, J Urol 138:623-626, 1987.
612. Viskens D, Van Hove C, Fransen G et al: Phyllodes type of atypical prostatic hyperplasia, Acta Chir Belg 91:22-26, 1991.
613. Yokota T, Yamashita Y, Okuzono Y et al: Malignant cystosarcoma phyllodes of prostate, Acta Pathol Jpn 34:663-668, 1984.
614. Young JF, Jensen PE, Wiley CA: Malignant phyllodes tumor of the prostate: a case report with immunohistochemical and ultrastructural findings, Arch Pathol Lab Med 116:296-299, 1992.
615. Yum M, Miller JC, Agrawal BL: Leiomyosarcoma arising in atypical fibromuscular hyperplasia (phyllodes tumor) of the prostate with distant metastasis, Cancer 68:910-915, 1991.
616. Bostwick DG, Halling AC, Jones EC et al: Prostatic phyllodes tumor: proposed grading system based on clinicopathologic study of seven cases and review of the literature, manuscript submitted for publication, 1996.
617. Casiraghi O, Martinez-Madrigal F, Mostofi FK et al: Primary prostatic Wilms' tumor, Am J Surg Pathol 15:885-890, 1991.
618. Johnson DE, Chalbaud R, Ayala AG: Secondary tumors of the prostate, J Urol 112:507-508, 1974.
619. Zein TA, Huben R, Lane W et al: Secondary tumors of the prostate, J Urol 133:615-616, 1985.
620. Grignon DJ, Ro JY, Ayala AG: Malignant melanoma with metastasis to adenocarcinoma of the prostate, Cancer 63:196-198, 1989.
621. Stein BS, Kendall AR: Malignant melanoma of the genitourinary tract, J Urol 132:859-868, 1984.
622. Parr NJ, Grigor KM, Ritchie AWS: Metastatic carcinoid tumour involving the prostate, Br J Urol 70:103-104, 1992.
623. Berry NE, Reese L: Malignant melanoma which had its first clinical manifestations in the prostate gland, J Urol 69:286-287, 1953.
624. Thompson GJ, Albers DD, Broders AC: Unusual carcinomas involving the prostate gland, J Urol 69:416-418, 1953.
625. Albers DD, Stephenson PL: Metastatic carcinoma of the prostate from silent carcinoma of the stomach. A case report, J Okla State Med Assoc 55:78-81, 1962.
626. Dowd JB: Carcinoma of the pancreas presenting as obstructing cancer of the prostate, Lahey Clin Bull 13:214-215, 1964.
627. Karolyi P, Endes P, Krasznai G et al: Bizarre leiomyoma of the prostate, Virchows Arch A Pathol Anat Histopathol 412:383-387, 1988.
628. Regan JB, Barrett DM, Wold LE: Giant leiomyoma of the prostate, Arch Pathol Lab Med 111:381-383, 1987.
629. Leonard A, Baert L, Van Praet F et al: Solitary leiomyoma of the prostate, Br J Urol 60:184-187, 1988.
630. Persaud V, Douglas LL: Bizarre (atypical) leiomyoma of the prostate gland, West Indian Med J 31:217-220, 1982.
631. Wunsch PH, Muller HA: Hemangiopericytoma of the prostate: a light microscopic study of an unusual tumor, Pathol Res Pract 172:334-336, 1982.
632. Chen KTK: Hemangiopericytoma of the prostate, J Surg Oncol 35:42-45, 1987.
633. Reyes JW, Shinozuka H, Garry P et al: A light and electron microscopic study of a hemangiopericytoma of the prostate with local extension, Cancer 40:1122-1127, 1977.
634. Dennis PJ, Lewandowski AE, Rohner TJ Jr et al: Pheochromocytoma of the prostate: an unusual location, J Urol 141:130-132, 1989.
635. Maluf HM, King ME, DeLuca FR et al: Giant multilocular prostatic cystadenoma: a distinctive lesion of the retroperitoneum in men. A report of two cases, Am J Surg Pathol 15:131-137, 1991.
636. Lim DJ, Hayden RT, Murad T et al: Multilocular prostatic cystadnoma presenting as a large complex pelvic cystic mass, J Urol 149:856-859, 1993.
637. Watanabe J, Konishi T, Takeuchi H et al: A case of giant prostatic cystadenoma, Acta Urol Jap 36:1077-1079, 1990.
638. Levy DA, Gogate PA, Hampel N: Giant multilocular prostatic cystadenoma: a rare clinical entity and review of the literature, J Urol 150:1920-1922, 1993.
639. Waring PM, Newland RC: Prostatic embryonal rhabdomyosarcoma in adults. A clinicopathologic review, Cancer 69:755-762, 1992.
640. Ghavimi F, Herr H, Jereb B et al: Treatment of genitourinary rhabdomyosarcoma in children, J Urol 132:313, 1984.
641. Loughlin KR, Retik AB, Weinstein HJ et al: Genitourinary rhabdomyosarcoma in children, Cancer 63:1600-1606, 1989.
642. Asmar L, Gehan EA, Newton WA et al: Agreement among and within groups of pathologists in the classification of rhabdomyosarcoma and related childhood sarcomas. Report of an international study of four pathology classifications, Cancer 74:2579-2588, 1994.
643. Boyle ET Jr, Reiman HM, Kramer SA et al: Embryonal rhabdomyosarcoma of bladder and prostate: nuclear DNA patterns studied by flow cytometry, J Urol 140:1119-1121, 1988.
644. Raney RB Jr, Gehan EA, Hays DM et al: Primary chemotherapy with or without radiation therapy and/or surgery for children with localized sarcoma of the bladder, prostate, vagina, uterus, and cervix. A comparison of the results in Intergroup Rhabdomyosarcoma Studies I and II, Cancer 66:2072-2081, 1990.
645. Verga G, Parigi GB: Conservative surgery of bladder-prostate rhabdomyosarcoma in children: results after long-term follow-up, J Pediatr Surg 28:1016-1018, 1993.
646. Witherow R, Molland E, Oliver T et al: Leiomyosarcoma of prostate and superficial soft tissue, Urology 15:513, 1980.
647. Cheville JC, Dundore PA, Nascimento AG et al: Leiomyosarcoma of the prostate. Report of 23 cases, Cancer 76:1422-1427, 1995.
648. Ramos A, Davis C, Sesterhenn I et al: Preliminary findings in 20 prostatic leiomyosarcomas, Mod Pathol 6:67A, 1993.
649. Chin W, Fay R, Ortega P: Malignant fibrous histiocytoma of prostate, Urology 27:363-365, 1986.
650. Bain GO, Danyluk JM, Shnitka TK et al: Malignant fibrous histiocytoma of prostate gland, Urology 26:89-91, 1985.

651. Smith DM, Manivel C, Kapps D et al: Angiosarcoma of the prostate: report of 2 cases and review of the literature, J Urol 135:382-384, 1986.
652. Ekfors TO, Aho HJ, Kekomaki M: Malignant rhabdoid tumor of the prostatic region. Immunohistological and ultrastructural evidence for epithelial origin, Virchows Arch A Pathol Anat Histopathol 406:381-388, 1985.
653. Proppe KH, Scully RE, Rosai J: Postoperative spindle cell nodules of genitourinary tract resembling sarcomas: a report of eight cases, Am J Surg Pathol 8:101-108, 1984.
654. Huang WL, Ro JY, Grignon DJ et al: Postoperative spindle cell nodule of the prostate and bladder, J Urol 143:824-826, 1990.
655. Ro JY, El-Naggar AK, Amin MB et al: Pseudosarcomatous fibromyxoid tumor of the urinary bladder and prostate. Immunohistochemical, ultrastructural, and DNA flow cytometric analyses of nine cases, Hum Pathol 24:1203-1210, 1993.
656. Tetu B, Ro JY, Ayala AG et al: Atypical spindle cell lesions of the prostate, Semin Diagn Pathol 5:284-293, 1988.
657. Hafiz MA, Toker C, Sutula M: An atypical fibromyxoid tumor of the prostate, Cancer 54:2500-2504, 1984.
658. Sahin AA, Ro JY, El-Naggar AK et al: Pseudosarcomatous fibromyxoid tumor of the prostate, Am J Clin Pathol 96:253-258, 1991.
659. Young RH, Scully RE: Pseudosarcomatous lesions of the urinary bladder, prostate gland, and urethra: a report of three cases and review of the literature, Arch Pathol Lab Med 111:354-358, 1987.
660. Bostwick DG, Mann RB: Malignant lymphomas involving the prostate. A study of 13 cases, Cancer 56:2932-2938, 1985.
661. Suzuki H, Nakada T, Iijima Y et al: Malignant lymphoma of the prostate. Report of a case, Urol Int 47:172-175, 1991.
662. Ewing J: Neoplastic diseases, ed 4, Philadelphia, 1940, WB Saunders.
663. Fukase N: Hyperplasia of the rudimentary lymph nodes of the prostate, Surg Gynecol Obstet 35:131-136, 1922.
664. Fell P, O'Connor M, Smith JM: Primary lymphoma of prostate presenting as bladder outflow obstruction, Urology 29:555-559, 1987.
665. Ben-Ezra J, Sheibani K, Kendrick FE et al: Angiotropic large cell lymphoma of the prostate gland: an immunohistochemical study, Hum Pathol 17:964-966, 1986.
666. Banerjee SS, Harris M: Angiotropic lymphoma presenting in the prostate, Histopathology 12:667-683, 1988.
667. Peison B, Benisch B, Nicora B et al: Acute urinary obstruction secondary to pseudolymphoma of prostate, Urology 10:478-479, 1977.
668. Humphrey PA, Vollmer RT: Extramedullary hematopoiesis in the prostate, Am J Surg Pathol 15:486-490, 1991.
669. Viadana E, Bross IDJ, Pickren JW: An autopsy study of the metastatic patterns of human leukaemias, Oncology 35:87-96, 1978.
670. Cachia PG, McIntyre MA, Dewar AE et al: Prostatic infiltration in chronic lymphatic leukaemia, J Clin Pathol 40:342-345, 1987.
671. Sridhar KN, Woodhouse CRJ: Prostatic infiltration in leukaemia and lymphoma, Eur Urol 9:153-156, 1983.
672. Thalhammer F, Gisslinger H, Chott A et al: Granulocytic sarcoma of the prostate as the first manifestation of a late relapse of acute myelogenous leukemia, Ann Hematol 68:97-99, 1994.
673. Frame R, Head D, Lee R et al: Granulocytic sarcoma of the prostate. Two cases causing urinary obstruction, Cancer 59:142-146, 1987.
674. Yasuda N, Ohmori S-I, Usui T: IgD myelomas involving the prostate, Am J Hematol 47:65-66, 1994.
675. Benson RC Jr, Segura JW, Carney JA: Primary yolk-sac (endodermal sinus) tumor of the prostate, Cancer 41:1395-1398, 1978.
676. Dalla Palma P, Dante S, Guazzieri S et al: Primary endodermal sinus tumor of the prostate: report of a case, Prostate 12:255-261, 1988.
677. Arai Y, Watanabe J, Kounami T et al: Retroperitoneal seminoma with simultaneous occurrence in the prostate, J Urol 139:382-385, 1988.
678. Michel F, Gattengo B, Roland J et al: Primary nonseminomatous germ cell tumor of the prostate, J Urol 135:597-599, 1986.
679. Prym P: Spontanheilung eines bosartigen, wahrscheinlich Chorionepitheliomatosen gewachses im Hodem, Virchows Arch A Pathol Anat Histopathol 265:239-244, 1927.
680. Dvoracek C: Primarni chorionepitheliom prostaty s gynekomastii, Cas Lak Cesk 88:198-202, 1949.
681. Beckman EN, Pintado SO, Leonard GL et al: Endometriosis of the prostate, Am J Surg Pathol 9:374-379, 1985.
682. Deguchi T, Doi T, Ehara H et al: Detection of micrometastatic prostate cancer cells in lymph nodes by reverse transcriptase-polymerase chain reaction, Cancer Res 53:5350-5354, 1993.
683. Mansi JL, Berger U, Wilson P et al: Detection of tumor cells in bone marrow patients with prostatic carcinoma by immunocytochemical techniques, J Urol 139:545-550, 1988.
684. Wood DP Jr, Banks ER, Humphreys S et al: Identification of bone marrow micrometastases in patients with prostate cancer, Cancer 74:2533-2540, 1994.
685. Moreno JG, Croce CM, Fisher R et al: Detection of hematogenous micrometastases in patients with prostate cancer, Cancer Res 52:6110-6112, 1992.

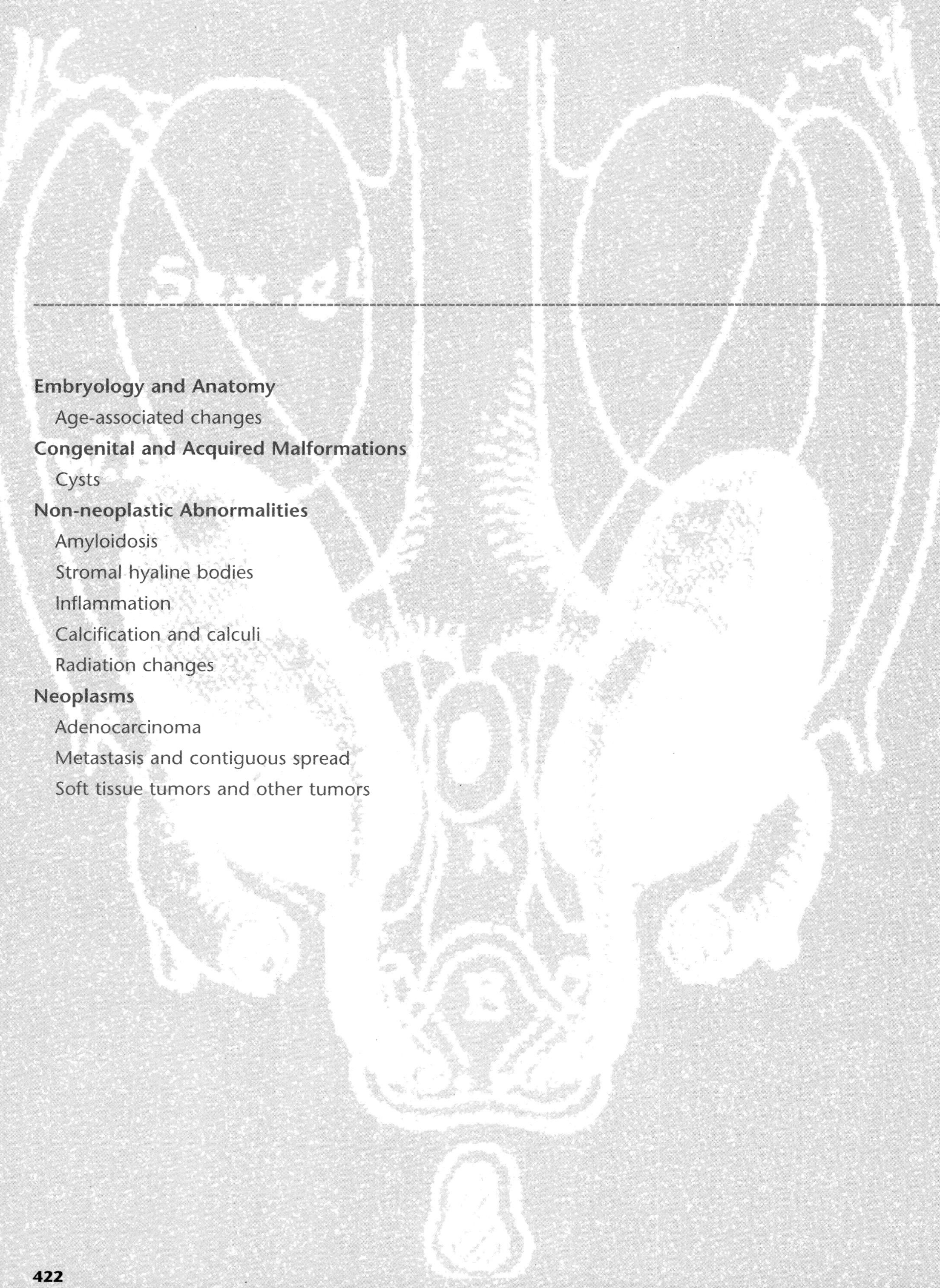

Embryology and Anatomy

Age-associated changes

Congenital and Acquired Malformations

Cysts

Non-neoplastic Abnormalities

Amyloidosis

Stromal hyaline bodies

Inflammation

Calcification and calculi

Radiation changes

Neoplasms

Adenocarcinoma

Metastasis and contiguous spread

Soft tissue tumors and other tumors

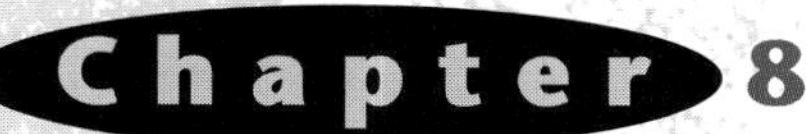

SEMINAL VESICLES

DAVID G. BOSTWICK

The seminal vesicles were described by the Italian anatomist Berengario a Carpi in 1521. These paired androgen-dependent accessory sex glands were first regarded simply as storage sites for semen, but their milky alkaline secretions are now known to constitute the majority of the ejaculate, promoting sperm function and providing a variety of potent antibacterial factors to the male genital tract.[1-3] Infections, cysts, and neoplasms of the seminal vesicles are rare, in sharp contrast with their anatomic neighbor, the prostate.

EMBRYOLOGY AND ANATOMY

Under the influence of testosterone, the seminal vesicles appear during the thirteenth week of development as outpouchings of the lower mesonephric ducts. They are bounded by the prostate distally, the base of the bladder anteriorly, and Denonvilliers' fascia and the rectum posteriorly. Their anatomic position in this region is variable, and they are sometimes found within or adherent to the posterior capsule of the prostate gland. The seminal vesicles may be palpable on digital rectal examination, and, when adherent to the prostate, may be mistaken for prostatic nodularity or induration. Approximately 5% of prostate biopsies for nodularity contain fragments of seminal vesicle epithelium, a potential source of diagnostic confusion (Fig. 8-1).[4] In adults, the seminal vesicles average 6 cm long and 2 cm wide, with a capacity of up to 4.5 ml, although there is wide variation in size, shape, and volume.[3]

The muscular wall of the seminal vesicles consists of a thick circumferential coat of smooth muscle, which contracts during ejaculation. Contraction is regulated by excitatory adrenergic and modulatory neuropeptide-Y-encephalin-peptidergic nerve fibers.[3] Tangential cuts through this wall frequently reveal irregular clusters of epithelial tubules, which may be mistaken for adenocarcinoma.

The ducts of the seminal vesicles merge with the ampullae of the vasa deferentia on each side to form the ejaculatory ducts, and these structures compose a functional unit that develops slowly until the onset of puberty.[3] These ducts immediately enter the central zone of the prostate and converge as they approach their outlets at either side of the verumontanum in the prostatic sinus of the prostatic urethra.

Histologically, the seminal vesicular mucosa consists of complex papillary folds and irregular convoluted lumens lined with nonciliated, pseudostratified tall columnar epithelium. The cells are predominantly secretory, containing microvesicular lipid droplets and characteristic lipofuscin pigment granules. The pigment is golden-brown and refractile, increasing in amount with age. These cells also contain androgen receptors, similar to the prostatic epithelium. Secretory products include glycoproteins, protein kinase inhibitor, protein C inhibitor, fructose, prostaglandins, ascorbic acid, sperm motility factor, transferrin, lactoferrin, lysozyme, and metallothionein. Secretion is regulated by nerves from the pelvic plexus, which are cholinergic post-ganglionic, sympathetic, and possibly parasympathetic.[3,5,6] Up to 85% of the seminal fluid originates in the seminal vesicles, and the semen volume varies from 2 to 5 ml. It takes 3 days for the epithelium to refill the seminal vesicles after ejaculation.

AGE-ASSOCIATED CHANGES

The seminal vesicles begin to shrink in the seventh decade.[7] The tall columnar cells lining the mucosa in young men are replaced over time by flattened cuboidal cells, comprising only 50% of the epithelium in men in the fifth decade of life and 2% in octagenarians. With advancing age, the stroma of the seminal vesicles becomes hyalinized and fibrotic.

The flattening of the epithelium is accompanied by striking nuclear abnormalities, and highly atypical cells are present in about 75% of older men (Fig. 8-2).[8-13] These cells have large irregular hyperchromatic nuclei with coarse chromatin and prominent nucleoli. Multinucleated cells are also present, as well as giant ring-shaped nuclei with large intranuclear cytoplasmic inclusions. Mitotic figures are absent. These nuclear abnormalities, not observed before age 20, are probably degenerative

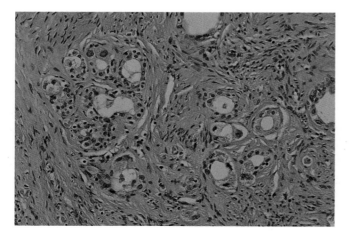

8-1. Tangential needle biopsy through the seminal vesicles, which may be mistaken for adenocarcinoma.

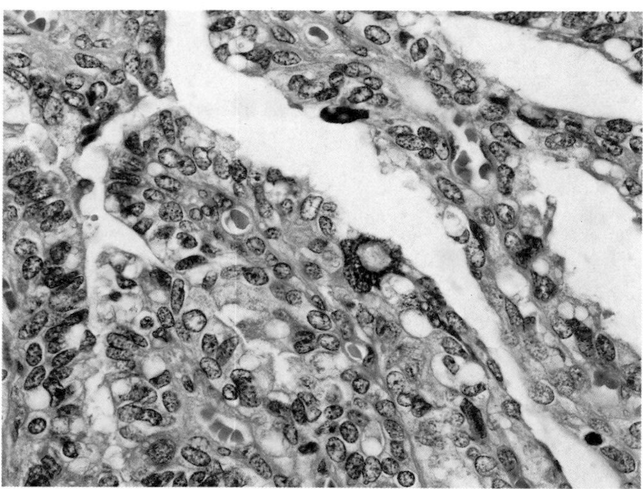

8-2. Seminal vesicle from an 80-year-old man showing distinctive highly atypical epithelial cells.

changes reflecting hormonal influences. When encountered in needle biopsies, such "pseudomalignant" cytologic atypia may lead to a mistaken diagnosis of prostate cancer. Difficulty may also be encountered in cytologic evaluation of fluids obtained by prostatic massage because seminal vesicular cells are frequently shed intact into the lumens. The distinctive lipochrome pigment aids in their recognition.[10-12] Cells in prostatic aspirates derived from the seminal vesicles and ejaculatory ducts may be cytologically indistinguishable. DNA ploidy analysis reveals aneuploidy in 6.7% of seminal vesicles.[13] Consequently, DNA analysis of prostate cancer specimens may yield false-positive results if contaminated by seminal vesicle tissue. It is uncertain why there is such a low level of aneuploidy in an organ with frequent and substantial cytologic atypia.

Seminal vesicular cells are found as contaminants of cervical smears in 10% of specimens with spermatozoa, and may be diagnostically confusing.[14] These cells contain foamy cytoplasm, scant pigment, vesicular hyperchromatic nuclei, sieve-like chromatin pattern, and mild anisokaryosis.

CONGENITAL AND ACQUIRED MALFORMATIONS

Malformations of the seminal vesicles are frequently associated with abnormal development of other mesonephric derivatives, although isolated hypoplasia, agenesis, and cysts have been reported.[15] Unilateral absence of one seminal vesicle may be associated with ipsilateral renal agenesis. Unilateral agenesis is often associated with decreased semen volume, hypospermia or azoospermia, impaired sperm motility, acidic ejaculate, and absence of fructose and coagulation activity. Up to 37.5% of these men are infertile, implying that the single vas is abnormal. Bilateral dilation or absence of the seminal vesicles is sometimes observed in patients with cystic fibrosis, reportedly caused by an unexplained failure of development.[16] Unilateral duplication of the seminal vesicles is an unusual anomaly. Seminal vesicle surgery is usually undertaken for evaluation of congenital malformations.

Maldevelopment of the ureteric bud results in ureteral ectopy, with the ureters terminating in the seminal vesicles, prostatic urethra, vas deferens, epididymis, or ejaculatory ducts. Ureteral ectopy is frequently seen in association with ipsilateral renal dysgenesis or contralateral renal hypertrophy, and the seminal vesicles become enlarged and dilated with accompanying ureterocele.

CYSTS

Seminal vesicle cysts are rare and may be congenital or aquired. Symptoms are vague, including perineal pain during ejaculation or defecation, dysuria, urinary retention, and recurrent epididymitis. Congenital cysts are associated with ipsilateral renal agenesis in 80% of cases and commonly with ureteral ectopia or agenesis (Zinner's syndrome), with more than 100 reported cases.[17-27] These paired anomalies are caused by the close association of the ureteric bud and mesonephric duct during embryogenesis; the ureteric bud is more cephalad, and the elongated ureter may fail to connect with and stimulate the differentiation of the nephrogenic blastema. Other cases of congenital cysts are associated with ipsilateral absence of the testis[28] or hemivertebra.[29] Congenital cysts of the seminal vesicle are usually detected in patients between 18 and 41 years of age, the period of maximal sexual and reproductive activity; all have arisen in white patients except for one black patient.[30] The cyst is usually unilateral and unilocular, lateral to the midline, up to three times larger than the normal seminal vesicle, and considerably smaller than müllerian duct cysts (Table 8-1). Enlargement is caused by insufficient drainage with accumulation of seminal fluid. This unilocular cyst contains viscous pale white fluid, similar to the usual secretions of the seminal vesicles, and is lined with a cuboidal or flattened epithelium with a fibrous wall of variable thickness. Massive enlargement has been called *hydrocele* or *hydrops*.[31] Bilateral congenital cysts are rare and may be associated with absent vasa deferentia.[32]

Acquired cyst is usually associated with inflammation and obstruction of the ejaculatory ducts and seminal vesicles (Fig. 8-3). This fluctuant cyst may be palpable on digital rectal examination, and often contains red cells, white cells, and spermatozoa. The epithelial lining is inflamed or sloughed, depending on the duration and severity of inflammation. In one case, endoscopic removal of a small calculus lodged at the orifice of the ipsilateral ejaculatory duct caused complete resolution of a 14 cm seminal vesicle cyst, evidence for an obstructive etiology and demonstration of the utility of preoperative imaging techniques to detect stones.[33] Echinococcal

TABLE 8-1.
DIFFERENTIAL DIAGNOSIS OF SEMINAL VESICLE CYST

Type of Cyst	Location	Size	Contains Sperm
Seminal vesicle cyst	Lateral	Large	Yes
Diverticulum of ejaculatory duct of ampulla	Lateral	Variable	Yes
Prostatic cyst	Lateral	Variable	No
Müllerian duct cyst	Midline	Large	No

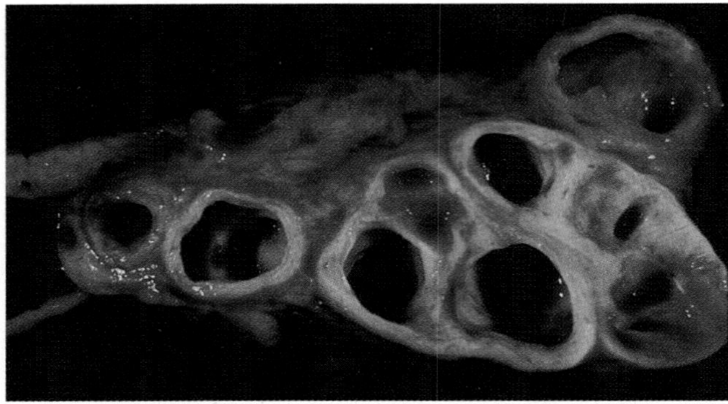

8-3. Incidental acquired cyst of the seminal vesicles found at autopsy in a 70-year-old man.

(hydatid) cyst can occur in the retrovesicular region, invariably in association wth infection in another organ.[34] Megavesicles are characterized by marked dilation of the seminal vesicles. The cause of megavesicles is unknown, but this condition is sometimes seen in diabetics.[35] Cystadenoma is a benign neoplasm mimicking aquired cyst (see later in this chapter).

The differential diagnosis of seminal vesicle cyst includes prostatic cyst, ejaculatory duct diverticulum, and cystic dilation of wolffian and müllerian duct remnants (see Table 8-1).[35,36] The cysts may produce hydronephrosis caused by displacement of the lower ureter toward the midline with obstruction. Radiographic evaluation of seminal vesicle cyst includes vasoseminovesiculography, ultrasonography, computerized tomography, and magnetic resonance imaging.[21,37] Aspiration of congenital or aquired cysts relieves symptoms, but surgical removal or marsupialization is preferred.

NON-NEOPLASTIC ABNORMALITIES

AMYLOIDOSIS

Localized amyloidosis of the seminal vesicles (senile seminal vesicle amyloidosis) is observed at autopsy in 5% to 8% of men between 46 and 60 years of age, 13% to 23% between 61 and 75 years, and 21% to 34% over 75 years.[38-40] It often extends bilaterally along the ejaculatory ducts, forming linear or massive nodular subepithelial deposits of amorphous eosinophilic fibrillar material (Fig. 8-4). Basement membrane thickening is observed, and deposits may be seen within the vesicular lumens, occasionally causing significant luminal narrowing. Rare cases are associated with calcification or a florid foreign body giant cell reaction.[41] By contrast, systemic amyloidosis infrequently affects the seminal vesicles, involving vascular walls, smooth muscle, and stroma. Vesicular amyloidosis is usually asymptomatic, but may cause hematospermia, chronic perineal pain, or mimic seminal vesiculitis.[42,43] It cannot be visualized by imaging studies except for pelvic magnetic resonance imaging, and may mimic tumor invasion from bladder or prostate cancer.[44-46] Localized and systemic amyloidosis may coexist.[47]

Special stains that confirm the diagnosis of amyloid include Congo red, which appears red by light microscopy with apple-green polarization birefringence; methylene blue, which reveals green polarization birefringence; crystal violet and toluidine blue, which impart a metachromatic appearance to the deposits; and periodic acid-Schiff (PAS) and Alcian blue stains, which are weakly to moderately positive. The composition of localized seminal vesicle amyloid is histochemically unique (permanganate-sensitive, non-AA, non-B2M, non-pre-albumin type), apparently derived from secretory protein of the seminal vesicles; amyloid at other sites is derived from light chains or serum amyloid protein.[38,41,47-49]

STROMAL HYALINE BODIES

Small 15 to 20 μm eosinophilic hyaline bodies are sometimes observed within the muscular wall of the seminal vesicles, vas deferens, and prostate, and are designated stromal hyaline bodies (Fig. 8-5).[9,50,51] These round to oval structures probably result from degeneration of smooth muscle fibers, and transition forms can be seen arising from smooth muscle cells. They stain red with Masson trichrome and pink with PAS, but fail to stain with PTAH, methyl green pyronine, Feulgen, Alcian blue at pH 2.5, or Congo red.

INFLAMMATION

Seminal vesiculitis is associated with infection and inflammation of adjacent organs, including the prostate, bladder, ejaculatory ducts, vas deferens, and epididymis.[52] Acute vesiculitis is usually caused by retrograde infection with or without indwelling catheter, ureteral or ejaculatory duct stenosis or anatomic anomaly, calculi, or surgical trauma (Fig. 8-6). Studies in rats have shown that the seminal vesicles are highly resistant to infection unless their secretory capability is decreased as occurs with androgen deprivation.[53] Antibiotic therapy is usually effective, employing the same agents used for acute prostatitis; biopsies are rarely obtained in such cases and may be contraindicated because of complications of abscess formation and stricture. Protracted acute and chronic seminal vesiculitis results in atrophy and ejaculatory duct stricture. Abscess presents with irritative voiding symptoms, fever, and pain in the scrotum, testis, perineum, or rectum; ultrasonography, computerized coaxial tomography, and magnetic resonance imaging are useful in verifying the diagnosis and directing transurethral incision and drainage.[54,55]

Chronic vesiculitis is associated with chronic prostatitis, and both respond poorly to antibiotic therapy. Prior to the antibiotic era, the most common cause of vesiculitis was tuberculosis, which resulted in perineal fistula, fibrous adhesions, ejaculatory duct stricture, and massive circumferential calcification of the walls of the seminal vesicles at the site of previous necrotizing granulomas. Seminal vesicle dilation and congestion may occur after prostatectomy, resulting in persistent dysuria.[56]

Schistosomiasis, usually secondary to *S. haematobium* infection of the bladder, involves the seminal vesicles more commonly than the prostate. Viruses, fungi, and parasites

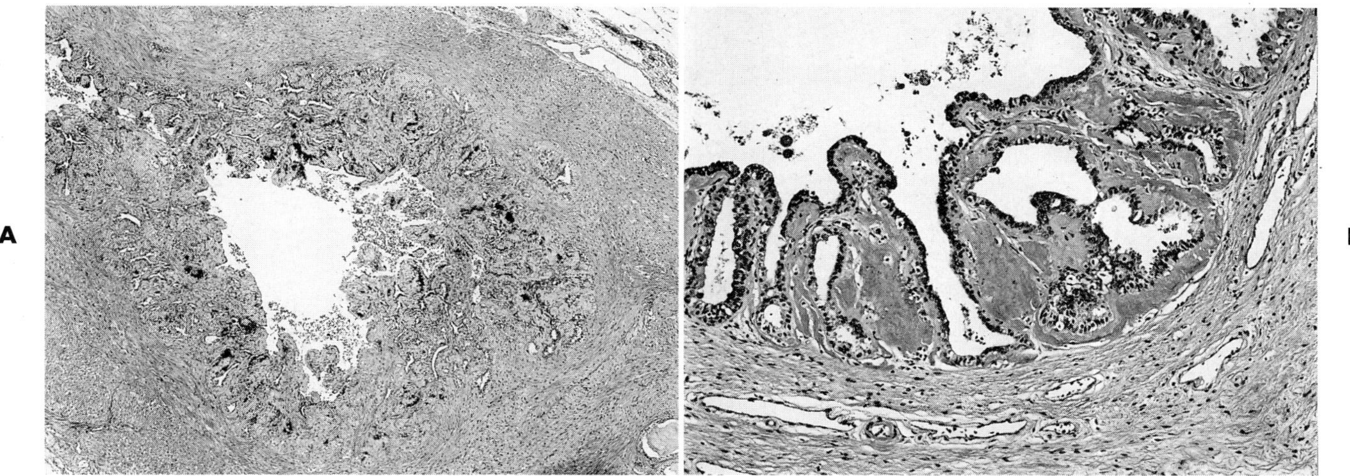

8-4. Amyloidosis of seminal vesicles (A) and ejaculatory ducts (B).

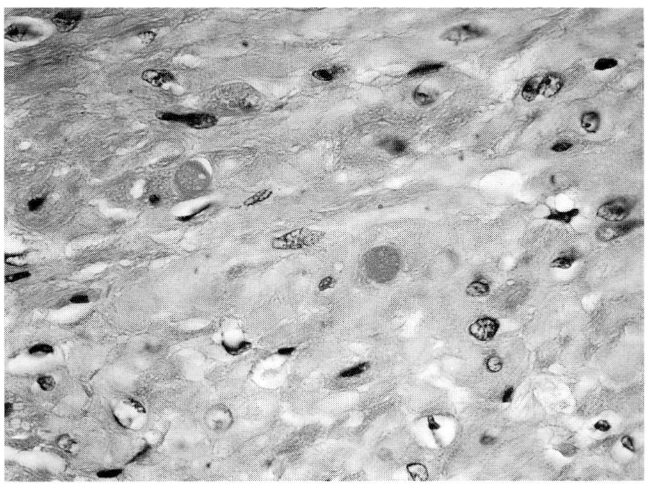

8-5. Stromal hyaline bodies within the muscular wall of the seminal vesicles.

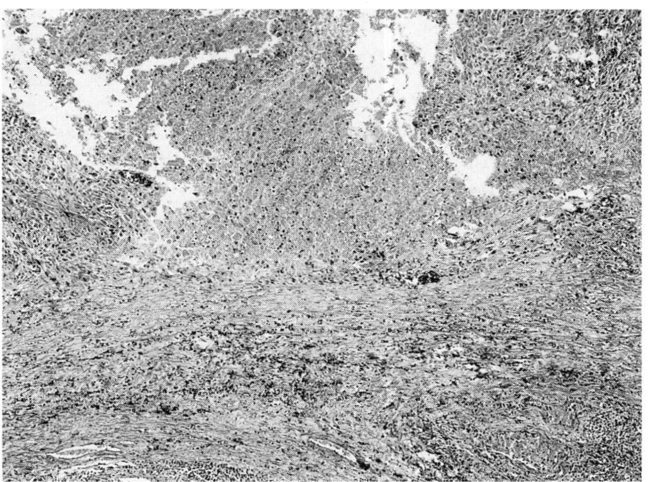

8-6. Patchy acute seminal vesiculitis.

are rare causes of seminal vesiculitis. Echinococcal cyst of the seminal vesicles and prostate has been reported.[34]

Surgery for seminal vesiculitis is unnecessary unless complicated by abscess, fistula, or stricture. In the early 1900s, the seminal vesicles were thought to be the cause of inflammatory rheumatoid disease, and perineal seminal vesiculotomy was popular at that time. This was also the treatment of choice for vesicular tuberculosis until the advent of antibiotic therapy.

CALCIFICATION AND CALCULI

Calcification often follows seminal vesiculitis, particularly with tuberculosis. Patients with long histories of diabetes mellitus or uremia also develop dystrophic calcification of the seminal vesicles and other mesonephric derivatives. Most foci of calcification are idiopathic and asymptomatic, and imaging studies of the pelvis may detect them incidentally (Fig. 8-7). Calcification may be unilateral or bilateral and usually coexists with calcification of the vas deferens.[57-65] Calcification is present with the muscular wall, often forming concentric rings; the mucosa is rarely involved. Osseous metaplasia is also rarely observed in the wall (see Fig. 8-7).

Calculi are more frequent in the seminal vesicles than in the vas deferens, appearing as brown stones of variable number up to 1 cm in diameter (Fig. 8-8). They usually consist of phosphate and carbonate salts. The mechanism of formation is uncertain, but may be caused by reflux of urine up the ejaculatory ducts.[66,67]

RADIATION CHANGES

Radiation therapy for prostatic carcinoma causes atrophy and fibrosis of the seminal vesicles and perivesicular fat in 89% of patients.[68] The golden-brown lipochrome pigment characteristic of the seminal vesicle epithelium is retained. Magnetic resonance imaging shows decreased luminal fluid and stromal fibrosis in about 37% of cases.[69]

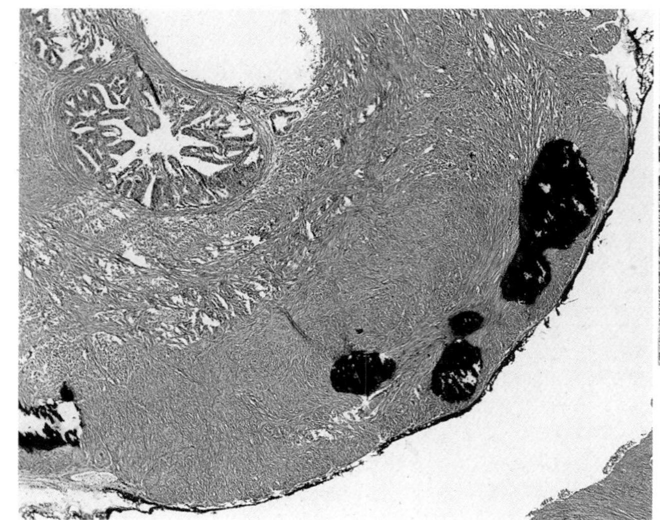

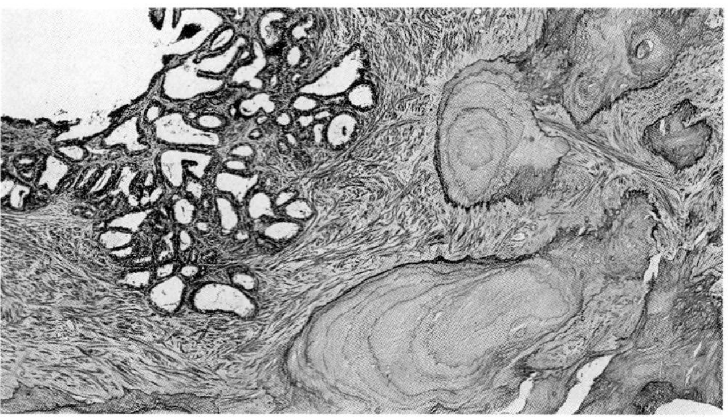

8-7. **A**, Idiopathic mural calcification of the seminal vesicle in a patient undergoing radical prostatoseminovesiculectomy for prostatic adenocarcinoma. **B**, Osseous metaplasia.

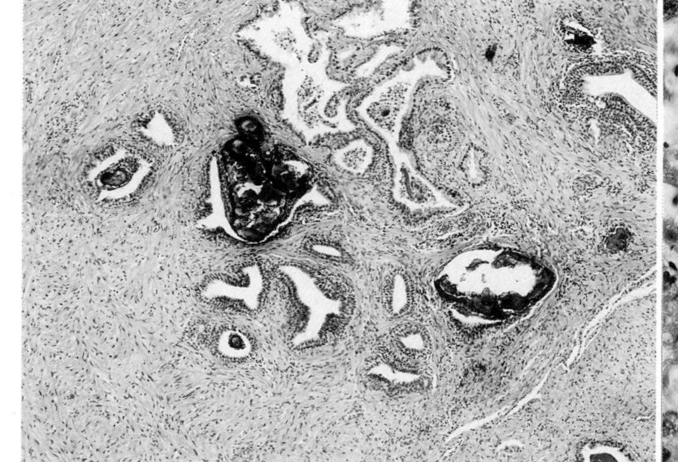

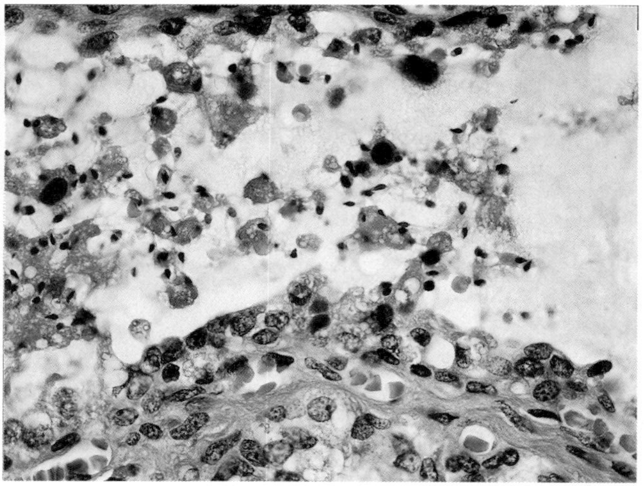

8-8. **A**, Calculi within the seminal vesicular lumen. **B**, Sperm within the seminal vesicular lumens.

NEOPLASMS

The seminal vesicles are frequently involved secondarily by tumors originating elsewhere, particularly prostatic carcinoma. However, fewer than 100 primary neoplasms of the seminal vesicles have been reported. Clinical documentation of many is poor, and the pathologic diagnosis is often questionable.

ADENOCARCINOMA

Adenocarcinoma is the most common primary malignancy of the seminal vesicles, but is extremely rare, with fewer than 40 acceptable cases reported.[70-73] Mean patient age is 62 years (range, 17 to 90 years), and presenting symptoms include urinary obstruction and hematospermia.[71,74] Seminovesiculography and computerized tomography are useful in identifying these tumors.

The diagnosis of seminal vesicle adenocarcinoma requires the following: (1) tumor located primarily in the seminal vesicle; (2) no evidence of carcinoma in the prostate, bladder, or colon; (3) architectural features of adenocarcinoma, usually with papillary or sheet-like growth and mucinous differentiation; (4) in situ adenocarcinoma in the adjacent seminal vesicle epithelium; (5) cytoplasmic immunoreactivity for carcinoembryonic antigen (CEA); and (6) absence of staining for prostate-specific antigen and prostatic acid phosphatase. With high-stage, poorly differentiated adenocarcinoma, the precise site of origin may be impossible to determine. Tumor cells may be hobnail, columnar, or polygonal, with clear cytoplasm and rarely lipofuscin. Radical surgery and external beam radiation therapy have been employed in many cases, but the prognosis is poor. Androgen deprivation therapy may also be of value.[75,76]

Two cases of noninvasive, well-differentiated adenocarcinoma have been reported within seminal vesicle cysts, including one in a 19-year-old with an aquired cyst[74] and another in a 17-year-old with congenital cyst

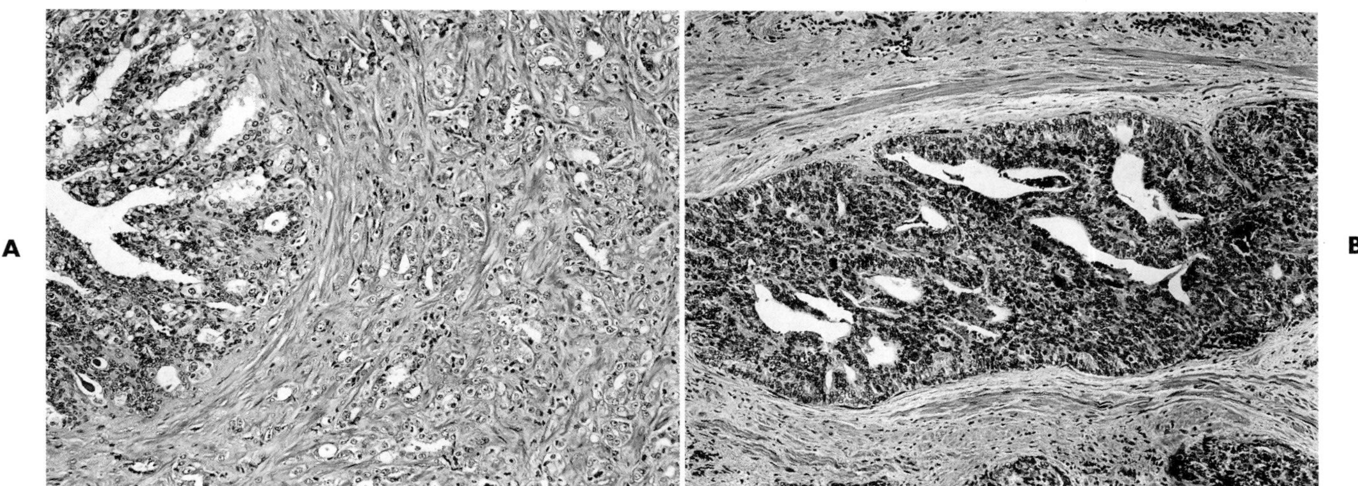

8-9. Prostatic adenocarcinoma invading the seminal vesicles (**A**) and fill the ejaculatory ducts (**B**).

and ipsilateral renal agenesis.[77] A case of combined seminal vesicle adenocarcinoma, prostatic adenocarcinoma, and carcinosarcoma was recently reported with autopsy documentation.[78] Ohmori et al described a primary adenocarcinoma of the seminal vesicles that expressed CA-125 immunoreactivity and showed serologic evidence of this marker, which fluctuated with growth and recurrence of the cancer.[79]

Adenocarcinoma of the seminal vesicles and prostate can be induced experimentally in Lobund-Wistar rats using a combination of testosterone proprionate and nitrosamine compounds. A recently described system for grading these tumors stratifies them into three groups: in situ, invasive without desmoplasia, and invasive with desmoplasia.[80]

METASTASIS AND CONTIGUOUS SPREAD

Seminal vesicle involvement by prostatic adenocarcinoma is common, observed in about 12% of radical prostatectomy specimens from patients with cancer clinically confined to the prostate (Fig. 8-9). There are three patterns of seminal vesicle invasion: direct spread along the ejaculatory duct complex into the seminal vesicles, prostatic capsular perforation followed by extension into the periprostatic soft tissues and spread into the seminal vesicles, and isolated deposits of cancer in the seminal vesicles (see Chapter 7).[81-84]

Bulky urothelial carcinoma of the bladder may also invade the seminal vesicles by direct extension or mucosal spread.[85] Direct extension is usually observed in cancer of the trigone and inferoposterior wall and indicates pathologic stage T4 cancer. Mucosal involvement by in situ urothelial carcinoma is rare, present in only 1% of cases. It spreads along the mucosa of the prostatic urethra, the prostatic and ejaculatory ducts, and seminal vesicles by intraepithelial replacement and pagetoid spread along the basement membrane. Rectal adenocarcinoma occasionally invades the seminal vesicles and prostate, and may cause diagnostic difficulty. Metastases to the seminal vesicles from other organs have only been reported in autopsy series, although a surgical case of seminoma metastatic to the retrovesicular space with entrapment of one seminal vesicle was recently described.[86]

SOFT TISSUE TUMORS AND OTHER TUMORS

A variety of benign soft tissue tumors have been described in the seminal vesicles, including leiomyoma[87,88] and fibroma. There is a spectrum of mixed epithelial-stromal neoplasms arising in the seminal vesicle, analogous to fibroadenoma and phyllodes tumor in the breast and prostate, and these have been referred to as cystadenoma,[89-92] cystomyoma,[93] low-grade phyllodes tumor,[94] benign mesenchymoma,[95] adenomyosis,[96] and mesonephric hamartoma.[97] Cystadenoma is a rare benign tumor composed of cysts lined with a simple columnar epithelium with chronically inflamed loose fibrous stroma or fibromuscular stroma (Fig. 8-10). The cysts are grossly multiloculated, ranging in size from 5 to 15 cm in diameter. Ultrasound and computed tomography scan reveal a characteristic "honeycombing" pattern.[98] The patients' average age is 60 years, and most cases are incidental findings at autopsy.[89-92] One case of cystadenoma did not recur in the 25 years after the initial resection (DG Bostwick, unpublished observation).[91]

Phyllodes tumor consists of a mixture of variably cellular stroma and glandular elements (Fig. 8-11). The density and cytologic features of the stroma determine whether the tumor is a fibroadenoma, low-grade phyllodes tumor, or high-grade phyllodes tumor (cytosarcoma phyllodes). Features considered predictive of malignancy of phyllodes tumor in the breast may apply in the seminal vesicles, including infiltrating margins, stromal atypia, increased numbers of mitotic features, and overgrowth of glands by stroma; however, too few cases have been reported in the seminal vesicles to determine prognosis based on histologic features alone. One case of low-grade phyllodes tumor displayed stromal pleomorphism without mitotic activity; 2 years

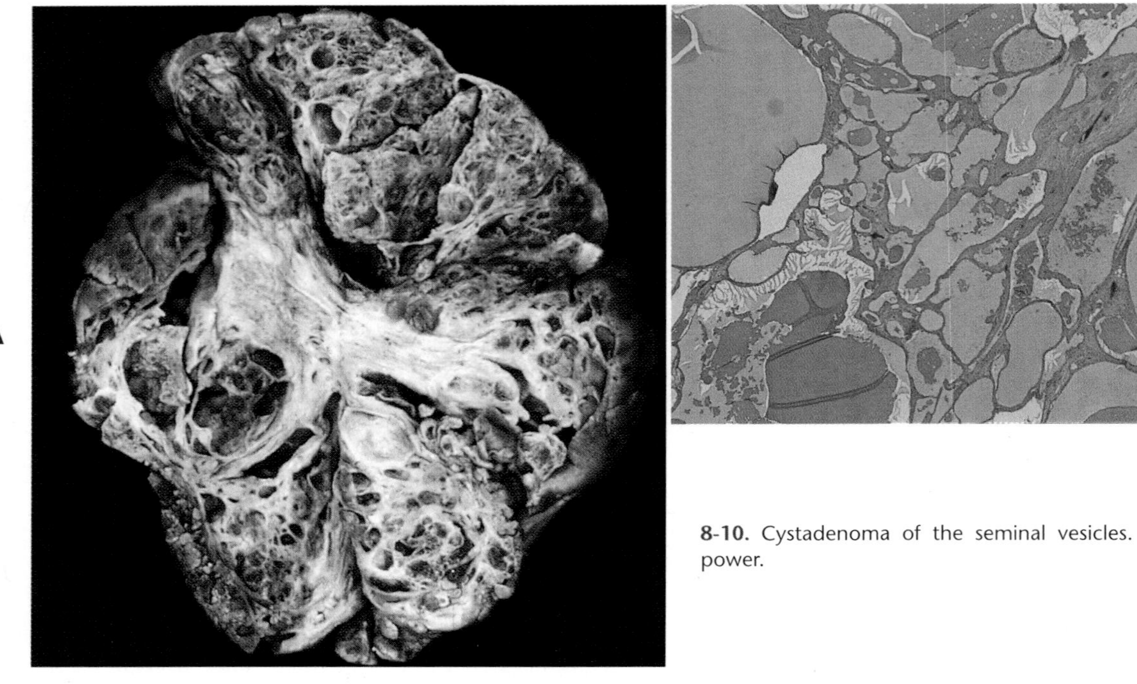

8-10. Cystadenoma of the seminal vesicles. A, gross; B, low power.

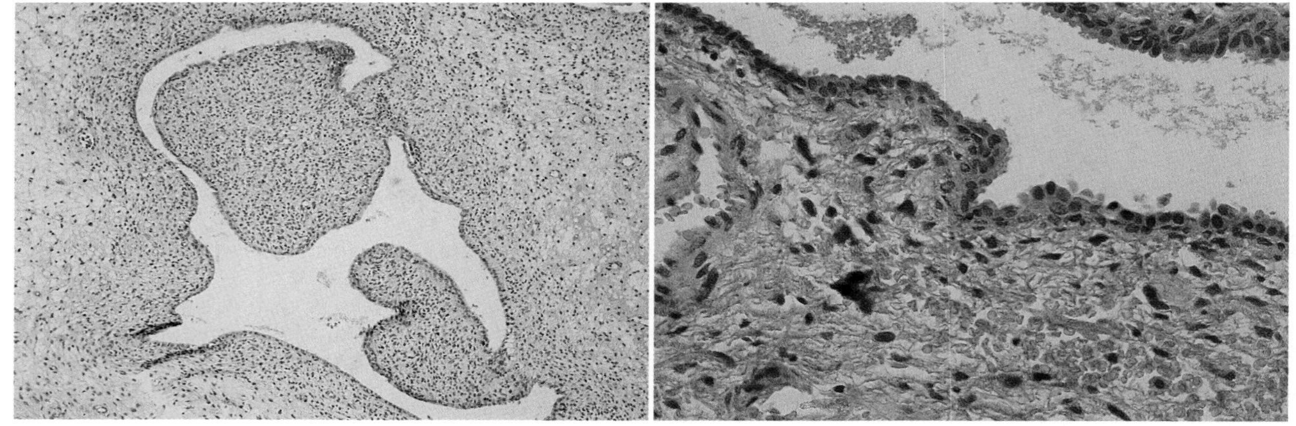

8-11. Cystosarcoma phyllodes of the seminal vesicle. At low magnification (**A**), there is a proliferation of slit-like epithelial spaces with a cellular stroma. At high magnification (**B**), the stromal cells display varying degrees of cytologic atypia.

after excision, the tumor recurred in the pelvis, but did not recur with 18-month follow up after second excision.[99] The authors preferred the descriptive term *cystic epithelial-stromal tumor* rather than *cystosarcoma* or *atypical cystadenoma* pending study of additional cases with long-term follow up. Another report described a benign tumor consisting of glands with epithelium arranged in leaf-like clefts and slits with subepithelial stromal condensation.[91] Two cases of cystosarcoma phyllodes have been reported, including one that metastasized to the lungs after 5 years despite radical surgery.[94,100] This tumor was considered malignant because of its expansive and destructive growth pattern, densely cellular stroma, moderate stromal atypia, focal hemorrhage and necrosis, and numerous mitotic figures. Heterologous differentiation was not apparent histologically or ultrastructurally, although desmin reactivity was observed in 30% of the stromal cells, particularly in the looser myxoid regions, suggesting muscular differentiation.[94]

Other sarcomas of the seminal vesicle are also rare and usually present with symptoms of pelvic pain, urinary obstruction, rectal obstruction, and symptoms from distant metastases. Unlike prostatic sarcoma, seminal vesicle sarcoma rarely presents with hematuria unless the tumor is large and advanced. These tumors grow locally and compress adjacent pelvic organs such as the prostate, bladder, and rectum. Tripathi and Dick reviewed 46 cases of primary urogenital sarcoma encountered at multiple Boston hospitals between 1923 and 1968 and found only one sarcoma (leiomyosarcoma) of the seminal vesicle.[101]

Schned et al reviewed 11 reported cases of primary sarcoma of the seminal vesicle, including leiomyosarcoma, fibrosarcoma, liposarcoma colliding with prostatic carcinoma, "primary sarcoma," "large cell alveolar sarcoma," "pleomorphic cell sarcoma," "malignant myoblastoma," leiomyoma of vascular origin with "some suggestion of malignant potential," "round cell sarcoma," and "fibrosarcoma with evidence of smooth muscle differentiation by electron microscopy."[102] Amirkhan et al recently reported a high-grade leiomyosarcoma of the right seminal vesicle arising in a 68-year-old man with urinary obstructive symptoms, low back pain, and impending rectal obstruction.[103] The tumor appeared to arise from the muscular wall of the seminal vesicle and displayed immunoreactivity for muscle-specific actin, smooth muscle actin, and focally for keratin AE1/AE3. The patient was well 13 months after radical surgery. Other malignant soft tissue tumors of the seminal vesicle include angiosarcoma[104,105] and fibrosarcoma.[87]

Rare primary germ cell tumors have been reported in the seminal vesicles, presumably caused by midline entrapment of primitive germ cells in the fetus. Primary choriocarcinoma was reported in a 28-year-old forming a hemorrhagic 12 cm diameter mass; at autopsy, the testes were normal on serial sectioning and no other primary site was found.[106] Primary seminoma was found in a 48-year-old, which required cystoprostatectomy; the testes were clinically normal.[107]

Primary carcinoid tumor has also been reported in the seminal vesicles.[108]

REFERENCES

1. Clavert A, Cranz C, Bollack C: Functions of the seminal vesicle, Andrologia 22(Suppl 1):185-192, 1990.
2. Ramchandani P, Banner MP, Pollack HM: Imaging of the seminal vesicles, Sem Roentgen 28:83-91, 1993.
3. Aumuller G, Riva A: Morphology and functions of the human seminal vesicle, Andrologia 24:183-196, 1992.
4. Coyne JD, Kealy WF, Annis P: Seminal vesicle epithelium in prostatic needle biopsy specimens, J Clin Pathol 40:932, 1987.
5. Suzuki T, Yamanaka H, Nakajima K et al: Immunohistochemical study of metallothionein in human seminal vesicles, Tohoku J Exp Med 167:127-134, 1992.
6. Lange W, Unger J: Peptidergic innervation within the prostate gland and seminal vesicles, Urol Res 18:337-340, 1990.
7. Terasaki T, Watanabe H, Kamoi K et al: Seminal vesicle parameters at 10-year intervals measured by transrectal ultrasonography, J Urol 150:914-916, 1993.
8. Arias-Stella J, Takano-Moron J: Atypical epithelial changes in the seminal vesicle, Arch Pathol 66:761-766, 1958.
9. Kuo PM, Gomez LG: Monstrous epithelial cells in human epididymis and seminal vesicles. A pseudomalignant change, Am J Surg Pathol 5:483-490, 1981.
10. Koivuniemi A, Tyrkku J: Seminal vesicle epithelium in fine-needle aspiration biopsies of the prostate as a pitfall in the cytologic diagnosis of carcinoma, Acta Cytologica 20:116-119, 1976.
11. Droese M, Voeth C: Cytologic features of seminal vesicle epithelium in aspiration biopsy smears of the prostate, Acta Cytologica 20:120-125, 1976.
12. Mesonero CE, Oertel YC: Cells from ejaculatory ducts and seminal vesicles and diagnostic difficulties in prostatic aspirates, Mod Pathol 4:723-726, 1991.
13. Arber DA, Speights VO: Aneuploidy in benign seminal vesicle epithelium: an example of the paradox of ploidy studies, Mod Pathol 4:687-689, 1991.
14. Meisels A, Ayotte D: Cells from the seminal vesicles: contaminants of the V-C-E smear, Acta Cytologica 20:211-219, 1976.
15. Dominguez C, Boronat F, Cunat E et al: Agenesis of seminal vesicles in infertile males: ultrasonic diagnosis, Eur Urol 20:129-132, 1991.
16. Olson JR, Weaver DK: Congenital mesonephric defects in male infants with mucoviscidosis, J Clin Path 22:725-730, 1969.
17. Rappe BJM, Meuleman EJH, Debruyne FMJ: Seminal vesicle cyst with ipsilateral renal agenesis, Urol Int 50:54-56, 1993.
18. Fuselier HA, Peters DH: Cyst of seminal vesicle with ipsilateral renal agenesis and ectopic ureter: case report, J Urol 116:833-835, 1976.
19. Reddy YN, Winter CC: Cyst of the seminal vesicle: a case report and review of the literature, J Urol 108:134-135, 1972.
20. Zinner A: Ein Fall von intravesikaler Samenblasenzyste, Wien Med Wochenschr 64:605-607, 1914.
21. King BF, Hattery RR, Lieber MM et al: Congenital cystic disease of the seminal vesicle, Radiol 178:207-211, 1991.
22. Ejeckam GC, Govatsos S, Lewis AS: Cyst of seminal vesicle associated with ipsilateral renal agenesis, Urology 24:372-374, 1984.
23. Schnitzer B: Ectopic ureteral opening into seminal vesicle: a report of four cases, J Urol 93:576-581, 1965.
24. Beeby DI: Seminal vesicle cyst associated with ipsilateral renal agenesis: case report and review of literature, J Urol 112:120-122, 1974.
25. Juhl M, Larsen KE, Nielsen HV: Bilateral cystic seminal vesicles associated with unilateral renal agenesis, Eur Urol 9:319-320, 1983.
26. Karamcheti A, Berg G: Seminal vesicle cyst associated with ipsilateral renal agenesis, Urology 12:572-574, 1978.
27. Donohue RE, Greenslade NF: Seminal vesicle cyst and ipsilateral renal agenesis, Urology 2:66-69, 1973.
28. Das S, Amar AD: Ureteral ectopia into cystic seminal vesicle with ipsilateral dysgenesis and monorchia, J Urol 124:574-575, 1980.
29. Sheih C-P, Liao Y-J, Li Y-W et al: Seminal vesicle cyst associated with ispilateral renal malformation and hemivertebra. Report of 2 cases, J Urol 150:1214-1215, 1993.
30. Rajfer J, Eggleston JC, Sanders RC et al: Fever and prostatic mass in a young man, J Urol 119:555-558, 1978.
31. Hart JB: A case of cyst or hydrops of the seminal vesicle, J Urol 86:137-141, 1961.
32. Ornstein MH, Kershaw DR: Cysts of the seminal vesicle are Müllerian in origin, J R Soc Med 78:1050-1051, 1985.
33. Conn IG, Peeling WB, Clements R: Complete resolution of a large seminal vesicle cyst. Evidence for an obstructive aetiology, Br J Urol 69:636-639, 1992.
34. DeKlotz RJ: Echinococcal cyst involving the prostate and seminal vesicles: a case report, J Urol 115:116-117, 1976.

35. Pryor JP, Hendry WF: Ejaculatory duct obstruction in subfertile males: analysis of 87 patients, Fertil Steril 56:725-730, 1991.
36. Hendry WF, Pryor JP: Müllerian duct (prostatic utricle) cyst: diagnosis and treatment in subfertile males, Br J Urol 69:79-82, 1992.
37. Gevenois PA, Van Sinoy ML, Sintzoff SA Jr et al: Cysts of the prostate and seminal vesicles: MR imaging findings in 11 cases, AJR Am J Roentgenol 155:1021-1024, 1990.
38. Pitkanen P, Westermark P, Cornwell GG III et al: Amyloid of the seminal vesicles: a distinctive and common localized form of senile amyloidosis, Am J Pathol 110:64-69, 1983.
39. Bursell S: Beitrag zur Kenntis der Para-amyloidose in urogenitalen System unter besonderer Berucksichtigung der Sog. Senilen Amyloidose in den Samenblaschen und ihres Verhaltnisses zum Samenblaschen-pigment, Ups Lakaref Forh 47:313-326, 1942.
40. Goldman H: Amyloidosis of seminal vesicles and vas deferens, Arch Pathol 75:106-110, 1963.
41. Khan SM, Birch PJ, Bass PS et al: Localized amyloidosis of the lower genitourinary tract: a clinicopathological and immunohistochemical study of nine cases, Histopathol 21:143-147, 1992.
42. Carris GK, McLaughlin AP, Gittes RF: Amyloidosis of the lower genitourinary tract, J Urol 115:423-426, 1976.
43. Krane RJ, Klugo RC, Olsson CA: Seminal vesicle amyloidosis, Urology 2:70-72, 1973.
44. Ramchandani P, Schnall MD, LiVolsi VA et al: Senile amyloidosis of the seminal vesicles mimicking metastatic spread of prostatic carcinoma on MR images, AJR Am J Roentgenol 161:99-100, 1993.
45. Kaji Y, Sugimura K, Nagaoka S et al: Amyoid deposition in seminal vesicles mimicking tumor invasion from bladder cancer: MR findings, J Comp Assist Tomogr 16:989-991, 1992.
46. Terris MK, McNeal JE, Stamey TA: Invasion of the seminal vesicles by prostatic cancer: detection with transrectal sonography, AJR Am J Roentgenol 155:811-815, 1990.
47. Coyne JD, Kealy WF: Seminal vesicle amyloidosis: morphological, histochemical and immunohistochemical observations, Histopathology 22:173-177, 1993.
48. Seidman JD, Shmookler BM, Connolly B et al: Localized amyloidosis of seminal vesicles: report of three cases in surgically obtained material, Mod Pathol 2:671-675, 1989.
49. Cornwell GG III, Westermark GT, Pitkanen P et al: Seminal vesicle amyloid: the first example of exocrine cell origin of an amyloid fibril precursor, J Pathol 167:297-303, 1992.
50. Madara JL, Haggitt RC, Federman M: Intranuclear inclusions of the human vas deferens, Arch Pathol Lab Med 102:648-650, 1978.
51. Kovi J, Jackson MA, Akberzie ME: Unusual smooth muscle change in the prostate, Arch Pathol Lab Med 103:204-205, 1979.
52. Krishnan R, Heal MR: Study of seminal vesicles in acute epididymitis, Br J Urol 67:632-637, 1991.
53. Maglione M, Nardi A, Cranz C et al: Acute vesiculitis and its prostatic complications caused by *E. coli* in the rat, Urol Res 14:265-266, 1986.
54. Fox CW Jr, Vaccaro JA et al: Seminal vesicle abscess: the use of computerized coaxial tomography for diagnosis and therapy, J Urol 139:384-385, 1988.
55. Chandra I, Doringer E, Sarica K et al: Bilateral seminal vesicle abscesses, Eur Urol 20:164-166, 1991.
56. Cytron S, Baniel J, Kessler O et al: Seminal vesicle congestion as a cause of postprostatectomy dysuria, Eur Urol 24:327-331, 1993.
57. George S: Calcification of the vas deferens and the seminal vesicles, JAMA 47:103-105, 1906.
58. Kretschmer HL: Calcification of the seminal vesicles, J Urol 7:67-71, 1922.
59. Marks JH, Ham DP: Calcification of the vas deferens, AJR Am J Roentgenol 47:859-863, 1942.
60. Wilson JL, Marks JH: Calcification of the vas deferens, its relations to diabetes mellitus and arteriosclerosis, N Engl J Med 245:321-325, 1951.
61. Culver GH, Tannenhaus J: Calcification of the vas deferens in diabetes, JAMA 173:648-651, 1960.
62. Camiel MR: Calcification of vas deferens associated with diabetes, J Urol 86:634-636, 1961.
63. Grunebaum M: The calcified vas deferens, Isr J Med Sci 7:311-314, 1971.
64. Silber SJ, McDonald FD: Calcification of the seminal vesicles and vas deferens in a uremic patient, J Urol 105:542-544, 1971.
65. Bacic J, Kuzmic M: Spermolithiasis, Int Urol Nephrol 7:235-239, 1975.
66. Wilkinson AG: Case report: calculus in the seminal vesicle, Pediatr Radiol 23:327, 1993.
67. Li YK: Diagnosis and management of large seminal vesicle stones, Br J Urol 68:322-323, 1991.
68. Bostwick DG, Egbert BM, Fajardo JL: Radiation injury of the normal and neoplastic prostate, Am J Surg Pathol 6:541-551, 1982.
69. Chan TW, Kressel HY: Prostate and seminal vesicles after irradiation: MR appearance, JMRI 1:503-511, 1991.
70. Tanaka T, Takeuchi T, Oguchi K et al: Primary adenocarcinoma of the seminal vesicle, Hum Pathol 18:200-202, 1987.
71. Benson RC Jr, Clark WR, Farrow GM: Carcinoma of the seminal vesicle, J Urol 132:483-485, 1984.
72. Dalgaard JB, Giertsen JC: Primary carcinoma of the seminal vesicle, Acta Pathol Microbiol Scand 39:255-267, 1956.
73. Chinoy RF, Kulkarni JN: Primary papillary adenocarcinoma of the seminal vesicle, Indian J Cancer 30:82-84, 1993.
74. Atobe T, Naoe S, Taguchi K et al: Primary seminal vesicle carcinoma in a 19-year-old male, Gan No Rinsho 30:205-207, 1984.
75. Williamson RCN, Slade N, Feneley RCL: Seminal vesicle tumours, J Royal Soc Med 71:286-288, 1978.
76. Gohji K, Kamidono S, Okada S: Primary adenocarcinoma of the seminal vesicle, Br J Urol 72:514-515, 1993.
77. Okada Y, Tanaka H, Takeuchi H et al: Papillary adenocarcinoma in a seminal vesicle cyst associated with ipsilateral renal agenesis: a case report, J Urol 148:1543-1545, 1992.
78. Zenklusen HR, Weymuth G, Rist M et al: Carcinosarcoma of the prostate in combination with adenocarcinoma of the prostate and adenocarcinoma of the seminal vesicles. A case report with immunocytochemical analysis and review of the literature, Cancer 66:998-1001, 1990.
79. Ohmori T, Okada K, Tabei R et al: CA125-producing adenocarcinoma of the seminal vesicle, Pathology Inter 44:333-337, 1994.

80. Slayter MV, Anzano MA, Kadomatsu K et al: Histogenesis of induced prostate and seminal vesicle carcinoma in Lobund-Wistar rats: a system for histological scoring and grading, Cancer Res 54:1440-1445, 1994.
81. Ohori M, Scardino PT, Lapin SL et al: The mechanisms and prognostic significance of seminal vesicle involvement by prostate cancer, Am J Surg Pathol 17:1252-1261, 1993.
82. Mukamel E, DeKernion JB, Hannah J et al: The incidence and significance of seminal vesicle invasion in patients with adenocarcinoma of the prostate, Cancer 59:1535-1538, 1987.
83. Villers AA, McNeal JE, Redwine EA et al: Pathogenesis and biological significance of seminal vesicle invasion in prostatic adenocarcinoma, J Urol 143:1183-1187, 1990.
84. Epstein JI, Carmichael M, Walsh PC: Adenocarcinoma of the prostate invading the seminal vesicle: definition and relation of tumor volume, grade, and margins of resection to prognosis, J Urol 149:1040-1045, 1993.
85. Ro JY, Ayala AG, el-Nagger A et al: Seminal vesicle involvement by in situ and invasive transition cell carcinoma of the bladder, Am J Surg Pathol 11:951-958, 1987.
86. Rooney MT, Patterson DE, Bostwick DG: Retrovesicular seminoma with evidence of regressed primary testicular tumor, J Urol Pathol 1996 (in press).
87. Buck AC, Shaw RE: Primary tumours of the retro-vesicle region with special reference to mesenchymal tumours of the seminal vesicles, Br J Urol 44:47-50, 1972.
88. Gentile AT, Moseley HS, Quinn SF et al: Leiomyoma of the seminal vesicle, J Urol 151:1027-1029, 1994.
89. Lundhus E, Bundgaard N, Sorensen FB: Cystadenoma of the seminal vesicle. A case report, Scand J Urol Nephrol 18:341-342, 1984.
90. Damjanov I, Apic R: Cystadenoma of seminal vesicles, J Urol 111:808-809, 1974.
91. Soule EH, Dockerty MB: Cystadenoma of the seminal vesicle, a pathologic curiosity. Report of a case and review of the literature concerning benign tumors of the seminal vesicle, Mayo Clinic Proc 26:406-414, 1951.
92. Mazzucchelli L, Studer UE, Zimmermann A: Cystadenoma of the seminal vesicle: case report and literature review, J Urol 147:1621-1624, 1992.
93. Plaut A, Standard S: Cystomyoma of seminal vesicle, Annals Surg 199:253-261, 1944.
94. Fain JS, Cosnow I, King BF et al: Cystosarcoma phyllodes of the seminal vesicle, Cancer 71:2055-2061, 1993.
95. Islam M: Benign mesenchymoma of seminal vesicles, Urology 13:203-205, 1979.
96. Fujisawa M, Ishigami J, Kamidono S et al: Adenomyosis of the seminal vesicle with hematospermia, Hinyokika Kiyo Acta Urol Jap 39:73-76, 1993.
97. Kinas H, Kuhn M: Mesonephric hamartoma of the seminal vesicle: a rare cause of a retrovesical mass, NY State J Med 87:48-49, 1987.
98. Lagalla R, Zappasodi F, Lo Casto A et al: Cystadenoma of the seminal vesicle: US and CT findings, Abdom Imaging 18:298-300, 1993.
99. Mazur MT, Myers JL, Maddox WA: Cystic epithelium-stromal tumor of the seminal vesicle, Am J Surg Pathol 11:210-217, 1987.
100. Laurila P, Leivo I, Makisalo H et al: Müllerian adenosarcomalike tumor of the seminal vesicle. A case report with immunohistochemical and ultrastructural observations, Arch Pathol Lab Med 116:1072-1076, 1992.
101. Tripathi VNP, Dick VS: Primary sarcoma of the urogenital system in adults, J Urol 101:898-904, 1969.
102. Schned AR, Ledbetter JS, Selikowitz SM: Primary leiomyosarcoma of the seminal vesicle, Cancer 57:2202-2206, 1986.
103. Amirkhan RH, Mohlberg KH, Wiley EL et al: Primary leiomyosarcoma of the seminal vesicle, Urology 44:132-135, 1994.
104. Chiou RK, Limas C, Lange PH: Hemangiosarcoma of the seminal vesicle: case report and literature review, J Urol 134:371-373, 1985.
105. Lamont JS, Hesketh PJ, De Las Morenas A et al: Primary angiosarcoma of the seminal vesicle, J Urol 146:165-167, 1991.
106. Fairey AE, Mead GM, Murphy D et al: Primary seminal vesicle choriocarcinoma, Br J Urol 71:756-757, 1993.
107. Adachi Y, Rokujyo M, Kojima H et al: Primary seminoma of the seminal vesicle: report of a case, J Urol 146:857-859, 1991.
108. Soyer P, Rougier P, Gad M et al: Primary carcinoid tumor of the seminal vesicles: CT and MR findings, J Belge Radiol 74:117-119, 1991.

Embryologic Development and Normal Anatomy

Congenital Anomalies

- Urethral valves
- Urethral diverticula
- Duplication of urethra
- Congenital urethral polyps

Non-neoplastic Diseases

- Urethritis
- Caruncle
- Polypoid urethritis
- Nephrogenic adenoma
- Malakoplakia
- Amyloidosis
- Condylomata acuminata
- Metaplasia of urothelium
- Ectopic prostatic tissue and prostatic urethral polyps

Neoplastic Diseases

- Benign neoplasms
  - Papilloma
  - Inverted papilloma
- Malignant neoplasms
  - Urothelial carcinoma in association with carcinoma of urinary bladder
  - Primary urethral carcinoma
  - Bladder neck carcinoma
  - Urethral carcinoma in women
  - Adenocarcinoma
  - Other histologic types of carcinoma
  - Malignant melanoma
  - Mesenchymal neoplasms

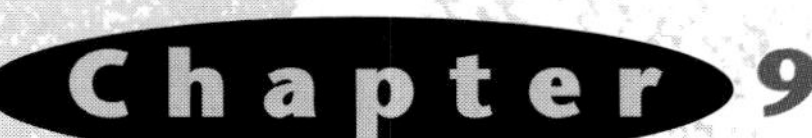

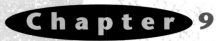

URETHRA

VICTOR E. REUTER

EMBRYOLOGIC DEVELOPMENT AND NORMAL ANATOMY

The urethra conveys urine from the urinary bladder to the exterior through the external urethral meatus. In males it also serves as a conduit for semen. The epithelium of the urethra is derived from the urogenital sinus, which is formed when the endodermal cloaca divides into the rectum dorsally and the urogenital sinus ventrally, separated by the urorectal septum.[1] In females the epithelium of the urethra is derived from endoderm of the urogenital sinus, while the surrounding connective tissue and smooth muscle arise from splanchnic mesenchyme. In males the epithelium also is derived from the urogenital sinus, except in the fossa navicularis where it is derived from ectodermal cells migrating from glans penis. As in females the connective tissue and smooth muscle surrounding the male urethra is derived from splanchnic mesenchyme.

In men the urethra is 15 to 20 cm long and is divided into three anatomical segments (Fig. 9-1). The prostatic urethra is approximately 3 to 4 cm long and begins at the internal urethral orifice at the bladder neck and extends through the prostate to the prostatic apex.[2] Most prostatic ducts open along the posterior and lateral walls of the prostatic urethra, adjacent to the urethral crest, which is a longitudinal ridge along the dorsal wall of the prostatic urethra. In the central part of the urethral crest is an eminence called the *verumontanum* or *colliculus seminalis*. In the verumontanum is a slitlike opening that leads to an epithelium-lined sac called the *prostatic utricle*, a müllerian vestige. The ejaculatory ducts empty into the urethra on either side of the prostatic utricle. The membranous urethra is the shortest segment, only 1 cm long. It extends from the prostatic apex to the bulb of the penis, traversing the musculature of the urethral sphincter and inferior fascia of the urogenital diaphragm. Cowper's glands, small bulbourethral glands, are located on the left and right sides of the membranous urethra and secrete into it.[2-6] The penile urethra is the longest segment (10 to 15 cm) and extends from the lower surface of the urogenital diaphragm to urethral meatus in the glans penis. The orifices of the bulbourethral glands are located on the lateral surfaces of the proximal (bulbous) portion of the penile urethra. The penile urethra is surrounded by the corpus spongiosum along its scattered length. Scattered mucus-secreting periurethral glands (Littre's glands) are present at the periphery of the penile urethra except anteriorly.

The female urethra is approximately 4 cm long (Fig. 9-2). At its periphery are paraurethral glands (Skene's glands), which empty into the urethra through two ducts near the external urethral orifice.

The type of epithelium lining the urethra varies along its length.[2-4] In general, urothelium lines the prostatic urethra; pseudostratified columnar epithelium lines the membranous segment and most of the penile urethra, and nonkeratinized stratified squamous epithelium lines the fossa navicularis and external urethral orifice. In females the proximal one third of the urethra is lined by urothelium and the distal two thirds by nonkeratinized stratified squamous epithelium. However, it should be remembered that most urethral tissue submitted for surgical pathologic examination is diseased or altered by instrumentation, both of which may cause metaplastic changes.

The lymphatic drainage of the male urethra arises from a rich mucosal network that extends the entire length of the urethra.[5] This network is continuous proximally with that of the prostate and urinary bladder and distally with that of the penis. The lymphatics of the prostatic and bulbomembranous segments drain to the obturator and medial external iliac lymph nodes, while those of the distal penile urethra drain to the superficial inguinal nodes. In females the proximal urethra drains to the external iliac, hypogastric, and obturator lymph nodes. The distal urethral lymphatics communicate freely with vulvar lymphatics and drain to the superficial inguinal nodes.

CONGENITAL ANOMALIES

URETHRAL VALVES

Several congenital anomalies affect the urethra but are rarely encountered by surgical pathologists. Urethral valves are mucosal folds that project into the urethral lumen and may cause obstruction, hematuria, or inflammatory symptoms, although they are usually asymptomatic.[7,8] Urethral valves are usually covered by normal

9-1. Anatomy of the male urethra.

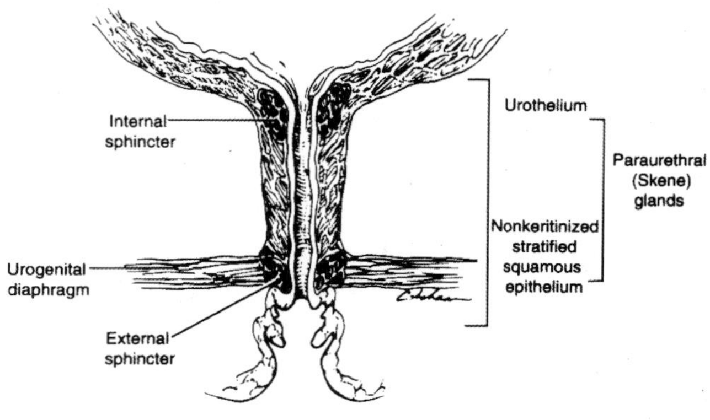

9-2. Anatomy of the female urethra.

urothelium but may be inflamed. The submucosa may also be inflamed and edematous. The so-called posterior urethral valves, usually seen in adult males, are associated with bladder neck hypertrophy.[7]

URETHRAL DIVERTICULA

Urethral diverticula are uncommon and are often overlooked or misinterpreted. The overwhelming majority occur in women.[9-12] They may be asymptomatic but can present with irritative symptoms or dribbling, sometimes with localized pain. On physical examination diverticula present as a paraurethral mass that can sometimes be palpated through the vagina. It is thought that urethral diverticula may be either acquired or congenital, but there are no clear morphologic criteria to make this distinction. The majority of urethral diverticula in adults are acquired as sequelae of infection and trauma, or obstruction, dilation, and inflammation of a paraurethral gland.[11-12]

Diverticula are usually lined by urothelium, although it often undergoes squamous or glandular metaplasia. Nephrogenic adenoma may also arise in diverticula.[13] The submucosa often is edematous and inflamed. Most patients with clinically apparent urethral diverticula have a major complication, such as infection, lithiasis with subsequent obstruction, or carcinoma (Fig. 9-3).[11,14] The percentage of urethral diverticula that develop cancer is unclear, with reported incidences ranging from 2% to 15% of symptomatic diverticula.[15,16] Carcinomas that develop in this setting are usually squamous cell carcinoma or adenocarcinoma but may also be urothelial.[17] Adenocarcinoma may be of the conventional type[18,19] or of the clear cell type (see the section on clear cell adenocarcinoma later in this chapter).

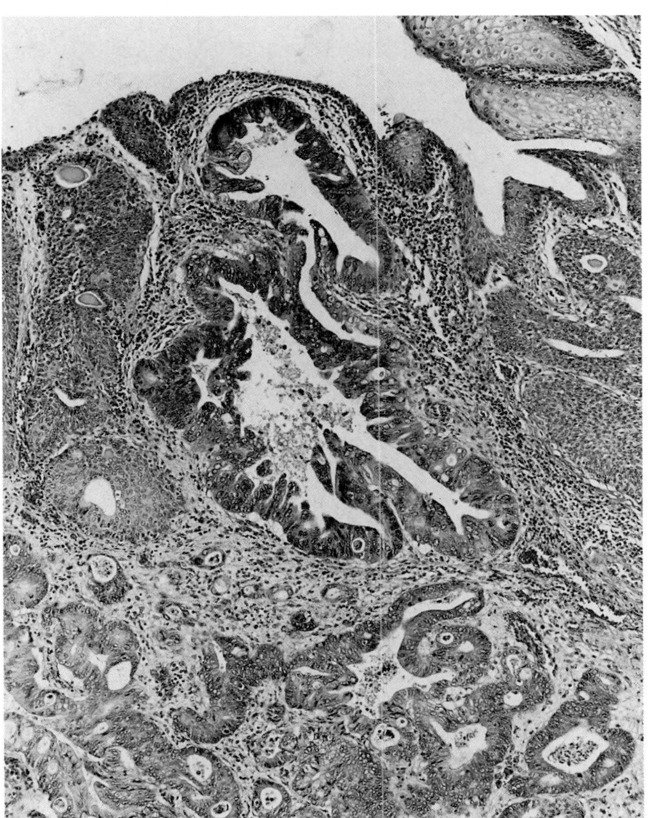

9-3. Adenocarcinoma arising in a urethral diverticulum. These tumors commonly have enteric morphologic features. Note area of squamous metaplasia in the diverticulum, a common finding.

DUPLICATION OF URETHRA

Duplication of the urethra is rare and usually comes to the attention of pathologists at autopsy.[20-22] The first description of a case of duplication of the urethra is attributed to Aristotle. Duplication of the urethra may be complete, extending from the bladder to the dorsum of the penis,[21] or partial, extending from the dorsal surface or, less commonly, the ventral surface of the penis and ending blindly. In only 15% of cases of duplicated urethra, whether complete or partial, is there connection with the functional urethra. Most cases are asymptomatic, but the most common complication is infection. Patients may have urinary obstruction caused by compression of the functional urethra by a mass of desquamated material in the blind accessory urethra. In other cases patients may complain of incontinence or double urinary stream.

CONGENITAL URETHRAL POLYPS

Also known as fibroepithelial polyps, congenital urethral polyps, a rare lesion, occur exclusively in males.[23-29] Usually patients come to clinical attention between the ages of 3 and 9, but rarely are infants or adults.[7] For this reason it has been suggested that they are secondary to poorly understood congenital defects in the urethral wall. Congenital urethral polyps usually arise in the prostatic urethra, adjacent to the verumontanum (posterior urethral polyps). Signs and symptoms include hematuria, difficulty voiding, urinary retention, and infection. The symptoms are similar to other obstructing urethral lesions, including urethral valves, strictures, and lithiasis.

Morphologically, congenital urethral polyps are covered by urothelium that may be inflamed, ulcerated, or exhibit squamous metaplasia. This differs from the more common prostatic urethral polyps occurring in adults, which are covered by prostatic epithelium (see the section titled Ectopic Prostatic Tissue and Prostatic Urethral Polyps below).

Anterior urethral polyps are extremely rare lesions arising in the membranous or penile urethra.[29] They produce the same symptoms and have the same morphology as posterior polyps. The subepithelial stroma consists of loose fibrous tissue that may be highly vascular and may contain a few fascicles of smooth muscle. If the lesion has a long stalk, it may "telescope" into the bladder and produce bladder outlet obstruction.

NON-NEOPLASTIC DISEASES

URETHRITIS

Urethritis is defined morphologically as an inflammatory response in the urethra. Men are often asymptomatic and the diagnosis is made by the presence of a urethral discharge and the finding of polymorphonuclear leukocytes in the urethral smear. Women are often symptomatic; the symptoms are similar to those of cystitis, including dysuria, urinary urgency, and urinary frequency.[30,31] A urethral smear will also aid in the diagnosis in women. Urethritis may be caused by sexually transmissible agents such as *Neisseria gonorrhoeae, Chlamydia trachomatis, Gardnerella vaginalis, Ureaplasma urealyticum, Mycoplasma hominis, Trichomonas vaginalis*, and *Candida* species. In women, urethritis secondary to *Neisseria, Trichomonas*, or *Candida* rarely occurs without a concomitant cervical infection.[31]

Reiter's syndrome is characterized by the triad of urethritis, conjunctivitis, and arthritis.[32] The etiology is uncertain, but it is usually preceded by an enteric or venereal infection. The syndrome occurs predominantly in men between the ages of 18 and 40, but women occasionally are affected. Urethritis is the most common initial symptom. Other urologic manifestations of Reiter's syndrome include prostatitis and hemorrhagic cystitis. In the acute phase the mucosa appears congested and may contain shallow ulcers. Symptoms commonly subside within 2 to 4 weeks, but recur at irregular intervals in 50% to 75% of cases. It is important to recognize that the involved organ systems may be symptomatic at different times so this syndrome should always be included in the differential diagnosis of urethritis in young adults.

CARUNCLE

Urethral caruncle is a pedunculated or sessile polypoid lesion in the distal urethra in women, near the meatus. Grossly, it has a fleshy, pink-red appearance and bleeds readily (Fig. 9-4). Patients may be asymptomatic, although commonly they experience dysuria, urinary frequency, or obstructive symptoms.[33-35] Three histologic groups are described: papillomatous, angiomatous, and granulomatous. This separation is based on the most prominent component of the lesion (surface epithelial, vascular, and inflammatory, respectively), but this distinction has no apparent clinical relevance. The surface epithelium may be transitional or squamous and is invariably inflamed (Fig. 9-5). A few caruncles covered by metaplastic columnar epithelium have been reported. The epithelium may be hyperplastic and constitute the bulk of the lesion. The underlying stroma is richly vascular and inflamed, occasionally containing glandular elements thought to be derived from Skene's glands.

Rarely, the stroma of urethral caruncles may contain atypical mesenchymal cells, mimicking a sarcoma (inflammatory pseudotumor) (Fig. 9-6).[36] Recognition of the mixed inflammatory infiltrate and rich vascularity, in

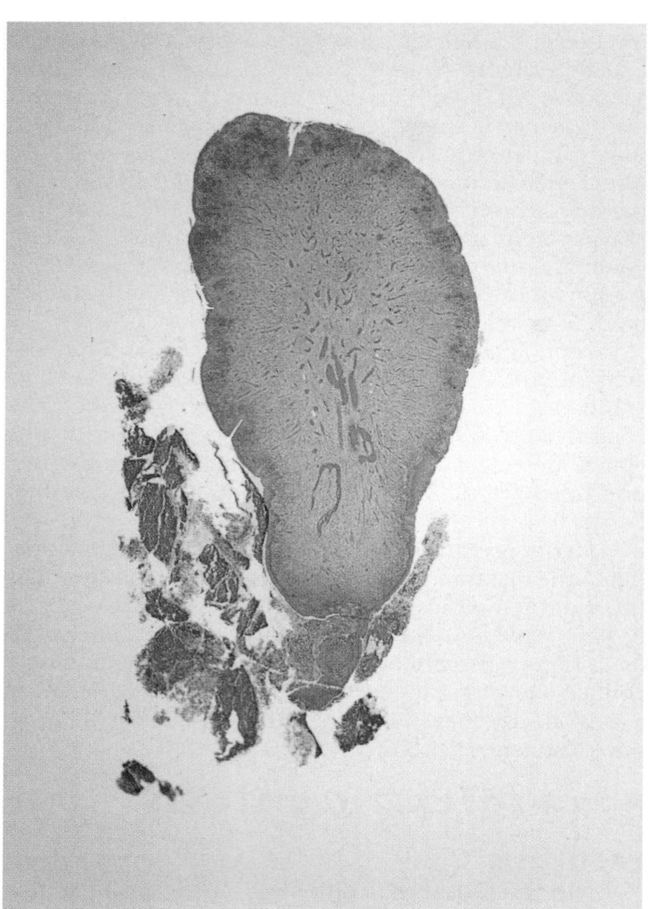

9-4. Macroscopic appearance of caruncle. This reactive erythematous polypoid mass may be confused with a true neoplasm at the time of urethroscopy.

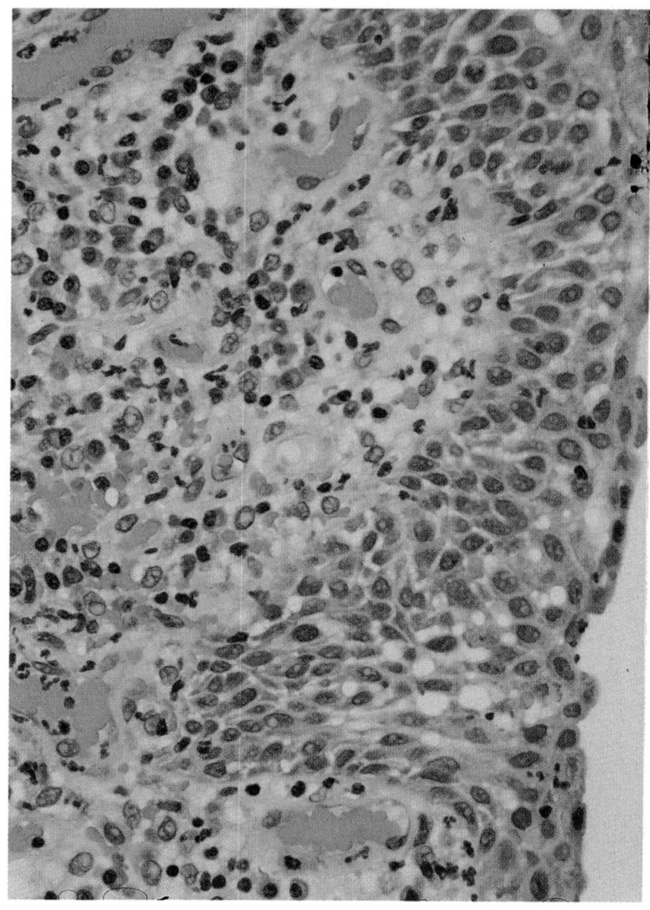

9-5. Caruncle. Inflamed mucosa and lamina propria with extravasated red blood cells and prominent vascularity.

combination with the clinical setting, should establish the correct diagnosis. Inflammatory pseudotumor may appear spontaneously or follow a pelvic surgical procedure by weeks or months (postoperative spindle cell nodule) and present not only as a polypoid lesion but also as a paraurethral mass.[37] Like other pseudosarcomatous lesions of the urothelial tract, the atypical spindle cells are reactive myofibroblasts, which may be cytokeratin and/or actin positive by immunohistochemistry. Epithelial membrane antigen is invariably negative. Electron microscopy is very helpful in establishing the myofibroblastic component of the lesion.

POLYPOID URETHRITIS

Polypoid urethritis is the urethral counterpart of polypoid cystitis, although an association with indwelling catheters has not been noted with urethral lesions.[38,39] Polypoid urethritis is a non-neoplastic inflammatory lesion that usually resolves spontaneously after removal of the inflammatory stimulus. It is commonly found in the prostatic urethra near the verumontanum, appearing as single or multiple polypoid or papillary growths. Morphologically, these are characterized by abundant edematous stroma containing distended blood vessels and a chronic inflammatory infiltrate (Fig. 9-7). The overlying urothelium may be ulcerated or exhibit metaplastic and proliferative changes such as squamous metaplasia, Brunn's nests, or urethritis cystica.[38,39]

Polypoid urethritis does not usually recur after resection unless the cause of the irritation persists. At the time of urethroscopy it may be confused with a papillary urothelial tumor, although experienced urologists will recognize it as a benign, reactive, or low-grade lesion and rarely confuse it with high-grade, aggressive neoplasm.

NEPHROGENIC ADENOMA

Similar to Brunn's nests and urethritis cystica, nephrogenic adenoma is a reactive, proliferative lesion that occurs along the entire urothelial tract as a consequence of local irritation.[40-42] It is most common in the urinary bladder but occasionally arises in the urethra. Nephrogenic adenoma is thought to arise through metaplasia of the urothelium in response to an inflammatory stimulus or local injury, and some researchers prefer the term *nephrogenic metaplasia*. Often these lesions are incidental findings at surgery for other reasons. The most common symptom is hematuria. They appear grossly as flattened, erythematous areas or as discrete papillae. Microscopically, the latter architecture consists of complex papillary structures covered by cuboidal epithelium with basophilic or eosinophilic cytoplasm which may be vacuolated. The nuclei are round to oval, hyperchromatic,

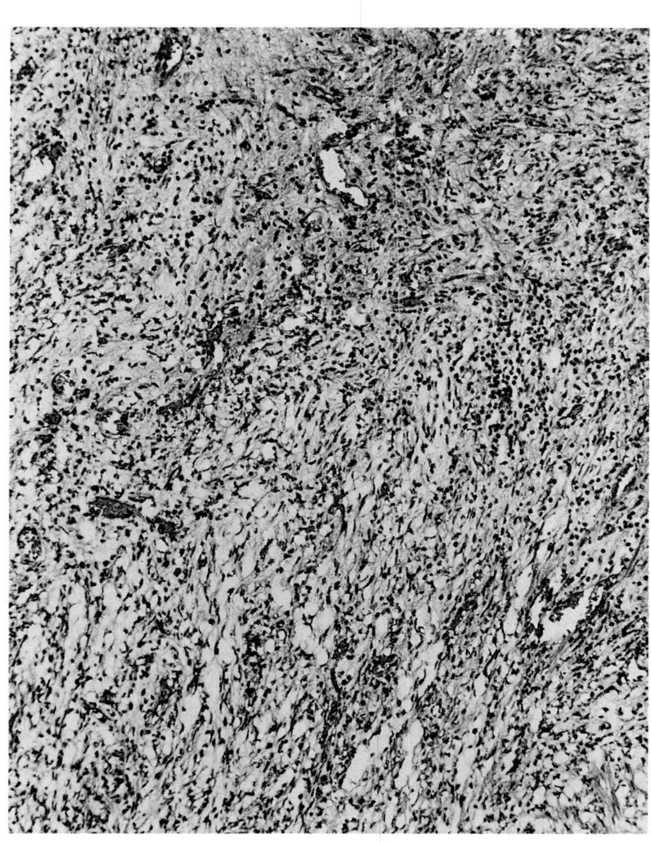

9-6. Inflammatory pseudotumor (postoperative spindle cell nodule). Patient developed a hemorrhagic polypoid mass several months after an endoscopic procedure. Note myxoid background, scattered inflammatory cells, and prominent vascularity.

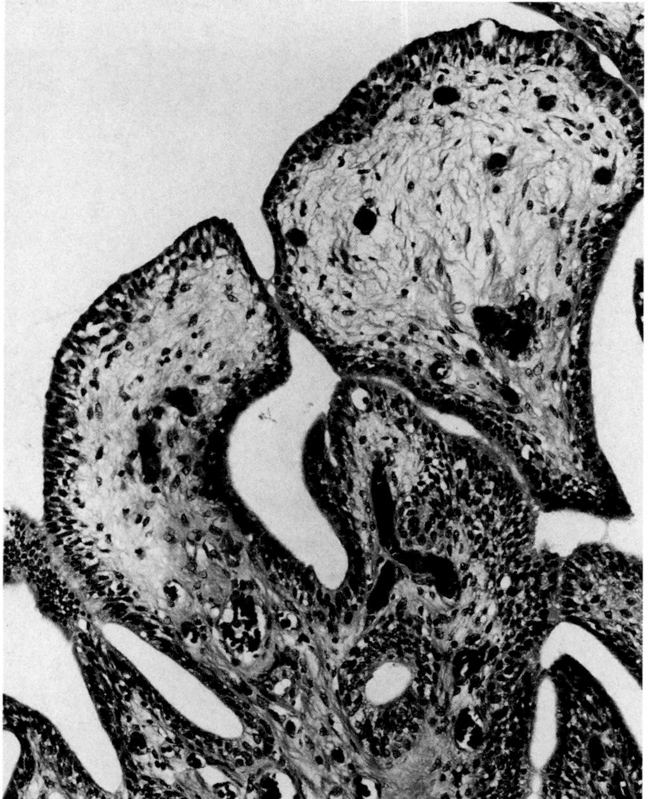

9-7. Polypoid urethritis. This reactive fibroepithelial lesion results from chronic local insult.

centrally located, and may contain small nucleoli. Mitotic figures are uncommon. The same epithelium may form discrete tubules in the underlying stroma. These have distinct lumina that are usually empty but may contain deeply eosinophilic secretions or pale basophilic material (Fig. 9-8). These tubules are thought to arise through a process of invagination from the surface epithelium, much like Brunn's nests. Each is surrounded by a distinct basement membrane.[39] Infrequently, cuboidal cells are present in the stroma singly or in small groups lacking a visible lumen, or they may have a signet ring cell appearance. The luminal secretions may be periodic acid–Schiff-positive, diastase resistant, or mucicarminophilic, but intracytoplasmic mucin is less frequent. Neither prostate-specific antigen nor prostatic acid phosphatase is present in the epithelium. The lesion often appears infiltrative and may be confused with adenocarcinoma, especially in cases lacking a papillary component and composed primarily of tubules in the stroma. The surrounding stroma may be edematous and inflamed, but there is no desmoplastic reaction to the epithelial cells.

There is no convincing evidence that nephrogenic adenoma is a preneoplastic condition, although rare cases coincidentally coexist with or precede the development of carcinoma.[42] Nevertheless, it is possible that both have common predisposing conditions and consequently may develop independently. For example, nephrogenic adenoma and adenocarcinoma have been reported in association with urethral diverticulum.[13] Like other proliferative lesions of the urothelium, nephrogenic adenoma may recur after resection if the inflammatory stimulus is not removed.

MALAKOPLAKIA

Malakoplakia is a rare condition that mainly affects the urothelial tract but that has also been described in other sites such as the testes, gastrointestinal tract, and retroperitoneum.[43-45] Although it may occur anywhere along the urothelial mucosa, most cases occur in the urinary bladder, and urethral involvement is rare.[46-47] Women are affected more often than men, in a ratio of 4:1. Patients usually present with irritative symptoms or urinary obstruction and endoscopy may reveal an erythematous plaquelike lesion or a polypoid or nodular mass that is clinically suggestive of a neoplasm. Microscopically, malakoplakia is characterized by a mixed inflammatory infiltrate dominated by histiocytes with abundant granular, eosinophilic cytoplasm (von Hansemann cells). Within the cytoplasm are Michaelis-Gutmann bodies which are laminated calcospherites, basophilic and targetoid in appearance, and 5 to 10 µm in diameter. These stain for iron as well as calcium and may occasionally be found within the stroma. The overlying urothelium may be ulcerated, hyperplastic, or may

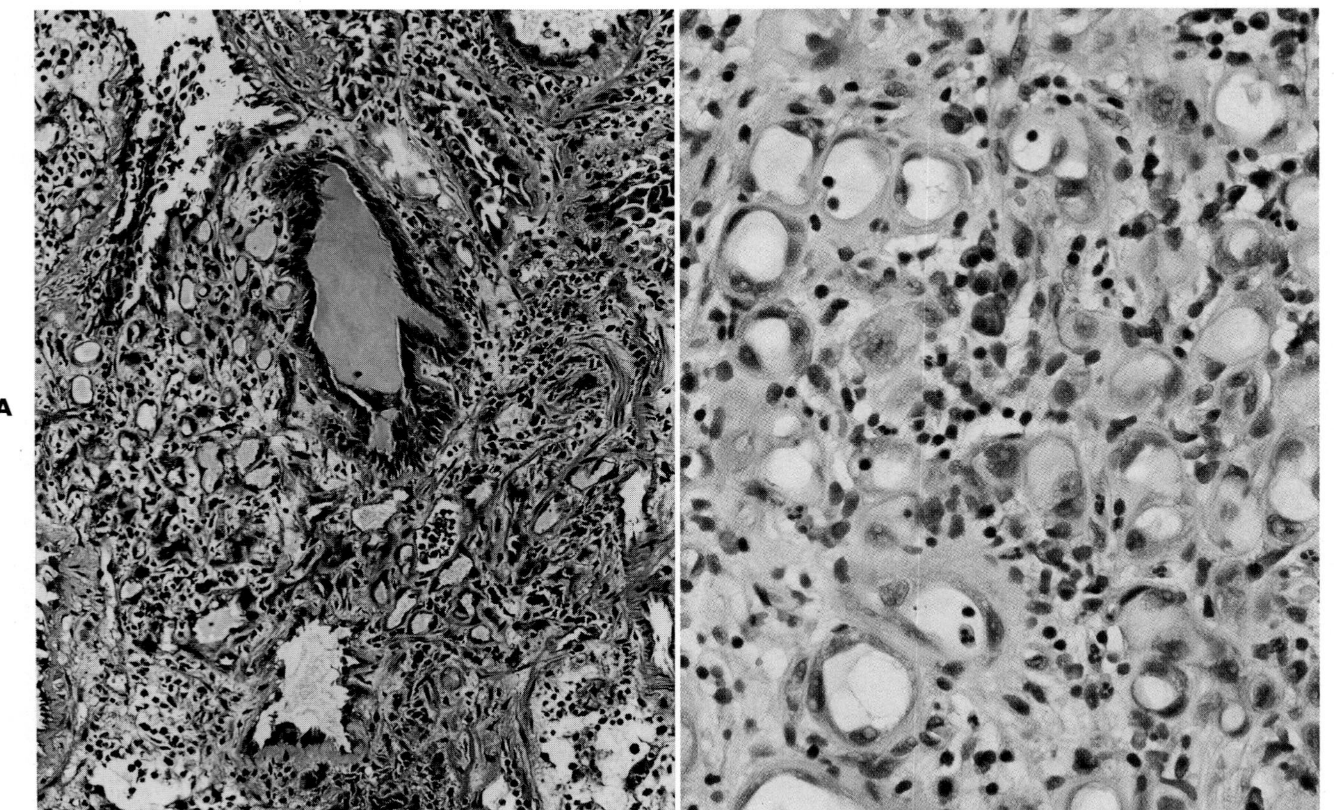

9-8. Nephrogenic "adenoma." **A**, Low power. **B**, High power. Note the small tubules which may be confused with adenocarcinoma infiltrating the periurethral prostatic tissue.

exhibit metaplastic change. In chronic lesions the characteristic infiltrate may be replaced by fibrosis and scar.

The etiology of malakoplakia is unknown, although current knowledge suggests that it is an unusual response to infection, perhaps the result of a disturbed immune response or abnormal macrophage or lysosomal function in the host.[43-45]

AMYLOIDOSIS

The urothelial mucosa can be involved in cases of systemic amyloidosis but rarely is the primary site of disease.[48-51] In descending order of frequency, amyloid deposits have been described in the urinary bladder, ureter, renal pelvis, and urethra. The usual clinical presentation is hematuria, although dysuria, partial obstruction, or a deviated urinary stream have also been reported. At cystoscopy the lesion may appear anywhere along the urethra as an elevated plaque or mass that is commonly confused with a neoplasm. The overlying mucosa may be ulcerated or hyperemic. The amyloid deposits appear as eosinophilic, homogeneous material within the lamina propria, often extending into the underlying muscle and connective tissue. Perivascular amyloid deposits are uncommon in tumoral amyloidosis but common in systemic amyloidosis. Inflammation is usually absent except adjacent to ulcerated mucosa. Special stains, such as Congo red, crystal violet, or van Gieson's solution of trinitrophenol and acid fuchsin, are useful in establishing the diagnosis. Localized lesions may be managed by transurethral resection, but cases with diffuse involvement and intractable symptoms may require radical surgery.[52]

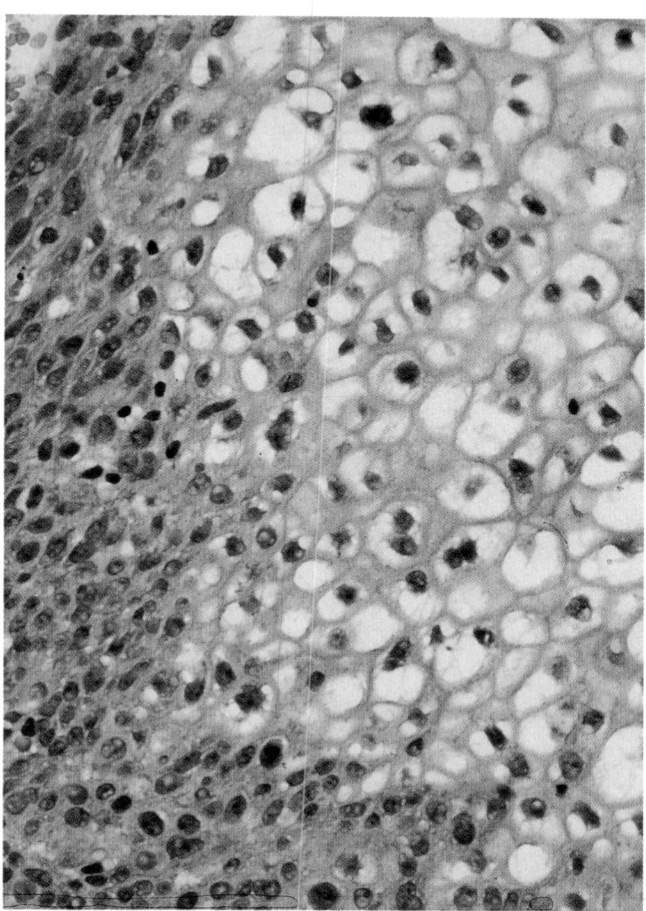

9-9. Condyloma acuminatum. Cells contain irregular nuclei with perinuclear haloes.

CONDYLOMATA ACUMINATA

Condylomata acuminata are common, sexually transmitted infectious lesions caused by human papillomavirus. They usually occur on the mucocutaneous surfaces of the external genitalia, perineum, or anus, but extension into the urethra occurs in up to 20% of cases.[53-55] The lesions are often multifocal or diffuse. Macroscopically, they are smooth, pink-tan, and often papillary. Flat condylomata may be difficult to visualize cystoscopically. Microscopically, the lesions consist of papillary fronds or flat mucosa containing hyperplastic squamous epithelium which can be hyperkeratotic. The squamous epithelial cells typically have clear perinuclear halos and the nuclei are eccentrically placed, hyperchromatic, and pleomorphic (koilocytic atypia) (Fig. 9-9). Many cases can be diagnosed by these morphologic features alone, although in subtle cases the diagnosis can be confirmed by immunohistochemistry, viral culture, in situ hybridization, or polymerase chain reaction.[56-59] The antibodies presently available to identify human papillomavirus are rather insensitive; in situ hybridization and polymerase chain reaction are more reliable, even from paraffin-embedded sections. The human papillomavirus sero types most commonly found in urothelial condylomata are 6, 11, 16, and 18. These often coincide with the type in the patient's sexual partner.[56-58]

Condylomata of the urinary tract may cause hematuria and irritative symptoms. Surgical management may be by transurethral resection, laser, or cryotherapy or a more radical procedure, depending on the extent of disease. It is important to remember that condylomata may undergo transformation to verrucous or infiltrating squamous cell carcinoma.[55,57,58]

METAPLASIA OF UROTHELIUM

Urothelium frequently undergoes squamous or glandular metaplasia as a response to chronic inflammatory stimuli like urinary tract infection, diverticula, calculi, or repeated instrumentation (Fig. 9-3). This is very common and is not preneoplastic per se. Nevertheless, under certain conditions carcinoma may arise in metaplastic epithelium, as in adenocarcinoma or squamous carcinoma arising in diverticula. Glandular metaplasia is more common in the urinary bladder but may occur along the urethra. The morphology of the metaplastic urothelium is usually tall columnar with goblet cells strikingly similar to enteric epithelium.

ECTOPIC PROSTATIC TISSUE AND PROSTATIC URETHRAL POLYPS

Prostatic acinar epithelium may line the urothelial tract focally. This is seen mostly in adult males but occasionally occurs at younger ages.[60-65] This process is most

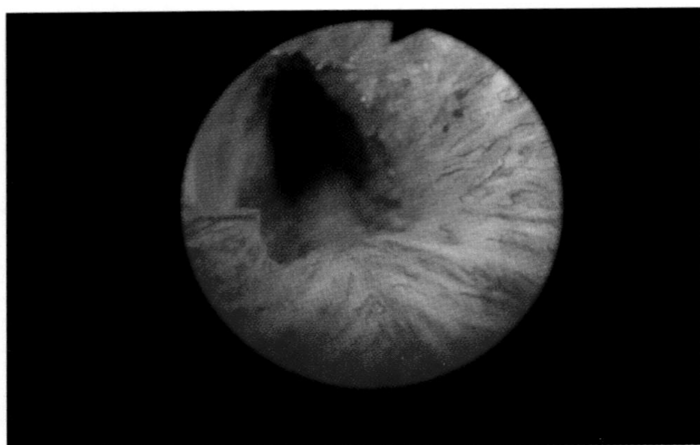

9-10. Prostatic urethral polyp. Endoscopically, the small papillae are clearly identifiable.

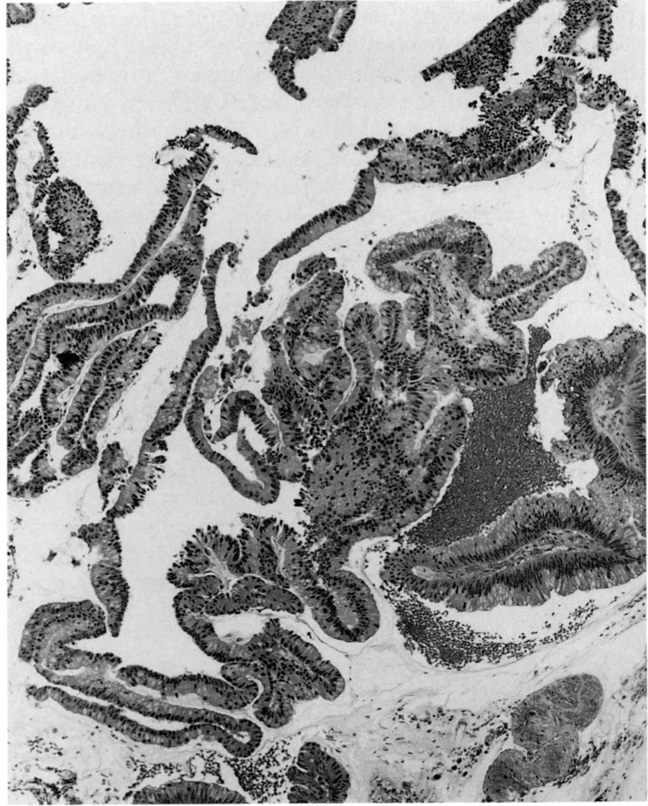

9-12. Urethral implant from urachal adenocarcinoma. After partial cystectomy, patient developed urethral mucosal implants, which were treated by transurethral resection. Given the low-grade nature of this lesion, it was confused with a prostatic urethral polyp until the pathologist compared it with the original lesion and performed immunohistochemical stains for prostate-specific antigen, which were negative.

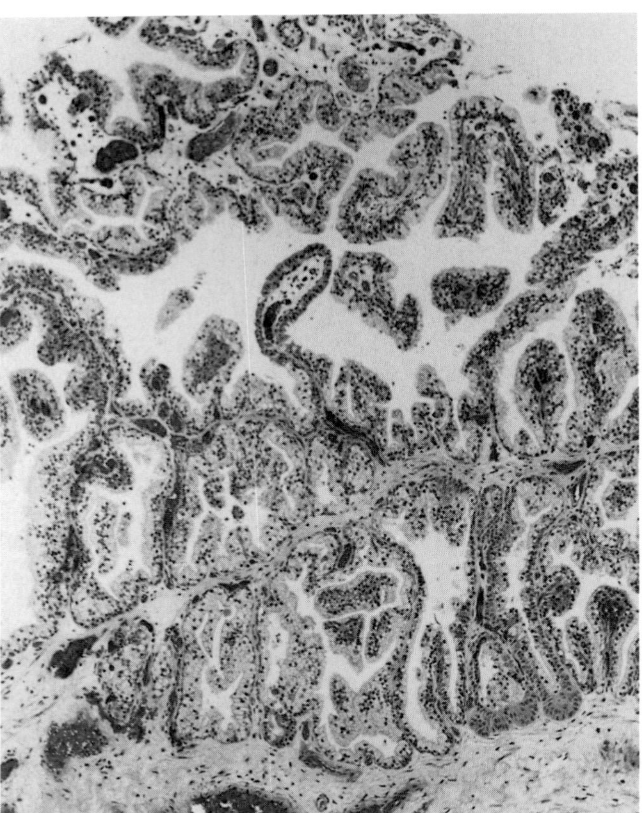

9-11. Prostatic urethral polyp. The urothelium of the prostatic urethra is replaced by papillary fronds lined by benign prostatic acinar cells.

common in the prostatic urethra (prostatic urethral polyp) but has also been described at the bladder neck, bulbous, and penile urethra.[66-68] This ectopic tissue is usually asymptomatic and discovered at urethroscopy for other causes. Hematuria is the most common symptom. Cystoscopically, the lesions appear as discrete small papillary growths, which may be solitary or extensive, producing a velvetlike coating of the mucosa (Fig. 9-10). The papillary fronds contain a thin fibrovascular core and are covered by prostatic acinar epithelium with abundant clear or faintly eosinophilic apical cytoplasm and a small basally located round or oval nucleus without visible nucleolus (Fig. 9-11). Occasionally, foci of residual urothelium are intermingled with the prostatic epithelium. Immunohistochemical stains for prostate-specific antigen are positive.[62,64,66]

The etiology of this phenomenon is controversial. Prostatic urethral polyps probably result from hyperplasia and overgrowth of the overlying urothelium by prostatic acinar epithelium. It is important to carefully examine the underlying prostatic urethral tissue because there may be an associated acinar-type prostatic adenocarcinoma. Also, the cytological features of the epithelial cells must be evaluated since prostatic adenocarcinoma may extend to the mucosal surface and take on a papillary growth pattern. Rarely, low-grade papillary adenocarcinoma of the bladder or urachus may seed the prostatic urethra, mimicking a prostatic urethral polyp (Fig. 9-12). The origin of ectopic prostatic tissue in the penile urethra is less clear and may represent implantation, metaplasia, or an embryologic abnormality (Fig. 9-13). These lesions are benign and, if symptomatic, should be managed con-

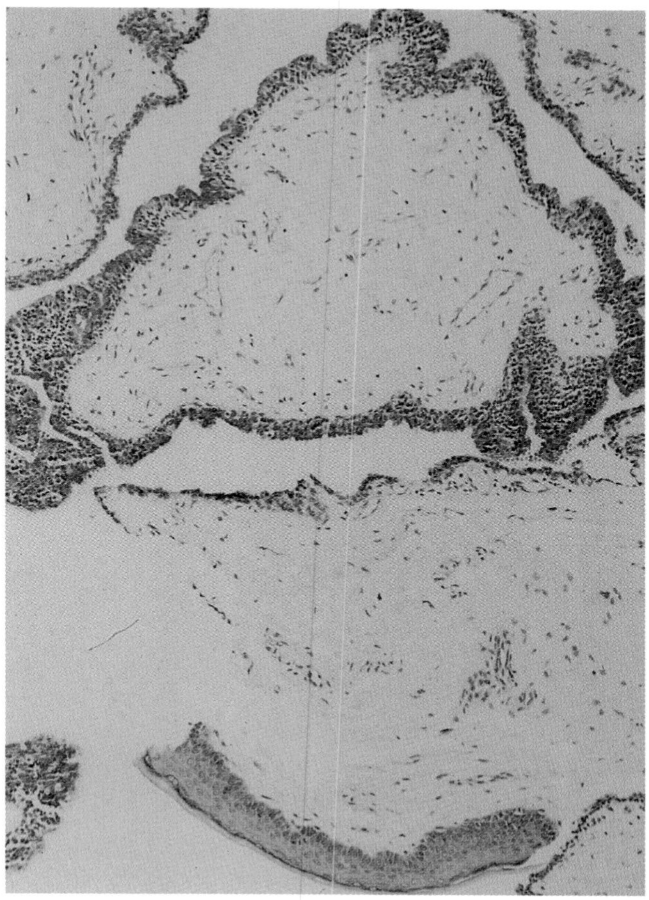

9-13. Benign polyp arising at the fossa navicularis. Immunohistochemical stain for prostatic acid phosphatase is positive.

servatively by urethroscopic resection or electrocauterization. Urologists commonly see these lesions during endoscopic evaluation for other causes and seldom perform biopsies on them unless they believe that they are the source of the patient's symptoms.

NEOPLASTIC DISEASES

BENIGN NEOPLASMS

Papilloma

Papilloma, like other papillary urothelial tumors, rarely arises de novo within the urethra. The definition of papilloma has evolved over the years.[69,70] These benign tumors are characterized by discrete papillary projections with thin fibrovascular cores covered by hyperplastic urothelium. The urothelial cells maintain their polarity perpendicular to the basement membrane and have abundant eosinophilic cytoplasm, which commonly contains perinuclear vacuoles. The nuclei are elongated or round, depending on the plane of sectioning. They may be slightly enlarged compared with normal urothelium but show little or no pleomorphism. The chromatin pattern is homogeneous, and nucleoli are absent or small and sparse. Mitotic figures are usually absent, although a few normal mitotic figures may be observed in the basal layer. The thickness of the epithelium (the number of cell layers) is variable.[69,70]

The main feature of this neoplasm is its discrete nature and the lack of cytologic evidence of malignancy. As defined here, these tumors would fall into the category of grade I papillary urothelial carcinoma under the morphologic criteria of the World Health Organization. There is substantial evidence that these criteria are too restrictive and do not reflect the biologic potential of the lesions.[70] There is no question that papilloma may recur and occasionally (approximately 10%) increase in grade. Nevertheless, it is incapable of invasion (progression) without increasing in grade, that is, acquiring cytologic evidence of malignancy. In this way it is analogous to adenoma of the colon which is clearly a neoplastic growth with a capacity to recur and, occasionally, to transform into carcinoma. For this reason urothelial papilloma should be managed with transurethral resection alone. Patients must undergo surveillance because of the high incidence of development of new tumors.

Inverted papilloma

Inverted papilloma rarely occurs along the urethra, but when it does it shares all the morphologic features of the more common vesical inverted papilloma. Patients usually have hematuria, and on urethroscopy the lesions appear as polypoid or nodular growths with smooth, glistening surfaces. They range up to 2.5 cm in diameter[71,72] and are easily confused with carcinoma, even by experienced endoscopists. Microscopically, they are covered by compressed but benign urothelium and consist of invaginated, interconnected cords and nests of urothelium that proliferate and expand the lamina propria, giving the lesion its characteristic bulging or polypoid gross appearance.[71] The urothelial cells are cytologically benign but more closely packed than normal because of the endophytic growth pattern. Some cells may be spindle shaped, especially toward the center of the cords (Fig. 9-14). Occasionally, the centers of the cords become dilated, forming microcysts lined by flattened or cuboidal cells. Rarely, there is focal squamous metaplasia. The anastomosing cords of urothelium that make up this lesion result from invagination rather than invasion. There is no reactive fibrosis in the surrounding stroma. Mitotic figures are rare and, if present, are normal and in the basal layer. Inverted papilloma is well circumscribed.

The etiology of this lesion is controversial. Most investigators conclude that they are neoplasms, but others suggest that they are an unusual reactive, proliferative response to inflammation. They are not premalignant, although a few cases have been coincidentally associated with carcinoma.[72] Management of inverted papillomas should be limited to transurethral resection.

MALIGNANT NEOPLASMS

Urothelial carcinoma in association with carcinoma of urinary bladder

Secondary involvement of the urethra by urothelial carcinoma of the bladder is much more common than primary urethral carcinoma. As with vesical neoplasms, it

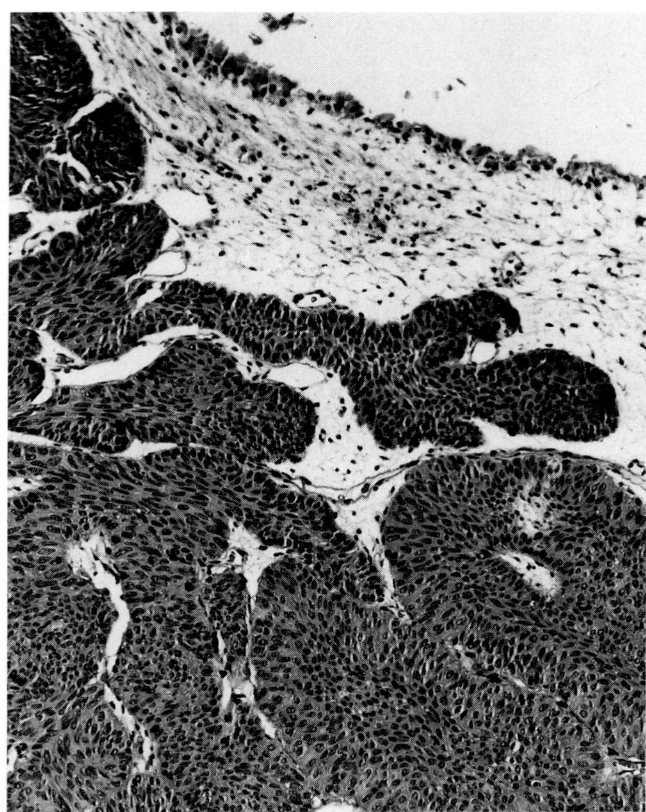

9-14. Inverted papilloma. Anastomosing nests and cords of urothelial cells extend into periurethral tissue but lack cytologic evidence of malignancy.

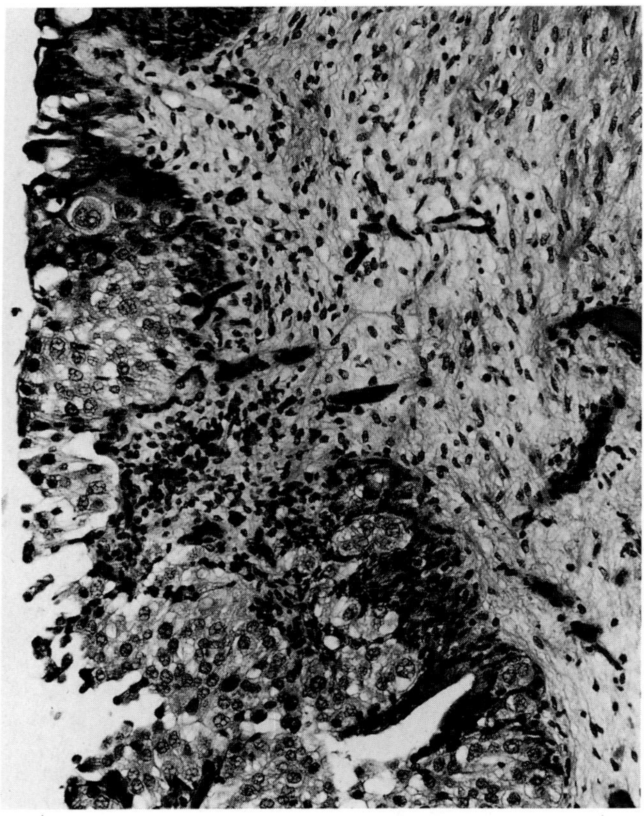

9-15. Urothelial carcinoma of the urinary bladder extending into the urethra. Tumor partially replaces the benign urothelium.

occurs more often in men. The reported incidence of urethral involvement varies according to the study design and the patient population. For example, an autopsy study by Gowing[73] reported an incidence of 20% in patients who had been treated with cystectomy for bladder cancer. Clinical series have reported the incidence of urethral involvement in patients with bladder cancer to be between 8% and 22%.[74-80] Recurrent urethral involvement by carcinoma is not an issue in female patients since total urethrectomy is part of the cystectomy procedure. In males a total urethrectomy is not performed routinely because of the increased morbidity caused by this procedure. It is standard to leave the membranous, bulbous, and penile urethra in place. Recurrence is possible in the immediate postoperative period or as late as 9 years after cystectomy. For this reason it is important for the clinician to routinely evaluate the urethra, whether by urethroscopy, cytology, flow cytometry, or a combination of these.[81,82] Most patients with invasive urethral recurrences die within 5 years. Urologists routinely assess the status of the prostatic urethra prior to cystectomy since most believe that patients with prostatic urethral involvement are not candidates for a "urethra-sparing" procedure.[80]

Multifocal papillary carcinoma and multifocal carcinoma in situ in the bladder predispose the patient to urethral involvement or subsequent recurrence. In a study of male patients, DePaepe et al[84] reported that 9 of 20 (45%) cases had prostatic duct involvement by urothelial carcinoma at the time of cystoprostatectomy. Carcinoma in situ of the bladder was observed in each of the 9 patients. In a similar study dealing with female patients, 4 of 22 patients (18%) had carcinoma in situ in the urethra. These four patients represented 24% of the patients with multifocal carcinoma in situ in the bladder.[84] Interestingly, three of these patients had carcinoma in situ extending into periurethral glands, and 17% of patients with invasive disease in the bladder also had stromal invasion in the urethra. This fact reconfirms that urethrectomy should be performed along with cystectomy in female patients.

Microscopically, secondary urethral involvement by urothelial carcinoma may take the form of papillary carcinoma or carcinoma in situ (Fig. 9-15). The tumors may be single or multiple and may occur at the surgical stump or anywhere along the urethra, including the meatus.[83-85]

Papillary urothelial carcinoma is characterized by papillary fronds lined by epithelial cells that show little or no orientation in relation to their basement membrane. The cells are crowded and have variable amounts of eosinophilic cytoplasm with an increased nuclear to cytoplasmic ratio. Nuclei are irregular and may contain nucleoli. Mitotic figures may be present, are sometimes atypical, and may be located well above the basal layer. Carcinoma in situ is characterized by flat mucosa containing simi-

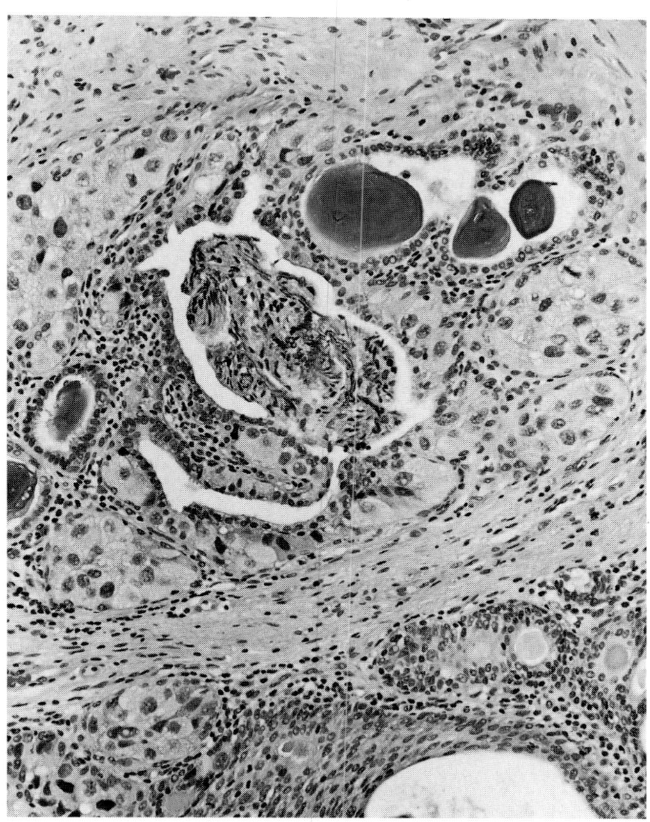

9-16. Urothelial carcinoma extending into prostatic ducts. Duct involvement must be distinguished from stromal invasion.

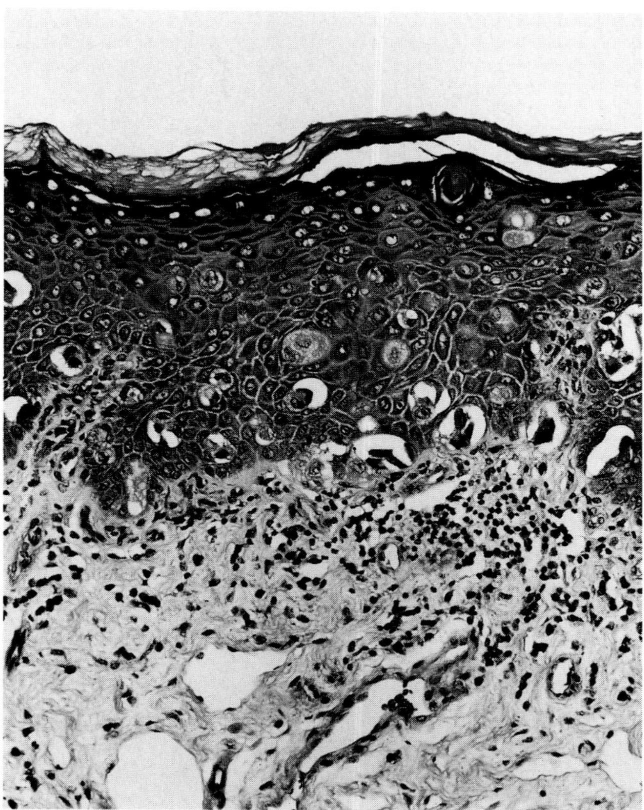

9-17. Pagetoid intramucosal spread of urothelial carcinoma in the membranous urethra. This pattern of spread is most commonly seen in association with multifocal urothelial carcinoma in situ in the urinary bladder.

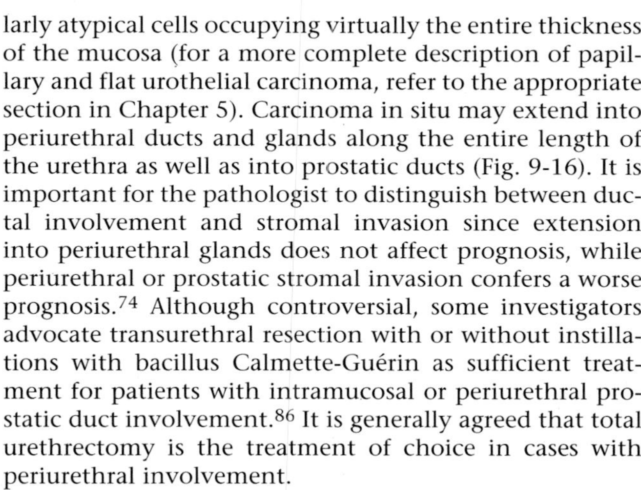

larly atypical cells occupying virtually the entire thickness of the mucosa (for a more complete description of papillary and flat urothelial carcinoma, refer to the appropriate section in Chapter 5). Carcinoma in situ may extend into periurethral ducts and glands along the entire length of the urethra as well as into prostatic ducts (Fig. 9-16). It is important for the pathologist to distinguish between ductal involvement and stromal invasion since extension into periurethral glands does not affect prognosis, while periurethral or prostatic stromal invasion confers a worse prognosis.[74] Although controversial, some investigators advocate transurethral resection with or without instillations with bacillus Calmette-Guérin as sufficient treatment for patients with intramucosal or periurethral prostatic duct involvement.[86] It is generally agreed that total urethrectomy is the treatment of choice in cases with periurethral involvement.

A subtle but important morphologic pattern of urothelial carcinoma in the urethra is intramucosal pagetoid spread (Fig. 9-17). This pattern occurs most frequently in association with multifocal carcinoma in situ of the bladder and is characterized by individual or small groups of carcinoma cells percolating through an otherwise benign urothelium.[83,87,88] The carcinoma cells may have minimal or abundant cytoplasm but have large rounded or irregular hyperchromatic nuclei with prominent nucleoli and closely resemble the cells of Paget's disease of the breast. The surrounding urothelium often undergoes squamous metaplasia. The tumor cells are unreactive for S-100 protein and prostate-specific antigen but express the Lewis-X blood group antigen. Occasionally they may be weakly mucicarmine-positive. This variant of carcinoma in situ may be seen in the surface urothelium, metaplastic squamous epithelium, or periurethral or prostatic ducts. It is rare in primary urethral carcinoma. For this reason, when encountered in a urethral biopsy, the differential diagnosis for this pattern should include urothelial carcinoma arising in the urinary bladder, malignant melanoma, and periurethral or prostatic adenocarcinoma.[89]

Primary urethral carcinoma

Primary carcinoma of the urethra is rare. The incidence is higher in women than in men[78] and the age distribution is similar to that of other urothelial carcinomas (mean incidence in the seventh decade of life). In general, tumors arising proximally (prostatic urethra in males, proximal third in females) have the morphology of typical urothelial cancer, whereas distal carcinomas (membranous, bulbous, or penile in men, distal two thirds in women) are likely to be squamous cell carcinomas. These findings coincide with the epithelial lining in those sites, although

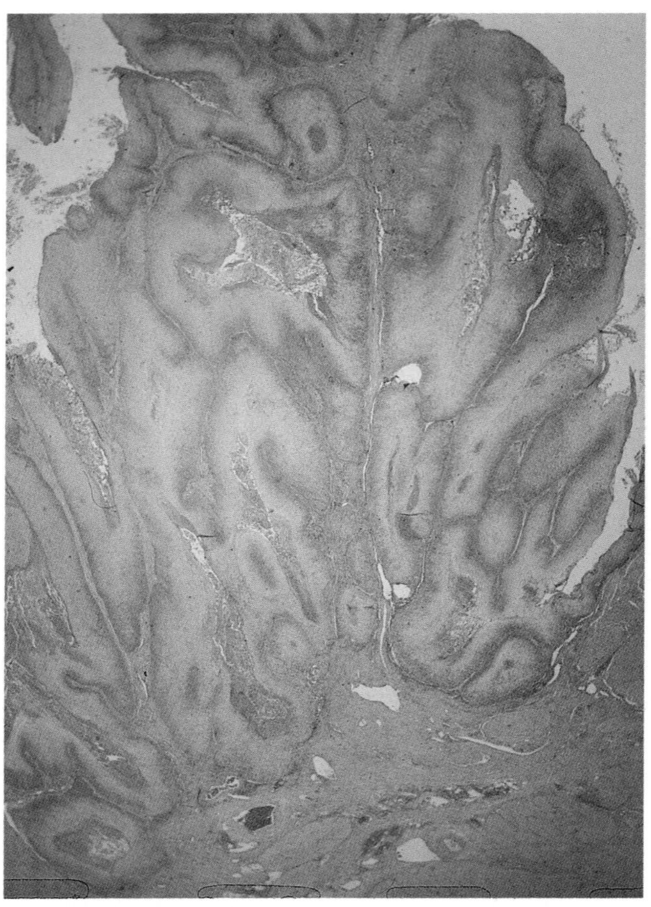

9-18. Verrucous carcinoma. Tall compressed mucosal papillae with a broad infiltrative base. These lesions tend to arise in the distal urethra.

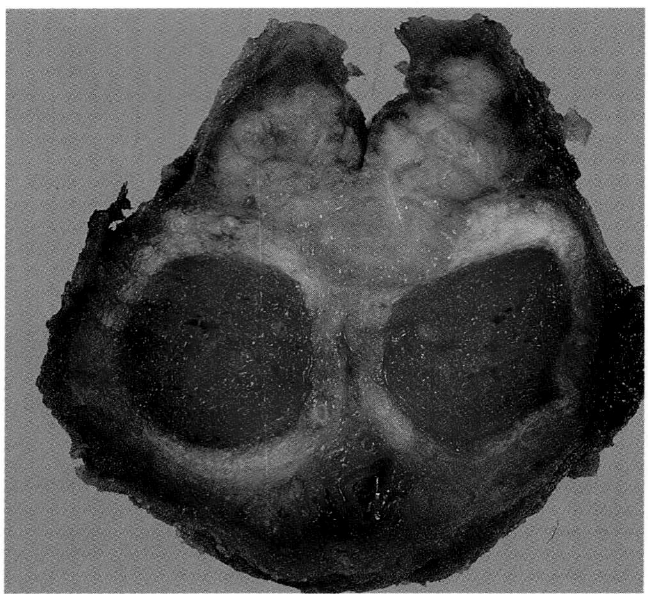

9-19. Squamous carcinoma of penile urethra. The tumor invades through the corpus spongiosum, into the septum but spares the corpora cavernosa (pT2). *(From Reuter VE, Melamed M: The lower urinary tract. In Sternberg S, ed: Diagnostic surgical pathology, ed 2, New York, 1994, Raven Press; with permission).*

TABLE 9-1.
PATHOLOGIC STAGING OF URETHRAL TUMORS

TNM		Ray et al[77]
Ptis	Carcinoma in situ	
		0
pTa	Noninvasive papillary, polypoid, or verrucous	
pT1	Invasion of submucosa	A
pT2	Invasion of corpus spongiosum or cavernosum	B
pT3	Invasion of corpus cavernosum or beyond prostate capsule or anterior vagina or bladder neck	
		C
pT4	Invasion into other adjacent organs	

it must be remembered that the morphology and anatomic distribution of "normal" mucosa may be quite variable. This is especially true in patients with irritative symptoms in whom squamous and glandular metaplasia are quite common. Moreover, it may be morphologically impossible to differentiate moderate- to high-grade urothelial carcinoma from nonkeratinizing squamous cell carcinoma. Adenocarcinoma may arise anywhere along the urethra but is most commonly associated with diverticula, prostatic adenocarcinoma, or, in women, may arise in periurethral glands and extend to the urethral mucosa secondarily. The last is rarely seen in men. Since the incidences of histologic types are different, primary carcinomas in males and females will be discussed separately.

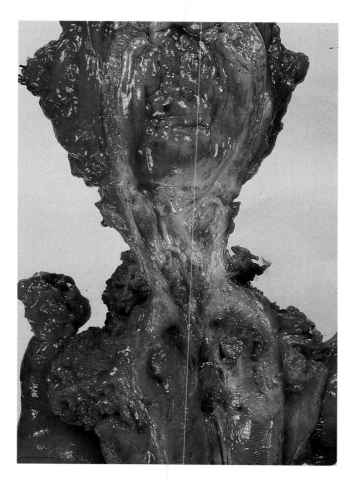

9-20. Squamous cell carcinoma arising in the bulbomembranous urethra. Tumors that arise at this site tend to be at an advanced stage at diagnosis. This lesion infiltrated the cavernous urethra, periurethral, and periprostatic soft tissues, requiring cystoprostaturethrectomy and total emasculation.

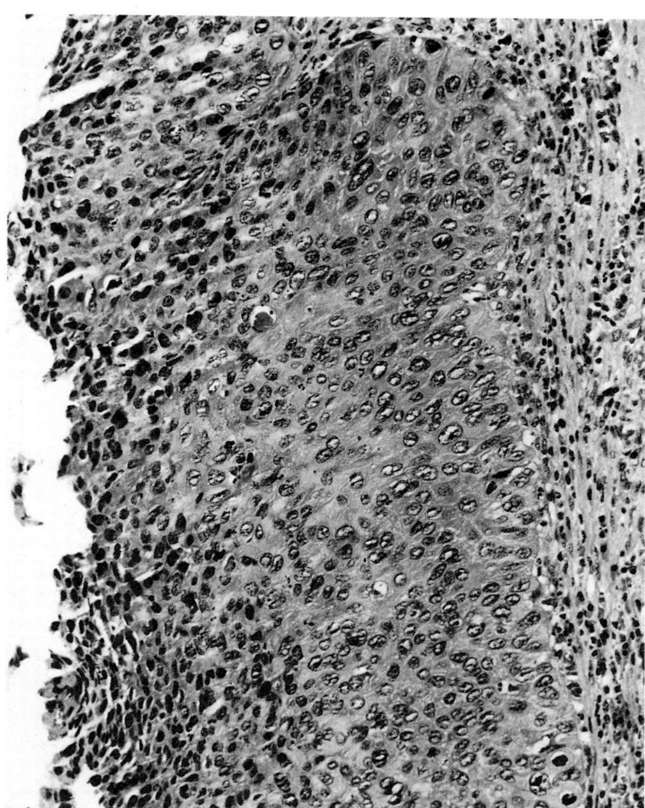

9-21. Squamous cell carcinoma in situ of penile urethra. The full thickness of the mucosa is replaced by high-grade neoplastic cells.

That primary urethral carcinoma is rare in males is underscored by the paper from Memorial Sloan-Kettering Cancer Center, an institution that treats hundreds of new bladder cancers each year, that reported only 23 urethral tumors in a series spanning 30 years.[77] Two were adenocarcinomas and the rest were either urothelial or squamous cell carcinomas. The symptoms are usually dysuria, hematuria, decrease in urinary stream, urinary obstruction, or fistula.[77,78,85] Histories of infection, diverticulum, fistula, or stricture are common. Ray et al[77] found that prognosis correlated with anatomic location and pathologic stage of the primary but not with grade or histologic subtype (Table 9-1). Stage for stage, cancer arising in the distal (bulbous and pendulous) urethra had a better prognosis than cancer arising in the membranous or prostatic urethra. In the former group 6 of 9 patients (67%) survived 5 years, while only 3 of 14 (21%) of the latter group survived 5 years. Tumors arising in the distal urethra are commonly diagnosed at an earlier stage. Well-differentiated squamous cell and verrucous carcinomas are common in the distal urethra (Fig. 9-18). Invasion into the vascular spaces of the corpus spongiosum (Fig. 9-19) or corpora cavernosa is common, and metastases, if present, will be to inguinal lymph nodes. Wide dissemination at the time of presentation is rare. Partial penectomy and inguinal lymph node dissection is usually the treatment of choice.

Tumors arising in the proximal urethra in males commonly present at a higher stage and can infiltrate into the prostatic stroma or pelvic soft tissues to the point that establishing adequate surgical margins of resection may be difficult (Fig. 9-20).[78] In these tumors the histologic distinction is difficult to ascertain between high-grade urothelial carcinoma and nonkeratinizing squamous cell carcinoma (Fig. 9-21). Metastases may be to inguinal or pelvic lymph nodes, and, if operable, treatment usually requires a cystoprostatectomy and urethrectomy. If the scrotal skin, soft tissues, or deep pelvic tissues are involved, total emasculation may be required, although this heroic surgical procedure rarely produces long-term survival.

Bladder neck carcinoma

There is a rare but important group of tumors arising in the proximal urethra that gives pathologists and clinicians many problems and of which little has been written. Some refer to them as *bladder neck carcinomas* (P.H. Lieberman, personal communication). They are moderate-grade to high-grade carcinomas, usually invading the bladder neck and prostate, especially the prostatic ducts.

The carcinoma has a vague glandular pattern and immunohistochemical stains for prostate-specific antigen may be weakly positive in isolated cells. Whether this is due to entrapped prostatic acinar cells or true positivity in tumor cells is unresolved. Serum prostate-specific antigen is usually within normal limits or slightly elevated (≤10 mg/dl). Metastases to bone are rare and, if present, are lytic. The differential diagnosis lies between urothelial carcinoma and high-grade prostatic adenocarcinoma arising in prostatic ducts. These tumors tend to be aggressive and follow a clinical course similar to urothelial tumors. Further research is necessary to develop a better understanding of these lesions.

Urethral carcinoma in women

Primary urethral carcinoma in women is also rare, although more common than in men.[90-93] The histories and symptoms of these patients are similar to those of male patients. In women urethral carcinoma is frequently initially misdiagnosed as caruncle. For this reason, a biopsy should be performed on any presumed caruncle that fails to respond to therapy or is associated with persistent bleeding. Approximately 75% of urethral carcinoma in women is nonkeratinizing or keratinizing squamous carcinoma and the remaining 25% to 30% are split between urothelial carcinoma and adenocarcinoma. Tumors arising in the distal third of the female urethra are commonly low-grade squamous cell or verrucous carcinoma (see Fig. 9-18). If invasive, metastases are usually to inguinal lymph nodes. Treatment usually consists of distal urethrectomy and inguinal lymph node dissection. Cancer arising in the proximal urethra is usually urothelial and typically metastasizes to pelvic lymph nodes. Treatment includes total urethrectomy as well as inguinal and pelvic lymph node dissection. Wide dissemination at presentation is quite rare, although metastases to regional lymph nodes are common. In two large series, approximately 28% of patients who underwent inguinal lymphadenectomy and approximately 50% of patients who underwent pelvic lymphadenectomy had metastases.[91,94] Histologic type and grade were not significant when corrected for stage.

Adenocarcinoma

Urethral adenocarcinoma is more common in women than in men.[78,95-100] Stage for stage, it has the same prognosis as squamous cell and urothelial carcinoma of the urethra. Adenocarcinoma may arise from the surface mucosa through metaplasia or from periurethral glands (Fig. 9-22, 9-23).[101-105] Those arising from the surface urothelium are usually associated with a chronic inflammatory insult, such as stricture, diverticulum, infection, or fistula (see Fig. 9-3) and present with irritative symptoms, hematuria, or urinary obstruction. On ure-

9-22. Adenocarcinoma of the female urethra presenting as an exophytic mass. It is easy to understand how a lesion such as this can lead to dysuria, hematuria, and urinary obstruction.

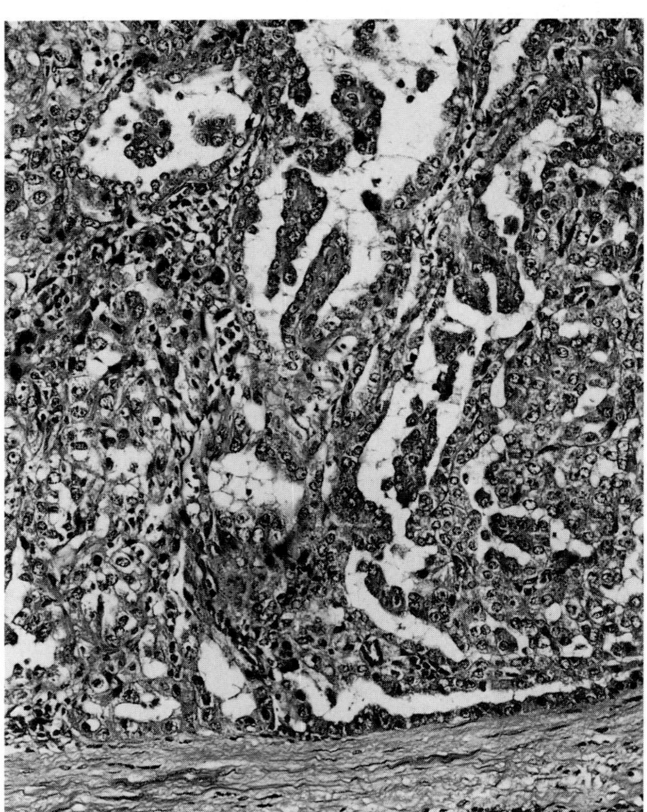

9-23. Papillary and solid adenocarcinoma arising in periurethral (Skene's) glands. The tumor cells have a high nuclear grade. A few cases such as this may express prostate-specific antigen.

throscopy they appear as papillary or polypoid masses. Microscopically, they are composed of simple or pseudostratified columnar epithelium with apical cytoplasm and basally located hyperchromatic nuclei. Occasionally the cytoplasm is vacuolated and contains mucin, giving the tumor a colonic appearance (Fig. 9-24). Rarely, urethral adenocarcinoma is frankly mucinous. High-grade lesions exhibit greater pleomorphism and numerous mitotic figures. Glandular metaplasia, urethritis cystica, and urethritis glandularis are often present in the adjacent mucosa. These tumors do not react with antibodies to prostate-specific antigen. They must be distinguished from the occasional case of intraurethral papillary prostatic adenocarcinoma, which usually arises adjacent to the verumontanum.[62] Papillary prostatic adenocarcinoma tends to have prominent eosinophilic nucleoli and to be associated with typical prostatic adenocarcinoma in the underlying periurethral prostatic tissue. Extension of other adenocarcinomas into the urethra, such as rectal adenocarcinoma in males or rectal, endometrial, endocervical, vaginal, or Bartholin's glands adenocarcinoma in females, must be considered in the differential diagnosis.

Adenocarcinoma of accessory glands. In males there are a few reports of adenocarcinomas arising in Cowper's glands and Littre's glands.[101-104] These diagnoses are very difficult because the tumor has usually destroyed the local anatomic landmarks and extended to or ulcerated the overlying mucosa. Adenocarcinoma arising in Cowper's glands is located in the bulbo-membranous region, while that arising from Littre's glands tends to originate toward the distal portions of the penile urethra but may arise at any point along its entire length. Both present with hematuria, dysuria, and progressive urinary obstruction. It is common for these patients to be treated for urethritis before the proper diagnosis is established. Microscopically, these neoplasms share features with adenocarcinoma arising from the urethral mucosa. The tumors may have a tubular or micropapillary growth pattern and the cells are either cuboidal or columnar with clear or eosinophilic cytoplasm and large, hyperchromatic nuclei. Intracytoplasmic mucin vacuoles or a frank mucinous component are uncommon. Cytoplasmic clearing, if present, is usually due to glycogen production (see the description on clear cell adenocarcinoma in the following section).

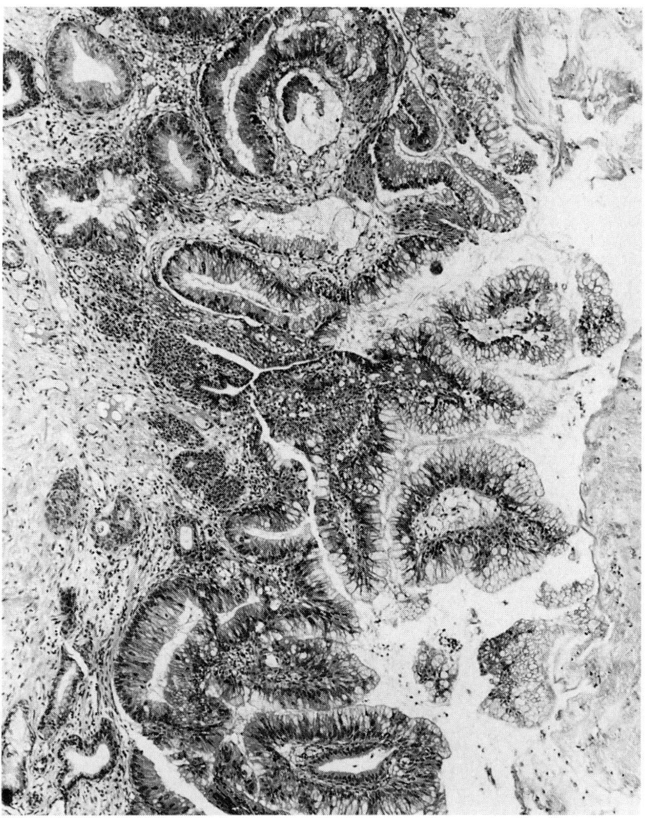

9-24. Villous adenoma arising in the area of the verumontanum. Note the intracytoplasmic and extracellular mucin.

In women adenocarcinoma arising from periurethral or Skene's glands displays the same symptoms as the accessory gland adenocarcinomas in men (see Fig. 9-22).[78,99,105] It may arise at any point in the urethra but is more common distally. In that location, patients often have a perineal mass that may be confused with an infected cyst or uterine prolapse. Microscopically, the tumors may have a glandular, papillary, or micropapillary architecture, and the tumor cells are either columnar or cuboidal with eosinophilic or clear cytoplasm (see Fig. 9-23). Cytoplasmic clearing is usually caused by glycogen deposition or, less frequently, intracytoplasmic mucin. Intraluminal mucin is common. The nuclei are large and hyperchromatic and often exhibit prominent nucleoli. It should be borne in mind that the diagnosis of adenocarcinoma arising in periurethral glands is usually very difficult because of extension or ulceration of the overlying urethral mucosa and obliteration of anatomic landmarks.[78,99] The best indication of periurethral gland origin is partial involvement of recognizable periurethral glands. Even then, this may represent downward extension from the surface. The prognosis in all cases of urethral adenocarcinoma, whether of surface or periurethral gland origin, is determined by the pathologic stage at the time of presentation rather than the site of origin.

Clear cell adenocarcinoma. Clear cell adenocarcinoma is an unusual variant of urethral adenocarcinoma that may arise from the mucosa or from periurethral glands.[99,106-111] It is also called *mesonephric adenocarcinoma*[108] and *glycogen-rich carcinoma*.[111] Its morphologic features are identical to those of clear cell adenocarcinoma of the genital tract. Nevertheless, Young and Scully[106] concluded that urethral clear cell adenocarcinomas arise through metaplasia of the surface mucosa or from periurethral glands rather than from müllerian or mesonephric origin.

Microscopically, clear cell adenocarcinomas may have tubular, papillary, micropapillary, acinar, or diffuse growth patterns (Fig. 9-23, 9-25). Commonly they exhibit a combination of growth patterns. The cells often have abundant, clear, or eosinophilic cytoplasm that contains glycogen and little or no mucin. Mucicarmine positivity is usually evident only in the luminal secretions. In a few

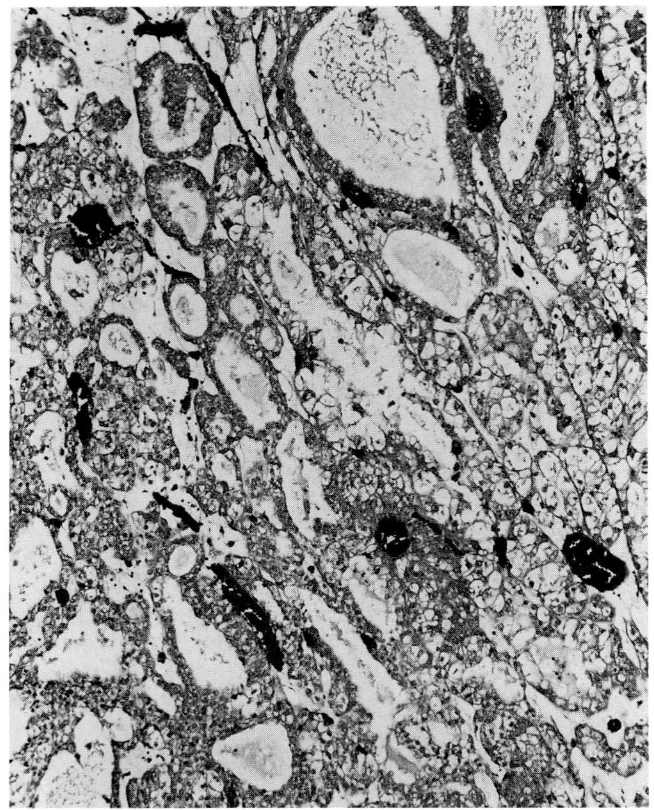

9-25. Clear cell adenocarcinoma. This tumor may arise from the surface mucosa or periurethral glands. Morphologically, it may be difficult to differentiate from clear cell adenocarcinomas arising in the female genital tract or metastatic from the kidney.

cases prostate-specific antigen and prostatic acid phosphatase immunoreactivity have been demonstrated in clear cell adenocarcinomas in women.[112-113] The nuclei are large, pleomorphic, and hyperchromatic and, if luminally located, give the tubules a distinctive hobnail appearance. Several cases have presented with paraneoplastic hypercalcemia similar to that seen with other clear cell tumors such as renal cell carcinoma.[106] Clear cell adenocarcinoma of the urethra is distinguished from gynecologic clear cell carcinoma and metastatic renal cell carcinoma by clinical history and diagnostic workup. Gynecologic clear cell adenocarcinoma tends to occur in younger patients exposed to nonsteroidal estrogens prior to birth. Cantrell et al[114] reported a case of papillary prostatic adenocarcinoma occupying the prostatic urethra and exhibiting clear cell features. The diffuse pattern may be confused with amelanotic melanoma. Also, clear cell adenocarcinoma must be distinguished from nephrogenic adenoma. Nephrogenic adenoma lacks the nuclear pleomorphism and hyperchromasia and infiltrative and destructive growth pattern seen in adenocarcinoma. Mitotic figures are rare in nephrogenic adenoma but usually are readily apparent in clear cell adenocarcinoma. This distinction may be difficult to establish on a small biopsy.

The prognosis of clear cell adenocarcinoma of the urethra is uncertain because of the rarity of this tumor and limited follow up in reported series. A series from M.D. Anderson Hospital suggests that these patients may have a somewhat better prognosis than those with adenocarcinomas of other types, although the numbers did not reach statistical significance.[99] In general, prognosis correlates with pathologic stage at presentation. Clinical management has varied, including transurethral resection, radical excision, and radiation therapy, or a combination of these.

Other histologic types of carcinoma

Other epithelial neoplasms arising within the urethra include adenosquamous carcinoma,[115] adenoid cystic carcinoma,[116] carcinoid,[117] and so-called cloacogenic carcinoma.[118,119] All have been single-case reports with limited follow-up. Their morphologic features are similar to their counterparts arising at other sites.

Malignant melanoma

Although very rare, the urethra is the most common site of origin of malignant melanoma in the urinary tract.[120-129] In 1988 Manivel and Fraley[121] reviewed the literature and found only 26 cases. The urethra is more commonly involved by spread from melanoma arising in the glans penis and vulva. Urethral melanoma occurs in males and females and has been described in black patients.[123,125] The tumor may be associated with melanosis, although precursor lesions are rarely identified. The majority of cases occur in older patients. Begun et al[120] reported a 13-year-old boy who developed melanoma, not of the urethra, but of the penis.

Patients usually present with hematuria, dysuria, deviated urinary stream, or urinary obstruction. Melanuria is an uncommon finding. Endoscopic examination reveals a nodular mucosal mass or masses that are usually pigmented and frequently ulcerated. As with other mucosal melanomas, the growth pattern is commonly lentiginous although all other patterns may be represented (Fig. 9-26). Mucosal melanoma is more likely to be amelanotic than cutaneous melanoma. Extensive radial growth is common, accounting for the frequency of local recurrence. Metastasis is usually to inguinal and pelvic lymph nodes and common in advanced lesions. Hematogenous spread to liver, lungs, and brain is common.

Treatment is surgical and includes urethrectomy or penectomy with regional lymph node dissection. The role of immunotherapy, radiation therapy, and chemotherapy remains uncertain.[126,128] Staging for urethral melanoma has not been standardized since most reports deal with isolated cases. Prognosis depends on the thickness of the lesion, similar to melanoma at other mucosal sites. Pathologists should carefully evaluate the status of the mucosal margin of resection because local recurrence at the surgical bed is common. Skip lesions involving the urinary bladder and ureter may occur and should be investigated prior to extirpative surgery.

Mesenchymal neoplasms

Leiomyoma is the most common mesenchymal neoplasm of the urethra, although no more than 30 cases have been reported.[130-135] Leiomyomas have also been

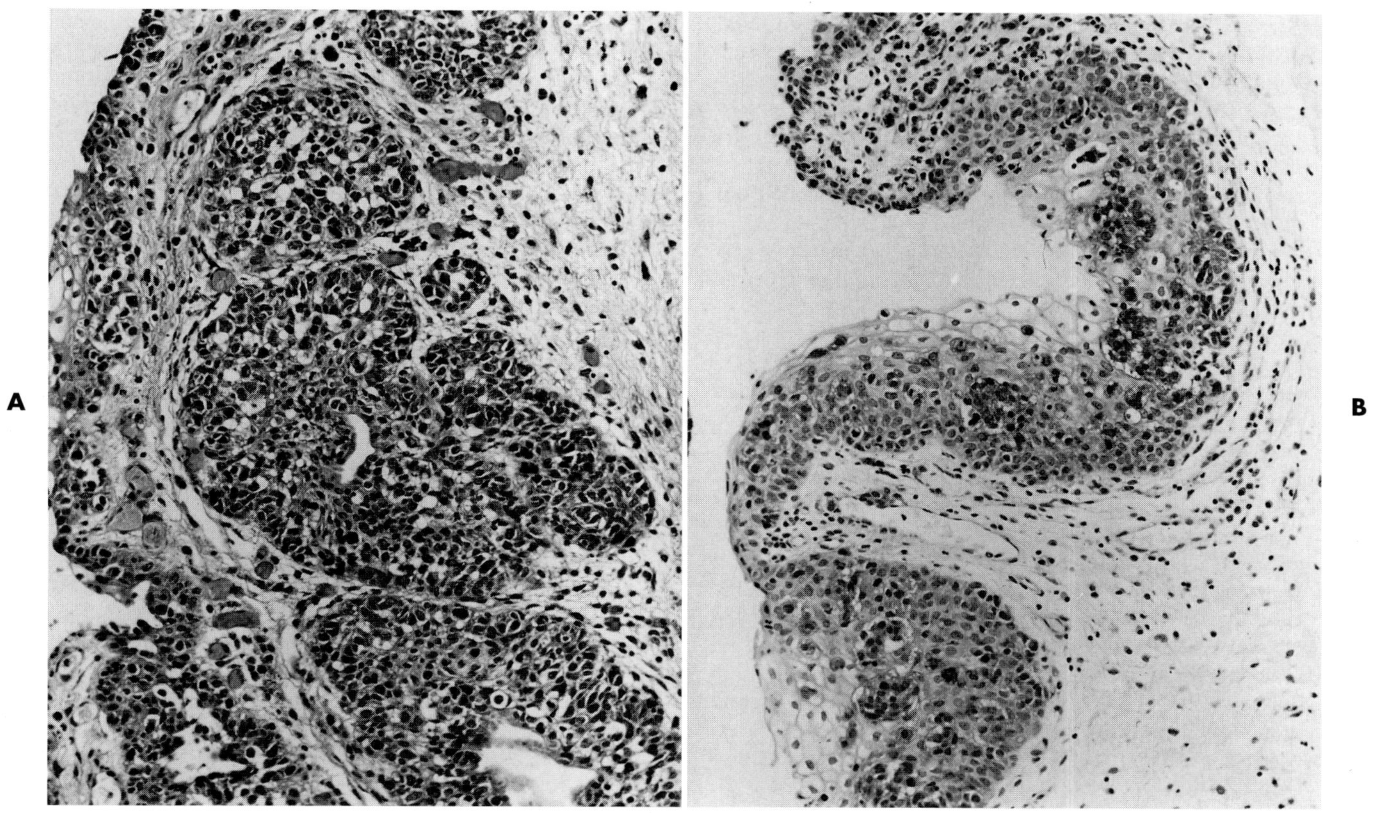

9-26. Urethral malignant melanoma. **A**, Neoplastic melanocytes occupy the surface mucosa and extend into periurethral glands. **B**, Tumor cells are immunoreactive with S-100 protein.

described involving the paraurethral soft tissue, but the exact site of origin of these is uncertain. Urethral leiomyomas range in size from 1 to 40 cm and may present as an asymptomatic mass or with dysuria and urinary obstruction.

Other nonepithelial neoplasms are rare in the urethra and periurethral soft tissues. These include hemangioma,[136-138] paraganglioma,[139-141] plasmacytoma,[142-144] and neurofibroma.[145] Lymphoma may involve the urethra but usually is a manifestation of systemic disease with only a few cases asserted to be primary in the urethra.[146,147]

While sarcomas have been described in the pelvic and paraurethral tissues, it is difficult to establish whether they truly are of urethral origin. Steeper and Rosai[148] described a mesenchymal tumor arising in the pelvis and perineal soft tissues of women and called it *aggressive angiomyxoma*. It consists of vascular fibromyxoid tissue and is locally infiltrative with a tendency to multiple recurrences. These patients may present with urinary obstruction or dysuria.

References

1. Moore KL, Persaud TVN: The urinary system. In The developing human, ed 5, Moore KL, ed: Philadelphia, 1993, WB Saunders.
2. Moore KL: The pelvis and perineum. In Moore KL, ed: Clinically oriented anatomy, ed 2, Baltimore, 1985, Williams & Wilkins.
3. Carroll PR, Dixon CM: Surgical anatomy of the male and female urethra, Urol Clin North Am 19:339-346, 1992.
4. Tanagho E: Anatomy of the lower urinary tract. In Walsh PC, Retik AB, Stamey TA et al, eds: Campbell's urology, ed 6, Philadelphia, 1992, WB Saunders.
5. Herr HW: Surgery of penile and urethral carcinoma. In Walsh PC, Retik AB, Stamey TA et al, eds: Campbell's urology, ed 6, Philadelphia, 1992, WB Saunders.
6. Herbut PA: Urological pathology, Philadelphia, 1952, Lea & Febiger.
7. Saraf PG, Valvo JR, Frank IN: Congenital urethral posterior valves in an adult, Urology 24:55-57, 1984.
8. Williams DI: Discussion on lower urinary obstruction, Arch Dis Child 37:132, 1962.
9. Coddington CC, Knab DR: Urethral diverticulum. A review, Obstet Gynecol Surv 38:357-364, 1983.
10. Newland DE, Patterson JH, Hofsess DW: Urethral diverticulum: a recondite disease, J Urol 103:174-175, 1970.
11. Davis HJ, Telinde RW: Urethral diverticula: an assay of 121 cases, J Urol 80:34-39, 1958.
12. Anderson MJF: The incidence of diverticula in the female urethra, J Urol 98:96-98, 1967.
13. Medeiros LJ, Young RH: Nephrogenic adenoma arising in urethral diverticula. A report of 5 cases, Arch Pathol Lab Med 113:125-128, 1989.

14. Bazzeed MA, Saad SM, Abou-el-Azm TA: Aquired urethral diverticula in the male, Urol Int 36:380-385, 1981.
15. Tesluk H: Primary adenocarcinoma of female urethra associated with diverticula, Urology 17:197-199, 1981.
16. Marshall S, Hirsch K: Carcinoma within urethral diverticula, Urology 10:161-163, 1977.
17. Srinivas V, Dow D: Transitional cell carcinoma in a urethral diverticulum with a calculus, J Urol 129:372-373, 1983.
18. Wheeler JS Jr, Flanigan RC, Hong HY et al: Female urethral diverticulum with clear cell adenocarcinoma, J Surg Oncol 49:66-71, 1992.
19. Cea PC, Ward JN, Lavengood RW Jr: Mesonephric adenocarcinomas in urethral diverticula, Urology 10:58-61, 1977.
20. Gross RE, Moore TC: Duplication of the urethra: report of two cases and summary of the literature, Arch Surg 60:749-753, 1950.
21. Olsen JG: Complete urethral duplication, J Urol 95:718-720, 1966.
22. Ortolano V, Nasrallah PF: Urethral duplication, J Urol 126:909-911, 1986.
23. Downs RA: Congenital urethral polyps of the prostatic urethra, Br J Urol 42:76-85, 1970.
24. Hanani Y, Hertz M, Jones P: Congenital urethral polyp in children, Urology 16:162-164, 1980.
25. Youssif M: Posterior urethral polyps in infants and children, Eur Urol 11:69-70, 1985.
26. Foster RS, Weigel JW, Mantz FA: Anterior urethral polyps, J Urol 124:145-146, 1980.
27. Bruijnes E, de Wall JG, Scholtmeijer RJ: Congenital polyp of the prostatic urethra in childhood. Report of 3 cases and review of literature, Urol Int 40:287-291, 1985.
28. Murphy DM, Guiney EJ: Polyp of the posterior urethra, Eur Urol 8:204-206, 1982.
29. Foster RS, Garrett RA: Congenital posterior urethral polyps, J Urol 136:670-672, 1986.
30. Wallin JE, Thompson SE, Zaidi A et al: Urethritis in women attending an STD clinic, Br J Vener Dis 57:50-54, 1981.
31. Swartz SL, Kraus SJ, Herrmann KL: Diagnosis and etiology of non-gonococcal urethritis, J Infect Dis 138:445-454, 1978.
32. Hoffman WW, Cheatum DE: Reiter's disease, Urol Surv 28:197-205, 1978.
33. Elbadawi A, Malhoski WE: Mucinous urethral caruncle, Urology 12:587-590, 1978.
34. Jarvi OH, Marin S: Intestinal mucosal heterotopia of an urethral caruncle, Acta Pathol Microbiol Immunol Scand A 90:213-219, 1982.
35. Willett GD, Lack EE: Periurethral colonic-type polyp simulating urethral caruncle. A case report, J Reprod Med 35:1017-1018, 1990.
36. Young RH, Scully RE: Clear cell adenocarcinoma of the bladder and urethra. A report of 3 cases and review of the literature, Am J Surg Pathol 9:816-826, 1985.
37. Proppe KH, Scully RE, Rosai J: Postoperative spindle-cell nodules of the genitourinary tract resembling sarcomas: a report of eight cases, Am J Surg Pathol 8:101-108, 1984.
38. Schinella R, Thurm J, Feiner H: Papillary pseudotumor of the prostatic urethra: proliferative papillary urethritis, J Urol 111:38-40, 1974.
39. Walker AN, Mills SE: Papillary and polypoid tumors of the prostatic urethra. In Damjanov I, Cohen AH, Mills SE et al, eds: Progress in reproductive and urinary tract pathology, New York, 1989, Field & Wood.
40. Bhagavan BS, Tiamson EM, Wenk RE et al: Nephrogenic adenoma of the urinary bladder and urethra, Hum Pathol 12:907-916, 1981.
41. Odze R, Begin LR: Tubular adenomatous metaplasia (nephrogenic adenoma) of the female urethra, Int J Gynecol Pathol 8:374-380, 1989.
42. Berger BW, Bhagavan SB, Reiner W et al: Nephrogenic adenoma: clinical features and therapeutic considerations, J Urol 126:824-826, 1981.
43. Lou TY, Teplitz C: Malakoplakia: pathogenesis and ultrastructural morphogenesis. A problem of altered macrophage (phagolysomal) response, Hum Pathol 5:191-207, 1974.
44. Damjanov I, Katz SM: Malakoplakia, Pathol Annu 16:103-126, 1981.
45. Stanton MJ, Maxted W: Malakoplakia: a study of the literature and current concepts of pathogenesis, diagnosis and treatment, J Urol 125:139-146, 1981.
46. McClure J: A case of urethral malakoplakia associated with vesical disease, J Urol 122:705-706, 1979.
47. Sharma TC Kagan H, Shiels JP: Malakoplakia of the male urethra, J Urol 125:885-886, 1981.
48. Ordóñez NG, Ayala AG, Gresik MV et al: Primary localized amyloidosis of male urethra (amyloidoma), Urology 14:617-619, 1979.
49. Constantian HM, Wyman P: Localized amyloidosis of the urethra: report of a case, J Urol 124:728-729, 1980.
50. Vasudevan P, Stein AM, Pinn VW et al: Primary amyloidosis of urethra, Urology 17:181-183, 1981.
51. Dounis A, Bourounis M, Mitropoulos D: Primary localized amyloidosis of the urethra, Eur Urol 11:344-345, 1985.
52. Bodner H, Retsky MI, Brown G: Primary amyloidosis of glans penis and urethra: resection and reconstruction, J Urol 125:586-588, 1981.
53. Debenedictis TJ, Marmar JL, Praiss DE: Intraurethral condylomas acuminata: management and review of the literature, J Urol 118:767-769, 1977.
54. Murphy WM, Fu YS, Lancaster WD et al: Papillomavirus structural antigens in condyloma acuminatum of the male urethra, J Urol 130:84-85, 1983.
55. Grussendorf-Conen EI, Deutz FJ, de Villiers EM: Detection of human papillomavirus-6 in primary carcinoma of the urethra in men, Cancer 60:1832-1835, 1987.
56. Melchers WJ, Schift R, Stolz E et al: Human papillomavirus detection in urine samples from male patients by the polymerase chain reaction, J Clin Microbiol 27:1711-1714, 1989.
57. Del Mistro A, Braunstein JD, Halwer M et al: Identification of human papillomavirus types in male urethral condylomata acuminata by in situ hybridization, Hum Pathol 18:936-940, 1987.
58. Weiner JS, Liu ET, Walther PJ: Oncogenic human papillomavirus type 16 is associated with squamous cell cancer of the male urethra, Cancer Res 52:5018-5023, 1992.
59. Mevorach RA, Cos LR, di Sant'Agnese PA et al: Human papillomavirus type 6 in grade I transitional cell carcinoma of the urethra, J Urol 143:126-128, 1990.

60. Remick DG Jr, Kumar NB: Benign polyps with prostatic-type epithelium of the urethra and the urinary bladder. A suggestion of histogenesis based on histologic and immunohistochemical studies, Am J Surg Pathol 8:833-839, 1984.
61. Craig JR, Hart WR: Benign polyps with prostatic-type epithelium of the urethra, Am J Clin Pathol 63:343-347, 1975.
62. Walker AN, Mills SE, Fechner RE et al: "Endometrial" adenocarcinoma of the prostatic urethra arising in a villous polyp. A light microscopic and immunoperoxidase study, Arch Pathol Lab Med 106:624-627, 1982.
63. Lubin J, Mark TM, Wirtschafter AR: Papillomas of prostatic urethra with prostatic-type epithelium: report of 8 cases, Mt Sinai J Med 51:218-221, 1984.
64. Satoh S, Ujiie T, Kubo T et al: Prostatic epithelial polyp of the prostatic urethra, Eur Urol 16:92-96, 1989.
65. Goldstein AM, Bragin SD, Terry R et al: Prostatic urethral polyps in adults: histopathologic variations and clinical manifestations, J Urol 126:129-131, 1981.
66. Heyderman E, Mandaliya KN, O'Donnell PJ et al: Ectopic prostatic glands in bulbar urethra. Immunoperoxidase study, Urology 29:76-77, 1987.
67. Hicks CC, Nicholas EM, Morgan JW: Hematuria from ectopic prostatic tissue in bulbous urethra, Urology 10:50-51, 1977.
68. Dejter SW Jr, Zuckerman ME, Lynch JH: Benign villous polyp with prostatic type epithelium of the penile urethra, J Urol 139:590-591, 1988.
69. Reuter VE, Melamed MR: The lower urinary tract. In Sternberg SS, ed: Diagnostic surgical pathology, ed 2, New York, 1994, Raven Press.
70. Jordan AM, Weingarten J, Murphy WM: Transitional cell neoplasms of the bladder: can biologic potential be predicted from histologic grading? Cancer 60:2766-2774, 1987.
71. De Meester LT, Farrow GH, Utz DS: Inverted papilloma of the urinary bladder, Cancer 36:505-513, 1975.
72. Renfer LG, Kelley J, Belville WD: Inverted papilloma of the urinary tract: histogenesis, recurrence and associated malignancy, J Urol 140:832-834, 1988.
73. Gowing NFC: Urethral carcinoma associated with cancer of the bladder, Br J Urol 32:428-430, 1960.
74. Schellhammer PF, Whitmore WF Jr: Urethral meatal carcinoma following cystourethrectomy for bladder carcinoma, J Urol 115:61-64, 1976.
75. Tobisu K, Tanaka Y, Mizutani T et al: Transitional cell carcinoma of the urethra in men following cystectomy for bladder cancer: multivariate analysis for risk factors, J Urol 146:1551-1553, 1991.
76. Richie JP, Skinner DG: Carcinoma in situ of the urethra associated with bladder carcinoma: the role of urethrectomy, J Urol 119:80-81, 1978.
77. Ray B, Canto AR, Whitmore WF Jr: Experience with primary carcinoma of the male urethra, J Urol 117:591-594, 1977.
78. Schellhammer PF: Urethral carcinoma, Semin Urol 1:82-89, 1983.
79. Schellhammer PF, Bean MA, Whitmore WF: Prostatic involvement by transitional cell carcinoma: pathogenesis, patterns and prognosis, J Urol 118:399-403, 1977.
80. Hardeman SW, Soloway MS: Urethral recurrence following radical cystectomy, J Urol 144:666-669, 1990.
81. Wolinska WH, Melamed MR, Schellhammer PF et al: Urethral cytology following cystectomy for bladder carcinoma, Am J Surg Pathol 1:225-234, 1977.
82. Hermansen DK, Badalament RA, Whitmore WF Jr et al: Detection of carcinoma in the post-cystectomy urethral remnant by flow cytometric analysis, J Urol 139:304-307, 1988.
83. Mahadevia PS, Alexander JE, Rojas-Corona R et al: Pseudosarcomatous stromal reaction in primary and metastatic urothelial carcinoma: a source of diagnostic difficulty, Am J Surg Pathol 13:782-790, 1989.
84. De Paepe ME, Andre R, Mahadevia P: Urethral involvement in female patients with bladder cancer. A study of 22 cystectomy specimens, Cancer 65:1237-1241, 1990.
85. Melicow MM, Roberts TW: Pathology and natural history of urethral tumors in males. Review of 142 cases, Urology 11:83-89, 1978.
86. Orihuela E, Herr HW, Whitmore WF Jr: Conservative treatment of superficial transitional cell carcinoma of prostatic urethra with intravesical BCG, Urology 34:231-237, 1989.
87. Tomaszewski JE, Korat OC, LiVolsi VA et al: Paget's disease of the urethral meatus following transitional cell carcinoma of the bladder, J Urol 135:368-370, 1986.
88. Begin LR, Deschenes J, Mitmaker B: Pagetoid carcinomatous involvement of the penile urethra in association with high-grade transitional cell carcinoma of the urinary bladder, Arch Pathol Lab Med 115:632-635, 1991.
89. Merino MJ, Livolsi VA, Lytton B: Penile Paget's disease and prostatic carcinoma, J Urol 120:121-122, 1978.
90. Grabstald H, Hilaris B, Henschke U et al: Cancer of the female urethra, JAMA 197:835-838, 1966.
91. Bracken RB, Johnson DE, Miller LS et al: Primary carcinoma of the female urethra, J Urol 116:188-192, 1976.
92. Johnson DE, O'Connell JR: Primary carcinoma of female urethra, Urology 21:42-45, 1983.
93. Roberts TW, Melicow MM: Pathology and natural history of urethral tumors in females, Urology 10:583-589, 1977.
94. Kamat MR, Kulkarni JN, Dhumale RG: Primary carcinoma of the female urethra: review of 20 cases, J Surg Oncol 16:105-106, 1981.
95. Yachia D, Turani H: Colonic-type adenocarcinoma of male urethra, Urology 37:568-570, 1991.
96. Bostwick DG, Lo R, Stamey TA: Papillary adenocarcinoma of the male urethra. Case report and review of the literature, Cancer 54:2556-2563, 1984.
97. Loo KT, Chan JK: Colloid adenocarcinoma of the urethra associated with mucosal in situ carcinoma, Arch Pathol Lab Med 116:976-977, 1992.
98. Lieber MM, Malek RS, Farrow GM et al: Villous adenocarcinoma of the male urethra, J Urol 130:1191-1193, 1983.
99. Meis JM, Ayala AG, Johnson DE: Adenocarcinoma of the urethra in women. A clinicopathologic study, Cancer 60:1038-1052, 1987.
100. Powell I, Cartwright H, Jano F: Villous adenoma and adenocarcinoma of female urethra, Urology 18:612-614, 1981.
101. Silverman ML, Eyre RC, Zinman LA et al: Mixed mucinous and papillary adenocarcinoma involving male urethra, probably originating in periurethral glands, Cancer 47:1398-1402, 1981.
102. Sacks SA, Waisman J, Apfelbaum HB et al: Urethral adenocarcinoma (possibly originating in the glands of Littre), J Urol 113:50-55, 1975.

103. Bourque JL, Charghi A, Gauthier GE et al: Primary carcinoma of Cowper's gland, J Urol 104:854-856, 1970.
104. Keen MR, Golden RL, Richardson JF et al: Carcinoma of Cowper's gland treated with chemotherapy, J Urol 104:854-856, 1970.
105. Taylor RN, Lacey CG, Shuman MA: Adenocarcinoma of Skene's duct associated with a systemic coagulopathy, Gynecol Oncol 22:250-256, 1985.
106. Young RH, Scully RE: Pseudosarcomatous lesions of the urinary bladder, prostate gland, and urethra. A report of 3 cases and review of the literature, Arch Pathol Lab Med 111:354-358, 1987.
107. Assimos DG, O'Conor VJ Jr: Clear cell adenocarcinoma of the urethra, J Urol 131:540-541, 1984.
108. Altwein JE, Schafer R, Hohenfellner R: Mesonephric carcinoma of the female urethra, Eur Urol 1:248-250, 1975.
109. Rivard DJ, Waisman SS: Primary mesonephric carcinoma of the female urethra, J Urol 134:756-757, 1985.
110. Tanabe ET, Mazur MT, Schaeffer AJ: Clear cell adenocarcinoma of the female urethra: clinical and ultrastructural study suggesting a unique neoplasm, Cancer 49:372-378, 1982.
111. Hull MT, Eglen DE, Davis T et al: Glycogen-rich clear cell carcinoma of the urethra: an ultrastructural study, Ultrastruct Pathol 11:421-427, 1987.
112. Spencer JR, Brodin AG, Ignatoff JM: Clear cell adenocarcinoma of the urethra: evidence for origin within paraurethral ducts, J Urol 143:122-125, 1990.
113. Svanholm H, Andersen OP, Rohl H: Tumour of female paraurethral duct. Immunohistochemical similarity with prostatic carcinoma, Virchows Arch A Pathol Anat Histopathol 411:395-398, 1987.
114. Cantrell BB, Leifer G, DeKlerk DP et al: Papillary adenocarcinoma of the prostatic urethra with clear-cell appearance, Cancer 48:2661-2667, 1981.
115. Saito R: An adenosquamous carcinoma of the male urethra with hypercalcemia, Hum Pathol 12:383-385, 1981.
116. Aronson P, Ronan SG, Briele HA et al: Adenoid cystic carcinoma of female periurethral area. Light and electron microscopic study, Urology 20:312-315, 1982.
117. Sylora HO, Diamond HM, Kaufman M et al: Primary carcinoid tumor of the urethra, J Urol 114:150-153, 1975.
118. Díaz-Cano SJ, Rios JJ, Rivera-Hueto F et al: Mixed cloacogenic carcinoma of male urethra, Histopathology 20:82-84, 1992.
119. Lucman L, Vadas G: Transitional cloacogenic carcinoma of the urethra, Cancer 31:1508-1510, 1973.
120. Begun FP, Grossman HB, Diokno AC et al: Malignant melanoma of the penis and male urethra, J Urol 132:123-125, 1984.
121. Manivel JC, Fraley EE: Malignant melanoma of the penis and male urethra: 4 case reports and literature review, J Urol 139:813-816, 1988.
122. Weiss J, Elder D, Hamilton R: Melanoma of the male urethra: surgical approach and pathological analysis, J Urol 128:382-385, 1982.
123. Pow-Sang JM, Klimberg IW, Hackett RL et al: Primary malignant melanoma of the male urethra, J Urol 139:1304-1306, 1988.
124. Oldbring J, Mikulowski P: Malignant melanoma of the penis and male urethra. Report of 9 cases and review of the literature, Cancer 59:581-587, 1987.
125. Sanders TJ, Venable DD, Sanusi ID: Primary malignant melanoma of the urethra in a black man: a case report, J Urol 135:1012-1014, 1986.
126. Katz JI, Grabstald H: Primary malignant melanoma of the female urethra, J Urol 116:454-457, 1976.
127. Yoshida K, Tsuboi N, Akimoto M: Primary malignant melanoma of female urethra: report of a case and review of the literature, Hinyokika Kiyo 32:105-111, 1986.
128. Nissenkorn I, Servadio C, Avidor I et al: Malignant melanomas of female urethra, Urology 29:562-565, 1987.
129. Kim CJ, Pak K, Hamaguchi A et al: Primary malignant melanoma of the female urethra, Cancer 71:448-451, 1993.
130. Oi RH, Poirier-Brode KY: Leiomyoma of the female urethra, J Reprod Med 22:259-260, 1979.
131. Mooppan MM, Kim H, Wax SH: Leiomyoma of the female urethra, J Urol 121:371-372, 1979.
132. Lake MH, Kossow AS, Bokinsky G: Leiomyoma of the bladder and urethra, J Urol 125:742-743, 1981.
133. Ohtani M, Yanagizawa R, Shoji F et al: Leiomyoma of the male urethra, Eur Urol 8:372-373, 1982.
134. Di Cello V, Saltutti C, Mincione GP et al: Paraurethral leiomyoma in women, Eur Urol 15:290-293, 1988.
135. Cheng C, Mac-Moune Lai F, Chan PS: Leiomyoma of the female urethra: a case report and review, J Urol 148:1526-1527, 1992.
136. Steinhardt G, Perlmutter A: Urethral hemangioma, J Urol 137:116-117, 1987.
137. Sharma SK, Reddy MJ, Joshi VV et al: Capillary hemangioma of male urethra, Br J Urol 53:277, 1981.
138. Barua R, Munday RN: Intravascular angiomatosis in female urethral mass. Masson intravascular hemangioendothelioma, Urology 21:191-193, 1983.
139. Badalament RA, Kenworthy P, Pellegrini A et al: Paraganglioma of urethra, Urology 38:76-78, 1991.
140. Cholhan HJ, Caglar H, Kremzier JE: Suburethral paraganglioma, Obstet Gynecol 78:555-558, 1991.
141. Bryant KR, Thompson IM, Ortiz R et al: Urethral paraganglioma presenting as a urethral polyp, J Urol 130:571-572, 1983.
142. Witjes JA, de Vries JD, Scharfsma HE et al: Extramedullary plasmacytoma of the urethra: a case report, J Urol 145:826-828, 1991.
143. Mark JA, Pais VM, Chong FK: Plasmacytoma of the urethra treated with transurethral resection and radiotherapy, J Urol 143:1010-1011, 1990.
144. Campbell CM, Smith JA Jr, Middleton RG: Plasmacytoma of the urethra, J Urol 127:986, 1982.
145. Eidelman A, Reif R: Periurethral myxoid neurofibroma, J Urol 125:746-747, 1981.
146. Melicow MM, Lattes R, Pierre-Louis C: Lymphoma of the female urethra masquerading as a caruncle, J Urol 108:748-750, 1972.
147. Touhami H, Brahimi S, Kubisz P et al: Non-Hodgkin's lymphoma of the female urethra, J Urol 137:991-992, 1987.
148. Steeper TA, Rosai J: Aggressive angiomyxoma of the female pelvis and perineum: report of nine cases of a distinctive type of gynecologic soft tissue neoplasm, Am J Surg Pathol 7:463-475, 1983.

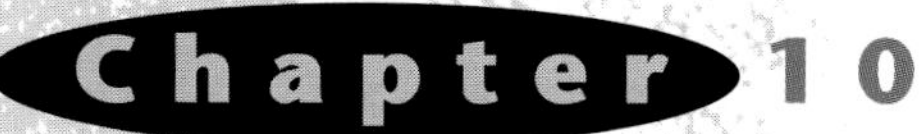

NON-NEOPLASTIC DISEASES OF THE TESTIS

MANUEL NISTAL
RICARDO PANIAGUA

EMBRYOLOGY AND ANATOMY OF TESTIS

EMBRYOLOGY

DEVELOPMENT OF TESTIS

Testicular differentiation is a sequential process that occurs when the human embryo has a 46XY chromosomal constitution. The testis determining factor gene (located on the Y chromosome and designated as the SRY gene) is responsible for testicular differentiation.[1]

In the fourth week of gestation, the urogenital ridges appear as two parallel prominences along the posterior abdominal wall. These prominences give rise to two important pairs of structures: the genital ridges arise from the medial prominence and the mesonephric ridges from the lateral.

The genital ridges are the first primordium of the gonad and stand out as a pair of prominences about the midline. In 30- to 32-day embryos, each genital ridge is lateral to the aorta and medial to the mesonephric duct (Fig. 10-1). The celomic epithelium forming the genital ridges grows as cordlike structures to create the primary sex cords. Immediately beneath the celomic epithelium there are several mesonephric ductuli and glomeruli.

Initially the genital ridges are devoid of germ cells. In the third week, primordial germ cells appear in the extraembryonal mesoderm lining the posterior wall of the yolk sac, near the allantoic evagination. They are ovoid and 12 to 14 μm in diameter, and they are easily detected histochemically by their high content of alkaline phosphatase. Their nuclei are spherical and possess one or two prominent central nucleoli. The cytoplasm contains mitochondria with tubular cristae, lysosomes, microfilaments, lipid inclusions, numerous ribosomes, and abundant glycogen granules. Attracted by chemotactic factors, the primordial germ cells migrate along the mesenchyme of the mesentery, reaching the genital ridge by 32 to 35 days. At that time the center of the gonad begins to be occupied by a cordlike proliferation of cells arising from the mesonephros, the primordial sex cords (Fig. 10-2).[2] These replace the primary sex cords which then atrophy. The primordial sex cords branch from the dorsal toward the ventral part of the genital ridges and become the most voluminous part of the gonad. The primordial germ cells colonize these cords, separated from the gonadal stroma by a basement membrane. At the beginning of the sixth week the male and female gonads appear identical.

During the sixth week the primordial sex cords branch radially toward the celomic epithelium, now reduced to one to three cell layers. The most posterior sex cords,

10-1. Longitudinal section of a fetus showing the relationships among the primitive gonad, mesonephros, and metanephros.

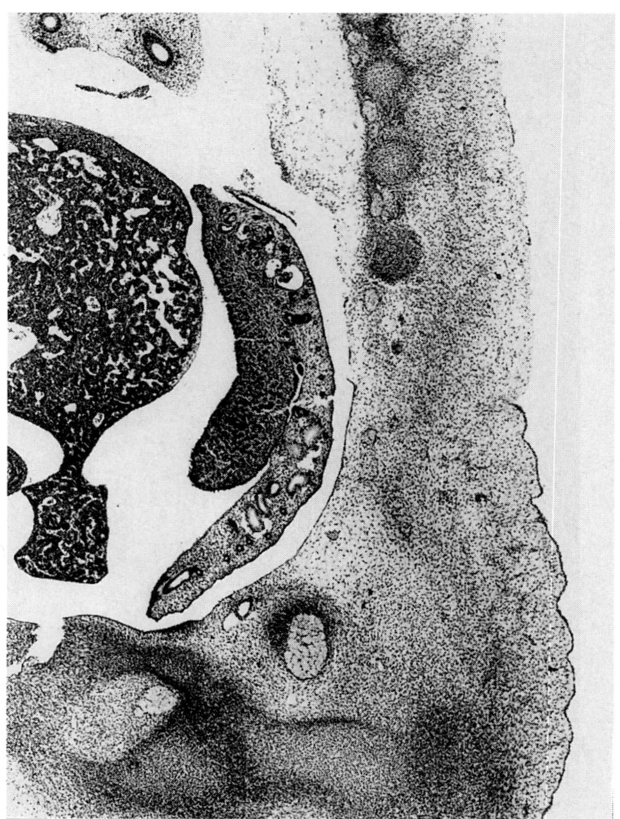

10-2. Longitudinal section of a fetus. The primitive gonad is closely associated with the mesonephros which shows some ductules and glomeruli.

those closest to the renal glomeruli, give rise to the rete testis. At the same time the incorporation of mesonephric cells into the sex cords is arrested, the connection between the testis and mesonephros becomes thinner, and the testis acquires a circular outline on transverse sections (Fig. 10-3).

Previously, a major role in gender differentiation was attributed to the H-Y antigen. Today there is a more precise understanding of the genetic control of gender differentiation.[3] The command for testicular differentiation is given by a small DNA fragment located on the distal portion of the short arm of the Y chromosome. This is known as the testicular differentiation factor gene and acts on somatic cells but not on germ cells.[4] Normal male development also requires the cooperation of genes on the X chromosome. Further, the differentiation of a normal male phenotype requires additional genes located on autosomes. In humans there are at least 19 genes involved in gender determination.[5]

Sertoli cells arise from somatic sex cord cells. These cells produce antimüllerian hormone, which has two principal effects: stimulation of Sertoli cell proliferation, and thus the testicular sex cord configuration, and inhibition of the entry of germ cells into meiosis. The intercord gonadal blastema gives rise to the Leydig cells (Fig. 10-4, 10-5).

DEVELOPMENT OF UROGENITAL TRACT

The development of the urogenital tract begins at the stage of the undifferentiated gonad, with the appearance of two different pairs of ducts: the wolffian ducts and the müllerian ducts.

The wolffian ducts are formed in the mesonephros in the third week of gestation when the cranial region of the segmented intermediate mesoderm gives rise to 10 pairs of tubules—the nephric tubules—which are metamerically arranged. These tubules form the pronephros. On each side of the body the tubules converge to form a longitudinal duct that opens in the celomic cavity. In the fourth week the pronephros disappears and is replaced by another tubular system (derived from the intermediate mesoderm that is not segmented) which forms the mesonephros. The medial ends of the mesonephric tubules do not open to the celomic cavity but are connected to glomeruli on one end and to the wolffian duct on the other. At the end of the second month of gestation the mesonephros is replaced by the metanephros or definitive kidney. However, in the male, the most caudal mesonephric tubules and the wolffian duct persist. The former give rise to the ductuli efferentes, and the latter forms the ductus epididymidis, the ductus deferens, the seminal vesicle, and the ejaculatory duct.

Both müllerian ducts originate from a longitudinal invagination of the celomic epithelium in the anterolateral

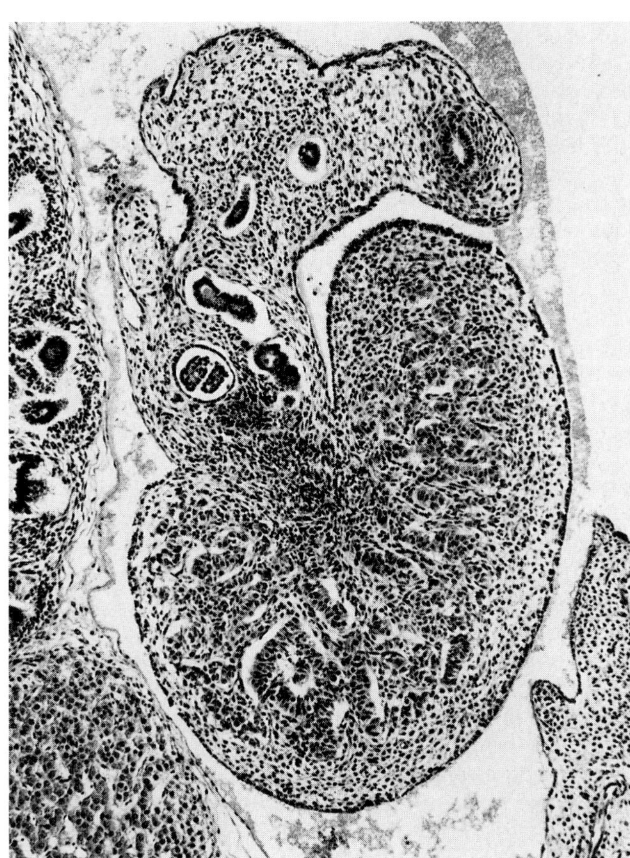

10-3. The testis consists of radially arranged sex cords. Mesenchyme separates the celomic epithelium from the sex cords.

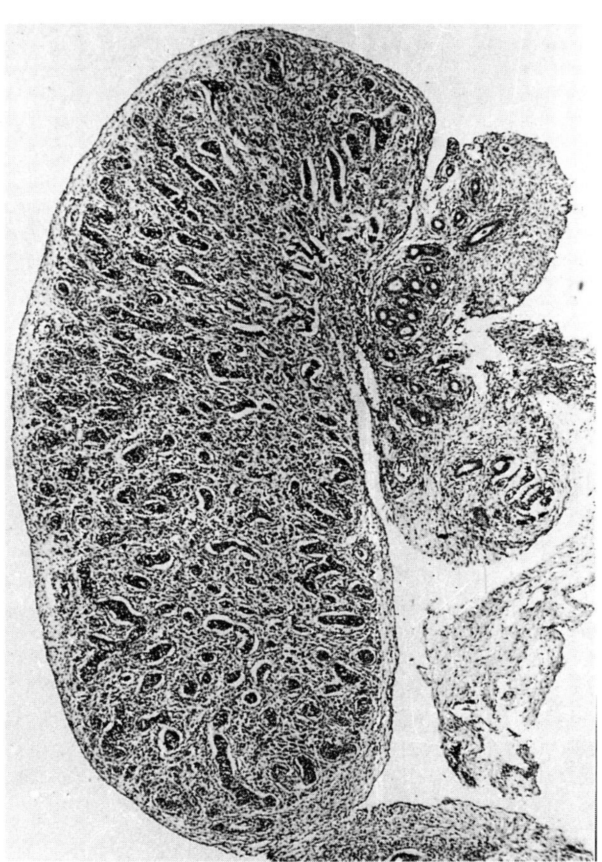

10-4. Longitudinal section of testis at the thirteenth week of gestation. More than half of the testicular parenchyma is occupied by Leydig cells.

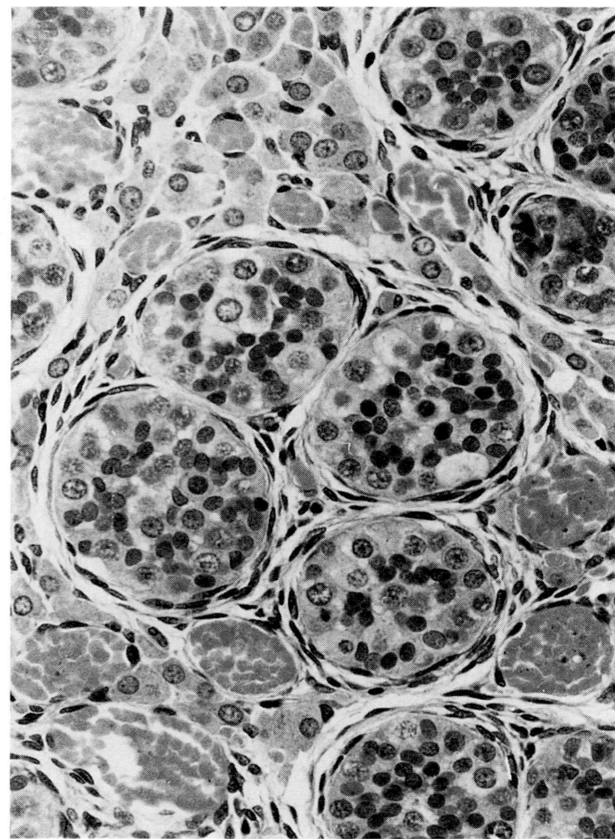

10-5. Testis from a 24-day-old fetus. The seminiferous tubules contain Sertoli cells (small, dark nuclei) and gonocytes (round cells with larger nuclei with central nucleoli). At this time, the interstitium still contains numerous Leydig cells.

aspect of the genital ridge. The cranial end of each duct is a funnel which opens in the celomic cavity. Each duct runs parallel and lateral to the respective wolffian duct and as they pass caudally, the müllerian duct crosses over the wolffian duct and lies medial to it. Finally, the two müllerian ducts fuse into the uterovaginal duct. This elongates caudally to the posterior aspect of the urogenital sinus, forming the müllerian tubercle. The wolffian ducts terminate at either side of this tubercle.

The remaining structures of the male genital system are derived from the urogenital sinus. Its epithelium, which has an endodermal origin, forms the prostate, the urethra, and the bulbourethral and periurethral glands. The primitive urogenital sinus derives from the cloaca, a structure appearing at the end of the first month, consisting of a dilation of the terminal portion of the primitive posterior intestine. The cloaca is closed by the cloacal membrane. In the third week mesenchyme proliferates in the outer aspect of the cloacal membrane to form the cloacal folds and the cloacal eminence. In the sixth week the cloacal folds enlarge to form the genital (or urethral) folds while the cloacal eminence forms the genital tubercle. External to each genital fold another mesenchymal thickening develops into the genital prominences or genital swellings.

In the fifth week a septum forms, dividing the cloaca into two compartments. The anterior compartment is the primitive urogenital sinus, which is covered by the urogenital membrane. The posterior compartment is the anorectal canal, which is covered by the anal membrane. The primitive urogenital sinus then divides into two new compartments: superior and inferior. The superior compartment is the vesical-urethral canal, which later forms the urinary bladder and the urethra. The inferior compartment is the definitive urogenital sinus.

Differentiation of the prostate and external genitalia requires dihydrotestosterone, a hormone derived from testosterone in the target tissues by the action of the enzyme 5 alpha-reductase. Dihydrotestosterone causes the enlargement of the genital tubercle to form the glans penis, the thickening of the genital folds and their fusion to form the penile shaft, the migration of the urethral orifice to the tip of the glans, the fusion of the genital swellings to form the scrotum, and the differentiation of the prostate from the urogenital sinus. The first effects of dihydrotestosterone are observed at approximately the seventieth day and include the fusion of the labioscrotal folds and closure of the middle raphe. The urethral groove is closed at about the seventieth day, and the external genitals are completely developed between the eighteenth and the twentieth weeks. In addition to dihydrotestosterone, further development of the male genital system requires the action of antimüllerian hormone and testosterone (Fig. 10-6).[6] Antimüllerian hormone, secreted by the Sertoli cells, is a glycoprotein polymer consisting of 72 kDa subunits linked by disulfide bonds.[7] It is detected by 56 days and is present throughout the fetal period and after birth, dropping to undetectable levels at the onset of puberty.[8] Antimüllerian hormone causes the involution of the ipsilateral müllerian duct, beginning by 53 to 63 days at the caudal pole and progressing rapidly. Remnants of the müllerian ducts include the appendix testis at the cranial end, and the prostatic utricle at the caudal end. Antimüllerian hormone also stimulates the development of the tunica albuginea, formed by the insertion of mesenchyme between the celomic epithelium and the primordial sex cords, with deposition of collagen fibers in several layers that parallel the testicular surface.

Testosterone is synthesized by the Leydig cells. These cells first appear among the sex cords in the eighth week of gestation and their number increases to 48 million per pair of testes by the thirteenth to sixteenth weeks,[9] at that time occupying about 50% of the testicular volume. The relative number of Leydig cells decreases from the sixteenth week to the twenty-fourth week due to the rapid enlargement of the testis during this period. However, the absolute number of Leydig cells remains constant. From the twenty-fourth week to birth, the number of Leydig cells decreases to 18 million per pair of testes in the newborn. Testosterone synthesis begins after the fifty-sixth day of gestation, but significant levels are detected only after the seventy-first day. Testosterone stimulates differentiation of the ductus epididymidis, ductus deferens, and seminal vesicle.

The actions of these three hormones occur at precise moments in development. Failure in the amount or tim-

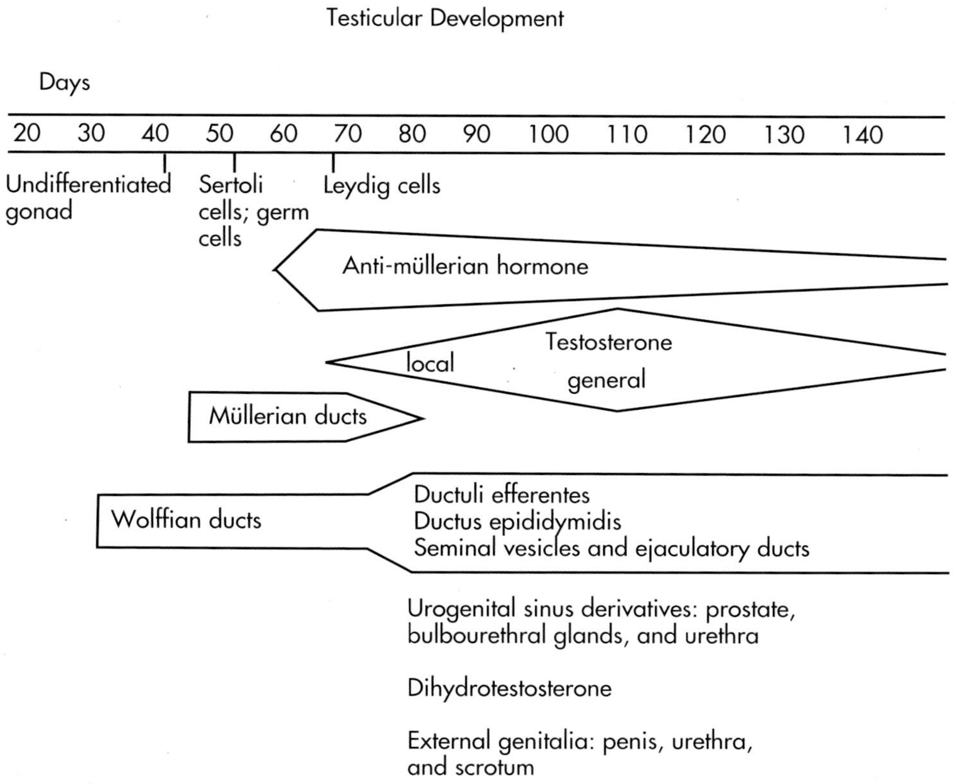

10-6. Development of the genital system during the first months of intrauterine life.

ing of secretion, or in the responsiveness of target tissues causes most malformations in intersex conditions.[10]

TESTICULAR DESCENT

Testicular descent is the result of hormonal and mechanical actions which are not yet completely understood. Three steps are recognized: nephric displacement, transabdominal descent, and inguinal descent. In nephric displacement the gonad detaches from the metanephros in the seventh week. The second step, transabdominal descent, occurs in the twelfth week and consists of the displacement of the testis toward the deep inguinal ring. The third step, inguinal descent, occurs between the seventh month and birth.[11] Clinically the term testicular descent often refers only to this last step, in which the testis passes from the abdominal cavity to the scrotum.

Testicular descent is directed by the gubernaculum testis, which appears in the sixth week as an elongate condensation of mesenchymal cells extending from the genital ridge to the presumptive inguinal region.[12,13] At this level in the abdominal wall, the gubernacular cells persist as simple mesenchyme while the remaining abdominal wall cells differentiate into muscle. These mesenchymal cells give rise to the inguinal canal. Thus, the testis lies on a continuous column of mesenchyme, the plica gubernaculi, which joins the testis to the future scrotal region. The periphery of this mesenchymal tissue is invaded by the processus vaginalis, which develops from persistent simple mesenchyme. Once the inguinal canal and the plica gubernaculi are formed, development slows. In the seventh month, the processus vaginalis undergoes active growth, the cremasteric muscle develops from the mesenchyme outside the processus vaginalis, and the distal end of the gubernaculum enlarges markedly. Gubernacular enlargement is caused by both hyperplasia and hypertrophy, together with the absorption of a great volume of water by the glycosaminoglycans of the matrix.[14] The tissue is reminiscent of Wharton's jelly of the umbilical cord. By this time the testis-epididymis complex is pear shaped and its largest component is the gubernaculum. The testis and epididymis slide through the inguinal canal behind the gubernaculum. Simultaneously, development of the processus vaginalis is completed and the gubernaculum begins to shorten, the epididymis develops further, and the testicular blood vessels and ductus deferens lengthen.[15]

Testicular descent is a complex process integrating several essential factors, including normal function of the hypothalamic-pituitary-testicular hormonal axis, and normal development of the abdominal musculature, gubernaculum, and processus vaginalis.[16,17] The critical role of normal hormonal function is supported by clinical and experimental observations: destruction of the hypophysis in laboratory animals impedes testicular descent; anencephalic fetuses usually have undescended testes; many cryptorchid patients have transitory neonatal hypogonadism; and some undescended testes descend after treatment with human chorionic gonadotropin or gonadotropin releasing hormone. Adequate intraabdominal pressure is another requisite.[18,19] In prune belly syndrome, bilateral cryptorchidism is associated with urologic malformations and absence of the abdominal wall musculature. In a variant of this syndrome termed *pseudo–prune belly syndrome,* there is a positive correlation between the development of the abdominal wall musculature and testicular descent.[20] Development of the processus vaginalis also plays a critical role in testicular descent. This structure grows within the gubernaculum; if it is partially replaced by fibrous tissue, the testis will follow other directions in its descent and end in an ectopic location. If fibrous tissue completely replaces the gubernaculum, the processus vaginalis and cremasteric muscle fail to develop fully, and descent of the testis is mechanically blocked.[20]

The hormonal requirements for testicular descent are not clear.[21] It was assumed that antimüllerian hormone is required for transabdominal descent; male pseudohermaphrodites with müllerian remnants have undescended testes and antimüllerian hormone levels are low in infants with cryptorchid testes.[22] However, female rabbits immunized against antimüllerian hormone had male offspring with persistent müllerian structures but without cryptorchidism.[23] In the absence of antimüllerian hormone, male mice developed descended testes.[24] Androgens are involved in inguinal descent, although the target of androgen action is yet uncertain.[23]

Testosterone secretion peaks in the fourteenth week of gestation and then decreases slowly during the remainder of fetal life. Its secretion is influenced by other hormones, including human chorionic gonadotropin and luteinizing hormone. The former passes to the fetus from the mother in a ratio of 1:30, and fetal production is proportional to the number of Leydig cells. Chorionic gonadotropin–dependent testosterone secretion plays an important role in genital differentiation; enzymatic deficiency in androgen synthesis results in incomplete virilization and cryptorchidism. Luteinizing hormone appears after the tenth week and peaks in the eighteenth week, declining slowly thereafter until birth. Luteinizing hormone appears to be necessary for androgen secretion in the second half of fetal life, accounting for the association of cryptorchid testes and normally virilized external genitalia in anencephalic fetuses.

An influence of androgens on the gubernaculum, which possess a low content of androgen receptors,[25] has been proposed.[26,27] Serum testosterone levels increase before the rapid development of the gubernaculum and testicular descent occur. Cryptorchidism is more frequent in children with deficient gonadotropin secretion or impaired androgen function. In contrast, with complete testicular feminization syndrome about 10% of children have testicular descent and 75% of testes are in the inguinal canal. In addition, antiandrogens only impede testicular descent in 50% of cases.[28] Androgens might also act indirectly by the influence of a calcitonin-gene related peptide (CGRP),[29] a neuromuscular transmitter that causes neuronal masculinization in the spinal nucleus of the genito-femoral nerve and would guide the gubernaculum toward the scrotum. However, several features contradict this opinion: CGRP alone is not sufficient to induce testicular descent in mice; CGRP liberation is not increased by androgens; and, more importantly, the human gubernaculum is devoid of muscle cells.[30] At present, major attention is addressed to descendin, an androgen-independent testicular paracrine factor that seems to initiate the enlargement of the gubernaculum for testicular descent.[31]

After birth, the gubernaculum and the processus vaginalis regress. The gubernaculum is replaced by fibrous tissue which forms the scrotal ligament. The cephalic segment of the processus vaginalis atrophies after testicular descent. An exaggerated resorption of the processus vaginalis with pulling up of the testis could induce a testis that has descended normally to ascend and become cryptorchid.[32]

PREPUBERTAL TESTIS

The testis is a dynamic structure from birth to puberty, an important consideration in interpreting biopsies from children. All testicular components undergo waves of proliferation and differentiation prior to puberty.[33] The three waves of germ cell proliferation occur in the neonatal period, in infancy, and at puberty.[34] The last gives rise to complete spermatogenesis. There also are three waves of Leydig cell proliferation (fetal, neonatal, and pubertal); the last corresponds to the pubertal wave of germ cell proliferation.

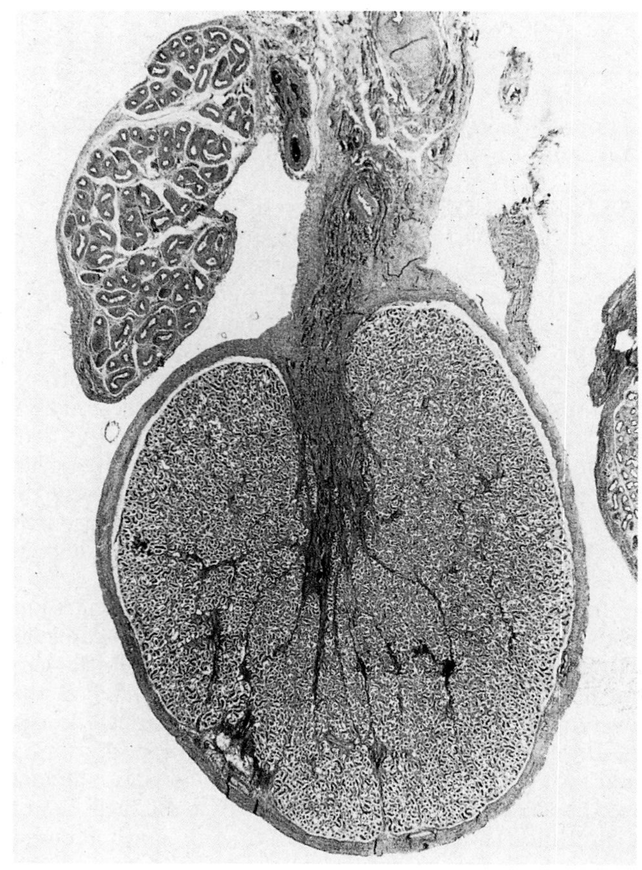

10-7. Intratesticular septa divide the testis into testicular lobules converging in the mediastinum testis.

DEVELOPMENT OF TESTIS FROM BIRTH TO PUBERTY

The testis at birth

The newborn testis is covered by a thin tunica albuginea from which the intratesticular septa arise. These divide the testis into lobules containing the seminiferous tubules and testicular interstitium (Fig. 10-7). The seminiferous tubules are 60 to 65 μm in diameter and are filled with Sertoli cells and germ cells, with no apparent lumen. Sertoli cells are the most abundant, with 26 to 28 cells per tubular profile (Fig. 10-8).[35] They form a pseudostratified epithelium and have elongate to ovoid nuclei with darker chromatin than that of mature Sertoli cells and one or two small peripheral nucleoli. The cytoplasm contains abundant rough endoplasmic reticulum and Golgi complexes. No specialized intercellular junctions appear between Sertoli cells but desmosome-like junctions are present between Sertoli cells and germ cells.[36]

Two types of germ cells are present at birth: gonocytes and spermatogonia. Gonocytes are usually located near the centers of the tubules, with voluminous nuclei and large central nucleoli.[35] Spermatogonia are mainly located on the basal lamina, with smaller nuclei and less cytoplasm than gonocytes; the nucleoli are peripheral and very small. At birth most spermatogonia correspond to the adult type A (see discussion on the adult testis in this chapter) (Fig. 10-9).

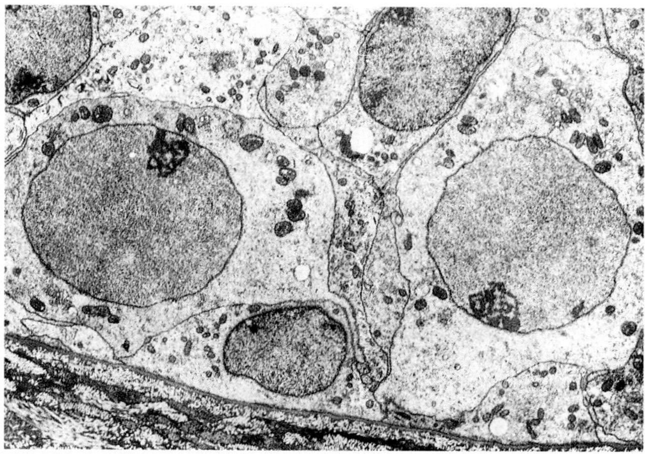

10-9. Spermatogonia have abundant cytoplasm with regular nuclei with eccentric nucleoli. The cytoplasm contains mitochondria joined by electron-dense bars.

10-8. The seminiferous tubules contain two types of germ cells, gonocytes and spermatogonia. The gonocytes have large nuclei with large, central nucleoli. The spermatogonia have smaller nuclei and pale cytoplasm. Leydig cells are present in the interstitium.

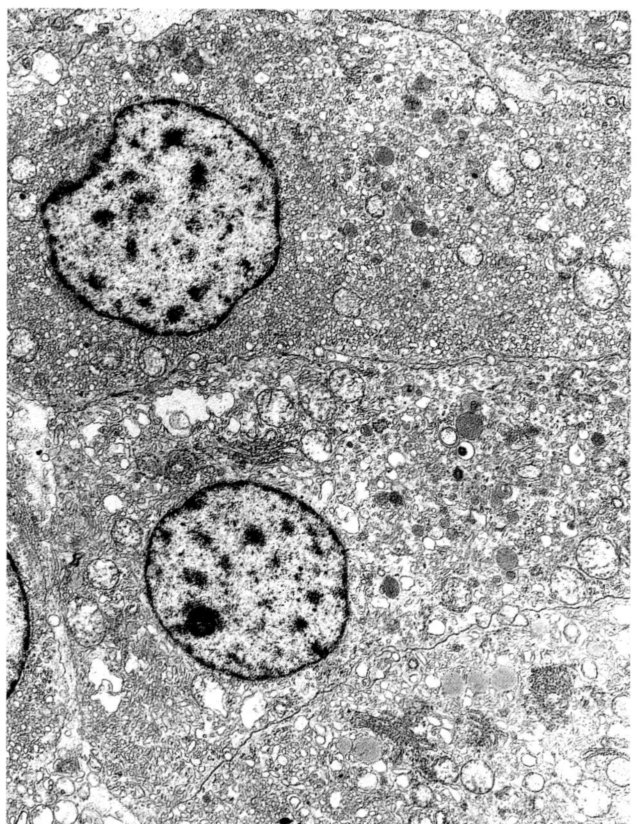

10-10. Leydig cells have eccentric, round nuclei; abundant smooth endoplasmic reticulum and mitochondria; lysosomes; and stacks of rough endoplasmic reticulum cisternae.

The testicular interstitium contains fetal Leydig cells, which resemble adult Leydig cells but lack Reinke's crystalloids (Fig. 10-10).[37,38] Additionally, mast cells, macrophages, and foci of hematopoietic cells are present.[39]

The first wave of testicular development occurs during the neonatal period and involves germ cells and Leydig cells. These changes are caused by a significant increase in secretion of both follicle stimulating hormone and luteinizing hormone during the third postnatal month.[40-42] Testicular weight and volume increase. Luteinizing hormone stimulates the Leydig cells to produce testosterone,[37,43] which stimulates the transformation of gonocytes to spermatogonia of the Ad type. Afterward, some of these divide to form Ap spermatogonia (see discussion on the adult testis in this chapter). Six months after birth, no gonocytes are present.

The testis in infancy

From the sixth month to approximately the second half of the third year of life, the testis is in a resting period, which is broken by the beginning of the second wave of germ cell proliferation.[44] The number of Ap spermatogonia increases and B spermatogonia (derived from Ap spermatogonia) are observed (Fig. 10-11). In some normal testes of this age, meiotic primary spermatocytes and round spermatids are observed. This spermatogenic attempt fails and many degenerated germ cells may be observed in this period.[45,46]

The cause of this second wave of germ cell proliferation is unknown; there is no elevation of follicle stimulating hormone or luteinizing hormone levels between 6 months and 10 years of life. After the sixth year there is a slight increase in adrenal androgens, but testicular testosterone levels increase only after the tenth year.[47,48] By the third year most Leydig cells have degenerated. From about 18 million Leydig cells at birth, only 60,000 remain in 6-year-old boys. At this age testosterone levels are similar to those of girls,[47] and most androgens are of adrenal origin.

The testis in childhood

At about 9 years, the third and definitive wave of spermatogenesis begins,[49,50] coinciding with a significant elevation of luteinizing hormone. This is followed by a further major increase in the levels of this hormone

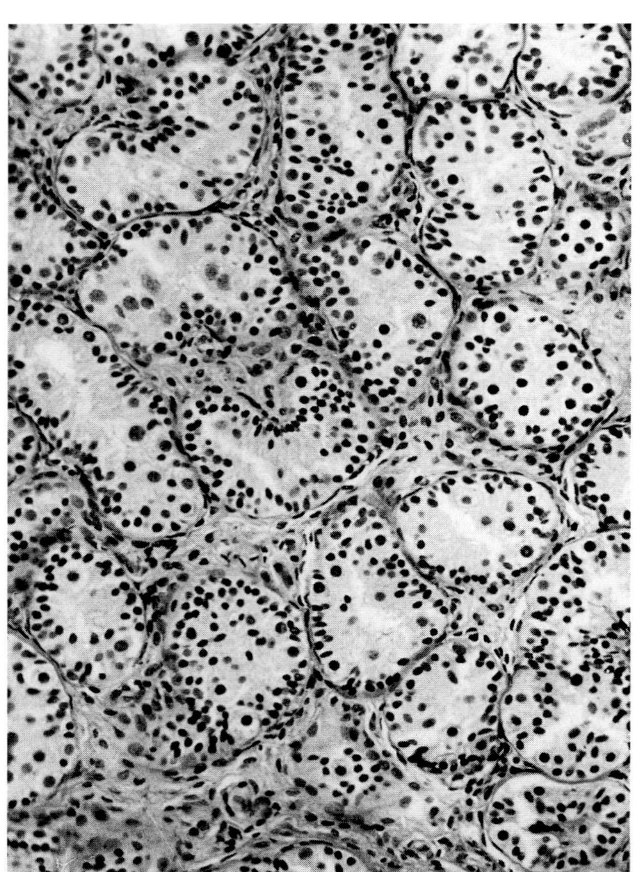

10-11. Testis from a 4-year-old boy. Each seminiferous tubule profile shows at least one spermatogonium. Primary spermatocytes can be seen in the centers of some tubules.

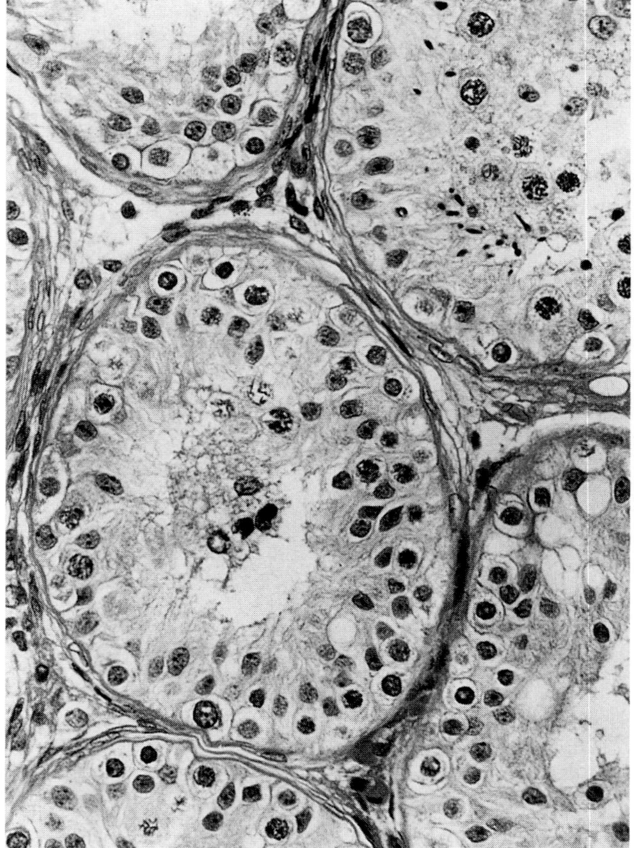

10-12. Testis from an 11-year-old boy. Germ cell development varies from tubule to tubule. The number of spermatogonia is less than that in adulthood. Residual immature Sertoli cells contain elongated nuclei with small nucleoli. Leydig cells are scant.

between 13 and 15 years of age. Luteinizing hormone induces fibroblast-like Leydig cell precursors to differentiate into mature Leydig cells.[51] By the end of puberty the population of Leydig cells per testis has risen to about 786 million.[52] Leydig cells secrete androgens, which, together with the rise in follicle stimulating hormone between 11 and 14 years of age, cause Sertoli cell maturation, germ cell development, and the appearance of tubular lumens[36] (Fig. 10-12), increasing the size of the testes between the ages of 11½ and 12½.[53-55] At 13½ years, before the testis reaches adult size, spermatozoa are present, secondary sex characteristics are completely developed, and the epiphyses close.[56-59]

INTERPRETATION OF TESTICULAR BIOPSY FROM PREPUBERTAL TESTES

Testicular biopsy is useful for diagnosing patients with ambiguous genitalia, a history of leukemia or lymphoma whose testes underwent rapid enlargement, or precocious testicular maturation of unknown cause. In other situations the value of testicular biopsy is less established. For example, the value of biopsy of cryptorchid testes during orchiopexy is controversial. Evaluation of biopsies of prepubertal testes should involve assessment of several features, including mean tubular diameter, and the number of germ cells, Sertoli cells, and Leydig cells per tubular profile, per unit area or unit volume, or per testis.

Mean tubular diameter

The mean tubular diameter is an excellent indicator of the development of the seminiferous epithelium. In the prepubertal testis it depends principally on the Sertoli cells and thus indicates whether they are adequately stimulated by follicle stimulating hormone and responsive to this stimulus. Tubular diameter varies throughout childhood, being smallest in the fourth year of life, slowly enlarging up to 9 years of age, and rapidly enlarging thereafter up to 15 years (Fig. 10-13).

The most frequent abnormality in the prepubertal testes is a low mean tubular diameter. This is seen in undescended testes as well as in hypogonadotropic or hypergonadotropic hypogonadism. In the latter the lesion is due to anomalous Sertoli cell responsiveness to follicle stimulating hormone.[60]

There are three levels of severity of low tubular diameter: slight tubular hypoplasia (up to 10% reduction relative to the diameter normal for the age), marked tubular hypoplasia (from 10% to 30% reduction), and severe tubular hypoplasia (more than 30% reduction). In many biopsies, giant malformed tubules, referred to as *megatubules* or *ring-shaped tubules*, are found. This histological appearance results from dense packing of helical tubules. Such tubules usually contain eosinophilic bodies or microliths. The presence of megatubules suggests the child will be infertile as an adult.

Germ cell number

Germ cells may be counted by several methods. The most common is calculation of the tubular fertility index, which is the mean number of germ cells per tubular profile. The number of germ cells per tubular profile is calculated by counting the germ cells in a light microscopic field and dividing this by the number of tubular profiles in the same field. In the first 6 months of postnatal life the normal testis has four germ cells per tubular profile. The tubular fertility index reflects the percentage of tubular profiles containing germ cells. In newborns, 68% of tubular profiles contain at least one germ cell. From birth to 3 years this decreases to 50%, followed by a progressive increase to 100% at puberty.[44] If the numbers of gonocytes and spermatogonia are calculated separately, it is possible to know when the transformation of gonocytes into spermatogonia occurs. A more complete measure of germ cell number is calculation of the total germ cell number per testis. This is more difficult because it requires morphometric assessment of intratubular volume and careful clinical measurement of the three axes of the testis.

Three levels of severity of germinal hypoplasia are recognized: slight (tubular fertility index higher than 50), marked (tubular fertility index between 50 and 30), and severe (tubular fertility index less than 30) (see Fig. 10-13). Marked and severe germinal hypoplasia are usually associated with marked or severe tubular hypoplasia, in most cases resulting from tubular dysgenesis. It also is useful to determine whether the seminiferous tubules devoid of germ cells are randomly distributed. If they are grouped, they are probably from the same lobule or group of lobules which never will develop normally.

Sertoli cell number

The number of Sertoli cells per tubular profile varies during childhood as a result of very slow Sertoli cell proliferation from 4 years to 12 years[35] and the redistribution of Sertoli cells as the seminiferous tubules become longer and broader. The pseudostratified pattern characteristic of Sertoli cells at birth changes slowly to a columnar pattern at puberty (see Fig. 10-13). Testicular biopsies may reveal hypoplasia or hyperplasia of Sertoli cells; hyperplasia is usually pronounced and a sign of tubular dysgenesis, often detected during the first year of life and/or the beginning of puberty.[60]

Leydig cell number

Calculation of Leydig cell number during infancy is difficult due to the scant population at this age.[51] Semithin sections or immunohistochemistry to detect cells containing testosterone may be helpful.[52] Selection of the appropriate denominator to express Leydig cell population is another problem. The most frequent measures are Leydig cell number per tubular profile, per unit area, or total number per testis.[53]

Low numbers of Leydig cells are observed in undescended testes, hypogonadotropic hypogonadism, some variants of male pseudohermaphroditism, and in anencephalic fetuses. High numbers of Leydig cells occur in congenital Leydig cell hyperplasia,[61] triploid fetuses,[62] variants of precocious puberty, and several syndromes such as leprechaunism and Beckwith-Wiedemann syndrome.

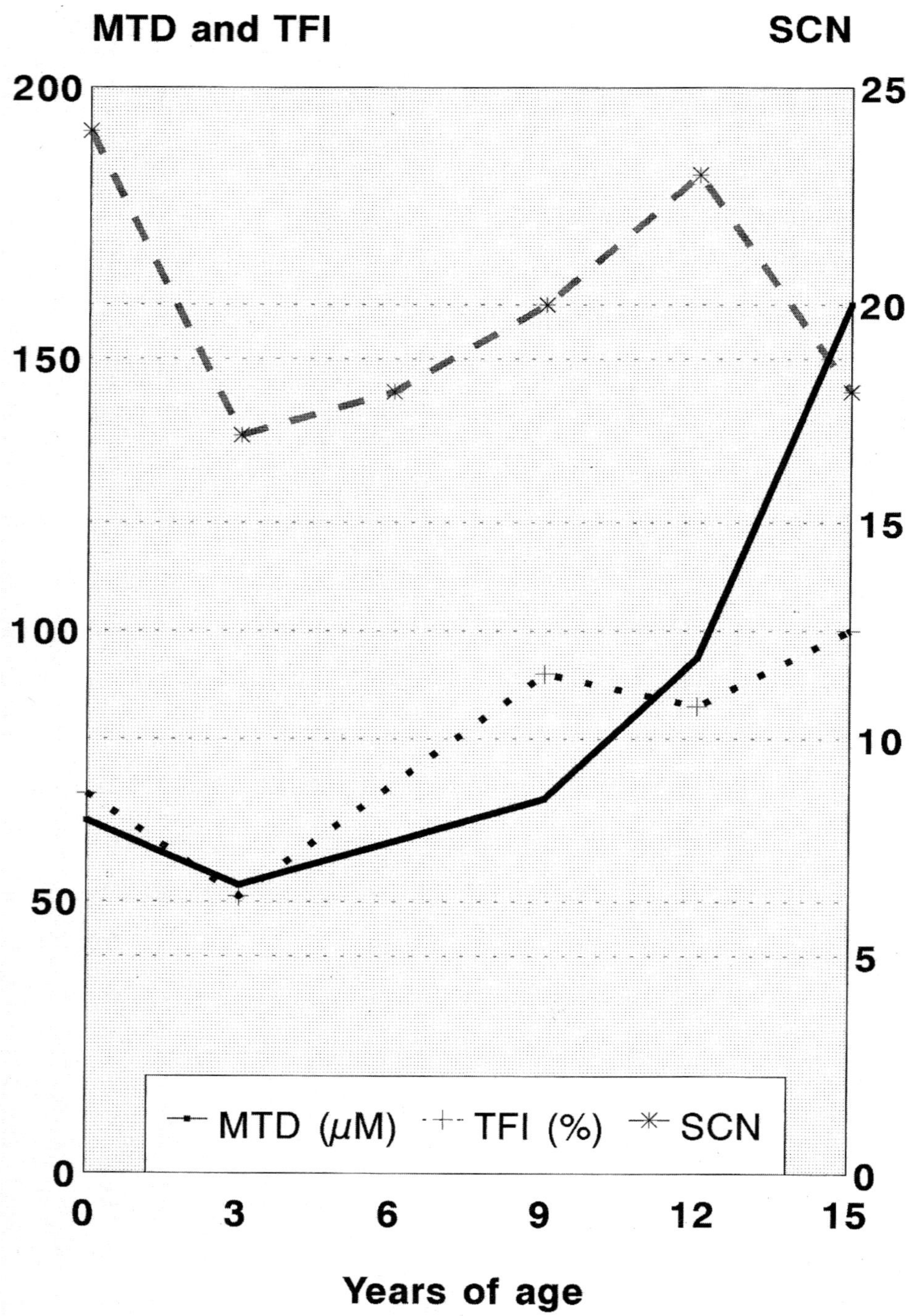

10-13. Changes in the mean tubular diameter (MTD), tubular fertility index (TFI), and Sertoli cell number per tubular profile (SCN) from birth to puberty.

ADULT TESTIS

ANATOMY

The adult testis is an egg-shaped organ that hangs in the scrotum from the spermatic cord, the retroepididymal surface, and the scrotal ligament. The mean weights in caucasian men are 21.6 ± 0.4 g for the right testis, and 20 ± 0.4 g for the left. The mean testicular diameters are 4.6 cm (range, 3.6 to 5.5 cm) for the longest axis and 2.6 cm (range, 2.1 to 3.2 cm) for the shortest axis.[63-66]

SUPPORTING STRUCTURES

The tunica albuginea and the interlobular septa make up the connective tissue framework of the testis. The tunica albuginea consists of three connective tissue lay-

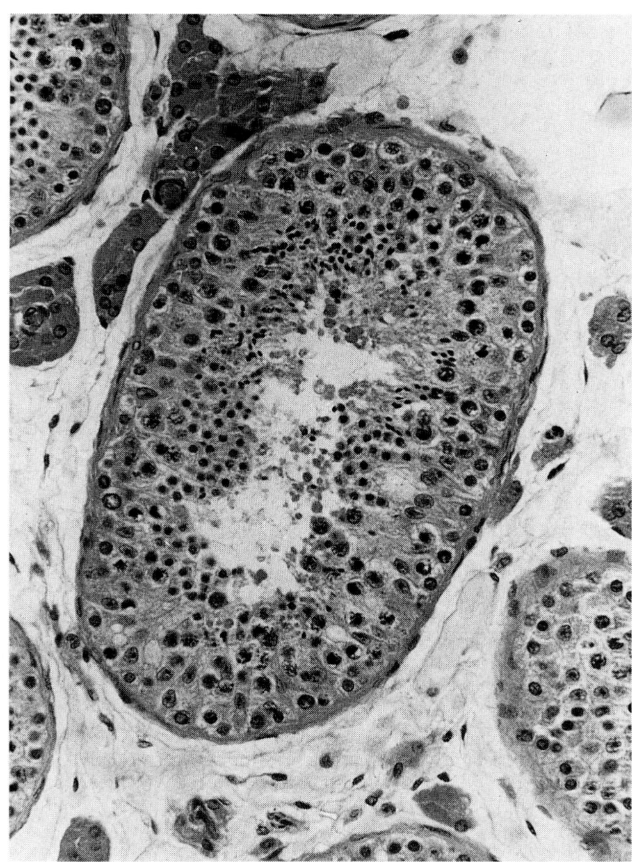

10-14. Seminiferous tubule with complete spermatogenesis.

ers, and its outer surface is covered by mesothelium. From the outer to the inner layers, the amount of collagen fibers decreases while the cellularity increases. The fibers and cells in the two outermost layers form planes parallel to the testicular surface. The cells include fibroblasts, myofibroblasts, and mast cells. The myofibroblasts are more numerous in the posterior of the testis. The thickness of the tunica albuginea increases with age from 400 to 450 µm in young men to more than 900 µm in elderly men.[67] It acts as a semipermeable membrane which is important in regulating testicular volume. The innermost layer, the tunica vasculosa, consists of cellular connective tissue containing blood and lymphatic vessels. The interlobular septa consist of fibrous connective tissue containing blood vessels supplying the testicular parenchyma. The interlobular septa divide the testis into approximately 250 pyramidal lobules with their bases at the tunica albuginea and vertices at the mediastinum testis. Each lobule contains two to four seminiferous tubules and numerous Leydig cells.[68]

SEMINIFEROUS TUBULES

Adult seminiferous tubules are 180 to 200 µm in diameter and about 540 m long (range, 299 to 981 m).[69] They are highly convoluted and tightly packed within the lobules. The tubular lining of germ cells and Sertoli cells is surrounded by a lamina propria (tunica propria) (Fig. 10-14).

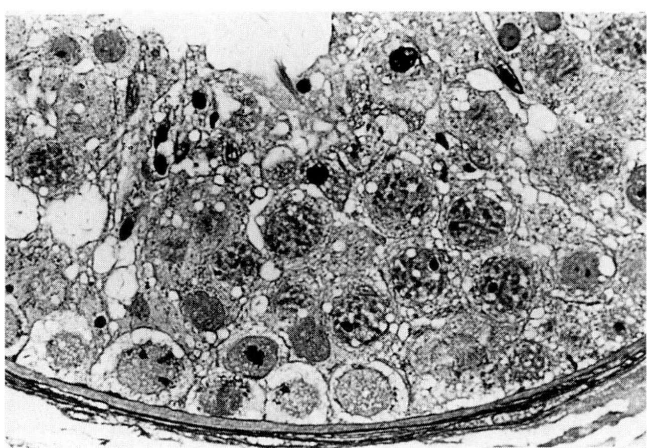

10-15. Germ cell development progresses from the basal lamina toward the lumen of the tubule. Each germ cell type forms a different layer in the seminiferous epithelium and may be identified by its nuclei. Spermatogonia are basal cells with pale cytoplasm, round nuclei, and eccentric nucleoli. Above these cells, the Sertoli cell nuclei can be recognized by their large central nucleoli. The inner layers consist of primary spermatocytes with the chromatin pattern characteristic of meiosis. Near the top are young spermatids with round nuclei and maturing spermatids with elongate, dark nuclei.

Sertoli cells

Sertoli cells are columnar cells that extend from the basal lamina to the tubular lumen with 10 to 12 cells per tubular profile. They are easily identified by their nuclear characteristics. The nucleus is located near the basal lamina and has a triangular shape with indented outline, pale chromatin, and a large central nucleolus (Fig. 10-15). Charcot-Böttcher crystals and lipid droplets often are visible in the cytoplasm.[70-73]

Ultrastructurally, Sertoli cells have characteristic nucleoli, plasma membranes, and cytoplasmic components. The nucleolus has a tripartite structure with a round fibrillar center, a compact granular portion, and a three-dimensional net composed of intermingled fibrillar and granular portions.[74-76] The plasma membrane has two types of intercellular junctions which are developed at puberty: junctions between adjacent Sertoli cells and Sertoli cell–germ cell junctions.[77] The inter-Sertoli cell junctions are tight-junction complexes which are the morphologic basis for the blood-testis barrier and divide the seminiferous epithelium into the basal compartment (which contains spermatogonia and newly formed primary spermatocytes) and the adluminal compartment (which contains primary spermatocytes, secondary spermatocytes, and spermatids). These junctions permit each compartment to have its own microenvironment for spermatogenic development.[78-80] The Sertoli cell–germ cell junctions persist from the primary spermatocyte stage through spermatozoon release. Recent studies using freeze-fracture techniques indicate that these desmosome and gap-type junctions are morphologically similar to desmosomes but with points of occlusion between adjacent membranes. These junctions have also occasionally been observed with spermatogonia.[81]

TABLE 10-1.
SERTOLI CELL–LEYDIG CELL REGULATORY INTERACTIONS

Paracrine Factor	Origin	Receptor	Action
Androgens	Leydig cell	Sertoli cell	Regulate-maintain function and differentiation
POMC peptides	Leydig cell	Sertoli cell	Decrease FSH actions
ß endorphin	Leydig cell	Sertoli cell	Decrease steroidogenesis
Gn-RH-like factor	Sertoli cell	Leydig cell	Decrease steroidogenesis
estrogens	Sertoli cell	Leydig cell	Decrease steroidogenesis
TGFα	Sertoli cell	Leydig cell	Decrease steroidogenesis
IL-1	Sertoli cell	Leydig cell	Decrease steroidogenesis
IGF-1	Sertoli cell	Leydig cell	Increase steroidogenesis
Inhibin	Sertoli cell	Leydig cell	Increase steroidogenesis

POMC, proopiomelanocortin; Gn-RH, gonadotropin-releasing hormone; TGF, transforming growth factor; IL-1, interleukin 1; IGF-1, insulin-like growth factor 1; FSH, follicle stimulating hormone.

Sertoli cell cytoplasm contains abundant smooth endoplasmic reticulum, elongate mitochondria, annulate lamellae, lysosomes, residual bodies, glycogen granules, microtubules, vimentin filaments around the nucleus,[82] actin filaments in the ectoplasmic specializations that surround germ cells,[83] lipid droplets in amounts that vary with the seminiferous epithelium cycle,[84] and Charcot-Böttcher crystals (structures several microns long, formed of multiple, parallel lamina of protein) and scant, rough endoplasmic reticulum and ribosomes.[85]

The number of Sertoli cells decreases with age from about 250 million per testis in young men to 125 million in men older than 50 years.[86,87] There is a positive correlation between the number of Sertoli cells and daily sperm production.[88] Sertoli cells synthesize factors that stimulate the proliferation and maturation of germ cells; regulate the function of other cells, such as Leydig cells (Table 10-1) and peritubular cells[89]; contribute to hormonal regulation (inhibin secretion); and form the tubular fluid. Sertoli cells also secrete various proteins into the tubular lumen which become parts of the tubular fluid (Table 10-2). These include androgen binding protein, which is reabsorbed by the epididymal epithelium; transferrin, which transports iron necessary for mitochondrial cytochromes of spermatocytes and other germ cells of the adluminal compartment[90]; ceruloplasmin, which transports copper necessary for coenzymes and ferroxidase; and sulfated glycoprotein 1, which transports sphingolipids. Other proteins, such as folate binding protein and biotin binding protein, are involved in the transport of Sertoli cell secretions.

Germ cell proliferation produces a continuous displacement of differentiating germ cells toward the tubular lumen. This movement leads to changes in the configuration of the Sertoli cell cytoplasm and intercellular junctions, requiring the synthesis of plasminogen activator and other proteases by Sertoli cells.[91] Sertoli cells also have an endocrine function, secreting inhibin. Sertoli cells stimulate the proliferation and differentiation of other testicular

TABLE 10-2.
MAJOR SERTOLI CELL SECRETORY PRODUCTS

Products	Functions and/or Characteristics
Transport binding proteins	
Androgen binding protein	Androgen transport
Transferrin	Iron transport
Ceruloplasmin	Copper transport
Sulfated glycoprotein 1	Sphingolipid binding
Regulatory proteins	
Inhibin	Endocrine-paracrine agent
Müllerian duct inhibitory agent	Development
Sulfated glycoprotein 2	Sperm coating immunosuppressant
Growth factors	
TGFα	Growth stimulation
TGFß	Growth inhibition
IGF-1	Maintenance growth differentiation
IL-1	Growth regulation
Metabolites	
Lactate-pyruvate	Energy metabolites
Estrogens	Steroid hormone endocrine paracrine
Proteases/inhibitors	
Plasminogen activator	Plasminogen activation
Cyclic protein 2	Cathepsin activity
α_2 macroglobulin	Protease inhibitor
Extracellular matrix components	
Laminin	
Collagens IV and I	
Proteoglycans	

TGF, Transforming growth factor; IGF-1, insulin-like growth factor 1; IL-1, interleukin 1.

cells by secretion of paracrine factors and local trophic agents. The best known of these is insulin-like growth factor 1, which stimulates meiosis. Sertoli cells also secrete seminiferous growth factor, Sertoli cell–secreted growth factor, transforming growth factors alpha and beta, interleukin 1,[92] and insulin-like growth factor 2. The proliferation of germ cells seems to be stimulated by interleukin 1 while insulin-like growth factor 2 promotes the metabolism of these cells. In addition, Sertoli cells possess receptors for several factors such as nerve growth factor, which is produced by spermatocytes and young spermatids, underscoring the complexity of the Sertoli cell–germ cell relationship. Sertoli cells also produce several components of the wall of the seminiferous tubule, including laminin, type IV collagen, and heparin sulfate-rich proteoglycans.

Germ cells

The germ cells of the adult testis include spermatogonia, primary and secondary spermatocytes, and spermatids (see Fig. 10-15).

Spermatogonia. There are two types of spermatogonia: A and B. Type A spermatogonia are about 12 μm in diameter, rest on the basal lamina, and are surrounded by the cytoplasm of adjacent Sertoli cells. The nuclei of type A spermatogonia are spherical, contain several peripheral nucleoli, and have four different patterns: Ad (dark), Ap (pale), Al (long), and Ac (cloudy).[93,94] The cytoplasm of these spermatogonia contains a moderate amount of ribosomes, small ovoid mitochondria joined by electron-dense bars, and Lubarsch's crystals. Lubarsch's crystals are several microns long and are composed of numerous 8 to 15 nm parallel filaments intermingled with ribosome-like granules.

Ad spermatogonia are thought to be the stem cells in spermatogenesis. Some of them replicate their DNA and, during replication, acquire the Al pattern. Afterward, they divide to make another Ad (maintaining the stem cell reservoir) and an Ap spermatogonium. During their replication, Ap spermatagonia become Ac spermatagonia and then divide to form two type B spermatagonia.[95-97]

Type B spermatogonia are the most numerous and their contact with the basal lamina is less extensive than that of type A spermatogonia. Their nuclei usually are more distant from the basal lamina than those of type A spermatogonia and contain one or two large central nucleoli. Their cytoplasm contains more ribosomes than type A spermatogonia and intermitochondrial bars are usually not observed. Type B spermatogonia divide to form primary spermatocytes.

Primary spermatocytes. Interphase primary spermatocytes lose contact with the basal lamina and inhabit cavities formed by the Sertoli cell cytoplasm. Their cytoplasm contains more rough endoplasmic reticulum than that of spermatogonia, and the Golgi complex is more developed.[98] Meiotic primary spermatocytes are readily identified by their chromatin pattern. The leptotene spermatocyte, with filamentous chromatin, leaves the basal compartment, migrates to an intermediate compartment, and then to the adluminal compartment. In the zygotene spermatocyte the chromosomes are shorter and pairing of homologous chromosomes begins. Ultrastructural studies show coarse chromatin masses in which synaptonemal complexes and sex pairs may be observed. The nucleolus acquires a peculiar appearance with segregation of the fibrillar and granular portions. Associated with the nucleolus is the round body, which contains proteins but no nucleic acids.[75] In pachytene spermatocytes the homologous chromosomes are completely paired, and by electron microscopy the chromatin masses appear larger and less numerous than in zygotene spermatocytes. In diplotene spermatocytes the paired homologous chromosomes begin to separate and remain joined by the points of interchange (chiasmata); neither synaptonemal complexes nor sex pairs are observed. The diakinesis spermatocyte shows maximal chromosome shortening and the chiasmata begin to resolve by displacement toward the chromosomal ends. The nuclear envelope and the nucleolus disintegrate. The spermatocyte completes the other phases of the first meiotic division (metaphase, anaphase, and telophase) forming two secondary spermatocytes; the first meiotic division lasts 24 days.[99]

Secondary spermatocytes are haploid cells, smaller than primary spermatocytes, and show coarse chromatin granules and abundant rough endoplasmic reticulum cisternae.[100] These cells rapidly undergo the second meiotic division and within 8 hours give rise to two spermatids. The newly formed spermatids differ from secondary spermatocytes, having smaller nuclei with homogeneously distributed chromatin.

Spermiogenesis. The transformation of spermatids into spermatozoa is called *spermiogenesis*. During this process pronounced changes occur in the nucleus and cytoplasm.[101] The nucleus becomes progressively darker and elongate.[102] The cytoplasm develops the acrosome and flagellum,[103] the mitochondria cluster around the first portion of the spermatozoon tail, and the remaining cytoplasm is phagocytosed by Sertoli cells.[104,105] By electron microscopy there are four transient stages of spermatid development: Golgi, cap, acrosome, and maturation. These correspond to those defined by light microscopy of nuclear morphology: Sa, Sb, Sb_1, Sb_2, Sc, Sd_1, and Sd_2.[106,107] These phases may be grouped as early (or round) spermatids, which comprise the stages with round nuclei (Sa and Sb), and as late (or elongate) spermatids, which comprise the stages with elongate nuclei (Sc and Sd). Mature spermatids (Sd_2) are the spermatozoa that are released into the tubular lumen (spermiation). All the germ cells derived from the same stem cell remain interconnected by cytoplasmic bridges that ensure synchronous maturation during the spermatogenic process.[108]

Cycle of seminiferous epithelium. At first glance the arrangement of the germ cells in the seminiferous tubules appears disorderly. However, closer study reveals that these cells are grouped into six successive associations, designated I to VI. In contrast with other mammals, in humans the volume occupied by each association is small, so that several associations may be observed in the same tubular profile. Stereological studies have shown that the successive associations are organized helically along the length of the seminiferous tubule.[73,109,110] Each association persists for a specific number of days (I, 4.8 days; II, 3.1 days; III, 1 day; IV, 1.2 days; V, 5 days; and

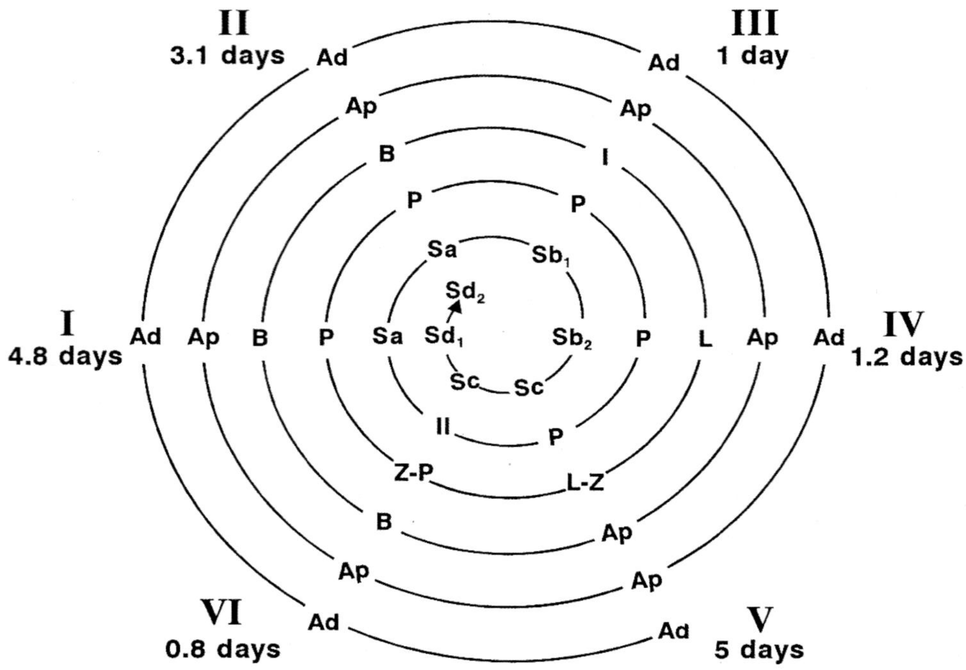

10-16. The six different germ cell associations of the seminiferous epithelium and the sequence of spermatogenesis. Completion of spermatogenesis requires more than four cycles and lasts for approximately 74 days. Each association is indicated by Roman numerals with its corresponding duration. Ad: dark type of A spermatogonia; Ap: pale type of a spermatogonia; B: B spermatogonia; I: interphase primary spermatocyte; L: leptotene primary spermatocyte; Z: zygotene primary spermatocyte; P: pachytene primary spermatocyte; II: secondary spermatocyte (only in stage VI). S_a, S_{b1}, S_{b2}, S_c, S_{d1}, and S_{d2} represent the progressive stages of spermatid differentiation into spermatozoa.

VI, 0.8 days). Each association successively transforms into the following one. Finally, at the end of association VI, the cycle is repeated, to complete the spermatogenic process which requires 4.6 cycles.[111] Because each cycle lasts 15.9 days, the transformation of spermatogonium into spermatozoon takes 74 days (Fig. 10-16).

Tunica propria

The seminiferous tubule is surrounded by a 6 µm lamina propria (tunica propria) consisting of a basal lamina, myofibroblasts, fibroblasts, collagen and elastic fibers, and extracellular matrix.[112,113]

The basal lamina is the inner layer in contact with the seminiferous epithelium and contains laminin and type IV collagen synthesized by the Sertoli cells. External to the basal lamina, there are five to seven layers of flattened, elongate, peritubular cells which have important secretory functions (Table 10-3).[114] The cells forming the three to five innermost layers are myofibroblasts containing numerous actin, myosin, and desmin filaments. These cells play an important role in the rhythmic tubular contractions that propel the spermatozoa toward the rete testis.[115,116] The two outermost cell layers consist of fibroblasts without desmin filaments and with less actin and myosin than the myofibroblasts.

Collagen fibers are present among the peritubular cells and are abundant between the basal lamina and the peritubular cells. Elastic fibers are mainly located at the periphery of peritubular cells. Since elastic fibers appear

TABLE 10-3.
MAJOR PERITUBULAR CELL SECRETORY PRODUCTS

Products	Functions
P-mod-S	Paracrine regulatory agent
Plasminogen activator inhibitor	Inhibition of plasminogen activator activity
Fibronectin	Extracellular matrix component
Collagen I	Extracellular matrix component
Proteoglycans	Extracellular matrix component
TGFα	Growth stimulation/EGF-like
TGFß	Growth inhibition
IGF-1	Maintenance growth differentiation

TGF, Transforming growth factor; IGF-1, insulin-like growth factor 1; EGF, epidermal growth factor.

at puberty, their absence in adults is a sign of tubular immaturity or dysgenesis.[117] The extracellular matrix contains proteoglycans and fibronectin. In addition, the tubular wall contains capillaries and Leydig cells. These are very similar to the interstitial Leydig cells and are named *peritubular Leydig cells*. Seminiferous tubules undergo contraction in vitro when treated with noradrenaline or acetylcholine. Conversely, isoproterenol

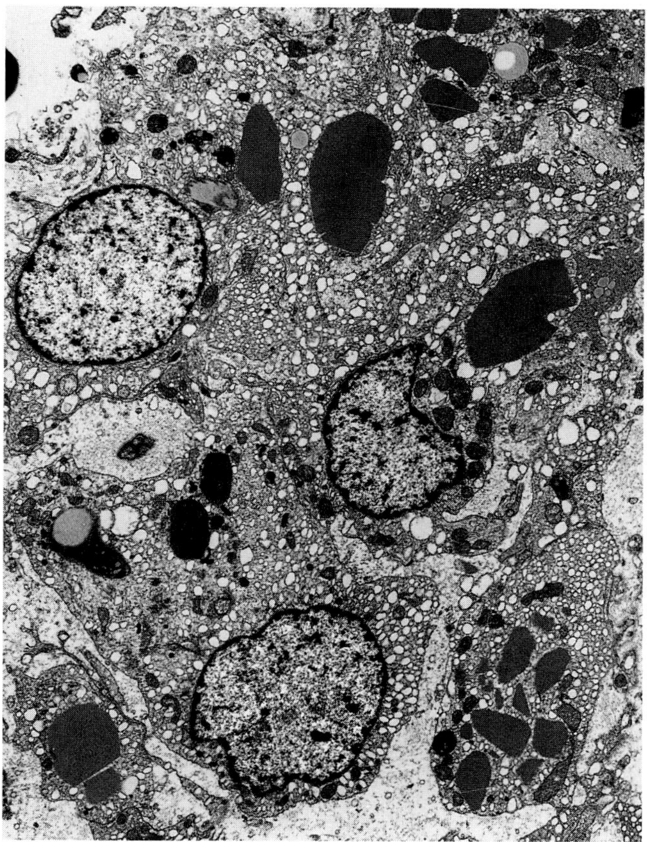

10-17. Leydig cells with round nuclei, abundant smooth endoplasmic reticulum, and Reinke's crystalloids.

causes relaxation of the tubular wall. These findings indicate that the myofibroblasts contain alpha and beta adrenergic and muscarinic receptors.[118]

TESTICULAR INTERSTITIUM

The interstitium between the seminiferous tubules contains Leydig cells, macrophages, mast cells, blood vessels, lymphatic vessels, and nerves, accounting for 25% to 40% of testicular volume.[119]

Leydig cells

Leydig cells are distributed singly or in clusters. Most are in the testicular interstitium, although they may also be found in the tubular tunica propria, mediastinum testis, tunica albuginea, epididymis, and spermatic cord. Extratesticular Leydig cells are usually seen within or near nerve trunks.[120-122]

Leydig cells have spherical eccentric nuclei with one or two eccentric nucleoli and thick nuclear membranes. Their cytoplasm is abundant, eosinophilic, and contains lipid droplets, lipofuscin granules (residual bodies), and Reinke's crystalloids (Fig. 10-17). Reinke's crystalloids are found only in the Leydig cells of adults and, although long believed to occur exclusively in humans, have also been observed in the wild bush rat. Reinke's crystalloids are up to 20 μm long and 2 to 3 μm wide, consisting of a complicated meshwork of 5 nm filaments with a trigonal lattice arrangement. Depending on the plane of section, three basic aspects of this lattice can be discerned. Frequently, the crystalloids display pale lines, considered to be potential planes of cleavage. The filaments are grouped into 19-nm-wide hexagons visible on cross section. In some areas there are aggregates of electron-dense, rod-shaped structures. Some Leydig cells contain other types of paracrystalline inclusions, the most common of which consists of multiple, parallel-folded lamina.[123]

TABLE 10-4.
MAJOR LEYDIG CELL SECRETORY PRODUCTS

Products	Functions and/or Characteristics
Androgens	Steroid hormone/endocrine paracrine agent
POMC peptides	Opiates/POMC regulatory agents
Inhibin	Endocrine-paracrine regulatory agents
IGF-1	Maintenance growth differentiation

POMC, proopiomelanocortin; IGF-1, insulin-like growth factor 1.

Leydig cells contain abundant, well-developed, smooth endoplasmic reticulum, pleomorphic mitochondria with tubular cristae, lysosomes, and peroxisomes. Leydig cells react with antibodies to S-100 protein and neuron-specific enolase.[124]

The number of Leydig cells per testis decreases with age; the testes of 60-year-old men contain about half as many as those of 20-year-old men.[125-128] Mitotic figures are seen occasionally in normal Leydig cells.[129]

Leydig cells are the target cell of luteinizing hormone, in response to which they produce testosterone and other androgens necessary for maintenance of spermatogenesis and many structures of the male genital tract, as well as other tissues such as bone, muscles, and skin.[130-133] Testosterone acts on the Sertoli cells, either directly[134] or via the P-mod-S factor secreted by the myofibroblasts in the tunica propria.[135-137] Leydig cells also secrete numerous nonsteroidal factors, including oxytocin, which acts on myofibroblasts and stimulates seminiferous tubule contraction; beta endorphin, which inhibits Sertoli cell proliferation and function; and others with less known actions such as angiotensin, proopiomelanocortin, and alpha melanocyte stimulating hormones (Table 10-4). Leydig cells are associated with both cholinergic and adrenergic nerve fibers.[138] Varicosities containing synaptic vesicles in the proximity of Leydig cells and nerve endings in direct contact with Leydig cells have been reported, although the functional significance of this innervation is unknown.[139]

Macrophages and mast cells

Macrophages are a normal component of the testicular interstitium. Their population varies with age, from very low in infancy to increasing in puberty.[140] In adults macrophages often are found beside Leydig cells, suggesting a functional relationship between them. Macrophages secrete factors such as interleukin 1, that stimulate germ cell proliferation. Mast cells are a normal component of the testicular interstitium where they are often found near blood vessels. Their number increases in several diseases.[141]

Blood and lymphatic vessels

The testis is supplied by the testicular artery, which arises from the abdominal aorta. In the spermatic cord, the testicular artery gives rise to two or three branches that obliquely penetrate the tunica albuginea testis and to multiple branches that run along the interlobular septa of the testis.[142] These centripetal arteries lead to the mediastinum testis. Along their course the centripetal arteries give off branches that abruptly reverse direction; these are called *centrifugal arteries*. Both the centripetal and centrifugal arteries develop pronounced spiral architectures at puberty.[143,144] The centrifugal arteries branch farther in the testicular interstitium, giving rise to arterioles and these to capillaries which form intertubular plexuses, some of which are apposed to the tunica propria.[145,146] The mediastinum testis is poorly vascular.

The inner two thirds of the testicular parenchyma is drained by veins that follow the interlobular septa to the mediastinum testis (centripetal veins). The outer third is drained by veins that lead to the tunica albuginea (centrifugal veins). Both centripetal and centrifugal veins join to form the pampiniform plexus, which drains the testis via the spermatic cord.

Lymphatic vessels are poorly developed in the testis and limited to the interlobular septa,[147] where they accompany arterioles and venules. Prelymphatic vessels have been reported in the interstitium and probably drain interstitial fluid into the true interlobular lymphatic vessels.

Nerves

The nerve fibers that form the superior spermatic plexus accompany the testicular artery and, following its branches, enter the testes and give rise to the nerves of the interstitium. Most of the nerve fibers are vasomotor and end in arterioles; others end in the vicinity of or in contact with Leydig cells, or reach the tunica propria and end close to Sertoli cells.[148] Afferent nerve endings form corpuscles similar to those of Meissner and Pacini in the tunica albuginea.

RETE TESTIS

The rete testis is a network of channels and cavities that connect the seminiferous tubules with the efferent ductules. Differences in configuration and size of channels and cavities distinguish the three portions of the rete testis: septal (intralobular), composed of the tubuli recti; mediastinal, composed of a network of interconnected channels; and extratesticular, composed of dilated cavities (up to 3 mm in diameter), termed the *bullae retis*.

The tubuli recti are short tubules (0.5 to 1 mm long) that connect the seminiferous tubules to the mediastinal rete, although some seminiferous tubules may connect directly to the mediastinal rete, principally those in the central region of the testis. The tubuli recti are lined by cuboidal epithelium. There are approximately 1500 tubuli recti (or their analogous seminiferous tubule segments). The tubuli recti in the cranial, central, and anterior testis are perpendicular to the mediastinal rete testis channel into which they drain, while those in the caudal testicular region are parallel to their respective channels. The transitional segments between the seminiferous tubules and the tubuli recti are formed by modified Sertoli cells.[149]

The epithelium of the mediastinal rete testis consists of flattened cells interspersed with small areas of columnar cells. Both cell types have single centrally located cilia and numerous microvilli on their free surfaces, and contain keratin and vimentin filaments.[150] There are interdigitations between adjacent cells. The epithelium rests on a basal lamina surrounded by a layer of myoid cells and a more peripheral layer of fibroblasts and collagen and elastic fibers.

The rete channels and cavities are traversed by the chordae rete, columns 15 μm to 100 μm long and from 5 μm to 40 μm wide, arranged obliquely to the long axis of the cavity. The chordae consist of fibrous connective tissue with fibroblasts and are covered by flattened epithelium; the widest chordae contain capillaries. The rete testis probably has the following functions: damping differences in pressure between the seminiferous tubules and ductuli efferentes; reabsorption of protein and potassium from tubular fluid; and, occasionally, phagocytosis of spermatozoa.

CONGENITAL ANOMALIES OF TESTIS

ALTERATIONS IN NUMBER, SIZE, AND LOCATION

ANORCHIDISM

Types

Anorchidism refers to the absence of one (monorchidism) or both testes (testicular regression syndrome). Monorchidism is estimated to occur in about 4.5% of cryptorchid testes,[151] 40% of the testes that are impalpable in physical examination,[152] or 1 in 5000 males. Bilateral anorchidism occurs in approximately 1 in 20,000 males.[153]

Monorchidism. The hormonal pattern in prepubertal patients with monorchidism does not differ from that of normal children, whereas children lacking both testes have elevated levels of gonadotropins and fail to respond to stimulation with human chorionic gonadotropin.[153-155] Although the human chorionic gonadotropin stimulation test is often positive in children with bilateral cryptorchidism, it has been negative in some children with bilateral intraabdominal cryptorchidism. Basal levels of follicle stimulating hormone and luteinizing hormone may be normal in these children.[156]

For unknown reasons, the left testis is more frequently absent (68.7%) than the right. The contralateral scrotal

TABLE 10-5.
TESTICULAR REGRESSION SYNDROMES

	Embryonal Period		Fetal Period		
	EARLY	LATE	EARLY	MIDDLE	LATE
Müllerian structures	vestigial	differentiated	differentiated-vestigial	vestigial	vestigial
Wolffian structures	vestigial	vestigial	vestigial-differentiated	differentiated	differentiated
External genitalia	female	female	ambiguous	ambiguous-male	male

testis usually undergoes compensatory hypertrophy and its volume is over 2 cm^3.[157] Compensatory hypertrophy has also been reported in association with an abdominal cryptorchid testes.[158]

The absence of testicular parenchyma should be confirmed before diagnosing monorchidism. At exploration, the finding of a ductus deferens ending near or in a hypoplastic epididymis is not sufficient for the diagnosis of monorchidism. The only acceptable finding is blindly ending spermatic vessels. If inguinoscrotal exploration fails to find these vessels, intraabdominal exploration is required to ensure against an undescended testis and avoid the development of a testicular tumor.[159] All remnants found at exploration should be removed.[160]

Testicular regression syndrome (anorchidism). Testicular regression syndrome refers to a variety of conditions, including agonadism, anorchidism, testicular agenesis, rudimentary testes, hypoplastic testes, and embryonal testicular dysgenesis.[161] These have in common the complete absence or involution of both testes[162] but differ in the time of testicular disappearance during development. The most frequent of these are Swyer's syndrome (see discussion on gonadal dysgenesis in this chapter), true agonadism, rudimentary testes, bilateral anorchidism, vanishing testes syndrome, and Leydig cell–only syndrome (Table 10-5).

True agonadism (46XY gonadal agenesis syndrome). Patients with true agonadism have ambiguous external genitalia, fusion of the labia, and short vagina, reflecting very early testicular regression, between the eighth and twelfth weeks of embryonal development. The internal genitalia consist of rudimentary uterine tubes, and if gonadal remnants are present these consist of fibrous strands. Some cases are familial.[163]

Rudimentary testes syndrome. Patients with rudimentary testes syndrome have a normal male phenotype. Müllerian remnants are absent and wolffian derivatives usually are found.[164] The testes are cryptorchid and very small, less than 0.5 cm long. Seminiferous tubules are few. Testicular regression occurs between the fourteenth and twentieth weeks of gestation. This syndrome has been reported in several members of the same family,[165] suggesting genetic transmission, but this is not a constant feature.[166,167]

Congenital bilateral anorchidism. Congenital bilateral anorchidism occurs in 1 in 20,000 newborns. The patients have normal male external genitalia, but the internal genitalia consist only of normal wolffian derivatives without müllerian derivatives, suggesting that testes were present and functionally active up to approximately the twentieth week of gestation.

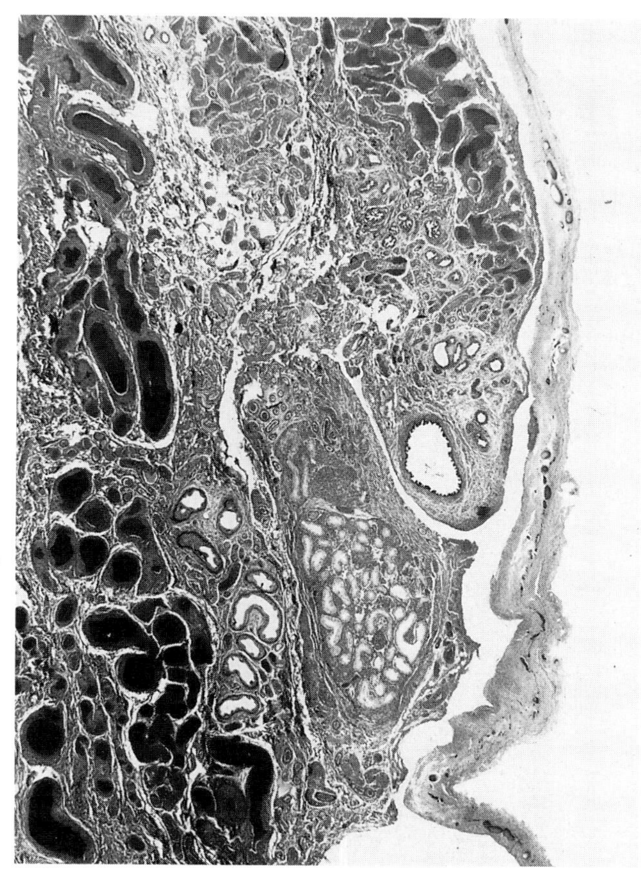

10-18. Vanishing testes syndrome. The testis consists of a small group of seminiferous tubules. Several sections of the epididymis, together with numerous blood vessels of the pampiniform plexus, also are visible.

Vanishing testes syndrome. This term refers to the disappearance of both testes between the last months of intrauterine life and the beginning of puberty.[166-170] Since testicular regression occurs after the seventh month, exploration finds the vas deferens in the inguinal canal or high in the scrotum; it may be accompanied by epididymis and, less frequently, by testicular remnants consisting of small groups of seminiferous tubules (Fig. 10-18). These patients develop hypergonadotropic hypogonadism after puberty, with gynecomastia, infantile phallus, hypoplastic scrotum, and impalpable prostate. The condition sometimes has a genetic cause.[171]

Leydig cell–only syndrome. Patients with Leydig cell–only syndrome have anorchidism without eunuchoidism with normal male phenotype and external genitalia, although meticulous surgical exploration fails to find testicular remnants. Study of serial sections from the spermatic cord reveals clusters of Leydig cells.[172] Detection of testosterone in spermatic vein blood indicates that these ectopic Leydig cells are functionally active and synthesize testosterone in amounts sufficient to cause the differentiation of a male phenotype but insufficient to support complete development of secondary sex characteristics.

Macroscopic and microscopic findings

The morphology of the spermatic cord is similar in monorchidism and testicular regression syndrome occurring after the twentieth week of gestation.[173-175] Grossly, a small, firm mass is found at the end of the cord (Fig. 10-19). Histologic examination reveals vas deferens, epididymis, or small groups of seminiferous tubules in 69% to 83% of cases.[176] Vas deferens is the most constant finding (79%), followed by epididymis (36%) and seminiferous tubules (5% to 13%). The spermatic vessels are abnormally small in 83% of cases.[160,177] Areas of dystrophic calcification, hemosiderin deposition, or giant cell reaction may be found within the mass in place of the testis. Other findings include arterial and venous vessels (88%), fat (44%), and nerves that may resemble a traumatic neuroma (56%).

Etiology

The histologic findings suggest that most cases of unilateral and bilateral anorchidism are produced during the fetal period, after the testis has inhibited the müllerian ducts and induced differentiation of the wolffian duct derivatives. Two hypotheses account for the disappearance of the testes: a primary anomaly of the gonad and atrophy secondary to a vascular lesion, such as thrombosis or intrauterine torsion. The presence of macrophages with hemosiderin and dystrophic calcification support the latter hypothesis. Absence of one testis may be associated with malformations of the urogenital system such as absence of the kidney, cystic seminal vesicles, and ipsilateral renal dysgenesis.[178,179]

POLYORCHIDISM

Polyorchidism is a rare condition, with only approximately 80 reported cases.[180] It was first described in a postmortem study in 1880,[181] and the first case treated surgically and confirmed histologically was reported in

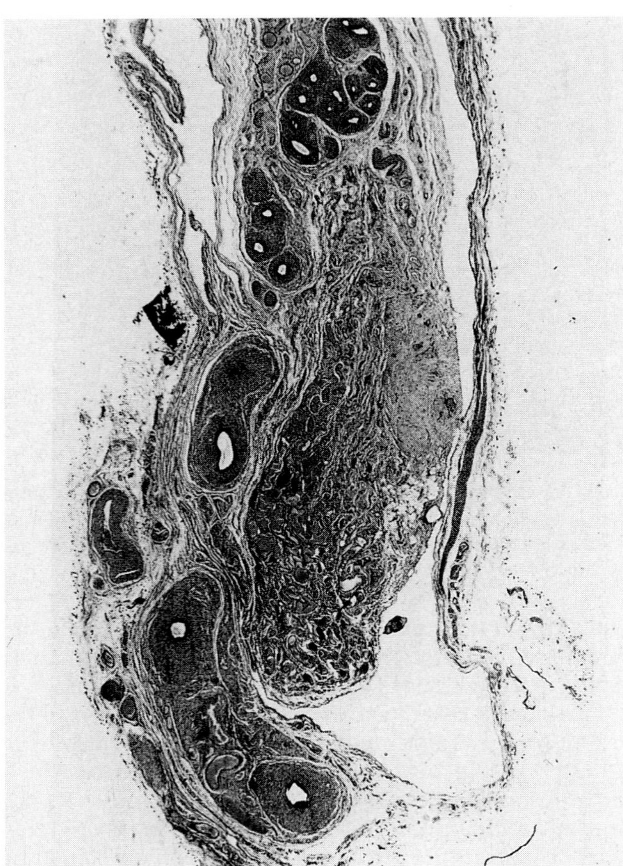

10-19. Spermatic cord in anorchidism. Fibrous connective tissue containing dystrophic calcifications surrounds the distal end of the vas deferens and replaces the testis.

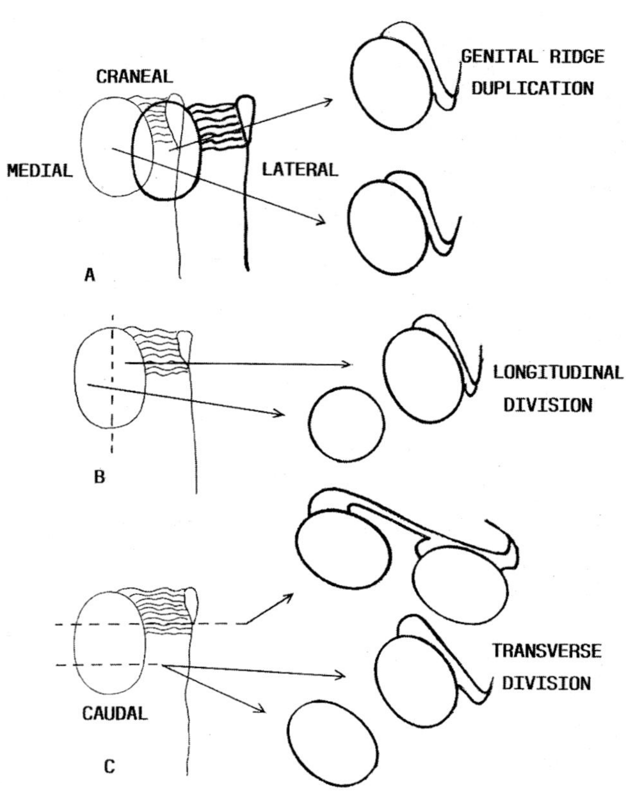

10-20. Possible mechanisms of polyorchidism. **A**, Genital ridge duplication gives rise to two testes with their respective epididymides. **B**, Longitudinal division of the genital ridge. The testis derived from the medial region has no epididymis. **C**, Transverse division of the genital ridge. The resulting testes either share a single epididymis or one testis is devoid of epididymis.

1895.[182] Although three testes is most frequent, four testes have been reported in three patients,[183-185] and one case with five testes was reported without histologic confirmation.[186] Age at diagnosis varies from newborn to 74 years, with a mean of 17 years. Testicular duplication is usually an incidental finding during surgery for inguinal hernia, cryptorchidism, or testicular torsion, but has also been detected in patients with infertility or unexplained fertility after bilateral vasectomy.[187] The extra testis is often intrascrotal (75%) and less frequently is inguinal (20%) or retroperitoneal (5%).[188,189] Testicular maldescent (14%), inguinal hernia (30%), hydrocele, varicocele, and contralateral cryptorchidism[190-192] are the most frequently associated anomalies. Testicular torsion (13%)[192,193] and testicular cancer (5.4%) are occasional complications. Although the extra testis may be histologically normal,[194-196] it usually is not[190,197] and displays lesions such as Sertoli cell–only tubules, hypospermatogenesis, or maturation arrest. The lack of spermatogenesis has been attributed to the anomalous location of the testis and the absence of communication between the testis and the excretory ducts.[198]

The embryologic origin of polyorchidism remains uncertain and the following have been proposed to account for the variety of findings in different cases (Fig. 10-20):

1. Longitudinal division of all the structures of the genital ridge and mesonephric ducts. Each of the two testes resulting from the duplication would have its own excretory ducts and develop active spermatogenesis.[182,187,199-201]
2. Longitudinal division of the genital ridge. Of the two resulting testes, the medial would lose its connection with the mesonephric ducts and undergo atrophy.
3. High transverse division of the genital ridge. The two resulting portions would be in continuity with the mesonephric ducts which give rise to the efferent ductules. Each testis may have its own ductus epididymidis or share a common one, but there is a single vas deferens for both.[196,202]
4. Low transverse division of the genital ridge. The more caudal testis has no excretory ducts.[192]

The differential diagnosis of polyorchidism includes most pathologic conditions that enlarge the scrotum and spermatic cord: spermatocele, hydrocele, cysts and tumors of the spermatic cord, crossed testicular ectopia, adrenal cortical ectopia, and splenogonadal fusion. Intrascrotal rhabdomyosarcoma, testicular teratoma, and seminoma have been reported in patients with polyorchidism.[203,204]

TESTICULAR HYPERTROPHY (MACROORCHIDISM)

Macroorchidism may be unilateral or bilateral and may be associated with chromosomal anomalies or endocrine alterations. An increase in the testicular parenchyma occurs in several conditions,[205] including compensatory hypertrophy, benign idiopathic macroorchidism, Martin-Bell syndrome (fragile X chromosome), and various forms of precocious puberty.

Compensatory hypertrophy

Compensatory hypertrophy has been observed in monorchidism,[206] cryptorchidism (Fig. 10-21),[207] and after testicular injury. Hypertrophy persists and may increase during childhood and puberty but ceases after puberty; the hypertrophic testis then becomes normal or remains slightly enlarged.[208,209] The degree of hypertrophy is determined by three factors: the volume of the remaining testicular parenchyma, the age at which the injury occurred, and the functional ability of the descended testis.[210] Compensatory hypertrophy results from an alteration in the hypophyseal hormonal feedback mechanism, followed by an increase in secretion of follicle stimulating hormone, evidence that the contralateral testis is normal. In monorchidism the testis is initially normal.[152] When a 50% reduction of testicular mass occurs (probably before birth), the endocrine feedback changes and the resulting secretion of follicle stimulating hormone (before or immediately after birth) causes accelerated growth of the contralateral testis. In cryptorchidism the reduction in testicular mass is less severe than in monorchidism, and the scrotal testis may also be abnormal, inducing a lesser compensatory hypertrophy. Compensatory hypertrophy develops between birth and 3 years of age, and the testis may reach a volume twice that of normal when the other testis is absent.[158]

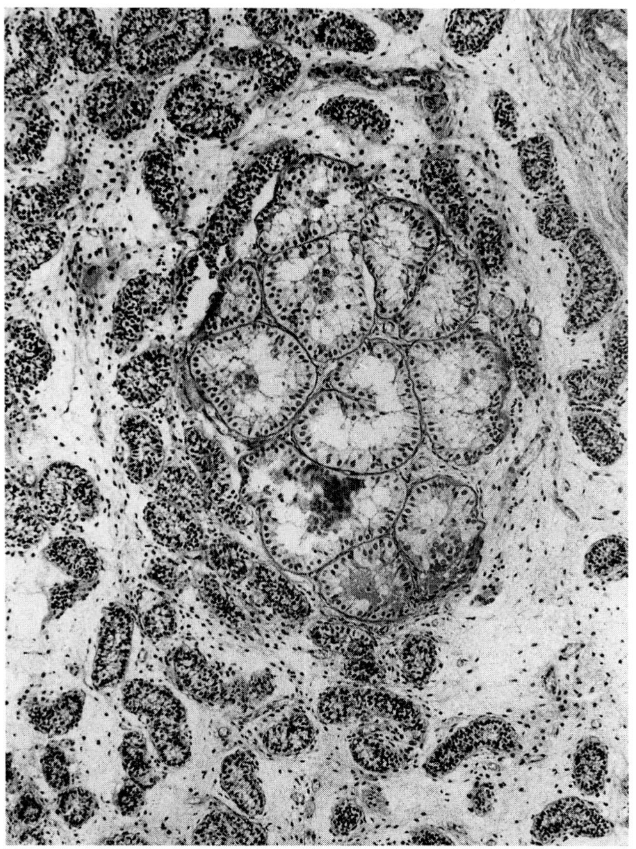

10-21. Contralateral scrotal testis from a cryptorchid patient showing a group of large seminiferous tubules that stand out from the surrounding small tubules.

Idiopathic benign macroorchidism

Some prepubertal and pubertal patients have pronounced unilateral[211] or bilateral[212-214] testicular hypertrophy in the absence of other pathologic findings. This probably results from altered hormonal receptivity in the testicular parenchyma. Morphometric studies have shown that the testicular enlargement is chiefly due to increase in the length of the seminiferous tubules,[215] although increases in tubular diameter and Sertoli cell number have also been observed. In addition, Leydig cell hyperplasia and deficient spermatogenesis are frequent findings in adult life. Since the development of the two testes may be asynchronous during puberty, some unilateral macroorchidism may represent cases in which these differences are unusually exaggerated.

Martin-Bell syndrome (fragile X chromosome)

Macroorchidism is often associated with other anomalies, such as psychomotor retardation and facial dysmorphia, in a syndrome caused by a fragile site in the long arm of the X chromosome.[216] First described by Martin and Bell in 1943,[217] multiple variants have been reported.[218-224] In addition to facial malformations (high forehead, large ears, and prognathism) and mental retardation, macroorchidism (testicular volume greater than 25 ml) is present in more than 75% of adult patients.[225] In men with this syndrome, the average testicular volume is more than 70 ml (four times greater than normal). The penis also is larger than normal and both abnormalities often are apparent in infancy. The scrotum is also enlarged and prematurely pigmented. This precocious genital development is difficult to explain because the hypothalamic-pituitary axis is normal, but it may be caused by increased sensitivity to stimulation by follicle stimulating hormone.[226]

Testicular biopsies from adults may be normal or show interstitial edema and hypospermatogenesis (Fig. 10-22). Usually there is normal testicular parenchyma with some areas showing tubules with reduced spermatogenesis and Sertoli cell hyperplasia (Fig. 10-23) or tubules containing only immature Sertoli cells. Morphometry indicates that the testicular enlargement is chiefly the result of lengthening of seminiferous tubules.[215] The low number of spermatids is attributed to atrophy caused by compression by the tubular fluid.[227] Meiotic anomalies have been excluded.[228] The fragile X syndrome occurs in 1 in 1500 newborns and is second in frequency only to Down syndrome as a cause of mental retardation.[229-231] However, this chromosomal anomaly is not always associated with mental retardation or macroorchidism, and there are men with fragile-X syndrome who are otherwise normal.[232]

Precocious puberty

Some cases of bilateral macroorchidism are caused by primary testicular abnormalities, such as familial testo-

10-22. Martin-Bell syndrome (fragile X chromosome). Seminiferous tubules showing variable degrees of dilation and atrophy from a testis more than 8 cm long.

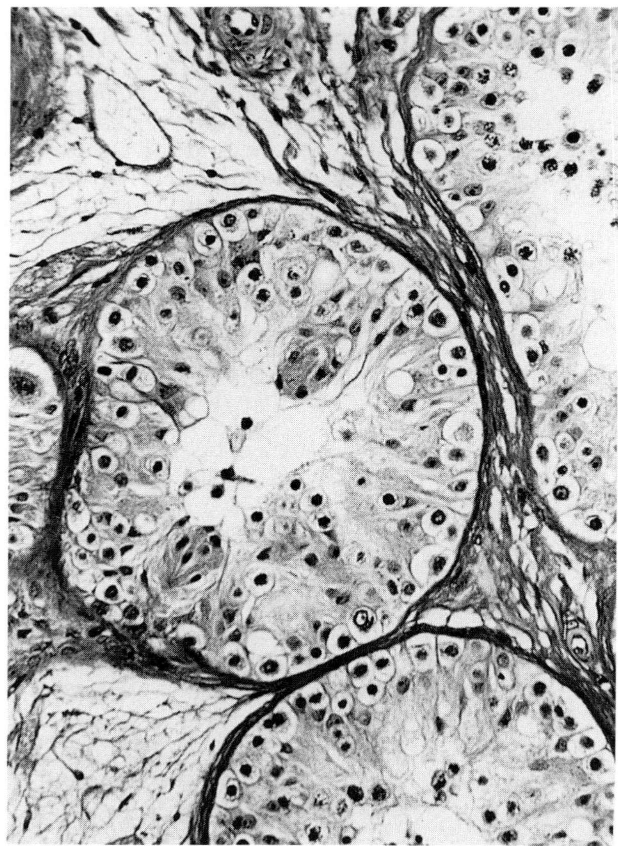

10-23. Martin-Bell syndrome (fragile X chromosome). Seminiferous tubules showing marked hypospermatogenesis. Two groups of dysgenetic Sertoli cells are seen near the lumen.

toxicosis and Leydig cell tumor, while others are secondary to other endocrine disorders. These include lesions of the hypothalamic-hypophyseal axis (precocious puberty, follicle stimulating hormone–secreting pituitary adenomas, and hyperprolactinemia and hypoprolactinemia); thyroid gland (hypothyroidism); adrenal glands (virilizing adrenal carcinoma, congenital adrenal hyperplasia, and Nelson's syndrome); and human chorionic gonadotropin–secreting tumors.

Familial testotoxicosis. Familial testotoxicosis is a form of sexual precocity characterized by early differentiation of Leydig cells and spermatogenesis in the absence of stimulation by pituitary gonadotropin. This is a primary testicular abnormality and has an autosomal dominant inheritance.[233,234] Ultrastructural studies confirm an adult Leydig cell pattern and complete spermatogenesis, although many spermatids are abnormal.[235]

Leydig cell tumor. Leydig cell tumor may cause precocious puberty. The testis is enlarged by the tumor and by the maturation of seminiferous tubules adjacent to the tumor, as a result of androgen secretion by tumor cells. In most cases the contralateral testis is not enlarged.

Other forms of precocious puberty. In other forms of precocious puberty due to different causes (constitutional or idiopathic, secondary to disorders of the central nervous system, associated with phacomatosis or McCune-Albright syndrome, and von Recklinghausen syndrome), pubertal development begins before 9 years of age, with bilateral testicular enlargement and development of secondary sex characteristics. In McCune-Albright syndrome, testicular maturation is induced by the steroid secretion of the testis itself, causing early maturation of the hypothalamic-hypophyseal-testicular axis.[236] Testicular hypertrophy associated with follicle stimulating hormone–secreting pituitary adenomas,[237] hyperprolactinemia or hypoprolactinemia, or hypothyroidism[238] is easily corrected with adequate hormonal treatment. Most children with virilizing carcinoma of the adrenal gland have small testes, although testicular hypertrophy has been reported in some cases, because of the adrenal secretion that causes maturation of the seminiferous tubules.[239] In untreated or inadequately treated congenital adrenal hyperplasia, both testes may be markedly enlarged by masses of cells resembling adrenal cortical cells. Similar lesions may be found in Nelson's syndrome. Paraneoplastic precocious puberty secondary to human chorionic gonadotropin–secreting tumors causes slight testicular enlargement, and the most important histologic finding is Leydig cell hyperplasia.

Congenital Leydig cell hyperplasia

Congenital Leydig cell hyperplasia is uncommon and may be diffuse or nodular. The diagnosis of diffuse Leydig cell hyperplasia requires Leydig cell quantitation by

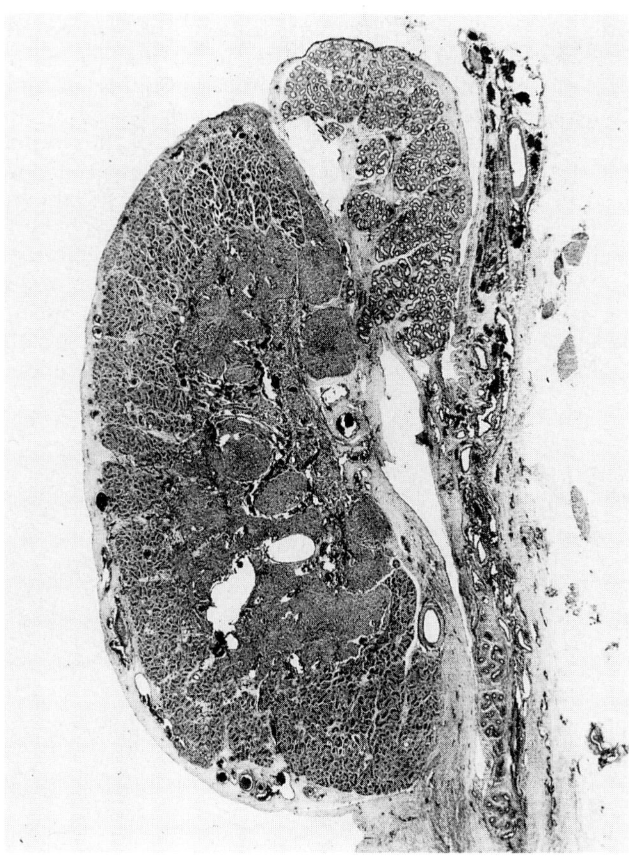

10-24. Congenital Leydig cell hyperplasia. Multiple nodules of dysgenetic Leydig cells are present in the mediastinum testis as well as deep in the parenchyma.

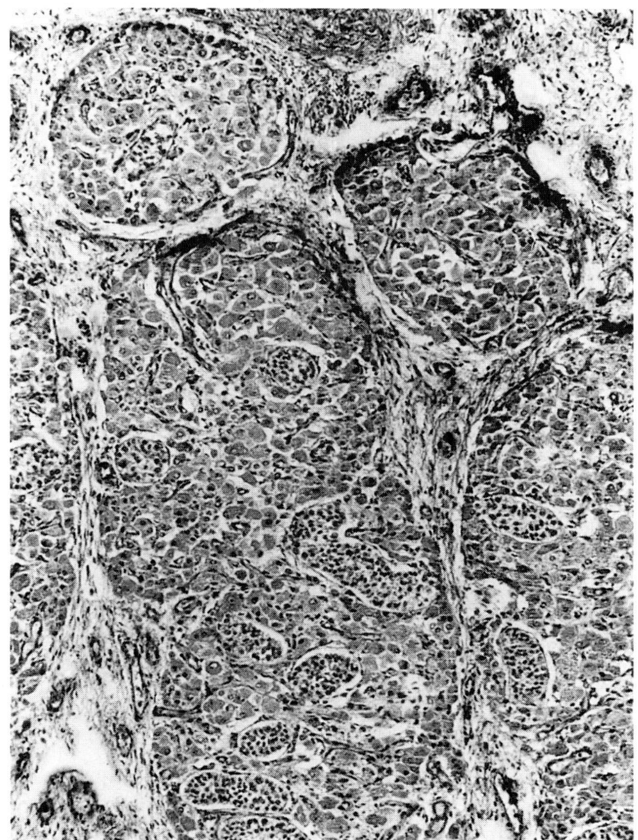

10-25. Congenital Leydig cell hyperplasia. Fetal Leydig cells form large clusters surrounding groups of seminiferous tubules.

morphometry, using normal newborn testes as controls. Nodular Leydig cell hyperplasia is characterized by the presence of unencapsulated nodules of Leydig cells in the mediastinum testis, adjacent testicular parenchyma, and the connective tissue among the efferent ductules (Fig. 10-24, 10-25).

The differential diagnosis of nodular Leydig cell hyperplasia includes intratesticular adrenal rest and bilateral Leydig cell tumor. Intratesticular adrenal rests are rare (except for patients with adrenogenital syndrome) and encapsulated, consisting of radially arranged cells with vesicular nuclei and small nucleoli displacing the rete testis or seminiferous tubules. Leydig cell tumors may be bilateral, poorly circumscribed, and surrounded by testicular parenchyma, features making them difficult to distinguish from Leydig cell hyperplasia. However, Leydig cell tumors are rarely congenital, while those occurring in infancy often induce precocious maturation of the adjacent seminiferous tubules and early macrogenitosomia.

Leydig cell hyperplasia is caused by large quantities of human chorionic gonadotropin entering in the fetal circulation. Diabetic mothers, particularly those with hypertension, may develop hyperplacentosis; the resulting edema in the placental villi alters the vascular permeability and allows the passage of human chorionic gonadotropin to the fetus. Congenital Leydig cell hyperplasia decreases rapidly during the first months of postnatal life, after maternal human chorionic gonadotropin is gone. Combined diffuse and nodular Leydig cell hyperplasia has been reported in several malformative syndromes and in infants with Rh isoimmunization.[240]

TESTICULAR ECTOPIA AND TESTICULAR FUSION

Testicular ectopia

A testis is ectopic when it is in a location outside of the normal path of descent. Unlike cryptorchid testes, ectopic testes have nearly normal size and are accompanied by a spermatic cord that is normal or even longer than normal and by a normal scrotum.[241] Testicular ectopia is classified according to location[242-246]; in decreasing order of frequency the major types are:

1. *Interstitial or inguinal superficial ectopia*. This is the most frequent form and may be confused with inguinal cryptorchidism. After passing through the outer genital opening, the testis ascends to the anterior-superior iliac spine and remains on the aponeurosis of the major oblique muscle. These testes often are more nearly normal histologically than are cryptorchid testes.
2. *Femoral or crural ectopia*. After passing through the inguinal canal, the testis lodges in the high crural cone in Scarpa's triangle.
3. *Perineal*. The testis located between the raphe and the genitocrural fold.
4. *Transverse or crossed ectopia*. Both testes descend through the same inguinal canal and lodge in the same scrotal pouch. Each possesses its own vascular supply, epididymis, and vas deferens. In addition, there is ipsilateral inguinal hernia.[247-253]
5. *Pubopenile ectopia*. The ectopic testis is on the back of the penis, near the symphysis pubis.[254]
6. *Pelvic ectopia*. The testis is in the pelvis, usually in the depth of Douglas's cul-de-sac.
7. Other unusual testicular locations include retroumbilical and craniolateral to the inner inguinal opening between the outer and inner oblique muscles. Rarely, the testis and its spermatic cord may protrude through a defect in the scrotal skin, a condition called *testicular exstrophy*.[255]

Testicular fusion

Testicular fusion is a rare anomaly characterized by fusion of the testes to form a single structure, usually in the midline. Each has its own epididymis and vas deferens. This anomaly often is associated with other malformations such as fusion of the adrenal glands or horseshoe kidney.

HAMARTOMATOUS TESTICULAR LESIONS

CYSTIC DYSPLASIA

Cystic dysplasia of the testis is a congenital lesion characterized by cystic transformation of an excessively developed rete testis, which may extend to the tunica albuginea of the opposite pole.[256] The seminiferous tubules may be dilated and atrophic; this is more evident after puberty. The epididymis is usually not involved.[257] The cysts arise in the septal and mediastinal rete testis (Fig. 10-26), interconnect and contain acellular, eosinophilic, periodic acid–Schiff positive material. They are lined by cuboidal cells that resemble those of the normal rete testis.[258-260] The connective tissue between the cysts is scant and histologically similar to the interstitial connective tissue. The lesions vary from small groups of cysts limited to the region of the mediastinum testis to cysts extending throughout the testis. In extensive cases, residual seminiferous tubules occupy only a small crescent beneath the tunica albuginea, and the testis is grossly spongy. Cystic dysplasia occurs in normally descended

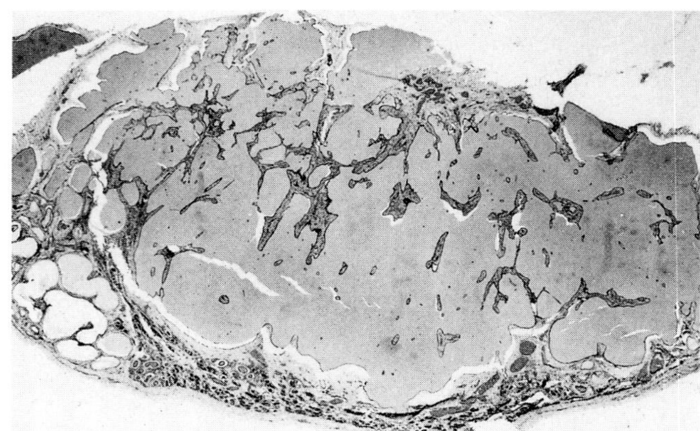

10-26. Cystic dysplasia of the testis. There is cystic transformation of both the rete testis and the adjacent seminiferous tubules.

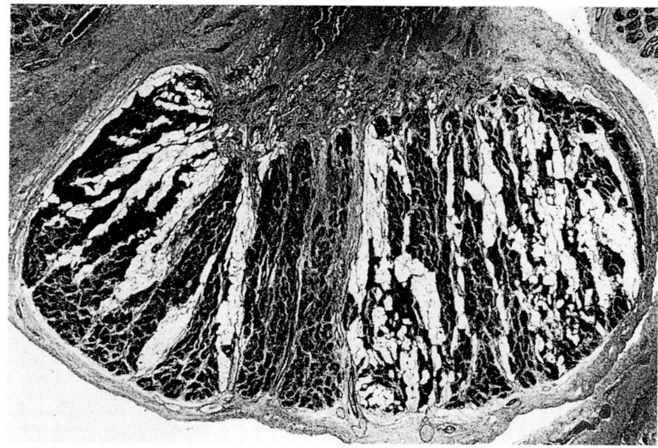

10-27. Congenital testicular lymphangiectasis. Lymphatic vessels of the testicular parenchyma are markedly dilated and elongated.

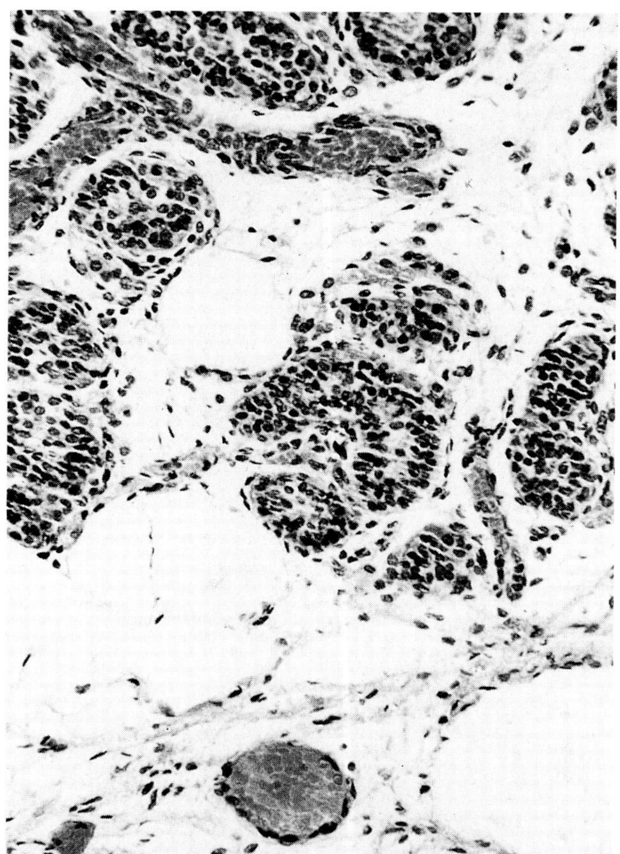

10-28. Congenital testicular lymphangiectasis. Ectatic lymphatic vessels compress the seminiferous tubules.

and cryptorchid testes in infants and adults, and it may affect one or both testes.[261] In adults the residual parenchyma often shows complete tubular sclerosis or hypospermatogenesis with intratubular accumulation of spermatozoa and Leydig cell pseudohyperplasia.

Testicular cystic dysplasia is frequently associated with severe anomalies of the urinary system. Renal agenesis,[261-263] renal dysplasia,[261] hydroureter, and urethral stenosis[264] have been reported ipsilateral to the cystic dysplasia. The etiology and pathogenesis of cystic dysplasia are unknown, but because the rete testis is a mesonephric derivative and most of the associated renal malformations may be caused by failure in the induction of the renal blastema by the mesonephros, cystic dysplasia may be the result of an abnormal mesonephros.

The normal rete testis has no lumen during childhood; the lumen is formed during puberty. The adult rete testis is not only a conduit for the passage of tubular fluid and spermatozoa but also actively reabsorbs part of this fluid and adds ions, proteins and steroids to it.[265] Malfunction of the rete testis cells may cause formation of excessive fluid of abnormal composition; a condition morphologically similar to cystic dysplasia of the rete testis is induced in fowl by sodium intoxication or administration of the salt-retaining hormone, deoxycorticosterone acetate.[266]

CONGENITAL TESTICULAR LYMPHANGIECTASIS

Congenital testicular lymphangiectasis is characterized by abnormal and excessive development of lymphatic vessels in the tunica albuginea, mediastinum testis, interlobular septa, and testicular interstitium.[267,268] Ultrastructurally, these dilated vessels are similar to normal lymphatic capillaries, although some are markedly dilated and the testicular interstitium is slightly edematous (Fig. 10-27). Testicular lymphangiectasis occurs in both cryptorchid and scrotal testes; in one of the latter cases, the patient had Noonan's syndrome. The disease does not seem to affect the seminiferous tubules, and low numbers of spermatogonia and reduced tubular diameters are observed only in cryptorchid testes. The epididymis and spermatic cord are not affected, nor has congenital testicular lymphangiectasis been associated with pulmonary, intestinal, or systemic lymphangiectasis.

In the fetal period, lymphatics are visible only immediately beneath the tunica albuginea and in the interlobular septa.[269] During childhood the number and size of the septal lymphatics begins to decrease[270]; by adulthood they are inconspicuous.[271] In lymphangiectasis the septal lymphatics are large and often massively dilated (Fig. 10-28). Lymphangiectasis has been found only in children's testes, suggesting that these dilated vessels undergo involution at puberty or that the pubertal development of the seminiferous tubules masks the lymphangiectasis.

TESTICULAR PARENCHYMAL ECTOPIA

SEMINIFEROUS TUBULE ECTOPIA

The presence of seminiferous tubules within the tunica albuginea is rare and usually is an incidental histologic finding.[272] Such ectopic tubules have been found in approximately 0.8% of pediatric autopsies and 0.3% of adult autopsies. The lower incidence in adults may be explained by proportionally lesser sampling. The lesions range from microscopic to a few millimeters in diameter and may be visible as minute bulges in which multiple

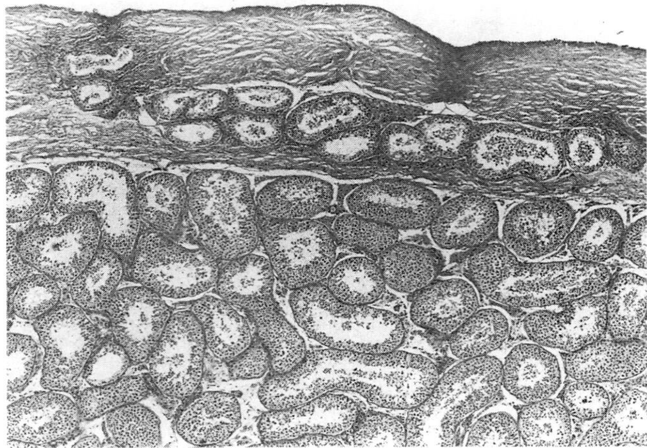

10-29. Ectopic seminiferous tubules within the tunica albuginea.

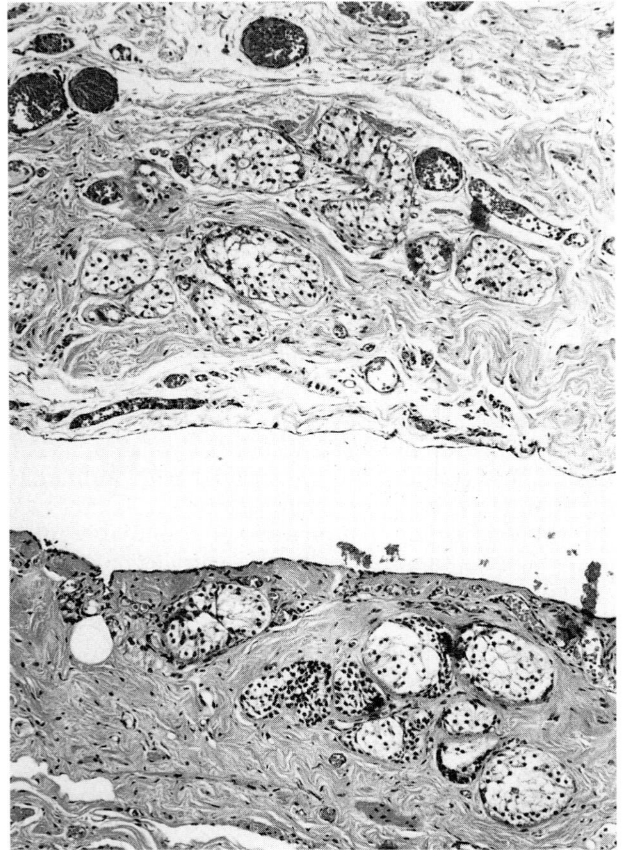

10-30. Ectopic seminiferous tubules in the wall of a hernia sac.

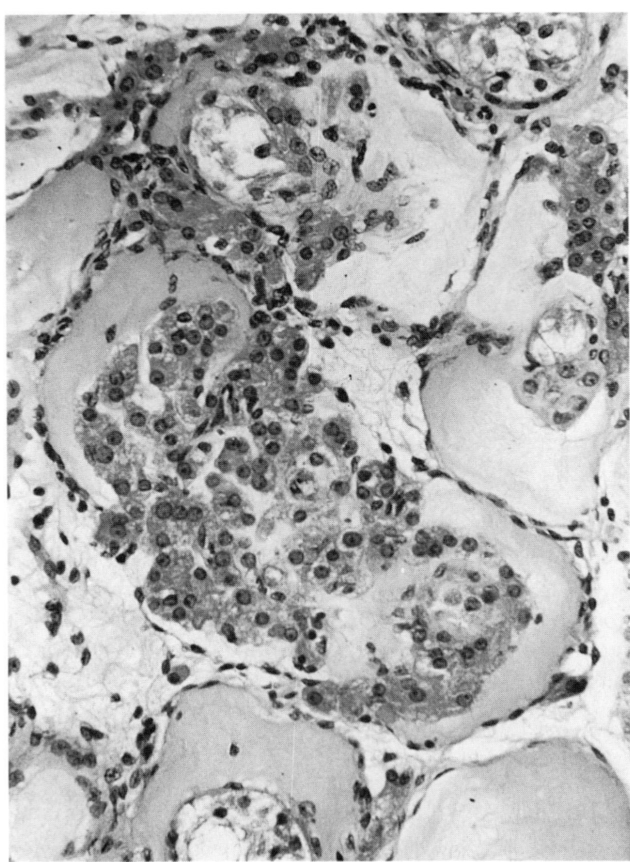

10-31. Ectopic Leydig cells within sclerotic seminiferous tubules.

small vesicles protrude through a thin tunica albuginea. Histologically, these protrusions consist of groups of seminiferous tubules in the tunica albuginea, sometimes accompanied by Leydig cells. In children the ectopic tubules resemble normal ones. In adults the tubules are usually slightly dilated, although some may be sclerotic. Serial sections reveal continuity with the rest of the tubular system (Fig. 10-29).

Ectopia of seminiferous tubules is probably congenital, although it has been found in elderly men.[273] It does not appear to be the result of trauma. The malformation probably arises in the sixth week of gestation, when the primordial sex cords have formed and are branching toward the gonadal surface,[274] and the developing testis is covered by only one to three layers of celomic epithelium.[275] Later the tunica albuginea forms around the sex cords and under the celomic epithelium. Failure of insertion of the tunica albuginea between the sex cords and celomic epithelium could entrap seminiferous tubules.

Ectopia differs from testicular dysgenesis, a distinctive form of male pseudohermaphroditism with müllerian remnants. The following features, characteristic of ectopic seminiferous tubules, distinguish it from other conditions: normal thickness and collagenization of the tunica albuginea, absence of interstitial tissue resembling ovarian stroma (characteristic of testicular dysgenesis), and clear delimitation of the tunica albuginea and testicular parenchyma (see discussion on male pseudohermaphroditism with müllerian remnants in this chapter).

In a unique case there were multiple clusters of seminiferous tubules in the wall of a hernia sac which accompanied an undescended testis removed from an adult (Fig. 10-30). The ectopic tubules were not surrounded by tunica albuginea and were similar to those in the cryptorchid testicular parenchyma with a seminiferous epithelium consisting of dysgenetic Sertoli cells only.

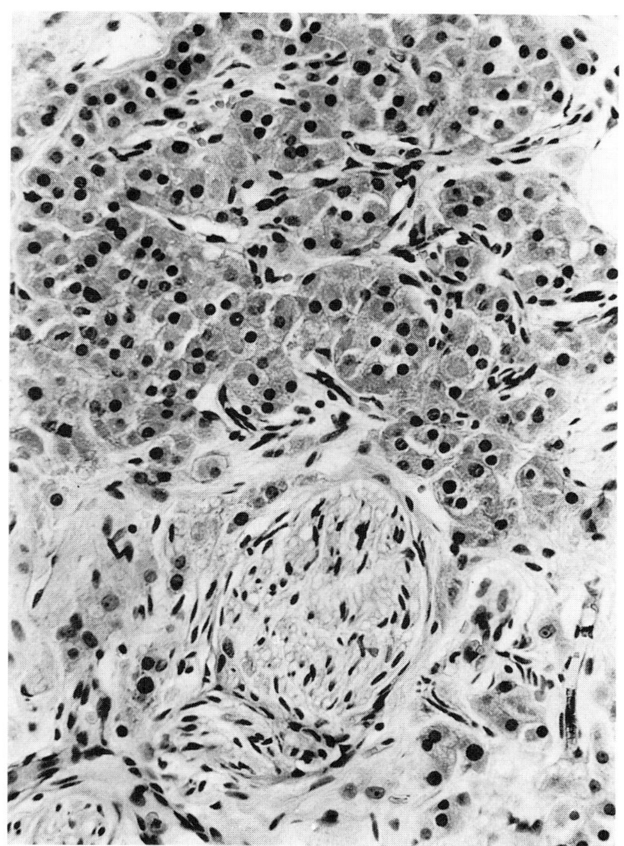

10-32. Ectopic Leydig cells around small nerves in the spermatic cord.

LEYDIG CELL ECTOPIA

Leydig cells occur normally in the testicular interstitium (interstitial Leydig cells) and in the walls of the seminiferous tubules (peritubular Leydig cells). However, clusters of Leydig cells are often observed at other locations in the testis or in the epididymis or spermatic cord.[275,276]

Ectopic Leydig cells may be found in the interlobular septa,[277-279] rete testis, tunica albuginea,[280-282] or within sclerotic seminiferous tubules.[279,283-285] Intratubular Leydig cells are found only in tubules with advanced atrophy and marked thickening of the tunica propria, including the tubules in adult cryptorchid testes and those of men with Klinefelter's syndrome (Fig. 10-31). Immunohistochemical studies suggest that the endocrine function of these cells is very low.[286] Several theories have been offered to account for these ectopic cells, including in situ differentiation, migration from the testicular interstitium, and trapping of peritubular Leydig cells in the tunica propria during its thickening.[287] Leydig cells are commonly found in the epididymis[286] and spermatic cord[279,288,289]; 26 of 64 autopsies had such foci.[290] Extratesticular Leydig cells usually form small groups within or adjacent to nerves (Fig. 10-32).[277,290]

UNDESCENDED TESTES

Testicular descent is not always complete at birth, and about 3.2% of term newborns have incompletely descended testes. Most of these descend within 3 months and only 0.8% of infants have incompletely descended testes 12 months after birth. Spontaneous testicular descent is exceptional after the first year.

In 5% of these cases there is no testis. The other cases include true cryptorchidism, testicular ectopia, and retractile testis. True cryptorchidism includes abdominal, inguinal, and high scrotal testes that cannot be moved to the scrotum. Ectopic testes are those located out of the normal path of testicular descent; the most frequent site is a superficial inguinal pouch. Other, more rarely observed locations include the abdominal wall, the upper thigh, the perineum, and the base of the penis. Retractile testes may be moved to the scrotum at exploration and account for about one third of undescended testes. Exceptionally, a descended testis may become a cryptorchid testis as a consequence of anomalous reabsorption of the processus vaginalis.[291]

TRUE CRYPTORCHIDISM

Patients with true cryptorchidism account for about 25% of cases of empty scrotum. These testes most frequently are found in the inguinal canal or upper scrotum; arrest within the abdomen is less frequent. Cryptorchidism is slightly more frequent on the right than the left and in approximately 18% of cases is bilateral. There is a family history of cryptorchidism in 14% of cases.

There are multiple causes of testicular maldescent, including anatomical anomalies of the gubernaculum testis, hormonal dysfunction (hypogonadotropic hypogonadism), mechanical impairment (short spermatic cord, underdeveloped vaginal process), dysgenesis (primary anomaly of the testis), and heredity.

The cryptorchid testis is usually smaller than the contralateral testis and this difference often is discernible at 6 months of age.[292] One third of cryptorchid testes are soft.

Etiology and pathogenesis

Cryptorchidism progressively damages the seminiferous epithelium, and for this reason it is desirable to move the cryptorchid testis to the scrotum at an early age to prevent irreversible damage. Although there have been a number of biopsy studies in the first years of life, there is no agreement about the severity of the damage or the time of its onset.[293-295] The most common abnormalities are a low number of spermatogonia and decreased tubular diameter. Three mechanisms seem to be involved in the process:

1. *Primary testicular anomaly*. Cryptorchid testes may bear an anomalous germ cell population, as was suggested many years ago.[296] More than 40% of cryptorchid patients have a marked decrease in the tubular fertility index,[297] even with nearly normal numbers of spermatogonia; these cells also have abnormal DNA contents.[298]
2. *Lesions secondary to transient perinatal hypogonadotropic hypogonadism*. Cryptorchid patients do not have the gonadotropin elevation that normally occurs between 60 and 90 days after birth, and this deficiency of luteinizing hormone could cause Leydig cell involution. The subsequent androgen deficiency could account for the failure of gonocytes to differentiate into spermatogonia.[293,299,300]

3. *Injury caused by increased temperature.* This was suggested in the past on the basis of experimental studies in laboratory animals. In follow-up biopsies from testes that were descended surgically or with hormonal treatment, the sole parameter that improved during childhood was the tubular diameter. Because this depends on Sertoli cells, it may be that temperature is more important for Sertoli cells than for spermatogonia.[297]

Histology

Prepubertal testes. Based on the tubular fertility index and the mean tubular diameter, most testicular biopsies from cryptorchid testes of children may be classified in one of three groups:

Type I (testes with slight alterations). The testicular fertility index is higher than 50, and mean tubular diameter is normal or slightly (less than 10%) decreased. Approximately 31% of cryptorchid testes are in this group (Fig. 10-33).

Type II (testes with marked germinal hypoplasia). The testicular fertility index is between 30 and 50, and the mean tubular diameter is 10% to 30% lower than normal. The spermatogonia are distributed irregularly and most are in tubular profiles that are grouped suggesting testicular lobules. These comprise approximately 29% of cryptorchid testes (Fig. 10-34).

Type III (testes with severe germinal hypoplasia). The testicular fertility index is less than 30, and the mean tubular diameter less than 30% of normal. Many of the spermatogonia are giant spermatogonia with dark nuclei (Fig. 10-35). These testes often contain ring-shaped tubules, megatubules (with or without eosinophilic bodies or microliths) (Fig. 10-36), and focal granular changes in the Sertoli cells. The testicular interstitium is wide and edematous (Fig. 10-37). These comprise about 40% of cryptorchid testes.

The seminiferous tubules of testes with type II or III lesions show a thickened lamina propria during childhood and, at puberty, Sertoli cell hyperplasia.[301] Patients with bilateral cryptorchidism have a higher incidence of type II and III lesions than those with unilateral cryptorchidism.

Type I lesions are comparable to those seen in experimental cryptorchidism, normal testes in which lesions were induced by increased temperature.[302] Testes with type II or III lesions bear variable degrees of dysgenesis, which in addition to germ cells involves Sertoli cells, myofibroblasts, and Leydig cells. The dysgenesis of these other cell types is evident only after puberty. In about

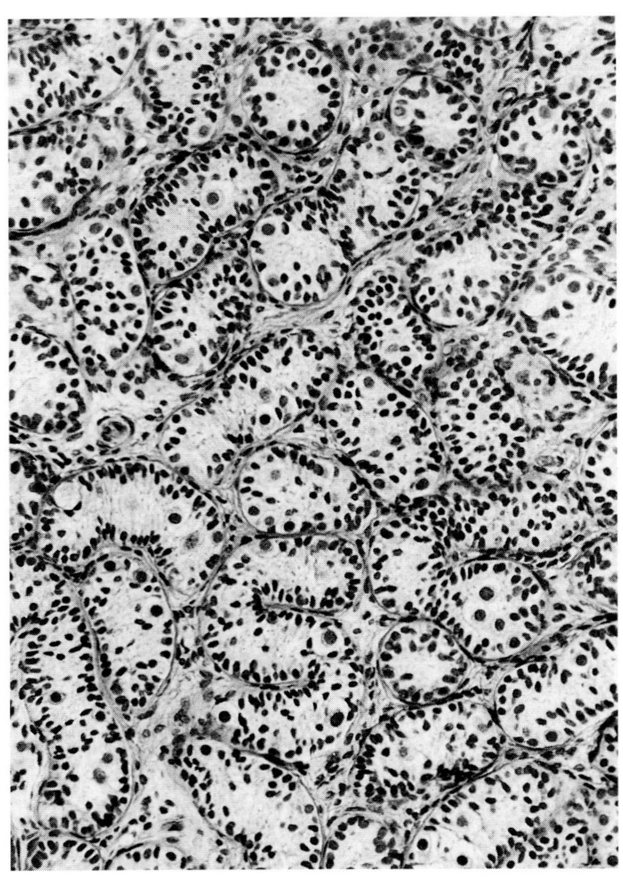

10-33. Cryptorchidism. Seminiferous tubules with type I lesions showing slightly decreased diameters and a normal tubular fertility index.

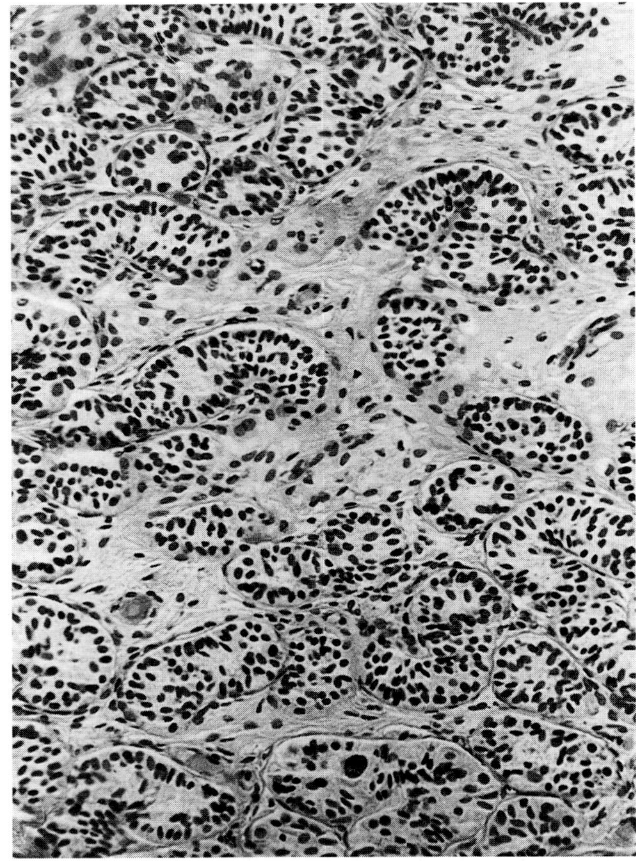

10-34. Cryptorchidism. Seminiferous tubules with type II lesions showing markedly decreased diameters and an irregular distribution of germ cells.

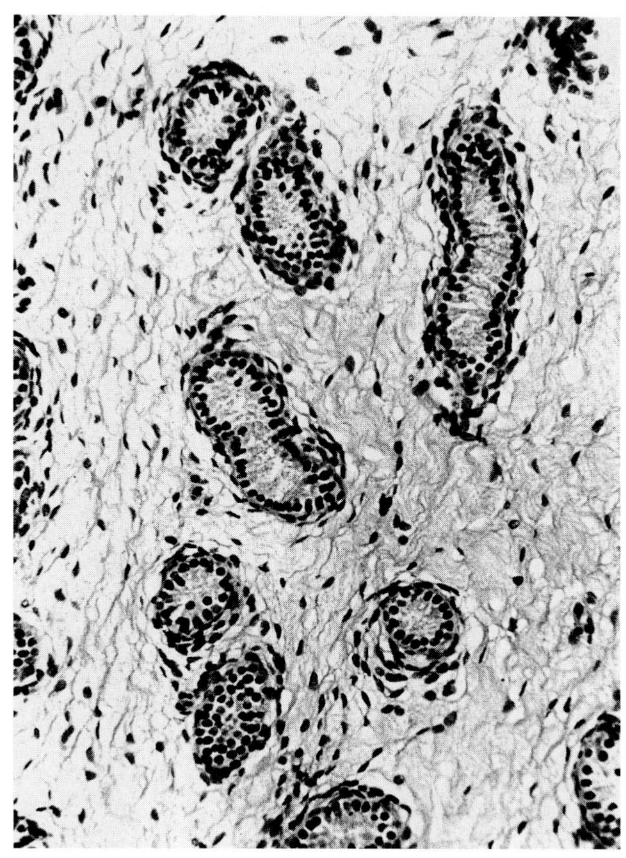

10-35. Cryptorchidism. Seminiferous tubules with type III lesions showing severe reduction in both tubular diameter and tubular fertility index.

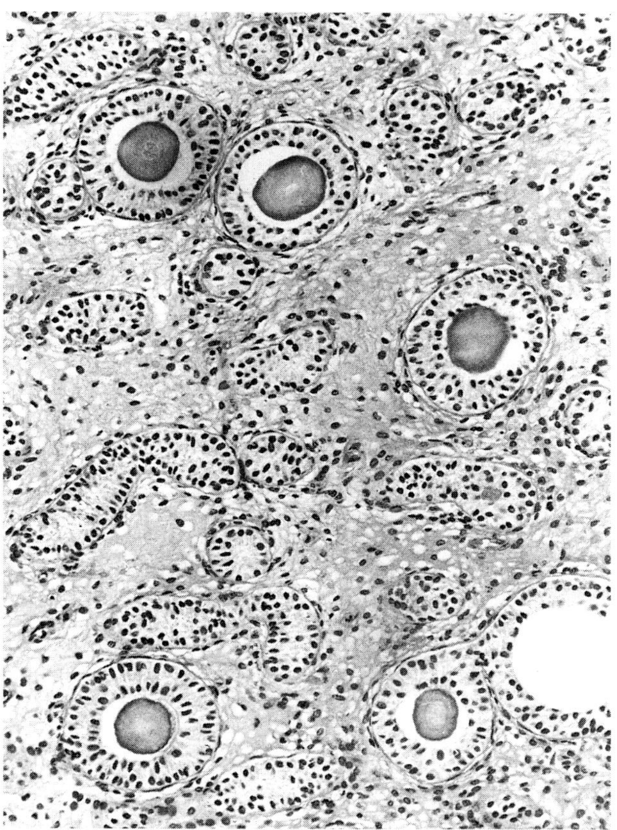

10-36. Cryptorchidism. Lamellated eosinophilic bodies surrounded by a double layer of Sertoli cells in a cryptorchid testis with type III lesions.

25% of cases the contralateral scrotal testis also has histologic lesions of variable severity.

Adult testes. Most pubertal and adult cryptorchid testes have abnormalities in all testicular structures. The seminiferous tubules have decreased diameters and deficient spermatogenesis. In decreasing order of frequency, the most common germ cell lesions are tubules with Sertoli cells and spermatogonia only, tubules with Sertoli cells (dysgenetic) only, tubular sclerosis, and mixed tubular atrophy. The lamina propria has few elastic fibers and increased collagen fibers.[303] Sertoli cells are present in increased numbers and do not mature normally except in tubules with spermatogonia.[301] Often groups of tubules containing only Sertoli cells with a prepubertal pattern (very small diameter and total absence of maturation) are present and are considered hypoplastic or dysgenetic zones (Fig. 10-38). Areas of apparent Leydig cell hyperplasia are frequent, and many of these cells contain vacuolated lipid-laden cytoplasm.

The rete testis is hypoplastic in most cases and lined by columnar epithelium with rare areas of flattened cells. Cystic dilation is common and adenomatous hyperplasia has been found in some cases (Fig. 10-39). Near the rete testis the testicular parenchyma frequently contains metaplastic fat (Fig. 10-40). The epididymal tubules are poorly developed and the peritubular tissue is immature.

OBSTRUCTED TESTES

These testes are located in the superficial inguinal pouch (Denis-Browne pouch) and are considered ectopic by some authors and cryptorchid by others.[304,305] Histologic studies reveal that most obstructed testes bear the same lesions as true cryptorchid testes. Type I lesions are observed in half, type II in more than one third, and the remainder show type III lesions. The higher proportion of type I lesions suggests a better prognosis than in true cryptorchid testes.

RETRACTILE TESTES

Retractile testes may be variants of cryptorchidism, but most authors believe that these testes are normal and exclude them from studies of cryptorchidism.[306,307] Retractile testes may not always be movable to the lower scrotum (70 to 75 mm from the pubic tubercle) and are smaller than scrotal testes in 50% of cases. Approximately 50% of retractile testes remain high after age 6 when cremasteric activity declines.[308] During childhood both tubular diameter and tubular fertility index decrease.[307] Adults with retractile testes that descended spontaneously but late may be fertile[309] or infertile.[310] Usually there is germ cell atrophy, which varies in severity from lobule to lobule.[307] Regular examination of retractile testes is advisable during childhood,

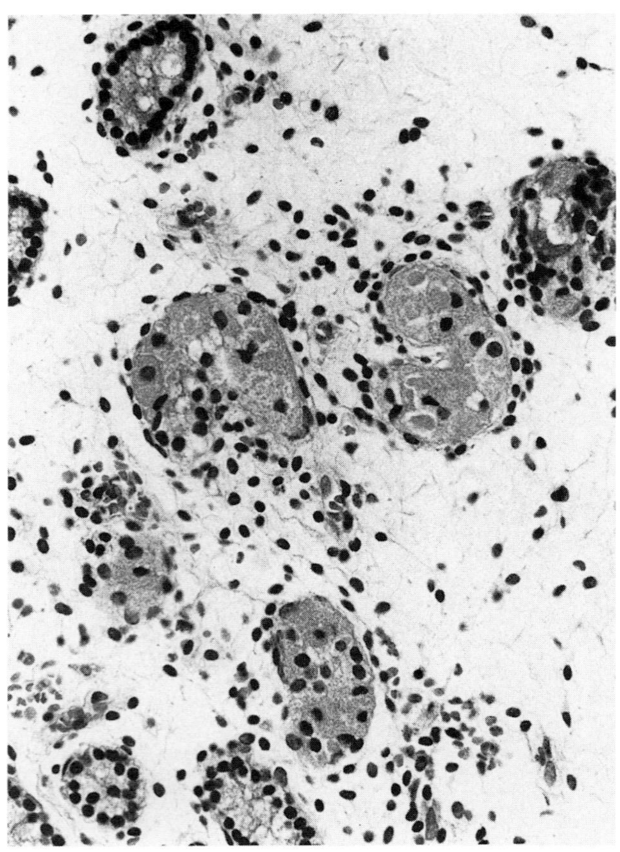

10-37. Cryptorchidism. Type III lesions in which the interstitium is expanded by edema. The cytoplasm of the Sertoli cells contains numerous eosinophilic granules of variable size.

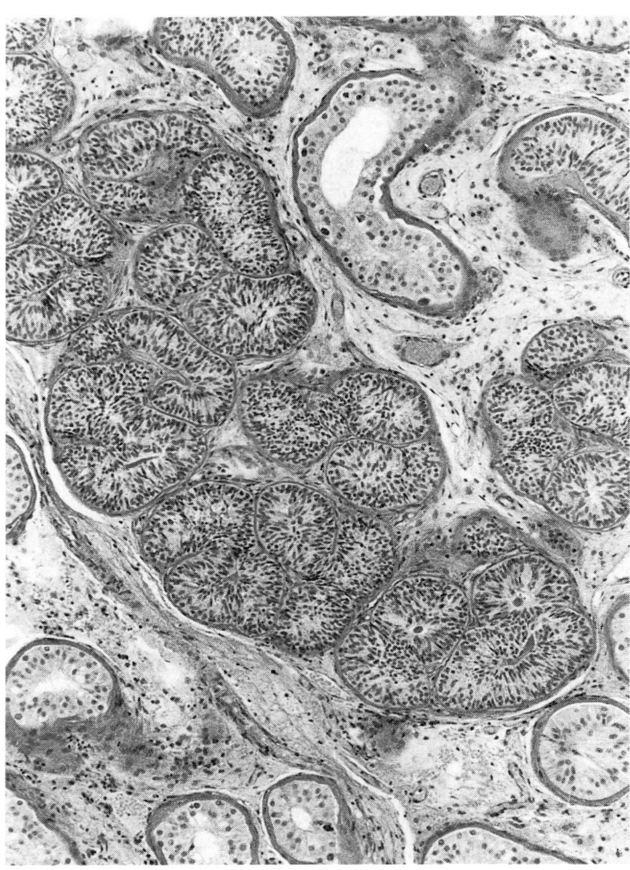

10-38. Cryptorchidism. Adult testis containing compact groups of small seminiferous tubules with pseudostratified epithelium and without lumens.

and if complete testicular descent does not occur, orchiopexy should be done.

CONGENITAL ANOMALIES ASSOCIATED WITH UNDESCENDED TESTES

Often, cryptorchidism is part of the Klinefelter's, Noonan's, Kallmann's, Prader-Willi, and prune belly syndromes. Undescended testes may also be associated with trisomies 13, 18, or 21, and the Aarskog-Scott and Rubinstein-Taybi syndromes. Cryptorchidism is more frequent in patients with omphalocele, myelomeningocele, and gastroschisis. Most cryptorchid patients have a persistent processus vaginalis and inguinal hernia; other urologic anomalies are present in 10.5% of patients and the most frequent are hypospadias, complete duplication of the urinary tract, nonobstructive ureteral dilation, kidney malrotation, and posterior urethral valves.

Sperm excretory duct anomalies occur in 36% to 79% of cryptorchid patients.[311,312] These have been classified into three types:[313]

1. *Ductal fusion anomalies* (25% of cases). These consist of anomalous fusion of the caput epididymidis to the testis or segmental atresia of the epididymis and vas deferens. This is chiefly associated with intraabdominal or high scrotal cryptorchid testes.
2. *Ductal suspension anomalies* (59% of cases). The caput epididymidis is attached to the testis while the corpus and the cauda epididymidis are separated from the testis by a mesentery. A variant consists of an excessively long cauda epididymidis that descends along the inguinal duct to the scrotum.
3. *Anomalies associated with absent or vanishing testes* (16% of cases).

COMPLICATIONS OF CRYPTORCHIDISM

The main complications of cryptorchidism are testicular cancer, infertility, testicular torsion, and psychologic problems.

Testicular cancer

Approximately 0.8% of 1-year-old males have cryptorchidism, but about 10% of testicular cancer patients have had cryptorchidism. The risk of testicular cancer in cryptorchid males is 4 to 10 times higher than that of the general population. The most frequent tumor in undescended testes is seminoma.[314,315] No matter how early it is done, orchiopexy does not decrease the risk of cancer, although it facilitates early detection since

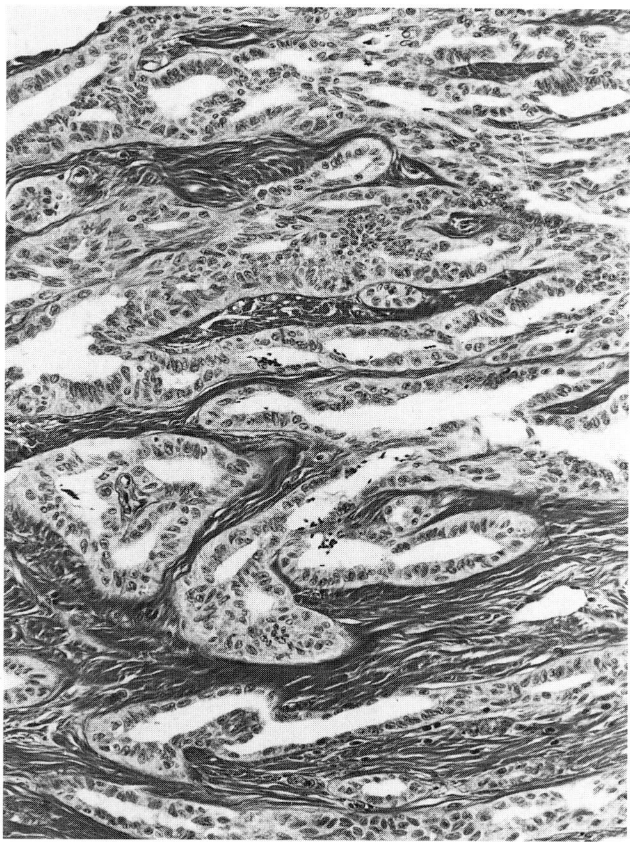

10-39. Cryptorchidism. Adult testis in which the rete testis is lined by hyperplastic tall columnar epithelium. Spermatozoa are visible in the channels of the rete testis.

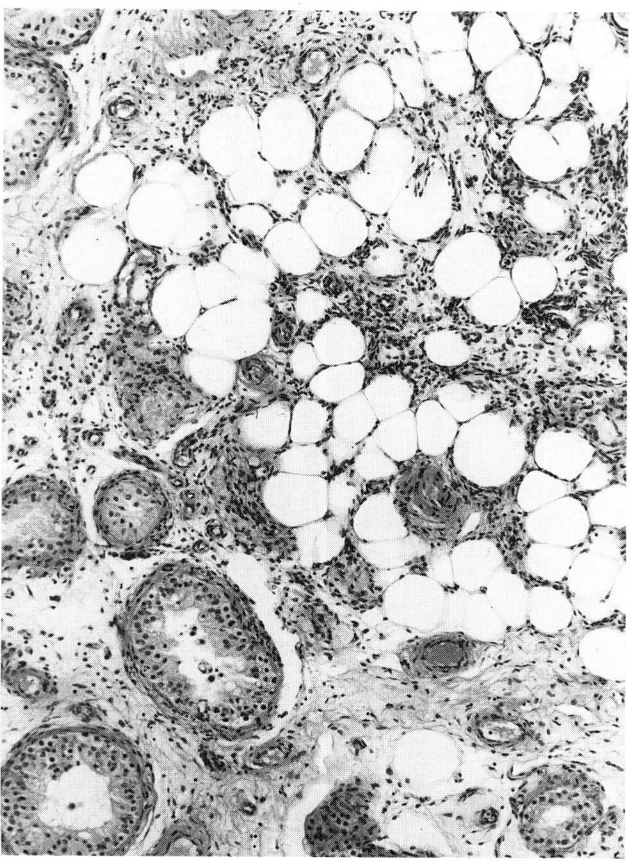

10-40. Cryptorchidism. Adult testis containing metaplastic fat cells between the seminiferous tubules and the rete testis.

the intrascrotal testis is palpable. One in five testicular tumors arises in properly descended testes contralateral to cryptorchid testes, suggesting that there is a primary testicular anomaly in cryptorchidism. Intraabdominal testes have a higher incidence of tumors[315] (Fig. 10-41).

Infertility

Infertility is the most frequent problem caused by cryptorchidism. In a series of patients seeking help with infertility, nearly 9% had had cryptorchidism.[316] Infertility is influenced by several factors, the most profound of which is bilaterality. Only 16%[317] to 25%[318] of men with bilateral cryptorchidism have normal sperm counts (20 million/ml or greater). The highest sperm counts occur with testes in the superficial inguinal pouch. Patients with bilaterally impalpable testes are usually azoospermic.[318] Fertility rates in unilateral cryptorchidism vary from 25% to 81%.[319]

The age of orchiopexy may influence fertility, although this has not been proven. In patients older than 4 years, orchiopexy does not enhance fertility.[320] The most important prognostic factor is the tubular fertility index.[321]

BENEFIT OF TESTICULAR BIOPSY IN CRYPTORCHIDISM

Testicular biopsy at orchiopexy has been useful for research, but the data provided by these biopsies are of insufficient clinical relevance to justify routine biopsy. With regard to future fertility, even in the best cases when the number of spermatogonia is nearly normal, spermatogenesis may never occur, due to deficient spermatogonium development during childhood, failure of spermatogenesis at puberty, or obstruction of sperm excretory ducts.

In childhood the chance of a biopsy finding an occult cancer is low because intratubular germ cell neoplasia is not diffusely distributed throughout the testis in children. The situation is different in adults because intratubular germ cell neoplasia is present in 2% to 3% of cases and it is diffuse.[322,323] When intratubular germ cell neoplasia is detected in a child, further examination of the testis and rebiopsy after puberty are recommended.[324] In adults, if intratubular germ cell neoplasia is unilateral, orchiectomy should be done, but if it is bilateral, radiation may be used to eradicate the intratubular germ cell neoplasia while maintaining Leydig cell function.[325]

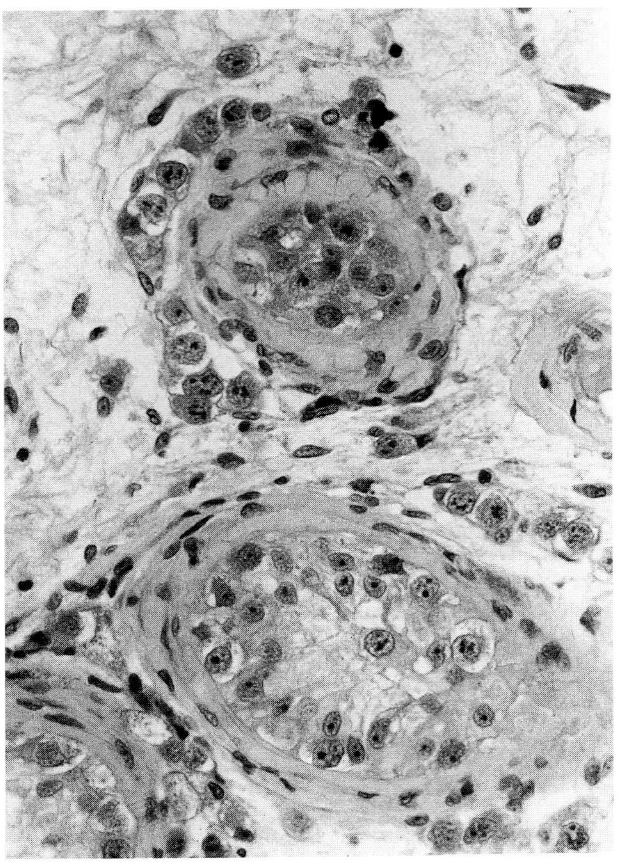

10-41. Cryptorchidism. Microinfiltrative germ cell neoplasia. Cells with pale cytoplasm and round nuclei containing one or two prominent nucleoli are present within and around seminiferous tubules.

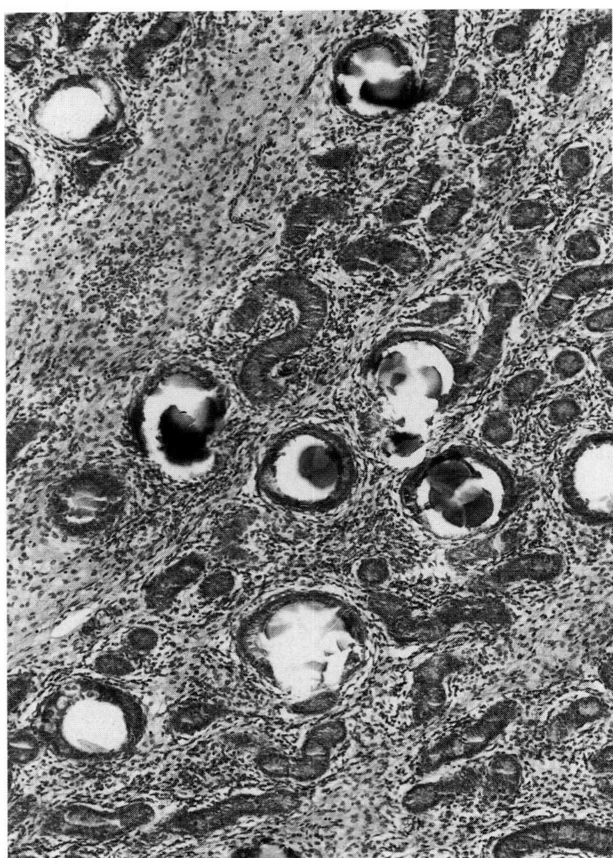

10-42. Testicular microlithiasis. Infantile cryptorchid testis with type III lesions and numerous microliths within the seminiferous tubules.

TESTICULAR MICROLITHIASIS

Testicular microlithiasis is characterized by the presence of numerous calcifications diffusely distributed through the testicular parenchyma. The number and size of these calcifications often is great enough to be detected radiographically or by ultrasound.[326] Isolated testicular microliths have been reported in undescended testes, prepubertal Klinefelter's syndrome, male pseudohermaphroditism, and rarely in otherwise normal scrotal testes. Testicular microlithiasis occurs in 0.3% of cryptorchid testes and is slightly more common in prepubertal than adult testes. In adults it usually is diagnosed when men seek help for infertility, pain, or testicular asymmetry.[327]

In the prepubertal testis, microliths are surrounded by a double layer of Sertoli cells and are up to 300 µm in diameter. When they are very large, the seminiferous epithelium may be destroyed and the microlith is surrounded by peritubular cells (Fig. 10-42). Testes with microlithiasis have subnormal mean tubular diameters and tubular fertility indices.[328] In adult testes with microliths there is incomplete spermatogenesis. Some seminiferous tubules with microliths are cystically dilated (Fig. 10-43). Microliths arise as extratubular eosinophilic bodies which mineralize and pass into the tubular lumen.[329] Microlithiasis may be a disorder of the tunica propria. Also, testicular microlithiasis occasionally is associated with pulmonary microlithiasis and with calcifications in the parasympathetic nervous system.[330]

GONADAL DYSGENESIS

Gonadal dysgenesis refers to disorders characterized by amenorrhea and streak gonads in phenotypically female patients. In adults, streak gonads are elongate masses of fibrous tissue resembling ovarian stroma (Fig. 10-44). They may contain hilar cells and rete or epithelial cords with variable degrees of maturation and may result from failure of gonadal formation, failure of gonadal differentiation to ovary, and failure of gonadal differentiation to testis. Some streak gonads contain a few ovocytes or primordial follicles, but all germ cells disappear at puberty. Patients with streak gonads have a hypoplastic uterus and fallopian tubes. Four types of gonadal dysgenesis have been described: 46XY pure, 46XX pure, 45X0, and mixed gonadal dysgenesis.

46XY GONADAL DYSGENESIS

46XY gonadal dysgenesis (Swyer's syndrome) is characterized by female phenotype, absence of Turnerian stigmata, and female external genitalia, sometimes with fused labia majora, hypertrophic clitoris, and hypospadias. The

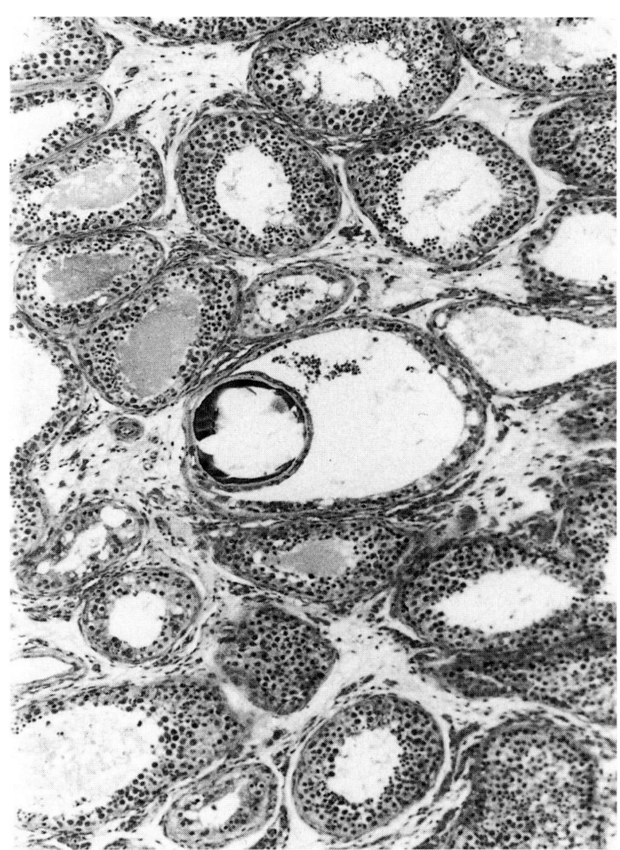

10-43. Testicular microlithiasis. Seminiferous tubules with dilated lumens in a patient biopsied for infertility. The central tubule contains a microlith which developed in the tubular wall and protrudes into the lumen.

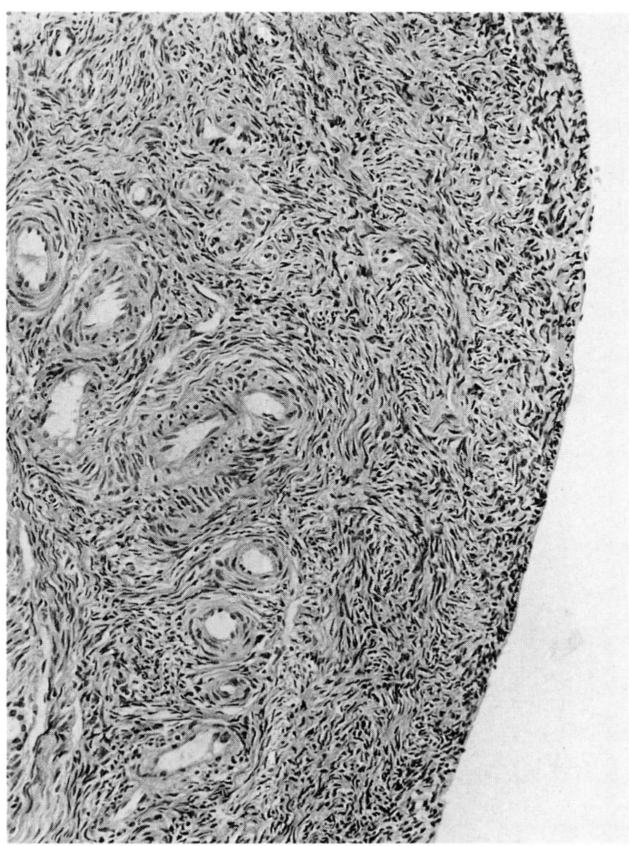

10-44. Gonadal dysgenesis. Streak of fibroblastic stroma resembling ovarian cortex.

breasts develop at puberty. Sexual infantilism persists in adulthood, and eunuchoidism and amenorrhea appear. These patients have elevated serum gonadotropin levels and low serum estradiol. Some also have myotonic dystrophia or mental retardation,[331,332] and cases with chronic renal insufficiency have been reported.[333,334]

Histologically, there are two different types of streak gonads: one composed of an ovarian-type stroma with sclerohyaline nodules, the other composed of undifferentiated stroma with numerous tubules and channels resembling the rete testis. These findings suggest that ovarian differentiation was canceled in the first type and testicular differentiation failed in the second type. The first is similar to the gonad of 45X0 Turner's syndrome while the second resembles the gonad of mixed gonadal dysgenesis.[335] The clitoromegaly may be caused by androgens secreted by hyperplastic Leydig cells in the streak gonad.

This disorder may be caused by lack of the testicular differentiation factor, the gene for which is located on the Y chromosome.[336] The gene may have been lost, inactivated, or deprived, or some cofactor involved in testicular differentiation may be lacking.[337,338] The consequence of failure would be very early gonadal alteration (sixth to eighth week of gestation). With the subsequent absence of müllerian inhibiting factor, testosterone, and dihydrotestosterone, a female phenotype would develop.

Most cases are sporadic, although the syndrome has been reported in several members of the same family,[339-341] and several forms of inheritance (X-linked, autosomal recessive, and male-limited autosomal dominant) have been proposed.[342] In addition to infertility, patients with 46XY gonadal dysgenesis have a high risk of germ cell tumors (Fig. 10-45). This risk is about 5% in the first decade of life and 25% to 30% overall.[343,344]

46XX GONADAL DYSGENESIS

Patients with 46XX gonadal dysgenesis have normal stature, well-developed external genitalia, and hypoplastic ovaries rather than streak gonads. The anomaly is usually detected when they present with primary amenorrhea or infertility. This syndrome is sporadic and familial, and it may be linked to a recessive autosomal gene or the X chromosome.[345]

45X0 GONADAL DYSGENESIS

Patients with 45X0 gonadal dysgenesis have the characteristic stigmata of Turner's syndrome, including short stature, pterygium coli, lymphedema, and cardiac malformations. The external genitalia are female and infantile; the gonads are typical streak gonads.

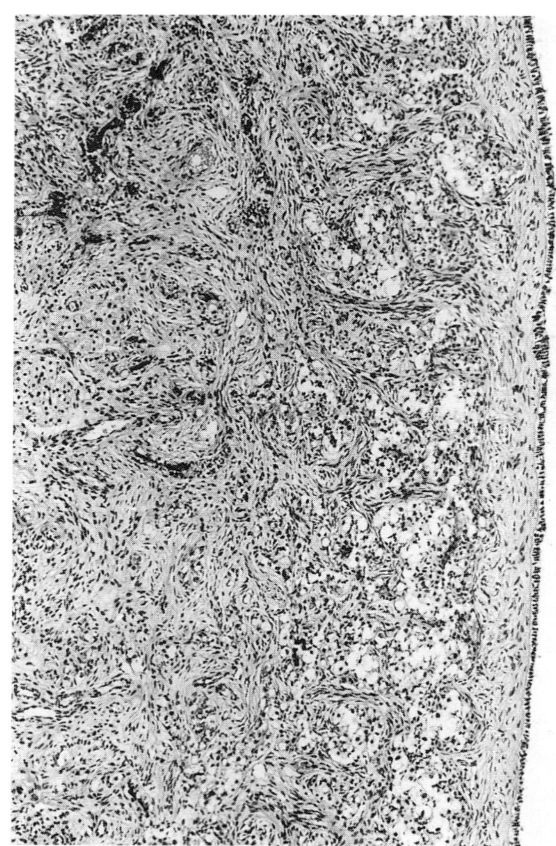

10-45. Gonadal dysgenesis. Streak gonad containing ill-defined small nodules parallel to the gonadal surface and composed of pale cells characteristic of gonadoblastoma.

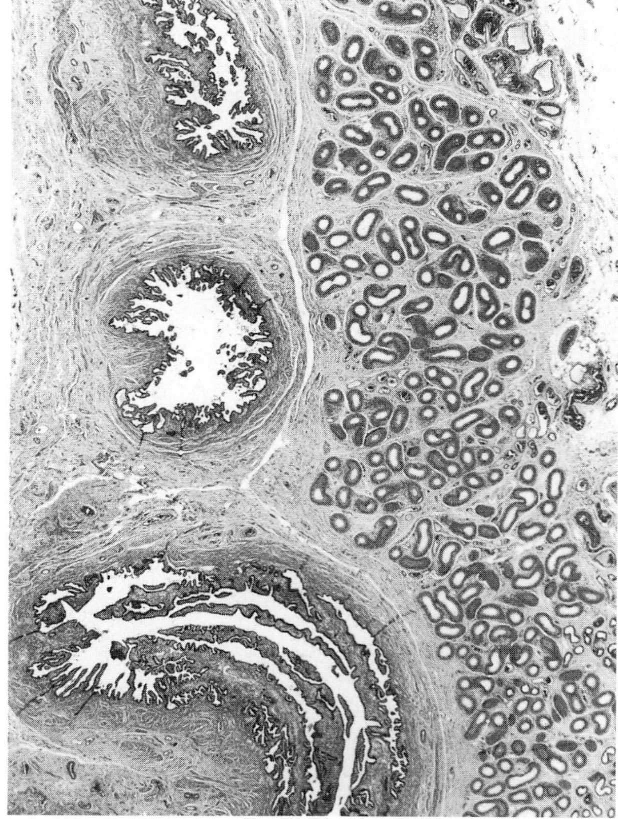

10-46. True hermaphroditism. Fallopian tube and epididymis in an adult hermaphrodite raised as a female.

MIXED GONADAL DYSGENESIS

Mixed gonadal dysgenesis is characterized by the presence of a streak gonad (alone or associated with a testis) and a contralateral testis (often cryptorchid) alone or associated with a streak gonad (see discussion on male pseudohermaphroditism with müllerian remnants in this chapter).

TRUE HERMAPHRODITISM

True hermaphroditism is a disorder of gonadal differentiation characterized by the presence in the same individual of both testicular and ovarian tissues. This condition is rare and usually difficult to diagnose, so only 25% of male hermaphrodites are diagnosed before age 20.[346] Failure to recognize this disorder may lead to surgical intervention for hernia repair or orchiopexy. Most hermaphrodites raised as males display symptoms for the first time at puberty because of breast development (95% of hermaphrodites have some degree of gynecomastia) or periodic hematuria (if they have a uterus ending in the urinary tract). Hermaphrodites raised as females come to medical attention for irregular menstruation or clitoromegaly. True hermaphroditism should be suspected in all children with ambiguous sex characteristics. The gonads of these patients are ovotestes, ovaries, or testes, in all possible combinations (Fig. 10-46).[347] About a dozen hermaphrodites raised as females have become mothers; paternity is much rarer.

Ovotestis is the most frequent gonadal type in true hermaphroditism. It is most frequent on the right side and is located in the abdomen (50% of cases), labioscrotal folds, inguinal canal, or at the external inguinal ring. The ovotestis has a bilobate or ovoid shape (Fig. 10-47). In the bilobate ovotestis the testis and ovary are connected by a pedicle, while in the ovoid ovotestis the ovarian tissue forms a crescent capping testicular parenchyma. The proportion of ovary to testis varies widely (Fig. 10-48, 10-49). At adulthood the ovarian follicles mature into corpora lutea or corpora albicantia (Fig. 10-50). The seminiferous tubules rarely develop complete spermatogenesis (Fig. 10-51). The interstitium usually contains Leydig cells.

The testis of hermaphrodites is most often on the right side (60%), located anywhere from the abdomen to the scrotum. These testes have low tubular fertility indices during childhood. After puberty the seminiferous tubules remain small, often containing only dysgenetic Sertoli cells, similar to the tubules of cryptorchid testes. Incomplete spermatogenesis has been reported in a few cases, but complete spermatogenesis is exceptional. The ovary of hermaphrodites is most frequently on the left

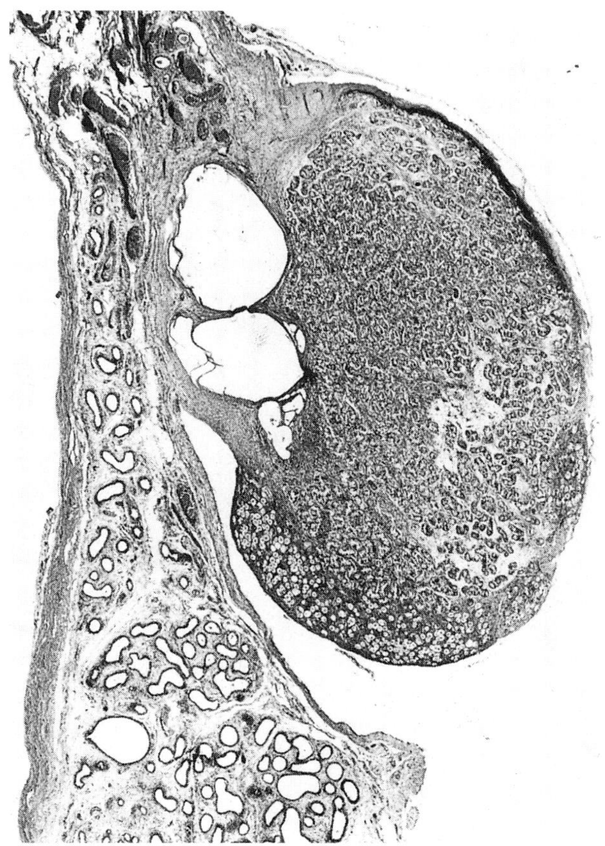

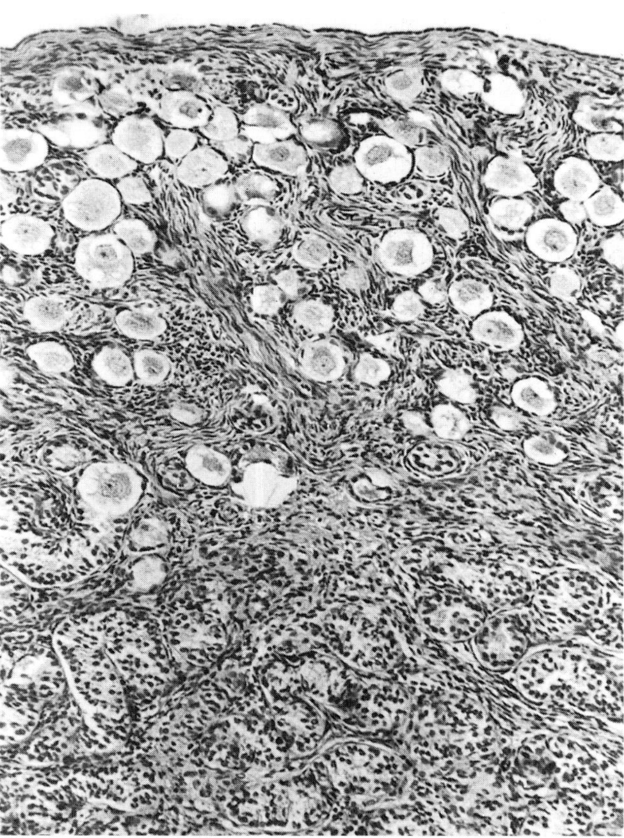

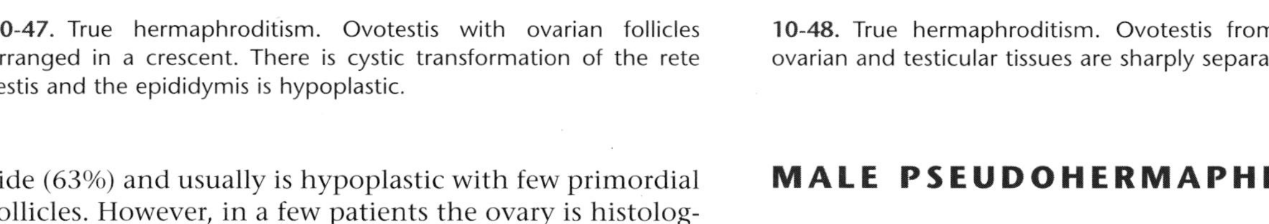

10-47. True hermaphroditism. Ovotestis with ovarian follicles arranged in a crescent. There is cystic transformation of the rete testis and the epididymis is hypoplastic.

10-48. True hermaphroditism. Ovotestis from a 2-year-old. The ovarian and testicular tissues are sharply separated.

side (63%) and usually is hypoplastic with few primordial follicles. However, in a few patients the ovary is histologically and functionally normal.

The karyotype is usually 46XX, although the following karyotypes (listed in decreasing order of frequency) have also been reported: 46XX/46XY; 46XY/47XXY; 46XY; 45X0/46XY. Because most hermaphrodites lack testicular differentiation factor, the presence of testicular tissue may result from mutation of an autosomal gene promoting testicular development.[348,349]

Management of true hermaphroditism depends on the patient's age at the time of diagnosis, the nature and location of the gonads, and the development of the external genitalia. Although bilateral castration may be justified in order to avoid the risk of neoplasia, gonadal preservation may be desirable until adulthood. In this case, if the patient is raised as a girl, puberty will occur spontaneously and there is a small chance of fertility.[350] However, the high risk of malignancy (estimated at 2.6%) should be taken into account. The most frequent tumors are gonadoblastoma, dysgerminoma, and yolk sac tumor.[347] The risk of cancer may be reduced if some precautions are taken, including removal of the testis if it has not descended and surveillance of the residual gonad with periodic ultrasound studies, especially in cases of chromosomal mosaicism.

MALE PSEUDOHERMAPHRODITISM

Normal male development requires adequate differentiation of the testes in the fetal period, synthesis and secretion of testicular hormones, and the proper response of target organs to these hormones. Antimüllerian hormone produced by Sertoli cells inhibits the development of müllerian derivatives which otherwise would form the uterus and fallopian tubes. Testosterone produced by Leydig cells stimulates differentiation of the wolffian ducts into male genital ducts. The conversion of testosterone into dihydrotestosterone by the enzyme 5 alpha reductase ensures the development of male external genitalia. Alterations in these processes may cause male pseudohermaphroditism.

IMPAIRED LEYDIG CELL ACTIVITY

Androgen synthesis deficiencies

These autosomal recessive syndromes are characterized by an error in testosterone synthesis resulting in incomplete or absent virilization. In some patients, cholesterol synthesis is also impaired and congenital adrenal hyperplasia is superimposed on the androgen deficiency. Deficient testosterone synthesis may result from abnormalities in enzymes involved in pregnenolone

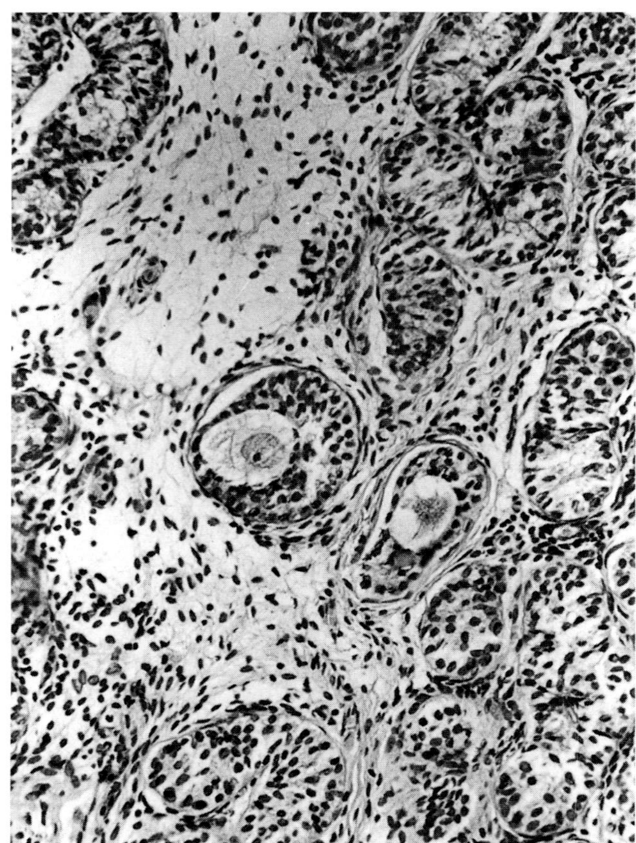

10-49. True hermaphroditism. Ovotestis with ovocytes within seminiferous tubules in the testicular parenchyma.

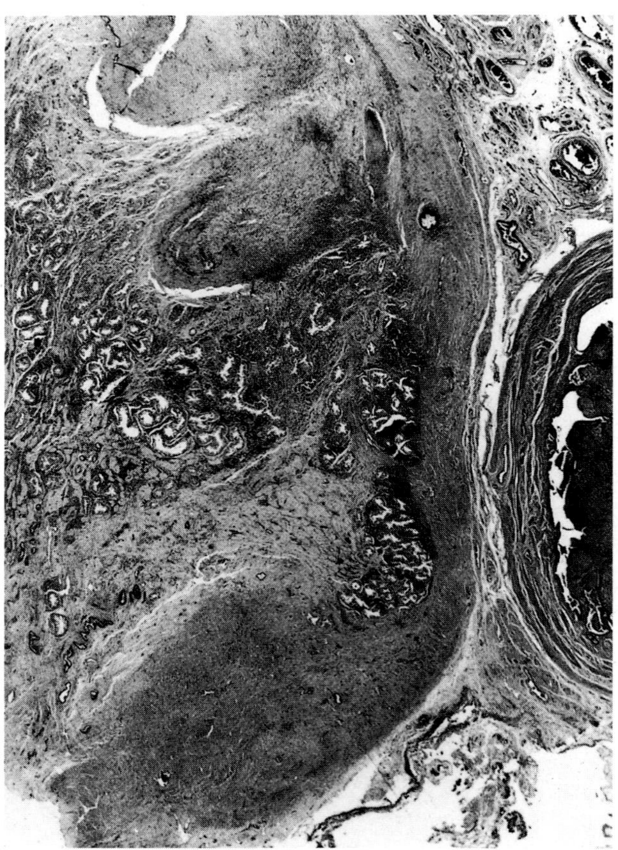

10-50. True hermaphroditism. Ovotestis with three corpora albicantia at the periphery, and seminiferous tubules with variable degrees of atrophy in the center.

formation; 3 beta hydroxysteroid dehydrogenase; 17 alpha hydroxylase; 17,20 desmolase; and 17 beta hydroxysteroid dehydrogenase (Fig. 10-52).

Pregnenolone formation deficiency. Conversion of cholesterol to pregnenolone requires the enzymes 20 alpha hydroxylase, 20,22 desmolase, and 22 alpha hydroxylase. Failure of any of these leads to deficits in cortisol, aldosterone, and testosterone. Most patients have female external genitalia and die shortly after birth. Autopsy reveals cryptorchid testes and adrenal gland lipoid hyperplasia.[351] The female phenotype persists in patients who survive.[352]

3 beta hydroxysteroid dehydrogenase deficiency. Patients with this defect have two main problems: a salt-loss syndrome produced by reduced aldosterone secretion and incomplete virilization.[353] At puberty, virilization increases and gynecomastia develops.[354]

17 alpha hydroxylase deficiency. This enzymatic defect impairs the synthesis of both cortisol and testosterone. Low cortisol levels stimulate adrenocorticotrophic hormone secretion, causing hypersecretion of aldosterone precursors and the development of hypertension and hypokalemia.[355] Patients usually have hypospadias and develop gynecomastia at puberty.[356]

17,20 desmolase deficiency. The enzyme 17,20 desmolase cleaves the side chain of 17 hydroxypregnenolone and 17 hydroxyprogesterone to form dehydroepiandrosterone and androstenedione, respectively. Varying degrees of 17,20 desmolase deficiency have been observed, resulting in varied development of the external genitalia, ranging from a female phenotype to a few instances of virilization with microphallus, bifid scrotum, and perineal hypospadias. In childhood the testes contain decreased numbers of spermatogonia.[357,358]

17 beta hydroxysteroid dehydrogenase deficiency. This enzyme transforms androstenedione into testosterone and also converts estrone into estradiol. The enzymatic defects are sex linked. Most patients have a female phenotype at birth and are raised as girls but at puberty undergo virilization. One or both testes may be cryptorchid or are located in the labia majora. Normal spermatogenesis has never been observed. The most common testicular patterns are hypoplasia or absence of germ cells and Leydig cell hyperplasia.[359] The germ cell injury was initially attributed to cryptorchidism, but it is now thought to be a primary testicular lesion because even very young patients lack germ cells.[360]

Leydig cell hypoplasia

This variant of male pseudohermaphroditism is defined by insufficient testosterone secretion[361] and

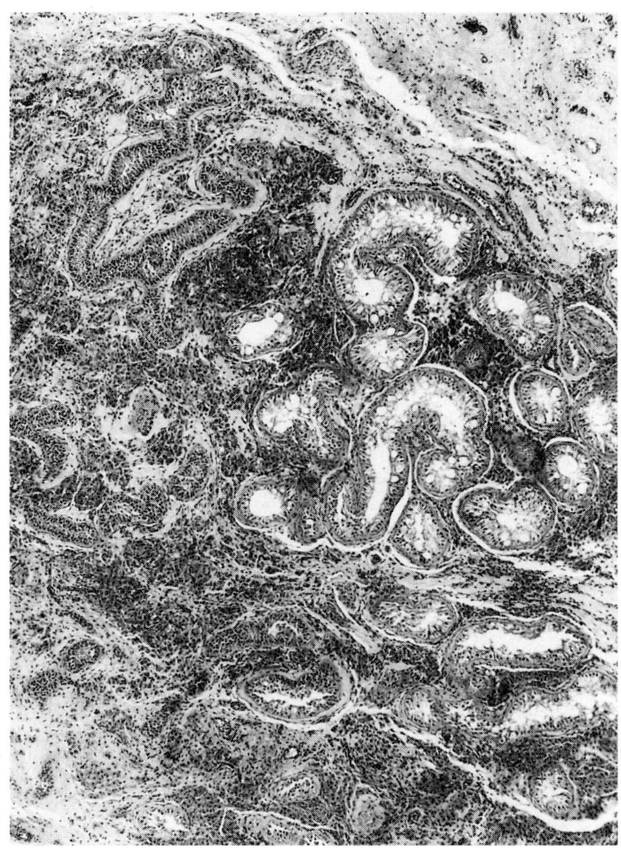

10-51. True hermaphroditism. Detail of the ovotestis in Fig 10-50. Some seminiferous tubules are slightly dilated and the apical cytoplasm of Sertoli cells is vacuolated. Some tubules are completely sclerotic or form compact cords composed of dysgenetic Sertoli cells.

the following characteristics: predominance of female external genitalia, absence of male secondary sex characteristics at puberty, absence of uterus and fallopian tubes and presence of epididymis and ductus deferens, 46XY karyotype, lack of response to the human chorionic gonadotropin stimulation test, absence of an enzymatic defect in testosterone synthesis, and small undescended testes that are gray and mucoid on section.[362-365]

The testes contain small seminiferous tubules with Sertoli cells, spermatogonia, and thickened basement membranes. Leydig cells are rare or absent, in contrast with the Leydig cell hyperplasia seen in other types of male pseudohermaphroditism, such as those arising from defects in androgen synthesis or in androgen action on peripheral tissues.[366,367] Leydig cell hypoplasia accounts for low serum testosterone levels, lack of virilization, and lack of spermatogenesis. The absence of müllerian derivatives suggests normal function of Sertoli cells, which synthesize müllerian inhibiting factor. The cause of Leydig cell hypoplasia is unknown, but the proposed possibilities include a deficit in Leydig cell precursors, a deficit in luteinizing hormone or human chorionic gonadotropin receptors, and an inadequate response of these receptors.

The age at diagnosis varies from 4 months to 35 years. The syndrome is sporadic and familial.[368,369] A mild form of Leydig cell hypoplasia has been observed in a family of brothers with consanguine parents; these patients had male external genitalia, hypergonadotropic hypogonadism, and testes with a few incompletely differentiated Leydig cells.[370,371]

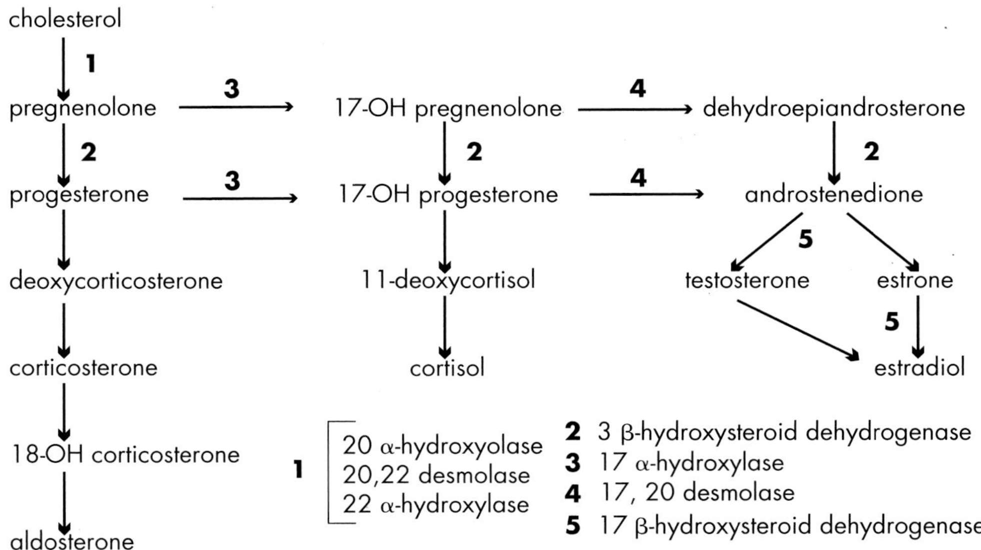

10-52. Enzymatic defects in impaired testosterone biosynthesis.

IMPAIRED ANDROGEN METABOLISM IN PERIPHERAL TISSUES

Androgen insensitivity syndromes

Resistance to androgen stimulation is the cause of several syndromes with varied phenotypes: female (testicular feminization syndrome),[372] male but ambiguous (Reifenstein's syndrome), and normal male except for gynecomastia and infertility.[373] These syndromes are caused by total or partial lack of response of the target organs to androgens,[374] due to the absence, diminution, or impairment of androgen receptors or to a postreceptor anomaly.[367] The gene for the androgen receptor is on the X chromosome and X-linked transmission occurs in two thirds of cases. The karyotype is usually 46XY, but 47XXY and several mosaicisms have been observed.[375]

Testicular feminization syndrome. This form of male pseudohermaphroditism is characterized by a female phenotype and the presence of testes. Its frequency is estimated at between 1 in 20,000 and 1 in 64,000 newborns. Complete and incomplete forms have been described.

The size of the testes varies from small to large. The testes are tan-brown and nodular with yellow specks, containing small seminiferous tubules without lumens which usually contain only Sertoli cells[376,377] (Fig. 10-53, 10-54). In one third of patients both Sertoli cells and spermatogonia are present.[378] In patients with partial androgen sensitivity the seminiferous tubules are more developed and may have some spermatogenesis. Ultrastructurally, the Sertoli cells lack Charcot-Böttcher crystals and annulate lamellae; inter-Sertoli cell specialized junctions are poorly developed, and in cryofracture studies the arrangement of intermembrane particles has an immature pattern.[379] Leydig cells are abundant, but few contain Reinke's crystalloids. Often there are areas resembling ovarian stroma in the testicular interstitium.

In about 25% of cases the testes contain grossly visible yellowish nodules that stand out from the surrounding testicular parenchyma. Histologically, these consist of small seminiferous tubules with immature Sertoli cells and hyalinized lamina propria lacking in elastic fibers (Fig. 10-55) and numerous Leydig cells among the tubules. These have been referred to as *Sertoli-Leydig cell hamartomas*.

Approximately 60% of cases have small cystic structures closely apposed to the testes, and about 80% of patients have thick bundles of smooth muscle fibers resembling myometrium near the testis. True myometrium has been demonstrated in only one case. Hypoplastic fallopian tubes are present in about one third of cases. If present the epididymis is rudimentary. Approximately 10% of the testes from patients with testicular feminization syndrome develop cancer. The frequency

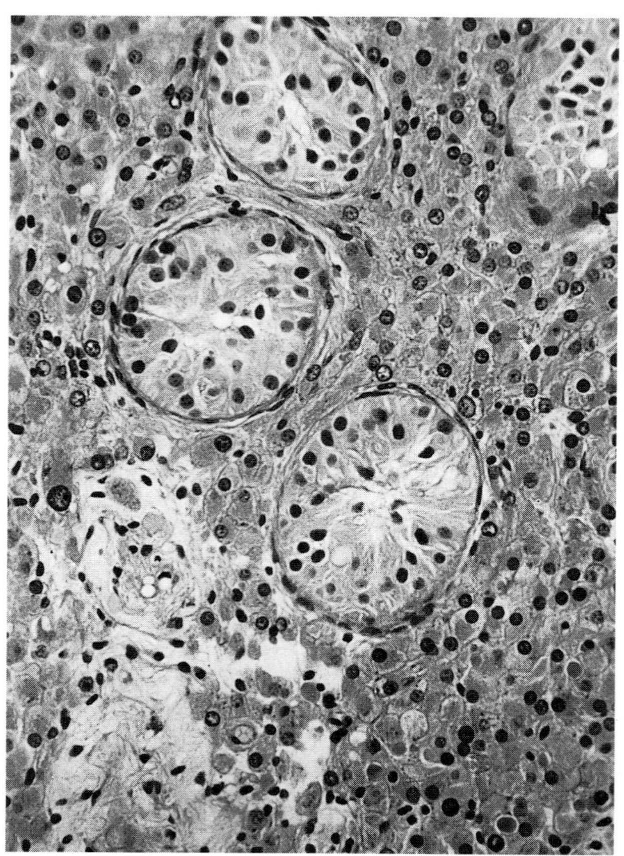

10-53. Testicular feminization syndrome. Seminiferous tubules containing only dysgenetic Sertoli cells, surrounded by Leydig cells.

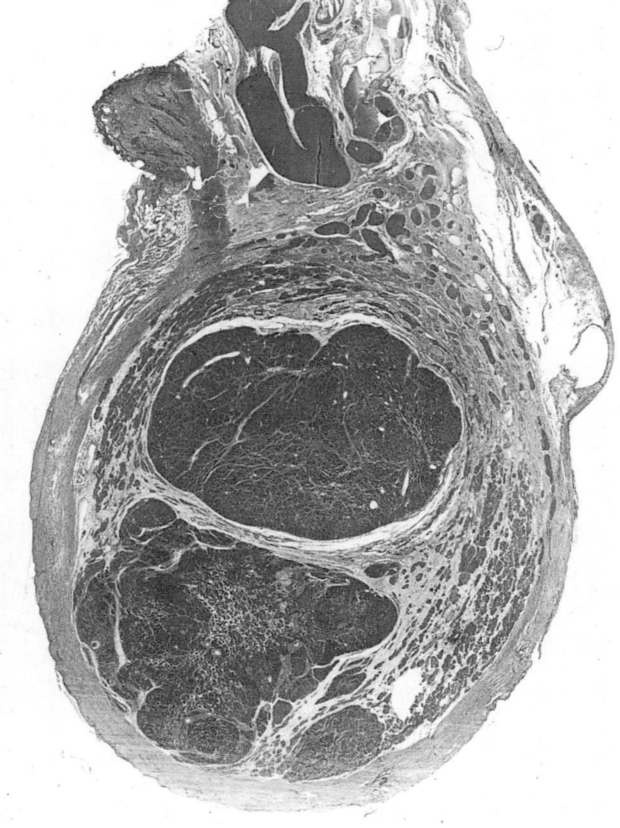

10-54. Testicular feminization syndrome. Transverse section of a testis that shows multiple, well-delimited nodules.

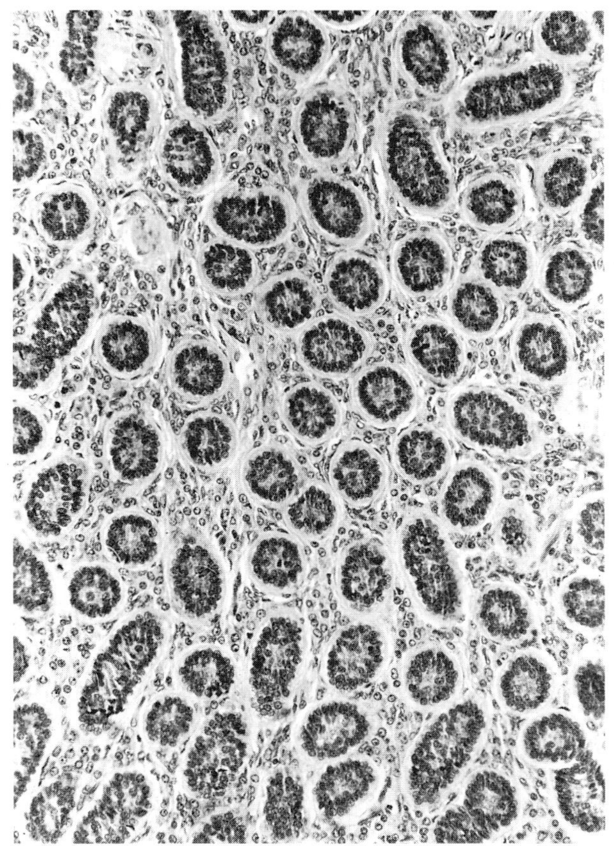

10-55. Testicular feminization syndrome. Hamartomatous proliferation of tubules surrounded by thick basement membranes and Leydig cells.

increases with age, but tumors rarely appear before puberty. These tumors include intratubular germ cell neoplasia,[377] several types of germ cell tumors, and sex cord tumors.[380] Thus, the gonads should be removed immediately after puberty.

Complete testicular feminization syndrome. Complete testicular feminization syndrome is rarely diagnosed during childhood except in patients who present with hernia, inguinal tumor, or with a family history of pseudohermaphroditism. Primary amenorrhea is the principal presentation in adults.

The testes may be in the abdomen, inguinal duct, or labia majora and, during the first years of life, may be normal histologically except for decreased tubular diameter and low tubular fertility index. After age 5, the germ cells decrease dramatically and the few remaining spermatogonia are concentrated in clusters of seminiferous tubules. The testicular interstitium contains numerous spindle cells arranged in bundles and, during the first year of life, Leydig cells with abundant eosinophilic or vacuolated cytoplasm. At puberty the patients have female external genitalia; a short, blind-ended vagina; feminine breast development; and scarce pubic and axillary hair. Serum testosterone is at the normal male level and luteinizing hormone is markedly increased.

Incomplete testicular feminization syndrome. Patients with incomplete testicular feminization differ from those with the complete form, having partial fusion of labioscrotal folds, a definitive introitus, clitoromegaly, pubic and axillary hair, male skeletal development, and poor breast development.[381-383]

There are three syndromes of androgen resistance associated with incomplete testicular feminization: Gilbert-Dreyfus syndrome, the symptoms of which include a normal male habitus, small phallus, hypospadias, incomplete development of wolffian derivatives, and gynecomastia[384]; Reifenstein's syndrome, characterized by hypospadias, weak or absent virilization, testicular atrophy, gynecomastia, azoospermia, and infertility[385]; and Rosewater syndrome, which is present in infertile men whose only abnormal feature is gynecomastia.[386]

5 alpha reductase deficiency

This disorder is a variant of male pseudohermaphroditism caused by a lack of the enzyme 5 alpha reductase and the subsequent failure of conversion of testosterone into dihydrotestosterone. The karyotype is 46XY.[387]

During childhood the patients have a clitoriform penis, bifid scrotum, urogenital sinus, and testes in either the inguinal ducts or the labioscrotal folds. Müllerian derivatives are absent. At puberty they develop a male phenotype with development of the penis and scrotum. Adults have erections, ejaculations, and normal libido; scanty body hair and beard; very small prostates; and lack temporal hairline recession (male pattern baldness). Serum levels of follicle stimulating hormone, luteinizing hormone, and testosterone are increased, but dihydrotestosterone is decreased.[388]

The testes contain small seminiferous tubules, most lacking lumens. The seminiferous epithelium usually consists of immature Sertoli cells,[389] although spermatogenesis has been observed occasionally. The testicular interstitium contains increased numbers of Leydig cells.

The disorder is autosomal recessive and has been observed in many consanguineous families from the Dominican Republic.[390]

DEFECTIVE REGRESSION OF MÜLLERIAN DUCTS

This group of male pseudohermaphrodites is characterized by the presence of both müllerian derivatives and unilateral or bilateral testicular dysgenesis. These two features depend on antimüllerian hormone gene mutations and end-organ insensitivity.[391-394]

In normal development, antimüllerian hormone is responsible for inhibition of the ipsilateral müllerian duct and collagenization of the tunica albuginea. Patients with deficient secretion of this hormone also may have androgen deficiency. Three variants of defective müllerian duct regression have been reported: mixed gonadal dysgenesis, dysgenetic male pseudohermaphroditism, and persistent müllerian duct syndrome.

Mixed gonadal dysgenesis

Mixed gonadal dysgenesis (asymmetric gonadal differentiation) is characterized by the presence of a testis

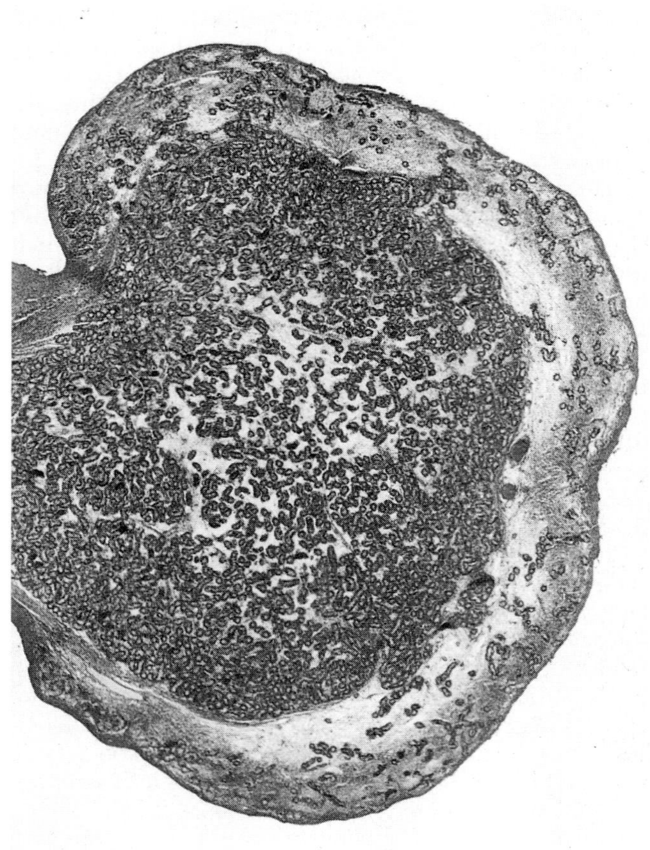

10-56. Testicular dysgenesis. The gonad comprises a central portion showing a testicular pattern and a peripheral band consisting of poorly collagenized connective tissue that contains seminiferous tubules that reach the gonadal surface.

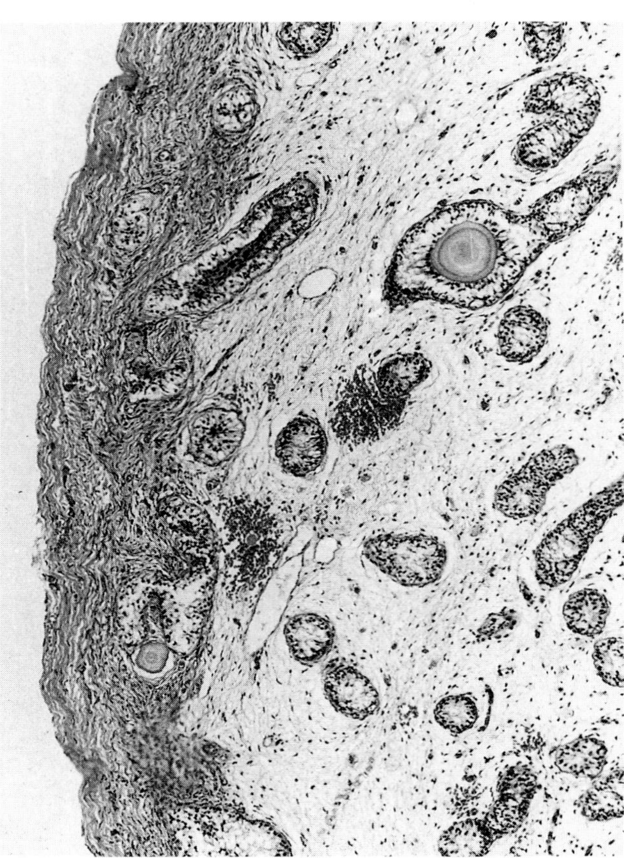

10-57. Poorly collagenized tunica albuginea containing seminiferous tubules of variable shape and size. Eosinophilic bodies can be recognized within and around the tubules.

on one side of the body and a streak gonad on the other.[395] If the gonads are intraabdominal, the labioscrotal folds may appear as either normal labia or empty scrotal sacs. In the former the syndrome cannot be recognized in the newborn, unless a peniform clitoris is present. If the gonad is descended, it is usually a testis. Müllerian derivatives such as fallopian tubes are usually associated with the streak gonad (95% of cases) but may also be associated with the testis (74%). A hypoplastic uterus and a poorly developed vagina are frequent findings.

This syndrome accounts for about 15% of intersex conditions. Some patients are raised as males, although their external genitalia are usually ambiguous as a result of fetal virilization. The penis is clitoriform and the urethra opens in the perineum. Most have cryptorchid testes and are raised as girls, becoming virilized at puberty. Infertility is a common symptom.[396] Many patients with mixed gonadal dysgenesis have Turnerian features in accord with their 45X0/46XY karyotype. Approximately 81% of patients have one Y chromosome.

The testes show the characteristic lesions of testicular dysgenesis (Fig. 10-56).[397] The tunica albuginea is variably thickened and resembles ovarian stroma with a storiform arrangement of fibers and cells. The testicular parenchyma may contain seminiferous tubules in a disorderly arrangement (Fig. 10-57). The seminiferous tubules are small and contain few germ cells during childhood. At adulthood, spermatogenesis, if present at all, is deficient. Light microscopy indicates a wide spectrum of testicular lesions, ranging from those of patients with 46XY pure gonadal dysgenesis to the testicular lesions of patients with true hermaphroditism. The testes in mixed gonadal dysgenesis are incapable of müllerian duct inhibition and allow complete differentiation of wolffian derivatives, virilization of external genitalia, and, in most cases, testicular descent. The risk of germ cell neoplasia reaches 50% in the third decade of life, usually beginning with a gonadoblastoma. The testes should be removed after puberty (Fig. 10-58, 10-59).

Dysgenetic male pseudohermaphroditism

Dysgenetic male pseudohermaphroditism is a disorder of sexual differentiation characterized by bilateral dysgenetic testes, persistent müllerian structures, and cryptorchidism. This syndrome is considered a variant of

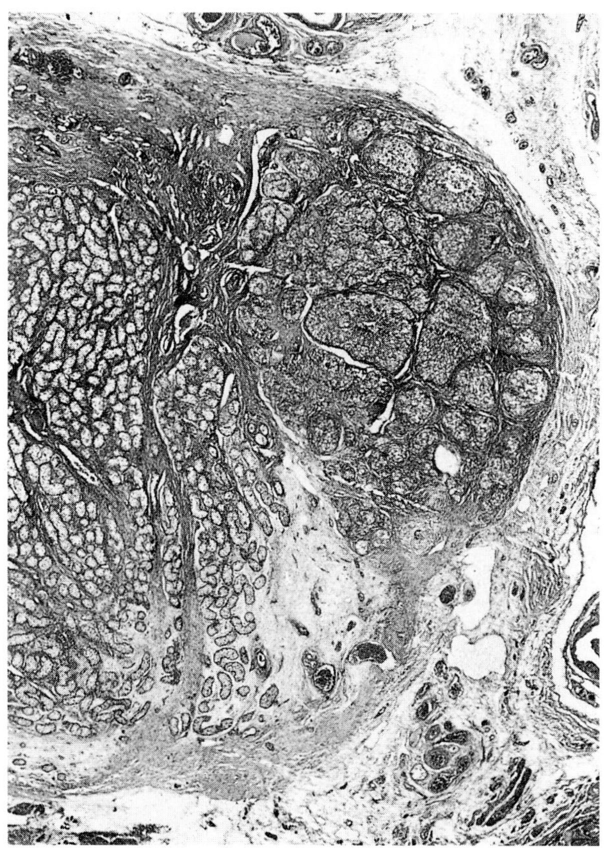

10-58. Testicular dysgenesis. A neoplasm composed of well-circumscribed small clusters of cells is present in the tunica albuginea.

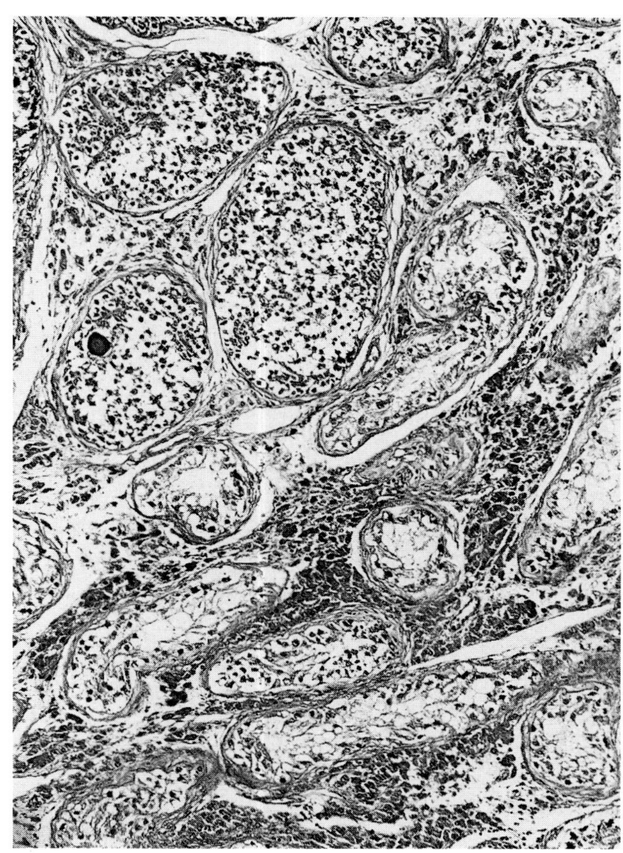

10-59. Well-circumscribed solid nests of cells form a gonadoblastoma in the periphery of a dysgenetic testis of an adult.

mixed gonadal dysgenesis.[391,398] The karyotype may be 46XY or 45/X0/46XY, and Turnerian stigmata may be present. A uterus and fallopian tubes are present, and both are usually hypoplastic (Fig. 10-60). The testes show the lesions characteristic of testicular dysgenesis, with few germ cells during childhood. In adults, spermatogenesis is poorly developed and the testicular interstitium shows Leydig cell hyperplasia.

Persistent müllerian ducts syndrome

Persistent müllerian ducts syndrome has many names, including *male with uterus, tubular hermaphroditism, persistent oviduct syndrome*, and *hernia uteri inguinalis*.[399] It is a rare form of pseudohermaphroditism with müllerian derivatives in an otherwise phenotypically normal male, and is the most characteristic form of isolated antimüllerian hormone deficiency.

Although the external genitalia are male, one (35% of cases) or both testes (75% of cases) are cryptorchid. The syndrome usually also includes inguinal hernia contralateral to the undescended testis, with a uterus and fallopian tubes within the hernia sac (Fig. 10-61).[400] Several cases with transverse testicular ectopia with persistent müllerian duct structures have been reported.[401,402] Patients usually have inguinal hernia, but others have cryptorchidism, infertility,[403] and testicular tumor.[404]

In childhood the testes have a low tubular fertility index and decreased tubular diameter. In adults the tunica albuginea is variably thickened, contains connective tissue resembling ovarian stroma, and may contain tubular structures, alterations typical of testicular dysgenesis. The seminiferous tubules are usually atrophic and hyalinized. Tubules with reduced spermatogenesis or patterns suggesting mixed atrophy (seminiferous tubules with spermatogenesis intermingled with Sertoli cell–only tubules) have also been reported. The Leydig cells appear hyperplastic. Azoospermia or oligozoospermia are common and paternity is exceptional.

The syndrome is sporadic or familial with autosomal recessive or X-linked inheritance.[405,406] These patients have a higher risk of testicular tumors than that attributed to cryptorchidism,[407] and all types of germ cell tumors have been observed.[408]

OTHER FORMS OF MALE PSEUDOHERMAPHRODITISM

Many dysmorphic syndromes are associated with incomplete virilization of the external genitalia. The best known are Smith-Lemli-Opitz syndrome, characterized by microcephaly, cleft palate, and hypospadias; Meckel's syndrome, characterized by encephalocele, microphthalmia, cleft palate, and hypospadias; Opitz's syndrome,

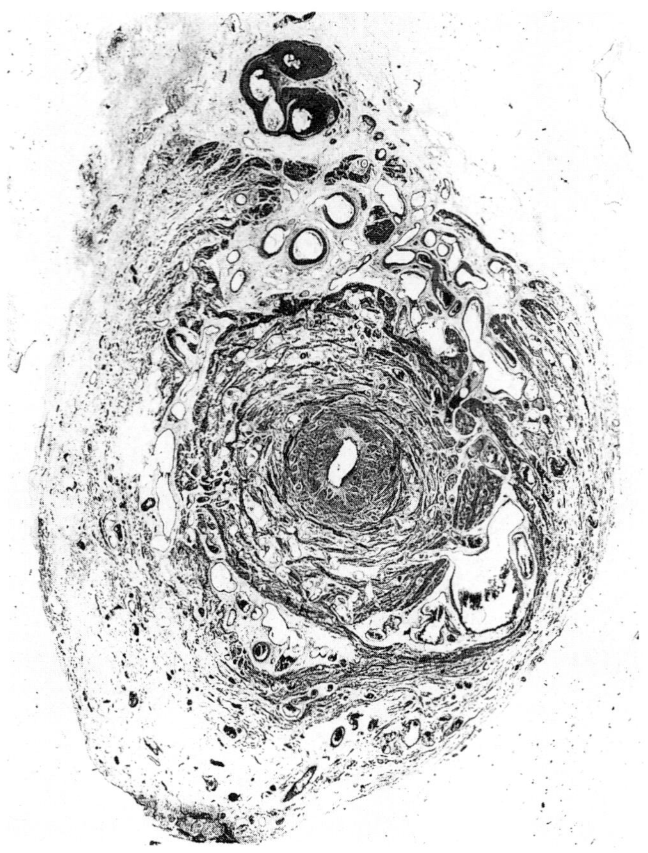

10-60. Dysgenetic male pseudohermaphroditism. Transverse section of a hypoplastic uterus. Its tunica adventitia contains a convoluted vas deferens.

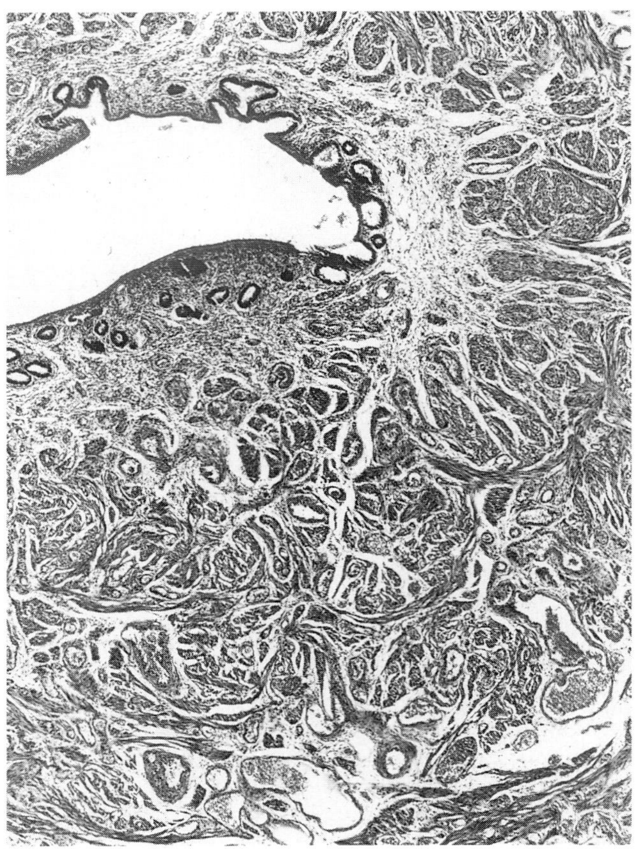

10-61. Persistent müllerian ducts syndrome. Uterine wall showing an atrophic endometrium and a hypoplastic myometrium in a hernia sac.

characterized by hypertelorism and hypospadias; branchio-skeletal-genital syndrome; Down syndrome and other trisomies; and Denis-Drash syndrome.

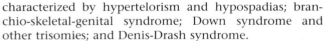

In Denis-Drash syndrome, male pseudohermaphroditism is associated with nephroblastoma and renal insufficiency.[409] The pseudohermaphroditism is usually either mixed gonadal dysgenesis, dysgenetic male pseudohermaphroditism, 46XY pure gonadal dysgenesis, or true hermaphroditism.[410] The most common nephropathy is diffuse mesangial sclerosis.[411] This syndrome is explained by the relationship of the kidney and testis during embryonal development and suggests an anomaly in the urogenital ridge.[412]

INFERTILITY

TESTICULAR BIOPSY

Interest in testicular biopsy to diagnose infertility arose in the 1940s[413,414] and most of the diagnostic terms used today were created then.[415] These terms are usually descriptive and, except for a few of them (normal testes, Sertoli cell–only tubules, tubular hyalinization, for example), do not specify the degree of tubular abnormality that is evaluated by each pathologist subjectively. The terms *maturation arrest* and *hypospermatogenesis* have been applied to biopsies in more than 50% of cases of infertility,[416-418] but the criteria for these vary widely among pathologists.

Two forms of maturation arrest have been described: spermatogenic arrest; and spermatocytic arrest, or its equivalent, meiotic arrest. True spermatogenic arrest is rare because germ cell maturation usually does not arrest at the level of a defined germ cell type.[419] To avoid confusion the term *irregular hypospermatogenesis* has been proposed[420] for testicular biopsies with decreased numbers of germ cells, subclassified as slight, moderate, or severe. However, this diagnosis is little help to clinicians. The reported frequency of spermatocytic (meiotic) arrest in infertile men varies from 12%[421] to 32.1%[422] and is present in one or both testes of about 18% of oligozoospermic or azoospermic patients.[423] If it is observed in only one testis, the contralateral testis may show histologic changes ranging from normal spermatogenesis to hyalinized tubules.

Disorganization of the seminiferous epithelium is another frequent diagnosis in testicular biopsy studies,[415,424,425] but this term is rejected by many pathologists. Actual disorganization of the seminiferous epithelium is unlikely and has not been demonstrated in ultrastructural studies.

In most cases the apparent disorganization is an artifact induced by handling or fixation.[426]

The term *tubular blockage* was introduced by Meinhard and co-workers[425] for testes with at least 50% of seminiferous tubules devoid of central lumens and showing spatial disorganization of germ cells. This morphology was found in 28% of testicular biopsies from infertile men, mainly those with obstructive azoospermia.[427] Although this appearance can result from improper fixation,[428] the accumulation of Sertoli cells and immature germ cells in the centers of tubules suggests a specific lesion, a variant of germ cell sloughing.

This diagnostic confusion decreased the interest and trust of urologists and andrologists in the study of testicular biopsies. Subsequent studies attempted to correlate semen spermatozoa concentration with testicular size and biochemical findings, such as serum levels of follicle stimulating hormone, and testicular biopsy was undertaken only in a limited number of oligozoospermic and azoospermic patients.[426,429,430] However, these studies were also discouraging because follicle stimulating hormone was found to correlate poorly with numbers of spermatozoa in the semen but better with numbers of spermatogonia in the seminiferous tubules,[431] and normal numbers of spermatozoa can be produced by relatively small testes while some large testes have no spermatogenesis.[432]

The development of morphometry caused a resurgence of interest in biopsies, and many semiquantitative[420,433-435] and quantitative[436-441] studies were carried out. The greatest achievements of these studies were enhancement of the reproducibility of results and better evaluation of the reversibility of lesions. Morphometry emerged as the best method to objectively evaluate the seminiferous epithelium.[442] The scoring method of Johnsen,[434] estimation of the germ cell/Sertoli cell ratio for each germ cell type,[437] and calculation of germ cell number per unit length of seminiferous tubules[436] are reliable and useful.

Several methods are available to evaluate the Leydig cell population, including the mean number of Leydig cells per seminiferous tubule and per Leydig cell cluster, the mean number of Leydig cell clusters per seminiferous tubule, the ratio of Leydig cell area to seminiferous tubule area,[443] and the ratio of Leydig cells to Sertoli cells.[444] These methods have shown that the appearance of Leydig cell hyperplasia described in many conditions is false and that true Leydig cell hyperplasia is extremely rare.

Optimal interpretation of testicular biopsies depends on the surgical technique by which the tissue sample is taken, the care and delicacy with which the specimen is manipulated, and proper fixation and processing of the tissue. The size of the biopsy should not be greater than a grain of rice; that is, no diameter should be greater than 3 mm. This amounts to about 0.12% of the testicular volume (normal volume is approximately 20 ml). The biopsy should be bilateral because in more than 28% of patients the findings differ between the testes. At the time of the biopsy the testicular axes should be measured as the basis of quantitative studies. The tissue should be taken opposite to the rete testis through a 4 to 5 mm incision in the tunica albuginea. The parenchyma herniates through the incision and can be carefully snipped off. If only light microscopy is to be performed, the specimen should be fixed in Bouin's fluid for 24 hours. The examination of testicular biopsies includes qualitative and quantitative evaluation of the testis and correlation between the biopsy and spermiogram.

QUALITATIVE AND QUANTITATIVE EVALUATION

Light microscopic study immediately reveals whether the lesion is focal or diffuse. If focal the percentage of tubules showing each lesion (Sertoli cell–only, hyalinization, tubular hypoplasia, etc.) should be calculated. It is useful to evaluate elastic fibers with a special stain because this highlights groups of small tubules that may be missed with hematoxylin and eosin. About 20 to 30 tubular profiles should be studied (this is usually possible when five or six histological sections are available). The diameter of each tubular profile should be measured, and the numbers of spermatogonia, primary spermatocytes, young spermatids (also called *round spermatids* or S_a + S_b *spermatids*), mature spermatids (also called *elongated* or S_c + S_d *spermatids*), Sertoli cells, and, in some cases, peritubular cells counted. The presence of tubular diverticula,[445,446] the maturation of Sertoli cells, and morphologic anomalies in germ cells, principally spermatids, should also be noted. Evaluation of the testicular interstitium should include the number of Leydig cells per tubule (or number of Leydig cell clusters per tubule), the presence of angiectasis (phlebectasis), and the occurrence of peritubular or perivascular inflammation. Normal values are tabulated in Table 10-6. For a clear and rapid understanding of the results, data can be presented using cartesian axes (see Fig. 10-69, 10-78).

TABLE 10-6.
TESTICULAR PARAMETERS IN NORMAL ADULT TESTES

Values per cross-sectioned tubule	Means ± SD
SEMINIFEROUS TUBULES	
Mean tubular diameter (μm)	193 ± 8
Number of spermatogonia	21 ± 4
Number of primary spermatocytes	31 ± 6
Number of young (S_a + S_b) spermatids	37 ± 7
Number of mature (S_c + S_d) spermatids	25 ± 4
Number of Sertoli cells	10.4 ± 2
Number of Sertoli cell vacuoles	0.8 ± 0.3
Lamina propria thickness (μm)	5.3 ± 1
Number of peritubular cells	21 ± 4
TESTICULAR INTERSTITIUM	
Number of Leydig cell clusters per tubule	1.2 ± 0.3
Number of Leydig cells per tubule	5 ± 0.2

COMMON LESIONS

The most frequently observed lesions are Sertoli cell–only tubules, tubular hyalinization, alterations in spermatogenesis in either the adluminal or basal compartments of seminiferous tubules, and mixed tubular atrophy.

Sertoli cell–only syndrome

Sertoli cell–only syndrome includes all azoospermias in which the seminiferous epithelium consists only of Sertoli cells and, occasionally, isolated spermatogonia. To better understand this syndrome, it is necessary to consider the morphological and functional changes induced in the Sertoli cell by hypophyseal gonadotropin secretion during puberty. During childhood, Sertoli cells are pseudostratified and their nuclei are dark, small, and round or elongate, with regular outlines and one or two small peripherally placed nucleoli. The cytoplasm lacks specialized organelles.[447] Adult Sertoli cells have characteristically pale, triangular nuclei with irregular, indented outlines. The nucleoli are large and have tripartite structures. The cytoplasm contains abundant smooth endoplasmic reticulum, and specialized structures including annulate lamellae, Charcot-Böttcher crystals, and there are specialized junctional complexes with other Sertoli cells. The pubertal increase in both length and width of the seminiferous tubules replaces the infantile pseudostratified pattern with a simple columnar distribution.

Five variants of Sertoli cell–only syndrome are identified by Sertoli cell morphology, degree of development of the seminiferous tubules, and the presence or absence of interstitial lesions.[448] These variants are designated by the appearance of the predominant Sertoli cell population: immature Sertoli cells, dysgenetic Sertoli cells, adult Sertoli cells, involuting Sertoli cells, and dedifferentiated Sertoli cells. Each type is associated with other tubular and interstitial alterations (Table 10-7).

TABLE 10-7.
DIFFERENTIAL DIAGNOSIS IN THE SERTOLI CELL–ONLY SYNDROME

TESTIS PATTERN	VARIANTS OF THE SERTOLI CELL–ONLY SYNDROME				
	Immature Sertoli cells	**Dysgenetic Sertoli cells**	**Adult Sertoli cells**	**Involuting Sertoli cells**	**Dedifferentiated Sertoli cells**
Tubular diameter	Very decreased	Decreased	Decreased	Decreased	Decreased
Tubular lumen	Small or absent	Small or absent	Normal	Normal	Normal
Lamina propria thickness	Thin	Enlarged	Normal or enlarged	Normal or enlarged	Enlarged
Elastic fibers in lamina propria	Absent	Decreased	Normal	Normal	Normal
Sertoli cells					
Number	Very increased	Increased	Normal or increased	Normal or increased	Increased
Distribution	Pseudostratified	Pseudostratified	Columnar	Columnar	Columnar or pseudostratified
Nuclear shape	Ovoid	Round or ovoid	Triangular	Lobated	Round
Nuclear outline	Regular	Regular	Few indented	Very indented	Regular
Chromatin	Dark	Pale with granules	Pale	Pale	Pale
Nucleolus	Small, peripheral	Developed, central	Developed, central	Developed, central	Small, central, or peripheral
Vacuoles	Absent	Present	Present	Abundant	Abundant
Lipids	Absent	Absent	Present	Abundant	Abundant
Vimentin filaments	Basal	Basal	Basal and perinuclear	Basal and perinuclear	Basal
Interstitium	Scanty	Increased	Normal	Normal/fibrosis	Fibrosis
Leydig cells	Absent	Pleomorphic, vacuolated, increased or decreased	Normal	Decreased, many lipofuscin granules	Decreased, many lipofuscin granules
Clinical symptoms	Hypogonadotropic hypogonadism	Infertility	Infertility, orchitis	Infertility, hypergonadotropic hypogonadism, chemotherapy or radiotherapy	Treatment with estrogens, antiandrogens or cisplatinum, chronic hepatopathy

The most frequent types of Sertoli cell–only syndrome in infertility patients are dysgenetic Sertoli cells, adult Sertoli cells, and involuting Sertoli cells. The clinical manifestations are similar, including normal external genitalia, well-developed secondary male characteristics, azoospermia, elevated serum follicle stimulating hormone level, normal or elevated serum luteinizing hormone level, and normal or slightly low testosterone. These clinical and histologic features were long thought to constitute a single syndrome, del Castillo's syndrome, but recent ultrastructural, histochemical, immunohistochemical, and cytogenetic studies have shown that this results from a variety of syndromes that may have primary or secondary causes (Table 10-7).[449-453]

Some patients with either the adult Sertoli cell or dysgenetic Sertoli cell variants have a few spermatozoa in their spermiograms. This discrepancy between the oligozoospermia and the biopsy histology is caused by mixed testicular atrophy. As a result of sampling error, testicular biopsy often is not representative of the testicular pathology in these cases.

Sertoli cell–only syndrome with immature Sertoli cells. The Sertoli cells in adult testes with this variant of Sertoli cell–only syndrome have an immature prepubertal appearance with pseudostratification. The number of cells per tubular profile is greater than normal. Spermatogonia, if present, are not capable of producing primary spermatocytes. Other tubular and interstitial features suggest immaturity, including small tubular diameters (less than 80 µm), tubules lacking central lumens, thin lamina propria lacking elastic fibers, and interstitium lacking mature Leydig cells.[454-456]

This syndrome is caused by deficiency of both follicle stimulating hormone and luteinizing hormone. This deficit begins in childhood and is responsible for the lack of maturation of the Sertoli cells, tubular walls, and interstitium. Subsequently there is no renewal or differentiation of germ cells, and these eventually disappear. When these patients have been treated with hormones, the biopsy may show thickening and hyalinization of the tubular basement membrane.

Sertoli cell–only syndrome with dysgenetic Sertoli cells. Dysgenetic Sertoli cells begin pubertal differentiation but variably deviate from normal maturation so that the morphology of dysgenetic Sertoli cells differs among tubules and even among Sertoli cells within the same tubule. Nuclei usually have both mature features (pale chromatin and a centrally located, tripartite nucleolus) and features of immaturity (ovoid or round shape; regular outline; and small, dense chromatin granules).[457] Most tubules lack central lumens or have very small ones. The number of Sertoli cells is elevated and the mean tubular diameter is below 150 µm (Fig. 10-62). The tubular wall contains few elastic fibers[458] and is variably hyalinized. The interstitium contains a variable number of Leydig cells (normal, decreased, or apparently increased), many of which are pleomorphic with abundant paracrystalline inclusions.[459]

Most patients have normal or slightly subnormal testosterone levels and elevated levels of follicle stimulating hormone and luteinizing hormone. This syndrome can be observed in men with cryptorchid testes, men with idiopathic infertility,[460] and men with Y chromosome anomalies.[461]

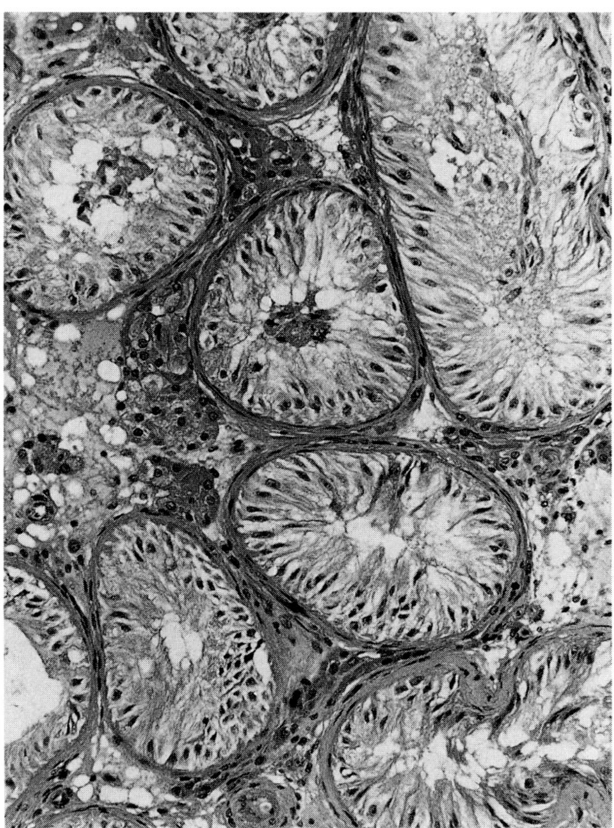

10-62. Sertoli cell–only syndrome with dysgenetic Sertoli cells. Seminiferous tubules show a slightly thickened tunica propria. The Sertoli cells are increased in number and have elongate nuclei and abundant apical cytoplasm.

Sertoli cell–only syndrome with mature Sertoli cells. In this variant most Sertoli cells appear mature, but they are present in increased numbers (14 ± 0.8 Sertoli cells per tubular profile). The seminiferous tubules have small diameters, but larger than in the two variants described above, and central lumens are visible. The cytoplasm contains abundant vacuoles that communicate with the tubular lumen (Fig. 10-63). The lateral cell surfaces have many infoldings and extensive specialized junctions with other Sertoli cells (from the basement membrane to the apical cytoplasmic portion). Lipid droplets derived from phagocytosis of spermatid tubulobulbar complexes and dead germ cells are scant.[450] Vimentin filaments are abundant in the basal and perinuclear cytoplasm.[462] The lamina propria is normal or slightly thickened. Leydig cells are normal.

Serum testosterone levels are normal or nearly normal and follicle stimulating hormone and luteinizing hormone levels are elevated.[463-465] This syndrome is probably caused by failure of migration of primordial germ cells from the primitive yolk sac to the gonadal ridge.[466] A similar histologic pattern can be induced experimentally by inhibiting germ cell migration with busulfan. A

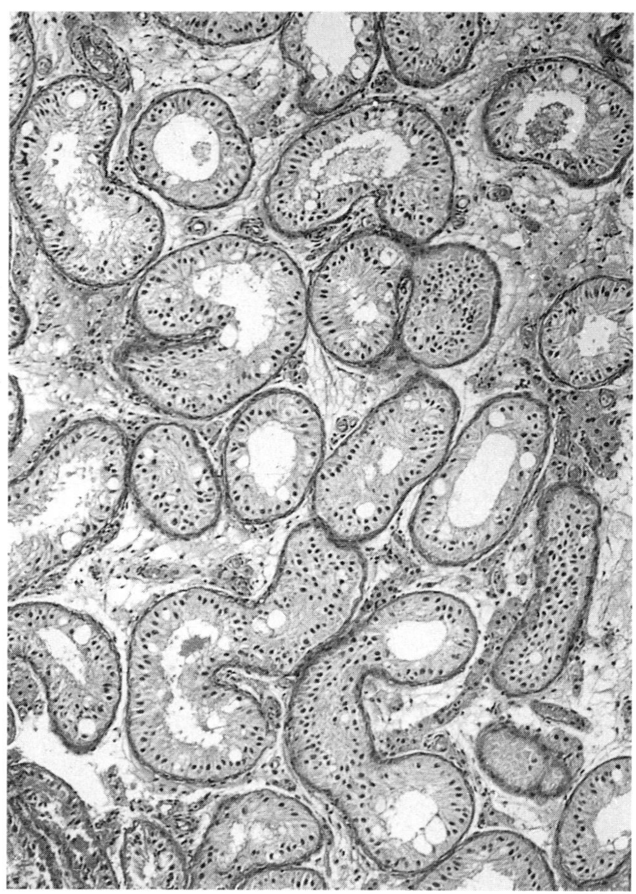

10-63. Sertoli cell–only syndrome with mature Sertoli cells. The seminiferous tubules are lined by adult Sertoli cells, many with cytoplasmic vacuoles.

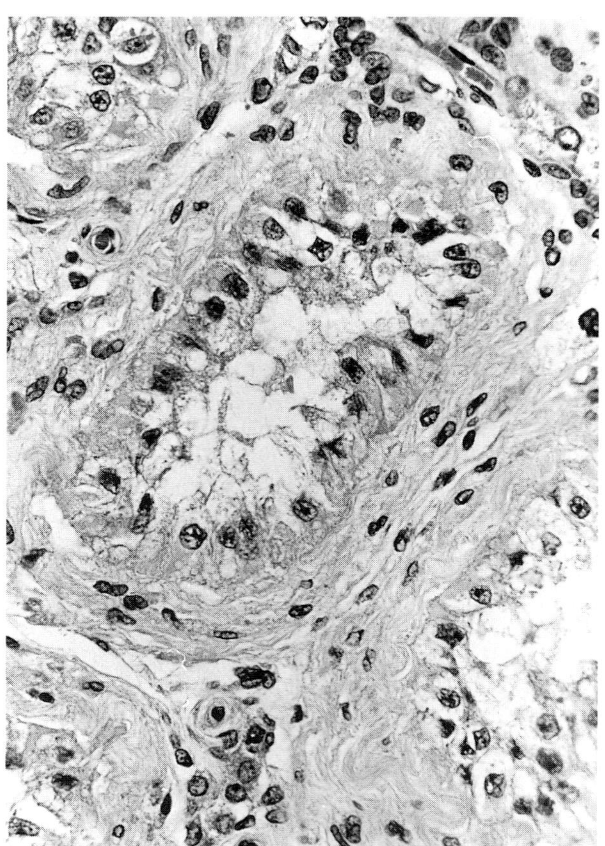

10-64. Sertoli cell–only syndrome with involuting Sertoli cells. The Sertoli cell nuclei are hyperchromatic and have irregular outlines.

history of viral orchitis in some patients suggests a viral etiology for this syndrome.

Sertoli cell–only syndrome with involuting Sertoli cells. Testes with this variant of Sertoli cell–only syndrome apparently are beginning to atrophy. This atrophy involves the germ cells, which disappear, and the Sertoli cells, which undergo atrophic changes. Many Sertoli cell nuclei have lobulated shapes with very irregular outlines and coarse chromatin granules and the nucleoli are less prominent than normal. The seminiferous tubules have central lumens, decreased diameters, and variable thickening of the basement membrane (Fig. 10-64). Elastic fibers are present in normal amounts. The Leydig cells are variably involuted.

This syndrome has multiple causes, including irradiation, or toxic therapies such as cancer chemotherapy or treatment for nephrotic syndrome.[467] It is not usually possible to determine the etiology from the appearance of the biopsy. The changes in the tubular walls are more pronounced in patients with histories of cyclophosphamide treatment, combination chemotherapy, or radiotherapy. The testicular interstitium can be fibrotic in patients treated with cisplatinum or cyclophosphamide.[468]

Sertoli cell–only syndrome with dedifferentiated Sertoli cells. The presence of immature-appearing Sertoli cells in otherwise mature tubules is the most striking feature of this variant. The Sertoli cells appear abnormally numerous due to shortening of the tubular length, and their nuclei are either round or elongate. The round nuclei have single, small, central or peripheral nucleoli; the elongate nuclei have dense chromatin masses and small peripheral nucleoli.

The tubular wall is thickened and contains elastic fibers, increased amounts of collagen fibers, and elevated numbers of peritubular cells as a result of tubular shortening. The mean tubular diameter is markedly decreased (less than 150 μm). The testicular interstitium contains few Leydig cells, and these appear dedifferentiated or contain increased amounts of lipofuscin.

This variant has been observed in biopsies from patients receiving hormonal treatment for prostatic cancer, estrogen treatment for transsexuality, and cancer chemotherapy with cisplatinum. There is a correlation between the degree of Sertoli cell dedifferentiation and the dose and the time of treatment with estrogen or antiandrogen. Brief treatment induces germ cell loss and inconspicuous Sertoli cell changes; long-term treatment causes pronounced Sertoli cell changes: initial nuclear rounding followed by nuclear elongation with development of dark chromatin masses.[469] Eventually the nuclei

TABLE 10-8.
DIFFERENTIAL DIAGNOSIS IN TUBULAR HYALINIZATION

	Dysgenesis	Hormonal deficit	Ischemia	Excretory duct obstruction	Postinflammatory hyalinization	Physical or chemical agents	Immunologic hyalinization
Hyalinized tubule size	Minimum	Minimum	Minimum	Very decreased	Minimum	Very decreased	Minimum
Tubular lumen	Absent	Absent	Absent	Present	Absent	Absent	Absent
Peritubular cells	Decreased	Decreased	Decreased	Increased	Decreased or increased	Decreased	Decreased or increased
Elastic fibers	Decreased	Normal	Normal	Normal	Normal	Normal	Normal
Leydig cells	Increased or decreased, pleomorphic	Absent	Absent	Normal	Pseudohyperplasia	Decreased	Normal or decreased
FSH	Increased	Decreased	Increased	Increased	Increased	Increased	Increased
LH	Increased	Decreased	Increased	Increased	Increased	Increased	Increased
Testosterone	Normal or decreased	Decreased	Normal or decreased	Normal	Normal	Normal or decreased	Decreased

FSH, Follicle stimulating hormone; LH, luteinizing hormone.

come to resemble those of infantile Sertoli cells, even in their pseudostratified distribution. At the same time the tubules hyalinize and peritubular cells increase while Leydig cells decrease.[470,471]

Estrogens act on the pituitary, by inhibiting luteinizing hormone secretion, and on Leydig cells.[472] The action of gonadotropin releasing hormone agonist analogues is only on the pituitary, and cisplatinum acts only on the testis.

Tubular hyalinization

A few azoospermic patients have diffuse hyalinization of seminiferous tubules. The incidence of this lesion is difficult to estimate since these patients usually are not biopsied because their testes are small. Hyalinization of seminiferous tubules is the endpoint of tubular atrophy and includes absence of both germ cells and Sertoli cells with alterations in the lamina propria and Leydig cells. Its etiology can be determined from several histologic features and clinical data, including:

1. General histologic appearance: extent and topography of the hyalinized tubules and presence of isolated tubules containing germ cells or Sertoli cells only (dysgenetic, adult, involuting, or dedifferentiated).
2. Appearance of atrophic tubules: all tubules showing the same pattern or variable atrophy, tubular diameter, trophism of peritubular cells, presence of elastic fibers, degree of collagenization of the lamina propria, and presence of cell remnants or unusual cells in the tubules.
3. Appearance of the interstitium: number and morphology of Leydig cells, vascular lesions, and lymphoid infiltrates.
4. Chronology of testicular shrinkage.

The most common causes of tubular hyalinization include dysgenesis, hormonal deficit, ischemia, obstruction, inflammation, physical or chemical agents, and autoimmunity. The differential diagnosis is given in Table 10-8.

Dysgenetic hyalinization. Dysgenetic hyalinization is a diffuse lesion in which most tubules are uniformly hyalinized (Fig. 10-65). The tubules lack seminiferous epithelium and have a reduced number of peritubular cells. The few preserved tubules usually contain only Sertoli cells, although a few tubules with spermatogenesis rarely are present. Dysgenetic hyalinization is seen in Klinefelter's syndrome and in testes that remained cryptorchid through puberty.

Tubular hyalinization is pronounced in Klinefelter's syndrome, and from infancy the seminiferous tubules are small, containing reduced numbers of Sertoli cells and few or no spermatogonia. At puberty the dysgenetic Sertoli cells fail to mature and they disappear. The tubules collapse, giving the appearance of phantom tubules.[473] The peritubular cells fail to differentiate and their number is low.[474] They form a discontinuous ring around the hyalinized tubules and are incapable of synthesizing elastic fibers and other components of the lamina propria. Dysgenesis also involves the interstitium; the Leydig cells exhibit a characteristic adenomatous pattern, although their total number is decreased. The morphology of the Leydig cells is not uniform, and there are shrunken, normal, and large forms. Most contain reduced amounts of lipofuscin granules and lipid droplets. Reinke's crystalloids are uncommon and paracrystalline inclusions are abundant.[459] In spite of the hyperplastic adenomatous appearance of the Leydig cells, testosterone secretion is markedly decreased and the resulting hypogonadism is the most important clinical feature of Klinefelter's syndrome.

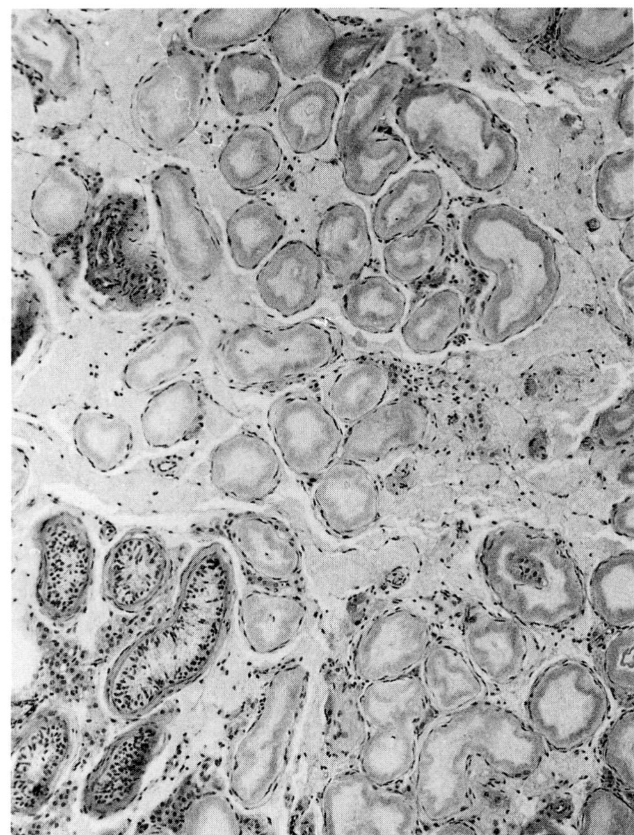

10-65. Dysgenetic hyalinization. Fully hyalinized testicular tubules together with tubules containing only dysgenetic Sertoli cells. There are few peritubular cells.

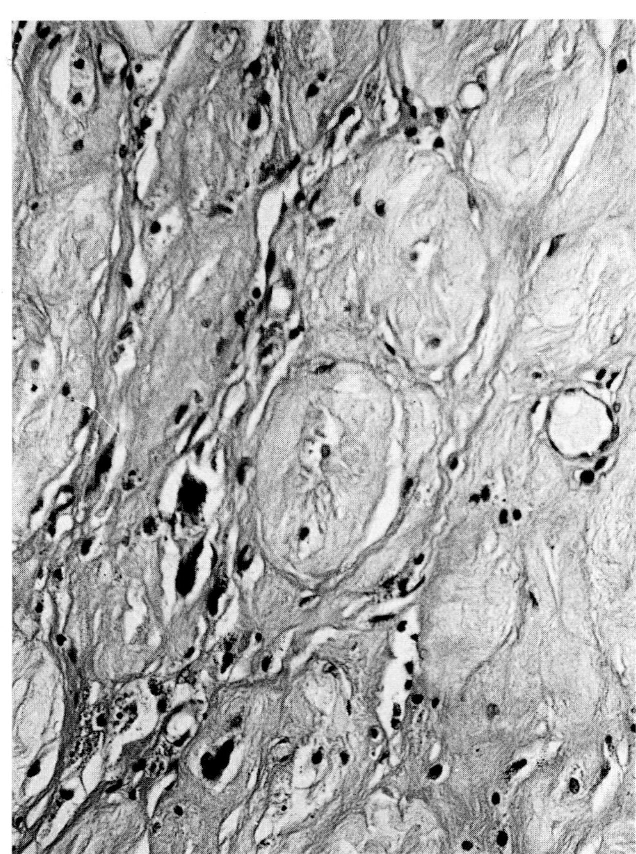

10-66. Tubular hyalinization secondary to ischemia. Only a few peritubular cells and hemosiderin-laden macrophages can be recognized. Leydig cells are not visible.

Tubular hyalinization in the cryptorchid testis is also dysgenetic. However, in contrast to the atrophic collapse seen in Klinefelter's syndrome, the profiles of the hyalinized tubules in cryptorchidism resemble targets. This results from the arrangement of the peritubular cells into two layers, suggesting an atrophic process that has evolved over a longer period than in Klinefelter's syndrome or a lower degree of dysgenesis.[475] Elastic fibers are diminished.[458] In the interstitium the Leydig cells appear hyperplastic, forming large aggregates, although their absolute number is decreased. Leydig cell pleomorphism is less intense than in Klinefelter's syndrome. Many Leydig cells have abundant vacuolated cytoplasm. Whereas tubular hyalinization in Klinefelter's syndrome is secondary to the effect of pubertal gonadotropin secretion on dysgenetic tubules, tubular hyalinization in cryptorchidism probably results from increased testicular temperature. However, other mechanisms are also involved in cryptorchid tubular hyalinization, including obstruction of sperm excretory ducts (anomalies in these ducts are frequent in cryptorchidism) and ischemia (principally in testes that could only be incompletely descended).

Hyalinization caused by hormonal deficit. Hormonal deficit causes diffuse tubular hyalinization, although the tubules may be recognized for a time as epithelial cords surrounded by hyaline material. Sertoli cells, a few spermatogonia, and rare primary spermatocytes may be identified in these cords. When hyalinization is complete, only the elastic fibers in the lamina propria echo the structure of the previously normal adult testis. Peritubular myofibroblasts decreased in number and form a ring at the periphery of the lamina propria. Leydig cells disappear as hyalinization progresses and the few remaining have pyknotic nuclei and shrunken cytoplasm with abundant lipofuscin granules.

This process manifests clinically as a postpubertal hypogonadotropic hypogonadism and is usually caused by lesions in or near the pituitary, such as pituitary adenoma, craniopharyngioma, and trauma to the cranial base or sella turcica (see discussion on hypogonadotropic hypogonadism in this chapter).

Ischemic hyalinization. Ischemic atrophy is usually caused by torsion of the spermatic cord, vascular injury during inguinal surgery,[476] polyarteritis nodosa, and severe arteriosclerosis.[477] Except for cases caused by torsion of the cord, these patients usually are not seen in infertility clinics.

Torsion of the spermatic cord often is not listed among the causes in large series of infertile patients. However, follow-up of men with torsion reveals marked alteration in their spermiograms. Several hypotheses have been offered to explain the low number of sperm produced by

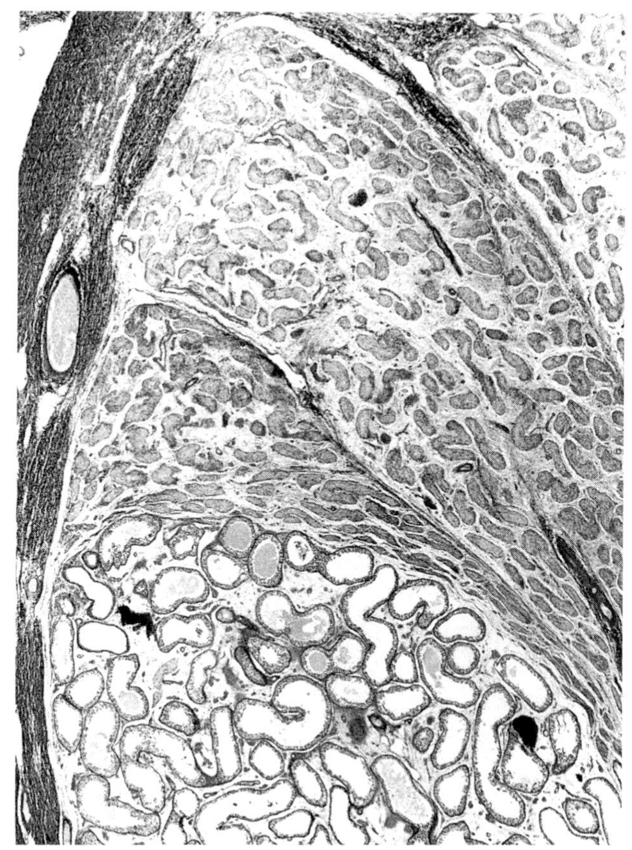

10-67. Postobstructive hyalinization. Testis from a patient with epididymal cyst. The testicular parenchyma shows lobules with tubular hyalinization and lobules with marked tubular dilatation.

10-68. Autoimmune hyalinization. The outline of the hyalinized tubules is unclear. The testicular interstitium is collagenized while the Leydig cells are preserved.

the contralateral normal testis; the most promising include response to the release of antigens by the ischemic testis and primary lesions of the contralateral testis.[478]

Testicular anoxia caused by torsion rapidly produces severe lesions that are irreversible without adequate treatment. Eight hours after torsion there is intense hemorrhagic infarction of the seminiferous epithelium. Chronic anoxia leads to tubular hyalinization and loss of Leydig cells (Fig. 10-66).

Postobstructive hyalinization. Obstruction of the sperm excretory ducts may cause atrophy of seminiferous tubules. In order to produce tubular hyalinization, the obstruction must be close to the testis because the efferent ductules in the head of the epididymis absorb about 90% of tubular fluid and protect the testis from excessive pressure. Obstructive tubular hyalinization is usually focal and secondary to varicocele and other disorders involving dilation of the channels of the rete testis. These may be congenital, as in epididymis-testis dissociation, or acquired, as in rete testis dilation secondary to epididymal atrophy caused by arteritis, arteriosclerosis, or androgen insufficiency. Obstructive tubular hyalinization also occurs in the seminiferous tubules at the periphery of the testis in patients who have had orchitis.[479]

Obstructive hyalinization has a mosaic distribution; lobules of completely hyalinized tubules are intermingled with lobules of normal tubules (Fig. 10-67). The diameter of the hyalinized tubules is not as small as in the other causes of hyalinization and the tubules occasionally contain Sertoli cells. In the centers of many of the tubules there is a small lumen or a vacuole; the latter in the cytoplasm of a residual Sertoli cell.[480] The lamina propria is very thick and contains hypertrophic peritubular cells and abundant extracellular material. Finally, the peritubular cells dedifferentiate and only fibroblasts remain.[481] The interstitium contains a normal number of Leydig cells, forming small clusters, some of which are among hyalinized tubules. This is not seen in other patterns, such as ischemic hyalinization. In addition, dilated veins with eccentrically hyalinized walls can be seen in testes associated with varicocele.

Postinflammatory hyalinization. Many infections of the testis cause irreversible lesions in the seminiferous epithelium. In bacterial infections the epididymis is usually involved, resulting in obstructive azoospermia. In viral infections the testis is often affected, even without symptoms. Two types of viral orchitis often cause infertility: mumps orchitis and Coxsackie B virus orchitis.

Tubular atrophy caused by viral infection has a mosaic topography in which hyalinized and normal tubules are intermingled. In fully hyalinized tubules the only recognizable cells are peritubular cells which form an incomplete, peripheral ring around the hyalinized material. The presence of elastic fibers in these tubules distinguishes this from dysgenetic hyalinization. Leydig cells form clusters of variable size, but their total number is normal. In bacterial infections the pattern of tubular hyalinization is variable.

Hyalinization caused by physical or chemical agents. Radiation and a wide variety of chemicals cause tubular hyalinization. Lengthy cancer chemotherapy in combination with radiotherapy invariably causes hyalinization. Children's testes are more sensitive to radiation than adults'. Radiation for testicular leukemic infiltrates frequently causes hyalinization. In addition to tubular hyalinization, radiation induces dense interstitial fibrosis and loss of peritubular cells, obscuring the borders between the interstitium and the tubules. This makes the tubules hard to see in hematoxylin-eosin-stained sections. Leydig cells are atrophic and few. Ischemia secondary to radiation-induced vascular injury also contributes to hyalinization.

In tubular hyalinization associated with cancer chemotherapy, in addition to drugs' direct toxicity in the seminiferous epithelium (see discussion on Sertoli cell–only syndrome with involuting Sertoli cells in this chapter), nutritional deficiencies cause hypogonadotropic hypogonadism.[473,482]

Autoimmune hyalinization. Some tubular atrophy of unknown etiology may be caused by an autoimmune response. This appears to occur in hypogonadism associated with disorders in other endocrine glands such as Addison's disease associated with gonadal insufficiency, adrenal-thyroid-gonadal insufficiency, and the association of diabetes, hypogonadism, adrenal insufficiency, and hypothyroidism. The testicular lesions are morphologically similar to those seen in the seminiferous tubules at the periphery of germ cell tumors and in testes

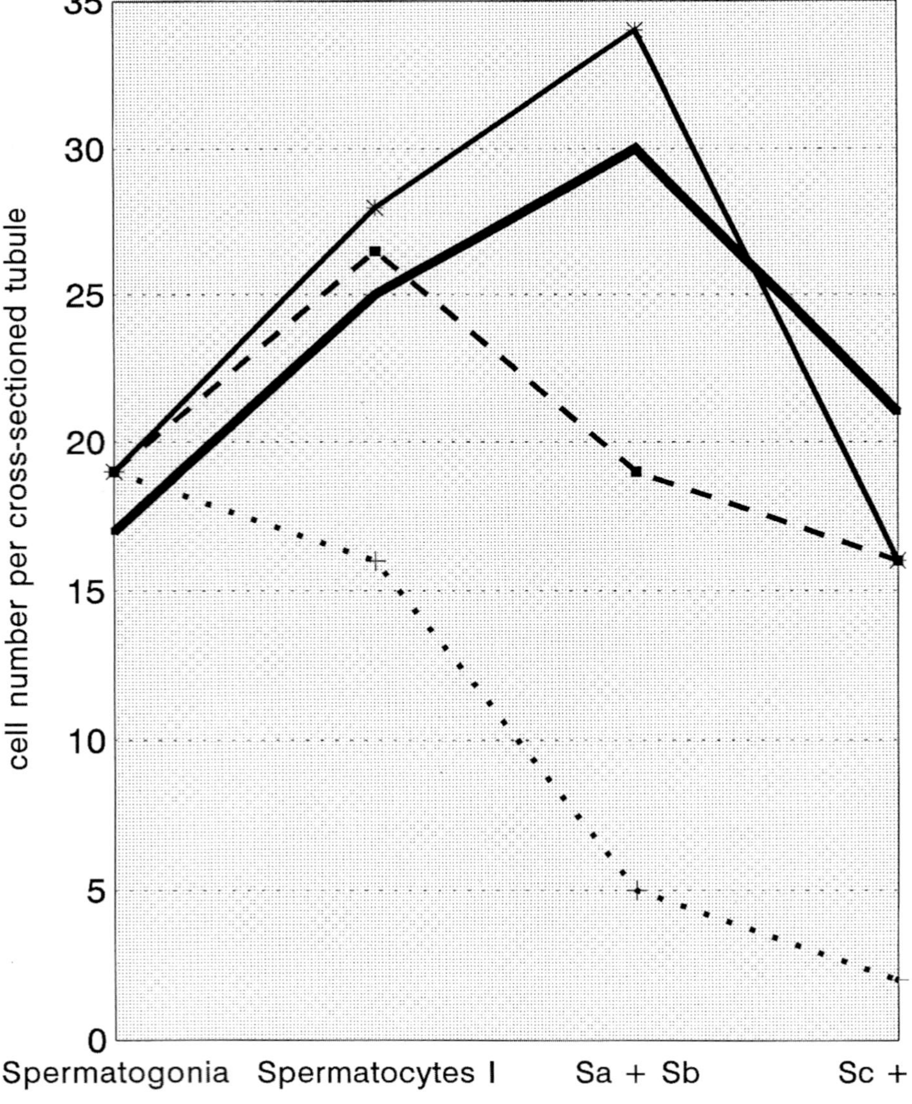

10-69. Germ cell numbers per cross-sectioned tubule in patients with lesions in the adluminal compartment of seminiferous tubules. *Thick line,* lowest values in normal control testes; *thin line,* patients with young spermatid sloughing; *discontinuous line,* patients with late spermatocyte I sloughing; *dotted line,* patients with early spermatocyte I sloughing.

with burnt-out seminoma. In the initial stages of hyalinization associated with germ cell neoplasms, the tubules are small and contain intratubular germ cell neoplasia and dedifferentiating Sertoli cells, and the lamina propria is infiltrated by lymphocytes and plasma cells. In the final stages the intratubular cells have degenerated, the inflammatory infiltrate has disappeared, and the seminiferous tubules are replaced by areas of hypocellular or acellular fibrosis (Fig. 10-68). It should be noted that autoimmune hyalinization is not the most common type of hyalinization associated with testicular tumors; the obstructive and ischemic variants are more common.

Diffuse lesions in spermatogenesis

Histophysiologic studies have distinguished two compartments in the seminiferous epithelium: basal and adluminal. The blood-testis barrier separates these, and each contains different cell types with diverse hormonal and nutritional requirements. On this basis, lesions may be classified as involving only the basal or adluminal compartments or both the basal and adluminal compartments. The following discussion of spermatogenic lesions uses this new concept of tubular pathophysiology, conserving as much as possible of the classic terminology.

Lesions in basal compartment of seminiferous tubules. This category includes all infertile testes with normal numbers of spermatogonia per tubular profile, but decreased numbers of the other types of germ cells. A descriptive term for this disorder is *immature germ cell sloughing*.

A few immature germ cells are normally found in the lumens of the seminiferous tubules, a finding[483] that correlates with their presence in the ejaculates of fertile men.[484] When these cells make up more than 4% of the cells in the ejaculate it is abnormal and the result of premature sloughing of spermatids and, in some cases, of spermatocytes.[485,486] Some authors have attempted to establish a correlation between the number of sloughed immature germ cells and the severity of lesions of the seminiferous epithelium by light[487] and electron[488] microscopy.

Lesions in adluminal compartment of seminiferous tubules. Lesions in the adluminal compartment are classified according to the most abundant type of sloughed germ cell: young spermatids, late primary spermatocytes, or early primary spermatocytes.

Young spermatid sloughing. Lesions are diagnosed as young spermatid sloughing when the ratio of elongate ($S_c + S_d$) spermatids to round ($S_a + S_b$) spermatids is lower than normal (Fig. 10-69). The implication of this pattern is that many round spermatids are incapable of further differentiation and are sloughed (Fig. 10-70). Since spermatogonial proliferation and meiosis occur

10-70. Seminiferous tubules with normal diameters and slight young spermatid sloughing.

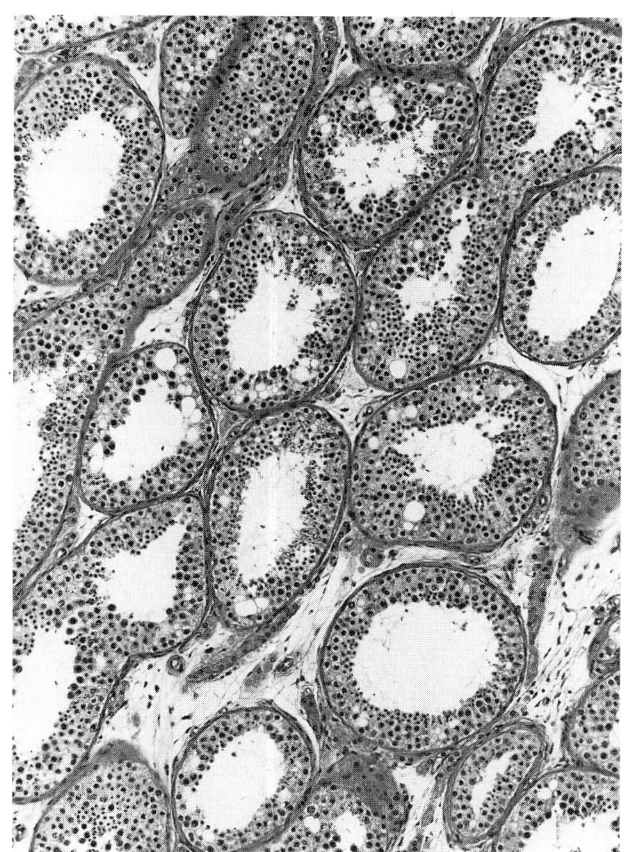

10-71. Seminiferous tubules with marked dilation of their lumens. Germ cell development is arrested at the primary spermatocyte level in some tubules.

normally, it appears that endocrine, paracrine, and autocrine factors function normally and the mechanism is local. An alteration in the apical Sertoli cell cytoplasm, resulting in a precocious desquamation, may be the cause. Increased intratubular pressure may be the underlying cause, since many of these patients have obstructive azoospermia or oligozoospermia. Failure of spermatid differentiation into spermatozoa has also been linked to structural defects in the cytoskeletal proteins.[462]

Late primary spermatocyte sloughing. In this condition, spermatogenesis develops normally up to the level of interphase primary spermatocytes, and these are present in normal numbers. Afterward, these spermatocytes degenerate without achieving meiosis and slough into the tubular lumen. All types of spermatid are greatly reduced in numbers (see Fig. 10-69). When biopsies of these testes are not properly fixed, the seminiferous tubules may have a targetlike appearance, with numerous cells in the lumen, an appearance sometimes referred to as *tubular blockage*. Another descriptive term, *spermatogenic arrest*, also has been applied to this morphology. The latter term is inadequate because some spermatids are present, and the number of primary spermatocytes is not increased as would occur if the transformation of spermatocyte into spermatid were blocked without spermatocyte sloughing (Fig. 10-71). *Late primary spermatocyte sloughing* more accurately names this condition and is preferred. Primary spermatocyte sloughing occurs at the pachytene or diplotene stage of meiosis. The mechanism is controversial, an anomaly in the meiotic process[489] or a Sertoli cell lesion are the leading theories. The first requires that true meiotic arrest occurs. Although meiotic alterations and histologic findings of true spermatocytic arrest have been reported in some patients with chromosomal anomalies,[423,490] patients with these anomalies have a wide variety of histologic abnormalities and may even have normal testes. Moreover, these patients often have different lesions in each testis.[491] This suggests that in true maturation arrest caused by chromosomal anomalies, the abnormal genome hinders the normal meiotic process in some spermatocytes but not in all.[492] The high frequency of other lesions in the contralateral testis also weighs against a genetically mediated primary meiotic anomaly.

The Sertoli cells of testes with late primary spermatocyte sloughing have many vacuoles in their apical cytoplasm. The tubular lumen (except for tubules containing desquamated cells) is wide, suggesting excessive tubular fluid. Excessive intratubular pressure may hinder fluid

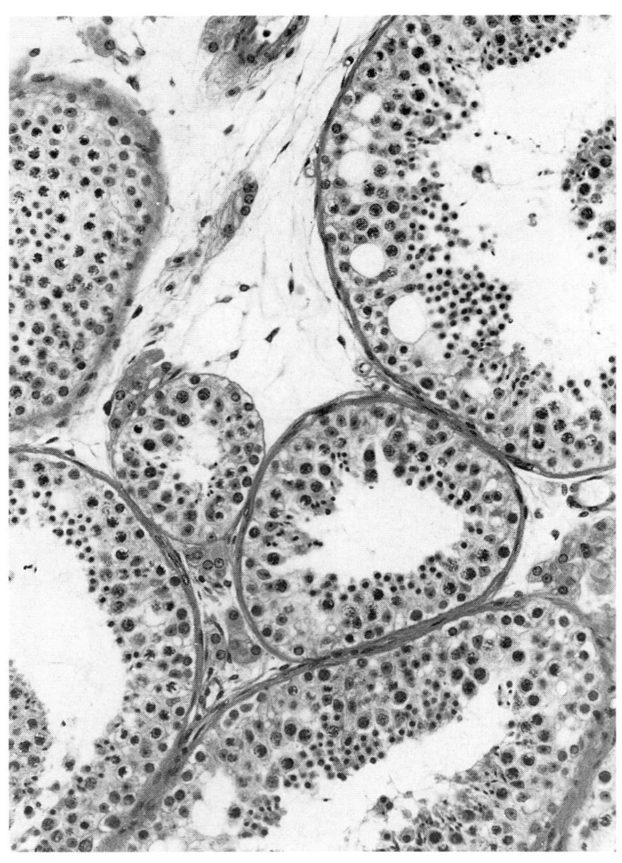

10-72. The toothed pattern of the seminiferous epithelium with germ cells protruding toward the tubular lumen is caused by the supranuclear vacuolation of Sertoli cells. The smallest tubular formation corresponds to a seminiferous tubule diverticulum.

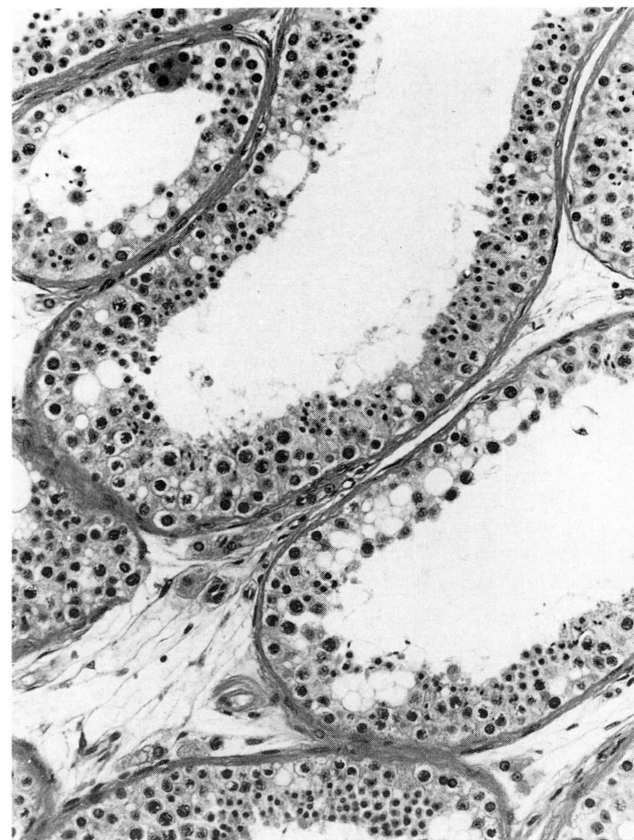

10-73. Seminiferous tubules with dilated lumens and variable lesions in the adluminal compartment. The lesions that are usually designated as primary spermatocyte arrest or hypospermatogenesis are probably secondary to Sertoli cell damage. Note apical vacuoles in Sertoli cells.

transport from the basal to the apical Sertoli cell cytoplasm, causing failure of the specialized Sertoli cell–germ cell junction system. These junctions contain cytoplasmic actin filaments that are anchored in the plasma membrane by vinculin. Defective synthesis of vinculin may alter cellular adhesion, promoting germ cell sloughing.[493] Ultrastructural studies of these testes reveal alterations in these Sertoli cells.[494-496]

Early primary spermatocyte sloughing. This lesion is characterized by the presence of a normal number of spermatogonia and a decreased number of primary spermatocytes (see Fig. 10-69). The seminiferous tubules may contain a few spermatids. The term *early primary spermatocyte sloughing* does not imply an early meiotic lesion which, as explained above,[423] is quite rare.[486] Rather, this term refers to the early stage of meiosis (initiation of pachytene) at which the primary spermatocytes are sloughed. The Sertoli cells may show vacuolation of the apical cytoplasm as an expression of germ cell loss (Fig. 10-72). This lesion often is more severe than that in testes with late primary spermatocyte sloughing and is considered to be the result of Sertoli cells' failure in maintaining the adluminal compartment.

In addition to quantitative data about germ cell numbers, a number of qualitative features may be diagnostically helpful in cases of spermatocyte sloughing, although they are not always present. These include an increase in tubular diameter as well as in the number of diverticula; Sertoli cells with their adherent germ cells protrude into the lumen, giving it an indented outline (see Fig. 10-72) deposition of eosinophilic (slightly periodic acid–Schiff positive) material on the inner surface of the seminiferous epithelium, results in an abnormally sharp tubular outline. Apical vacuolation of the Sertoli cell cytoplasm (Fig. 10-73) and an accumulation of spermatids in the lumens are seen in some tubules (Fig. 10-74).

Etiology. More than 70% of testes with lesions in the adluminal compartment show patchy abnormalities. The severity of the lesions varies among groups of tubules from different lobules. A mosaic pattern of clusters of tubules with different lesions is typical of obstruction. The obstruction may be complete or partial and may be at different levels: vas deferens, epididymis, or intratesticular excretory ducts (for causes, see discussion on azoospermia and obstructive oligozoospermia in this chapter).

Intratesticular obstruction in the rete testis or seminiferous tubules usually causes severe oligozoospermia and, rarely, azoospermia.

Rete testis obstruction. Varicocele is the most frequent cause of obstruction of the rete testis. More than

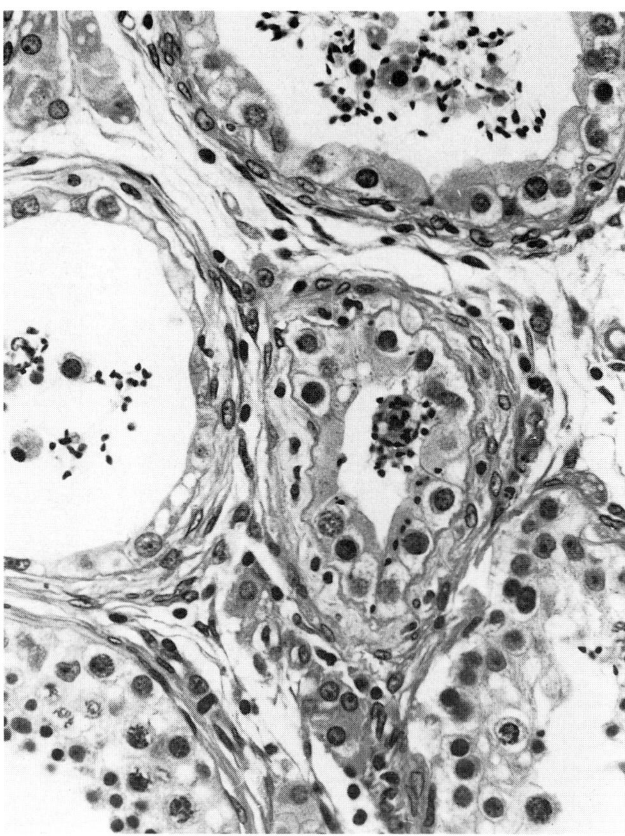

10-74. Group of seminiferous tubules, probably in the same lobule, showing variable degrees of luminal dilation and a seminiferous epithelium consisting of spermatogonia and cuboidal Sertoli cells. Abundant spermatozoa are present in the tubular lumens.

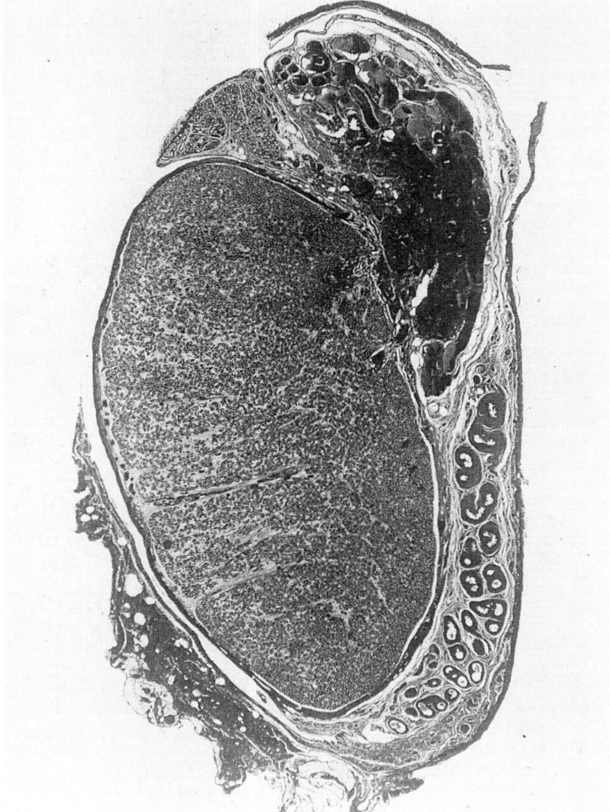

10-75. Rete testis obstruction. Autopsy specimen from a young adult man with history of varicocele. The veins in the pampiniform plexus are intensely ectatic, compressing the initial segments of the efferent ductiles.

50% of testes with varicocele have a mosaic pattern of tubular lesions, together with marked dilation and eccentric mural fibrosis of intratesticular veins. In normal testes the walls of veins are extremely thin and the lumens nearly collapsed. Varicocele patients also often have spermatozoa with characteristically elongate heads with thin bases.[497] Initially the abnormalities are confined to the testis ipsilateral to the varicocele, but eventually both testes are affected, although the abnormalities are more severe in the ipsilateral. The elevated pressure in pampiniform plexus is transmitted to the veins within the testis, principally to the centripetal veins that cross the testicular mediastinum and drain the testis (Fig. 10-75).[498] The dilated centripetal veins compress the intratesticular sperm excretory ducts, explaining the mosaic distribution of the tubular lesions (Fig. 10-76).[499]

Seminiferous tubule obstruction. Obstruction at the level of the seminiferous tubule can be dysgenetic or postorchitic. A dysgenetic cause may be suspected in specimens with a mosaic distribution of lesions and seminiferous tubules with small diameters, thickened lamina propria, and an unusual seminiferous epithelium consisting only of cuboidal Sertoli cells and spermatozoa that clog the lumens (Fig. 10-77). The diagnosis is confirmed if study of serial sections demonstrates continuity between these tubules and tubules with conserved spermatogenesis. The structure of seminiferous tubules has been observed by scanning electron microscopy at such points of continuity.[500] This tubular stenosis appears to be due to a primary anomaly of Sertoli cells and peritubular cells.

Postorchitic obstruction should be suspected in cases of tubular atrophy with a mosaic pattern without dysgenetic tubules or varicocele. Some of these patients have histories of orchitis associated with parotiditis[501]; in others the only findings are oligozoospermia and small testes. Testicular biopsy, sampling only the testicular periphery, reveals only the consequences of obstruction, lesions similar to those observed with varicocele. However, some postinflammatory changes should also be present, including hyalinized tubules, dilated tubules lined by cuboidal Sertoli cells or with complete spermatogenesis. Occasionally there are small perivascular or peritubular inflammatory infiltrates and angiectasis.

Other causes. About 30% of testes with diffuse lesions of the adluminal compartment do not have a mosaic distribution of lesions, perhaps related to the alteration in

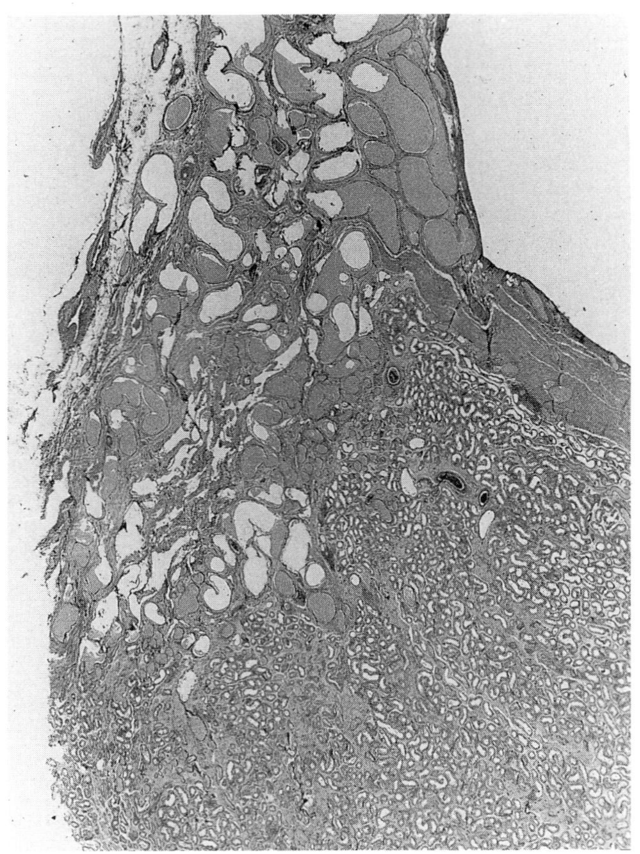

10-76. Rete testis obstruction. Cross-sectioned testis showing irregularly outlined rete testis cavities among dilated veins. The testicular parenchyma shows variable degrees of atrophy between lobules.

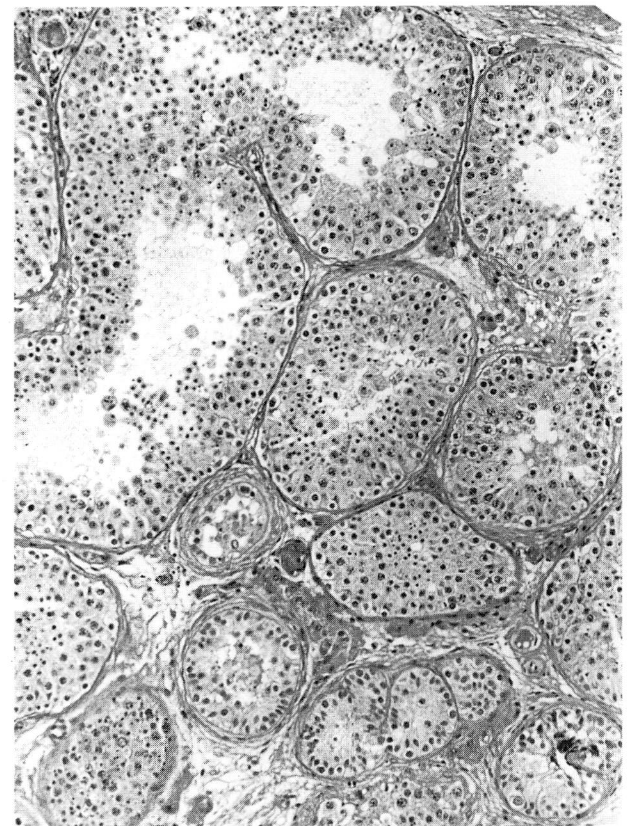

10-77. Seminiferous tubule obstruction. The seminiferous tubule in the center of the picture, which has a normal histologic pattern, is surrounded by dilated tubules and small tubules with thickened basement membranes. Both tubule types have well-preserved germ cell development. In addition, there is a group of three tubules with a hypoplastic or dysgenetic pattern.

spermatid transport, which is discussed at the end of this section (functional azoospermia and oligozoospermia).

Lesions in basal and adluminal compartment of seminiferous tubules. Lesions in the basal and adluminal compartments of seminiferous tubules are the most frequent histological findings in testicular biopsies from infertile men. These testes may be classified into two major subgroups: hypospermatogenesis and spermatogonial maturation arrest (Fig. 10-78).

Hypospermatogenesis. ***Types.*** Hypospermatogenesis is defined as reduced numbers of both spermatogonia and primary spermatocytes, with the primary spermatocytes outnumbering the spermatogonia. Most seminiferous tubules contain few spermatids. About 8% of patients with hypospermatogenesis have focal tubular hyalinization.[502] Two variants of hypospermatogenesis have been distinguished quantitatively: pure hypospermatogenesis and hypospermatogenesis associated with sloughing of primary spermatocytes.

Pure hypospermatogenesis is defined as a proportionate decrease in the numbers of all types of germ cells. The number of spermatogonia per tubular profile is lower than 17 and usually higher than 10. The number of primary spermatocytes is equal to or higher than that of the spermatogonia. The number of round spermatids is higher than that of primary spermatocytes, and the number of elongated spermatids is similar to that of spermatogonia (Fig. 10-79).

Hypospermatogenesis associated with primary spermatocyte sloughing is characterized by two features: low numbers of

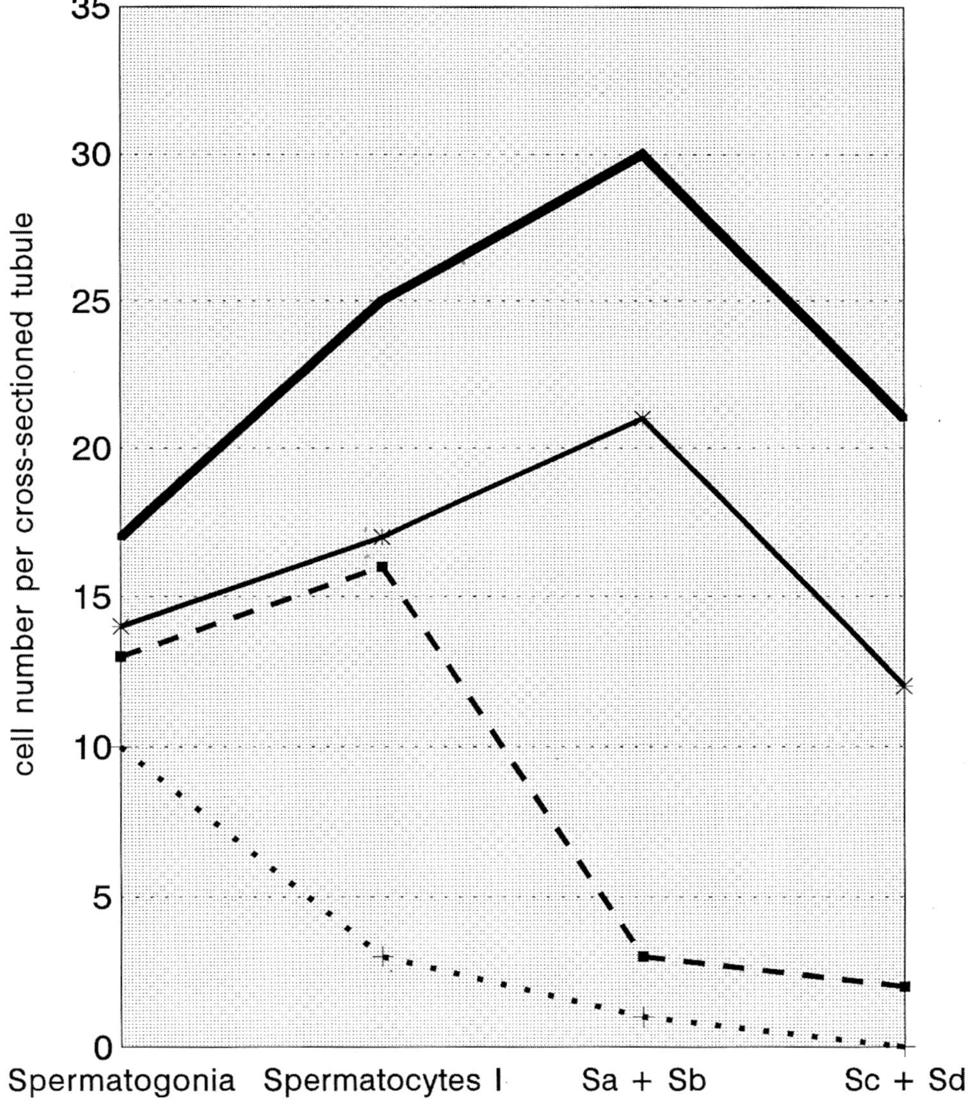

10-78. Germ cell numbers per cross-sectioned tubule in patients with lesions in the basal and adluminal compartments of seminiferous tubules. *Thick line,* lowest values in normal control testes; *thin line,* patients with hypospermatogenesis; *discontinuous line,* patients with spermatocyte I sloughing associated with hypospermatogenesis; *dotted line,* patients with spermatogonial maturation arrest.

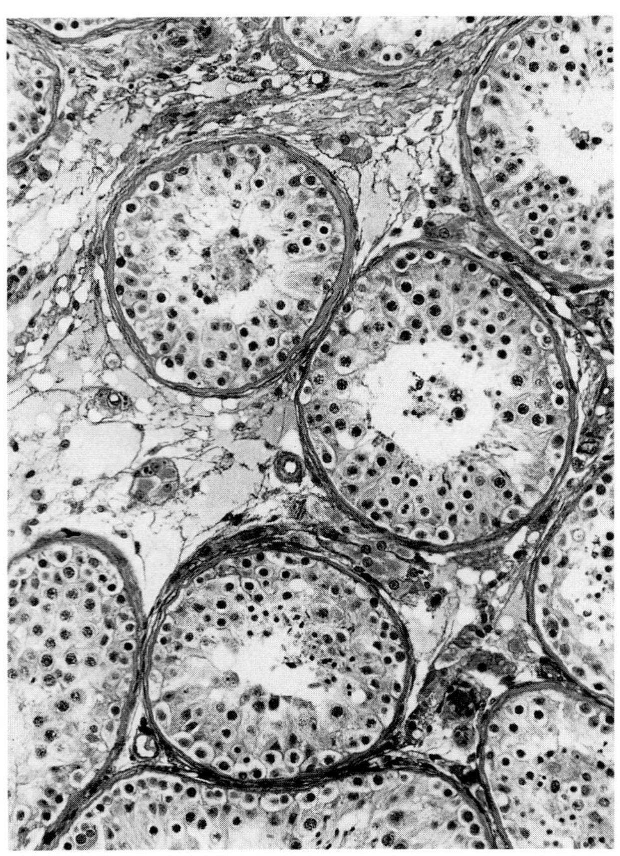

10-79. Pure hypospermatogenesis. Seminiferous tubules with thickened tunica propria and decreased numbers of all germ cell types.

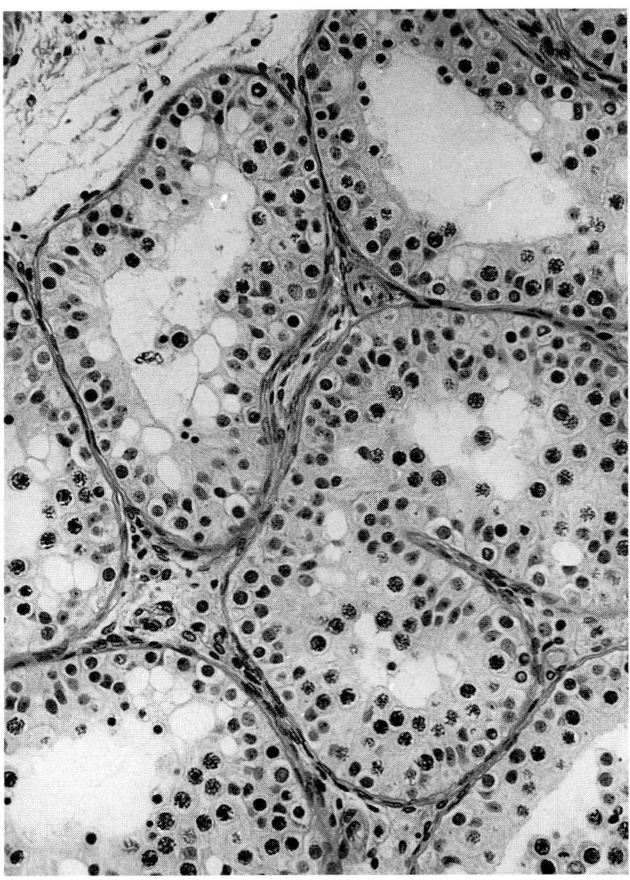

10-80. Hypospermatogenesis associated with primary spermatocyte sloughing. The number of spermatogonia and primary spermatocytes is proportionally reduced. Spermatids are few.

spermatogonia and primary spermatocytes (with spermatocytes more numerous than spermatogonia) and degeneration and sloughing of many primary spermatocytes, the remaining primary spermatocytes giving rise to the few spermatids remaining in the tubules (Fig. 10-80). Quantitative studies show reduced proliferation of spermatogonia and failure of primary spermatocytes to complete the first meiotic division. Both processes are controlled by factors synthesized by Sertoli cells, so the disease is attributed to failure of Sertoli cell function. The presence of angiectasis in more than one third of cases suggests that this may be secondary to varicocele.

Hypospermatogenesis may result from hormonal dysfunction, congenital germ cell deficiency, Sertoli cell dysfunction, Leydig cell dysfunction, androgen insensitivity, exposure to chemical or physical agents, and vascular malfunction.

Although complete spermatogenesis may be observed in men with low levels of follicle stimulating hormone and luteinizing hormone, production of normal numbers of spermatozoa requires normal gonadotropin levels. Hypospermatogenesis is found in patients with deficits in follicle stimulating hormone, isolated insufficiency of luteinizing hormone, biologically inactive luteinizing hormone, hyperprolactinemia, and adrenal and thyroid dysfunction (see discussion on hypogonadism secondary to endocrine gland dysfunction in this chapter).

Biopsy of cryptorchid patients after orchiopexy reveals that spermatogonial proliferation is decreased and germ cell development is insufficient in adulthood even if the number of spermatogonia was normal in infancy. It is likely that this poorly understood primary anomaly of germ cells also is present in some cases of hypospermatogenesis.

For many years primary germ cell deficiency was considered the most common cause of hypospermatogenesis; today it is known that Sertoli cell failure is the cause of many cases of germ cell deficiency. This conclusion is based on several findings. The Sertoli cells of many infertile patients are markedly abnormal, with increases in glycogen granules[503] and in acid phosphatase activity[450]; decrease in lipid droplets; and alterations in the cytoskeleton,[504] the nucleus,[505] and cytoplasmic organelles.[506] In some cases the Sertoli cells show abnormal maturation, with elongated nuclei containing coarse chromatin masses instead of triangular-shaped nuclei with pale chromatin. Anomalies in Sertoli cell follicle stimulating hormone receptors have been found in idiopathic oligozoospermia associated with elevated levels of follicle stimulating hormone.[507] Thus, when the basal

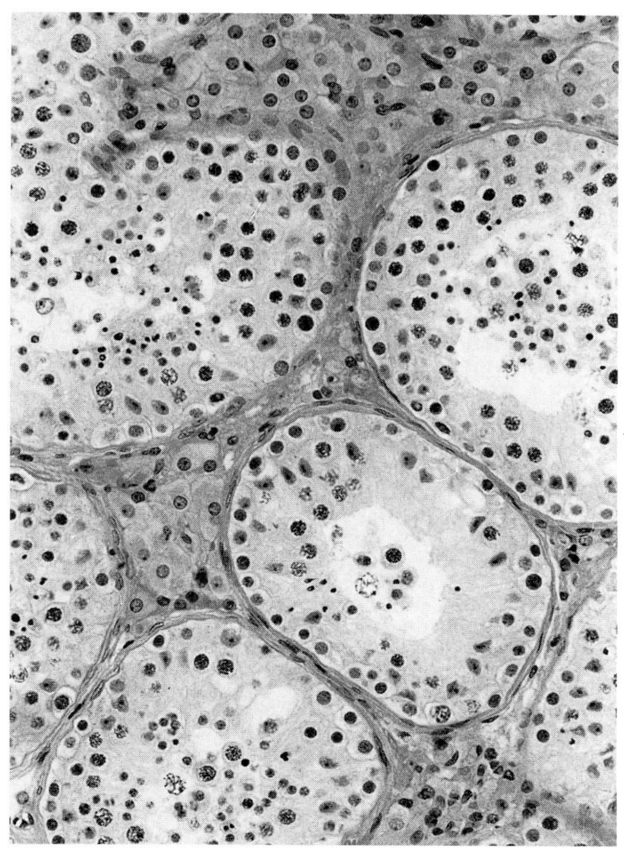

10-81. Hypospermatogenesis due to androgen receptor defect. Seminiferous tubules with hypospermatogenesis associated with diffuse Leydig cell hyperplasia.

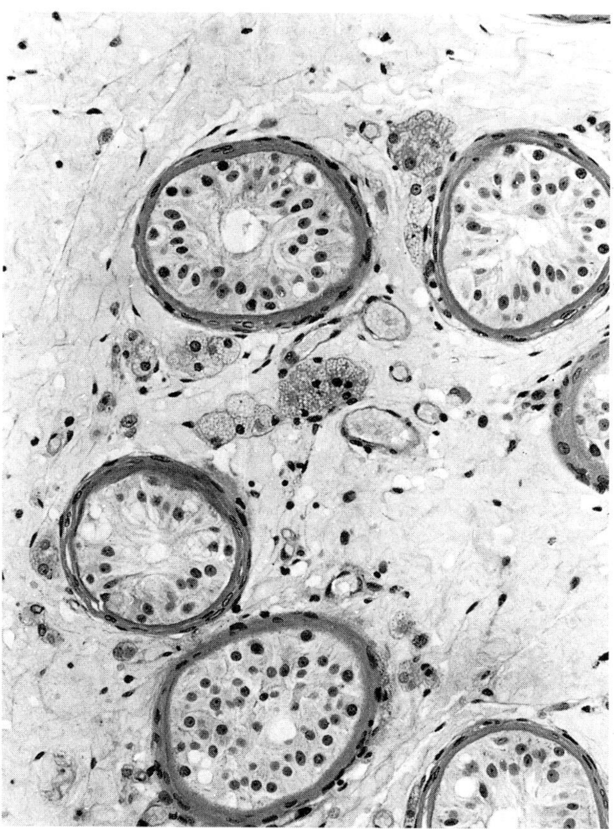

10-82. Spermatogonial maturation arrest. Small seminiferous tubules with thickened walls. The seminiferous epithelium consists of spermatogonia and Sertoli cells. The interstitium contains small groups of microvacuolated Leydig cells.

compartment is normal and the adluminal compartment is abnormal, or both compartments are abnormal, the cause of the lesion usually lies in the Sertoli cells.

Testosterone synthesis by Leydig cells is necessary for normal spermatogenesis,[508] and abnormal Leydig cell function is a frequent finding in idiopathic oligozoospermia.[509,510] Leydig cell dysfunction should be suspected when the cells appear diffusely hyperplastic in a pattern reminiscent of Klinefelter's syndrome. These patients have elevated serum luteinizing hormone levels with depletion of rapid-release testosterone, revealing a lack of early response of the Leydig cells to gonadotropin releasing hormone stimulation. The ratio of testosterone to luteinizing hormone in the plasma indicates the degree of Leydig cell dysfunction. A decreased ratio with normal testosterone level suggests a compensated dysfunction. Patients with a ratio of less than 1:5 and normality in the other parameters have the potential for complete spermatogenesis.[510]

Some patients with severe oligozoospermia or azoospermia have a defect in androgen receptor responsiveness similar to that in Reifenstein's syndrome.[511,512] The abnormality may arise from a genetic defect in the eight exons that code for this receptor or from posttranslational errors.[513,514] Histologically, the testis is similar to that observed with Leydig cell dysfunction, or in mixed atrophy, although the mechanism causing the Leydig cell hyperplasia is quite different (Fig. 10-81). Peripheral resistance to testosterone action alters the regulation of the hypothalamic-hypophyseal-testicular axis, and luteinizing hormone and testosterone levels are elevated. Androgen insensitivity causes between 10%[515] and 40%[516] of all cases of severe oligozoospermia or azoospermia. In such cases spermatogenesis improves with administration of tamoxifen citrate[516] or clomiphene citrate.[517] Calculation of the index of androgen insensitivity can be helpful: plasma luteinizing hormone (mIU/ml) X plasma testosterone levels (ng/ml). In patients with androgen insensitivity, the index is higher than 200 (normal is about 102).

The number of chemicals implicated in infertility increases daily. A detailed history is invaluable in evaluating these patients. The same is true of physical agents such as prolonged exposure to heat, ionizing radiation, or microwave radiation.[518]

Varicocele is commonly associated with infertility.[496,519-521] Varicocele is found in 15% of the general population but is present in 30% to 40% of infertile men. The mechanism by which varicocele affects fertility is unknown. Clinical varicoceles may occur without a testicular lesion (or only phlebectasis) and subclinical varicocele may be associated with severe spermatogenic lesions. Increased testicular temperature[522,523] and compression of intratesticular sperm excretory ducts by dilated veins[499] are the most plausible mechanisms by which varicocele may cause infertility.

Spermatogonial maturation arrest. Spermatogonial maturation arrest is a disorder diagnosed when the testicular biopsy shows fewer than 17 spermatogonia per tubular profile, with fewer primary spermatocytes than spermatogonia. Spermatids are usually absent. The most frequent causes, in descending order, are cryptorchidism, alcoholism or exposure to other toxic substances, anticancer chemotherapy, and hypogonadotropic hypogonadism. In the cryptorchid testis the most typical findings are reduced numbers of spermatogonia, giant spermatogonia, pseudohyperplasia of Leydig cells, and diminution of elastic fibers in the tubule walls (Fig. 10-82). In chronic alcoholism, tubular diameters are reduced, basement membranes are thickened, and there are more spermatogonia than in cryptorchid testes. Chemotherapy causes involution of Sertoli cells which develop very irregular nuclear outlines, thickening of the lamina propria, and great reduction in spermatogonia. Patients with hypogonadotropic hypogonadism have seminiferous tubules with infantile Sertoli cells and lamina propria that lacks elastic fibers.

Focal lesions in spermatogenesis (mixed atrophy)

Mixed atrophy is a descriptive term for the coexistence, in the same testis, of tubules containing only Sertoli cells and tubules with complete or incomplete spermatogenesis.[524] This disorder includes patchy failure of spermatogenesis and partial del Castillo's syndrome.

The extent of Sertoli cell–only tubules varies widely. The tubules with spermatogenesis may be normal or partially atrophic. Tubular hyalinization is occasionally seen (Fig. 10-83). Mixed atrophy is more common than suggested by the literature, many cases having been included under other diagnoses, such as "hypospermatogenesis with a severe germ cell depletion in such a way that some Sertoli-cell-only tubules are seen,"[426] and "Sertoli cell–only syndrome with focal spermatogenesis."[525]

Serial sections from testes with mixed atrophy reveal that the two different types of tubules are grouped according to their histologic pattern, suggesting that their distribution is by testicular lobules. In cases of mixed atrophy, the percentage of tubules with spermatogenesis, the degree of spermatogenic development in these tubules, and the primary or secondary nature of the lesion should be reported. Correlation of the first two with the spermiogram gives an indication of prognosis and knowledge of the nature of the lesion often suggests the best treatment.

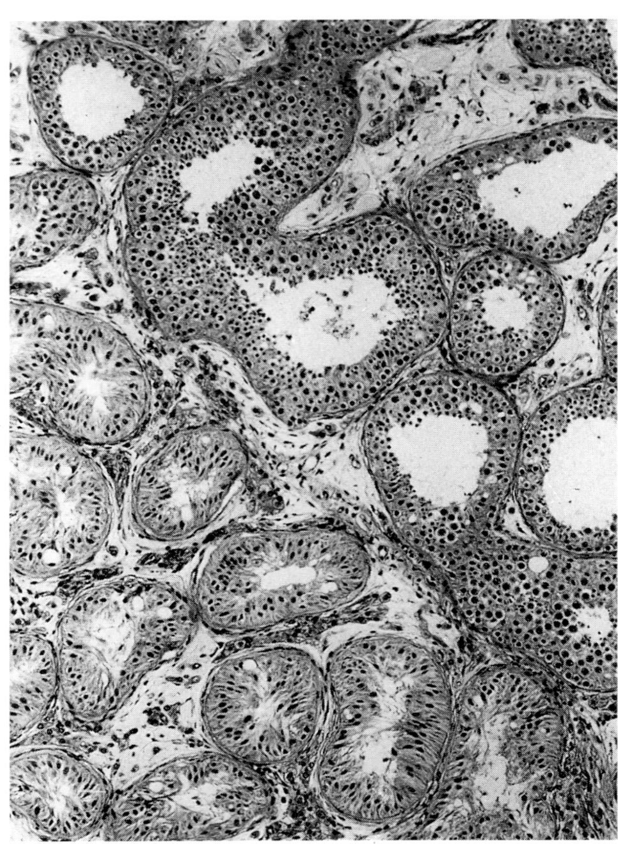

10-83. Mixed atrophy. Seminiferous tubules with spermatogenesis adjoining Sertoli cell–only tubules. A connective tissue septum with small blood vessels separates the two areas.

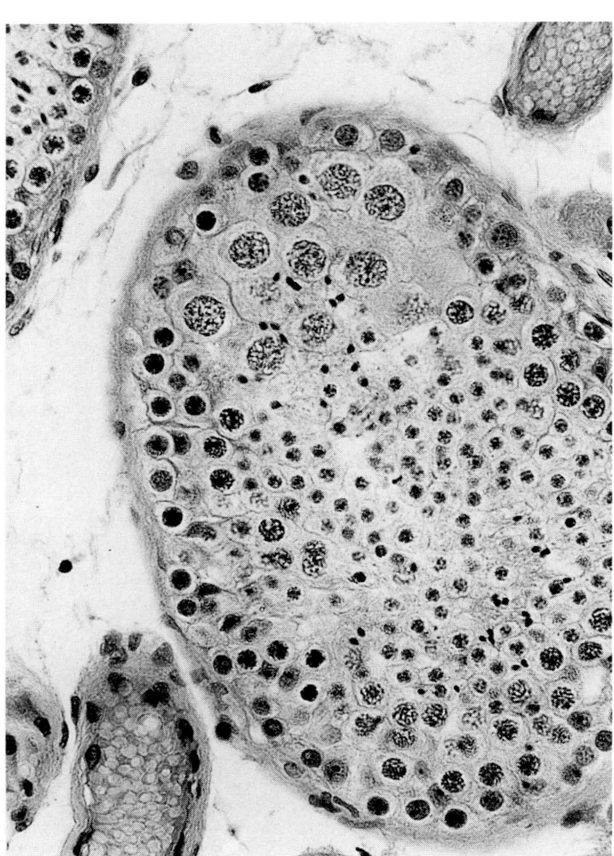

10-84. Megalospermatocytes. Seminiferous tubule containing a group of very large primary spermatocytes with fine chromatin and eosinophilic cytoplasm.

Mixed atrophy (probably primary) is observed in both the cryptorchid and contralateral descended testis in patients with cryptorchidism (even if orchiopexy was done in infancy), in men with retractile testes, and in patients with chromosomal anomalies such as Down's syndrome, 47/XYY karyotype, 46/XX karyotype, giant Y chromosome, and Klinefelter's syndrome with chromosomal mosaicism. Mixed atrophy has also been reported in men with partial androgen insensitivity and some male pseudohermaphrodites. Secondary mixed atrophy is sometimes seen in patients with varicocele and following chemotherapy.

GERM CELL ANOMALIES IN INFERTILE PATIENTS

In addition to abnormalities in the seminiferous tubules, examination of the biopsy should include morphology of the germ cells.

Giant spermatogonia

Giant spermatogonia are a normal component of the seminiferous epithelium. These cells may be altered spermatogonia in the S or G_2 phases of the cell cycle. They rest on the basal lamina and have pale cytoplasm and a pale, ovoid nucleus, at least 13 μm in diameter. The frequency of these cells in normal and infertile men is about 0.65 cells per 50 tubular profiles, although their number is usually higher in mixed atrophy. These cells, which should not be mistaken for intratubular germ cell neoplasia, are also present in normal numbers in the tubules at the periphery of germ cell tumors.[526]

Dislocated spermatogonia

Normally, spermatogonia are seen away from the basal lamina only in the transition zone between the seminiferous tubules and the tubuli recti. Similar dislocated spermatogonia have been found throughout the testis in old age,[527] in infertile patients with a variety of lesions, and after long-term estrogen therapy.[528]

Megalospermatocytes

Megalospermatocytes are large primary spermatocytes, arrested in the leptotene stage (Fig. 10-84). Joined by cytoplasmic bridges, they form small groups.[529] These cells may be clones of synchronously degenerating spermatocytes.[530] They are frequently found in elderly men and are a nonspecific finding in infertile patients.

Multinucleate spermatids

The presence of spermatids with multiple nuclei (from 2 to 86) is frequent in old age.[531] Similar cells with fewer nuclei have also been reported in infertility due to cryptorchidism,[532] hyperprolactinemia, and in idiopathic infertility (Fig. 10-85).

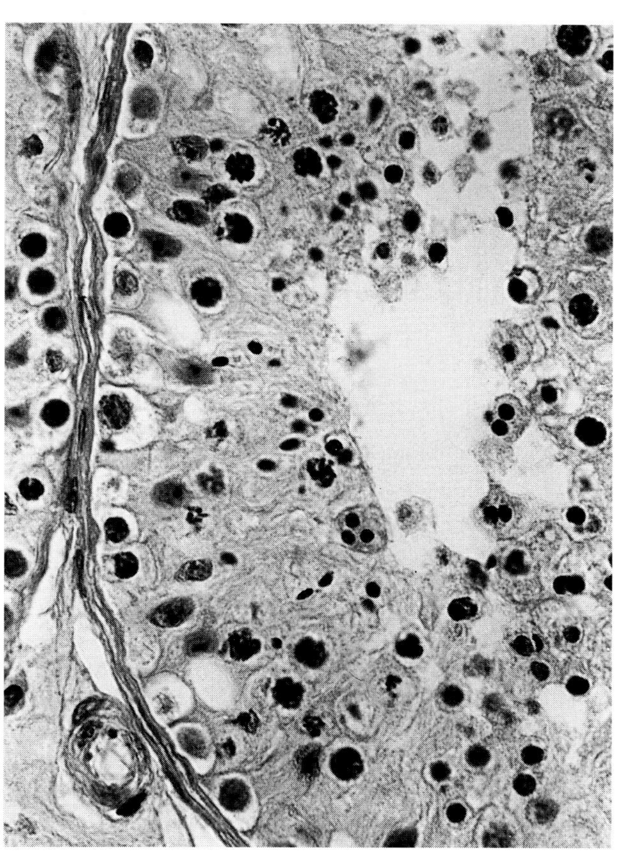

10-85. Multinucleate spermatids.

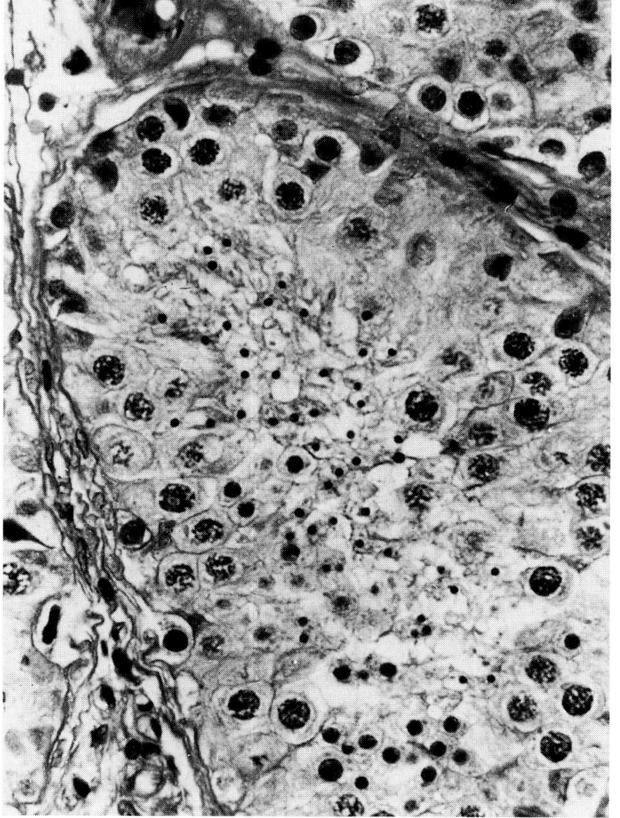

10-86. Biopsy showing spermatids with small spherical nuclei, a finding characteristic of round spermatozoa lacking acrosomes. The remaining germ cells are morphologically normal.

Malformed spermatids

Although spermatozoal abnormalities are not usually studied by testicular biopsy, there are three teratospermic syndromes that are easily identified in testicular biopsies by the morphology of elongate (S_c and S_d) spermatids: excessively elongate nuclei (characteristic of varicocele); small and spherical nuclei (characteristic of round spermatozoa lacking acrosomes) (Fig. 10-86); and excessively abundant cytoplasmic remnants (characteristic of spermatozoa with short and thick tails).[533]

Morphologically abnormal spermatozoa

Ultrastructural study of spermatozoa is sometimes necessary to determine the cause of male infertility. A number of morphologically abnormal spermatozoa are seen in all semen, even from fertile men, but abnormal spermatozoa are very numerous in infertile patients. Ultrastructural study is advised in all cases of asthenospermia, in teratospermia when the number of spermatozoa showing the same morphological anomaly is high, and in cases with apparently normal spermatozoa that fail to fertilize in vitro. The classification of ultrastructural anomalies in spermatozoa is based on light microscopic findings[534] of lesions in the head and tail.

Anomalies of spermatozoal head. These are defined by changes in the shape of the head, and usually involve both the nucleus and acrosome. Some anomalies, such as pear-shaped, candle-shaped, or egg-shaped heads,[535,536] are regarded as minor variants of normal. More significant abnormalities are the elongate, microcephalic, macrocephalic, and crater-defect forms.

The most frequent abnormal head shape is an elongate head with a narrow base (tapered head spermatozoa). This anomaly is frequently associated with varicocele.[537]

Microcephalic spermatozoa have spherical (globozoospermia) or irregularly shaped heads. The former have spherical nuclei with poorly condensed chromatin and lack acrosomes, postacrosomic sheaths, and nuclear rings (Fig. 10-87). Most cases are sporadic, but this lesion has been reported in two pairs of infertile brothers.[538,539] Microcephalic spermatozoa with irregularly shaped heads have small and irregularly shaped acrosomes that usually are not in contact with the nucleus. This anomaly may be congenital or secondary to heat exposure or hashish smoking. In both types of microcephaly the loss of connection between the acrosomic vesicle and the spermatozoal head is attributed to a deficiency in basic proteins of the sperm perinuclear theca, which promote nuclear

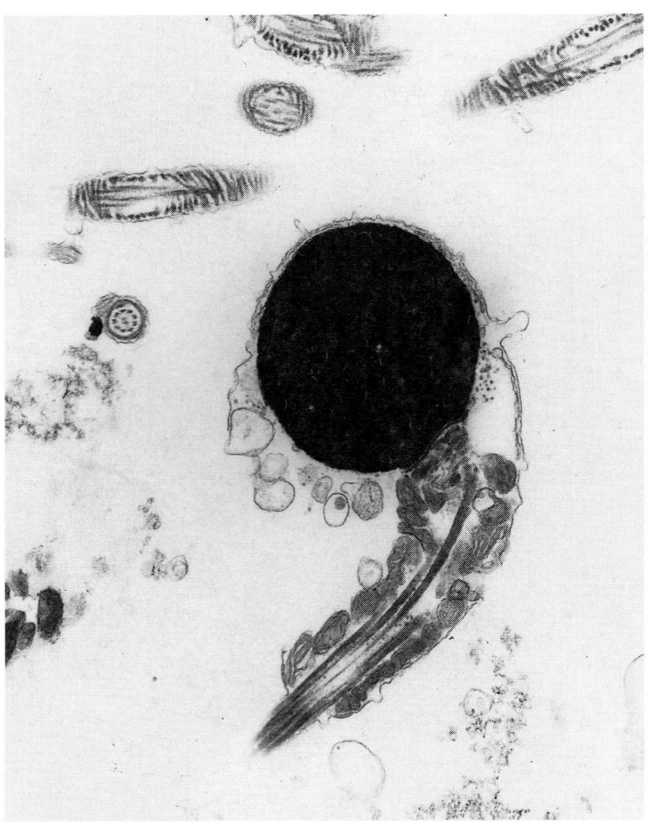

10-87. Microcephalic spermatozoon with a spherical nucleus lacking an acrosome. The cross-sectioned principal piece shows no axonemal ultrastructural anomaly.

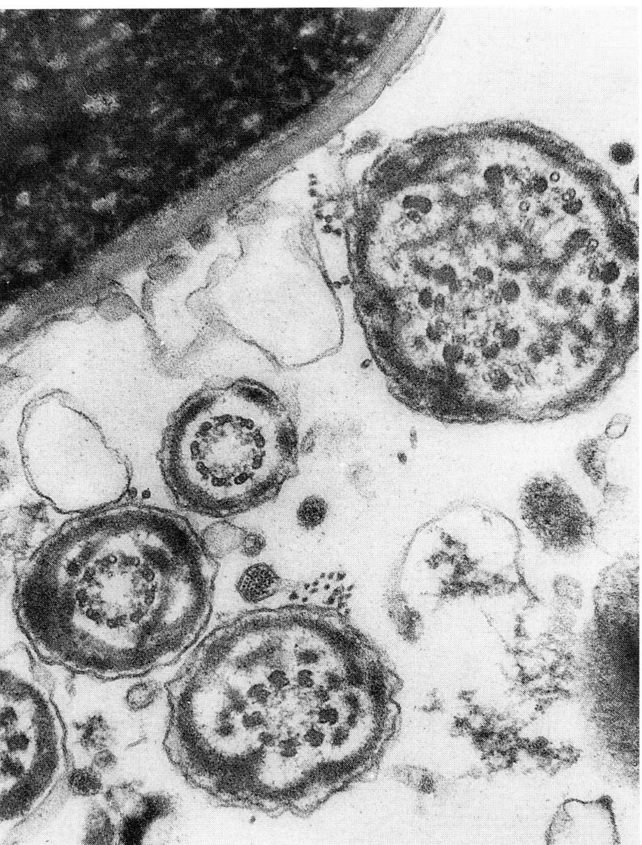

10-88. Tail stump spermatozoal malformation. Cross sections of the principal pieces from several spermatozoa. The most constant anomaly is the absence of the central pair of microtubules in the axoneme. A spermatozoon shows excessive amounts of microtubules, outer dense fibers, and fibrous sheath material.

envelope organization and adhesion of the acrosomic vesicle.[540]

Macrocephalic spermatozoa have enlarged, irregularly shaped heads; deficient chromatin condensation; and multiple tails.[541,542]

Irregularly shaped spermatozoa are characterized by irregularity in the shape of the nucleus or acrosome.[543] In the crater-defect syndrome, there is an invagination of the nuclear envelope into which the acrosome penetrates. The tail is morphologically normal and motility is only slightly reduced. Other anomalies include double-headed spermatozoa and spermatozoa with two nuclei sharing a single acrosome.[544]

Anomalies of spermatozoal tail. Spermatozoal tail anomalies are classified as generalized abnormalities of the tail or as anomalies in defined tail components such as the connecting piece, the axoneme, or periaxonemal structures.[545]

Generalized abnormalities of the tail. ***Cytoplasmic remnants.*** The presence of cytoplasmic droplets in some spermatozoa is thought to be the result of deficient maturation in the epididymis. The cytoplasmic remnant may be located either around the intermediate piece or surrounding the head. These spermatozoa also have other flagellar anomalies.

Bent tail. A bend in the tail may occur at the level of the connecting piece or the intermediate piece. In bends of the connecting piece the tail is laterally implanted and forms an angle with a nucleus that displays a thin base. In bends of the intermediate piece the bend is associated with cytoplasmic droplets, malposition of mitochondria, and loss of parallel arrangement of the dense outer fibers.

Coiled tail. Spermatozoa with a coiled tail have a perinuclear cytoplasmic remnant containing a flagellum that is coiled around the nucleus. This is frequently associated with abnormalities of the dense outer fibers and axoneme.

Tail stump. The tail stump category also includes short-thick tail and absence of the central pair of flagellar microtubules.[546] Some spermatozoa with a short and thick tail have no principal piece, and the intermediate piece usually lacks organized flagellar components. Other short-thick-tailed spermatozoa have thickened intermediate pieces that contain disorganized accumulations of fibrous sheath fragments or a rudimentary intermediate piece and a principal piece with an irregularly thickened fibrous sheath.[547] These malformations are associated with the absence of the central pair of flagellar microtubules (Fig. 10-88).[548]

Multiple tails. The presence of more than two tails is associated with macrocephalic spermatozoa.[542]

Anomalies of connecting piece. In the syndrome of decapitated spermatozoa the flagella are released to the tubular lumen and the nuclei are phagocytosed by Sertoli cells. Semen analysis shows only flagella. The spermatozoa do not possess normal heads, but there is a knoblike cytoplasmic thickening that connects with an intermediate piece showing variable disorganization of the mitochondrial sheath.[549] There are two variants of decapitated spermatozoa, which are caused by developmental failure in the postnuclear region, resulting in the absence of the basal plate and the implantation fossa, and flagellar implantation failure, due either to a chemical abnormality of the filamentous material between the capitulum and the basal plate or to a defect in flagellar migration toward the caudal pole of the spermatid nucleus.[550]

Anomalies in axoneme and periaxonemal structures. Abnormalities of the axoneme are usually associated with those of the periaxonemal structures. Axonemal anomalies are also observed in the cilia of the respiratory mucosa in the immotile cilia syndrome.[551] The most frequent abnormalities are absence of microtubule doublets and peripheral junctions, the central microtubule complex, the outer dynein arms, the central junctions, the two dynein arms, and the inner dynein arm plus the peripheral junctions (Fig. 10-89). Spermatozoa lacking the two dynein arms or the peripheral junctions are immotile. Reduced motility is seen in spermatozoa with only one dynein arm.

Periaxonemal abnormalities include mitochondrial sheath defects[552]; malposition of the annulus; alteration in number, shape, or length of the outer dense fibers; and absence, thickening, or disruption of the fibrous sheath.[553,554]

CORRELATION BETWEEN TESTICULAR BIOPSY AND SPERMIOGRAM

For effective therapy, it is important to know whether or not the azoospermia or oligozoospermia is the result of obstruction.[430,555]

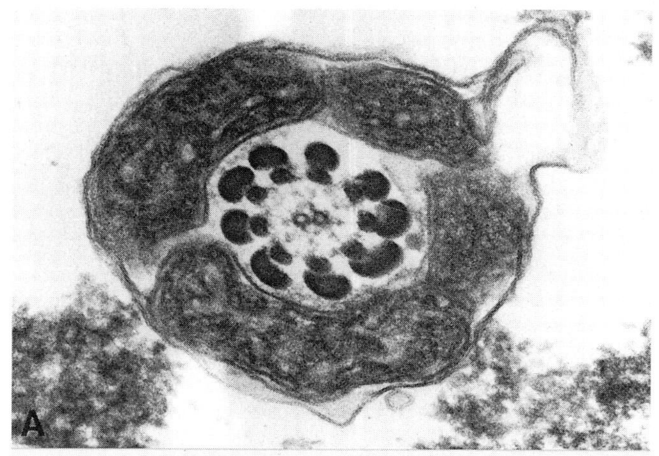

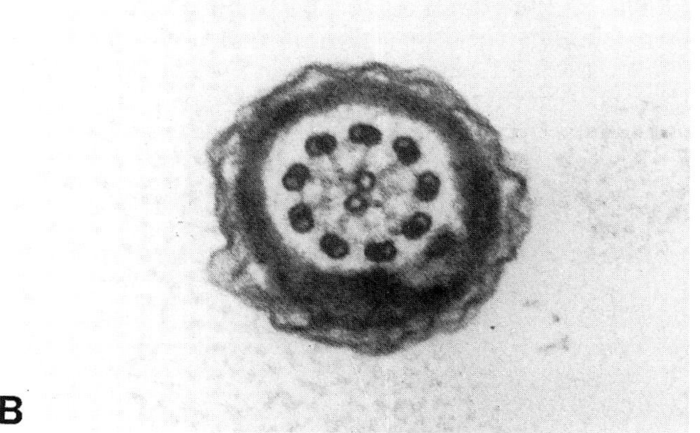

10-89. Cross section of the intermediate (**A**) and principal (**B**) pieces from spermatozoa lacking in dynein arms.

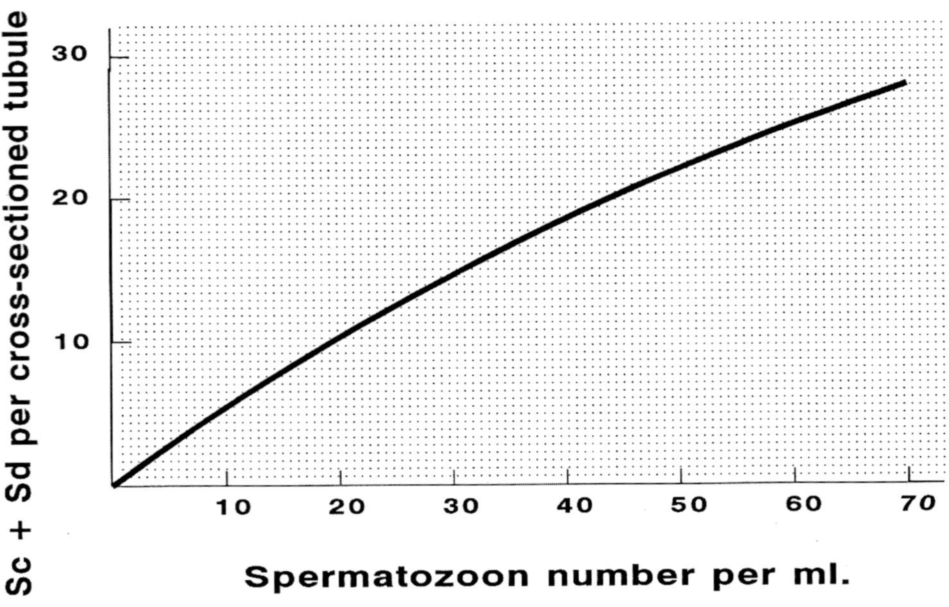

10-90. Power curve showing the correlation between the number of spermatozoa in the spermiogram and the number of adult spermatids (Sc + Sd) per tubular profile. If the number of mature (Sc + Sd) spermatids is correlated with that spermatozoa in the spermiogram, the oligozoospermia is of the pure secretory type. If the number of mature spermatids is higher than that of spermatozoa, the disorder is either an obstructive azoospermia with "normal" testicular biopsy or a mixed, obstructive, secretory oligozoospermia.

Obstructive azoospermia and oligozoospermia

Azoospermia caused by obstruction is usually easily diagnosed but difficulty arises with oligospermia. Obstruction of the ductal system should be suspected when there are fewer than 20 mature spermatids (S_c + S_d) per tubular profile and more than 10 million spermatozoa in the spermiogram (Fig. 10-90).[556,557] Obstructive azoospermia is implicated in 7.4% to 14.3% of male infertility.

Classification of obstructive azoospermia by location. Obstruction is classified as proximal, distal, and mixed according to the distance from the testis to the point of obstruction in the ductal system.

Proximal obstruction. Obstruction is considered proximal when the lesion lies between the seminiferous tubules and the distal end of the ampulla of the vas deferens. Epididymal obstruction, principally of the caput-corpus transition zone, accounts for 66% of cases. Rarely, there is a defective connection between the rete testis and epididymal ductuli efferentes. Since their seminal vesicles are normal, men with proximal obstruction have normal volumes of semen (the testicular contribution to semen is about 5% of the total volume).

Distal obstruction. Distal obstructions are located between the ampulla of the ductus deferens and the junction of the ejaculatory ducts and urethra. These patients may present with sacral, perineal, or scrotal pain on ejaculation. Rectal examination often reveals enlarged seminal vesicles. The volume of semen is low and it consists of watery fluid which fails to coagulate. Seminal vesicle secretions are lacking. The concentration of prostatic secretions, such as acid phosphatase and citric acid, is increased due to the lack of semen dilution. Vasography may help in the diagnosis since higher segments fail to fill.[558]

Mixed obstruction. The term *mixed obstruction* refers to the congenital absence of the vas deferens or lack of patency of this duct. Most patients with congenital absence of vas deferens have low volumes of semen due to abnormalities of the seminal vesicles. The vas deferens and seminal vesicles are mesonephric duct derivatives, so mixed obstruction may include congenital anomalies in both structures, with hypoplasia or agenesis of seminal vesicles in 33% of cases. Since 66% of patients have seminal vesicles, agenesis or obstruction of the ejaculatory ducts has been proposed to account for the low volume of semen in most cases of mixed obstruction.

Etiology of obstructive azoospermia. Obstructive azoospermia may be caused by congenital or acquired lesions.

Congenital azoospermia. In about 1% of cases of azoospermia, there is bilateral absence or atresia of both vasa deferentia. Approximately 36% of cryptorchid patients also have anatomical anomalies in the epididymis or vas deferens. These are classified in the box on page 517.

Agenesis of all mesonephric duct derivatives. Agenesis of all mesonephric duct derivatives is a rare disorder that gives rise to varied anatomical anomalies, depending on the stage of embryonic development at which the mesonephric duct derivatives disappear. If failure occurs before the fourth week the ipsilateral kidney and ureter are absent, although the testis may be present, or there are other renal anomalies. If failure occurs in the

CONGENITAL ANOMALIES OF THE MALE MESONEPHRIC DUCTS

I. Agenesis of all mesonephric duct derivatives
II. Epididymis
 Agenesis of the epididymis
 Testis-epididymis dissociation
 Failure in the connection of ductuli efferentes–ductus epididymidis
 Cysts of the epididymis
 Anomalies in epididymal configuration
  Elongate epididymis
  Angulate epididymis
  Free epididymis
III. Ductus deferens
 Agenesis of the ductus deferens
 Persistent mesonephric duct
IV. Seminal vesicle
 Agenesis of the seminal vesicle
 Cysts of the seminal vesicle
 Opening of the ureter into the seminal vesicle
V. Ejaculatory duct
 Agenesis of the ejaculatory duct

fourth week, and the ureteral bud is already formed, the ureter and kidney may develop normally. If failure occurs between the fourth and thirteenth weeks, there is a variable constellation of anomalies which most frequently include normal development of the testis and globus major and hypoplasia of the other excretory duct segments, or agenesis of an excretory duct segment (epididymis, ductus deferens, or seminal vesicle).

Epididymal anomalies. The most frequent epididymal anomalies are absence of the epididymis, testis-epididymis dissociation, defective connection of vas deferens and epididymis, epididymal cysts, and anatomic abnormalities of the epididymis.

Complete absence of the epididymis is frequent in monorchidism and anorchidism. In place of the epididymis is a small mass of cellular connective tissue with abundant blood vessels at the blind end of the vas deferens. Partial absence is more frequent than complete. Absence of the body of the epididymidis gives rise to a characteristic malformation called *bilobate epididymis*. This varies from simple strangulation to complete separation of the head and tail. These anomalies are often associated with absence of the vas deferens.

Testis-epididymis dissociation is found in 1% of cases of obstructive azoospermia and is usually associated with cryptorchidism.

Defects in connection between the vas deferens and epididymis are rarely complete. In the complete form microdissection shows that some of the 5 to 30 efferent ductules in the epididymis are short and end blindly.

Epididymal cysts usually arise from blindly ending efferent ductules and contain spermatozoa. These spermatoceles retain their epithelial lining, although it becomes atrophic. Some epididymal cysts arise from embryonal remnants, do not contain spermatozoa, and are lined by columnar or pseudostratified epithelium. Large epididymal cysts require removal and must be excised with great care to avoid damaging the efferent ductules which would cause an obstruction. Epididymal cysts are present in about 5% of males, and the incidence is high (21%) in patients who were exposed to diethylstilbestrol during gestation.

Anomalies in epididymal configuration, altering its shape and location, are frequent in cryptorchidism patients and uncommon in men with descended testes. The most common malformations are elongate epididymis, angulate epididymis, and free epididymis. Elongate epididymis is found in approximately 68% of undescended testes. The length of the epididymis may be several times that of the testis, and, in abdominal or inguinal cryptorchidism, the epididymis extends several centimeters below the testis. Angulate epididymis is characterized by a long epididymis that has a sharp bend in the body, with or without stenosis. With free epididymis all or part of the epididymis is unattached to the testis. The most common variant is epididymis with free tail.

Vas deferens anomalies. There are two anomalies of the vas deferens: congenital absence and persistent mesonephric duct.

Congenital absence of the vas deferens is unilateral or bilateral absence of either the whole vas deferens or only a segment of it. Obviously, azoospermia occurs with bilateral absence. The frequency of this malformation varies among patient populations. In autopsy series the incidence is 0.5%, but it is 1% to 1.3% in infertile men[559] and 10% to 70% in patients with obstructive azoospermia. Unilateral complete absence is three times more frequent than bilateral and absence of only a segment is even more frequent. The affected segment may be absent or reduced to a fibrous cord. Absence of the vas deferens may be associated with other malformations of the sperm excretory ducts or the urinary system. The most frequent malformations of the excretory ducts are absence of the ejaculatory ducts (33% of cases) and, less frequently, absence of seminal vesicles. About 71% of patients with bilateral absence of the vas deferens have partial aplasia of the epididymis. The most frequent malformations of the urinary system are absence of the ipsilateral kidney and other renal anomalies. Complete or partial absence of the vas deferens occurs frequently in patients with cystic fibrosis.

Persistent mesonephric duct consists of the ureter joined to the vas deferens, forming a single duct that opens in an ectopic orifice between the trigone and the verumontanum. This malformation may be associated with cystic transformation or absence of the seminal vesicle. The kidney may be normal or dysplastic.

Anomalies of seminal vesicle and ejaculatory duct. The most frequent anomalies are agenesis of the seminal vesicles or ejaculatory ducts, cyst of the seminal vesicle, and ectopic opening of the ureter into the seminal vesicle. The last is the most common and often is associated with ipsilateral renal dysplasia.

Acquired azoospermia. Inflammation and trauma are the main causes of acquired azoospermia. Epididymitis is a frequent cause of acquired azoospermia; *Chlamydia trachomatis*[560,561] and *Escherichia coli* are currently the most common infectious causes. Infections with *Neisseria gonorrhoeae* and mycobacteria also are implicated, and nonspecific epididymitis is important. Aside from elective vasectomy, the most frequent traumatic causes of azoospermia are surgical accidents during herniorrhaphy in children,[562] orchiopexy, varicocelectomy, hydrocelectomy, and deferentography.[563] Obstructive azoospermia may also result from blockage of the ejaculatory ducts following transurethral resection or as a result of chronic urethral catheterization.

Testicular and epididymal lesions resulting from obstruction of sperm excretory ducts. The effects of lesions on the testis and epididymis resulting from obstructed sperm excretory ducts depend on the location, origin (congenital or acquired), and duration of the obstruction.

Location of obstruction. Obstruction at the level of the ampullae of the vas deferens, seminal vesicles, or ejaculatory ducts usually does not cause significant lesions in the testis or epididymis. More proximal obstruction at the levels of the vas deferens, epididymis, or testis-epididymis junction usually cause severe lesions in both the sperm excretory ducts and testicular parenchyma. Obstruction of the vas deferens causes increased pressure within the ductus epididymis. As a result, the epididymal lumen dilates, the epithelium atrophies, and fluid containing few spermatozoa and some spermiophages accumulates in the lumen. The most dilated epididymal segment is the head. The ductuli efferentes often become cystically dilated and filled with spermatozoa and macrophages. From the reabsorption and lysosomal degradation of this protein-rich fluid, the epithelium accumulates lipofuscin granules. Macrophages and lymphocytes often are present in the intertubular connective tissue.[564]

Etiology of obstruction. Obstruction secondary to congenital absence of the vas deferens usually causes little testicular injury, mainly dilation of the seminiferous tubules and an increase in the number of mature ($S_c + S_d$) spermatids.[565] Lesions resulting from vasectomy are more important. Increased intraluminal pressure in the epididymis[566] may give rise to pain (late postvasectomy syndrome).[567] The spermatogenic rhythm in the testis is slower than before vasectomy, and lesions characteristic of testicular obstruction develop, including thickening of the lamina propria and fibrosis of the interstitium.[568]

Duration of obstruction. In acquired obstruction the testicular lesions worsen with time. Obstruction in the head of the epididymis leads to the disappearance of all germ cells in the adluminal compartment of the seminiferous tubules. The tubules become dilated and the Sertoli cells vacuolated. Testicular alterations after vasectomy may not be related to the duration of the obstruction but to the initial injury, and they may disappear with time as the intraluminal pressure decreases.[569] However, if a significant amount of time has elapsed after vasectomy, the possibility of attaining a normal spermiogram with vasovasostomy is very low. Vasal patency is restored in most cases, but the paternity rates are markedly lower (25% to 51%)[570] than normal (85%).[571]

Functional azoospermia and oligozoospermia

Some azoospermic patients have testicular biopsies with minimal histologic abnormality or minor tubular dilation without detectable excretory duct obstruction. These findings are characteristic of two main conditions: Young's syndrome and alterations in spermatozoal transport.

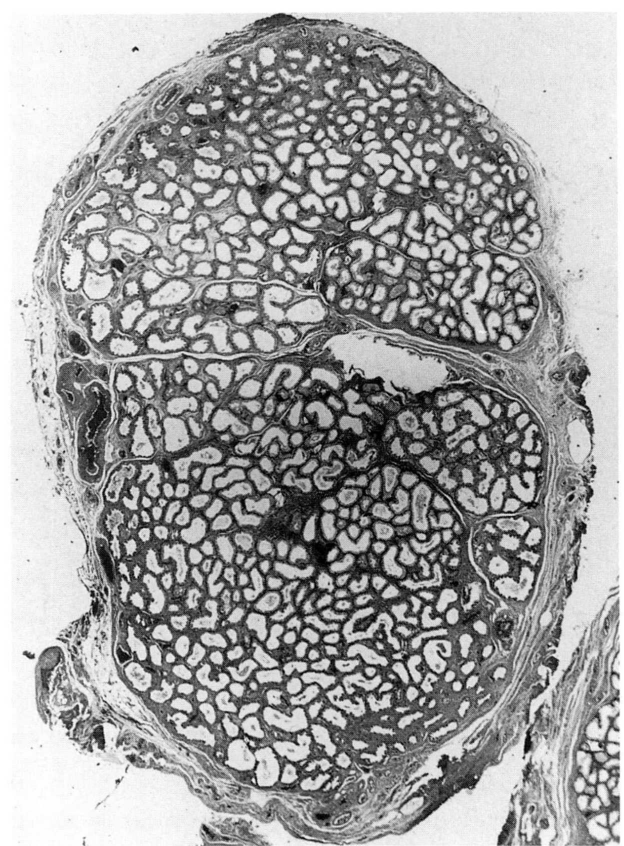

10-91. Young's syndrome. Caput epididymidis showing marked dilation of the efferent ductules.

Young's syndrome. Young's syndrome is defined by the following constellation of findings: azoospermia, sinusitis, bronchitis or bronchiectasis, and normal spermatozoal flagella.[572] The incidence is probably higher than that recorded in the literature, and Young's syndrome should be suspected in all patients with obstructive azoospermia without histories of epididymitis or scrotal trauma. These patients have a lesion at the junction of the head and body of the epididymis which gives the epididymis a characteristic gross appearance. The head of the epididymis is distended, the ductuli efferentes contain yellowish fluid and numerous spermatozoa, while the remaining epididymal segments are normal (Fig. 10-91). The ductus epididymidis is blocked by a thick fluid.[573] Young's syndrome should be distinguished from other causes of infertility also associated with chronic sinusitis and pulmonary infections, including ciliary dyskinesia and cystic fibrosis. Ciliary dyskinesia consists of morphological, biochemical, and functional alterations in cilia and flagella, and includes several diseases such as immotile cilium syndrome, Kartagener's syndrome, and miscellaneous syndromes characterized by less well defined abnormalities of cilia and flagella.[574] In Young's syndrome, sinusitis and pulmonary infections develop in childhood and stabilize or improve in adolescence; in these other conditions, the pulmonary damage increases with age and the cilia and flagella are ultrastructurally abnormal.[575]

Alterations in spermatozoal transport. Normally, spermatozoa detach from the Sertoli cells and are transported through the intratesticular and extratesticular excretory ducts, where they are stored, mainly in the tail of the epididymis, and, finally, released from the body by ejaculation or are eliminated by phagocytosis. Only about 50% of spermatozoa are ejaculated. While the release of spermatozoa from the body is intermittent, their transport through the sperm excretory ducts is continuous. Transport is accomplished by the myoid cells in the walls of the seminiferous tubules and ductuli efferentes and the smooth muscle cells in the walls of the ductus epididymidis and vas deferens. These cells cause peristaltic contraction, propelling spermatozoa along the length of the epididymis in an average of 12 days (range, 1 to 21 days). The walls of the seminiferous tubules and extratesticular excretory ducts are under hormonal and neural control. The myoid cells in the seminiferous tubules have oxytocinic, alpha 1-beta adrenergic, and muscarinic receptors. Unmyelinated nerve fibers penetrate the tubular lamina propria, pass among the myoid cells, and end near the Sertoli cells.[576] Along their length these nerve fibers have varicosities containing sympathetic vesicles.

The ductus epididymidis is innervated by sympathetic adrenergic nerve fibers that end among the smooth muscle cells. Several hormones, including oxytocin, vasopressin, and prostaglandins, act on the musculature of the ductus epididymidis. The peristaltic contractions begin in the head and propagate toward the tail. The frequency and amplitude of contractions varies from region to region, higher in frequency near the head and of maximal amplitude in the initial portion of the tail. The progressive increase in amplitude parallels the progressive increase in the thickness of the muscular wall and the requirement for greater force to propel the fluid as it becomes progressively more viscous with a higher concentration of spermatozoa. The distal portion of the tail is usually at rest because it is the main reservoir of spermatozoa between ejaculations. Several times daily, vigorous contractions of the distal tail impel the spermatozoa from the tail toward the vas deferens.

INFERTILITY AND CHROMOSOMAL ANOMALIES

Other than in Klinefelter's syndrome and Down's syndrome, chromosomal abnormalities are unlikely to be suggested by physical examination of the infertile man. Most are suspected only after examination of the testicular biopsy and then confirmed cytogenetically. In some cases infertility may be the consequence of a chromosomal anomaly; in others infertility and chromosomal anomaly coexist but are not causally linked.

ABNORMALITIES OF SEX CHROMOSOMES

Klinefelter's syndrome

Genetic and clinical aspects. Klinefelter's syndrome is characterized by an abnormal number of X chromosomes and primary gonadal insufficiency. The original description was of a man with eunuchoidism, gynecomastia, small testes, mental retardation, and elevated levels of serum gonadotropin.[577] The frequency of this syndrome varies according to the population studied: 1 in 1000 to 1 in 1400 of surviving newborns, 1 in 100 of patients in mental institutions, and 3.4 in 100 of infertile men.

In 80% of cases the karyotype is 47XXY. The remaining 20% have chromosomal mosaicism with at least two X chromosomes. The most common are XY/XXY, XY/XXXY, XX/XXY, XY/XO/XXY, XX/XXY/XXXY, and XXXY/XXXXY. The 47XXY lesion is due to nondysjunction in sex chromosome migration during the first or second meiotic division of the spermatocyte or ovule or during the first mitotic division of the zygote.[578] Study of the Xg antigen in blood revealed that in 73% of cases the extra X chromosome is from the mother. Advanced maternal age increases the incidence of children with the 47XXY karyotype.

In 47XXY patients, the most common clinical findings are:

1. Eunuchoid phenotype with increased stature. The increased height is due to a disproportionate lengthening of the lower extremities. The ratio of span to height is less than 1.
2. Incomplete virilization. This is variable and ranges from normal development to absence of secondary sex characteristics.
3. Gynecomastia, usually bilateral, is present in 50% of patients.
4. Mental retardation.

Other commonly associated conditions include chronic bronchitis; varicose veins; cervical rib; kyphosis; scoliosis or pectus excavatum; and a high incidence of hypothalamic, hypophyseal, thyroid, and pancreatic dysfunctions.[579]

The external genitalia usually are normally developed. The testes are usually less than 2.5 cm long, although in some cases of chromosomal mosaicism they are of normal size. The incidence of cryptorchidism is low in 47XXY patients but increased in mosaicism.[580]

Histologically, the testes show the classic picture of tubular dysgenesis with small hyalinized seminiferous tubules lacking elastic fibers and pseudoadenomatous clustering of Leydig cells (Fig. 10-92, 10-93).[577] Most biopsies show some tubules with a few Sertoli cells.[581] These cells may be dysgenetic (pseudostratified distribution of nuclei, which are dark and elongate and contain small peripherally placed nucleoli in tubules without apparent lumens) or exhibit an involutional pattern (irregular nuclei with a columnar distribution in tubules with lumens). Sex chromatin may only be observed in dysgenetic Sertoli cells.[582] This suggests that either there is testicular mosaicism of the X chromosome or both X chromosomes are heterochromatinized. In mosaicism the Sertoli cell–only tubules may be more numerous than sclerotic ones.

The reduced testicular volume gives an appearance of Leydig cell hyperplasia,[583] although quantitative studies have shown that the total number of Leydig cells is lower than normal.[584] Many of the Leydig cells are pleomorphic and some are multivacuolated. Immature

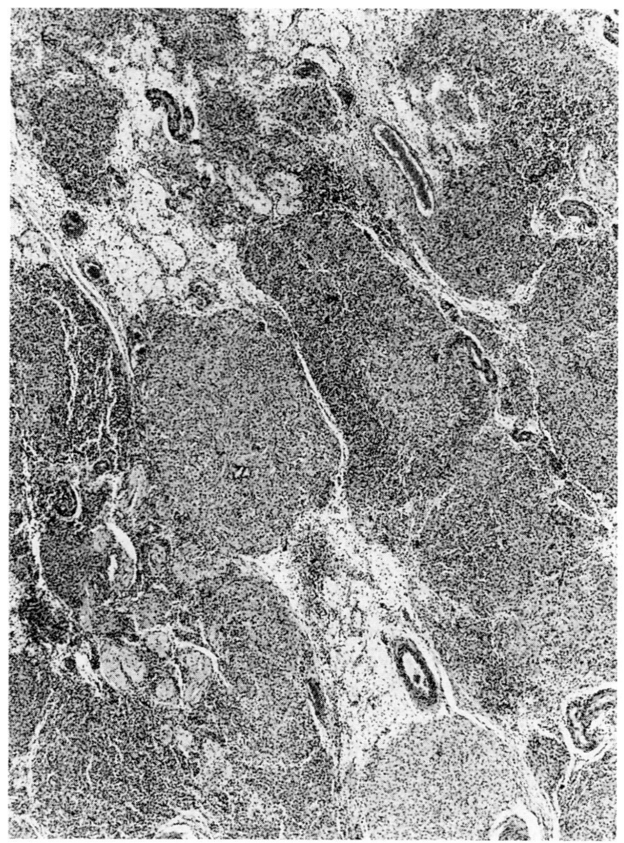

10-92. Klinefelter's syndrome. Leydig cell nodules mingle with hyalinized tubules.

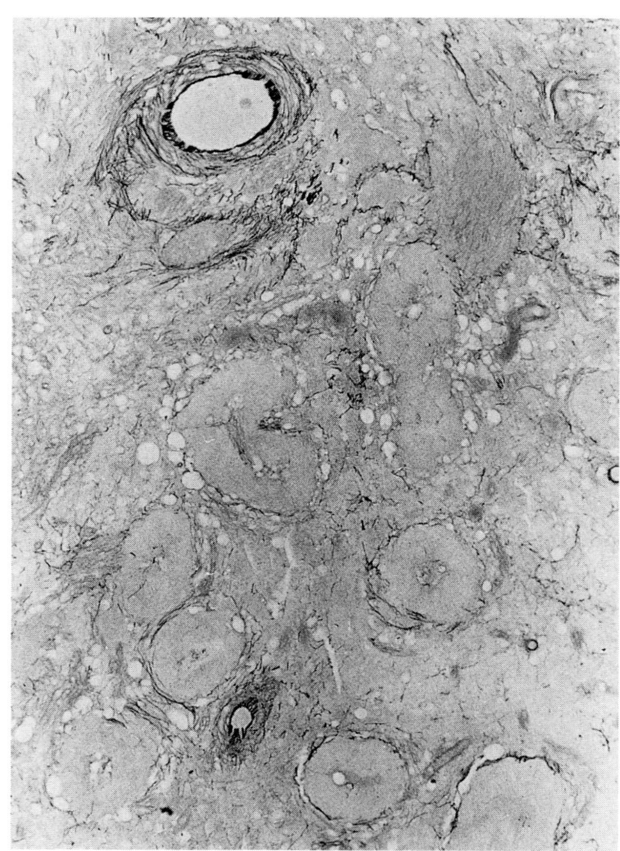

10-93. Klinefelter's syndrome. Most of the seminiferous tubules have no elastic fibers as demonstrated with the orcein staining method. The positive staining of the inner elastic membrane in an artery serves as a positive control.

fibroblast-like Leydig cells may be present. The abnormally differentiated Leydig cells have nuclei with coarse masses of dense chromatin, deep infoldings of the nuclear envelope, multiple paracrystalline inclusions instead of Reinke's crystalloids, multilayered concentric cisternae of smooth endoplasmic reticulum, large masses of microfilaments, and scant lipid droplets.[585] Sex chromatin is apparent in 40% to 70% of Leydig cells. Leydig cell function is insufficient and androgen levels are less than 50% of normal. Basal follicle stimulating hormone and luteinizing hormone levels are markedly increased.[579,586,587] In a few patients the testicular damage is less severe than in XXY patients, with some tubules showing spermatogenesis and less prominence of Leydig cells.[588] Exceptionally, complete spermatogenesis and even paternity have been reported.[589]

The XX/XXY karyotype is the most frequent variant of Klinefelter's syndrome with chromosome mosaicism. In this condition the clinical abnormalities may be attenuated. Gynecomastia is present in 33% of cases, compared with a frequency of 55% in men with the 47XXY karyotype. Azoospermia is found in 50% of cases (93% in XXY men). The testes are larger and spermatogenesis is more developed than in men with XXY because there are spermatogonia with normal karyotypes.

The incidence of the 48XXYY karyotype is estimated to be 0.04 per 1000 live births.[590-593] This karyotype may be associated with aggressive character, antisocial behavior, more severe mental retardation, and a higher frequency of congenital malformations than the 47XXY karyotype. Men with the 48XXYY karyotype also have characteristic dermatoglyphics with increases in arches, decreases in total finger ridge count, and ulnar triradiuses associated with pictures in the hypothenar region.[594] Concentric lamellae of smooth endoplasmic reticulum in Leydig cells is a characteristic finding.[595] Men with the 48XXXY or 49XXXYY karyotypes often have skeletal malformations, principally radioulnar synostosis, and cryptorchidism.[596] Men with the 49XXXXY karyotype have, in addition to the characteristic symptoms of 47XXY Klinefelter's syndrome, other abnormalities including severe mental retardation, hypoplasia of external genitalia, cardiac malformations, radioulnar synostosis, microcephaly, and high arched palate.[597]

Association with malignant tumors. Patients with Klinefelter's syndrome have a higher incidence of malignant tumors than the general population. The association was first discovered with breast carcinoma,[598] with an incidence 20 times greater than in the general male population,[599] and is related to hormonal stimula-

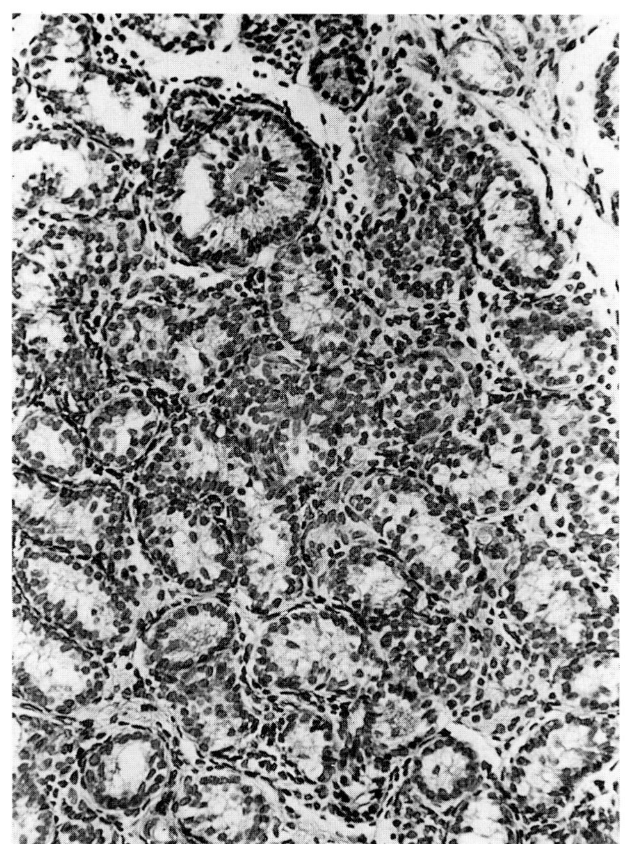

10-94. Klinefelter's syndrome in infantile testis. Seminiferous tubules with decreased diameter and absence of germ cells. A ring-shaped tubule is present.

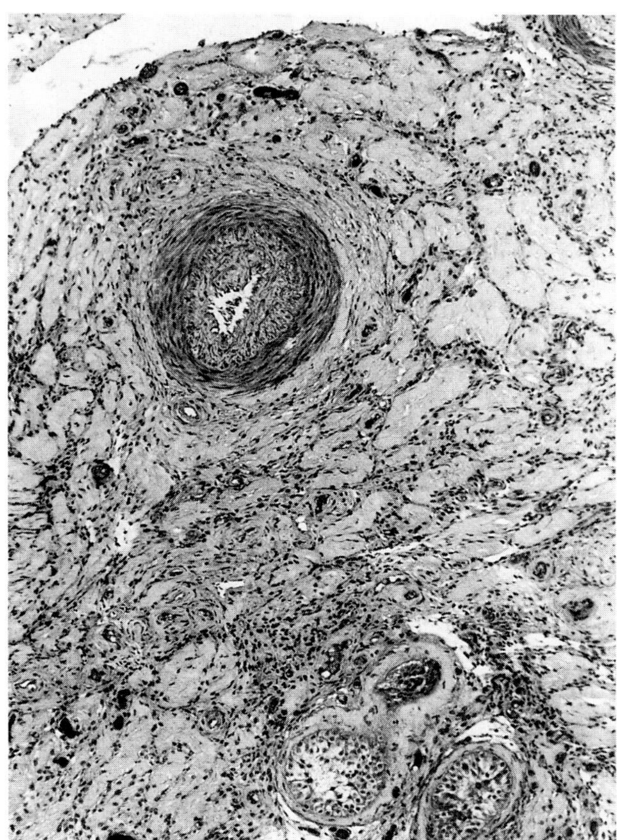

10-95. Klinefelter's syndrome with hypogonadotropic hypogonadism. Diffuse tubular hyalinization associated with absence of Leydig cells. Only tubules with dysgenetic Sertoli cells are present.

tion.[600] Although testicular germ cell tumors are rare in these patients,[601] extragonadal germ cell tumors are 30 to 40 times more frequent than in the general population. Most occur in the mediastinum (about 71%) and are less frequent in the pineal gland, central nervous system, and retroperitoneum. The most frequent types are teratoma and choriocarcinoma; embryonal carcinoma and seminoma are rare.[602-604] The extragonadal origin of germ cell tumors has been attributed to abnormal germ cell migration from the yolk sac. The high incidence has been attributed to elevated hormone levels and the chromosomal anomaly.[605] In a patient with the XY/XXY chromosomal mosaic and bronchogenic carcinoma, cultured XXY fibroblasts transformed 3 times more frequently than the patient's XY fibroblasts when exposed to SV40 virus, and 3 to 10 times more frequently than fibroblasts from normal men.[606]

Other tumors reported in patients with Klinefelter's syndrome (lymphomas, leukemias, bronchogenic carcinoma, urothelial carcinoma of the bladder, adrenal carcinoma, prostatic adenocarcinoma, and testicular Leydig cell tumor) do not seem to have a higher incidence than in the general population.[607,608]

Occurrence in childhood. Early identification of this syndrome in children is possible when there is systematic cytogenetic study of newborns with positive sex chromatin or mental retardation.[609] Several clinical symptoms suggest Klinefelter's syndrome, including mental retardation, psychiatric problems, excessive stature or span, and small testes.[610] Testicular biopsy reveals scant or absent germ cells. Quantitative studies indicate that the number of germ cells in 47XXY fetuses is significantly lower than in normal 46XY fetuses. The seminiferous tubules have reduced diameters, particularly those devoid of germ cells. The number of Sertoli cells per tubular profile is decreased. Megatubules, ring-shaped tubules, and intratubular eosinophilic bodies are common (Fig. 10-94). In some cases of Klinefelter's syndrome associated with Down's syndrome, tubular hyalinization is observed in childhood. The interstitium is wide and contains few Leydig cell precursors. If one testis is undescended, its histology does not differ from that of the contralateral testis. The testicular pattern remains constant throughout childhood.[611] At puberty, before maturation of the tunica propria occurs, the seminiferous tubules rapidly hyalinize and Leydig cell precursors differentiate into Leydig cells.

Association with hypogonadotropic hypogonadism. Klinefelter's syndrome is often associated with pituitary disorders such as panhypopituitarism[612] or incomplete hypopituitarism.[613] Deficits in follicle stimulating hormone,[614] luteinizing hormone,[615] or both[616,617] have been reported. The cause of this association is unknown, and diverse etiologies such as trauma, immunologic disorders, and genetic deficiencies have been postulated. Alternately, it may be due to exhaustion of pituitary gonadotropin-secreting cells after years of gonadotropin releasing hormone stimulation.[613]

In patients deficient in both gonadotropins, testicular biopsy shows diffuse tubular hyalinization and marked reduction in or absence of Leydig cells. The histological picture is very similar to that of hypogonadotropic hypogonadism occurring after puberty except for the presence of isolated tubules containing only dysgenetic Sertoli cells and the absence of elastic fibers in the hyalinized tubular walls (Fig. 10-95).[617] The biopsy of patients with a deficit only in follicle stimulating hormone is similar to that of the dysgenetic Sertoli cell variant of the Sertoli cell–only syndrome, although some hyalinized tubules are present. The testicular biopsy of patients deficient only in luteinizing hormone resembles that of men with Klinefelter's syndrome.

46XX males

Men with the 46XX karyotype have clinical features similar to Klinefelter's syndrome, including small testes, small or normal penis, azoospermia, gynecomastia, and minimal development of secondary sex characteristics. However, in these men body proportions are harmonious, stature is normal or slightly low, and intelligence is normal. The incidence of hypospadias is elevated.[618] The incidence of 46XX males is 1 in 9000 live births, accounting for about 0.2% of infertile men.[619,620] Males with 46XX karyotype have hypergonadotropic hypogonadism with elevated levels of follicle stimulating hormone and, to a lesser degree, elevated luteinizing hormone, with normal or slightly decreased testosterone.

During childhood, biopsy of 46XX males has shown decreased numbers of germ cells.[621,622] Biopsies from adults show one of three patterns: histology similar to that of 47XXY men including diffuse tubular hyalinization with prominent Leydig cells[623]; Sertoli cell–only tubules[624,625]; or both patterns intermingled with less prominent Leydig cells. The last is the most frequent (Fig. 10-96). Ultrastructural studies reveal an increase in intermediate filaments and absence of annulate lamellae in Sertoli cells,[626] and absence of Reinke's crystalloids and abundance of intracytoplasmic and intranuclear paracrystalline inclusions in Leydig cells.[624]

The cause of this syndrome remains controversial. All hypotheses are based on the indispensable role of the Y chromosome in testicular development and attempt to

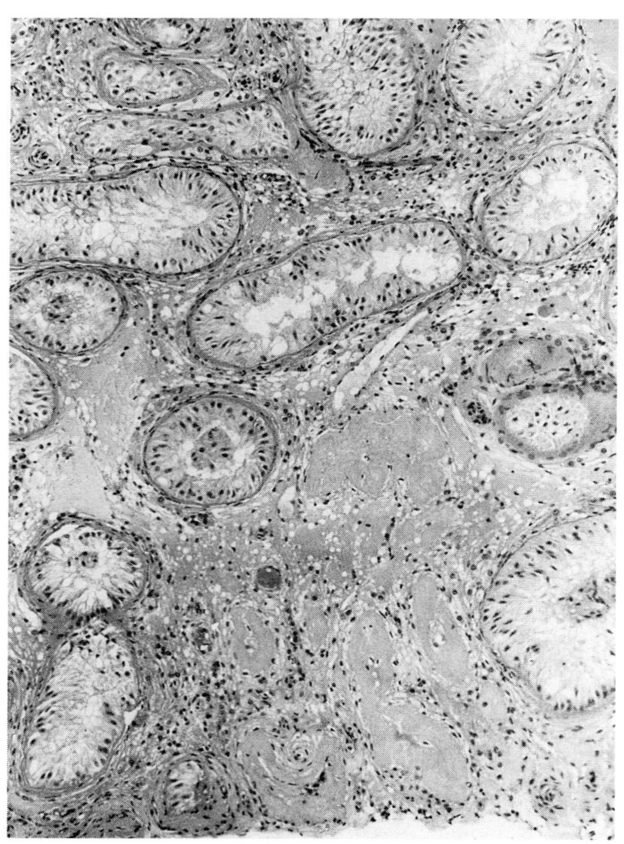

10-96. Testis of 46XX male shows Sertoli cell–only tubules around a group of hyalinized tubules.

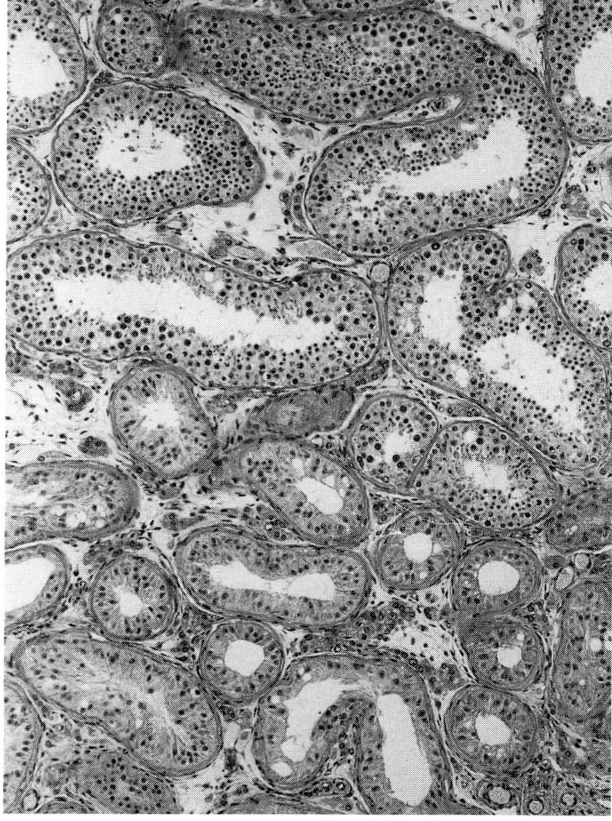

10-97. Testis of 47XYY syndrome shows mixed tubular atrophy. Seminiferous tubules showing spermatogenesis and Sertoli cell–only tubules are seen together.

explain the apparent absence of this chromosome. Current hypotheses are:

1. Translocation of the short arm of the Y chromosome. In most XX males, the Y-specific sequences may be located on X chromosomes.[627,628] This suggests that the testis determining factor gene (sex determining region Y or SRY) is transferred to the X chromosome of the father by an X-Y interchange during meiosis.[629]
2. Mosaicism. If chromosomal mosaicism is established by mitotic nondysjunction of sex chromosomes during the first stages of embryonic development, the Y chromosome might be restricted to a very low number of cells including some testicular cells but not lymphocytes on which karyotype analyses are performed. Y chromosome–specific DNA sequences have been found in XX male cells from the skin and testis using the polymerase chain reaction technique.[630]
3. Genetic mutation. It has been reported that the SRY gene cannot be detected in some 46XX males. It is possible that these men have undergone mutation in unknown X chromosomal or autosomal genes, this mutation promoting testicular differentiation.[631]

47XYY syndrome

47XYY syndrome was first described in 1961 in the father of a girl with Down's syndrome.[632] The only clinical findings were that he was unusually tall and had pustular acne. Study of other cases suggests that these men are predisposed to psychopathic personalities and antisocial behavior, although most have normal personalities and are socially adapted. The incidence of this chromosomal anomaly is 1.5 in 1000 live births[633] and rises to 3% in men from mental institutions and prisons. These men have normal external genitalia and secondary sex characteristics. Fertility is decreased,[634] although many have been fathers, including the man of the original description. Usually, testicular biopsy reveals mixed tubular atrophy: tubules with spermatogenesis associated with Sertoli cell–only tubules (Fig. 10-97).[635,636] The tubules with spermatogenesis may show normal spermatogenesis or have lesions in the adluminal or basal compartments. The variability in germ cell development is apparently due to elimination of those germ cells that could not pair their sex chromosomes during the first or second meiotic divisions[637] or, later, during the round spermatid stage.[638] Spermatocytes that succeed in forming trivalent chromosomes are initially viable.[639] The ultimate segregation of trivalents yields aneuploid and euploid cells in equal numbers. The Sertoli cell–only tubules are attributed to spermatogonial damage by substances released from degenerate spermatocytes.[640] These men have normal serum levels of testosterone and luteinizing hormone. The latter may be slightly increased in 47XYY men with severe spermatogenic alterations.[641]

Men with three and four Y chromosomes have been reported. Men with the 48XYYY karyotype are tall and have a normal male phenotype, slight mental retardation, azoospermia and, during childhood, frequent infections of the upper respiratory tract.[642] Testicular biopsy shows Sertoli cell–only tubules, severe hyalinization of the tubular basement membrane, and diffuse Leydig cell hyperplasia. Men with 49XYYYY have no important

TABLE 10-9.
PATHOLOGIC FINDINGS IN INFERTILE MEN WITH Y CHROMOSOME ANOMALIES IN THE Y_Q11 REGION

Karyotype	External genitalia	Testicular lesions	Associated anomalies
$46XY_q$	Small testes	Tubular hyalinization, Sertoli cell–only, spermatogenetic maturation arrest	Low stature, mental retardation, gynecomastia
46XYnf 45X0	Small and soft testes, small penis, ambiguous genitalia, cryptorchidism, hypospadias	Tubular hyalinization, Sertoli cell–only, Leydig cell hyperplasia, decreased spermatid number	Low stature, gynecomastia
46Xr(Y) 45X0	Small testes, cryptorchidism, hypospadias	Sertoli cell–only, spermatogenetic arrest in premeiotic spermatocytes	Low stature
$46Xt(Y_p11,Y_q11)$ 45X0	Small and soft testes, hypospadias	Spermatogenetic arrest in premeiotic spermatocytes, decreased spermatid number	Low stature
$46Yt(X_p22,Y_q11)$	Small testes, small penis	Spermatogenetic arrest in premeiotic spermatocytes	Mental retardation, digital anomalies, facial dysmorphism
$46XY_qt(Y_q11\text{-qter},A)$	Normal or small testes	Spermatogenetic arrest in premeiotic spermatocytes	
$46Xt(Y_q11\text{-pter},A)$	Normal or hypoplastic testes, cryptorchidism, hypospadias	Sertoli cell–only, immature seminiferous tubules	

physical anomalies either (except for cases of chromosomal mosaicism). Slight mental retardation, infertility, and antisocial behavior are the most significant clinical findings.[643]

Structural anomalies of Y chromosome

The Y chromosome is essential for sex determination and spermatogenesis; abnormalities in it often lead to infertility. The relationship between Y chromosome abnormalities and infertility is best understood in azoospermic men with alterations in the Y_q11 region in the distal region of the euchromatic part of the long Y arm, the location of a male fertility gene complex called *azoospermia factor*. Six different partial deletions of this region have been found in azoospermic patients (Table 10-9).

Monocentric deleted Y_q chromosome. Partial deletion of the distal portion of the euchromatic Y_q11 region is associated with azoospermia due to the loss of the azoospermia factor. These men have normal external genitalia although the testes are small,[644] normal testosterone and luteinizing hormone levels, and increased follicle stimulating hormone serum levels. Testicular biopsy shows Sertoli cell–only tubules or hyalinized tubules. The number of Leydig cells is normal. These findings suggest that the azoospermia factor is required for early spermatogenesis.[645] If the breakpoint of Y_q11 is proximal to the centromere, patients are short because the gene that controls stature is close to that for the azoospermia factor.[646]

Dicentric Y_q isochromosomes. Sterility is frequent in men with dicentric Y_q isochromosomes. This anomaly is usually associated with a 45X cell line. The proportion of this line varies among patients and among cell types (fibroblast or lymphocyte). When the point of breakage and fusion of the two Y chromosomes is in the distal region Y_q11, and the second centromere is inactivated, the Y isochromosome is of normal size but does not stain with quinacrine, and thus is called a *nonfluorescent Y chromosome* (Ynf). Since the breakpoint is in the Y_q11 region, the azoospermia factor function is altered. Development of the external genitalia varies from ambiguous to normal and is probably related to the extent of the XO present.[647] Testicular biopsies are similar to those of men with monocentric deleted Y_q chromosomes (Fig. 10-98).[648,649]

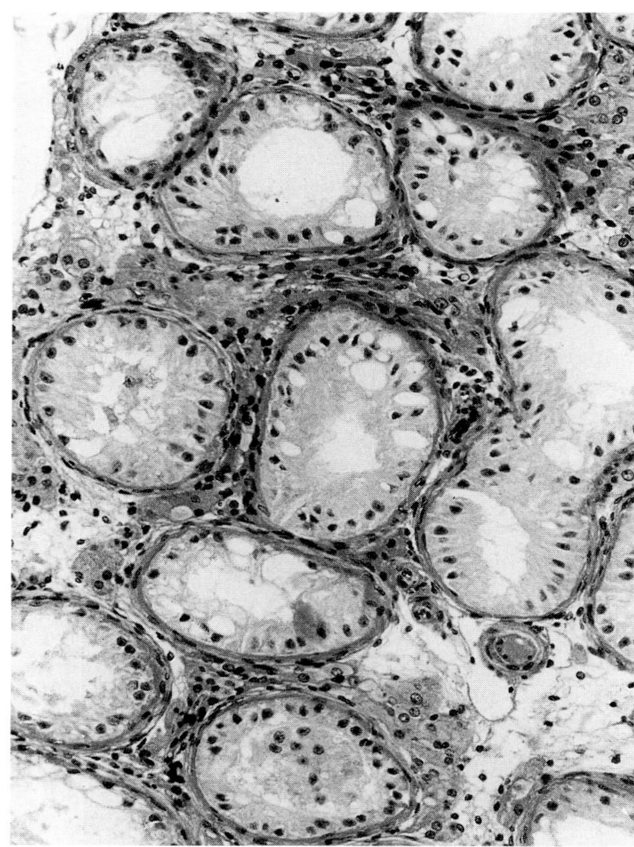

10-98. Testis of dicentric Y_q isochromosome shows seminiferous tubules with Sertoli cells only and slight Leydig cell hyperplasia.

Ring Y chromosome. Men with ring Y chromosomes have normal male phenotype, azoospermia, and, in some cases, short stature. Most have a mosaic karyotype with a 45X line. In some cases the testicular biopsy resembles that of men with monocentric deleted Y_q chromosome but in others shows premeiotic arrest of spermatocyte maturation.[650] This is attributed to difficulties in pairing the X and Y chromosomes during meiosis.

Y/Y translocation chromosome. Patients with this anomaly have small soft testes and primary spermatocyte maturation arrest, due to defective pairing of the X and Y chromosomes. The karyotype may be a mosaic with a 45X line.[651]

Translocation of Y chromosome to X chromosome. Most frequently, this translocation is cytogenetically undetectable and the patients are found in series of infertile patients with 46XX karyotype.[652] The phenotype is similar to that of men with Klinefelter's syndrome except for shorter stature, absence of mental retardation, and smaller teeth. Testicular biopsy shows Sertoli cell–only tubules. Men with cytogenetically detectable translocations have short stature, small testes, tubular hyalinization, and prominent clustered Leydig cells similar to Klinefelter's syndrome.

Autosomal translocation of Y chromosome. Translocation of the distal heterochromatic portion of the Y chromosome to the short arm of an acrocentric chromosome occurs occasionally. The fertility of these men depends on the point of breakage. If this occurs in the X_q12 heterochromatic region, the patient has a male phenotype and is fertile. If the point of breakage is in the Y_q11 region, patients are infertile and have small testes. The seminiferous tubules may show only Sertoli cells, spermatogenic arrest in early stages of meiosis, or an infantile pattern.[653,654]

Interstitial microdeletion in Y_q11. In a number of azoospermic patients with interstitial deletions in the Y_q11 region, the deletions are so small that they cannot be demonstrated by cytogenetic methods, requiring molecular biology techniques.[655] Testicular biopsy in one patient showed Sertoli cell–only tubules.[656]

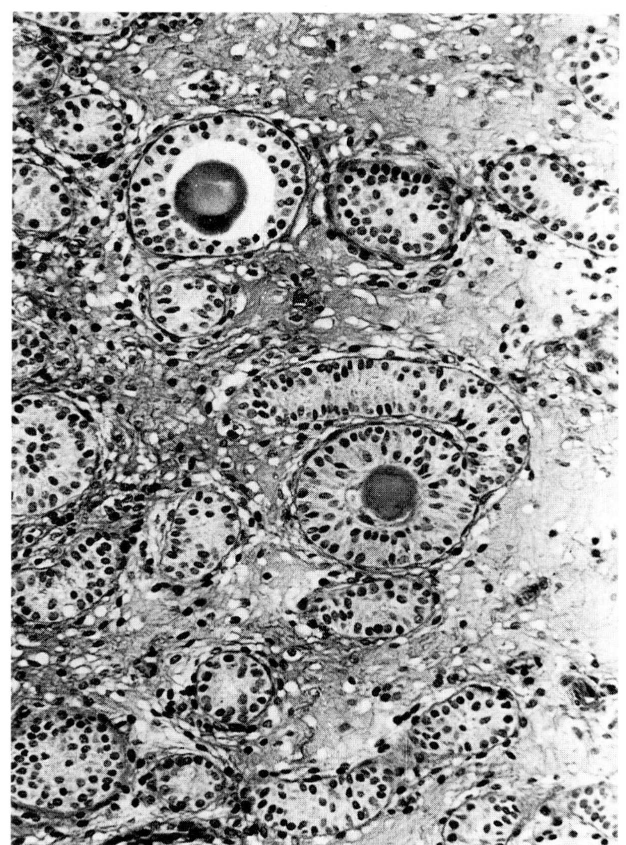

10-99. Prepubertal testis in Down's syndrome. There are megatubules, ring-shaped tubules, and small tubules. The germ cell number is very low in all these tubules. Eosinophilic bodies or microliths are present in some tubules.

ANOMALIES IN AUTOSOMES

The most frequent autosomal abnormalities in infertile men are Down's syndrome, Prader-Willi syndrome, and a variety of chromosomal translocations and inversions.

Down's syndrome

In addition to trisomy of chromosome 21 and the characteristic appearance, patients with Down's syndrome usually have cryptorchidism, small testes, and hypoplasia of the penis and scrotum. Adults have oligozoospermia or azoospermia secondary to a primary testicular deficiency. Levels of follicle stimulating hormone and luteinizing hormone are elevated while testosterone is normal or slightly diminished.[657] These patients have increased risk of cancer, including leukemia, central nervous system tumors, retinoblastoma, and testicular tumors.[658]

Histologic studies of prepubertal testes from autopsies show decreases in both tubular diameter and tubular fertility index. Eosinophilic bodies or microliths may be present in some tubules (Fig. 10-99). Adult testes have deficient spermatogenesis and mixed atrophy, with some tubules showing complete spermatogenesis and others containing only Sertoli cells.

Prader-Willi syndrome

Prader-Willi syndrome is characterized by hypogonadism, obesity, muscular hypotonia, mental and physical retardation, and acromicria.[659] Other frequent findings include strabismus and non–insulin-dependent diabetes mellitus. The incidence is estimated at 1 in 25,000 live births and is 60% higher in males. Patients have low serum levels of follicle stimulating hormone, luteinizing hormone, testosterone, and estradiol. The penis and testes are hypoplastic, and cryptorchidism is present in about 70% of cases (bilateral in 45% of cases).[660] During infancy and childhood the testes have reduced tubular diameters; adults have an infantile pattern.[661] This syndrome is caused by an anomaly of chromosome 15, usually in the 15_p, 11–12 band. Other chromosomal anomalies include robertsonian translocations, reciprocal translocations, small supernumerary metacentric chromosomes, and partial deletion of the long arm of chromosome 15.

Chromosomal translocations and inversions

Chromosomal translocations and inversions in infertile men are classified into three groups.

1. Balanced translocations. This includes robertsonian translocations, centric fusions, and reciprocal translocations. The most frequent robertsonian translocations are in chromosomes 13 to 15, 21, and 22. It accounts for about 0.6% of male infertility. The most frequent centric fusions are between chromosomes 14 and 21, and 13 and 14.[662] The most frequent reciprocal translocation is between chromosomes 11 and 22, with an incidence of about 0.3%.
2. Inversions. Infertile patients with chromosomal inversions comprise 0.01% of infertile men.
3. Other anomalies observed in infertile men include translocations such as insertion. Rarely trisomies other than Down's syndrome or monosomies are seen.

PRIMARY HYPOGONADISM WITHOUT CHROMOSOMAL ANOMALIES

Several different syndromes share an association with hypergonadotropic hypogonadism. Histologically, all resemble Klinefelter's syndrome, although no sex chromatin is found in Leydig cells.[663] Myotonic dystrophy, progressive muscular dystrophy, Werner syndrome, Alström syndrome, Weinstein's syndrome, Sohval-Soffer syndrome, and Noonan's syndrome are the best known.

Myotonic dystrophy accounts for approximately 30% of men with muscular disorders, and about 80% of these also have testicular atrophy. The muscular abnormality involves the distal muscles of the extremities. In addition, patients may have premature baldness, posterior subcapsular cataracts, cardiac conduction defects, impotence, gynecomastia (rarely), and dementia (at later stages). The disease is linked to an autosomal gene with variable penetrance. The hypogonadism is hypergonadotropic in most cases. Testicular biopsy shows small seminiferous tubules with hyalinized basement membranes, and prominent Leydig cells. Morphologic and hormonal findings suggest primary failure of Sertoli cells. In some patients the hypogonadism is hypogonadotropic, and the testes show an infantile pattern.

Progressive muscular dystrophy is a multisystem X-linked disease. It is usually associated with gonadal atrophy caused by a defective locus in chromosome 19. Patients rarely live more than 20 years. The incidence is approximately 1 in 4000 live births.

Werner syndrome (progeria) is characterized by short stature, prematurely graying hair, baldness, cataracts, atrophy and calcification of muscle and fat, wrinkling of the skin, keratosis, osteoporosis, telangiectasis, atheroma, diabetes mellitus, gynecomastia, and hypergonadotropic hypogonadism. The life span of fibroblasts and other cells is shortened in this syndrome.

Alström syndrome is characterized by retinitis pigmentosa, nerve deafness, obesity, diabetes, and hypergonadotropic hypogonadism.

Weinstein's syndrome is characterized by hypergonadotropic hypogonadism, deafness, blindness, and metabolic anomalies (hyperuricemia, hypertriglyceridemia, and hyperprebetalipoproteinemia).

Sohval-Soffer syndrome is characterized by mental retardation, multiple skeletal anomalies, hypergonadotropic hypogonadism, azoospermia, and gynecomastia.

Noonan's syndrome is characterized by multiple malformations reminiscent of Turner's syndrome, including short stature, pterygium coli and cubitus valgus, although there is a normal male karyotype. Cryptorchidism is present in about 70% of cases and is usually bilateral. During childhood, testicular biopsy shows a low tubular fertility index. Puberty is often delayed, and at adulthood hypogonadotropic or hypergonadotropic hypogonadism occurs. Ultrastructural studies have revealed morphologic anomalies in germ cells.[664] Although spermatogenesis is generally impaired, some patients have been fertile.

SECONDARY IDIOPATHIC HYPOGONADISM

Hypogonadotropic hypogonadism or hypogonadism of hypothalamic-hypophyseal origin is classified according to whether the hypothalamic-hypophyseal failure occurs before or after puberty. Eunuchoidism, present only in the former group, is the basis of the distinction. The most frequent types of hypogonadism caused by hypothalamic-hypophyseal failure are isolated gonadotropin deficit, hypogonadism associated with anosmia, isolated deficit of follicle stimulating hormone, isolated deficit of luteinizing hormone (Pasqualini's or fertile eunuch syndrome), hypogonadism associated with ataxia, and Laurence-Moon-Bardet-Biedl syndrome.

CONSTITUTIONAL DELAYED PUBERTY

Constitutional delayed puberty is characterized by delayed sexual maturation in otherwise healthy males. Patients are short and usually have family histories of delayed puberty. Puberty usually begins at 13 to 14 years of age and progresses over 2 years. If a 14-year-old boy has not begun pubertal changes (testicular enlargement, growth in height, and development of secondary sex characteristics), delayed puberty should be suspected.[665] Simple pubertal delay, which will be overcome naturally in a short time without treatment, must be distinguished from hypogonadotropic hypogonadism. The latter should be suspected when any of the following symptoms are present in the patient or his family: a midline defect, anosmia, or pubic hair without testicular development. Hormonal assays may also assist in diagnosis. If a patient between 16 and 18 years old has prepubertal gonadotropin levels, he probably has hypogonadotropic hypogonadism.

ISOLATED GONADOTROPIN DEFICIT

A variant of hypogonadotropic hypogonadism, isolated gonadotropin deficit is characterized by defects in the synthesis or release of follicle stimulating hormone and luteinizing hormone; other hypophyseal functions are normal. Patients have a eunuchoid phenotype, with small testes and penis, scanty body hair and beard, high-pitched voices, and poorly developed muscles. Although most cases are sporadic, X-linked inheritance has also been reported. Patients have very low levels of follicle stimulating hormone, luteinizing hormone, testosterone,

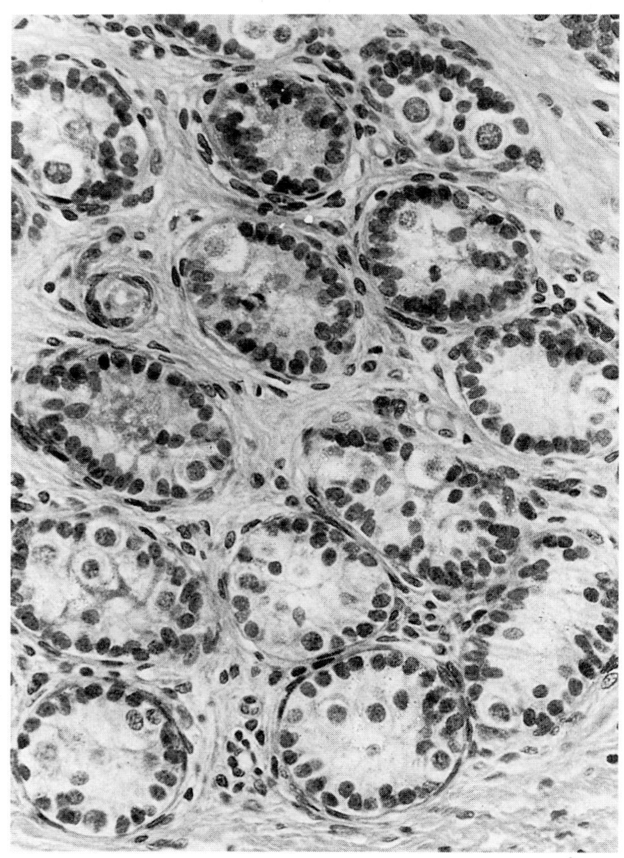

10-100. Isolated gonadotropin deficit. Seminiferous tubules with a prepubertal diameter showing several hypertrophic spermatogonia.

and estrogens. Clomiphene citrate fails to stimulate hormonal secretion.[666]

Testicular biopsy reveals an appearance similar to that of children. The seminiferous tubules have neither lumens nor elastic fibers in their lamina propria (Fig. 10-100). Sertoli cells are immature, and no differentiated Leydig cells are seen. Spermatogonia are rare. In some patients, the testicular pattern is similar to that of Sertoli cell–only testes with immature Sertoli cells.[667]

HYPOGONADISM ASSOCIATED WITH ANOSMIA

Hypogonadism associated with anosmia is also known as Maestre de San Juan,[668] Kallman's,[669] or De Morsier[670] syndromes. The two most important features are hypogonadotropic hypogonadism and anosmia. Members of affected families may have both features or only one. Associated abnormalities include olfactory bulb agenesis, cryptorchidism, mental retardation, color blindness, facial asymmetry, nerve deafness, epilepsy, shortening of the fourth metacarpal, tarsal navicular fibrous dysplasia, familial cerebellar ataxia, diabetes mellitus, hyperlipidemia, gynecomastia, cleft lip, maxilla or palate, unilateral renal aplasia, and cardiovascular abnormalities. The syndrome may be X linked or autosomal.

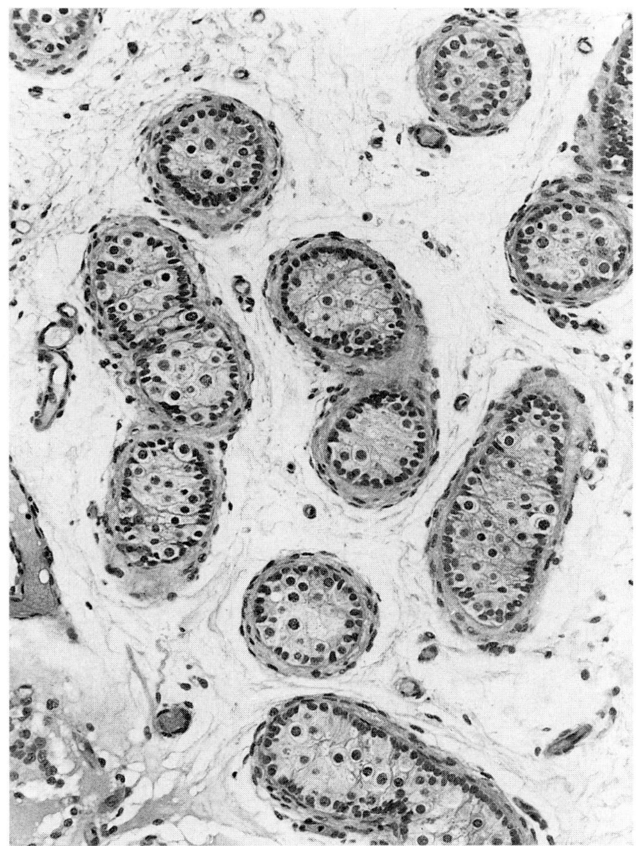

10-101. Hypogonadism associated with anosmia. Marked hyalinization of the tubular walls in a previously treated patient. The seminiferous epithelium shows isolated spermatogonia and primary spermatocytes. Leydig cells are absent.

Patients are classified into two groups according to the complete or partial lack of gonadotropin releasing hormone. Complete absence of gonadotropin releasing hormone is diagnosed by the absence of spontaneous pulses of luteinizing hormone, follicle stimulating hormone, and testosterone during a 24-hour period. These patients show an increase in follicle stimulating hormone only after gonadotropin releasing hormone administration.[671] The testes are histologically infantile, but the diameter of the seminiferous tubules is particularly low. The tubules lack lumens and contain immature Sertoli cells and isolated spermatogonia.[672] The interstitium is wide and consists of acellular connective tissue containing no recognizable Leydig cell precursors (Fig. 10-101).[673] Partial absence of gonadotropin releasing hormone is diagnosed by the presence of spontaneous pulses of luteinizing hormone, follicle stimulating hormone, and testosterone during a 24-hour period.

Autopsy studies in patients with anosmia and hypogonadism have found agenesis of the olfactory bulbs, which may be complete or partial and unilateral or bilateral, together with an apparently normal hypophysis, and a normal or hypoplastic hypothalamus. This syndrome is the least severe form of the holoprosencephaly-hypopituitarism complex, a spectrum of developmental anomalies associated with impaired midline cleavage of the embryonic forebrain, aplasia of the olfactory bulbs and tracts, and midline dysplasia of the face. Testicular seminoma has been reported in a patient with anosmia and hypogonadotropic hypogonadism.[674]

ISOLATED DEFICIT OF FOLLICLE STIMULATING HORMONE

This rare syndrome is characterized by azoospermia or oligozoospermia in normally virilized patients with normal sexual potency. Serum levels of luteinizing hormone and testosterone are normal, but levels of follicle stimulating hormone are very low or undetectable. The clomiphene stimulation test gives variable results. The gonadotropin releasing hormone test induces a normal response only of luteinizing hormone. Testicular biopsy shows maturation arrest at the spermatocyte level, hypospermatogenesis, or a partial Sertoli cell–only pattern.[675] Gonadotropin treatment increases spermatozoal numbers in most cases and fertility may be induced.

ISOLATED DEFICIT OF LUTEINIZING HORMONE

Also known as *Pasqualini's* or *fertile eunuch* syndrome,[676,677] this is characterized by hypogonadism secondary to luteinizing hormone deficit with preservation of spermatogenesis. Patients have eunuchoid habitus, small testes, decreased libido, female distribution of pubic hair, and high-pitched voices. Other frequent findings include gynecomastia, anosmia, ocular lesions, and pituitary tumors.[678] Levels of follicle stimulating hormone are normal, but luteinizing hormone and testosterone levels are very low. The clomiphene test is usually negative and gonadotropin releasing hormone stimulation increases luteinizing hormone and, to a

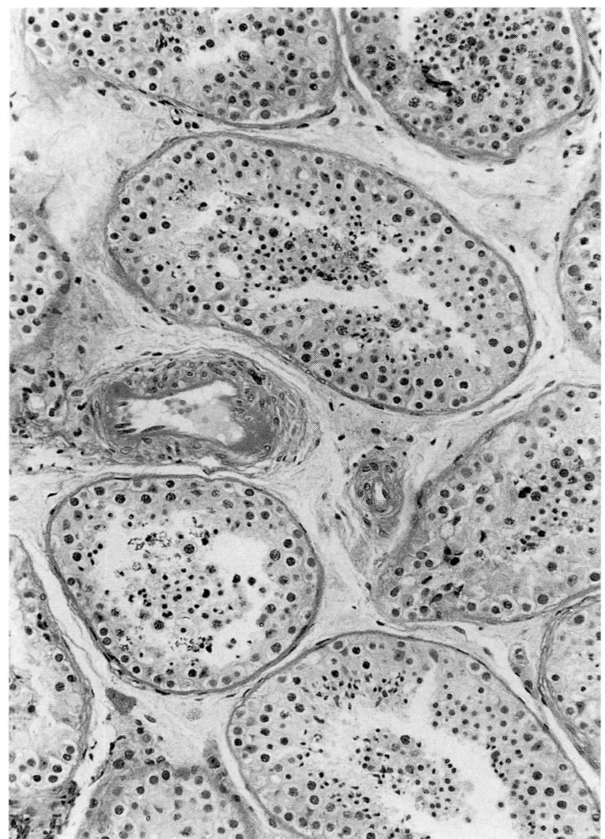

10-102. Isolated deficiency of luteinizing hormone. Most of the seminiferous tubules show complete spermatogenesis in contrast with the absence of differentiated interstitial Leydig cells. An artery shows subendothelial hyalinization.

lesser degree, follicle stimulating hormone. Testicular biopsy shows seminiferous tubules with normal or slightly decreased diameters and complete spermatogenesis; however, the numbers of all germ cell types are below normal. Leydig cells are rare or absent (Fig. 10-102).

LAURENCE-MOON-BARDET-BIEDL SYNDROME

This syndrome is characterized by obesity, infantilism, short stature, diabetes insipidus, mental retardation, retinitis pigmentosa, polydactyly, and syndactyly. It is more frequent in males than in females. Men with this syndrome are infertile, and about 74% show hypogonadism. The testes have a prepubertal development, the scrotum is hypoplastic or bifid, and the penis is small. Cryptorchidism is found in 42% of males and is bilateral in 28%.

HYPOGONADOTROPIC HYPOGONADISM ASSOCIATED WITH DERMATOLOGIC DISEASES

Hypogonadotropic hypogonadism is associated with a variety of skin diseases giving rise to a variety of syndromes. Lynch's syndrome, associated with ichthyosis and frequently with cryptorchidism, often is familial. Rud's syndrome is associated with ichthyosis, mental retardation, and epilepsy. In Rothmund-Thomson syndrome (congenital poikiloderma) and in Zinsser-Cole-Engman syndrome (congenital dyskeratosis) hypogonadism is frequent although not constant.

HYPOGONADOTROPIC HYPOGONADISM ASSOCIATED WITH ATAXIA

Hypogonadism is common in patients with ataxia, and this association has been described in the following syndromes:

1. Louis-Bar syndrome consists of cerebellar ataxia, mucocutaneous telangiectasis, skeletal growth retardation, and, frequently, respiratory tract infections. Inheritance is autosomal recessive. The testes are infantile, and the hypophysis contains abnormal cells with increased size and telescoped inclusions.
2. Marie's ataxia is frequently associated with hypogonadotropic hypogonadism.
3. In Friedreich's ataxia most cases have hypogonadotropic hypogonadism, although cases of hypergonadotropic hypogonadism have also been reported.
4. Other syndromes with hypogonadotropic hypogonadism are the Kraus-Ruppert, Carpenter's, Biedmond, Börjeson's, and Richards-Rundle syndromes.

HYPOGONADISM SECONDARY TO ENDOCRINE DYSFUNCTION AND OTHER DISORDERS

Maintenance of spermatogenesis requires the harmonious cooperation of several endocrine glands and the proper functioning of other organs and tissues. The most important endocrine problems associated with testicular disorders involve the hypophysis, thyroid gland, adrenal glands, pancreas, liver, kidney, and intestines.

HYPOPHYSIS

Hypopituitarism

The important role of the hypophysis in the control of testicular function is discussed elsewhere in this chapter. This section deals with hypogonadism resulting from destruction of the hypophysis by primary or secondary hypothalamic tumors; infiltration by adjacent tumor; and trauma, infection, and lesions in the hypophysis or its neighborhood (such as adenomas, cysts, and aneurysms of the inner carotid artery). Many of these cause panhypopituitarism with varied symptoms.[679]

Clinical manifestations of hypogonadism in patients with pituitary lesions vary according to whether the lesion arises in childhood or after puberty. In prepubertal hypopituitarism the testes retain an infantile appearance in adulthood, and proliferation of spermatogonia and development of primary spermatocytes rarely occur. Biopsy shows variable hyalinization of the tubules. In postpubertal

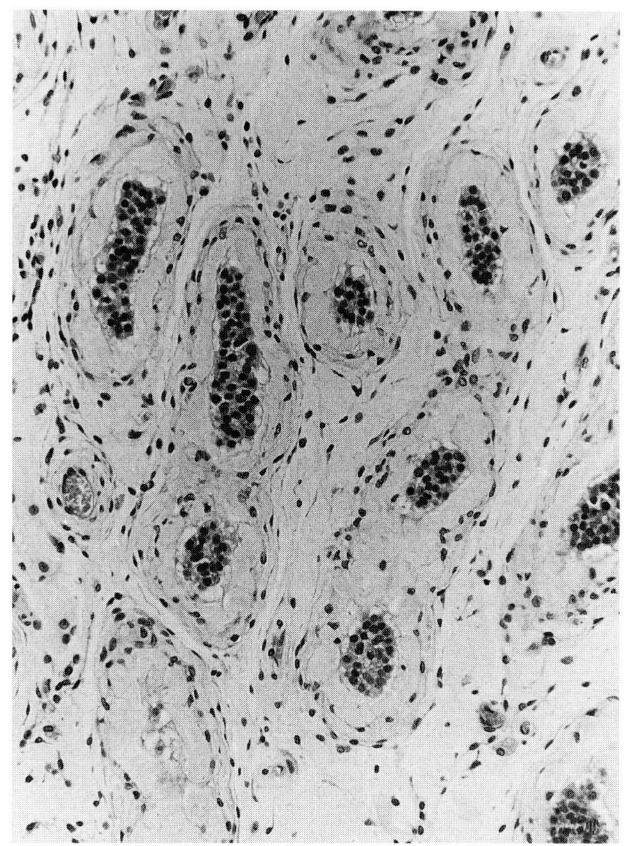

10-103. Hypopituitarism. Partial tubular hyalinization with a marked decrease in Leydig cells. The remaining seminiferous epithelium consists of Sertoli cells and isolated spermatogonia.

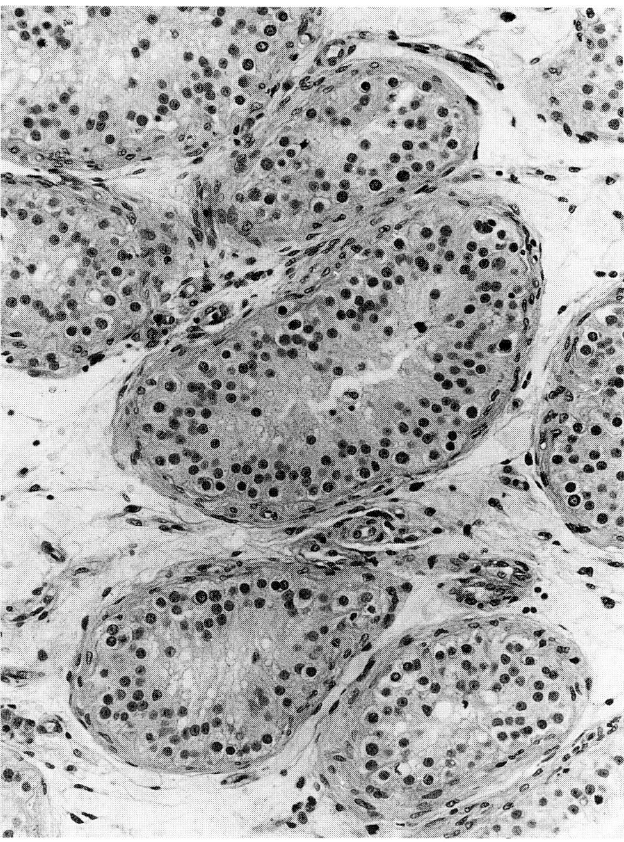

10-104. Hypogonadism caused by estrogen therapy for prostate cancer. The seminiferous epithelium consists of isolated spermatogonia and dedifferentiated Sertoli cells with spherical nuclei; small nucleoli; and a pseudostratified, infantile, distribution. The interstitium contains few Leydig cells.

hypopituitarism the appearance ranges from complete spermatogenesis to tubular hyalinization (Fig. 10-103). The presence of elastic fibers in the tubule walls indicates that pubertal maturation occurred before the development of hypopituitarism. Leydig cells have pyknotic nuclei and retracted cytoplasm with abundant lipofuscin.

There are rare cases in which pituitary adenomas secrete both follicle stimulating hormone and luteinizing hormone, inducing testosterone hypersecretion and elevated sperm counts.[680] Follicle stimulating hormone–secreting pituitary adenomas associated with large testes and increased serum inhibin concentrations have been reported.[681]

Hyperprolactinemia

In men hyperprolactinemia causes impairment of spermatogenesis, impotence, loss of libido, and depressed serum testosterone. Some patients seek treatment because of oligozoospermia and infertility. Hyperprolactinemia is associated with dysfunction of Leydig cell prolactin receptors.[682] Spermiograms usually show oligozoospermia and an elevated level of fructose,[683] although not all males with hyperprolactinemia have subnormal testicular function.[684]

Testicular biopsy reveals variable testicular atrophy. The most frequent lesion is in the tubular adluminal compartment, with degenerative changes in the apical cytoplasm of the Sertoli cells, sloughing of young spermatids,[683] and increased lipid droplets in Leydig cells.[685] In boys two different conditions associated with abnormal prolactin secretion have been reported: hyperprolactinemia, testicular enlargement, and primary hypothyroidism; and prolactin deficiency, obesity, and enlarged testes.

THYROID GLAND

Infertility caused by thyroid gland malfunction is rare but reversible. It accounts for about 0.6% of male infertility. Testicular function is impaired more by hypothyroidism than by hyperthyroidism. Patients with hyperthyroidism may have gynecomastia, impotence, and infertility. Levels of follicle stimulating hormone and luteinizing hormone are normal or increased, with elevated sex hormone binding globulin, increased testosterone concentration, reduced non–sex hormone binding globulin bound testosterone, and little or no change in free testosterone.[686,687] The number and motility of spermatozoa are reduced. Testicular biopsy reveals hypospermatogenesis or incomplete maturation arrest.

Prepubertal hypothyroidism may impair testicular function by causing precocious or delayed puberty. In delayed puberty, hypothyroidism leads to hypogonadotropic hypogonadism, with testes showing an incomplete maturation arrest and, in severe myxedematous hypothyroidism, hydrocele.[688] In experimental hypothyroidism, testicular enlargement is frequently associated with increased spermatid production.[689] Primary hypothyroidism in adults causes hypogonadotropic hypogonadism with decreased libido, sexual potency, semen volume, and number and motility of spermatozoa.[690] The cause of testicular damage is decreased gonadotropins or hyperprolactinemia.[691]

ADRENAL GLAND

Congenital adrenal hyperplasia

Infertility is frequent in patients with minor forms of congenital adrenal hyperplasia, and these patients often seek care for infertility. Patients with deficient activity of 21 hydroxylase or 11 beta hydroxylase usually have complete spermatogenesis but with reduced numbers of all germ cell types. The most characteristic histologic finding is a decrease in Leydig cells.[692-694] In untreated patients the testes become enlarged by "tumors" of the adrenogenital syndrome, which consist of cells similar to adrenal cortical cells.[695-697]

Adrenal cortical carcinoma

Adrenal carcinoma is often associated with excessive secretion of several hormones, causing hyperaldosteronism, Cushing's syndrome, virilization, or feminization. In childhood, virilizing tumors produce precocious pseudopuberty. In adults these tumors cause marked spermatogenic depletion, caused by conversion of the great amounts of dehydroepiandrosterone produced by the tumor into estrogens. Feminizing tumors present more striking clinical characteristics, including progressive loss of secondary sex characteristics, followed by feminization caused by elevated estrogens. The testes atrophy due to the inhibitory effect of estrogens on pituitary gonadotropins. Similar symptoms may be observed in patients with prostatic carcinoma treated with estrogens (Fig. 10-104) and in other conditions with excessive estrogen production, such as Sertoli cell or Leydig cell tumors.

Cushing's syndrome

Patients with Cushing's syndrome or diseases that require long-term corticoid therapy, such as ulcerative colitis, rheumatoid arthritis, or asthma, have reversible reduction of fertility and hypogonadotropic hypogonadism.

PANCREAS

Diabetes mellitus

The alterations in carbohydrate, lipid, and protein metabolism characteristic of diabetes mellitus involve the genital system. Gonadal impairment depends on the type of diabetes and the time of development of the disease (infancy and childhood, puberty, or adulthood).[698] The testicular lesions in newborns from diabetic mothers are discussed in the section on congenital anomalies of the testis.[699]

Puberty may be delayed in diabetic patients, although the cause is unknown. Other gonadal alterations appear at puberty, and adult diabetic men who have not been adequately treated may have infertility and sexual dysfunction. Spermiograms reveal low numbers and motility of spermatozoa.[700] Serum levels of follicle stimulating hormone and luteinizing hormone are normal or slightly increased. Prolactin levels are increased and testosterone levels are low or near normal.

The seminiferous tubules have reduced diameters, thickening of the lamina propria, and alterations in the adluminal compartment. These consist of degenerative changes in the Sertoli cell apical cytoplasm and sloughing of immature germ cells. The major lesions are in the interstitial connective tissue and Leydig cells. The small interstitial blood vessels show diabetic microangiopathy: enlargement and duplication of the basal lamina, pericyte degeneration, and endothelial cell alterations. The number of fibroblasts and the amounts of collagen fibers and ground substance are increased in the interstitial connective tissue.[701] Leydig cells show abundant lipid droplets and lysosomes.

The tubular lesions have been attributed to low serum testosterone levels, probably due to both defi-

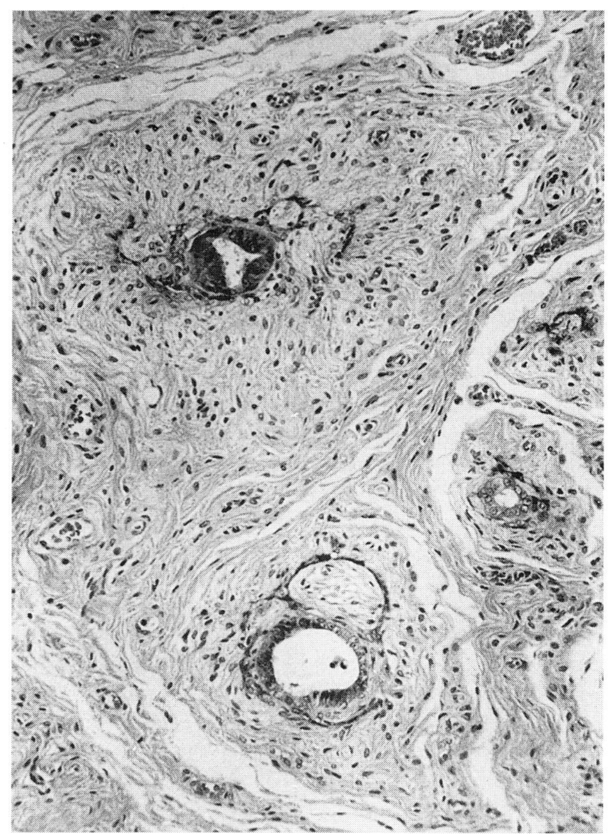

10-105. Epididymis in cystic fibrosis. The ductus epididymidis has a narrow lumen. Its epithelium is of variable height and is surrounded by an indistinct lamina propria.

cient Leydig cell stimulation by insulin and abnormal carbohydrate metabolism of the Sertoli cells. Sexual dysfunction is present in more than half of patients and consists of impotence, decreased libido, disorders in intercourse, and retrograde ejaculation. The causes of impotence are multiple, including microangiopathy and macroangiopathy, hormonal deficiencies, psychological factors, and autonomic neuropathy affecting the parasympathetic system. Neuropathy is probably chiefly responsible for erectile failure in diabetic men.[702]

Cystic fibrosis

Although cystic fibrosis (mucoviscidosis) was recognized as a disease prior to 1940, its effects on male genitalia were not recognized until the 1970s. This may be explained by improvement in medical care during childhood, allowing the survival of many patients to adulthood, and recognition of cystic fibrosis in patients who had been diagnosed with chronic bronchitis with hepatic or digestive dysfunction.

Most patients with cystic fibrosis have infertility due to obstruction; the most frequent findings are atresia or absence of the vas deferens and incomplete development of the ductus epididymidis or seminal vesicles.[703]

Histologic studies in children, even at early ages, reveal that the vas deferens and ductus epididymidis are absent or reduced to small ductuli with reduced or absent lumens and thin poorly muscular walls (Fig. 10-105). The testes are normal during childhood. In adulthood they show hypospermatogenesis and spermatid malformations. The spermiogram is characteristic of obstructive azoospermia with acid pH, decreased semen volume and fructose concentration, and increased citric acid and acid phosphatase.[704]

The disease is a genetic disorder with autosomal recessive inheritance. The impaired gene (cystic fibrosis gene) is on chromosome 7.[705] Congenital bilateral obstructive azoospermia secondary to the bilateral absence of the vas deferens, even in absence of other symptoms, is often a *forme fruste* of cystic fibrosis.[706] Before initiating treatment for infertility, the possibility that the patient is a carrier of the cystic fibrosis gene should be evaluated.[707] Malformations of the genital system play the most important role in infertility in cystic fibrosis.[708] The lesions begin in the tenth week of gestation when the wolffian duct forms the sperm excretory ducts.[709] Variable penetrance of the cystic fibrosis gene accounts for the diversity of malformations affecting different regions of the male genital system.

LIVER

Hypogonadism is frequent in the final stages of severe chronic liver diseases, including alcoholism, nonalcoholic liver disease, and hemochromatosis.

Hypogonadism, liver disease, and excessive alcohol consumption

The association of testicular atrophy with gynecomastia and hepatic cirrhosis is well known and is referred to as the Silvestrini-Corda syndrome.[710,711]

Alcohol has a direct toxic effect on Leydig cells. Acute alcohol intoxication suppresses serum testosterone levels in voluntary nonalcoholic men and in laboratory animals. Chronic alcohol ingestion, even in the absence of cirrhosis, causes hypogonadism with symptoms of Leydig cell failure: testicular atrophy, infertility, decreased libido, impotence, and decreased size of the prostate and seminal vesicles.[712] Chronic alcoholic patients with cirrhosis also have symptoms of hyperestrogenism, including gynecomastia, female escutcheon, and female type of fat distribution.

Most chronic alcoholic patients, with or without cirrhosis, have significant testicular lesions. The seminiferous tubules have reduced diameters, thickened lamina propria, and decreased or absent germ cells. Leydig cells are reduced in number and contain abundant lipofuscin granules. The spermiogram correlates with the variability of histologic findings, usually showing a marked reduction in the number and motility of spermatozoa and an increase in the percentage of morphologically abnormal spermatozoa.[713,714] About 20% of patients initially have an increase in serum testosterone; with advanced disease, the testosterone level decreases. The initial increase is due to elevation in sex hormone binding globulin concentration and reduced testosterone metabolism by the liver.[715] Serum estrogen levels also increase, due to increased conversion of testosterone to estrogen in peripheral adipose and muscular tissues.[716]

Nonalcoholic liver disease and infertility

Nonalcoholic liver diseases impair gonadal function according to the severity of the disease.[717] These patients have decreased levels of total and biologically active free testosterone. Hormonal alterations are not as severe as in alcoholic patients, underscoring direct action of alcohol on the Leydig cell. In alpha 1 antitrypsin deficiency, testicular function and fertility are conserved; only in advanced stages of the disease do minor biochemical alterations occur.[718] In Alagille's syndrome (intrahepatic biliary duct hypoplasia), hypogonadism is associated with cholestasis; frequent vertebral, cardiac, and facial malformations; and mental retardation. Hypogonadism is manifest by small testes, delayed puberty and, in the adult, lack of germ cell development.

Hemochromatosis and infertility

Patients with hemochromatosis have a hereditary alteration in iron metabolism causing increased iron deposition in skeletal and cardiac muscle and in the epithelial cells of the liver, stomach, pancreas, hypophysis, and adrenal glands. Eventually, hepatic, pancreatic, and cardiac function are impaired. Hypogonadism may be the first symptom when the disease develops in early adult life. The hypogonadism is hypogonadotropic with low testosterone levels. Testicular biopsy reveals atrophy with decreased tubular diameter, progressive disappearance of spermatogenesis, and increased lipofuscin granules in the Leydig cells. Hemosiderin is not usually deposited in the testes.

KIDNEY

Chronic renal insufficiency is associated with disturbed endocrine function in the pituitary, thyroid, and parathyroid glands, and testis. The associated sexual dysfunction consists of erectile impotence, diminution of libido and semen volume, oligozoospermia or azoospermia, and infertility. In children, skeletal development and puberty are delayed.[719]

Hormonal studies reveal elevated levels of follicle stimulating hormone, luteinizing hormone, and prolactin, but testosterone levels are low.[720] Testicular biopsy shows seminiferous tubules with reduced diameters and reduced or absent germ cells.[721,722] The interstitium contains a normal number of Leydig cells and increased numbers of macrophages. Additionally, patients with chronic renal insufficiency due to glomerulonephritis have thickening of the tubular lamina propria and a decreased number of Leydig cells.

The cause of gonadal dysfunction is uncertain and probably involves several factors, including impaired testicular steroidogenesis,[723] decreased clearance of pituitary hormones,[724] and secretory defects of the pituitary and hypothalamus.[725] Hemodialysis does not improve testicular function. The response to renal transplantation is not immediate and is related to the glomerular filtration rate. Patients with rates lower than 50 ml/min develop atrophy of the seminiferous epithelium.[723]

CHRONIC INFLAMMATORY BOWEL DISEASE

Hypogonadism is a frequent finding in men with celiac disease and results in clinical symptoms in 5% to 10% of untreated patients. Celiac disease causes infertility in some cases. Spermiograms show reduced motility and numerous morphologic abnormalities in spermatozoa. Hormonal studies show elevated levels of follicle stimulating hormone in more than 25% of men with celiac disease. Luteinizing hormone also is increased in more than 50% of these men. Response of follicle stimulating hormone and luteinizing hormone to gonadotropin releasing hormone stimulation is excessive. The causes of this pituitary derangement are unknown. Sperm anomalies are not always corrected by a gluten-free diet.

Studies in patients with ulcerative colitis and regional enteritis have shown low sperm counts, impaired motility, and ultrastructural alterations, including nuclear pleomorphism and chromatin malcondensation and decondensation. The alterations apparently are related to the extent of the intestinal lesions and the severity of symptoms and not to sulfasalazine treatment.[726]

CHRONIC ANEMIA

Thalassemia major is often associated with endocrine disorders, principally delayed puberty and hypogonadism. Hypogonadism is probably due to hemosiderosis from multiple transfusions and is hypogonadotropic in most patients.[727] Patients with sickle cell anemia have marked alterations in sexual maturation, often with a eunuchoid habitus, scant development of secondary sex characteristics, and hypogonadotropic hypogonadism.

POLYGLANDULAR INSUFFICIENCY

Failure of multiple endocrine glands is more common in women than in men, and gonadal involvement is infrequent. Male hypogonadism has been observed in thyroid and adrenal hypofunction. Gonadal insufficiency is present in some men with combined Addison's disease and diabetes mellitus and in men with hypoadrenalism, hypothyroidism, and diabetes. The most frequent association is hypogonadism with Addison's disease. Hypergonadotropic hypogonadism is present in more than 25% of patients with primary adrenal insufficiency. These patients have atrophic testes with seminiferous tubules with reduced diameters and immunoglobulin deposits in the basement membranes. In most patients with Addison's disease the hypogonadism is hypogonadotropic. The cause of hypogonadism is unknown, although an autoimmune mechanism has been postulated.[728,729]

ADRENAL LEUKODYSTROPHY

Adrenal leukodystrophy is a sex-linked recessive disorder principally affecting the central nervous system and the adrenal cortex, causing destruction of the white matter and adrenal insufficiency. It results from accumulation of cholesterol esters containing an elevated proportion of long chain fatty acids.[730] The disease is most frequent in children between 5 and 15 years of age. A less severe variant has been reported as the adrenomyeloneuropathic form. Hypogonadotropic hypogonadism is evident after puberty in patients with clinical adrenal insufficiency and pronounced neurologic involvement. The most common histologic finding in the testis are lamellar-lipid cytoplasmic inclusions in Leydig cells. Similar inclusions are found in the adrenal cortex microglial, endoneural, and Schwann cells.[731,732]

INFERTILITY RESULTING FROM PHYSICAL AND CHEMICAL AGENTS

OCCUPATIONAL EXPOSURE

The relationship between infertility and exposure to occupational and environmental agents is well known. Spermatogenic injury was first linked to exposure to carbon disulfide and dibromochloropropane; today the list of physical agents and substances with noxious effects on spermatogenesis is extensive.[733]

Carbon disulfide

Carbon disulfide is used as a solvent in the production of viscose rayon. Continuous exposure is toxic to the nervous system, and causes a decrease in spermatogenesis and libido and an increase in follicle stimulating hormone and luteinizing hormone.[733,734]

Dibromochloropropane

Dibromochloropropane is used as a soil fumigant to control nematodes. Lengthy exposure causes azoospermia, oligozoospermia, and increased follicle stimulating hormone and luteinizing hormone levels, as well as Y-chromosome nondysjunction.[735]

Lead

Of the two natural forms of lead, organic and inorganic, the inorganic form is more dangerous. Exposure to inorganic lead, which is used by workers in smelting, battery, and stained-glass plants, causes direct spermatogenic damage. The patients have asthenospermia, teratospermia, and oligozoospermia.[736,737]

Oral contraceptive manufacture

Workers in pharmaceutical plants using synthetic estrogens and progestins develop hyperestrogenism, with gynecomastia, decreased libido, and impotence.[738]

Radiation

Ionizing radiation causes alterations in spermatogenesis and hormonal regulation of the testis. Some patients recover fertility a few years after exposure.[739] The effects of nonionizing radiation are less severe; however, reduced libido and reduced numbers of spermatozoa have been reported in men exposed to microwaves.[740]

Heat

The normal intratesticular temperature is 31°C to 33°C, about 4°C to 6°C lower than core body temperature. Conditions causing higher testicular temperature, such as varicocele and cryptorchidism, are known to cause testicular damage. These patients have a decreased number of spermatozoa and an elevated percentage of spermatozoa with abnormal forms and low motility.[741] Primary spermatocytes at the end of the pachytene stage appear to be the cells most sensitive to heat. The mechanism by which heat produces testicular lesions is unknown; hyperthermia affects the activity of enzymes such as ornithine decarboxylase[742] and carnitine acetyl transferase,[743] both necessary for metabolism and proliferation of the seminiferous epithelium.[744] The synthesis of DNA and RNA by germ cells also depends on temperature. It has been reported that DNA synthesis by spermatogonia and preleptotene primary spermatocytes is higher at 31°C than at 37°C. RNA and protein synthesis are normal at temperatures from 28°C to 37°C, but decrease markedly at 40°C.[745]

Other agents

Other agents implicated in testicular damage include anesthetic gases, arsenic, benzene, boron, cadmium, carbaryl, chlordecone, chloroprene, dinitrotoluene, toluene diamine, ethylene dibromide, manganese, methyl mercury, pesticides, pentachlorophenol, solvents (hydrocarbons and glycol ethers), 2,3,8-tetrachlorodibenzo-p-dioxin, and vinyl chloride.[746,747]

CANCER THERAPY

As cancer treatment has become more effective, fertility problems have been recognized in young patients who have been cured of cancer.[748]

Radiotherapy

The testicular parenchyma is one of the most radiosensitive tissues of the body and the germ cells are the most radiosensitive cells of the testis. Experimental irradiation of volunteers with a single dose has shown that late spermatogonia (Ap and B spermatogonia) are more radiosensitive than early spermatogonia (Ad spermatogonia). Whereas Ap and B spermatogonia can be destroyed with doses of 0.3 Gy (1 Gy = 100 rad), B spermatogonia tolerate doses higher than 4 Gy. Type A spermatogonia, spermatids, and spermatozoa are 100, 200, and 10,000 times less radiosensitive than B spermatogonia, respectively. Doses higher than 6 Gy produce a Sertoli cell–only testicular pattern, with seminiferous tubules with reduced diameters and hyalinized lamina propria. Leydig cells tolerate up to 8 Gy and Sertoli cells up to 60 Gy, although Sertoli cells show ultrastructural alterations and increased phagocytosis of germ cell remnants after low doses of radiation.

Even with the best protection, the contralateral testis absorbs from 0.2 to 1.4 Gy when the opposite testis is irradiated,[749] a dose sufficient to cause temporary azoospermia. Even with gonadal protection, irradiation of the iliac or inguinal lymph nodes for Hodgkin's disease or other lymphomas exposes the testes to about 5 Gy.[750] Restoration of testicular function is time dependent[751] and at least 2 years are needed for recovery.[752]

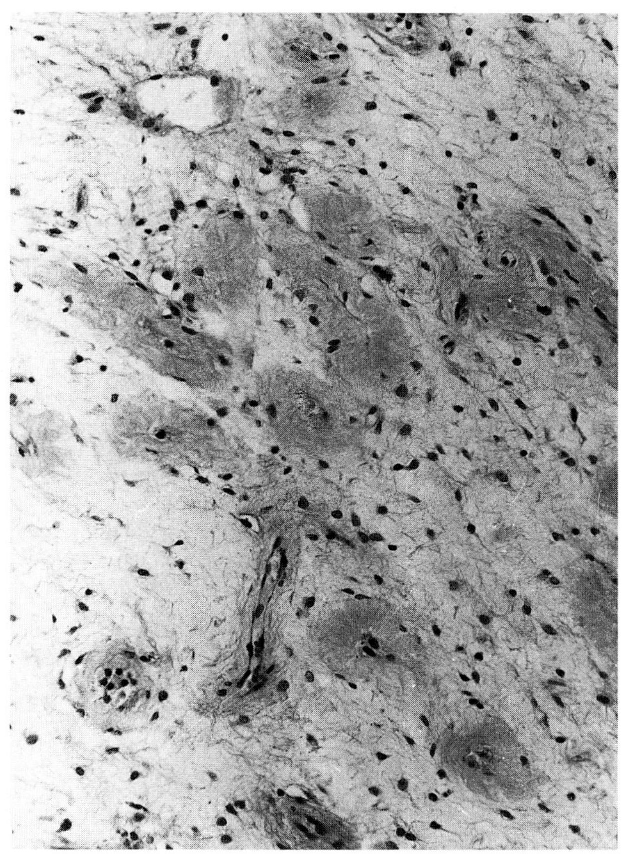

10-106. Radiation effect: diffuse tubular hyalinization with pronounced collagenization of the testicular interstitium. The specimen is from a patient who underwent radiotherapy after testicular recurrence of acute lymphoblastic leukemia.

Prepubertal testes also are sensitive to radiotherapy. Patients treated for Wilms' tumors may have delayed puberty and, at adulthood, azoospermia or oligozoospermia with elevated levels of follicle stimulating hormone. This suggests that Leydig cells also are damaged. A special case is that of children with acute lymphocytic leukemia involving the testis. Radiotherapy with doses of 20 to 25 Gy, either alone or with chemotherapy, causes irreversible damage to the seminiferous tubules and Leydig cells. These patients develop azoospermia and hypogonadotropic hypogonadism with low serum testosterone (Fig. 10-106).

Chemotherapy

The widespread use of cancer chemotherapy has revealed a number of collateral effects, including gonadotoxicity. Combination chemotherapy makes it difficult to ascertain which agents are responsible for the azoospermia and Leydig cell dysfunction that follow. Comparative studies of chemotherapy for acute lymphoblastic leukemia,[753] extragonadal solid tumors,[754] Hodgkin's disease,[755] Ewing's sarcoma, and other soft tissue sarcomas[756] in children and pubertal boys have led to the conclusion that alkylating agents cause the most severe testicular damage. Alkylating agents destroy the seminiferous epithelium and induce tubular atrophy, shrinking the testis and increasing follicle stimulating hormone serum levels. These agents also impair Leydig cell function, causing low testosterone, normal or elevated serum levels of luteinizing hormone, and an exaggerated response of luteinizing hormone to gonadotropin releasing hormone administration.[757] The testicular damage may be increased by the action of other agents (Fig. 10-107).

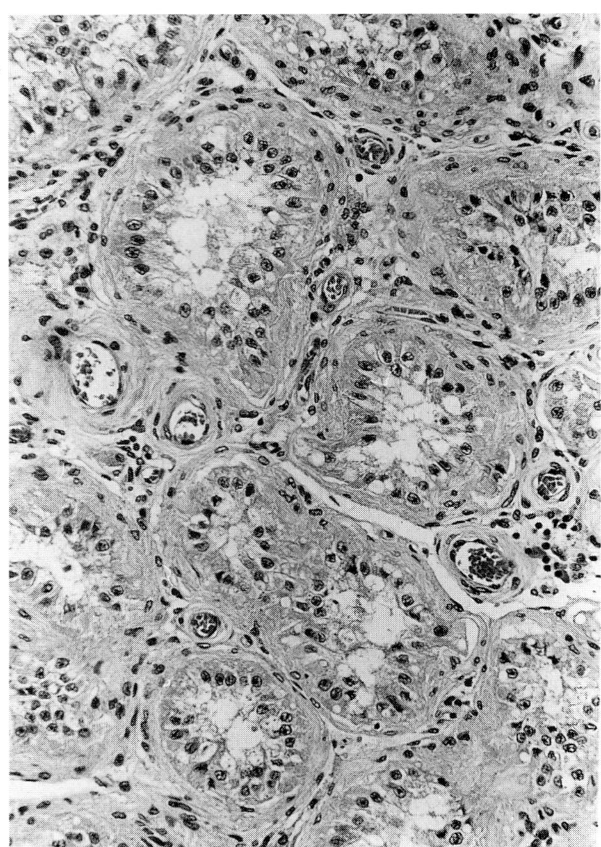

10-107. Chemotherapy effect: Sertoli cell–only tubules with thickened walls in a patient with Hodgkin's disease.

Cyclophosphamide appears to be responsible for most permanent or temporary azoospermias after chemotherapy. This agent acts directly on the spermatogenic stem cells,[756] and recovery depends on the number of surviving cells.[468] In children, cyclophosphamide decreases seminiferous tubule diameter and germ cell number; the nuclei are enlarged in the residual spermatogonia. Puberty may progress, even during treatment, and the adult testis may show a Sertoli cell–only pattern.[753] In adults, cyclophosphamide treatment may cause irreversible testicular damage. Administered alone, a dose of 20,000 mg/m^2 produces permanent azoospermia in 50% of men. If cyclophosphamide is administered with doxorubicin, vincristine, dacarbazine, or dactinomycin (drugs that alone do not cause azoospermia), doses of 7500 mg/m^2 cause azoospermia in 50% of patients.

Procarbazine, used to treat Hodgkin's disease, causes permanent azoospermia in 30% of patients, even when not combined with alkylating agents. Patients treated with a combination of cyclophosphamide and procarbazine in the COPP protocol (cyclophosphamide, vincristine, procarbazine, and prednisone) do not recover spermatogenesis even if the cyclophosphamide dose does not exceed 4800 mg/m^2.

Chemotherapy without alkylating agents or procarbazine, such as the ABVD (doxorubicin, bleomycin, vinblastine, and dacarbazine) or VBM (vinblastine, bleomycin, and methotrexate) regimens, produces reversible azoospermia in 36% of patients. The alternating use of MOPP (mechlorethamine, vincristine, procarbazine, and prednisone) and ABVD treatments causes testicular dysfunction in 87% of patients, but spermatogenesis recovers in 40%.

In all of these cases, recovery takes years and cannot be predicted by serum levels of follicle stimulating hormone, which, in most cases, remain elevated for many years. A worrisome, poorly understood complication of chemotherapy is the development of congenital anomalies in descendants.[758]

An important consideration to be taken into account in patients with testicular cancer or Hodgkin's disease is the existence of testicular dysfunction before treatment. In some series,[759] dysfunction is present at diagnosis in more than 50% of patients; its causes are unknown. Proposed mechanisms include primary germ cell deficiency, release of toxic substances by tumor cells, and alterations in the hypothalamic-hypophyseal-testicular axis.

Surgery

Sexual function is often lost in patients who undergo bilateral retroperitoneal lymph node dissection for nonseminomatous testicular cancer. Up to 90% lose antegrade ejaculation, although libido, erection, and orgasm are normal. The loss of antegrade ejaculation is due to removal or injury of sympathetic ganglia and the hypogastric nervous plexus during surgery. Unilateral surgery, especially if the left side is not operated on, reduces this complication.[760,761] Hypospermatogenesis sometimes occurs after surgery for rectal cancer, perhaps due to vascular compromise.[762]

INFERTILITY IN PATIENTS WITH SPINAL CORD INJURIES

Paraplegic patients, frequently young adults, have decreased fertility.[762] The explanation is complex, and five main factors may be involved: impotence; ejaculatory dysfunction; infection of the urinary tract that migrates into the genital tract, adversely affecting sperm morphology and motility; endocrine abnormalities; and anomalies in testicular morphology and/or sperm morphology.[763,764]

In most cases testicular size and serum levels of follicle stimulating hormone, luteinizing hormone, testosterone, prolactin, and 17 beta estradiol are normal. Testicular biopsy shows only slight alteration in 50% of patients in some series,[763,765] although histologic abnormalities were found in 95% of patients in another series.[766] In the abnormal testes, the seminiferous epithelium contains numerous groups of sloughing degenerating cells that are mainly spermatids. The elongate spermatids show ultrastructural anomalies in the head, principally in the acrosome. The number of Sertoli cells per tubular profile is increased.[565]

Testicular hyperthermia is probably responsible for these lesions. Hyperthermia may result from damage to sympathetic innervation by an injury above T11. This would cause dilation of testicular blood vessels and impair sweating, with an increase in testicular temperature of approximately 1°C. Another hypothesis proposes that testicular hyperthermia is due to extended contact with adjacent body tissues during prolonged time in a wheelchair.[767] The greater the extent of the spinal cord lesion, the worse the prognosis for fertility, especially if the injury is in the high lumbar and low thoracic segments.[768]

INFLAMMATION AND INFECTION

Infectious agents may reach the testis and epididymis through the blood vessels, lymphatic vessels, sperm excretory ducts, or directly from the environment through a wound. Infections transmitted through the blood mainly affect the testis and cause orchitis, while infections ascending through the spermatic ductal system usually cause epididymitis. Acute inflammation is accompanied by enlargement of the testis or epididymis. The tunica albuginea is covered by a fibrinous exudate, and the testicular parenchyma is yellowish or brownish. Bacterial infections may cause abscesses. In some cases the infection begins to heal and the lesions are repaired by granulation tissue and fibrosis; in others the infection may persist as an active process for a long time, chronic orchidoepididymitis.

ORCHITIS

VIRAL ORCHITIS

The most frequent causes of viral orchidoepididymitis are mumps virus and Coxsackie B virus. Other viral infections that occasionally cause acute orchitis include influenza, infectious mononucleosis, echovirus, lymphocytic choriomeningitis, adenovirus, bat salivary gland virus, smallpox, varicella, vaccinia, rubella, dengue, and phlebotomus fever. Subclinical orchitis probably occurs during other viral infections.

Mumps orchidoepididymitis complicates 14% to 35% of adult mumps cases and is bilateral in 20% to 25% of cases. In about 85% of these the epididymis also is involved but epididymal involvement alone is rare.[769] Clinical symptoms of orchitis usually appear 4 to 6 days after symptoms of parotiditis but orchitis may also appear without parotid involvement.[770] The testicular involvement is multifocal and consists of acute inflammation of the interstitium and seminiferous tubules. The tubular lining is destroyed, and eventually only hyalinized tubules and clusters of Leydig cells remain (Fig. 10-108).[771] With time, the testes shrink and become soft. If the infection is bilateral, the patient usually is infertile, with azoospermia or severe oligozoospermia. If only one testis was affected, the sperm concentration may be normal or slightly decreased and fertility is maintained. Occasionally the testicular damage is so severe that testicular endocrine function is impaired, causing hypergonadotropic hypogonadism with low testosterone levels and regression of secondary sex characteristics. Mumps orchidoepididymitis is infrequent in childhood.

BACTERIAL ORCHITIS

Most bacterial orchitis is associated with bacterial epididymitis. Orchitis secondary to suppurative epididymitis caused by *Escherichia coli* is most common.[772] By light microscopy the tubules are effaced by intense acute inflammation. Chronic orchitis with microabscesses is caused by *E. coli*, streptococci, staphylococci, pneumococci, *Salmonella enteritidis*,[773] and *Actinomyces israelii*.[774] In some cases of chronic bacterial orchitis, the testis contains an inflammatory infiltrate similar to that of idiopathic granulomatous orchitis, but lacking intratubular giant cells. Rarely, as in Whipple's disease, large numbers of bacilli are present in histiocytes in the interstitium, vascular walls, and seminiferous tubules.

The most frequent complications of pyogenic bacterial orchidoepididymitis are scrotal pyocele and chronic draining scrotal sinus. Small fragments of testicular parenchyma may be eliminated through the scrotal skin, clinically known as *fungus testis*. Another complication is testicular infarct, resulting from compression or thrombosis of the veins of the spermatic cord, in the scrotal neck or superficial inguinal ring.[775]

GRANULOMATOUS ORCHIDOEPIDIDYMITIS

Most chronic orchidoepididymitis is associated with granulomas in the testis. Specific causes may often be determined by special stains, cultures, or serologic tests,

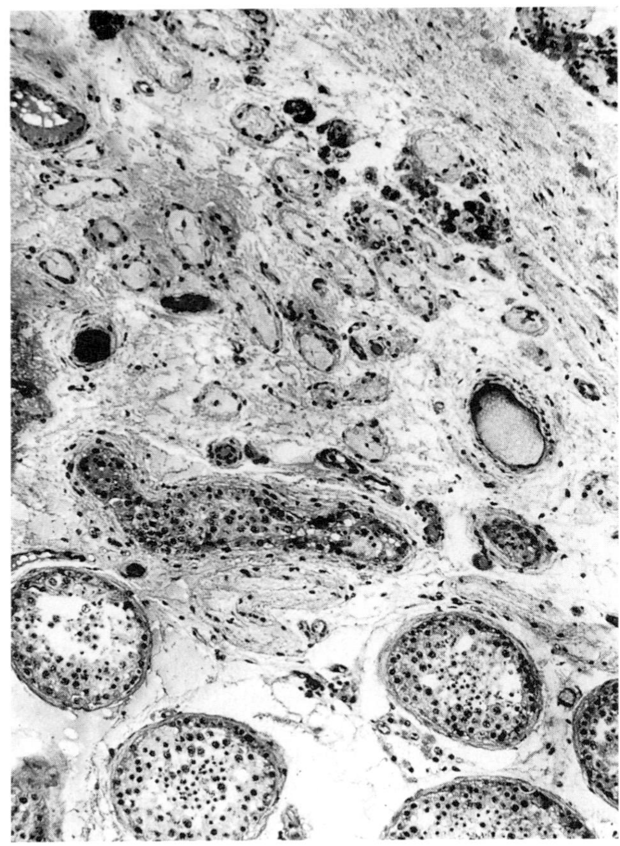

10-108. End result of mumps orchitis. Seminiferous tubules with partially preserved spermatogenesis adjacent to completely hyalinized tubules.

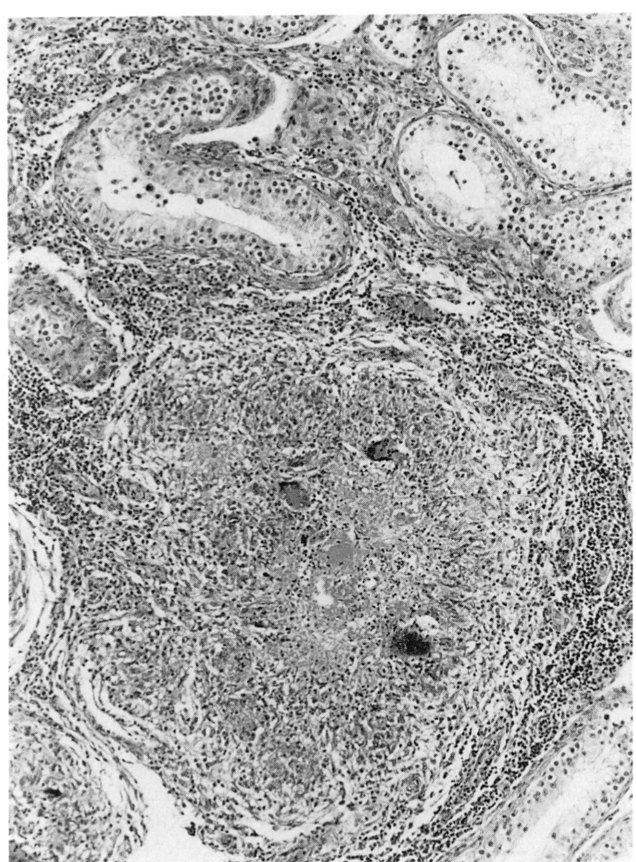

10-109. Tuberculous orchitis with focal destruction of seminiferous tubules and interstitium. Several giant cells and numerous epithelioid cells and lymphocytes surround a zone of necrosis.

and include tuberculosis, syphilis, leprosy, brucellosis, mycoses, and parasitic diseases. In sarcoidosis and idiopathic granulomatous orchitis the agent is unknown.

Tuberculosis

The incidence of tuberculous orchidoepididymitis declined after the development of effective antibiotics, but it has recently undergone resurgence among people who have emigrated from countries with high incidences of tuberculosis and the increasing population of immunologically compromised patients.

Most tuberculous orchidoepididymitis is associated with involvement elsewhere in the genitourinary system.[776] Tuberculous epididymitis usually is the result of ascent from tuberculous prostatitis, which, in turn, is often secondary to renal tuberculosis. The pattern of spread is different in children; more than half have advanced pulmonary tuberculosis and the testis is infected through the blood.[777] More than 50% of patients with renal tuberculosis develop tuberculous epididymitis and orchitis occurs in approximately 34% of patients with genital tuberculosis, usually secondary to epididymal tuberculosis. It has been suggested that some tuberculous orchidoepididymitis is sexually transmitted.[778] Tuberculous orchidoepididymitis occurs mainly in adults: 72% of patients are older than 35 years of age, and 18% of patients are older than 65 years. The symptoms may be minor, involving testicular enlargement and scrotal pain. Fever is infrequent and constitutional symptoms may be absent.[779]

Histologically, there are typical caseating and noncaseating granulomas that destroy the seminiferous tubules and interstitium (Fig. 10-109). In immunosuppressed patients the granulomas consist of epithelioid histiocytes and a few lymphocytes with rare giant cells. Acid-fast bacilli tend to be more numerous in immunosuppressed patients.

Syphilis

Syphilitic orchitis may be congenital or acquired. In congenital orchitis, both testes are enlarged at birth. The histological findings are similar to those of the interstitial orchitis of the acquired syphilis. If diagnosis is delayed until puberty, the testis often shows retraction and fibrosis (Fig. 10-110). In adults, acquired orchitis is a complication of the tertiary stage of syphilis and has two characteristic histologic patterns, interstitial inflammation and gumma.

Early in the disease, patients with interstitial orchitis have painless testicular enlargement. Grossly, the testicular parenchyma is gray with translucent areas. Histologically, plasma cells are abundant. The inflammation begins in the mediastinum testis and testicular septa,

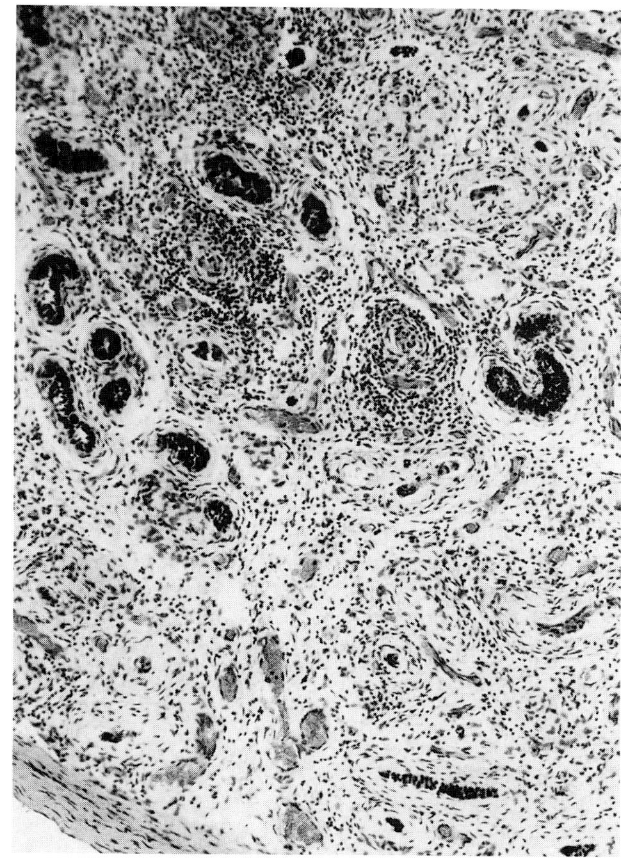

10-110. Congenital syphilitic orchitis with diffuse tubular atrophy and dense interstitial infiltrates consisting of plasma cells and lymphocytes.

later extending around the seminiferous tubules which lose their epithelium and undergo sclerosis. Initially the arteries show an obliterans type of endarteritis. Small gummas may be present. Eventually, the inflammation subsides and is replaced by fibrosis. The epididymis is usually not affected.

Gummatous orchitis is characterized by the presence of one or multiple well-delineated grossly gray-yellow zones of necrosis.[780] Histologically, the ghostly silhouettes of seminiferous tubules are visible within the gummas. Around the gumma there is an inflammatory infiltrate consisting of lymphocytes, plasma cells, and a few giant cells. In most cases spirochetes may be demonstrated histochemically with stains such as the Warthin-Starry silver stain.

Leprosy

The testis may be infected in patients with lepromatous or borderline leprosy. The frequent involvement of the testis in lepromatous leprosy is related to the low intrascrotal temperature which promotes the growth of the bacilli. The orchitis is usually bilateral, although the degree of testicular involvement may differ between the testes. Occasionally, testicular infection may be the sole indication of the infection, and the diagnosis may be made by testicular biopsy.[781]

The histologic findings in the testis vary with the duration of the infection. Initially there are a perivascular lymphocytic infiltrate and numerous interstitial macrophages that contain many acid-fast bacilli. Later the seminiferous tubules undergo atrophy, the Leydig cells cluster, and the blood vessels show endarteritis obliterans. Finally, the testis is replaced by fibrous tissue with a few lymphocytes and macrophages containing acid-fast bacilli. Most patients with lepromatous leprosy are infertile, even if the orchitis was clinically mild.[782]

Brucellosis

Brucellosis remains common in some parts of the world, such as the Middle East. Orchitis occurs in some patients and may be the first sign of the disease. Brucellosis should be suspected when testicular enlargement occurs in patients with undulating fever, malaise, sweats, weight loss, and headache.[783] Occasionally this may mimic a testicular tumor. Histologically, there is a dense lymphohistiocytic infiltrate with occasional noncaseating granulomas in the interstitium. The seminiferous tubules are infiltrated by inflammatory cells and undergo atrophy.

Sarcoidosis

Sarcoidosis is a systemic granulomatous disease of unknown etiology, preferentially affecting young black adults. The genitourinary tract is involved in only 0.2% of clinical cases and 5% of autopsy cases. Fewer than 30 cases of primary epididymal involvement have been reported, and only six of these also involved the testis.[784] Testicular sarcoidosis is usually unilateral and nodular.[784] It often is asymptomatic and found at autopsy.[785] The testis contains noncaseating granulomas similar to sarcoid granulomas at other locations. Before diagnosing testicular sarcoidosis, other granulomatous lesions should be excluded, including tuberculosis, sperm granuloma, granulomatous orchitis, and seminoma. Some seminomas show an intense sarcoidlike reaction, and examination of multiple histologic sections may be necessary to find diagnostic foci of seminoma. An association of mediastinal sarcoidosis and testicular cancer has been reported.[786]

MALAKOPLAKIA

Malakoplakia is a chronic inflammatory disease that was initially described in the bladder[787] and subsequently in many other organs. The testis (alone or together with the epididymis) is involved in 12% of cases of malakoplakia of the urogenital system.[788] Grossly, the testis is enlarged and has a brown-yellow parenchyma,[789] often with abscesses. Malakoplakia causes tubular destruction that is associated with an interstitial infiltrate of macrophages with eosinophilic cytoplasm which may contain Michaelis-Gutmann bodies (Fig. 10-111).[790,791]

The differential diagnosis includes idiopathic granulomatous orchitis and Leydig cell tumor. Inflammation in idiopathic granulomatous orchitis includes intratubular multinucleate giant cells; in malakoplakia, it is difficult to identify the tubular outlines and giant cells are usually absent. Leydig cell tumors are not usually associated with inflammation but contain mononucleate or binucleate cells with abundant eosinophilic cytoplasm. Reinke's crystalloids are identifiable in 40% of Leydig cell tumors but absent in malakoplakia, and Michaelis-Gutmann bodies are not present in Leydig cell tumors.

ORCHIDOEPIDIDYMITIS CAUSED BY FUNGI AND PARASITES

Fungal orchitis is rare; most cases are associated with blastomycosis, coccidioidomycosis, histoplasmosis, or cryptococcosis.[792] The genital tract may be involved in widespread blastomycosis. In decreasing order, the organs most frequently affected are prostate, epididymis, testis, and seminal vesicles. Grossly, there often are small abscesses that may have caseous centers. Fungi, 8-15 µm in diameter, with double refringent contours, are present in the giant cells in the granulomas and stain positively with periodic acid–Schiff and methenamine silver procedures. Coccidioidomycosis is endemic in California, the southwestern United States, and Mexico, and it may present as an epididymal disease after remission of the systemic symptoms. The granulomas are similar to those of tuberculosis and contain 30 to 120 µm sporangia with endospores which stain with periodic acid–Schiff. Dissemination of histoplasmosis and cryptococcosis frequently occurs after steroid therapy and may give rise to granulomatous orchitis with extensive necrosis.[793] *Histoplasma capsulatum* is 1 to 5 µm in diameter and may be demonstrated with silver stains. *Cryptococcus* is identified by its thick wall, which stains with mucicarmine. Most parasites that reach the genital tract, such as *Phyllaria* and *Schistosoma,* are in the spermatic cord, and the testicular lesions are secondary to vascular injury by these parasites. Testicular lesions have also been reported in patients with visceral leishmaniasis, congenital and acquired toxoplasmosis,[794] and *Echinococcus* infection.[795]

IDIOPATHIC GRANULOMATOUS ORCHITIS

Idiopathic granulomatous orchitis is a chronic inflammatory lesion of older adults. The most prominent clinical symptom is testicular enlargement suggesting a malignant tumor. Most patients give a history of scrotal trauma, 66% have symptoms of urinary tract infection with negative cultures, and 40% have sperm granulomas in the epididymis. An autoimmune etiology has been suggested.

The testis is enlarged, with a nodular cut surface and areas of necrosis or infarction. There are two histologic forms according to whether the lesion is predominantly

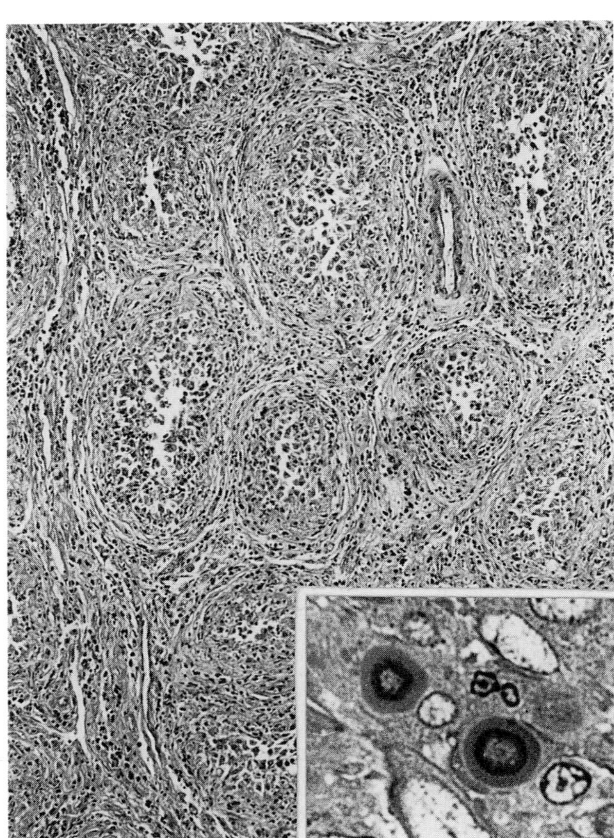

10-111. Malakoplakia. Macrophages with eosinophilic cytoplasm are present in the interstitium and in the seminiferous tubules. *Inset*: detail of Michaelis-Gutmann bodies in a semithin section.

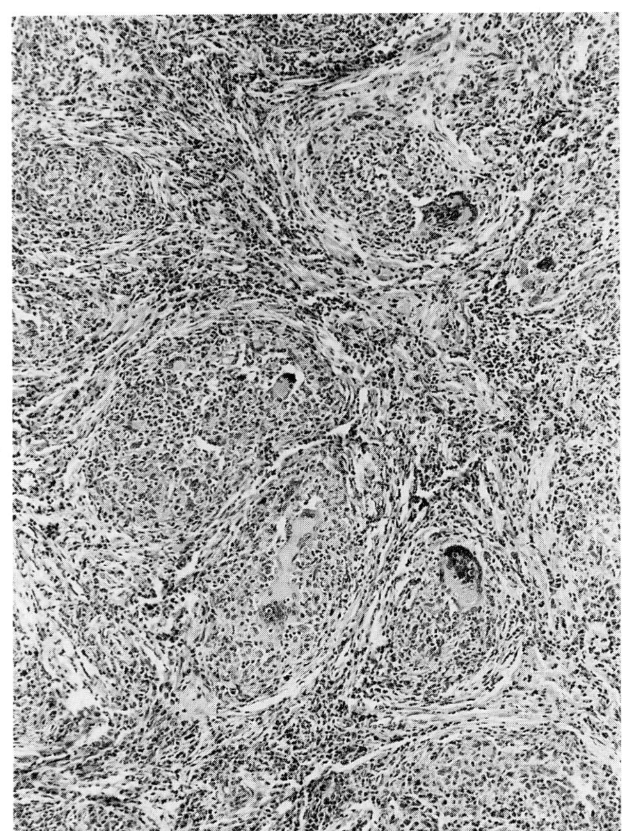

10-112. Idiopathic granulomatous orchitis showing seminiferous tubules with peritubular fibrosis. Numerous lymphocytes and macrophages are present in the interstitium and within the seminiferous tubules. Multinucleated giant cells are present in some tubules.

in the tubules (tubular orchitis) or in the interstitium (interstitial orchitis). In tubular orchitis the germ cells degenerate and the Sertoli cells have vacuolated cytoplasm and vesicular nuclei. Plasma cells and lymphocytes infiltrate the wall of the seminiferous tubule, forming concentric rings. Multinucleated giant cells are present in the tubular lumens and sometimes in the interstitium (Fig. 10-112). Vascular thrombosis and arteritis are common. In interstitial orchitis the inflammation is predominantly interstitial. Ultimately, tubular atrophy and interstitial fibrosis prevail in both forms. The two forms may arise via different immune mechanisms.[796] Tubular orchitis histologically resembles experimental orchitis caused by injection of serum from animals with orchitis, while interstitial orchitis resembles orchitis produced by the transfer of cells from immunized animals.

The differential diagnosis of idiopathic granulomatous orchitis is infectious orchitis caused by bacteria, spirochetes, fungi, or parasites. A useful clue in the tubular form is the presence of giant cells within seminiferous tubules. Focal orchitis caused by immune complexes has been reported in young men[797-799] and may cause infertility.[800]

TESTICULAR PSEUDOLYMPHOMA

Pseudolymphoma is a benign reactive process with a lymphoid cell proliferation so intense that it may be mistaken for lymphoma. Testicular pseudolymphoma shows inflammatory infiltrates with numerous lymphocytes and plasma cells and these infiltrates destroy, totally or partially, the testicular parenchyma (Fig. 10-113).[801]

The differential diagnosis includes lymphoma, various forms of orchitis, and seminoma. The diagnosis of lymphoma may be excluded by the lack of atypia and mixed population of inflammatory cells. Syphilitic orchitis also contains a plasma cell–rich inflammatory infiltrate, but pseudolymphoma does not have other characteristic features of syphilitic orchitis, such as endarteritis obliterans, and spirochetes cannot be demonstrated by special stains. The lack of granulomas or significant numbers of macrophages, together with the negative results of specific histochemical stains, also helps to exclude idiopathic granulomatous orchitis, tuberculosis, leprosy, sarcoidosis, and fungal infections. Finally, although the presence of a prominent inflammatory infiltrate and, in many cases, numerous lymphoid follicles, may suggest the diagnosis of seminoma, the presence of seminoma cells should be easily demonstrated with Best's carmine or periodic acid–Schiff stains. The term *plasma cell granuloma* refers to a reactive process characterized by the presence of polyclonal adult plasma cells, which are absent in testicular plasmacytoma.

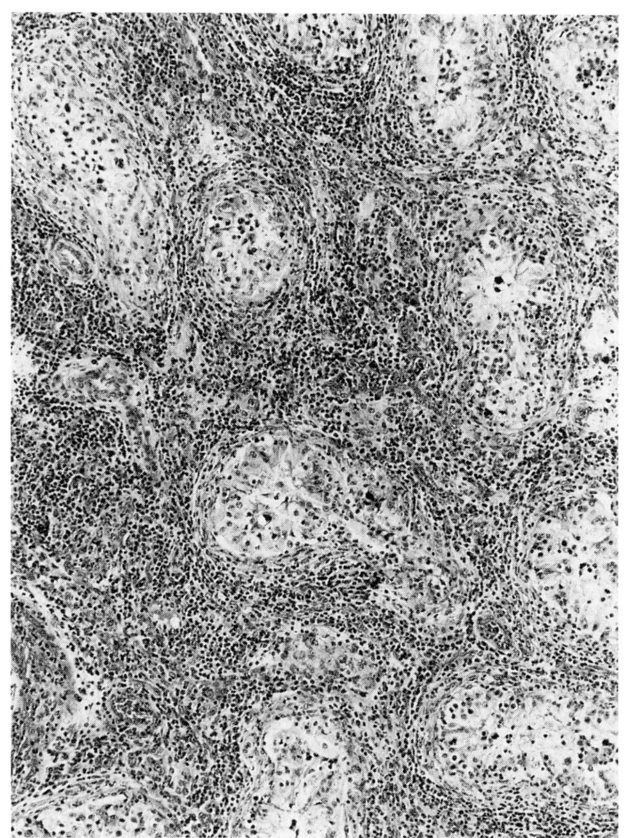

10-113. Testicular pseudolymphoma with dense interstitial infiltrates of mature lymphocytes, which also infiltrate the walls of the seminiferous tubules.

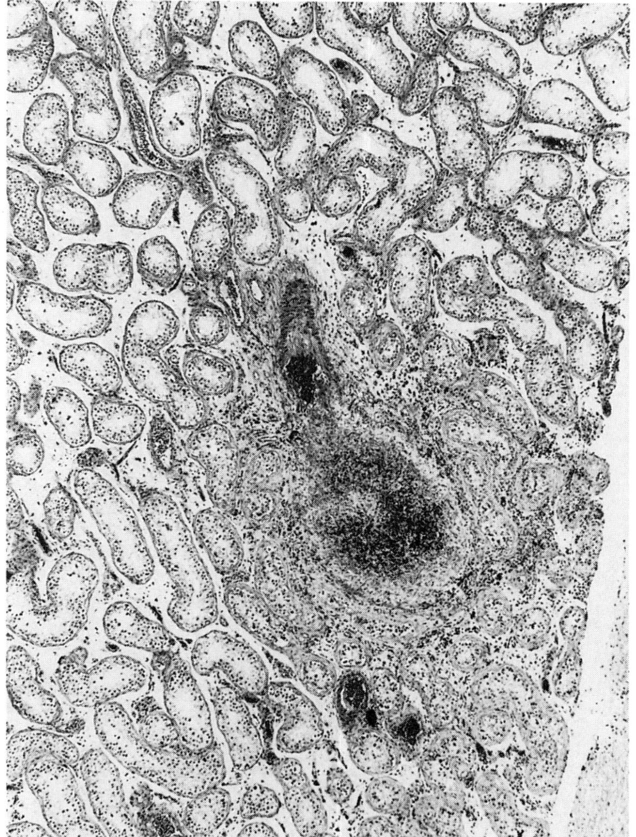

10-114. Polyarteritis nodosa with necrotizing arteritis.

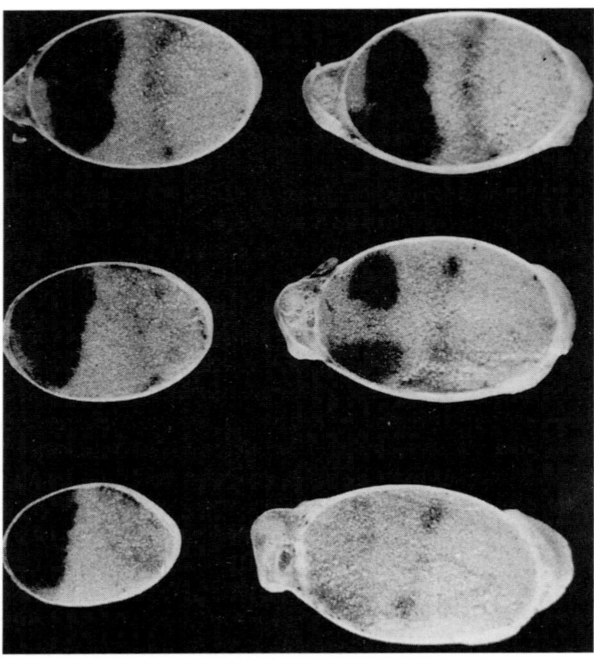

10-115. Serial sections of a testis with focal hemorrhagic infarct.

POLYARTERITIS NODOSA

The testicular arteries may be affected in systemic disorders such as rheumatoid arthritis, Schönlein-Henoch purpura, and polyarteritis nodosa.[802] Approximately 60% to 80% of patients with polyarteritis nodosa have testicular or epididymal involvement, but only 2% to 18% are diagnosed during life. In only a few cases has testicular or epididymal polyarteritis nodosa been the first manifestation of the disease.[803,804]

The testis usually shows arterial lesions in different stages of evolution: fibrinoid reaction, inflammatory reaction, thrombosis, or aneurysm. The parenchyma initially has zones of infarction (Fig. 10-114) and later develops tubular sclerosis with interstitial fibrosis. A histologic and immunohistochemical picture similar to polyarteritis nodosa may occasionally be observed in the testis or the epididymis without lesions elsewhere and is referred to as isolated arteritis of the testis and epididymis. These lesions differ from classic polyarteritis, lacking vascular thrombosis, aneurysms, and infarcts. The etiology of isolated arteritis is unknown. The prognosis of isolated necrotizing arteritis is excellent. The histologic finding of necrotizing arteritis in the testis or epididymis should be followed by clinical, hematologic, and biochemical studies to exclude systemic polyarteritis nodosa.[805,806]

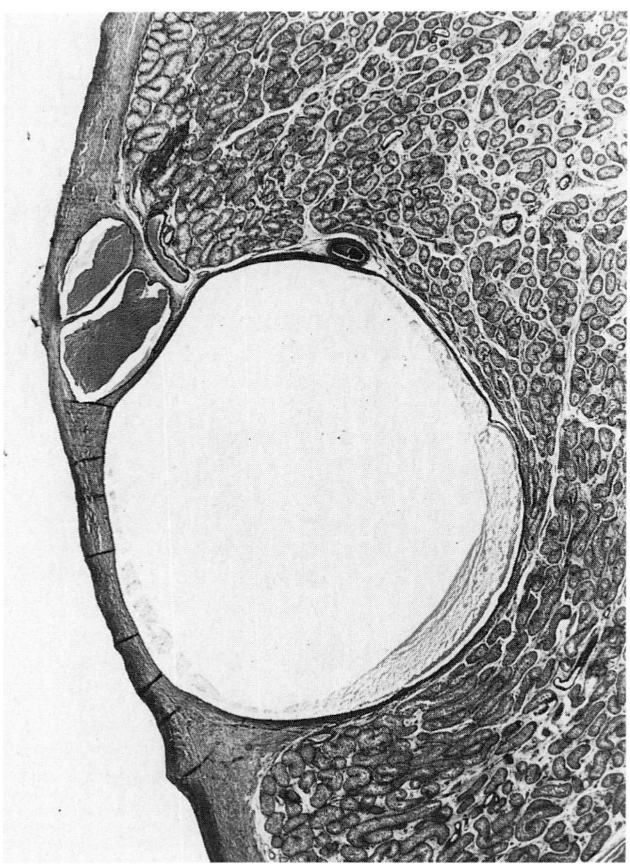

10-116. Multilocular cyst in the tunica albuginea. The largest cavity protrudes into the testicular parenchyma.

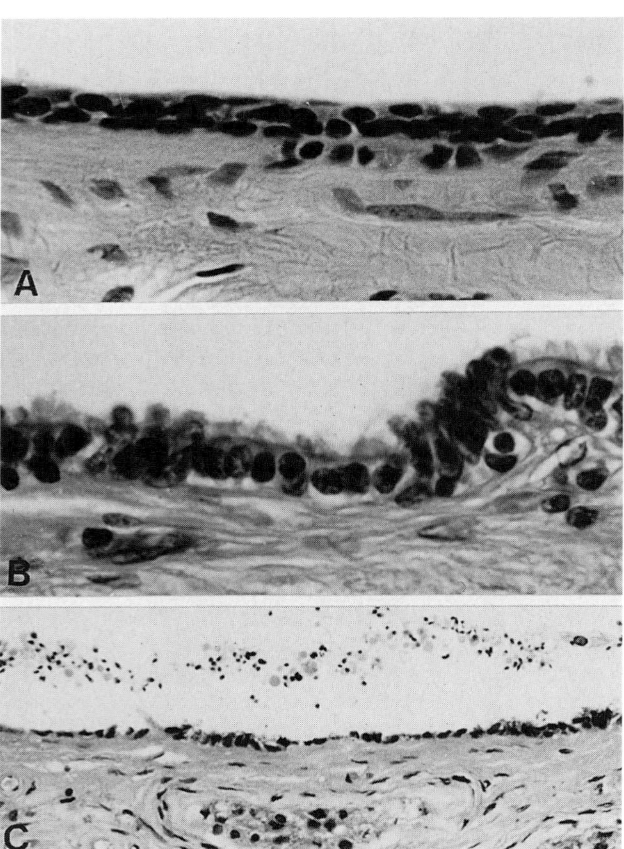

10-117. The epithelium lining tunica albuginea cysts is either cuboidal pseudostratified (**A**) or ciliated columnar (**B**). Rete testis cysts are lined by flattened or columnar epithelium (**C**) and contain spermatozoa.

TESTICULAR INFARCT

Torsion of the spermatic cord is the most frequent cause of testicular infarct. If surgical intervention is delayed more than 8 hours, the testis is usually not viable and should be removed; rare cases of incomplete torsion may have a better prognosis. Trauma[807] and lesions of the vessels of the spermatic cord also may cause testicular infarction (Fig. 10-115). Ischemic atrophy is a risk of inguinal surgery, including herniorrhaphy, varicocelectomy, and hydrocelectomy. The incidence of atrophy after inguinal herniorrhaphy varies from 0.06% in primary herniorrhaphy[808] to 7.9% after surgery for recurrent hernia,[809] depending on the difficulty and extent of the hernia. Atrophy occurs in some cases of thrombosis of the vena cava or spermatic artery.[810] Focal infarction of the testis has been associated with polycythemia, sickle cell disease, and trauma.[811,812] Focal infarction may also be spontaneous. Clinical symptoms of testicular infarcts mimic a testicular tumor, and the diagnosis often is made only after orchiectomy.

OTHER TESTICULAR DISEASES

CYSTIC MALFORMATIONS

Cystic malformations of the tunica albuginea and testicular parenchyma were first described in the nineteenth century[813] and were long considered rare and mainly present in the tunica albuginea.[814,815] With the systematic use of ultrasonography, the incidence of cysts has been found to be much higher[816]; non-neoplastic cysts are found in from 2.1%[817] to 9.8%[818] of testes.

Cysts of the tunica albuginea are usually incidental findings in patients in the fifth or sixth decades of life.[819] They are located in the anterior-lateral aspect of the testis and may be unilocular or multilocular.[819] They range from 2 to 4 mm, and contain clear fluid without spermatozoa. The cysts may be embedded within the connective tissue of the tunica albuginea, protrude from the inner surface of the tunica albuginea into the testicular parenchyma, or protrude from the outer surface forming a blue lump in the tunica albuginea (Fig. 10-116). The epithelium lining the cysts may be either simple columnar or stratified cuboidal and is supported by a thin layer of collagenized connective tissue. The columnar epithelium usually includes some ciliated cells,[820] and the cuboidal epithelium is composed of two layers of nonciliated cells (Fig. 10-117).

Cysts of the rete testis are identified by a distinctive epithelial lining of areas of flattened cells intermingled with areas of columnar cells. Spermatozoa are frequently found within the cysts (Fig. 10-117*C*).[821] Rete testis cysts are not always attached to the rete and can be found at a distance from it.

Simple cysts of the testis constitute the remaining intraparenchymal cysts. These are usually lined by cuboidal epithelium and contain no spermatozoa.[822-824] They range from 2 to 18 mm in diameter.[825]

The origin of the three types of testicular cysts has been discussed for years. Previously, traumatic[826] and inflammatory[827] origins have been attributed to tunica albuginea cysts, but most now believe that they are derived from embryonic remnants of the mesonephric ducts[820,828] or mesothelial cells embedded in the tunica albuginea during embryogenesis.[819,829,830] Simple cysts of the testis may also have a mesothelial origin, but it is possible that some arise from ectopic rete testis epithelium. These cysts are unrelated to epidermoid cyst, differing in their ultrasonographic[831,832] and histologic features (see discussion on testicular tumors in this chapter). Ultrasound studies indicate that testicular cysts have little potential for growth.[831,833] Presently, excision is recommended only in children when their presence may impair testicular development.[834]

HYPERPLASIA OF RETE TESTIS

The epithelium of the rete testis is usually flattened with scattered areas of columnar cells. It may undergo diffuse transformation into tall, columnar epithelium in patients receiving estrogen, patients with chronic hepatic insufficiency, and in some uncommon disorders that are known as hyperplasia of the rete testis.

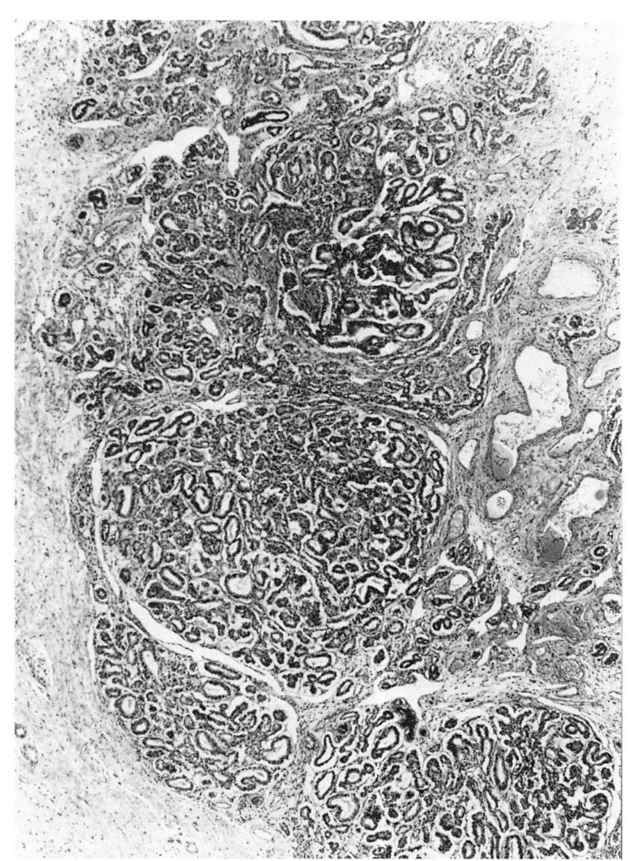

10-118. Adenomatous hyperplasia of the rete testis, forming multiple nodules in the mediastinum testis.

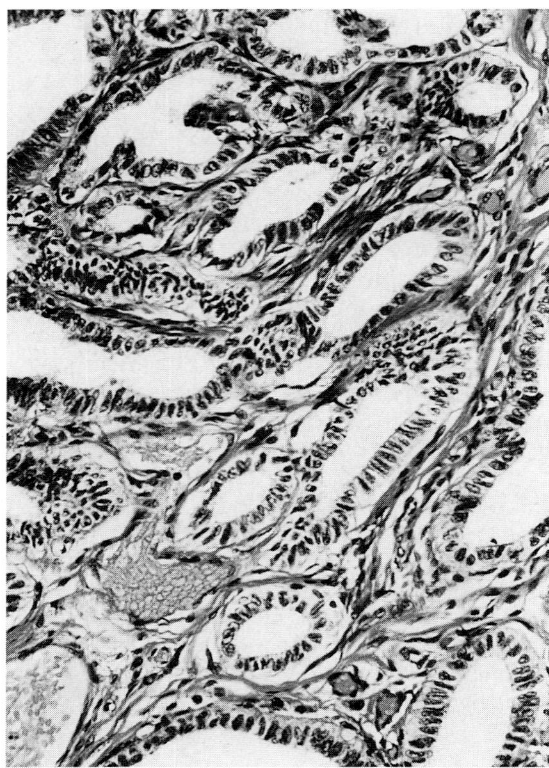

10-119. Adenomatous hyperplasia of the rete testis. The epithelium is columnar and is supported by a well-collagenized stroma.

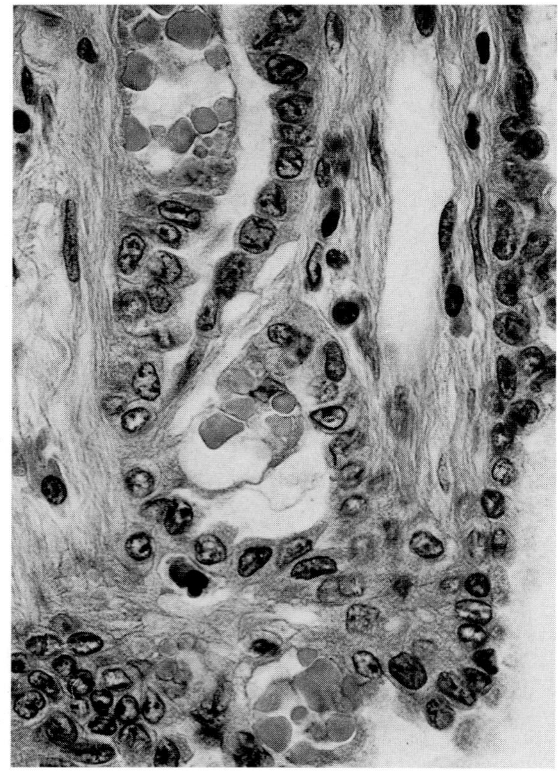

10-120. Rete testis hyperplasia with hyaline globules. The cells containing globules protrude into the lumens of the rete testis channels.

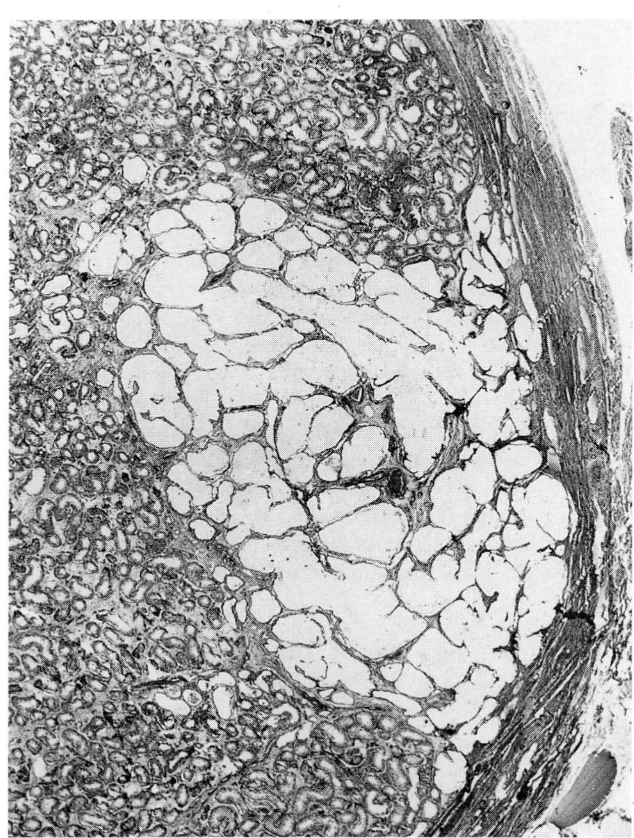

10-121. Cystic transformation of the rete testis secondary to a lesion in the caput epididymidis in a patient with chronic epididymitis.

ADENOMATOUS HYPERPLASIA

This lesion is characterized by diffuse or nodular proliferation of tubular or papillary structures derived from the rete testis.[835] Congenital and acquired forms are recognized. Bilateral congenital adenomatous hyperplasia was reported in a newborn. The mediastinum testis was enlarged and filled with cordlike or ductlike epithelial structures identical to rete testis epithelium,[836] forming a mass equal to one third of the testicular volume.

Acquired adenomatous hyperplasia of the rete testis is a benign unilateral or bilateral condition that is usually an incidental finding in autopsy specimens or testes resected from adults for other reasons. The rete epithelium forms nodules and glandlike structures that are not encapsulated (Fig. 10-118). The cells are tall and columnar (Fig. 10-119) and ultrastructurally resemble normal rete testis cells. The seminiferous tubules are slightly atrophic. In some cases a few spermatozoa have been observed in the lumens of the glandular structures.

Adenomatous hyperplasia of the rete testis should be differentiated from rete testis tumors. Benign tumors of the rete, such as solid adenoma, papillary adenoma, and cystadenoma, form circumscribed masses unlike the diffuse proliferation in adenomatous hyperplasia. Rete testis adenocarcinoma is an aggressive tumor with

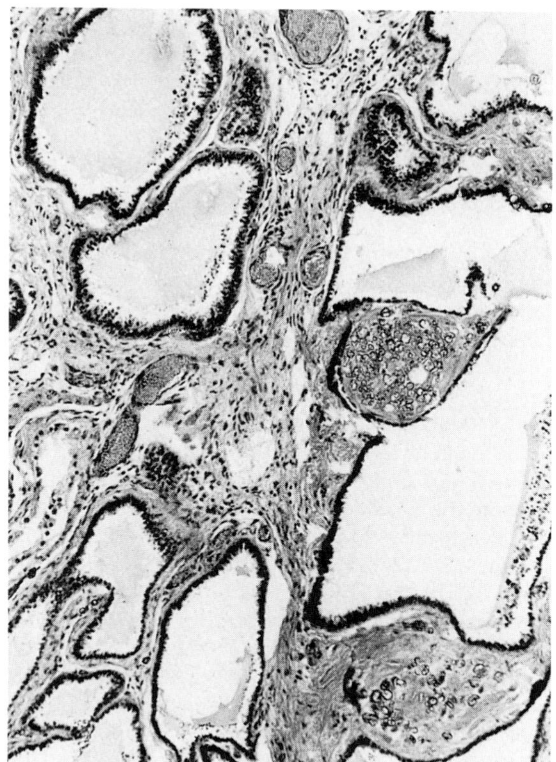

10-122. Renal dialysis-associated cystic transformation of the rete testis is characterized by pronounced dilation of the rete testis with columnar transformation of the rete testis epithelium.

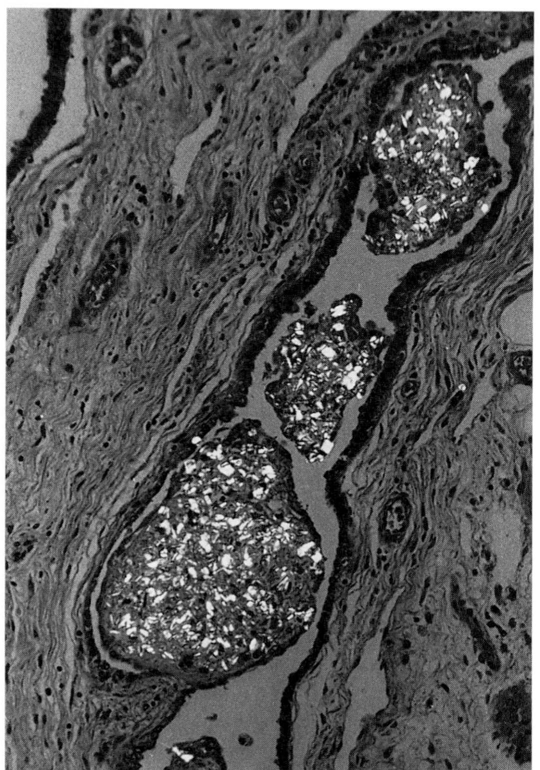

10-123. Renal dialysis-associated cystic transformation of the rete testis with oxalate crystals shown by polarized light.

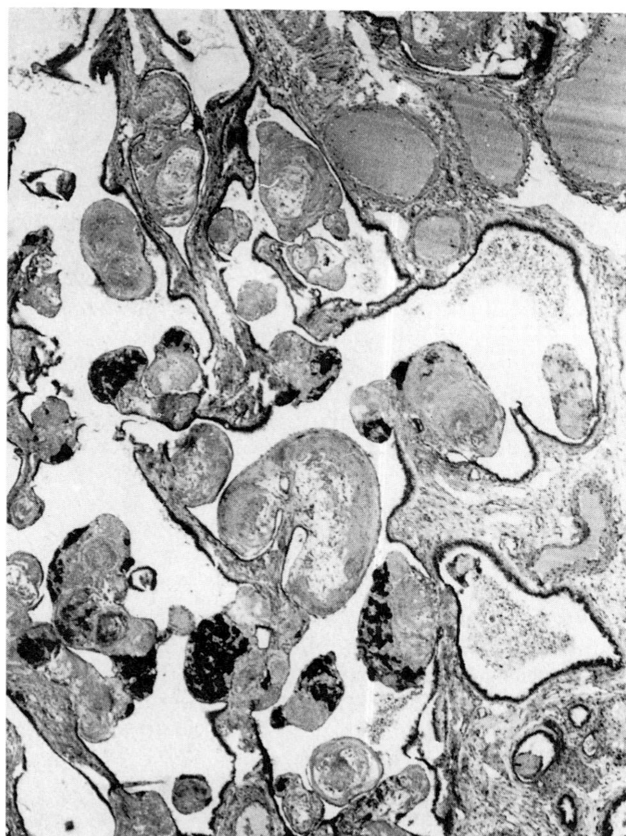

10-124. Nodular proliferation of calcifying connective tissue in the rete testis. The rete testis channels are dilated, and polypoid excrescences protrude into them.

numerous mitotic figures, and it infiltrates the adjacent structures.[837]

HYPERPLASIA WITH HYALINE GLOBULES

This reactive lesion is characterized by the presence of intracytoplasmic accumulations of hyaline eosinophilic globules in the epithelial cells of the rete testis. The epithelium may be hyperplastic, but it does not display mitotic figures or nuclear atypia. The hyaline globules may be up to 10 μm in diameter (Fig. 10-120). This lesion mainly occurs in testes with germ cell tumors. Yolk sac tumor infiltrating the rete testis may closely resemble this type of rete testis hyperplasia. Positive immunoreactions for alpha fetoprotein and placenta-like alkaline phosphatase, as well as nuclear atypia, are helpful to distinguish germ cell neoplasia from rete testis hyperplasia.[838]

HYPERPLASIA WITH CYSTIC TRANSFORMATION

Several disorders cause dilation of the rete testis and may have an impact on the seminiferous epithelium. These may be extratesticular, such as obstruction occurring near the head of the epididymis (Fig. 10-121), or intratesticular, such as the irregular dilation of seminiferous tubules occurring in patients with long-term varicocele or chronic renal failure.

Cystic transformation of the rete testis secondary to renal failure is observed in patients on dialysis. The histologic findings are reminiscent of the acquired cystic disease of kidney that occurs in these patients (Fig. 10-122).[839] Associated with the cystic dilation and hyperplasia of the epithelial lining are deposits of proteinaceous material containing calcium oxalate crystals, which are easily identified by their birefringence under polarized light (Fig. 10-123). These crystals, without any inflammatory reaction, are also observed beneath the rete testis epithelium in the mediastinum testis. The epithelial cells of the efferent ductules have variable height and contain numerous eosinophilic granules. The ductal lumens are dilated and contain amorphous and/or crystalline deposits. A foreign body giant cell reaction may be seen in ductules that are partially destroyed.

NODULAR PROLIFERATION OF CALCIFYING CONNECTIVE TISSUE IN RETE TESTIS

This lesion is characterized by the presence of multiple nodules that originate from the rete testis lining and adjacent connective tissue, protruding into the channels of the rete testis (Fig. 10-124). These consist of cellular connective tissue covered by several layers of fibrinlike material, which, in turn, is covered by rete testis epithelium. The nodules may be totally or partially calcified (Fig. 10-125).[840] The lesion is an incidental finding in autopsies of patients with impaired peripheral perfusion.

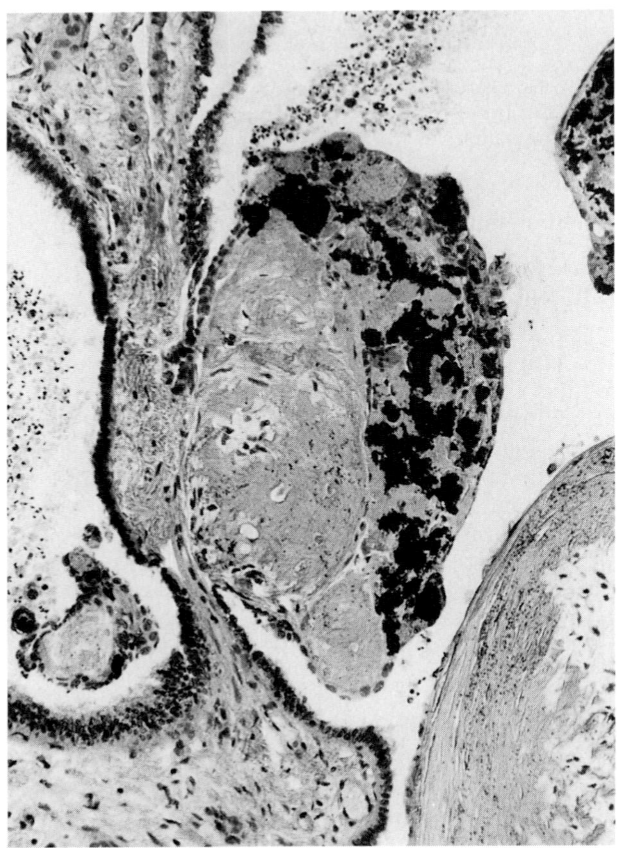

10-125. Nodular proliferation of calcifying connective tissue in the rete testis. Detail of a polypoid formation showing large calcium deposits.

REFERENCES

1. Sinclair AH, Berta P, Palmer MS et al: A gene from the human sex determining region encodes a protein with homology to a conserved DNA-binding motif, Nature 346:240-244, 1990.
2. Satoh M: Histogenesis and organogenesis of the gonad in human embryos, J Anat 177:85-107, 1991.
3. Davis RM: Localization of male determining factors in men: a thorough review of structural anomalies of the Y chromosome, J Med Genet 18:161-195, 1981.
4. Bishop CE, Guellaen G, Geldwerth D et al: Single-copy DNA sequences specific for the human Y chromosome, Nature 309:253-255, 1984.
5. Blyth B, Duckett JW: Gonadal differentiation: a review of the physiological process and influencing factors based on recent experimental evidence, J Urol 145:689-694, 1991.
6. Cunha GR: Development of the male urogenital tract. In Rajfer J, ed: Urologic endocrinology, Philadelphia, 1986, WB Saunders.
7. Jost A, Magre S: Control mechanisms of testicular differentiation, Philos Trans R Soc Lond (Biol) 322:55-61, 1988.
8. Forest MG, Sizonenko PC, Cathiard AM et al: Hypophysogonadal function in humans during the first year of life. I. Evidence for testicular activity in early infancy, J Clin Invest 53:819-824, 1974.
9. Whitehead RH: The embryonic development of the interstitial cells of Leydig, Am J Anat 3:167-187, 1904.
10. Cunha GR, Alarid ET, Turner T et al: Normal and abnormal development of the male urogenital tract. Role of androgens, mesenchymal epithelial interactions and growth factors, J Androl 13:465-475, 1992.
11. Wensing CJG: The embryology of testicular descent, Horm Res 30:144-152, 1988.
12. Heyns CF, De Klerk DP: The gubernaculum during testicular descent in the pig fetus, J Urol 133:694-699, 1985.
13. Heyns CF: The gubernaculum during testicular descent in the human fetus, J Anat 153:93-112, 1987.
14. Heyns CF, Human HJ, De Klerk DP: Hyperplasia and hypertrophy of the gubernaculum during testicular descent in the fetus, J Urol 135:1043-1047, 1986.
15. Frey HL, Rajfer J: Epididymis does not play an important role in the process of testicular descent, Surg Forum 33:618-619, 1982.
16. Baumans V, Dijkstra G, Wensing CJG: The role of nonandrogenic testicular factor in the process of testicular descent in the dog, Int J Androl 6:541-542, 1983.
17. Hutson JM: A biphasic model of the hormonal control of testicular descent, Lancet 2:419-422, 1985.
18. Backhouse KM: The gubernaculum testis Hunteri, testicular descent and maldescent, Ann R Coll Surg Engl 35:227-233, 1964.
19. Frey HL, Rajfer J: Role of the gubernaculum and intraabdominal pressure in the process of testicular descent, J Urol 131:574-579, 1984.

20. Backhouse KM: Mechanism of testicular descent, Karger Prog Reprod Biol Med 10:16-23, 1984.
21. Habenicht UF, Neuman NF: Hormonal regulation of testicular descent, Adv Anat Embryol Cell Biol 81:1-55, 1983.
22. Hutson JM, Donahoe PK: The hormonal control of testicular descent, Endocr Rev 7:270-283, 1986.
23. Tran D, Picard JY, Vigier B et al: Persistence of müllerian ducts in male rabbits passively immunized against bovine anti-müllerian hormone during fetal life, Dev Biol 116:160-167, 1986.
24. Behringer RR, Finegold JM, Cate LR: Müllerian-inhibiting substance function during mammalian sexual development, Cell 79:415-425, 1994.
25. Radhakrishnam J, Morikawa Y, Donahoe PK et al: Observations on the gubernaculum during descent of the testis, Invest Urol 16:365-368, 1979.
26. Frey HL, Peng S, Rajfer J: Synergy of abdominal pressure and androgens in testicular descent, Biol Reprod 29:1233-1239, 1983.
27. Elder JS, Isaachs JT, Walsh P: Androgenic sensitivity of the gubernaculum testis. Evidence for hormonal/mechanical interactions in testicular descent, J Urol 127:170-175, 1982.
28. Husmann PA, Levy JB: Current concepts in the pathophysiology of testicular undescent, Urology 46:267-276, 1995.
29. Park WH, Hutson JM: The gubernaculum shows rhythmic contractility and active movement during testicular descent, J Pediatr Surg 26:615-617, 1991.
30. Yamanaka J, Metcalf SA, Hutson JM et al: Testicular descent II. Ontogeny and response to denervation of calcitonin gene-related peptide receptors in neonatal rat gubernaculum, Endocrinology, 132:280-284, 1993.
31. Van der Schoot P, Vigier B, Prepin J et al: Development of the gubernaculum and processus vaginalis in freemartinism: further evidence in support of a specific fetal testis hormone governing male-specific gubernaculum development, Anat Rec 241:211-224, 1995.
32. Belman AB: Acquired undescended (ascendent) testis: effects of human chorionic gonadotropin, J Urol 140:1189-1190, 1988.
33. Vilar O: Histology of the human testis from neonatal period to adolescence, Adv Exp Med Biol 10:95-111, 1970.
34. Müller J, Skakkebaek NE: Fluctuations in the number of germ cells during late foetal and early postnatal periods in boys, Acta Endocrinol 105:271-274, 1984.
35. Cortes D, Müller J, Skakkebaek NE: Proliferation of Sertoli cells during development of the human testis assessed by stereological methods, Int J Androl 10:589-596, 1987.
36. Nistal M, Abaurrea MA, Paniagua R: Morphological and histometric study of human Sertoli cells from birth to the onset of puberty, J Anat 134: 351-363, 1982.
37. Prince FP: Ultrastructural evidence of mature Leydig cells and Leydig cell regression in the neonatal human testis, Anat Rec 228:405-417, 1990.
38. Hadziselimovic F: Ultrastructure of normal and cryptorchid testis development, Adv Anat Embryol Cell Biol 53:47-50, 1977.
39. Nistal M, Santamaría L, Paniagua R: Mast cells in the human testis and epididymis from birth to adulthood, Acta Anat 139:535-552, 1984.
40. Faiman C, Reyes FI, Winter JSD: Serum gonadotropin patterns during the perinatal period in man and in the chimpanzee, INSERM 32:281-298, 1974.
41. Forest MG, Sizonenko PC, Cathiard AM et al: Hypophysogonadal function in humans during the first year of life. 1. Evidence for testicular activity in early infancy, J Clin Invest 53:819-824, 1974.
42. Bidlingmaier F, Dörr HG, Eisenmenger W et al: Testosterone and androstenedione concentrations in human testis and epididymis during the first two years of life, J Clin Endocrinol Metab 57:311-315, 1983.
43. Codesal J, Regadera J, Nistal M et al: Involution of human fetal Leydig cells. An immunohistochemical, ultrastructural and quantitative study, J Anat 172:103-114, 1990.
44. Müller J, Skakkebaek NE: Quantification of germ cells and seminiferous tubules by stereological examination of testicles from 50 boys who suffered from sudden death, Int J Androl 6:143-156, 1983.
45. Paniagua R, Nistal M: Morphological and histometric study of human spermatogonia from birth to the onset of puberty, J Anat 139: 535-552,1984.
46. Codesal J, Santamaría L, Paniagua R et al: Proliferative activity of human spermatogonia from fetal period to senility measured by cytophotometric DNA quantification, Arch Androl 22:209-215, 1989.
47. Frasier SD, Horton R: Androgens in the peripheral plasma of prepubertal children and adults, Steroids 8:777-784, 1966.
48. Forti G, Santoro S, Andrea-Grisolia G et al: Spermatic and peripheral plasma concentration of testosterone and androstenedione in prepubertal boys, J Clin Endocrinol Metab 53:883-886, 1981.
49. Lee VMK, Burger HG: Pituitary testicular axis during puberal development. In De Kretser DM, Burger HG, Hudson B, eds: The pituitary and testis. Clinical and experimental studies, Heidelberg, 1983, Springer.
50. Méndez JA, Emery JL: The seminiferous tubules of the testis before, around and after birth, J Anat 128:601-607, 1979.
51. Mancini Re, Vilar O, Lavieri JC et al; Development of Leydig cells in the normal human testis. A cytological, cytochemical and quantitative study, Am J Anat 112:203-214, 1963.
52. Nistal M, Paniagua R, Regadera J et al: A quantitative morphologic study of human Leydig cells from birth to adulthood, Cell Tissue Res 246:229-236, 1986.
53. Zachmann M, Kind HP, Häfliger H et al: Testicular volume during adolescence. Cross-sectional and longitudinal studies, Helv Paediatr Acta 29:61-72, 1974.
54. Waaler PE, Thorsen T, Stoa KF et al: Studies in normal male puberty, Acta Paediatr Scand Suppl 249:3-36, 1974.
55. Burr FM, Sizonenko PC, Kaplan SL et al: Hormonal changes in puberty. I. Correlation of serum luteinizing hormone and follicle stimulating hormone with stages of puberty, testicular size, and bone age in normal boys, Pediatr Res 4:25-35, 1970.
56. Daniel WA, Feinstein RA, Howard-Peebles P et al: Testicular volumes of adolescents, J Pediatr 101: 1010-1012, 1982.
57. Nielsen CT, Skakkebaek NE, Richardson DW et al: Onset of the release of spermatozoa (spermarche) in boys in relation to age, testicular growth, pubic hair, and height, J Clin Endocrinol Metab 62:532-535, 1986.

58. Winter JSD, Faiman C: Pituitary-gonadal relations in male children and adolescents, Pediatr Res 6:126-135, 1972.
59. Hansen P, With TH: Clinical measurement of the testes in boys and men, Acta Med Scand 226(suppl):457-465, 1952.
60. Nistal M, Paniagua R, Abaurrea MA et al: Hyperplasia and the immature appearance of Sertoli cells in primary testicular disorders, Hum Pathol 13:3-12, 1982.
61. Nistal M, González-Peramato P, Paniagua R: Congenital Leydig cell hyperplasia, Histopathology 12:307-317, 1988.
62. Doshi N, Surti UI, Szulman AE: Morphologic anomalies in triploid liveborn fetuses, Hum Pathol 14:716-723, 1983.
63. Behre HM, Nashan D, Nieschlag E: Objective measurement of testicular volume by ultrasonography: evaluation of the technique and comparison with orchidometer estimates, Int J Androl 12:395-403, 1989.
64. Diamond JM: Ethnic differences. Variation in human testis size, Nature 320:488-489, 1986.
65. Handelsman DJ, Stara S: Testicular size: the effects of aging, malnutrition, and illness, J Androl 6:144-151, 1985.
66. Prader A: Testicular size: assessment and clinical importance, Triangle 7:240-243, 1966.
67. Sosnik H: Studies of the participation of the tunica albuginea and rete testis (TA and RT) in the quantitative structure of human testis, Gegenbaurs Morphol Jahrb 131:347-356, 1985.
68. Trainer TD: Histology of the normal testis, Am J Surg Pathol 11:107-171, 1987.
69. Lennox B, Ahmad RN, Mack WS: A method for determining the relative total length of the tubules in the testis, J Pathol 102:229-238, 1970.
70. Fawcett DW, Burgos MH: The fine structure of Sertoli cells in the human testis, Anat Rec 124:401-402, 1956.
71. Nagano T: Some observations on the fine structure of the Sertoli cell in the human testis, Z Zellforsch 73:89-106, 1966.
72. Schulze C: On the morphology of the human Sertoli cell, Cell Tissue Res 153:339-355, 1974.
73. Schulze W, Rehder V: Organization and morphogenesis of the human seminiferous epithelium, Cell Tissue Res 237:395-407, 1984.
74. Fawcett DW: The mammalian spermatozoon, Dev Biol 44:394-436, 1975.
75. Paniagua R, Nistal M, Amat P et al: Ultrastructural observations on nucleoli and related structures during human spermatogenesis, Anat Embryol 174:301-306, 1986.
76. Bustos-Obregón E, Esponda P: Ultrastructure of the nucleus of human Sertoli cells in normal and pathological testes, Cell Tissue Res 152:467-475, 1974.
77. Sáez JM, Avallet O, Lejeune H et al: Cell-cell communication in the testis, Horm Res 36:104-115, 1991.
78. Dym M: The fine structure of the monkey (Macaca) Sertoli cell and its role in maintaining the blood-testis barrier, Anat Rec 175:639-656, 1973.
79. Fawcett DW, Leak LV, Heidger PM: Electron microscopic observations on the structural components of the blood testis barrier, J Reprod Fertil Suppl 10:105-122, 1979.
80. Russell LD, Peterson RN: Sertoli cell junctions: morphological and functional correlates, Int Rev Cytol 94:177-211, 1985.
81. Russell LD: Morphological and functional evidence for Sertoli–germ cell relationship. In Russell LD, Griswold MD, eds: The Sertoli cell, Clearwater, Fla, 1993, Cache River Press.
82. Ritzen EM, Hansson V, French FS: The Sertoli cell. In Burger H, De Kretser DM eds: The testis. New York, 1981, Raven Press.
83. Pfeiffer DC, Vogl AW: Evidence that vinculin is codistributed with actin bundles in ectoplasmic ("junctional") specializations of mammalian Sertoli cells, Anat Rec 231:89-100, 1991.
84. Paniagua R, Rodríguez MC, Nistal M et al: Changes in the lipid inclusion/Sertoli cell cytoplasm area ratio during the cycle of the human seminiferous epithelium, J Reprod Fertil 80:335-341, 1987.
85. Bawa SR: Fine structure of the Sertoli cell of the human testis, J Ultrastruct Res 9:459-474, 1963.
86. Paniagua R, Martín A, Nistal A et al: Testicular involution in elderly men: comparison of histologic quantitative studies with hormone patterns, Fertil Steril 47:671-679, 1987.
87. Schulze W, Schulze C: Multinucleate Sertoli cells in aged human testes, Cell Tissue Res 217:259-266, 1981.
88. Johnson L, Petty CC, Neaves WB: Influence of age on sperm production and testicular weights in men, J Reprod Fertil 70:211-218, 1984.
89. Lejeune H, Skalli M, Chatelain PG et al: The paracrine role of Sertoli cells on Leydig cell function, Cell Biol Toxicol 8:73-83, 1992.
90. Petrie RG, Morales CR: Receptor-mediated endocytosis of testicular transferrin by germinal cells of the rat testis, Cell Tissue Res 267:45-55, 1992.
91. Parvinen M, Vihko, Toppari J: Cell interactions during the seminiferous epithelial cycle, Int Rev Cytol 104:115-151, 1986.
92. Khan SA, Schmidt K, Hallin P et al: Human testis cytosol and ovarian follicular fluid contain high amounts of interleukin-1-like factor(s), Mol Cell Endocrinol 58:221-230, 1988.
93. Paniagua R, Nistal M, Amat P et al: Quantitative differences between variants of A spermatogonia in man, J Reprod Fertil 77:669-673, 1986.
94. Rowley MJ, Berlin JD, Heller CG: The ultrastructure of the four types of human spermatogonia, Z Zellforsch 112:139-157, 1971.
95. Nistal M, Codesal J, Paniagua R et al: Decrease in the number of Ap and Ad spermatogonia and the Ap/Ad ratio with advancing age, J Androl 8:64-68, 1987.
96. Paniagua R, Codesal J, Nistal M et al: Quantification of cell types throughout the cycle of the human seminiferous epithelium and their DNA content, Anat Embryol 176:225-230, 1987.
97. Schulze W: Normal and abnormal spermatogonia in the human testis, Fortschr Androl 7:33-45, 1981.
98. Nistal M, Paniagua R, Esponda E: Development of the endoplasmic reticulum during human spermatogenesis, Acta Anat 108:238-249, 1980.
99. Heller CG, Clermont Y: Kinetics of the germinal epithelium in man, Recent Prog Horm Res 20:545-571, 1964.
100. Holstein AF, Roosen-Runge EC: Atlas of human spermatogenesis, Berlin, 1981, Grosse-Verlag.

101. De Kretser DM: Ultrastructural features of human spermiogenesis, Z Zellforsch 98:477-505, 1969.
102. Fawcett DW, Anderson WA, Phillips DM: Morphogenetic factors influencing the shape of the sperm head, Dev Biol 26:220-251, 1971.
103. Fawcett DW, Phillips DM: The fine structure and development of the neck region of the mammalian spermatozoon, Anat Rec 165:153-184, 1969.
104. Bruecker H, Schafe E, Holstein AF: Morphogenesis and fate of the residual body in human spermiogenesis, Cell Tissue Res 240:303-309, 1985.
105. Chemes H: The phagocytic function of Sertoli cells. A morphological, biochemical, and endocrinological study of lysosomes and acid phosphatase localization in the rat testis, Endocrinology 119:1673-1681, 1986.
106. Clermont Y: Renewal of spermatogonia in man, Am J Anat 118:509-524, 1966.
107. Holstein AF: Ultrastructural observations on the differentiation of spermatids in man, Andrologia 8:157-165, 1976.
108. Dym M, Fawcett DW: Further observations on the numbers of spermatogonia, spermatocytes and spermatids connected by intercellular bridges in the mammalian testis, Biol Reprod 4:195-215, 1971.
109. Schulze W: Evidence of a wave of spermatogenesis in the human testis, Andrologia 14:200-207, 1982.
110. Schulze W, Reimer M, Rehder V et al: Computer aided three-dimensional reconstructions of the arrangement of primary spermatocytes in human seminiferous tubules, Cell Tissue Res 244:1-8, 1986.
111. Clermont Y: The cycle of the seminiferous epithelium in man, Am J Anat 112:35-51, 1963.
112. Bustos-Obregón E: Ultrastructure and function of the lamina propia of mammalian seminiferous tubules, Andrologia 8:179-185, 1976.
113. De Kretser DM, Kerr JB, Paulsen CA: The peritubular tissue in the normal and pathological human testis: an ultrastructural study, Biol Reprod 12:317-324, 1975.
114. Christl HW: The lamina propria of vertebrate seminiferous tubules: a comparative light and electron microscopic investigation, Andrologia 22:85-94, 1990.
115. Ross MH, Long IR: Contractile cells in human seminiferous tubules, Science 153:1271-1273, 1966.
116. Virtanen I, Kallojoki M, Narvanen O: Peritubular myoid cells of human and rat testis are smooth muscle cells that contain desmin-type intermediate filaments, Anat Rec 215:10-20, 1986.
117. De Menczes AP: Elastic tissue in the limiting membrane of the human seminiferous tubules, Am J Anat 150:349-374, 1977.
118. Miyake K, Yamamoto M, Narita H et al: Evidence for contractility of the human seminiferous tubule confirmed by its response to noradrenaline and acetylcholine, Fertil Steril 46:734-737, 1986.
119. Johnson L, Petty CS, Neves WB: Age-related variations in seminiferous tubules in men. A stereologic evaluation, J Androl 7:316-322, 1986.
120. Nelson AA: Giant interstitial cells and extraparenchimal interstitial cells of the human testis, Am J Pathol 14:831-841, 1938.
121. Okkels M, Sand K: Morphological relationship between testicular nerves and Leydig cells in man, J Endocrinol 2:38-49, 1940.
122. Schulze C: Sertoli cells and Leydig cells in man, Adv Anat Embryol Cell Biol 88:1-104, 1984.
123. Paniagua R, Amat P, Nistal M et al: Ultrastructure of Leydig cells in human ageing testes, J Anat 146:173-183, 1986.
124. Schulze W, Davidoff MS, Ivell R et al: Neuron-specific enolase-like immunoreactivity in human Leydig cells, Andrologia 23:279-283, 1991.
125. Kaler LW, Neaves WB: Attrition of the human Leydig cell population with advancing age, Anat Rec 192:513-518, 1978.
126. Kothari LK, Gupta AS: Effect of ageing on the volume, structure and total Leydig cell content of human testis, Int J Fertil 19:140-146, 1974.
127. Mori H, Hiromoto N, Nakahara M et al: Stereological analysis of Leydig cell ultrastructure in aged humans, J Clin Endocrinol Metab 55:634-641, 1982.
128. Nistal M, Santamaría L, Paniagua R et al: Multinucleate Leydig cells in normal human testes, Andrologia 18:268-272, 1986.
129. Amat P, Paniagua R, Nistal M et al: Mitosis in adult human Leydig cells, Cell Tissue Res 243:219-221, 1986.
130. Neaves WB, Johnson L, Porter JC et al: Leydig cell numbers, daily sperm production and serum gonadotropin levels in ageing men, J Clin Endocrinol Metab 55:756-763, 1984.
131. Neaves WB, Johnson L, Petty CS: Age-related change in numbers of other interstitial cells in testes of adult men: evidence on the fate of Leydig cells lost with increasing age, Biol Reprod 33:259-269, 1985.
132. Sharpe RM, Maddocks S, Millar M et al: Testosterone and spermatogenesis. Identification of stage-specific, androgen-regulated proteins secreted by adult rat seminiferous tubules, J Androl 13:172-184, 1992.
133. Parvinen M: Regulation of the semininiferous epithelium, Endocr Rev 3:404-417, 1982.
134. Paniagua R, Rodríguez MC, Nistal M et al: Changes in surface area and number of Leydig cells in relation to the 6 stages of the cycle of the human seminiferous epithelium, Anat Embryol 178:423-427, 1988.
135. Anthony CT, Rosselli M, Skinner MK: Actions of the testicular paracrine factor (P-Mod-S) on Sertoli cell transferrin secretion througout pubertal development, Endocrinology 129:353-360, 1991.
136. Norton JN, Skinner MK: Regulation of Sertoli cell function and differentiation through the actions of a testicular paracrine factor P-Mod-S, Endocrinology 124:2711-2719, 1989.
137. Skinner MK: Cell-cell interactions in the testis, Endocr Rev 12:45-77, 1991.
138. Prince FP: Ultrastructural evidence of indirect and direct autonomic innervation of human Leydig cells: comparison of neonatal, childhood and pubertal ages, Cell Tissue Res 269:383-390, 1992.
139. Nistal M, Paniagua R: Leydig cell differentiation induced by stimulation with HCG and HMG in two patients affected with hypogonadotropic hypogonadism, Andrologia 11:211-222, 1979.
140. Hutson JC: Changes in the concentration and size of testicular macrophages during development, Biol Reprod 43:885-890, 1990.

141. Maseki Y, Mikaye K, Mitsuya H et al: Mastocytosis occurring in testes from patients with idiopathic male infertility, Fertil Steril 36:814-817, 1981.
142. Jarow JP, Ogle A, Kaspar J et al: Testicular artery ramification within the inguinal canal, J Urol 147:1290-1292, 1992.
143. Kormano M, Suoranta H: Microvascular organization of the adult human testes, Anat Rec 170:31-40, 171.
144. Suoranta M: Changes in the small blood vessels of the adult human testis in relation to age and to some pathological conditions, Virchows Arch A Pathol Anat Histopathol 352:165-181, 1971.
145. Takayama H, Tomoyoshi T: Microvascular architecture of rat and human testes, Invest Urol 18:341-344, 1981.
146. Suzuki F, Nagano T: Microvasculature of the human testis and excurrent duct system. Resin-casting and scanning electron-microscopic studies, Cell Tissue Res 243:79-89, 1986.
147. Holstein AF, Orlandini GE, Moller R: Distribution and fine structure of the lymphatic system in the human testis, Cell Tissue Res 200:15-27, 1979.
148. Nistal M, Paniagua R, Aburrea MA: Varicose axons bearing "synaptic" vesicles on the basal lamina of the human seminiferous tubules, Cell Tissue Res 226:75-82, 1982.
149. Jonte G, Holstein AF: On the morphology of the transitional zones from the rete testis into the ductuli efferentes and from the ductuli efferentes into the ductus epididymidis, investigations on the human testis and epididymis, Andrologia 19:398-412, 1978.
150. Dinges HP, Zatloukal K, Schmid C et al: Co-expression of cytokeratin and vimentin filaments in rete testis and epididymis. An immunohistochemical study, Virchows Archiv A Pathol Anat Histopathol 418:119-127, 1991.
151. Kogan SJ: Cryptorchidism. In Kelalis PP, King LR, Belman AB, eds: Clinical pediatric urology, ed 2, vol 2, Philadelphia, 1985, WB Saunders.
152. Oesch I, Ransley PG: Unilaterally impalpable testis, Eur Urol 13:324-325, 1987.
153. Levitt SB, Kogan SJ, Schnider KM et al: Endocrine tests in phenotypic children with bilateral impalpable testes can reliably predict "congenital" anorchism, Urology 11:11-17, 1978.
154. Aynsley-Green A, Zachman M, Illig R et al: Congenital bilateral anorchia in childhood: a clinical, endocrine, and therapeutic evaluation of twenty-one cases, Clin Endocrinol 5:381-391, 1976.
155. Rivarola MA, Bergada C, Cullen M: HCG stimulation test in prepubertal boys with cryptorchidism, in bilateral anorchia, and in male pseudohermaphroditism, J Clin Endocrinol Metab 31:526-530, 1970.
156. Jarow JP, Berkovitz GD, Migeon CJ et al: Elevation of serum gonadotropins establishes the diagnosis of anorchism in prepubertal boys with bilateral cryptorchidism, J Urol 136:277-279, 1986.
157. Koff SA: Does compensatory testicular enlargement predict monorchism? J Urol 146:632-633, 1991.
158. Huff DS, Snyder HM, Hadziselimovic F et al: An absent testis is associated with contralateral testicular hypertrophy, J Urol 148:627-628, 1992.
159. Brothers LR, Weber CH, Ball TP: Anorchism versus cryptorchidism; the importance of a diligent search for intraabdominal testes, J Urol 119:207-209, 1971.
160. Plotzker ED, Rushton HG, Belman AB et al: Laparoscopy for nonpalpable testes in childhood: is inguinal exploration also necessary when vas and vessels exit the inguinal ring? J Urol 148:635-638, 1992.
161. Edman CD, Winter AJ, Porter JC et al: Embryonic testicular regression: a clinical spectrum of XY agonadal individuals, Obstet Gynecol 2:208-217, 1977.
162. Coulam CB: Testicular regression syndrome, Obstet Gynecol 53:44-49, 1979.
163. Wright JE: The "atrophic" testicular remnant, Pediatr Surg Int 1:229-231, 1986.
164. Bergada C, Cleveland WW, Jones HW Jr et al: Variants of embryonic testicular dysgenesis: bilateral anorchia and the syndrome of rudimentary testes, Acta Endocrinol 40:521-536, 1962.
165. Najjar SS, Takla RJ, Nassar VH: The syndrome of rudimentary testes: occurrence in live siblings, J Pediatr 84:119-122, 1974.
166. Glass AR: Identical twins discordant for the "rudimentary testes" syndrome, J Urol 127:140-141, 1982.
167. Acquafredda A, Vassal J, Job JC: Rudimentary testes syndrome revisited, Paediatrics 2:209-214, 1987.
168. Tosi SE, Morin LS: The vanishing testis syndrome. Indications for conservative therapy, J Urol 115:758, 1976.
169. Sparnon A, Guiney EJ, Puri P: The vanishing testis, Pediatr Surg Int 1:227-228, 1986.
170. Abeyaratne MR, Aherne WA, Scott JES: The vanishing testis, Lancet 2:822-824, 1969.
171. Simpson JL, Horwith M, Morrillo-Cucci G: Bilateral anorchia: discordance in monozygotic twins, Birth Defects 7:196-200, 1971.
172. Amelar RD: Anorchism without eunochoidism, J Urol 76:174, 1956.
173. Honoré M: Unilateral anorchism. Report of 11 cases with discussion of etiology and pathogenesis, Urology 11:251-254, 1978.
174. Nistal M, Paniagua R, Regadera J et al: Hyperplasia of spermatic cord nerves: a sign of testicular absence, Urology 29:411-415, 1987.
175. Salle B, Hedinger C, Nicole R: Significance of testicular biopsies in cryptorchidism in children, Acta Endocrinol 58:67-76, 1968.
176. Kogan SJ, Gill B, Bennett B et al: Human monorchism: a clinicopathological study of unilateral absent testes in 65 boys, J Urol 135:758-761, 1986.
177. Smith NM, Byard RW, Bourne AJ: Testicular regression syndrome, a pathological study of 77 cases, Histopathology 19:269-272, 1991.
178. Das S, Amar AD: Ureteral ectopia into cystic seminal vesicle with ipsilateral renal dysgenesis and monorchia, J Urol 124:574-575, 1980.
179. Matsuoka LY, Wortsman J, McConnachie P: Renal and testicular agenesis in a patient with Darier's disease, Am J Med 78:873-877, 1985.
180. Thum G: Polyorchidism: case report and review of literature, J Urol 145:370-372, 1991.
181. Ahlfeld F: Die Missbildungen des Menschen, Leipzig, 1880, Grunow.
182. Lane WA: A case of supernumerary testis, Trans Clin Soc Lond 28:59-60, 1895.

183. Baker LL, Hajek PC, Burkhard TK et al: Polyorchidism: evaluation by MR, AJR Am J Roentgenol 148:305-307, 1987.
184. Singh A, Sobti MK: Polyorchidism, Br J Urol 61:458-459, 1988.
185. Snow BW, Tarry WF, Duckett JW: Polyorchidism: an unusual case, J Urol 133:483-484, 1985.
186. Day GH: One man with five testes: report of case, JAMA 71:2055-2057, 1918.
187. Hakami M, Mosavy SH: Triorchidism with normal spermatogenesis: an unusual cause for failure of vasectomy, Br J Surg 62:633, 1975.
188. Giyanani VL, McCarthy J, Venable DD et al: Ultrasound of polyorchidism: case report and literature review, J Urol 138:863-864, 1987.
189. Hancock RA, Hodgins TE: Polyorchidism, Urology 24:303-307, 1984.
190. Pelander WM, Luna G, Lilly JR: Polyorchidism: case report and literature review, J Urol 119:705-706, 1978.
191. Gandia VM, Arrizabalaga M, Leiva O et al: Polyorchidism discovered as testicular torsion associated with undescended atrophic contralateral testis. A surgical solution, J Urol 137:743-744, 1987.
192. Verdú TF, Pérez-Bustamante I, Jiménez CM: Poliorquia. Revisión y aportación de un nuevo caso, Actas Urol Esp 10:277-278, 1986.
193. Feldman S, Drach GW: Polyorchidism discovered as testicular torsion, J Urol 130:976-977, 1983.
194. Khan C: Polyorchidism with normal spermatogenesis, Br J Urol 61:100-103, 1988.
195. Smart RH: Polyorchidism with normal spermatogenesis, J Urol 107:278, 1972.
196. Nocks BN: Polyorchidism with normal spermatogenesis and equal sized testes. A theory of embryonal development, J Urol 120:638-640, 1978.
197. Garat JM, Marina S, Sole-Balcells F et al: Polyorchidie, J d'Urologie, 87:175-176, 1981.
198. Mallafre JM, Janeiro MR, Corominas S et al: Testiculo supernumerario. Comunicación de un caso y revisión de la literatura, Arch Esp Urol 42:166-168, 1989.
199. Al-Hibbal Z, Izzidien AY: Polyorchidism: case report and review of the literature, J Pediatr Surg 19:212-214, 1984.
200. Darrow RP, Humes JJ: Polyorchidism: a case report, J Urol 72:53-54, 1954.
201. Thiessen NW: Polyorchidism: report of a case, J Urol 49:710-711, 1943.
202. Nistal M, Paniagua R, Martín-Lopez R: Polyorchidism in a newborn: case report and review of the literature, Pediatr Pathol 10:601-607, 1990.
203. Grechi G, Zampi GC, Selli C et al: Polyorchidism and seminoma in a child, J Urol 123:291-292, 1980.
204. Scott KW: A case of polyorchidism with testicular teratoma, J Urol 124:930-932, 1980.
205. Takihara H, Consentino MJ, Sakatoku J et al: Significance of testicular size measurement in andrology. II. Correlation of testicular size with testicular function, J Urol 137:416-418, 1987.
206. Huff DS, Wu HY, Snyder H et al: Evidence in favor of the mechanical (intrauterine torsion) theory over the endocrinopathy (cryptorchidism) theory in the pathogenesis of testicular agenesis, J Urol 146:630-631, 1991.
207. Laron Z, Zilka E: Compensatory hypertrophy of testicle in unilateral cnyptorchidism, J Clin Endocrinol Metab 29:1409-1413, 1969.
208. Laron Z, Dickerman Z, Prager-Lewin R et al: Plasma LH and FSH response to LRH in boys with compensatory testicular hypertrophy, J Clin Endocrinol Metab 40:977-981, 1975.
209. Laron Z, Dickerman Z, Ritterman I et al: Follow up of boys with unilateral compensatory testicular hypertrophy, Fertil Steril 33:297-300, 1980.
210. Zachman M, Prader A, Kind HP et al: Testicular volume during adolescence, Helv Paediatr Acta 29:61-72, 1974.
211. Lee PA, Marshall FF, Greco JM et al: Unilateral testicular hypertrophy: an apparently benign occurrence without cryptorchidism, J Urol 127:329-331, 1982.
212. Nisula BC, Loriaux DL, Sherins RJ et al: Benign bilateral testicular enlargement, J Clin Endocrinol Metab 38:440-445, 1974.
213. Breen DH, Braunstein GD, Neufeld N et al: Benign macroorchidism in a pubescent boy, J Urol 125:589-591, 1981.
214. Truwit CHL, Jackson M, Thompson IM: Idiopathic macroorchidism, J Clin Ultrasound 17:200-205, 1989.
215. Nistal M, Martínez-García F, Regadera J et al: Macroorchidism: light and electron microscopic study of four cases, Hum Pathol 23:1011-1018, 1992.
216. Lubs HA: A marker X chromosome, Am J Hum Genet 21:231-234, 1969.
217. Martin JP, Bell J: A pedigree of mental defect showing sex-linkage, J Neurol Psychiatr 6:154-157, 1943.
218. Turner G, Daniel A, Frost M: X-linked mental retardation, macroorchidism, and the X_q 27 fragile site, J Pediatr 96:837-841, 1980.
219. Turner G, Eastman C, Casey J et al: X-linked mental retardation associated with macroorchidism, J Med Genet 12:367-371, 1975.
220. Cantú JM, Scaglia HE, González-Didi M et al: Inherited congenital normofunctional testicular hyperplasia and mental deficiency. A corroborative study, Hum Genet 12:367-371, 1975.
221. Ruvalcaba RHA, Myhre SA, Roosen-Runge EC et al: X-linked mental deficiency megalotestes syndrome, JAMA 238:1646-1650, 1977.
222. Sutherland GR, Ashforth PLC: X-linked mental retardation with macroorchidism and the fragile site at X_q 27 or 28, Hum Genet 48:117-120, 1979.
223. Howard-Peebles PN, Stoddard GR: Familial-X-linked mental retardation with a marker X chromosome and its relationship to macroorchidism, Clin Genet 17:125-128, 1980.
224. Hecht JT, Moore CM, Scott CI: A recognizable syndrome of sex-linked mental retardation, large testes and marker X chromosome, South Med J 74:1493-1495, 1981.
225. Sutherland GR: The fragile X chromosome, Int Rev Cytol 81:107-143, 1983.
226. Berkowitz GD, Wilson DP, Carpenter NJ et al: Gonadal function in men with the Martin-Bell (fragile X) syndrome, Am J Med Genet 23:227-239, 1986.
227. Johannisson R, Rehder H, Wendt V et al: Spermatogenesis in two patients with the fragile X syndrome. I. Histology: light and electron microscopy, Hum Genet 76:141-147, 1987.

228. Johannisson R, Froster-Iskenius U, Saadallah N et al: Spermatogenesis in two patients with the fragile X syndrome, Hum Genet 79:231-234, 1988.
229. Gerald PS: X-linked mental retardation and an X-chromosome marker, N Engl J Med 303:696-697, 1980.
230. Webb TP, Bundey SE, Thake AI et al: Population incidence and segregation ratios in Martin-Bell syndrome, Am J Hum Genet 23:573-580, 1986.
231. Vuelckel MA, Philip N, Piquet C et al: Study of a family with a fragile site on the X chromosome at Xq 27-28 without mental retardation, Hum Genet 81:353-357, 1989.
232. Rudelli RD, Jenkins EC, Wisniewscki K et al: Testicular size in fetal fragile X syndrome, Lancet 1:1221-1222, 1983.
233. Wierman ME, Beardsworth DE, Mansfield MJ: Puberty without gonadotropins: a unique mechanism of sexual development, N Engl J Med 312:65-72, 1985.
234. Rosenthal SM, Grumbach MM, Kaplan SL: Gonadotropin-independent familial sexual precocity with premature Leydig and germinal cell maturation (familial testotoxicosis): effects of a patent luteinizing hormone-releasing factor agonist and metroxyprogesterone acetate therapy in four cases, J Clin Endocrinol Metab 57:571-579, 1983.
235. Gondos B, Egli CA, Rosenthal SM et al: Testicular changes in gonadotropin-independent familial male sexual precocity. Familial testotoxicosis, Arch Pathol Lab Med 109:990-995, 1985.
236. Giovannelli G, Bernasconi S, Banchini G: McCune-Albright syndrome in a male child: a clinical and endocrinologic enigma, J Pediatr 92:220-226, 1978.
237. Heseltine D, White MC, Kendall-Taylor P et al: Testicular enlargement and elevated serum inhibin concentrations occurs in patients with pituitary macroadenomas secreting follicle stimulating hormone, Clin Endocrinol 31:411-423, 1989.
238. Cordero GL, Gracia R, Nistal M et al: Hipotiroidismo y maduración testicular precoz, Rev Clin Esp 128:83-88, 1973.
239. Drago JR, Olstein JS, Tesluk H et al: Virilizing adrenal cortical carcinoma with hypertrophy of spermatic tubules in childhood, Urology 14:70-75, 1979.
240. Nistal M, González-Peramato P, Paniagua R: Congenital Leydig cell hyperplasia, Histopathology 12:307-317, 1988.
241. Campbell MF: Anomalies of the testicle. In Campbell MF, Harrisson JH eds: Urology, ed 3, Philadelphia, 1986, WB Saunders.
242. Dieckmann KP, Düe W, Fiedler U: Perineale Hodenektopie, Urologe [A] 27:358-362, 1988.
243. Murphy DM, Butler MR: Preperitoneal ectopic testis: a case report, J Pediatr Surg 20:93-94, 1985.
244. Paramo PG, Nacarino L, Polo G: Ectopia epidídimo-perineal, Arch Esp Urol 24:61-63, 1971.
245. Tramoyeres A, Esteve J, Fernández A et al: Testículo ectópico perineal, Arch Esp Urol 33:357, 1980.
246. Wattenberg CA, Rape MG, Beare JB: Perineal testicle, J Urol 62:858-861, 1949.
247. Doraiswamy NV: Crossed ectopic testis. Case report and review, Z Kinder Chir 38:264-268, 1983.
248. Fujita J: Transverse testicular ectopia, Urology 16:400-402, 1980.
249. Miura T, Takahashi G: Crossed ectopic testis with common vas deferens, J Urol 134:1206-1208, 1985.
250. Gornall PG, Pender DJ: Crossed testicular ectopia detected by laparoscopy, Br J Urol 59:283, 1987.
251. Peters JH, Sing S: Transverse testicular ectopia: a case report, Del Med J 59:333-335, 1987.
252. Beasley SW, Auldist AW: Crossed testicular ectopia in association with double incomplete testicular descent, Aust N Z J Surg 55:301-303, 1985.
253. Dogruyol H, Özcan M, Balkan E: Two rare genital abnormalities: crossed testicular and scroto-testicular ectopia, Br J Urol 70:201-203, 1992.
254. Middleton GW, Beamon CR, Gillenwater JY: Two rare cases of ectopic testes, J Urol 115:445-446, 1976.
255. Heyns CF: Exstrophy of the testis, J Urol 144:724-725, 1990.
256. Leissring JC, Oppenheimer ROF: Cystic dysplasia of the testis: a unique anomaly studied by microdissection, J Urol 110:362-363, 1973.
257. Cho CS, Kosek J: Cystic dysplasia of the testis: sonographic and pathologic findings, Radiology 156:777-778, 1985.
258. Roosen-Runge EC, Holstein AF: The human rete testis, Cell Tissue Res 189:409-433, 1978.
259. Bustos-Obregón E, Holstein AF: The rete testis in man: ultrastructural aspects, Cell Tissue Res 175:1-15, 1976.
260. Dym M: The mammalian rete testis. A morphological examination, Anat Rec 186:493-524, 1976.
261. Nistal M, Regadera J, Paniagua R: Cystic dysplasia of the testis: light and electron microscopic study of three cases, Arch Pathol Lab Med 108:579-583, 1984.
262. Fischer JE, Jewett TC, Nelson ST et al: Ectasia of the rete testis with ipsilateral renal agenesis, J Urol 128:1040-1043, 1982.
263. Glantz L, Hansen K, Caldamone A et al: Cystic dysplasia of the testis, Hum Pathol 24:1141-1145, 1993.
264. Tesluk H, Blankenberg TA: Cystic dysplasia of testis, Urology 29:47-49, 1987.
265. Tuck RR, Setchell BP, Waites GMH et al: The composition of fluid collected by micropuncture and catheterization from the seminiferous tubules and rete testis of rats, Eur J Physiol 318:225-243, 1970.
266. Siller WG, Deward WA, Whitehead CC: Cystic dilatation of the seminiferous tubules in the fowl: a sequel of sodium intoxication, J Pathol 107:191-197, 1972.
267. Nistal M, Paniagua R, Bravo MP: Testicular lymphangiectasis in Noonan's syndrome, J Urol 131:759-761, 1984.
268. Nistal M, García-Rojo M, Paniagua R: Congenital testicular lymphangiectasis in children with otherwise normal testes, Histopathology 17:335-338, 1990.
269. Ostroverkhova VG: Macro-microscopischeskoe issledovanie vnutriorgannoi limfaticheskoi sistemy muzhskoi polovoi zhelezy (Macro-microscopic study of intraorgan lymphatic system of male gonad in man), Arch Anat Gist Embriol 39:59-65, 1960.
270. Holstein AF, Orlandini GE, Moeller R: Distribution and fine structure of the lymphatic system in the human testis, Cell Tissue Res 200:15-20, 1979.
271. Fawcett DW, Heidger PM, Leak V: Lymph vascular system of the interstitial tissue of the testis as revealed by electron microscopy, J Reprod Fertil 19:109-119, 1969.
272. Nistal M, Paniagua R, León L, Regadera J: Ectopic seminiferous tubules in the tunica albuginea of normal and dysgenetic testes, Appl Pathol 3:123-128, 1985.

273. Schmidt SS, Minckler TM: Pseudocysts of the tunica albuginea: benign invasion by testicular tubules, J Urol 138:151, 1987.
274. Nistal M, Paniagua R: Development of the testis from birth to puberty. In Nistal M, Paniagua R, eds: Testicular and epididymal pathology, New York, 1984, Thieme-Stratton.
275. Okkels H, Sand K: Morphological relationship between testicular nerves and Leydig cells in man, J Endocrinol 2:38-46, 1940.
276. Regadera J, Cobo P, Martínez-García C et al: Testosterone immunoexpression in human Leydig cells of the tunica albuginea testis and spermatic cord. A quantitative study in normal fetuses, young adults, elderly men and patients with cryptorchidism, Andrologia 25:115-122, 1993.
277. Nelson AA: Giant interstitial cells and extraparenchymal interstitial cells of the human testis, Am J Pathol 14:831-841, 1938.
278. Halley JBW: The infiltrative activity of Leydig cells, J Pathol Bact 81:347-353, 1961.
279. Halley JBW: Relation of Leydig cells in the human testicle to the tubules and testicular function, Nature 185:865-866, 1960.
280. McDonald JH, Calams JA: A histological study of extraparenchymal Leydig-like cells, J Urol 79:850-858, 1958.
281. Berbingler H: Über die Zwischenzellen des Hodens, Verh D Path Ges 18:186-197, 1921.
282. Brack E: Zur pathologischen Anatomie der Leydig Zelle, Virchows Arch Path Anat Physiol 240:127-143, 1923.
283. Schulze C, Holstein AF: Leydig cells within the lamina propria of seminiferous tubules in four patients with azoospermia, Andrologia 10:444-452, 1978.
284. Mori H, Shiraishi T, Matsumoto K: Ectopic Leydig cells in seminiferous tubules of an infertile human male with a chromosomal aberration, Andrologia 10:434-443, 1978.
285. Mori H, Tamai M, Fushimi H et al: Leydig cells within the spermatogenic seminiferous tubules, Hum Pathol 18:1227-1231, 1987.
286. Regadera J, Codesal J, Paniagua R et al: Immunohistochemical and quantitative study of interstitial and intratubular Leydig cells in normal men, cryptorchidism, and Klinefelter's syndrome, J Pathol 164:299-306, 1991.
287. Priesel A: Über das Verhalten von Hoden und Nebenhoden bei angeborenem Fehlen des Ductus deferens, zugleich zur Frage des Vorkommens von Zwischenzellen in menschliche Nebenhoden, Virchows Arch Path Anat Physiol 249:246-304, 1924.
288. Berger L: Sur l'existence de glands sympathicotropes dans l'ovaire et le testicule humains; leur rapport avec la glande interstitielle du testicule, Compt Rend Acad Sci París 175:907-909, 1922.
289. Peters KH: Zur Ultrastrusktur der Leydigzellen im Funiculus spermaticus des Menschen, Verh Anat Ges 71:555-559, 1977.
290. Nistal M, Paniagua R: Histogenesis of human extraparenchymal Leydig cells, Acta Anat 105:188-197, 1979.
291. Schiffer KA, Kogan SJ, Reda EF et al: Acquired undescended testis, AJDC 141:106-107, 1987.
292. Cendron M, Huff DS, Keating MA et al: Anatomical, morphological and volumetric analysis: a review of 759 cases of testicular maldescent, J Urol 149:570-573, 1993.
293. Huff DS, Hadziselimovic F, Snyder HMC et al: Early postnatal testicular maldevelopment in cryptorchidism, J Urol 146:624-626, 1991.
294. Kogan S, Tennenbaum S, Gill B et al: Efficacy of orchiopexy by patient age 1 year for cryptorchidism, J Urol 144:508-509, 1990.
295. Thorup J, Cortes D, Nielsen H: Clinical and histopathologic evaluation of operated maldescended testes after luteinizing hormone-releasing hormone treatment, Pediatr Surg Int 8:419-422, 1993.
296. Farrington GH: Histologic observations in cryptorchidism: the congenital germinal-cell deficiency of the undescended testis, J Pediatr Surg 4:606-613, 1969.
297. Nistal M, Paniagua R, Díez-Pardo JA: Histologic classification of undescended testes, Hum Pathol 11:666-673, 1980.
298. Codesal J, Paniagua R, Queizán A et al: Cytophotometric DNA quantification in human spermatogonia of cryptorchid testes, J Urol 149:382-385, 1993.
299. Christiansen P, Müller J, Buhl S et al: Hormonal treatment of cryptorchidism—hCG or GnRH—a multicentre study, Acta Paediatr 81:605-608, 1992.
300. Bica DTG, Hadsizelimovic F: Busereline treatment of cryptorchidism: a randomized, double-blind, placebo-controlled study, J Urol 148:617-621, 1992.
301. Paniagua R, Martínez-Onsurbe P, Santamaría L et al: Quantitative and ultrastructural alterations in the lamina propria and Sertoli cells in human cryptorchid testes, Int J Androl 13:470-487, 1990.
302. Karpe B, Plöen L, Hagenäs L et al: Recovery of testicular functions after surgical treatment of experimental cryptorchidism in the rat, Int J Androl 4:145-160, 1981.
303. Gotoh M, Miyake K, Mitsuya H: Elastic fibers in tunica propria of undescended and contralateral scrotal testes from cryptorchid patients, Urology 30:359-363, 1987.
304. Nistal M, Paniagua R, Queizán A: Histologic lesions in undescended ectopic obstructed testes, Fertil Steril 43:455-462, 1985.
305. Herzog B, Steigert M, Hadziselimovic F: Is a testis located at the superficial inguinal pouch (Denis Browne pouch) comparable to a true cryptorchid testis? J Urol 148:622-623, 1992.
306. Ito H, Katauni Z, Kuwamura K et al: Changes in the volume and histology of retractile testes in prepubertal boys, Int J Androl 9:161-169, 1986.
307. Nistal M, Paniagua R: Infertility in adult males with retractile testes, Fertil Steril 41:395-403, 1984.
308. Wyllie GW: The retractile testis, Med J Aust 140:403-405, 1984.
309. Puri P, Nixon HH: Bilateral retractile testes—subsequent effects on fertility, J Pediatr Surg 12:563-566, 1967.
310. Rasmussen TB, Ingerslev HJ, Hostrup H: Natural history of the maldescended testis, Horm Res 30:164-166, 1988.
311. Elder JS: Epididymal anomalies associated with hydrocele/hernia and cryptorchidism: implications regarding testicular descent, J Urol 148:624-626, 1992.
312. Scorer CG, Farrington GH: Congenital deformities of the testis and epididymis, New York, 1971, Appleton-Century-Crofts.
313. Mollaeian M, Mehrabi V, Elahi V: Significance of epididymal and ductal anomalies associated with undescended testis, Urology 43:857-860, 1994.

314. Abrat RP, Reddi VB, Sarembock LA: Testicular cancer and cryptorchidism, Br J Urol 70:656-659, 1992.
315. Giwercman A, Müller J, Skakkebaek NE: Cryptorchidism and testicular neoplasia, Horm Res 30:157-163, 1988.
316. Larizza C, Antiba A, Palazzi J et al: Testicular maldescent and infertility, Andrologia 22:285-288, 1990.
317. Cortes D, Thorup J: Histology of testicular biopsies taken at operation for bilateral maldescended testes in relation to fertility in adulthood, Br J Urol 68:285-291, 1991.
318. Puri P, O'Donnell B: Semen analysis in patients operated on for impalpable testes, Br J Urol 66:646-647, 1990.
319. Kogan SJ: Fertility in cryptorchidism: an overview in 1987, Eur J Pediatr 146(suppl 2):S21, 1987.
320. Okuyama A, Nonomure N, Nakamura M et al: Surgical management of undescended testis: retrospective study of potential fertility in 274 cases, J Urol 142:749-751, 1989.
321. Cendron M, Keating MA, Huff DS et al: Cryptorchidism, orchiopexy and infertility: a critical long-term retrospective analysis, J Urol 142:559-562, 1989.
322. Pedersen KV, Boisen P, Zetterlund CG: Experience of screening for carcinoma-in-situ of the testis among young men with surgically corrected maldescended testes, Int J Androl 10:181-185, 1987.
323. Berthelsen JG, Skakkebaek NE: Distribution of carcinoma-in-situ in testes from infertile men, Int J Androl Suppl 4:172-184, 1981.
324. Giwercman A, Clausen OPF, Skakkebaek NE: Carcinoma-in-situ of the testis: aneuploid cells in semen, Br Med J 296:1762-1764, 1988.
325. Giwercman A, Müller J, Skakkebaek NE: Cryptorchidism and testicular neoplasia, Horm Res 30:157-163, 1988.
326. Smith SW, Brammer HM, Henry M et al: Testicular microlithiasis: sonographic features with pathologic correlation, AJR Am J Roentgenol 157:1003-1004, 1991.
327. Sasagawa I, Nakada T, Kazama T et al: Testicular microlithiasis in male infertility, Urol Int 43:368-369, 1988.
328. Priebe CJ, Garret R: Testicular calcification in a 4-year-old boy, Pediatrics 46:785-789, 1970.
329. Nistal M, Martínez-García C, Paniagua R: The origin of testicular microliths, Int J Urol 18:221-229, 1995.
330. Coetzee T: Pulmonary alveolar microlithiasis with involvement of the sympathetic nervous system and gonads, Thorax 25:637-642, 1970.
331. Schipper JA, Delemarre- VD, Waal HA et al: Testicular dysgenesis and mental retardation in two incompletely masculinized XY-siblings, Acta Paediatr Scand 80:125-128, 1991.
332. Hoffman RP, Steele MW, Lee PA et al: 46 XY siblings with inadequate virilization and CNS deficiency, Horm Res 29:207-210, 1988.
333. Haning RV Jr, Chesney RW, Moorthy AV et al: A syndrome of chronic renal failure and XY gonadal dysgenesis in young phenotypic females without genital ambiguity, Am J Kidney Dis 6:40-48, 1985.
334. Harkins PG, Haning RV Jr, Shapiro SS: Renal failure with XY gonadal dysgenesis: report of the second case, Obstet Gynecol 56:751-752, 1980.
335. Vilain E, Jaubert F, Fellous M et al: Pathology of 46,XY pure gonadal dysgenesis: absence of testis differentiation associated with mutations in the testis-determining factor, Differentiation 52:151-159, 1993.
336. De la Chapelle A: The Y-chromosomal and autosomal testis-determining genes, Development Suppl 101:33-38, 1987.
337. Behzadian MA, Tho SP, McDonough PG: The presence of the testicular determining sequence, SRY, in 46, XY females with gonadal dysgenesis (Swyer syndrome), Am J Obstet Gynecol 165:1887-1890, 1991.
338. Jager RJ, Anvret M, Hall K et al: A human XY female with a frame shift mutation in the candidate testis determining gene SRY, Nature 348:452-454, 1990.
339. Brosnan PG, Lewandowski RC, Toguri AG et al: A new familial syndrome of 46 XY gonadal dysgenesis with anomalies of ectodermal and mesodermal structures, J Pediatr 97:586-590, 1980.
340. Sternberg WH, Barclay DL, Klopfer HW: Familial XY gonadal dysgenesis, N Engl J Med 278:695-700, 1968.
341. Chemke J, Carmichael R, Stewart JM et al: Familial XY gonadal dysgenesis, J Med Genet 7:105-111, 1970.
342. Simpson JL, Blagowidow N, Martin AO: XY gonadal dysgenesis: genetic heterogeneity based upon clinical observations, H-Y antigen status and segregations analysis, Hum Genet 58:91-97, 1981.
343. Mann JR, Corkery JJ, Fisher HJW et al: The X linked recessive form of XY gonadal dysgenesis with high incidence of gonadal cell tumors: clinical and genetic studies, J Med Genet 20:264-270, 1983.
344. Simpson JL, Photopulos G: The relationship of neoplasia to disorders of abnormal sexual diferentiation, Birth Defects 12:15-50, 1976.
345. Portuondo JA, Neyro JL, Benito JA et al: Familial 46, XX gonadal dysgenesis, Int J Fertil 32:56-58, 1987.
346. Aaronson IA: True hermaphoditism. A review of 41 cases with observations on testicular histology and function, Br J Urol 57:775-779, 1985.
347. Nichter LS: Seminoma in a 46 XX true hermaphrodite with positive H-Y antigen. A case report, Cancer 53:1181-1184, 1984.
348. Toublanc JE, Boucekkine C, Abbas N et al: Hormonal and molecular genetic findings in 46, XX subjects with sexual ambiguity and testicular differentiation, Eur J Pediatr 152(suppl2):S70-S75, 1993.
349. Greenfield SP: Familial 46XX males coexisting with familial 46,XX true hermaphrodites in same pedigree, J Pediatr 110:244-248, 1987.
350. Nihoul-Fekete C, Lortat-Jacob S, Cachin O et al: Preservation of gonadal function in true hermaphroditism, J Pediatr Surg 19:50-55, 1984.
351. Prader A, Gurtner HP: Das syndrom des Pseudohermaphroditismus masculinus bei kongenitaler Nebennierensiden-Hyperplasie ohne Androgenüberproduktion, Helvet Pediatr Acta 10:397-412, 1955.
352. Kirkland RT, Kirkland JL, Johnson CM et al: Congenital lipoid adrenal hyperplasia in an eight-year-old phenotype female, J Clin Endocrinol 36:488-496, 1973.
353. Bongiovanni AM: Unusual steroid pattern in congenital adrenal hyperplasia: deficiency of 3 beta-hydroxysteroiddehydrogenase, J Clin Endocrinol 21:860-862, 1961.
354. Parks GA, Bermudez JA, Anast CS et al: Pubertal boy with the 3 beta-hydroxysteroiddehydrogenase defect, J Clin Endocrinol 33:269-278, 1971.

355. Biglieri EG, Herron MA, Brust N: 17 alpha-hydroxylation deficiency in man, J Clin Invest 45:1946-1954, 1966.
356. Sabage MO, Chausain JL, Evain D et al: Endocrine studies in male pseudohermaphroditism in childhood and adolescence, Clin Endocrinol 8:219-231, 1978.
357. Zachmann M, Vollman JA, Hamilton W et al: Steroid 17,20 desmolase deficiency, Clin Endocrinol 1:369-385, 1972.
358. Goebelsmann U, Davajan V, Isreal R et al: Male pseudohermaphroditism consistent with 17-20 desmolase deficiency, Gynecol Invest 5:60-64, 1974.
359. Millan M, Audi L, Martínez-Mora J et al: 17 ketosteroid reductase deficiency in an adult patient without gynecomastia but with female psychosexual orientation, Acta Endocrinol 102:633-640, 1983.
360. Dumic M, Plavsic V, Fattorini I et al: Absent spermatogenesis despite early bilateral orchidopexy in 17-ketoreductase deficiency, Horm Res 22:100-106, 1985.
361. Berthezene F, Forest MG, Grimaud JA et al: Leydig-cell agenesis. A cause of male pseudohermaphroditism, N Engl J Med 295:969-972, 1976.
362. Brown DM, Markland C, Dehner LP: Leydig cell hypoplasia: a cause of male pseudohermaphroditism, J Clin Endocrinol Metab 46:1-7, 1978.
363. Eil C, Austin RM, Sesterhenn I et al: Leydig cell hypoplasia causing male pseudohermaphroditism: diagnosis 13 years after prepubertal castration, J Clin Endocrinol Metab 58:441-448, 1984.
364. Lee PA, Rock JA, Brown TR et al: Leydig cell hypofunction resulting in male pseudohermaphroditism, Fertil Steril 37:675-679, 1982.
365. Park IJ, Burnett LS, Jones HW et al: A case of male pseudohemaphroditism associated with elevated LH, normal FSH and low testosterone possibly due to the secretion of an abnormal LH molecule, Acta Endocrinol 83:173-181, 1976.
366. Wilson JD, Harrod MJ, Goldstein JL et al: Familial incomplete male pseudohermaphroditism, type I. Evidence for androgen resistance and variable clinical manifestations in a family with the Reifenstein syndrome, N Engl J Med 290:1097-1103, 1974.
367. Griffin JE, Durrant JL: Quantitative receptor defects in families with androgen resistance; failure of stabilization of the fibroblast cytosol androgen receptor, J Clin Endocrinol Metab 55:465-474, 1982.
368. Pérez-Palacios G, Scaglia HE, Kofman-Alpharo S et al: Inherited male pseudohermaphroditism due to gonadotropin unresponsiveness, Acta Endocrinol 98:148-155, 1981.
369. Saldanha PH, Arnhold IJP, Mendonça BB et al: A clinicogenetic investigation of Leydig cell hypoplasia, Am J Med Genet 26:337-344, 1987.
370. Toledo SPA, Arnhold IJP, Luthold W et al: Leydig cell hypoplasia determining familial hypergonadotropic hypogonadism. In Papadatos CJ, Bartsocas CS, eds: Endocrine genetics and genetics of growth. Progress in clinical and biological research, vol 200, New York, 1985, Alan R Liss.
371. Arnhold IJP, Mendonça BB, Bloise W et al: Male pseudohermaphroditism resulting from Leydig cell hypoplasia, J Pediatr 106:1057-1060, 1985.
372. Morris JM: The syndrome of testicular feminization in male pseudohermaphrodites, Am J Obstet Gynecol 65:1192-1211, 1953.
373. Schulster A, Ross L, Scommegna A: Frequency of androgen insensitivity in infertile phenotypically normal men, J Urol 130:699-701, 1983.
374. Rutgers JL, Scully RE: The androgen insensitivity syndrome (testicular feminization). A clinicopathologic study of 43 cases, Int J Gynecol Pathol 10:126-145, 1991.
375. Gerli M, Migliorini G, Bocchini V et al: A case of complete testicular feminization and 47 XXY karyotype, J Med Genet 16:480-483, 1879.
376. Müller J: Morphometry and histology of gonads from twelve children and adolescents with the androgen insensitivity (testicular feminization) syndrome, J Clin Endocrinol Metab 59:485-789, 1984.
377. Müller J, Skakkebaek NE: Testicular carcinoma in situ in children with the androgen insensitivity (testicular feminization) syndrome, Br Med J 288:1419-1420, 1984.
378. Nistal M, De la Roza C, Cano J: Síndrome de feminización testicular completa, Patología 12:119-125, 1979.
379. Aumuller G, Peter ST: Inmunohistochemical and ultrastructural study of Sertoli cells in androgen insensitivity, Int J Androl 9:99-108, 1986.
380. O'Dowd J, Gaffney EF, Young RH: Malignant sex cord stromal tumor in a patient with the androgen insensitivity syndrome, Histopathology 16:279-282, 1990.
381. Lubs HA Jr, Vilar O, Bergenstal DM: Familial male pseudohermaphroditism with labial testes and partial feminization: endocrine studies and genetic aspects, J Clin Endocrinol Metab 19:1110-1120, 1959.
382. Sultan C, Picard JY, Josso N et al: Incomplete androgen insensitivity syndrome: partially masculinized genitalia in two patients with absence of androgen receptor in cultured fibroblasts, Clin Endocrinol 19:565-574, 1983.
383. Gunasegaram R, Loganath A, Peh KL et al: Altered hypothalamic-pituitary-testicular function in incomplete testicular feminization syndrome, Aus N Z J Obstet Gynecol 24:288-292, 1984.
384. Gilbert-Dreyfus S, Sebaoum CIA, Belaisch J: Etude d'un cas familial d'androgynoïdisme avec hypospadias grave, gynécomastie et hyperoestrogénie, Ann Endocrinol 18:93-101, 1957.
385. Reifenstein EC Jr: Hereditary familial hypogonadism, Clin Res 3:86-89, 1947.
386. Rosewater S, Gwinup G, Hamwi GJ: Familial gynecomastia, Ann Intern Med 63:377-385, 1965.
387. Imperato-McGinley J, Guerrero J, Gautier T et al: Steroid 5 alpha-reductase deficiency in man. An inherited form of male pseudohermaphroditism, Science 186:1213-1215, 1974.
388. Schmidt JA, Schweikert, HU: Testosterone and epitestosterone metabolism of single hairs in 5 patients with 5 alpha-reductase-deficiency, Acta Endocrinol 113:588-592, 1986.
389. Okon E, Livni N, Rösler A et al: Male pseudohermaphroditism due to 5 alpha-reductase deficiency, Arch Pathol Lab Med 104:363-367, 1980.
390. Peterson RE, Imperato-McGinley J, Gautier T et al: Male pseudohermaphroditism due to steroid 5 alpha-reductase deficiency, Am J Med 62:170-191, 1977.
391. Josso N, Fekete C, Cachin O et al: Persistence of müllerian ducts in male pseudohermaphroditism, and its relationship to cryptorchidism, Clin Endocrinol 19:247-258, 1983.

392. Josso N, Boussin L, Knebelmann B et al: Anti-Müllerian hormone and intersex states, Trends Endocrinol Metab 2:227-233, 1991.
393. Josso N, Cate RL, Picard JY et al: Anti-Müllerian hormone, the Jost factor, Recent Prog Horm Res 48:1-59, 1993.
394. Josso N, Picard JY, Imbeaud S et al: The persistent müllerian duct syndrome: a rare cause of cryptorchidism, Eur J Pediatr 152(suppl 2):S76-S78, 1993.
395. Sohval AR: Hermaphroditism with atypical or "mixed" gonadal dysgenesis. Relationship to gonadal neoplasm, Am J Med 36:281-292, 1964.
396. Zäh W, Kalderon AE, Tucci JR: Mixed gonadal dysgenesis, Acta Endocrinol 197(suppl):3-39, 1975.
397. Robboy SJ, Miller T, Donahoe PK et al: Dysgenesis of testicular and streak gonads in the syndrome of mixed gonadal dysgenesis. Perspective derived from a clinicopathologic analysis of twenty-one cases, Hum Pathol 13:700-716, 1982.
398. Rajfer J, Mendelsohn G, Arnheim J et al: Dysgenetic male pseudohermaphroditism, J Urol 119:525-527, 1978.
399. Nilson O: Hernia uteri inguinalis beim Manne, Acta Chir Scand 83:231-240, 1939.
400. Sheehan SJ, Tobbia IN, Ismail MA et al: Persistent müllerian duct syndrome. Review and report of 3 cases, Br J Urol 57:548-551, 1985.
401. Beheshti M, Churchill BM, Hardy BE et al: Familial persistent müllerian duct syndrome, J Urol 131:968-969, 1984.
402. Mouli K, McCarthy P, Ray P et al: Persistent müllerian duct syndrome in a man with transverse testicular ectopia, J Urol 139:373-375, 1988.
403. Hershlag A, Spitz IM, Hochner-Celnikier D et al: Persistent müllerian structures in infertile male, Urology 28:138-141, 1986.
404. Malayaman D, Armiger G, D'Arcangues C et al: Male pseudohermaphroditism with persistent müllerian and wolffian structures complicated by intra-abdominal seminoma, Urology 24:67-69, 1984.
405. Sloan WR, Walsh PC: Familial persistent müllerian duct syndrome, J Urol 115:459-461, 1976.
406. Carré-Eusèbe D, Imbeaud S, Harbison M et al: Variants of the anti-müllerian hormone gene in a compound heterozygote with the persistent müllerian duct syndrome and his family, Hum Genet 90:389-394, 1992.
407. Nistal M, Paniagua R, Isorna S et al: Diffuse intratubular undifferentiated germ cell tumor in both testes of a male subject with a uterus and ipsilateral testicular dysgenesis, J Urol 124:286-289, 1980.
408. Snow BW, Rowland RG, Seal GM et al: Testicular tumor in a patient with persistent müllerian duct syndrome, Urology 26:495-497, 1985.
409. Drash A, Sherman F, Hartmann WH et al: A syndrome of pseudohermaphroditism, Wilms' tumor, hypertension and degenerative renal disease, J Pediatr 76:585-593, 1970.
410. Rajfer J: Association between Wilms tumor and gonadal dysgenesis, J Urol 125:388-390, 1981.
411. McCoy FE, Franklin WA, Aronson AJ et al: Glomerulonephritis associated with male pseudohermaphroditism and nephroblastoma, Am J Surg Pathol 7:387-395, 1983.
412. Heppe RK, Koyle MA, Beckwith JB: Nephrogenic rests in Wilms tumor patients with the Drash syndrome, J Urol 145:1225-1228, 1991.
413. Charny CW: Testicular biopsy, its value in male sterility, JAMA 115:1429-1432, 1940.
414. Charny CW, Meranze DR: Testicular biopsy. Further studies in male infertility, Surg Gynecol Obstet 74:836-842, 1942.
415. Nelson WO: Interpretation of the testicular biopsy, JAMA 151:449-452, 1953.
416. Pesce C: Testicular biopsy in the evaluation of male infertility, Semin Diagn Pathol 4:264-274, 1987.
417. Wong TW, Straus FH II, Warner NE: Testicular causes of infertility, Arch Pathol 95:151-159, 1973.
418. Wong TW, Straus FH II, Warner NE: Pretesticular causes of infertility, Arch Pathol 98:1-8, 1974.
419. Guarch R, Pesce C, Puras A et al: A quantitative approach to the classification of hypospermatogenesis in testicular biopsies for infertility, Hum Pathol 23:1032-1037, 1992.
420. Honoré LJ: Testicular biopsy for infertility: a review of sixty-eight cases with a simplified histologic classification of lesions, Int J Fertil 24:49-52, 1979.
421. Girgis SM, Etriby A, Ibrahim AA et al: Testicular biopsy in azoospermia: a review of the last ten years. Experience of over 800 cases, Fertil Steril 20:467-477, 1969.
422. Wong TW, Straus FH II, Warner NE: Posttesticular causes of infertility, Arch Pathol 95:160-164, 1973.
423. Söderström KO, Suominen J: Histopathology and ultrastructure of meiotic arrest in human spermatogenesis, Arch Pathol Lab Med 104:476-482, 1980.
424. Charny CW: Reflections on testicular biopsy, Fertil Steril 14:610-616, 1963.
425. Meinhard E, McRae CU, Chisholm GD: Testicular biopsy in evaluation of male infertility, Br Med J 3:577-581, 1973.
426. Levin HS: Testicular biopsy in the study of male infertility. Its current usefulness, histologic techniques, and prospects for the future, Hum Pathol 10:569-584, 1979.
427. Bairati A, Della Morte E, Giarola A et al: Testicular biopsy of azoospermic men with vas deferens malformation using two different techniques, Arch Androl 17:67-78, 1986.
428. Narbaitz R, Tolnai G, Jolly E et al: Ultrastructural studies on testicular biopsies from eighteen cases of hypospermatogenesis, Fertil Steril 30:679-686, 1978.
429. Fossati P, Asfour M, Blacker C et al: Serum and seminal gonadotropins in normal and infertile men: correlations with sperm count, prolactinemia, and seminal prolactin, Arch Androl 2:247-252, 1979.
430. Johnson L, Petty CS, Neaves WB: The relationship of biopsy evaluations and testicular measurements to over-all daily sperm production in human testes, Fertil Steril 34:36-40, 1980.
431. De Kretser DM, Burger HG, Hudson B: The relationship between germinal cells and serum FSH levels in males with infertility, J Clin Endocrinol Metab 38:787-793, 1974.
432. Silber SJ: Microsurgery for vasectomy reversal and vaso-epididymostomy, Urology 23:505-524, 1984.
433. Makler A, Abramovici H: The correlation between sperm count and testicular biopsy using a new scoring system, Int J Fertil 23:300-304, 1978.
434. Johnsen SG: Testicular biopsy score count—a method for registration of spermatogenesis in human testes: normal values and results in 335 hypogonadal males, Hormones 1:2-25, 1970.

435. Meyer JM, Roos M, Rumpler Y: Statistical study of a semiquantitative evaluation of testicular biopsies, Arch Androl 20:71, 1988.
436. Steinberger E, Tjioe DY: A method for quantitative analysis of human seminiferous epithelium, Fertil Steril 19:960-970, 1968.
437. Rowley MJ, Heller CG: Quantitation of the cells of the seminiferous epithelium of human testis employing Sertoli cells as a constant, Z Zellforsch 115:461-472, 1971.
438. Skakkebaek NE, Hammen R, Philip J et al: Quantification of human seminiferous epithelium. III. Histological studies in 44 infertile men with normal chromosome complements, Acta Pathol Microbiol Scand (A) 81:97-111, 1973.
439. Skakkebaek NE, Hulten M, Philip J: Quantification of human seminiferous epithelium. IV. Histological studies in 17 men with numerical and structural autosomal aberrations, Acta Pathol Microbiol Scand (A) 81:112-124, 1973.
440. Skakkebaek NE, Heller CG: Quantification of human seminiferous epithelium. I. Histological studies in twenty-one fertile men with normal chromosome complements, J Reprod Fertil 32:179-189, 1983.
441. Zuckerman Z, Rodriguez-Rigau LJ, Weiss DB et al: Quantitative analysis of the seminiferous epithelium in human testicular biopsies, and the relation of spermatogenesis to sperm density, Fertil Steril 30:448-455, 1978.
442. Johnson L, Zane RS, Petty CS: Quantification of the human Sertoli cell population: its distribution, relation to germ cell numbers, and age related decline, Biol Reprod 31:785-795, 1984.
443. Weiss DB, Rodriguez-Rigau LJ, Smith KD et al: Quantitation of Leydig cells in testicular biopsies of oligospermic men with varicocele, Fertil Steril 30:305-309, 1978.
444. Heller CG, Lalli MF, Pearson JE et al: A method for the quantification of Leydig cells in man, J Reprod Fertil 25:177-184, 1971.
445. Averback P, Wight DGD: Seminiferous tubule hypercurvature: a newly recognized common syndrome of human male infertility, Lancet 1:181-183, 1979.
446. Averback P: Branching of seminiferous tubules associated with hypofertility and chronic respiratory infection, Arch Pathol Lab Med 104:361-362, 1980.
447. Nistal M, Abaurrea MA, Paniagua R: Morphological and histometric study on the human Sertoli cells from birth to the onset of puberty, J Anat 134:351-363, 1982.
448. Nistal M, Jiménez F, Paniagua R: Sertoli cell types in Sertoli-cell-only syndrome: relationships between Sertoli cell morphology and aetiology, Histopathology 16:173-180, 1990.
449. Schulze C, Holstein AF, Schirren C et al: On the morphology of the human Sertoli cells under normal conditions and in patients with impaired fertility, Andrologia 8:167-178, 1976.
450. Chemes HE, Dym, M, Fawcet DW et al: Pathophysiological observations of Sertoli cells in patients with germinal aplasia or severe germ cell depletion. Ultrastructural findings and hormone levels, Biol Reprod 17:108-123, 1977.
451. Terada T, Hatakeyama S: Morphological evidence for two types of idiopathic "Sertoli-cell-only" syndrome, Int J Androl 14:117-126, 1991.
452. Goslar HG, Hilscher B, Haider SG et al: Enzyme histochemical studies on the pathological changes in human Sertoli cells, J Histochem Cytochem 30:1268-1274, 1982.
453. Fabbrini A, Re M, Spera G: Behaviour of glycogen and related enzymes in the Sertoli cell syndrome, Experientia 25:647-651, 1969.
454. Nistal M: Testículo humano. Hypoplasia túbulo intersticial difusa (hipogonadismo hipogonadotrópico), Arch Esp Urol 3:252-280, 1973.
455. Nistal M, Paniagua R: Leydig cell differentiation induced by stimulation with HCG and HMG in two patients affected with hypogonadotropic hypogonadism, Andrologia 11:211-222, 1979.
456. De Kretser DM: The fine structure of the immature human testis in hypogonadotrophic hypogonadism, Virchows Arch B Cell Pathol 1:283-296, 1968.
457. Nistal M, Paniagua R, Abaurrea MA et al: Hyperplasia and the immature appearance of Sertoli cells in primary testicular disorders, Hum Pathol 13:3-12, 1982.
458. Gotoh M, Miyake K, Mitsua H: Elastic fibers in tunica propria of undescended and contralateral scrotal testes from cryptorchid patients, Urology 30:359-363, 1987.
459. Paniagua R, Nistal M, Bravo MP: Leydig cell types in primary testicular disorders, Hum Pathol 15:181-190, 1984.
460. Mack WS, Scott LS, Ferguson-Smith MA et al: Ectopic testis and the undescended testis: a histological comparison, J Pathol Bacteriol 82:439-443, 1961.
461. Taniuchi I, Mizutani S, Namiki M et al: Short arm dicentric Y chromosome in a sterile man: a case report, J Urol 146:415-416, 1991.
462. Aumüller G, Schulze C, Viebahn C: Intermediate filaments in Sertoli cells, Microsc Res Tech 20:50-72, 1992.
463. Christiansen P: Urinary gonadotropins in the Sertoli-cell-only syndrome, Acta Endocrinol 78:180-191, 1975.
464. Hammar M, Berg AO: Impaired Leydig cell function *in vitro* in testicular tissue from human males with "Sertoli cell only" syndrome, Andrologia 17:37-41, 1985.
465. Okuyama A, Nonomura N, Koh E et al: Testicular FSH and HCG receptors in Sertoli-cell-only syndrome, Arch Androl 23:119-124, 1989.
466. Del Castillo EB, Trabucco A, De la Balze FA: Syndrome produced by absence of the germinal epithelium without impairment of the Sertoli or Leydig cells, J Clin Endocrinol Metab 7:493-497, 1947.
467. Rothman MC, Sims SA, Stotts CI: Sertoli cell only syndrome in 1982, Fertil Steril 38:388-390, 1982.
468. Buchanan JD, Fairley KF, Barrie JU: Return of spermatogenesis after stopping cyclophosphamide therapy, Lancet 2:156-157, 1975.
469. Decensi AU, Guarneri D, Marroni P et al: Evidence for testicular impairment after long-term treatment with a luteinizing hormone-releasing hormone agonist in elderly men, J Urol 142:1235-1238, 1989.
470. Sapino A, Pagani A, Godano A et al: Effects of estrogens on the testis of transsexuals: a pathological and immunocytochemical study, Virchows Arch A Pathol Anat Histol 411:409-414, 1987.
471. Schulze C: Response of the human testis to long-term estrogen treatment: morphology of Sertoli cells, Leydig cells and spermatogonial stem cells, Cell Tissue Res 251:31-43, 1988.
472. Daehlin L, Tomic R, Damber JE: Depressed testosterone release from testicular tissue *in vitro* after withdrawal of oestrogen treatment in patients with prostatic carcinoma, Scand J Urol Nephrol 22:11-13, 1988.

473. Söderström KO: Tubular hyalinization in human testes, Andrologia 18:97-103, 1986.
474. Martín R, Santamaría L, Nistal M et al: The peritubular myofibroblasts in the testes from normal men and men with Klinefelter's syndrome. A quantitative, ultrastructural, and immunohistochemical study, J Pathol 168:59-66, 1992.
475. Santamaría L, Martínez-Onsurbe P, Paniagua R et al: Laminin, type IV collagen, and fibronectin in normal and cryptorchid human testes. An immunohistochemical study, Int J Androl 13:470-487, 1990.
476. Wantz GI: Testicular atrophy as a sequela of inguinal herniorrhaphy, Int Surg 71:159-163, 1986.
477. Regadera J, Nistal M, Paniagua R: Testis epididymis, and spermatic cord in elderly men. Correlation of angiographic and histologic studies with systemic arteriosclerosis, Arch Path Lab Med 109:663-667, 1985.
478. Nistal M, Martínez C, Paniagua R: Primary testicular lesions in the twisted testis, Fertil Steril 57: 381-386, 1992.
479. Morgan AD: Inflammation and infestation of the testis and paratesticular structures. In Pugh RCB, ed: Pathology of the testis, Oxford, 1976, Blackwell.
480. Mirsch IH, Choi H: Quantitative testicular biopsy in congenital and acquired genital obstruction, J Urol 143:311-312, 1990.
481. Santamaría L, Martín R, Nistal M et al: The peritubular myoid cells in the testes from men with varicocele. An ultrastructural, immunohistochemical and quantitative study, Histopathology 21:423-433, 1992.
482. Potashnic G, Ben-Aderet N, Israeli R et al: Suppressive effects of 1,2-dibromo-3-3-chloropropane on human spermatogenesis, Fertil Steril 30:444-447, 1978.
483. Barton M, Wiesner BP: Significance of testicular exfoliation in male infecundity, Br Med J 1:958-962, 1952.
484. Belsey MAR, Eliasson AJ, Gallegos KS et al: Laboratory manual for the examination of human semen and semen-cervical mucus interaction. In Paulsen CA, Prasad MNR, eds: VHO special program in human reproduction, Singapore, 1980, Press Concern.
485. Sigg C, Hornstein OP: Zytologische Klassifikation von reifer Keimzellen im Luftgetrockneten Ejakulatausstrich beim spermatologischen Syndrom der vermehrten Desquamation von Zellen der Spermatogenese (VDZS), Andrologia 19:378-391, 1987.
486. Breucker H, Hofmann N, Holstein AF: Transformed spermatocytes constituting the ejaculate of an infertile man, Andrologia 20:526-535, 1988.
487. Riedel HH: Die Differenzierung der "Rundzellen" in menschlichen Ejakulat. Inaugural dissertation, Hamburg, 1976.
488. Holstein C: Morphologie freier unreifer Keimzellen im menschlichen Hoden, Nebenhoden und Ejaculat, Andrologia 15:7-25, 1983.
489. Amelar RD, Dubin L: Other factors affecting male sterility. In Amelar RD, Dubin L, Walsh PC, eds: Male infertility, Philadelphia, 1977, WB Saunders.
490. Kula K: Hyperactivation of early steps of spermatogenesis compromises meiotic insufficiency in men with hypergonadotropism. A possible quantitative assay for high FSH/low testosterone availabilities, Andrologia 23:127-133, 1991.
491. Hendry WF, Polani PE, Pugh RCB et al: 200 infertile males: correlation of chromosome, histological, endocrine and clinical studies, Br J Urol 47:899-908, 1976.
492. Matsuda T, Horii Y, Hayashi K et al: Quantitative analysis of seminiferous epithelium in subfertile carriers of chromosomal translocations, Int J Fertil 36:344-351, 1991.
493. Grove BD, Vogl AW: Sertoli cell ectoplasmic specializations: a type of actin-associated adhesion junction? J Cell Sci 93:309-323, 1989.
494. Meyer JM, Maetz JL, Rumpler Y: Cellular relationship impairment in maturation arrest of human spermatogenesis: an ultrastructural study, Histopathology 21:25-33, 1992.
495. Baccetti B, Burrini AG, Capitani S et al: Studies on varicocele. I. Submicroscopical and endocrinological features, J Submicrosc Cytol Pathol 23:659-665, 1991.
496. Cameron DF, Snydle FE: Ultrastructural surface characteristics of seminiferous tubules from men with varicocele, Andrologia 14:425-433, 1982.
497. MacLeod J: Seminal cytology in the presence of varicocele, Fertil Steril 16:735-757, 1965.
498. Takihara M, Sakatoku J, Cockett ATK: The pathophysiology of varicocele in male infertility, Fertil Steril 55:861-868, 1991.
499. Nistal M, Paniagua R, Regadera J et al: Obstruction of the tubuli recti and ductuli efferentes by dilated veins in the testes of men with varicocele and its possible role in causing atrophy of the seminiferous tubules, Int J Androl 7:309-323, 1984.
500. Yamamoto M, Hashimoto J, Takaba H et al: Scanning electron microscopic study on the shape of infertile seminiferous tubules: a hypothesis of pathogenesis of idiopathic male infertility, Int J Fertil 33:265-272, 1988.
501. Gall EA: The histopathology of acute mumps orchitis, Am J Pathol 23:637-651, 1947.
502. Gulizia S, Vicari E, Aleffi A et al: Abnormal germ cell exfoliation in semen of hypogonadotrophic patients during a hCG treatment, Andrologia 13:74-77, 1981.
503. Sigg S: Klassifizierung tubulärer Hodenatrophien bei Sterilitätabklärungen, Schweiz Med Wochenschr 35:1284-1293, 1979.
504. Martinova Y, Kantcheva L, Tzvetkov D: Testicular ultrastructure in infertile men, Arch Androl 22:103-122, 1989.
505. Bustos-Obregón E, Esponda P: Ultrastructure of the nucleus of human Sertoli cells in normal and pathological testes, Cell Tissue Res 152:467-475, 1974.
506. De Kretser DM, Kerr JB, Paulsen CA: Evaluation of the ultrastructural changes in the human Sertoli cell in testicular disorders and the relationship of the changes to the levels of serum FSH, Int J Androl 4:129-144, 1981.
507. Namiki M, Koide T, Okuyama A et al: Abnormality of testicular FSH receptors in infertile men, Acta Endocrinol 106:548-555, 1984.
508. Gerris J, Comhaire F, Hellemans P et al: Placebo-controlled trial of high-dose mesterolone treatment of idiopathic male infertility, Fertil Steril 55:603-607, 1991.
509. Stecker JF, Lloyd JW: Leydig and Sertoli cell function in normal and oligospermic males: a preliminary report, Fertil Steril 29:204-208, 1978.

510. Giagulli VA, Vermeulen A: Leydig cell function in infertile men with idiopathic oligospermic infertility, J Clin Endocrinol Metab 66:62-67, 1988.
511. Aiman J, Griffin JE, Gazak JM et al: Androgen insensitivity as a cause of infertility in otherwise normal men, N Engl J Med 300:223-227, 1979.
512. Aiman J, Griffin JE: The frequency of androgen receptor deficiency in infertile men, J Clin Endocrinol Metab 54:725-732, 1982.
513. Akin JW: The use of clomiphene citrate in the treatment of azoospermia secondary to incomplete androgen resistance, Fertil Steril 59:223-224, 1993.
514. Akin JW, Behzadian A, Tho SPT et al: Evidence for a partial deletion in the androgen receptor gene in a phenotypic male with azoospermia, Am J Obstet Gynecol 165:1891-1894, 1991.
515. Schulster A, Ross L, Scommegna A: Frequency of androgen insensitivity in infertile phenotypically normal men, J Urol 130:699-701, 1983.
516. Gooren L: Improvement of spermatogenesis after treatment with the antiestrogen tamoxifen in a man with the incomplete androgen insensitivity syndrome, J Clin Endocrinol Metab 68:1207-1210, 1989.
517. Sokol RZ, Steiner BS, Bustillo M et al: A controlled comparison of the efficacy of clomiphene citrate in male infertility, Fertil Steril 49:865-870, 1988.
518. Schrag SD, Dixon RL: Occupational exposures associated with male reproductive dysfunction, Ann Rev Pharmacol Toxicol 25:567-592, 1985.
519. Takihara H, Cosentino MJ, Sakaratoku J et al: Significance of testicular size measurement in andrology. II. Correlation of testicular size with testicular function, J Urol 137:416-419, 1987.
520. Chehval MJ, Purcell MH: Deterioration of semen parameters over time in men with untreated varicocele: evidence of progressive testicular damage, Fertil Steril 57:174-177, 1992.
521. Agger P, Johnsen SG: Quantitative evaluation of testicular biopsies in varicocele, Fertil Steril 29:52-57, 1978.
522. Dubin L, Hotchkiss RS: Testis biopsy in subfertile men with varicocele, Fertil Steril 20:50-57, 1969.
523. Etriby A, Girgis SM, Hefnawy H et al: Testicular changes in subfertile males with varicocele, Fertil Steril 18:666-671, 1967.
524. Hatakeyama S, Takizawa T, Kawara Y: Focal atrophy of the seminiferous tubule in the human testis, Acta Pathol Jpn 29:901-905, 1979.
525. Sigg C, Hedinger C: Quantitative and ultrastructural study on germinal epithelium in testicular biopsies with "mixed atrophy," Andrologia 13:412-424, 1981.
526. Sigg C, Hedinger C: The frequency and morphology of "giant spermatogonia" in the human testis, Virchows Arch B Cell Pathol 44:115-134, 1983.
527. Paniagua R, Nistal M, Amat P et al: Seminiferous tubule involution in elderly men, Biol Reprod 36:939-947, 1987.
528. Bergmann M, Nashan D, Nieschlag E: Pattern of compartmentation in human seminiferous tubules showing dislocation of spermatogonia, Cell Tissue Res 256:183-190, 1989.
529. Miething A: Intercellular bridges between megalospermatocytes in the human testis, Andrologia 23:91-97, 1991.
530. Holstein AF, Eckmann C: Megalospermatocytes: indicators of disturbed meiosis in man, Andrologia 18:601-609, 1986.
531. Nistal M, Codesal J, Paniagua R: Multinucleate spermatids in aging human testes, Arch Androl 16:125-129, 1986.
532. Vegni-Talluri M, Bigliardi E, Soldani P: Unusual incidence of binucleate spermatids in human cryptorchidism, J Submicrosc Cytol 10:357-361, 1978.
533. Aumüller G, Fuhrmann W, Krause W: Spermatogenetic arrest with inhibition of acrosome and sperm tail development, Andrologia 19:9-17, 1987.
534. David G, Bisson JP, Czyglik F et al: Anomalies morphologiques du spermatozoide humain. Propositions pour un système de classificatión, J Gynecol Obstet Biol Reprod 4:17-36, 1975.
535. Holstein AF: Morphologische Studien an abnormen Spermatiden und Spermatozoen des Menschen, Virchows Arch A Pathol Anat Histol 367:92-112, 1975.
536. Holstein AF, Schirren C: Classification of abnormalities in human spermatids based on recent advances in ultrastructural research on spermatid differentiation. In Fawcett DW, Bedford JM eds: The spermatozoon. Maturation, mobility, surface properties and comparative aspects, Baltimore, 1979, Urban and Schwarzenberg.
537. Portuondo JA, Calabozo M, Echanojauregui AD: Morphology of spermatozoa in fertile man with and without varicocele, J Androl 4:312-315, 1983.
538. Kullander S, Rausing A: On round headed human spermatozoa, Int J Fertil 2:33-40, 1975.
539. Nistal M, Paniagua R: Morphogenesis of round headed human spermatozoa lacking acrosomes in a case of severe teratozoospermia, Andrologia 10:49-51, 1978.
540. Escalier D: Failure of differentiation of the nuclear-perinuclear skeletal complex in the round-headed human spermatozoa, Int J Dev Biol 34:287-297, 1990.
541. Escalier D: Human spermatozoa with large heads and multiple flagella: a quantitative ultrastructural study of 6 cases, Biol Cell 48:65-74, 1983.
542. Nistal M, Paniagua R, Herruzo A: Multi-tailed spermatozoa in a case with asthenospermia and teratospermia, Virchows Arch B Cell Pathol 26:111-118, 1977.
543. Baccetti B, Burrini AG, Collodel G et al: Crater defect in human spermatozoa, Gamete Res 22:249-255, 1989.
544. Matano Y: Ultrastructural study of human binucleate spermatids, J Ultrastruct Res 34:123-134, 1971.
545. Dadoune JP: Ultrastructural abnormalities of human spermatozoa, Hum Reprod 3:311-318, 1988.
546. Barthelemy C, Tharanne MJ, Lebos C et al: Tail stump spermatozoa: morphogenesis of the defect. An ultrastructural study of sperm and testicular biopsy, Andrologia 22:417-425, 1990.
547. Alexandre C, Bisson JP, David G: Asthenozoospermie totale avec anomalie ultraestructurale du flagelle dans deux fréres stériles, J Gyn Obst Biol Reprod 7:31-38, 1978.
548. Nistal M, Paniagua R, Herruzo A: Absence de la paire centrale du complexe axonemique dans une tératospermie avec flagelles courts et épais, J Gynecol Obstet Biol Reprod 8:47-50, 1979.
549. Perotti ME, Giarola A, Gioria M: Ultrastructural study of the decapitated sperm defect in an infertile man, J Reprod Fertil 63:543-549, 1981.

550. Zamboni L: Sperm structure and its relevance to infertility, Arch Pathol Lab Med 116:325-344, 1992.
551. Afzelius BA, Eliasson R, Hohnsen O et al: Lack of dynein arms in immotile human spermatozoa, J Cell Biol 66:225-232, 1975.
552. Schieferstein G, Wolburg H, Adam W: Stiff-tail-order Mittelstück-Syndrome, Andrologia 1:5-8, 1987.
553. Haidl G, Becker A, Henkel R: Poor development of outer dense fibres as a major cause of tail abnormalities in the spermatozoa of asthenoteratozoospermic men, Hum Reprod 6:1431-1438, 1991.
554. Chemes HE, Brugo S, Zanchetti F et al: Dysplasia of the fibrous sheath: an ultrastructural defect of human spermatozoa associated with sperm immotility and primary sterility, Fertil Steril 48:664-669, 1987.
555. Makler A, Geresh I: An attempt to explain occurrence of patent reproductive tract in azoospermic males with tubular spermatogenesis, Int J Fertil 24:246-250, 1979.
556. Silber SJ, Rodriguez-Rigau LJ: Quantitative analysis of testicular biopsy: determination of partial obstruction and prediction of sperm count after surgery for obstruction, Fertil Steril 36:480-485, 1981.
557. Nistal M, Codesal J, Santamaría L et al: Correlation between spermatozoon numbers in spermiogram and seminiferous epithelium histology in testicular biopsies from subfertile men, Fertil Steril 48:507-509, 1987.
558. Pryor JP, Hendry WF: Ejaculatory duct obstruction in subfertile males: analysis of 87 patients, Fertil Steril 56:725-730, 1991.
559. Dubin L, Amelar RD: Etiologic factors in 1294 consecutive cases of male infertility, Fertil Steril 22:469-480, 1971.
560. Auroux M, De Mouy DM, Acar JF: Male fertility and positive chlamydial serology. A study of 61 fertile and 82 subfertile men, J Androl 8:197-200, 1987.
561. Hillier SL, Rabe LK, Muller CH et al: Relationship of bacteriologic characteristics to semen indices in men attending an infertility clinic, Obstetr Gynaecol 75:800-804, 1990.
562. Sandhu DPS, Osborn DE, Munson KW: Relationship of azoospermia to inguinal surgery, Int J Androl 15:504-506, 1992.
563. Ross LS, Suzanne Flom L: Azoospermia. A complication of hydrocele repair in a fertile population, J Urol 146:852-853, 1991.
564. Rajalakshmi M, Ratna Kumar BV, Ramakrishnan PR et al: Histology of the epididymis in men with obstructive infertility, Andrologia 22:319-326, 1990.
565. Hirsch IH, McCue P, Allen J et al: Quantitative testicular biopsy in spinal cord injured men: comparison to fertile controls, J Urol 146:337-341, 1991.
566. Pardanini DS, Patil NG, Pawar HN: Some gross observations of the epididymides following vasectomy: a clinical study, Fertil Steril 27:267-270, 1976.
567. McMahon AJ, Buckley J, Taylor A et al: Chronic testicular pain following vasectomy, Br J Urol 69:188-191, 1992.
568. Jarow JP, Budin RE, Dym M et al: Quantitative pathologic changes in the human testis after vasectomy. A controlled study, N Engl J Med 313:1252-1256, 1985.
569. Jenkins IL, Muir VY, Blacklock NJ et al: Consequences of vasectomy: an immunological and histological study related to subsequent fertility, Br J Urol 51:406-410, 1979.
570. Marmar JL: The status of vasectomy reversals, Int J Fertil 36:352-357, 1991.
571. Urry RL, Heaton JB, Moore M et al: A fifteen-year study of alterations in semen quality occurring after vasectomy reversal, Fertil Steril 53:341-345, 1990.
572. Young D: Surgical treatment of male infertility, J Reprod Fertil 23:541-542, 1970.
573. Handelsman DJ, Conway AJ, Boylan LM et al: Young's syndrome: obstructive azoospermia and chronic sinopulmonary infections, N Engl J Med 310:3-4, 1984.
574. Neville E, Brewis RAL, Yeates WK et al: Respiratory tract disease and obstructive azoospermia, Thorax 38:929-930, 1983.
575. Hendry WF, Knight RK, Whitfield HN: Obstructive azoospermia: respiratory function tests, electron microscopy and the results of surgery, Br J Urol 50:598-604, 1978.
576. Nistal M, Paniagua R, Abaurrea MA: Varicose axon-bearing "synaptic" vesicles on the basal lamina of the human seminiferous tubules, Cell Tissue Res 226:75-82, 1982.
577. Klinefelter HF Jr, Reifenstein EC Jr, Albright F: Syndrome characterized by gynecomastia, aspermatogenesis without aleydigism and increased excretion of follicle-stimulating hormone, J Clin Endocrinol 2:615-627, 1942.
578. Ohno S: Control of meiotic process. In Troen P, Nankin HR, eds: The testis in normal and infertile men, New York, 1977, Raven Press.
579. Hsueh WA, Hsu TH, Federman DD: Endocrine features of Klinefelter's syndrome, Medicine 57:447-461, 1978.
580. Becker KL: Clinical and therapeutic experiences with Klinefelter's syndrome, Fertil Steril 23:568-578, 1972.
581. Mor C, Ben-Bassat M, Leiba S: Leydig and Sertoli cells. Their five structures in three cases of Klinefelter's syndrome, Arch Pathol Lab Med 106:228-230, 1982.
582. Frohland A, Skakkebaek NE: Dimorphism in sex chromatin pattern of Sertoli cells in adults with Klinefelter's syndrome: correlation with two types of "Sertoli-cell-only" tubes, J Clin Endocrinol Metab 33:683-687, 1971.
583. Ahmad KN, Dykes JRW, Ferguson-Smith MA et al: Leydig cell volume in chromatin-positive Klinefelter's syndrome, J Clin Endocrinol Metab 33:517-520, 1971.
584. Nistal M, Santamaría L, Paniagua R: Quantitative and ultrastructural study of Leydig cells in Klinefelter's syndrome, J Pathol 146:323-331, 1985.
585. Rubin P, Mattei A, Cesarini JP et al: Étude en microscopie électronique de la cellule de Leydig dans la maladie de Klinefelter en périodes pre, per et postpubertaires, Ann Endocrinol 32:671-681, 1971.
586. Gabrilove JC, Freiberg EK, Nicolis GC: Testicular function in Klinefelter's syndrome, J Urol 124:825-828, 1980.
587. Wellen JJ, Smals AGH, Rijken JCW et al: Testosterone and Δ_4 androstenedione in the saliva of patients with Klinefelter's syndrome, Clin Endocrinol 18:51-59, 1983.
588. Gómez-Acebo J, Parrilla R, Abrisqueta JA et al: Fine structure of spermatogenesis in Klinefelter's syndrome, J Clin Endocrinol Metab 28:1287-1292, 1968.
589. Steinberger E, Smith KD, Perloff WH: Spermatogenesis in Klinefelter's syndrome, J Clin Endocrinol Metab 25:1325-1330, 1965.
590. Muldal S, Ockey CH: The "double male." A new chromosome constitution in Klinefelter's syndrome, Lancet 2:492-493, 1960.

591. Ellis JR, Miller OJ, Penrose LS et al: A male with XXYY chromosomes, Ann Hum Genet 25:145-152, 1961.
592. Borgaonkar DS, Muler E, Char F: Do the 48 XXYY males have a characteristic phenotype? Clin Genet 1:272-277, 1970.
593. Bloomgarden ZT, Delozier CD, Cohen MP et al: Genetics and endocrine findings in a 48 XXYY male, J Clin Endocrinol Metab 50:740-743, 1980.
594. Uchida IA, Miller JR, Soltan HC: Dermatoglyphics associated with the XXYY chromosome complement, Am J Hum Genet 16:284-289, 1964.
595. Nistal M, Paniagua R, Lopez-Pajares I: Ultrastructure of Leydig cells in Klinefelter's syndrome with 48 XXYY karyotype, Virchows Arch B Cell Pathol 28:39-46, 1978.
596. Ferguson-Smith MA, Johnston AW, Handmaker S: Primary amentia and microorchidism associated with an XXXY sex-chromosome constitution, Lancet 2:184-187, 1960.
597. Fraccaro M, Kaijser K, Lindsten J: A child with 49 chromosomes, Lancet 2:899-902, 1960.
598. Jackson AW, Muldal S, Ockey CH et al: Carcinoma of the male breast in association with Klinefelter's syndrome, Br Med J 1:223-225, 1965.
599. Scheike O: Male breast cancer, Acta Pathol Microbiol Scand 251(suppl):13-35, 1975.
600. Mies R, Fischer H, Pfeiff B et al: Klinefelter's syndrome and breast cancer, Andrologia 14:317-321, 1982.
601. Isurugi K, Imao S, Hirose K et al: Seminoma in Klinefelter's syndrome with 47 XXY, 15s+ karyotype, Cancer 39:2041-2047, 1977.
602. Vanfleteren E, Steeno O: Klinefelter's syndrome and mediastinal teratoma, Andrologia 13:573-577, 1981.
603. Gohji K, Goto A, Takenaka A et al: Extragonadal germ cell tumor in the retrovesical region associated with Klinefelter's syndrome: a case report and review of literature, J Urol 141:133-136, 1989.
604. McNeil MM, Leong A, Sage RE: Primary mediastinal embryonal carcinoma in association with Klinefelter's syndrome, Cancer 47:343-345, 1981.
605. Sogge MR, McDonald SD, Cofold PB: The malignant potential of the dysgenetic germ cell in Klinefelter's syndrome, Am J Med 66:515-518, 1979.
606. Mukerjee D, Bowen J, Anderson DE: Simian papovavirus 40 transformation of cells from cancer patient with XY/XXY mosaic Klinefelter's syndrome, Cancer Res 30:1769-1772, 1970.
607. Pascual J, Liaño F, García-Villanueva A et al: Isolated primary aldosteronism in a patient with adrenal carcinoma and XY/XXY mosaic Klinefelter's syndrome, J Urol 144:1454-1456, 1990.
608. Penchansky L, Krause JR: Acute leukemia following a malignant teratoma in a child with Klinefelter's syndrome, Cancer 50:684-689, 1982.
609. Ferguson-Smith MA: The prepubertal testicular lesion in chromatin-positive Klinefelter's syndrome (primary microorchidism). As seen in mentally handicapped children, Lancet 1:219-222, 1959.
610. Lanman JT, Skalarin BS, Cooper HL et al: Klinefelter's syndrome in a ten-month-old mongolian idiot, N Engl J Med 263:887-888, 1960.
611. Gracia R, Martín-Álvarez L, Figols J et al: Síndrome de Klinefelter XXY en el periodo prepuberal. Estudio de ocho observaciones, An Esp Pediatr 7:510-523, 1974.
612. Maisey DN, Mills IH, Middleton H et al: A case of Klinefelter's syndrome with acquired hypopituitarism, Acta Endocrinol 105:126-129, 1984.
613. Smals AGH, Kloppenborg PWC: Klinefelter's syndrome with hypogonadotropic hypogonadism, Br Med J 1:839-839, 1977.
614. Rabinowitz D, Cohen MM, Rosenmann E et al: Chromatin-positive Klinefelter's syndrome with undetectable peripheral FSH levels, Am J Med 59:584-590, 1975.
615. Shirai M, Matsuda S, Mitsukawa S: A case of hypogonadotrophic hypogonadism with an XY/XXY chromosome mosaicism, Tohoku J Exp Med 114:131-139, 1974.
616. Carter JN, Wisseman DGH, Lee HB: Klinefelter's syndrome with hypogonadotrophic hypogonadism, Br Med J 1:212, 1977.
617. Nistal M, Paniagua R, Abaurrea MA et al: 47, XXY Klinefelter's syndrome with low FSH and LH levels and absence of Leydig cells, Andrologia 12:426-433, 1980.
618. Fuse H, Ito H, Minagawa H et al: A case of XX-male syndrome, Jpn J Fertil Steril 27:77-82, 1982.
619. Maeda O, Nakamura M, Namiki M et al: 45X/46XX boy with hypospadias: case report, J Urol 135:1249-1251, 1986.
620. De la Chapelle A, Hortling H, Niemi M et al: XX sex chromosomes in a human male. First case, Acta Med Scand Suppl 412:25-38, 1964.
621. De la Chapelle A: Analytic review: nature and origin of males with XX sex chromosomes, Am J Hum Genet 24:71-105, 1972.
622. Kovacs K, Singer W, Casal G: Leydig cell ultrastructure in an XX male, J Urol 112:651-654, 1974.
623. Nistal M, Barreiro E, Herruzo A et al: Varón con cariotipo 46 XX, Arch Esp Urol 28:263-272, 1975.
624. Nistal M, Paniagua R: Ultrastructure of testicular biopsy from an XX male. Virchows Arch B Cell Pathol 31:45-55, 1979.
625. Romani F, Terquem A, Dadoune JP: Le testicule chez l'homme 46, XX: A propos d'une observation ultrastructural, J Gynecol Obstet Biol Reprod 6:1049-1059, 1977.
626. Sasagawa I, Terada T, Katayama T et al: Ultrastructure of the testis man XX-male with normal plasma testosterone, Andrologia 18:361-367, 1986.
627. Butler MG, Walzak MP, Sanger WG et al: A possible etiology of the infertile 46 XX male subject, J Urol 130:154-156, 1983.
628. Muller U, Donlon T, Schmid M et al: Deletion mapping of the testis determining locus with DNA probes in 46 XX males and in 46 XY and 46 X dic (Y) females, Nucleic Acid Res 14:6489-6505, 1986.
629. Fuse H, Satomi S, Kazama T et al: DNA hybridization study using Y-specific probes in an XX-male, Andrologia 23:237-239, 1991.
630. Yoshida M, Kakizawa Y, Moriyama N et al: Deoxyribonucleic acid and cytological detection of Y-containing cells in a XX hypospadic boy with polyorchidism, J Urol 146:1356-1358, 1991.
631. Fukutani K, Kajiwara T, Nagafuchi S et al: Detection of the testis determining factor in a XX man, J Urol 149:126-128, 1993.

632. Sanberg AA, Koepf GF, Ishihara T et al: XYY human male, Lancet 2:888-889, 1961.
633. Cleveland WW, Arias D, Smith GE: Radioulnar synostosis, behavioral disturbance, and XYY chromosomes, J Pediatr 74:103-106, 1969.
634. Baghdassarian A, Bayard F, Borgaonkar DS et al: Testicular function in XYY men, Johns Hopkins Med J 136:15-24, 1975.
635. Skakkebaek NE, Hulten M, Jacobsen P et al: Quantification of human seminiferous epithelium. II. Histological studies in eight 47, XYY men, J Reprod Fertil 32:391-401, 1973.
636. Speed RM, Faed MJW, Batstone PJ et al: Persistence of two Y chromosomes through meiotic prophase and metaphase I in an XYY man, Hum Genet 87:416-420, 1991.
637. Miklos GLG: Sex chromosome pairing and male fertility, Cytogenet Cell Genet 13:558-577, 1974.
638. Burgoyne PS, Sutcliffe MJ, Mahadevaiah SK: The role of unpaired sex chromosomes in spermatogenetic failure, Andrologia 24:17-20, 1992.
639. Burgoyne PS: Evidence for an association between univalent Y chromosomes and spermatocyte loss in XYY mice and men, Cytogenet Cell Genet 23:84-89, 1979.
640. Hulten M: Meiosis in XYY men, Lancet 1:717-718, 1970.
641. Nielsen J, Johnsen SG: Pituitary gonadotrophins and 17-ketosteroids in patients with the XYY syndrome, Acta Endocrinol 72:191-196, 1973.
642. Hori N, Kato T, Sugimura Y et al: A male subject with 3 Y chromosomes (48, XYYY): a case report, J Urol 139:1059-1061, 1988.
643. Sirota L, Zlotogora Y, Shabtai F et al: 49 XYYYY. A case report, Clin Genet 19:87-93, 1981.
644. Tiepolo L, Zuffardi O: Localization of factors controlling spermatogenesis in the nonfluorescent portion of the human Y chromosome long arm, Hum Genet 34:119-124, 1976.
645. Hartung M, Devictor M, Codaccioni JL et al: Y_q deletion and failure of spermatogenesis, Ann Genet 31:21-26, 1988.
646. Kosztolanyi G, Trixler M: Y_q deletion with short stature, abnormal male development, and schizoid character disorder, J Med Genet 20:393-394, 1983.
647. Daniel A: Y isochromosomes and rings. In Sandberg AA ed: The Y chromosome, Part B: clinical aspects of Y chromosome abnormalities, New York, 1985, Alan R Liss.
648. Chandley AC, Ambros P, McBeath S et al: Short arm dicentric Y chromosome with associated statural defect in a sterile man, Hum Genet 73:350-353, 1986.
649. Giraud F, Mattei JF, Lucas C et al: Four new cases of dicentric Y chromosomes, Hum Genet 36:249-260, 1977.
650. Chandley AC, Edmond P: Meiotic studies on a subfertile patient with a ring Y chromosome, Cytogenetics 10:295-304, 1971.
651. Wahlström J: Y/Y translocations and their cytologic and clinical manifestation. In Sandberg AA ed: The Y chromosome, Part B: clinical aspects of Y chromosome abnormalities, New York, 1985, Alan R Liss.
652. Petit C, De la Chapelle A, Levilliers J et al: An abnormal terminal X-Y interchange accounts for most but not all cases of human XX maleness, Cell 49:595-602, 1987.
653. Andersson M, Page DC, Pettay D et al: Y; autosome translocations and mosaicism in the aetiology of 45,X maleness: assignment of fertility factor to distal Y_q ll, Hum Genet 79:2-7, 1988.
654. Andersson M, Page DC, Brown LG et al: Characterization of a (Y;4) translocation by DNA hybridization, Hum Genet 78:377-381, 1988.
655. Vogt P, Keil R, Köhler M et al: Genome analysis: from sequence to function. In Collins J, Driesel AJ eds: Adv in Mol Gen 4:277-280, 1991.
656. Johnson MD, Tho SPT, Behzadian A et al: Molecular scanning of Y_q 11 (interval 6) in men with Sertoli-cell-only syndrome, Am J Obstet Gynecol 161:1732-1737, 1989.
657. Sasagawa I, Nakada T, Hashimoto T et al: Hormone profiles and contralateral testicular histology in Down's syndrome with unilateral testicular tumor, Arch Androl 30:93-98, 1993.
658. Johannisson R, Gropp A, Winking H et al: Down syndrome in the male. Reproductive pathology and meiotic studies, Hum Genet 63:132-138, 1983.
659. Prader A, Labhart A, Willi H: Ein syndrom von Adipositas, Kleinwuchs, Kryptorchismus, und Oligophrenie nach myotonieartigen Zustand in Neugeborenenalter, Schweiz Med Wochenschr 86:1260-1261, 1956.
660. Uehling D: Cryptorchidism in the Prader-Willi syndrome, J Urol 124:103-104, 1980.
661. Martín-Zurro A, Sánchez-Franco F, Cerdán-Vallejo A et al: Síndrome de Prader-Willi, Rev Clin Esp 125:5-15, 1972.
662. Pellestor F, Sele B, Jalbert H: Chromosome analysis of spermatozoa from a male heterozygous for a 13; 14 Robertsonian translocation, Hum Genet 76:116-120, 1987.
663. Nistal M, Paniagua R: Hypogonadism due to primary testicular failure. In Nistal M, Paniagua R, eds: Testicular and epididymal pathology, New York, 1984, Thieme-Stratton.
664. Nistal M, Paniagua R, Pallardo LF: Testicular biopsy and hormonal study in a male with Noonan's syndrome, Andrologia 15:415-425, 1983.
665. Pallardo LF, Santiago M, Cerdán A et al: Algunos aspectos del eunucoidismo hipogonadotrópico, Med Clin 59:390-396, 1972.
666. Boyar R, Finkelstein J, Roffwang H et al: Synchronization of augmented luteinizing hormone secretion with sleep during puberty, N Engl J Med 287:582-586, 1972.
667. Nistal M, Paniagua R: Hypogonadism due to secondary testicular failure. In Nistal M, Paniagua R eds: Testicular and epididymal pathology, New York, 1984, Thieme-Stratton.
668. Maestre de San Juan A: Falta total de nervios olfatorios con anosmia en un individuo en quien existía una atrofia congénita de los testículos y miembro viril, Siglo Médico 131:211-214, 1856.
669. Kallmann FJ, Shoenfeld WA, Barrera SE: The genetic aspects of primary eunuchoidism, Am J Ment Defic 48:203-236, 1944.
670. De Morsier G, Gauthier G: La dysplasie olfacto-genitale, Pathol Biol 11:1267-1271, 1963.
671. Happ J, Ditscheid W, Krause U: Pulsatile gonadotropin-releasing therapy in male patients with Kallmann's syndrome or constitutional delay of puberty, Fertil Steril 43:599-608, 1985.

672. Enríquez L, Díaz-Rubio M, Zamarrón A et al: Hipogonadismo hipogonadotrópico con anosmia, Rev Clin Esp 131:383-392, 1973.
673. Pervaiz N, Hagedoorn J, Mininberg DT: Electron microscopic studies of testes in Kallmann syndrome, Urology 14:267-269, 1979.
674. Albers DD, Males JL: Seminoma in hypogonadotropic hypogonadism associated with anosmia (Kallmann's syndrome), J Urol 126:57-58, 1981.
675. Al-Ansari AAK, Khalil TH, Kelani Y et al: Isolated follicle-stimulating hormone deficiency in men: successful long-term gonadotropin therapy, Fertil Steril 42:618-626, 1984.
676. Pasqualini RQ, Bur GE: Hypoandrogenic syndrome with spermatogenesis, Fertil Steril 6:144-157, 1955.
677. Pasqualini RQ, Bur GE: Síndrome hipoandrogénico con gametogénesis conservada: clasificación de la insuficiencia testicular, Rev Asoc Med Argent 64:6-10, 1950.
678. McCullagh EP, Beck JC, Schaffenburg CA: A syndrome of eunuchoidism with spermatogenesis, normal urinary FSH, and low-normal ICSH ("fertile eunuchs"), J Clin Endocrinol Metab 13:489-509, 1953.
679. Veldjuis JB, Hammond JM: Endocrine function after spontaneous infarction of the human pituitary. Report, review and reappraisal, Endocr Rev 1:100-107, 1980.
680. Zárate A, Fonseca ME, Mason M et al: Gonadotropin-secreting pituitary adenoma with concomitant hypersecretion of testosterone and elevated sperm count. Treatment with LRH agonists, Acta Endocrinol 113:29-34, 1986.
681. Heseltine D, White MC, Kendall-Taylor P et al: Testicular enlargement and elevated serum inhibin concentrations occur in patients with pituitary macroadenomas secreting follicle stimulating hormone, Clin Endocrinol 31:411-423, 1989.
682. Bouhdiba M, Leroy-Martin B, Peyrat J Ph et al: Immunohistochemical detection of prolactin and its receptors in human testis, Andrologia 21:223-228, 1989.
683. Cameron DF, Murray FT, Drylie D: Ultrastructural lesions in testes from hyperprolactinemic men, J Androl 5:285-293, 1984.
684. Eggert-Kruse W, Schwalbach B, Gerhard I et al: Influence of serum prolactin on semen characteristics and sperm function, Int J Fertil 36:243-251, 1991.
685. Murray FT, Cameron DF, Ketchum C: Return of gonadal function in men with prolactin-secreting tumors, J Clin Endocrinol Metab 59:79-85, 1984.
686. Ford HC, Cooke RR, Keightley EA et al: Serum levels of free and bound testosterone in hyperthyroidism, Clin Endocrinol 36:187-192, 1992.
687. Hudson RW, Edwards AL: Testicular function in hyperthyroidism, J Androl 13:117-124, 1992.
688. De La Balze F, Arillaga F, Mancini RE et al: Male hypogonadism in hypothyroidism: A study of six cases, J Clin Endocrinol Metab 22:212-222, 1962.
689. Cooke PS: Thyroid hormones and testis development: a model system for increasing testis growth and sperm production, Ann NY Acad Sci 637:122-132, 1991.
690. Corrales-Hernández JJ, Miralles García JM, García-Díez LC: Primary hypothyroidism and human spermatogenesis, Arch Androl 25:21-27, 1990.
691. Buitrago JMG, García-Díez LC: Serum hormones and seminal parameters in males with thyroid disturbance, Andrologia 19:37-41, 1987.
692. Bonaccorsi AC, Adler I, Figueiredo JG: Male infertility due to congenital adrenal hyperplasia: testicular biopsy findings, hormonal evaluation, and therapeutic results in three patients, Fertil Steril 47:664-670, 1987.
693. Burke EF, Gilbert E, Uehling DT: Adrenal rest tumors of the testes, J Urol 109:649-652, 1973.
694. Oberman AS, Flatau E, Luboshitzki R: Bilateral testicular adrenal rests in a patient with 11-hydroxylase deficient congenital adrenal hyperplasia, J Urol 149:350-352, 1993.
695. Cutfield RG, Bateman JM, Odell WD: Infertility caused by bilateral testicular masses secondary to congenital adrenal hyperplasia (21-hydroxylase deficiency), Fertil Steril 40:809-814, 1983.
696. Cara JF, Moshang T Jr, Bongiovanni AM et al: Elevated 17-hydroxyprogesterone and testosterone in a newborn with-3-beta-hydroxysteroid dehydrogenase deficiency, New Engl J Med 313:618-621, 1985.
697. Sasano H, Masuda T, Ojima M et al: Congenital 17 alpha-hydroxylase deficiency: a clinico-pathologic study, Hum Pathol 18:1002-1007, 1987.
698. Dinulovic D, Radonjic G: Diabetes mellitus/male infertility, Arch Androl 25:277-293, 1990.
699. Nistal M, Gonzalez-Peramato P, Paniagua R: Congenital Leydig cell hyperplasia, Histopathology 12:307-317, 1988.
700. García-Díez LC, Corrales-Hernández J, Hernández-Díaz J et al: Semen characteristics and diabetes mellitus: significance of insulin in male infertility, Arch Androl 26:219-227, 1991.
701. Cameron DF, Murray FT, Drylie DD: Interstitial compartment pathology and spermatogenic disruption in testes from impotent diabetic men, Anat Rec 213:53-62, 1985.
702. Quadri R, Veglio M, Flecchia D et al: Autonomic neuropathy and sexual impotence in diabetic patients: analysis of cardiovascular reflexes, Andrologia 21:346-352, 1989.
703. Denning CR, Sommers SC, Herbert J et al: Infertility in male patients with cystic fibrosis, Pediatrics 41:7-17, 1968.
704. Feigelson J, Pecau Y: Anomalies du sperme, des defférents et de l'epididyme dans la mucoviscidose, Presse Med 15:523-525, 1986.
705. Osborne L, Knight RA, Santis G et al: A mutation in the second nucleotide binding fold of the cystic fibrosis gene, Am J Hum Genet 48:608-612, 1991.
706. Schellen TMCM, Van Stratten A: Autosomal recessive hereditary congenital aplasia of the vasa deferentia in four siblings, Fertil Steril 35:401-404, 1980.
707. Anguiano A, Oates RD, Amos JA et al: Congenital bilateral absence of the vas deferens. A primary genital form of cystic fibrosis, JAMA 267:1794-1797, 1992.
708. Olson JR, Weaver DK: Congenital mesonephric defects in male infants with mucoviscidosis, J Clin Pathol 22:725-730, 1969.
709. Holsclaw DS, Perlmutter AD, Jockin H et al: Genital abnormalities in male patients with cystic fibrosis, J Urol 106:568-574, 1971.
710. Silvestrini R: La reviviscenza mammaria nell'uomo affecto da cirrosi del Laennec, Riforma Med 42:701-704, 1926.

711. Corda L: Sulla c.d. reviviscenza della mammella maschile nella cirrosi epatica (nota preventiva), Minerva Med 5:1067-1069, 1925.
712. Van Thiel DH, Lester R, Sherins RJ: Hypogonadism in alcoholic liver disease: evidence for a double defect, Gastroenterology 67:1188-1199, 1974.
713. Comathi C, Balasubramanian K, Vijayabhanu N et al: Effect of chronic alcoholism on semen—studies on lipid profiles, Int J Androl 16:175-181, 1993.
714. Galvao-Teles A, Gonçalves L, Carvalho H et al: Alterations of testicular morphology in alcoholic disease, alcoholism, Clin Exp Res 7:144-149, 1983.
715. Terasaki T, Nowlin DM, Pardridge WM: Differential binding of testosterone and oestradiol to isoforms of sex hormone binding globulin: selective alteration of estradiol binding in cirrhosis, J Clin Endocrinol Metab 67:639-643, 1988.
716. Gluud C, Copenhagen Study Group for liver diseases: Serum testosterone concentration in men with alcoholic cirrhosis: background for variation, Metabolism 36:373-378, 1987.
717. Zifroni A, Schiavi RC, Schaffner F: Sexual function and testosterone levels in men with nonalcoholic liver disease, Hepatology 14:479-482, 1991.
718. Handelsman DJ, Conway AJ, Boylan LM et al: Testicular function and fertility in men with homozygous alpha-1 antitrypsin deficiency, Andrologia 18:406-412, 1986.
719. Van Steenbergen MW, Wit JM, Donckerwolcke RAMG: Testosterone esters advance skeletal maturation more than growth in short boys with chronic renal failure and delayed puberty, Eur J Pediatr 150:676-680, 1991.
720. Blackman MR, Weintraub BD, Kourides IA et al: Discordant elevation of the common alpha subunit of the glycoprotein hormones compared to beta subunits in serum of uremic patients, J Clin Endocinol Metab 53:39-48, 1981.
721. Holsdsworth S, Atkins RC, De Kretser DM: The pituitary testicular axis in men with chronic renal failure, N Engl J Med 296:1245-1249, 1977.
722. Elias AN, Vaziri ND, Farooqui S et al: Pathology of endocrine organs in chronic renal failure. An autopsy analysis of 66 patients, Int J Artif Organs 7:251-256, 1984.
723. Lim VS, Fang VS: Gonadal dysfunction in uremic men. A study of the hypothalamo-pituitary-testicular axis before and after renal transplantation, Am J Med 58:655-662, 1975.
724. Enmanouel DS, Lindheimer MD, Katz AI: Pathogenesis of endocrine abnormalities in uremia, Endocrinol Rev 1:28-44, 1980.
725. Cowden EA, Ratcliffe WA, Ratcliffe JG et al: Hypothalamic-pituitary function in uremia, Acta Endocrinol 98:488-495, 1981.
726. Hrudka F, Singh A: Sperm nucleomalacia in men with inflamatory bowel disease, Arch Androl 13:37-57, 1984.
727. Pintor C, Loche S, Puggioni R et al: Adrenal and testicular function in boys affected by thalassemia, J Endocrinol Invest 7:147-149, 1984.
728. Trence DL, Morley JE, Handwerger BS: Polyglandular autoimmune syndromes, Am J Med 77:107-116, 1984.
729. Barkan AL, Kelch RP, Marshall JC: Isolated gonadotropin failure in the polyglandular autoimmune syndrome, N Engl J Med 312:1535-1540, 1985.
730. Graham GE, MacLeod PM, Lillicrap DP et al: Gonadal mosaicism in a family with adreno-leukodystrophy. Molecular diagnosis of carrier status among daughters of a gonadal mosaic when direct detection of the mutation is not possible, J Inhert Metabol Dis 15:68-74, 1992.
731. Libber SM, Migeon CJ, Brown FR et al: Adrenal and testicular function in 14 patients with adrenoleukodystrohpy or adrenomyeloneurophaty, Horm Res 24:1-8, 1986.
732. Powers JM, Schaumburg HH: The testis in adreno-leukodystrophy, Am J Pathol 102:90-98, 1981.
733. Meyer CR: Semen quality in workers exposed to carbon disulfide compared to a control group from the same plant, J Occup Med 23:435-439, 1981.
734. Wagar G, Tolonen M, Stenman UH et al: Endocrinologic studies in men exposed occupationally to carbon disulfide, J Toxicol Environ Health 7:363-371, 1981.
735. Kapp RW Jr, Picciano DJ, Jacobson CB: Y-chromosomal nondysjunction in dibromochloropropane-exposed workmen, Mutat Res 64:47-51, 1979.
736. Lancranjan I, Popescu HI, Gavanescu O et al: Reproductive ability of workmen occupationally exposed to lead, Arch Environ Health 30:396-401, 1975.
737. Cullen MR, Kayne RD, Robins JM: Endocrine and reproductive dysfunction in men associated with occupational inorganic lead intoxication, Arch Environ Health 39:431-440, 1984.
738. Harrington JM: Occupational exposure to synthetic estrogens: some methodological problems, Scand J Work Environ Health 8:167-171, 1992.
739. Ash P: The influence of radiation on fertility in man, Br J Radiol 53:271-278, 1980.
740. Lancrajan I, Maicanescu M, Rafaila E et al: Gonadal function in workmen with long term exposure to microwaves, Health Phys 29:381-383, 1975.
741. Mieusset R, Bujan L, Mansat A et al: Effects of artificial cryptorchidism on sperm morphology, Fertil Steril 47:150-155, 1987.
742. Peñafiel R, Solano F, Gramdes A: The effect of hyperthermia on ornithine decarboxylase activity in different rat tissues, Biochem Pharmacol 37:497-502, 1988.
743. Amendola R, Cordelli E, Mauro F et al: Effects of L-acetyl-carnitine (LAC) on the post-injury recovery of mouse spermatogenesis monitored by flow cytometry. Recovery after hyperthermic treatment, Andrologia 23:135-140, 1991.
744. Casillas ER, Erickson BJ: The role of carnitine in spermatozoa metabolism. Substrate induced elevations in the acetylation state of carnitine and coenzyme A in bovine and monkey spermatozoa, Biol Reprod 12:275-283, 1975.
745. Okuyama A, Koh E, Kondoh N et al: *In vitro* temperature sensitivity of DNA, RNA, and protein synthesis throughout puberty in human testis, Arch Androl 26:7-13, 1991.
746. Donat H, Matthies J, Schwarz I: Fertilität bei Exponierten gegenüber Pffanzenschutz- und Schädlingsbe-Kämpfungsmitteln, Andrologia 22:401-407, 1990.
747. Ernst E, Lauritsen JG: Effect of organic and inorganic mercury on human sperm motility, Pharmacol Toxicol 68:440-444, 1991.
748. Nicholson HS, Beyrne J: Fertility and pregnancy after treatment for cancer during childhood or adolescence, Cancer 71:3392-3399, 1993.

749. Hahn EW, Feingold SM, Simpson L et al: Recovery from aspermia induced by low-dose radiation in seminoma patients, Cancer 50:337-340, 1982.
750. Speiser B, Rubin P, Casarett G: Aspermia following lower truncal irradiation in Hodgkin's disease, Cancer 32:692-698, 1973.
751. Freund I, Zenzes MA, Müller RP et al: Testicular function in eight patients with seminoma after unilateral orchidectomy and radiotherapy, Int J Androl 10:447-455, 1987.
752. Fosså SD, Almaas B, Jetne V et al: Paternity after irradiation for testicular cancer, Acta Radiol Oncol 25:33-36, 1986.
753. Müller J, Hertz H, Skakkebaek NE: Development of the seminiferous epithelium during and after treatment for acute lymphoblastic leukemia in childhood, Horm Res 30:115-120, 1988.
754. Matus-Ridley M, Nicosia SV, Meadows AT: Gonadal effects of cancer therapy in boys, Cancer 55:2353-2363, 1985.
755. Brämswig JH, Heimes U, Heiermann E et al: The effects of different cumulative doses of chemotherapy on testicular function, Cancer 65:1298-1302, 1990.
756. Meistrich ML, Wilson G, Brown BW et al: Impact of cyclophosphamide on long-term reduction in sperm count in men treated with combination chemotherapy for Ewing and soft tissue sarcomas, Cancer 70:2703-2712, 1992.
757. Friedman NM, Plymate SR: Leydig cell dysfunction and gynaecomastia in adult males treated with alkylating agents, Clin Endocrinol 12:553-556, 1980.
758. Green DM, Zevon MA, Lowrie G et al: Congenital anomalies in children of patients who received chemotherapy for cancer in childhood and adolescence, N Engl J Med, 325:141-146, 1991.
759. Viviani S, Ragni G, Santoro A et al: Testicular dysfunction in Hodgkin's disease before and after treatment, Eur J Cancer 27:1389-1392, 1991.
760. Fosså SD, Ous S, Åbyholm T et al: Posttreatment fertility in patients with testicular cancer. Part 1, Br J Urol 57:204-209, 1985.
761. Nijman JM, Schraffordt Koops H, Oldhoff J et al: Sexual function after bilateral retroperitoneal lymph node dissection for nonseminomatous testicular cancer, Arch Androl 18:255-267, 1987.
762. Murphy JB, Lipschultz LI, Vervoort SM: Infertility in the spinal cord injured male, World J Urol 4:83-87, 1986.
763. Perkash I, Martin DE, Warner H et al: Reproductive biology of paraplegics: results of semen collection, testicular biopsy and serum hormone evaluation, J Urol 134:284-288, 1985.
764. Siösteen A, Steen Y, Forssman L et al: Auto-immunity to spermatozoa and quality of semen in men with spinal cord injury, Int J Fertil 38:117-122, 1993.
765. Leriche A, Berard E, Vauzelle JL et al: Histological and hormonal testicular changes in spinal cord patients, Paraplegia 15:274-279, 1977-78.
766. Holstein AF, Sauerwein D, Schirren U: Spermatogenese bei Patienten mit traumatischer Querschnittähmung, Urologe [A] 24:208-215, 1985.
767. Brindley GS: Deep scrotal temperature and the effect on it of clothing, air, temperature, activity, posture and paraplegia, Br J Urol 54:49-55, 1982.
768. Chapelle PA, Roby-Brami A, Yakovleff A et al: Neurological correlations of ejaculation and testicular size in men with a complete spinal cord section, J Neurol Neurosurg Psychiatry 51:197-202, 1988.
769. Shulman A, Shohat B, Gillis D et al: Mumps orchitis among soldiers: frequency, effect on sperm quality, and sperm antibodies, Fertil Steril 57:1344-1346, 1992.
770. Diehl K, Hondl H: Mumps orchitis: symptoms and treatment possibilities, Z Urol Nephrol 83:243-247, 1990.
771. Charny CW, Meranze DR: Pathology of mumps orchitis, J Urol 60:140-146, 1948.
772. Mikuz G, Damjanov I: Inflammation of the testis, epididymis, peritesticular membranes and scrotum, Pathol Annu 1:101-128, 1982.
773. Ejlertsen T, Jensen HK: Orchitis and testicular abscess formation caused by non-typhoid salmonellosis, APMIS 98:294-298, 1990.
774. Jani AN, Casibang V, Mufarrij W: Disseminated actinomycosis presenting as a testicular mass. A case report, J Urol 143:1012-1014, 1990.
775. Eisner DJ, Goldman SM, Petronis J et al: Bilateral testicular infarction caused by epididymitis, AJR Am J Roentgenol 157:517-519, 1991.
776. Almagro UA, Tresp M, Sheth NK: Tuberculous epididymitis occurring 35 years after renal tuberculosis, J Urol 141:1204-1205, 1989.
777. Cabral DA, Johnson HW, Coleman GU et al: Tuberculous epididymitis as a cause of testicular pseudomalignancy in two young children, Pediatr Infect Dis J 4:59-62, 1985.
778. Wolf JS Jr, McAninch JW: Tuberculous epididymo-orchitis. Diagnosis by fine needle aspiration, J Urol 145:836-838, 1991.
779. Stein AL, Miller DB: Tuberculous epididymo-orchitis. A case report, J Urol 129:613, 1983.
780. Persaud V, Rao A: Gumma of testis, Br J Urol 49:142-143, 1977.
781. Akhtar M, Alli MA, Mackey DM: Lepromatous leprosy presenting as orchitis, Am J Clin Pathol 73:712-715, 1980.
782. Kumar B, Raina A, Ktaur S et al: Clinicopathological study of testicular involvement in leprosy, Indian J Lepr 54:48-55, 1982.
783. Reisman EM, Colquitt LA, Childers J et al: Brucella orchitis: a rare cause of testicular enlargement, J Urol 143:821-822, 1990.
784. Ryan DM, Lesser BA, Crumley LA et al: Epididymal sarcoidosis, J Urol 149:134-136, 1993.
785. Singer AJ, Gavrell GJ, Leidich RB et al: Genitourinary involvement of systemic sarcoidosis confined to testicle, Urology 35:422-444, 1990.
786. Blacher EJ, Maynard JF: Seminoma and sarcoidosis: an unusual association, Urology 26:288-289, 1985.
787. Michaelis L, Gutmann C: Ueber Einschlüsse in Blastumoren, Ztschr Klin Med 47:208-215, 1902.
788. McClure J: A case of malacoplakia of the epididymis associated with trauma, J Urol 124:934-935, 1980.
789. Saraf P, di Sant'Agnese P, Valvo J et al: An unusual case of malacoplakia involving the testis and prostate, J Urol 129:149-151, 1983.
790. Díaz-González R, Leiva D, Navas-Palacios JJ et al: Testicular malacoplakia, J Urol 127:325-328, 1982.

791. Nistal M, Rodríguez Echandía EL, Paniagua R: Septate junctions between digestive vacuoles in human malakoplakia, Tissue Cell 10:137-142, 1978.
792. Orr WA, Mulholland SG, Walzak MP Jr: Genitourinary tract involvement with systemic mycosis, J Urol 107:1047-1050, 1972.
793. James CL, Lomax-Smith JD: Cryptococcal epididymoorchitis complicating steroid therapy for releasing polychondritis, Pathology 23:256-258, 1991.
794. Nistal M, Santana A, Paniagua R et al: Testicular toxoplasmosis in two men with the acquired immunodeficiency syndrome (AIDS), Arch Pathol Lab Med 110:744-746, 1986.
795. Strohmaier WL, Bichler KH, Wilbert DM et al: Alveolar echinococcosis with involvement of the ureter and testes, J Urol 144:733-734, 1990.
796. Sato K, Hirokawa K, Hatakeyama S: Experimental allergic orchitis in mice. Histopathological and immunological studies, Virchows Arch A Pathol Anat Histopathol 392:147-158, 1981.
797. Suominen J, Söderström KO: Lymphocytic infiltration in human testicular biopsies, Int J Androl 5:461-466, 1982.
798. Salomon F, Saremaslani P, Jacob M et al: Immune complex orchitis in infertile men. Immunoelectron microscopy of abnormal basement membrane structures, Lab Invest 47:555-567, 1982.
799. Lehmann D, Emmons LR: Immunological phenomena observed in the testis and their possible role in infertility, Am J Reprod Immunol 19:43-52, 1989.
800. El-Demiry MI, Hargreave TB, Bussuttil A: Immunocompetent cells in human testis in health and disease, Fertil Steril 48:470-479, 1987.
801. Gowing NFC: Malignant lymphoma of the tetis. In Pugh RCB, ed: Pathology of the testis, Oxford, 1976, Blackwell.
802. O'Regan S, Robitaille P: Orchitis mimicking testicular torsion in Henoch-Schönlein's purpura, J Urol 126:834-835, 1981.
803. Dahl EV, Baggenstoss AH, DeWeerd JH: Testicular lesions of periarteritis nodosa, with special reference to diagnosis, Am J Med 28:222-228, 1960.
804. Teichman JMH, Mattrey RF, Demby AM et al: Polyarteritis nodosa presenting as acute orchitis. A case report and review of the literature, J Urol 149:1139-1140, 1993.
805. Huisman TK, Collins WT, Voulgarakis GR: Polyarteritis nodosa masquerading as a primary testicular neoplasm. A case report and review of the literature, J Urol 114:1236-1238, 1990.
806. Shurbaji MS, Epstein JI: Testicular vasculitis. Implication for systemic disease, Hum Pathol 19:186-189, 1988.
807. Tomomasa H, Oshio S, Ameniya H et al: Testicular injury. Late results of semen analyses after orchiectomy, Arch Androl 29:59-63, 1992.
808. Wantz GE: Testicular atrophy as a sequela of inguinal hernioplasty, Int Surg 71:159-163, 1986.
809. Rutledge RH: Cooper's ligament repair for adult groin hernias, Surgery 87:601-610, 1980.
810. Roach R, Messing E, Starling J: Spontaneous thrombosis of left spermatic vein: report of 2 cases, J Urol 134:369-373, 1985.
811. Nistal M, Palacios J, Regadera J et al: Postsurgical focal testicular infarct, Urol Int 41:149-151, 1986.
812. Nawrocki JD, Cook AJ: Localised infarction of the testis, Br J Urol 69:541, 1992.
813. Cooper AP: Observations on the structure and diseases of the testis, London, 1930, McDowall.
814. Jenkins RH, Deming CL: Cysts of the testicle, New Engl J Med 213:57-59, 1935.
815. Sethney HT, Albers DD: Tunica albuginea cyst: rare testicular mass, Urology 15:285-286, 1980.
816. Leung ML, Gooding GAW, Williams RD: High-resolution sonography of scrotal contents in asymptomatic subjects, AJR Am J Roentgenol 143:161-164, 1984.
817. Haas GP, Shumaker BP, Cerny JC: The high incidence of benign testicular tumors, J Urol 138:1219-1220, 1987.
818. Gooding GAW, Leonhardt W, Stein R: Testicular cysts. US findings, Radiology 163:537-538, 1987.
819. Nistal M, Iñiguez L, Paniagua R: Cysts of the testicular parenchyma and tunica albuginea, Arch Pathol Lab Med 113:902-906, 1989.
820. Bryant J: Efferent ductule cyst of tunica albuginea, Urology 27:172-173, 1986.
821. Tejada E, Eble JN: Simple cyst of the rete testis, J Urol 139:376-377, 1988.
822. Tosi SE, Richardson JR: Simple cyst of the testis: case report and review of literature, J Urol 114:473-475, 1975.
823. Schmidt SS: Congenital simple cysts of the testis: a hitherto undescribed lesion, J Urol 96:236-238, 1966.
824. Takihara H, Valvo JR, Tokuhara M et al: Intratesticular cysts, Urology 20:80-82, 1982.
825. Hamm B, Fobbe F, Loy V: Testicular cysts: differentiation with US and clinical findings, Radiology 168:19-23, 1988.
826. Frater K: Cysts of the tunica albuginea (cysts of the testis), J Urol 21:135-136, 1929.
827. Arcadi JA: Cysts of the tunica albuginea testis, J Urol 68:631-632, 1952.
828. Mennemeyer RP, Mason JT: Non-neoplastic cystic lesions of the tunica albuginea: an electron microscopic and clinical study of 2 cases, J Urol 121:373-375, 1979.
829. Mancilla-Jiménez R, Matsuda GT: Cysts of the tunica albuginea: report of 4 cases and review of the literature, J Urol 114:730-733, 1975.
830. Warner KE, Noyes DT, Ross JS: Cysts of the tunica albuginea: a report of 3 cases with a review of the literature, J Urol 132:131-132, 1984.
831. Köbarth K, Kratzik CH: High resolution ultrasonography in the diagnosis of simple intratesticular cysts, J Urol 70:546-549, 1992.
832. Rifkin MD, Jacobs JA: Simple testicular cyst diagnosed preoperatively by ultrasound, J Urol 129:982-983, 1983.
833. Kratzik C, Hainz A, Kuber W et al: Surveillance strategy for intratesticular cysts: preliminary report, J Urol 143:313-315, 1990.
834. Altadonna V, Snyder HM, Rosenberg HK et al: Simple cysts of the testis in children: preoperative diagnosis by ultrasound and excision with testicular preservation, J Urol 140:1505-1507, 1988.
835. Nistal M, García-Villanueva M, Sánchez J: Displasia quística del testículo: anomalia en la diferenciación del parénquima testicular por probable fallo en la conexión entre los conductos de origen mesonéfrico y los cordones testiculares, Arch Esp Urol 29:431-444, 1976.

836. Nistal M, Paniagua R: Adenomatous hyperplasia of the rete testis, J Pathol 154:343-346, 1988.
837. Hartwick RWJ, Ro JY, Srigley JR et al: Adenomatous hyperplasia of the rete testis. A clinicopathologic study of nine cases, Am J Surg Pathol 15:350-357, 1991.
838. Ulbright TM, Gersell DJ: Rete testis hyperplasia with hyaline globule formation. A lesion simulating yolk sac tumor, Am J Surg Pathol 15:66-74, 1991.
839. Nistal M, Santamaría L, Paniagua R: Acquired cystic transformation of the rete testis secondary to renal failure, Hum Pathol 20:1065-1070, 1989.
840. Nistal M, Paniagua R: Nodular proliferation of calcifying connective tissue in the rete testis: a study of three cases, Hum Pathol 20:58-61, 1989.

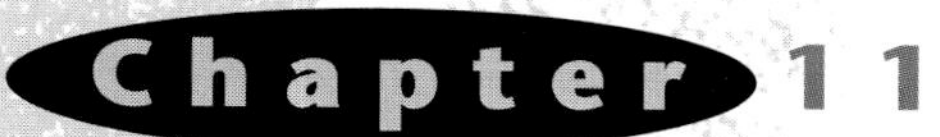

NEOPLASMS OF THE TESTIS

THOMAS M. ULBRIGHT

Despite an average weight of only 19 grams,[1] the testis is responsible for a complex array of neoplasms. The rapidly proliferating spermatogenic cells of the testis are the progenitors for the majority of testicular tumors, 95% of which are of germ cell derivation. These highly malignant tumors usually occur in young men but can be cured by current therapies; therefore, accurate diagnosis is essential. The supporting cells and interstitial cells of the testis are the progenitors for the rare sex-cord stromal tumors that are responsible for a disproportionate number of diagnostic problems. Some of these tumors are true neoplasms whereas others may represent hamartomatous lesions.[2,3] There are important associations among some of these nongerminal lesions with clinical syndromes that may be detected by testicular pathology.[4-6] Thus, it is important to recognize testicular tumors and their clinical significance.

STAGING

At present, there is no uniformly accepted system of staging for testicular cancer. Most staging systems are loosely based on the original method of Boden and Gibb,[7] which recognized an early, localized stage (confined to the testis), a stage of early dissemination (retroperitoneal lymph node involvement), and an advanced stage of dissemination (supradiaphragmatic involvement). Most of the controversy concerns the subdivision of the stage of retroperitoneal spread into clinically significant categories. A summary of several staging systems is provided in Table 11-1.[7-15] Staging may also be based on clinical and radiographic assessment of the patient or on pathologic examination of retroperitoneal lymph nodes. The methodology of staging must be explicitly stated.

PATTERNS OF METASTASIS

Testicular neoplasms, as exemplified by germ cell tumors, usually metastasize first to retroperitoneal lymph nodes. Seminoma tends to metastasize in an orderly pattern through lymphatics, whereas choriocarcinoma usually spreads by hematogenous routes. The other germ cell tumors, such as embryonal carcinoma, tend to have a lymphatic pattern of spread, although hematogenous spread can also be seen. There tends to be selective lymph node involvement with early stage tumors that depends on whether the right or left testis is involved. For right-sided tumors, the interaortocaval nodes, usually at about the level of the second lumbar vertebra, tend to be involved first, although right paracaval and precaval involvement may also occur.[8,9] In early stage involvement from right-sided tumors, there is an absence of both suprahilar nodal involvement and involvement of the left paraaortic nodes below the inferior mesenteric artery.[9] For left-sided tumors, the left paraaortic nodes, in an area bounded by the left ureter, left renal vein, aorta, and origin of the inferior mesenteric artery, are first involved.[8] Suprahilar nodal metastases may be seen in early stage disease from left-sided testicular tumors, in contrast to right-sided lesions.[9] As metastases become more widespread, right-sided lesions develop suprahilar and contralateral spread and left-sided tumors develop interaortocaval and precaval involvement, as well as a greater frequency of suprahilar involvement. As the volume of retroperitoneal disease increases, retrograde involvement of iliac and inguinal nodes may be seen.[9] Inguinal nodal involvement may also be seen when the primary tumor has extended to the scrotal skin or a transcrotal approach was used for the primary resection. The extension of the primary tumor to the epididymis also correlates with the development of external iliac nodal spread. Eventually, supradiaphragmatic spread occurs to the mediastinum and supraclavicular and cervical lymph nodes, tending to involve the left supraclavicular nodes much more commonly than the right.[16] Hematogenous spread is most commonly reflected by lung, liver, central nervous system, and bone involvement.[17]

GROSS EXAMINATION

The gross examination and proper handling of the orchiectomy specimen is often neglected, and many diagnostic problems at the microscope can be traced to poor processing of the gross specimen. Under the best circumstances the testis and accompanying tunics and spermatic cord should be received fresh, dissected, and allowed to thoroughly fix before tissue blocks are submitted. What generally happens, however, is the urologist places the radical orchiectomy specimen intact into fixative, and only hours later is the specimen dissected. The testicular tunics do not permit ready penetration of fixative, so this approach results in autolytic changes in the neoplasm. It would be preferable for the urologist to make a single, virtually through and through incision in the specimen before placing it into fixative if it is not feasible to immediately send it to the laboratory.

A radical orchiectomy specimen consists of the testis, tunica vaginalis, and a portion of spermatic cord. The specimen should be weighed, measured in three dimensions, and the length of the cord noted. The tunica vaginalis should be incised, any abnormalities described, the quantity and nature of any intratunical fluid recorded, and the tunica albuginea carefully inspected and palpated for penetration by neoplasm. The testis should then be bisected in the plane of its long axis, through the testicular hilum, by a long, sharp knife. Fresh tissues may then be harvested for special studies such as cytogenetics, flow cytometry, electron microscopy, and oncogene analysis. Photographs may be obtained, and then multiple, serial, parallel cuts at 3 mm intervals should be made, leaving the tunica albuginea intact posteriorly to keep the specimen together. The specimen should then be placed in a generous volume of the pathologist's preferred fixative (10% neutral buffered formalin is suitable) and allowed to thoroughly fix prior to further processing.

After fixation, the neoplasm should be described and measured, with particular attention to the relationships to the tunica albuginea and the testicular hilum. Multiple blocks of neoplasm should be submitted, because many tumors are quite heterogeneous. Blocks of all of the different-appearing areas must be submitted and hemorrhagic and necrotic areas must be included in the samples. A minimum of one block of neoplasm for every

TABLE 11-1.
STAGING SYSTEM FOR TESTICULAR CANCER

TNM System[10] (American Joint Committee [AJC])	Stage Grouping for AJC-TNM System	TNM System (UICC)[11]	Boden/Gibb[7]	Memorial Sloan Kettering Cancer Center	Royal Marsden[8,9]	M.D. Anderson[13]	Skinner[14]	Massachusetts General Hospital[15]
Tx—Unknown status of testis T0—No apparent primary (includes scars) Tis—Intratubular tumor, no invasion T2—Beyond tunica albuginea or into epididymis T3—Spermatic cord T4—Scrotum Nx—Unknown nodal status N0—No regional node involvement N1—Single node ≤2 cm N2—Single node 2-5 cm or multiple nodes ≤5 cm N3—Any nodes >5 cm Mx—Unknown status of distant metastases M0—No distant metastases M1—Distant metastases	Stage 0—Tis N0, M0 Stage I—Any T Stage II—Any T, N1-N3, M0 Stage III—Any T, Any N, M0	T0—No apparent primary T1—Testis only (excludes rete testis) T2—Beyond the tunic albuginea T3—Rete testis or epididymal involvement T4—Spermatic cord a—Spermatic cord b—Scrotum N0—No nodal involvement N1—Ipsilateral regional nodal involvement N2—Contralateral or bilateral abdominal or groin nodes N3—Palpable abdominal nodes or fixed groin nodes N4—Juxtaregional nodes M0—No distant metastases M1—Distant metastases present	A—Testis only B—Regional nodal metastases C—Spread beyond retroperitoneal nodes	A—Testis and adnexa only B—Infradiaphragmatic nodal metastases B1—<5 cm B2—5 to 10 cm B3—>10 cm C—Spread beyond retroperitoneal nodes	I—Testis only (I^m continued positive serologic evidence of tumor after orchiectomy) II—Infradiaphragmatic nodal involvement IIA—<2 cm IIB—2 to 5 cm IIC—>5 cm III—Supraclavicular or mediastinal involvement IV—Extranodal metastases IVL—Lung metastases IVH—Liver metastases	I—Testis only IIA—Negative lymphangioma but pathologically positive retroperitoneal nodes IIB—Positive lymphangiogram IIIA—Supraclavicular nodes IIIB1—Gynecomastia, lacking gross tumor IIIB2—Lung metastasis (no more than 5 nodules per lung and not >2 cm) IIIB3—Advanced lung IIIB4—Advanced abdominal or obstructive uropathy IIIB5—Visceral disease, excluding lung	A—Testis only B—Infradiaphragmatic B1—<6 nodes, no extranodal extension B2—>6 nodes or any node >2 cm B3—Bulky disease (>5 cm) C—Supradiaphragmatic involvement	I—Testis only II—Retroperitoneal involvement IIA—<2 cm IIB—≥2 cm III—Supraclavicular and mediastinal IV—Disseminated disease

TNM - tumor, nodes, metastases; UICC - International Union Against Cancer

From Ulbright TM, Roth LM: Testicular and paratesticular tumors. In Sternberg SS, ed: Diagnostic surgical pathology, ed 2, New York, 1994, Raven Press; by permission.

centimeter of maximum tumor dimension is a general rule of thumb; however, it is prudent to submit blocks quite generously if the gross appearance suggests seminoma, because the discovery of nonseminomatous elements will usually change the therapy. Hence, small seminomas should be submitted whole, and at least 10 blocks of larger tumors (or one block for every centimeter of maximum tumor dimension, whichever is the larger number) should be submitted. The non-neoplastic testis should also be sampled, as well as a block to include the testicular hilum. The epididymis should be incised by multiple, parallel cuts perpendicular to its long axis, any abnormalities should be noted, and the appropriate blocks should be submitted. The resection margin of the spermatic cord should be submitted separately, as well as blocks from the proximal and mid-cord.

GERM CELL TUMORS

CLASSIFICATION

About 95% of testicular neoplasms are of germ cell origin. The classification of testicular germ cell tumors presented in the box on this page is a modification of the classification of the World Health Organization (WHO)[18] and contrasts with the classification frequently employed in Great Britain, which stems from the work of the British Testicular Tumour Panel (BTTP).[19] The fundamental tenet of the WHO-based classification is that these neoplasms are of germ cell derivation but with differentiation to various embryonic, adult, or extra-embryonic tissues. Hence, embryonal carcinoma resembles the undifferentiated cells of the embryonic plate; yolk sac tumor resembles structures of the embryonic yolk sac of the rodent, as well as the extra-embryonic mesenchyme and allantoic membranes; teratoma resembles either adult type (mature teratoma) or embryonic type (immature teratoma) somatic tissues; and seminoma consists of cells resembling primitive, fetal gonocytes (the primordial germ cells). Conversely, the BTTP system is based on the erroneous notion that nonseminomatous tumors are derived from displaced, nonorganized embryonic blastomeres and, hence, are all teratomatous.[20] This concept results in two fundamental divisions—seminomas and teratomas. Table 11-2 compares the WHO-based system and the BTTP system.[21,22] The BTTP system classifies histologically disparate lesions under a common nomenclature, which makes comparative studies impossible.[11] The WHO-based classification is therefore preferable.

HISTOGENESIS

The histogenesis of testicular germ cell tumors, while still controversial, has been clarified by recent observations. Perhaps most important is the recognition that all forms of testicular germ cell tumor, with the notable exception of spermatocytic seminoma, are derived from a common precursor, which Skakkebaek[23-26] originally recognized and described as *carcinoma-in-situ* of the testis. The preferred term for this lesion, given the nonepithelial nature of the constituent cells, is *intratubular germ cell neoplasia of the unclassified type* (IGCNU).[27,28] This lesion consists of an initially basilar proliferation of seminoma-

CLASSIFICATION OF TESTICULAR TUMORS

Germ Cell Tumors

- Precursor Lesion
  - Intratubular germ cell neoplasia (carcinoma in situ)
- Tumors of One Histologic Type
  - Seminoma
    - Variant: Seminoma with syncytiotrophoblastic cells
  - Spermatocytic seminoma
    - Variant: Spermatocytic seminoma with a sarcomatous component
  - Embryonal carcinoma
  - Yolk sac tumor (endodermal sinus tumor)
  - Choriocarcinoma
  - Teratoma
    - Mature teratoma
      - Dermoid cyst
    - Immature teratoma
    - Teratoma with an overtly malignant component
    - Monodermal variants
      - Carcinoid (pure and with teratomatous elements)
      - Primitive neuroectodermal tumor
- Tumors of More than One Histologic Type
  - Mixed germ cell tumors (specify individual components and estimate their amount as a percentage)
    - Polyembryoma
    - Diffuse embryoma

Sex Cord-Stromal Tumors

- Leydig cell tumor
- Sertoli cell tumor
  - Typical
  - Sclerosing
  - Large cell calcifying
- Granulosa cell
  - Adult
  - Juvenile
- Mixed sex cord–stromal tumors
- Unclassified sex cord–stromal tumors

Mixed Germ Cell/Sex Cord–Stromal Tumors

- Gonadoblastoma
- Others

Tumors of the Rete Testis

- Adenocarcinoma
- Adenoma
- Adenomatous hyperplasia

Tumors of Hematopoietic Origin

- Lymphoma
- Plasmacytoma
- Leukemia

Miscellaneous

- Epidermoid cyst
- Mesenchymal tumors
- Metastatic tumors

TABLE 11-2.
COMPARISON OF NOMENCLATURES BETWEEN THE WHO-BASED SYSTEM AND THE BRITISH TESTICULAR TUMOUR PANEL (BTTP) CLASSIFICATION

Modified WHO Classification	BTTP Classification
Tumors of One Histologic Type	
Seminoma	Seminoma
Spermatocytic seminoma	Spermatocytic seminoma
Embryonal carcinoma	Malignant teratoma, undifferentiated (MTU)
Yolk sac tumor (adult type)	MTU
Yolk sac tumor (childhood type)	Yolk sac tumor
Teratoma	
Mature	Teratoma, differentiated (TD)
Immature	TD
With an overtly malignant component	Malignant teratoma, intermediate (MTI)
Choriocarcinoma (pure)	
Mixed Germ Cell Tumors	
Embryonal carcinoma & mature and/or immature teratoma	MTI
Yolk sac tumor & mature and/or immature teratoma	MTI
Seminoma and teratoma	Combined tumor (seminoma & TD)
Seminoma & embryonal carcinoma	Combined tumor (seminoma & MTU)
Choriocarcinoma & embryonal carcinoma	Malignant teratoma, trophoblastic (MTT)
Choriocarcinoma & teratoma	MTT
Choriocarcinoma & seminoma	Combined tumor (MTT & seminoma)

Adapted from Mostofi FK: Comparison of various clinical and pathological classifications of tumors of testes, Semin Oncol 6:26-30, 1979 and Pugh RCB, Parkinson C: The origin and classification of testicular germ cell tumours, Int J Androl 4(Suppl):15-25, 1981. Table reprinted from Ulbright TM, Roth LM: Testicular and paratesticular neoplasms. In Sternberg SS, ed: Diagnostic surgical pathology, ed 2, New York, 1994, Raven Press.

like cells with clear cytoplasm, and enlarged, hyperchromatic nuclei, which may have one or two prominent nucleoli. Genetic changes in IGCNU include anomalies of the short arm of chromosome 12, commonly in the form of an isochromosome of the short arms—i(12p).[29] As might be expected, the derivative invasive germ cell tumors also have anomalous overrepresentation of 12p, either in the form of i(12p) or other cytogenetic anomalies.[30,31] Deletions from the short arm of chromosome 11 have also been implicated as an early event in testicular germ cell neoplasia.[32]

The cells of IGCNU and seminoma appear to be identical according to the light microscopy of the two cell types, their ultrastructure,[33,34] the immunohistochemical reactions with monoclonal antibodies M_2A[35] and TRA-1-60[36] and antibodies directed against placental-like alkaline phosphatase[37-39] and glutathione-S-transferase (isoenzyme pi),[40] the DNA content,[41] the common presence of i(12p),[42] the number of nucleolar organizer regions,[43] and the lectin binding patterns.[44]

The identity of IGCNU and seminoma implies that seminoma is also a precursor for other germ cell tumors. This interpretation is supported by a number of observations. First, pure testicular seminoma may subsequently develop nonseminomatous elements according to histologic examination or elevation of serum alpha-fetoprotein. Autopsy studies of patients who died of metastatic germ cell neoplasm following resections of pure testicular seminoma have demonstrated nonseminomatous elements in 30% to 40% of cases.[17,45] By light microscopy, seminoma may appear to transform either to embryonal carcinoma or to yolk sac tumor.[46,47] Also, 10% to 20% of seminomas contain syncytiotrophoblastic cells, and some trophoblastic hormone-containing cells in seminoma are not easily distinguished histologically from the surrounding seminoma cells.[48-50] Ultrastructural studies of seminoma have demonstrated evidence of epithelial differentiation (seminoma with early carcinomatous features) in some light microscopically typical cases.[51] Furthermore, the DNA content of seminoma is consistently higher than in nonseminomatous germ cell tumors,[41,42,52] suggesting that nonseminomatous tumors evolve from seminoma as a consequence of gene loss, perhaps caused by loss of cancer suppressor genes. Karyotypic analyses have shown a striking tendency for certain chromosomes to be in parallel excess or deficiency in seminoma and the nonseminomatous germ cell tumors.[42] These data indicate that seminoma may transform to nonseminomatous tumors.

Transformation of IGCNU to nonseminomatous tumors may occur within the seminiferous tubules or at the time of extratubular extension of IGCNU. The common occurrence of seminoma with nonseminomatous elements also supports transformation from invasive seminoma, but the occurrence of pure embryonal carcinoma, yolk sac tumor, or choriocarcinoma, associated with IGCNU, is consistent with either of the other two mechanisms of transformation. IGCNU adjacent to

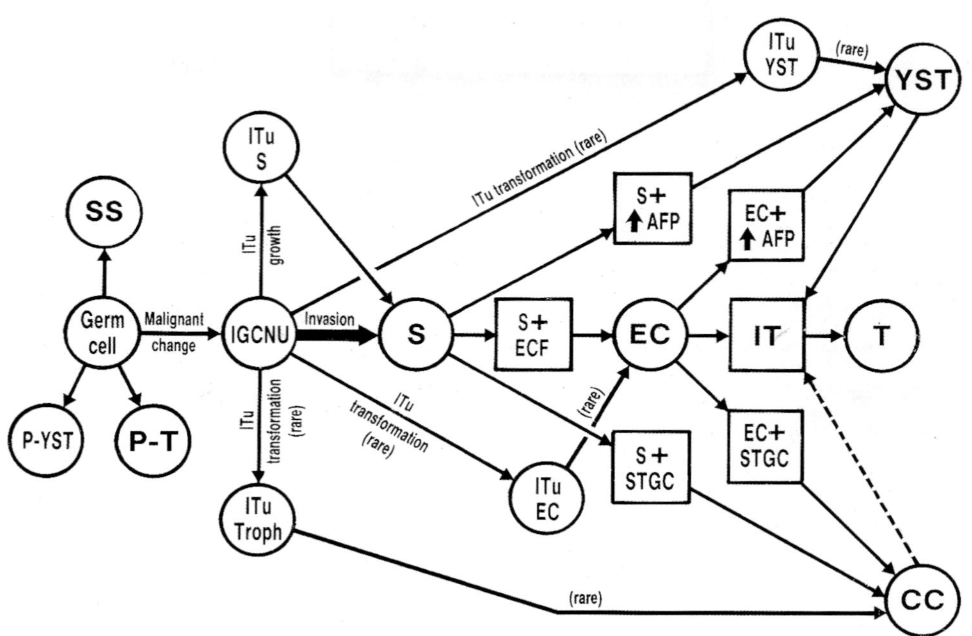

11-1. New model of germ cell tumor histogenesis, based on the tetrahedron model of Srigley et al.[51] In this model, seminoma plays a pivotal role as a precursor to many other forms of germ cell tumor, although nonseminomatous tumors may develop directly from IGCNU. There are transitional forms of some neoplasms. Abbreviations: AFP, alpha-fetoprotein; CC, choriocarcinoma; EC, embryonal carcinoma; ECF, early carcinomatous features; IGCNU, intratubular germ cell neoplasia, unclassified; IT, immature teratoma; Itu, intratubular; P-T, pediatric teratoma; P-YST, pediatric yolk sac tumor; S, seminoma; SS, spermatocytic seminoma; STGC, syncytiotrophoblastic giant cells; T, teratoma; Troph, trophoblastic cells; YST, yolk sac tumor; broken arrow indicates more speculative step. *(From Ulbright TM, Roth LM: Testicular and paratesticular neoplasms. In Sternberg SS, ed: Diagnostic surgical pathology, ed 2, New York, 1994, Raven Press, by permission of Raven Press; adapted from Srigley JR, Toth P, Edwards V: Diagnostic electron microscopy of male genital tract tumors, Clin Lab Med 7:91-115, 1987.)*

seminoma or nonseminomatous tumors shares certain chromosomal abnormalities with the invasive tumor, and these abnormalities differ depending on whether the adjacent tumor is seminomatous or nonseminomatous,[53] an observation that supports the occurrence of genetic transformation within the tubules before morphological change. These observations led to a revised model of testicular germ cell tumor histogenesis, based on the tetrahedron model proposed by Srigley et al (Fig. 11-1).[51]

EPIDEMIOLOGY

Germ cell tumors of the testis (with the exception of spermatocytic seminoma) occur almost exclusively in young males, with the incidence accelerating rapidly following puberty and peaking close to 30 years of age (Fig. 11-2). There is a smaller peak in early childhood, but the peak of testicular cancer in elderly men corresponds to lymphomatous involvement of the testis rather than to germ cell tumors (see Fig. 11-2). White males have a much higher frequency of testicular germ cell tumors than do nonwhite males, with the exception of the Maori of New Zealand who have an incidence comparable to white populations.[54,55] Native Hawaiians, Native Alaskans, and Native Americans are at higher risk than other nonwhites.[56] Denmark and Switzerland have the highest rates of testicular cancer, about 9 cases per 100,000 males per year, compared with the rate in the United States white population of about 6 per 100,000 males. The rates in Africans and Asians are generally about 1 per 100,000 males.[57] The incidence of testicular germ cell tumors has increased steadily in the United States during the twentieth century,[58] and a similar trend has been noted in several other countries,[59] including Denmark,[60] England,[61] Scotland,[62] New Zealand,[55] and Australia.[63]

Numerous studies have confirmed a higher frequency of testicular germ cell tumors in professional workers or those of higher socioeconomic class compared to laborers or those of lower socioeconomic class.[55,56,64-68] Higher frequency has also been found in those with occupational exposure to fertilizers, phenols, heat, smoke, or fumes;[69] in farm workers, draftsmen, and those in food manufacture and preparation;[65] in leather workers;[70,71] in policemen exposed to hand-held radar;[72] in aircraft repairmen;[73] in motor vehicle mechanics;[55] in electrical workers, fishermen, paper and printing workers, and foresters;[64] and in physicians.[55] Other studies have suggested other etiologies, including in-utero exposure to estrogenic compounds,[74,75] various HLA-haplotypes,[76-83] a family history of breast cancer,[84] early puberty,[84] early birth order,[74] ichthyosis,[85] Marfan syndrome,[86] the Li-Fraumeni syndrome,[87] and dysplastic nevus syndrome.[88] Most of these associations, however, are weak and fail to

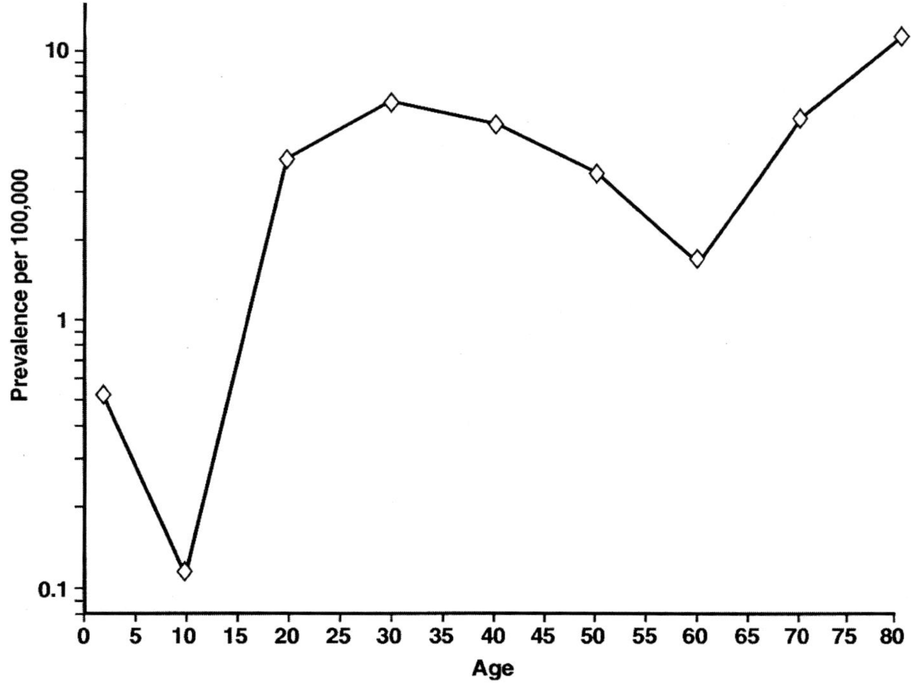

11-2. Prevalence of testicular tumors according to patient age. Note a small peak in infancy, nadir at age 10 years, and rapid rise after puberty. The peak incidence occurs at 25 to 30 years. The late peak corresponds to nongerminal tumors, mainly lymphoma.

TABLE 11-3.
ESTIMATED INCREASED RISKS OF TESTICULAR GERM CELL TUMORS ASSOCIATED WITH CERTAIN CONDITIONS

Condition	Estimated Increased Risk	References
Cryptorchidism	3.5–5X	96, 98
Prior testicular germ cell tumor	5–10X	1, 99–101
Family history (first degree male relative)	5.5X	102, 103
Gonadal dysgenesis with a Y-chromosome	50X*	1, 104, 105
Androgen insensitivity syndrome	15X	1, 3, 106–108

*Includes cases of gonadoblastoma.

account for the general increase in testicular germ cell tumors. It is hypothesized that important causative factors in testicular cancer occur in the antenatal period, with a protective effect noted in Denmark for men born during the Nazi occupation.[59] The use of alcohol and tobacco, prior vasectomy, and radiation exposure have not been associated with testicular germ cell tumors.[54,89,90] Despite the weak correlation of most etiologic factors with testicular germ cell tumors,[54,91] four contributing factors are proven: cryptorchidism, prior testicular germ cell tumor, family history of testicular germ cell tumors, and certain somatosexual ambiguity syndromes. An estimate of the increased risks associated with these disorders is provided in Table 11-3.

Cryptorchidism

An increased frequency of cryptorchidism, varying from 6.5% to 14.5%, has been found in patients with testicular germ cell tumors,[58,75,92-97] which has led to increased risk calculations of 2.5 to 35 times higher among cryptorchid patients.[93-96,98,109-114] Such risk does not manifest prior to 20 years of age[98] and is probably most accurately assessed as 3.5 to 5.0 times increased over a control population.[96,98] If cryptorchidism is unilateral, the noncryptorchid testis is also at increased risk for a testicular germ cell tumor, although at a lower rate than the cryptorchid testis.[56,109,111,115,116] Ectopia alone cannot explain the association of cryptorchidism and testicular germ cell tumor, a fact reinforced by the failure of orchidopexy to reduce the risk[97,109,117] (although there is probably insufficient experience with orchidopexy in the very young to rule out an ameliorating effect[56]). It is possible that cryptorchidism is a marker of patients with a general defect in genitourinary embryogenesis and that cryptorchid testes are dysgenetic,[118] as supported by abnormalities of the external genitalia or sex chromosomes in some cryptorchid patients with germ cell tumor.[119] Patients with cryptorchidism and testicular germ cell tumor appear to have a disproportionate risk for seminoma.[92,113,120,121]

About 2% to 8% of patients with cryptorchidism have IGCNU,[122-124] and at least 50% of such patients develop germ cell tumor within 5 years.[23] Giwercman et al[125] cite a 2.8% frequency of IGCNU in the cryptorchid population, a four-fold increase over the general population of young men. Thus, bilateral testicular biopsy at 18 to 20 years of age is recommended for cryptorchid patients.[126] A negative result is excellent evidence of no increased risk,[122] and a positive biopsy should prompt orchiectomy of the affected testis. In testes with extreme atrophy, the biopsy should be directed to sample the region near the rete testis.[127] Nodules composed of small tubules lined by Sertoli cells, often with central deposits of basement membrane, are commonly identified in cryptorchid testes, as well as in noncryptorchid testes. These Sertoli cell nodules have been termed *Pick's adenoma* but are not true neoplasms.[128,129]

Prior testicular germ cell tumor

A second germ cell tumor occurs in the remaining testis of 2% to 5% of patients with a previous germ cell tumor.[100,130-136] Similarly, there is a 4.5% to 6.6% frequency of IGCNU in the opposite testis of patients with a germ cell tumor.[99-101,136] There is no apparent increased risk in the absence of IGCNU on biopsy.[137] If the residual testis is either atrophic[138] or cryptorchid, the risk is even greater,[101] with a 23% frequency of IGCNU.[99] Almost 50% of cases of contralateral IGCNU would be missed if contralateral biopsies were restricted to patients with atrophy or cryptorchidism.[101] A recent study suggested that atrophy rather than maldescent is the important predictor of contralateral IGCNU.[138] Young age at onset of the first tumor and bilateral cryptorchidism also appear to be associated with an increased risk of bilateral occurrence.[100] About 50% of second primary tumors of the testis occur 3 to 5 years after the diagnosis of the initial germ cell tumor,[132,139] but intervals of more than a decade can occur.[140] Concordant or discordant histologies may occur, with some tendency for concordance of pure seminoma.[132] The risk of bilateral tumors in patients with a germ cell tumor is increased about four-fold with a positive family history.[141,142] Chemotherapy treatment of the first tumor decreases the risk of a contralateral tumor.[134,135] An increased frequency of rare alleles of the Ha-*ras*1 oncogene is seen in patients with testicular germ cell tumors, and such rare alleles are associated with bilaterality and early age of onset.[143]

Family history

First degree male relatives of patients with germ cell tumor of the testis have a 5.5 times greater risk of a testicular germ cell tumor than the general population.[102,103] Also, a family history of testicular germ cell tumor is associated with an 8% to 14% frequency of bilaterality[102,141] compared to the 2% to 5% frequency in the general population of patients with testicular germ cell tumors.[130-133] The occurrence of an unexpected number of testicular germ cell tumors in the relatives of children with soft tissue sarcomas has raised the question of whether testicular germ cell tumors may represent part of the spectrum of the Li-Fraumeni cancer syndrome.[144] It remains controversial, however, if p53 mutations commonly occur in testicular germ cell tumors. p53 protein is identified in some cases,[145,146] and one study identified gene mutations,[147] whereas no such mutations were identified in others.[148,149] Immunohistochemical demonstration of p53 protein may therefore indicate overexpression of nonmutated protein.

Intersex syndromes

Patients with some intersex syndromes are at increased risk for germ cell tumors. Patients with gonadal dysgenesis in the presence of a Y-chromosome, including patients with pure 46XY gonadal dysgenesis (Swyer's syndrome), mixed gonadal dysgenesis, and dysgenetic male pseudohermaphroditism, commonly develop gonadal germ cell tumors.[104,105,150] About 25% to 30% of such patients develop gonadoblastoma,[104,105] and this may serve as the precursor lesion for the development of an invasive germ cell tumor. IGCNU is also present in about 8% of children and adolescents with gonadal dysgenesis.[151] Because an invasive tumor may develop in childhood, gonadectomy is indicated as soon as the diagnosis is established. Male pseudohermaphrodites with the androgen insensitivity syndrome develop a malignant germ cell tumor in 5% to 10% of cases.[3,106-108,152] The tumor usually develops after puberty, and this may permit delayed gonadectomy until full feminization has occurred, although this remains controversial because of an occasional case of invasive germ cell tumor developing at an early age. Delay of prophylactic gonadectomy beyond the early postpubescent period in patients with the androgen insensitivity syndrome is risky,[106] with a 22% frequency of malignant germ cell tumor in such patients beyond 30 years of age.[153] Not all testicular masses in patients with the androgen insensitivity syndrome are germ cell tumors; these patients commonly develop hamartomatous nodules composed of Sertoli cell–lined tubules with intervening clusters of Leydig cells in the interstitium, as well as pure Sertoli cell adenomas.[3,104,108]

Infertility

Patients with infertility have about a 1% frequency of testicular germ cell tumor.[33,99] It is not clear, however, if infertility is a risk factor for germ cell tumor that is independent of cryptorchidism or gonadal dysgenesis.[154]

INTRATUBULAR GERM CELL NEOPLASIA

Grossly, the testis with IGCNU may be unremarkable or appear atrophic and fibrotic. Microscopically, intratubular germ cell neoplasia consists of a proliferation of

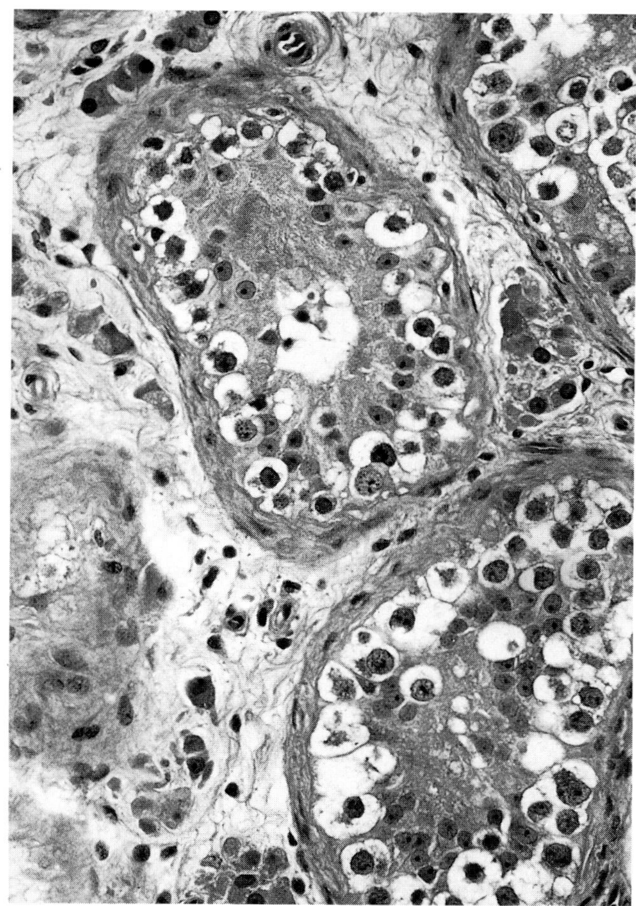

11-3. IGCNU in seminiferous tubules.

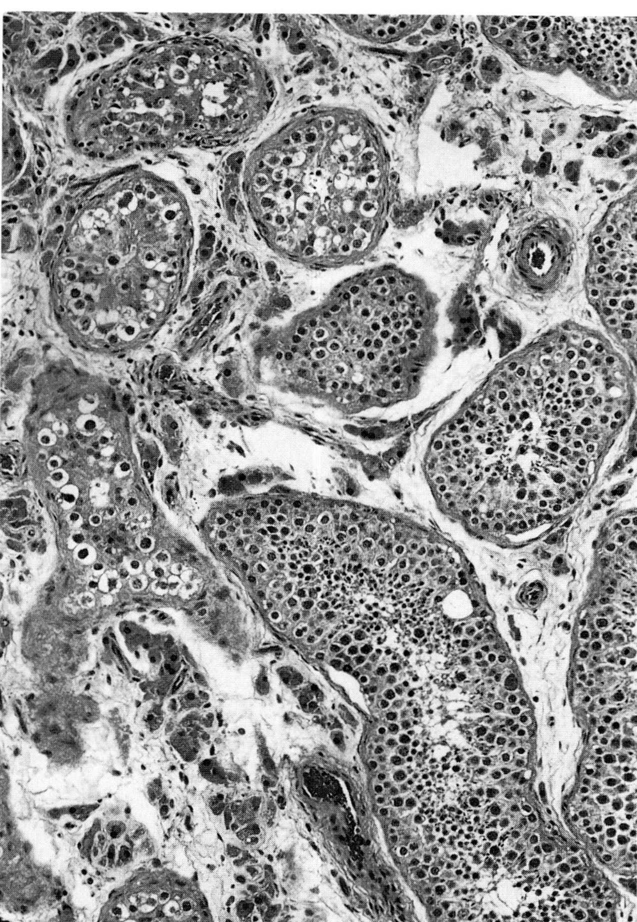

11-4. Patchy distribution of IGCNU. Tubules lacking IGCNU have spermatogenesis and are adjacent to tubules with IGCNU and lacking spermatogenesis.

malignant germ cells, which may be a specific neoplastic type, such as intratubular embryonal carcinoma or intratubular spermatocytic seminoma, or may consist of undifferentiated germ cells resembling primitive gonocytes. The primitive gonocyte-like form of intratubular germ cell neoplasia is typically confined to the basilar aspect of the seminiferous tubules and is associated with all types of germ cell tumors, except for spermatocytic seminoma. It is called *intratubular germ cell neoplasia of the unclassified type* (IGCNU). The cells of IGCNU have enlarged, hyperchromatic nuclei, often with one or two prominent nucleoli, thickened nuclear membranes, and clear cytoplasm (Fig. 11-3). The median nuclear diameter of the cells of IGCNU is 9.7 μm, compared with a median nuclear diameter in spermatogonia of 6.5 μm.[155] Spermatogenesis in the affected tubules is usually decreased or absent, and the tubules may have a thickened peritubular basement membrane. Sertoli cells are often displaced luminally (see Fig. 11-3). The distribution of IGCNU is characteristically patchy, and adjacent profiles of seminiferous tubules may appear unremarkable, with intact spermatogenesis (Fig. 11-4). Leydig cell hyperplasia may occur in the interstitium. IGCNU often spreads into the rete testis in a "pagetoid" fashion, intermixing with non-neoplastic epithelium.[156] The strong similarity of the cells of seminoma and IGCNU suggests that IGCNU could be termed intratubular seminoma; however, this term may falsely connote that IGCNU is the precursor lesion only for seminoma rather than for virtually all postpubertal germ cell tumors. By convention, the term *intratubular seminoma* is reserved for those proliferations of IGCNU-like cells that fill and distend seminiferous tubules. Skakkebaek and co-workers used the term *carcinoma-in-situ* for IGCNU; although *carcinoma-in-situ* does correctly imply the tendency of this lesion to progress to invasive germ cell tumor, it is histogenetically inaccurate because the cells of IGCNU are not of epithelial type.[33,157,158]

Special studies

Glycogen is present in the cytoplasm of 98% of cases of IGCNU (Fig. 11-5),[159] and its demonstration is diagnostically helpful but nonspecific because non-neoplastic spermatogonia and Sertoli cells may also contain glycogen.[160] Equally sensitive but more specific for IGCNU are immunostains directed against placental alkaline

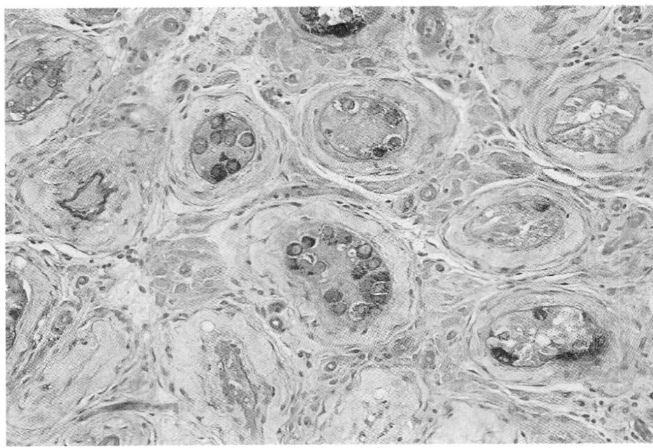

11-5. Cytoplasmic glycogen in IGCNU, periodic acid–Schiff stain.

phosphatase, which highlight a placental-like alkaline phosphatase (PLAP) with a predominantly cytoplasmic membrane pattern of distribution in virtually every case (Fig. 11-6).[160,161] Only rarely (less than 1%) are isolated non-neoplastic spermatocytes (which are unlikely to be confused with IGCNU) PLAP-positive, with spermatogonia being PLAP-negative.[162] IGCNU has also been found to react with monoclonal antibodies M_2A, 43-9F, and TRA-1-60 and with antibodies directed against glutathione-S-transferase, isoenzyme pi.[35,36,40,163-165] By electron microscopy, IGCNU has evenly dispersed chromatin, intricate nucleoli, and sparse cytoplasmic organelles with prominent glycogen deposits. Occasional rudimentary intercellular junctions may be identified.[33,158,166-168] These features are essentially the same as those of seminoma.[169] The DNA content of IGCNU is similar to that of seminoma, usually in the triploid and hypotetraploid range.[41,170] IGCNU, like many invasive germ cell tumors, contains isochromosome 12p.[29] The positive reactions for PLAP and TRA-1-60 of IGCNU support the idea that IGCNU resembles fetal gonocytes.[36,38,171]

Differential diagnosis

IGCNU should be distinguished from the specific forms of intratubular germ cell neoplasia. Intratubular seminoma fills and distends the tubules, whereas IGCNU is restricted to the basilar area, although the cells are identical. Intratubular seminoma is usually seen in conjunction with invasive seminoma.

Prognosis

The practical importance of IGCNU is its progression to an invasive germ cell tumor (either seminomatous or nonseminomatous) in about 50% of cases within 5 years after identification.[172] Also, only a fraction of patients remain free of an invasive tumor by 7 or 8 years of follow-up[173] (Fig. 11-7), although some patients may not develop a tumor for more than 15 years.[125] Furthermore, there is no documented case of spontaneous regression of typical IGCNU.[125] IGCNU is identified with increased frequency in patients with cryptorchidism,[33,122-124,126] a previous history of a testicular germ cell tumor,[136,137,174,175] gonadal

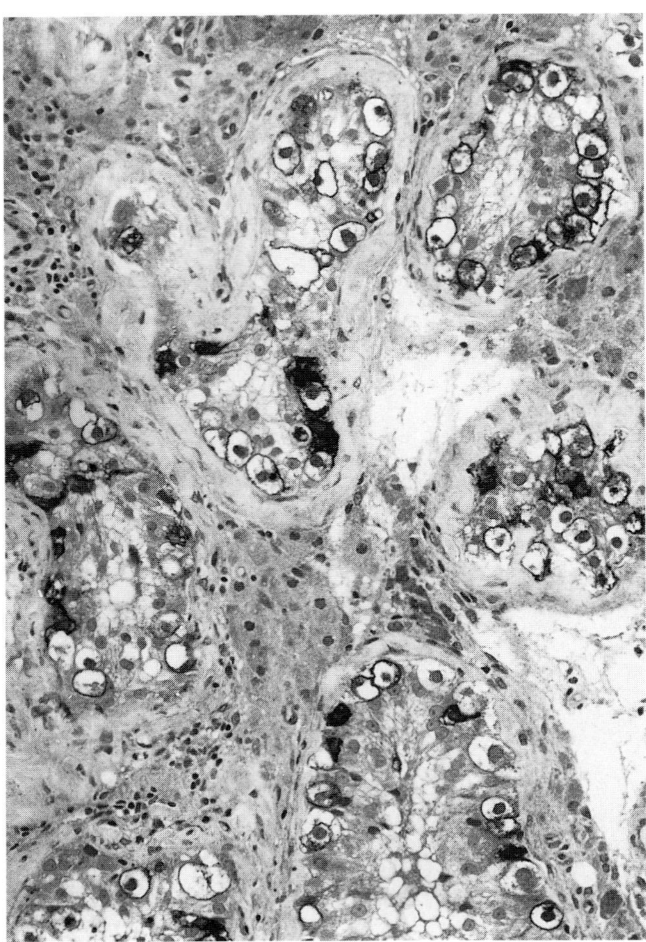

11-6. Anti-placental alkaline phosphatase demonstrates intense, cytoplasmic membrane-associated reactivity in IGCNU. Focal cytoplasmic staining is also present.

dysgenesis,[176] androgen insensitivity syndrome,[177] and infertility.[24,175,178] IGCNU is also identified in the residual seminiferous tubules of virtually every postpubertal patient with an invasive testicular germ cell tumor with the exception of spermatocytic seminoma.[23,159,179-181]

The association of IGCNU with pediatric germ cell tumors is controversial, with some studies reporting an absence of IGCNU in prepubertal patients with yolk sac tumor[182] or teratoma,[183] but recent case reports describing IGCNU in a few pediatric tumors.[170,184-186] These reports described cells with the characteristic morphology and immunoreactivity of IGCNU, and, in one instance, with triploidy for chromosome 1 that contrasted with the tetraploidy of the invasive tumor.[170,184] Nonetheless the association of the pediatric tumors with IGCNU is much less constant than the association of postpubertal tumors with IGCNU.

Biopsy diagnosis

Testicular biopsies are a sensitive method for detecting IGCNU. Fixatives such as Bouin's, B-5, and Stieve's enhance cytologic detail and permit easier detection of IGCNU compared to formalin fixation. Berthelsen and

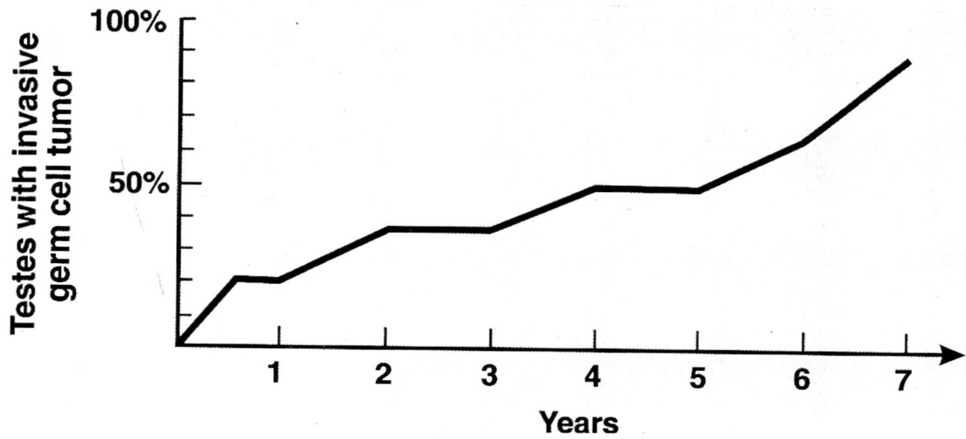

11-7. Follow-up of patients with IGCNU on biopsy. About 90% have invasive tumor after 7 years.

Skakkebaek concluded that one or two 3 mm biopsies of a testis harboring IGCNU will detect virtually every case.[187] In cases of severe atrophy, with obliteration of many tubules, it may be necessary to sample the region near the hilum where IGCNU is often preserved within the epithelium of the rete testis.[127] Bilateral biopsy is indicated because IGCNU occurs bilaterally in up to 30% to 40% of cases with infertility.[24,178] Potential populations for screening biopsies include patients with cryptorchidism, a prior testicular germ cell tumor, somatosexual ambiguity in the presence of a Y-chromosome, and, less strongly, oligospermic infertility.[125,155] IGCNU in a biopsy from a patient with retroperitoneal germ cell tumor probably indicates the regression of a prior invasive tumor that had metastasized to the retroperitoneum.[188,189] Therefore, a patient with presumed primary germ cell tumor of the retroperitoneum may benefit from testicular biopsy[125].

Treatment

Because of the high rate of progression of IGCNU to invasive testicular germ cell tumor, these patients should receive appropriate ablative treatment. Unilateral IGCNU is usually managed by orchiectomy, and bilateral IGCNU may be treated by bilateral orchiectomy or radiation. Chemotherapy, often given to patients with metastatic disease from a contralateral testicular tumor, may ablate IGCNU in the residual testis but is not a consistently effective means of therapy.[155,190-192]

SEMINOMA

Clinical features

Seminoma is the most common form of pure testicular germ cell tumor, and pure seminoma accounts for almost 50% of all cases of testicular germ cell tumor.[193,194] It occurs in patients with an average age of 40 years,[193] which is about 10 years older than those patients with nonseminomatous germ cell tumor[46,193]; African-Americans may have an earlier age of onset.[195] Seminoma is extremely rare before puberty.[196,197] Most patients with seminoma present with a painless testicular mass, but there may be a dull, aching sensation. Occasionally, patients (2% to 3%) with seminoma present with symptoms of metastases, usually back pain caused by retroperitoneal metastases; gastrointestinal bleeding, bone pain, central nervous system dysfunction, dyspnea and cough, and other symptoms are rare presenting complaints.[8] Gynecomastia may occur as a result of elevation of serum human chorionic gonadotropin because of intermingled syncytiotrophoblastic elements in seminoma and is rarely a presenting feature; also, very rarely, a paraendocrine form of exophthalmos can be a presenting complaint.[198,199] Although symptoms of metastases are unusual presenting complaints in patients with seminoma, about 30% have metastases at the time of diagnosis.[193]

Patients with seminoma usually lack serum alpha-fetoprotein and human chorionic gonadotropin elevations that occur commonly in patients with nonseminomatous germ cell tumor. Alpha-fetoprotein levels should be normal, although concomitant liver disease (including seminomatous metastases to the liver) may cause modest alpha-fetoprotein elevation.[200] Most oncologists regard significant alpha-fetoprotein elevation in a patient with apparently pure testicular seminoma as evidence of nonseminomatous elements and treat accordingly. About 10% to 20% of patients with clinical stage I pure testicular seminoma have elevated serum human chorionic gonadotropin, and 25% or more with advanced seminoma have human chorionic gonadotropin elevations.[201] At initial diagnosis, 7% to 25% of patients with seminoma have elevated human chorionic gonadotropin.[202-207] If blood is sampled from the testicular vein, 80% of patients have elevated human chorionic gonadotropin.[208] Such elevation reflects the presence of intermingled syncytiotrophoblastic elements in these tumors, and the elevations are generally modest. Elevations of serum human chorionic gonadotropin exceeding 40 IU/L are correlated with a worse prognosis,[209] although this is controversial.[202] Elevation of serum levels of lactate dehydrogenase, PLAP, and neuron-specific enolase may also occur in patients with seminoma. Such elevations, however, are neither specific nor especially sensitive,[201,209-212] which limits their clinical utility.

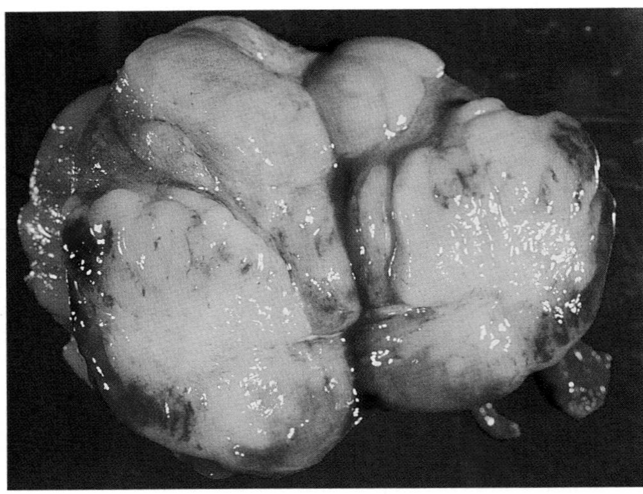

11-8. Cut surface of a seminoma demonstrating a cream-colored, multinodular neoplasm bulging from the surrounding testicular parenchyma.

Pathologic findings

Grossly, seminoma is usually cream to tan and often multi-nodular (Fig. 11-8), with occasional yellow foci of necrosis. Infrequently, necrosis is extensive. In some cases the tumor is diffuse, fleshy, and encephaloid, similar to testicular lymphoma (Fig. 11-9). In contrast to lymphoma, however, only about 10% of seminomas extend into paratesticular structures.[213] Intraparenchymal hemorrhage may cause red discoloration.[28] The cut surface of seminoma usually bulges from the surrounding parenchyma (see Fig. 11-8). Punctate foci of hemorrhage often correspond to intermingled foci of syncytiotrophoblastic elements.[214] A fibrous consistency is uncommon but results when prominent fibrous septa develop in the tumor.

Microscopically, seminoma is usually arranged in a diffuse, sheet-like pattern interrupted by branching, fibrous septa containing an inflammatory infiltrate consisting chiefly of lymphocytes but often containing plasma cells and eosinophils (Fig. 11-10). Distinct nodules of seminoma may be apparent, sometimes with confluent growth imparting a lobulated pattern. In some cases, a prominent cord-like arrangement of cells is present (Fig.

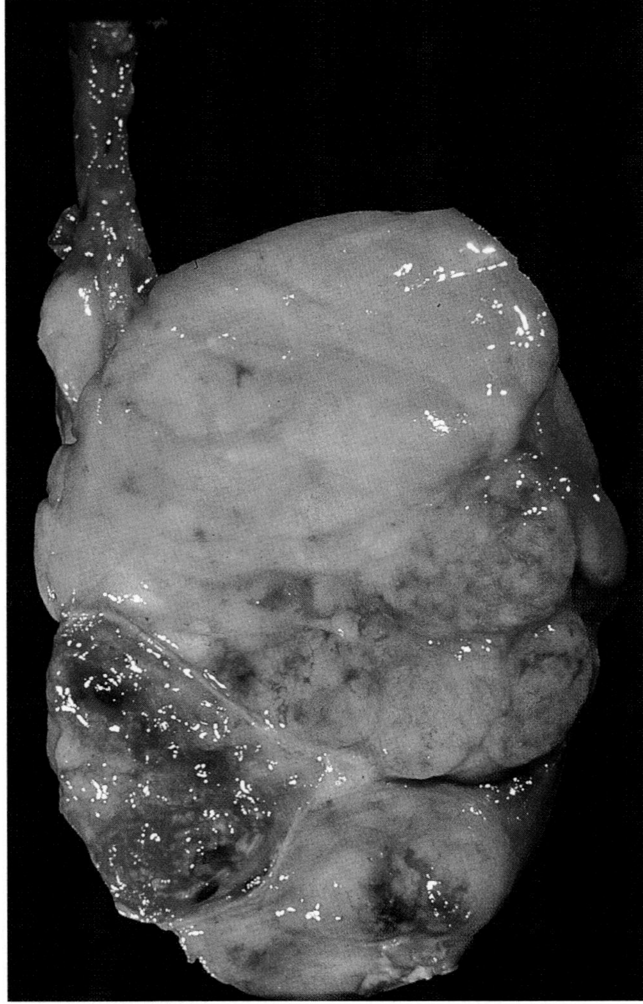

11-9. Seminoma with a diffusely fleshy, encephaloid appearance and foci of hemorrhage. *(Courtesy of RH Young, MD.)*

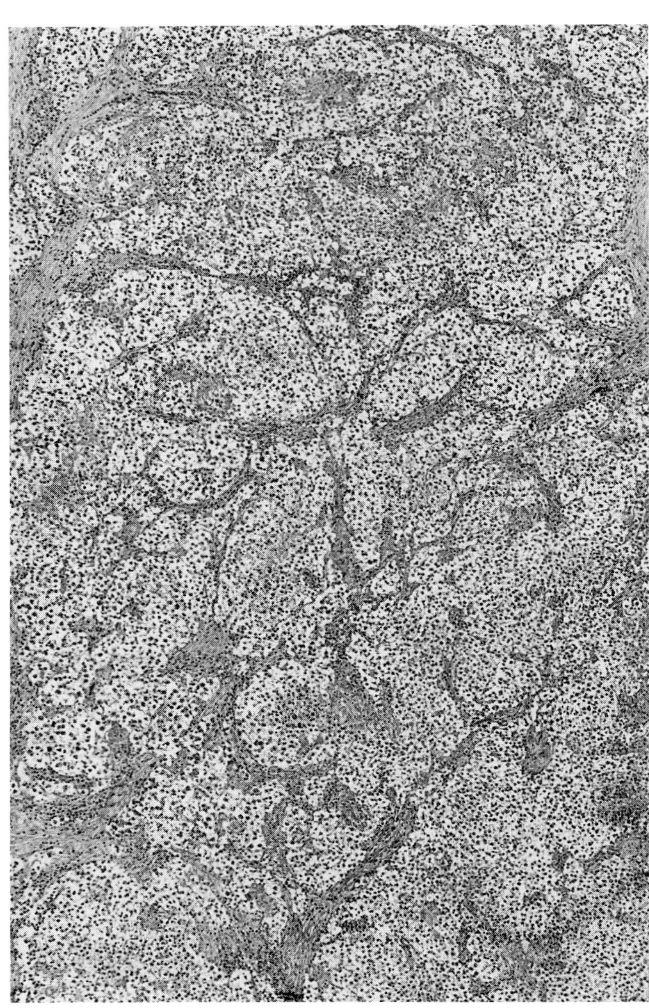

11-10. Sheet-like pattern of seminoma is interrupted by branching, fibrous trabeculae.

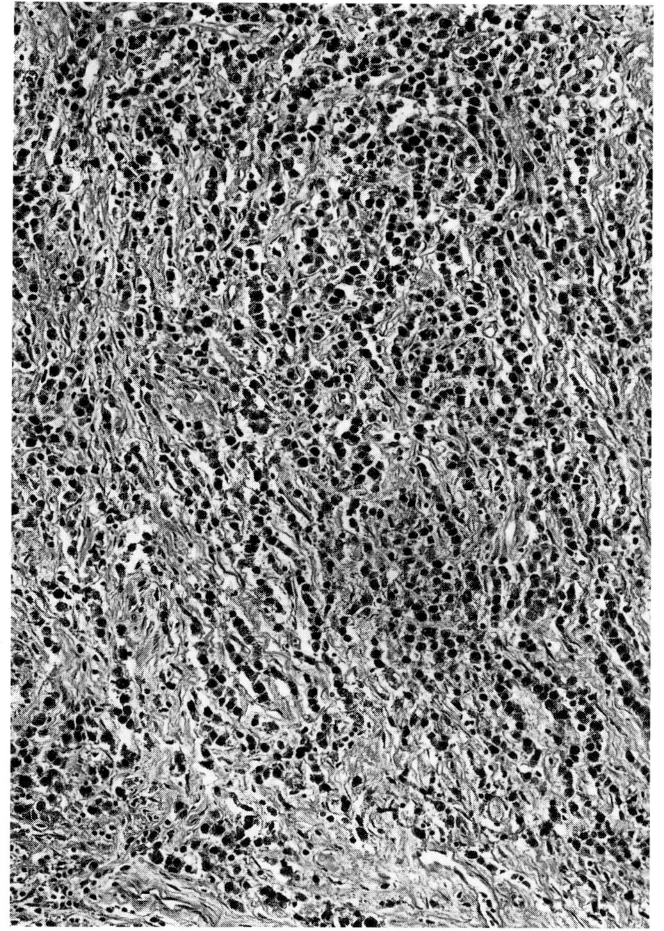

11-11. Prominent cord-like pattern of seminoma.

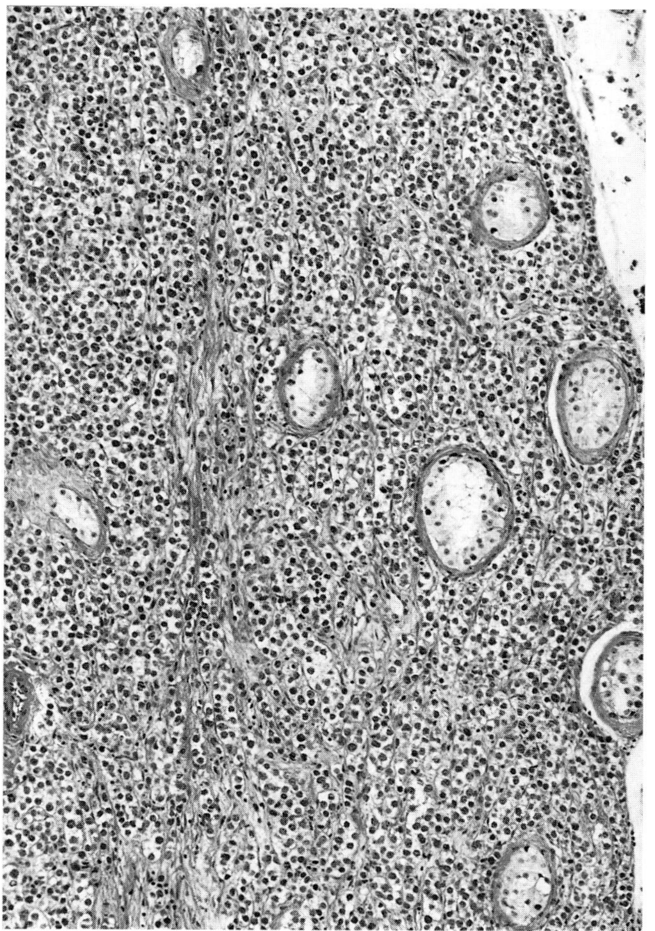

11-12. Interstitial growth of seminoma preserves some seminiferous tubules at the periphery of the tumor.

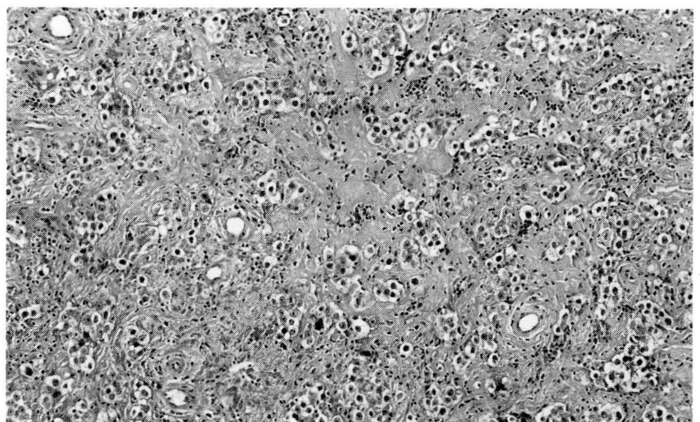

11-13. Scarring in seminoma creates a pattern of small nests and solid pseudotubules separated by hyalinized stroma.

11-11), often at the periphery of nodules showing a sheet-like pattern. Foci of interstitial growth may be seen, with preservation of seminiferous tubules; this pattern is usually most apparent at the periphery of neoplastic nodules (Fig. 11-12). In rare seminomas, an interstitial growth pattern may predominate, with well-preserved seminiferous tubules even in the central portions of the neoplasm. This growth pattern is much more common, however, in testicular lymphoma (see page 627).

With time, many seminomas develop foci of scarring. Hyalinized deposits of collagen may separate the neoplastic cells into small nests resembling solid pseudotubules (Fig. 11-13). Extensive collagen deposits may result in broad scars with only a few scattered neoplastic cells. Rarely, seminoma may show a distinctly tubular pattern in which a palisade-like arrangement of neoplastic cells occurs at the periphery of tubule-like structures, which may contain loosely cohesive neoplastic cells in their lumens (Fig. 11-14).[215-217]

Seminoma may also develop intercellular edema with separation of neoplastic cells and formation of microcystic spaces (Fig. 11-15). These spaces are generally irregular in outline and frequently contain visible edema fluid and intracystic exfoliated neoplastic cells that contrast with the cleaner, more round and regular microcystic spaces commonly identified in yolk sac tumor (see page 593). Foci of coagulative necrosis are present in about half of seminomas and may be extensive in a minority of cases.[218]

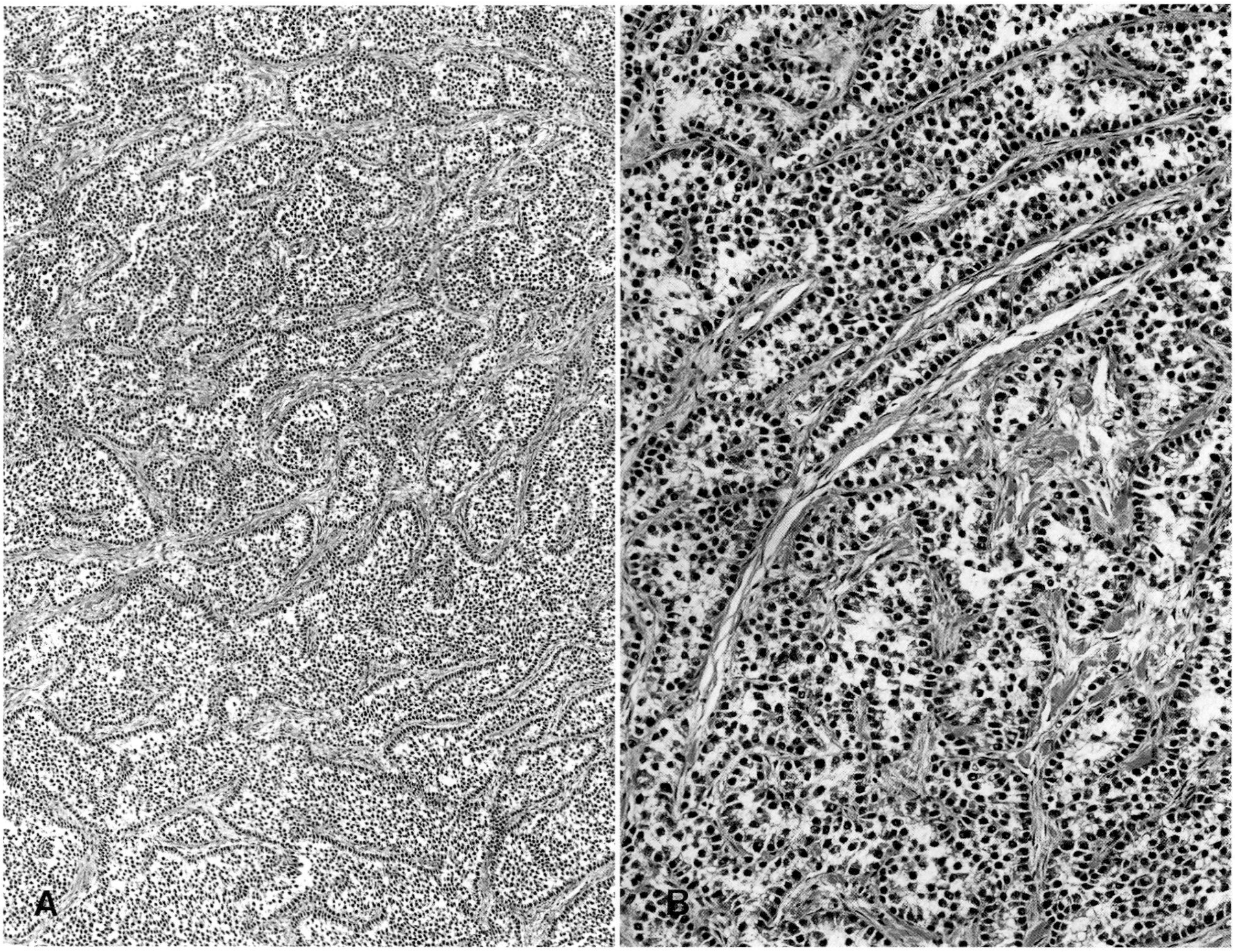

11-14. **A**, Tubular pattern of seminoma, with palisade-like arrangement of cells at the periphery of tubular structures. **B**, Higher magnification shows loosely cohesive seminoma cells within central spaces of "tubules." *(Courtesy of RH Young, MD.)*

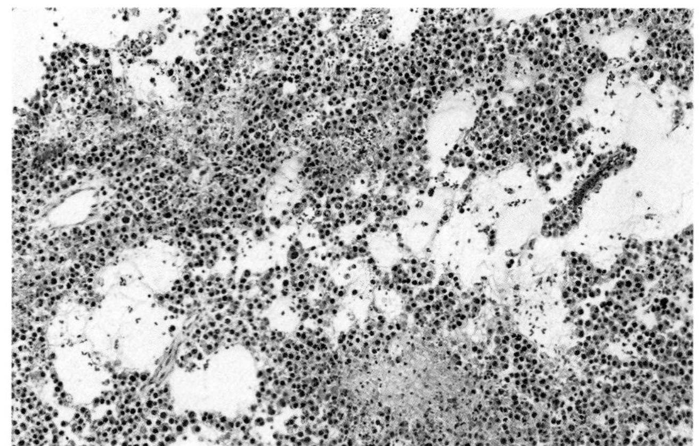

11-15. Edema in seminoma creating an irregular, microcystic pattern.

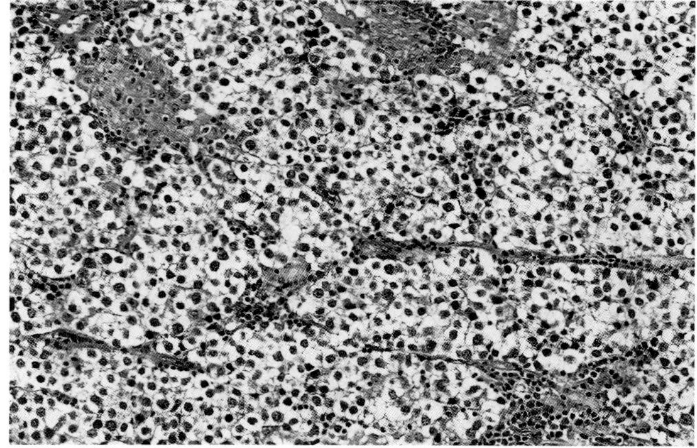

11-16. Lymphocytes (*bottom*) and small granulomas (*top*) in seminoma.

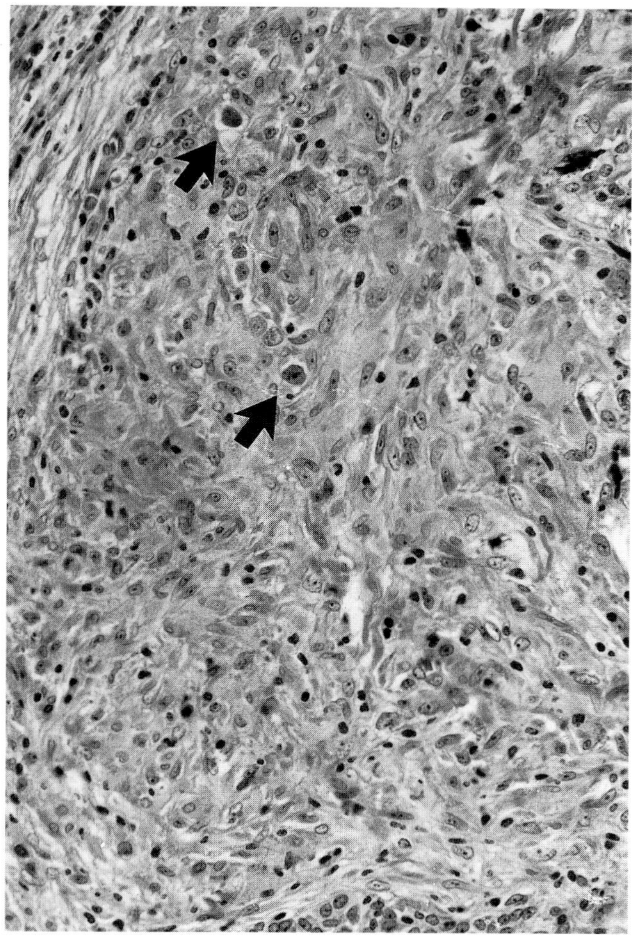

11-17. Extensive granulomatous reaction in seminoma, leaving only two residual tumor cells near center and top (*arrows*).

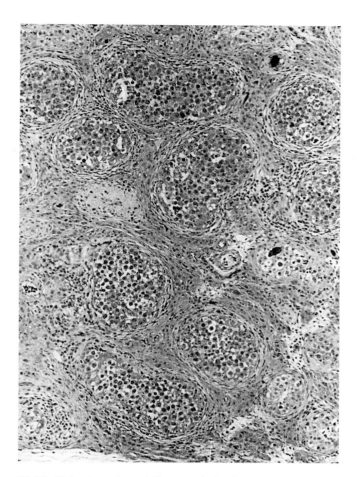

11-18. Distension of seminiferous tubules by seminoma cells is referred to as "intratubular seminoma."

A lymphocytic infiltrate is a virtually constant feature of seminoma, and is usually most dense in perivascular areas and around fibrous trabeculae, which also contain many capillaries (Fig. 11-16). Lymphocytes are also frequently intermingled with the seminoma cells elsewhere. A florid lymphoid reaction, with formation of germinal centers, occurs in a minority of cases, but most of the lymphocytes in seminomas are T-cells.[219-224] Ultrastructural studies have demonstrated a cytolytic effect of the lymphocytes on the seminoma cells,[224] correlating with the observation of some investigators of a better prognosis in cases associated with a prominent lymphocytic reaction.[225]

A variable granulomatous reaction occurs in up to 50% of seminomas. In most cases, this reaction consists of small clusters of epithelioid histiocytes scattered among neoplastic cells (see Fig. 11-16); Langhans'-type giant cells and other multinucleate giant cells may be present. Intratubular collections of epithelioid histiocytes may also be seen. Rarely, the granulomatous reaction can be extensive and virtually efface the neoplasm (Fig. 11-17); in such cases, it may be difficult to distinguish a florid granulomatous reaction in a seminoma from granulomatous orchitis, and careful search for residual seminoma and IGCNU is indicated.

Seminoma often proliferates within the tubular system of the testis, distending the seminiferous tubules as "intratubular seminoma" (Fig. 11-18).[156] Intratubular spread into the rete testis may produce a complicated pattern in which seminomatous cells undermine the epithelium of the rete testis in a pagetoid fashion (Fig. 11-19). An identical picture may be produced by the spread of IGCNU into the rete testis.[156] Such intrarete spread is unlikely to be misinterpreted as a primary carcinoma of the rete testis or papillary pattern of embryonal carcinoma if the characteristic appearance of the seminoma cells and the compressed epithelium of the rete testis are appreciated. Seminoma with ossification of the fibrous trabeculae has been described.[226]

The cells of seminoma are generally clear to lightly eosinophilic, measuring 15 to 25 μm in diameter. The nuclei are uniform, round to oval, usually central or slightly eccentric, with finely granular chromatin and one or two prominent nucleoli (Fig. 11-20). The nuclear membranes are irregularly thickened. The cell borders are well-defined in adequately fixed specimens (see Fig. 11-20).

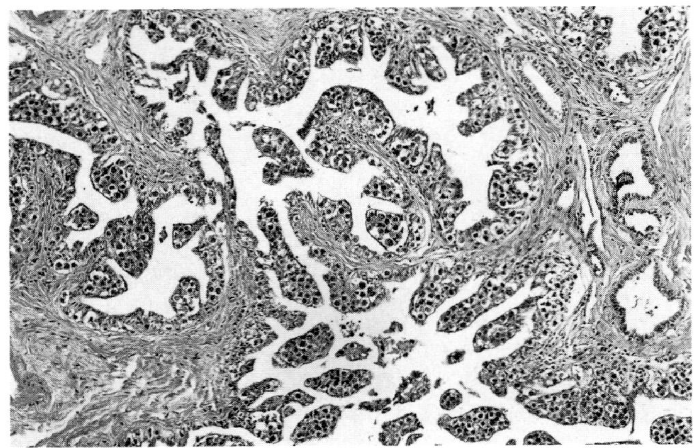

11-19. Pagetoid spread of intratubular seminoma into the rete testis.

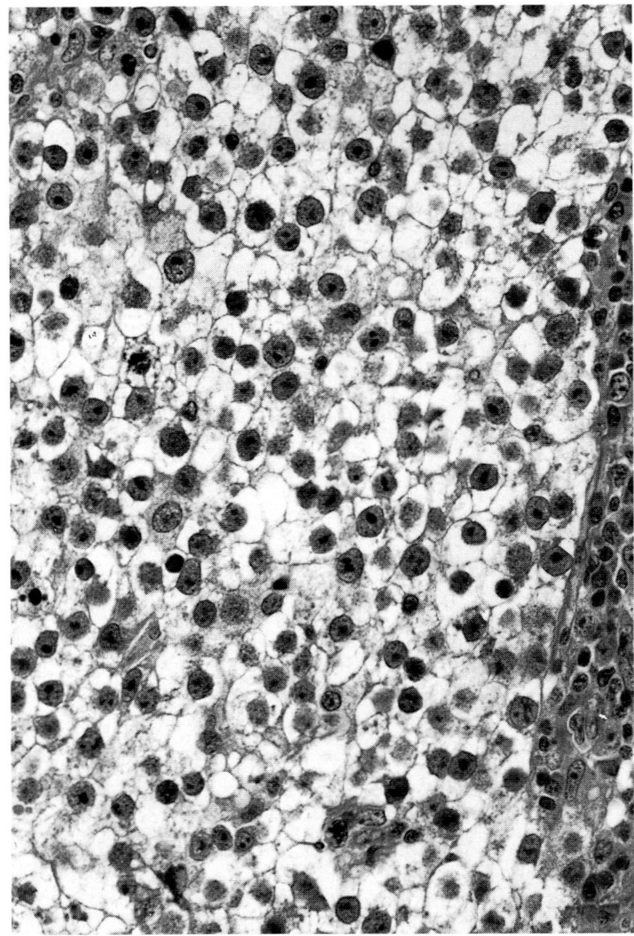

11-20. Seminoma cells with clear cytoplasm, well-defined cell borders, and round nuclei with one or two prominent nucleoli. Lymphocytes are along right edge.

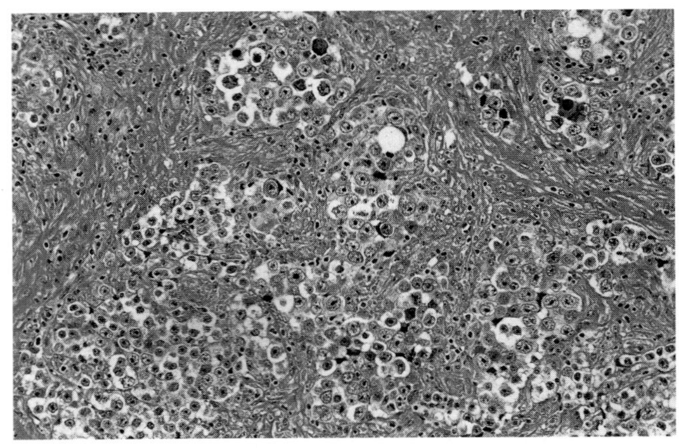

11-21. Seminoma with zones of increased nuclear atypia. Note the larger size of the cells and the poorly defined cell borders in the groups at the center and right compared with those at the left.

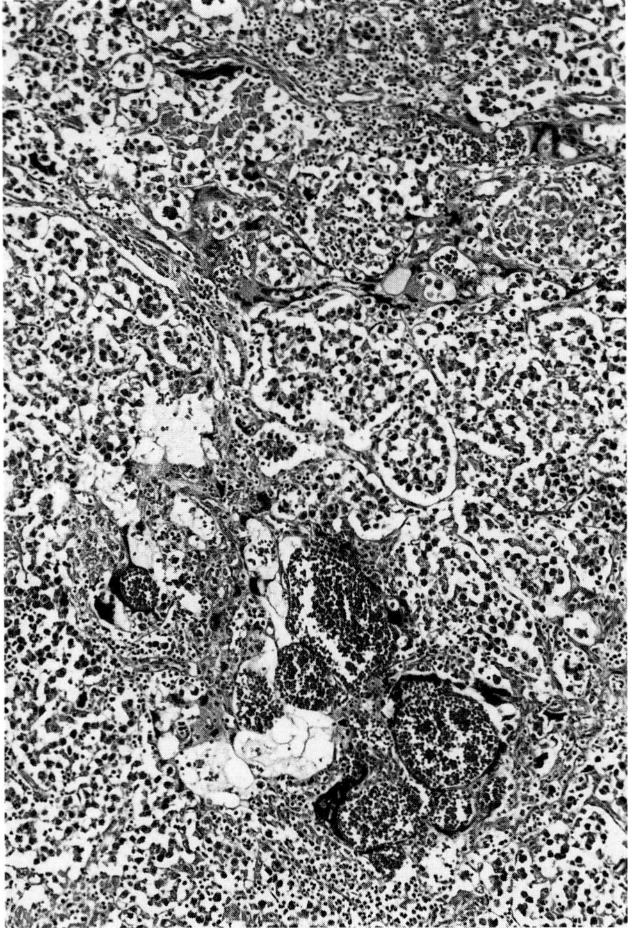

11-22. Seminoma with syncytiotrophoblastic cells. Intracytoplasmic lacunae contain erythrocytes.

Abundant cytoplasm separates the nuclei so that overlapping nuclei are not seen. Glycogen is present in the cytoplasm of most cases, although prolonged exposure to some aqueous fixatives may result in loss of cytoplasmic glycogen. Occasionally, seminoma displays foci of increased cellular atypia with less well-defined cytoplasmic boundaries, darker cytoplasm, and enlarged, crowded nuclei (Fig. 11-21). Such changes may be seen in association with early necrosis and contain pyknotic nuclear fragments. Such isolated foci, in the absence of distinct epithelial differentiation, should not militate against a diagnosis of seminoma.

Mitotic figures in seminoma are prominent, and, in the past, when present in sufficient numbers they were considered as evidence of anaplastic seminoma.[110] Now it is clear that the practice of using an average of three mitoses per high power field identified far too many seminomas as anaplastic[227] and, more importantly, there is evidence that high mitotic rate seminoma behaves no differently than seminoma with a lower mitotic rate.[228,229] Furthermore, there is no immunohistochemical difference between typical and anaplastic seminomas.[229] Although some seminomas behave more aggressively than most seminomas, there are no established criteria for the recognition of such cases; use of the term *anaplastic seminoma* is therefore discouraged.

Seminoma with syncytiotrophoblastic cells

Syncytiotrophoblastic cells are present in 10% to 20% of seminomas.[49] The morphology of these cells is variable, ranging from typical syncytiotrophoblastic cells having cytoplasmic lacunae and multinucleation (Fig. 11-22) to large mononucleate or binucleate cells, which may not be easily distinguished from the background of seminoma cells but which are highlighted by immunostains directed against human chorionic gonadotropin.[230] Intermediate between these extremes are cells containing multiple nuclei in a mulberry pattern. Syncytiotrophoblastic cells are often located close to capillaries, and microhemorrhages may be seen in these foci. Unlike choriocarcinoma, the syncytiotrophoblastic cells are not intermingled with a cytotrophoblastic component nor do they form a nodular aggregate of variably differentiated trophoblastic cells. Instead, they are randomly scattered as single cells or very small groups.

Special studies

Glycogen is usually prominent in seminoma (Fig. 11-23), and almost all cases show immunoreactivity for PLAP, generally in a peripheral, membranous staining pattern (Fig. 11-24); cytoplasmic staining may also be identified.[39,160,231,232] Many seminomas also express cytokeratin immunoreactivity, although such staining may only be demonstrable using frozen sections.[233] The most common cytokeratins in seminoma are cytokeratins 8 and 18 of Moll's catalog, although others, including cytokeratins 4, 17, and 19, can be identified occasionally.[233] Epithelial membrane antigen is not expressed in seminoma,[39,213] and the combination of positivity for PLAP and negativity for epithelial membrane antigen and cytokeratin (AE1/AE3) in formalin-fixed, paraffin-embedded tissue appears to be a relatively specific pattern for seminoma.[234] Vimentin, lactate dehydrogenase, and neuron specific enolase may be present in seminoma[39,233,235] but are not specific findings. A minority of seminomas may stain for Leu-7, alpha-1-antitrypsin, desmin, and neurofilament protein.[39,233] Desmoplakins and desmoglein are usually present in seminoma.[233,236] The syncytiotrophoblastic cells of seminoma contain human chorionic gonadotropin,[39,48-50,237] and some cells containing human chorionic gonadotropin may not have an overtly syncytiotrophoblastic appearance in routine sections.[48,49]

Ultrastructurally, seminoma has closely apposed cytoplasmic membranes, which usually show only sparse, primitive, intercellular junctions. The cellular organelles consist of scattered mitochondria, occasional cisternae of smooth and rough endoplasmic reticulum, ribosomes, and polyribosomes, occasional membrane-bound lysosome-like structures, and occasional Golgi bodies; glycogen may be present in large quantities but may also be sparse. It is common for the cytoplasmic organelles to be polarized eccentrically in the cytoplasm. The nuclei are round and have

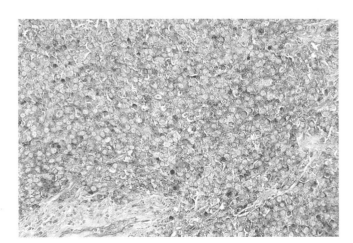

11-23. Periodic acid–Schiff positivity in a seminoma, indicating abundant glycogen.

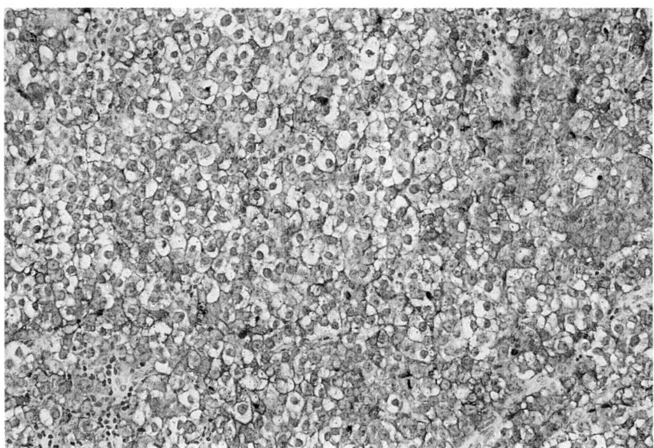

11-24. Seminoma showing a membranous pattern of immunoreactivity for placental alkaline phosphatase.

evenly dispersed chromatin and intricate, large nucleoli.[51,238,239] Occasional seminomas that are typical-appearing at the light microscopic level may show evidence of epithelial differentiation, with small, extra-cellular lumens, microvilli, and well-defined junctional complexes.[51] Such cases, despite transitional morphology at the ultrastructural level, appear to behave as typical seminoma.[51]

The DNA content of seminoma is generally in the triploid to hypotetraploid range and is greater than that of non-seminomatous tumors.[41,52,240] Evolution of seminoma to other types of germ cell tumors may occur as a result of the loss of as yet unidentified cancer suppressor genes.[41,52,240,241] The DNA content of seminoma with syncytiotrophoblasts does not differ from seminoma lacking syncytiotrophoblasts, supporting seminoma classification.[242] Decreased expression of m-RNA from the retinoblastoma gene has been identified in seminoma, but the gene itself appears intact.[243,244] As in many testicular germ cell tumors, seminoma frequently contains an isochromosome derived from the short arms of chromosome 12—i(12p).[245,246] Numerous other cytogenetic abnormalities have also been described.[245] The role of oncogenes in the evolution of seminoma is not yet clear; several studies have implicated roles for the ras family,[245] C-myc,[247] N-myc,[243,248] C-kit,[249] and hst-1[249] oncogenes. Mutations in the p53 tumor suppressor gene have also been implicated.[145,147]

Differential diagnosis

Seminoma can be misinterpreted as the solid pattern of embryonal carcinoma, especially in poorly fixed preparations. The formation of glands, true tubules, or papillae argues against the diagnosis of seminoma. The nuclei of seminoma are more uniform and round, less crowded, and more evenly spaced than those of embryonal carcinoma, which are pleomorphic, irregularly shaped, crowded, and appear to abut or even overlap. The cytoplasmic borders of seminoma are well defined, and those of embryonal carcinoma are poorly defined. Embryonal carcinoma lacks the regular fibrous septa of many seminomas. Cytokeratin reactivity is usually weaker and PLAP reactivity stronger in seminoma than in embryonal carcinoma. Alpha-fetoprotein is occasionally positive in embryonal carcinoma and is negative in seminoma. Monoclonal antibody 43-9F is reported to be strongly reactive in embryonal carcinoma and negative or only weakly positive in seminoma,[165] but additional experience is necessary to confirm this finding. The distinction of seminoma from spermatocytic seminoma is discussed on page 585.

Yolk sac tumor with a solid pattern may mimic seminoma. Such cases are usually distinguished from seminoma by the presence of typical patterns of yolk sac tumor and the tendency for microcyst formation in the solid areas. Edematous seminoma, however, may also produce a microcystic pattern, but the cystic spaces are more irregular in shape and contain edema fluid and exfoliated neoplastic cells, features that are not seen in yolk sac tumor. Hyaline globules and intercellular basement membrane are common in yolk sac tumor but are rare in seminoma.[250] Fibrous septa and a lymphoid infiltrate are not usual features of yolk sac tumor. Alpha-fetoprotein is negative in seminoma and usually positive in yolk sac tumor; cytokeratin is often negative or weak in seminoma (in routinely processed tissues), whereas it is almost always strongly positive in yolk sac tumor.

Lymphoma must be distinguished from seminoma; most patients with testicular lymphoma are older than 50 years, whereas patients with seminoma are usually younger.[251-256] Bilateral involvement is more likely in lymphoma than seminoma.[252,254-257] Lymphoma usually infiltrates interstitially, preserving the seminiferous tubules,[254,255,258] whereas interstitial infiltration is rarely prominent except at the periphery of seminoma. IGCNU is seen in seminoma but not lymphoma. Lymphoma often is more pleomorphic than seminoma and may be composed of cells with cleaved and irregularly shaped nuclei, which stand in contrast to the round and relatively uniform nuclei of seminoma. The cytoplasm of lymphoma is usually amphophilic and less distinct than that of seminoma. Immunostains directed against PLAP are usually positive in seminoma and negative in lymphoma, whereas leukocyte common antigen shows opposite results.[39,234]

Rarely, seminoma with a tubular pattern may be confused with Sertoli cell tumor, a neoplasm that frequently has a tubular architecture.[215,216] The cytoplasmic clarity in seminoma is caused by glycogen whereas lipid is responsible for this appearance in Sertoli cell tumor. Most Sertoli cell tumors have low-grade cytologic atypia, which contrasts with the high-grade atypism of seminoma. IGCNU is present in almost all seminomas but is not associated with Sertoli cell tumor. Tubular patterns in seminoma are usually focal but may be widespread in Sertoli cell tumor.[216]

Treatment and prognosis

Patients with early seminoma (clinical stage I or nonbulky stage II) are currently treated with orchiectomy and radiation to the paraaortic and paracaval nodes, often with ipsilateral pelvic nodal radiation[259-261] (although this may not be necessary[262]). Prophylactic mediastinal radiation is not recommended. More than 95% of patients in clinical stage I are cured.[259-261] Most recurrences arise outside of the radiated field, in the mediastinum, cervical lymph nodes, or lungs.[261,263] About 87% of patients with nonbulky retroperitoneal metastases are cured.[264,265] Chemotherapy is currently recommended for patients with bulky retroperitoneal involvement or in more advanced stages. *Bulky* is defined variously in different studies as metastases greater than 5 cm, 6 cm, or 10 cm in diameter. Survival of about 80% has been reported in cases at this advanced stage.[8,266]

A prominent lymphocytic reaction has been associated with an improved prognosis.[267,268] Elevation of serum human chorionic gonadotropin levels may indicate a worse prognosis,[205,209,269] although there are contradictory results in the literature.[202,270] It would be useful to identify a subset of seminoma with a poor prognosis at an early stage because it is likely that initial treatment with standard forms of chemotherapy would improve the outcome in such a group. It is also likely that the poor prognosis relates to the tendency of such cases to transform to nonseminomatous tumors, given the high frequency of nonseminomatous tumors at autopsy in patients who died following resection of pure testicular seminoma.[17,45] The worse prognosis associated with high human chorionic gonadotropin levels in seminoma may indicate that such cases are more likely to undergo transformation.

SPERMATOCYTIC SEMINOMA

Clinical features

Historically, spermatocytic seminoma was considered a variant of seminoma. Today it is recognized as a unique clinicopathologic entity with morphology and clinical features distinct from seminoma and other germ cell tumors.[271] Originally described by Masson in 1946,[272] spermatocytic seminoma is an unusual testicular tumor that represents only 1% to 2% of testicular germ cell tumors[193] and occurs twenty times less frequently than seminoma.[273] Unlike other germ cell tumors, it occurs only in the testis, more frequently on the right side.[274-276] Also, unlike other testicular germ cell tumors, spermatocytic seminoma is not associated with cryptorchidism,[273] IGCNU,[181] or other types of germ cell tumors. It occurs as a pure lesion, except in rare cases in which it is associated with a sarcoma.[275,277-279] Spermatocytic seminoma is bilateral in about 9% of cases,[273] almost five times as frequently as seminoma.

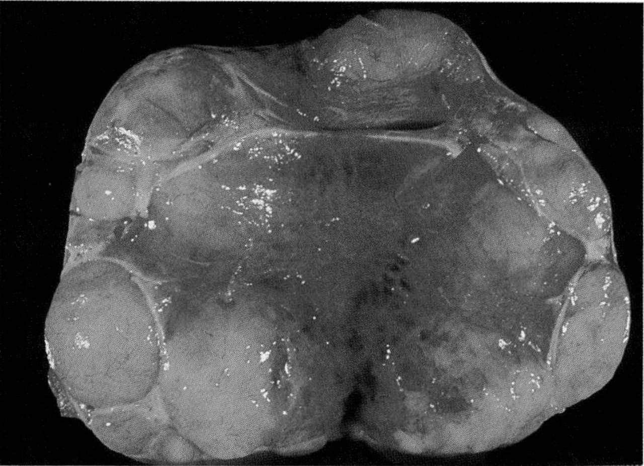

11-25. Cut surface of spermatocytic seminoma showing a multinodular, myxoid tumor. *(Courtesy of RH Young, MD.)*

Most patients with spermatocytic seminoma are older than patients with other types of testicular germ cell tumors. In three series of spermatocytic seminoma, the average age varied from 52 to 58 years,[193,275,280] compared to an average of 40 years for patients with seminoma.[193] Most patients with spermatocytic seminoma present with painless, often long-standing testicular enlargement.[273,275] Most patients are white, but occurrence in African-Americans and Asians has been reported.[275] Serum marker studies (alpha-fetoprotein, human chorionic gonadotropin, lactate dehydrogenase) are negative.

Pathologic features

Grossly, spermatocytic seminoma ranges from 3 to 15 cm in diameter,[273] and has a variable appearance, with zones of fleshy, white tissue, mucoid change, friability, hemorrhage, and cystic change (Fig. 11-25). A multinodular appearance is common, and paratesticular extension may uncommonly occur.[275,281] Several

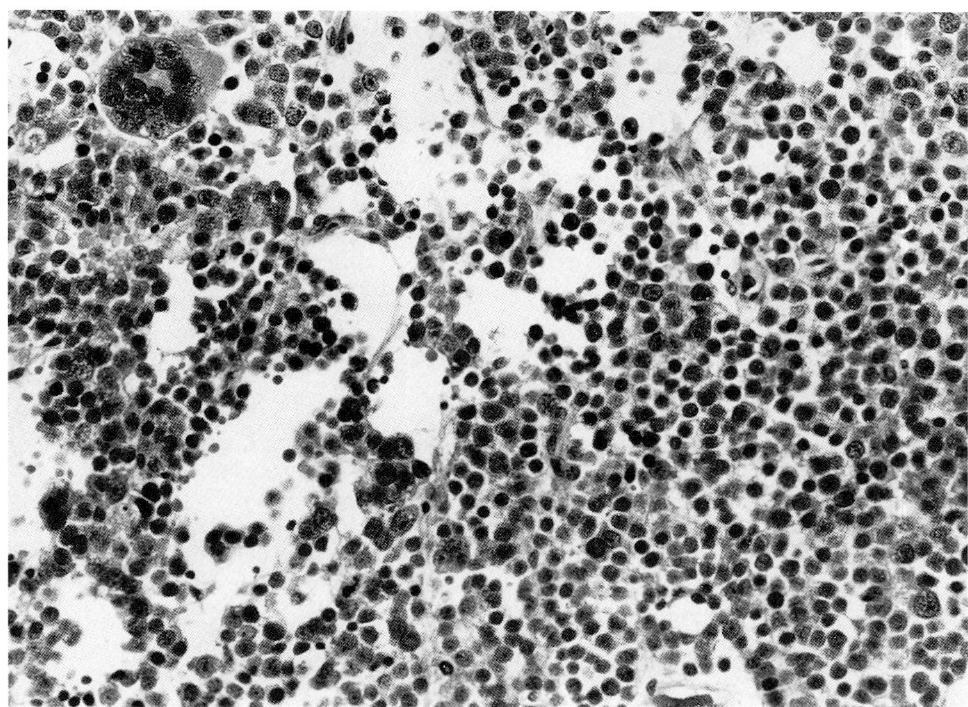

11-26. Edematous microcystic spaces interrupt sheets of cells in spermatocytic seminoma. Note multinucleate neoplastic giant cell.

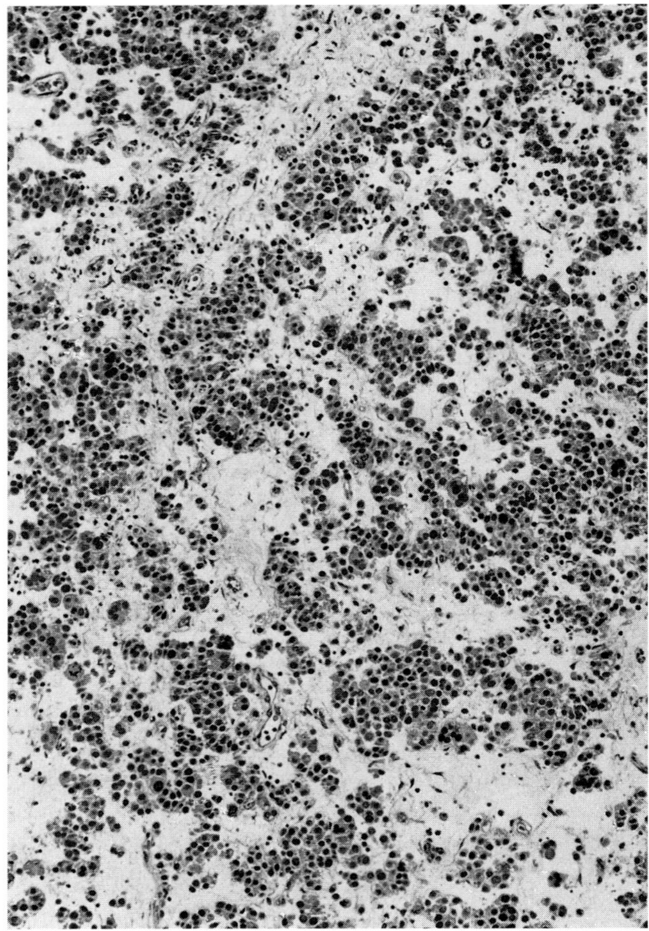

11-27. Small clusters of spermatocytic seminoma cells are separated by edematous stroma.

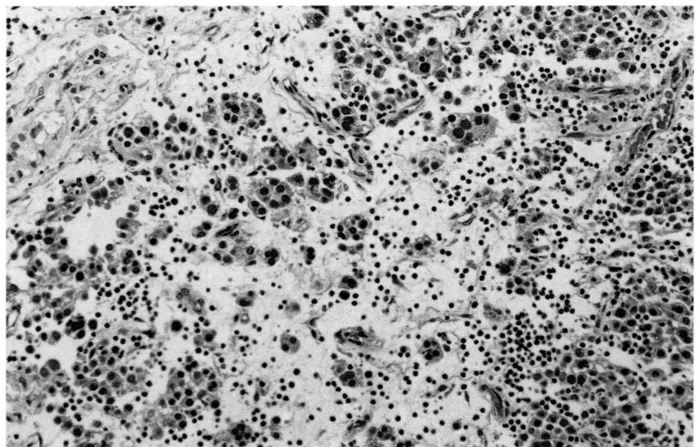

11-28. Unusual spermatocytic seminoma with a prominent lymphocytic infiltrate.

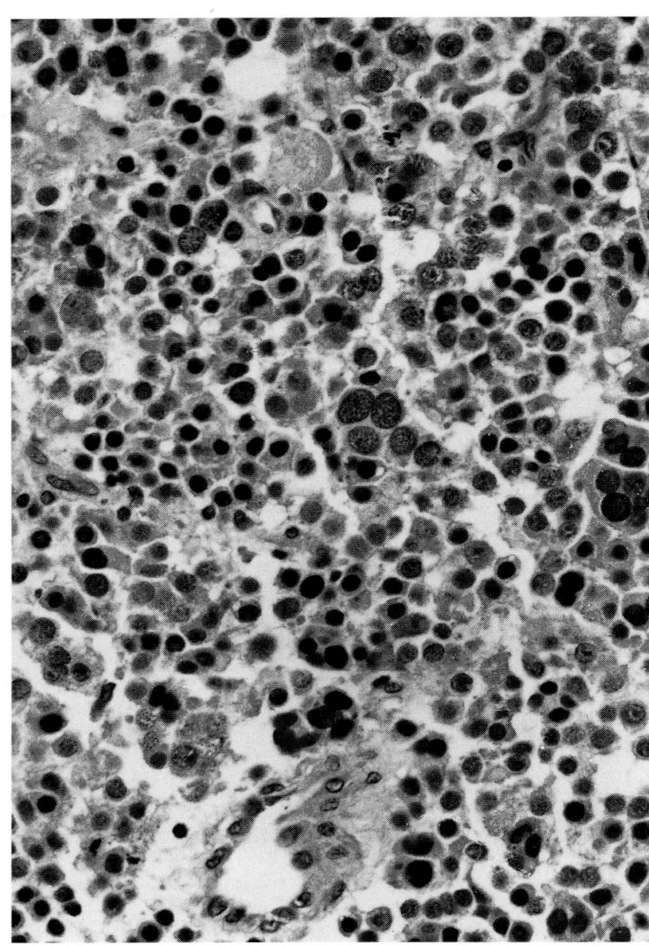

11-29. The characteristic polymorphous cell population of spermatocytic seminoma. Most of the cells are small or intermediate in size; intermediate cells at center have filamentous chromatin.

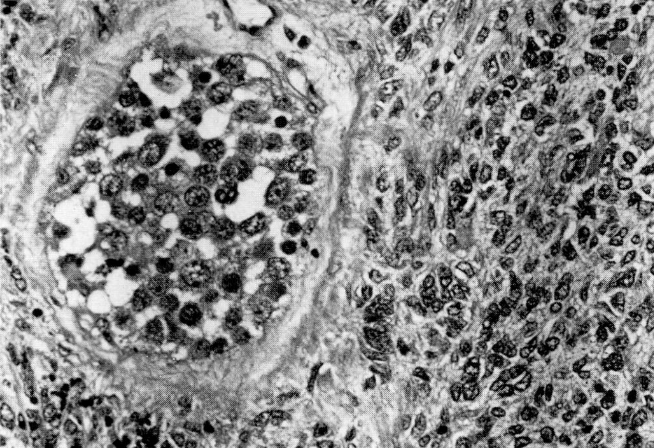

11-30. Embryonal rhabdomyosarcoma in a spermatocytic seminoma. The spermatocytic seminoma in this field is intratubular (*left*). *(Courtesy of RH Young, MD.)*

patterns may be identified, often including a diffuse, sheet-like pattern that may be interrupted by pseudoglandular or microcystic areas caused by edema (Fig. 11-26). A well-defined cord-like or small nested pattern is most commonly seen in association with edematous areas (Fig. 11-27). A lymphoid infiltrate is rarely seen (Fig. 11-28), and granulomatous reactions are absent, unlike seminoma. The microscopic hallmark of spermatocytic seminoma is a polymorphous population of cells (Fig. 11-29), which consists of three major types: a small, lymphocyte-like cell 6 to 8 μm in diameter; an intermediate-sized cell averaging 15 to 20 μm in diameter; and giant cells, some of which may be multinucleate (Fig. 11-30), averaging 50 to 100 μm in diameter. The smallest cell has smudged, degenerate-appearing chromatin and scant eosinophilic to basophilic cytoplasm. The intermediate-sized cell has a round nucleus, usually with granular chromatin and scant cytoplasm. In some intermediate-sized cells, the chromatin has a distinctive filamentous appearance that is similar to the chromatin of meiotic-phase, non-neoplastic spermatocytes (spireme chromatin) (see Fig. 11-28). The giant cells are uninucleate or multinucleate and may show spireme chromatin. The borders between the cells, in contrast to seminoma, are generally indistinct. Intratubular growth is common and probably gives rise to separate invasive foci that cause the common multinodular or lobulated pattern of the tumor.

Special studies

In contrast to seminoma, spermatocytic seminoma lacks glycogen. Most immunohistochemical markers are negative, including vimentin, actin, desmin, alpha-fetoprotein, human chorionic gonadotropin, carcinoembryonic antigen, and leukocyte common antigen.[274,275,282,283] Stains for placental alkaline phosphatase are also generally negative, although rare, focal positivity for PLAP may occur in isolated clusters of cells.[275,283] Cytokeratin stains are also usually negative, although perinuclear, dot-like positivity for cytokeratin 18 can be seen occasionally.[233,274]

Ultrastructurally, spermatocytic seminoma may show intercellular bridges similar to those described in spermatocytes, as well as leptotene stage-type chromosomes—that is, filamentous chromosomes with lateral fibrils.[284,285] These features suggest meiotic phase differentiation, but their presence and specificity are disputed.[286] Adjacent cells occasionally show macula adherens type junctions, and a Golgi body is a variably prominent feature. Other features include scattered mitochondria, occasional profiles of rough endoplasmic reticulum, nuclei with prominent nucleoli, and a thin basement membrane surrounding nests of tumor cells.[284,286]

Flow cytometric studies of spermatocytic seminoma have demonstrated variable DNA content, including hyperdiploidy, peritriploidy, diploidy, peridiploidy, tetraploidy, and aneuploidy.[181,283,286] No haploid population has ever been found, weighing against the concept that spermatocytic seminoma is postmeiotic. These variable results probably reflect the heterogeneous population of these neoplasms because static cytophotometry of spermatocytic seminoma has demonstrated a diploid or near diploid DNA content in the small cell component, and a DNA content ranging up to 42C in the giant cell population, with intermediate values in the intermediate-sized cells.[287] One study suggested that the cells of spermatocytic seminoma arise following cycles of polyploidization, refuting the notion of a meiotic phase tumor.[288]

Treatment and prognosis

There is only one credible case of a metastasizing spermatocytic seminoma,[289] and prior reports of metastases reflect misdiagnoses of testicular lymphoma.[276] Therefore, orchiectomy alone is adequate treatment[273]; adjuvant therapy is not indicated and may be harmful.

Differential diagnosis

The major differential diagnosis of spermatocytic seminoma is seminoma. A summary of features helpful in this distinction is listed in Table 11-4.

Spermatocytic seminoma with sarcoma

Recently, several cases of spermatocytic seminoma associated with sarcoma were reported.[275,277-279] Some of the patients gave histories of stable testicular masses that underwent rapid enlargement or became painful.[277,278] Some patients had symptoms secondary to metastases.[277] Grossly, many of the tumors were hemorrhagic, necrotic, and had a whorled appearance on cut surface.[277,278] Microscopically, the sarcoma was often admixed with the spermatocytic seminoma and was usually described as an undifferentiated, spindle cell sarcoma or embryonal rhabdomyosarcoma (see Fig. 11-30).[275,277-279] In contrast to pure spermatocytic seminoma, over half of the reported cases of spermatocytic seminoma with sarcoma have metastasized, frequently with a fatal outcome.[277-279] Metastases were in a hematogenous distribution, with the lung being the most common metastatic site.

EMBRYONAL CARCINOMA

Although very common in mixed germ cell tumors (occurring in 87% of nonseminomatous germ cell tumors[193]), embryonal carcinoma is an unusual form of pure testicular germ cell tumor, constituting only 2.3% of cases in a referral practice.[291] A decline in the reported proportion of pure embryonal carcinoma among testicular germ cell tumors is largely attributable to the recognition of foci of yolk sac tumor in such cases, leading to their categorization as mixed germ cell tumors. This finding reflects the capacity of embryonal carcinoma to differentiate into other forms of testicular neoplasia, as verified by experimental observations including tissue culture.[292-296] Embryonal carcinoma expresses the stage specific embryonic antigen (SSEA) indicative of a primitive, undifferentiated stage of development, SSEA-3, but not SSEA-1, which indicates a more mature phenotype.[297]

Clinical features

The peak incidence of embryonal carcinoma occurs at about 30 years of age,[193] and it is quite unusual in prepubertal children.[197,298,299] It presents as a testicular mass,

TABLE 11-4.
COMPARISON OF THE CLINICAL AND PATHOLOGIC FEATURES OF SPERMATOCYTIC SEMINOMA WITH TYPICAL SEMINOMA

	Spermatocytic Seminoma	Typical Seminoma
Proportion of germ cell tumors	2%	40% to 50%
Sites	Testis only	Testis, ovary (dysgerminoma), mediastinum, pineal, RP
Associated with cryptorchidism	No	Yes
Bilaterality	9%	2%
Association with other forms of germ cell tumor	No	Yes
Association with IGCNU	No	Yes
Association with sarcoma	Rare	No
Composition	3 cell types, with denser cytoplasm, round nuclei	1 cell type, often clear cytoplasm, less regular nuclei
Intercellular edema	Common	Uncommon
Stroma	Scanty	Prominent
Lymphoid reaction	Rare to absent	Prominent
Granulomas	Absent	Often prominent
Growth pattern	Intratubular > interstitial	Interstitial > intratubular
Glycogen	Absent to scant	Abundant
PLAP staining	Absent to scant	Prominent
hCG staining	Absent	Present in 10%
Metastases	Quite rare	Common

hCG, human chorionic gonadotropin; IGCNU, intratubular germ cell neoplasia, unclassified; PLAP, placental-like alkaline phosphatase; RP, retroperitoneum

Adapted from Damjanov I: Tumors of the testis and epididymis. In Murphy WM, ed: Urological pathology, Philadelphia, 1989, W.B. Saunders and Scully RE: Spermatocytic seminoma of the testis: a report of 3 cases and review of the literature, Cancer 14:788-794, 1961. Reprinted from Ulbright TM, Roth LM: Testicular and paratesticular neoplasms. In Sternberg SS, ed: Diagnostic surgical pathology, ed 2, New York, 1994, Raven Press.

with gynecomastia or symptoms of metastases occurring in about 10% of cases.[300] Rare cases present with sudden death caused by massive tumor thrombo-emboli to the lungs.[301,302] However, metastases are clinically evident in about 40% of patients at presentation, and two thirds of patients who are pathologically staged have metastases.[300]

Serum alpha-fetoprotein elevation in embryonal carcinoma[203] is undoubtedly the result of misclassification of mixed germ cell tumors (embryonal carcinoma and yolk sac tumor), and it is unusual for morphologically pure embryonal carcinoma to be associated with serum alpha-fetoprotein elevation.[291] Many embryonal carcinomas are associated with syncytiotrophoblastic cells, accounting for serum human chorionic gonadotropin elevation in 60% of cases.[203] PLAP and lactate dehydrogenase levels may also be elevated.[303]

Pathologic features

Grossly, embryonal carcinoma is usually poorly circumscribed and gray-white with prominent areas of hemorrhage and necrosis (Fig. 11-31). Microscopically, there are three major patterns, all of which are composed of cohesive groups of primitive, anaplastic epithelial cells. In the solid pattern, the cells are arranged in diffuse sheets (Fig. 11-32). In the tubular or glandular pattern, well-defined, gland-like or tubule-like structures are formed by epithelium varying from cuboidal to columnar (Fig. 11-33). The luminal spaces are cleft-like or round. In the papillary pattern, the papillae may or may not have stromal cores (Fig. 11-34). Prominent foci of eosinophilic, coagulative necrosis are common in all forms of embryonal carcinoma. Cells with smudged, hyperchromatic nuclei are distinctive but nonspecific (see Fig. 11-32, 11-35). Such cells are considered to be degenerate, but they may be misinterpreted as syncytiotrophoblasts, thereby leading to a misdiagnosis of choriocarcinoma. Unlike syncytiotrophoblasts, however, these degenerate embryonal carcinoma cells lack human chorionic gonadotropin and are not usually associated with hemorrhage.

Rarely, embryonal carcinoma has a blastocyst-like pattern with central vesicle-like spaces.[214] A double-lay-

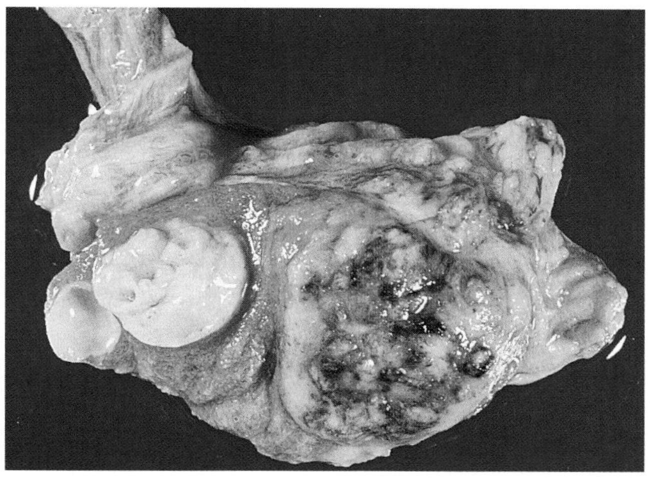

11-31. Embryonal carcinoma with areas of necrosis and hemorrhage.

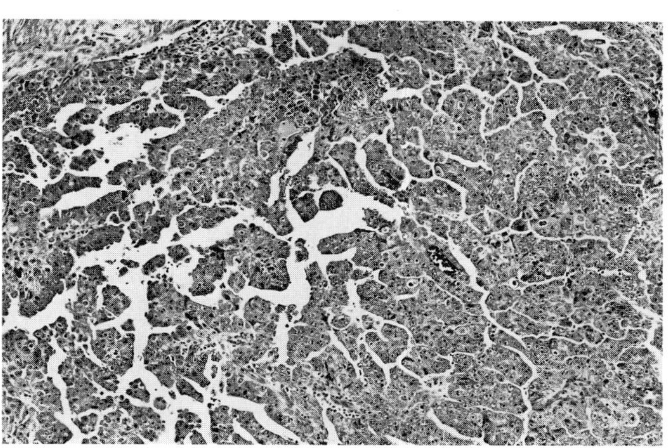

11-34. Embryonal carcinoma, papillary pattern.

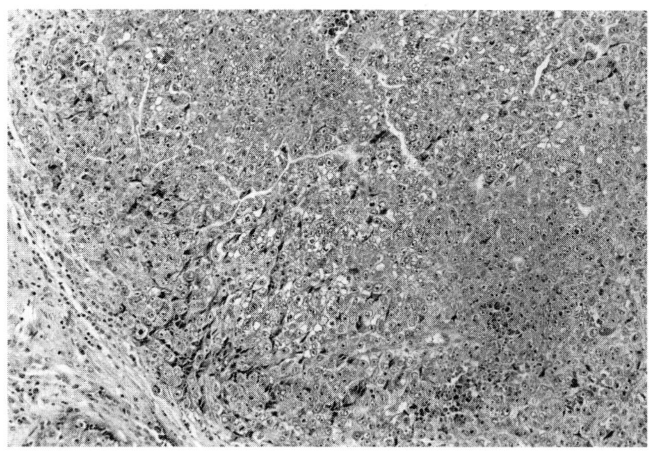

11-32. Solid pattern of embryonal carcinoma. Note darkly staining, degenerate cells.

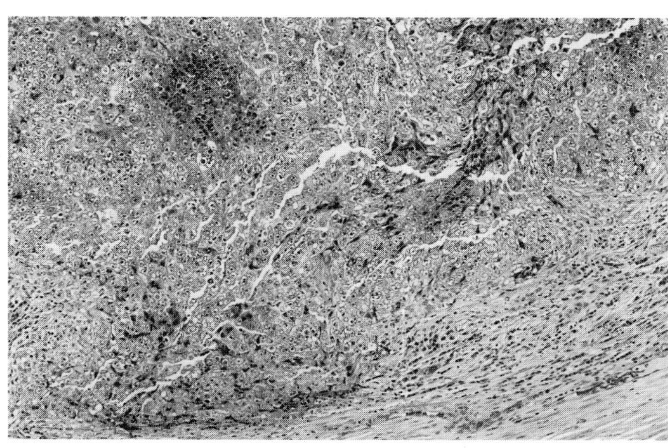

11-35. Solid pattern of embryonal carcinoma with degenerate smudged cells and focal necrosis.

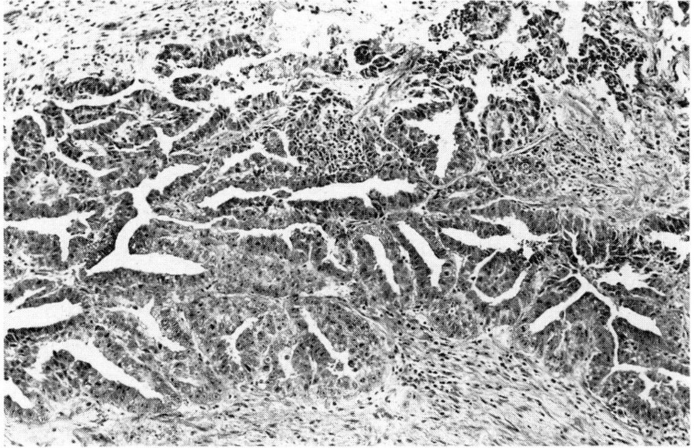

11-33. Embryonal carcinoma, glandular pattern.

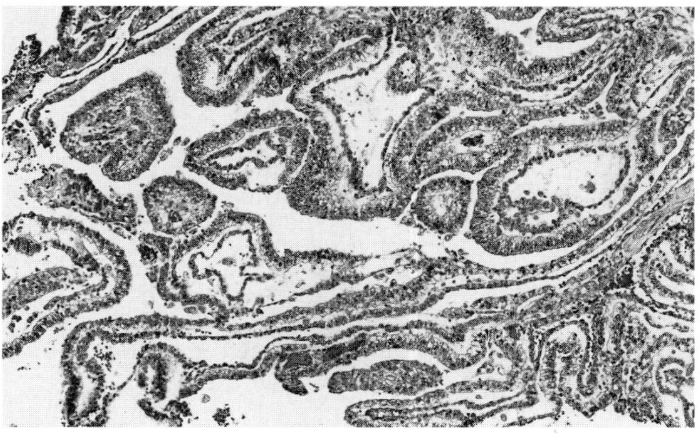

11-36. The "double-layered pattern of embryonal carcinoma," consisting of ribbons of embryonal carcinoma with a parallel layer of flattened cells. This is classified as a mixed germ cell tumor, consisting of embryonal carcinoma and yolk sac tumor (the flattened layer).

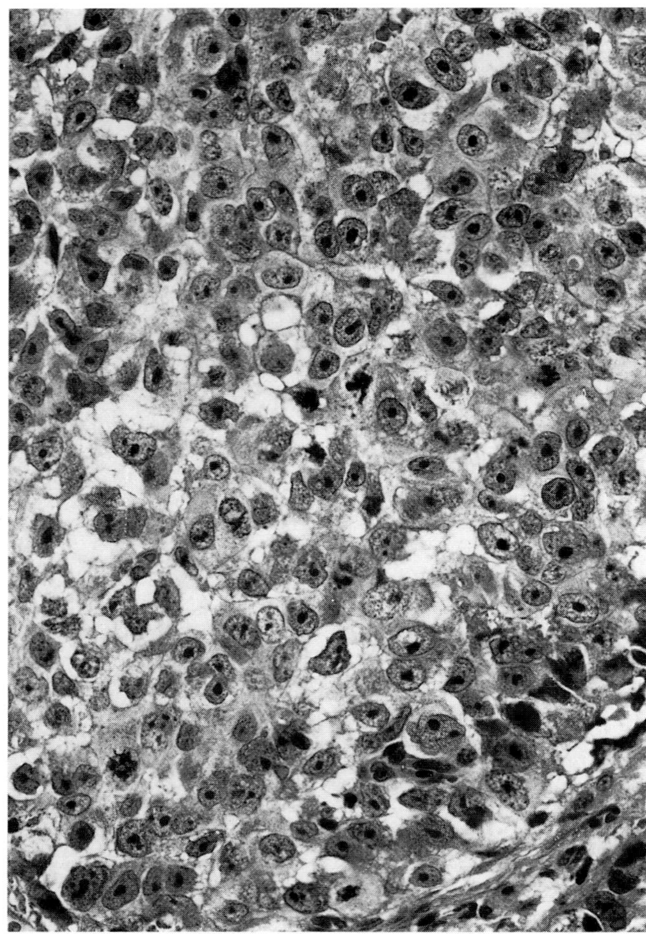

11-37. Embryonal carcinoma resembling seminoma. Note the ill-defined cell borders and large, crowded, vesicular nuclei with large nucleoli.

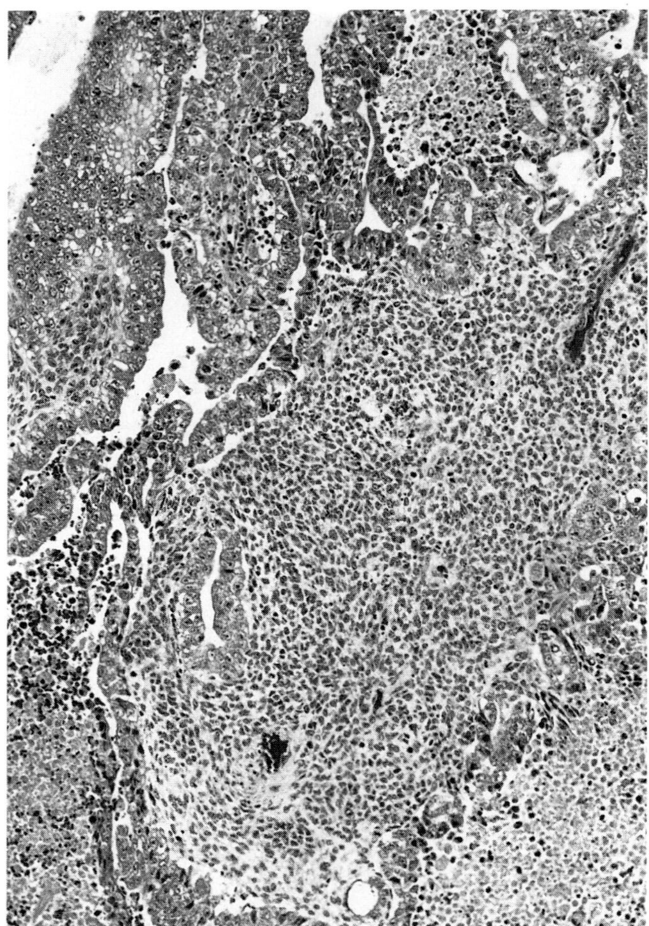

11-38. Neoplastic stroma in an embryonal carcinoma. Classification of such cases as pure embryonal carcinoma or embryonal carcinoma and teratoma is controversial.

ered pattern of embryonal carcinoma has also been described in which a papillary arrangement of embryonal carcinoma is accompanied by a parallel layer of flattened neoplastic epithelium (Fig. 11-36).[304] It appears, though, that this pattern represents embryonal carcinoma with yolk sac tumor and should therefore be regarded as a mixed germ cell tumor.

At high magnification, the cells of embryonal carcinoma have variably staining, abundant cytoplasm and large, vesicular, irregular nuclei with prominent macronucleoli (Fig. 11-37). The cell borders are ill-defined, unlike seminoma, and the nuclei are often crowded, appearing to abut or overlap. Karyorrhectic fragments are frequent in the background, and the mitotic rate is high.

The capacity of embryonal carcinoma to form a minor amount of undifferentiated neoplastic stroma is widely recognized (Fig. 11-38).[18,213] The rationale for this is that embryonal carcinoma is a primitive neoplasm recapitulating an early phase of embryonic development, and the formation of such stroma is consistent with this concept. Nonetheless, there are inconsistencies with respect to diagnosing such cases as embryonal carcinoma or embryonal carcinoma and teratoma.[194] Based on the experience of the BTTP, no significant prognostic difference was noted in embryonal carcinoma with or without a stromal component, but those data were obtained in an era before chemotherapy.[19] It seems rational to permit a minor amount of undifferentiated stroma in neoplasms that are diagnosed as pure embryonal carcinoma, but it would be important to validate this approach by comparing the clinical courses of patients with embryonal carcinoma with and without a stromal component who are managed by modern methods. The alternative approach is to regard such cases as embryonal carcinoma and immature teratoma.

Embryonal carcinoma is often associated with intratubular embryonal carcinoma, which is typically extensively necrotic, having a comedocarcinoma-like appearance (Fig. 11-39). Such necrotic foci may undergo dystrophic calcification leading to the formation of so-called *hematoxylin-staining bodies*.[305] Scarring and intratubular hematoxylin-staining bodies may be

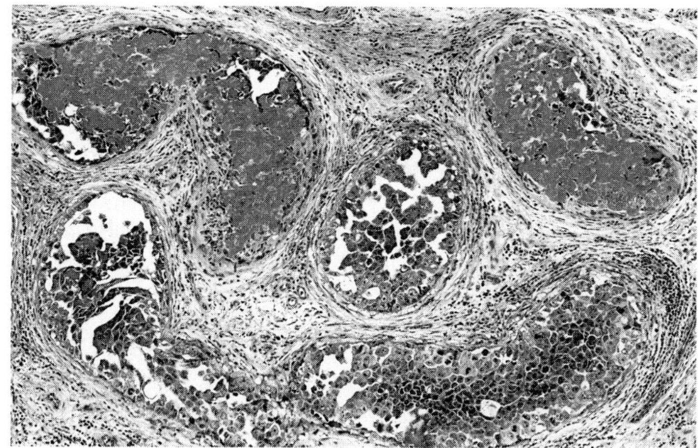

11-39. Intratubular embryonal carcinoma with characteristic abundant necrosis.

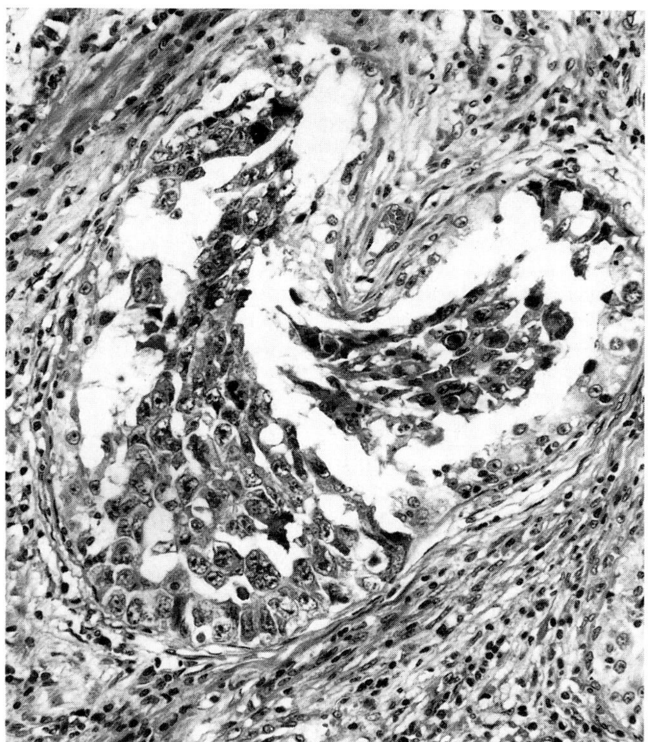

11-40. Intratubular embryonal carcinoma can be reliably distinguished from vascular invasion if there are residual Sertoli cells (*seen at bottom*).

the only residual findings in a regressed germ cell tumor.[305]

The identification of vascular invasion in nonseminomatous germ cell tumors (including embryonal carcinoma) is important in deciding whether patients with clinical stage I tumors are appropriate candidates for surveillance only management. Embryonal carcinoma is the angioinvasive element in the majority of cases when such invasion is present, but there are some pitfalls in deciding if vascular invasion is present. First, intratubular

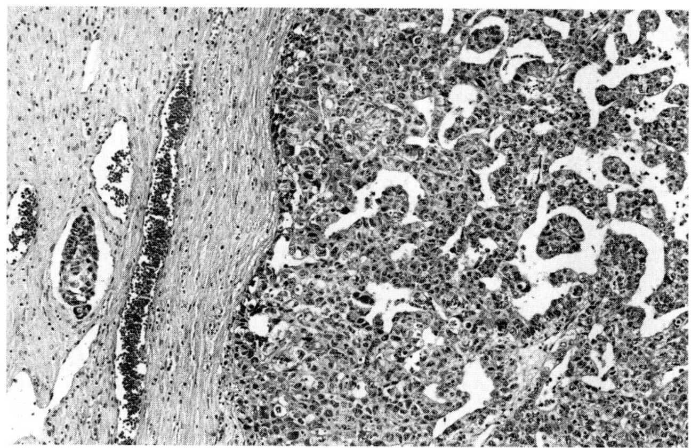

11-41. Vascular invasion at the periphery of a nodule of embryonal carcinoma.

neoplasm can closely resemble intravascular neoplasm. The presence of residual Sertoli cells in a possible vessel is good evidence that it is a tubule (Fig. 11-40). Second, stringent criteria must be applied so that invaded tissue spaces are clearly lined by endothelial cells before regarding them as vessels. Third, germ cell tumors, and especially embryonal carcinoma, are quite cellular and friable, leading to artifactual, knife-implantation of tumor cells into vascular spaces. Such implants, however, are loosely cohesive and unassociated with vascular thrombosis, whereas legitimate vascular invasion is characterized by neoplasm conforming to the shape of the vessel, which may also show evidence of thrombosis. Commonly, artifactual vascular implants are also associated with implants on the surfaces of tissues. It is usually easiest to appreciate vascular invasion a short distance away from the periphery of the neoplasm rather than within the tumor (Fig. 11-41).

Special studies

Immunohistochemically, only a small percentage of pure embryonal carcinomas demonstrate alpha-fetoprotein positivity, but such positivity is more common in the embryonal carcinoma component of mixed germ cell tumors[157,306]—a fact that likely represents early biochemical transformation to a yolk sac tumor component in cases of mixed germ cell tumor before morphological differentiation. PLAP-positivity occurs in 86% to 97% of cases of embryonal carcinoma[39,162,307] but is usually patchy and weaker than in seminoma. Several different cytokeratin classes are present in embryonal carcinoma, most prominently cytokeratins 8 and 18, but also cytokeratin 19, and occasionally cytokeratins 4 and 17.[308] Most authors, therefore, report strong and diffuse positivity for cytokeratins in the majority of embryonal carcinomas, including routinely processed cases (Fig. 11-42).[39,309] Epithelial membrane antigen is negative in almost all embryonal carcinomas,[39] creating a characteristic immunohistochemical profile: cytokeratin-positive, PLAP-positive, and epithelial membrane antigen negative. This profile can be of great clinical value in distinguishing embryonal carcinoma in an extragonadal

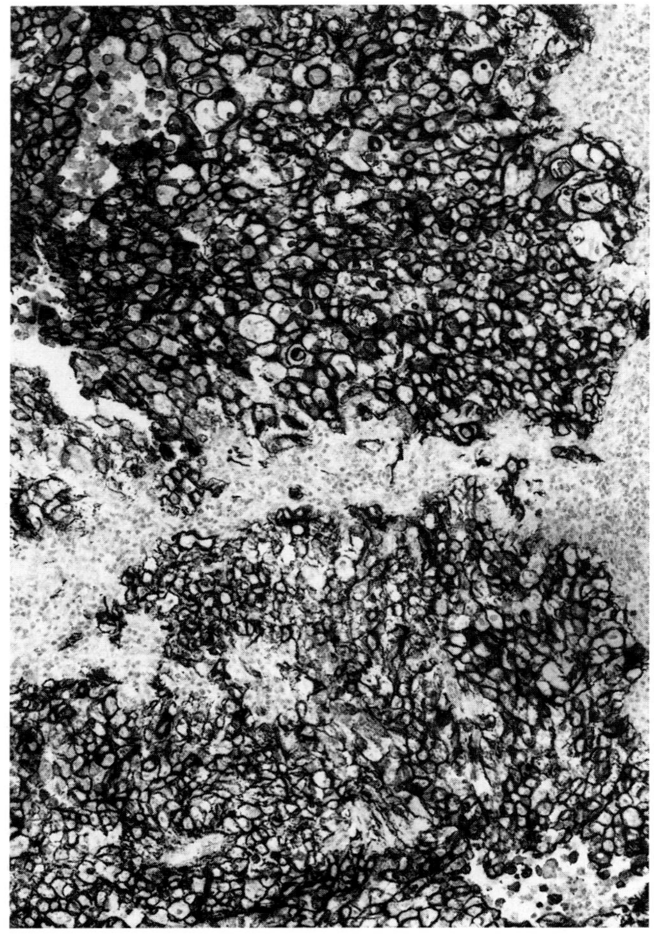

11-42. Intense cytoplasmic immunoreactivity for cytokeratin in embryonal carcinoma.

site (either a metastasis or an extratesticular primary) from a poorly differentiated carcinoma of nongerminal origin (typically, cytokeratin-positive, PLAP-variable [but most commonly negative], and epithelial membrane antigen positive).[234] Ki-1, the antigen that, in part, defines anaplastic large cell lymphoma, may also be present in embryonal carcinoma,[310] indicating the necessity for caution and additional supportive evidence before accepting a Ki-1–positive, poorly differentiated malignant neoplasm as an anaplastic large cell lymphoma. Reactivity with monoclonal antibody 43-9F has been reported as positive in embryonal carcinoma but weak or absent in seminoma, choriocarcinoma, and most cases of yolk sac tumor.[165] Occasionally, embryonal carcinoma will also stain for alpha-1-antitrypsin, Leu-7, vimentin, lactate dehydrogenase, human placental lactogen, and ferritin.[39,157,235,311] The product of the p53 tumor suppressor gene is often identifiable in embryonal carcinoma, perhaps indicating the occurrence of point mutations in the p53 gene,[145,146] although the absence of mutations with molecular biologic techniques may indicate that this is the result of nonmutated overexpression.[148,149]

Ultrastructurally, embryonal carcinoma usually resembles a poorly differentiated, primitive adenocarcinoma with poorly defined lumens in solid areas and well-defined, large lumens in glandular areas.[51] The lumens are bordered by cells having well-defined junctional complexes with characteristically long tight junctions.[312] Short microvilli project into the luminal spaces, and the cytoplasm contains ribosomes, a prominent Golgi body, rough endoplasmic reticulum, teleolysosomes, mitochondria, glycogen, and occasional lipid droplets. The nuclei are large, deeply indented, often contain cytoplasmic inclusions, and have large nucleoli with complex nucleolonema.[51]

Embryonal carcinoma has a DNA index ranging from 1.4 to 1.6 times normal, which is significantly less than that of seminoma.[41,52] Embryonal carcinoma often contains isochromosome (12p), and increased copy numbers of i(12p) have correlated with a more aggressive clinical course.[246] The presence of i(12p) in a poorly differentiated carcinoma, either metastatic or a primary neoplasm of an extragonadal site, may be a useful means of separating embryonal carcinoma from other poorly differentiated neoplasms.[313] The detection of i(12p) can be accomplished on interphase cells obtained from fresh biopsy samples by fluorescent in situ hybridization.[314] A characteristic deletion—del(12)(q13-q22)—has also been identified in nonseminomatous testicular germ cell tumors.[315] Mutations in the *N-ras* proto-oncogene, localized to chromosome 12, have often been identified in embryonal carcinoma and in other testicular germ cell tumors.[316] Expression of a variety of other oncogenes has been reported in cell lines of embryonal carcinoma and teratoma.[317]

Differential diagnosis

The distinction of embryonal carcinoma from seminoma was discussed on page 587. The distinction of embryonal carcinoma from yolk sac tumor depends on the presence, in yolk sac tumor, of one of several distinctive patterns (see page 593), and the larger and more pleomorphic nature of the neoplastic cells in embryonal carcinoma. Yolk sac tumors often contain hyaline globules and intercellular basement membrane, which are almost always lacking in embryonal carcinoma,[250] and alpha-fetoprotein is much more likely to be present in yolk sac tumors than in embryonal carcinoma. Because embryonal carcinoma may transform into yolk sac tumor, there are foci where the distinction is arbitrary. Such cases, however, invariably show areas of both neoplastic types. The smudged, degenerate cells common in embryonal carcinoma may be misinterpreted as syncytiotrophoblasts, causing a misdiagnosis of choriocarcinoma. These cells, however, lack human chorionic gonadotropin, and the background is usually not hemorrhagic, unlike true choriocarcinoma. Large cell lymphoma usually occurs in older patients, lacks the epithelial patterns commonly identified in embryonal carcinoma, has an interstitial growth pattern, is not associated with IGCNU, and is PLAP- and cytokeratin-negative and leukocyte common antigen positive, features that contrast with those of embryonal carcinoma.[234]

Treatment and prognosis

The treatment of nonseminomatous germ cell tumors, including embryonal carcinoma, depends on the clinical stage of the patient; there is a lack of consensus about the best approach in some cases. For patients with clinical stage I tumor, the lack of consensus is most apparent. Orchiectomy is required in all instances for therapy and diagnosis. However, one school of thought advocates nerve-sparing retroperitoneal lymph node dissection,[318] tailored to excise the commonly involved nodal groups ipsilateral to the affected testis, in order to prove the absence of retroperitoneal metastases (pathologic stage I).[319] If nodal involvement is not identified by retroperitoneal lymph node dissection, no additional treatment is required. About 10% of such patients relapse, but almost all are salvaged by combination chemotherapy.[319] If there are nodal metastases, such patients may either be followed (with the thought that retroperitoneal lymph node dissection was both diagnostic and therapeutic) or receive adjuvant chemotherapy, depending on such factors as the extent of nodal involvement and the reliability of the patient. Survival is greater than 95% for this group.[319]

Another school of thought advocates simple follow-up of patients with clinical stage I nonseminomatous germ cell tumor (the "surveillance only" approach), because only 30% to 40% ultimately relapse (most of whom would have had clinically occult metastases identified on retroperitoneal lymph node dissection). Relapse can be detected early by serum marker elevation, and almost all relapsing patients can be salvaged by standard chemotherapy. This approach avoids unnecessary retroperitoneal lymph node dissection in 60% to 70% of patients who are cured by orchiectomy alone. A review of 560 clinical stage I patients managed by surveillance only found that 97% were tumor-free and that 72% required no therapy after orchiectomy.[320] However, there may be certain patients with clinical stage I tumors in whom the risk of relapse is excessive, making them inappropriate candidates for surveillance only. These patients may be identified by a careful, multifactorial analysis of the orchiectomy specimen. Factors that correlate with relapse or occult retroperitoneal metastases include: lymphovascular invasion,[300,320-331] large proportion of embryonal carcinoma,[325,331,332] pure embryonal carcinoma,[324,333] absence of a yolk sac tumor component,[333,334] prominent neovascularization,[335] embryonal carcinoma in the absence of teratoma,[320] less than 50% teratoma,[322,325] the presence of choriocarcinoma,[327] high S-phase values as determined by flow cytometry,[333] and highly aneuploid tumor stemlines.[336,337] A preorchiectomy alpha-fetoprotein value exceeding 80 ng/ml[325] and an abnormally slow decline in alpha-fetoprotein values following orchiectomy[328] have also correlated with relapse.

Patients having clinically apparent, nonbulky retroperitoneal involvement (clinical stage II) are usually managed by retroperitoneal lymph node dissection with either close follow-up or a limited course of adjuvant therapy. Survival in excess of 95% is expected.[319] For patients with bulky clinical stage II or more advanced tumor, treatment is combination chemotherapy followed by surgical resection of residual masses if the serum markers have normalized. Survival of 70% to 80% is expected.[8,338] Specimens resected after chemotherapy must be carefully evaluated pathologically to determine the need for additional chemotherapy.[339]

A number of studies have been conducted in order to identify prognostic factors in patients with nonseminomatous testicular germ cell tumors. The most important factors are tumor stage, the extent of serum marker elevation, the age of the patient (older being worse), the presence of choriocarcinoma, and the proliferative fraction by flow cytometry.[338,340-343]

YOLK SAC TUMOR

Yolk sac tumor is the most recently recognized testicular germ cell tumor. For years, ovarian yolk sac tumor was misclassified, along with ovarian clear cell carcinoma, as *mesonephroma*. Teilum[344] recognized the identity between testicular and ovarian yolk sac tumor and the frequent admixture of the testicular lesion with other forms of germ cell tumor. This observation permitted the classification of yolk sac tumor as a form of germ cell neoplasm and removal of the ovarian lesion from the mesonephroma category. Subsequently, Teilum recognized the resemblance of the mesenchyme of yolk sac tumor to the extraembryonic mesenchyme of development and the glomeruloid structures to the endodermal sinuses of the rat placenta.[345,346]

Clinical features

Yolk sac tumor is the most common testicular neoplasm in prepubertal children, accounting for 82% of testicular germ cell tumors and the majority of all testicular neoplasms.[197] It occurs in children from birth to 9 years of age, with a median age of about 18 months.[347,348] Unlike yolk sac tumor in adults, those in children are almost always pure without other germ cell tumor components. Postpubertal patients with yolk sac tumor fall within the usual spectrum of age for nonseminomatous testicular germ cell tumor, ranging from 15 to 45 years and averaging 25 to 30 years; rare cases have been reported in elderly patients.[349] Prospective studies of nonseminomatous germ cell tumors have shown that yolk sac tumor elements are present in 44% of cases.[350]

The usual epidemiologic associations of testicular germ cell tumor do not apply to childhood yolk sac tumor. There is no association with cryptorchidism, and the predilection for whites more than other races is lacking.[351]

Children with yolk sac tumor almost always present with a painless testicular mass; clinical evidence of metastasis is quite rare at presentation, occurring in only 6% of cases.[347] Adults with yolk sac tumor in a mixed germ cell tumor are more likely to have lower stage disease than those without a yolk sac tumor component, and the absence of a yolk sac tumor component in a mixed germ cell tumor may be a positive predictor of occult metastases with clinical stage I tumors.[329] Almost all patients with yolk sac tumor have a significant elevation of serum alpha-fetoprotein, varying from hundreds to thousands of nanograms per milliliter.[352,353] Embryonal carcinoma or enteric elements of teratoma may cause minor elevation of serum alpha-fetoprotein, but this is unusual.[291,352]

Pathologic features

Grossly, yolk sac tumor in children appears as solid, gray-white to tan, homogeneous nodules with myxoid or gelatinous cut surfaces (Fig. 11-43); cystic change may be present. In adults, because the yolk sac tumor is usually a component of a mixed germ cell tumor, the appearance is quite heterogeneous, with frequent areas of hemorrhage, necrosis, and cystic change (Fig. 11-44). Numerous patterns are seen in yolk sac tumor and commonly include hybrid, incomplete, and transitional forms. The patterns, modified from the enumeration of Talerman,[354] include:

1. Microcystic (honeycomb, reticular, vacuolated)
2. Endodermal sinus (perivascular)
3. Papillary
4. Solid
5. Glandular/alveolar
6. Myxomatous
7. Sarcomatoid
8. Macrocystic
9. Polyvesicular vitelline
10. Hepatoid
11. Parietal

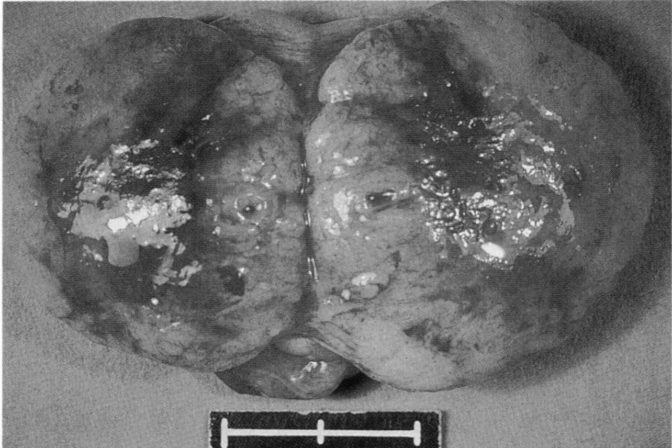

11-43. Infantile yolk sac tumor consists of a myxoid, tan nodule with focal hemorrhage.

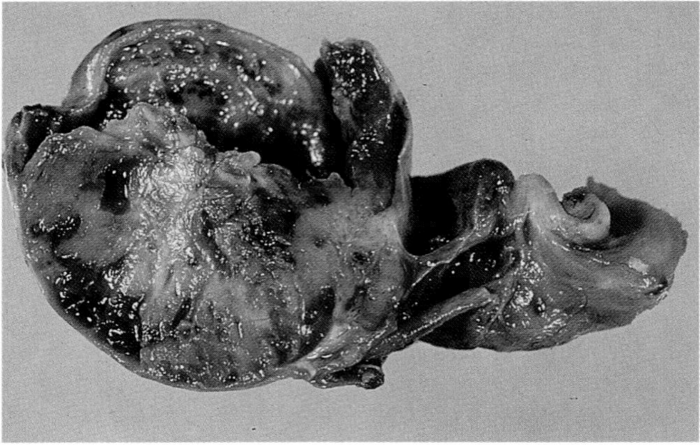

11-44. Adult yolk sac tumor showing hemorrhage, cystic degeneration, and myxoid change. *(From: Ulbright TM, Roth LM: Testicular and paratesticular neoplasms. In Sternberg SS, ed: Diagnostic surgical pathology, ed 2, New York, 1994, Raven Press; by permission of Raven Press.)*

The microcystic pattern is most common and is characterized by intracellular vacuoles creating attenuated lengths of cytoplasm connected in a spiderweb-like array (Fig. 11-45). In some cases, the cells are arranged in cords and surround extracellular spaces (Fig. 11-46). The cells often resemble lipoblasts, with compressed nuclei secondary to the vacuoles, although the vacuoles do not contain lipid. The microcystic pattern is often seen with a myxoid stroma and blends with the myxomatous pattern (Fig. 11-47). The solid pattern is also commonly intermingled with the microcystic (Fig. 11-48).

The endodermal sinus pattern consists of a central vessel rimmed by fibrous tissue, which is, in turn, surrounded by malignant epithelium. This structure is contained within a cystic space, which is often lined by flattened tumor cells (Fig. 11-49). Oblique cuts of these structures result in fibrovascular cores of tissue, which are

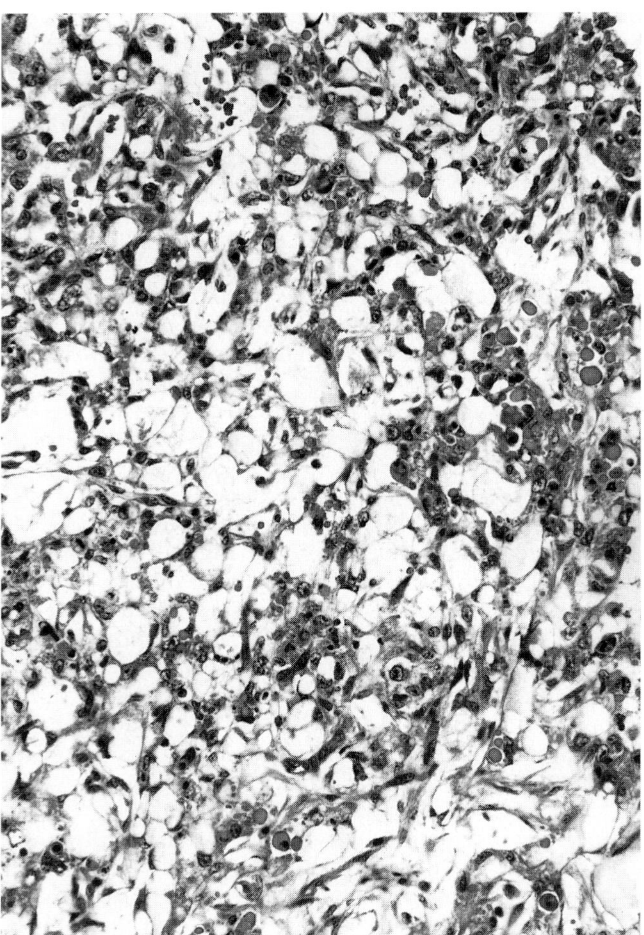

11-45. Microcystic pattern of yolk sac tumor resulting from intracellular vacuoles.

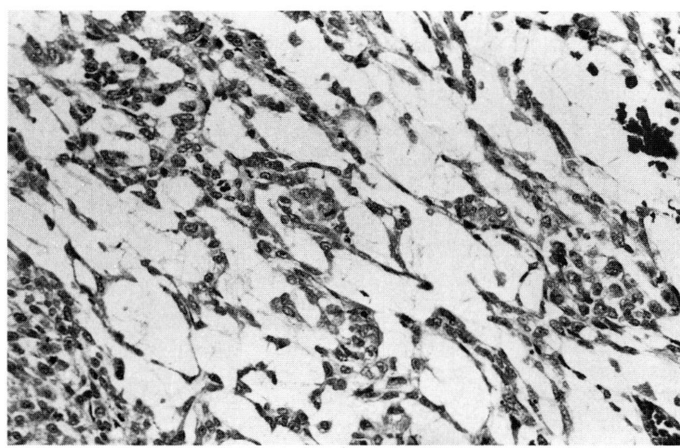

11-46. Microcystic pattern of yolk sac tumor created by cords of cells surrounding extracellular space (also referred to as reticular pattern).

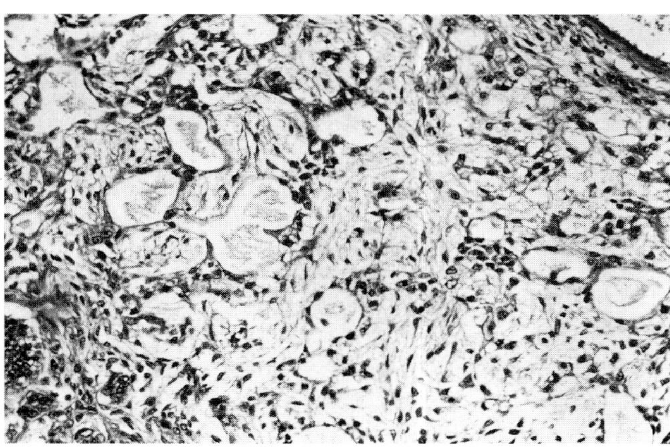

11-47. Blending of microcystic and myxoid patterns of yolk sac tumor. Neoplastic cells appear to "bud" from microcystic structures and blend into a myxoid stroma.

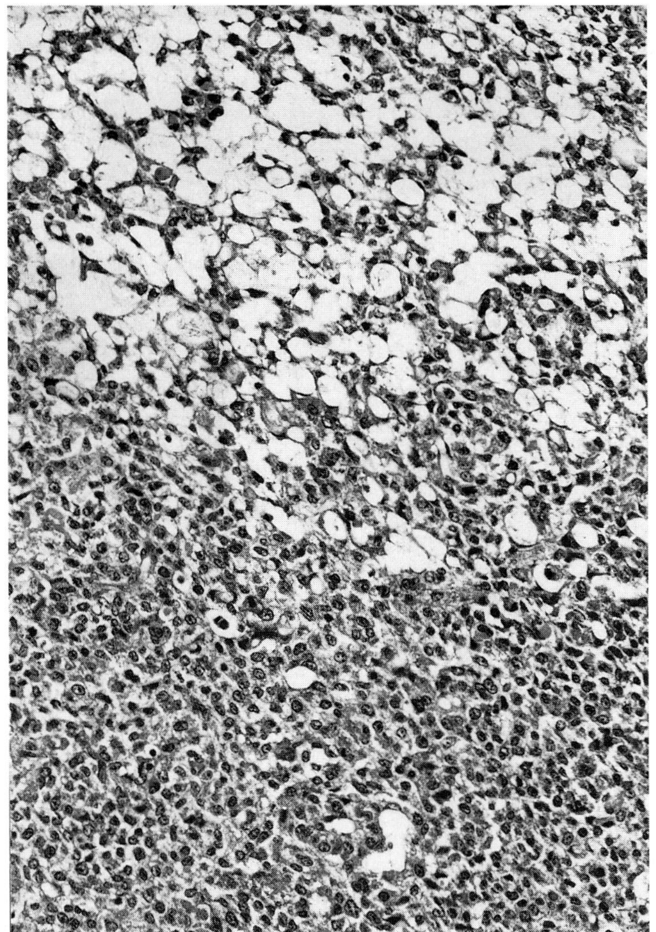

11-48. Mixture of solid and microcystic patterns in yolk sac tumor.

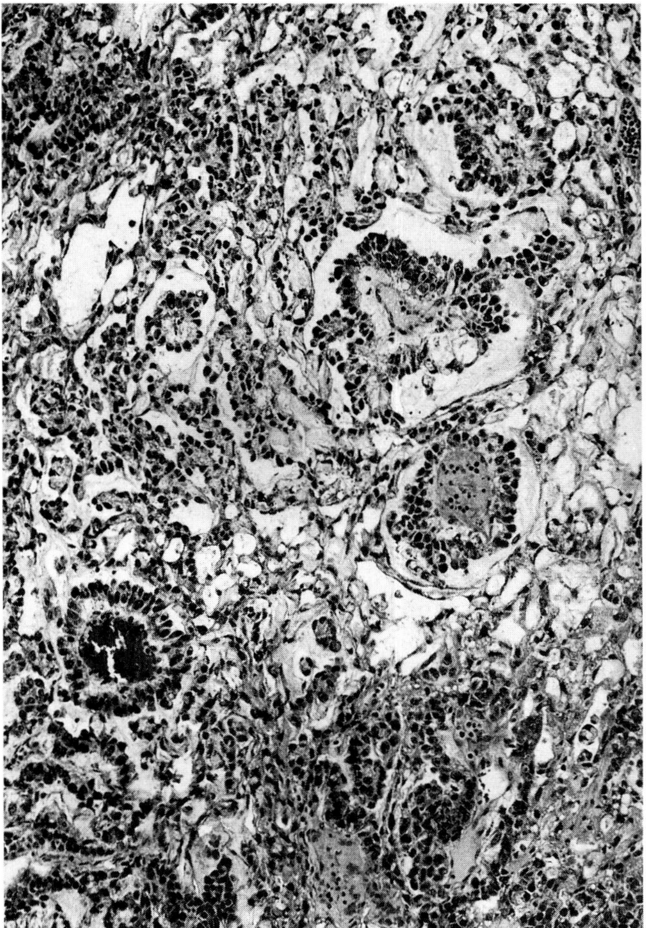

11-49. Endodermal sinus pattern of yolk sac tumor. Several endodermal sinus-like structures are present in this field.

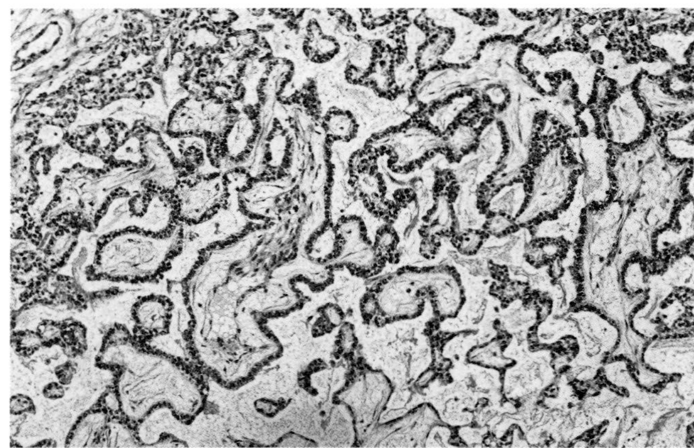

11-50. Oblique sections of endodermal sinus-like structures result in ellipsoid configurations with festoons of malignant epithelium at the periphery and a complex labyrinthine pattern of interconnecting, extracellular spaces.

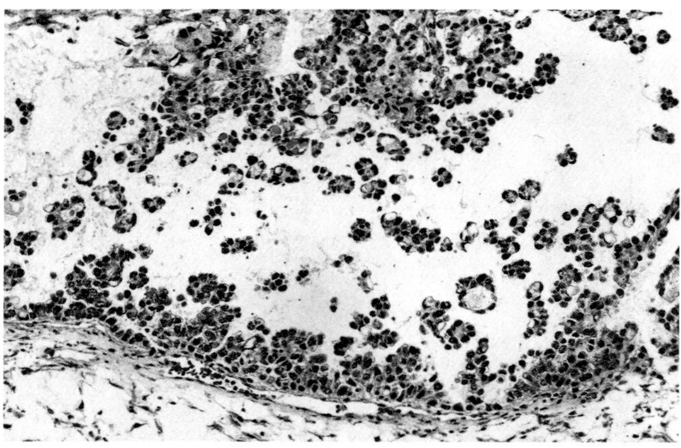

11-51. Papillary yolk sac tumor with lining of cuboidal cells projecting into a cystic space.

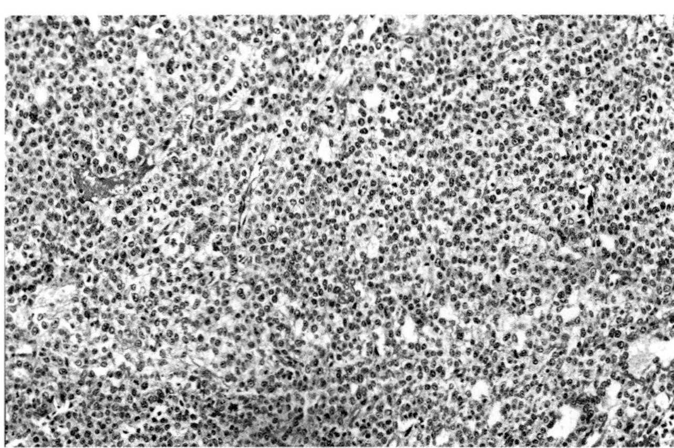

11-52. Solid pattern of yolk sac tumor composed of cells with clear cytoplasm and distinct borders. Note focal microcystic change.

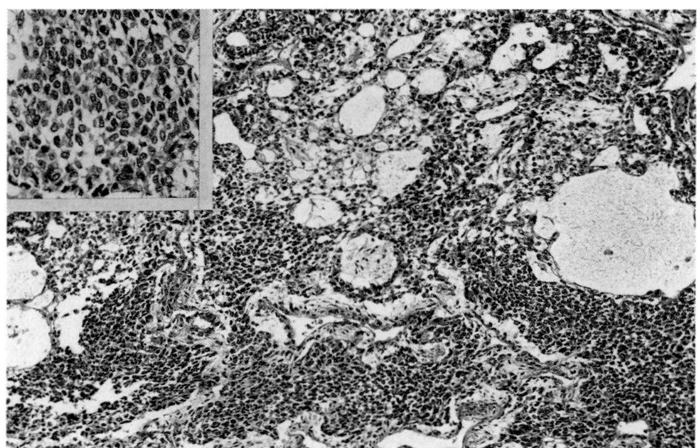

11-53. Solid areas in yolk sac tumor, composed of small, blastematous cells, mixed with a microcystic pattern. Inset shows blastematous cells.

"draped" or "festooned" by malignant cells with an accompanying complex (labyrinthine) arrangement of anastomosing extracellular spaces (Fig. 11-50). Some authors call this pattern a *perivascular* or a *festoon* pattern. The endodermal sinus-like structure is sometimes termed a *glomeruloid* or *Schiller-Duval* body.[346]

The papillary pattern has papillae, with or without fibrovascular cores, which project into cystic spaces (Fig. 11-51). The cells are often cuboidal to low columnar, with a hobnail configuration caused by the nucleus producing an apical cytoplasmic bulge. Exfoliated clusters of neoplastic cells may be present in the cystic spaces. The papillary pattern may blend with the endodermal sinus pattern.

The solid pattern is quite common and may resemble seminoma, consisting of sheets of uniform cells with lightly staining to clear cytoplasm and well-defined borders (Fig. 11-52); however, the lymphoid component and fibrous septa of seminoma are usually absent. Some solid patterns have prominent thin-walled blood vessels, and focal microcysts may also be seen in an otherwise solid pattern (see Fig. 11-48, 11-52). In some cases, the solid pattern has small cells with scant cytoplasm resembling blastema (see Fig. 11-53); such foci are intimately intermingled with classic patterns of yolk sac tumor.

Well-defined glands, often with enteric features, are common in yolk sac tumor, present in 34% of cases in one series (Fig. 11-54).[250] The glands may be contiguous with vesicles typical of the polyvesicular vitelline pattern, or may appear in a background of myxomatous, microcystic, or solid patterns. Usually the glands are simple, round, and tubular, but may show an elaborate branching pattern or become quite intricate and complex (Fig. 11-55). Unlike the glands of teratoma, the glands of yolk sac tumor are not associated with other teratomatous components and lack the smooth muscle component that is common but not invariable in teratoma.[355] In many cases, the nuclei of the glands are more bland than those of the surrounding yolk sac tumor. The glands may show basal subnuclear vacuolation, reminiscent of the early secretory pattern of the endometrium; and predominantly glandular yolk sac tumor in the ovary has been called *endometrioid-like* to emphasize its resemblance to

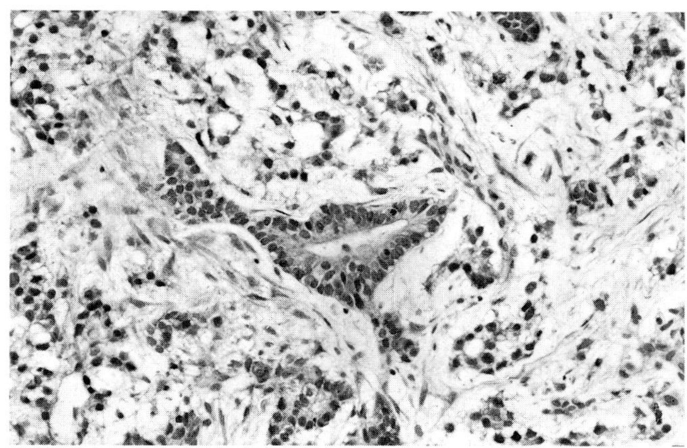

11-54. Glandular structures in the microcystic (reticular) pattern of yolk sac tumor.

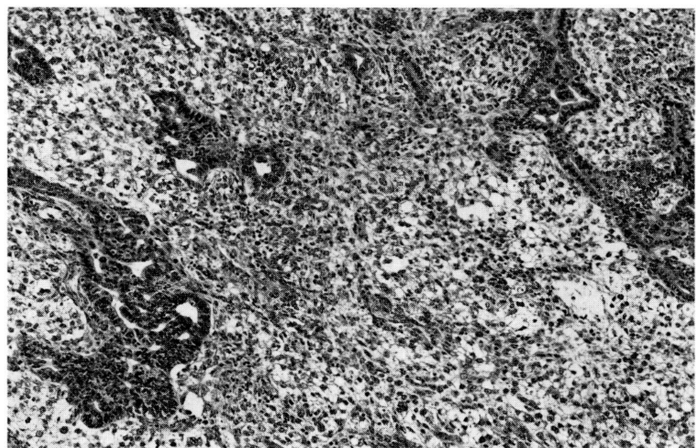

11-55. Complex glands in the solid pattern of yolk sac tumor.

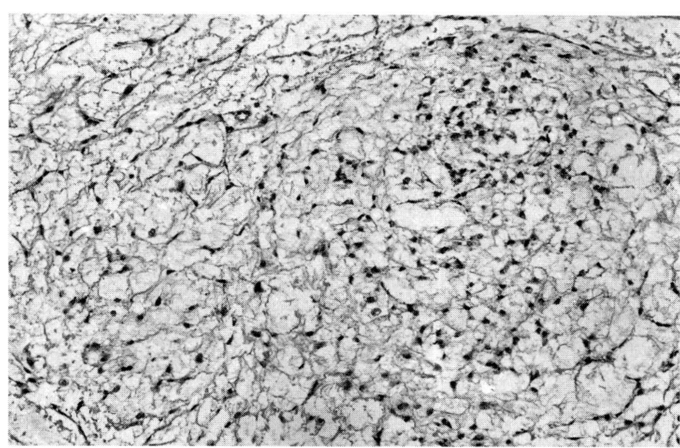

11-56. Stellate and spindle cells are dispersed in a myxoid stroma in the myxomatous pattern of yolk sac tumor.

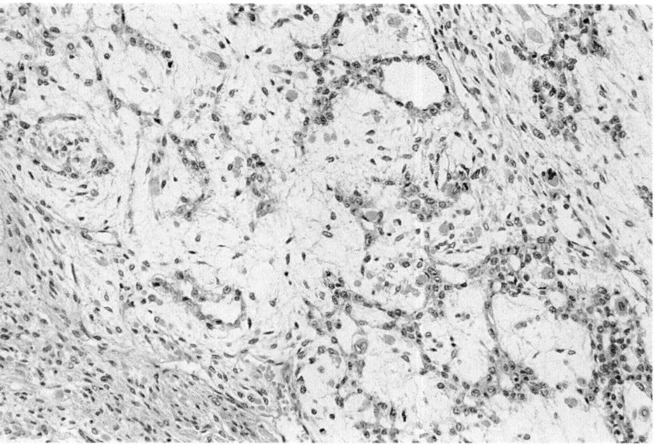

11-57. Rhabdomyoblastic cells intermingle with spindle cells in the myxomatous portion of this yolk sac tumor.

endometrioid carcinoma.[356] Purely or predominantly glandular testicular yolk sac tumor is more rare than in the ovary, but may be associated with a high serum alpha-fetoprotein.[357] Purely glandular yolk sac tumor is more common following chemotherapy and is therefore usually found in metastases.

The myxomatous pattern is common, consisting of neoplastic epithelioid to spindle cells dispersed in a stroma that is rich in mucopolysaccharide, staining only lightly with hematoxylin and eosin (Fig. 11-56). A prominent vascular network is common, and Teilum described this pattern as "angioblastic mesenchyme," which he felt was homologous with the extraembryonic mesenchyme (the magma reticulare) of development.[358] Myxomatous foci commonly merge with other patterns, and hybrids of microcystic and myxomatous patterns are more the rule than the exception. By light microscopy, the spindle cells appear to arise from solid or microcystic foci by budding from them and blending into the surrounding myxoid stroma (see Fig. 11-47). Intense cytokeratin immunoreactivity within these cells supports derivation from the epithelial component of yolk sac tumor.[359] These cells are, in fact, pluripotential cells with the capacity to form differentiated mesenchymal tissue such as skeletal muscle, cartilage, and bone,[359] thus blurring the distinction between yolk sac tumor and teratoma (Fig. 11-57). Classification of such elements as yolk sac tumor is justified by the recognition that the surrounding tissues are typical yolk sac tumor.

The sarcomatoid pattern is uncommon, consisting of a cellular proliferation of spindle cells in continuity with other yolk sac tumor patterns, most commonly the microcystic pattern. The sarcomatoid pattern is distinguished from the solid pattern by the spindle cell nature of the component cells. Despite the sarcomatoid appearance, the spindle cells usually express cytokeratin. It is likely that embryonal rhabdomyosarcoma arising in testicular germ cell tumor derives from differentiation of sarcomatoid spindle cells to rhabdomyoblastic cells.[360] The occasional intimate admixture of embryonal rhabdomyosarcoma with yolk sac tumor supports this hypothesis.

The macrocystic pattern appears to arise from coalescence of microcystic spaces to form large, round to irregular cysts, and the surrounding pattern is often microcystic.

In the polyvesicular vitelline pattern (Fig. 11-58), vesicle-like structures are lined by flattened, innocuous-appearing epithelium, with a myxoid to fibrous stroma. Sometimes the vesicles have a central constriction, resembling a dumbbell or figure 8. Teilum[361] compared these vesicles to the embryonic subdivision of the primary yolk sac into the secondary yolk sac. At the point of constriction, the epithelium may change from flattened to cuboidal or columnar; the latter often has enteric features, including an apical brush border. Alpha-fetoprotein is often present in the epithelial lining of the vesicles, and hyaline globules are occasionally seen within the epithelial cells. In some cases, a transition from microcystic pattern to polyvesicular vitelline pattern can be identified. The bland cytologic appearance of the polyvesicular vitelline pattern may falsely suggest benignancy, but the presence of other patterns should prevent this pitfall. The polyvesicular pattern is less common in testicular yolk sac tumor than in its ovarian counterpart.

A hepatoid pattern also occurs in about 20% of yolk sac tumors and consists of small clusters of polygonal, eosinophilic cells arranged in sheets or trabeculae (Fig. 11-59).[250,362] The cells have round, vesicular nuclei with prominent nucleoli and contain abundant alpha-fetoprotein; hyaline globules are common in hepatoid foci as are bile canaliculi, although bile is not present.[214,363] Hepatoid foci are scattered randomly in yolk sac tumor and usually are minor components; rarely, a more diffuse hepatoid pattern may be seen, although a prominent hepatoid pattern is more common in ovarian tumors.[364]

The parietal pattern has extensive deposits of extracellular basement membrane, with only scattered neoplastic cells in an abundant, eosinophilic matrix (Fig. 11-60). It is considered the extreme end of parietal differentiation (see discussion on p. 599) in which basement membrane is deposited in the extracellular space in a variety of yolk sac tumor patterns. In a true parietal-pattern yolk sac tumor, any underlying yolk sac tumor pattern is effaced by the basement membrane deposits. This is a very rare pattern, most often seen following chemotherapy.[365]

The frequency of the different patterns of yolk sac tumor is difficult to determine because of a lack of uni-

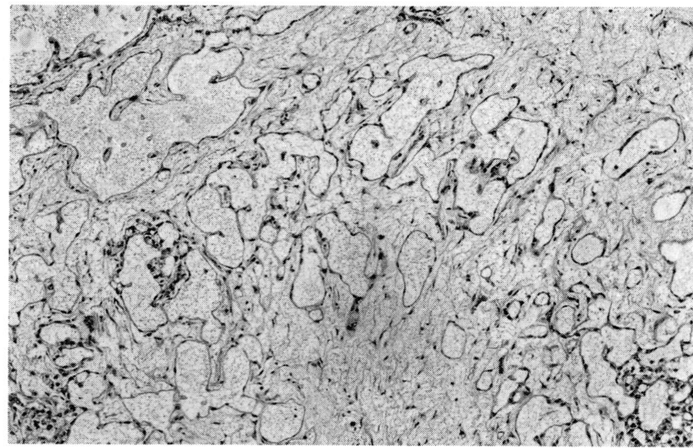

11-58. Polyvesicular vitelline pattern of yolk sac tumor.

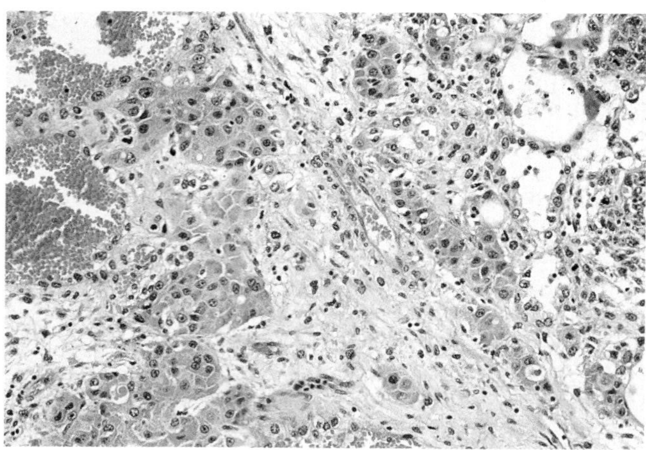

11-59. Hepatoid pattern of yolk sac tumor. Note islands of eosinophilic cells with round nuclei and prominent nucleoli adjacent to microcystic (reticular) pattern.

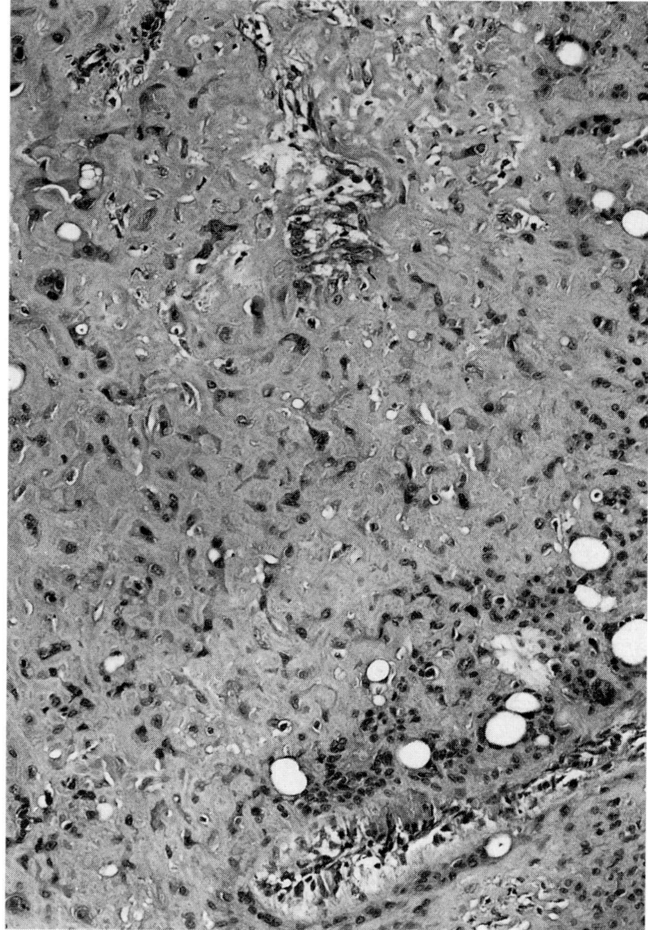

11-60. Diffuse basement membrane deposits characterize the parietal pattern of yolk sac tumor.

formity in classification. The microcystic, solid, and myxomatous patterns are most common, with glandular, macrocystic, endodermal sinus, hepatoid, and papillary patterns also occurring frequently. The polyvesicular vitelline pattern is less common, and sarcomatoid and parietal patterns are unusual. If only four patterns are employed for classification, the frequency of the patterns diminishes from reticular to solid to endodermal sinus to polyvesicular vitelline. Jacobsen[304] noted a vacuolated network in 91% of yolk sac tumors, microcystic pattern in 67%, myxomatous pattern in 51%, macrocystic pattern in 44%, solid pattern in 27%, hepatoid areas in 23%, labyrinthine formations in 17%, and endodermal sinus-like structures in 9%.

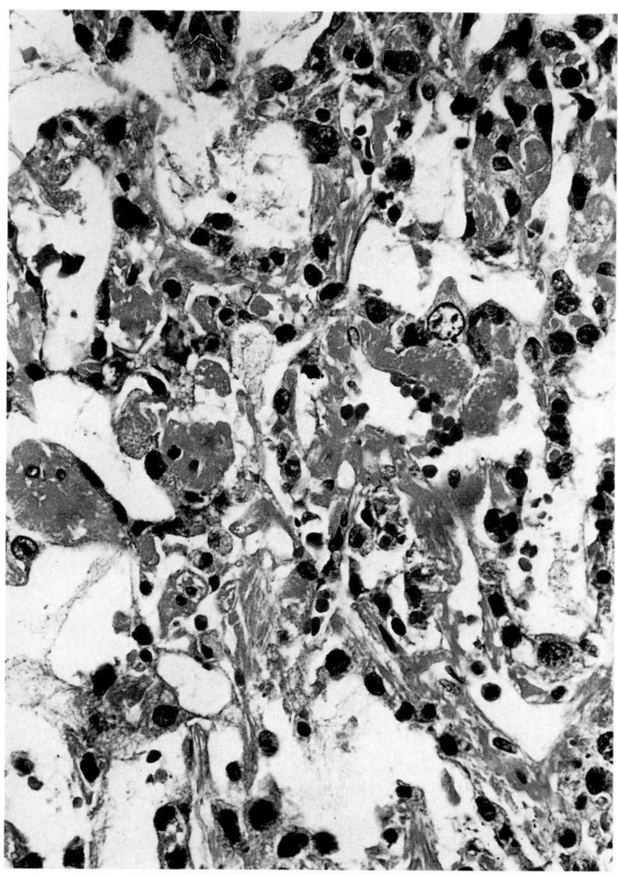

11-61. Bands and irregularly shaped deposits of basement membrane constitute parietal differentiation in this microcystic (reticular) pattern of yolk sac tumor. *(From Ulbright TM, Roth LM: Recent developments in the pathology of germ cell tumors, Semin Diagn Pathol 4:304-319, 1987.)*

A general feature of yolk sac tumor is the deposition of extracellular basement membrane, identified in 92% of cases.[250] These deposits generally are irregularly shaped, eosinophilic bands between the neoplastic cells (Fig. 11-61) and have been referred to as parietal differentiation because of the synthesis of a thick basement membrane (known as *Reichert's membrane*) by the parietal layer of the embryonic yolk sac of the rat.[250,361] Such intercellular basement membrane, although not specific for yolk sac tumor, is characteristic and can be helpful in diagnosis, particularly in small biopsy samples taken from extratesticular tumors. Another characteristic but nonspecific feature in most yolk sac tumors is the presence of intracellular, round, hyaline globules of variable size (from 1 micron to more than 50 microns in diameter) (Fig. 11-62). These globules are PAS-positive and diastase-resistant and may be present in the extracellular space following cell necrosis. Occasionally these globules may stain positively for alpha-fetoprotein, but most do not. The hyaline globules and basement membrane deposits of yolk sac tumor are separate and distinct findings, although they have sometimes been confused in the literature.

Hematopoietic elements, usually erythroblasts, are present in a minority of testicular yolk sac tumors, usually in vascular spaces or stromal tissues.

Special studies

Immunohistochemically, most yolk sac tumors show cytoplasmic alpha-fetoprotein; the frequency varies from 50% to 100% depending on the technique employed and the number of blocks examined.[39,50,157,366] Positivity is characteristically patchy (Fig. 11-63); intense staining is

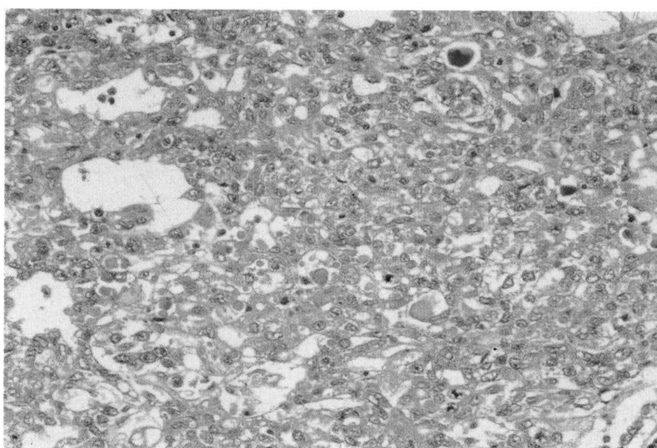

11-62. Solid and microcystic patterns of yolk sac tumor with eosinophilic hyaline globules.

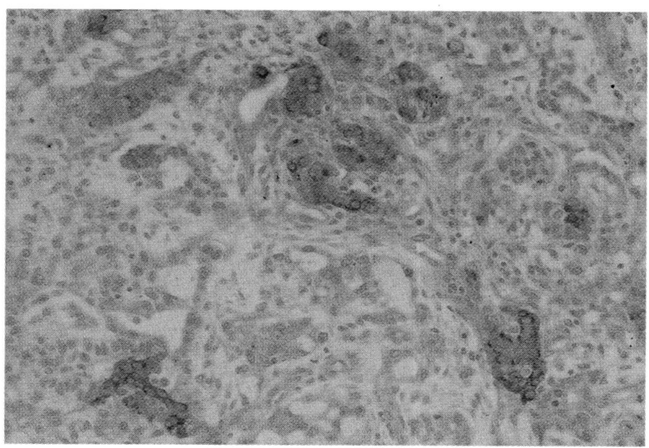

11-63. Patchy immunoreactivity for alpha-fetoprotein in a yolk sac tumor.

usually present in hepatoid foci. Adult yolk sac tumor stains more frequently for alpha-fetoprotein than childhood cases.[157] Positivity for alpha-1-antitrypsin occurs in about 50% of cases,[39,50] and the enteric glands of yolk sac tumor may stain for carcinoembryonic antigen.[39,250,311] Cytokeratin is present in virtually all cases,[39,367] and vimentin is present in the spindle cells of myxomatous and sarcomatoid patterns.[367] Albumin, ferritin, neuron specific enolase, and Leu-7 are present in a variable number of cases.[39,311] From 39% to 85% of yolk sac tumors are reported as positive for PLAP,[39,160,162] and epithelial membrane antigen is usually negative.[39] p53 may be identified in yolk sac tumor,[145] and laminin is present in areas of parietal differentiation.[250] Experimental antibodies directed against cell surface antigens of a yolk sac tumor cell line have marked yolk sac tumors.[368]

Ultrastructurally, yolk sac tumors show clusters of epithelial cells joined by junctional complexes. Apical microvilli may be seen in some cases, as well as extracellular lumens. Basement membrane material can be identified in the extracellular space, and flocculent material is present within dilated cisternae of endoplasmic reticulum, often with a central lucent zone.[51,250,369,370] Cytoplasmic glycogen may be conspicuous.[369,371] The nuclei are usually irregular, with complex nucleolonema. Glands have microvilli with glycocalyceal bodies and long anchoring rootlets.[250] Densely osmiophilic, cytoplasmic, nonmembrane bound, round bodies correspond to the hyaline globules observed at the light microscopic level.

Unlike adult cases, childhood yolk sac tumors lack i(12p) on karyotypic analysis.[372] About 30% of childhood yolk sac tumors are diploid, with peritetraploid values in the remainder,[42] whereas adult tumors are almost invariably nondiploid.[42] These results may be related to the paucity or absence of IGCNU in childhood yolk sac tumors.[182]

Differential diagnosis

In the differential diagnosis of yolk sac tumor, the solid pattern must be distinguished from seminoma, an issue that is addressed on page 596. The distinction of yolk sac tumor from embryonal carcinoma has less clinical significance but is based on the distinctive patterns of yolk sac tumor and the less pleomorphic, less atypical nature of the neoplastic cells. Embryonal carcinoma probably transforms to yolk sac tumor,[373] so there are transitional forms that are difficult to categorize. Juvenile granulosa cell tumor (see page 623) may mimic yolk sac tumor; both may be seen in very young children, but juvenile granulosa cell tumor usually is seen in children under 5 months of age,[374] whereas yolk sac tumor occurs in older children, the peak being at 17 to 18 months of age.[347,348] Histologically, both tumors may show microcystic, macrocystic, and solid patterns, as well as high mitotic rates and cellular atypia. The presence of other patterns is a key to recognizing yolk sac tumor; intracellular alpha-fetoprotein does not occur in juvenile granulosa cell tumor but may be seen in pediatric yolk sac tumor.[28] There is limited information concerning the immunohistochemistry of testicular juvenile granulosa cell tumor,[375] but it appears to have variable, often weak to absent, cytokeratin reactivity and strong vimentin positivity,[376,377] compared with strong cytokeratin reactivity in yolk sac tumors. However, such qualitative differences are unlikely to be diagnostic. Serum alpha-fetoprotein levels may be physiologically elevated in infants under 6 months of age,[378] and should not be overinterpreted to support the diagnosis of yolk sac tumor rather than juvenile granulosa cell tumor. A hyperplastic reaction of the rete testis with hyaline globules may be induced by invasion of the rete testis by a neoplasm, thus simulating yolk sac tumor.[379] The arborizing pattern of the rete testis and the bland nature of the hyperplastic cells should prevent this misinterpretation, although immunostains may also be of value.[379]

Treatment and prognosis

Adult patients with yolk sac tumor are treated in a fashion similar to that outlined on page 593, although the presence of a yolk sac tumor component in a patient with clinical stage I tumor has been associated with a decreased likelihood of occult metastases.[329,380] Patients with metastatic yolk sac tumor do not respond as well to chemotherapy as patients with other forms of metastatic nonteratomatous testicular germ cell tumor and therefore seem to have a worse prognosis.[381] Eighty percent to 90% of children with testicular yolk sac tumor have pathologic stage I tumor,[347,382] and current trends are to expectantly follow patients with clinical stage I tumors (including postorchiectomy alpha-fetoprotein levels) rather than perform retroperitoneal lymph node dissection.[383] Retroperitoneal lymph node dissection may not be the optimal therapy given an increased frequency of hematogenous metastases to the lung, and the occurrence of retroperitoneal involvement in only 4% to 14% of cases.[384] These data indicate that childhood yolk sac tumors behave in a more indolent fashion than nonseminomatous germ cell tumors in adult patients,[385] although some investigators believe that retroperitoneal involvement is more common than usually stated in childhood yolk sac tumors, and that dissemination in the absence of alpha-fetoprotein elevation may occur more commonly in childhood cases, thereby making early relapse difficult to detect.[386]

The prognosis of childhood yolk sac tumor is good, with a 5-year survival of 91%.[299] Differences in prognosis with respect to age in children[348] are no longer identified,[299,347] perhaps as a result of contemporary therapies. The greater chemoresistance of yolk sac tumor in adult patients is reflected in a higher frequency of yolk sac tumor metastases at autopsy in patients in the chemotherapeutic era compared to the prechemotherapeutic era.[387]

TERATOMA

Clinical features

Teratoma is the second most common form of testicular germ cell tumor in children (yolk sac tumor is the most common), accounting for 14% to 18% of cases.[197,348] In children, testicular teratoma occurs as a pure neoplasm, at a mean age of 20 months,[348] and is most commonly found during routine physical examination or by a parent. Testicular teratoma in children older than 4 years of age is unusual.[348] This tumor is associated with a variety of congenital anomalies, including spina bifida, retrocaval ureter, hemihypertrophy, and hernia,[388] but most cases lack such an association. In contrast, teratoma usually occurs in adults as a component of a mixed germ cell tumor and is present in more than half of all mixed germ cell tumors and in approximately 25% of all nonseminomatous germ cell tumors.[194,389]

The metastatic potential of pure testicular teratoma has been a source of confusion. Children with pure teratoma are not reported to have metastases.[390,391] Conversely, postpubertal patients have a definite risk of metastases, even with pure mature teratoma. Hence, there are reports of pure mature teratoma metastasizing as pure mature teratoma[392-395] and, interestingly, pure mature teratoma associated with metastases of nonteratomatous type, such as embryonal carcinoma.[390] The most likely explanation for these observations is that postpubertal patients with pure mature teratoma developed their neoplasm by evolution from IGCNU, a supposition supported by the frequent identification of IGCNU in seminiferous tubules adjacent to pure teratoma of the testis in postpubertal patients.[183] It is therefore likely that nonteratomatous malignant elements were initially a component of many postpubertal teratomas, but transformation of such elements to teratoma (or their regression) occurred prior to orchiectomy. Metastasis of nonteratomatous elements with subsequent transformation at the metastatic site to teratomatous elements could explain the phenomenon of mature teratoma metastasizing as mature teratoma; failure to transform at the site of metastasis could explain the situation of mature teratoma associated with metastases of nonteratomatous type. Mostofi and Sesterhenn[48] suggest that some mature teratomas may directly metastasize because they have identified vascular invasion in the testis by such elements. Whatever the mechanism, it is important to recognize that a postpubertal patient with a pure mature testicular teratoma is at risk for metastasis, and the term *pure mature teratoma* cannot be equated with benignity. The reported absence (or paucity) of IGCNU in prepubertal patients with testicular teratoma[183] may account for the absence of metastases in this group of patients.

Most patients with testicular teratoma present with a testicular mass, although postpubertal patients may have symptoms secondary to metastases. Serum marker elevation may occur in postpubertal patients because of intermixed yolk sac tumor or syncytiotrophoblastic cells; in addition, mild alpha-fetoprotein elevation may occur in patients with pure teratoma secondary to synthesis of alpha-fetoprotein by endodermal glandular structures of teratomatous type.[48,50,311]

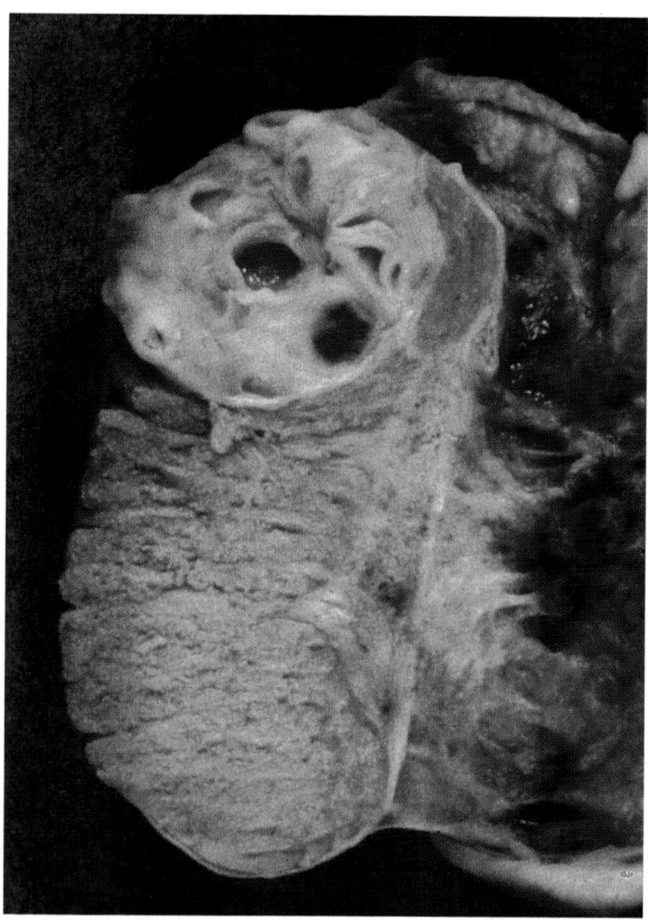

11-64. Mature teratoma with several cysts and gray-white cartilage.

Pathologic features

Grossly, teratoma has a variable appearance. Mature teratoma often contains multiple cysts, generally under 1 cm in diameter, which contain watery to mucoid fluid (Fig. 11-64). Semitranslucent nodules of gray-white cartilage may be present, and a fibromuscular stroma may be seen among the cartilaginous and cystic structures. In other areas, the tumor may be solid. Fleshy, encephaloid, and hemorrhagic areas usually correspond to foci of immaturity, which, if extensive, may justify a diagnosis of teratoma with an overtly malignant component. Such foci in postpubertal patients may also represent intermixed nonteratomatous elements.

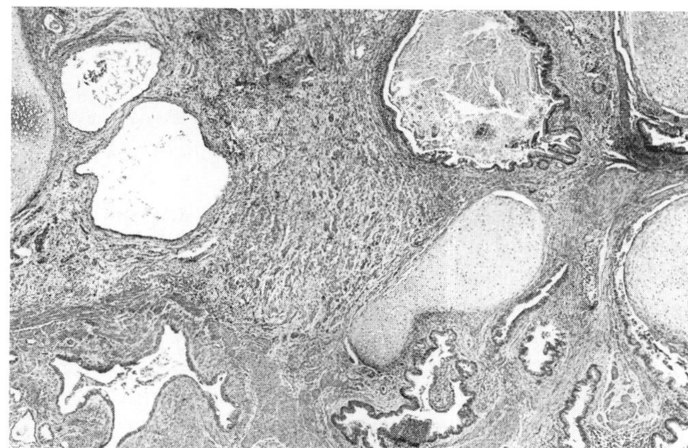

11-65. Mature teratoma with islands of hyaline cartilage, glandular structures lined by enteric-type epithelium, and fibromuscular stroma.

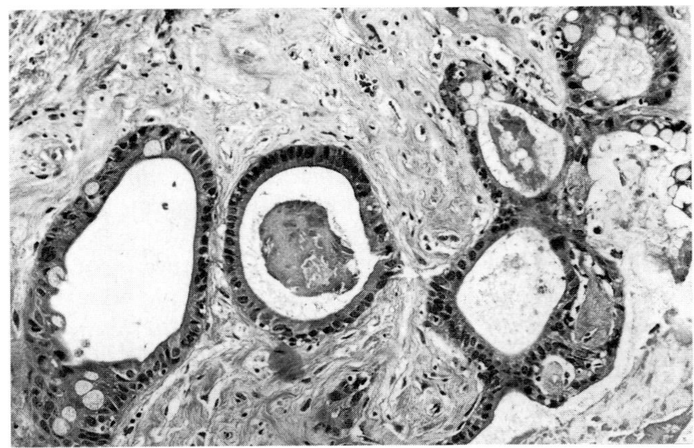

11-66. Mature enteric-type glands in the fibrous stroma of teratoma.

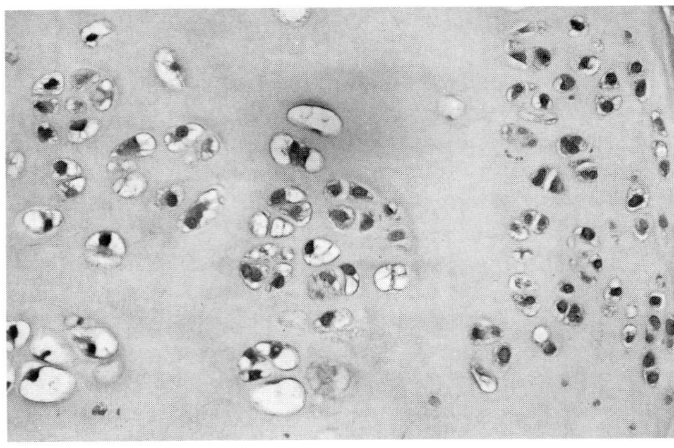

11-68. Cytologic atypia of hyaline cartilage in mature teratoma.

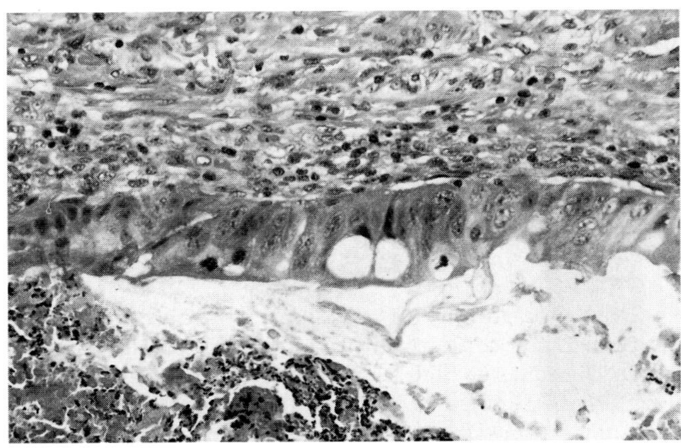

11-67. Cytologic atypia of enteric-type epithelium in mature teratoma.

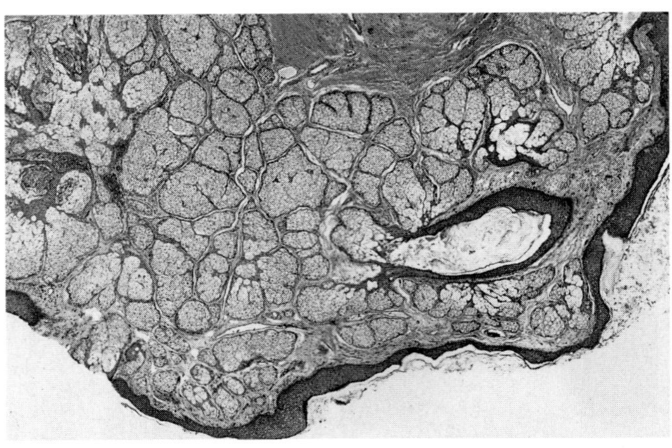

11-69. The wall of a dermoid cyst, with keratinizing, squamous epithelium and sebaceous glands.

Microscopically, mature teratoma consists of a variety of somatic-type tissues (Fig. 11-65), commonly including cartilage, smooth and skeletal muscle, neuroglia, enteric-type glands (Fig. 11-66), squamous epithelial islands and cysts, respiratory epithelium, and urothelial islands. Less commonly, bone and pigmented choroidal epithelium and rarely kidney, liver, pancreas, or prostatic-type tissues are present. These tissues are considered mature, but it is quite common to find significant cytologic atypia, especially in postpubertal patients (Fig. 11-67, 11-68). This atypia correlates with the presence of aneuploidy in mature testicular teratoma.[396] There is no evidence that the grading of the degree of atypia, based on qualitative assessment of nuclear enlargement, hyperchromasia, and mitotic rate, has any prognostic significance, but it may be useful to characterize the atypia as low or high grade for both the epithelial and mesenchymal components.

Dermoid cyst is very rare and represents a subset of mature teratoma that grossly forms a unicystic mass filled with grumous, keratinous debris and which may contain hair. It is analogous to its ovarian counterpart and may have a similar mural protuberance.[397,398] Microscopically, a cyst, filled with keratin and lined by epidermis containing hair follicles, sebaceous glands, and other appendigeal structures, is identified (Fig. 11-69). Some authors also include as dermoid cyst those cases that have a minority of nonectodermal tissues such as cartilage, smooth muscle, adipose tissue and bone, as long as the lesion is unicystic and the components are histologically benign.[213,399] The distinction from mature teratoma may be difficult if cases with noncutaneous structures are considered valid; the presence of IGCNU, as well as cytologic atypia, is indication for classification as mature teratoma. Metastasis from a pure dermoid cyst of the testis has not been reported.[213,398,399]

Immature elements are required for the diagnosis of immature teratoma. Such elements are easily recognized when they consist of highly immature tissues such as neuroepithelium, blastema, or embryonic tubules. Neuroepithelium consists of small, hyperchromatic cells arranged in tubules and rosettes (Fig. 11-70). Blastema consists of nodular collections of oval cells with scant cytoplasm and hyperchromatic nuclei (Fig. 11-71); such blastematous elements may be mixed with embryonic tubules lined by cuboidal cells with scant, inconspicuous cytoplasm.

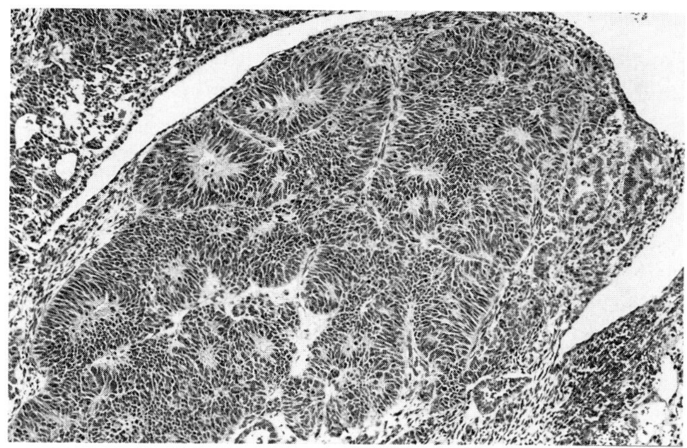

11-70. Immature neuroepithelium in an immature teratoma. This is a high-grade immature element.

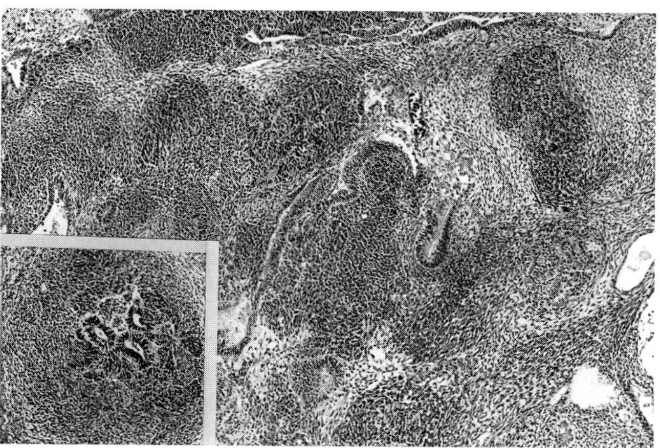

11-71. Cellular nodules of blastema with glands in an immature teratoma. Inset shows characteristic mixture of glands and blastema resembling nephroblastoma.

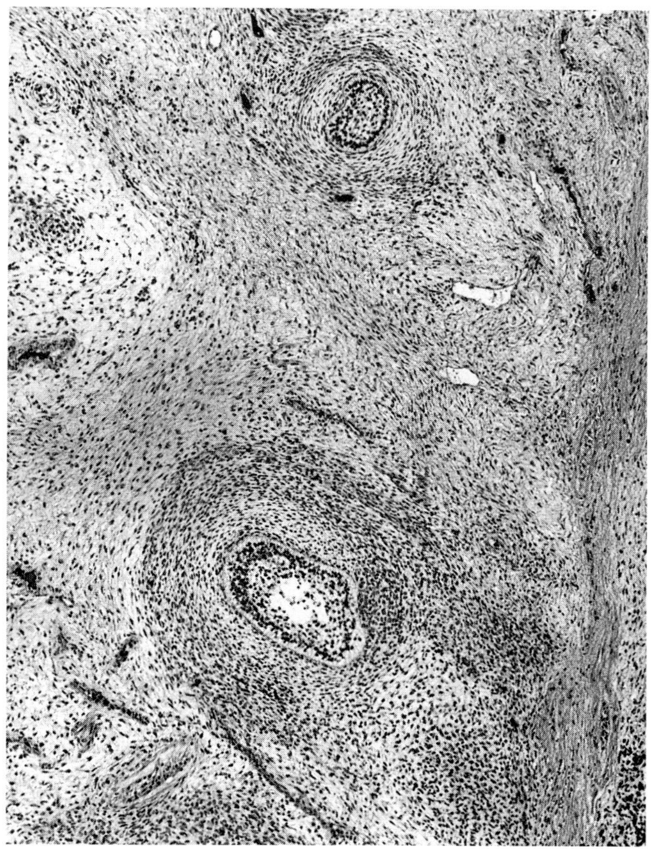

11-72. Low grade immature teratoma, with modestly cellular stroma around islands of epithelium.

When intermixed, these two components resemble a primitive blastomatous neoplasm such as nephroblastoma or pulmonary blastoma (see Fig. 11-71). Lower grade immature elements may consist of a hypercellular or a myxomatous, hypocellular mesenchyme (Fig. 11-72). This low grade immature stroma often is arranged concentrically around islands of epithelium, resembling developing smooth muscle in the embryonic gastrointestinal or respiratory system (see Fig. 11-72). As in the grading of atypia in mature teratoma, it is not clear if the grading of immature elements is prognostically useful. It is, nonetheless, recommended that a qualitative grading be performed, with an estimate of the amount (rare, focal, diffuse) and the degree of immaturity (low grade or high grade) so that some insight into this question can be gained. The lack of evidence that grading has significance likely stems from the common admixture of the postpubertal teratoma with other germ cell elements that behave more aggressively and hence determine the natural history of the neoplasm.

Teratoma with an overtly malignant component has also been classified as teratoma with malignant transformation. The latter term, however, connotes an unacceptable notion that teratoma in the absence of such a transformation is not malignant. An overtly malignant component in a teratoma may have either a mature or immature appearance. Carcinoma of somatic type, representing the destructive growth of epithelium with a mature phenotype, is recognized by its invasive features. It forms masses of cytologically malignant epithelium or irregularly configured, infiltrating cords or nests associated with a desmoplastic reaction. Adenocarcinoma, squamous cell carcinoma, and undifferentiated carcinoma may occur. Sarcoma may also occur but, because invasion of mesenchymal elements is not as easily appreciated as with epithelium, it may be confused with atypical teratomatous mesenchyme. It seems reasonable that growth beyond a certain size connotes an independently evolving neoplasm, but a threshold has not been established. My personal guideline is to diagnose a sarcoma when a substantial portion of a 4X field is occupied by a pure proliferation of a single type of highly atypical mesenchyme, but this is arbitrary. Similarly, teratoma with malignant transformation can be recognized in immature teratoma by the pure overgrowth of immature elements, using the guidelines described above. It is therefore justifiable to diagnose primitive neuroectodermal tumor with a pure overgrowth of neuroepithelium; a blastomatous, Wilm's tumor–like neoplasm with overgrowth of blastema and primitive tubules, and embryonal rhabdomyosarcoma with a pure overgrowth of primitive rhabdomyoblastic cells (Fig. 11-73). Similar primitive elements may be admixed with other teratomatous components, a finding within the spectrum of immature teratoma; hence, the emphasis on a pure proliferation of such elements in this type of overgrowth.

The clinical significance of teratoma with an overtly malignant component is not clear. Patients with such tumors probably more commonly develop chemoresistant nongerm cell neoplasms following chemotherapy.[400,401] However, Ahmed et al[402] were unable to document a poor prognosis in five patients with testicular germ cell tumors having malignant transformation of teratomatous elements. The identification of such a neoplasm after chemotherapy is associated with a guarded prognosis.[400,402]

Special studies

Immunohistochemical staining of teratomatous elements yields results expected for the nature of the particular tissue.[367,403] Alpha-fetoprotein may be present within glands of enteric or respiratory type,[50,311] as well as within liver-like tissue[48]; therefore, pure teratoma may be associated with modestly elevated serum alpha-fetoprotein. Alpha-1-antitrypsin, CEA, and ferritin may also be produced by teratomatous epithelium,[311] and PLAP-positivity may be expressed in glands of a minority of teratomas.[160,162,231]

Mature teratoma often has aneuploid DNA content, frequently in the hypotriploid range.[404,405] The i(12p) marker chromosome may also be found in testicular teratoma.[246] These data support the derivation of postpubertal teratoma from IGCNU.

Differential diagnosis

It is important to distinguish dermoid and epidermoid cysts from mature teratoma because they are benign.[213,398,399,406,407] Dermoid cyst consists of an epidermal-lined cyst with adnexal structures in the wall; an epidermoid cyst consists of an epidermal-lined cyst lined by keratinizing squamous epithelium but lacks associated adnexal structures. Unlike mature teratoma in postpubertal patients, these cysts do not display cytologic atypia, and, at least with epidermoid cyst, there is a documented absence of IGCNU.[183] Immature elements are not present in dermoid or epidermoid cysts.

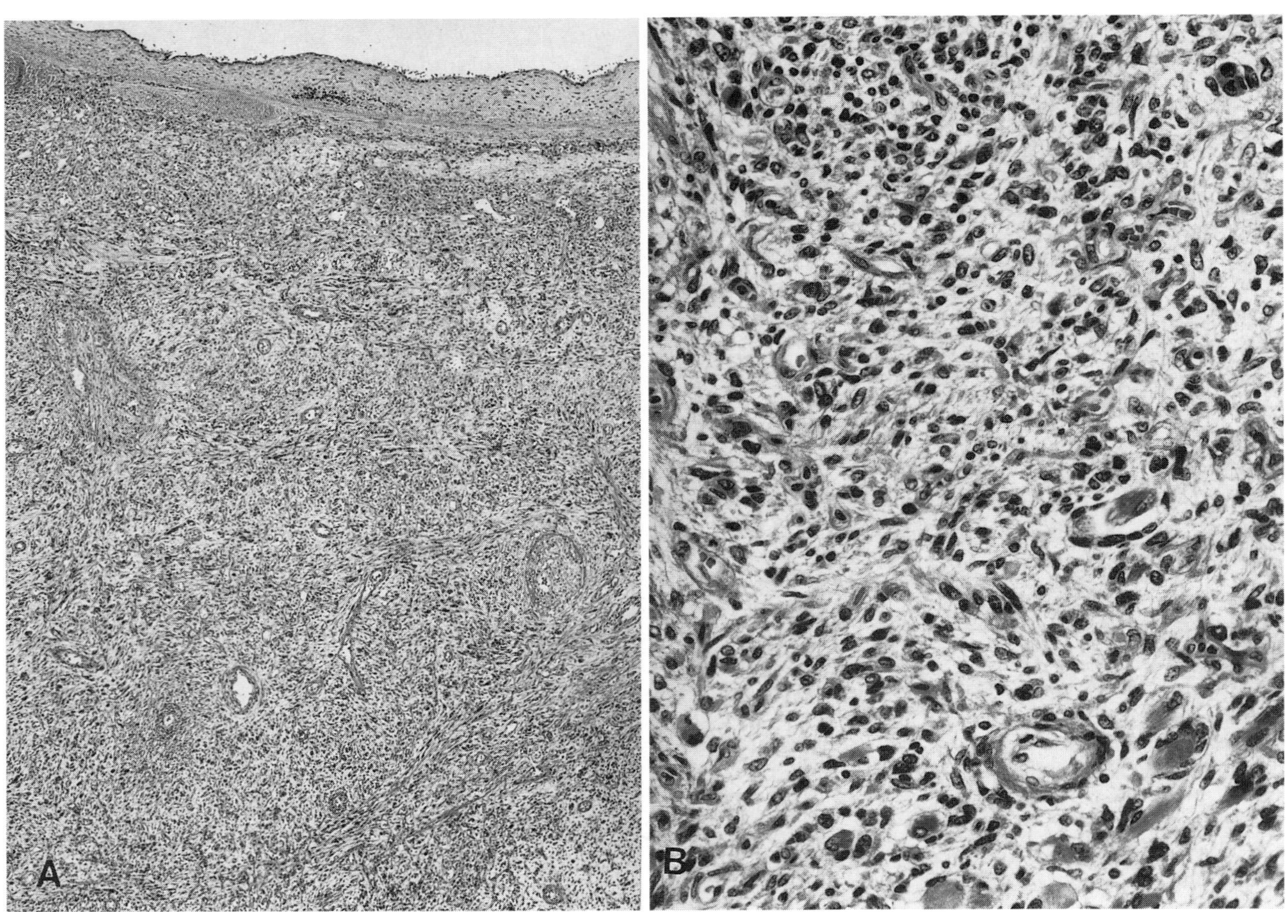

11-73. Embryonal rhabdomyosarcoma in teratoma. **A**, Low magnification shows overgrowth by rhabdomyoblasts. The wall of a cyst remains at top. **B**, High magnification shows primitive spindle and oval small cells with differentiated rhabdomyoblasts.

Treatment and prognosis

The prognosis of patients with pure testicular teratoma is variable. Prepubertal patients are cured by orchiectomy, with no reports of metastases;[390,391] however, it is recommended that clinical staging be performed. Postpubertal patients with pure mature teratoma have a guarded prognosis. Johnson et al[408] performed orchiectomy and retroperitoneal lymph node dissection in 18 patients with mature teratoma, some of whom also had a seminomatous component, and reported 100% 5-year survival. Conversely, 2 of 12 adult patients with pure teratoma reported by the British Testicular Tumour Panel died of nonteratomatous metastases.[390] Dixon and Moore[409] reported 70% 5-year survival for patients with teratoma, with or without seminoma.

Carcinoid tumor

Carcinoid tumor of the testis is considered a monodermal form of teratoma; and in support of this concept, about 15% to 25% of testicular carcinoid tumors are associated with other teratomatous elements.[410-412] These rare tumors constitute 0.17% of testicular tumors in the files at the Armed Forces Institute of Pathology.[411] They occur in older patients, with a median age of 45 to 50 years,[411,412] with some cases reported in elderly men.[410,413] Most patients present with a testicular mass; carcinoid syndrome is uncommon (occurring in about 12% of cases) but correlates with increased metastatic potential.[412] It is more common to identify serotonin in tissue or serum, or its metabolites in urine, than for clinical carcinoid syndrome to occur.[412] Alpha-fetoprotein and human chorionic gonadotropin levels are normal in these patients.

Grossly, testicular carcinoids are solid, yellow to tan, and well-circumscribed, varying from 0.8 to 8 cm in diameter (Fig. 11-74).[410,412] Associated cystic spaces may represent a teratomatous component; calcification occurs in about 10% of cases.[412] Microscopically, a pattern of mid-gut carcinoid tumor is the usual finding, with solid nests and acini of cells in a fibrous to hyalinized stroma (Fig. 11-75). The cells have eosinophilic, granular cytoplasm and round nuclei with a punctate or "peppery" chromatin pattern. Vascular invasion or extratesticular extension occurs in about 20% of testicular carcinoids, but does not correlate with clinical malignancy in most instances.[412] Argyrophil and argentaffin stains are typically positive, and luminal mucin can be identified in some cases. Rarely a trabecular carcinoid pattern may occur.[413] Serotonin, substance P, chromogranin, neuron specific enolase, gastrin, vasoactive intestinal polypeptide, neurofilament protein, and cytokeratin have been identified in testicular carcinoid,[412,414,415] and one would expect to find positivity for other substances typical of mid-gut carcinoid tumors.[416] Ultrastructurally, the tumor cells contain pleomorphic neurosecretory granules typical of mid-gut carcinoid tumors.[410,412,414] Flow cytometry of three cases demonstrated aneuploid DNA values that were near diploid and S-phase values of under 5%.[412]

It is prognostically important to differentiate primary carcinoid tumor of the testis from metastasis to the testis. The occurrence of other teratomatous elements in some testicular carcinoid tumors is an indication of their primary nature. The occurrence of bilateral involvement, multifocal tumor, microvascular invasion, or extratesticular spread favor carcinoid tumor metastatic to the testis rather than primary testicular carcinoid. Primary carcinoid has a good prognosis; Berdjis and Mostofi[411] reported metastases in 2 of 12 patients, and Zavala-Pompa et al[412] reported metastases in 11.6% of patients. Large size (average diameter of metastasizing tumors = 7.3 cm vs average diameter of nonmetastasizing tumors = 2.9 cm) and the carcinoid syndrome were the strongest predictors of metastasis,[412] whereas mitotic activity, vascular invasion, and tumor necrosis had no predictive value.[412] Most cases are cured by orchiectomy. The course of patients with metastatic testicular carcinoid tumor is often indolent, and the utility of retroperitoneal lymph node dissection is unknown.

Primitive neuroectodermal tumor

Primitive neuroectodermal tumor of the testis, like carcinoid tumor, is considered a monodermal form of testicular teratoma. This neoplasm probably results from overgrowth of neuroepithelial elements that are a common component of immature testicular teratoma. It is best to reserve the term *primitive neuroectodermal tumor of the testis* for rare cases that are a pure proliferation of such elements,[28,417-419] and to diagnose cases with residual teratomatous elements as teratoma with areas of primitive neuroectodermal tumor. The literature, however, has included both types of cases in descriptions of primitive neuroectodermal tumor. Clinically, these cases have occurred in patients 20, 30, and 51 years old.[417,419,420] Gray-white, partially necrotic tumors were identified. Microscopically, the tumors contain small, hyperchromatic, poorly differentiated neural-type cells arranged in rosettes or tubules.[417,419] Neurosecretory granules may be identified ultrastructurally.[419] Immunohistochemical studies utilizing neural markers may be useful. The differential diagnosis includes other small cell tumors, including metastatic small cell carcinoma of the lung, malignant lymphoma, and overgrowth of a blastematous

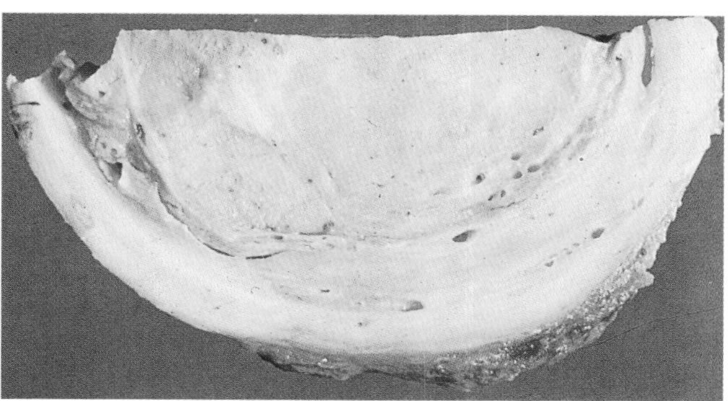

11-74. Testicular carcinoid tumor. Note well-circumscribed yellow nodule with white, fibrotic areas. *(Courtesy of DJ Gersell, MD; from Ulbright TM, Roth LM: Testicular and paratesticular neoplasms. In Sternberg SS, ed: Diagnostic surgical pathology, ed 2, New York, 1994, Raven Press; with permission of Raven Press.)*

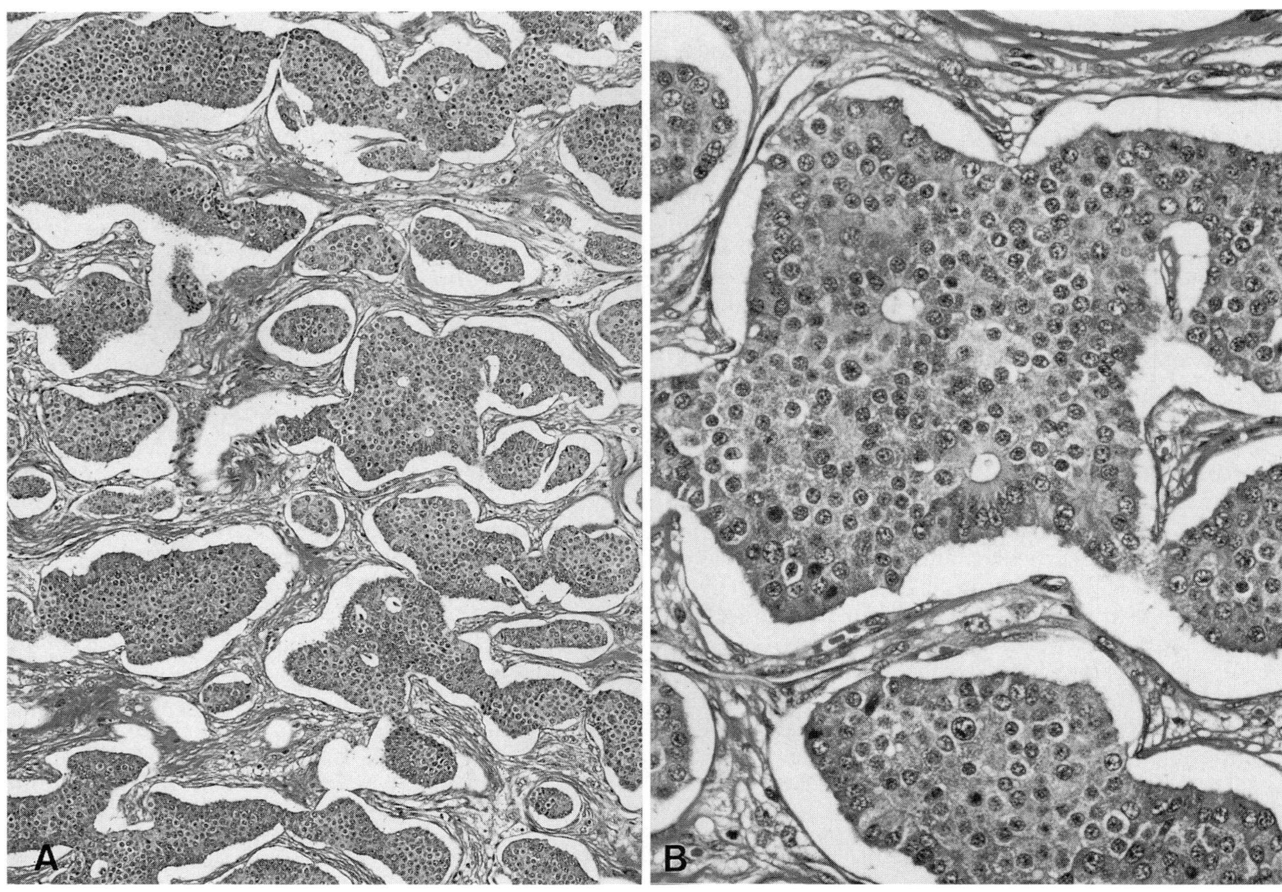

11-75. **A**, Typical insular pattern in testicular carcinoid tumor. There is artifactual retraction around nests of cells. **B**, Focal gland formation and punctate chromatin.

component of immature teratoma. Ultrastructural or immunohistochemical results allow separation of most alternative diagnoses, although clinical information may be required in the differential with metastatic small cell carcinoma.[419] The few reported cases of primitive neuroectodermal tumor of the testis have behaved aggressively.

CHORIOCARCINOMA

Clinical features

Choriocarcinoma is an uncommon component of mixed germ cell tumors (present in 15% of cases[350]), and pure choriocarcinoma is extremely rare in the testis, representing only 0.3% of testicular tumors in a registry of 6,000 cases.[213] Most patients with choriocarcinoma present with symptoms secondary to metastases, unlike other testicular tumors in which a palpable mass is the usual presenting complaint. Often the testicular tumor remains occult even after the diagnosis of metastatic choriocarcinoma. Typically, metastases are in a hematogenous distribution, often affecting the lungs, brain, and gastrointestinal tract, although retroperitoneal lymph node involvement may occur. Most patients are in the second and third decades, and choriocarcinoma has not been reported prior to puberty.[197] Serum levels of human chorionic gonadotropin may be highly elevated, resulting in secondary hormonal manifestations such as gynecomastia and thyrotoxicosis, caused by cross reactivity of human chorionic gonadotropin with thyroid stimulating hormone.[268,358,421]

Pathologic features

Grossly, the testis may be externally normal; the cut surface usually shows a hemorrhagic and necrotic nodule (Fig. 11-76), although in some instances regression of the primary lesion has occurred, with residual scarring as the only evidence of prior neoplasm. Classically, choriocarcinoma consists of a random mixture of mononucleate cells with clear to lightly staining cytoplasm (cytotrophoblasts) and multinucleate cells, often with smudged or degenerate-appearing nuclei and densely eosinophilic cytoplasm (syncytiotrophoblasts) (Fig. 11-77). The syncytiotrophoblasts may have intracytoplasmic lacunae containing an eosinophilic precipitate or erythrocytes. The area surrounding a choriocarcinoma is almost always hemorrhagic, and the central portions of the neoplasm are hemorrhagic and necrotic. Extensive sampling of such tumors may be necessary to demonstrate the diagnostic cell types, typically at the periphery (Fig. 11-78). In the best organized examples of choriocarcinoma the syncytiotrophoblasts appear to surround or "cap" masses of

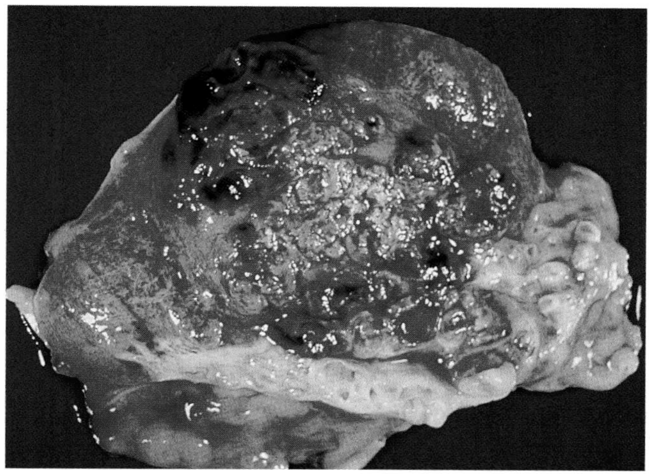

11-76. Choriocarcinoma of the testis. Note hemorrhagic, granular lesion.

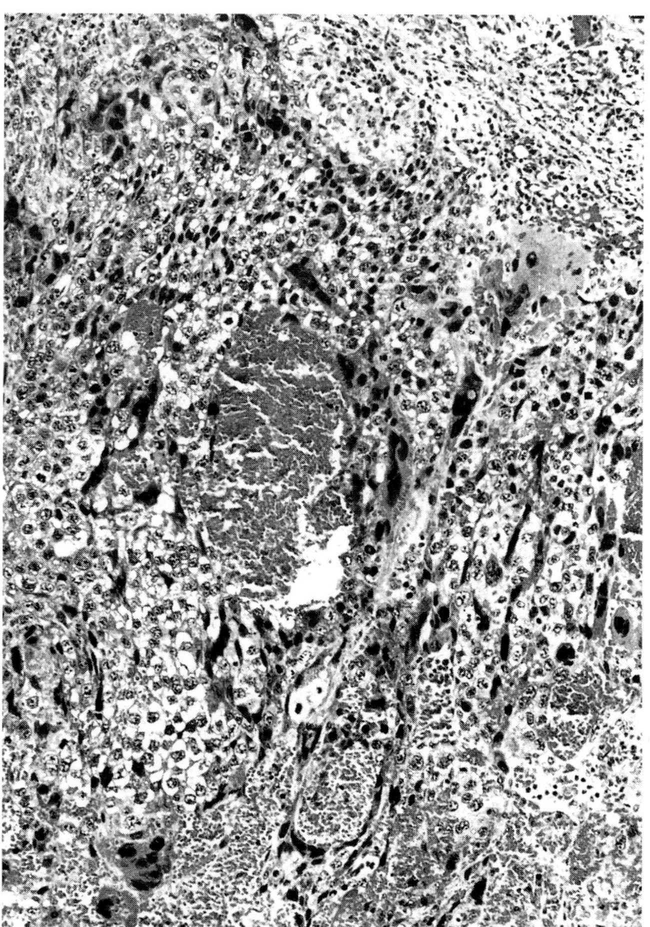

11-77. Characteristic mixture of syncytiotrophoblast and cytotrophoblast in choriocarcinoma. The background is hemorrhagic.

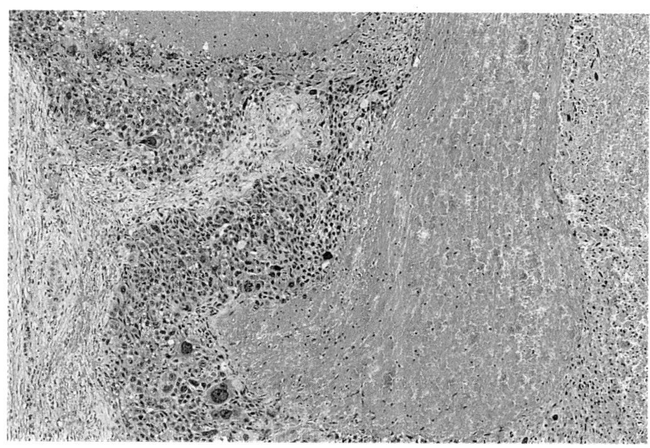

11-78. Choriocarcinoma forms a rim around pools of blood and fibrin.

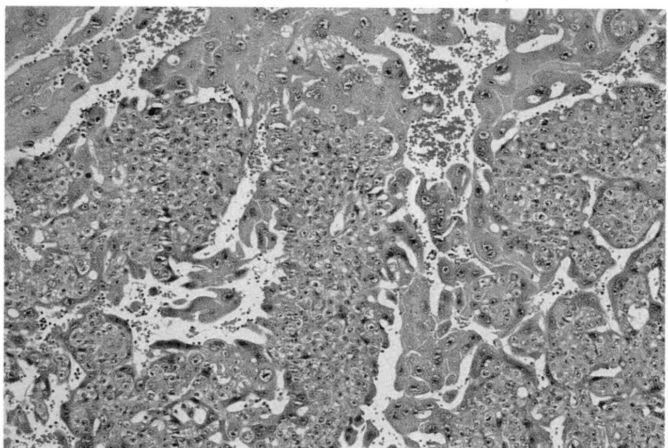

11-79. Choriocarcinoma with syncytiotrophoblast capping cytotrophoblast in a villus-like architecture.

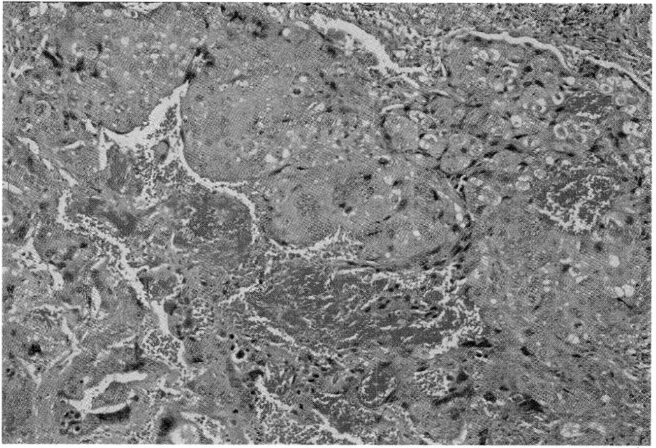

11-80. Choriocarcinoma in which the syncytiotrophoblast is inconspicuous, appearing as intermingled, smudged cells. Note the hemorrhage and typical syncytiotrophoblast at the bottom.

cytotrophoblasts, similar to immature placental villi (Fig. 11-79). However, in some cases the syncytiotrophoblastic cells are inconspicuous, with relatively scant cytoplasm and a degenerate appearance (Fig. 11-80). In other cases, a biphasic pattern of intermingled syncytiotrophoblasts and cytotrophoblasts is not readily apparent; instead, there occurs a nodular proliferation of atypical trophoblastic cells of varying size. These are usually mononucleate and occasionally binucleate trophoblasts, and the background remains hemorrhagic (Fig. 11-81). Angioinvasive foci are commonly identified in all variants.

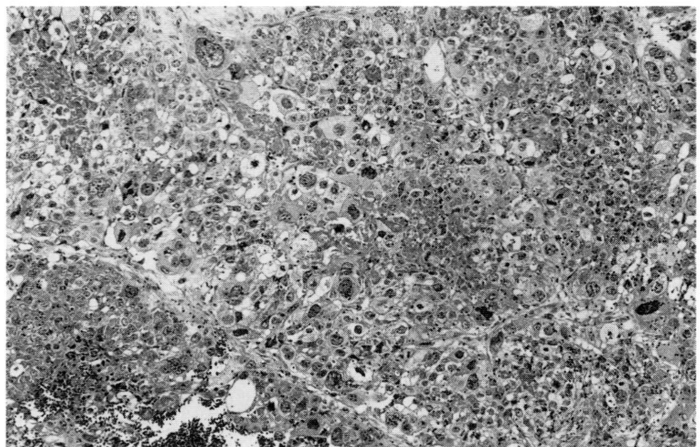

11-81. Unusual pattern of choriocarcinoma in which a spectrum of trophoblastic cells appears in a hemorrhagic background.

Some trophoblastic proliferations in the testis are not readily classified as choriocarcinoma, including occasional cases of mononucleate trophoblastic proliferations. In some instances these cells resemble cytotrophoblasts and line hemorrhagic cysts (Fig. 11-82*A*); in other instances there is a nodule of cells resembling intermediate trophoblastic cells of the placenta (Fig. 11-82*B*). Further, mononucleate, squamoid trophoblastic cells with only rare mitotic figures may line cystic spaces (Fig. 11-83). Trophoblastic proliferations such as these should not necessarily be categorized as choriocarcinoma because it is not clear that they are clinically aggressive. Instead, they should be reported descriptively until their clinicopathologic features can be elaborated and an appropriate nomenclature devised.

Special studies

Immunostains for human chorionic gonadotropin are useful in establishing the diagnosis of a trophoblastic pro-

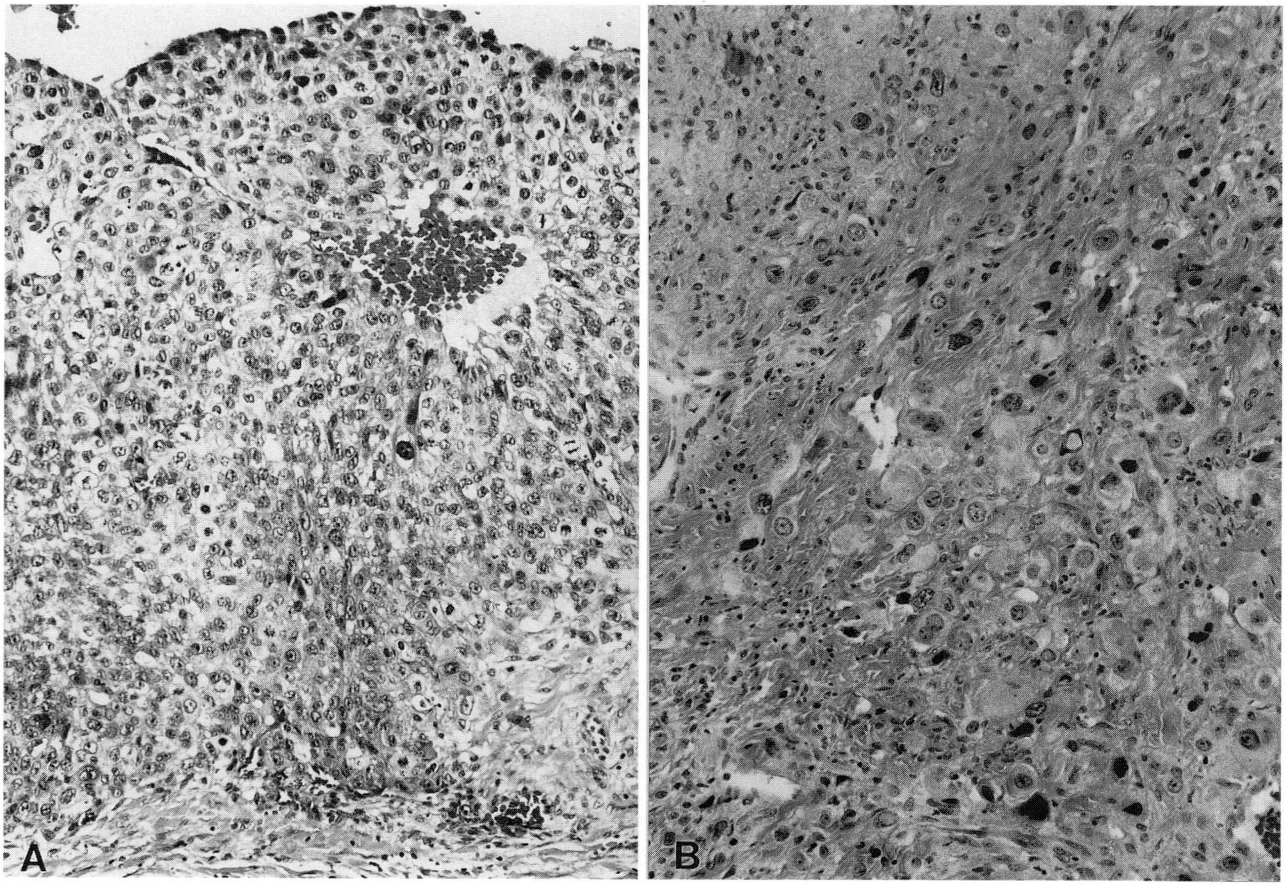

11-82. A, Trophoblastic proliferation in which cytotrophoblast-like cells line a hemorrhagic cyst. **B**, Cells resembling intermediate trophoblast in a fibrous stroma.

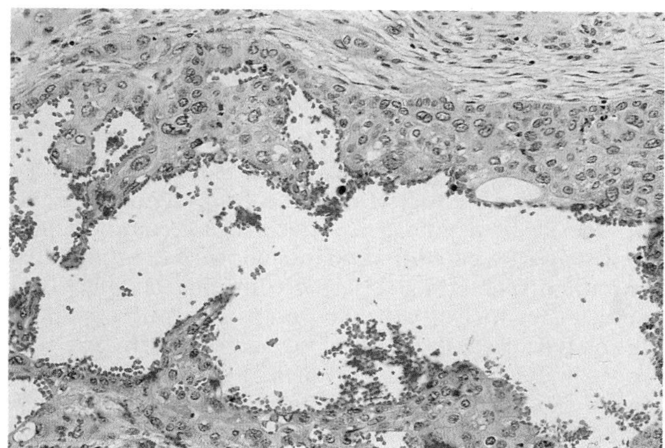

11-83. Squamoid, mononucleate trophoblastic cells line a hemorrhagic cyst.

liferation, including choriocarcinoma. Positivity for human chorionic gonadotropin is strongest in syncytiotrophoblastic cells and in large mononucleate trophoblastic cells that may represent transitional forms between cytotrophoblasts and syncytiotrophoblasts.[39,50,422] Cytotrophoblasts generally have only weak or absent staining for human chorionic gonadotropin. Similarly, pregnancy-specific beta-1-glycoprotein and human placental lactogen may be identified in syncytiotrophoblasts and intermediate-sized trophoblasts but are not seen in the cytotrophoblastic population.[422] About one half of choriocarcinomas stain for PLAP,[39] and carcinoembryonic antigen can be identified in both syncytiotrophoblasts and cytotrophoblasts in about 25% of cases.[39,423] Cytokeratin is readily identifiable in both the syncytiotrophoblastic and cytotrophoblastic components of choriocarcinoma,[39,214] including cytokeratins 7, 8, 18, and 19 of Moll's catalog.[424] Epithelial membrane antigen positivity is noted in about half of choriocarcinomas, usually within syncytiotrophoblasts,[39] whereas most other nonteratomatous germ cell tumors of the testis do not express epithelial membrane antigen.

Ultrastructurally, the multinucleate syncytiotrophoblastic cells have prominent cisternae of rough endoplasmic reticulum, which often contain electron dense material, together with interdigitating microvilli on the cell surface.[51,425] Cytotrophoblasts lack the prominent rough endoplasmic reticulum but have numerous free cytoplasmic ribosomes. Desmosomes are identified with all cell types.

Differential diagnosis

Other types of germ cell tumor may contain trophoblasts, but they are scattered as individual cells or small nests and lack the biphasic pattern of choriocarcinoma. For example, the syncytiotrophoblasts that occur in many seminomas are randomly distributed as separate cells and small islands without accompanying cytotrophoblasts. Neither is there a distinct nodule of trophoblasts of varying sizes as may be seen in some cases of choriocarcinoma. Embryonal carcinoma may show degenerate cells that mimic choriocarcinoma with a poorly defined syncytiotrophoblastic component. The lack of hemorrhage and human chorionic gonadotropin in such cases distinguishes them from choriocarcinoma. Rare cases of embryonal carcinoma may show transformation to choriocarcinoma[426]; however, if the background is hemorrhagic and the admixed multinucleate cells contain human chorionic gonadotropin, choriocarcinoma should be diagnosed.

Treatment and prognosis

Choriocarcinoma tends to metastasize prior to detection of the primary lesion, and most patients have advanced stage tumor at the time of diagnosis. Choriocarcinoma often shows a less orderly pattern of metastasis than other germ cell tumors, frequently skipping the retroperitoneum and metastasizing in a hematogenous pattern to the lungs and liver.[213,389] The prognosis of choriocarcinoma is therefore worse than other germ cell tumors. It is also likely that mixed germ cell tumors with a proportion of choriocarcinoma have a worse prognosis, but it remains unclear how much choriocarcinoma in such cases is required for a worsening in prognosis. This concept is supported by several studies demonstrating a poorer prognosis in patients with nonseminomatous germ cell tumors who had elevated serum human chorionic gonadotropin levels,[268,427,428] and in those with choriocarcinoma in mixed germ cell tumors.[268,427,429,430] Patients with choriocarcinoma can achieve substantial tumor-free survival with chemotherapy.[268]

MIXED GERM CELL TUMOR

Mixed germ cell tumors are composed of more than one type of germ cell tumor element, including one or more nonseminomatous elements, and are thus classified as nonseminomatous tumors, even if seminoma is the chief component. Mixed germ cell tumors are quite common, accounting for about one third of germ cell tumors and 69% of all nonseminomatous germ cell tumors of the testis.[193] Virtually any combination of elements may be present. Common combinations include embryonal carcinoma and teratoma; embryonal carcinoma and seminoma; embryonal carcinoma, yolk sac tumor, and teratoma; embryonal carcinoma, teratoma, and choriocarcinoma; embryonal carcinoma, teratoma, and seminoma; and teratoma and seminoma.[193] Although seminoma with syncytiotrophoblastic cells is histopathologically a mixed germ cell tumor, it is classified as a variant of seminoma rather than a mixed, nonseminomatous neoplasm because the natural history and treatment appear to be similar to that of seminoma.

Clinical features

Patients with mixed germ cell tumor have the same clinical features as those with nonseminomatous germ cell tumor, and most present with a testicular mass. Those with a predominance of embryonal carcinoma in mixed germ cell tumor average 28 years of age, whereas patients with a predominance of seminoma average 33 years.[431]

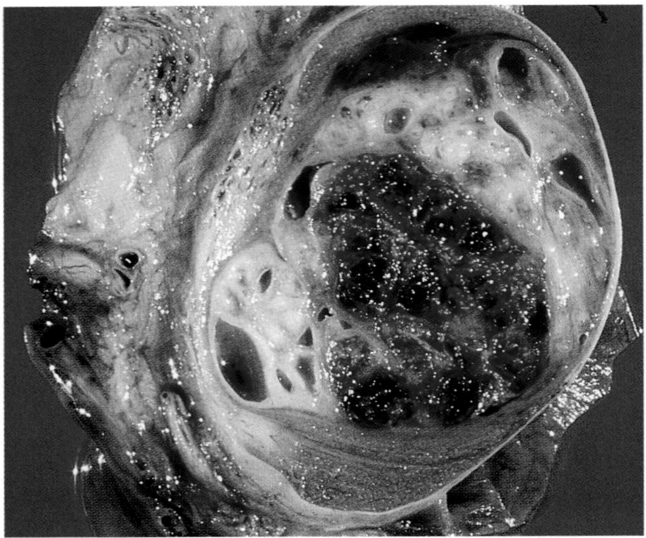

11-84. Variegated appearance of mixed germ cell tumor, with hemorrhagic, cystic, and fleshy areas.

Alpha-fetoprotein and human chorionic gonadotropin elevation occurs in about 60% and 55% of patients with mixed germ cell tumor, respectively.[201]

Pathologic features

Grossly, mixed germ cell tumor is often variegated because of the mixture of different components (Fig. 11-84). Foci of hemorrhage and necrosis are common. The microscopic features are similar to those of the individual components described elsewhere in this chapter. It is common for foci of yolk sac tumor with microcystic or vacuolated patterns to be contiguous with areas of embryonal carcinoma, and such foci are easily overlooked (Fig. 11-85). A double-layered pattern of embryonal carcinoma has been described in which ribbons of columnar embryonal carcinoma cells are accompanied by a parallel ribbon of flattened tumor cells.[304,432] The intense alpha-fetoprotein immunoreactivity of this flattened cell layer, together with its morphology, indicates yolk sac tumor differentiation, and this pattern should therefore be classified as a form of mixed germ cell tumor (embryonal carcinoma and yolk sac tumor).

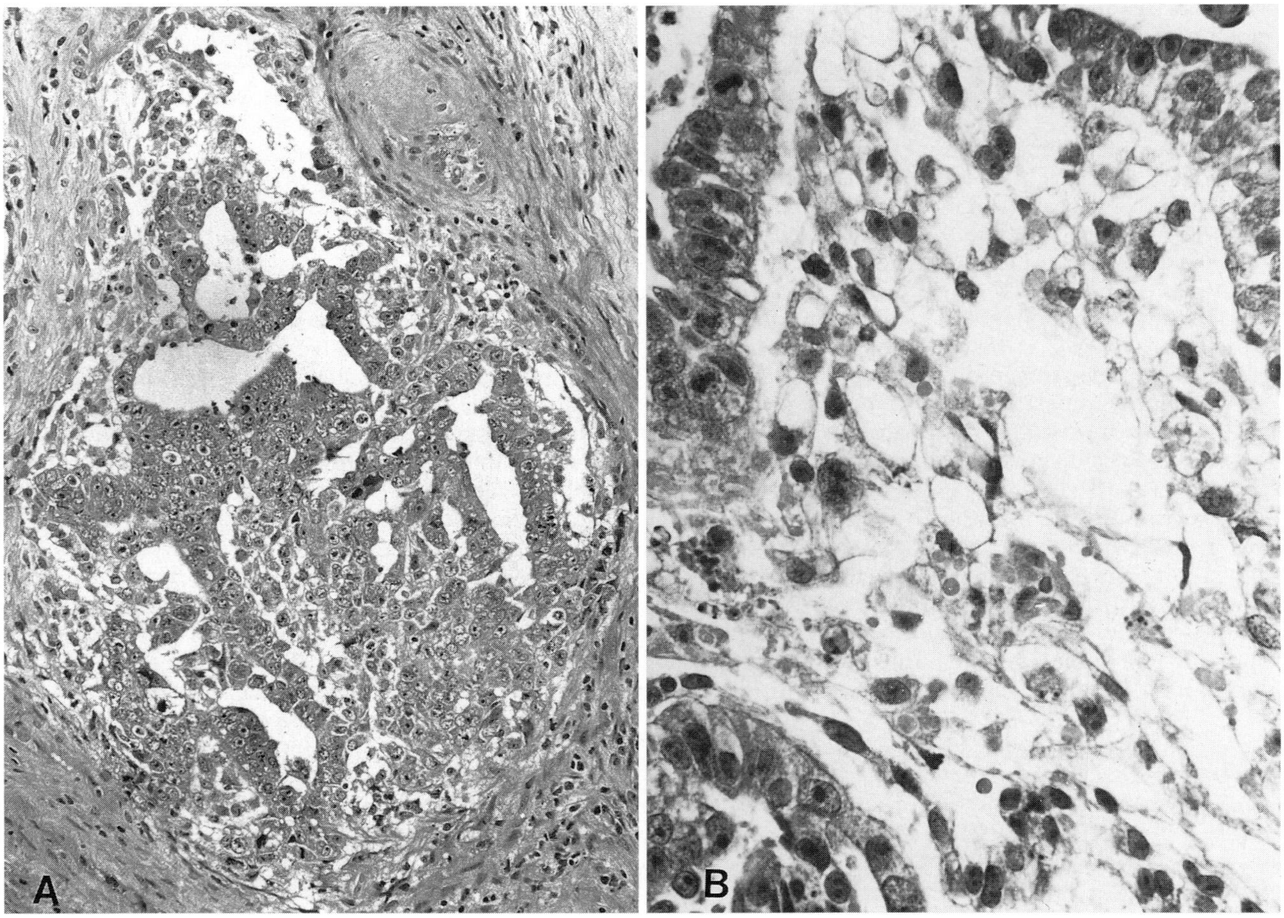

11-85. **A**, Low power appearance of small, vacuolated cells representing yolk sac tumor, occurring with embryonal carcinoma. **B**, High power of another case showing vacuolated cells of yolk sac tumor adjacent to embryonal carcinoma.

Polyembryoma and diffuse embryoma

Polyembryoma is a distinct form of mixed germ cell tumor that recapitulates small embryoid bodies. The embryoid body consists of a central core of cuboidal to columnar, sometimes stratified, embryonal carcinoma cells, a ventral yolk sac tumor component forming a yolk sac–like vesicle, and a dorsal amnion-like space (Fig. 11-86).[433,434] The embryoid body is surrounded by loose, myxomatous, richly vascular tissue, similar to extraembryonic mesenchyme, which is also commonly identified in yolk sac tumor (see Fig. 11-86). Because of the yolk sac tumor component, patients with polyembryoma may have substantial alpha-fetoprotein elevation.[433] In some cases, intestinal and squamous differentiation of the amniotic epithelium is present, as well as hepatic differentiation in the yolk sac–like zone.[433] Imperfectly formed embryoid bodies are occasionally seen in mixed germ cell tumors, consisting of small nodular collections of embryonal carcinoma admixed with yolk sac tumor, surrounded by a myxomatous to fibrous stroma (Fig. 11-87). Diffuse embryoma consists of a sheet-like admixture of embryonal carcinoma and yolk sac tumor (Fig. 11-88).[435] The behavior and treatment of polyembryoma and diffuse embryoma is similar to other mixed germ cell tumors with these components.

Treatment and prognosis

Patients with mixed germ cell tumors are managed like patients with nonseminomatous tumors. Tumors consisting of embryonal carcinoma and teratoma are less likely to metastasize than tumors having the same volume of embryonal carcinoma but lacking a teratomatous component, suggesting that the ability of embryonal carcinoma to differentiate is associated with a decrease in metastatic potential.[436] A similar observation has been made for cases having a yolk sac tumor component, with a decrease in metastatic potential.[329]

REGRESSION OF GERM CELL TUMOR

Some patients with extragonadal germ cell tumor lack clinical evidence of a primary testicular tumor.[437-440] Some have primary extragonadal germ cell tumor, especially those with tumor confined to the mediastinum or pineal region without retroperitoneal involvement. Accumulating evidence indicates that retroperitoneal tumor, frequently thought in the past to be a common

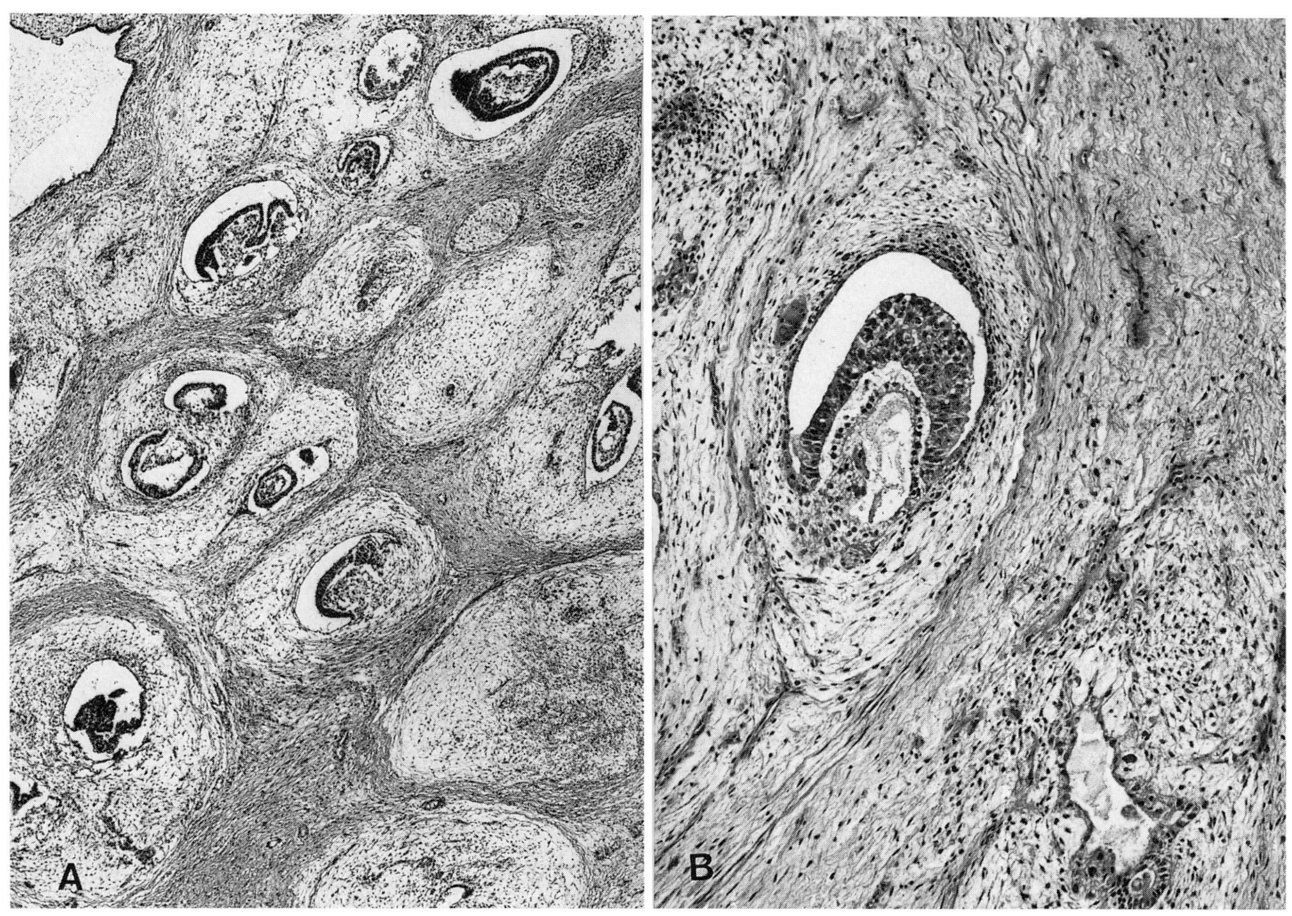

11-86. **A**, Polyembryoma consists of embryoid bodies in a myxoid stroma. **B**, Embryoid body composed of a central core of embryonal carcinoma, a "ventral" yolk sac tumor component, and a "dorsal" amnion.

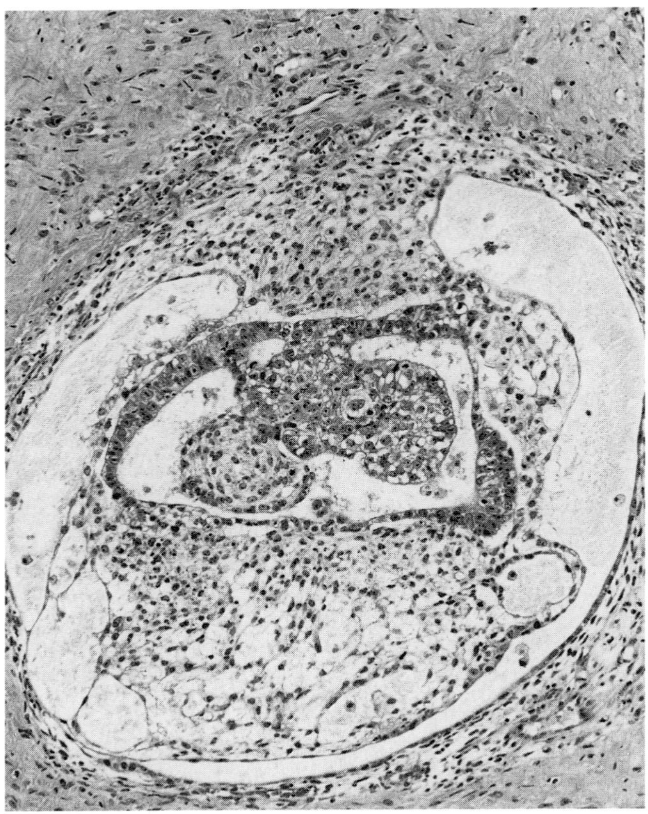

11-87. Complex embryoid body.

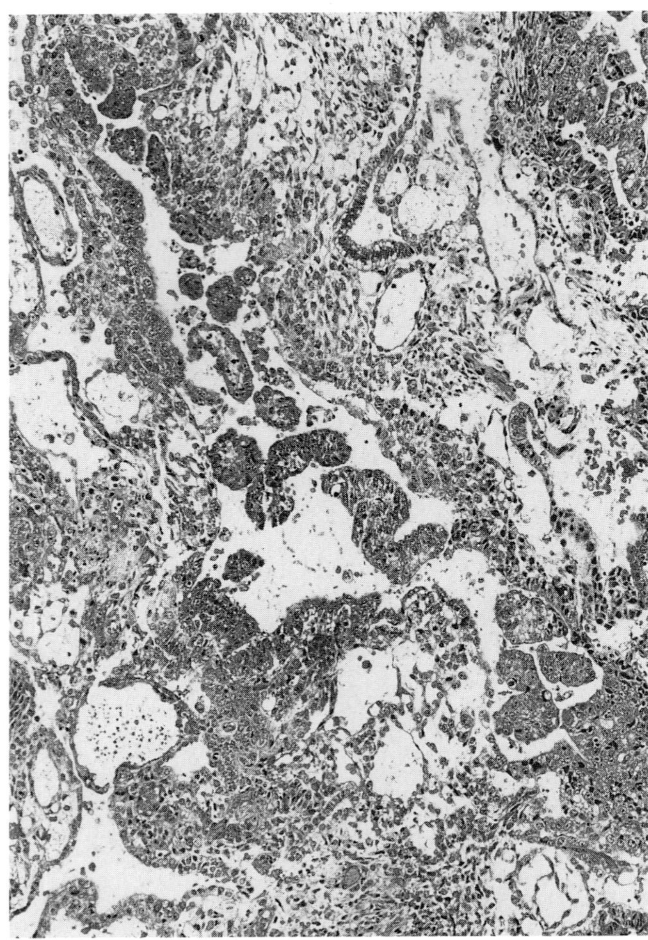

11-88. Diffuse embryoma consists of an approximately equal mixture of embryonal carcinoma and yolk sac tumor.

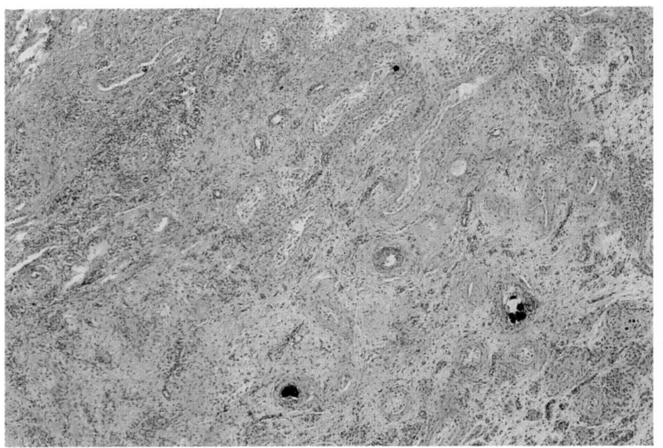

11-89. Regressed germ cell tumor consisting of scarring with lymphocytes, siderophages, and intratubular calcifications.

site of primary extragonadal germ cell tumor, is often caused by a regressed testicular primary.[188,440] Examination of the testis in such cases often demonstrates foci of testicular scarring and IGCNU.[188] This phenomenon of primary testicular tumor regression in the presence of metastases is documented in autopsy studies, and almost 10% of patients who die of metastatic testicular germ cell tumor show "burnt out" primary tumors.[441] Choriocarcinoma is especially likely to produce widespread metastases and yet regress in the testis, leaving only residual fibrous tissue and hemosiderin-laden macrophages. Other germ cell tumors may also regress, and regression can be recognized as zones of scarring with adjacent intratubular calcifications (or hematoxylin-staining bodies), resulting from intratubular karyorrhectic debris from the necrotic neoplasm and superimposed dystrophic calcification (Fig. 11-89).[118] Siderophages and IGCNU are often identified as well. Teratomatous components are less likely to regress and are therefore often seen adjacent to scars.

POSTCHEMOTHERAPY SPECIMENS

Chemotherapy in patients with metastatic testicular germ cell tumor often results in a marked decrease in tumor size, although large masses may persist. Persistent masses are often surgically excised, and the pathologic findings are of prime importance in determining the future treatment for these patients.[339]

Following chemotherapeutic cytoreduction, residual masses may consist of necrosis (often associated with a xanthomatous reaction), fibrosis, and viable-appearing germ cell tumor histologically similar to the original tumor or with an altered morphology. Additionally,

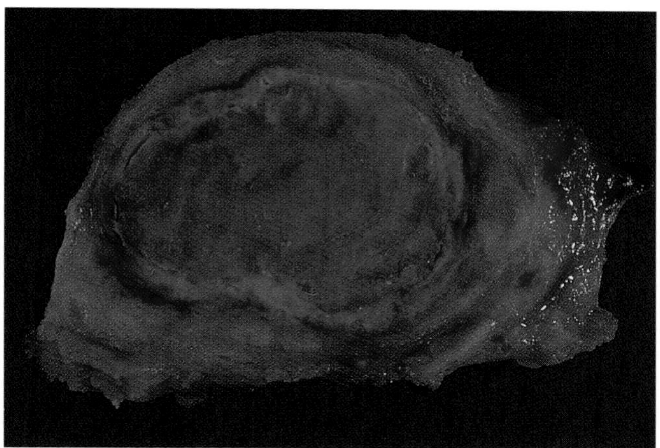

11-90. Tumor necrosis following chemotherapy. A tan, granular nodule is surrounded by a yellow band and an outer shell of fibrosis.

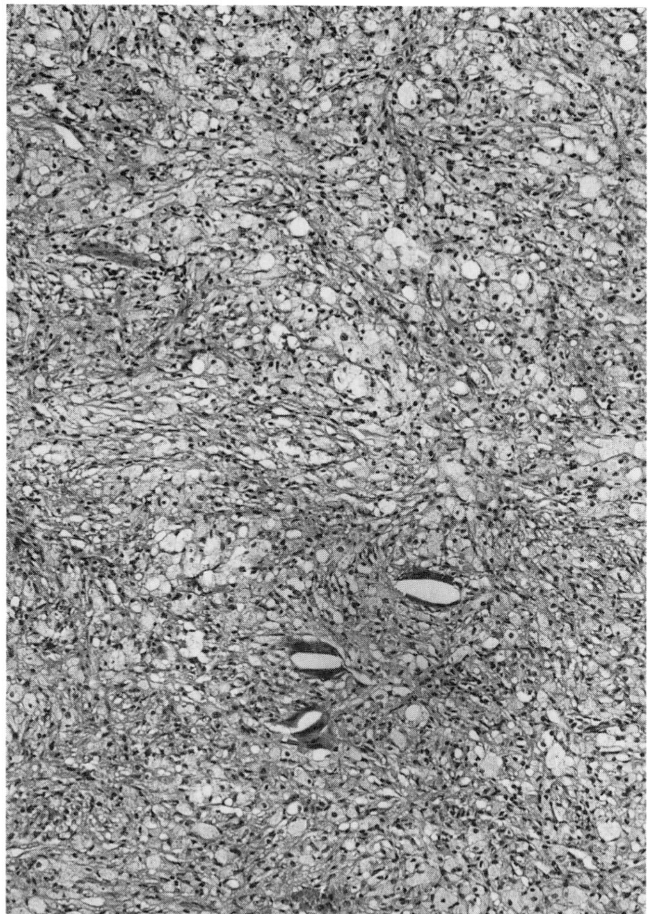

11-91. The fibroxanthomatous reaction seen after chemotherapy. Note cholesterol clefts with giant cell reaction.

malignant neoplasms with somatic-type differentiation (for example, sarcoma and carcinoma) may occur.[339,400] Patients with necrosis, fibrosis, and mature (although often atypical-appearing) teratomatous lesions following chemotherapy are not usually treated with additional

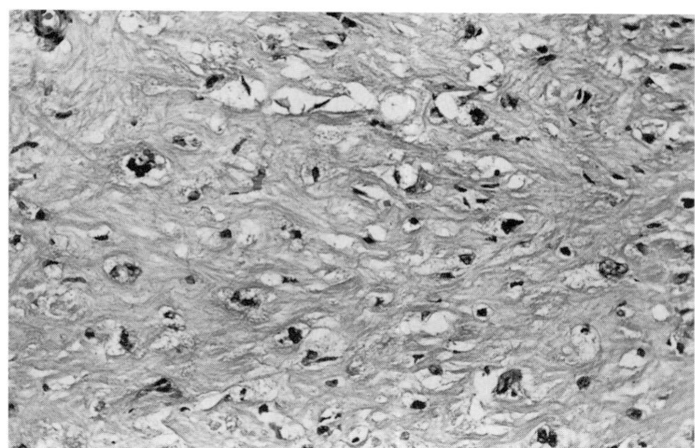

11-92. Scattered atypical and degenerate spindle and polygonal cells in dense fibrous tissue following chemotherapy.

chemotherapy; conversely, those who have persistent embryonal carcinoma, yolk sac tumor, choriocarcinoma, or seminoma are candidates for second-line (salvage) chemotherapy. The treatment of postchemotherapy sarcoma and carcinoma is problematic and often ineffective, but is usually by surgical resection. In one study of 101 patients with advanced, nonseminomatous germ cell tumor treated with cisplatin-based chemotherapy and resection of residual masses, 51% had necrosis or fibrosis; 37% had residual mature teratoma; and 12% had residual malignant, nonteratomatous germ cell tumor.[442]

Necrotic foci in postchemotherapy resections often appear as tan, granular nodules surrounded by a thin yellow rim (Fig. 11-90). Microscopically, there is central, coagulative necrosis consisting of eosinophilic debris with ghostlike outlines of necrotic tumor cells. These areas of necrosis usually lack prominent karyorrhectic debris. Surrounding the areas of necrosis are infiltrates of macrophages with abundant, foamy cytoplasm, accounting for the grossly visible yellow rim. The nuclei of these cells may be mildly atypical, which, in conjunction with the clear cytoplasm, can lead to a misinterpretation of seminoma.[339] The absence of significant atypia and the lack of mitotic figures are usually sufficient to permit separation without resorting to special stains for glycogen, placental alkaline phosphatase, and macrophage markers. An active fibroblastic proliferation may be intermingled with the foamy macrophages, creating a fibroxanthomatous reaction (Fig. 11-91).

Grossly, fibrosis in postchemotherapy resections is firm and white and, microscopically, consists of scattered spindle cells set in dense collagenous tissue. Some spindle cells may be enlarged and cytologically atypical but do not form fascicles and are scattered randomly, creating a hypocellular appearance (Fig. 11-92). Some of these fibrous lesions apparently represent postchemotherapy persistence of the hypocellular, mesenchymal component of yolk sac tumor, based on the identification of this yolk sac tumor pattern in the orchiectomy

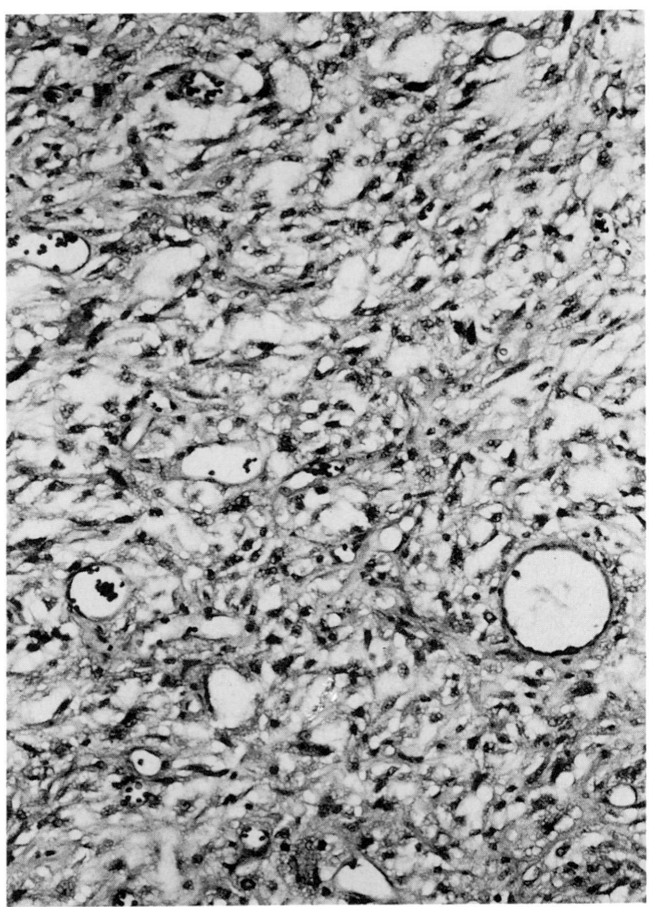

11-93. Cellular spindle cell proliferation with prominent vessels and a myxoid background following chemotherapy.

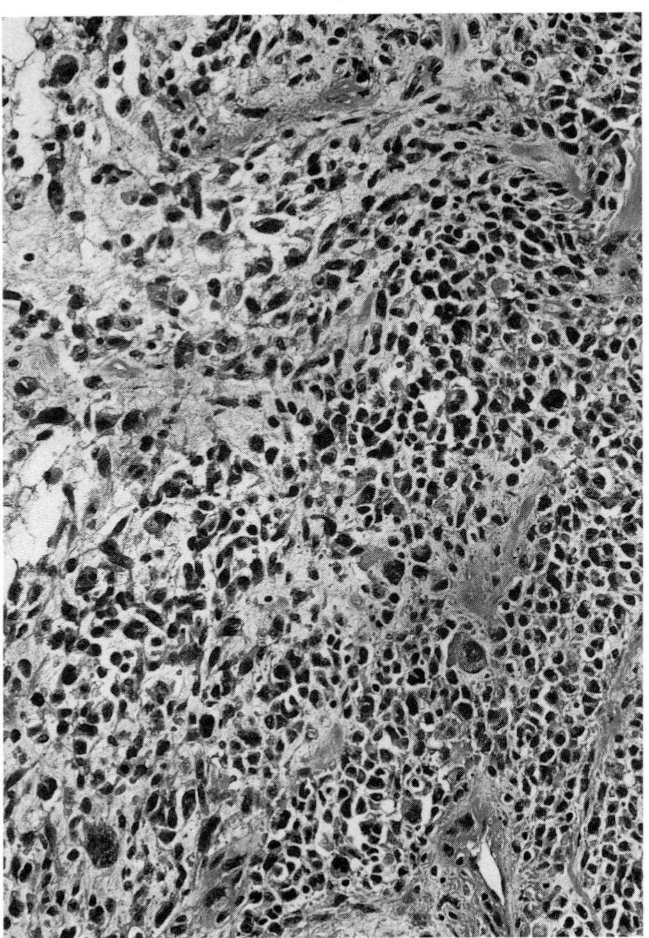

11-94. Rhabdomyosarcoma following chemotherapy.

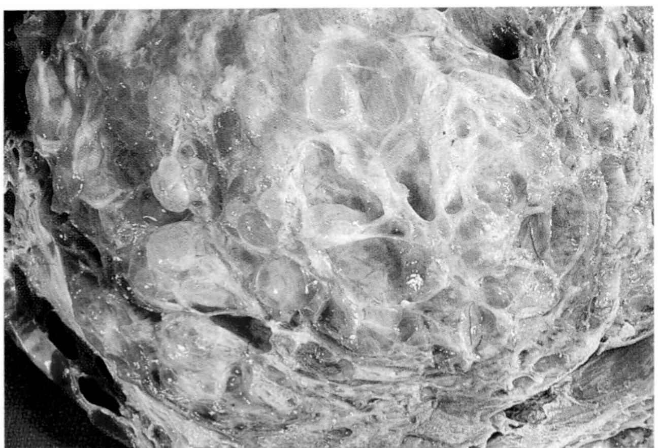

11-95. Metastatic mature teratoma following chemotherapy, showing the characteristic multicystic appearance.

specimen and the intense cytokeratin reactivity of the spindle cells.[360] It is probably best, however, to consider the hypocellular, collagenous lesions as fibrosis rather than creating clinical confusion by characterizing it as persistence of a yolk sac tumor component.

Some spindle cell lesions observed after chemotherapy display increased cellularity and mitotic activity with a more myxomatous background; these are apparently derived from the mesenchymal component of yolk sac tumor (Fig. 11-93).[360] Alpha-fetoprotein positivity is usually absent in these lesions (alpha-fetoprotein is also absent from the spindle cell component of the primary lesion),[360] although rare transitional cases show persistent foci of an epithelioid, microcystic pattern of yolk sac tumor. Some of these sarcomatoid proliferations differentiate to embryonal rhabdomyosarcoma (Fig. 11-94). The prognosis of patients with high-grade spindle cell lesions in postchemotherapy resections is poor.[360]

Teratomatous lesions following chemotherapy are common and are readily diagnosed by those aware of the phenomenon of metastatic teratoma following orchiectomy for mixed germ cell tumor or pure nonteratomatous germ cell tumor.[443] Metastatic teratoma appears as a multicystic mass with intervening fibrous tissue (Fig. 11-95); the cysts usually contain clear, serous fluid. Microscopically, there are often glands, squamous nests, islands of cartilage, smooth and striated muscle, and intervening fibrous stroma. Significant cytologic atypia can be identi-

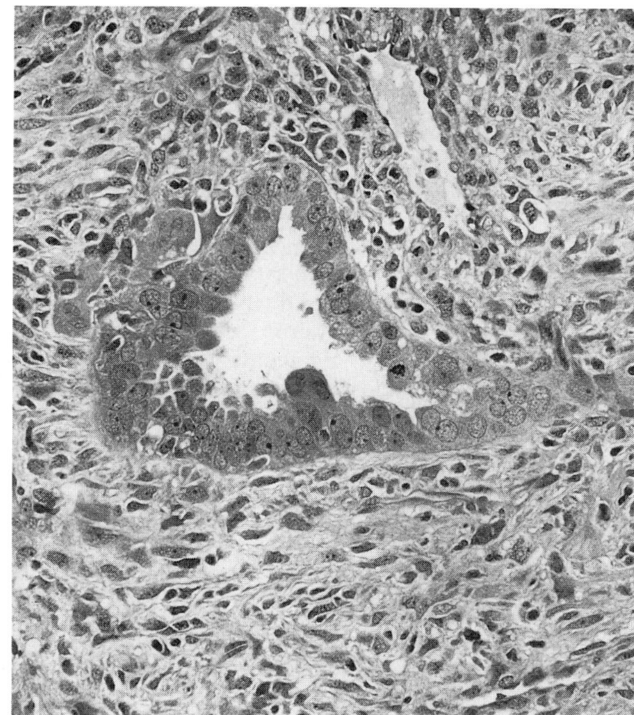

11-96. High-grade epithelial atypia in a teratomatous gland embedded in sarcomatous stroma.

fied in these tumors.[444] Glandular epithelium, although confined to round, noninvasive glands, may be stratified with enlarged, hyperchromatic, and mitotically active nuclei that raise a concern for embryonal carcinoma (Fig. 11-96). However, the primitive, vesicular nuclei and macronucleoli of embryonal carcinoma are absent. These glands often have intestinal differentiation, with goblet cells and eosinophilic absorptive cells. Squamous nests and cartilage may also display cytologic atypia. Stromal invasion by highly atypical elements indicates a diagnosis of carcinoma or sarcoma; criteria for invasion are the same as in primary teratoma with an overtly malignant component.

Metastatic mature teratoma may be life-threatening. Mature teratoma may undergo progressive enlargement, according to serial radiographic studies, and may impinge on vital structures, especially in the mediastinum. This has been described as the *growing teratoma syndrome*[445-448] and is justification for complete excision of metastatic teratomatous tumor whenever feasible.[446] Although classified as mature teratoma, these tumors contain cells with a malignant genotype (as well as phenotype) based on karyotypic and ploidy studies.[334,396,449] Consequently, such lesions should be surgically excised before evolution to a more aggressive clone of cells results in overgrowth with a malignancy of teratomatous origin.[404,405,449] Despite the cytologic atypia that occurs in metastatic teratomatous lesions following polychemotherapy, the atypia does not appear to have prognostic significance in the absence of evolution to an invasive malignant neoplasm.[444]

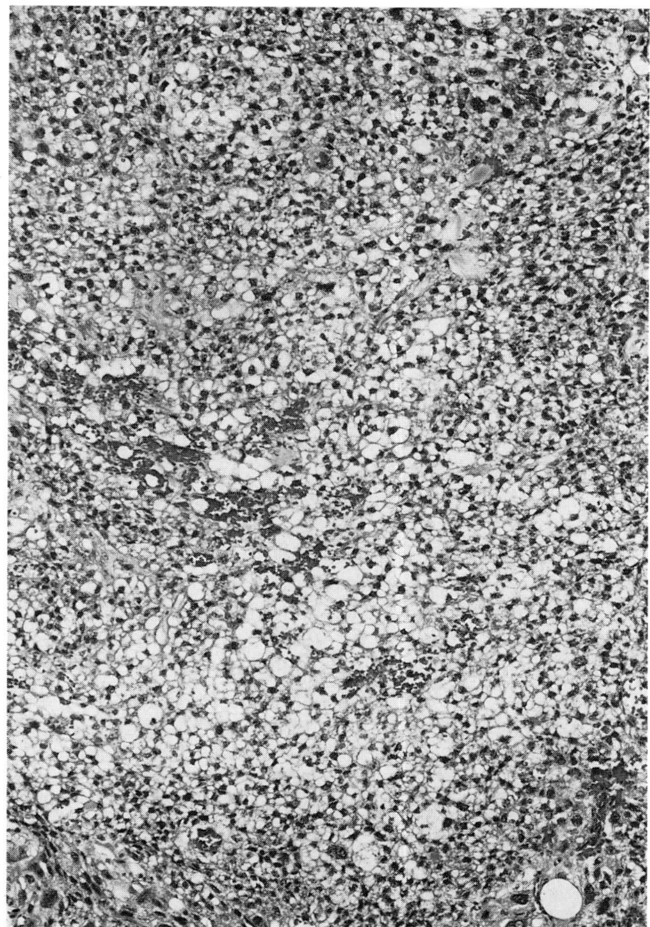

11-97. Monophasic (atypical) choriocarcinoma following chemotherapy.

A variety of somatic-type, teratomatous malignancies are identified in postchemotherapy resections. These consist of fleshy or necrotic areas among fibrous tissue and cysts. Embryonal rhabdomyosarcoma is the most common such malignancy (and some cases are probably derived from yolk sac tumor rather than teratoma), and others include chondrosarcoma, adenocarcinoma, undifferentiated carcinoma, and undifferentiated sarcoma.[400] The prognosis in such cases is poor.

The morphology of persistent, postchemotherapy, nonteratomatous germ cell tumor is usually similar to that of primary testicular neoplasms. However, exceptions to this rule occur, particularly with trophoblastic proliferations. Unlike the biphasic proliferation of syncytiotrophoblast and cytotrophoblast in classic choriocarcinoma, the trophoblastic proliferations commonly identified in postchemotherapy resections often lack definite syncytiotrophoblast. Instead, cytotrophoblast-like and intermediate trophoblast-like cells may be identified in the absence of syncytiotrophoblast (Fig. 11-97). Mazur et al[450] described this pattern in patients treated for gestational choriocarcinoma as *atypical choriocarcinoma*. In some cases, the trophoblastic cells are exclusively mononuclear and form the epithelial lining of cysts, closely mimicking teratomatous cysts composed of atypical squamous epithelium (Fig. 11-98).[451] The distinction between cystic atypical choriocarcinoma and teratoma is probably not clinically important if there is no evidence of invasion and the mitotic rate is low, and it may cause confusion if diagnosed as a form of choriocarcinoma. The significance of altered trophoblastic proliferations in postchemotherapy resections has yet to be determined. At Indiana University, we recommend additional chemotherapy for patients in whom it is feasible and who have solid nodules of monophasic trophoblastic cells that are mitotically active (see Fig. 11-97). For trophoblastic lesions that resemble teratomatous cysts, treatment is similar to that of teratoma and includes surgical excision and follow-up. Rare cells may express human chorionic gonadotropin in these monophasic, postchemotherapy tumors, but immunohistochemistry is usually unimpressive.[451] This staining pattern correlates with low or absent serum levels of human chorionic gonadotropin.[451]

The outcome of patients undergoing excision of persistent masses following chemotherapy for metastatic testicular germ cell tumor varies depending on the pathologic findings. Eighty-eight percent of patients with only necrosis in retroperitoneal lymph node dissections were well on follow-up.[452] Similarly, only 1 of 25 patients (4%) with fibrosis relapsed on follow-up.[453] Residual mature teratoma is also associated with a good prognosis; a combination of three series reported benign follow-up in 90% of 42 cumulative patients.[453-455] Conversely, seven of nine patients with malignant, somatic-type neoplasms developed recurrent tumor following resection.[444] For patients with persistent, apparently viable germ cell tumor other than teratoma in postchemotherapy resections, the prognosis is guarded. Those who do well include patients who have complete surgical excision of persistent tumor, who have received only primary chemotherapy before resection, and who also receive postresection chemotherapy; patients with retroperitoneal tumor who meet these criteria have a 70% disease-free survival.[456] Patients who have persistent retroperitoneal germ cell tumor other than teratoma after salvage therapy and who are completely resected have a 40% disease-free survival.[456] Inability to completely resect viable germ cell tumor other than teratoma after primary or salvage chemotherapy carries a poor prognosis, with only 9% remaining clinically tumor free.[456]

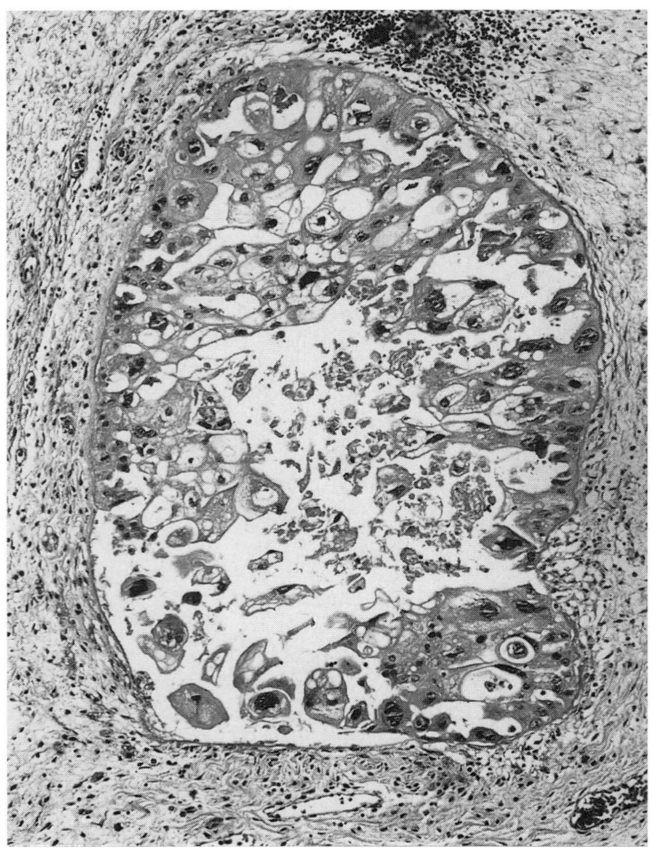

11-98. Cyst lined by atypical trophoblastic cells with squamoid features following chemotherapy. This alone would not be an indication for additional chemotherapy.

SEX CORD–STROMAL TUMORS

Sex cord–stromal tumors make up only about 4% of testicular neoplasms.[110,457] These include Leydig cell tumor, Sertoli cell tumor, granulosa cell tumor, and sex cord–stromal tumors of mixed and unclassified (indeterminate) types. Many authors also include within the sex cord–stromal tumor category those hamartomatous or hyperplastic lesions of the testis in patients with the adrenogenital syndrome, Nelson's syndrome, and the androgen insensitivity syndrome, which are derived from interstitial cells and Sertoli cells. In this chapter these lesions are discussed with the neoplasm they most closely resemble—Leydig cell tumor (for the adrenogenital syndrome and Nelson's syndrome) and Sertoli cell tumor (for the androgen insensitivity syndrome).

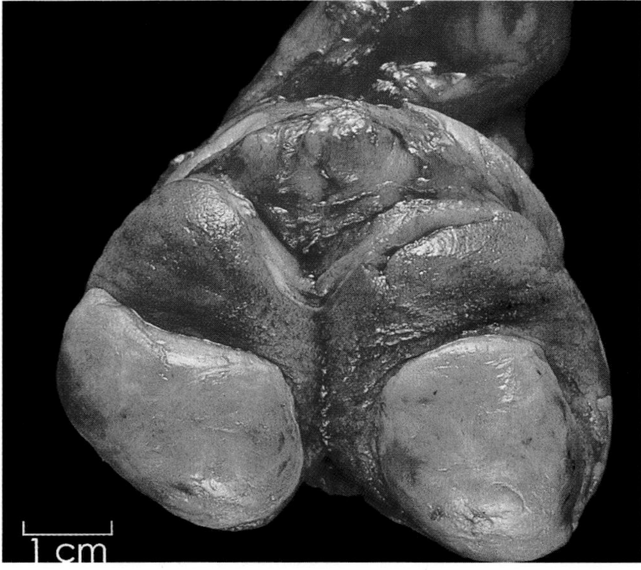

11-99. Leydig cell tumor.

LEYDIG CELL TUMOR

Clinical features

Leydig cell tumor accounts for about 3% of testicular neoplasms.[458] It has two age peaks, with about 20% of cases occurring in children[459] (most commonly between 5 and 10 years of age[460] but not in infants under 2 years[461]) and 80% occurring in adults (most commonly between 20 and 60 years[458]). Children usually present with significantly smaller tumors because of the early clinical detection of androgen production manifest by isosexual pseudoprecocity, the presenting feature in virtually all pediatric cases.[458] Such patients may not have palpable tumors and testicular ultrasound or differential testicular vein sampling for androgens may be required for clinical diagnosis. About 10% of children have gynecomastia superimposed on virilization.[460] Adults, in whom neoplastic androgen production is much less readily detected than in children, most commonly present with a testicular mass, with about 30% of patients developing gynecomastia.[458] Bilateral involvement occurs in about 3% of cases.[458] Leydig cell tumor shares some of the epidemiologic features of testicular germ cell tumors, occurring more commonly in patients with cryptorchidism, testicular atrophy, and infertility, and occurring almost exclusively in white patients.[462] Familial occurrence is described.[463]

Pathologic features

Most Leydig cell tumors appear as yellow, brown, or tan, solid, sometimes lobulated, intratesticular nodules, infrequently with areas of necrosis or hemorrhage (Fig. 11-99). The majority are 2 to 5 cm in diameter, but some exceed 10 cm[458]; children more often have Leydig cell tumors less than 1 cm in diameter. Extratesticular extension occurs in about 10% of cases.[458] A variety of light microscopic patterns may be seen; the solid, sheet-like pattern is most common (Fig. 11-100), but pseudoglandular, cord-like (trabecular), and compact nested patterns may also be present, often in the same neoplasm. It is common for nodular aggregates of tumor cells to be separated by edematous or fibrous stroma (Fig. 11-101). The cells are

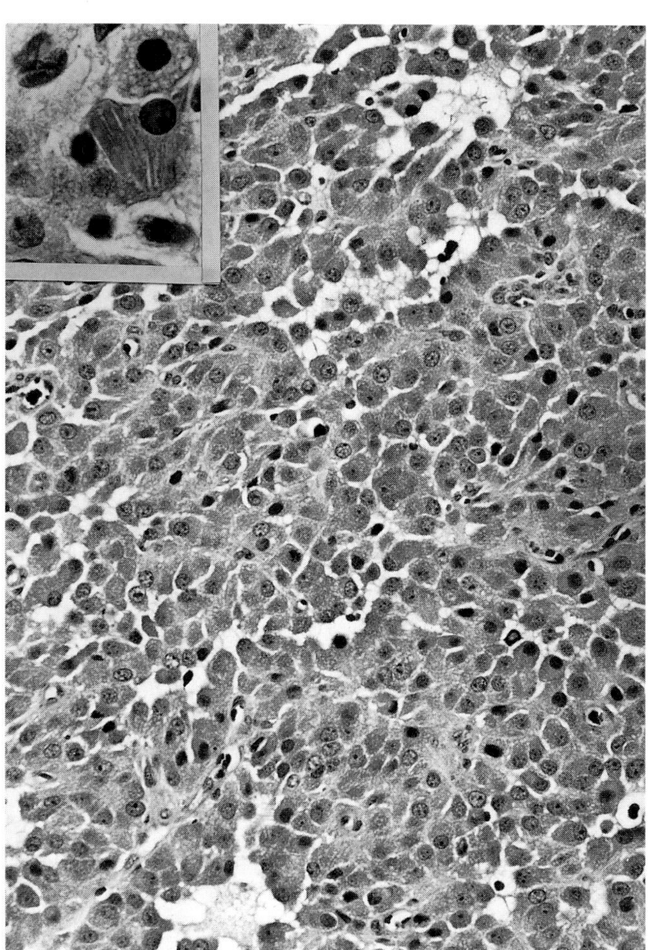

11-100. Sheets of cells in a Leydig cell tumor with microcysts. Inset demonstrates intracytoplasmic crystals of Reinke.

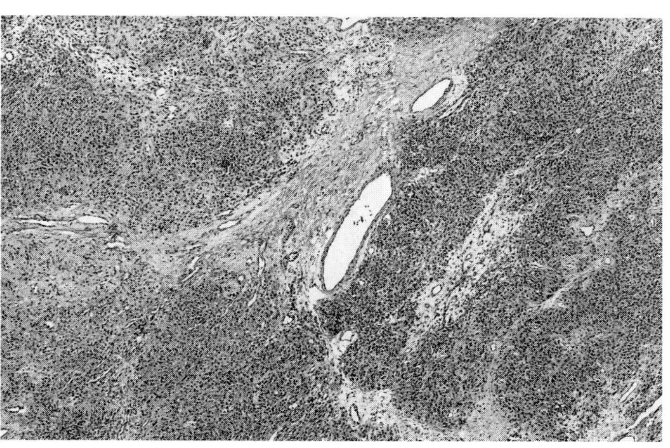

11-101. Nodular pattern in Leydig cell tumor.

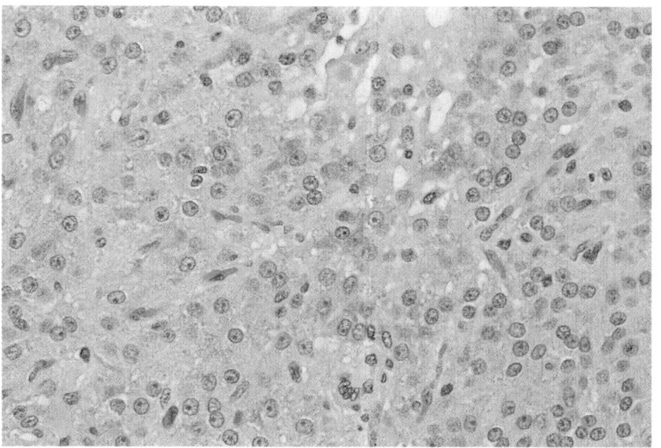

11-102. Leydig cell tumor with intracytoplasmic lipofuscin. Note the eosinophilic cytoplasm and round nuclei with moderate-sized nucleoli.

polygonal, with abundant, eosinophilic cytoplasm, round, variably sized nuclei, and prominent, central nucleoli (Fig. 11-102). Finely granular lipofuscin pigment is present in the cytoplasm of tumors from postpubertal patients (see Fig. 11-102) (usually giving a tan to brown gross appearance) and careful search allows for the identification of rod-shaped, intracytoplasmic crystals of Reinke in up to 40% of cases (see Fig. 11-100).[457] Spindle-shaped stromal cells rarely occur as a minor component, probably reflecting the embryonic derivation of Leydig cells from undifferentiated gonadal stroma. Neoplasms composed chiefly of spindle cells with a minority of neoplastic Leydig cells are best categorized as unclassified or indeterminate stromal tumors.[464] Cytoplasmic accumulation of lipid imparts a clear, finely vacuolated appearance resembling the adrenal cortical zona fasciculata in some cases (Fig. 11-103). Mitotic figures are usually infrequent, and a rate of 3 or more per 10 high power fields is a feature that suggests malignancy (see below). Rare foci of ossification have been described,[465,466] including one malignant case.[466] The presence of ossification and calcification in a presumed Leydig cell tumor should also raise the possibility of large cell calcifying Sertoli cell tumor (see page 619). Adipose metaplasia may rarely occur.[467] Androgenic hormones may be identified by immunohistochemistry of Leydig cell tumor, and vimentin is the dominant cytoplasmic intermediate filament.[468] One case with enkephalin immunoreactivity has been described.[469] Ultrastructurally, Leydig cell tumor has features of steroid hormone synthesizing cells, including abundant lipid droplets, prominent cisternae of smooth endoplasmic reticulum, and mitochondria with tubular cristae.[470,471] Reinke crystals appear as sharply demarcated geometric shapes, such as hexagons and rhomboids, which have a lattice-like substructure.[472]

Treatment and prognosis

About 10% of Leydig cell tumors are clinically malignant, but this subset cannot be easily distinguished on pathologic examination. Pathologic features associated with malignancy include more than 3 mitoses per 10 high power fields, nuclear atypia, infiltrative borders, necrosis, large tumor size, and vascular invasion (Fig. 11-104).[458] Older patients are more likely to have malignant Leydig cell tumors,[473] whereas malignant behavior before puberty has not been reported.[458,459] Gynecomastia is more common with benign Leydig cell

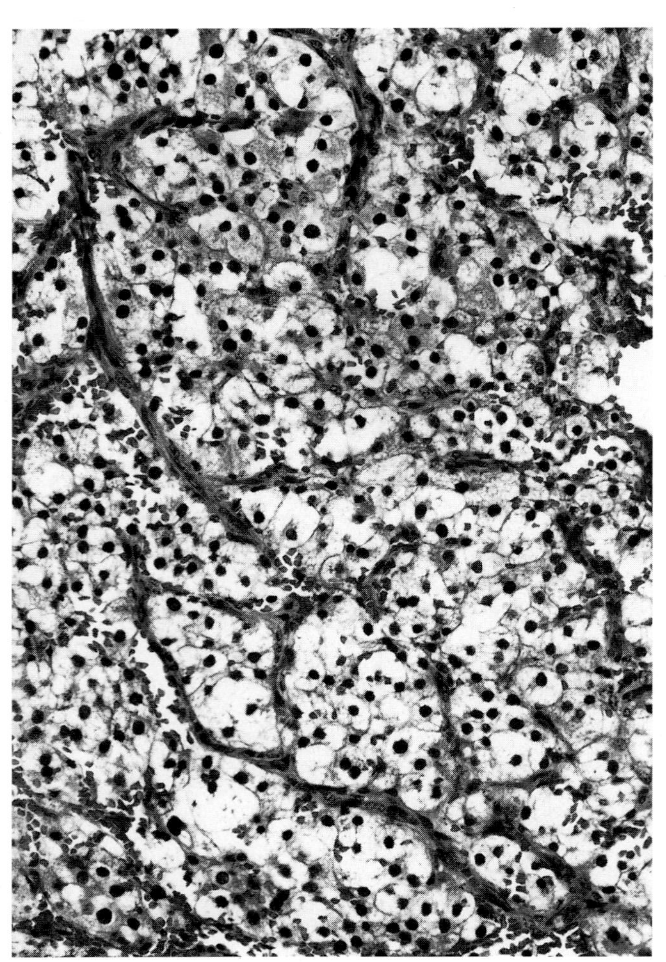

11-103. Leydig cell tumor with clear cells, which was initially interpreted as seminoma.

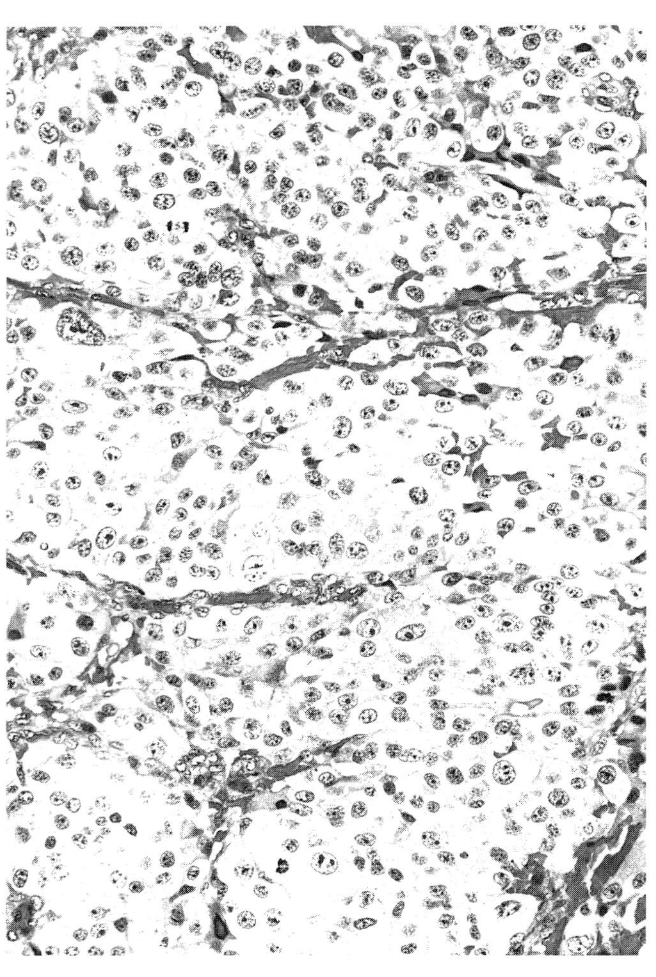

11-104. Metastasizing Leydig cell tumor with cellular pleomorphism and mitotic figures.

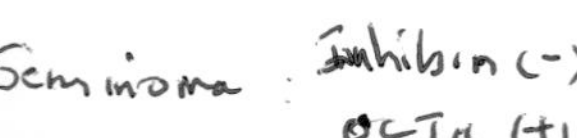

tumor.[458] Radiation and chemotherapy are not effective in the treatment of malignant Leydig cell tumor; retroperitoneal lymphadenectomy remains the mainstay of management in such cases. Mean survival of patients with malignant Leydig cell tumor is about 4 years,[473] but some patients may develop metastases more than 10 years after orchiectomy.

Differential diagnosis

Several entities should be considered in the differential diagnosis of Leydig cell tumor.[457] Leydig cell hyperplasia, although usually diffuse, may form nodules that mimic Leydig cell tumor. However, this is an interstitial, nondestructive process that preserves seminiferous tubules. It may be seen in patients with elevated gonadotropin levels, including patients with elevated human chorionic gonadotropin levels. Apparent Leydig cell hyperplasia occurs in many cases of testicular atrophy because of a normal population of Leydig cells in a greatly reduced testicular volume. It is seen in Klinefelter's syndrome where other pathologic features of that disorder are present and help with the diagnosis. Patients who have the adrenogenital syndrome[2,474] or Nelson's syndrome[475] (Cushing's syndrome associated with occult pituitary adenoma that becomes clinically evident with high levels of adrenocorticotrophin after bilateral adrenalectomy) may develop testicular nodules that closely resemble Leydig cell tumor. These nodules appear to be hyperplastic and are usually distinguished from Leydig cell tumor by their multifocality, bilaterality, uniform absence of Reinke crystals, and tendency for prominent lipofuscin deposits.[457] Clinical history is often of value.

Large cell calcifying Sertoli cell tumor, an entity that is associated with Carney's syndrome, may resemble Leydig cell tumor because the neoplastic cells are usually polygonal with abundant eosinophilic cytoplasm.[5,476-480] However, unlike Leydig cell tumor, large cell calcifying Sertoli cell tumor is often bilateral, multifocal, lacks Reinke crystals, is frequently associated with calcifications (and sometimes ossification), and may show intratubular growth.[457] Malakoplakia may resemble Leydig cell tumor but has intratubular infiltrates of eosinophilic histiocytes and cytoplasmic calcifications that are not seen in Leydig cell tumor. Young and Talerman[457] reported metastatic prostate carcinoma to the testis mimicking Leydig cell tumor, but immunostains against prostate specific antigen and prostatic acid phosphatase were positive, resolving the differential diagnosis. Leydig cell tumor with prominent cytoplasmic clarity may be misinterpreted as seminoma, but the clarity is caused by lipids rather than glycogen; there is no association with IGCNU, and the characteristic lymphoid infiltrate and granulomatous reaction of seminoma are not present.

SERTOLI CELL TUMOR

Clinical features

Sertoli cell tumor is rare, accounting for about 1% of testicular neoplasms. It can occur at virtually any age but is most common in middle age. Most patients present with a testicular mass,[460] but estrogen production by the tumor can cause gynecomastia or impotence, which can be the presenting complaints.[464] Isolated gynecomastia may be the initial manifestation of Sertoli cell tumor in a child; children with Leydig cell tumor, in contrast, do not develop gynecomastia without virilization.[460] Patients with Peutz-Jeghers syndrome have been reported with testicular Sertoli cell tumor,[6] but it is not clear if these were ordinary Sertoli cell tumors or something else. One boy with Peutz-Jeghers syndrome was found to have sex cord tumors with annular tubules in the testis,[481] and similar lesions have been described in the testes of patients with the androgen insensitivity syndrome.[482] The experience with ovarian tumors in patients with the Peutz-Jeghers syndrome suggests the possibility that many of the testicular lesions in these cases may be sex cord tumor with annular tubules[483,484]; alternatively, some of these cases may be large cell calcifying Sertoli cell tumor. Estrogen production by such lesions is implied by the development of gynecomastia in boys with the Peutz-Jeghers syndrome and testicular neoplasm.[6]

Pathologic features

Grossly, Sertoli cell tumor usually is a solid, gray or white nodule, usually under 3 cm in diameter, although large tumors may occur but should raise a concern for malignancy (Fig. 11-105).[485] Microscopically, solid tubules in a fibrous stroma are typical (Fig. 11-106). Frequently, the cells have cytoplasmic vacuolization, creating a microcystic pattern (Fig. 11-107). In some cases, the tubules may have distinct lumens rather than appearing as solid tubular arrays; in other cases, the cells may be arranged as solid nests (Fig. 11-108) or cords. The cells often have clear cytoplasm caused by abundant cellular lipid, and the nuclei are oval, often with moderate-sized nucleoli. Both cytokeratin and vimentin may be demonstrated immunohistochemically; epithelial membrane antigen yields variable results,[367,468,485-487] and NSE positivity has been described in several cases.[485] Features of steroid synthesizing cells are identified ultrastructurally, including abundant cisternae of smooth endoplasmic reticulum and numerous intracytoplasmic lipid droplets. Adjacent cells are connected by desmosomes.[488] Charcot-Böttcher filaments (perinuclear arrays of filaments) are considered pathognomonic of Sertoli cell differentiation. They have been identified in ovarian Sertoli cell tumor[489]

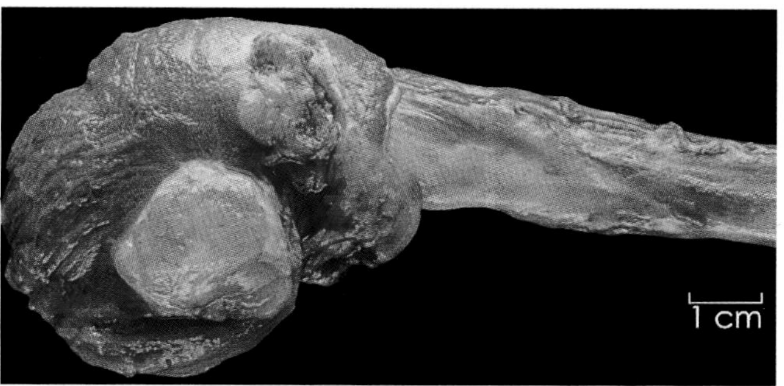

11-105. Sertoli cell tumor.

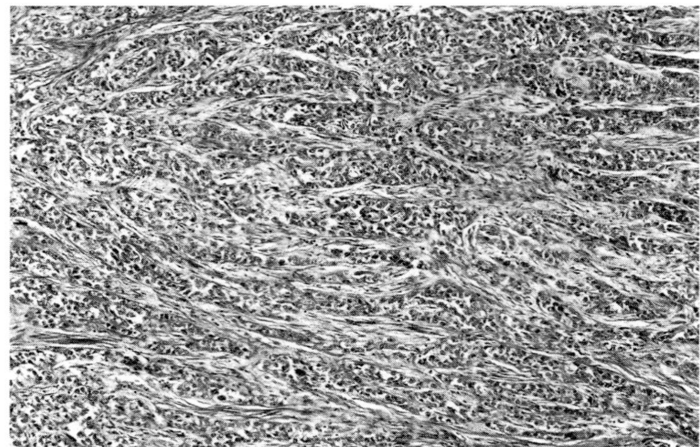

11-106. Sertoli cell tumor composed of solid tubules.

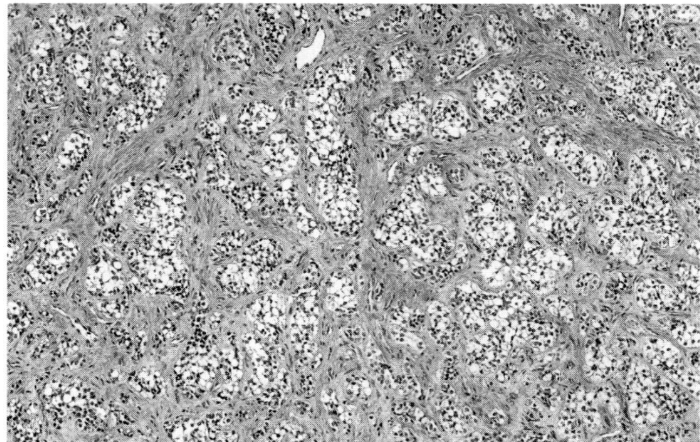

11-107. Sertoli cell tumor with cytoplasmic vacuolization.

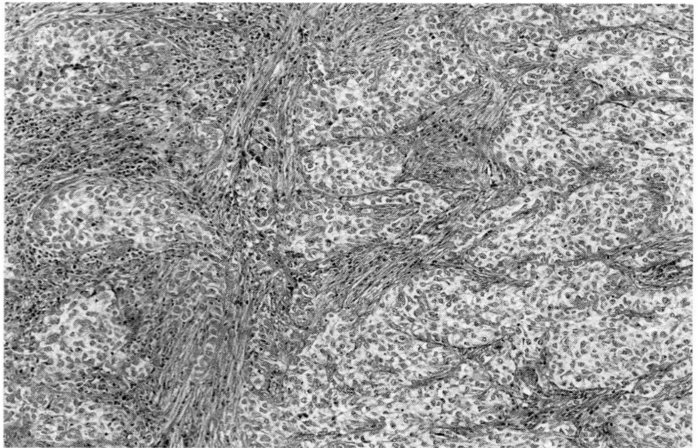

11-108. Solid nests in a Sertoli cell tumor.

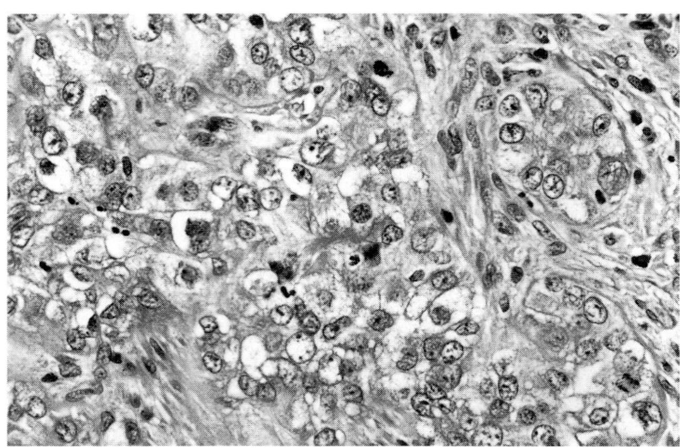

11-109. Metastasizing Sertoli cell tumor with nuclear atypia and mitotic figures.

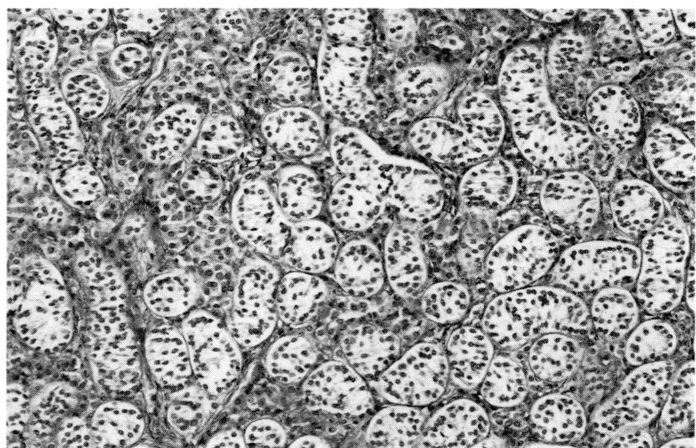

11-110. Nodule of Sertoli cell-lined tubules and Leydig cells in a patient with the androgen insensitivity syndrome.

and in large cell calcifying Sertoli cell tumor,[476,477,480] but most reports of testicular Sertoli cell tumor have not mentioned their presence.

Malignant behavior in Sertoli cell tumor, as in Leydig cell tumor, may be difficult to predict from pathologic features alone. Features that correlate with an increased likelihood of malignancy include cytologic atypia and pleomorphism, invasive borders, mitotic activity, vascular invasion, and large tumor size (Fig. 11-109).[485,490-493] About 10% of Sertoli cell tumors are malignant, and in contrast with Leydig cell tumor malignant cases may occur in children.[93,464,485] Gynecomastia appears to be more common with malignant tumors than benign tumors.[485]

Differential diagnosis

Sertoli cell tumor must be distinguished from the rare seminoma with a tubular pattern,[215] a differential diagnosis discussed on page 584. Patients with the androgen insensitivity syndrome (also known as the testicular feminization syndrome) may develop multiple hamartomatous testicular nodules composed of closely spaced tubules lined by Sertoli cells but, in contrast with true Sertoli cell tumor, these lesions also have intervening Leydig cells within the interstitium (Fig. 11-110).[3,104] About 25% of patients with androgen insensitivity syndrome also develop multifocal, bilateral Sertoli cell adenomas composed of pure proliferations of Sertoli cell-lined tubules.[3] These lesions are indistinguishable from

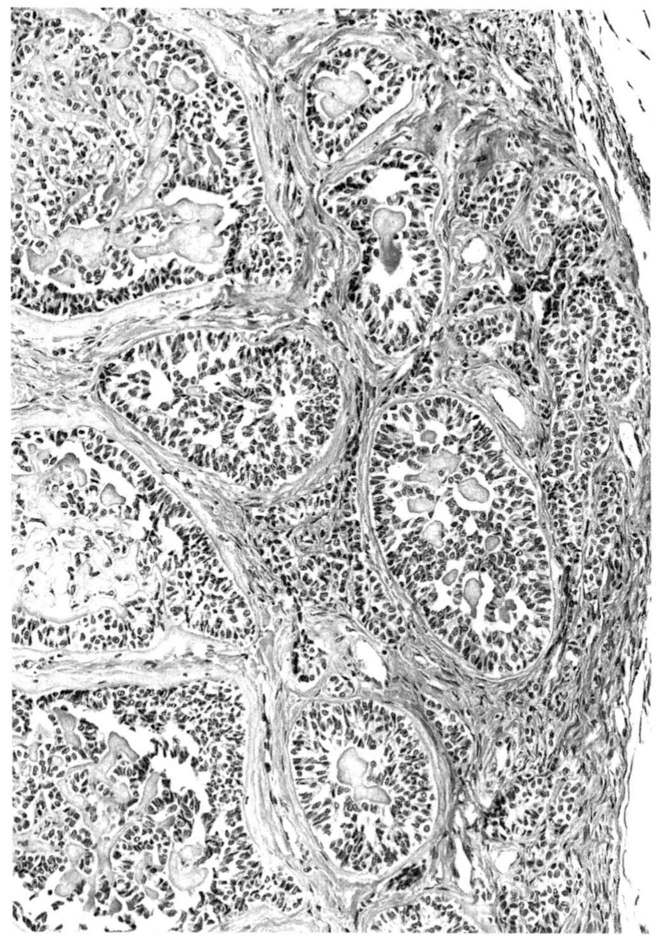

11-111. Sex cord tumor with annular tubules. (Illustration from an ovarian case.)

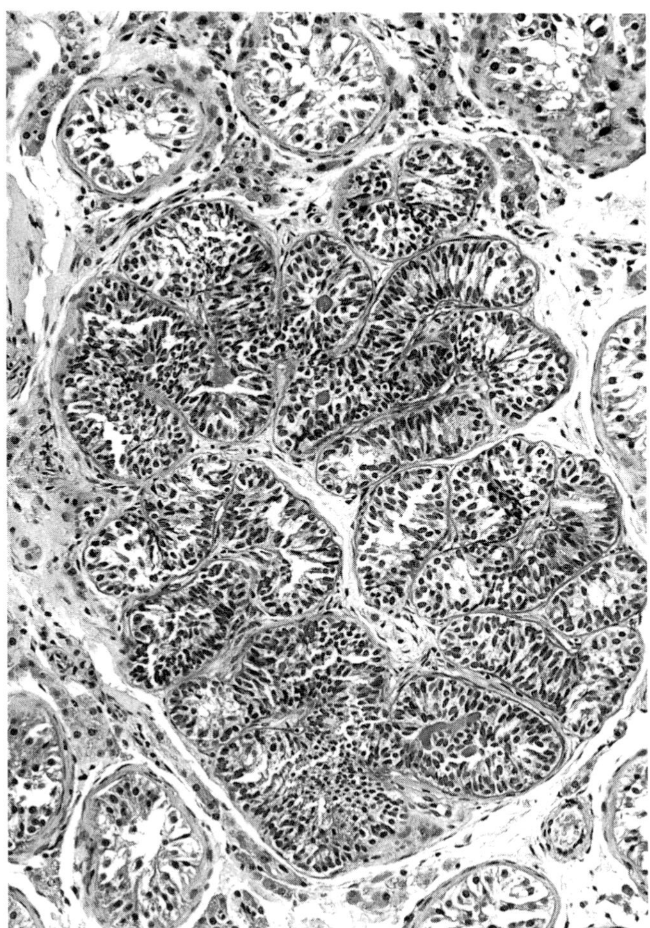

11-112. Sertoli cell nodule in a cryptorchid testis.

well-differentiated Sertoli cell tumor, and it is uncertain if they are neoplastic or hamartomatous. Malignant behavior in pure Sertoli cell proliferations in patients with androgen insensitivity syndrome have not been reported, thus the term *Sertoli cell adenoma* is appropriate even though it connotes a neoplastic process.[3,104] A recent unique case of a malignant sex cord–stromal tumor in a patient with androgen insensitivity syndrome did not have the features of a typical Sertoli cell adenoma and more closely resembled juvenile granulosa cell tumor, although ultrastructure supported Sertoli cell differentiation.[494] Patients with androgen insensitivity syndrome may also develop lesions resembling the sex cord tumor with annular tubules,[482] a lesion more commonly identified in the ovary, especially in patients with Peutz-Jeghers syndrome.[483,484] These distinctive lesions are composed of nests of Sertoli-like cells arranged around hyaline cylinders of basement membrane (Fig. 11-111).

Microscopic, nonencapsulated nodules composed of small tubules lined by Sertoli cells are common in orchiectomy specimens, and may be more common in cryptorchid testes (Fig. 11-112).[128,129] These Sertoli cell nodules often contain central accumulations of basement membrane, which can be seen in continuity with thickened peripheral basement membrane surrounding the tubules. In contrast to true Sertoli cell tumor, these are invariably incidental microscopic findings. In patients with germ cell tumor, they may be colonized by IGCNU, simulating gonadoblastoma (Fig. 11-113). Occasional Sertoli cell nodules may also contain spermatogenic cells, unlike Sertoli cell tumor.

Sclerosing Sertoli cell tumor

Sclerosing Sertoli cell tumor is a recently described variant of Sertoli cell tumor that occurs in patients with an average age of 35 years and a range of 18 to 80 years.[495] All patients present with a testicular mass without associated hormonal symptoms. Grossly, sclerosing Sertoli cell tumor consists of solid, white to yellow-tan nodules. Microscopically, it is composed of cords, solid or hollow tubules, and nests of Sertoli cells set in a densely collagenous stroma (Fig. 11-114). The nuclei vary from large and vesicular to small and hyperchromatic, and the cytoplasm is pale and sometimes vacuolated. Mitotic activity and cytologic atypia were significant in only 1 of the 10 reported cases, but, despite this finding, all cases

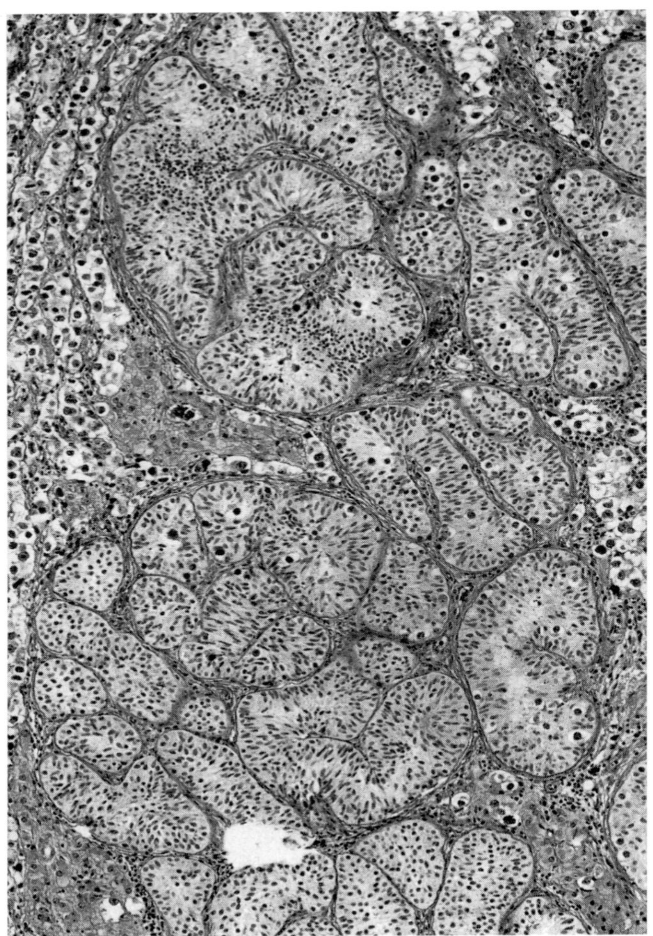

11-113. Sertoli cell nodule partially populated by IGCNU cells and surrounded by seminoma.

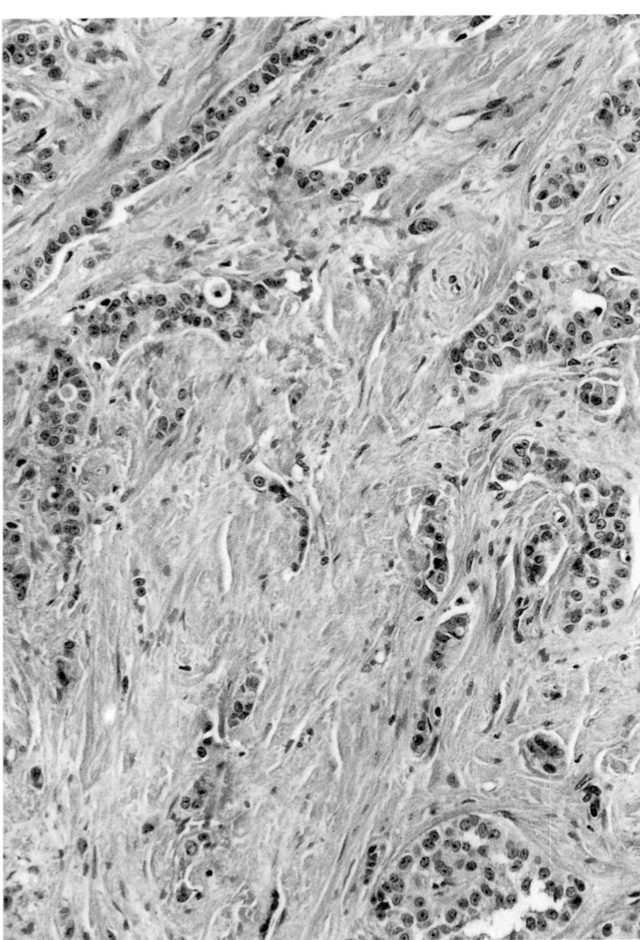

11-114. Cord-like and small nested patterns in a sclerosing Sertoli cell tumor. Note densely collagenous stroma.

had a benign outcome.[495] Vimentin is present in the neoplastic cells. The cord-like pattern may be misinterpreted as trabecular carcinoid tumor, but most primary carcinoids have an insular pattern and may be associated with teratomatous elements. The presence of a cord-like or tubular pattern with vacuolated cells may suggest adenomatoid tumor, a paratesticular rather than intratesticular lesion that is strongly cytokeratin positive, unlike the sclerosing Sertoli cell tumor.[495]

Large cell calcifying Sertoli cell tumor

Large cell calcifying Sertoli cell tumor is another variant of Sertoli cell tumor, which has some unique clinical associations.[4,5,476-480,496] It may be the lesion that has been described in patients with the Peutz-Jeghers syndrome, although it seems more likely that those cases, like the ovarian cases of Peutz-Jeghers syndrome, are examples of the sex-cord tumor with annular tubules. It is now apparent that large cell calcifying Sertoli cell tumor is a component of the Carney syndrome in which patients develop lentigines of the face, myxomas of the heart, skin, soft tissue, and elsewhere, myxoid fibroadenomas of the breast, blue nevi of the skin, pigmented nodules of the adrenal cortex associated with Cushing's syndrome, growth hormone producing adenomas of the pituitary gland, and psammomatous melanotic schwannomas.[4,5,480,496-499] Because 40% or so of large cell calcifying Sertoli cell tumors are associated with the Carney syndrome, its diagnosis should prompt consideration of this association because of the potential life-threatening complications of cardiac myxoma. The majority of patients with large cell calcifying Sertoli cell tumor are under 20 years of age, with a mean age of 16 years.[4,457] A testicular mass is the usual presenting complaint but gynecomastia and isosexual pseudoprecocity may also occur[476,478]; the hormones responsible for these manifestations may be produced by the neoplasm or by associated nodules of hyperplastic Leydig cells.

Grossly, large cell calcifying Sertoli cell tumor is usually tan or yellow with associated gritty calcification and is often multifocal, with a 40% frequency of bilaterality.[5,496] Microscopically, there are nests and cords of cells with abundant, eosinophilic cytoplasm in a myxoid to collagenous stroma, which is calcified or even ossified in about one half of cases (Fig. 11-115). Intratubular neoplasm and calcification are common. Nuclei are usually round and may have prominent nucleoli, but mitotic figures are usually rare. Malignant behavior is unusual;

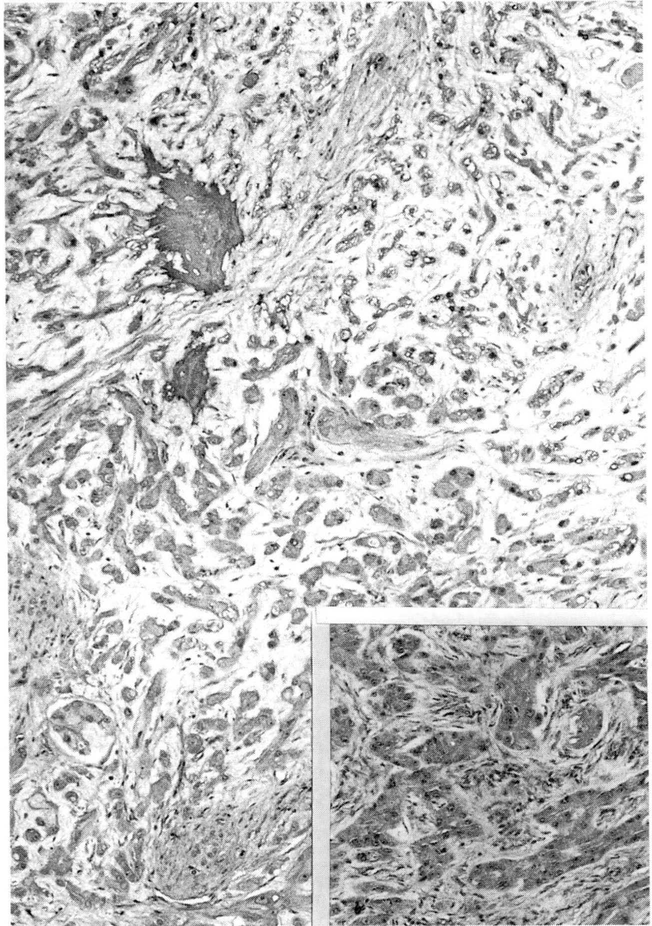

11-115. Large cell calcifying Sertoli cell tumor. Note focal calcification (*top right*). Inset shows neoplastic cells at high magnification.

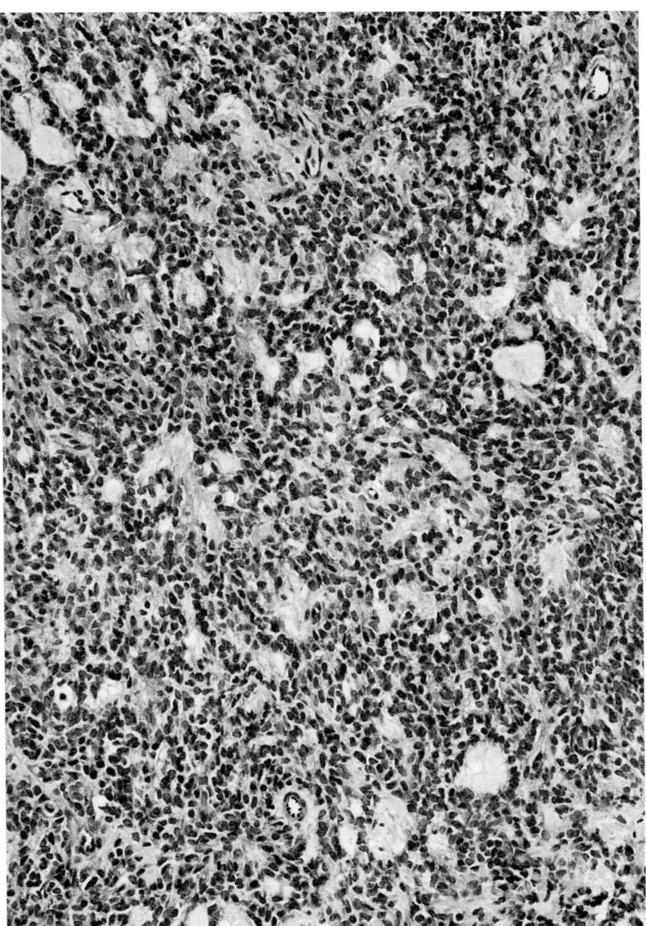

11-116. Testicular granulosa cell tumor of the adult type with Call-Exner bodies.

Proppe and Scully[5] identified a malignant large cell calcifying Sertoli cell tumor with numerous mitotic figures. A case seen in consultation at Indiana University had no histological features of malignancy but metastasized to lymph nodes. Ultrastructural studies of large cell calcifying Sertoli cell tumor have demonstrated Charcot-Böttcher filaments and other features of Sertoli cells.[476,480] The main differential diagnostic problem posed by large cell calcifying Sertoli cell tumor is separation from Leydig cell tumor (see page 619).

GRANULOSA CELL TUMOR, ADULT TYPE

There are two major types of granulosa cell tumor of the testis: adult and juvenile. The adult type is quite rare,[500-505] occurring in patients from 16 to 76 years of age,[457] and is frequently associated with hyperestrogenism, often causing gynecomastia.[504] Grossly, the adult type may be solid, cystic, or both, and is typically yellow to gray.[457,502] Gross hemorrhage and necrosis may correlate with malignant behavior.[505] Microscopically, the patterns of the common granulosa cell tumor of the ovary may be identified, including microfollicular (Fig. 11-116), macrofollicular, trabecular, gyriform, insular, and diffuse patterns. Call-Exner bodies are characteristic of the microfollicular pattern. The cells have scant, lightly staining cytoplasm, and the nuclei are pale, round to oval, and frequently grooved. Mitotic figures are usually infrequent but there may rarely be up to 6 per 10 high power fields.[505] Vimentin is usually present and cytokeratins 8 and 18 may be identified,[376,500,503] although one study reported an absence of cytokeratin reactivity in five of five cases[505]; epithelial membrane antigen is negative.[376,500,503,505] Ultrastructural studies have shown results similar to ovarian granulosa cell tumor.[501,503] Most reported cases have been benign, but malignant behavior is a possibility.[504,505] Large tumor size (>7 cm), vascular invasion, hemorrhage, and necrosis are considered useful in identifying cases with the greatest risk of malignant behavior.[505]

GRANULOSA CELL TUMOR, JUVENILE TYPE

Juvenile granulosa cell tumor of the testis is similar in appearance to its ovarian counterpart but occurs in a more restricted age range, with almost all patients under 5 months of age.[374,506,507] There are no well-established risk factors, although a disproportionate number occur in patients with either gonadal dysgenesis or anomalies of sex chromosomes, including patients with X/XY mosaicism.[150,508,509]

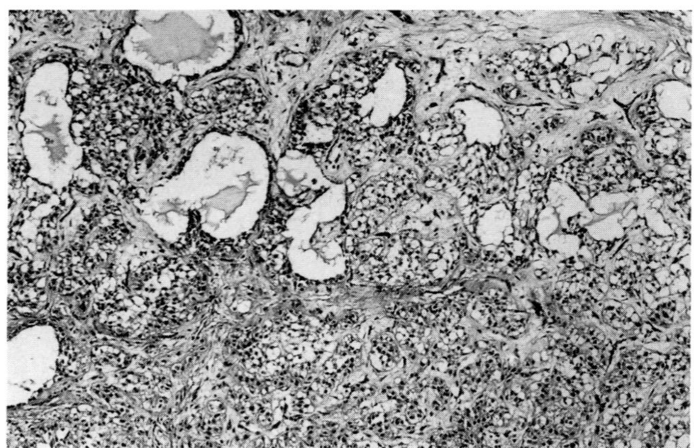

11-117. Juvenile granulosa cell tumor with follicle-like structures filled with watery to mucoid secretion. Note microcystic pattern.

A testicular mass is invariably the presenting feature. Grossly, it consists of a solid to cystic, gray to yellow nodule.[374] The cystic foci are filled with mucoid to watery fluid. Microscopically, juvenile granulosa cell tumor has solid, cellular zones admixed with follicle-like, cystic structures filled with watery, faintly mucicarminophilic fluid (Fig. 11-117). The solid areas may display prominently hyalinized, collagenous stroma. The neoplastic cells have abundant pale to eosinophilic cytoplasm with round, hyperchromatic nuclei and identifiable nucleoli.[374,457] Mitoses may be prominent, but malignant behavior has not been reported, another feature that differs from ovarian juvenile granulosa cell tumor.

Immunohistochemical studies reveal cytokeratin and vimentin reactivity of the granulosa-like cell, which is present both within follicle-like structures and in nests within the stroma.[375] In addition, a peri-"follicular" spindle cell demonstrates reactivity with vimentin and muscle-specific actin, and focally with desmin.[375] The histogenesis of this tumor is controversial, with some favoring Sertoli cell derivation rather than granulosa cell differentiation[375] (Talerman A, personal communication, 1993). Because of

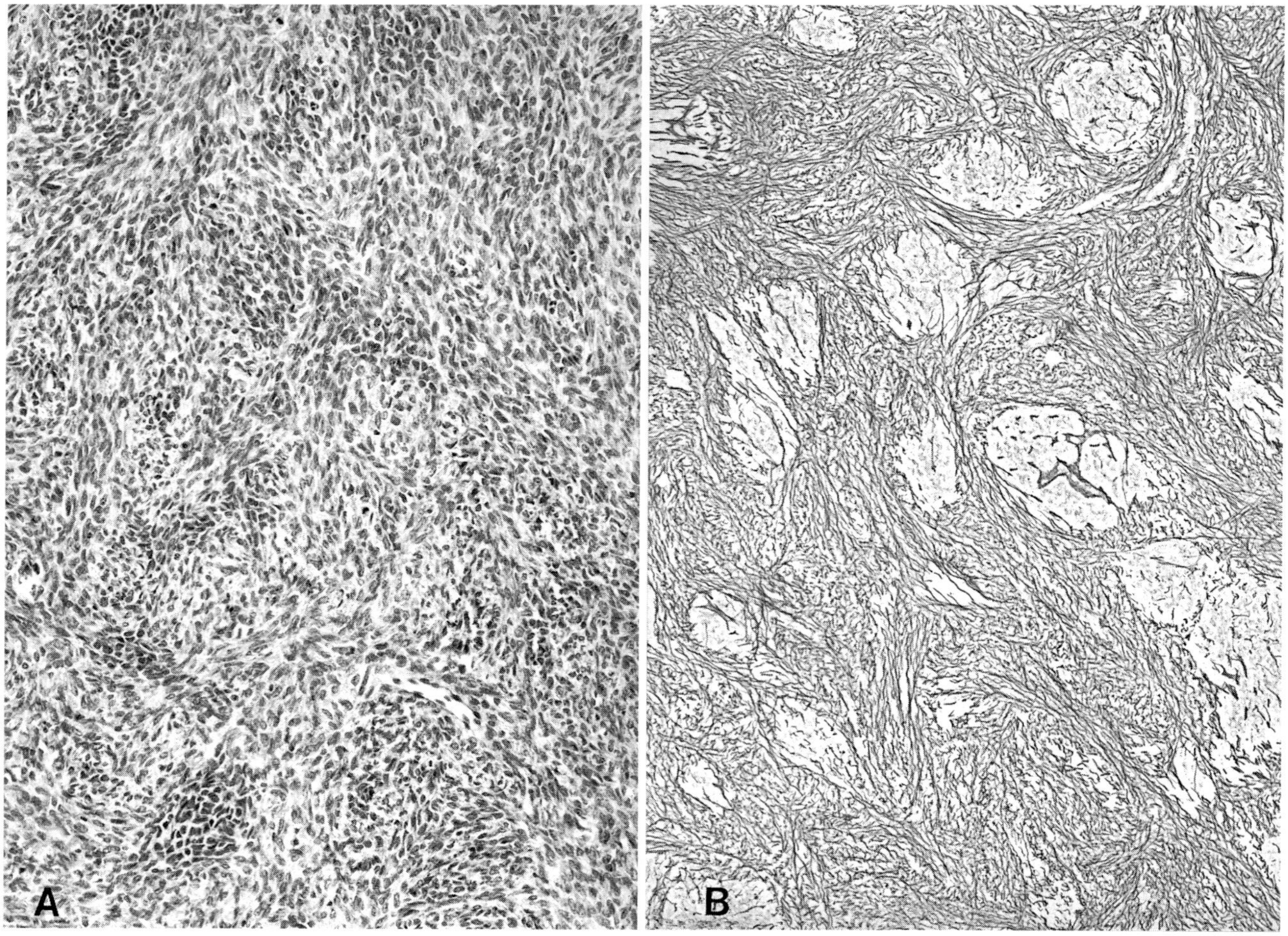

11-118. **A**, Unclassified sex cord–stromal tumor. Darkly staining nests represent sex cord elements. **B**, Reticulin stain accentuates the reticulin-free sex cord elements surrounded by the reticulin-rich stromal component.

the exclusive occurrence in infants and young children, and the solid and cystic pattern, juvenile granulosa cell tumor may be confused with testicular yolk sac tumor. This differential diagnosis is discussed on page 600.

MIXED AND UNCLASSIFIED SEX CORD–STROMAL TUMORS

A sizable group of sex cord–stromal neoplasms of the testis show admixtures of various forms of differentiation or incomplete differentiation. Such cases are classified as mixed or unclassified sex cord–stromal tumors, respectively. An example of a mixed sex cord–stromal tumor is adult granulosa cell tumor with tubules lined by Sertoli cells. Unclassified sex cord–stromal tumors consist of proliferations of incompletely differentiated sex cord or stromal elements, which cannot be further characterized at the light microscopic level. These neoplasms are heterogeneous and have been grouped into a "wastebasket" category. Mixed and unclassified sex cord–stromal tumors occur at all ages, with 50% of cases occurring in children.[510] They usually present as a testicular mass, and 15% of cases are associated with gynecomastia.[457] Most consist of gray, tan, or yellow solid nodules of variable size. Both epithelial (sex cord) and stromal differentiation may be apparent at the light microscopic level (Fig. 11-118), and reticulin stains may enhance the different elements, surrounding groups of sex cord–like cells and individual stromal cells (see Fig. 11-118). In other cases, the stromal component may be dominant, consisting of a relatively pure spindle cell proliferation with a sarcomatoid appearance. Such cases may have many mitoses and a pleomorphic appearance, and such features indicate malignancy. The demonstration of epithelial features by electron microscopy and immunohistochemistry suggests that some of these stromal tumors are spindled forms of epithelial origin.[511] In other cases, the presence of myofilaments in spindled stromal tumors suggests origin from myofibroblastic cells of the testicular interstitium, especially the peritubular myoid cells.[512] Such cases should probably be classified as pure mesenchymal tumors (see page 630) rather than unclassified sex cord–stromal tumors. Mixed and unclassified sex cord–stromal tumors behave in a benign fashion in children under 10 years of age, but metastases develop in 20% of older patients.[510] The presence of cellular atypia and pleomorphism, a high mitotic rate, necrosis, vascular invasion, invasive margins, and large tumor size are features that identify patients at risk for metastases. These tumors are usually managed by radical orchiectomy, with retroperitoneal lymph node dissection reserved for patients with clinical evidence of metastatic involvement or high risk pathologic features.

MIXED GERM CELL AND SEX CORD–STROMAL TUMORS

GONADOBLASTOMA

Clinical features

Gonadoblastoma is composed of a mixture of seminoma-like cells and sex cord cells having features of Sertoli cells, with Charcot-Böttcher filaments in the cytoplasm.[513,514] Gonadoblastoma usually arises in abnormal, dysgenetic gonads of patients with an intersex syndrome; 80% are phenotypically female, and 20% are phenotypically male, but ambiguous genitalia occur in many cases.[515] Phenotypically male patients present in childhood or early adolescence with cryptorchidism, hypospadias, or other anomalies of the external genitalia, and gynecomastia. Surgical exploration of the cryptorchid testes often demonstrates persistence of female-type internal genital structures stemming from failure of involution of the müllerian ductal system.[108] Bilateral involvement by gonadoblastoma occurs in about one third of cases.[515] Karyotypic analysis of the patients, regardless of sexual phenotype, almost always reveals a Y-chromosome, with 46XY and 45X/46XY occurring most commonly.[108]

Pathologic features

Grossly, gonadoblastoma usually forms solid, yellow and tan nodules with gritty calcifications. Microscopically, the nodules usually consist of well-defined,

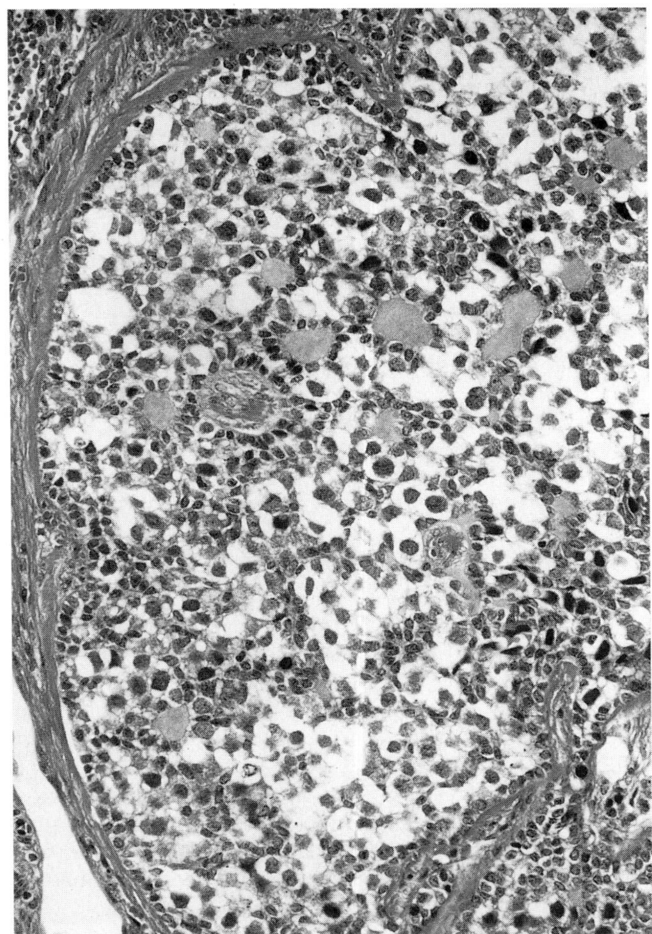

11-119. Gonadoblastoma composed of a mixture of seminoma-like cells with clear cytoplasm and small, dark sex cord cells. The sex cord cells form palisades at the periphery of the tumor and around eosinophilic matrix.

rounded nests of large, pale seminoma-like cells admixed with small, dark, angular, sex cord cells that may form a peripheral palisade around the cellular nests (Fig. 11-119). Foci of hyalinized basement membrane can be seen in the center of these nests and at the periphery. Calcifications appear initially on this basement membrane and may become quite prominent. In some gonadoblastomas, a trabecular growth pattern of seminoma-like cells and sex cord cells may occur in tandem. In the stroma adjacent to gonadoblastoma, collections of Leydig-like cells lacking Reinke crystals may be seen in about two thirds of cases.[108,515]

Treatment and prognosis

Gonadoblastoma is a premalignant lesion from which invasive germ cell tumors can develop; most are seminoma, but any nonseminomatous germ cell tumor may occur.[515] Excision of a gonad with gonadoblastoma prior to development of an invasive lesion is curative. Bilateral gonadectomy is indicated because of the dysgenetic nature of the gonads and the high frequency of bilaterality of gonadoblastoma.

Differential diagnosis

Sertoli cell nodule with colonization by IGCNU may be misinterpreted as gonadoblastoma (see page 622, Fig. 11-113). However, this lesion is microscopic rather than macroscopic, and the associated gonad is not dysgenetic. In some cases, the colonization by IGCNU is focal, and the seminoma-like cells are not uniformly distributed throughout the Sertoli cell nodule, whereas gonadoblastoma contains seminoma-like cells, which are an integral and diffusely distributed component. This distinction is important because the diagnosis of gonadoblastoma implies an underlying dysgenetic gonad and much higher risk of bilateral gonadal involvement by a premalignant lesion. In contrast, a patient with a Sertoli cell nodule with IGCNU probably has a risk of bilateral involvement similar to that of any patient with IGCNU in one testis, approximately 2% to 5% of cases.

OTHER MIXED GERM CELL SEX CORD–STROMAL TUMORS

Mixed germ cell and sex cord–stromal neoplasms other than gonadoblastoma are quite rare.[516] Such tumors have been reported in adults between 30 and 69 years of age and present as asymptomatic testicular masses; the features of gonadal dysgenesis or an intersex syndrome are absent in these cases.[516] Grossly, the tumors are usually fleshy, solid, and gray-white, although some may show foci of cystic degeneration. Microscopically, there are sheets or nests of germ cells admixed with dark sex cord–like cells, which may form distinct areas similar to granulosa cell tumor and Sertoli cell tumor. The germ cell component in these cases has been described as seminoma-like, but in three cases seen in consultation at Indiana University, these cells appeared more like nonneoplastic spermatogonia, having a uniform, fine chromatin and lacking the vesicular nuclei and large nucleoli of seminoma. In one case, Charcot-Böttcher filaments provided evidence of Sertoli cell differentiation in the sex cord–stromal component.[517] The discrete, small nests typical of gonadoblastoma are not identified, and the surrounding testis does not have dysgenetic features. Further, overgrowth of germ cell elements in the form of a typical germ cell tumor has not been reported nor have metastases been reported, although the rarity of these neoplasms makes generalizations from the available data tenuous.[516] Treatment consists of orchiectomy followed by careful follow-up. Assessment of the retroperitoneum by radiographic techniques is probably also prudent.

NEOPLASMS OF THE RETE TESTIS

ADENOCARCINOMA

Adenocarcinoma of the rete testis is very rare, occurring in patients between 31 and 91 years of age and reported exclusively in whites.[518] Many patients present with symptoms of hydrocele or with testicular pain and swelling. The initial clinical impression is often epididymitis or hydrocele. Grossly, there is a white to tan, yellow, or brown, ill-defined mass near the testicular hilum, often with extension into paratesticular structures. Microscopically, the tumor displays solid, papillary, and glandular patterns. The tumor often has an intraluminal component, which distends the spaces of the rete, as well as a component that infiltrates the supporting stroma of the rete testis (Fig. 11-120). Ideally, a transition from benign to malignant epithelium is seen in the lining of the rete testis.[518] The solid pattern is often punctuated by slit-like lumens (see Fig. 11-120), and a spindle cell pattern rarely occurs.[519] Lymphatic metastases occur most commonly and initially involve retroperitoneal lymph nodes; sometimes there is involvement of the skin of the scrotum or perineum.[520] The prognosis is poor, with only 36% of patients being tumor-free on follow-up.[518]

The differential diagnosis includes carcinoma and low malignant potential tumors of ovarian epithelial type (see Chapter 12); these occur more commonly in the paratesticular area, probably from metaplasia of the mesothelium, but also rarely occur within the testis, perhaps from mesothelial inclusions. It is likely that some cases of papillary serous tumor of low malignant potential have been reported as adenocarcinoma of the rete testis,[518] thus leading to an overly optimistic prognosis for rete testis carcinoma. Psammoma bodies, squamous metaplasia, or mucinous cell type should raise the question of müllerian-type neoplasms. The differential is probably not of great importance except when it involves the distinction of a low malignant potential tumor from an invasive carcinoma. Mesothelioma should also be considered, and immunohistochemical studies to distinguish between adenocarcinoma and mesothelioma may help in difficult cases. Prostatic carcinoma may involve the rete testis, but the clinical history and immunostains for prostate specific antigen should allow identification.

ADENOMA

Adenoma of the rete testis is rare, consisting of papillary or glandular proliferations of cytologically bland cells. These cases are too rare to draw conclusions.[521-523]

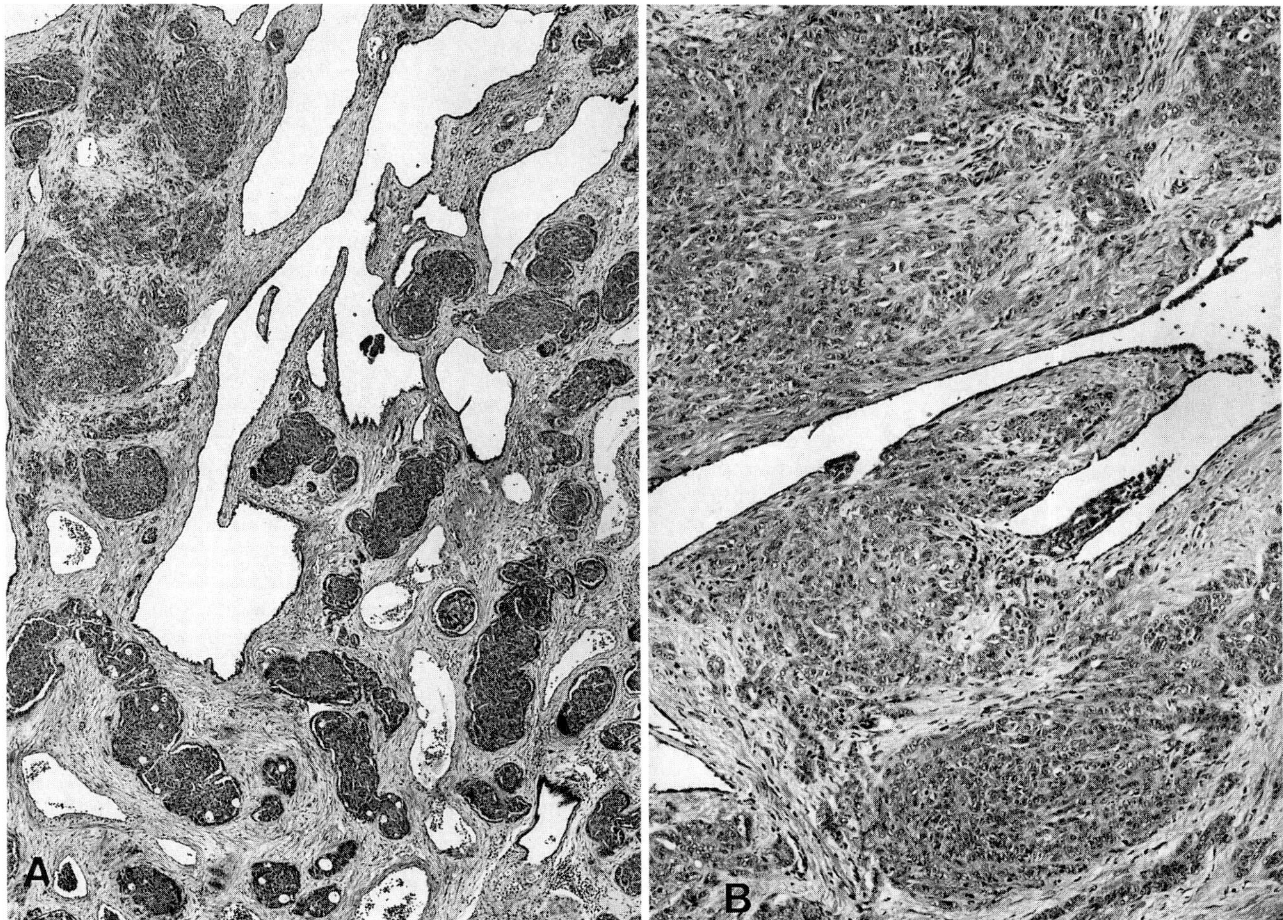

11-120. **A**, Rete testis carcinoma with solid pattern. Nests of carcinoma cells are within distended spaces of the rete testis; stromal invasion is at upper left. **B**, Tumor infiltrates stroma between dilated luminal spaces of rete testis. *(Courtesy of Lucien E. Nochomovitz, MD.)*

ADENOMATOUS HYPERPLASIA

Hartwick et al described nine cases of adenomatous hyperplasia of the rete testis in patients ranging from 30 to 74 years of age; in three cases the hyperplasia produced grossly evident, solid and cystic masses in the testicular hilum.[524] Microscopically, there were tubulopapillary proliferations of bland cells within the distended rete testis. Whether these cases are distinct from adenoma is unclear; they do not appear to be similar to the hyperplastic reaction of the rete testis typically seen in cases of germ cell tumor.[379]

NEOPLASMS OF LYMPHOID AND HEMATOPOIETIC CELLS

LYMPHOMA

Lymphoma in the testis usually represents secondary spread from lymph nodes,[254,256] although there are occasional cases that meet the criteria for primary testicular lymphoma.[254,258,525] The criteria include principal involvement of the testis and absence of nodal involvement after careful staging.[254] However, these restrictions may be inadequate for recognizing lymphoma originating in the testis. The tendency of apparently primary testicular lymphoma to progress rapidly after excision supports the belief that many "testicular" lymphomas originated elsewhere but spread to the testis and became clinically evident.[254,256,526,527] Consistent clonal rearrangements of the immunoglobulin light chain genes in synchronous, bilateral testicular lymphoma likely indicates occult dissemination of lymphoma with seeding of the testes,[528] and argues against primary bilateral testicular lymphoma. The poor survival of patients with bilateral lymphoma provides additional support for this view.[525] In many studies of testicular lymphoma, it is not clear if the tumor is primary extranodal lymphoma or lymphoma that originated elsewhere and subsequently spread to the testis, making interpretation of this literature difficult.

Clinical features

Patients with testicular lymphoma are usually older than those with germ cell tumors, with a mean age of about 60 years[251-256,525]; 50% of testicular neoplasms occurring in patients over age 60 are lymphoma.[457] Although most patients present secondary to a testicular mass, systemic symptoms such as fever, sweats, and weight loss also occur.[254] Bilateral testicular involvement occurs in about 20% of cases,[252,254-256,529] and is usually metachronous but may also be synchronous.

Pathologic features

Grossly, testicular lymphoma forms a fleshy, white-gray to pink mass that often diffusely replaces the testicular parenchyma (Fig. 11-121). Foci of necrosis may be conspicuous. It may be difficult to distinguish grossly from seminoma, although extension into the paratesticular structures suggests lymphoma rather than seminoma.[258,525] Microscopically, lymphoma usually has an interstitial pattern, with neoplastic cells surrounding but not replacing seminiferous tubules deep within the tumor (Fig. 11-122). Transtubular migration of the neoplastic cells may occur, and there may rarely be conspicuous intratubular involvement (Fig. 11-123). Despite interstitial growth, the seminiferous tubules may eventually be destroyed and replaced by tumor, so the absence of an interstitial pattern does not exclude lymphoma. Most testicular lymphomas in adults are diffuse large cell type[221,251,253-255,525,527] of B-cell immunophenotype[221,251,525]; some show the characteristic features of an immunoblastic lymphoma, with large, vesicular nuclei with prominent central nucleoli.[251,525,527] In children, Burkitt's lymphoma is the most common lymphoma in the testis[529] and shows the characteristic features, including small, mitotically active cells with round nuclei having several small nucleoli intermixed with macrophages containing phagocytosed nuclear debris. Rare cases of Burkitt's lymphoma of the testis have occurred in adults,[530] and Hodgkin's disease involving the testis is rare.[525,529,531]

Prognosis

The stage of testicular lymphoma is the most important prognostic factor. In patients with stage I disease, there is a 60% 5-year tumor-free survival, whereas patients with more advanced stage disease have only a 17% 5-year tumor-free survival.[525] Histologic classification is also prognostically useful[255]; in a multivariate analysis, lymphoma with sclerosis had a significantly better outcome, and, for unclear reasons, so did right-sided testicular lymphoma.[525]

Differential diagnosis

A major differential diagnostic consideration in testicular lymphoma is seminoma, which is addressed on page 584. Chronic orchitis may also be confused with lymphoma but contains a heterogenous cell population, consisting of lymphocytes, plasma cells, and neutrophils without atypia. Reactive lymphoid hyperplasia within the testis is a rare condition and has been described as testicular "pseudolymphoma"[532]; its distinction from lymphoma is based on the same criteria used at other sites.

PLASMACYTOMA

Plasmacytoma of the testis is rare and usually occurs in older patients with an established diagnosis of multiple myeloma.[533-535] Even more rarely, however, testicular plasmacytoma may be an apparently isolated finding, and, in such cases, the patient must be carefully worked up and followed for multiple myeloma.[535] Autopsy studies of patients with multiple myeloma demonstrate about a 2% frequency of testicular involvement, but the majority of such involvement remains clinically inapparent.[457] Grossly, plasmacytoma often appears as a soft, fleshy, gray-white, and hemorrhagic intratesticular mass. Micro-

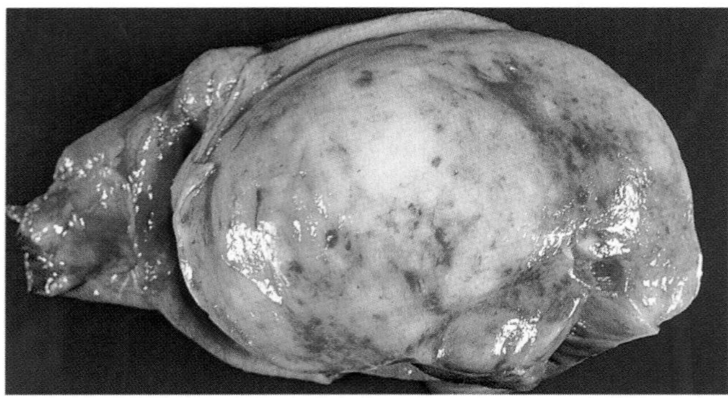

11-121. Lymphoma in the testis. Note fleshy, pink to cream-colored tumor.

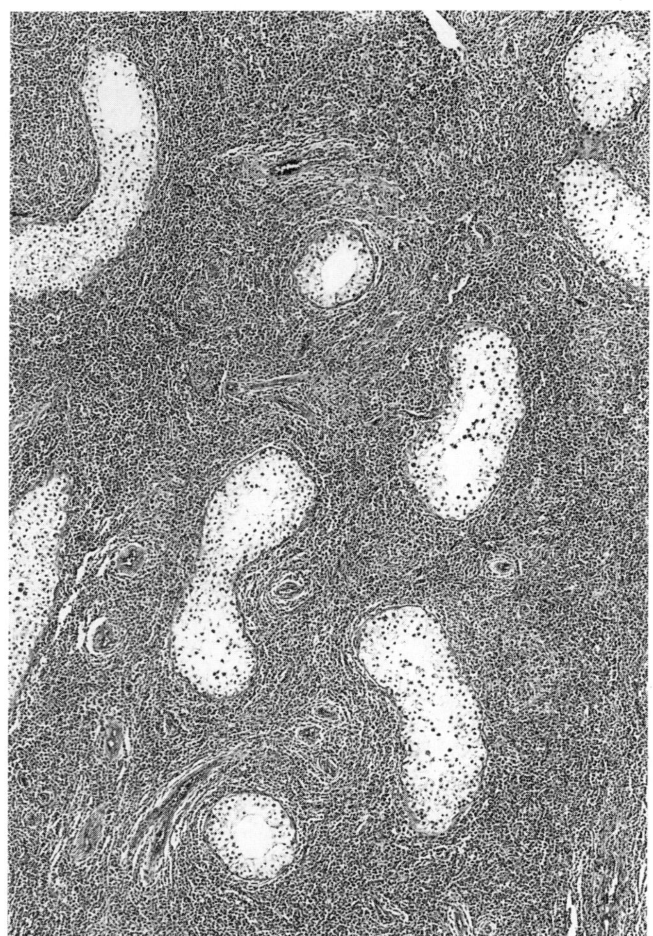

11-122. Typical interstitial pattern of lymphoma, with preservation of seminiferous tubules.

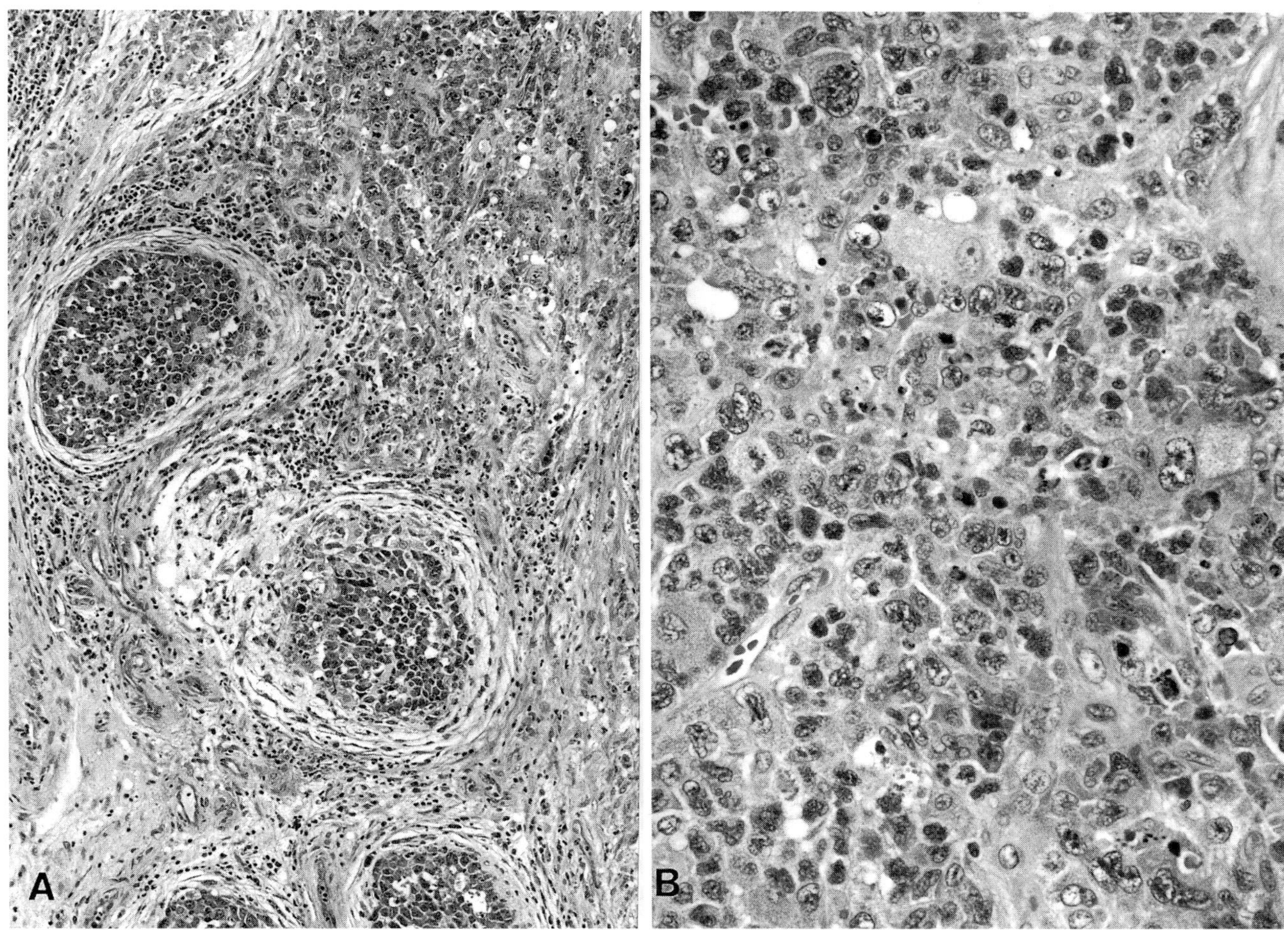

11-123. **A**, Unusual growth pattern of large cell lymphoma within seminiferous tubules. **B**, Higher magnification shows large, irregular nuclei.

scopically, sheets of variably differentiated neoplastic plasma cells are identified. Unlike chronic orchitis, a polymorphic cell population is absent and immunohistochemical studies of the plasma cells demonstrate immunoglobulin light chain restriction.[534,535]

LEUKEMIA

Leukemic infiltrates occur commonly in the testis, with frequency rates at autopsy between 40% and 65% of patients with acute leukemia and 20% to 35% of patients with chronic leukemia.[531,536] Acute lymphoblastic leukemia is especially prone to testicular involvement, and the testis may be a sanctuary site for leukemic cells such that testicular biopsy may detect leukemic infiltrates during periods of otherwise complete remission. The detection of leukemia in the testis in such cases occurs in 5% to 10% of patients and is predictive of subsequent systemic relapse.[537-539] The leukemic testis is usually not enlarged and the diagnosis is established by biopsy of patients at risk. Occasionally, diffuse testicular enlargement or induration or a testicular mass may be observed.[539] Bilateral involvement is common. Exceptionally, leukemia may initially present as testicular enlargement.[457] Microscopically, leukemia shows an interstitial pattern of infiltration similar to lymphoma. The neoplastic cells are characteristic of the particular type of leukemia. It may not be possible to morphologically distinguish between some types of lymphoma and leukemia, and clinical information regarding peripheral blood involvement and bone marrow studies are required. The distinction between neoplastic monocytic and myelocytic infiltrates and lymphoid neoplasia may require histochemical and immunohistochemical studies. Rarely, granulocytic sarcoma occurs in the absence of leukemia, although subsequent leukemia is expected.[540]

MISCELLANEOUS LESIONS

EPIDERMOID CYSTS

Epidermoid cysts are lined by squamous epithelium and filled with keratin. They characteristically occur in patients in the second to fourth decades of life[406] and are usually located at the periphery of the testis, close to the tunica albuginea. The pathogenesis is unknown and may be caused by monodermal or one-sided development of teratoma, squamous metaplasia of displaced mesothelial inclusions, or embryonically displaced inclusions of squamous epithelium derived from anlagen of scrotal skin. If the origin is teratomatous, the cyst must have a fundamentally different pathogenesis from typical mature teratoma because it is not associated with IGCNU, unlike teratoma in postpubertal patients.[183]

Grossly, epidermoid cysts usually are 2 to 3 cm in diameter[457] and are filled with white to yellow, friable, often pungent, keratinous material (Fig. 11-124). Microscopically, there is a squamous epithelial lining with a granular cell layer and a fibrous wall of variable thickness (Fig. 11-125). The lining is often compressed to just a few flattened layers of cells. Unlike dermoid cysts, there are no adnexal structures in the wall of the cyst. It is important to examine the surrounding testis for teratomatous or other germ cell tumor elements and IGCNU in the seminiferous tubules; any of these findings would cause reclassification of the lesion as mature teratoma. There are rare, problematic cases in which an epidermoid cyst is an apparent incidental finding in a testis with separate nodules of seminoma, and it is uncertain if these cases should be managed as seminoma (with incidental epidermoid cyst) or as mixed germ cell tumor consisting of seminoma and mature teratoma.

Epidermoid cysts are benign lesions that require no additional therapy following orchiectomy.[406,407] In rare cases where testicular preservation is considered essential, it may be justifiable to perform an enucleation of the cyst with a rim of surrounding testis with frozen section examination to determine the presence of teratoma or other germ cell tumor.[541] In most patients, however, orchiectomy is preferred.

MESENCHYMAL TUMORS

A variety of mesenchymal tumors of the testis arise from interstitial mesenchymal cells, endothelium, and probably peritubular myoid cells.[420,512] It may be difficult to separate some of these from unclassified sex cord–stromal tumor, but that distinction should be based on the absence of recognizable sex cord or epithelial differentiation. Thus, neurofibroma,[542] hemangioma[543-545] (including epithelioid hemangioma[546]), leiomyoma,[547] hemangioendothelioma,[548] osteosarcoma,[549,550] leiomyosarcoma,[551] fibrosarcoma,[550] and rhabdomyosarcoma[552-554] of the testis have been reported. Some of these may represent overgrowth of teratomatous elements of a germ cell tumor, particularly those occurring in younger patients. I have seen two cases of pure testicular embryonal rhabdomyosarcoma associated with IGCNU, and one other case has been reported in the literature,[544] suggesting that some testicular sarcomas are of teratomatous origin.

METASTASES TO THE TESTIS

Metastases to the testis are most commonly identified in patients with known malignancies, and the most common sites of origin are the prostate (35%), lung (19%), skin (melanoma, 9%), colon (9%), kidney (7%), and elsewhere (20%).[555] It is likely that the predominance of the prostate in this ranking represents a selection bias resulting from routine examination of orchiectomy specimens from patients with prostatic carcinoma.[556] Rarely metastases to the testis may present as apparent primary testic-

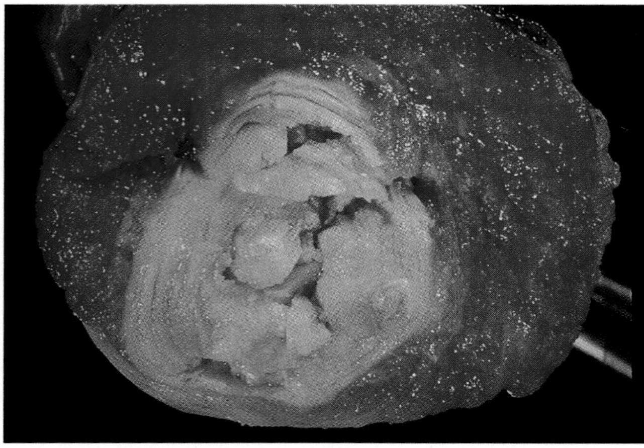

11-124. Epidermoid cyst filled with lamellated keratin. *(Courtesy of SF Cramer, MD; from Ulbright TM, Roth LM: Testicular and paratesticular neoplasms. In Sternberg SS, ed: Diagnostic surgical pathology, ed 2, New York, 1994, Raven Press; with permission of Raven Press.)*

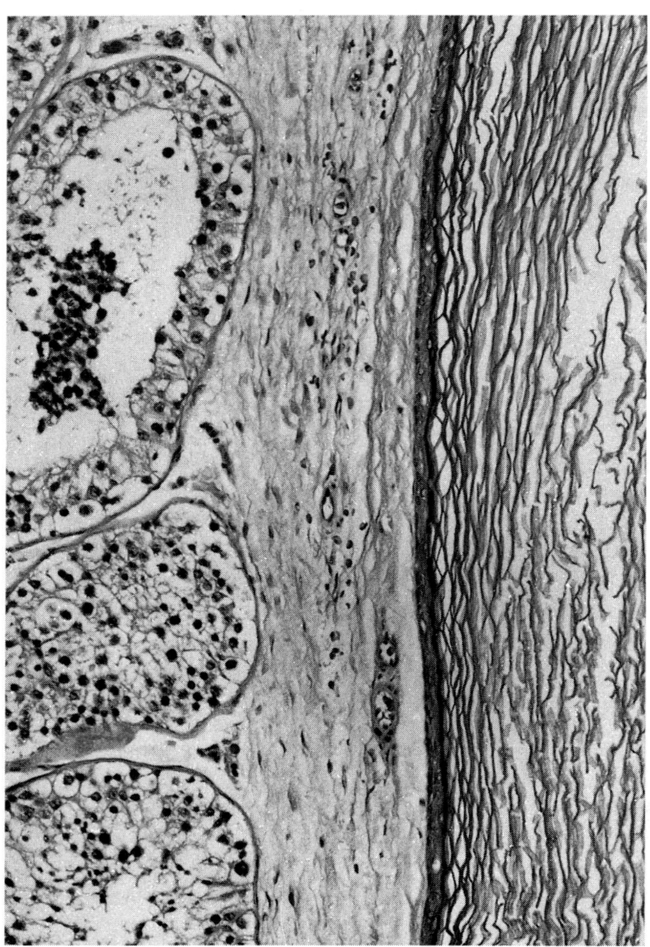

11-125. Epidermoid cyst showing a thin, compressed layer of stratified squamous epithelium lining a space filled with keratin. Note the absence of IGCNU in the surrounding seminiferous tubules.

ular tumors, including those originating in the prostate, lung, gastrointestinal tract (stomach and colon), skin (melanoma), pancreas, and liver, as well as carcinoid tumor.[457,555,557] Misinterpretation of metastatic carcinoma as embryonal carcinoma or Leydig cell tumor may occur,[555] or metastatic carcinoid may be misinterpreted as primary testicular carcinoid.[411] An extensive interstitial pattern, prominent microvascular involvement, multifocality, and bilaterality are features that favor metastasis rather than primary testicular tumor[555,556] (Fig. 11-126); the clinical history may also be of value because patients with metastatic lesions to the testis are older (average age 57 years) than patients with a germ cell tumor such as embryonal carcinoma (average age 30 years). However, patients with metastatic stomach and small intestinal cancer fall within the usual age range of those with testicular germ cell tumor.[558] Serum alpha-fetoprotein and human chorionic gonadotropin levels are much more likely to be elevated in patients with germ cell tumor. The absence of IGCNU in the surrounding seminiferous tubules increases the probability of a metastatic tumor, as do epithelial membrane antigen positivity and PLAP-negativity.[234] Other immunohistochemical studies may prove useful, including prostate-specific antigen and melanoma-specific antigen (HMB 45).

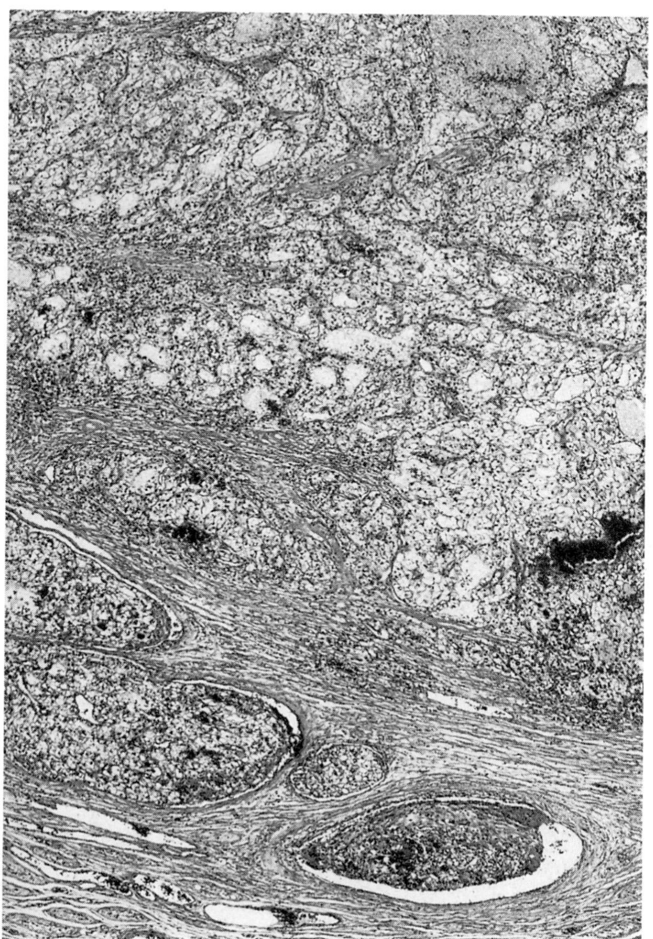

11-126. Renal cell carcinoma metastatic to the testis. Numerous vascular spaces containing tumor (*bottom*) raise the suspicion of metastasis.

References

1. Giwercman A, Müller J, Skakkebaek NE: Prevalence of carcinoma in situ and other histopathological abnormalities in testes from 399 men who died suddenly and unexpectedly, J Urol 145:77-80, 1991.
2. Rutgers JL, Young RH, Scully RE: The testicular "tumor" of the adrenogenital syndrome. A report of six cases and review of the literature on testicular masses in patients with adrenocortical disorders, Am J Surg Pathol 12:503-513, 1988.
3. Rutgers JL, Scully RE: The androgen insensitivity syndrome (testicular feminization): a clinicopathologic study of 43 cases, Int J Gynecol Pathol 10:126-145, 1991.
4. Buchino JJ, Uhlenhuth ER: Large-cell calcifying Sertoli cell tumor, J Urol 141:953-954, 1989.
5. Proppe KH, Scully RE: Large-cell calcifying Sertoli cell tumor of the testis, Am J Clin Pathol 74:607-619, 1980.
6. Wilson DM, Pitts WC, Hintz RL et al: Testicular tumors with Peutz-Jeghers syndrome, Cancer 57:2238-2240, 1986.
7. Boden G, Gibb R: Radiotherapy and testicular neoplasms, Lancet 2:1195-1197, 1951.
8. Richie JP: Neoplasms of the testis. In Walsh PC, Retik AB, Stamey TA, Vaughan ED, Jr, eds: Campbell's urology, Philadelphia, 1992, W.B. Saunders.
9. Donohue JP: Metastatic pathways of nonseminomatous germ cell tumors, Semin Urol 2:217-229, 1984.
10. American Joint Committee on Cancer: In Beahrs OH, Henson DE, Hutter RVP, Kennedy BJ, eds: Manual for staging of cancer, ed 4, Philadelphia, 1992, J.B. Lippincott.
11. Mostofi FK: Comparison of various clinical and pathological classifications of tumors of testes, Semin Oncol 6:26-30, 1979.
12. Hendry WF, Barrett A, McElwain TJ et al: The role of surgery in the combined management of metastases from malignant teratomas of testis, Br J Urol 52:38-49, 1980.
13. Johnson DE: Clinical staging. In Donohue JP, ed: Testis tumors, Baltimore, 1983, Williams and Wilkins.
14. Skinner DG: Non-seminomatous testis tumors: a plan of management based on 96 patients to improve survival in all stages by combined therapeutic modalities, J Urol 115:65-69, 1969.
15. Shipley WU: The role of radiation in the management of adult germinal testis tumors. In Einhorn LH, ed: Testicular tumors, New York, 1980, Masson.
16. Richie JP: Diagnosis and staging of testicular tumors. In Skinner DG, Lieskovsky G, eds: Diagnosis and management of genitourinary cancer, Philadelphia, 1988, W.B. Saunders.
17. Bredael JJ, Vugrin D, Whitmore WF Jr: Autopsy findings in 154 patients with germ cell tumors of the testis, Cancer 50:548-551, 1982.
18. Mostofi FK, Sobin LH: Histological typing of testicular tumors (International histological classification of tumors, No. 16), Geneva, 1977, World Health Organization.
19. Pugh RCB: Testicular tumours—introduction. In Pugh RCB, ed: Pathology of the testis, Oxford, 1976, Blackwell Scientific.

20. Willis RA: Pathology of tumours, ed 4, London, 1967, Butterworths.
21. Pugh RCB, Parkinson C: The origin and classification of testicular germ cell tumours, Int J Androl 4(Suppl):15-25, 1981.
22. Ulbright TM, Roth LM: Testicular and paratesticular neoplasms. In Sternberg SS, ed: Diagnostic surgical pathology, ed 2, New York, 1994, Raven Press.
23. Skakkebaek NE, Berthelsen JG, Giwercman A et al: Carcinoma-in-situ of the testis: possible origin from gonocytes and precursor of all types of germ cell tumours except spermatocytoma, Int J Androl 10:19-28, 1987.
24. Skakkebaek NE: Carcinoma in situ of the testis: frequency and relationship to invasive germ cell tumours in infertile men, Histopathology 2:157-170, 1978.
25. Skakkebaek NE: Abnormal morphology of germ cells in two infertile men, Acta Pathol Microbiol Scand [A] 80:374-378, 1972.
26. Skakkebaek NE: Possible carcinoma-in-situ of the undescended testis, Lancet 2:516-517, 1972.
27. Scully RE: Intratubular germ cell neoplasia (carcinoma in situ): what it is and what should be done about it, World Urol Update Ser Lesson 17:1982.
28. Young RH, Scully RE: Testicular tumors, Chicago, 1990, ASCP Press.
29. Vos A, Oosterhuis JW, de Jong B et al: Cytogenetics of carcinoma in situ of the testis, Cancer Genet Cytogenet 46:75-81, 1990.
30. Geurts van Kessel A, Suijkerbuijk RF, Sinke RJ et al: Molecular cytogenetics of human germ cell tumours: i(12p) and related chromosomal anomalies, Eur Urol 23:23-28, 1993.
31. Atkin NB, Fox MF, Baker MC et al: Chromosome 12-containing markers, including two dicentrics, in three i(12p)-negative testicular germ cell tumors, Genes Chromosom Cancer 6:218-221, 1993.
32. Lothe RA, Hastie N, Heimdal K et al: Frequent loss of 11p13 and 11p15 loci in male germ cell tumours, Genes Chromosom Cancer 7:96-101, 1993.
33. Gondos B, Migliozzi JA: Intratubular germ cell neoplasia, Semin Diagn Pathol 4:292-303, 1987.
34. Schulze C, Holstein AF: On the histology of human seminoma: development of the solid tumor from intratubular seminoma cells, Cancer 39:1090-1100, 1977.
35. Giwercman A, Marks A, Bailey D et al: M2A—a monoclonal antibody as a marker for carcinoma-in-situ germ cells of the human adult testis, Acta Pathol Microbiol Immunol Scand [A] 96:667-670, 1988.
36. Giwercman A, Andrews PW, Jorgensen N et al: Immunohistochemical expression of embryonal marker TRA-1-60 in carcinoma in situ and germ cell tumors of the testis, Cancer 72:1308-1314, 1993.
37. Jacobsen GK, Norgaard-Pedersen B: Placental alkaline phosphatase in testicular germ cell tumours and carcinoma-in-situ of the testis: an immunohistochemical study, Acta Pathol Microbiol Immunol Scand [A] 92:323-329, 1984.
38. Koide O, Iwai S, Baba K et al: Identification of testicular atypical germ cells by an immunohistochemical technique for placental alkaline phosphatase, Cancer 60:1325-1330, 1987.
39. Niehans GA, Manivel JC, Copland GT et al: Immunohistochemistry of germ cell and trophoblastic neoplasms, Cancer 62:1113-1123, 1988.
40. Klys HS, Whillis D, Howard G et al: Glutathione S-transferase expression in the human testis and testicular germ cell neoplasia, Br J Cancer 66:589-593, 1992.
41. El-Naggar AK, Ro JY, McLemore D et al: DNA ploidy in testicular germ cell neoplasms: histogenetic and clinical implications, Am J Surg Pathol 16:611-618, 1992.
42. de Jong B, Oosterhuis JW, Castedo SM et al: Pathogenesis of adult testicular germ cell tumors. A cytogenetic model, Cancer Genet Cytogenet 48:143-167, 1990.
43. Delahunt B, Mostofi FK, Sesterhenn IA et al: Nucleolar organizer regions in seminoma and intratubular malignant germ cells, Mod Pathol 3:141-145, 1990.
44. Malmi R, Söderström KO: Lectin histochemistry of embryonal carcinoma, APMIS 99:233-243, 1991.
45. Johnson DE, Appelt G, Samuels ML et al: Metastases from testicular carcinoma. Study of 78 autopsied cases, Urology 8:234-239, 1976.
46. Friedman NB, Moore RA: Tumors of the testis: a report on 922 cases, Mil Surgeon 99:573-593, 1946.
47. Czaja JT, Ulbright TM: Evidence for the transformation of seminoma to yolk sac tumor, with histogenetic considerations, Am J Clin Pathol 97:468-477, 1992.
48. Mostofi FK, Sesterhenn IA: Pathology of germ cell tumors of testes, Prog Clin Biol Res 203:1-34, 1985.
49. von Hochstetter AR, Sigg C, Saremaslani P et al: The significance of giant cells in human testicular seminomas. A clinico-pathological study, Virchows Arch A Pathol Anat Histopathol 407:309-322, 1985.
50. Jacobsen GK, Jacobsen M: Alpha-fetoprotein (AFP) and human chorionic gonadotropin in testicular germ cell tumours: a prospective immunohistochemical study, Acta Pathol Microbiol Scand [A] 91:165-176, 1983.
51. Srigley JR, Mackay B, Toth P et al: The ultrastructure and histogenesis of male germ neoplasia with emphasis on seminoma with early carcinomatous features, Ultrastruct Pathol 12:67-86, 1988.
52. Oosterhuis JW, Castedo SM, de Jong B et al: Ploidy of primary germ cell tumors of the testis. Pathogenetic and clinical relevance, Lab Invest 60:14-21, 1989.
53. Oosterhuis JW, Gillis AJ, van Putten WJ et al: Interphase cytogenetics of carcinoma in situ of the testis. Numeric analysis of the chromosomes 1, 12 and 15, Eur Urol 23:16-21, 1993.
54. Forman D, Gallagher R, Moller H et al: Aetiology and epidemiology of testicular cancer: report of consensus group, Prog Clin Biol Res 357:245-253, 1990.
55. Pearce N, Sheppard RA, Howard JK et al: Time trends and occupational differences in cancer of the testis in New Zealand, Cancer 59:1677-1682, 1987.
56. Swerdlow AJ: The epidemiology of testicular cancer, Eur Urol 23(suppl 2):35-38, 1993.
57. Cancer incidence in five continents, vol 5, Lyon, France, 1987, International Agency for Research on Cancer.
58. Schottenfeld D, Warshauer ME, Sherlock S et al: The epidemiology of testicular cancer in young adults, Am J Epidemiol 112:232-246, 1980.
59. Moller H: Clues to the aetiology of testicular germ cell tumours from descriptive epidemiology, Eur Urol 23:8-13, 1993.

60. Osterlind A: Diverging trends in incidence and mortality of testicular cancer in Denmark, 1943-1982, Br J Cancer 53:501-505, 1986.
61. Pike MC, Chilvers CE, Bobrow LG: Classification of testicular cancer in incidence and mortality statistics, Br J Cancer 56:83-85, 1987.
62. Boyle P, Kaye SB, Robertson AG: Changes in testicular cancer in Scotland, Eur J Cancer Clin Oncol 23:827-830, 1987.
63. Stone JM, Cruickshank DG, Sandeman TF et al: Trebling of the incidence of testicular cancer in Victoria, Australia (1950-1985), Cancer 68:211-219, 1991.
64. Swerdlow AJ, Skeet RG: Occupational associations of testicular cancer in south east England, Br J Ind Med 45:225-230, 1988.
65. McDowall ME, Balarajan R: Testicular cancer mortality in England and Wales 1971-1980: variations by occupation, J Epidemiol Community Health 40:26-29, 1986.
66. Ross RK, McCurtis JW, Henderson BE et al: Descriptive epidemiology of testicular and prostatic cancer in Los Angeles, Br J Cancer 39:284-292, 1979.
67. Graham S, Gibson R, West D et al: Epidemiology of cancer of the testis in Upstate New York, J Natl Cancer Inst 58:1255-1261, 1977.
68. Davies JM: Testicular cancer in England and Wales: some epidemiological aspects, Lancet 1:928-932, 1981.
69. Haughey BP, Graham S, Brasure J et al: The epidemiology of testicular cancer in Upstate New York, Am J Epidemiol 130:25-36, 1989.
70. Marshall EG, Melius JM, London MA et al: Investigation of a testicular cancer cluster using a case-control approach, Int J Epidemiol 19:269-273, 1990.
71. Anonymous: Testicular cancer in leather workers—Fulton County, New York, MMWR 38:105-106, 1989.
72. Davis RL, Mostofi FK: Cluster of testicular cancer in police officers exposed to hand-held radar, Am J Ind Med 24:231-233, 1993.
73. Ducatman AM, Conwill DE, Crawl J: Germ cell tumors of the testicle among aircraft repairmen, J Urol 136:834-836, 1986.
74. Swerdlow AJ, Huttly SR, Smith PG: Prenatal and familial associations of testicular cancer, Br J Cancer 55:571-577, 1987.
75. DePue RH, Pike MC, Henderson BE: Estrogen exposure during gestation and risk of testicular cancer, J Natl Cancer Inst 71:1151-1155, 1983.
76. Majsky A, Abrahamova J, Korinkova P et al: HLA system and testicular germinative tumours, Oncology 36:228-231, 1979.
77. Carr BI, Bach FH: Possible association between HLA-Aw24 and metastatic germ-cell tumours, Lancet 1:7156-7157, 1979.
78. Pollack MS, Vugrin D, Hennessy W et al: HLA antigens in patients with germ cell cancers of the testis, Cancer Res 42:2470-2473, 1982.
79. Dieckmann KP, von Keyserlingk HJ: HLA association of testicular seminoma, Klin Wochenschr 66:337-339, 1988.
80. Kratzik C, Aiginger P, Kuzmits R et al: HLA-antigen distribution in seminoma, HCG-positive seminoma and nonseminomatous tumours of the testis, Urol Res 17:377-380, 1989.
81. Oliver RT: HLA phenotype and clinicopathological behaviour of germ cell tumours: possible evidence for clonal evolution from seminomas to nonseminomas, Int J Androl 10:85-93, 1987.
82. DeWolf WC, Lange PH, Einarson ME et al: HLA and testicular cancer, Nature 277:216-217, 1979.
83. Dieckmann KP, Klan R, Bunte S: HLA antigens, Lewis antigens, and blood groups in patients with testicular germ-cell tumors, Oncology 50:252-258, 1993.
84. Moss AR, Osmond D, Bacchetti P et al: Hormonal risk factors in testicular cancer: a case control study, Am J Epidemiol 124:39-52, 1986.
85. Lykkesfeldt G, Bennett P, Lykkesfeldt AE et al: Testis cancer. Ichthyosis constitutes a significant risk factor, Cancer 67:730-734, 1991.
86. Dexeus FH, Logothetis CJ, Chong C et al: Genetic abnormalities in men with germ cell tumors, J Urol 140:80-84, 1988.
87. Li FP, Fraumeni JF Jr: Testicular cancers in children: epidemiologic characteristics, J Natl Cancer Inst 48:1575-1582, 1972.
88. Sigg C, Pelloni F: Dysplastic nevi and germ cell tumors of the testis—a possible further tumor in the spectrum of associated malignancies in dysplastic nevus syndrome, Dermatologica 176:109-110, 1988.
89. Nienhuis H, Goldacre M, Seagroatt V et al: Incidence of disease after vasectomy: a record linkage retrospective cohort study, BMJ 304:743-746, 1992.
90. Hewitt G, Logan CJ, Curry RC: Does vasectomy cause testicular cancer? Br J Urol 71:607-608, 1993.
91. Van den Eeden SK, Weiss NS, Strader CH et al: Occupation and the occurrence of testicular cancer, Am J Ind Med 19:327-337, 1991.
92. Halme A, Kellokumpu-Lehtinen P, Lehtonen T et al: Morphology of testicular germ cell tumours in treated and untreated cryptorchidism, Br J Urol 64:78-83, 1989.
93. Lanson Y: Epidemiology of testicular cancers, Prog Clin Biol Res 203:155-159, 1985.
94. Javadpour N, Bergman S: Recent advances in testicular cancer, Curr Probl Surg 15(Feb):1-64, 1978.
95. Henderson BE, Benton B, Jing J et al: Risk factors for cancer of the testis in young men, Int J Cancer 23:598-602, 1979.
96. Pottern LM, Brown LM, Hoover RN et al: Testicular cancer risk among young men: role of cryptorchidism and inguinal hernia, J Natl Cancer Inst 74:377-381, 1985.
97. Pike MC, Chilvers C, Peckham MJ: Effects of age at orchidopexy on risk of testicular cancer, Lancet 1:1246-1248, 1986.
98. Giwercman A, Grindsted J, Hansen B et al: Testicular cancer risk in boys with maldescended testis: a cohort study, J Urol 138:1214-1216, 1987.
99. Giwercman A, Berthelsen JG, Muller J et al: Screening for carcinoma-in-situ of the testis, Int J Androl 10:173-180, 1987.
100. Dieckmann KP, Loy V: Prevalence of bilateral testicular germ cell tumors and early detection by testicular intraepithelial neoplasia, Eur Urol 23(Suppl 2):22-23, 1993.
101. Loy V, Dieckmann KP: Prevalence of contralateral testicular intraepithelial neoplasia (carcinoma in situ) in patients with testicular germ cell tumour. Results of the German multicentre study, Eur Urol 23:120-122, 1993.

102. Fuller DB, Plenk HP: Malignant testicular germ cell tumors in a father and two sons. Case report and literature review, Cancer 58:955-958, 1986.
103. Tollerud DJ, Blattner WA, Fraser MC et al: Familial testicular cancer and urogenital developmental anomalies, Cancer 55:1849-1854, 1985.
104. Rutgers JL, Scully RE: Pathology of the testis in intersex syndromes, Semin Diagn Pathol 4:275-291, 1987.
105. Hughesdon PE, Kumarasamy T: Mixed germ cell tumours (gonadoblastomas) in normal and dysgenetic gonads: case reports and review, Virchows Arch A Pathol Anat Histopathol 349:258-280, 1970.
106. Manuel M, Katayama KP, Jones HW: The age of occurrence of gonadal tumors in intersex patients, Am J Obstet Gynecol 124:293-306, 1976.
107. Morris JM: The syndrome of testicular feminization in male pseudohermaphrodites, Am J Obstet Gynecol 65:1192-1211, 1953.
108. Rutgers JL: Advances in the pathology of intersex syndromes, Hum Pathol 22:884-891, 1991.
109. Senturia YD: The epidemiology of testicular cancer, Br J Urol 60:285-291, 1987.
110. Mostofi FK: Testicular tumors: epidemiologic, etiologic, and pathologic features, Cancer 32:1186-1201, 1973.
111. Swerdlow AJ, Huttly SRA, Smith PG: Testicular cancer and antecedent disease, Br J Cancer 55:97-103, 1987.
112. Brendler H: Cryptorchidism and cancer, Prog Clin Biol Res 203:189-196, 1985.
113. Miller A, Seljelid R: Histopathologic classification and natural history of malignant testis tumors in Norway, 1959-1963, Cancer 28:1054-1062, 1971.
114. Whitaker RH: Neoplasia in cryptorchid men, Semin Urol 6:107-109, 1988.
115. Gilbert JB, Hamilton JB: Studies in malignant testis tumors: III—incidence and nature of tumors in ectopic testes, Surg Gynecol Obstet 71:731-743, 1940.
116. Johnson DE, Woodhead DM, Pohl DR et al: Cryptorchidism and testicular tumorigenesis, Surgery 63:919-922, 1968.
117. Batata MA, Chu FCH, Hilaris BS et al: Testicular cancer in cryptorchids, Cancer 49:1023-1030, 1982.
118. Fram RJ, Garnick MB, Retik A: The spectrum of genitourinary abnormalities in patients with cryptorchidism, with emphasis on testicular carcinoma, Cancer 50:2243-2245, 1982.
119. Cortes D, Thorup J, Frisch M et al: Examination for intratubular germ cell neoplasia at operation for undescended testis in boys, J Urol 151:722-725, 1994.
120. Collins DH, Pugh RCB: Classification and frequency of testicular tumours, Br J Urol 36(suppl):1-11, 1964.
121. Morrison AS: Cryptorchidism, hernia, and cancer of the testis, J Natl Cancer Inst 56:731-733, 1976.
122. Giwercman A, Muller J, Skakkebaek NE: Carcinoma in situ of the undescended testis, Semin Urol 6:110-119, 1988.
123. Pedersen KV, Bolesen P, Zetter-Lund CG: Experience of screening for carcinoma-in-situ of the testis among young men with surgically corrected maldescended testes, Int J Androl 10:181-185, 1987.
124. Krabbe S, Skakkebaek NE, Berthelsen JG et al: High incidence of undetected neoplasia in maldescended testes, Lancet 1:999-1000, 1979.
125. Giwercman A, von der Maase H, Skakkebaek NE: Epidemiological and clinical aspects of carcinoma in situ of the testis, Eur Urol 23:104-110, 1993.
126. Giwercman A, Bruun E, Frimodt-Moller C et al: Prevalence of carcinoma-in-situ and other histopathologic abnormalities in testes of men with a history of cryptorchidism, J Urol 142:998-1002, 1989.
127. Nistal M, Codesal J, Paniagua R: Carcinoma in situ of the testis in infertile men. A histological, immunocytochemical, and cytophotometric study of DNA content, J Pathol 159:205-210, 1989.
128. Stalker AL, Hendry WT: Hyperplasia and neoplasia of the Sertoli cell, J Pathol Bacteriol 64:161-168, 1952.
129. Hedinger CE, Huber R, Weber E: Frequency of so-called hypoplastic or dysgenetic zones in scrotal and otherwise normal human testes, Virchows Arch A Pathol Anat Histol 342:165-168, 1967.
130. Scheiber K, Ackermann D, Studer UE: Bilateral testicular germ cell tumors: a report of 20 cases, J Urol 138:73-76, 1987.
131. Dieckmann KP, Boeckmann W, Brosig W et al: Bilateral testicular germ cell tumors. Report of nine cases and review of the literature, Cancer 57:1254-1258, 1986.
132. Kristianslund S, Fossä SD, Kjellevold K: Bilateral malignant testicular germ cell cancer, Br J Urol 58:60-63, 1986.
133. Osterlind A, Berthelsen JG, Abildgaard N et al: Incidence of bilateral testicular germ cell cancer in Denmark, 1960-1984: preliminary findings, Int J Androl 10:203-208, 1987.
134. Bokemeyer C, Schmoll HJ, Schoffski P et al: Bilateral testicular tumours: prevalence and clinical implications, Eur J Cancer 29A:874-876, 1993.
135. Bokemeyer C, Schmoll HJ, Schoffski P et al: Bilateral testicular tumours: prevalence and clinical implications, Eur J Cancer 29A:874-876, 1993.
136. Dieckmann KP, Loy P, Buttner P: Prevalence of bilateral testicular germ cell tumours and early detection based on contralateral testicular intra-epithelial neoplasia, Br J Urol 71:340-345, 1993.
137. von der Maase H, Rorth M, Walbom-Jorgensen S et al: Carcinoma in situ of contralateral testis in patients with testicular germ cell cancer: study of 27 cases in 500 patients, BMJ 293:1398-1401, 1986.
138. Harland SJ, Cook PA, Fossa SD et al: Risk factors for carcinoma in situ of the contralateral testis in patients with testicular cancer. An interim report, Eur Urol 23:115-118, 1993.
139. Zingg EJ, Zehntner C: Bilateral testicular germ cell tumors, Prog Clin Biol Res 203:673-680, 1985.
140. Ware SM, Heyman J, Al-Askari S et al: Bilateral testicular germ cell malignancy, Urology 19:366-372, 1982.
141. Dieckmann KP, Becker T, Jonas D et al: Inheritance and testicular cancer. Arguments based on a report of 3 cases and a review of the literature, Oncology 44:367-377, 1987.
142. Hayakawa M, Mukai K, Nagakura K et al: A case of simultaneous bilateral germ cell tumors arising from cryptorchid testes, J Urol 136:470-472, 1986.
143. Ryberg D, Heimdal K, Fossa SD et al: Rare Ha-ras1 alleles and predisposition to testicular cancer, Int J Cancer 53:938-940, 1993.

144. Hartley AL, Birch JM, Kelsey AM et al: Are germ cell tumors part of the Li-Fraumeni cancer family syndrome? Cancer Genet Cytogenet 42:221-226, 1989.
145. Bartkova J, Bartek J, Lukas J et al: p53 protein alterations in human testicular cancer including pre-invasive intratubular germ-cell neoplasia, Int J Cancer 49:196-202, 1991.
146. Ulbright TM, Orazi A, de Riese W et al: The correlation of p53 protein expression with proliferative activity and occult metastases in clinical stage I non-seminomatous germ cell tumors of the testis, Mod Pathol, 1994 (in press).
147. Ye DW, Zheng J, Qian SX et al: p53 gene mutations in Chinese human testicular seminoma, J Urol 150:884-886, 1993.
148. Heimdal K, Lothe RA, Lystad S et al: No germline TP53 mutations detected in familial and bilateral testicular cancer, Genes Chromosom Cancer 6:92-97, 1993.
149. Peng HQ, Hogg D, Malkin D et al: Mutations of the p53 gene do not occur in testis cancer, Cancer Res 53:3574-3578, 1993.
150. Gourlay WA, Johnson HW, Pantzar JT et al: Gonadal tumors in disorders of sexual differentiation, Urology 43:537-540, 1994.
151. Ramani P, Yeung CK, Habeebu SSM: Testicular intratubular germ cell neoplasia in children and adolescents with intersex, Am J Surg Pathol 17:1124-1133, 1993.
152. Collins GM, Kim DU, Logrono R et al: Pure seminoma arising in androgen insensitivity syndrome (testicular feminization syndrome): a case report and review of the literature, Mod Pathol 6:89-93, 1993.
153. Morris JM, Mahesh VB: Further observations on the syndrome, "testicular feminization," Am J Obstet Gynecol 87:731-748, 1963.
154. Swerdlow AJ, Huttly SR, Smith PG: Testis cancer: post-natal hormonal factors, sexual behaviour and fertility, Int J Cancer 43:549-553, 1989.
155. Giwercman A, Skakkebaek NE: Carcinoma-in-situ (gonocytoma-in-situ) of the testis. In Burger H, de Kretser D, eds: The testis, ed 2, New York, 1989, Raven Press.
156. Perry A, Wiley EL, Albores-Saavedra J: Pagetoid spread of intratubular germ cell neoplasia into rete testis: a morphologic and histochemical study of 100 orchiectomy specimens with invasive germ cell tumors, Hum Pathol 25:235-239, 1994.
157. Mostofi FK, Sesterhenn IA, Davis CJ Jr: Immunopathology of germ cell tumors of the testis, Semin Diagn Pathol 4:320-341, 1987.
158. Sigg C, Hedinger C: Atypical germ cells of the testis. Comparative ultrastructural and immunohistochemical investigations, Virchows Arch A Pathol Anat Histopathol 402:439-450, 1984.
159. Coffin CM, Ewing S, Dehner LP: Frequency of intratubular germ cell neoplasia with invasive testicular germ cell tumors. Histologic and immunocytochemical features, Arch Pathol Lab Med 109:555-559, 1985.
160. Manivel JC, Jessuran J, Wick MR et al: Placental alkaline phosphatase immunoreactivity in testicular germ cell tumors, Am J Surg Pathol 11:21-29, 1987.
161. Burke AP, Mostofi FK: Intratubular malignant germ cells in testicular biopsies: clinical course and identification by staining for placental alkaline phosphatase, Mod Pathol 1:475-479, 1988.
162. Burke AP, Mostofi FK: Placental alkaline phosphatase immunohistochemistry of intratubular malignant germ cells and associated testicular germ cell tumors, Hum Pathol 19:663-670, 1988.
163. Giwercman A, Lindenberg S, Kimber SJ et al: Monoclonal antibody 43-9F as a sensitive immunohistochemical marker of carcinoma in situ of human testis, Cancer 65:1135-1142, 1990.
164. Bailey D, Baumal R, Law J et al: Production of monoclonal antibody specific for seminomas and dysgerminomas, Proc Nat Acad Sci USA 83:5291-5295, 1986.
165. Visfeldt J, Giwercman A, Skakkebaek NE: Monoclonal antibody 43-9F: an immunohistochemical marker of embryonal carcinoma of the testis, APMIS 100:63-70, 1992.
166. Nielsen H, Nielsen M, Skakkebaek NE: The fine structure of possible carcinoma-in-situ in the seminiferous tubules in the testis of four infertile men, Acta Pathol Microbiol Scand [A] 82:235-248, 1974.
167. Gondos B, Berthelsen JG, Skakkebaek NE: Intratubular germ cell neoplasia (carcinoma in situ): a preinvasive lesion of the testis, Ann Clin Lab Sci 13:185-192, 1983.
168. Albrechtsen R, Nielsen MH, Skakkebaek NE et al: Carcinoma in situ of the testis. Some ultrastructural characteristics of germ cells, Acta Pathol Microbiol Immunol Scand [A] 90:301-303, 1982.
169. Holstein AF, Körner F: Light and electron microscopical analysis of cell types in human seminoma, Virchows Arch A Pathol Anat Histopathol 363:97-112, 1974.
170. Hu LM, Phillipson J, Barsky SH: Intratubular germ cell neoplasia in infantile yolk sac tumor: verification by tandem repeat sequence in situ hybridization, Diagn Mol Pathol 1:118-128, 1992.
171. Jorgensen N, Giwercman A, Muller J et al: Immunohistochemical markers of carcinoma in situ of the testis also expressed in normal infantile germ cells, Histopathology 22:373-378, 1993.
172. Skakkebaek NE, Berthelsen JG, Muller J: Carcinoma-in-situ of the undescended testis, Urol Clin North Am 9:377-385, 1982.
173. Skakkebaek NE, Berthelsen JG, Visfeldt J: Clinical aspects of testicular carcinoma-in-situ, Int J Androl 4(suppl):153-162, 1981.
174. Berthelsen JG, Skakkebaek NE, von der Maase H et al: Screening for carcinoma in situ of the contralateral testis in patients with germinal testicular cancer, BMJ 285:1683-1686, 1982.
175. West AB, Butler MR, Fitzpatrick J et al: Testicular tumors in subfertile men: report of 4 cases with implications for management of patients presenting with infertility, J Urol 133:107-109, 1985.
176. Muller J, Skakkebaek NE, Ritzën M et al: Carcinoma in situ of the testis in children with 45,X/46,XY gonadal dysgenesis, J Pediatr 106:431-436, 1985.
177. Muller J, Skakkebaek NE: Testicular carcinoma in situ in children with the androgen insensitivity (testicular feminisation) syndrome, BMJ 288:1419-1420, 1984.
178. Pryor JP, Cameron KM, Chilton CP et al: Carcinoma in situ in testicular biopsies in men presenting with infertility, Br J Urol 55:780-784, 1983.

179. Jacobsen GK, Henriksen OB, von der Maase H: Carcinoma in situ of testicular tissue adjacent to malignant germ-cell tumors: a study of 105 cases, Cancer 47:2660-2662, 1981.
180. Skakkebaek NE: Atypical germ cells in the adjacent "normal" tissue of testicular tumours, Acta Pathol Microbiol Scand [A] 83:127-130, 1975.
181. Muller J, Skakkebaek NE, Parkinson MC: The spermatocytic seminoma: views on pathogenesis, Int J Androl 10:147-156, 1987.
182. Manivel JC, Simonton S, Wold SE et al: Absence of intratubular germ cell neoplasia in testicular yolk sac tumors in children, Arch Pathol Lab Med 112:641-645, 1988.
183. Manivel JC, Reinberg Y, Niehans GA et al: Intratubular germ cell neoplasia in testicular teratomas and epidermoid cysts. Correlation with prognosis and possible biologic significance, Cancer 64:715-720, 1989.
184. Jorgensen N, Muller J, Visfeldt J et al: Infantile germ cell tumors associated with carcinoma-in-situ of the testis, Onkologie 14(suppl 4):8, 1991 (abstract).
185. Stamp IM, Barlebo H, Rix M et al: Intratubular germ cell neoplasia in an infantile testis with immature teratoma, Histopathology 22:69-72, 1993.
186. Parkinson MC, Ramani P: Intratubular germ cell neoplasia in an infantile testis, Histopathology 23:99-100, 1993.
187. Berthelsen JG, Skakkebaek NE: Value of testicular biopsy in diagnosing carcinoma in situ testis, Scand J Urol Nephrol 15:165-168, 1981.
188. Daugaard G, von der Maase H, Olsen J et al: Carcinoma-in-situ testis in patients with assumed extragonadal germ-cell tumours, Lancet 2:528-530, 1987.
189. Chen KT, Cheng AC: Retroperitoneal seminoma and intratubular germ cell neoplasia, Hum Pathol 20:493-495, 1989.
190. von der Maase H, Giwercman A, Muller J et al: Management of carcinoma-in-situ of the testis, Int J Androl 10:209-220, 1987.
191. Bottomley D, Fisher C, Hendry WF et al: Persistent carcinoma in situ of the testis after chemotherapy for advanced testicular germ cell tumours, Br J Urol 66:420-424, 1990.
192. von der Maase H, Meinecke B, Skakkebaek NE: Residual carcinoma-in-situ of contralateral testis after chemotherapy, Lancet 1:477-478, 1988.
193. Jacobsen GK, Barlebo H, Olsen J et al: Testicular germ cell tumours in Denmark 1976-1980: pathology of 1058 consecutive cases, Acta Radiol Oncol 23:239-247, 1984.
194. von Hochstetter AR, Hedinger CE: The differential diagnosis of testicular germ cell tumors in theory and practice: a critical analysis of two major systems of classification and review of 389 cases, Virchows Arch A Pathol Anat Histopathol 396:247-277, 1982.
195. Moul JW, Schanne FJ, Thompson IM et al: Testicular cancer in blacks. A multicenter experience, Cancer 73:388-393, 1994.
196. Perry C, Servadio C: Seminoma in childhood, J Urol 124:932-933, 1980.
197. Kay R: Prepubertal testicular tumor registry, J Urol 150:671-674, 1993.
198. Taylor JB, Solomon DH, Levine RE et al: Exophthalmos in seminoma: regression with steroids and orchiectomy, JAMA 240:860-861, 1978.
199. Mann AS: Bilateral exophthalmos in seminoma, J Clin Endocrinol Metab 27:1500-1502, 1967.
200. Javadpour N: Management of seminoma based on tumor markers, Urol Clin North Am 7:773-781, 1980.
201. Rustin GJ, Vogelzang NJ, Sleijfer DT et al: Consensus statement on circulating tumour markers and staging patients with germ cell tumours, Prog Clin Biol Res 357:277-284, 1990.
202. Scheiber K, Mikuz G, Frommhold H et al: Human chorionic gonadotropin positive seminoma: is this a special type of seminoma with a poor prognosis, Prog Clin Biol Res 203:97-104, 1985.
203. Javadpour N: The role of biologic tumor markers in testicular cancer, Cancer 45:1755-1761, 1980.
204. Mann K, Siddle K: Evidence for free beta-subunit secretion in so-called human chorionic gonadotropin-positive seminoma, Cancer 62:2378-2382, 1988.
205. Dieckmann KP, Due W, Bauer HW: Seminoma testis with elevated serum beta-HCG—a category of germ cell cancer between seminoma and nonseminoma, Int Urol Nephrol 21:175-184, 1989.
206. Javadpour N: Tumor markers in testicular cancer—an update, Prog Clin Biol Res 203:141-154, 1985.
207. Chisolm GG: Tumour markers in testicular tumours, Prog Clin Biol Res 203:81-91, 1985.
208. Mumperow E, Hartmann M: Spermatic cord beta-human chorionic gonadotropin levels in seminoma and their clinical implications, J Urol 147:1041-1043, 1992.
209. Fossa A, Fossa SD: Serum lactate dehydrogenase and human chorionic gonadotropin in seminoma, Br J Urol 63:408-415, 1989.
210. Koshida K, Stigbrand T, Munck-Wikland E et al: Analysis of serum placental alkaline phosphatase activity in testicular cancer and cigarette smokers, Urol Res 18:169-173, 1990.
211. Kuzmits R, Schernthaner G, Krisch K: Serum neuron-specific enolase: a marker for response to therapy in seminoma, Cancer 60:1017-1021, 1987.
212. Gross AJ, Dieckmann KP: Neuron-specific enolase: a serum tumor marker in malignant germ-cell tumors, Eur Urol 24:277-278, 1993.
213. Mostofi FK, Price EB Jr: Tumors of the male genital system. Atlas of Tumor Pathology, 2nd Series, Fascicle 8, Washington D.C., 1973, Armed Forces Institute of Pathology.
214. Jacobsen GK, Talerman A: Atlas of germ cell tumours, Copenhagen, 1989, Munksgaard.
215. Young RH, Finlayson N, Scully RE: Tubular seminoma. Report of a case, Arch Pathol Lab Med 113:414-416, 1989.
216. Zavala-Pompa A, Ro JY, El-Naggar AK et al: Tubular seminoma: an immunohistochemical and DNA flow cytometric study of four cases, Am J Clin Pathol, 1994 (in press).
217. Talerman A: Tubular seminoma, Arch Pathol Lab Med 113:1204, 1989.
218. Thackray AC, Crane WAJ: Seminoma. In Pugh RCB, ed: Pathology of the testis, Oxford, 1976, Blackwell Scientific.
219. Bell DA, Flotte TJ, Bhan AK: Immunohistochemical characterization of seminoma and its inflammatory cell infiltrate, Hum Pathol 18:511-520, 1987.
220. Strutton GM, Gemmell E, Seymour GJ et al: An immunohistological examination of inflammatory cell infiltration in primary testicular seminomas, Aust N Z J Surg 59:169-172, 1989.

221. Wilkins BS, Williamson JM, O'Brien CJ: Morphological and immunohistological study of testicular lymphomas, Histopathology 15:147-156, 1989.
222. Bentley AJ, Parkinson MC, Harding BN et al: A comparative morphological and immunohistochemical study of testicular seminomas and intracranial germinomas, Histopathology 17:443-449, 1990.
223. Akaza H, Kobayashi K, Umeda T et al: Surface markers of lymphocytes infiltrating seminoma tissue, J Urol 124:827-828, 1980.
224. Wei YQ, Hang ZB, Liu KF: In situ observation of inflammatory cell-tumor cell interaction in human seminomas (germinomas): light, electron microscopic, and immunohistochemical study, Hum Pathol 23:421-428, 1992.
225. Dixon FJ, Moore RA: Tumors of the male sex organs. Atlas of Tumor Pathology, 1st series, Fascicles 31b & 32, Washington, D.C., 1952, Armed Forces Institute of Pathology.
226. Kahn DG: Ossifying seminoma of the testis, Arch Pathol Lab Med 117:321-322, 1993.
227. von Hochstetter AR: Mitotic count in seminomas—an unreliable criterion for distinguishing between classical and anaplastic types, Virchows Arch A Pathol Anat Histopathol 390:63-69, 1981.
228. Zuckman MH, Williams G, Levin HS: Mitosis counting in seminoma: an exercise of questionable significance, Hum Pathol 19:329-335, 1988.
229. Suzuki T, Sasano H, Aoki H et al: Immunohistochemical comparison between anaplastic seminoma and typical seminoma, Acta Pathol Jpn 43:751-757, 1993.
230. Hedinger C, von Hochstetter AR, Egloff B: Seminoma with syncytiotrophoblastic giant cells. A special form of seminoma, Virchows Arch A Pathol Anat Histopathol 383:59-67, 1979.
231. Uchida T, Shimoda T, Miyata H et al: Immunoperoxidase study of alkaline phosphatase in testicular tumor, Cancer 48:1455-1462, 1981.
232. Hustin J, Collettee J, Franchimont P: Immunohistochemical demonstration of placental alkaline phosphatase in various states of testicular development and in germ cell tumours, Int J Androl 10:29-35, 1987.
233. Fogel M, Lifschitz-Mercer B, Moll R et al: Heterogeneity of intermediate filament expression in human testicular seminomas, Differentiation 45:242-249, 1990.
234. Wick MR, Swanson PE, Manivel JC: Placental-like alkaline phosphatase reactivity in human tumors: an immunohistochemical study of 520 cases, Hum Pathol 18:946-954, 1987.
235. Murakami SS, Said JW: Immunohistochemical localization of lactate dehydrogenase isoenzyme 1 in germ cell tumors of the testis, Am J Clin Pathol 81:293-296, 1984.
236. Denk H, Moll R, Weybora W et al: Intermediate filaments and desmosomal plaque proteins in testicular seminomas and non-seminomatous germ cell tumours as revealed by immunohistochemistry, Virchows Arch A Pathol Anat Histopathol 410:295-307, 1987.
237. Bosman FT, Giard RWM, Kruseman ACN et al: Human chorionic gonadotrophin and alpha-fetoprotein in testicular germ cell tumors: a retrospective immunohistochemical study, Histopathology 4:673-684, 1980.
238. Janssen M, Johnston WH: Anaplastic seminoma of the testis: ultrastructural analysis of three cases, Cancer 41:538-544, 1978.
239. Min KW, Scheithauer BW: Pineal germinomas and testicular seminoma: a comparative ultrastructural study with special references to early carcinomatous transformation, Ultrastruc Pathol 14:483-496, 1990.
240. Damjanov I: Is seminoma a relative or a precursor of embryonal carcinoma, Lab Invest 60:1-3, 1989.
241. Rukstalis DB, DeWolf WC: Molecular biological concepts in the etiology of testicular and other urologic malignancies, Semin Urol 6:161-170, 1988.
242. Baretton G, Diebold J, DePascale T et al: Deoxyribonucleic acid ploidy in seminomas with and without syncytiotrophoblastic cells, J Urol 151:67-71, 1994.
243. Saksela K, Mäkelä TP, Alitalo K: Oncogene expression in small-cell lung cancer cell lines and a testicular germ-cell tumor: activation of the N-myc gene and decreased RB mRNA, Int J Cancer 44:182-185, 1989.
244. Strohmeyer T, Reissmann P, Cordon-Cardo C et al: Correlation between retinoblastoma gene expression and differentiation in human testicular tumors, Proc Natl Acad Sci U S A 88:6662-6666, 1991.
245. Castedo SM, de Jong B, Oosterhuis JW et al: Cytogenetic analysis of ten human seminomas, Cancer Res 49:439-443, 1989.
246. Delozier-Blanchet CD, Walt H, Engel E et al: Cytogenetic studies of human testicular germ cell tumours, Int J Androl 10:69-77, 1987.
247. Sikora K, Evan G, Watson J: Oncogenes and germ cell tumours, Int J Androl 10:57-67, 1987.
248. Misaki H, Shuin T, Yao M et al: Expression of myc family oncogenes in primary human testicular cancer, Nippon Hinyokika Gakkai Zasshi 80:1509-1513, 1989.
249. Strohmeyer T, Peter S, Hartmann M et al: Expression of the hst-1 and c-kit protooncogenes in human testicular germ cell tumors, Cancer Res 51:1811-1816, 1991.
250. Ulbright TM, Roth LM, Brodhecker CA: Yolk sac differentiation in germ cell tumors: a morphologic study of 50 cases with emphasis on hepatic, enteric and parietal yolk sac features, Am J Surg Pathol 10:151-164, 1986.
251. Nonomura N, Aozasa K, Ueda T et al: Malignant lymphoma of the testis: histological and immunohistological study of 28 cases, J Urol 141:1368-1371, 1989.
252. Hamlin JA, Kagan AR, Friedman NB: Lymphomas of the testicle, Cancer 29:1352-1356, 1972.
253. Hayes MM, Sacks MI, King HS: Testicular lymphoma. A retrospective review of 17 cases, S Afr Med J 64:1014-1016, 1983.
254. Paladugu RR, Bearman RM, Rappaport H: Malignant lymphoma with primary manifestation in the gonad: a clinicopathologic study of 38 patients, Cancer 45:561-571, 1980.
255. Turner RR, Colby TV, MacKintosh FR: Testicular lymphomas: a clinicopathologic study of 35 cases, Cancer 48:2095-2102, 1981.
256. Sussman EB, Hajdu SI, Lieberman PH et al: Malignant lymphoma of the testis: a clinicopathologic study of 37 cases, J Urol 118:1004-1007, 1977.
257. Duncan PR, Checa F, Gowing NF et al: Extranodal non-Hodgkin's lymphoma presenting in the testicle: a clinical and pathologic study of 24 cases, Cancer 45:1578-1584, 1980.

258. Talerman A: Primary malignant lymphoma of the testis, J Urol 118:783-786, 1977.
259. Hunter M, Peschel RE: Testicular seminoma. Results of the Yale University experience, 1964-1984, Cancer 64:1608-1611, 1989.
260. Babaian RJ, Zagars GK: Testicular seminoma: the M.D. Anderson experience: an analysis of pathological and patient characteristics, and treatment recommendations, J Urol 139:311-314, 1988.
261. Fossa SD, Aass N, Kaalhus O: Radiotherapy for testicular seminoma Stage I: treatment results and long-term post irradiation morbidity in 365 patients, Int J Radiat Oncol Biol Phys 16:383-388, 1989.
262. Brunt AM, Scoble JE: Para-aortic nodal irradiation for early stage testicular seminoma, Clin Oncol 4:165-170, 1992.
263. Horwich A, Dearnaley DP: Treatment of seminoma, Semin Oncol 19:171-180, 1992.
264. Doornbos JF, Hussey DH, Johnson E: Radiotherapy for pure seminoma of the testis, Radiology 116:401-404, 1975.
265. Thomas GM, Rider WD, Dembo AJ et al: Seminoma of the testis: results of treatment and patterns of failure after radiation therapy, Int J Radiat Oncol Biol Phys 8:165-174, 1982.
266. Peckham M: Testicular cancer, Acta Oncol 27:439-453, 1988.
267. Evensen JF, Fossä SD, Kjellevold K et al: Testicular seminoma: histological findings and their prognostic significance for stage II disease, J Surg Oncol 36:166-169, 1987.
268. Logothetis CJ, Samuels ML, Selig DE et al: Cyclic chemotherapy with cyclophosphamide, doxorubicin, and cisplatin plus vinblastine and bleomycin in advanced germ cell tumors: results with 100 patients, Am J Med 81:219-228, 1986.
269. Motzer RJ, Bosl GJ, Geller NL et al: Advanced seminoma: the role of chemotherapy and adjuvant surgery, Ann Intern Med 108:513-518, 1988.
270. Javadpour N: Human chorionic gonadotropin in seminoma, J Urol 131:407, 1984.
271. Eble JN: Spermatocytic seminoma, Hum Pathol 25:1035-1042, 1994.
272. Masson P: Etude sur le seminome, Rev Canad Biol 5:361-387, 1946.
273. Talerman A: Spermatocytic seminoma: clinicopathological study of 22 cases, Cancer 45:2169-2176, 1980.
274. Cummings OW, Ulbright TM, Eble JN et al: Spermatocytic seminoma: an immunohistochemical study, Hum Pathol 25:54-59, 1994.
275. Burke AP, Mostofi FK: Spermatocytic seminoma: a clinicopathologic study of 79 cases, J Urol Pathol 1:21-32, 1993.
276. Rosai J, Silber I, Khodadoust K: Spermatocytic seminoma. I. Clinicopathologic study of six cases and review of the literature, Cancer 24:92-102, 1969.
277. True LD, Otis CN, Delprado W et al: Spermatocytic seminoma of testis with sarcomatous transformation. A report of five cases, Am J Surg Pathol 12:75-82, 1988.
278. Floyd C, Ayala AG, Logothetis CJ et al: Spermatocytic seminoma with associated sarcoma of the testis, Cancer 61:409-414, 1988.
279. Matoska J, Talerman A: Spermatocytic seminoma associated with rhabdomyosarcoma, Am J Clin Pathol 94:89-95, 1990.
280. Batata MA, Chu FC, Hilaris BS et al: TNM staging of testis cancer, Int J Radiat Oncol Biol Phys 6:291-295, 1980.
281. Scully RE: Spermatocytic seminoma of the testis: a report of 3 cases and review of the literature, Cancer 14:788-794, 1961.
282. Cummings OW, Ulbright TM, Eble JN et al: Spermatocytic seminoma: an immunohistochemical study, Mod Pathol 5:51A, 1992 (abstract).
283. Dekker I, Rozeboom T, Delemarre J et al: Placental-like alkaline phosphatase and DNA flow cytometry in spermatocytic seminoma, Cancer 69:993-996, 1992.
284. Rosai J, Khodadoust K, Silber I: Spermatocytic seminoma. II. Ultrastructural study, Cancer 24:103-116, 1969.
285. Romanenko AM, Persidsky YV, Mostofi FK: Ultrastructure and histogenesis of spermatocytic seminoma, J Urol Pathol 1:387-395, 1993.
286. Talerman A, Fu YS, Okagaki T: Spermatocytic seminoma. Ultrastructural and microspectrophotometric observations, Lab Invest 51:343-349, 1984.
287. Takahashi H: Cytometric analysis of testicular seminoma and spermatocytic seminoma, Acta Pathol Jpn 43:121-129, 1993.
288. Takahashi H, Aizawa S, Konishi E et al: Cytofluorometric analysis of spermatocytic seminoma, Cancer 72:549-552, 1993.
289. Matoska J, Ondrus D, Hornäk M: Metastatic spermatocytic seminoma. A case report with light microscopic, ultrastructural, and immunohistochemical findings, Cancer 62:1197-1201, 1988.
290. Damjanov I: Tumors of the testis and epididymis. In Murphy WM, ed: Urological pathology, Philadelphia, 1989, W.B. Saunders.
291. Mostofi FK, Sesterhenn IA, Davis CJ Jr: Developments in histopathology of testicular germ cell tumors, Semin Urol 6:171-188, 1988.
292. Damjanov I, Andrews PW: Ultrastructural differentiation of a clonal human embryonal carcinoma cell line in vitro, Cancer Res 43:2190-2198, 1983.
293. Damjanov I, Clark RK, Andrews PW: Cytoskeleton of human embryonal carcinoma cells, Cell Differ 15:133-139, 1984.
294. Motoyama T, Watanabe H, Yamamoto T et al: Human testicular germ cell tumors in vitro and in athymic nude mice, Acta Pathol Jpn 37:431-448, 1987.
295. Pera MF, Blasco Lafita MJ, Mills J: Cultured stem-cells from human testicular teratomas: the nature of human embryonal carcinoma, and its comparison with two types of yolk-sac carcinoma, Int J Cancer 40:334-343, 1987.
296. Pera MF, Mills J, Parrington JM: Isolation and characterization of a multipotent clone of human embryonal carcinoma cells, Differentiation 42:10-23, 1989.
297. Damjanov I, Fox N, Knowles BB et al: Immunohistochemical localization of stage-specific embryonic antigens in human testicular germ cell tumors, Am J Pathol 108:225-230, 1982.
298. Mostofi FK: Pathology of germ cell tumors of testis: a progress report, Cancer 45:1735-1754, 1980.
299. Hawkins EP, Finegold MJ, Hawkins HK et al: Nongerminomatous malignant germ cell tumors in children: a review of 89 cases from the Pediatric Oncology Group, 1971-1984, Cancer 58:2579-2584, 1986.

300. Rodriguez PN, Hafez GR, Messing EM: Nonseminomatous germ cell tumor of the testicle: does extensive staging of the primary tumor predict the likelihood of metastatic disease, J Urol 136:604-608, 1986.
301. Saukko P, Lignitz E: Sudden death caused by malignant testicular tumors, Zeit Rechtsmed 103:529-536, 1990.
302. Aronsohn RS, Nishiyama RH: Embryonal carcinoma. An unexpected cause of sudden death in a young adult, JAMA 229:1093-1094, 1974.
303. Bosl GJ, Lange PH, Nochomovitz LE et al: Tumor markers in advanced non-seminomatous testicular cancer, Cancer 47:572-576, 1981.
304. Jacobsen GK: Histogenetic considerations concerning germ cell tumours. Morphological and immunohistochemical comparative investigation of the human embryo and testicular germ cell tumours, Virchows Arch A Pathol Anat Histopathol 408:509-525, 1986.
305. Azzopardi JG, Mostofi FK, Theiss EA: Lesions of testes observed in certain patients with widespread choriocarcinoma and related tumors, Am J Pathol 38:207-225, 1961.
306. Wittekind C, Wichmann T, Von Kleist S: Immunohistological localization of AFP and HCG in uniformly classified testis tumors, Anticancer Res 3:327-330, 1983.
307. Lamm DL, Wepsic HT, Feldman P et al: Importance of alpha-fetoprotein in patients with seminoma, Urology 10:233-235, 1977.
308. Lifschitz-Mercer B, Fogel M, Moll R et al: Intermediate filament protein profiles of human testicular non-seminomatous germ cell tumors: correlation of cytokeratin synthesis to cell differentiation, Differentiation 48:191-198, 1991.
309. Battifora H, Sheibani K, Tubbs RR et al: Antikeratin antibodies in tumor diagnosis: distinction between seminoma and embryonal carcinoma, Cancer 54:843-848, 1984.
310. Pallesen G, Hamilton-Dutoit SJ: Ki-1 (CD30) antigen is regularly expressed in tumor cells of embryonal carcinoma, Am J Pathol 133:446-450, 1988.
311. Jacobsen GK, Jacobsen M, Clausen PP: Distribution of tumor-associated antigens in the various histologic components of germ cell tumors of the testis, Am J Surg Pathol 5:257-266, 1981.
312. Ulbright TM, Goheen MP, Roth LM et al: The differentiation of carcinomas of teratomatous origin from embryonal carcinoma. A light and electron microscopic study, Cancer 57:257-263, 1986.
313. Motzer RJ, Rodriguez E, Reuter VE et al: Genetic analysis as an aid in diagnosis for patients with midline carcinomas of uncertain histologies, J Natl Cancer Inst 83:341-346, 1991.
314. Rodriguez E, Mathew S, Mukherjee AB et al: Analysis of chromosome 12 aneuploidy in interphase cells from human male germ cell tumors by fluorescence in situ hybridization, Genes Chromosom Cancer 5:21-29, 1992.
315. Samaniego F, Rodriguez E, Houldsworth J: Cytogenetic and molecular analysis of human male germ cell tumors: chromosome 12 abnormalities and gene amplification, Genes Chromosom Cancer 1:289-300, 1990.
316. Ganguly S, Murty VV, Samaniego F et al: Detection of preferential NRAS mutations in human male germ cell tumors by the polymerase chain reaction, Genes Chromosom Cancer 1:228-232, 1990.
317. Tesch H, Fürbass R, Casper J et al: Cellular oncogenes in human teratocarcinoma cell lines, Int J Androl 13:377-388, 1990.
318. de Bruin MJ, Oosterhof GO, Debruyne FM: Nerve-sparing retroperitoneal lymphadenectomy for low stage testicular cancer, Br J Urol 71:336-339, 1993.
319. Rowland RG, Foster RS, Donohue JP: Scrotum and testis. In Gillenwater JY, Grayhack JT, Howards SS et al, eds: Adult and pediatric urology, ed 3, St. Louis, 1996, Mosby–Year Book.
320. Sogani PC, Fair WR: Surveillance alone in the treatment of clinical Stage I nonseminomatous germ cell tumor of the testis (NSGCT), Semin Urol 6:53-56, 1988.
321. Moriyama N, Daly JJ, Keating MA et al: Vascular invasion as a prognosticator of metastatic disease in nonseminomatous germ cell tumors of the testis. Importance in "surveillance only" protocols, Cancer 56:2492-2498, 1985.
322. Fung CY, Kalish LA, Brodsky GL et al: Stage I nonseminomatous germ cell testicular tumor: prediction of metastatic potential by primary histopathology, J Clin Oncol 6:1467-1473, 1988.
323. Dunphy CH, Ayala AG, Swanson DA et al: Clinical stage I nonseminomatous and mixed germ cell tumors of the testis. A clinicopathologic study of 93 patients on a surveillance protocol after orchiectomy alone, Cancer 62:1202-1206, 1988.
324. Jacobsen GK, Rorth M, Osterlind K et al: Histopathological features in stage I non-seminomatous testicular germ cell tumours correlated to relapse. Danish Testicular Cancer Study Group, APMIS 98:377-382, 1990.
325. Wishnow KI, Johnson DE, Swanson DA et al: Identifying patients with low-risk clinical stage I nonseminomatous testicular tumors who should be treated by surveillance, Urology 34:339-343, 1989.
326. Javadpour N, Canning DA, O'Connell KJ et al: Predictors of recurrent clinical stage I nonseminomatous testicular cancer. A prospective clinicopathologic study, Urology 27:508-511, 1986.
327. Costello AJ, Mortensen PH, Stillwell RG: Prognostic indicators for failure of surveillance management of stage I nonseminomatous germ cell tumours, Aust N Z J Surg 59:119-122, 1989.
328. Fossä SD, Aass N, Kaalhus O: Testicular cancer in young Norwegians, J Surg Oncol 39:43-63, 1988.
329. Freedman LS, Parkinson MC, Jones WG et al: Histopathology in the prediction of relapse of patients with stage I testicular teratoma treated by orchidectomy alone, Lancet 2:294-298, 1987.
330. Sturgeon JF, Jewett MA, Alison RE et al: Surveillance after orchidectomy for patients with clinical stage I nonseminomatous testis tumors, J Clin Oncol 10:564-568, 1992.
331. Moul JW, McCarthy WF, Fernandez EB et al: Percentage of embryonal carcinoma and of vascular invasion predicts pathological stage in clinical stage I nonseminomatous testicular cancer, Cancer Res 54:362-364, 1994.
332. Moul JW, Foley JP, Hitchcock CL et al: Flow cytometric and quantitative histological parameters to predict occult disease in clinical stage I nonseminomatous testicular germ cell tumors, J Urol 150:879-883, 1993.

333. de Riese WT, Albers P, Walker EB et al: Predictive parameters of biologic behavior of early stage nonseminomatous testicular germ cell tumors, Cancer 74:1335-1341, 1994.
334. Castedo SM, de Jong B, Oosterhuis JW et al: Chromosomal changes in mature residual teratomas following polychemotherapy, Cancer Res 49:672-676, 1989.
335. Olivarez D, Ulbright T, de Riese W et al: Neovascularization in clinical stage A testicular germ cell tumor: prediction of metastatic disease, Cancer Res 54:2800-2802, 1994.
336. Allhoff EP, Liedkes S, Wittekind C et al: DNA content in NSGCT/CSI: a new prognosticator for biologic behaviour, J Cancer Res Clin Oncol 1(suppl):592, 1990 (abstract).
337. de Graaff WE, Sleijfer DT, de Jong B et al: Significance of aneuploid stemlines in testicular nonseminomatous germ cell tumors, Cancer 72:1300-1304, 1993.
338. Einhorn LH: Chemotherapy of disseminated testicular cancer. In Skinner DG, Lieskovsky G, eds: Diagnosis and management of genitourinary cancer, Philadelphia, 1988, W.B. Saunders.
339. Ulbright TM, Roth LM: A pathologic analysis of lesions following modern chemotherapy for metastatic germ cell tumors, Pathol Annu 25(Pt 1):313-340, 1990.
340. Mead GM, Stenning SP, Parkinson MC et al: The Second Medical Research Council study of prognostic factors in nonseminomatous germ cell tumors. Medical Research Council Testicular Tumour Working Party, J Clin Oncol 10:85-94, 1992.
341. Vogelzang NJ: Prognostic factors in metastatic testicular cancer, Int J Androl 10:225-237, 1987.
342. Stoter G, Sylvester R, Sleijfer DT et al: Multivariate analysis of prognostic variables in patients with disseminated nonseminomatous testicular cancer: results from an EORTC multi-institutional phase III study, Int J Androl 10:239-246, 1987.
343. Sledge GW Jr, Eble JN, Roth BJ et al: Relation of proliferative activity to survival in patients with advanced germ cell cancer, Cancer Res 48:3864-3868, 1988.
344. Teilum G: Gonocytoma: homologous ovarian and testicular tumors I: with discussion of "mesonephroma ovarii" (Schiller: Am J Cancer 1939), Acta Pathol Microbiol Scand 23:242-251, 1946.
345. Teilum G: "Mesonephroma ovarii" (Schiller)—an extraembryonic mesoblastoma of germ cell origin in the ovary and the testis, Acta Pathol Microbiol Scand 27:249-261, 1950.
346. Teilum G: Endodermal sinus tumors of the ovary and testis: comparative morphogenesis of the so-called mesonephroma ovarii (Schiller) and extraembryonic (yolk sac-allantoic) structures of the rat's placenta, Cancer 12:1092-1105, 1959.
347. Kaplan GW, Cromie WC, Kelalis PP et al: Prepubertal yolk sac testicular tumors—report of the testicular tumor registry, J Urol 140:1109-1112, 1988.
348. Brosman SA: Testicular tumors in prepubertal children, Urology 13:581-588, 1979.
349. Pierce GB, Bullock WK, Huntington RW: Yolk sac tumors of the testis, Cancer 25:644-658, 1970.
350. Talerman A: Endodermal sinus (yolk sac) tumor elements in testicular germ-cell tumors in adults: comparison of prospective and retrospective studies, Cancer 46:1213-1217, 1980.
351. Brown LM, Pottern LM, Hoover RN et al: Testicular cancer in the United States: trends in incidence and mortality, Int J Epidemiol 15:164-170, 1986.
352. Talerman A, Haije WG, Baggerman L: Serum alphafetoprotein (AFP) in patients with germ cell tumors of the gonads and extragonadal sites: correlation between endodermal sinus (yolk sac) tumor and raised serum AFP, Cancer 46:380-385, 1980.
353. Jacobsen GK: Alpha-fetoprotein (AFP) and human chorionic gonadotropin (HCG) in testicular germ cell tumours, Acta Pathol Microbiol Immunol Scand [A] 91:183-190, 1983.
354. Talerman A: Germ cell tumors. In Talerman A, Roth LM, eds: Pathology of the testis and its adnexa, New York, 1986, Churchill Livingstone.
355. Martinazzi M, Crivelli F, Zampatti C: Immunohistochemical study of hepatic and enteric structures in testicular endodermal sinus tumors, Bas Appl Histochem 32:239-245, 1988.
356. Clement PB, Young RH, Scully RE: Endometrioid-like variant of ovarian yolk sac tumor. A clinicopathological analysis of eight cases, Am J Surg Pathol 11:767-778, 1987.
357. Cohen MB, Friend DS, Molnar JJ et al: Gonadal endodermal sinus (yolk sac) tumor with pure intestinal differentiation: a new histologic type, Pathol Res Pract 182:609-616, 1987.
358. Teilum G: Special tumors of ovary and testis and related extragonadal lesions, Philadelphia, 1977, J. B. Lippincott.
359. Michael H, Ulbright TM, Brodhecker CA: The pluripotential nature of the mesenchyme-like component of yolk sac tumor, Arch Pathol Lab Med 113:1115-1119, 1989.
360. Ulbright TM, Michael H, Loehrer PJ et al: Spindle cell tumors resected from male patients with germ cell tumors: a clinicopathologic study of 14 cases, Cancer 65:148-156, 1990.
361. Teilum G: Classification of endodermal sinus tumor (mesoblastoma vitellinum) and so-called "embryonal carcinoma" of the ovary, Acta Pathol Microbiol Scand 64:407-429, 1965.
362. Jacobsen GK, Jacobsen M: Possible liver cell differentiation in testicular germ cell tumours, Histopathology 7:537-548, 1983.
363. Nakashima N, Fukatsu T, Nagasaka T et al: The frequency and histology of hepatic tissue in germ cell tumors, Am J Surg Pathol 11:682-692, 1987.
364. Prat J, Bhan AK, Dickersin GR et al: Hepatoid yolk sac tumor of the ovary (endodermal sinus tumor with hepatoid differentiation): a light microscopic, ultrastructural, and immunohistochemical study of seven cases, Cancer 50:2355-2368, 1982.
365. Damjanov I, Amenta PS, Zarghami F: Transformation of an AFP-positive yolk sac carcinoma into an AFP-negative neoplasm: evidence for in vivo cloning of the human parietal yolk sac carcinoma, Cancer 53:1902-1907, 1984.
366. Eglen DE, Ulbright TM: The differential diagnosis of yolk sac tumor and seminoma: usefulness of cytokeratin, alpha-fetoprotein, and alpha-1-antitrypsin immunoperoxidase reactions, Am J Clin Pathol 88:328-332, 1987.
367. Miettinen M, Virtanen I, Talerman A: Intermediate filament proteins in human testis and testicular germ-cell tumors, Am J Pathol 120:402-410, 1985.

368. Fujimoto J, Hata J, Ishii E et al: Differentiation antigens defined by mouse monoclonal antibodies against human germ cell tumors, Lab Invest 57:350-358, 1987.
369. Gonzalez-Crussi F, Roth LM: The human yolk sac and yolk sac carcinoma: an ultrastructural study, Hum Pathol 7:675-691, 1976.
370. Nogales-Fernandez F, Silverberg SG, Bloustein PA et al: Yolk sac carcinoma (endodermal sinus tumor): ultrastructure and histogenesis of gonadal and extragonadal tumors in comparison with normal human yolk sac, Cancer 39:1462-1474, 1977.
371. Roth LM, Gillespie JJ: Pathology and ultrastructure of germinal neoplasia of the testis. In Einhorn LH, ed: Testicular tumors: management and treatment, New York, 1980, Masson.
372. Oosterhuis JW, Castedo SM, de Jong B et al: Karyotyping and DNA flow cytometry of an orchidoblastoma, Cancer Genet Cytogenet 36:7-11, 1988.
373. Vogelzang NJ, Bronson D, Savino D et al: A human embryonal-yolk sac carcinoma model system in athymic mice, Cancer 55:2584-2593, 1985.
374. Lawrence WD, Young RH, Scully RE: Juvenile granulosa cell tumor of the infantile testis. A report of 14 cases, Am J Surg Pathol 9:87-94, 1985.
375. Groisman GM, Dische MR, Fine EM et al: Juvenile granulosa cell tumor of the testis: a comparative immunohistochemical study with normal infantile gonads, Pediatr Pathol 13:389-400, 1993.
376. Chadha S, van der Kwast TH: Immunohistochemistry of ovarian granulosa cell tumours: the value of tissue specific proteins and tumour markers, Virchows Arch A Pathol Anat Histopathol 414:439-445, 1989.
377. Biscotti CV, Hart WR: Juvenile granulosa cell tumors of the ovary, Arch Pathol Lab Med 113:40-46, 1989.
378. Wu JT, Book L, Sudar K: Serum alpha fetoprotein (AFP) levels in normal infants, Pediatr Res 15:50-52, 1981.
379. Ulbright TM, Gersell DJ: Rete testis hyperplasia with hyaline globule formation. A lesion simulating yolk sac tumor, Am J Surg Pathol 15:66-74, 1991.
380. Loehrer PJ Sr, Williams SD, Einhorn LH: Testicular cancer: the quest continues, J Natl Cancer Inst 80:1373-1382, 1988.
381. Logothetis CJ, Samuels ML, Trindade A et al: The prognostic significance of endodermal sinus tumor histology among patients treated for stage III nonseminomatous germ cell tumors of the testes, Cancer 53:122-128, 1984.
382. Sabio H, Burgert EO Jr, Farrow GM et al: Embryonal carcinoma of the testis in childhood, Cancer 34:2118-2121, 1974.
383. Carroll WL, Kempson RL, Govan DE et al: Conservative management of testicular endodermal sinus tumor in childhood, J Urol 13:1011-1014, 1985.
384. Kramer SA: Pediatric urologic oncology, Urol Clin North Am 12:31-42, 1985.
385. Marshall S, Lyon RP, Scott MP: A conservative approach to testicular tumors in children: 12 cases and their management, J Urol 129:350-351, 1983.
386. Kaplan WE, Firlit CF: Treatment of testicular yolk sac carcinoma in the young child, J Urol 126:663-664, 1981.
387. Nseyo UO, Englander LS, Wajsman Z et al: Histological patterns of treatment failures in testicular germ cell neoplasms, J Urol 133:219-220, 1985.
388. Gilman PA: The epidemiology of human teratomas. In Damjanov I, Knowles BB, Solter D, eds: The human teratomas: experimental and clinical biology, Clinton, NJ, 1983, Humana Press.
389. Barsky SH: Germ cell tumors of the testis. In Javadpour N, Barsky SH, eds: Surgical pathology of urologic diseases, Baltimore, 1987, Williams and Wilkins.
390. Pugh RCB, Cameron KM: Teratoma. In Pugh RCB, ed: Pathology of the testis, Oxford, 1976, Blackwell Scientific.
391. Kooijman CD: Immature teratomas in children, Histopathology 12:491-502, 1988.
392. Kusuda L, Leidich RB, Das S: Mature teratoma of the testis metastasizing as mature teratoma, J Urol 135:1020-1022, 1986.
393. Kedia K, Fraley EE: Adult teratoma of the testis metastasizing as adult teratoma: case report and review of literature, J Urol 114:636-639, 1975.
394. Cameron-Strange A, Horner J: Differentiated teratoma of testis metastasizing as differentiated teratoma in adult, Urology 33:481-482, 1989.
395. Wogalter H, Scofield GF: Adult teratoma of the testicle metastasizing as adult teratoma, J Urol 87:573-576, 1962.
396. Sella A, el Naggar A, Ro JY et al: Evidence of malignant features in histologically mature teratoma, J Urol 146:1025-1028, 1991.
397. Assaf G, Mosbah A, Homsy Y et al: Dermoid cyst of testis in five-year-old-child, Urology 22:432-434, 1983.
398. Dockerty MB, Priestly JT: Dermoid cysts of the testis, J Urol 48:392-400, 1942.
399. Burt AD, Cooper G, MacKay C et al: Dermoid cyst of the testis, Scott Med J 32:146-148, 1987.
400. Ulbright TM, Loehrer PJ, Roth LM et al: The development of non-germ cell malignancies within germ cell tumors. A clinicopathologic study of 11 cases, Cancer 54:1824-1833, 1984.
401. Mostofi FK: Histological change ostensibly induced by therapy in the metastasis of germ cell tumors of testis, Prog Clin Biol Res 203:47-60, 1985.
402. Ahmed T, Bosl GJ, Hajdu SI: Teratoma with malignant transformation in germ cell tumors in men, Cancer 56:860-863, 1985.
403. Trojanowski JQ, Hickey WF: Human teratomas express differentiated neural antigens: an immunohistochemical study with anti-neurofilament, anti-glial filament, and anti-myelin basic protein monoclonal antibodies, Am J Pathol 115:383-389, 1984.
404. Oosterhuis JW, de Jong B, Cornelisse CJ et al: Karyotyping and DNA flow cytometry of mature residual teratoma after intensive chemotherapy of disseminated nonseminomatous germ cell tumor of the testis: a report of two cases, Cancer Genet Cytogenet 22:149-157, 1986.
405. Molenaar WM, Oosterhuis JW, Meiring A et al: Histology and DNA contents of a secondary malignancy arising in a mature residual lesion six years after chemotherapy for a disseminanted nonseminomatous testicular tumor, Cancer 58:264-268, 1986.
406. Shah KH, Maxted WC, Chun B: Epidermoid cysts of the testis: a report of three cases and an analysis of 141 cases from the world literature, Cancer 47:577-582, 1981.

407. Price EB Jr: Epidermoid cysts of the testis: a clinical and pathologic analysis of 69 cases from the testicular tumor registry, J Urol 102:708-713, 1969.
408. Johnson DE, Bracken RB, Blight EM: Prognosis for pathologic Stage I non-seminomatous germ cell tumors of the testis managed by retroperitoneal lymphadenectomy, J Urol 116:63-68, 1976.
409. Dixon FJ, Moore RA: Testicular tumors: a clinicopathologic study, Cancer 6:427-454, 1953.
410. Talerman A, Gratama S, Miranda S et al: Primary carcinoid tumor of the testis: case report, ultrastructure and review of the literature, Cancer 42:2696-2706, 1978.
411. Berdjis CC, Mostofi FK: Carcinoid tumors of the testis, J Urol 118:777-782, 1977.
412. Zavala-Pompa A, Ro JY, El-Naggar A et al: Primary carcinoid tumor of the testis: immunohistochemical, ultrastructural, and DNA flow cytometric study of three cases with a review of the literature, Cancer 72:1726-1732, 1993.
413. Sullivan JL, Packer JT, Bryant M: Primary malignant carcinoid of the testis, Arch Pathol Lab Med 105:515-517, 1981.
414. Ordonez NG, Ayala AG, Sneige N et al: Immunohistochemical demonstration of multiple neurohormonal polypeptides in a case of pure testicular carcinoid, Am J Clin Pathol 78:860-864, 1982.
415. Ogawa A, Sugihara S, Nakazawa Y: A case of primary carcinoid tumor of the testis, Gan No Rinsho 34:1629-1634, 1988.
416. Lewin KJ, Ulich T, Yang K et al: The endocrine cells of the gastrointestinal tract: tumors, part II, Pathol Annu 21(Pt 2):181-215, 1986.
417. Aguirre P, Scully RE: Primitive neuroectodermal tumor of the testis. Report of a case, Arch Pathol Lab Med 107:643-645, 1983.
418. Nocks BN, Dann JA: Primitive neuroectodermal tumor (immature teratoma) of testis, Urology 22:543-544, 1983.
419. Nistal M, Paniagua R: Primary neuroectodermal tumour of the testis, Histopathology 9:1351-1359, 1985.
420. Evans HL: Unusual gonadal stromal tumor of the testis. Case report with ultrastructural observations, Arch Pathol Lab Med 101:317-320, 1977.
421. Giralt S, Dexeus F, Amato R et al: Hyperthyroidism in men with germ cell tumors and high levels of beta-human chorionic gonadotropin, Cancer 69:1286-1290, 1992.
422. Manivel JC, Niehans G, Wick MR et al: Intermediate trophoblast in germ cell neoplasms, Am J Surg Pathol 11:693-701, 1987.
423. Lind HM, Haghighi P: Carcinoembryonic antigen staining in choriocarcinoma, Am J Clin Pathol 86:538-540, 1986.
424. Clark RK, Damjanov I: Intermediate filaments of human trophoblast and choriocarcinoma cell lines, Virchows Arch A Pathol Anat Histopathol 407:203-208, 1985.
425. Pierce GB Jr, Midgley AR Jr: The origin and function of human syncytiotrophoblastic giant cells, Am J Pathol 43:153-173, 1963.
426. Motoyama T, Sasano N, Yonezawa S et al: Early stage of development in testicular choriocarcinomas, Acta Pathol Jpn 43:320-326, 1993.
427. Vaeth M, Schultz HP, von der Maase H et al: Prognostic factors in testicular germ cell tumours: experiences with 1058 consecutive cases, Acta Radiol Oncol 23:271-285, 1984.
428. Bosl GJ, Geller NL, Cirrincione C et al: Multivariate analysis of prognostic variables in patients with metastatic testicular cancer, Cancer Res 43:3403-3407, 1983.
429. Stoter G, Sylvester R, Sleijfer DT et al: A multivariate analysis of prognostic factors in disseminated non-seminomatous testicular cancer, Prog Clin Biol Res 269:381-393, 1988.
430. Seguchi T, Iwasaki A, Sugao H et al: Clinical statistics of germinal testicular cancer, Nippon Hinyokika Gakkai Zasshi 81:889-894, 1990.
431. Brawn PN: The origin of germ cell tumors of the testis, Cancer 51:1610-1614, 1983.
432. Okamoto T: A human vitelline component in embryonal carcinoma of the testis, Acta Pathol Jpn 36:41-48, 1986.
433. Nakashima N, Murakami S, Fukatsu T et al: Characteristics of "embryoid body" in human gonadal germ cell tumors, Hum Pathol 19:1144-1154, 1988.
434. Evans RW: Developmental stages of embryo-like bodies in teratoma testis, J Clin Pathol 10:31-39, 1957.
435. Cardoso de Almeida PC, Scully RE: Diffuse embryoma of the testis. A distinctive form of mixed germ cell tumor, Am J Surg Pathol 7:633-642, 1983.
436. Brawn PN: The characteristics of embryonal carcinoma cells in teratocarcinomas, Cancer 59:2042-2046, 1987.
437. Burt ME, Javadpour N: Germ-cell tumors in patients with apparently normal testes, Cancer 47:1911-1915, 1981.
438. Meares EM Jr, Briggs EM: Occult seminoma of the testis masquerading as primary extragonadal germinal neoplasm, Cancer 30:300-306, 1972.
439. Asif S, Uehling DT: Microscopic tumor foci in testes, J Urol 99:776-779, 1968.
440. Bohle A, Studer UE, Sonntag RW et al: Primary or secondary extragonadal germ cell tumors, J Urol 135:939-943, 1986.
441. Bär W, Hedinger C: Comparison of histologic types of primary testicular germ cell tumors with their metastases: consequences for the WHO and the British Nomenclatures, Virchows Arch A Pathol Anat Histopathol 370:41-54, 1976.
442. Fossä SD, Aass N, Ous S et al: Histology of tumor residuals following chemotherapy in patients with advanced nonseminomatous testicular cancer, J Urol 142:1239-1242, 1989.
443. Moran CA, Travis WD, Carter D et al: Metastatic mature teratoma in lung following testicular embryonal carcinoma and teratocarcinoma, Arch Pathol Lab Med 117:641-644, 1993.
444. Davey DD, Ulbright TM, Loehrer PJ et al: The significance of atypia within teratomatous metastases after chemotherapy for malignant germ cell tumors, Cancer 59:533-539, 1987.
445. Jeffery GM, Theaker JM, Lee AH et al: The growing teratoma syndrome, Br J Urol 67:195-202, 1991.
446. Gelderman WA, Scraffordt Koops H, Sleijfer DT et al: Late recurrence of mature teratoma in nonseminomatous testicular tumors after PVB chemotherapy and surgery, Urology 33:10-14, 1989.
447. Logothetis CJ, Samuels ML, Trindade A: The growing teratoma syndrome, Cancer 50:1629-1635, 1982.
448. Tongaonkar HB, Deshmane VH, Dalal AV et al: Growing teratoma syndrome, J Surg Oncol 55:56-60, 1994.

449. Looijenga LH, Oosterhuis JW, Ramaekers FC et al: Dual parameter flow cytometry for deoxyribonucleic acid and intermediate filament proteins of residual mature teratoma. All tumor cells are aneuploid, Lab Invest 64:113-117, 1991.
450. Mazur MT, Lurain JR, Brewer JI: Fatal gestational choriocarcinoma: clinicopathologic study of patients treated at a trophoblastic disease center, Cancer 50:1833-1846, 1982.
451. Ulbright TM, Loehrer PJ: Choriocarcinoma-like lesions in patients with testicular germ cell tumors. Two histologic variants, Am J Surg Pathol 12:531-541, 1988.
452. Donohue JP, Roth LM, Zachary JM et al: Cytoreductive surgery for metastatic testis cancer: tissue analysis of retroperitoneal masses after chemotherapy, J Urol 127:1111-1114, 1982.
453. Bracken RB, Johnson DE, Frazier OH et al: The role of surgery following chemotherapy in Stage III germ cell neoplasms, J Urol 129:39-43, 1983.
454. Einhorn LH, Williams SD, Mandelbaum I et al: Surgical resection in disseminated testicular cancer following chemotherapeutic cytoreduction, Cancer 48:904-908, 1981.
455. Vugrin D, Whitmore WF Jr, Sogani PC et al: Combined chemotherapy and surgery in treatment of advanced germ-cell tumors, Cancer 47:2228-2231, 1981.
456. Fox EP, Weathers TD, Williams SD et al: Outcome analysis for patients with persistent nonteratomatous germ cell tumor in postchemotherapy retroperitoneal lymph node dissections, J Clin Oncol 11:1294-1299, 1993.
457. Young RH, Talerman A: Testicular tumors other than germ cell tumors, Semin Diagn Pathol 4:342-360, 1987.
458. Kim I, Young RH, Scully RE: Leydig cell tumors of the testis. A clinicopathological analysis of 40 cases and review of the literature, Am J Surg Pathol 9:177-192, 1985.
459. Kaplan GW, Cromie WJ, Kelalis PP et al: Gonadal stromal tumors: a report of the Prepubertal Testicular Tumor Registry, J Urol 136:300-302, 1986.
460. Dilworth JP, Farrow GM, Oesterling JE: Non-germ cell tumors of testis, Urology 37:399-417, 1991.
461. Wheeler JE: Anatomy, embryology, and physiology of the testis and its ducts. In Hill GS, ed: Uropathology, New York, 1989, Churchill-Livingstone.
462. Dieckmann K-P, Loy V: Metachronous germ cell and Leydig cell tumors of the testis: do testicular germ cell tumors and Leydig cell tumors share common etiologic factors, Cancer 72:1305-1307, 1993.
463. Bokemeyer C, Kuczyk M, Schoffski P et al: Familial occurrence of Leydig cell tumors: a report of a case in a father and his adult son, J Urol 150:1509-1510, 1993.
464. Wheeler JE: Testicular tumors. In Hill GS, ed: Uropathology, New York, 1989, Churchill Livingstone.
465. Minkowitz S, Soloway H, Soscia J: Ossifying interstitial cell tumor of the testes, J Urol 94:592-595, 1965.
466. Balsitis M, Sokal M: Ossifying malignant Leydig (interstitial) cell tumour of the testis, Histopathology 16:599-601, 1990.
467. Santonja C, Varona C, Burgos FJ et al: Leydig cell tumor of testis with adipose metaplasia, Appl Pathol 7:201-204, 1989.
468. Miettinen M, Wahlstrom T, Virtanen I et al: Cellular differentiation in ovarian sex-cord-stromal and germ-cell tumors studied with antibodies to intermediate filament proteins, Am J Surg Pathol 9:640-651, 1985.
469. Descheemaeker T, Fontaine P, Racadot A et al: Enkephalin-like immunoreactivity in Leydig cell tumor, Ann Endocrinol 50:513-516, 1989.
470. Kay S, Fu Y-S, Koontz WW et al: Interstitial-cell tumor of the testis: tissue culture and ultrastructural studies, Am J Clin Pathol 63:366-376, 1975.
471. Sohval AR, Churg J, Suzuki Y et al: Electron microscopy of a feminizing Leydig cell tumor of the testis, Hum Pathol 8:621-634, 1977.
472. Sohval AR, Churg J, Gabrilove JL et al: Ultrastructure of feminizing testicular Leydig cell tumors, Ultrastruc Pathol 3:335-345, 1982.
473. Grem JL, Robins HI, Wilson KS et al: Metastatic Leydig cell tumor of the testis. Report of three cases and review of the literature, Cancer 58:2116-2119, 1986.
474. Srikanth MS, West BR, Ishitani M et al: Benign testicular tumors in children with congenital adrenal hyperplasia, J Pediatr Surg 27:639-641, 1992.
475. Johnson RE, Scheithauer B: Massive hyperplasia of testicular adrenal rests in a patient with Nelson's syndrome, Am J Clin Pathol 77:501-507, 1982.
476. Waxman M, Damjanov I, Khapra A et al: Large cell calcifying Sertoli tumor of the testis. Light microscopic and ultrastructural study, Cancer 54:1574-1581, 1984.
477. Horn T, Jao W, Keh PC: Large-cell calcifying Sertoli cell tumor of the testis: a case report with ultrastructural study, Ultrastruc Pathol 4:359-364, 1983.
478. Perez-Atayde AR, Nunez AE, Carroll WL et al: Large-cell calcifying Sertoli cell tumor of the testis. An ultrastructural, immunocytochemical, and biochemical study, Cancer 51:2287-2292, 1983.
479. Proppe KH, Dickersin GR: Large-cell calcifying Sertoli cell tumor of the testis: light microscopic and ultrastructural study, Hum Pathol 13:1109-1114, 1982.
480. Tetu B, Ro JY, Ayala AG: Large cell calcifying Sertoli cell tumor of the testis: a clinicopathologic, immunohistochemical, and ultrastructural study of two cases, Am J Clin Pathol 96:717-722, 1991.
481. Dubois RS, Hoffman WH, Krishnan TH et al: Feminizing sex cord tumors with annular tubules in a boy with Peutz-Jeghers syndrome, J Pediatr 101:568-571, 1982.
482. Ramaswamy G, Jagadha V, Tchertkoff V: A testicular tumor resembling the sex cord with annular tubules in a case of the androgen insensitivity syndrome, Cancer 55:1607-1611, 1985.
483. Scully RE: Sex cord tumor with annular tubules: a distinctive ovarian tumor of the Peutz-Jeghers syndrome, Cancer 25:1107-1121, 1970.
484. Young RH, Welch WR, Dickersin GR et al: Ovarian sex cord tumor with annular tubules: review of 74 cases including 27 with Peutz-Jeghers syndrome and four with adenoma malignum of the cervix, Cancer 50:1384-1402, 1982.
485. Jacobsen GK: Malignant Sertoli cell tumors of the testis, J Urol Pathol 1:233-255, 1993.
486. Aguirre P, Thor AD, Scully RE: Ovarian endometrioid carcinomas resembling sex cord–stromal tumors. An immunohistochemical study, Int J Gynecol Pathol 8:364-373, 1989.
487. Nielsen K, Jacobsen GK: Malignant Sertoli cell tumour of the testis: an immunohistochemical study and a review of the literature, APMIS 96:755-760, 1988.

488. Able ME, Lee JC: Ultrastructure of a Sertoli-cell adenoma of the testis, Cancer 23:481-486, 1969.
489. Tavassoli FA, Norris HJ: Sertoli cell tumors of the ovary: a clinicopathologic study of 28 cases with ultrastructural observations, Cancer 46:2281-2297, 1980.
490. Rosvoll R, Woodard JR: Malignant Sertoli cell tumor of the testis, Cancer 22:8-13, 1968.
491. Talerman A: Malignant Sertoli cell tumor of the testis, Cancer 28:446-454, 1971.
492. Morin LJ, Loening S: Malignant androblastoma (Sertoli cell tumor) of the testis: a case report with a review of the literature, J Urol 114:476-480, 1975.
493. Koppikar DD, Sirsat MV: A malignant Sertoli cell tumor of the testis, Br J Urol 45:213-217, 1973.
494. O'Dowd J, Gaffney EF, Young RH: Malignant sex cord–stromal tumour in a patient with androgen insensitivity syndrome, Histopathology 16:279-282, 1990.
495. Zukerberg LR, Young RH, Scully RE: Sclerosing Sertoli cell tumor of the testis: a report of 10 cases, Am J Surg Pathol 159:829-834, 1991.
496. Blix GW, Levine LA, Goldberg R et al: Large cell calcifying Sertoli cell tumor of the testis, Scand J Urol Nephrol 26:73-75, 1992.
497. Carney JA, Gordon H, Carpenter PC et al: The complex of myxomas, spotty pigmentation, and endocrine overactivity, Medicine 64:270-283, 1985.
498. Carney JA: Psammomatous melanotic schwannoma: a distinctive, heritable tumor with special associations, including cardiac myxoma and the Cushing syndrome, Am J Surg Pathol 14:206-222, 1990.
499. Carney JA, Toorkey BC: Myxoid fibroadenoma and allied conditions (myxomatosis) of the breast: a heritable disorder with special associations including cardiac and cutaneous myxomas, Am J Surg Pathol 15:713-721, 1991.
500. Düe W, Dieckmann KP, Niedobitek G et al: Testicular sex cord stromal tumour with granulosa cell differentiation: detection of steroid hormone receptors as a possible basis for tumour development and therapeutic management, J Clin Pathol 43:732-737, 1990.
501. Gaylis FD, August C, Yeldandi A et al: Granulosa cell tumor of the adult testis: ultrastructural and ultrasonographic characteristics, J Urol 141:126-127, 1989.
502. Talerman A: Pure granulosa cell tumour of the testis. Report of a case and review of the literature, Appl Pathol 3:117-122, 1985.
503. Nistal M, Läzaro R, Garcia J et al: Testicular granulosa cell tumor of the adult type, Arch Pathol Lab Med 116:284-287, 1992.
504. Matoska J, Ondrus D, Talerman A: Malignant granulosa cell tumor of the testis associated with gynecomastia and long survival, Cancer 69:1769-1772, 1992.
505. Jimenez-Quintero LP, Ro JY, Zavala-Pompa A et al: Granulosa cell tumor of the adult testis: a clinicopathologic study of seven cases and a review of the literature, Hum Pathol 24:1120-1126, 1993.
506. Nistal M, Redondo E, Paniagua R: Juvenile granulosa cell tumor of the testis, Arch Pathol Lab Med 112:1129-1132, 1988.
507. Pinto MM: Juvenile granulosa cell tumor of the infant testis: case report with ultrastructural observations, Pediatr Pathol 4:277-289, 1985.
508. Raju U, Fine G, Warrier R et al: Congenital testicular juvenile granulosa cell tumor in a neonate with X/XY mosaicism, Am J Surg Pathol 10:577-583, 1986.
509. Tanaka Y, Sasaki Y, Tachibana K et al: Testicular juvenile granulosa cell tumor in an infant with X/XY mosaicism clinically diagnosed as true hermaphroditism, Am J Surg Pathol 18:316-322, 1994.
510. Lawrence WD, Young RH, Scully RE: Sex cord–stromal tumors. In Talerman A, Roth LM, eds: Pathology of the testis and its adnexa, New York, 1986, Churchill Livingstone.
511. Miettinen M, Salo J, Virtanen I: Testicular stromal tumor: ultrastructural, immunohistochemical, and gel electrophoretic evidence of epithelial differentiation, Ultrastruc Pathol 10:515-528, 1986.
512. Greco MA, Feiner HD, Theil KS et al: Testicular stromal tumor with myofilaments: ultrastructural comparison with normal gonadal stroma, Hum Pathol 15:238-243, 1984.
513. Ishida T, Tagatz GE, Okagaki T: Gonadoblastoma: ultrastructural evidence for testicular origin, Cancer 37:1770-1781, 1976.
514. Roth LM, Eglen DE: Gonadoblastoma: immunohistochemical and ultrastructural observations, Int J Gynecol Pathol 8:72-81, 1989.
515. Scully RE: Gonadoblastoma. A review of 74 cases, Cancer 25:1340-1356, 1970.
516. Matoska J, Talerman A: Mixed germ cell–sex cord stroma tumor of the testis. A report with ultrastructural findings, Cancer 64:2146-2153, 1989.
517. Bolen JW: Mixed germ cell–sex cord stromal tumor. A gonadal tumor distinct from gonadoblastoma, Am J Clin Pathol 75:565-573, 1981.
518. Nochomovitz LE, Orenstein JM: Adenocarcinoma of the rete testis: review and regrouping of reported cases and a consideration of miscellaneous entities, J Urogenit Pathol 1:11-40, 1991.
519. Visscher DW, Talerman A, Rivera LR et al: Adenocarcinoma of the rete testis with a spindle cell component. A possible metaplastic carcinoma, Cancer 64:770-775, 1989.
520. Nochomovitz LE, Orenstein JM: Adenocarcinoma of the rete testis. Case report, ultrastructural observations, and clinicopathologic correlates, Am J Surg Pathol 8:625-634, 1984.
521. Altaffer LF III, Dufour DR, Castleberry GM et al: Coexisting rete testis adenoma and gonadoblastoma, J Urol 127:332-335, 1982.
522. Gupta RK: Benign papillary tumor of the rete testis, Ind J Cancer 11:480-481, 1974.
523. Yadav SB, Patil PN, Karkhanis RB: Primary tumors of the spermatic cord, epididymis, and rete testis, J Postgrad Med 15:49-52, 1969.
524. Hartwick RW, Ro JY, Srigley JR et al: Adenomatous hyperplasia of the rete testis. A clinicopathologic study of nine cases, Am J Surg Pathol 15:350-357, 1991.
525. Ferry JA, Harris NL, Young RH et al: Malignant lymphoma of the testis, epididymis, and spermatic cord. A clinicopathologic study of 69 cases with immunophenotypic analysis, Am J Surg Pathol 18:376-390, 1994.
526. Martenson JA Jr, Buskirk SJ, Ilstrup DM et al: Patterns of failure in primary testicular non-Hodgkin's lymphoma, J Clin Oncol 6:297-302, 1988.

527. Baldetorp LA, Brunkvall J, Cavallin-Ståhl E et al: Malignant lymphoma of the testis, Br J Urol 56:525-530, 1984.
528. Bentley RC, Devlin B, Kaufman RE et al: Genotypic divergence precedes clinical dissemination in a case of synchronous bilateral B-cell malignant lymphoma of the testes, Hum Pathol 24:675-678, 1993.
529. Doll DC, Weiss RB: Malignant lymphoma of the testis, Am J Med 81:515-524, 1986.
530. Root M, Wang TY, Hescock H et al: Burkitt's lymphoma of the testicle: report of 2 cases occurring in elderly patients, J Urol 144:1239-1241, 1990.
531. Givler RL: Testicular involvement in leukemia and lymphoma, Cancer 23:1290-1295, 1969.
532. Algaba F, Santaularia JM, Garat JM et al: Testicular pseudolymphoma, Eur Urol 12:362-363, 1986.
533. Senzaki H, Okada H, Izuno Y et al: An autopsy case of multiple myeloma accompanied by extensive nodular infiltration into the extraskeletal tissue, Gan No Rinsho 36:2491-2495, 1990.
534. Avitable AM, Gansler TS, Tomaszewski JE et al: Testicular plasmacytoma, Urology 34:51-54, 1989.
535. Oppenheim PI, Cohen S, Anders KH: Testicular plasmacytoma. A case report with immunohistochemical studies and literature review, Arch Pathol Lab Med 115:629-632, 1991.
536. Kuhajda FP, Haupt HM, Moore GW et al: Gonadal morphology in patients receiving chemotherapy for leukemia: evidence for reproductive potential and against a testicular tumor sanctuary, Am J Med 72:759-767, 1982.
537. Askin FB, Land VJ, Sullivan MP et al: Occult testicular leukemia: testicular biopsy at three years continuous complete remission of childhood leukemia: a Southwest Oncology Group study, Cancer 47:470-475, 1981.
538. Nesbit ME Jr, Robison LL, Ortega JA et al: Testicular relapse in childhood acute lymphoblastic leukemia: association with pretreatment patient characteristics and treatment: a report for Children's Cancer Study Group, Cancer 45:2009-2016, 1980.
539. Tiedemann K, Chessells JM, Sandland RM: Isolated testicular relapse in boys with acute lymphoblastic leukaemia: treatment and outcome, BMJ 285:1614-1616, 1982.
540. Economopoulos T, Alexopoulos C, Anagnostou D et al: Primary granulocytic sarcoma of the testis, Leukemia 8:199-200, 1994.
541. Goldstein AM, Mendez R, Vargas A et al: Epidermoid cysts of testis, Urology 15:186-189, 1980.
542. LiVolsi VA, Schiff M: Myxoid neurofibroma of the testis, J Urol 118:341-342, 1977.
543. Tada M, Takemura S, Takimoto Y et al: A case of cavernous hemangioma of the testis, Hinyokika Kiyo 35:1969-1971, 1989.
544. Nistal M, Paniagua R, Regadera J et al: Testicular capillary haemangioma, Br J Urol 54:433, 1982.
545. D'Esposito RF, Ferraro LR, Wogalter H: Hemangioma of the testis in an infant, J Urol 116:677-678, 1976.
546. Banks ER, Mills SE: Histiocytoid (epithelioid) hemangioma of the testis. The so-called vascular variant of "adenomatoid tumor," Am J Surg Pathol 14:584-589, 1990.
547. Honore LH, Sullivan LD: Intratesticular leiomyoma: a case report with discussion of differential diagnosis and histogenesis, J Urol 114:631-635, 1975.
548. Cricco CF Jr, Buck AS: Hemangioendothelioma of the testis: second reported case, J Urol 123:131-132, 1980.
549. Mathew T, Prabhakaran K: Osteosarcoma of the testis, Arch Pathol Lab Med 105:38-39, 1981.
550. Zukerberg LR, Young RH: Primary testicular sarcoma: a report of two cases, Hum Pathol 21:932-935, 1990.
551. Yachia D, Auslaender L: Primary leiomyosarcoma of the testis, J Urol 141:955-956, 1989.
552. Davis AE Jr: Rhabdomyosarcoma of the testicle, J Urol 87:148-154, 1962.
553. Ravich L, Lerman PH, Drabkin JW et al: Pure testicular rhabdomyosarcoma, J Urol 94:596-599, 1965.
554. Alexander F: Pure testicular rhabdomyosarcoma, Br J Cancer 22:498-501, 1968.
555. Haupt HM, Mann RB, Trump DL et al: Metastatic carcinoma involving the testis: clinical and pathologic distinction from primary testicular neoplasms, Cancer 54:709-714, 1984.
556. Bhasin SD, Shrikhande SS: Secondary carcinoma of testis—a clinicopathologic study of 10 cases, Ind J Cancer 27:83-90, 1990.
557. Richardson PG, Millward MJ, Shrimankar JJ et al: Metastatic melanoma to the testis simulating primary seminoma, Br J Urol 69:663-665, 1992.
558. Pienkos EJ, Jablokow VR: Secondary testicular tumors, Cancer 30:481-485, 1972.
559. Srigley JR, Toth P, Edwards V: Diagnostic electron microscopy of male genital tract tumors, Clin Lab Med 7:91-115, 1987.
560. Ulbright TM, Roth LM: Recent developments in the pathology of germ cell tumors, Semin Diagn Pathol 4:304-319, 1987.

Embryology and Normal Anatomy
- Embryology
- Anatomy

Congenital Anomalies
- Splenogonadal fusion
- Adrenal heterotopia and renal ectopia
- Wolffian and müllerian remnants
- Cystic fibrosis

Non-neoplastic Diseases
- Celes and cysts
- Inflammatory and reactive diseases
- Other non-neoplastic diseases

Neoplasms
- Benign neoplasms and pseudotumors
  - Lipoma
  - Adenomatoid hyperplasia
  - Adenomatoid tumor
  - Hamartoma
  - Osseous metaplasia of epididymis
  - Reactive mesothelial hyperplasia
  - Benign papillary mesothelioma
  - Fibrous pseudotumor
  - Leiomyosarcoma
  - Melanotic neuroectodermal tumor of infancy
  - Brenner tumor
  - Gonadal stromal tumor
  - Other benign tumors
- Malignant neoplasms
  - Liposarcoma
  - Rhabdomyosarcoma
  - Leiomyosarcoma
  - Malignant mesothelioma
  - Serous tumor of müllerian epithelium
  - Adenocarcinoma of epididymis
  - Malignant fibrous histiocytoma
  - Other sarcomas
  - Germ cell tumor
  - Malignant lymphoma and hematopoietic neoplasms
  - Neuroblastoma
  - Wilms' tumor
  - Metastases

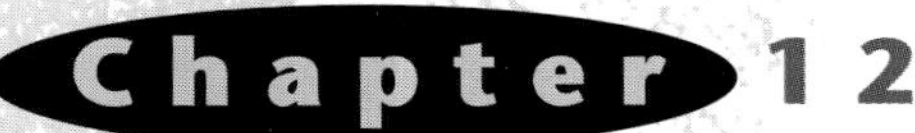

Chapter 12

SPERMATIC CORD AND TESTICULAR ADNEXA

DAVID G. BOSTWICK

The paratesticular region includes the testicular tunics, efferent ductules, epididymis, spermatic cord, and vas deferens. Numerous rare and interesting lesions arise in this region, including cysts, "celes," inflammatory diseases, embryonic remnants, neoplasms, and neoplasm-like proliferations (Table 12-1). In children one of the common neoplasms is paratesticular rhabdomyosarcoma. In adults the most common pathologic conditions in order of frequency are epididymitis, lipoma of the spermatic cord, adenomatoid tumor of the epididymis, and sarcoma of the spermatic cord.

TABLE 12-1.
PARATESTICULAR TUMORS AND CYSTS IN THE CANADIAN REFERENCE CENTER FOR CANCER PATHOLOGY, 1949–1986

	Number of Cases
CYSTS	
Mesothelial cyst	4
Epididymal cyst	1
BENIGN NEOPLASMS AND PSEUDOTUMORS	
Adenomatoid tumor	23
Nodular and diffuse fibrous proliferation	6
Leiomyoma	6
Cystadenoma of epididymis	3
Hamartoma of rete testis	1
Adenomatous hyperplasia of epididymis	1
Adenomatous hyperplasia of rete testis	1
Mixed gonadal stromal tumor	1
Adrenal cortical heterotopia	1
Rhabdomyoma	1
Miscellaneous soft-tissue tumors	8
MALIGNANT NEOPLASMS	
Primary	
Rhabdomyosarcoma	14
Liposarcoma	9
Leiomyosarcoma	7
Malignant mesothelioma	7
Malignant fibrous histiocytoma	3
Malignant mesenchymoma	1
Plasmacytoma	1
Papillary serous cystadenocarcinoma of low malignant potential	1
Sarcoma, not otherwise specified	3
Secondary	
Metastatic carcinoma	4
Metastatic carcinoid tumor	2
Metastatic non-Hodgkin's lymphoma	2

From Srigley JR, Hartwick RWH: Tumors and cysts of the paratesticular region, Pathol Annu 25(Part2):51–108, 1990 (review); with permission.

It is often difficult to diagnose paratesticular masses prior to or during surgery because of their varied morphologic appearance and rarity. An inguinal surgical approach is usually indicated when there is a suspicion of malignancy. The pathologist should document the anatomic site of origin and histologic classification of the lesion.

EMBRYOLOGY AND NORMAL ANATOMY

The paratesticular region contains numerous anatomically complex epithelial and mesenchymal structures, often within embryonic remnants (Fig. 12-1). The rete testis of the mediastinum of the testis, the first element of the wolffian collecting system, connects the seminiferous tubules and efferent ductules.

The most common abnormalities of the paratesticular region are benign and include hydrocele, lipoma, and inflammatory conditions such as epididymitis, but a variety of cystic and proliferative lesions also occur and are diagnostically challenging.

EMBRYOLOGY

The embryology of the testis and its adnexa is described in Chapter 10; herein is a brief summary of significant events in the development of paratesticular tissues. The testis and head of the epididymis arise from the genital ridge. The wolffian ducts, the male genital ducts, are paired tubes that are associated with the developing gonads and degenerating mesonephric tubules. The body and tail of the epididymis, the vas deferens, and the ejaculatory duct arise from the mesonephric tubules[1]; other degenerating tubules often persist as embryonic remnants, including the appendix epididymis, paradidymis,

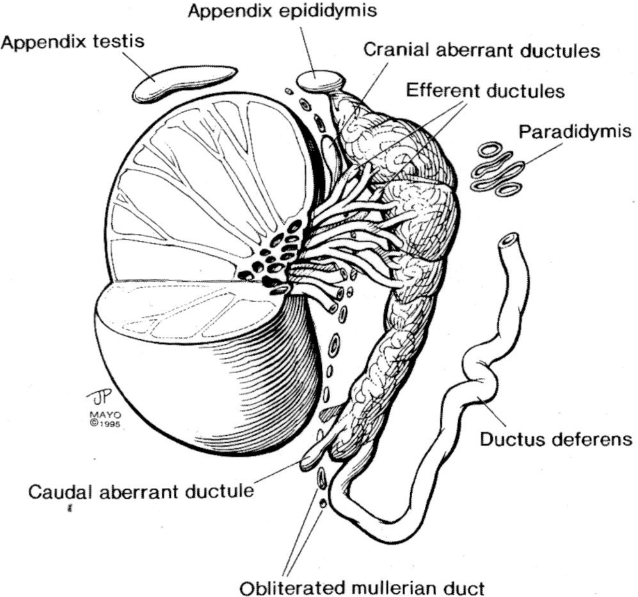

12-1. Anatomy of the testis and paratesticular adnexa, including embryonic remnants.

and cranial and caudal aberrent ductules (see Fig. 12-1). The paired vasa deferentia connect to the ejaculatory ducts within the prostate, which in turn have their outlets in the prostatic urethra adjacent to the müllerian tubercle. Blind diverticula of the distal vas deferens form the seminal vesicles. The müllerian duct, or paramesonephros, regresses in men but may persist as embryonic remnants, such as the appendix testis and prostatic utricle.

ANATOMY

Scrotum and testicular tunics

The sac of the scrotum is divided by a partial median septum into two compartments, each of which contains a testis and epididymis, and the lower portion of the spermatic cord. The scrotal wall consists of six layers; from the inside outward these are the tunica vaginalis, the internal spermatic fascia, the cremasteric muscle, the external spermatic fascia, the dartos muscle, and the skin. The tunica vaginalis is a thin mesothelium-covered layer of the parietal peritoneum, which also covers the white fibrous tunica albuginea of the testis and epididymis; it is initially in contact with the peritoneal cavity from which it arises but becomes isolated with regression of the processus vaginalis. The internal spermatic fascia is a continuation of the transversalis fascia, and the external fascia is a continuation of the external oblique aponeurosis. The cremasteric muscle consists of incomplete slips of muscle, usually in the upper part of the scrotal wall. The dartos muscle consists of smooth muscle embedded in loose areolar tissue. The scrotum is supplied by the external and internal pudendal, cremasteric, and testicular arteries. Lymphatic drainage is to the superficial inguinal lymph nodes.

Rete testis

The rete testis is formed by the convergence of the seminiferous tubules (see Chapter 10). The tubules follow a cranial and dorsal course through the fibrous connective tissue of the mediastinum testis, eventually merging into 12 to 20 ducts (the efferent ductules, or ductuli efferentes [Fig. 12-2]) that perforate the tunica vaginalis and

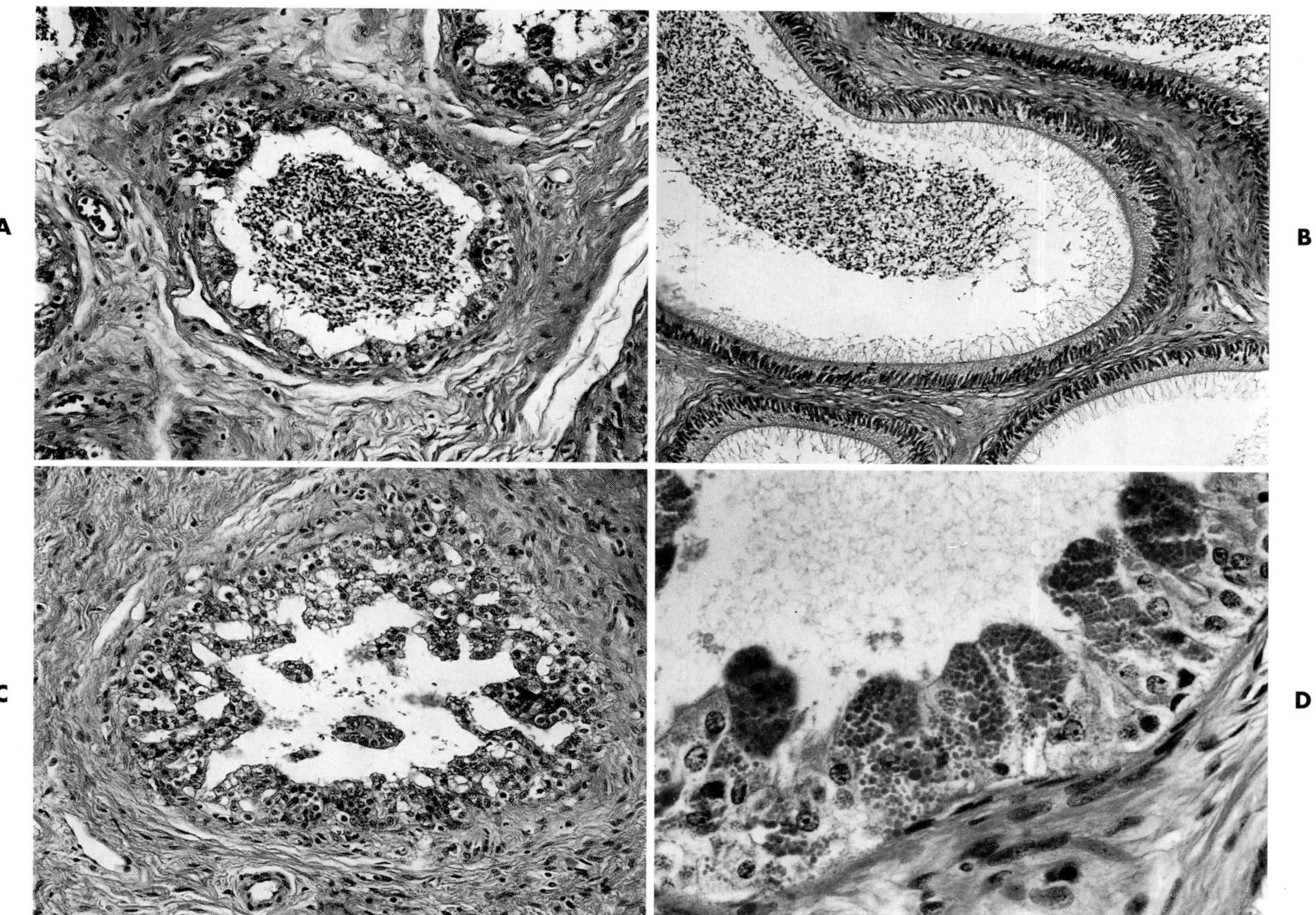

12-2. **A**, Normal efferent ductules with luminal sperm. **B**, Normal epididymis with luminal sperm. **C**, Cribriform hyperplasia of the efferent ductules. **D**, Coarse granular cytoplasmic change of the vas deferens. *(From Schned AR, Memoli VA: Coarse granular cytoplasmic change of the epididymis. An immunohistochemical and ultrastructural study, J Urol Pathol 2:213-222, 1994; with permission.)*

form the head of the epididymis at the upper pole of the testis. After puberty, elastic fibers are present in the muscular coat of the ductules, epididymis, and vas deferens.

Epididymis

The epididymis is a highly convoluted tubule that is attached to the dorsomedial portion of the testis, connecting the efferent ductules of the rete testis with the vas deferens. It is about 6 m long. The head consists of a series of conical masses, the lobules, each of which contain a single duct measuring 15 to 20 cm long; it is lined by tall columnar epithelium and invested with a thick layer of smooth muscle (see Fig. 12-2). The body of the epididymis is a single highly convoluted tube which increases in diameter distally to form the tail. The tail distally merges with the vas deferens. The epithelium may contain large multinucleated giant cells similar to those of the seminal vesicles and vas deferens (see discussion on vas deferens in the next section).[2,3] Cribriform hyperplasia is a recently described variant of normal efferent ductular and epididymal histology (see Fig. 12-2).[4-7] Coarse granular cytoplasmic change is uncommon (see Fig. 12-2). Prostate-type glands are rarely observed.[8]

Vas deferens (ductus deferens) and spermatic cord

The vas deferens is about 46 cm long, traversing the spermatic cord and inguinal canal to connect the tail of the epididymis with the ejaculatory ducts. In the spermatic cord it is invested with a thick muscular coat which includes the internal spermatic, cremasteric, and external spermatic fasciae; other structures of the spermatic cord include the pampiniform plexus, the testicular artery, lymphatics, and nerves. Upon exiting the spermatic cord, the vas deferens passes extraperitoneally, upward, and laterally in the pelvis, passes medial to the distal ureter and the posterior wall of the bladder, and terminates at an acute angle in a dilated ampulla, which, with the duct of the seminal vesicle, forms the ejaculatory duct. The vas deferens is supplied by its own artery, the artery of the vas deferens, which is usually a branch of the internal iliac or umbilical artery.

The vas deferens is lined by columnar epithelium in low folds. The epithelial cells often contain eosinophilic intranuclear inclusions[9-11] and there are occasional bizarre enlarged cells, similar to those of the seminal vesicles. The bizarre cells have marked variation in nuclear size, may contain periodic acid–Schiff positive, Alcian blue negative intranuclear inclusions and have characteristic yellow-brown lipofuscin cytoplasmic pigment, which increases in amount with age after puberty. The wall of the vas deferens consists of three layers of smooth muscle: the inner longitudinal, middle circular, and outer longitudinal layers. Elastic fibers appear in the muscular wall after puberty.

CONGENITAL ANOMALIES

Abnormal development of the paratesticular region may result in a variety of anomalies, including embryonic remnants, agenesis, atresia, ectopia, and cysts. There is an increased frequency of anomalies in boys with cryptorchidism and congenital rubella.[12-18] Bilateral anomalies result in sterility.[19-23]

Agenesis[24-26] and atresia[27,28] of the testis, epididymis, and vas deferens result from failure of development of the genital ridge, often with anomalies of other wolffian derivatives[29] and renal ectopia,[30] agenesis,[31-35] or dysplasia.[36] Congenital absence of the vas deferens may be autosomal recessive[37-40] and is often associated with cystic fibrosis (see discussion on cystic fibrosis in this chapter). Duplications may involve any structure of the adnexa but are rare.[33,35,41-44] Ectopic insertion of the ureteric bud in the epididymis, vas deferens, or seminal vesicles also may occur.[33,35,45-55] Congenital or developmental cysts of the epididymis are extremely rare[20,56-60] and may be associated with intrauterine exposure to diethylstilbesterol. The cysts are usually solitary but may be multiple and bilateral.

Ectopic epididymis may be found anterior to the testis, in the retroperitoneum, and within the kidney.[61]

SPLENOGONADAL FUSION

Splenogonadal fusion is a rare congenital anomaly in which there is fusion of the splenic and gonadal anlage. About 100 cases have been reported, usually on the left side (98%) in men (95%). Patients may present with nontender scrotal mass[62] or intestinal obstruction, but most cases are discovered incidentally at autopsy or surgery for cryptorchidism or inguinal hernia. About 57% are associated with other congenital anomalies, including peromelia, micrognathia, and cardiac anomalies.

There are two types of splenogonadal fusion. The continuous type is characterized by connection of the spleen and the splenogonad by a fibrous cord. The cord usually arises in the upper pole of the spleen, and may be retroperitoneal or anterior to the small bowel or colon. Splenic tissue may be present at both ends of the cord or stud the cord throughout its length. The discontinuous type of splenogonadal fusion has no connection between the spleen and splenogonad. The splenic tissue appears within the tunica albuginea or scrotum or along the vascular pedicle.

Splenogonadal fusion probably results from early fusion of the spleen and gonad during embryonic development, perhaps as the result of inflammation or adhe-

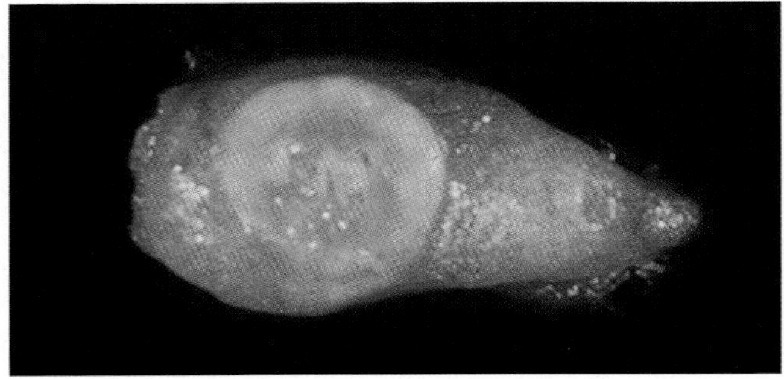

12-3. Heterotopic adrenal cortical tissue in the left spermatic cord forming a discrete yellow-orange nodule.

sions. The spleen develops during the fourth and fifth weeks of gestation, and rotates into proximity with the urogenital fold and developing gonadal mesoderm. During the eighth to tenth week, the gonads migrate caudally, probably accompanied by a portion of the spleen in cases of splenogonadal fusion. The limb buds and mandible are developing at the same time, accounting for the close association of splenogonadal fusion with peromelia and micrognathia.

Preoperative diagnosis of splenogonadal fusion by splenic scan may avoid unnecessary orchiectomy. Splenogonadal fusion and accessory spleen are important to consider when splenic ablation is needed.

ADRENAL HETEROTOPIA AND RENAL ECTOPIA

Adrenal cortical tissue may be present anywhere along the route of descent of the testis from the abdomen to the scrotum (Fig. 12-3). It is usually an incidental finding at inguinal herniorrhaphy or epididymoorchiectomy, present in up to 1% of children undergoing such operations. Adrenal cortical tissue has been identified in the inguinal hernia sac, spermatic cord[63] (see Fig. 12-3), epididymis,[64] and the rete testis. It may present as a small palpable tumor and appears as small yellow-orange nodules, usually near the inguinal ring. The lesions almost always consist of adrenal cortical tissue resembling zona glomerulosa and fasciculata. Rarely, they may contain medullary tissue. Involution during childhood is the rule, but exceptional cases persist and become functional, rarely harboring neoplasms or developing into "tumors" in adrenogenital syndrome and Nelson's syndrome. Removal of functional rests may result in adrenal insufficiency.

Ectopic renal tissue has rarely been observed in the scrotum, consisting of tubules and immature glomeruli.

WOLFFIAN AND MÜLLERIAN REMNANTS

Numerous embryonic remnants are found in the paratesticular area, including the appendix testis (hydatid of Morgagni), appendix epididymis, paradidymis, and vasa aberrans.[65]

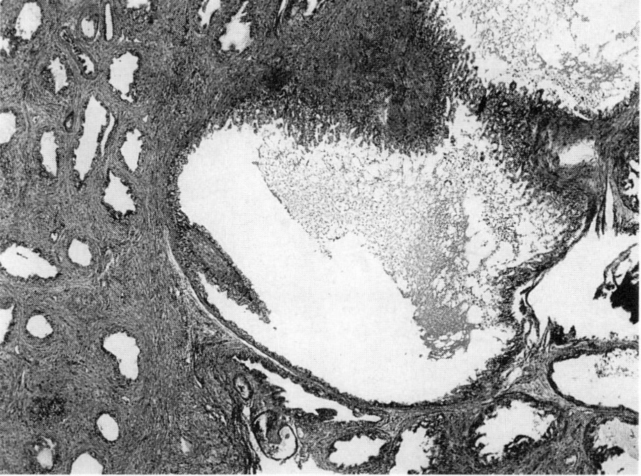

12-4. Small epididymal cyst which formed a palpable paratesticular mass.

Appendix testis (hydatid of Morgagni)

The appendix testis is present on more than 90% of testes at autopsy.[65] This structure is located at the superior pole of the testis adjacent to the epididymis. Grossly, it varies from 2 to 4 mm, appearing as a polypoid or sessile nodular excrescence. Microscopically, it contains a fibrovascular core of loose connective tissue covered by simple cuboidal or low columnar müllerian-type epithelium that is in continuity with the tunica vaginalis at the base. The fibrovascular core may contain tubular inclusions lined by similar cuboidal epithelium. Torsion of the appendix testis may be painful and mimic testicular torsion.[66,67]

Appendix epididymis (vestigial caudal mesonephric collecting tubule)

The appendix epididymis is present on about 35% of testicles examined at autopsy.[65] Grossly, it is a pedunculated spherical cystic or elongate structure arising from the anterosuperior pole of the head of the epididymis. Microscopically, it is lined by cuboidal to low columnar epithelium which may be ciliated and show secretory activity. The wall consists of loose connective tissue and is covered on its outer surface by flattened mesothelial cells that are continuous with the visceral tunica vaginalis. The appendix epididymis may become dilated by serous fluid and when enlarged, may mimic a tumor. Torsion may occur, sometimes in cryptorchidism.[67-69]

Paradidymis (organ of Giraldes)

This wolffian duct embryonic remnant consists of clusters of tubules lined by cuboidal to low columnar epithelium within the connective tissue of the spermatic cord, superior to the head of the epididymis.

Vasa aberrans (organ of Haller)

These wolffian duct remnants appear as clusters of tubules that are histologically similar to the paradidymis. They arise within the groove between the testis and epididymis. Torsion of the vas aberrans is rare.[67,70,71]

Other lesions associated with the epididymis

Other rare epididymal lesions have been described, including epididymal cyst (Fig. 12-4),[20,56-58,61] duplication,[33] and ectopic epididymal tissue associated with inguinal hernia.[61] Cyst and duplication may arise from the caudal vasa aberrantia.

Walthard's cell rest

This remnant, probably of müllerian origin, consists of solid and cystic nests of uniform epithelial cells with ovoid nuclei and characteristic longitudinal grooves.[72,73]

CYSTIC FIBROSIS

Cystic fibrosis is a genetic abnormality that often affects the testicular adnexa, resulting in infertility due to agenesis or atresia of mesonephric structures or anomalies of the testes (see Chapter 10).[19,27,74-83] Patients with congenital bilateral absence of vas deferens often have cystic fibrosis, although this finding may occur in patients without cystic fibrosis.[84-89]

NON-NEOPLASTIC DISEASES

CELES AND CYSTS

Hydrocele

A mesothelial-lined cyst, hydrocele results from accumulation of serous fluid between the parietal and visceral tunica vaginalis of the testis (Fig. 12-5). Congenital hydrocele occurs when a patent processus vaginalis within the spermatic cord communicates with the peritoneal cavity. The prevalence of congenital hydrocele is about 6% at birth and 1% in adulthood. Most cases of hydrocele are idiopathic but may be associated with inguinal hernia, scrotal trauma, epididymoorchitis, or tumors of the testis or paratesticular region.[12,59] Possible causes of idiopathic hydrocele include excessive secretion within the testicular tunics by parietal mesothelial cells, decreased reabsorption, and congenital absence of efferent lymphatics.

Hydrocele is lined by a single layer of cuboidal or flattened mesothelial cells, sometimes with prominent atypia,[90] with underlying connective tissue stroma. The luminal fluid is usually clear and serous unless complicated by infection or hemorrhage. The surface is often covered by fibrinous adhesions and inflammation, and subepithelial chronic inflammation and fibrosis may be present. In some cases, progressive fibrosis narrows or obliterates the cyst lumen, creating adhesions and multiple cysts. Spermatocele may rupture into the hydrocele sac.

Hematocele (hematoma)

Hematocele refers to the accumulation of blood in the space between the parietal and visceral tunica vaginalis, often in association with hydrocele (see Fig. 12-5). Long-standing hematocele becomes calcified and fibrotic, with numerous hemosiderin-laden macrophages. The causes of hematocele are similar to those for hydrocele.

Idiopathic hematoma may arise in the spermatic cord[91] or epididymis.[92]

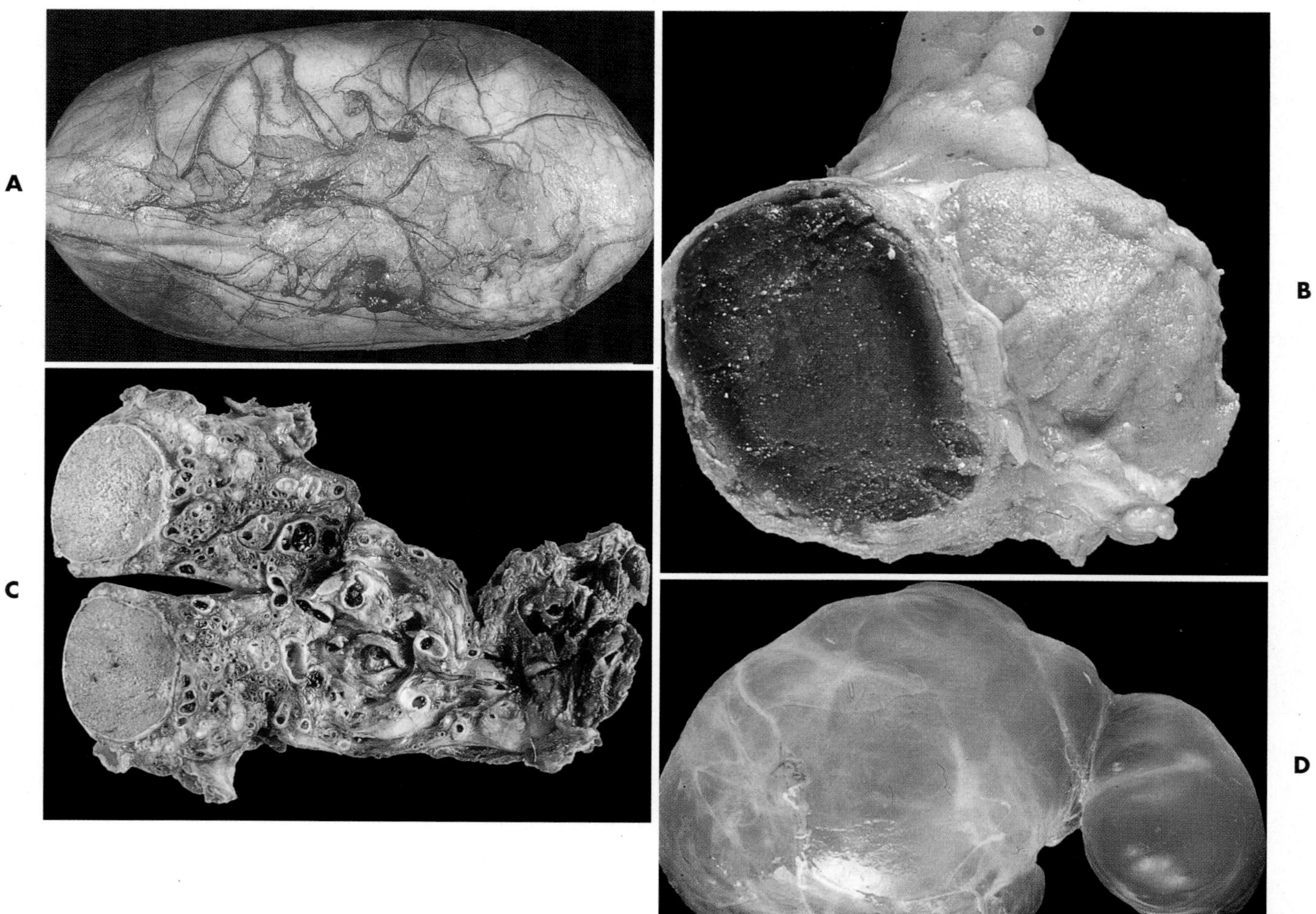

12-5. **A**, Hydrocele. **B**, Encapsulated hematocele. **C**, Varicocele. **D**, Spermatocele.

Varicocele

Varicocele is a mass of dilated tortuous veins of the pampiniform venous plexus of the spermatic cord which occurs posterior and superior to the testis, sometimes extending into the inguinal ring (see Fig. 12-5). The venous plexus normally empties into the internal spermatic vein near the internal inguinal ring; poor drainage and progressive dilation and elongation result from incompetent valves of the left internal spermatic vein which empties into the renal vein.[93] The right internal spermatic vein is less likely to be involved with varicocele because it drains directly into the inferior vena cava and is less likely to have incompetent valves.

Varicocele results from a number of conditions, but most cases are idiopathic. Unilateral varicocele in older men may indicate the presence of a renal tumor that has invaded the renal vein and occluded the spermatic vein drainage. Varicocele has been reported in association with maternal exposure to diethylstilbestrol.[94] Patients with varicocele sometimes present with testicular pain associated with sexual activity.

Long-standing varicocele causes testicular atrophy and infertility in the affected testis. Treatment consists of ligation of the internal spermatic vein at the level of the internal inguinal ring, and does not usually yield a pathologic specimen for analysis.

Spermatocele (acquired epididymal cyst)

Spermatocele is a dilation of an efferent ductule in the region of the rete testis or caput epididymis (see Chapter 10). The inner lining consists of a single layer of cuboidal to flattened epithelial cells which are often ciliated. The wall is composed of fibromuscular soft tissue, often with chronic inflammation, and the cyst may be unilocular or multilocular (see Fig. 12-5). Spermatocele is distinguished from hydrocele by the presence of spermatozoa within the cyst fluid, a distinction that can be made by aspiration cytology. Torsion is a rare complication of spermatocele.[95]

Benign papilloma may arise within the epithelial lining of spermatocele.[96] The papillae contain fibrovascular cores lined by a single layer of columnar epithelium with vacuolated cytoplasm. The epithelium appears cytologically benign, and there is no evidence of subepithelial invasion.

Mesothelial cyst

Mesothelial cyst arises within the tunica vaginalis, tunica albuginea, or, less commonly, the epididymis and spermatic cord.[60,97] The cyst may be single or multiple, measuring up to 2.5 cm in diameter and is lined by a single layer of uniform cuboidal to flattened attenuated mesothelial cells.

Mesothelial cyst of the tunica vaginalis arises from the connective tissue of the tunica. There may be nodular or diffuse proliferation of mesothelial cells, sometimes with squamous metaplasia. This cyst is probably an embryonic remnant or an inclusion of vaginalis mesothelium resulting from inflammation, trauma, or neoplasm, similar to mesothelial cyst of the tunica albuginea.

Mesothelial cyst of the tunica albuginea most often occurs in men over 40 years of age, but all ages are affected. It is usually located anterior and lateral to the testis, measuring up to 4 cm in diameter. The cyst is filled with clear or blood-tinged serous fluid, and the lining consists of typical mesothelial cells with a wall composed of hyalinized fibrous tissue.

Unilocular and multilocular mesothelial cyst of the spermatic cord is rare and probably arises from embryonic mesothelial remnants such as the processus vaginalis.

Epidermoid cyst (epidermal cyst)

Epidermoid cyst is common in the testis, comprising about 1% of testicular tumors, but it may also rarely arise in the paratesticular area and epididymis. Epidermoid cyst consists of a lining of benign keratinizing squamous epithelium and a wall composed of fibrous connective tissue, often with inflammation. Diligent search is required to exclude the presence of adnexal structures or teratomatous elements. Paratesticular epidermoid cyst may arise from squamous metaplasia of wolffian duct structures, displacement of squamous epithelium from the scrotal skin to paratesticular structures during embryogenesis, squamous metaplasia of mesothelial cyst, or monomorphic epidermal development of a teratoma. Epidermoid cyst in the paratesticular area does not recur after surgical excision. Some consider this tumor a cholesteatoma when it arises in the epididymis.[98]

Dermoid cyst (mature teratoma)

Dermoid cyst most often involves the testis and paratesticular structures, but it may occur in the spermatic cord and, very rarely, in the testicular tunics.[54,99] This cyst measures up to 4 cm in diameter and contains soft, cheesy yellow-white amorphous material with or without hair and calcifications. The cyst is lined by keratinized squamous epithelium, and the wall contains typical dermal adnexal structures such as pilosebaceous units, although these may be difficult to identify without thorough sectioning. Dermoid cyst does not recur or metastasize after excision.

Simple cyst of rete testis

Tejada and Eble[100] reported a simple cyst of the rete testis occurring in a 66-year-old man. This unilocular cyst measured 1 cm in diameter, was lined by normal rete testis tubular epithelium, and bulged into the testis proper.

INFLAMMATORY AND REACTIVE DISEASES

Epididymitis

Epididymitis may be acute or chronic, depending on the inciting agent and the duration of infection. It usually occurs in association with orchitis or after trauma but rarely is an isolated finding. Most cases result from retrograde spread by vesicoepididymal urine reflux, but hematogenous and lymphatic spread account for some cases. Congenital anomalies such as ureteral ectopia may cause epididymitis in infants. The surgical pathologist rarely receives specimens of these diseases. Urethral and epididymal smears and cultures are useful in identifying the causative infectious agent.

Acute epididymitis. Patients with acute epididymitis usually have unilateral painful enlargement of the epididymis and scrotum, more commonly on the right side, often involving the testicle (50% of cases have epididymoorchitis) and vas deferens (Fig. 12-6).[101-104] The epididymis is thickened, congested, and edematous, with white fibrinopurulent exudate in the tubules and stroma. Microabscesses and fistulae may occur, but rupture is uncommon. The tubules may be damaged or destroyed by the inflammation, sometimes with squamous metaplasia and regenerative changes.

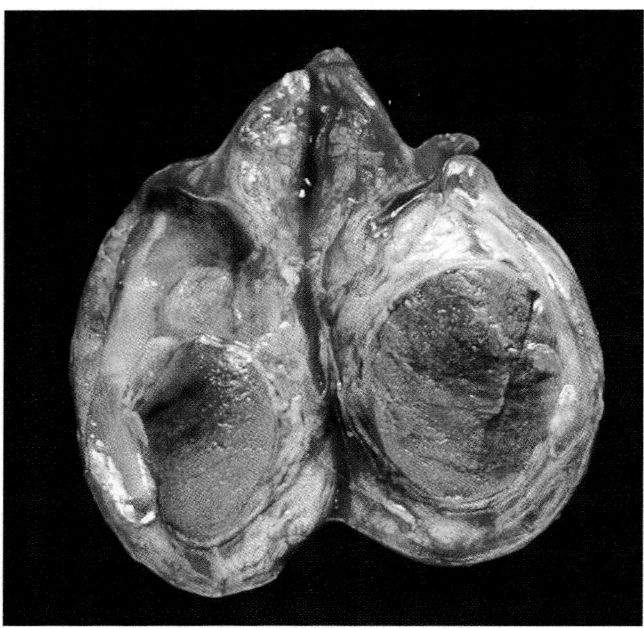

12-6. Acute epididymitis with associated testicular infarction.

Acute epididymitis is commonly caused by bacteria.[101,103,105,106] Coliforms account for most cases in children, whereas *Neisseria gonorrhoeae* and *Chlamydia trachomatis* are most frequent in young men, and *Escherichia coli* and *Pseudomonas* predominate in older men. Other bacteria that may cause acute epididymitis include *Klebsiella, Staphylococcus, Streptococcus pneumoniae, Neisseria meningitidis, Aerobacter aerogenes*, and *Haemophilus influenzae*. The epididymis is a reservoir for *N. gonorrhoeae*, and while infection may be asymptomatic, microabscesses and edema are common, usually without extensive necrosis. The round cytoplasmic inclusions of *C. trachomatis* are difficult to identify in hematoxylin-eosin stained sections, and immunohistochemical stains, culture, or genotypic studies are usually required.[106-108]

Clinical and histopathologic findings allow separation of some cases of chlamydial and bacterial epididymitis (Table 12-2). *C. trachomatis*–positive cases are clinically indolent, with minimally destructive periductal and intraepithelial inflammation with epithelial regeneration. Lymphoepithelial complexes and squamous metaplasia are sometimes present. *E. coli*–positive cases are characterized by scrotal pain, pyuria, leukocytosis, and highly destructive epididymitis with abscesses and xanthogranulomas.[106]

Viral causes of acute epididymitis include mumps and cytomegalovirus, similar to those causing orchitis (see Chapter 10).[109] Mumps epididymitis, present in 85% of

TABLE 12-2.
COMPARISON OF BACTERIAL AND CHLAMYDIAL EPIDIDYMITIS*

	Bacterial Epididymitis†	Chlamydial Epididymitis
CLINICAL FEATURES		
Patient age (yr)	59.8 (39–79)	42.8 (22–74)
Pain	Yes	Infrequent
LABORATORY FEATURES		
Pyuria	Frequent	Infrequent
Elevated ESR	Yes	No
Elevated C-Reactive Protein	Yes	No
PATHOLOGIC FEATURES		
Tissue Destruction	Yes	Minimal
Xanthogranulomas	Yes	Minimal
Abscesses and Necrosis	Yes	Minimal
Cytoplasmic Location of Antigens	Histiocytes	Epithelial Cells

*For details see Hori S, Tsutsumi Y: Histologic differentiation and bacterial epididymitis: nondestructive and proliferative versus destructive and abscess forming—immunohistochemical and clinicopathologic findings, Hum Pathol 26:402–407, 1995.
ESR, erythrocytic sedimentation rate.
†Usually *E.coli*.

cases of mumps orchitis, occurs before testicular involvement, usually appearing as unilateral scrotal swelling following parotiditis. The epididymis shows vascular congestion, edema, and interstitial lymphocytic inflammation; neutrophils are usually not a prominent feature. Cytomegaloviral epididymitis may occur in patients with AIDS.

Traumatic acute epididymitis is characterized by vascular congestion, petechial hemorrhages, and hematocele. Drugs such as amiodarone may also cause epididymitis.[110]

Chronic epididymitis. Although many cases of acute epididymitis resolve, some become chronic. The epididymis in chronic epididymitis is indurated and scarred, with cystically dilated tubules, marked fibrosis, chronic inflammation, and sperm granulomas (see discussion on sperm granuloma in this chapter). The epithelium shows reactive or metaplastic changes, often with cytoplasmic vacuolization and lumenal hyaline aggregates. Epididymitis nodosa, a proliferative lesion of the epididymis, may result from chronic inflammation or trauma, reminiscent of vasitis nodosa.[111] Coarse granular cytoplasmic changes appear in the epididymis in the setting of ductal obstruction or epididymal compression and probably result from heterophagic degradation of ductal contents, according to Schned and Memoli (see Fig. 12-2).[112] Calcification is common in chronic epididymitis,[113] and there may be a foreign body giant cell reaction. Xanthogranulomatous epididymitis may also occur.[114] Special stains for bacteria and fungi may be of value.

Specific causes of chronic epididymitis include tuberculosis, leprosy, malakoplakia, sarcoidosis, and sperm granuloma. The epididymis is the reservoir for tuberculous involvement in the male genital tract, with secondary testicular involvement and other local sites of involvement in about 80% of cases[115-117]; for example, 40% of cases of renal tuberculosis are accompanied by epididymal infection. Patients usually have painless scrotal swelling, but other signs and symptoms include unilateral or bilateral mass, infertility, and scrotal fistula. Caseating granulomatous inflammation is prominent, with fibrous thickening and enlargement of the epididymis and adjacent structures (Fig. 12-7). Rarely, miliary tuberculosis causes small punctate white lesions. The auramine-rhodamine stain is preferred over the Ziehl-Neelsen stain because of its greater sensitivity.

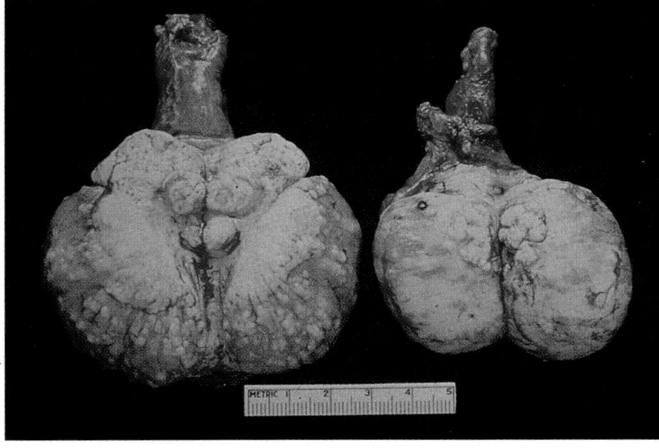

12-7. Tuberculosis of the epididymis and testis.

Lepromatous leprosy frequently involves the epididymis, usually following testicular involvement, but rarely spreads to the vas deferens.[118,119] Patients complain of painful scrotal swelling, and the epididymis and testes are thickened and enlarged. The inflammation consists chiefly of perivascular and perineural lymphocytic infiltrates, often with sheets of macrophages containing acid-fast bacilli set in a dense sclerotic stroma. Sterility results from testicular azoospermia rather than epididymal blockage. The dartos muscle of the testicular tunics shows a predilection for lepromatous myositis.

Malakoplakia of the epididymis is uncommon, usually occurring with testicular involvement.[120-122] Patients are asymptomatic or present with painful scrotal swelling or hydrocele. The histologic findings are similar to malakoplakia at other sites.

Sarcoidosis involves the genital tract in about 5% of cases at autopsy, but it is rarely symptomatic. The epididymis is the most common site of genital involvement.[123-127] Patients present with painful or painless scrotal swelling, which is bilateral in about 33% of cases. Non-necrotizing granulomatous inflammation is typical, similar to involvement at other sites. The main differential diagnostic consideration is sperm granuloma, but extravasated sperm are absent in sarcoidosis.

Epididymitis may also result from other fungi, bacteria, parasites, and viruses. *Histoplasma capsulatum* creates necrotizing inflammation and abscesses that mimic sperm granuloma; typical silver-stained 2 to 4 μm fungal spores are usually present.[128] *Coccidioides immitis* produces necrotizing and non-necrotizing granulomas of the epididymis and prostate; silver-stained fungal spherules measuring about 100 μm in diameter contain numerous endospores.[129] Systemic *Blastomyces dermatitidis* involves the epididymis in up to 30% of systemic cases, producing microabscesses that contain silver-stained budding fungal spores up to 15 μm in diameter with thick refractile capsules.[130] Other causes of epididymitis include *Paracoccidioides brasiliensis*, *Actinomyces*, *Sporothrix schenckii*,[131] *Schistosoma haematobium*,[132,133] *Treponema pallidum*, typhoid, brucellosis, rickettsia, and hydatid cyst. The degenerating worms of *Wucheria bancrofti* filariasis produce granulomas, often with prominent tissue and blood eosinophilia[134-136]; scrotal and penile elephantiasis results from lymphatic obstruction.

Sperm granuloma. Sperm granuloma is an exuberant foreign body giant cell reaction to extravasated sperm, and occurs in up to 42% of patients after vasectomy and 2.5% of routine autopsies.[137-140] Patients may have no symptoms but often present with a history of pain and swelling of the upper pole of the epididymis, spermatic cord, and, rarely, testis. Others have a history of trauma, epididymiditis, and orchitis. In some cases, sperm granuloma mimics testicular or spermatic cord tumor.[141]

Sperm granuloma appears as a solitary yellow nodule or multiple, small, indurated nodules measuring up to 3 cm in diameter. Foreign body–type granulomas are present, with necrosis in the early stages and progressive fibrosis in late stages (Fig. 12-8). Extravasated sperm are often present in large numbers, but they are quickly engulfed by macrophages (referred to as *spermiophages*) and eventually disappear. Yellow-brown ceroid pigment, a lipid degradation product of sperm, may persist, and is recognized by acid-fast stain or autofluorescence. Vasitis nodosa (see discussion on vasitis and vasitis nodosa in this chapter) occurs in about one third of cases of sperm granuloma.

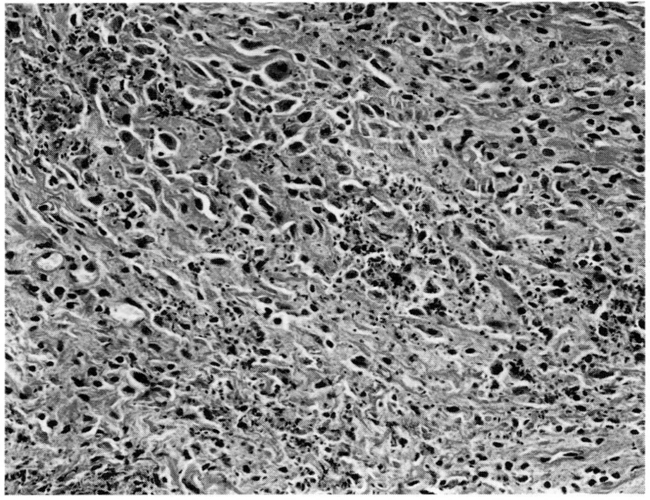

12-8. Sperm granuloma.

Disruption of the tubules and extravasation of sperm results in sperm granuloma, but isolated sperm may be present in the interstitium without significant inflammation. Cord ligation vasectomy accounts for most cases of sperm granuloma, whereas cauterization vasectomy rarely results in granuloma.[140] Experimental injection of ceroid pigment produces granulomatous inflammation, suggesting that destruction of sperm initiates the process. An autoimmune process has been proposed but is not favored.

Vasitis and vasitis nodosa

Inflammation of the vas deferens (vasitis, or deferentitis) usually occurs in association with epididymitis or posterior urethritis.[142,143] Vasitis nodosa is a benign ductular proliferation that produces nodular and fusiform enlargement of the vas deferens, often following vasectomy.[111,144-156] It resembles salpingitis isthmica nodosa and clinically mimics sperm granuloma.

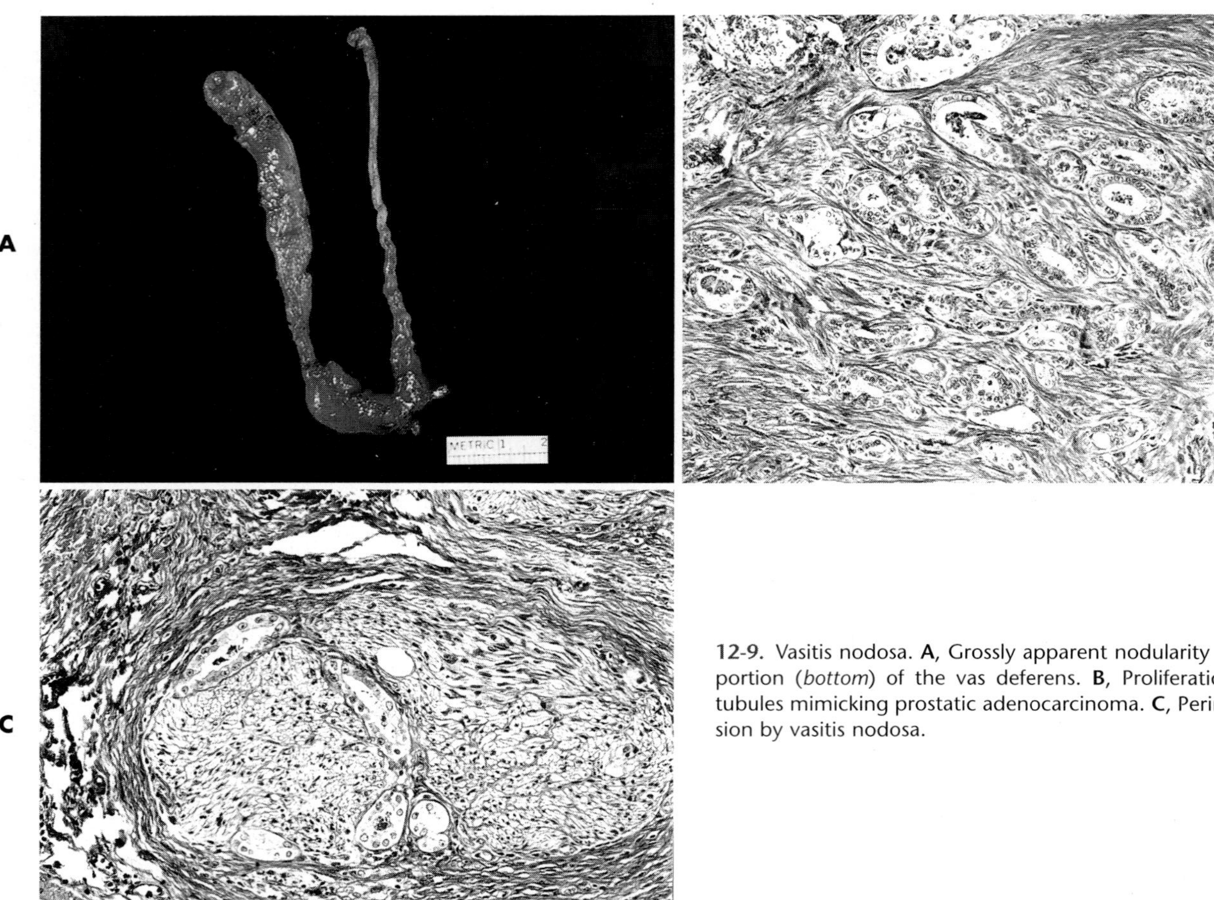

12-9. Vasitis nodosa. **A,** Grossly apparent nodularity in the midportion (*bottom*) of the vas deferens. **B,** Proliferation of small tubules mimicking prostatic adenocarcinoma. **C,** Perineural invasion by vasitis nodosa.

In vasitis nodosa, the vas deferens may be more than 1 cm in diameter, with diffuse enlargement or rounded, indurated masses punctuated by small lumens. The ductular proliferation is prominent and may be mistaken histologically for metastatic prostatic adenocarcinoma (Fig. 12-9). Chronic inflammation and fibrosis are always observed, although in variable amounts, and are sometimes accompanied by muscular hyperplasia of the wall. The ductules vary from discrete, round acinar structures to plexiform masses of irregular acini. The cells are cuboidal or low columnar, with a moderate amount of pale granular cytoplasm; central, large nuclei with uniform chromatin; and single enlarged nucleoli. Cilia may be present. Perineural invasion is common and often extensive and may be mistaken for malignancy[144,151,154]; benign vascular invasion may also occur.[145] Sperm granulomas are present in about 50% of cases, and sperm are often present in the acinar lumens of vasitis nodosa. As the number of sperm granulomas declines, the amount of ceroid pigment increases, resulting from lipid breakdown products of spermatozoa. A histologically similar process may occur in the epididymis, referred to by Schned and Selikowitz[111] as epididymitis nodosa.

Vasitis nodosa is a benign reactive process. Trauma or surgery results in epithelial rupture with a release of sperm into the soft tissues of the vas deferens, invariably invoking a prominent fibroinflammatory response.[152,156] However, some cases have no history of trauma and are idiopathic.

Funiculitis (inflammation of spermatic cord). Inflammation of the spermatic cord, or funiculitis, often accompanies vasitis, usually as the result of direct extension from the vas deferens, but isolated involvement may occur by hematogenous spread from other sites of inflammation. Funiculitis appears as painful enlargement of the spermatic cord. Tuberculous funiculitis is rare, presenting as multiple large, discrete masses or diffuse thickening with typical necrotizing granulomatous inflammation. Perforation of an incarcerated hernia may cause extravasation of fecal contents and vegetable fibers, resulting in an exuberant foreign body giant cell reaction in the cord. Sclerosing endophlebitis and thrombosis of the pampiniform plexus may accompany funiculitis, resulting in necrosis and gangrene.[157]

Meconium-induced inflammation

Prenatal or antenatal perforation of the colon may cause meconium leakage through the patent processus vaginalis into the scrotum, resulting in foreign body giant cell reaction, chronic inflammation, and scarring; this is also called *meconium periorchitis, meconium granuloma,* or *meconium vaginalisitis*.[158,159] Fewer than 30 cases have been reported, rarely in association with cystic fibrosis. Grossly, the tunica vaginalis contains a single mass or is studded with numerous orange or green nodules composed of chronically inflamed myxoid stroma, sometimes containing bile, cholesterol, or lanugo hairs within histiocytes. Hydrocele is often present.

Vasculitis

Systemic vasculitides may affect the epididymal and testicular vessels, sometimes resulting in hydrocele or swelling of the affected structures.[160-162] Polyarteritis nodosa is observed in these vessels at autopsy in 80% of affected patients, although clinical involvement is rare. Isolated epididymal or spermatic cord involvement has been reported.[163-166] Levine[167] found that there were no histopathologic differences between system vasculitis and isolated necrotizing vasculitis of testicular and epididymal tissue.

OTHER NON-NEOPLASTIC DISEASES

Torsion of spermatic cord and embryonic remnants

Torsion of the spermatic cord results in hemorrhagic infarction of the testis; this is described in detail in Chapter 10. Torsion of the embryonic remnants, discussed here, is a much rarer event that may clinically mimic torsion of the cord.

Torsion is a common abnormality of the appendix testis.[66,67] Patients complain of acute scrotal pain, often following vigorous exercise. About 90% of patients are boys between 10 and 12 years of age, but men of all ages are affected. Typical histologic features of torsion are present, including severe congestion, edema, and hemorrhagic infarction.

Torsion of the appendix epididymis is much less common than the appendix testis, and the histologic findings are similar.[67-69] Torsion of the vasa aberrantia is extremely rare, with fewer than 10 reported cases.[70,71]

Calculi and calcification

Acute and chronic epididymitis and vasitis predispose to calculus formation, usually in the epididymis, vas deferens, and scrotum (Fig. 12-10).[113,137,168] The calculi are composed of phosphates and carbonates and are brown stones up to 1 cm in diameter.

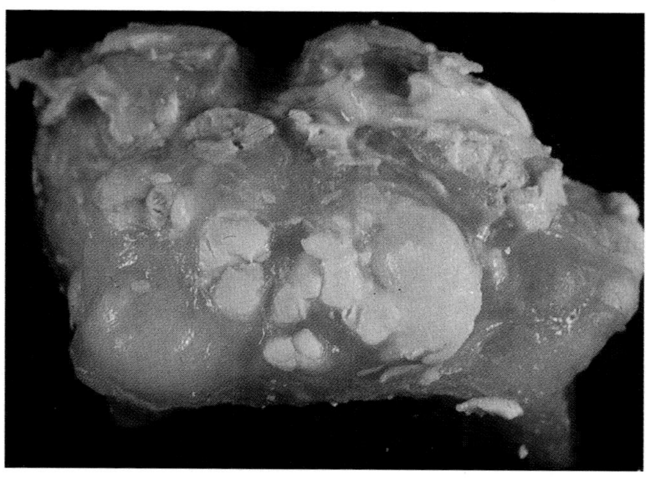

12-10. Idiopathic scrotal and epididymal calcinosis in an otherwise healthy 37-year-old man forming a multinodular mass measuring 3 cm in greatest dimension.

Idiopathic mural calcification of the vas deferens occurs in up to 15% of diabetics. These deposits in the smooth muscle are focal and variable in appearance, rarely with osseous metaplasia. Inflammation-induced calcifications are scattered throughout the smooth muscle, usually associated with chronic inflammation and fibrosis.

NEOPLASMS

BENIGN NEOPLASMS AND PSEUDOTUMORS

A variety of unusual tumors and tumorlike proliferations arise in the paratesticular region, often of uncertain histogenesis. Because of the rarity of many of these benign tumors, they may be erroneously considered malignant.

Lipoma

Lipoma is the most common paratesticular tumor, accounting for up to 90% of spermatic cord tumors (Fig. 12-11).[169-171] Lipoma usually occurs in adults but may be seen at all ages. Grossly, it is a circumscribed unencapsulated mass of lobulated yellow adipose tissue up to 30 cm in diameter and weighing as much as 3.2 kg.[172] The microscopic appearance is similar to lipoma at other sites, consisting of mature adipose tissue. Variants include angiolipoma, fibrolipoma,[172] fibromyxolipoma, myxolipoma, and myxoid myolipoma.[60] Hibernoma may also occur.[173]

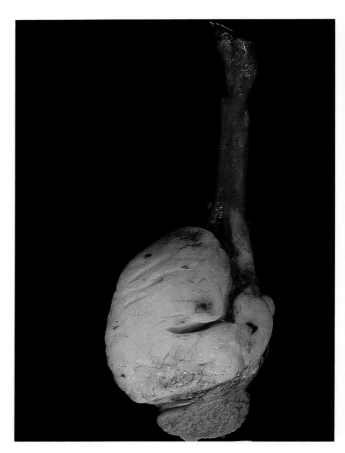

12-11. Lipoma of the cord dwarfing the testis.

Adenomatoid hyperplasia

Adenomatoid hyperplasia rarely occurs in the rete testis and epididymis (see Chapter 10). Srigley and Hartwick[60] described three cases involving the collecting duct epithelium of the rete testis, including two patients with testicular mass and one patient who underwent epididymo-orchiectomy for other reasons with incidental finding of adenomatous hyperplasia. Adenomatoid hyperplasia consists of a poorly circumscribed tubulopapillary proliferation of the rete testis or epididymis lined by uniform benign epithelial cells; there is no stromal invasion or other features of malignancy. Follow-up information was not available in reported cases, but this lesion is considered benign.

One case of adenomatoid hyperplasia involved the head of the epididymis in a 46-year-old man, measuring 1.5 cm in greatest dimension.[60] The lesion consisted of a proliferation of benign ductules and normal epididymal ducts. Many of the cells showed cytoplasmic clearing similar to that seen in papillary cystadenoma of the epididymis, but papillary-cystic architecture and circumscription were absent.

Adenomatoid tumor (benign nonpapillary mesothelioma)

Adenomatoid tumor is the most common tumor of the epididymis and cord and second in frequency only to lipoma in the paratesticular area; it accounted for 32% of paratesticular tumors in a series that excluded lipoma.[96,174] It also arises in the tunica vaginalis or tunica albuginea, and may be present in association with hydrocele.[60,174-189]

Adenomatoid tumor is usually seen in men between 20 and 50 years of age but has been reported in men as old as 79 years. Patients often present with a painless scrotal mass, but some lesions are found incidentally at epididymoorchiectomy or autopsy. Adenomatoid tumor consists of a firm circumscribed solid mass measuring up to 2 cm in greatest dimension, usually arising in the head of the epididymis or rarely in the lower pole of the epididymis, testicular tunics, or spermatic cord. The cut surface is homogeneous and white-gray (Fig. 12-12). The characteristic microscopic finding is irregular tubules, cell nests, and solid trabeculae of cuboidal to flattened epithelioid or endothelioid cells (see Fig. 12-12). The tumor cells are eosinophilic, with variably sized cytoplasmic vacuoles. In some cases, excessive vacuolization creates thin strands of cytoplasm spanning lumens; alternatively, it creates a signet ring cell pattern. Nuclei are small and vesicular with inconspicuous nucleoli. The stroma contains fibroblasts, blood vessels, and smooth muscle. Focal stromal hyalinization may be present, and the tumor may infiltrate the testis. Adenomatoid leiomyoma consists of adenomatoid tumor in association with prominent smooth muscle.[174]

Tumor cell cytoplasm contains hyaluronidase-sensitive acid mucopolysaccharides, similar to mesothelioma.[189] Immunohistochemistry reveals cytoplasmic immunoreactivity for cytokeratin in most cases, focal lumenal surface staining with epithelial membrane antigen in some cases,

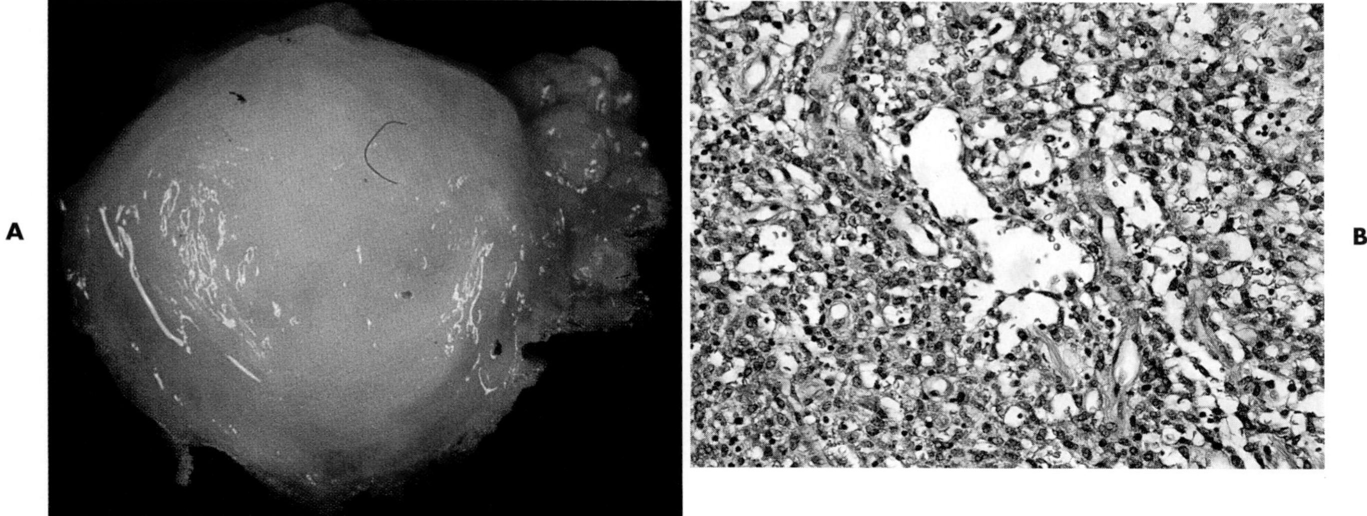

12-12. Adenomatoid tumor of the epididymis. **A**, Grossly, the tumor is a firm white-gray mass. **B**, Anastomosing tubules lined by cells with small nuclei and punctuated by thin-walled vessels.

and negative staining for carcinoembryonic antigen, vimentin, Factor VIII–related antigen, and *Ulex europaeus* agglutinin 1, although focal lumenal staining for Factor VIII has been occasionally reported.[183,188] Ultrastructural studies reveal mesothelial differentiation, including slender microvilli, intermediate filaments adjacent to the nuclei, intracellular canaliculi, desmosomes, basal lamina, and transition forms with features of both typical mesothelial cells and stromal spindle cells.[185,187,189] Mesothelial origin is likely for adenomatoid tumor because of the anatomic continuity between the surface mesothelium of the tunica vaginalis and tumor cells in some cases, as well as the identification of rare adenomatoid tumor in the abdominal peritoneum. The mesothelial theory of histogenesis has displaced earlier theories, including endothelial origin, mesonephric origin, and müllerian origin.

Despite the potential for local invasion, adenomatoid tumor is benign, with no metastatic potential. Intraoperative frozen section diagnosis allows local resection with preservation of the epididymis and testis. This tumor may recur if incompletely excised but does not recur after complete excision.

Hamartoma

One case of hamartoma of the rete testis arose in a 2-year-old as a testicular mass.[60] The tumor consisted of a disorganized cluster of tubules embedded in a loose connective tissue stroma. The tubules were lined by cells that were cytologically similar to normal rete testis. Hamartoma of the spermatic cord may be composed chiefly of smooth muscle (Fig. 12-13) or fibrous connective tissue.[190]

Osseous metaplasia of epididymis

Localized osseous metaplasia of the epididymis occurs sporadically or in association with fibrous pseudotumor, sometimes forming a mass that may be mistaken for a neoplasm.[60] Microscopically, it consists of trabecular bone set in connective tissue stroma.

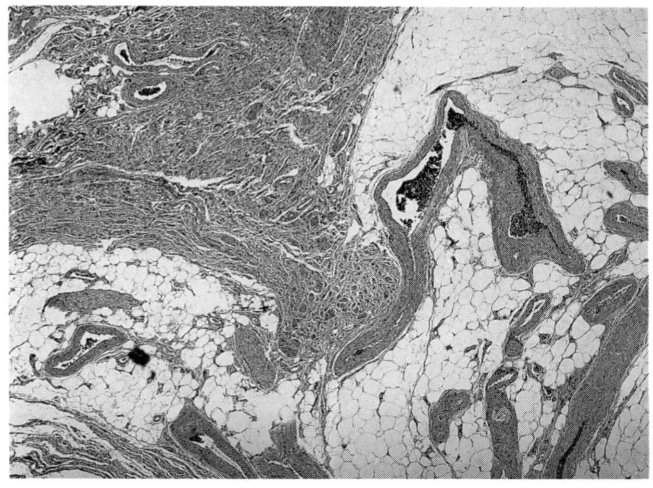

12-13. Smooth muscle hamartoma of the epididymis.

Reactive mesothelial hyperplasia

Reactive mesothelial hyperplasia appears as a small solid nodule of mesothelial cells, which is usually microscopic and clinically asymptomatic.[96,191] It probably arises as a result of mechanical irritation or inflammation. Reactive mesothelial hyperplasia has also been described in association with hydrocele, hematocele, inguinal hernia sac,[191] and fibrous pseudotumor.[96] Reactive hyperplasia consists of solid nests, tubules, simple papillae, or small cysts of cytologically benign mesothelium set in a fibrous stroma, often appearing beneath the surface mesothelium. Mild cytologic atypia may be present, and squamous metaplasia is rarely seen. Histologic mimics include benign papillary mesothelioma, malignant mesothelioma, and metastatic adenocarcinoma. Benign papillary mesothelioma usually has more complex papillary architecture.

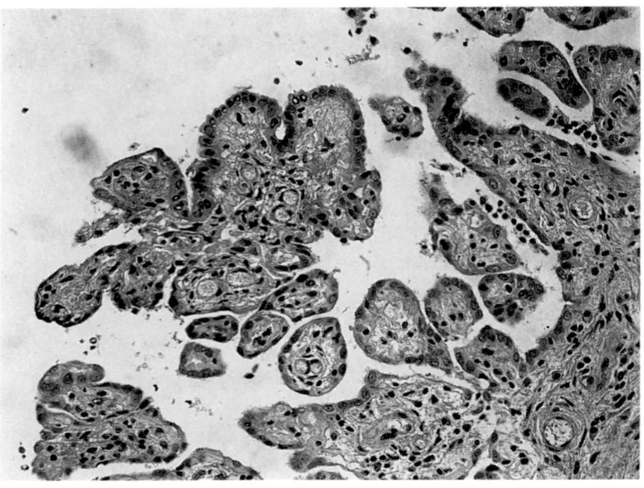

12-14. Benign papillary mesothelioma of the tunica vaginalis.

Malignant mesothelioma is also architecturally complex, often with nuclear atypia, increased mitotic activity, and stromal infiltration. Metastatic adenocarcinoma usually shows severe nuclear abnormalities which stand in contrast with the adjacent surface mesothelium; stains for neutral or hyaluronidase-resistant mucin may also be of value, with positive staining suggesting adenocarcinoma rather than mesothelioma.

Benign papillary mesothelioma

A rare tumor of the tunica vaginalis, benign papillary mesothelioma usually appears in young men.[192-194] Grossly, it consists of a hydrocele sac with papillary excrescences and cystic or solid areas. Microscopically, there are complex papillae covered by cuboidal, columnar, or flattened mesothelial cells with large vesicular nuclei and glassy eosinophilic cytoplasm (Fig. 12-14). There is no significant nuclear atypia. Careful search

A

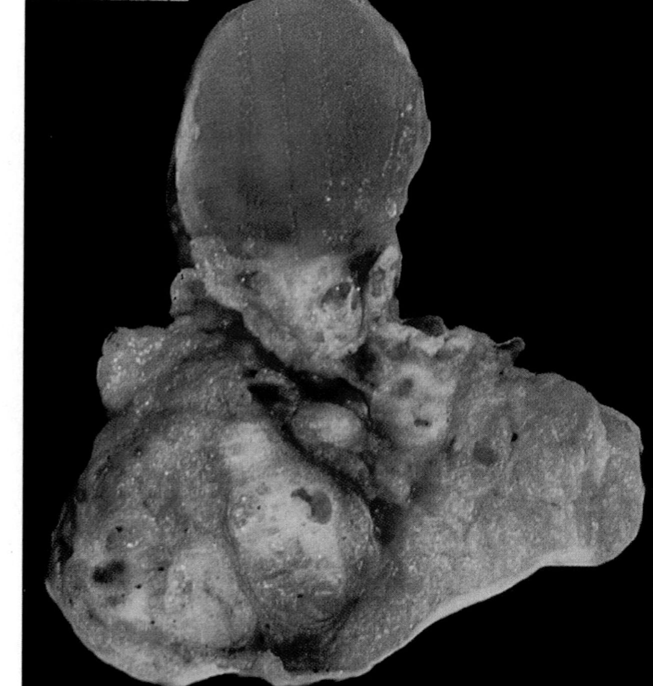

B

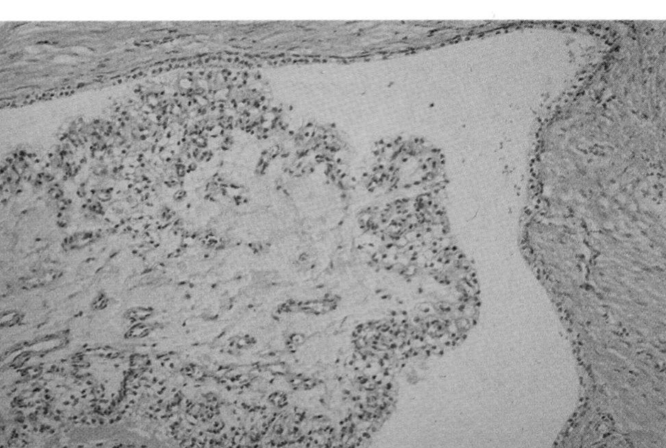

C

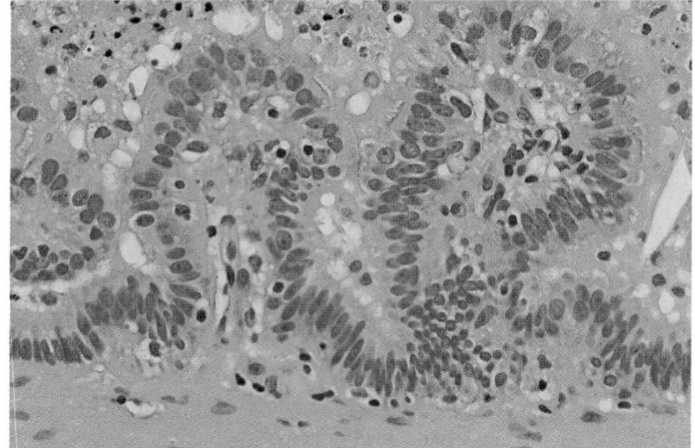

12-15. Papillary cystadenoma of the epididymis. **A**, Grossly, the tumor consists of a tan-brown mass. **B**, Cystic space containing well-formed papillae. This 35-year-old man has a history of von Hippel-Lindau disease, including bilateral renal cell carcinoma and cerebellar and retinal hemangioblastomas. **C**, A case of papillary cystadenoma from a patient without a history of von Hippel-Lindau disease. *(**A** and **B** courtesy Dr. Bernd Scheithauer.)*

should be made to determine if the papillary lining of the tumor is in continuity with the mesothelium of the adjacent tunica vaginalis. Psammoma bodies are often present. The tumor contains hyaluronidase-sensitive mucin, and ultrastructural study reveals mesothelial differentiation of tumor cells.

Papillary cystadenoma of epididymis

Papillary cystadenoma of the epididymis is a benign tumor that accounts for about one third of all primary epididymal tumors.[60,174,195-210] It occurs in males between 16 and 81 years of age, with a mean of 36 years. More than 50 cases have been reported, including one with coexistent adenomatoid leiomyoma. About 40% of cases of papillary cystadenoma of the epididymis are bilateral, and these appear as cystic masses in the head of the epididymis which measure up to 6 cm in diameter. The cut surface is gray-brown with yellow foci and often contains cyst fluid that varies from clear and colorless to yellow, green, or blood-tinged (Fig. 12-15). Microscopically, papillary cystadenoma consists of dilated ducts lined by papillae with a single or double layer of cuboidal to low columnar epithelium (see Fig. 12-15). The cells have characteristic clear glycogen-filled cytoplasm with secretory droplets and cilia at the surface. The papillary cores and cyst walls consist of fibrous connective tissue that may be hyalinized or inflamed, sometimes with a lipogranulomatous reaction. Solid cords of cells occasionally abut the cyst wall.

About two thirds of cases of papillary cystadenoma of the epididymis occur in patients with von Hippel-Lindau syndrome, and they are more frequently bilateral in this syndrome.[199,209] Other manifestations of von Hippel-Lindau syndrome include hemangioblastoma of the cerebellum, cerebrum, spinal cord, retina, pancreas, and urinary bladder; meningioma; syringomyelia; paraganglioma; renal cell carcinoma; pheochromocytoma; islet cell tumor; adrenal cortical adenoma; and a variety of cysts of the liver, kidney, adrenal, and pancreas.

Fibrous pseudotumor (nodular and diffuse fibrous proliferation)

Fibrous pseudotumor encompasses a wide variety of fibroproliferative lesions of the testicular tunics, epididymis, and spermatic cord.[60,211-215] This lesion has been referred to as chronic periorchitis, fibrous proliferation of the tunics, fibroma, nonspecific paratesticular fibrosis, nodular fibrous periorchitis, nodular fibropseudotumor, inflammatory pseudotumor, reactive periorchitis, and pseudofibromatous periorchitis. Early cases of spermatic cord and epididymal fibroma were probably fibrous pseudotumor.[216,217] This non-neoplastic fibroinflammatory reactive lesion clinically mimics testicular and paratesticular neoplasms. Patients are usually in the third decade of life, but age ranges from 7 to 95 years. It usually involves the tunics and may be associated with hydrocele, hematocele, or both. Less commonly, the epididymis or spermatic cord are involved. A history of epididymoorchitis, trauma, or inflamed hydrocele is often elicited.

Fibrous pseudotumor is a nodular or diffuse thickening of firm white tissue up to 9.5 cm in diameter, often with focal yellow calcifications (Fig.12-16). Histologically, it consists of granulation tissue with chronic inflammation, but long-standing tumors contain only paucicellular hyalinized fibrous connective tissue with calcification and ossification. Mostofi and Price[96] believed that 50% of cases of fibrous pseudotumor in the spermatic cord display the histologic findings of sclerosing lipogranuloma (Fig. 12-17) or sclerosing hemangioma, but still considered it reactive.

The differential diagnosis includes fibrous mesothelioma (solitary fibrous tumor), idiopathic fibromatosis, neurofibroma, and leiomyoma. Fibrous mesothelioma of the tunica vaginalis consists of cells with abundant eosinophilic cytoplasm set in a background of interlacing keratin-immunoreactive spindle cells. Ultrastructural studies indicate mesothelial origin for fibrous mesothelioma, unlike fibrous pseudotumor. Idiopathic fibromatosis may be seen in association with fibromatosis of the

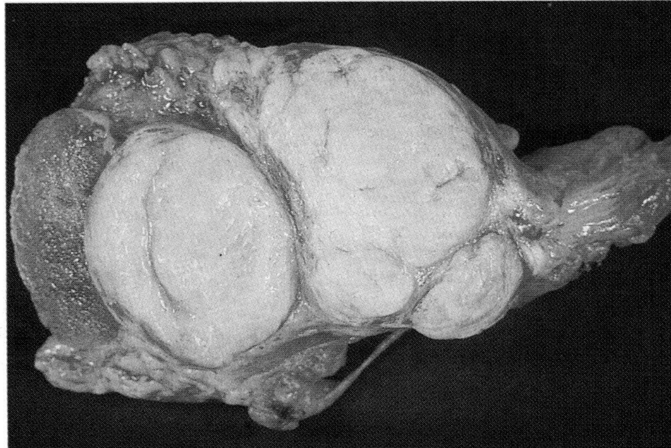

12-16. Fibrous pseudotumor of the testicular tunics.

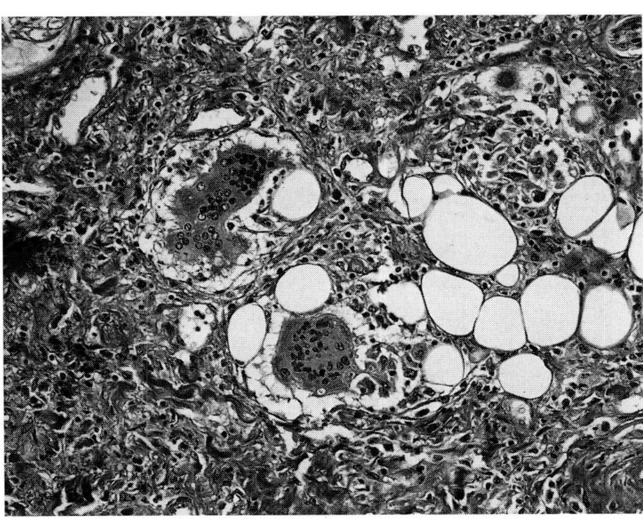

12-17. Sclerosing lipogranuloma of the spermatic cord.

retroperitoneum and tends to be more diffuse and less inflamed. Leiomyoma and neurofibroma are usually separated by light microscopy or by immunohistochemical evidence of smooth muscle or neural differentiation.

Leiomyoma

Reports of the relative frequency of leiomyoma to adenomatoid tumor of the epididymis vary from 1 in 9 to almost 1 in 1.[60] Men with genital leiomyoma range in age from 25 to 81 years, with a mean of 48 years.[60,174,218] Hydrocele or hernia sac are identified in up to 21% of cases, and up to 39% are bilateral. Leiomyoma appears as a round firm gray-white mass measuring up to 8 cm in diameter; the cut surface is homogeneous and whorled and bulges from the adjacent soft tissues (Fig. 12-18). It has typical microscopic features of leiomyoma, including interlacing fascicles of spindled smooth muscle cells with few or no mitotic figures. One case of leiomyoblastoma has been reported.[219] Differential diagnostic considerations include low-grade leiomyosarcoma and fibrous mesothelioma. The number of mitotic figures is reportedly the most reliable criterion for making this separation, but quantitative reporting in smooth muscle tumors of the epididymis and spermatic cord has not been consistent. Surgical excision of epididymal leiomyoma is curative.

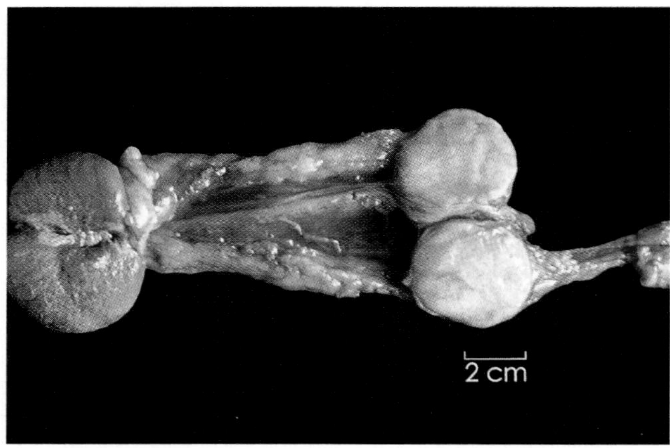

12-18. Leiomyoma of the vas deferens.

Leiomyoma is less common in the spermatic cord than the epididymis, with fewer than 20 reported cases.[220,221] Patient age is similar, although one case involved a premature infant with bilateral leiomyomas.

Melanotic neuroectodermal tumor of infancy (progonoma; retinal anlage tumor)

Melanotic neuroectodermal tumor of infancy most commonly arises in the jaw but has also been identified in the head of the epididymis and paratesticular region.[60,222-227] Patients range in age from newborn to 24 months, with a mean of about 7 months. The tumor is a solitary circumscribed solid blue-brown or black mass measuring up to 3 cm in diameter. Microscopically, it consists of cells with uniform round nuclei and abundant melanin granules lining small cystic spaces of variable size. Smaller round cells with hyperchromatic nuclei, prominent nucleoli, and minimal cytoplasm are observed within lumen spaces and the stroma. Tumor cells resemble neuroblasts and may form glomeruloid bodies, sometimes surrounded by a fibrous matrix set in a collagenous stroma.

Melanotic neuroectodermal tumor of infancy may replace the epididymis, but there are no reports of testicular or spermatic cord invasion. No recurrences or metastases have been identified, but the number of cases is small and the length of follow-up limited. Dehner[228] speculated that melanotic neuroectodermal tumor of infancy has the potential for local recurrence and regional lymph node involvement.

Brenner tumor

Brenner tumor of the testicular tunics is rare, occurring in men between 37 and 61 years of age. Ross[229] and Goldman[230] reported two cases that measured 0.6 and 2.7 cm in diameter and appeared as solid masses with smooth external surfaces. The tumors had typical histo-

A

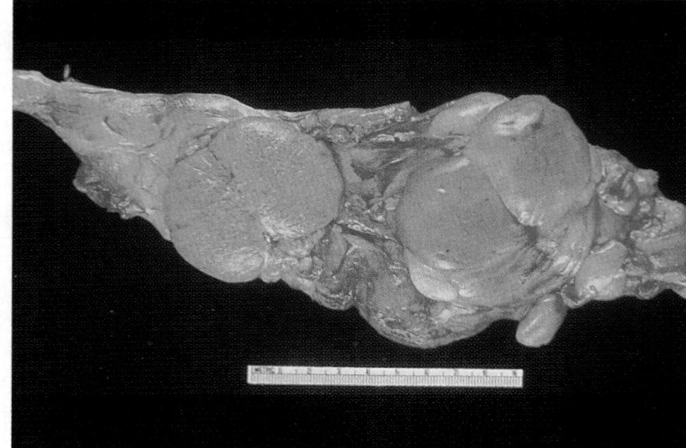

B

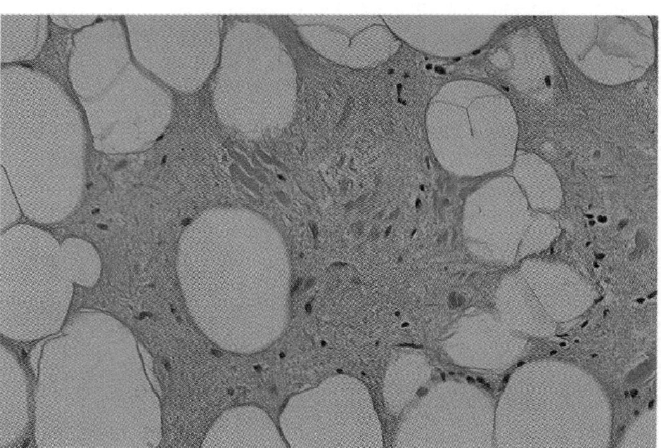

12-19. Liposarcoma of the spermatic cord. **A**, Grossly, the tumor consists of a multinodular mass of firm tan tissue. **B**, Delicate fibrosis and increased cellularity is observed within adipose tissue.

logic features of Brenner tumor, and origin from Walthard's cell rest was considered. Nogales et al[231] reported a mixed Brenner tumor–adenomatoid tumor of the tunica vaginalis appearing as a 3-cm partially cystic mass in a 37-year-old man. Most of the tumor was adenomatoid tumor, but scattered Brenner-type nests were seen throughout. Ultrastructural study revealed features typical of adenomatoid tumor and Brenner tumor. These authors favored a common histogenesis for both components.

Gonadal stromal tumor

Gonadal stromal tumor accounts for up to 3% of testicular tumors, and rare extratesticular examples have been reported.[232] One case of mixed gonadal stromal tumor arose in the tail of the epididymis in a 58-year-old man.[60] The tumor had features of both Sertoli and Leydig cell tumor without anaplasia, invasion, or lymphatic tumor emboli; orchiectomy revealed no evidence of testicular involvement.

Embryogenesis of the testis can account for extratesticular nests of germ cells and stromal cells. Microscopic foci of gonadal interstitial cells are occasionally observed in extratesticular sites such as the spermatic cord and epididymis in orchiectomy specimens removed for other reasons, and these may account for gonadal stromal tumor at such sites.[232]

Other benign tumors

Other rare benign paratesticular tumors include mucinous adenoid tumor,[233] neurofibroma,[234] and hemangioma[235] of the testicular tunics. Lymphangiectasia,[236] lymphangioma,[237,238] hemangioma,[239,240] and neurofibroma may arise in the spermatic cord or epididymis. There have been rare case reports of granular cell tumor,[241] paratesticular myxoma, carcinoid,[242] paraganglioma,[243] solitary fibrous tumor,[244] and rhabdomyoma[60] of the spermatic cord.

MALIGNANT NEOPLASMS

Liposarcoma

The most common sarcoma of the paratesticular region in adults is spermatic cord liposarcoma.[245-252] The mean patient age is 56 years, with a range from 16 to 90 years. Grossly, liposarcoma is a lobulated mass of yellow tissue that often resembles lipoma (Fig. 12-19). Microscopically, the most common pattern is well-differentiated liposarcoma (lipoma-like liposarcoma), often with prominent sclerosis. Myxoid liposarcoma and pleomorphic liposarcoma have also been described at this site.

Paratesticular liposarcoma is treated by radical orchiectomy with high ligation of the spermatic cord.[252] Hemiscrotectomy may be required in cases with inadequate surgical resection margins to avoid local recurrence. Lymphadenectomy is usually not indicated, especially with well-differentiated and myxoid liposarcoma. The role of radiation therapy and chemotherapy is uncertain. The majority of patients with paratesticular liposarcoma treated by resection with negative surgical margins are clinically free of tumor; however, 23% develop local recurrence, and less than 10% develop metastases, invariably in those with undifferentiated or high-grade liposarcoma.

The differential diagnosis of well-differentiated liposarcoma includes sclerosing lipogranuloma and lipoma. Myxoid liposarcoma should be distinguished from rhabdomyosarcoma and myxoid malignant fibrohistiocytoma. Pleomorphic liposarcoma may be difficult to distinguish from other types of high-grade sarcoma.

Rhabdomyosarcoma

Paratesticular rhabdomyosarcoma may arise in the testicular tunics, epididymis, or spermatic cord.[253-256] When the tumor is large or locally invasive, the exact site of origin cannot be determined. Rhabdomyosarcoma is the most common sarcoma of the paratesticular area in children, with a peak incidence at about 9 years, although it occurs at any age.

Grossly, rhabdomyosarcoma is an encapsulated white-gray mass with focal hemorrhage and cystic degeneration that measures up to 20 cm in diameter. Most are embryonal rhabdomyosarcoma, consisting of small, round cells with dark nuclei, scant cytoplasm, and variable numbers of cells showing myoblastic differentiation. The connective tissue stroma may be myxoid. Alveolar, botryoid, and pleomorphic patterns have rarely been observed at this site. Evidence of myoblastic differentiation is variable and includes histochemical demonstration of cytoplasmic filaments and cross striations; ultrastructural evidence of myofilaments and Z bands; and immunohistochemical demonstration of desmin, muscle-specific actin, and myoglobin. Rhabdomyosarcoma usually spreads to retroperitoneal lymph nodes, and patients without distant metastases are treated by radical inguinal orchiectomy with high ligation of the spermatic cord and ipsilateral or bilateral retroperitoneal or pelvic lymphadenectomy. Recent studies indicate that retroperitoneal lymphadenectomy can be avoided after radical inguinal orchiectomy when radiologic studies, such as computerized tomography, are negative. The extent of lymphadenectomy determines the likelihood of postoperative fertility. Locally invasive rhabdomyosarcoma, which involves the skin or arises with clinically suspicious inguinal lymph nodes, is treated by orchiectomy, scrotectomy, and inguinal lymphadenectomy. Long-term survival rates of greater than 80% are observed in patients receiving adjuvant radiation therapy and combination chemotherapy.

Leiomyosarcoma

Leiomyosarcoma is more common in the spermatic cord[257-259] than in the epididymis,[260,261] with more than 100 reported cases. It arises in patients of all ages, with a peak in the sixth and seventh decades; more than 80% of patients are over 40 years of age.

Grossly, leiomyosarcoma is a solid gray-tan mass involving the intrascrotal portion of the spermatic cord or epididymis. It consists of a spindle cell proliferation with typical features of leiomyosarcoma at other sites (see Fig. 12-19). Features that definitely separate low-grade leiomyosarcoma and leiomyoma are lacking, although the presence of necrosis, large number of mitotic figures,

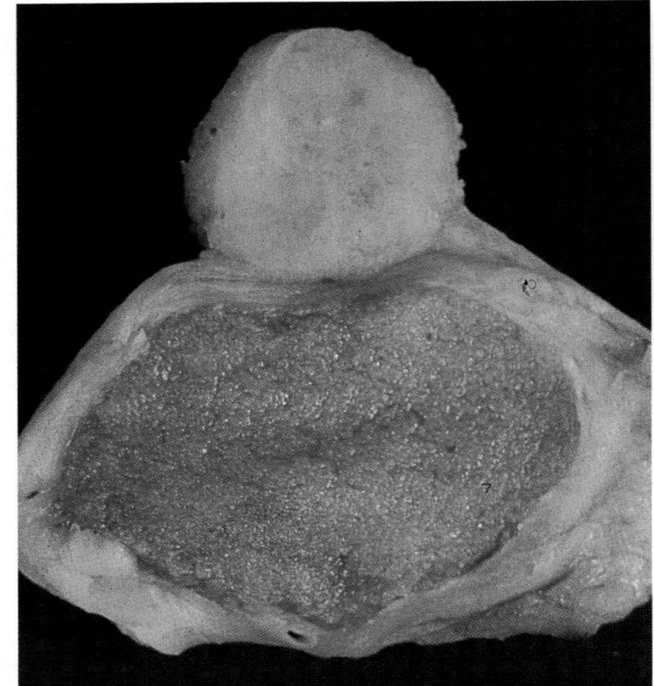

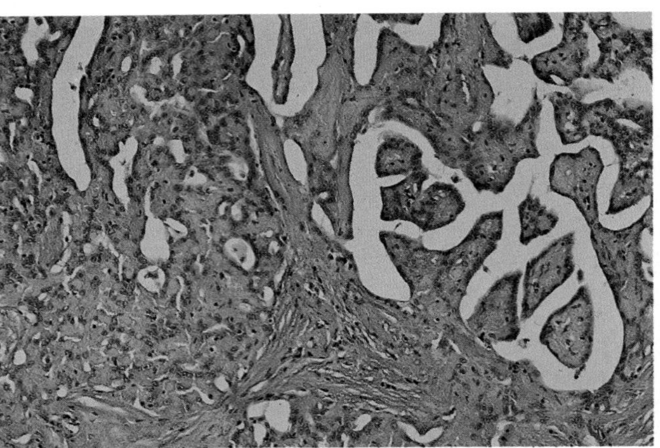

12-20. Malignant mesothelioma of the tunica vaginalis. **A**, Grossly, the tumor consists of a large exophytic papillary mass. **B**, Micropapillations are lined by flattened to cuboidal tumor cells. *(Courtesy Dr. Jan Kennedy.)*

nuclear pleomorphism, and marked cellularity suggest malignancy. Mostofi and Price[96] suggested that paratesticular leiomyosarcoma contains at least one or two mitotic figures per high power field.

Paratesticular leiomyosarcoma is treated by radical inguinal orchiectomy. The role of retroperitoneal lymphadenectomy is uncertain and is usually not recommended because of the propensity of leiomyosarcoma for hematogenous spread rather than lymphatic spread. Adjuvant radiation therapy and chemotherapy are considered palliative. Leiomyosarcoma may recur locally and metastasize, and about one third of patients die of metastases.

Malignant mesothelioma

Paratesticular malignant mesothelioma is rare, with less than 70 reported cases.[262-265] Most occur in the tunica vaginalis, with very few in the spermatic cord and epididymis. Mean patient age is about 55 years and ranges from 12 to 84 years. Primary peritoneal malignant mesothelioma may present as a mass in an inguinal hernia. Malignant mesothelioma of the tunica vaginalis may appear in pipe fitters with asbestos exposure, raising the possibility of asbestos as a contributory factor, similar to pleural and peritoneal mesothelioma.[263,264] One patient presented with bilateral mesothelioma of the tunica vaginalis.[265]

Grossly, malignant mesothelioma appears as multiple friable cystic and solid masses and small nodules studding the lining of a hydrocele sac, hernia sac, or the peritoneum (Fig. 12-20). Continuity between the tumor and adjacent mesothelium of the tunica vaginalis may be apparent, and there may be invasion of adjacent structures.

Histologically, paratesticular malignant mesothelioma is similar to mesothelioma at other sites, and may be epithelial, spindle cell, or biphasic, with a wide morphologic spectrum (see Fig. 12-20). The epithelial pattern is most common, accounting for about 75% of cases, and may be mixed with papillary, tubular, and solid areas. Spindle cells predominate in the sarcomatous pattern and may merge perceptively with solid epithelioid nests. Tumor cells are cuboidal or flattened, with variable amounts of eosinophilic cytoplasm and vesicular nuclei, often with prominent nucleoli. Mitotic figures are usually present. Morikawa et al[266] described an unusual case of malignant mesothelioma with squamous differentiation that involved the retroperitoneum.

Ancillary studies, including histochemical, immunohistochemical, and ultrastructural studies in paratesticular mesothelioma are similar to those for mesothelioma in other sites. Hyaluronidase-sensitive acid mucin may be present in tubular lumens or cell cytoplasm. Immunohistochemistry for low and high molecular weight keratin may be useful (usually positive), and carcinoembryonic antigen is usually negative. Ultrastructural features include slender microvilli, intercellular cannaliculi, desmosomes, perinuclear intermediate filaments, and basal lamina. Fine needle aspiration cytology is useful for diagnosis in some cases of malignant mesothelioma of the tunica vaginalis.[263] Preoperative diagnosis may prevent inappropriate scrotal surgery.

Malignant mesothelioma is aggressive, with a potential for late recurrence or metastasis. It recurs locally along the vas deferens or in the pelvis and usually spreads by lymphatic routes to pelvic, retroperitoneal, or distant lymph nodes. Radical inguinal orchiectomy is recommended with high ligation of the spermatic cord at the internal inguinal ring. Hemiscrotectomy or hemiscrotal irradiation may be useful to avoid local recurrence when a transscrotal incision is made. Primary retroperitoneal lymphadenectomy is often employed in patients with clinical or radiologic evidence of lymphatic metastases or in those without distant metastases. The utility of adjuvant chemotherapy is uncertain. About half of patients remain free of tumor up to 18 years after treatment.

The predominance of the epithelial or spindle cell component determines the differential diagnostic considerations. Epithelial malignant mesothelioma may be mistaken for reactive mesothelial hyperplasia, adenomatoid tumor, benign papillary mesothelioma, carcinoma of the rete testis, adenocarcinoma of the epididymis, paratesticular müllerian serous tumor, and metastatic adenocarcinoma. Paratesticular mesothelioma should be suspected in cases with in situ mesothelioma in the adjacent tunics, typical tubulopapillary architecture, and a lack of extrascrotal involvement. Spindle cell malignant mesothelioma should be distinguished from the variety of soft tissue sarcomas that arise at this site. Biphasic mesothelioma may be confused with stromal fibrosis, synovial sarcoma, and carcinosarcoma.

Serous tumor of müllerian epithelium (benign and malignant)

Rarely, müllerian epithelial tumors arise in the testis and paratesticular structures, probably from embryonic remnants such as the appendix testis.[60,267,268] Some early reports of adenocarcinoma of the testicular appendages apparently represent serous tumor of müllerian epithelium or malignant mesothelioma.

Papillary serous tumor of low malignant potential may occur in the tunica vaginalis, testis, and epididymis, and grossly and microscopically resembles its ovarian counterparts. Axiotos[268] reported a case in the testis with immunohistochemical and ultrastructural evidence of müllerian origin.

The differential diagnosis of serous tumor of müllerian epithelium includes papillary cystadenoma of the epididymis, benign papillary mesothelioma, malignant mesothelioma, adenocarcinoma of the rete testis or epididymis, and metastatic adenocarcinoma.

Adenocarcinoma of epididymis

Fewer than 30 reported cases of epididymal adenocarcinoma have been reported.[269-274] Mean patient age is 44 years, with a range from 5 to 78 years. The tumors measure up to 9 cm in diameter and may be multicystic or solid. About half are associated with hydrocele.

Microscopically, there are typical features of adenocarcinoma, including papillary, glandular, mucinous, and solid undifferentiated patterns. Squamous cell carcinoma may also be admixed. Of 15 cases with a mean of 12 months of follow-up, 7 patients died of metastatic carcinoma, 7 were free of tumor, and 1 died of unrelated causes.[60]

Malignant fibrous histiocytoma

Fewer than 20 reported cases of malignant fibrous histiocytoma involving the spermatic cord and paratesticular area have been reported.[60,275-280] Mean patient age is 64 years. Grossly, the tumor is solid gray or yellow-white, has a whorled cut surface, and measures up to 10 cm in diameter. Histologic patterns include myxoid, inflammatory, and pleomorphic malignant fibrous histiocytoma. Tanaka et al[276] described focal immunoreactivity for alpha-1-antitrypsin and alpha-1-antichymotrypsin in a case of spermatic cord malignant fibrous histiocytoma. In a recent review and case report, Eltorky et al[280] recommended extensive sampling of all paratesticular sarcomas such as malignant fibrous histiocytoma to exclude the presence of a germ cell component.

About one third of patients with malignant fibrous histiocytoma develop local recurrence or distant metastases. The treatment of choice is radical inguinal orchiectomy with high ligation of the spermatic cord. The value of adjuvant therapy is unknown.

Other sarcomas

More than 60 cases of spermatic cord and epididymal fibrosarcoma have been described,[281,282] but some of these probably represent other forms of sarcoma. Most occur in adults, but all ages may be affected. Some cases of fibrosarcoma reported in pediatric patients probably represent fibromatosis and its variants.[60] The gross and microscopic appearance of fibrosarcoma of the paratesticular area are similar to other sites. The differential diagnosis includes fibrous pseudotumor, malignant mesothelioma, leiomyosarcoma, malignant fibrous histiocytoma, and undifferentiated sarcoma. Of 16 patients with follow-up, 10 died of locally recurrent or metastatic tumor.

Most types of sarcoma have been described in the paratesticular area, including neurofibrosarcoma,[283] angiosarcoma,[284] malignant mesenchymoma,[285,286] chondrosarcoma,[287,288] and undifferentiated sarcoma. Peripheral neuroectodermal tumor has also been reported (Fig. 12-21).[289]

Germ cell tumor

A variety of germ cell tumors have been described in the paratesticular area, including seminoma,[290] embryonal carcinoma,[291] and teratoma.[271,292] The epididymis is

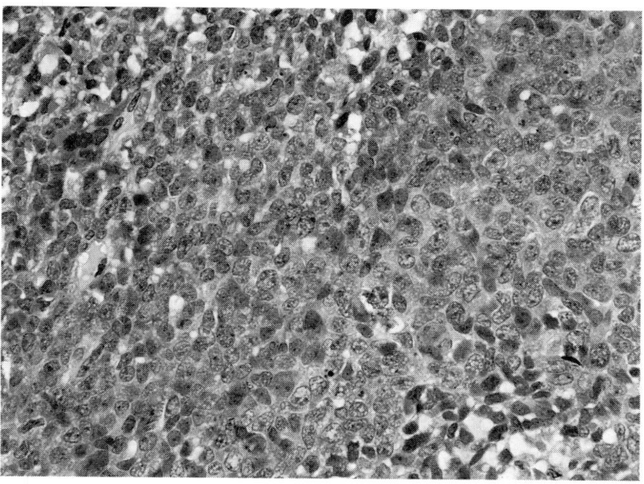

12-21. Peripheral neuroectodermal tumor of the spermatic cord. Tumor cells displayed MIC-2 immunoreactivity.

more commonly involved than the spermatic cord, but germ cell tumor at either site is rare. The demographic and pathologic features of paratesticular germ cell tumor are similar to those of the testis. These tumors probably arise from misplaced germinal elements.

Malignant lymphoma and hematopoietic neoplasms

Malignant lymphoma is the most common tumor of the testis in men over 50 years of age, yet paratesticular lymphoma is uncommon. Rare cases of primary epididymal or spermatic cord lymphoma have appeared.[293-300] Secondary lymphoma has been described in all sites of the paratesticular area, invariably in association with testicular involvement.

A case of plasmacytoma of the spermatic cord was described by Srigley and Hartwick.[60] The tumor arose in a 56-year-old man and did not involve the epididymis or testis. It was yellow, measured 3 cm in diameter, and showed typical features of plasmacytoma, including a proliferation of plasma cells with mild nuclear pleomorphism and hyperchromasia. The tumor recurred in the scrotum 3 years after diagnosis; 16 years later, the patient was diagnosed with multiple myeloma with lytic bone lesions.

Neuroblastoma

A single case of primary neuroblastoma of the spermatic cord has been reported.[301] A 7-year-old boy had metastatic neuroblastoma in ipsilateral retroperitoneal lymph nodes at diagnosis and was treated with paravertebral radiation therapy and cyclophosphamide. He was free of tumor after 8 years.

Wilms' tumor

Wilms' tumor rarely involves the spermatic cord.[302]

Metastases

Metastases to the paratesticular area are rare and usually arise from the prostate,[303-305] kidney,[306] and stomach (see Fig. 12-21).[307] Rare cases have originated from colonic adenocarcinoma[308,309] (Fig. 12-22), pancreatic adenocarcinoma, urothelial carcinoma,[310] ileal carcinoid, and malignant melanoma.[311] Patients with paratesticular metastases usually have a poor outcome.

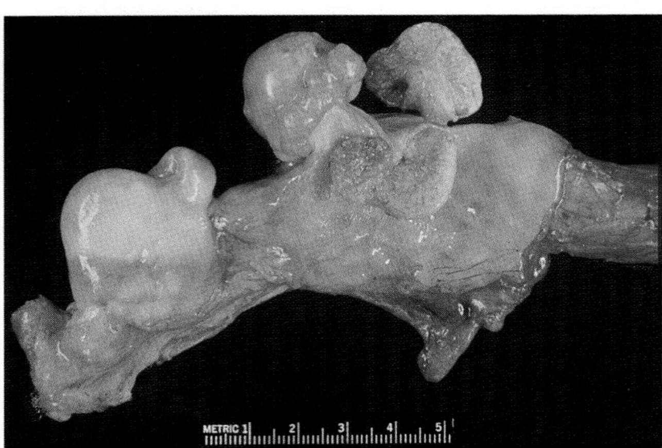

12-22. Hernia sac containing multiple nodules of metastatic colonic adenocarcinoma.

REFERENCES

1. Hadziselimovic F, Herzog B: The development and descent of the epididymis, Eur J Pediatr 152:S6-9, 1993.
2. Kuo T, Gomez LG: Monstrous epithelial cells in human epididymis and seminal vesicles. A pseudomalignant change, Am J Surg Pathol 5:483-490, 1981.
3. Nistal M, Santamaria L, Paniagua R: Multinucleate epithelial cells in the ductuli efferentes of human epididymis, Andrologia 22:591-596, 1990.
4. Sharp SC, Batt MA, Lennington WJ: Epididymal cribriform hyperplasia. A variant of normal epididymal histology, Arch Pathol Lab Med 118:1020-1022, 1994.
5. Abbott DP: Cribriform intra-tubular epididymal change and testicular atrophy, Histopathology 23:293, 1993 (letter).
6. Butterworth DM, Bisset DL: Cribriform intra-tubular epididymal change and adenomatous hyperplasia of the rete testis—a consequence of testicular atrophy? Histopathology 21:435-438, 1992.
7. Calder CJ, Aluwihare N, Graham CT: Cribriform intra-tubular epididymal change, Histopathology 22:406, 1993 (letter).
8. Bromberg WD, Kozlowski JM, Oyasu R: Prostate-type glands in the epididymis, J Urol 145:1273-1274, 1991.
9. Madara JL, Haggitt RC, Federman M: Intranuclear inclusions of the human vas deferens, Arch Pathol Lab Med 102:648-650, 1978.
10. Chakraborty J, Nelson L, Jhunjhunwala J et al: Intranuclear inclusion bodies in epithelial cells of human vas deferens, Arch Androl 2:1-12, 1979.
11. Tomaru A, Petrelli MP, Reid JD: Epithelial inclusions in the vas deferens: an electron microscopic study, J Urol 112:627-630, 1974.
12. Elder JS: Epididymal anomalies associated with hydrocele/hernia and cryptorchidism: implications regarding testicular descent, J Urol 148:624-626, 1992.
13. Johansen TE: Anatomy of the testis and epididymis in cryptorchidism, Andrologia 19:565-569, 1987.
14. Johansen TE: The anatomy of gubernaculum testis and processus vaginalis in cryptorchidism, Scand J Urol Nephrol 22:101-105, 1988.
15. Koff WJ, Scaletscky R: Malformations of the epididymis in undescended testis, J Urol 143:340-343, 1990.
16. Marshall FF, Shermeta DW: Epididymal abnormalities associated with undescended testis, J Urol 121:341-343, 1979.
17. Mininberg DT, Schlossberg S: The role of the epididymis in testicular descent, J Urol 129:1207-1208, 1983.
18. Priebe C Jr, Holahan JA, Ziring PR: Abnormalities of the vas deferens and epididymis in cryptorchid boys, J Pediatr Surg 14:834-838, 1979.
19. Casals T, Bassas L, Ruiz-Romero J et al: Extensive analysis of 40 infertile patients with congenital absence of the vas deferens: in 50% of cases only one CFTR allele could be detected, Hum Gene 95:205-211, 1995.

20. Crisp JC, Roberts PF: A case of bilateral cystadenoma of the epididymides presenting as infertility, Br J Urol 47:682, 1975.
21. Hall S, Oates RD: Unilateral absence of the scrotal vas deferens associated with contralateral mesonephric duct anomalies resulting in infertility: laboratory, physical and radiographic findings, and therapeutic alternatives, J Urol 150:1161-1164, 1993.
22. Rajalakshmi M, Kumar BV, Ramakrishnan PR et al: Histology of the epididymis in men with obstructive infertility, Andrologia 22:319-326, 1990.
23. Sivanesaratnam V: Male infertility due to absence of vas deferens, Eur J Obstet Gynecol Reprod Biol 14:31-35, 1982.
24. Padron RS, Mas J: Familial bilateral vas deferens agenesis, Int J Fertil 36:23-25, 1991.
25. Mercer S: Agenesis or atrophy of the testis and vas deferens, Can J Surg 22:245-246, 1979.
26. Nylander G, Persson BH: Bilateral agenesis of the vas deferens. Report of two cases with special reference to spermatogenesis and the epididymis, Acta Societatis Medicorum Upsaliensis, 73:221-228, 1968.
27. Gracey M, Campbell P, Noblett HR: Atretic vas deferens in cystic fibrosis, N Engl J Med 280:276, 1969.
28. Redman JF, Mooney DK: Fowler-Stephens orchiopexy in a patient with prune belly syndrome and segmental atretic vas deferens, Urology 41:130-131, 1993.
29. Emery CB, Goldstein AM, Morrow JW: Congenital absence of vas deferens with ipsilateral urinary anomalies, Urology 4:201-203, 1974.
30. Lurie A, Savir A, Lubin E: Non-fused crossed renal ectopia verified by radioisotope scanning and agenesis of the vas deferens on the ipsilateral side, Urol Int 26:45-50, 1971.
31. Deane AM, May RE: Absent vas deferens in association with renal abnormalities, Br J Urol 54:298-299, 1982.
32. Buresh WS, Caterine JM: Renal agenesis associated with a congenitally absent vas deferens, J Iowa Med Soc 69:97-98, 1979.
33. Gravgaard E, Garsdal L, Moller SH: Double vas deferens and epididymis associated with ipsilateral renal agenesis simulating ectopic ureter opening into the seminal vesicle, Scand J Urol Nephrol 12:85-87, 1978.
34. Ochsner MG, Brannan W, Goodier EH: Absent vas deferens associated with renal agenesis, JAMA 222:1055-1056, 1972.
35. Koyanagi T, Tsuji I, Kudo T et al: Double vas deferens associated with ipsilateral renal agenesis, simulating ectopic ureter, J Urol 108:631-634, 1972.
36. Hershman MJ, Dawson PM, Leung AW et al: Cystic dysplasia in ectopic kidney associated with absent vas deferens and congenital inguinal hernia, Urology 35:331-333, 1990.
37. Czeizel A: Congenital aplasia of the vasa deferentia of autosomal recessive inheritance in two unrelated sib-pairs, Hum Genet 70:288, 1985.
38. Gilgenkrantz S, Guillemin P, Kimmel B: On the familial occurrence of congenital bilateral absence of vas deferens, Clinical Genetics 37:159, 1990 (letter).
39. Kleczkowska A, Fryns JP, Steeno O et al: On the familial occurrence of congenital bilateral absence of vas deferens, Clinical Genet 35:268-271, 1989 (review).
40. Martin RA, Jones KL, Downey EC: Congenital absence of the vas deferens: recurrence in a family, Am J Med Genet 42:714-715, 1992.
41. Barrack S: Crossed testicular ectopia with fused bilateral duplication of the vasa deferential: an unusual finding in cryptorchidism. East Afr Med J 71:398-400, 1994 (review).
42. Binderow SR, Shah KD, Dolgin SE: True duplication of the vas deferens, J Pediatr Surg 28:269-270, 1993 (review).
43. Carr R: Apparent bilateral duplication of the vas deferens, Br J Urol 71:354, 1993.
44. Tolete-Velcek F, Bernstein MO, Hansbrough F: Crossed testicular ectopia with bilateral duplication of the vasa deferentia: an unusual finding in cryptorchism, J Pediatr Surg 23:641-643, 1988.
45. Aragona F, Ostardo E, Camuffo MC et al: Ectopia of the vas deferens into the ureter. Case report and review of the literature, Eur Urol 22:329-334, 1992 (review).
46. Ayyat F, Palmer MD, Tingley JO: Ectopic vas deferens communicating with lower ureter, Urology 19:423-426, 1982.
47. Boles E Jr., Lobe TE, Hamoudi A: Congenital vas deferens—ureteral connection, J Pediatr Surg 13:41-46, 1978.
48. Borger JA, Belman AB: Uretero-vas deferens anastomosis associated with imperforate anus: an embryologically predictable occurrence, J Ped Surg 10:255-257, 1975.
49. Glasser J, Lefleur R, Subramanyam B et al: Ectopic duplicated ureter opening into ipsilateral vas deferens, Urology 23:309-312, 1984.
50. Gotoh T, Takahashi Y, Kumagai A et al: Two cases of ectopic ureter opening into the ejaculatory duct: double vas deferens revisited, J Urol 130:550-552, 1983.
51. Johnson DK, Perlmutter AD: Single system ectopic ureteroceles with anomalies of the heart, testis and vas deferens, J Urol 123:81-83, 1980.
52. Mansson W, Brown I: Infertility due to congenital communication between vas deferens and refluxing triplicated ureter: successful insemination with sperm retrieved from urine. A case report, Scand J Urol Nephrol 22:71-73, 1988.
53. Redman JF, Sulieman JS: Bilateral vasal-ureteral communications, J Urol 116:808-809, 1976.
54. Sargent CR, Amis E Jr, Carlton C Jr: Ectopic ureter, ipsilateral vas deferens and seminal vesicle agenesis and associated dermoid cyst: a case report, J Urol 103:298-299, 1970.
55. Schwarz R, Stephens FD: The persisting mesonephric duct: high junction of vas deferens and ureter, J Urol 120:592-596, 1978.
56. Cooper TG, Raczek S, Yeung CH et al: Composition of fluids obtained from human epididymal cysts, Urol Res 20:275-280, 1992.
57. Rifkin MD, Brownstein PK: Abnormal echogenicity of the testicle caused by epididymal cysts, J Ultrasound Med 2:539-541, 1983.
58. Conley GR, Sant GR, Ucci AA et al: Seminoma and epididymal cysts in a young man with known diethylstilbestrol exposure in utero, JAMA 249:1325-1326, 1983.
59. Impieri M, Masoni T, Giusti F: Cystadenoma of the epididymis associated with hydrocele, Acta Urol Belg 50:373-375, 1982.
60. Srigley JR, Hartwick RWJ: Tumors and cysts of the paratesticular region, Pathol Annu 25(Part 2):51-108, 1990 (review).
61. Wollin M, Marshall FF, Fink MP et al: Aberrant epididymal tissue: a significant clinical entity, J Urol 138:1247-1250, 1987.

62. May JE, Bourne CW: Ectopic spleen in the scrotum: report of 2 cases, J Urol 111:120-123, 1974.
63. Bruning H, Kootstra G, Walther FJ et al: Ectopic adrenocortical tissue along the spermatic cord, Z Kinderchirurgie 39:269-270, 1984.
64. Freeman A: Adrenal cortical adenoma of the epididymis, Arch Pathol 39:336-337, 1945.
65. Rolnick D, Kawanoue S, Szanto P et al: Anatomic incidence of testicular appendages, J Urol 100:755-759, 1968.
66. Redman JF, O'Donnell PD: Simultaneous ipsilateral torsion of the appendices testis and epididymis, J Urol 117:255, 1977.
67. Skoglund RW, McRoberts JW, Ragde H: Torsion of testicular appendages: presentation of 43 new cases and a collective review, J Urol 104:598-605, 1970.
68. Krukowski ZH, Auld CD: Torsion of the appendix epididymis in a maldescended testis, Br J Urol 55:244-245, 1983.
69. Remzi D, Erkan I, Yazicioglu A: Torsion of appendix epididymis, N Y State J Med 80:646-647, 1980.
70. Ballesteros Sampol JJ, Munne A et al: A vas aberrans torsion, Br J Urol 58:97, 1986.
71. Virdi JS, Conway W, Kelly DG: Torsion of the vas aberrans, Br J Urol 66:435, 1990.
72. Nistal M, Iniguez L, Paniagua R et al: Tubular embryonal remnants in the human spermatic cord, Urol Int 42:260-264, 1987.
73. Hartz PM: Occurrence of Walthard cell rests or Brenner-like epithelium in the serosa of the epididymis, Am J Clin Pathol 17:654-659, 1947.
74. Mercier B, Verlingue C, Lissens W et al: Is congenital bilateral absence of vas deferens a primary form of cystic fibrosis? Analyses of the CFTR gene in 67 patients, Am J Hum Genet 56:272-277, 1995.
75. Meschede D, Eigel A, Horst J et al: Compound heterozygosity for the delta F508 and F508C cystic fibrosis transmembrane conductance regulator (CFTR) mutations in a patient with congenital bilateral aplasia of the vas deferens, Am J Hum Genet 53:292-293, 1993 (letter).
76. Oates RD, Amos JA: Congenital bilateral absence of the vas deferens and cystic fibrosis. A genetic commonality, World J Urol 11:82-88, 1993 (review).
77. Oates RD, Amos JA: The genetic basis of congenital bilateral absence of the vas deferens and cystic fibrosis, J Androl 15:1-8, 1994 (review).
78. Rigot JM, Lafitte JJ, Dumur V et al: Cystic fibrosis and congenital absence of the vas deferens, N Engl J Med 325:64-65, 1991 (letter).
79. Valman HB, France NE: The vas deferens in cystic fibrosis, Lancet 2:566-567, 1969.
80. Williams C, Mayall ES, Williamson R et al: A report on CF carrier frequency among men with infertility owing to congenital absence of the vas deferens, J Med Genet 30:973, 1993 (letter).
81. Anguiano A, Oates RD, Amos JA et al: Congenital bilateral absence of the vas deferens. A primarily genital form of cystic fibrosis, JAMA 267:1794-1797, 1992.
82. Goshen R, Kerem E, Shoshani T et al: Cystic fibrosis manifested as undescended testis and absence of vas deferens, Pediatrics 90:982-983, 1992.
83. Landing BH, Wells TR, Wang CI: Abnormality of the epididymis and vas deferens in cystic fibrosis, Arch Pathol 88:569-580, 1969.
84. Matfin G: Congenital bilateral absence of vas deferens in absence of cystic fibrosis, Lancet 345:200, 1995 (letter).
85. Anonymous: Congenital bilateral absence of the vas deferens and cystic fibrosis, Lancet 339:1328-1329, 1992 (editorial).
86. Augarten A, Yahav Y, Kerem BS et al: Congenital bilateral absence of vas deferens in the absence of cystic fibrosis, Lancet 344:1473-1474, 1994.
87. Bienvenu T, Beldjord C, Adjiman M et al: Male infertility as the only presenting sign of cystic fibrosis when homozygous for the mild mutation R117H, J Med Genet 30:797, 1993 (letter).
88. Dumur V, Gervais R, Rigot JM et al: Congenital bilateral absence of vas deferens in absence of cystic fibrosis, Lancet 345:200-201, 1995 (letter).
89. Durieu I, Bey-Omar F, Rollet J et al: Diagnostic criteria for cystic fibrosis in men with congenital absence of the vas deferens, Medicine 74:42-47, 1995.
90. Piscioli F, Polla E, Pusiol T et al: Pseudomalignant cytologic presentation of spermatic hydrocele fluid, Acta Cytol 27:666-670, 1983.
91. Helmling RL, Evans AT: Idiopathic hematoma of the spermatic cord. Case report, Ohio State Med J 63:484-485, 1967.
92. Nistal M, Martin L, Paniagua R: Idiopathic hematoma of the epididymis: presentation of three cases, Eur Urol 17:178-180, 1990.
93. Sayfan J, Halevy A, Shperber Y et al: The role of the spermatic cord layers in the development of varicoceles, J Urol 133:223-224, 1985.
94. Whitehead ED, Lieter E: Genital abnormalities and abnormal semen analyses in male patients exposed to diethylstilbestrol in utero, J Urol 125:47-50, 1981.
95. Jassie MP, Mahmood P: Torsion of spermatocele: a newly described entity with 2 cases, J Urol 133:683-684, 1985.
96. Mostofi FK, Price EBJ: Tumors of the male genital system, Atlas of tumor pathology, fascicle 8, 2nd series, Washington, D.C., 1973, Armed Forces Institute of Pathology.
97. Nistal M, Iniguez L, Paniagua R: Histological classification of spermatic cord cysts in relation to their histogenesis, Eur Urol 13:327-330, 1987.
98. Pingree LJ, Brown DE: Cholesteatoma of the epididymis, J Urol 56:454-455, 1951.
99. Bloom DA, DiPietro MA, Gikas PW et al: Extratesticular dermoid cyst and fibrous dysplasia of epididymis, J Urol 137:996-997, 1987.
100. Tejada E, Eble JN: Simple cyst of the rete testis, J Urol 139:376-378, 1988.
101. Berger RE, Alexander ER, Harnisch JP et al: Etiology, manifestation and therapy of acute epididymitis: prospective study of 50 cases, J Urol 121:751-756, 1979.
102. Furness G, Kamat MH, Kaminski Z et al: The etiology of idiopathic epididymitis, J Urol 106:387-392, 1971.
103. Mittemeyer BT, Lenox KW, Borski HA: Epididymitis. A review of 610 cases, J Urol 95:390-397, 1966.
104. Williams CB, Litvak AS, McRoberts JW: Epididymitis in infancy, J Urol 121:125-130, 1979.

105. Berner R, Schumacher RF, Zimmerhackl LB et al: Salmonella enteritidis orchitis in a 10-week-old boy, Acta Paediatrica 83:992-993, 1994.
106. Hori S, Tsutsumi Y: Histologic differentiation between chlamydial and bacterial epididymitis: nondestructive and proliferative versus destructive and abscess forming—immunohistochemical and clinicopathologic findings, Hum Pathol 26:402-407, 1995.
107. Melekos MD, Asbach HW: The role of chlamydiae in epididymitis, International Urol Nephrol 20:293-297, 1988.
108. Deguchi T, Kanematsu E, Iwata H et al: Chlamydia epididymitis diagnosed by genetic detection of *Chlamydia trachomatis* from epididymal aspirate by polymerase chain reaction, J Jpn Assoc Infect Dis 66:991-994, 1992.
109. Bostrom K: Patho-anatomical findings in a case of mumps with pancreatitis, myocarditis, orchitis, epididymitis and seminal vesiculitis, Virchows Arch A Pathol Anat Histopathol 344:111-118, 1968.
110. Gasparich JP, Mason JT, Greene HL et al: Amiodarone-associated epididymitis: drug-related epididymitis in the absence of infection, J Urol 133:971-972, 1985.
111. Schned AR, Selikowitz SM: Epididymitis nodosa. An epididymal lesion analogous to vasitis nodosa, Arch Pathol Lab Med 110:61-64, 1986.
112. Schned AR, Memoli VA: Coarse granular cytoplasmic change of the epididymis. An immunohistochemical and ultrastructural study, J Urol Pathol 2:213-222, 1994.
113. Raghavaiah NV: Epididymal calcification in genital filariasis, Urology 18:78-79, 1981.
114. Wiener LB, Riehl PA, Baum N: Xanthogranulomatous epididymitis: a case report, J Urol 138:621-622, 1987.
115. Cabral DA, Johnson HW, Coleman GU et al: Tuberculous epididymitis as a cause of testicular pseudomalignancy in two young children, Pediatr Infect Dis J 4:59-63, 1985.
116. Higashihara M, Nagata N, Takeuchi K et al: A case of tuberculous epididymitis associated with Addison's, Endocrinol Jpn 31:1-5, 1984.
117. Neelaranjitharajah PA: An unusual presentation of tuberculous epididymo-orchitis: case. Genitourin Med 62:61-62, 1986.
118. Ibrahiem AA, Awad HA, Metawi BA et al: Pathologic changes in testis and epididymis of infertile leprotic males, Int J Lepr Other Mycobact Dis 47:44-49, 1979.
119. Pareek SS, Tandon RC: Epididymal lesion in tuberculoid leprosy, Br Med J Clin Res Ed 291:313, 1985.
120. Povysil C: Extravesical malakoplakia, Arch Pathol 97:273-276, 1974.
121. Guccion JG, Thorgeirsson UP, Smith BH: Malacoplakia of epididymis, Urology 12:713-716, 1978.
122. McClure J: A case of malacoplakia of the epididymis associated with trauma, J Urol 124:934-935, 1980.
123. Amenta PS, Gonick P, Katz SM: Sarcoidosis of testis and epididymis, Urology 17:616-617, 1981.
124. McWilliams WA, Abramowitz L, Tiamson EM: Epididymal sarcoidosis: case report and review, J Urol 130:1201-1203, 1983.
125. Suzuki Y, Koike H, Tamura G et al: Ultrasonographic findings of epididymal sarcoidosis, Urol Int 52:228-230, 1994.
126. Yamamoto N, Hasegawa Y, Miyamoto K et al: Bilateral epididymal sarcoidosis. Case report, Scand J Urol Nephrol 26:301-303, 1992 (review).
127. Burke BJ, Parker SH, Hopper KD et al: The ultrasonographic appearance of coexistent epididymal and testicular sarcoidosis, J Clin Ultrasound 18:522-526, 1990.
128. Kauffman CA, Slama TG, Wheat LJ: Histoplasma capsulatum epididymitis, J Urol 125:434-435, 1981.
129. Conner WT, Drach GW, Bucher W Jr: Genitourinary aspects of disseminated coccidioidomycosis, J Urol 113:82-88, 1975.
130. Eickenberg H-U, Amin M, Lich RJ: Blastomycosis of the genitourinary tract, J Urol 113:650-652, 1975.
131. Selman SH, Hampel N: Systemic sporotrichosis: diagnosis through biopsy of epididymal, Urology 20:620-621, 1982.
132. Gelfand M, Ross CM, Blair DM et al: Schistosomiasis of the male pelvic organs. Severity of infection as determined by digestion of tissue and histologic methods in 300 cadavers, Am J Trop Med Hyg 19:779-784, 1970.
133. Honore LH, Coleman GU: Solitary epididymal schistosomiasis, Can J Surg 18:479-483, 1975.
134. Arora VK, Bhatia A: Adult filarial worm in fine needle aspirate of an epididymal nodule, Acta Cytol 33:421, 1989 (letter).
135. Clark WR, Lieber MM: Genital filariasis in Minnesota, Urology 28:518-520, 1986.
136. Jayaram G: Microfilariae in fine needle aspirates from epididymal lesions, Acta Cytol 31:59-62, 1987.
137. Coyne J, al-Nakib L, Goldsmith D et al: Secondary oxalosis and sperm granuloma of the epididymis, J Clin Pathol 47:470-471, 1994.
138. Cullen TH, Voss HJ: Sperm granulomata of the testis and epididymis, Br J Urol 38:202-207, 1966.
139. El-Beheiry AH, El-Akhras AI, El-Sayed AI et al: Epididymal sperm granuloma, Arch Androl 8:65-67, 1982.
140. Silber SJ: Sperm granuloma and reversibility of vasectomy, Lancet 2:588-589, 1977.
141. Dunner PS, Lipsit ER, Nochomovitz LE: Epididymal sperm granuloma simulating a testicular neoplasm, J Clin Ultrasound 10:353-355, 1982.
142. Carvalho TL, Ribeiro RD, Lopes RA: The male reproductive organs in experimental Chagas' disease. I. Morphometric study of the vas deferens in the acute phase of the disease, Exp Pathol 41:203-214, 1991.
143. Carvalho TL, Carraro AA, Lopes RA et al: The male reproductive organs in experimental Chagas' disease. II. Morphometric study of the vas deferens in the chronic phase of the disease, Exp Toxicolo Pathol 44:147-149, 1992.
144. Balogh K, Travis WD: The frequency of perineurial ductules in vasitis nodosa, Am J Clin Pathol 82:710-713, 1984.
145. Balogh K, Travis WD: Benign vascular invasion in vasitis nodosa, Am J Clin Pathol 83:426-430, 1985.
146. Basu D, Sakhuja P, Chaturvedi KU: Vasitis nodosa—a case report, Ind J Pathol Microbiol 36:69-71, 1993.
147. Bissada NK, Redman JF, Finkbeiner AE: Unusual inguinal mass secondary to vasitis, Urology 8:488-489, 1976.
148. Civantos F, Lubin J, Rywlin AM: Vasitis nodosa, Arch Pathol 94:355-361, 1972.
149. DeSchryver-Kecskemeti K, Balogh K, Neet KE: Nerve growth factor and the concept of neural-epithelial interactions. Immunohistochemical observations in two cases of vasitis nodosa and six cases of prostatic adenocarcinoma, Arch Pathol Lab Med 111:833-835, 1987.

150. Deshpande RB, Deshpande J, Mali BN et al: Vasitis nodosa (a report of 7 cases), J Postgrad Med 31:105-108, 1985.
151. Goldman RL, Azzopardi JG: Benign neural invasion in vasitis nodosa, Histopathology 6:309-315, 1982.
152. Hirschowitz L, Rode J, Guillebaud J et al: Vasitis nodosa and associated clinical findings, J Clin Pathol 41:419-423, 1988.
153. Kiser GC, Fuchs EF, Kessler S: The significance of vasitis nodosa, J Urol 136:42-44, 1986.
154. Kovi J, Agbata A: Benign neural invasion in vasitis nodosa, JAMA 228:1519, 1974 (letter).
155. Olson AL: Vasitis nodosa, Am J Clin Pathol 55:364-368, 1971.
156. Ralph DJ, Lynch MJ, Pryor JP: Vasitis nodosa due to torture, Br J Urol 72:515-516, 1993.
157. Elbadawi A, Khuri FJ, Cockett AT: Polypoid granulomatous and sclerosing endophlebitis of spermatic cord: new pathologic type of schistosomal funiculitis, Urology 13:309-314, 1979.
158. Heydenrych JJ, Marcus PB: Meconium granulomas of the tunica vaginalis, J Urol 115:596-598, 1976.
159. Dehner L, Scott D, Stocker J: Meconium peritonitis: a clinicopathologic study of four cases with a review of the literature, Hum Pathol 17:807-812, 1986.
160. McLean NR, Burnett RA: Polyarteritis nodosa of epididymis, Urology 21:70-71, 1983.
161. Nakauchi Y, Suehiro T, Kumon Y et al: Localized polyarteritis nodosa in the forearm and epididymis, Intern Med 33:48-52, 1994 (review).
162. Roy JB, Hamblin DW, Brown CH: Periarteritis nodosa of epididymis, Urology 10:62-63, 1977.
163. Halim A, Neild GH, Levine T et al: Isolated necrotizing granulomatous vasculitis of the epididymis and spermatic cord, World J Urol 12:357-358, 1994.
164. Karnauchow PN, Steele AA: Isolated necrotizing granulomatous vasculitis of the spermatic cords, J Urol 141:379-381, 1989.
165. Persellin ST, Menke DM: Isolated polyarteritis nodosa of the male reproductive system, J Rheumatol 19:985-988, 1992.
166. Womack C, Ansell ID: Isolated arteritis of the epididymis, J Clin Pathol 38:797-800, 1985.
167. Levine TS: Testicular and epididymal vasculitides. Is morphology of help in classification and prognosis? J Urol Pathol 2:81-88, 1994.
168. Ahlqvist J, Lahtiharju A, Elfving G: On intratubular calcification in the epididymis, Acta Pathologica et Microbiologica Scandinavica 65:541-544, 1965.
169. Kokotas NS, Papaharalambous ME: Lipoma of the spermatic cord in childhood, Br J Urol 55:572, 1983.
170. Rosenberg R, Williamson MR: Lipomas of the spermatic cord and testis: report of two cases, J Clin Ultrasound 17:670-674, 1989.
171. Lioe TF, Biggart JD: Tumours of the spermatic cord and paratesticular tissue. A clinicopathological study, Br J Urol 71:600-606, 1993.
172. Huben RP, Scarff JE, Schellhammer PF: Massive intrascrotal fibrolipoma, J Urol 129:154-155, 1983.
173. Fletcher CD, Cole RS, Gower RL et al: Hibernoma of the spermatic cord: the first reported case, Br J Urol 58:99-100, 1986.
174. Romanelli R, Sanna A: Adenomatoid leiomyoma and papillary cystadenoma of the epididymis, Pathologica 77:445-458, 1985.
175. Vyas KC, Khamesara HL, Gupta AS et al: Adenomatoid tumour of the spermatic cord, J Indian Med Assoc 88:15-16, 1990.
176. Soderstrom KO: Origin of adenomatoid tumor: a comparison between the structure of adenomatoid tumor and epididymal duct cells, Cancer 49:2349-2357, 1982.
177. Sidhu GS, Fresko O: Adenomatoid tumor of the epididymis: ultrastructural evidence of its biphasic nature, Ultrastruct Pathol 1:39-47, 1980.
178. Miller F, Lieberman MK: Local invasion in adenomatoid tumors, Cancer 21:933-939, 1968.
179. Halalau F, Laky D: Adenomatoid tumor of the epididymis. A case report, Morphologie et Embryologie 33:275-277, 1987.
180. Stephenson TJ, Mills PM: Adenomatoid tumours: an immunohistochemical and ultrastructural, J Pathol 148:327-335, 1986.
181. Morris JA, Oates K, Staff WG: Scanning electron microscopy of adenomatoid tumours, Br J Urol 58:183-187, 1986.
182. Sakai T, Nakada T, Kono T et al: Adenomatoid tumor of the epididymis with special reference to immunohistochemical study of 3 cases, Hinyokika Kiyo 35:1537-1542, 1989.
183. Detassis C, Pusiol T, Piscioli F et al: Adenomatoid tumor of the epididymis: immunohistochemical study of 8, Urol Int 41:232-234, 1986.
184. Nistal M, Paniagua R, Fuentes E et al: Histogenesis of adenomatoid tumour associated to pseudofibromatous, J Pathol 144:275-280, 1984.
185. Mucientes F: Adenomatoid tumor of the epididymis. Ultrastructural study of three, Path Res Pract 176:258-268, 1983.
186. Lodeville D, Zaroli A, Lampertico P: Adenomatoid tumor of the male genital tract: report of three cases, Pathologica 73:629-637, 1981.
187. Davy CL, Tang CK: Are all adenomatoid tumors adenomatoid mesotheliomas? Hum Pathol 12:360-369, 1981.
188. Nistal M, Contreras F, Paniagua R. Adenomatoid tumour of the epididymis: histochemical and ultrastructural study of 2 cases, Br J Urol 50:121-125, 1978.
189. Taxy JB, Battifora H, Oyasu R: Adenomatoid tumors: a light microscopic, histochemical, and ultrastructural study, Cancer 34:306-311, 1974.
190. Ritchie EL, Gonzalez-Crussi F, Zaontz MR: Fibrous hamartoma of infancy masquerading as a rhabdomyosarcoma of the spermatic cord, J Urol 140:800-801, 1988.
191. Rosai J, Dehner LP: Nodular meosthelial hyperplasia in hernia sacs. A benign reactive condition simulating a neoplastic process, Cancer 35:165-169, 1975.
192. Silberblatt JM, Gellman SZ: Mesotheliomas of spermatic cord, epididymis, and tunica vaginalis, Urology 3:235-237, 1974.
193. Chahla Y: Benign genital mesothelioma. Two case reports, Eur Urol 11:285-287, 1985.
194. Stein N, Henkes HD: Mesothelioma of the testicle in a child, J Urol 135:794-795, 1986.

195. Torikata C: Papillary cystadenoma of the epididymis. An ultrastructural and immunohistochemical study, J Submicrosc Cytol Pathol 26:387-393, 1994.
196. Calder CJ, Gregory J: Papillary cystadenoma of the epididymis: a report of two cases with an immunohistochemical study, Histopathology 23:89-91, 1993.
197. Kragel PJ, Pestaner J, Travis WD et al: Papillary cystadenoma of the epididymis. A report of three cases with lectin histochemistry, Arch Pathol Lab Med 114:672-675, 1990.
198. Billesbolle P, Nielsen K: Papillary cystadenoma of the epididymis, J Urol 139:1062, 1988.
199. Wernert N, Goebbels R, Prediger L: Papillary cystadenoma of the epididymis. Case report and review of the literature, Path Res Pract 181:260-264, 1986.
200. Kallie NR, Fisher GF, Harker JR: Papillary cystadenoma of the epididymis, Can J Surg 26:174-175, 1983.
201. Price E Jr: Papillary cystadenoma of the epididymis. A clinicopathologic analysis of 20 cases, Arch Pathol 91:456-470, 1971.
202. Pozza D, Masci P, Amodeo S et al: Papillary cystadenoma of the epididymis as a cause of obstructive azoospermia, Urol Int 53:222-224, 1994.
203. Greka HK, Morley AR, Evans D: Papillary cystadenoma of the epididymis, Br J Urol 57:356-357, 1985.
204. Witten FR, O'Brien DB, Sewell CW et al: Bilateral clear cell papillary cystadenoma of the epididymides, J Urol 133:1062-1064, 1985.
205. de Souza AJ, Bambirra EA, Bicalho OJ et al: Bilateral papillary cystadenoma of the epididymis as a component of von Hippel-Lindau's syndrome: report of a case presenting as infertility, J Urol 133:288-289, 1985.
206. Kedar GP, Bobhate SK, Kher AV: Papillary cyst adenoma of epididymis. A case report, Indian J Pathol Microbiol 27:309-310, 1984.
207. Hesp WL, Debruyne FM, Bogman MJ: Papillary cystadenoma of the epididymis, Neth J Surg 35:97-99, 1983.
208. Civil ID, Hackett AH: Papillary cystadenoma of the epididymis: a case report, Aust N Z J Surg 51:304-305, 1981.
209. Gruber MB, Healey GB, Toguri AG et al: Papillary cystadenoma of epididymis: component of von Hippel-Lindau, Urology 16:305-306, 1980.
210. Tsuda H, Fukushima S, Takahashi M et al: Familial bilateral papillary cystadenoma of the epididymis, Cancer 37:1831-1839, 1976.
211. Lam KY, Chan KW, Ho MH: Inflammatory pseudotumour of the epididymis, Br J Urol 75:255-257, 1995.
212. Yamashina M, Honma T, Uchijima Y: Myofibroblastic pseudotumor mimicking epididymal sarcoma. A clinicopathologic study of three cases, Path Res Pract 188:1054-1059, 1992.
213. Begin LR: Paratesticular (spermatic cord and tunica testis) fibroblastic/myofibroblastic proliferations, Am J Surg Pathol 17:530, 1993 (letter).
214. Hollowood K, Fletcher CD: Pseudosarcomatous myofibroblastic proliferations of the spermatic cord ("proliferative funiculitis"). Histologic and immunohistochemical analysis of a distinctive entity, Am J Surg Pathol 16:448-454, 1992.
215. Thompson JE, van der Walt JD: Nodular fibrous proliferation (fibrous pseudotumor) of the tunica vaginalis testis. A light, electron microscopic and immunocytochemical study of a case and a review of the literature, Histopathology 10:741-749, 1986.
216. Farkas A, Firstater M: Fibroma of the spermatic cord, Int Surg 57:578-579, 1972.
217. Lichtenheld FR, McCauley RT: Pseudofibroma of the epididymis, Mil Med 131:437-439, 1966.
218. deLuise VP, Draper JW, Gray G Jr: Smooth muscle tumors of the testicular adnexa, J Urol 115:685-688, 1976.
219. Tokunaka S, Taniguchi N, Hashimoto H et al: Leiomyoblastoma of the epididymis in a child, J Urol 143:991-993, 1990.
220. Taylor AM, Wijesuriya LI, Wong R et al: Leiomyoma of the spermatic cord, Br J Urol 75:101-102, 1995.
221. Sarma DP, Weilbaecher TG: Leiomyoma of the spermatic cord, J Surg Oncol 28:318-322, 1985.
222. Murayama T, Fujita K, Ohashi T et al: Melanotic neuroectodermal tumor of the epididymis in infancy: a case report, J Urol 141:105-106, 1989.
223. Denadai ER, Zerati Filho M, Verona CB et al: Tumor of the testicle: a case of melanotic neuroectodermal tumor of infancy, J Urol 136:117-118, 1986.
224. Frank GL, Koten JW: Melanotic hamartoma ("retinal anlage tumour") of the epididymis, J Pathol Bacteriol 93:549-554, 1967.
225. Jurincic-Winkler C, Metz KA, Klippel KF: Melanotic neuroectodermal tumor of infancy (MNTI) in the epididymis. A case report with immunohistological studies and special consideration of malignant features, Zentralbl Pathol 140:181-185, 1994.
226. Kanungo A, Chandi SM: Melanotic neuroectodermal tumor of the epididymis. A case report, Indian J Cancer 31:138-140, 1994.
227. Ricketts RR, Majmudarr B: Epididymal melanotic neuroectodermal tumor of infancy, Hum Pathol 16:416-420, 1985.
228. Dehner LP: Pediatric surgical pathology, Baltimore, 1987, Willams & Wilkins.
229. Ross L: Brenner-like tumor, Cancer 21:722-723, 1968.
230. Goldman R: A Brenner tumor of the testis, Cancer 26:853-855, 1970.
231. Nogales FF, Matill A, Ortega I et al: Mixed Brenner and adenomatoid tumor of the testis: an ultrastructural study and histogenetic consideration, Cancer 43:539-546, 1979.
232. Maurer R, Taylor CR, Schmuski O et al: Extratesticular gonadal stromal tumor in the pelvis. A case report with immunoperoxidase findings, Cancer 45:985-993, 1980.
233. Mukerjee MG, Norris M, Strum DP et al: Mucinous adenoid tumor of the paratesticular tissue, J Urol 115:472-475, 1976.
234. Levant B, Chetlin MA: Neurofibroma of the tunica albuginea testes, J Urol 59:1187-1188, 1948.
235. Pfitzenmaier NW, Wurster K, Kjelle-Schweigler M: Hemangioma of the tunica albuginea testis, Urol Int 30:237-241, 1975.
236. Kaido M, Iwai S, Ide Y et al: Epididymal lymphangiectasis, J Urol 150:1251-1252, 1993.
237. Huang PF, Farnum JB: Lymphangioma of the spermatic cord, J Tenn Med Assoc 80:270-272, 1987.

238. Arda S, Senocak ME, Buyukpamukcu N et al: Lymphangioma of the spermatic cord and tunica vaginalis in children, Eur Urol 21:253-255, 1992 (review).
239. Chetty R: Epididymal cavernous haemangiomas, Histopathology 22:396-398, 1993.
240. Chetty R, Bandid S, Freedman D: Cavernous haemangioma of the epididymis mimicking a testicular malignancy, Austr N Z J Surg 63:235-237, 1993.
241. Chung MD: Granular cell tumor of the spermatic cord: a case report with light and electron microscopic study, J Urol 120:379-381, 1978.
242. McGregor JR, Raweily EA, McLellan DR et al: Primary carcinoid tumour of the spermatic cord, Br J Urol 70:694, 1992.
243. Dharkar D, Kraft JR: Paraganglioma of the spermatic cord. An incidental finding, J Urol Pathol 2:89-93, 1994.
244. Fisher C, Bisceglia M: Solitary fibrous tumour of the spermatic cord, Br J Urol 74:798-799, 1994.
245. Certo LM, Avetta L, Hanlon JT et al: Liposarcoma of spermatic cord, Urology 31:168-170, 1988.
246. Dalla Palma P, Barbazza R: Well-differentiated liposarcoma of the paratesticular area: report of a case with fine-needle aspiration preoperative diagnosis and review of the literature, Diagn Cytopathol 6:421-426, 1990.
247. Goodman FR, Staunton MD, Rees HC: Liposarcoma of the spermatic cord, J Royal Soc Med 84:499-500, 1991.
248. Sonksen J, Hansen EF, Colstrup H: Liposarcoma of the spermatic cord. Case report, Scand J Urol Nephrol 25:239-240, 1991.
249. Pozza D, Masci P, D'Ottavio G et al: Spermatic cord liposarcoma in a young boy, J Urol 137:306-308, 1987.
250. Kent J. Giant liposarcoma of the spermatic cord, Med J Austr 148:602, 1988 (letter).
251. Johnson DE, Harris JD, Ayala AG: Liposarcoma of the spermatic cord, Urology 11:190-194, 1978.
252. Vorstman B, Block NL, Politano VA: The management of spermatic cord liposarcoma, J Urol 131:66-72, 1984.
253. Solivetti FM, D'Ascenzo R, Molisso A et al: Rhabdomyosarcoma of the funiculus, J Clin Ultrasound 17:521-522, 1989.
254. Nistal M, Fachal C, Paniagua R: Testicular carcinoma in situ associated with rhabdomyosarcoma of the spermatic cord, J Urol 142:358-360, 1989.
255. Fox T Jr, Collier RL: Rhabdomyosarcoma of the spermatic cord. A review and case presentation, Am Surg 33:483-489, 1967.
256. Hawkins HK, Camacho-Velasquez JV: Rhabdomyosarcoma in children. Correlations of form and prognosis in one institution's experience, Am J Surg Pathol 11:531-536, 1989.
257. Racalbuto A, Puleo S, Di Cataldo A et al: Leiomyosarcoma of the spermatic cord. Case report and review of the literature, Italian Journal of Surgical Sciences 18:279-285, 1988.
258. Kinjo M, Hokamura K, Tanaka K et al: Leiomyosarcoma of the spermatic cord. A case report and a brief review of literature, Acta Pathol Jpn 36:929-934, 1986.
259. de Bolla AR, Arkell DG: Leiomyosarcoma of the spermatic cord, Postgrad Med J 59:470-471, 1983.
260. Helm RH, Al-Tikriti S: Primary leiomyosarcoma of the epididymis, Br J Urol 58:99, 1986.
261. Davides KC, King LM, Paat F: Primary leiomyosarcoma of the epididymis, J Urol 114:642-644, 1975.
262. Reynard JM, Hasan N, Baithun SI et al: Malignant mesothelioma of the tunica vaginalis testis, Br J Urol 74:389-390, 1994.
263. Japko L, Horta AA, Schreiber K et al: Malignant mesothelioma of the tunica vaginalis testes: report of first case with preoperative diagnosis, Cancer 49:119-122, 1982.
264. Jones MA, Young RH, Scully RE: Malignant meosthelioma of the tunica vaginalis. A clinicopathologic analysis of 11 cases with review of the literature, Am J Surg Pathol 19:815-825, 1995.
265. McDonald RE, Sago AL, Novicki DE et al: Paratesticular mesotheliomas, J Urol 130:360-363, 1983.
266. Morikawa Y, Ishihara Y, Yanase Y et al: Malignant mesothelioma of tunica vaginalis with squamous differentiation, J Urol Pathol 2:95-102, 1994.
267. Young RH, Scully RE: Testicular and paratesticular tumors and tumor-like lesions of ovarian common epithelial and Müllerian types. A report of four cases and review of the literature, Am J Clin Pathol 86:146-156, 1986.
268. Axiotis C: Intratesticular serous papillary cystadenoma of low malignant potential: an ultrastructural and immunohistochemical study suggesting Müllerian differentiation, Am J Surg Pathol 12:56-66, 1988.
269. Kurihara K, Oka A, Mannami M et al: Papillary adenocarcinoma of the epididymis, Acta Pathol Jpn 43:440-443, 1993.
270. Nistal M, Revestido R, Paniagua R: Bilateral mucinous cystadenocarcinoma of the testis and epididymis, Arch Pathol Lab Med 116:1360-1363, 1992.
271. Salm R: Papillary carcinoma of the epididymis, J Pathol 97:253-259, 1969.
272. Yamamoto M, Miyake K, Mitsuya H et al: A case of primary carcinoma of the epididymis, Hinyokika Kiyo 33:1139-1142, 1987.
273. Wang TY, Chiang H, Huang JK et al: Papillary cystadenocarcinoma of the epididymis—report of a case, Chung Hua I Hsueh Tsa Chih, Chinese Med J 46:123-125, 1990.
274. Kher MM, Kherdekar MS, Grover S et al: Carcinoma of epididymis—report of a case, Indian J Cancer. 10:475-478, 1973.
275. Wise AG, Rao DM: Ultrasound appearances of malignant fibrous histiocytoma of the spermatic cord. A case report, Australas Radiol 32:512-514, 1988.
276. Tanaka T, Akazawa N, Ozaki Y et al: Malignant fibrous histiocytoma originating in the left spermatic cord with a review of 14 cases in the literature, Jpn J Clin Oncol 14:437-443, 1984.
277. Smailowitz Z, Kaneti J, Sober I et al: Malignant fibrous histiocytoma of the spermatic cord, J Urol 130:150-151, 1983.
278. Williamson JC, Johnson JD, Lamm DL et al: Malignant fibrous histiocytoma of the spermatic cord, J Urol 123:785-788, 1980.
279. Algaba F, Trias I, Castro C: Inflammatory malignant fibrous histiocytoma of the spermatic cord with eosinophilia, Histopathology 14:319-321, 1989.
280. Eltorky MA, O'Brien TF, Walzer Y: Primary paratesticular malignant fibrous histiocytoma. Case report and review of the literature, J Urol Pathol 1:425-429, 1993.
281. Dowling KJ, Lieb HE: Fibrosarcoma of epididymis, Urology 26:307-308, 1985.

282. McCormack M: Bilateral fibrosarcoma of the epididymis, J Clin Pathol 28:576-579, 1975.
283. Johnson DE, Kaesler KE, Mackay BM et al: Neurofibrosarcoma of spermatic cord, Urology 5:680-683, 1975.
284. Prince C: Malignant tumors of the spermatic cord: a brief review with presentation of a case of angioendothelioma, J Urol 47:793-797, 1942.
285. McCluggage WG, Lioe TF, Caughley LM: Malignant mesenchymoma of the spermatic cord, Histopathology 24:493-495, 1994.
286. Guy MS, Fishelovitz Y, Lifschitz-Mercer B et al: Malignant mesenchymoma of spermatic cord: a case report with intermediate filament typing, Isr J Med Sci 25:702-705, 1989.
287. Christenson PJ, O'Connell KJ: Metastatic extraosseous myxoid chondrosarcoma of spermatic cord, Urology 26:301-303, 1985.
288. MacDonald G Jr, D'Ambrosio P, Marshall DP: Chondrosarcoma of spermatic cord, Urology 9:439-441, 1977.
289. Aguirre P, Scully RE: Primitive neuroectodermal tumor of the testis. Report of a case, Arch Pathol Lab Med 107:643-645, 1983.
290. Dichmann O, Engel U, Jensen DB et al: Juxtatesticular seminoma, Br J Urol 66:324-325, 1990.
291. Leaf DN, Tucker GR, Harrison LH: Embryonal cell carcinoma originating in the spermatic cord: case report, J Urol 112:285-286, 1974.
292. Young TW: Malignant tumours of the spermatic cord. Case reports of a secondary teratoma and a primary fibrosarcoma, Br J Surg 56:260-262, 1969.
293. Moller MB: Non-Hodgkin's lymphoma of the spermatic cord, Acta Haematol 91:70-72, 1994 (review).
294. Glaholm J, Brada M, Horwich A: Hodgkin's disease of the epididymis and testis, J Royal Soc Med 82:558-559, 1989.
295. Zwanger-Mendelsohn S, Shreck EH, Doshi V: Burkitt lymphoma involving the epididymis and spermatic cord: sonographic and CT findings, AJR Am J Roentgenol 153:85-86, 1989.
296. Hautzer NW, Nikolai V: Primary lymphoma of the spermatic cord, Br J Urol 58:565-566, 1986.
297. Ferry JA, Harris NL, Young RH et al: Malignant lymphoma of the testis, epididymis, and spermatic cord. A clinicopathologic study of 69 cases with immunophenotypic analysis, Am J Surg Pathol 18:376-390, 1994.
298. Ginaldi L, De Pasquale A, De Martinis M et al: Epididymal lymphoma. A case report, Tumori 79:147-149, 1993.
299. Heaton JP, Morales A: Epididymal lymphoma: an unusual scrotal mass, J Urol 131:353-354, 1984.
300. Schned AR, Variakojis D, Straus F et al: Primary histiocytic lymphoma of the epididymis, Cancer 43:1156-1163, 1979.
301. Kreiger JN, Chasko SB, Keuhnelian JG: Paratesticular neuroblastoma associated with subependymal giant cell astrocytoma, J Urol 124:736-738, 1980.
302. Yadav K, Pathak IC: Wilms' tumour with left cord metastasis: short case report, Br J Urol 49:536-537, 1977.
303. Bahnson RR, Snopek TJ, Grayhack JT: Epididymal metastasis from prostatic carcinoma, Urology 26:296-297, 1985.
304. Wiebe B, Warnoe H, Klarlund M et al: Epididymal metastasis from prostatic carcinoma, Scand J Urol Nephrol 27:553-555, 1993.
305. Sarma DP, Weiner M, Weilbaecher TG: Epididymal metastasis from prostatic cancer, J Surg Oncol 24:322-324, 1983 (review).
306. de Riese W, Warmbold H, Aeikens B: Intrascrotal metastases from renal cell carcinoma, Int Urol Nephrol 18:449-452, 1986.
307. Ford ML, Tandan B: Metastatic tumor of the spermatic cord and testis from carcinoma of the stomach: a case report, South Med J 62:352-354, 1969.
308. Kanno K, Ohwada S, Nakamura S et al: Epididymis metastasis from colon carcinoma—a case report and a review of the literature, Jpn J Clin Oncol 24:340-344, 1994.
309. Parra RO, Boullier J, Mehan DJ: Malignant tumor of the colon metastatic to the epididymis as a first sign of recurrence of colon cancer, Mo Med 89:298-300, 1992.
310. Komeda Y, Kato M, Saito K: Spermatic cord metastasis from ureteral carcinoma, Urology 26:301-303, 1988.
311. Hammad FA: Metastatic malignant melanoma of the epididymis, Br J Urol 69:661, 1992.

Normal Anatomy and Histology

Congenital Abnormalities

Non-neoplastic Diseases of the Penis

- Inflammation
- Infections

Tumors and Tumorlike Conditions of the Penis

- Tumorlike conditions
  - Condyloma acuminata
  - Pearly penile papules
  - Penile cysts
  - Pseudoepitheliomatous keratotic and micaceous balanitis
  - Verruciform xanthoma
- Neoplastic diseases
  - Premalignant lesions
  - Malignant neoplasms
  - Squamous cell carcinoma

Diseases of the Scrotum

- Non-neoplastic diseases
  - Fournier's gangrene
  - Hidradenitis suppurativa
  - Idiopathic scrotal calcinosis
  - Lipogranuloma
  - Epidermal cyst
  - Fat necrosis
- Neoplastic diseases
  - Squamous cell carcinoma
  - Basal cell carcinoma
  - Paget's disease
  - Sarcoma

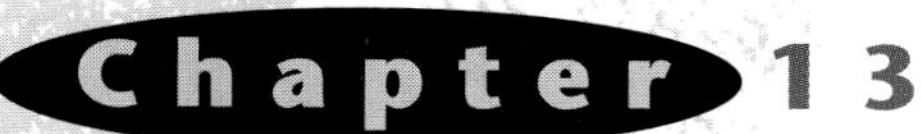

PENIS AND SCROTUM

JAE Y. RO
MAHUL B. AMIN
ALBERTO G. AYALA

NORMAL ANATOMY AND HISTOLOGY

The penis consists of three portions: the root, the body, and the glans. The root lies in the superficial perineal pouch and provides fixation and stability. The body constitutes the major part of the penis and is composed of three cylinders of spongy erectile tissues: the paired corpora cavernosa and the single corpus spongiosum. The two cavernous bodies lie on the dorsum of the penis and are surrounded by a double layer of dense fibrous connective tissue called *Buck's fascia* (tunica albuginea). The corpus spongiosum lies in the ventral aspect of the penis and surrounds the urethra in its center. The glans is the distal expansion of the corpus spongiosum; it is conical and normally covered by the loose skin of the prepuce. In the uncircumcised male the glans is covered by five to six layers of stratified nonkeratinizing squamous epithelium, which becomes keratinized in the circumcised male.

The foreskin of the penis is remarkably thin, dark, and loosely connected to the tunica albuginea. It has features of true skin but is devoid of subcutaneous adipose tissue. Sebaceous glands without associated hair follicles and sweat glands are present in the superficial dermis.

Histologically, the foreskin comprises five layers: epidermis, dermis, dartos, lamina propria, and squamous mucosa, which is a prolongation of the squamous mucosa of the glans and balanopreputial sulcus. The foreskin is a highly vascular tissue. Most of its blood supply is from the internal pudendal artery, which has three main branches: the deep artery, the bulbar artery, and the urethral artery. The venous return is through three channels: the cavernous veins, the deep veins, and the superficial dorsal veins. The lymphatic drainage of the penis is through the superficial and deep inguinal lymph nodes that drain to the external and common iliac nodes.

Histogenetically, the penis has two separate origins for its three erectile bodies. Genital tubercles are responsible for the corpora cavernosa. The urethra and corpus spongiosum are formed from the urogenital sinus and the urogenital folds.

The scrotum consists of skin; dartos muscle; and external spermatic, cremasteric, and internal spermatic fasciae. The internal fascia is loosely attached to the parietal layer of the tunica vaginalis. The epidermis covers the dermis, and the deepest layer of the dermis merges with the smooth muscle bundles of the dartos tunic. Although scattered fat cells are present, there is no subcutaneous adipose tissue layer. The dermis contains hair follicles and apocrine, eccrine, and sebaceous glands.

The scrotum contains the testes and the lower parts of the spermatic cords. The surface of the scrotum is divided into right and left halves by a cutaneous raphe, which continues ventrally to the inferior penile surface and dorsally along the midline of the perineum to the anus. The left side of the scrotum is usually lower because of the greater length of the left spermatic cord.

Embryologically, the scrotum originates from the genital swellings that meet ventral to the anus and unite forming the two scrotal sacs. A median raphe of fibrovascular connective tissue separates both halves. The scrotum derives its blood supply from the external and internal pudendal arteries, and additional blood comes to it from cremasteric and testicular arteries that traverse the spermatic cords. The lymphatic drainage of the scrotum is to the superficial inguinal nodes.

CONGENITAL ABNORMALITIES

Congenital absence of the upper wall of the urethra is known as epispadias. In this anomaly the urethral opening appears on the dorsum of the penis as a groove or cleft. The incidence of epispadias is 1 in 117,000 male births.[1,2] According to location, there are three types of epispadias: penopubic, penile, and glandular, the first being most frequent.[1] Urinary incontinence is frequently observed with penopubic epispadias and occasionally with penile type, but it is not associated with glandular epispadias.[2] Associated congenital anomalies include diastasis of the pubic symphysis, bladder exstrophy, renal agenesis, and ectopic pelvic kidney.[2-4]

Hypospadias is a developmental anomaly in which the urethra opens on the underside of the penile shaft or on the perineum (Fig. 13-1).[5,6] Hypospadias is frequently associated with chordee (Fig. 13-2) but can occur without chordee. The meatus most frequently occurs distally (71%) in the glans (13%), corona (43%), and distal shaft (34%). Midpenile (16%) and proximal (13%) locations make up the remainder. Proximal locations include the back of the penis, the area between the penis and the scrotum, the scrotum (see Fig. 13-1*B*), and the perineum.[5,6] The incidence of hypospadias is 1 per 300 live male births.[6,7] Associated anomalies include cryptorchidism and inguinal hernia. Association with anomalies of the upper urinary tract is uncommon unless other anomalies are present in other systems.[6-8]

A micropenis is a normally formed penis with a size 2 or more standard deviations below the mean. The ratio of the length of the penile shaft to its circumference is normal (Fig. 13-3). The corpora cavernosa may be severely hypoplastic. The scrotum is generally fused but often is diminutive, and the testes usually are small and frequently cryptorchid. A webbed or concealed penis often resembles a micropenis, but the penile shaft is of normal length. The three most common causes of micropenis are hypogonadotropic hypogonadism, hypergonadotropic hypogonadism (primary testicular failure), and idiopathic.[9,10]

A concealed penis is a normally developed penis that becomes buried in a suprapubic fat pad (Fig. 13-4). This anomaly may be congenital or idiopathic following circumcision. A concealed penis may be visualized by retracting skin lateral to the penile shaft.[11]

Aphallia (penile agenesis) results from failure of the genital tubercle to develop. The incidence is 1 in 10,000,000 live male births; only 70 cases have been reported.[12,13] The usual appearance is that of a well-developed scrotum with descended testes but no penile shaft. In most cases, the urethra opens at the anal verge adjacent to a small skin tag or, in other cases, opens into the rectum. Associated malformations include cryptorchidism, vesicoureteral reflux, horseshoe kidney, renal

13-1. **A**, Distal hypospadias with the urethal meatus at the junction of the glans and penile shaft. **B**, Proximal hypospadias with the urethral meatus at the base of scrotum.

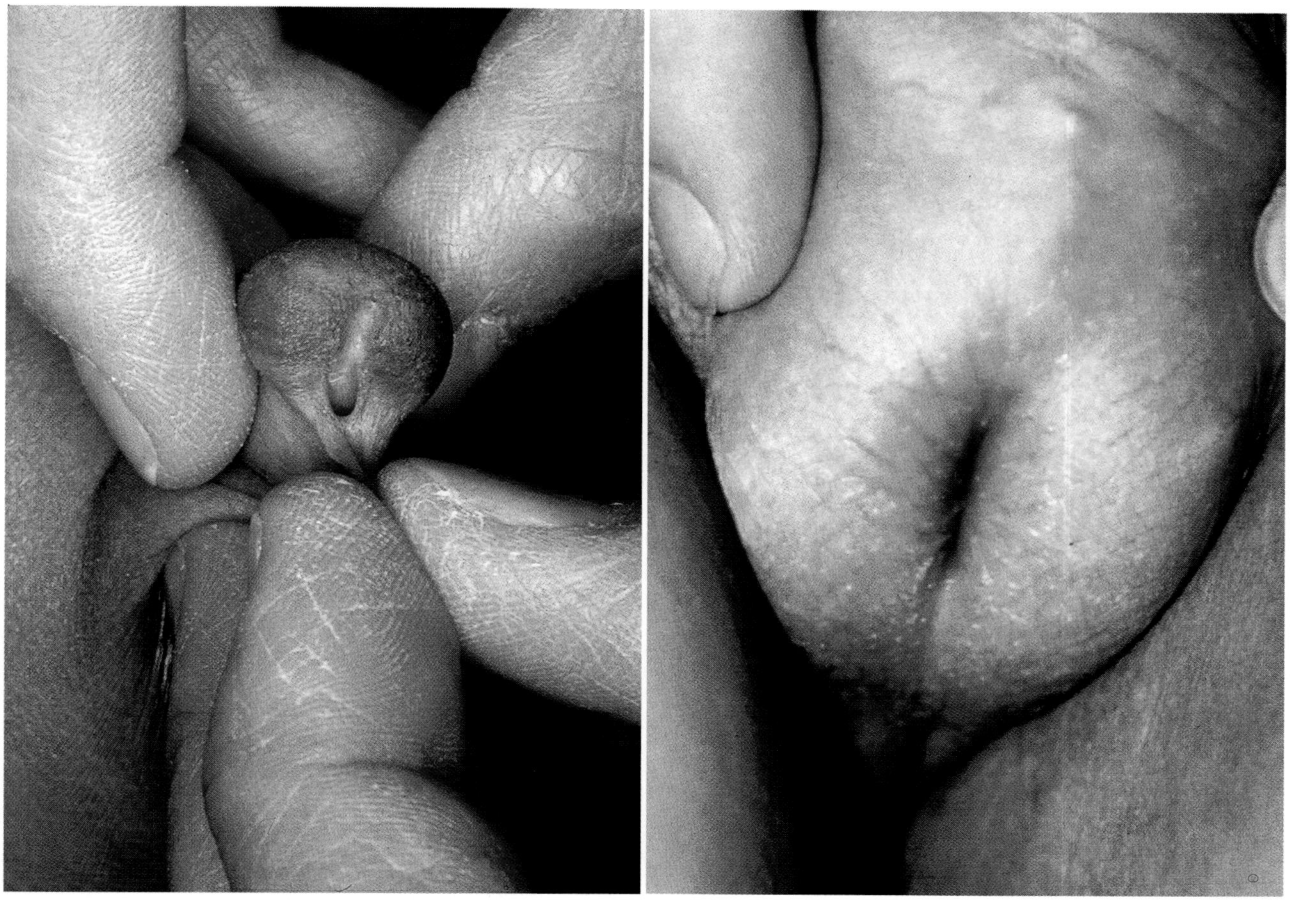

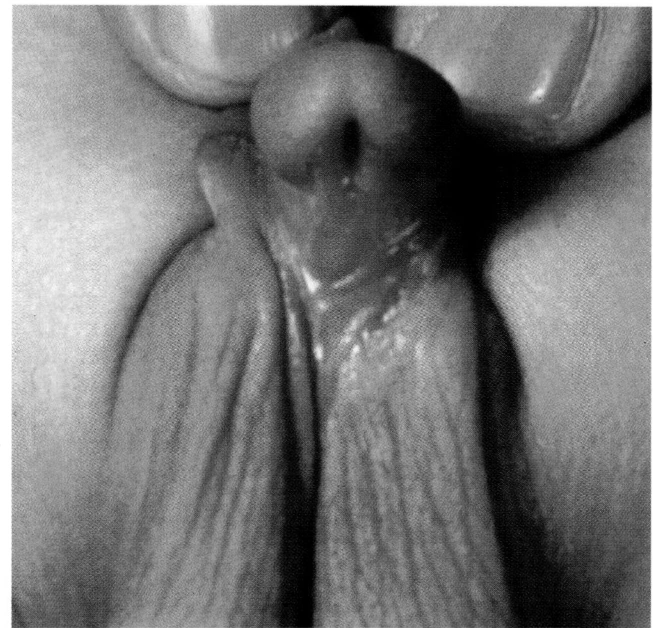

13-2. Hypospadias with chordee.

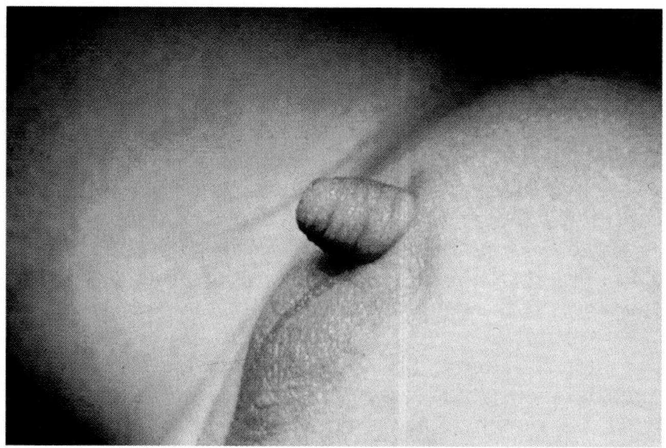

13-3. Micropenis.

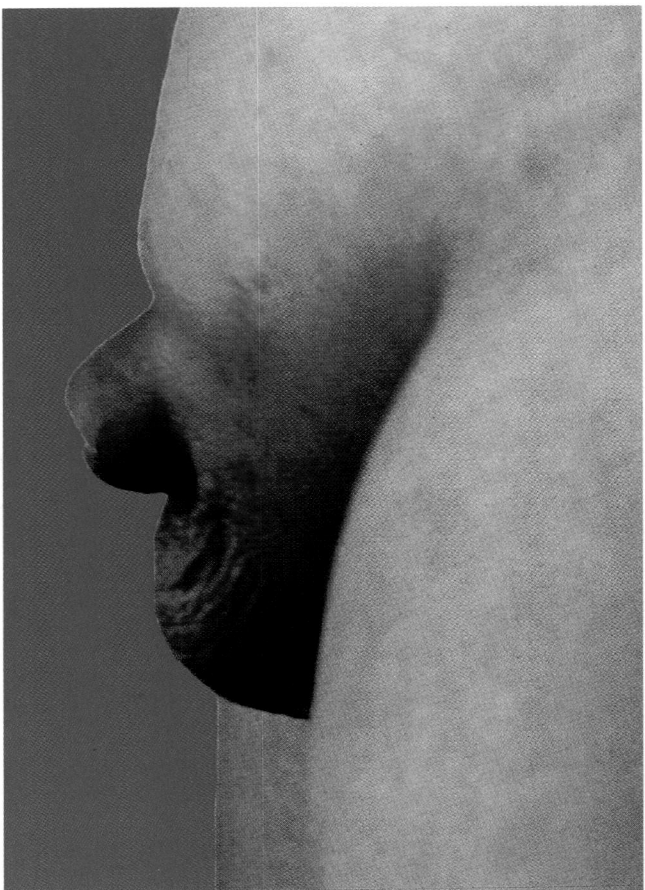

13-4. Concealed penis.

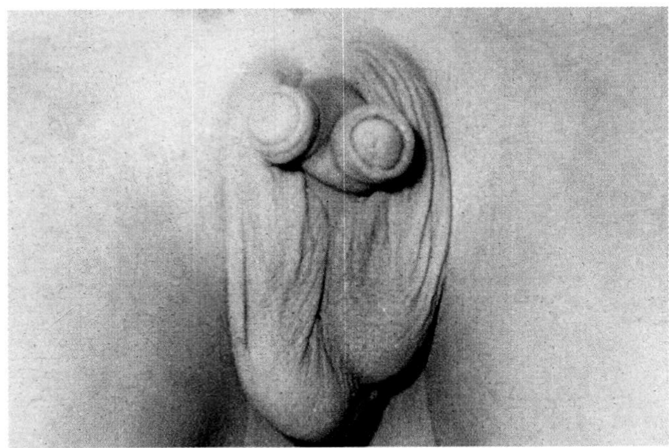

13-5. Diphallus.

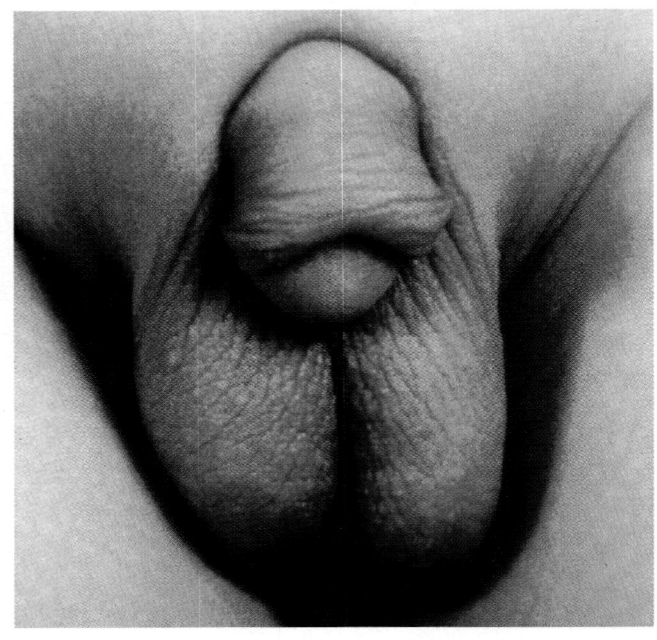

13-6. Scrotal engulfment.

agenesis, imperforate anus, and musculoskeletal and cardiopulmonary abnormalities.[12,13]

Diphallus, or duplication of the penis, is a rare anomaly that ranges from a small accessory penis to complete duplication (Fig. 13-5).[14] Associated anomalies include hypospadias, bifid scrotum, duplication of the bladder, renal agenesis or ectopia, and diastasis of the pubic symphysis. Anal and cardiac anomalies are also common.[14,15]

Chordee, a congenital or acquired bend of the penis, is caused by decreased elasticity in one or more of the fascial layers of the penis, leading to shortness of one corpus cavernosum when erection occurs. The bend may be ventral, dorsal, lateral, or complex. Chordee is most frequently associated developmentally with hypospadias when the mesenchyme distal to the meatus ceases to differentiate, creating a fan-shaped bend of dysgenetic fascia.[16] Acquired chordee may result from trauma or Peyronie's disease.[17]

Scrotal engulfment (penoscrotal transposition) results from incomplete migration of the inferomedial labioscrotal swelling (Fig. 13-6). This has been termed *bifid scrotum, doughnut scrotum, prepenile scrotum,* and *shawl scrotum.* Frequently it occurs in conjunction with perineal, scrotal, or penoscrotal hypospadias with chordee.[18,19]

Ectopic scrotum is rare and refers to the anomalous position of one hemiscrotum along the inguinal canal, most commonly the suprainguinal canal, although it may be within the infrainguinal canal or the perineum. Associated anomalies include cryptorchidism, inguinal hernia, exstrophy, popliteal pterygium syndrome, renal agenesis, renal dysplasia, and ectopic urethra.[20]

NON-NEOPLASTIC DISEASES OF THE PENIS

INFLAMMATION

Phimosis and paraphimosis

Phimosis is a condition in which the foreskin cannot be retracted behind the glans penis (Fig. 13-7). In adults and adolescents the foreskin can normally be retracted

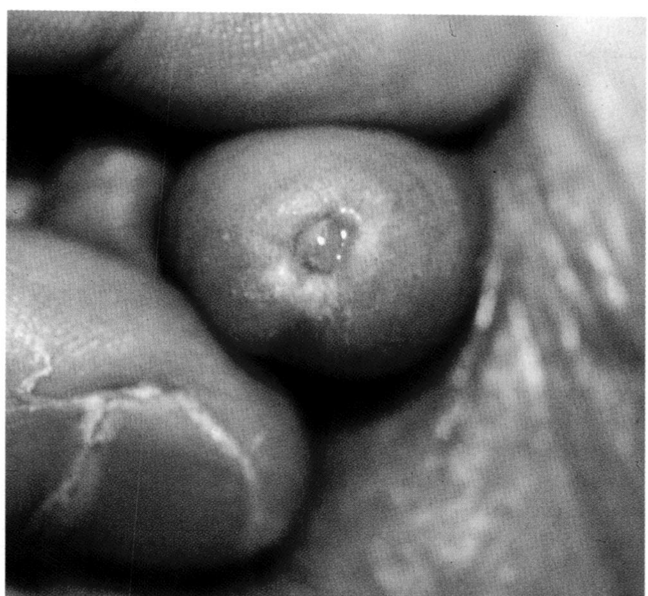

13-7. Phimosis. *(Courtesy of Dr. Julian Wan, State University of New York, Buffalo.)*

beyond the corona with relative ease, but it is important to note that in children less than 5 years old the foreskin is not retractable.[21,22] Phimosis may be seen in uncircumcised men at any age.

Phimosis may be congenital or acquired. Congenital phimosis is much rarer and is secondary to a small preputial orifice or to an abnormally long foreskin. Secondary phimosis usually results from an accumulation of smegma, which is due to poor hygiene and can lead to chronic inflammation, edema, and fibrosis. Balanoposthitis (inflammation of the glans and prepuce) and balanitis xerotica obliterans may cause phimosis.[22,23]

Circumcision is the treatment for phimosis, regardless of etiology. Surgical specimens from men should be carefully examined for areas of induration which might indicate dysplastic or neoplastic lesions.[22] Microscopically, phimotic prepuces show varying degrees of inflammation, fibrosis, edema, and vascular congestion, or they may be histologically normal. Lymphocytes and plasma cells are the predominant inflammatory components.[24] Patients with phimosis often complain of irritation, but significant pain is uncommon unless phimosis produces ballooning of the foreskin due to urinary obstruction.

Paraphimosis is a condition in which the foreskin has been retracted behind the glans penis and cannot be advanced back over the glans.[21,22] Constriction of the glans causes pain due to vascular engorgement and edema. Paraphimosis is often iatrogenic, occurring after examination of the penis or after urinary tract instrumentation. Rarer reported causes include *Plasmodium falciparum* malaria[25] and carcinoma metastatic to the penis.[26] Paraphimosis requires circumcision or an emergency dorsal slit procedure.[22]

Phimosis often coexists with penile carcinoma and is a risk factor for it (see the section on squamous cell carcinoma).[27,28]

BALANOPOSTHITIS: INFLAMMATION OF GLANS PENIS AND PREPUCE

- Balanoposthitis NOS
- Candidal balanitis
- Plasma cell balanitis (Zoon's balanitis)
- Balanitis xerotica obliterans (lichen sclerosus et atrophicus)
- Papulosquamous diseases
  - lichen planus
  - psoriasis
  - balanitis circinata of Reiter's syndrome
- Contact dermatitis
  - allergic
  - irritant
- Vesiculobullous diseases—may simulate balanitis clinically
  - cicatricial pemphigoid
  - fixed drug eruption

Balanoposthitis

Balanoposthitis (inflammation of the glans penis and prepuce) and balanitis (inflammation of the glans penis) occur most commonly in uncircumcised men.[29,30] The usual cause of balanoposthitis is poor hygiene. Failure to regularly retract and clean the foreskin leads to accumulation of smegma (desquamated epithelial cells and debris), which incites an inflammatory response, and may subsequently result in phimosis.

Balanoposthitis can also result from specific dermatologic lesions or infectious agents; these are summarized in the box above.[31] In a series of 86 patients with balanoposthitis and balanitis, 41% had no attributable etiologic factor; *Candida* species accounted for 30%, and beta-hemolytic streptococci were responsible for 11% of cases.[32]

Candidal balanoposthitis is discussed below in the section on infectious diseases of the penis. A discussion of papulosquamous and vesiculobullous diseases is beyond the scope of this textbook.

Plasma cell balanitis (Zoon's balanitis)

Plasma cell balanitis (Zoon's balanitis or balanitis circumscripta plasmacellularis) is a disorder that was first described in 1952 by Zoon.[33] The disease is not rare and is important because it clinically resembles erythroplasia of Queyrat or Bowen's disease of the glans penis.[34,35] Plasma cell balanitis is a benign disorder of unknown etiology that is thought to represent a reaction to a multitude of diverse stimuli. It is similar clinically and histologically to its vulvar counterpart, which is termed *vulvitis circumscripta plasmacellularis*.

Plasma cell balanitis affects only uncircumcised males.[36] It usually presents as a single large (2 cm or greater) bright red, moist patch on the glans or inner prepuce (Fig. 13-8). Rarely, multiple patches may be present, and in severe cases it may consist of extensive visibly eroded lesions. Because the clinical appearance of the lesion overlaps with candidal balanitis and erythroplasia of Queyrat, a biopsy is mandatory.

Histologically, the hallmark of plasma cell balanitis is a distinct upper dermal bandlike infiltrate containing numerous plasma cells (Fig. 13-9).[36,37] In some cases the number of plasma cells may be scant or moderate, and the histologic findings must be correlated with the clinical observations. The dermis also contains numerous dilated capillaries, adjacent to which may be extravasated erythrocytes or hemosiderin deposits. The overlying epidermis is thin and may occasionally be absent or partially separated from the dermis. The most distinctive feature within the epidermis is the presence of diamond, rhomboid, or flattened keratinocytes that are separated from one another by uniform intercellular edema.

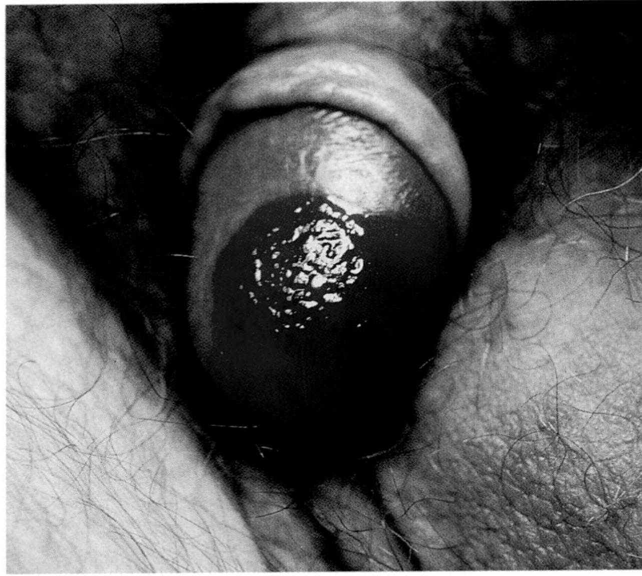

13-8. Zoon's balanitis. *(Courtesy of Dr. Hans Stricker, Henry Ford Hospital, Detroit, MI.)*

Currently, the treatment of choice is circumcision,[34,35] but laser surgery[38] and topical application of retin-A preparations or steroids have been employed with variable success.

Balanitis xerotica obliterans (lichen sclerosus et atrophicus)

Lichen sclerosus et atrophicus is an atrophic condition of the epidermis and dermal connective tissue that most commonly involves the genital and perianal skin of both males and females.[39] Extragenital lesions may accompany genital lesions, although they may also occur alone.[39] Balanitis xerotica obliterans is the term applied to lichen sclerosus et atrophicus of the glans penis and prepuce.[40]

Balanitis xerotica obliterans is commonly encountered in preputial resectates for phimosis in older men. In contrast, the prepubertal incidence in a series of 117 cases was 4%.[41] The idiopathic form of balanitis xerotica obliterans is not associated with phimosis and presents with the classic clinical and pathologic features. The cause of this classic form of balanitis xerotica obliterans is unknown, but recent evidence favors an autoimmune mechanism.[40,42-44] Patients with lichen

A

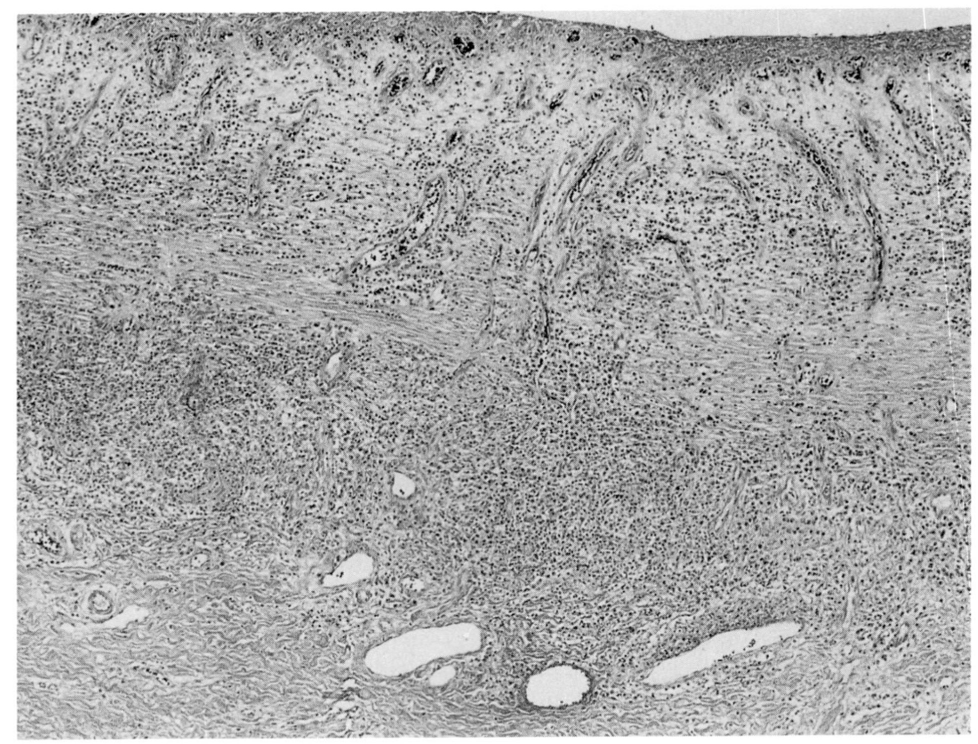

13-9. A, Zoon's balanitis (low power)

Continued.

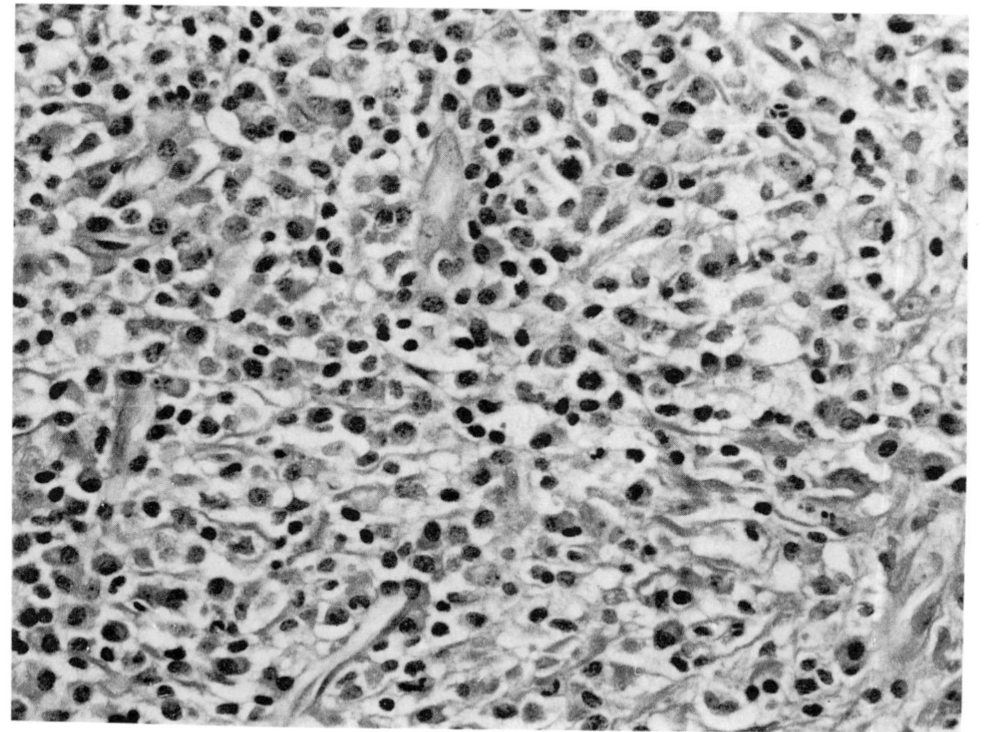

13-9, cont'd. B, Zoon's balanitis (high power).

sclerosus et atrophicus may have increased organ-specific antibodies (thyroid microsomal and parietal cell antibodies in women and smooth muscle and parietal cell antibodies in men).[42-44] Association with autoimmune diseases, including vitiligo and alopecia areata, further supports the premise that autoimmune pathogenetic mechanisms may play an important role in these lesions.

Clinically, balanitis xerotica obliterans presents as a well-defined and marginated white patch on the glans penis or prepuce that envelops or involves the urethral meatus (Fig. 13-10). It may also present as a lichenoid scale with a roughened surface. In longstanding cases, the lesion is firm due to the underlying fibrosis, which may cause phimosis in uncircumcised men. Most lesions occur on the glans penis or prepuce, but the shaft occasionally is involved. Urethral involvement may cause stricture.[45] Pruritus, pain, and dyspareunia are common in vulvar lichen sclerosus et atrophicus, but balanitis xerotica obliterans is mostly asymptomatic.

Histologically, active lesions of balanitis xerotica obliterans show pronounced orthokeratotic hyperkeratosis accompanied by striking atrophy of the epidermis, a distinctive combination of features. Basal cell vacuolation and clefting of the dermal-epidermal junction may also occur; in rare instances, there may be bullae.[46] Orthokeratotic plugging of cutaneous follicles, a feature of lichen sclerosus et atrophicus, is not seen in balanitis xerotica obliterans because of the absence of follicles in this area.[47] The upper dermis is markedly edematous and the collagen forms a homogenized band, beneath

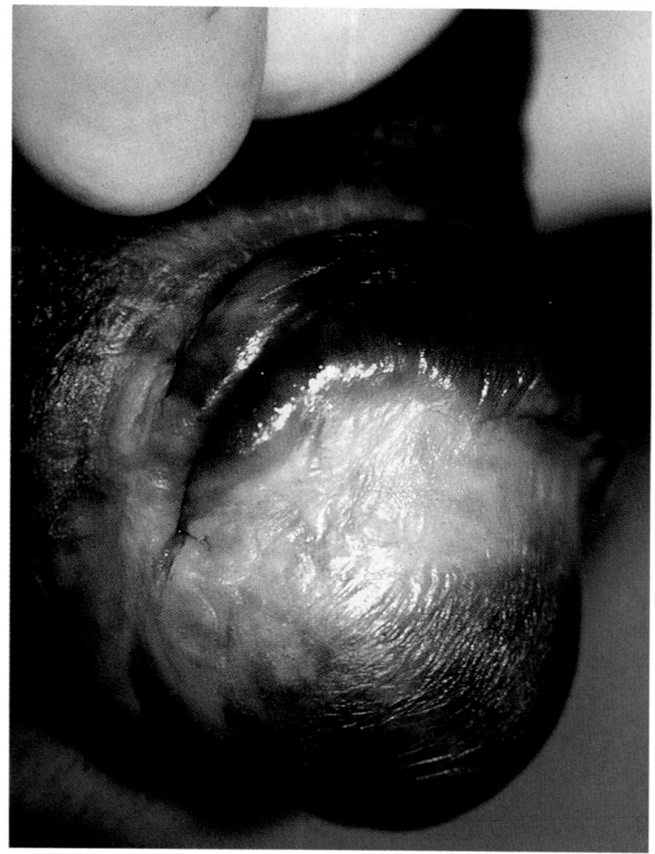

13-10. Balanitis xerotica obliterans.

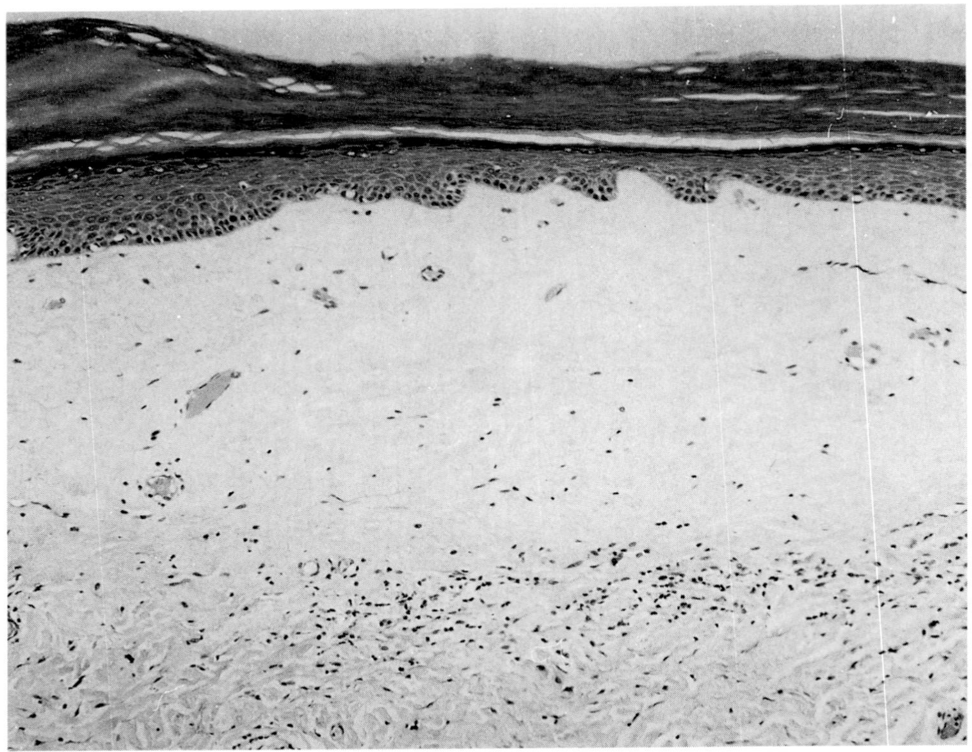

13-11. Balanitis xerotica obliterans showing homogeneous collagen in upper dermis with thin band of chronic inflammation just below.

which there may be a lymphoplasmacytic infiltrate (Fig. 13-11).

Over time, four principal changes occur: the basal layer of the epidermis becomes mature; the upper dermis is gradually replaced by sclerotic collagen; the inflammation in the middermis becomes patchy or absent and inflammation is seen in the superficial dermis; and areas of epithelial hyperplasia may alternate with atrophy. In rare cases, frank atypia may be evident. The chief differential diagnostic considerations are lupus erythematosus, morphea, and lichen planus.

The treatment of balanitis xerotica obliterans is often difficult. Circumcision; laser therapy; and topical administration of steroids, antifungal agents, and retinoids have been used with variable results.

Balanitis xerotica obliterans may precede, coexist with, or arise subsequent to the development of carcinoma. A few reports have associated balanitis xerotica obliterans with squamous cell carcinoma.[47-49]

Reiter's syndrome

In 1916 Reiter described a patient who developed systemic illness with polyarthritis, conjunctivitis, and nongonococcal urethritis after an episode of bloody diarrhea. Although this is not the first reported case, the syndrome characterized by the triad of arthritis, urethritis, and conjunctivitis is commonly referred to as Reiter's syndrome. More than two thirds of patients have associated mucocutaneous lesions, supporting the argument that Reiter's syndrome is better defined by a tetrad of symptoms that includes the mucocutaneous lesions.[50] More than 90% are male, with onset of symptoms in the third and fourth decades.[51] Epidemic (enteric) and endemic (urogenital) modes of presentation have been described, with the latter being much more common.[51-55] Patients frequently report histories of recent sexual contact with a new partner which is followed by the development of urethritis. The less common epidemic form is secondary to enteric infection and also occurs in children. Urethritis occurs in 90% of the postdysenteric or enteric form of the disease, so it should not be assumed that urethritis and Reiter's syndrome are sexually transmitted.

Chlamydia trachomatis probably is the most common cause for the sexually acquired form, although *Ureaplasma urealyticum*, *Shigella flexneri*, *Salmonella* species, *Campylobacter* species, *Yersinia enterocolitica*, and *Neisseria gonorrhoeae* have also been implicated.[53-56] Genetic susceptibility also plays an important role; 60% to 80% of patients are HLA-B27 positive. It is postulated that HLA-B27, either due to molecular mimicry or by virtue of its relation to antigens linked to genes controlling immune responses to certain infectious agents, produces an exaggerated or abnormal immune response to specific microbiologic agents that culminates in the inflammatory manifestations of the disease.[54,57]

Genital involvement occurs as part of the mucocutaneous manifestations of Reiter's syndrome and is common in the sexually acquired form of the disease. The lesions take two forms, known as balanitis circinata and

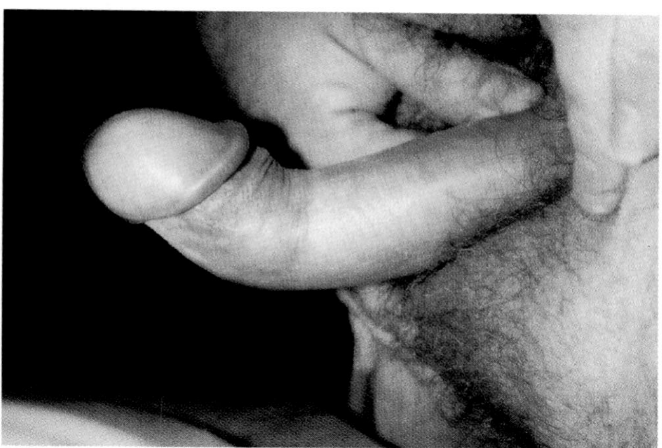

13-12. Peyronie's disease.

keratodermia blennorrhagica. Balanitis circinata is the more common and occurs in up to 85% of men with the sexually acquired form of the syndrome.[58] It is a painless lesion which begins as small red papules that enlarge centrifugally to form a circular or ringlike configuration. In circumcised men the lesion is hyperkeratotic and resembles the second lesion, keratodermia blennorhagica. Keratodermia blennorhagica is predominantly a cutaneous lesion, most commonly affecting the palms and soles. It begins as erythematous macules that enlarge to form hyperkeratotic papules with red halos. This form is clinically and histologically similar to psoriasis, and some cases of Reiter's syndrome progress to become indistinguishable from psoriatic arthritis.[58]

Histologically, the early lesions are indistinguishable from psoriasis vulgaris or pustular psoriasis, and they demonstrate psoriasiform hyperplasia, hyperkeratosis, parakeratosis, and neutrophilic exocytosis within the stratum corneum with formation of a spongiform pustule.[59] The spongiform pustule seen in the upper epidermis is the most characteristic histologic feature of Reiter's syndrome. The papillary dermis is thickened due to edema and may contain a neutrophilic perivascular infiltrate. In later stages the pustules are absent, and the epidermis shows nonspecific findings including acanthosis, hyperkeratosis, and focal parakeratosis. Reliable distinction of Reiter's syndrome from pustular psoriasis and psoriasis vulgaris may be extremely difficult and requires clinicopathologic correlation.

Peyronie's disease

Peyronie's disease (also called *plastic induration of the penis*, *fibrous sclerosis of the penis*, and *fibrous cavernitis*) presents with painful erection accompanied by distortion, bending, or constriction of the erect penis.[60] Observations resembling Peyronie's disease were made in 1561 by the Italian anatomist, Fallopius, but the first detailed description was by de la Peyronie, in a series of patients with deformities of the erect penis.

Peyronie's disease affects men between the ages of 20 and 80 years (median, 53 years) but is uncommon in men less than 40 years old. More than 66% of patients complain of painful erection. In patients without pain the presenting symptom is penile bending (Fig. 13-12), which varies in duration from an "overnight" appearance to a few months or, in some instances, a few years. Patients concerned about the presence of tumor may also seek attention after feeling a plaque. These lesions often are palpable as firm nodules or plaques on the dorsal surface of the erect penis. Examination of the flaccid penis may be unremarkable. Rarely, there may be multiple plaques. Some have suggested that Peyronie's disease may be related to fibromatosis because of its association with Dupuytren's contractures, palmar or plantar fibromatosis, in 10% to 20% of patients.[61] Others have suggested that it may be an inflammatory fibrotic reaction secondary to urethritis. Peyronie's disease also appears to be related to coital trauma and urethral instrumentation, and it has been associated with use of beta blockers, hypertension, diabetes, and immune reactions.[62-66] Although some earlier studies suggested a relationship between specific human leukocyte antigen types and Peyronie's disease, further studies have failed to corroborate this association.[67] Bivens et al[68] reported six patients with Peyronie's disease and carcinoid syndrome and suggested a causal role for elevated serum serotonin levels. Guerneri et al[69] found chromosomal aberrations in 9 of 14 cases.

The chief pathologic finding in Peyronie's disease is fibrosis of the tunica albuginea, not affecting the erectile tissue of the corpora cavernosa. Calcification and ossification may occur in the fibrous plaques. Histologically, Peyronie's disease begins with a perivascular inflammatory infiltrate in the loose connective tissue between the tunica albuginea and the sinusoids of the corpora cavernosa. Deposition of fibrin in the tunica albuginea may be the primary event, followed by inflammation, fibrosis, and collagenization. In surgical specimens the histologic features are less dramatic than the clinical presentation, and they often consist of a cellular proliferation resembling fibromatosis or merely fibrosis (Fig. 13-13). Studies have shown excessive amounts of type III collagen in the plaques.[70]

The clinical course is variable. The disease resolves spontaneously in less than one third of the patients, progresses in up to 40%, and remains stable in the rest.[71] Treatment has included surgical excision of the plaques, radiotherapy, and steroid injections. Prostheses may be required to restore potency.[72]

Heterotopic penile bone (os penis) is occasionally found in the plaques of Peyronie's disease, particularly in elderly men.[73] In children the presence of os penis is considered a congenital anomaly related to the normal occurrence of penile bone in numerous carnivorous animals, a feature lost in humans.[74,75] The bone is usually deposited just beneath the tunica albuginea.

Penile prosthesis

Penile prostheses are surgically implanted devices that aid in erection by providing penile rigidity.[76] Since their introduction in the early 1970s, the technology has greatly advanced, chiefly because of better understanding of erectile physiology and pathophysiology. These

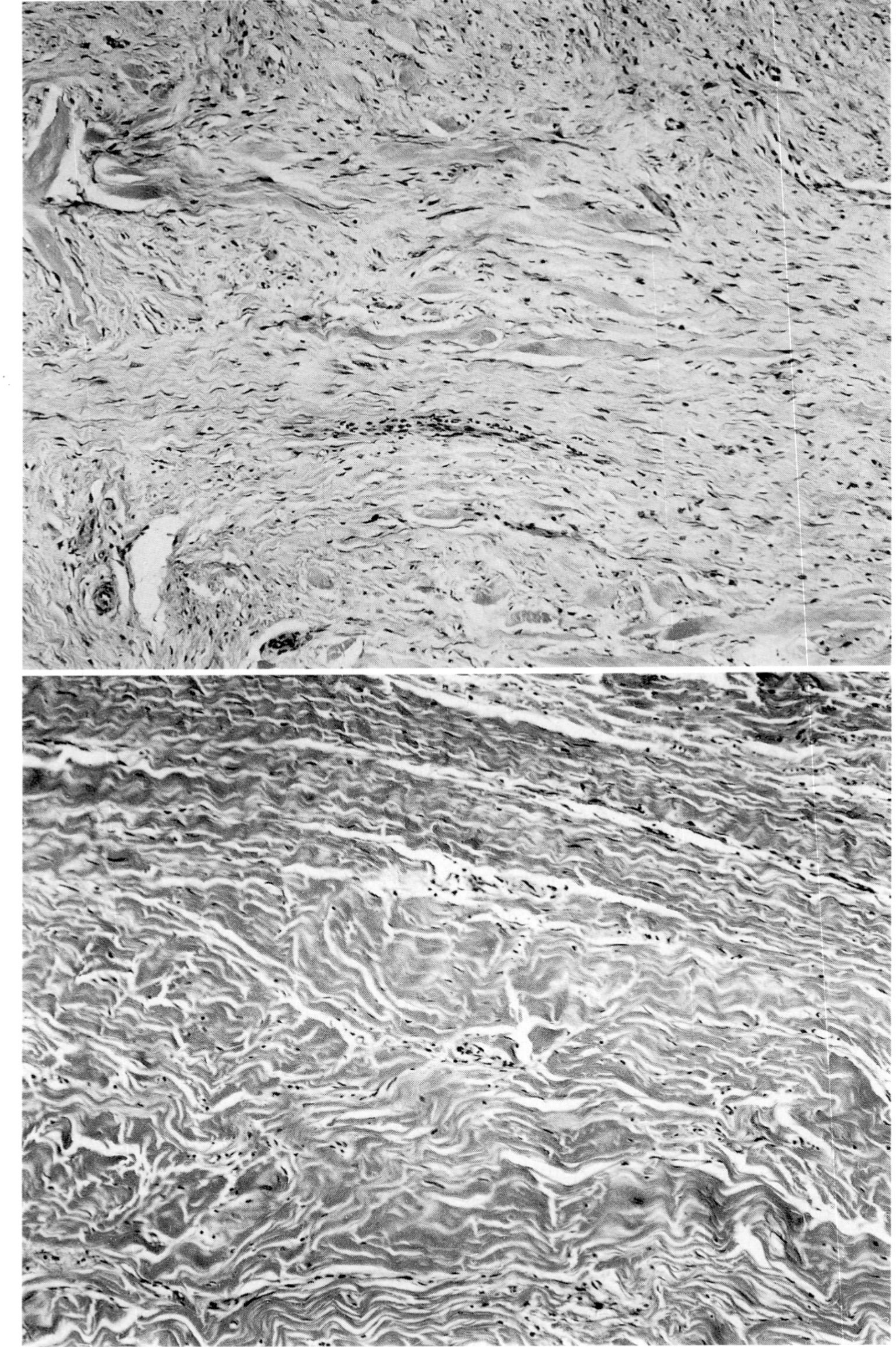

13-13. **A**, Peyronie's disease, cellular region. **B**, Peyronie's disease, densely collagenous region.

developments have resulted in widespread patient and physician acceptance of these devices, as well as a substantial reduction in complications.

The indications for prosthetic implantation are organic and psychogenic impotence; organic causes include diabetes, paraplegia, quadriplegia, and Peyronie's disease. Therapeutic advances in vascular surgery and pharmacotherapy are leading to a decreased use of penile prostheses in patients with organic causes, because other modalities offer better results.[76]

There are two general categories of penile prostheses: malleable devices and inflatable devices. These differ from one another in their construction and operation.[76-78] Malleable devices provide simplicity of implantation and have no mechanical parts to fail. They require very little manual dexterity as they need merely to be bent upward before use. They are disadvantageous because neither the size nor the rigidity of the penis changes. Inflatable devices are based on hydraulic principles that allow inflation for sexual intercourse with deflation in the detumescent phase. These devices are more difficult to implant and have limited lifespans due to eventual mechanical failure.

Complications of penile prostheses may occur during surgery (usually crural or corporal perforation), postoperatively (mainly infection or component failure), or may occur after some time due to device erosion. Although more than 90% of patients report satisfaction, the reoperative rate may be as high as 44%. Slightly lower rates have been reported recently and are expected to decline with improved designs and surgical advances.[79,80]

Priapism

Priapism is defined as prolonged erection unrelated to sexual desire. Typically, pain and tenderness result after 6 to 8 hours and are related to ensuing ischemia.

Priapism may be primary, secondary, or idiopathic. The secondary causes include genital trauma, thromboembolism, hemostasis and leukostasis (fat embolism, sickle cell anemia, leukemia), neurologic defects (anesthetic agents, spinal cord injury, and autonomic dysfunction), infiltration by cancer, pharmacologic effects (alcohol, drugs acting on central nervous system, total parenteral nutrition), and intracavernous injections for diagnostic procedures (papaverine hydrochloride, prostaglandin E, and phentolamine). Pohl et al[81] reviewed 230 cases from the literature; more than 33% were idiopathic; 21% were reactions to drugs and alcoholism, 12% were caused by trauma; 11% were caused by sickle cell anemia (an important cause of priapism in children), and less than 1% were due to neoplasms.

Data on pathologic findings in priapism are extremely limited. The corporeal tissue may be edematous, indurated, and ultimately sclerotic.[82] Ultrastructural examination reveals interstitial edema within 12 hours, destruction of sinusoidal endothelium and exposure of basement membrane with adherence of platelets by the end of 24 hours, and, finally, vascular thrombi associated with ischemic necrosis of smooth muscle tissue at 48 hours.[83]

Besides control of the precipitating factors, treatment includes: supportive therapy with analgesics, sedatives, and fluids; control of pain with penile block; irrigation of the corpora with saline or sympathomimetic drugs; and surgery for cavernosal shunt.[84]

INFECTIONS

Gonorrhea

Gonorrhea is caused by *Neisseria gonorrhoeae*, Gram-negative, nonmotile, non-spore-forming, biscuit-shaped diplococci. The term *gonorrhea* was coined by Galen in the second century and means "flow of semen," referring to the exudate of gonorrheal urethritis. The disease was recorded before the common era in descriptions by Hippocrates and Celcus. The latter treated gonorrheal strictures by catheterization.[85]

In men, gonorrhea typically produces urethritis with urethral discharge, which may be profuse, purulent, or scant (gleet), and burning micturition.[86,87] The disease is sexually acquired, and the risk of infection increases as the number of sexual partners increases. The penis is involved only as a complication of the disease, with cutaneous lesions, infection of median raphe, penile abscess, and gonococcal tysonitis (inflammation of the preputial glands).[88-90] The chief complication is urethral stricture. Laboratory tests are essential as the disease is frequently mimicked by, and coexists with, chlamydial infection. Standard diagnostic procedures include gram stain, culture, and microbial susceptibility testing.[86,87] The Centers for Disease Control and Prevention has given guidelines for its treatment, consisting primarily of antibiotic therapy.[91]

Syphilis

> Know syphilis in all its manifestations and relations, and all other things will be added unto you.
>
> Sir William Osler (1897)

Syphilis is one of the most fascinating diseases affecting humans and has been investigated and described by

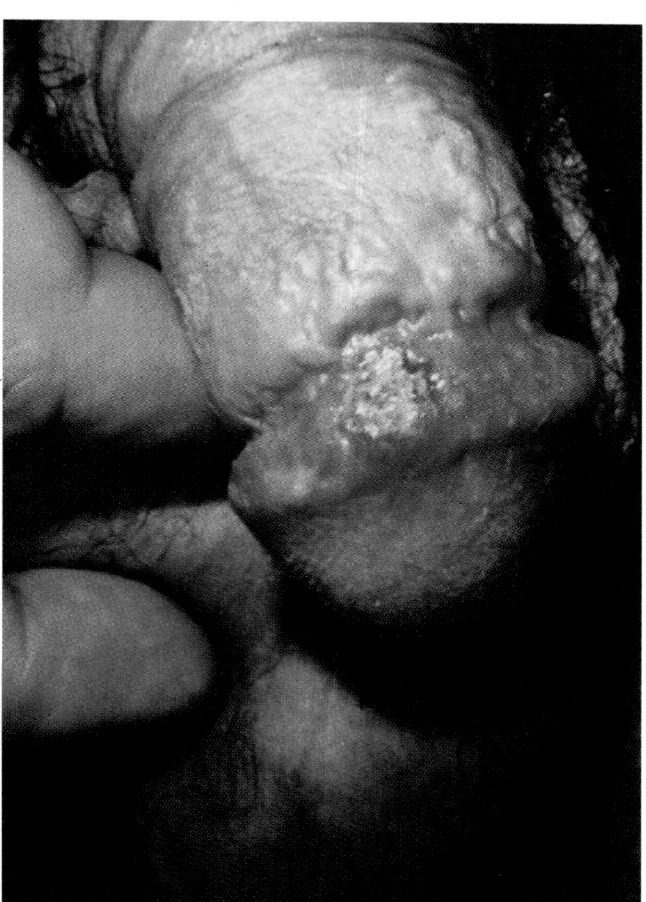

13-14. Syphilitic chancre.

clinical scholars, playwrights, and poets, including Fracastoro, who in 1530 wrote in his poem about the suffering shepherd Syphilis.[92] Although the disease was thought to be declining in incidence, it seems to be have made a comeback in recent years.[93-96] Syphilis is produced by *Treponema pallidum*, a microaerophilic Gram-negative spirochete, after a 9- to 90-day incubation period. In its classic form, untreated syphilis occurs in three stages: primary, secondary, and tertiary.

In the primary stage, penile involvement commences as a tiny papule, usually at the site of genital trauma on the glans penis, coronal sulcus, prepuce, frenulum, or shaft of the penis. In homosexual men the lesion may occur in the anal canal or rectum. The lesion progresses through the papular phase into an ulcerated chancre. The classical chancre is a single rounded, painless ulcer with clear cut margins and a clean, indurated base (Fig. 13-14). Lymphadenopathy develops within a week, and the nodes are typically painless, rubbery, and nonsuppurative. With or without therapy, the primary ulcer heals within 6 to 8 weeks.[92,93]

Dark-field microscopy forms the mainstay of diagnosis during this phase of the disease, because the antibody response lags.[93] Biopsy is usually not necessary but may be performed if the diagnosis of syphilis is not suspected. Histopathologic features include epidermal ulceration with acanthosis at the margins. The submucosa or dermis contains an inflammatory infiltrate of lymphocytes and plasma cells that is mostly diffuse but may be concentrated perivascularly and associated with pronounced proliferation of endothelial cells (Fig. 13-15).[92,97] Warthin-Starry or Levaditi stain reveals spirochetes in the epidermis or in the dermis around capillaries. The organisms typically have 8 to 12 convolutions, but reticulin fibers may mimic them and interpretation must be cautious.[97] The lymph nodes exhibit follicular hyperplasia with many plasma cells and endothelial proliferation. Special stains may also show many spirochetes in lymph nodes.

In secondary syphilis, penile involvement is usually part of the systemic mucocutaneous manifestations of this stage. The *T. pallidum* organisms circulate in the blood and lymphatic systems for 6 weeks to 6 months after the primary stage, producing symmetric skin lesions and generalized lymphadenopathy. The skin lesions are maculopapular, annular, and usually hyperpigmented. Condyloma latum and mucous patches are included in the constellation of mucocutaneous lesions. Smears from these lesions should be examined by dark-field microscopy for organisms. A biopsy may yield variable histological features and by itself is nonspecific, because in up to 25% of cases the plasma cell infiltrate and capillary endothelial proliferation typical of syphilis are absent.[98] The lesions lacking plasma cells and endothelial proliferation may mimic other cutaneous diseases, such as lichen planus or psoriasis. A pronounced lymphocytic response may also be mistaken for mycosis fungoides.[99] The epidermal changes include parakeratotic scales, acanthosis, ulceration, spongiosis, exocytosis, dyskeratosis, and basal vacuolation. Condyoma latum shows prominent epithelial hyperplasia that may become "pseudoepitheliomatous" with ulceration and exocytosis with neutrophils.[100]

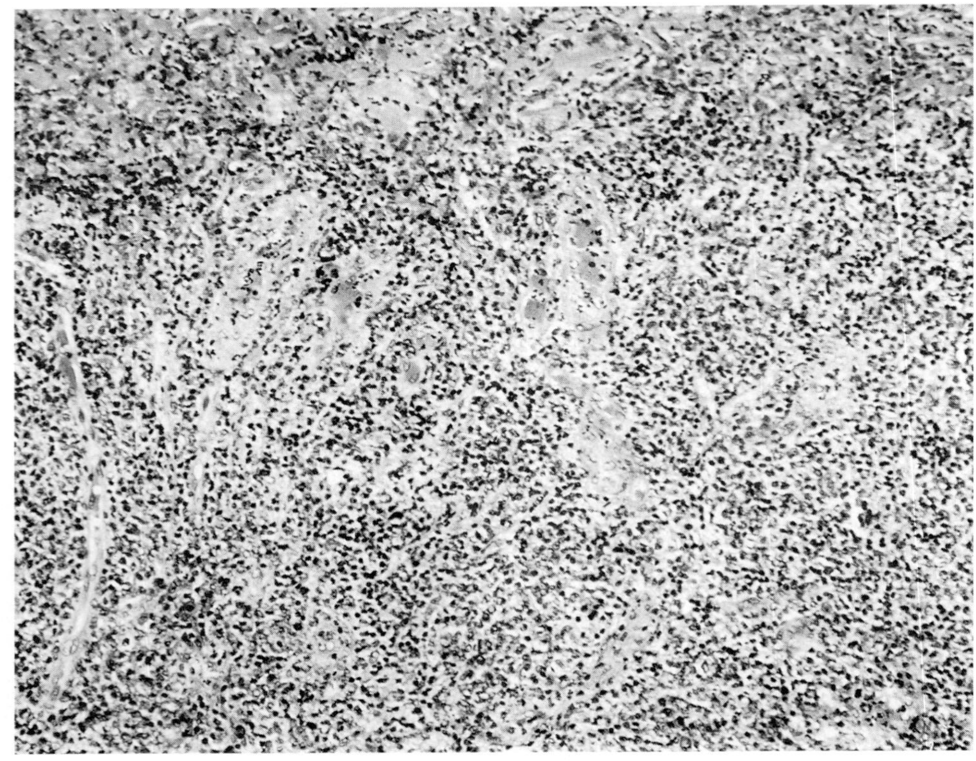

13-15. Syphilis: dense chronic inflammatory infiltrate with endothelial hyperplasia.

The third stage (tertiary syphilis) is characterized by granulomas referred to as gummata. These lesions may be nodular or gummatous, that is, accompanied by central necrosis. Nodular lesions lack tissue necrosis and are composed of "hard" granulomas accompanied by endothelial proliferation and perivascular inflammation. Central caseous necrosis heralds the gummatous phase, which has an intense inflammatory infiltrate in addition to the granulomas.

Therapy is stage dependent, consists predominantly of antimicrobial drugs, and is successful if it is timely. The Centers for Disease Control and Prevention recommend counseling all patients for risks and testing for human immunodeficiency virus (HIV) infection, which is also responsible for the reactivation of syphilis.

Herpes simplex

Herpes (from the Greek "to creep") simplex virus infection involving the genital system is an important sexually transmitted disease that may have a causal role in cervical carcinoma and has high morbidity and mortality in infants. The virus is a double-stranded DNA virus that has two subtypes: 1 and 2. Herpes simplex virus 1 produces oral lesions and herpes simplex virus 2 predominantly affects the genitalia; only 10% to 25% of herpes simplex virus 2 infections produce oral lesions.[101,102]

Clinical manifestations are more severe and fulminant in the first episode than in recurrent disease.[103,104] First episodes often have systemic symptoms (fever, malaise, and headache) and affect multiple extragenital and genital sites. Pain, itching, urethral discharge, dysuria, and tender lymphadenopathy are the most common local

A

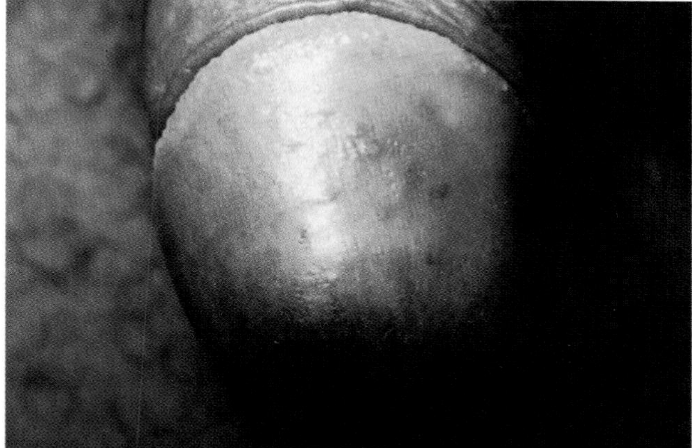

B

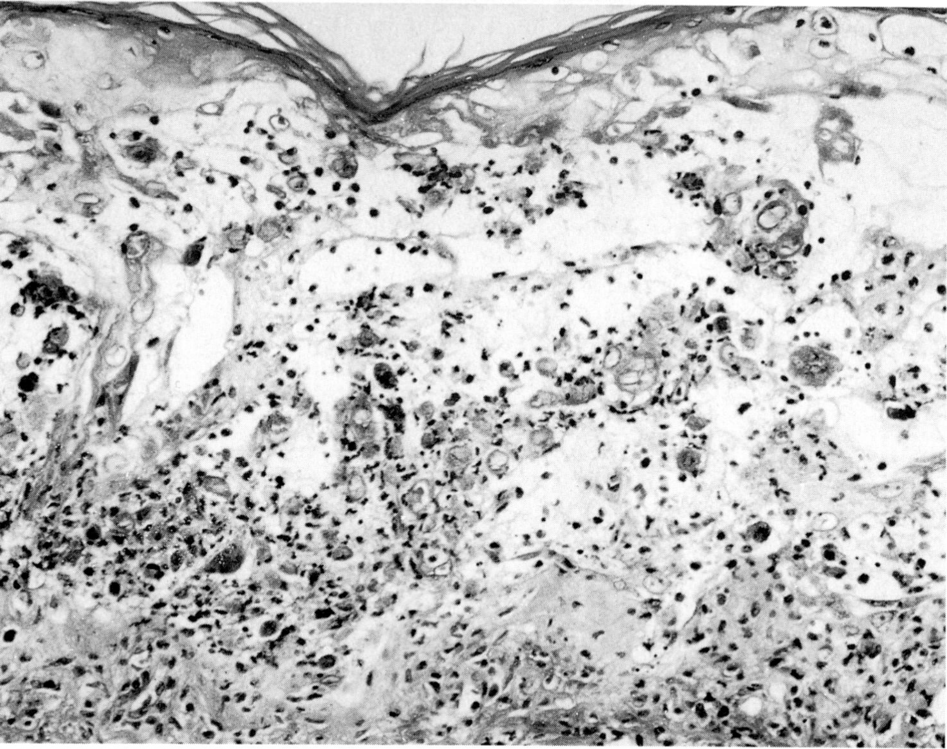

13-16. **A**, Herpes simplex. **B**, Herpes simplex vesicle.

symptoms. The genital lesions appear as multiple vesicles with erythematous bases that may coalesce, rupture, form pustules, and eventually form crusts (Fig. 13-16*A*). The clinical diagnosis may be confirmed by scraping the lesion and obtaining a Tzank smear (stained with Wright-Giemsa, toluidine blue, or Papanicolaou procedures), which reveals large multinucleated giant cells with ballooning degeneration and characteristic intranuclear inclusions. This method does not differentiate between herpes simplex virus and varicella-zoster infection. For this distinction, other techniques such as immunofluorescent antigen detection, virus isolation by culture, and serology are necessary.[105]

Histologically, herpes simplex and varicella-zoster lesions are identical, characterized by unilocular or multilocular intraepidermal vesicles produced by profound acantholysis (Fig. 13-16*B*).[106] The vesicles contain proteinaceous material and are surrounded by epidermal cells with reticular and ballooning degeneration, features that are hallmarks of herpes infection but absent in other vesiculobullous diseases, which may enter into the differential diagnosis. Cytopathic changes may be evident in adnexal and pilosebaceous structures, endothelial cells, and fibroblasts but are typically seen in the epidermal cells which exhibit chromatin margination and inclusion bodies (ranging from small demarcated acidophilic bodies to large, homogeneous, ground-glass acidophilic to basophilic bodies) surrounded by halos.

Complications of herpes, which also affect female sexual partners and infants, include neonatal complications; nervous system abnormalities (aseptic meningitis, encephalitis, radiculopathies)[107]; extragenital lesions on buttocks, groin, thighs, or other sites; disseminated infection causing arthritis, hepatitis, or hematologic disorders; superinfections; intractable nonhealing ulcers in patients with acquired immunodeficiency syndrome (AIDS); and possibly cervical cancer in women. Treatment options are limited. Acyclovir and phosphonoformate trisodi are effective in decreasing the intensity and duration of both primary and recurrent episodes but are not curative.[104]

Lymphogranuloma venereum

Lymphogranuloma venereum is a sexually transmitted disease caused by *Chlamydia trachomatis* subtypes L_1, L_2, and L_3. It was established as a clinicopathologic entity separate from other venereal diseases in 1913 by Durand, Nicolas, and Favre.[108] Lymphogranuloma venereum is sporadic in the United States and most European countries but is highly prevalent in Africa, Asia, and South America.

Like syphilis, lymphogranuloma venereum has three stages: a primary genital stage; a secondary inguinal stage characterized by acute lymphadenitis with bubo formation; and a rare chronic tertiary stage with genital ulcers, fistulas, elephantiasis, and rectal strictures.[109] After an incubation period of 3 days to 6 weeks, the lesion begins as a papule which transforms into a pustule and heals without treatment; therefore in 50% of patients the penile lesion may not be clinically examined. The pathognomonic clinical sign is the inguinal lymphadenopathy, commonly known as *bubo*. It is painful, usually unilateral (66%), and may enlarge to form an abscess and rupture (33%).[109-111]

The histologic features are nonspecific and nondiagnostic. The ulcer is coated with exudate and neutrophils; the base is composed of granulation tissue, with a mixed inflammatory infiltrate containing large mononuclear cells with occasional granulomas.[112] Giemsa stains may demonstrate purple chlamydial inclusions in the macrophages, but this procedure lacks specificity and sensitivity. The lymph nodes show follicular hyperplasia and elongated stellate abscesses similar to those of cat-scratch disease, tularemia, and fungal and atypical mycobacterial infections.

Culture of the organisms by aspirating the lymph nodes is the most specific method of detection but is technically difficult and costly. Frei's test is no longer used, but serologic tests have gained wide acceptance for diagnosis of lymphogranuloma venereum.[113] Antibiotics are effective if the diagnosis is achieved in a timely fashion.

Granuloma inguinale (donovanosis)

Granuloma inguinale is a chronic, progressive, sexually transmitted disease caused by *Calymmatobacterium granulomatis*, nonmotile, Gram-negative, pleomorphic intracellular bacilli of uncertain classification. Although rare in the United States, it is more prevalent in areas of Australia, India, the Caribbean, and Africa.[114,115]

Granuloma inguinale is only mildly contagious and affects the penis, anal region, and vulva. The incubation period varies from 8 to 80 days. The lesion starts as single or multiple small papules which subsequently form ulcers that bleed readily and have abundant beefy-red granulation tissue at their bases.[114-117] Ulcers are the hallmark of the disease and are typically nontender, indurated, and firm. A verrucous form occurs in the perianal region and may simulate carcinoma.[118,119]

Histologically, the lesions consist of a central ulcer bordered by acanthotic epidermis with features of pseudoepitheliomatous hyperplasia.[118,119] The dermis below the ulcer contains granulation tissue with vascular ectasia and endothelial proliferation, microabscesses with neutrophils, and large histiocytes (25 to 90 μm). These histiocytes have cytoplasmic vacuoles that contain dark particulate inclusions (Donovan bodies), seen best with Giemsa or Warthin-Starry stains.[120] Donovan bodies are often easier to see in smears than in histologic sections. Besides granuloma inguinale, other organisms may be evident within histiocytes in rhinoscleroma, histoplasmosis, and leishmaniasis; but the small size (1–2 μm) of *C. granulomatis* is an important distinguishing feature for granuloma inguinale.[121] The diagnosis must be established by microscopy because the bacilli are not readily cultured.[122] A recently developed serologic test using indirect immunofluorescence is available in some laboratories.[123] Antibiotic therapy is usually curative, although relapses may occur with early withdrawal of drugs.

Chancroid (soft chancre)

First described by Ricord in France in 1838, chancroid, a sexually transmitted disease, has recently increased in prevalence in the United States.[124,125] Chancroid causes painful acute ulcers, accompanied by painful lymphadenopathy in 50% of cases.[126] Chancroid is caused by *Haemophilus ducreyi*, Gram-negative, facultatively anaerobic, biochemically relatively inert bacteria that require an X factor for growth.

The ulcer develops following a 4- to 7-day incubation period, beginning as a tender erythematous papule which erodes, ulcerates, and becomes pustular. The ulcer is not indurated, but has undermined edges and is covered by grayish-yellow exudate. The lymphadenitis is unilateral and the lymph nodes may enlarge and rupture spontaneously.[125]

Histologically, the cutaneous findings are relatively distinctive, and form three zones: a surface zone containing exudate, fibrin, neutrophils, and debris at the base of the ulcer; a wide intermediate zone in which there is prominent vascular proliferation and ectasia with focal thrombosis; and a deep zone containing a dense infiltrate of lymphocytes and plasma cells.[127] The presumptive diagnosis based on the recognition of these typical zonal histologic features may be confirmed by demonstrating the bacteria by Giemsa, Gram, or methylene blue stains. The bacteria are more easily seen in smears than in histologic sections.[127] In smears the organisms have a "railroad track" or "school of fish" pattern of alignment of

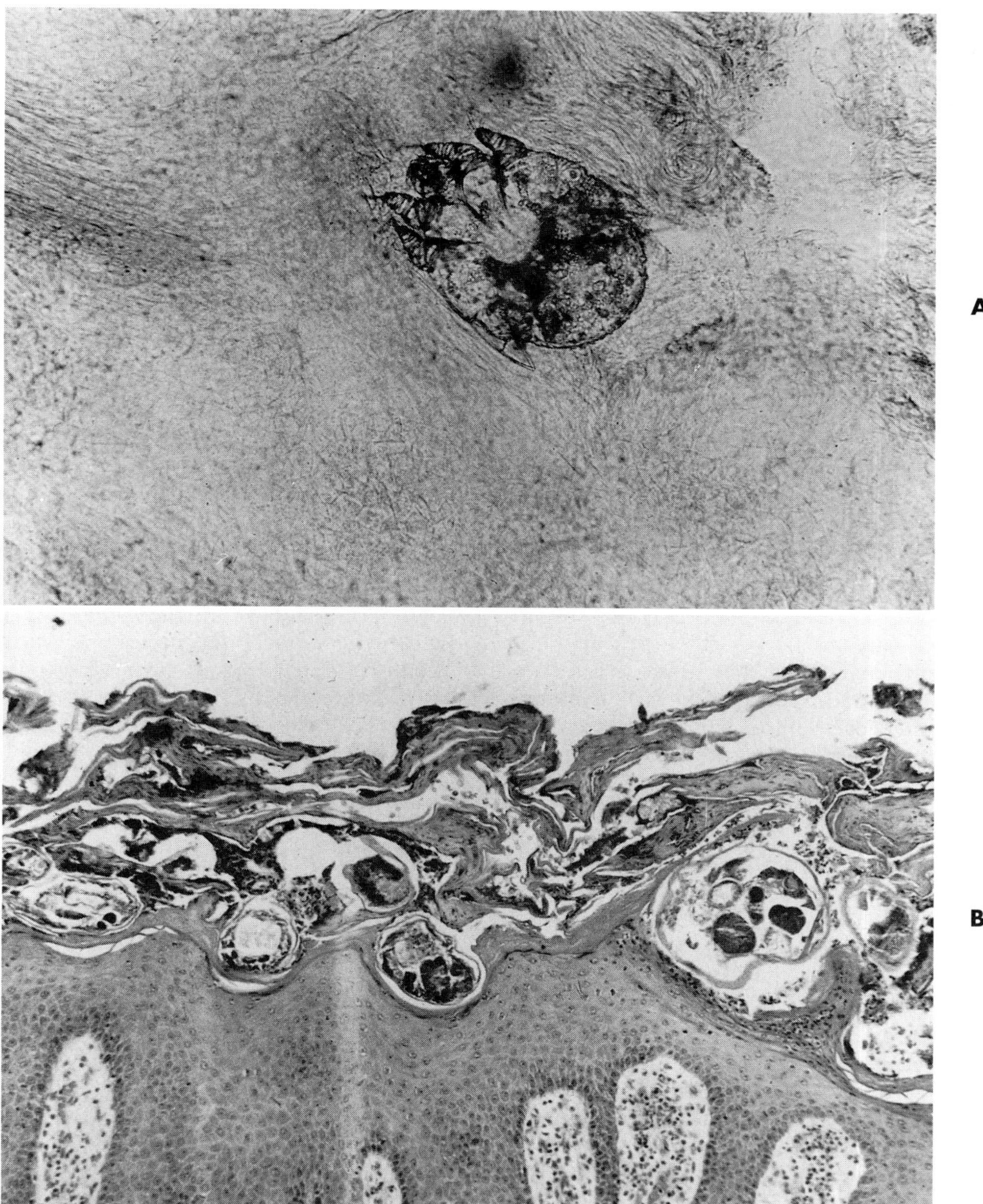

13-17. **A**, Scabies mite. **B**, Scabies burrow in the epidermis.

short rods.[128] The organisms may be cultured on a selective agar medium[129] and directly detected by polymerase chain reaction DNA amplification.[130]

There is evidence that chancroid is a risk factor for heterosexual spread of HIV.[131,132] Antibiotic therapy is usually curative, although cases associated with HIV infection do not respond as well.

Candidiasis

Candidiasis involves the penis as balanitis or balanoposthitis, visible clinically as bright red patches of inflammation with numerous minute pustules and erosions. Candidiasis is common in uncircumcised men, in whom heat and retained moisture within the preputial sac create a favorable environment.[133] Diabetes mellitus, lengthy antibiotic treatment, and immunosuppression are other predisposing factors.[134] *Candida albicans* is the most common species and may be identified in the curd-white exudate that often overlies the lesions. Microscopy of a wet-mount preparation with potassium hydroxide is sufficient for the diagnosis. A positive culture alone is not diagnostic because these fungi may colonize other forms of balanitis. Therapy consists of eliminating environmental factors predisposing to the infection, improving local hygiene, and topical antifungal agents. If local treatment fails, circumcision may be necessary. Patients may have concurrent candidal intertrigo. Severe life-threatening infections with formation of emphysematous lesions are rare.[135]

Scabies

Believed to be the first human disease with a known causative agent, scabies was discovered in 1687 to be due to the bite of the human itch mite (*Sarcoptes scabiei*).[136] Prolonged personal contact is required for transmission, and affliction of several members of a family or infection of sexual partners is likely.[137] Scabies may also be an undetected cause of recurrent staphylococcal or streptococcal infections.

Scabies is clinically characterized by severe itching that is more pronounced at night and may be severe enough to induce profound excoriation. In addition to the genitalia, the palms, wrists, feet, and elbows may be involved. Burrowing by female mites produces scaly red patches that may be papular, nodular, or excoriated. Vesicles may be visible at the ends of burrows.[137]

The diagnosis may be made by teasing the mite out from the burrow with a needle, or by scraping the skin with a sharp scalpel and examining the fragments with a microscope (Fig. 13-17*A*). A definite histopathologic diagnosis requires the demonstration of the mite or its products. The burrow is housed within the horny layer where the female mite, approximately 400 µm long, resides (Fig. 13-17*B*).[138-141] In the absence of the mite, eggs containing larvae or egg shells (chitin walls with marked eosinophilia and periodic acid–Schiff positivity) are diagnostic of scabies. Epidermal spongiosis and dermal eosinophilia are clues aiding recognition. Treatment consists of antipruritic agents and antiscabietic drugs which should also be administered to family members and sexual partners.[142]

Pediculosis pubis

Pediculosis pubis or phthiriasis is caused by infection with the *Pediculus pubis*, the crab louse, which along with head lice accounts for nearly 3 million cases annually in the United States. History and physical examination and a high index of suspicion are necessary to make a correct diagnosis.[143] Pediculosis should be suspected when there is itching of hair-bearing regions of the groin, scrotum, and thighs. Penile lesions may be evident as "blue spots." Transmission occurs with physical contact and contamination of clothing.[144] The lice and mites may be seen in the pubic hair with a magnifying lens. Treatment, essential for the patient, sexual partners, and close family members, consists of topical insecticide in cream or shampoo form and antibiotics, if necessary, for secondary infection.[145]

Molluscum contagiosum

Molluscum contagiosum is a fairly common viral mucocutaneous disorder caused by the molluscum contagiosum virus, a large brick-shaped DNA pox virus.[146] The lesion was named in 1817 by Bateman for its pedunculated gross appearance and contagious nature which is due to the milky contents of the lesion.

The incubation period is 2 to 7 weeks, and the lesions appear as multiple, discrete, dome-shaped, 3 to 6 mm papules (Fig. 13-18) with small central umbilications through which milky-white contents may be extruded under pressure.[147] Molluscum contagiosum occurs in children, adolescents, young adults, and in immunocompromised patients (including AIDS patients). In immunocompromised patients, there may be hundreds of lesions which fail to involute.

Histologically, the characteristic low-power picture is of a cup-shaped invagination of acanthotic epidermis into the dermis (Fig. 13-19).[148,149] The basal layer is uninvolved, but the cells of the stratum malpighii acquire cytoplasmic inclusions that progressively enlarge as they reach the surface. The inclusions, known as molluscum bodies (Henderson-Patterson bodies), contain viral particles. The inclusions initially are eosinophilic but gradually acquire basophilia and granularity as they enlarge

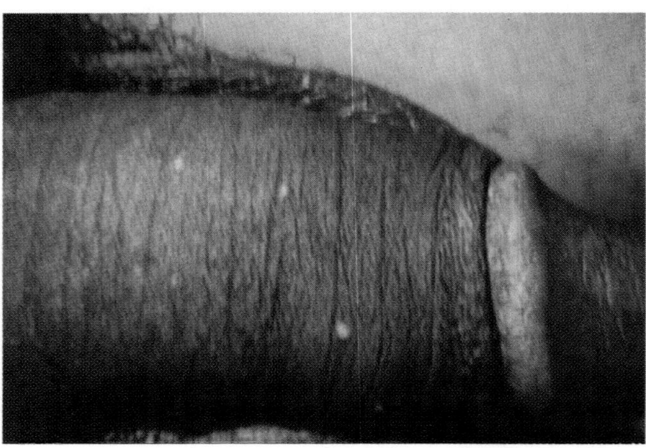

13-18. Molluscum contagiosum.

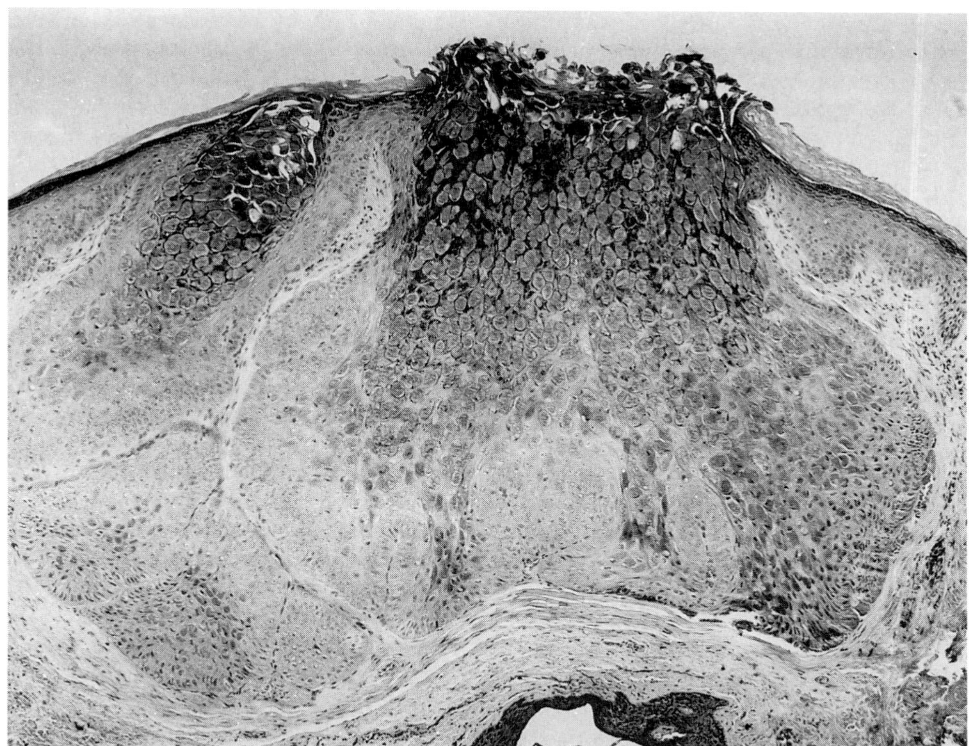

13-19. Molluscum contagiosum showing epidermal crater filled with molluscum bodies.

and displace the nucleus. The stratum corneum ultimately ruptures releasing the molluscum bodies through a central crater. The underlying dermis usually lacks significant inflammation unless the molluscum bodies and epidermal contents rupture into it.[150]

Most lesions regress spontaneously within 6 to 12 months, but treatment is necessary to prevent autoinoculation and transmission to others. Treatment consists of curettage with application of podophyllin or silver nitrate, or laser vaporization.

Erythrasma

Erythrasma is a superficial, asymptomatic, noninflammatory disease caused by a diphtheroid organism, *Corynebacterium minutissimum*.[151] The lesions are often overlooked, appearing as sharply delineated, round to oval patches or plaques with fine scales in intertriginous areas (the genitocrural form). Examination with a Wood's light (ultraviolet light in the ultraviolet A range) reveals the characteristic coral-red fluorescence. The histologic abnormalities are limited to the stratum corneum, where hyperkeratosis and small Gram-positive bacilli are seen.[152,153] The basal epidermis and dermis lack specific histologic changes. The disease is more common in tropical and subtropical climates and treatment with antibiotics is effective.

Penile lesions in AIDS

Almost all sexually transmitted diseases are common in AIDS patients. These include gonorrhea, syphilis, herpes, candidiasis, chancroid, molluscum contagiosum, human papilloma virus, scabies, Reiter's syndrome, and others.[154-158] In patients with AIDS, these diseases are generally more severe, of longer duration, and less responsive to therapy than in other patients.

Kaposi's sarcoma, multiple squamous carcinomas, and multifocal carcinoma in situ are malignancies of penile skin associated with AIDS.[159-162] Condyloma acuminata and squamous cell carcinoma in situ are also reported in the perianal region of homosexual males. Finally, Foscarnet (trisodium phosphonoformate hexahydrate), an agent used therapeutically for herpes and cytomegalovirus infections in AIDS patients, may induce penile ulcers, mimicking an infectious disease.[163,164]

TUMORS AND TUMORLIKE CONDITIONS OF THE PENIS

TUMORLIKE CONDITIONS

Condyloma acuminata

The most common tumorlike lesion of the penis is condyloma acuminata, an infection caused by human papilloma virus. Condyloma acuminata, typically a disease of young adults, has reached epidemic proportions during the last decade.[165,166] The incidence of condyloma is reported to be around 5% among adults aged 20 to 40 years.[167,168] The great majority of these lesions are sexually transmitted. Men whose sexual partners have human papilloma virus–related cervical lesions have an increased (50% to 85%) incidence of penile condyloma.[169] When genital condyloma is seen in children, sexual abuse should be suspected.[170] After the initial infection, autoinfection is common. The incubation period for penile condyloma varies from several weeks to months or even years.[171] Condylomas are most often located on the corona of the glans, the penile meatus, or at the fossa navicularis urethrae, but they also occur on the scrotal skin and perineum (Fig. 13-20).[171] Condylomas are flat, delicately papillary or warty cauliflowerlike lesions. Histologically, there are proliferations of squamous epithelium with an acanthotic and papillomatous architecture, showing orderly epithelial maturation (Fig. 13-21*A*). Hyperkeratosis, parakeratosis, and koilocytic atypia are common (Fig. 13-21*B*).[172] Although cytologic atypia is usually minimal in penile condyloma, and mitotic figures are confined to the basal layer, treatment with podophyllin or lasers can cause bizarre cytologic changes that may raise the question of malignancy.[173] To avoid an erroneous diagnosis of carcinoma, information should be obtained regarding treatment. Human papillomavirus can be demonstrated in condyloma by in-situ hybridization or immunohistochemistry.[174-177] Human papillomaviruses 6 and 11 are common in typical condyloma without dysplasia, but human papillomaviruses 16, 18, 31, and 33 are common in dysplastic condyloma.[174-176] Although condylomas may regress spontaneously, they persist in approximately 50% of cases. The lesions are usually treated with topical podophyllin or laser and, in the great majority of cases, respond to treatment.[177] The relationship of human papillomavirus infection to carcinogenesis is discussed later in this chapter

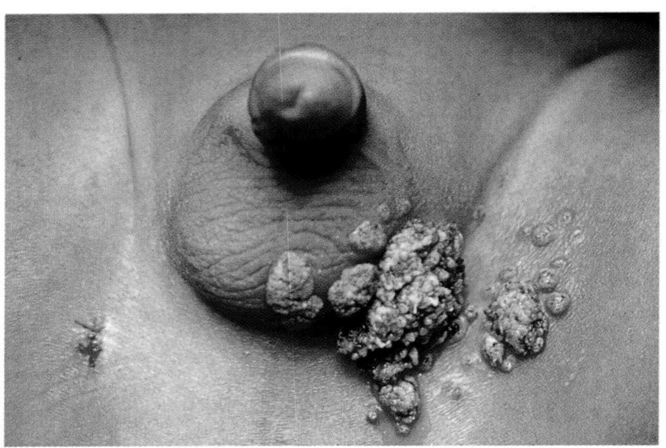

13-20. Condyloma acuminatum. *(Courtesy of Dr. Julian Wan, State University of New York, Buffalo.)*

Pearly penile papules

Pearly penile papules, also called hirsutoid papillomas, are common penile lesions without clinical significance that are present in approximately 10% to 20% of males.[178] These lesions are thought to be embryologic remnants of an organ that is well developed in other mammals. They must also be distinguished from the preputial glands (Tyson's glands). Pearly penile papules are typically 1 to 3 mm in diameter. They appear as yellow-white papules on

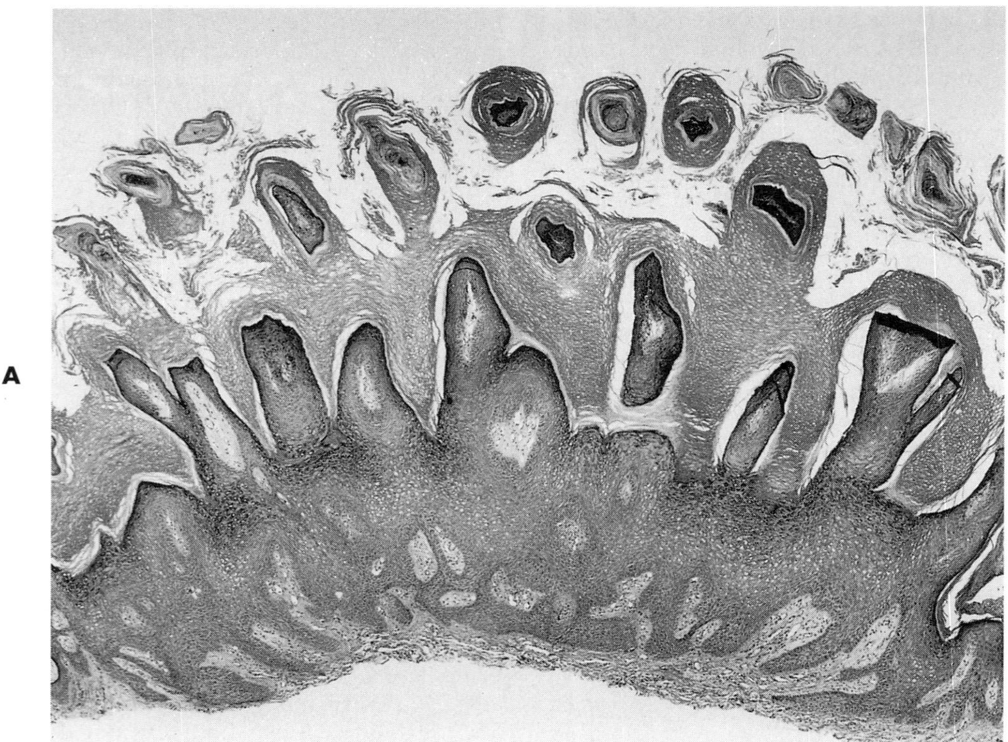

13-21. **A**, Condyloma acuminatum with marked papillomatosis and hyperkeratosis.

Continued.

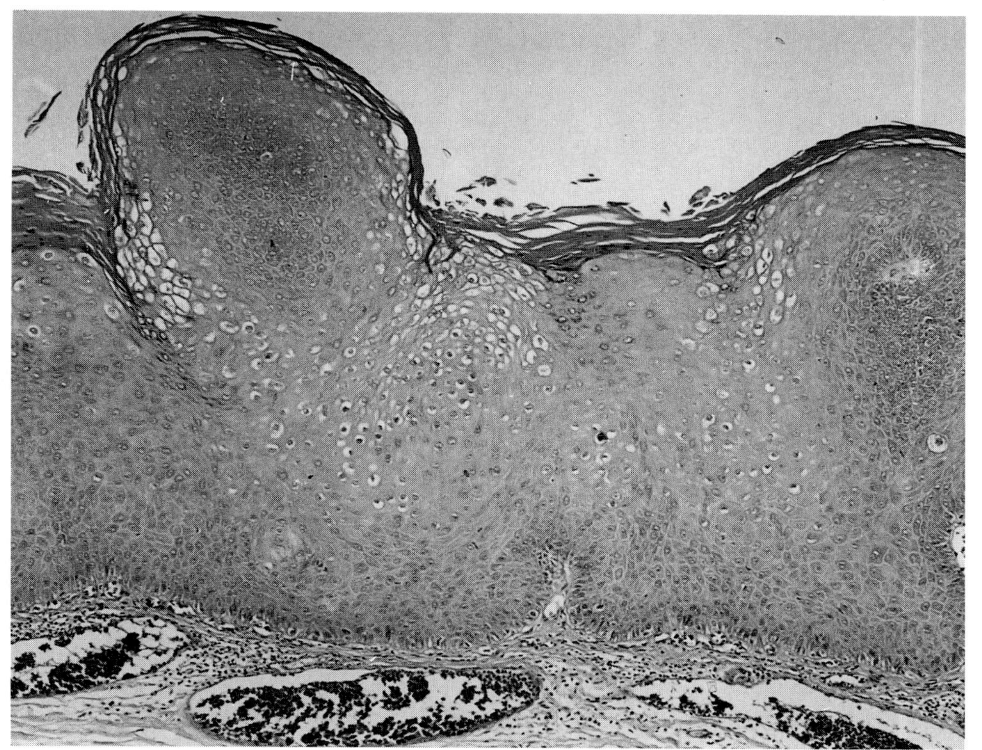

13-21, cont'd. B, Condyloma acuminatum with koilocytic atypia.

the corona or, rarely, on the frenulum of the penis.[179] The individual lesions are domelike, resembling hair, and are usually arranged in a row. Histologically, they show epithelial thickening over a central fibrovascular core resembling angiofibroma, and they lack glandular elements.[180] Pearly penile papules are associated with no known infectious agent and have no potential for malignant transformation; they require no treatment.

Penile cysts

Epidermal cysts are the most common cystic lesions of the penis and usually occur on the penile shaft. They vary in size from 0.1 to 1 cm in diameter.[181] Mucoid cysts of the penis arise from ectopic urethral mucosa.[182] They are lined by stratified columnar epithelium with mucous cells and are filled with mucoid material. Usually located on the prepuce or the glans, most are unilocular and range from 0.2 to 2 cm in diameter. Median raphe cysts arise during embryogenesis from incomplete closure of the genital fold. These cysts are lined by pseudostratified columnar epithelium and may be unilocular or multilocular.[181,183,184]

Pseudoepitheliomatous keratotic and micaceous balanitis

This is a rare lesion that appears as hyperkeratotic, micaceous growths on the glans penis.[185] It was first described by Lortat-Jacob and Civatte[186] as a rare scaling, raised lesion of the glans penis characterized by acanthosis, hyperkeratosis, and pseudoepitheliomatous hyperplasia. Pseudoepitheliomatous keratotic and micaceous balanitis often recurs and may be a precursor of verrucous carcinoma.

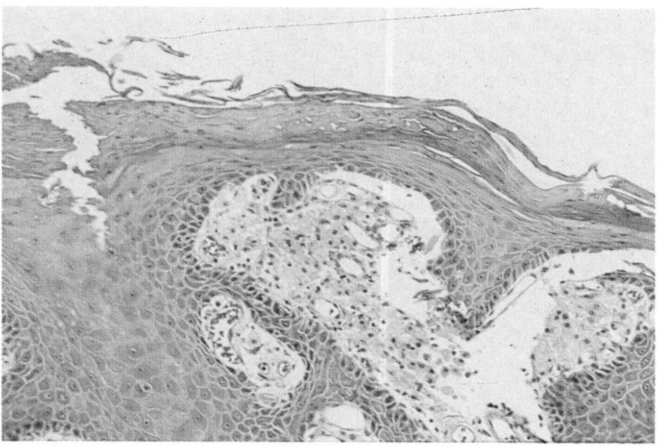

13-22. Verruciform xanthoma with infiltrate of foamy histiocytes.

Verruciform xanthoma

Verruciform xanthoma is a warty lesion characterized by acanthosis, hyperkeratosis, and parakeratosis with long rete ridges associated with a neutrophilic infiltrate. A variable (often prominent) xanthomatous infiltrate occupies the dermis between the rete ridges (Fig. 13-22). This lesion is usually encountered in the oral cavity, and only four genital lesions have been described (two penile and two vulvar).

NEOPLASTIC DISEASES

Premalignant lesions

One of the major areas of confusion in the nomenclature of penile lesions is the terminology of premalignant epithelial proliferations. The terms, *erythroplasia of Queyrat*, *Bowen's disease*, and *bowenoid papulosis* have been used to describe lesions that are histologically similar but have different clinical presentations and biologic behaviors (Table 13-1).[45,187] Whether erythroplasia of Queyrat and Bowen's disease are the same lesion or are different clinicopathologic entities remains controversial. Some have recommended that these two names be replaced by terms such as *intraepithelial neoplasia* or *carcinoma in situ*.[188-190]

Erythroplasia of Queyrat. Although originally described by Tarnovsky in 1891, it was in 1911 that Queyrat[191] applied the term *erythroplasia* to bright red, well-defined, minimally raised, glistening, velvety, and

TABLE 13-1.
DISTINGUISHING FEATURES OF THREE DIFFERENT PRENEOPLASTIC CONDITIONS

Features	EQ	BD	BP
Site	glans, prepuce	penile shaft	penile shaft
Age	5th and 6th decade	4th and 5th decade	3rd and 4th decade
Lesion	erythematous plaque	scaly plaque	papules
Hyperkeratosis	-	+	+
Maturation	-	-	+
Sweat gland involvement	-	-	+
Pilosebaceous involvement	-	+	-
Progress to carcinoma	10%	5% to 10%	-
Association with internal cancer	-	+	-
Spontaneous regression	-	-	+

EQ, erythroplasia of Queyrat; BD, Bowen's disease; BP, bowenoid papulosis.

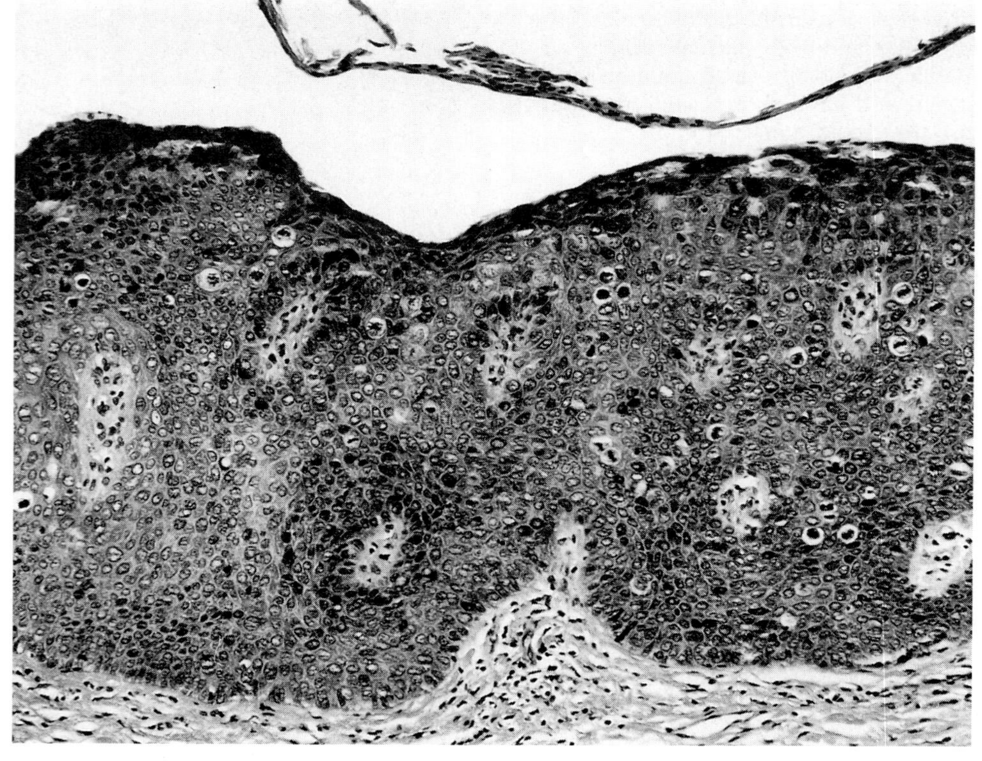

13-23. Erythroplasia of Queyrat showing severe nuclear abnormalities and acanthosis.

persistent plaques on the glans penis and the prepuce.[191] Erythroplasia of Queyrat has been reported among patients within a wide range of ages but usually occurs in men in the fifth and sixth decades of life. In the 100 cases studied by Graham and Helwig,[192] the median age was 51 years. Circumcision protects against the development of erythroplasia of Queyrat, as it does against invasive squamous carcinoma of the penis (see the discussion on squamous cell carcinoma in this chapter).

Clinically, erythroplasia of Queyrat is a shiny, elevated, red, velvety, erythematous plaque located on the glans penis or the prepuce.[192,193] The lesion may also involve the urethral meatus, frenulum, or neck of the penis. In more than 50% of patients, erythroplasia of Queyrat is a solitary lesion.[192] Histologically, it is a full-thickness alteration of the squamous epithelium with loss of polarity, large hyperchromatic nuclei, dyskeratosis, multinucleated cells, and numerous typical and atypical mitotic figures (Fig. 13-23). The underlying stroma contains a band of chronic inflammation and vascular proliferation. About 10% of patients with erythroplasia of Queyrat progress to invasive squamous cell carcinoma and 2% develop distant metastases.[192] A number of different diseases may produce penile lesions that are clinically similar to erythroplasia of Queyrat. These include

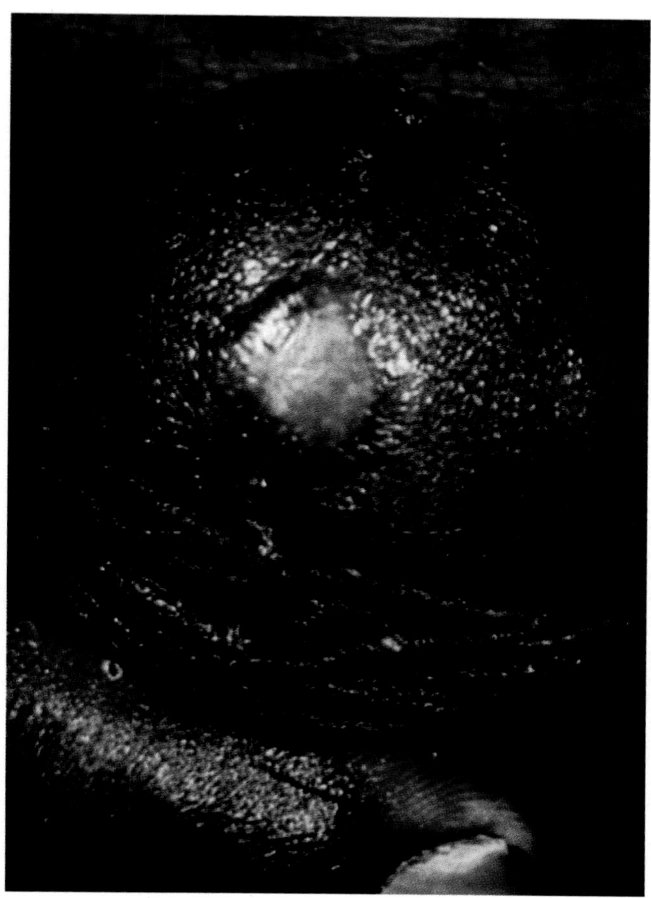

13-24. Bowen's disease.

Zoon's balanitis, other inflammatory processes, and penile manifestations of benign dermatoses such as drug eruption, psoriasis, and lichen planus.

Bowen's disease. Bowen's disease was first described by Bowen in 1912 and the term has been used to designate squamous cell carcinoma in situ of both sun-exposed and sun-protected skin. The term *Bowen's disease* is used to denote a lesion histologically similar to erythroplasia of Queyrat when it involves the shaft of the penis or when the lesion does not have the red clinical appearance of erythroplasia of Queyrat.[45,187,188,194] Bowen's disease occurs most often in men in the fourth and fifth decades of life, a decade earlier than erythroplasia of Queyrat.[194] Typically it is a crusted, sharply demarcated scaly plaque (Fig. 13-24). Rarely, Bowen's disease forms papillomatous lesions.[195] Histologically, it shows features virtually identical to those of erythroplasia of Queyrat (Fig. 13-25). Although some authors have pointed to minor histologic differences, these are mainly the result of differing anatomic locations.[187] Bowen's disease is hyperkeratotic and commonly involves pilosebaceous units, features that are not seen in erythroplasia of Queyrat because erythroplasia of Queyrat occurs in the mucocutaneous epithelium (see Table 13-1).[188,192,196]

The incidence of progression to invasive squamous cell carcinoma is similar (approximately 5%-10%) for erythroplasia of Queyrat and Bowen's disease. They are considered separate entities because of differences in their natural histories. It has been believed that up to 33% of patients with Bowen's disease develop visceral cancers (often respiratory, gastrointestinal, or urogenital).[192] In contrast, erythroplasia of Queyrat has no such association.[192,197-199] The distinction has become less clear because more recent studies of Bowen's disease have cast doubt on the association of Bowen's disease with visceral cancers.[188]

Bowenoid papulosis. The term *bowenoid papulosis* was first used by Wade et al[200] in 1978 to describe lesions on the penile shaft or perineum in young men. Histologically, bowenoid papulosis closely resembles squamous cell carcinoma in situ. However, it is multicentric and has an indolent clinical course.[196,201] In all reported cases the lesions either responded to conservative treatment (local excision, topical or laser treatment) or regressed spontaneously.[196,202] Bowenoid papulosis is considered the male counterpart to multifocal vulvovaginal dysplasia in young women.[203]

Bowenoid papulosis usually occurs in young men, as shown in a study of 51 cases in which the mean age was 29.5 years.[196] In that series the lesions occurred most commonly on the penile shaft and were usually multicentric papules ranging in size from 2 to 10 mm.[196] The papules sometimes coalesce to form plaques resembling condyloma acuminata.

Histologically, bowenoid papulosis is characterized by varying degrees of hyperkeratosis, parakeratosis, irregular acanthosis, and papillomatosis (Fig. 13-26).[196] Although scattered atypical keratinocytes and mitotic figures may be seen even in the top layers of the epithelium, there is usually more maturation of keratinocytes in bowenoid papulosis than in Bowen's disease or erythroplasia of

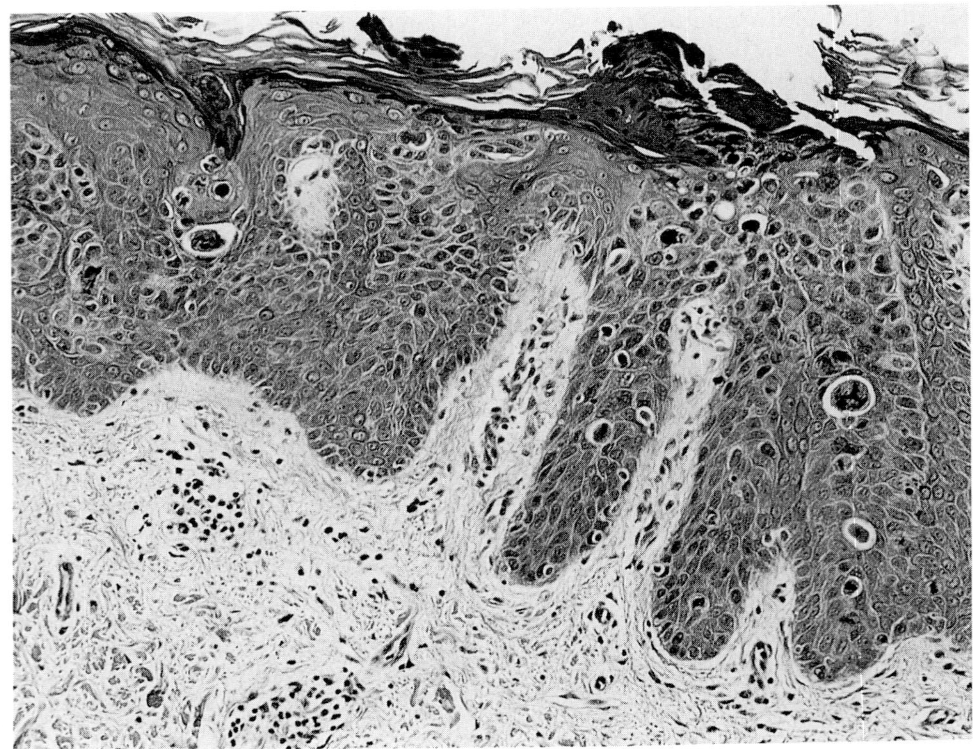

13-25. Bowen's disease with marked nuclear pleomorphism and abnormal mitotic figures.

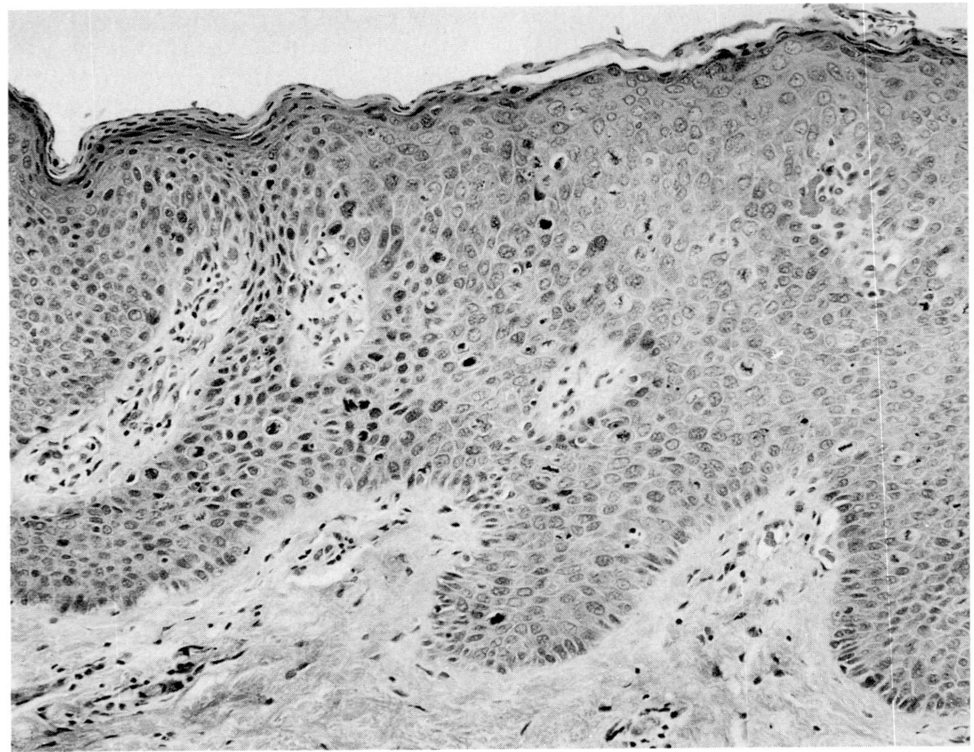

13-26. Bowenoid papulosis with close histological resemblance to Bowen's disease and erythroplasia of Queyrat.

Queyrat. Patterson et al[196] pointed out that the atypical keratinocytes in bowenoid papulosis involve the upper parts of sweat glands, usually sparing pilosebaceous units (see Table 13-1). This pattern is reversed in Bowen's disease.[196] The minor histologic differences between bowenoid papulosis and Bowen's disease and erythroplasia of Queyrat do not allow for an accurate diagnosis on the basis of histologic findings alone. Bowenoid papulosis should be suspected when a young man has multiple skin lesions that range histologically from dysplasia to squamous carcinoma in situ on the penile shaft.

The etiology of bowenoid papulosis is unknown, but viral, immunologic, and chemical causes have been suggested.[196] Human papillomavirus DNA has been demonstrated in several cases of bowenoid papulosis.[204,205] Follow-up data from the reported cases indicate that the behavior of bowenoid papulosis differs significantly from that of Bowen's disease or erythroplasia of Queyrat. Spontaneous regression has been reported in a number of cases. Neither progression to invasive carcinoma nor association with visceral cancer has been observed in any of the cases.[206]

Malignant neoplasms

Cancer of the penis is uncommon, affecting approximately 1 in 100,000 men and accounting for less than 0.5% of all neoplasms in men in North America and Europe.[190,207] In some countries, such as Uganda, Brazil, Jamaica, Mexico, and Haiti, penile cancer is far more common, comprising as much as 10% to 12% of malignancies in men.[207-210] Worldwide more than 95% of penile cancers are squamous cell carcinoma. Sarcomas account for most of the remaining 4% to 5%. Rarely, other cancers, such as melanoma and basal cell carcinoma arise in the penis. More frequently, urothelial carcinoma arises in the penile urethra; this is discussed in chapter 9.

Squamous cell carcinoma

A variety of factors, including lack of circumcision, poor hygiene, phimosis, and viruses are suspected or proven risk factors for squamous cell carcinoma of the penis.[207,211] Squamous cell carcinoma is extremely unusual among individuals who were circumcised in infancy; for example, it is rare among Jews, who practice circumcision shortly after birth.[212] Circumcision in late childhood or adolescence seems to confer some, but not full, protection;[213-215] a higher incidence of penile squamous cell carcinoma has been reported in Muslims, who are circumcised later in childhood.[215] In India more than 95% of penile carcinomas occur among Hindus, who do not customarily undergo circumcision.[213] Although the data indicate that circumcision at birth provides excellent protection against penile cancer, it appears that equally low incidence rates can be achieved in uncircumcised males who practice good hygiene. The very low rate of penile carcinoma in Northern European countries, where males are not circumcised but where good hygiene is practiced, supports this conclusion.[216]

Almost 50% of patients with penile carcinoma also have phimosis.[217] Experimental evidence suggests that smegma may play an important role in penile carcinogenesis.[207] Retention of smegma or its derivatives is thought to have an irritating effect on penile epithelium, and in phimosis this effect may be exacerbated.[207] *Mycobacterium smegmatis* may be a factor in carcinogenesis by direct effect or by converting smegma sterols into carcinogenic sterols.

A viral etiology has also been suggested for penile carcinoma.[218-225] Human papillomaviruses 16 and 18 have been demonstrated in approximately 50% of penile carcinoma.[220-225] Studies that found an increase in the incidence of cervical cancer among spouses or ex-spouses of men with penile carcinoma support the hypothesis that a sexually transmitted agent plays a causative role.[226] This remains controversial.[227] Human papillomavirus infection may play a role in the development of penile cancer, but this neoplasm probably has a multifactorial etiology. Although an early report demonstrated the presence of human papillomavirus 6,[228] human papillomavirus 16 is more frequently implicated.[229] Human papillomavirus 16 has been found in bowenoid papulosis[230] and in an early penile carcinoma associated with a cutaneous horn.[231] Nucleic acid analysis by in-situ hybridization for human papillomavirus 16 or 18 has demonstrated this virus in both primary and metastatic penile cancers.[223,232] Human papillomaviruses 11 and 30 have also been associated with penile carcinoma. Ultraviolet radiation also may play a carcinogenic role for some of the squamous cell carcinomas of the penis and scrotum. The best information comes from patients with psoriasis who have been treated with oral 8-methoxy-psoralen and ultraviolet A phototherapy or ultraviolet B.[233]

Penile carcinoma usually occurs in older men.[234-240] Although patient age at diagnosis ranges from 20 to 90 years, squamous cell carcinoma rarely affects men younger than 40 years.[240,241] This may be changing, however. In a 1992 study from the United States, 22% of the patients were younger than 40 years and 7% were younger than 30 years.[240] In the United States men of African ancestry are affected more often than whites, by a ratio of almost 2:1.

Patients usually have an exophytic or ulcerated mass. Penile pain, discharge, difficulty in voiding, and lymphadenopathy can also be presenting symptoms.[207] The majority of cancers arise in the glans or the prepuce.[207,240] The penile shaft and the urethral meatus are rare sites for squamous cell carcinoma (Table 13-2).[236-241]

TABLE 13-2.
PRIMARY SITES OF SQUAMOUS CARCINOMA OF THE PENIS

Site(s)	Frequency (%)
Glans	48
Prepuce	21
Glans, prepuce, and shaft	14
Glans and prepuce	9
Coronal sulcus	6
Shaft	2

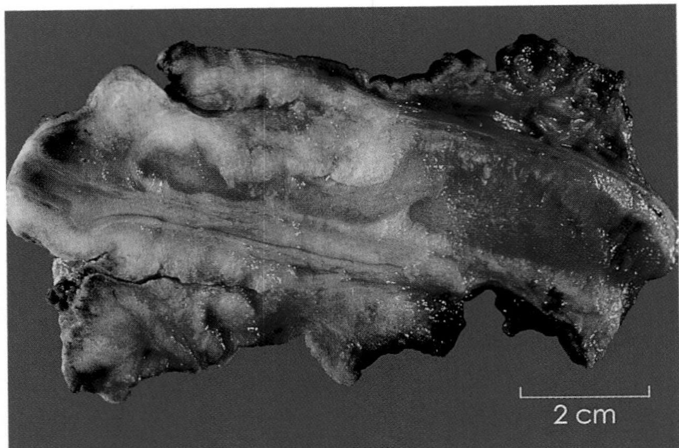

13-27. Squamous cell carcinoma of penis. The glans and prepuce are eroded and replaced by a fungating mass, which invades the corpus cavernosum (sagittal section in plane of urethra).

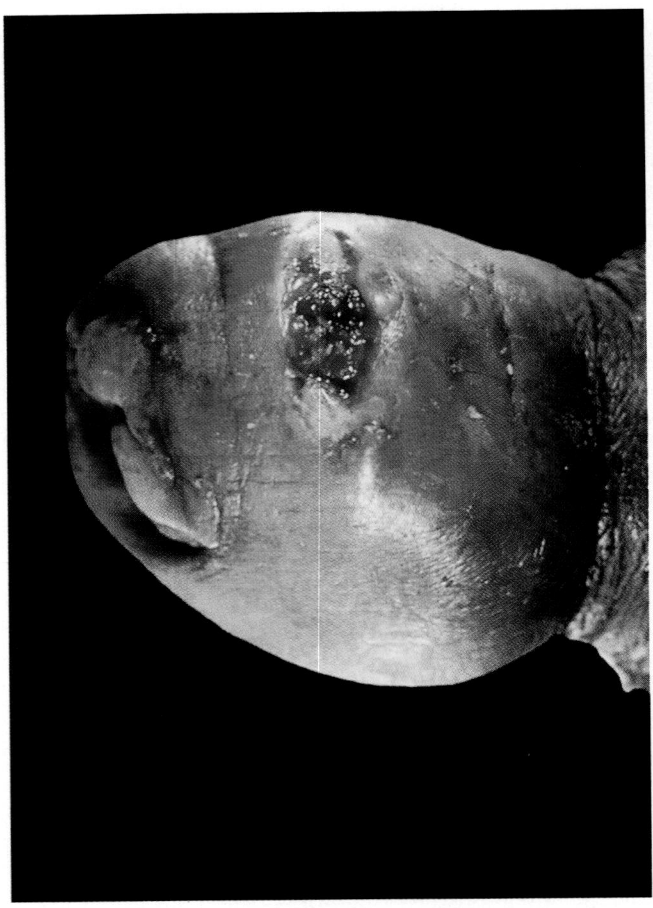

13-28. Squamous cell carcinoma of penis has eroded through the foreskin of this uncircumcised penis.

TABLE 13-3.
GRADING OF SQUAMOUS CARCINOMA (MODIFIED BRODERS' SYSTEM)

Grade		Histologic Features
1	Well	Prominent intercellular bridges Prominent keratin pearl formation Minimal cytologic atypia Rare mitotic figures
2/3	Moderate	Occasional intercellular bridges Fewer keratin pearls Increased mitotic activity Moderate nuclear atypia
4	Poorly	Marked nuclear pleomorphism Numerous mitotic figures Necrosis No keratin pearls

There are two main types of penile carcinoma: the fungating/exophytic type and the ulcerating/infiltrating type (Fig. 13-27, 13-28). There is no special histologic grading system for penile squamous cell carcinoma; the grading system for cutaneous squamous cell carcinoma is used. In this modified Broders' grading system (Table 13-3),[242] the degree of keratinization is the most important feature. Most squamous cell carcinomas are low grade at the time of biopsy. Well-differentiated squamous cell carcinoma shows fingerlike downward projections of atypical squamous cells that originate from a thickened, hyperkeratotic, papillomatous epidermis (Fig. 13-29).

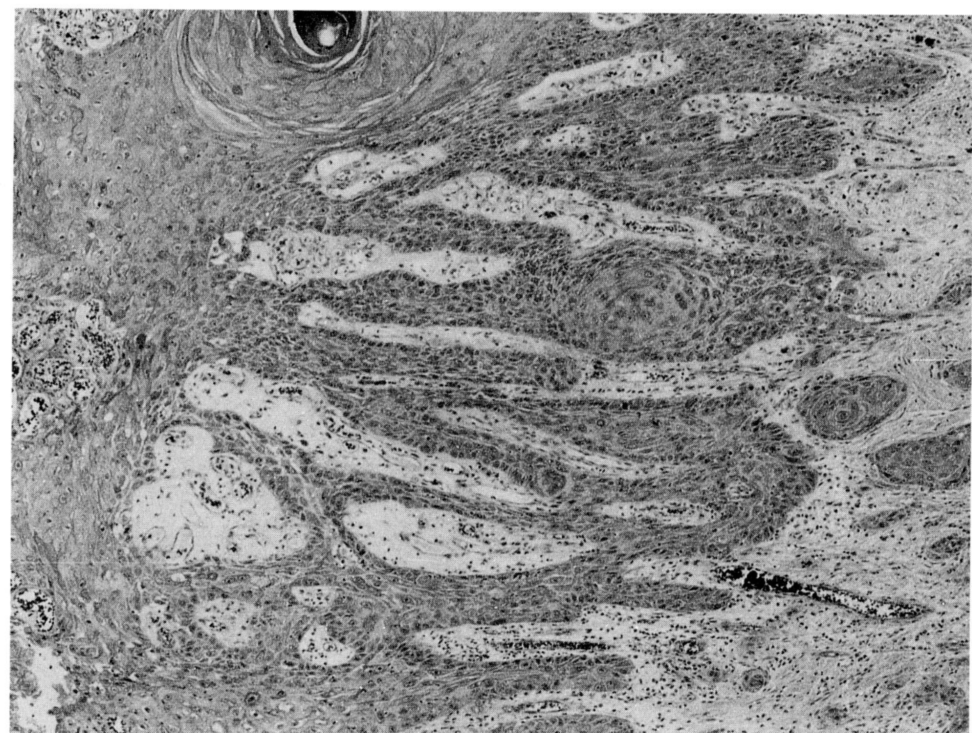

13-29. Fingerlike projections of well-differentiated squamous cell carcinoma extend into the dermis.

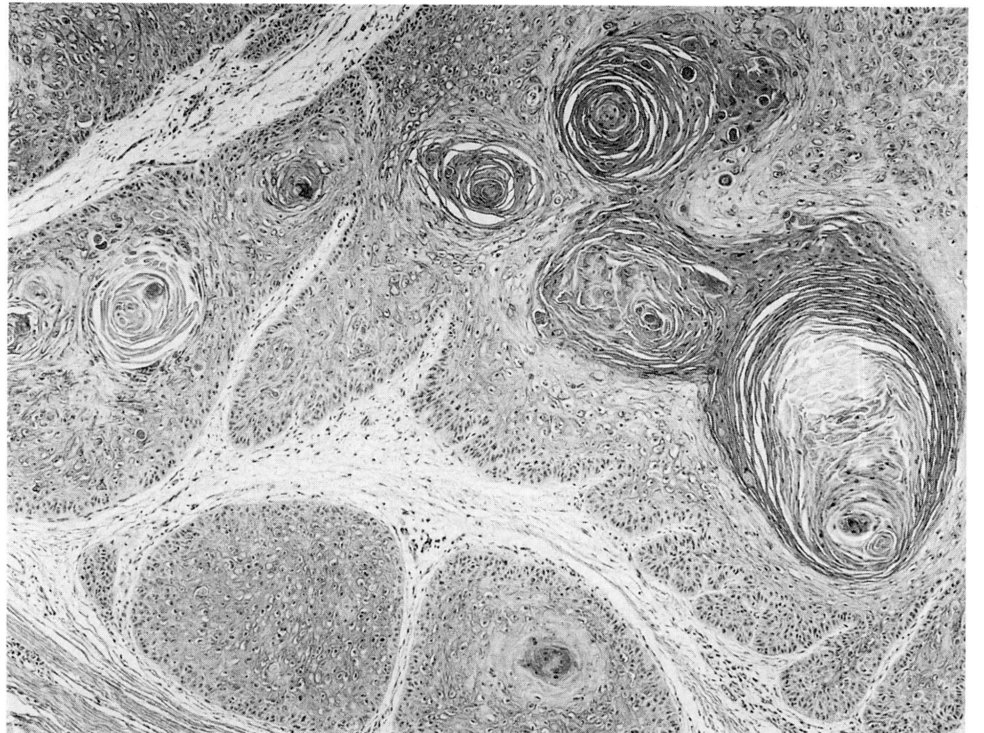

13-30. A, Squamous cell carcinoma forming keratin pearls.

Continued.

B

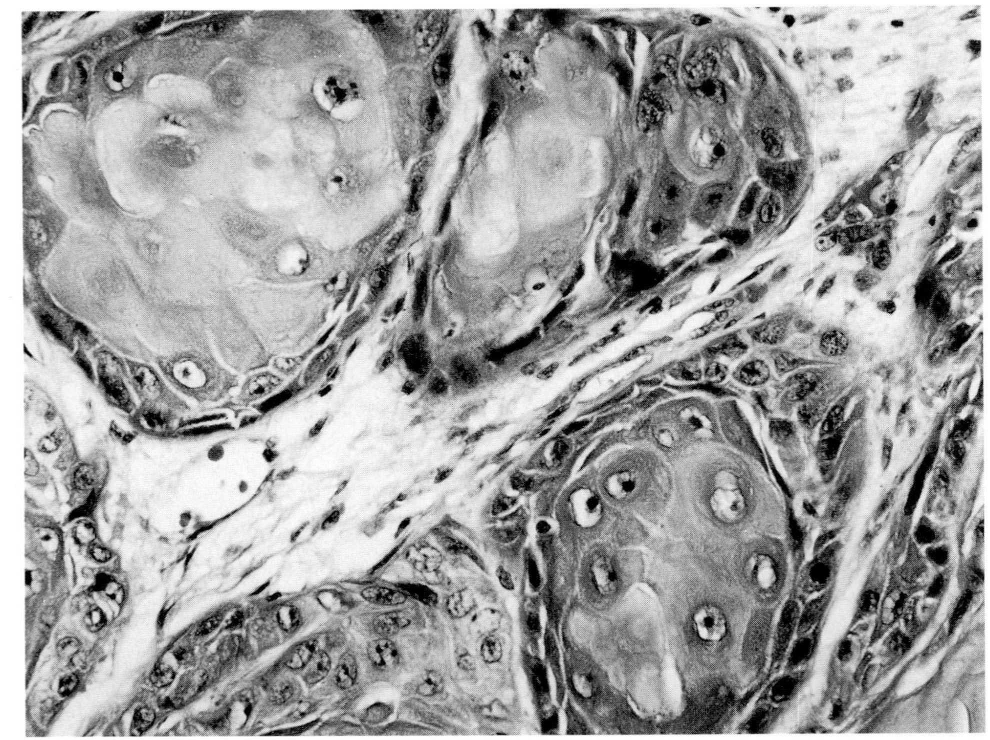

13-30, cont'd. B, Squamous cell carcinoma of penis at higher magnification showing glassy cytoplasm of keratinizing cells.

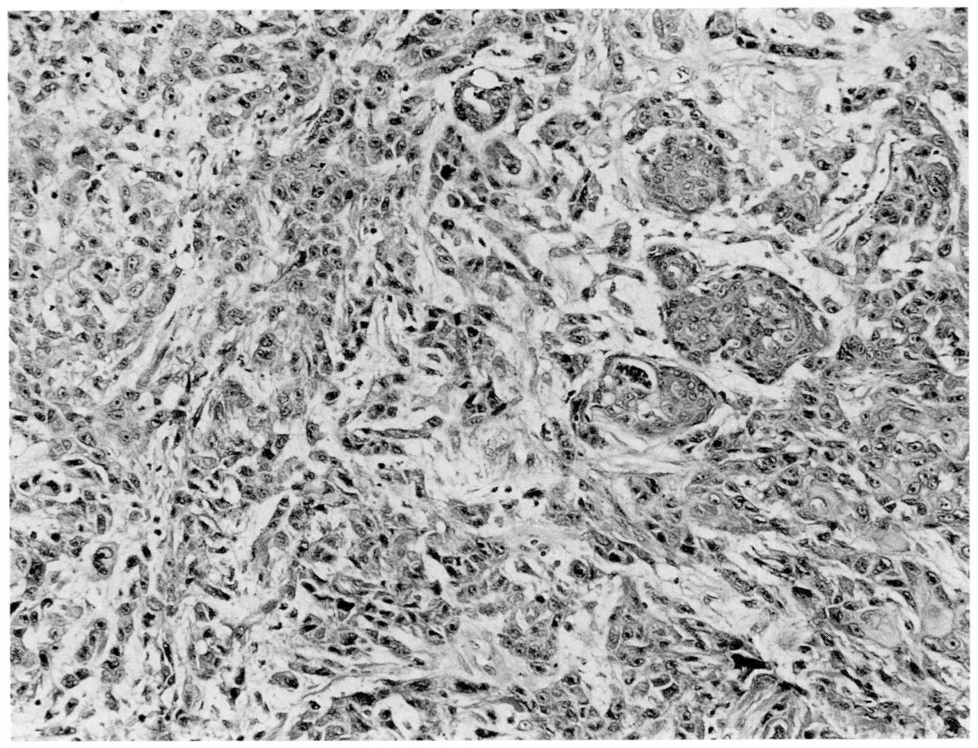

13-31. Squamous cell carcinoma infiltrating the penis as small nests of cells.

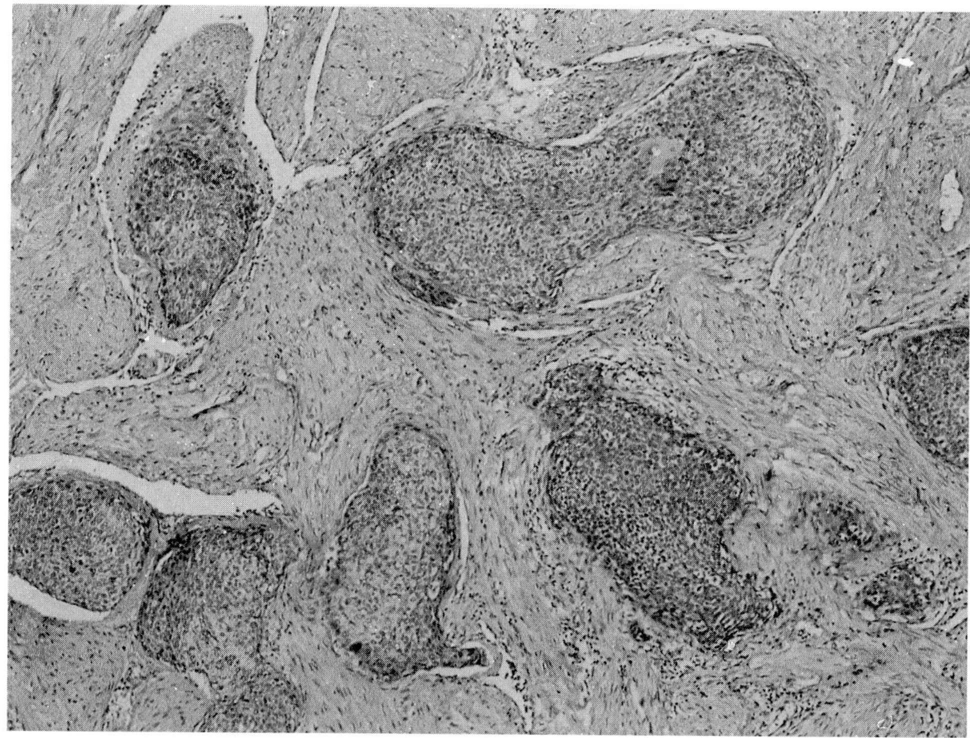

13-32. Deeply invasive poorly differentiated squamous cell carcinoma.

These projections often resemble nests of cells within the dermis. Concentrically arranged masses of cells often surround accumulations of anucleate keratin known as keratin pearls (Fig. 13-30*A*). These represent a disorganized attempt by the malignant cells to undergo differentiation. Intercellular bridges often are prominent (Fig. 13-30*B*). Well-differentiated lesions (grade 1) have limited atypia, consisting of nuclear enlargement and pleomorphism and the presence of one or more large nucleoli. Mitotic figures can usually be found but are rare. Individual cells may become dyskeratotic with deeply eosinophilic cytoplasm. Usually the dermis along the tumor margin contains a dense lymphocytic or mixed inflammatory infiltrate. Poorly differentiated squamous cell carcinoma (grade 3) forms few or no keratin pearls (Fig. 13-31), but it has marked nuclear pleomorphism and hyperchromasia and may have areas of necrosis and superinfection. Mitotic figures are usually numerous, and poorly differentiated tumors are generally deeply invasive (Fig. 13-32). Moderately differentiated carcinoma (grade 2) shows histologic differentiation intermediate between grades 1 and 3 with moderate nuclear atypia, and more mitotic activity and fewer keratin pearls than grade 1.

Maiche et al[243] proposed a scoring system for grading squamous cell carcinoma of the penis on the basis of four criteria: the degree of keratinization, the number of mitotic figures per high power field (x 400), the degree of nuclear atypia, and the presence of inflammatory cells (see box on page 702). They reported that this grading system was practical and showed a correlation between histologic grade and stage.[243] In their series, patients with stage I and II disease had grade 1 and 2 tumors more frequently than patients with stage III and IV carcinoma. The highest proportion of poorly differentiated grade 4 cancer was found in patients with stage IV disease. Maiche et al also found that the histologic grade appeared to be a valuable prognostic factor. The 5- and 10-year relative survival rates were highest among patients with grade 1 tumors and lowest among those with grade 4 cancer. There was no significant difference in the survival rates between patients with grade 2 and 3 cancer.[243]

Cubilla et al[244] divided penile carcinoma into superficially spreading squamous cell carcinoma, vertical growth squamous cell carcinoma, verrucous carcinoma (discussed separately in this chapter), and multicentric carcinoma. Superficially spreading carcinoma occurred most frequently. Inguinal lymph node metastases were found in 82% of patients with vertical growth carcinoma, 42% of those with superficially spreading carcinoma, and 33% of men with multicentric carcinoma.

Squamous cell carcinoma can extend deeply, with invasion into the lymphatic system or the corpora cavernosa. Although most patients present in clinical stages I or II, controversy exists regarding the role of prophylactic bilateral inguinal node dissection.[245-252] Palpation of the inguinal lymph nodes is approximately 70% to 85% sensitive and 50% specific in detecting metastases. If clinical evaluation of the groin lymph nodes is delayed several weeks after excision of the primary tumor, the false-

MAICHE ET AL'S SCORING SYSTEM FOR SQUAMOUS CELL CARCINOMA OF PENIS

Degree of keratinization
- Points
  - 0: No keratin pearls. Keratin in < 25% of cells
  - 1: No keratin pearls. Keratin in 25% to 50% of cells
  - 2: Keratin pearls incomplete or keratin in 50% to 75% of cells
  - 3: Keratin pearls complete or keratin in > 75% of cells

Mitotic activity
- Points
  - 0: 10 or more mitotic cells/field
  - 1: 6–9 mitotic cells/field
  - 2: 3–5 mitotic cells/field
  - 3: 0–2 mitotic cells/field

Cellular atypia
- Points
  - 0: All cells atypical
  - 1: Many atypical cells/field
  - 2: Moderate number of atypical cells/field
  - 3: Few atypical cells/field

Inflammatory cells
- Points
  - 0: No inflammatory cells present
  - 1: Inflammatory cells (lymphocytes) present

Grade 1: 8-10 points
Grade 2: 5-7 points
Grade 3: 3-4 points
Grade 4: 0-2 points

From Maiche Ag, Pyrhonen S, Karkinen M: Histological grading of squamous cell carcinoma of the penis. A grading system, Br J Urol 67:522-526, 1991.

TABLE 13-4. JACKSON'S STAGING SYSTEM FOR SQUAMOUS CELL CARCINOMA OF PENIS

Stage	Description
I	Confined to glans, prepuce, or both
II	Extending onto penile shaft or corpora
III	Operable inguinal lymph node metastases
IV	Inoperable inguinal lymph node metastases, adjacent structure involvement and/or distant metastases

From Jackson SM: The treatment of carcinoma of the penis, Br J Surg 53:33-35, 1966.

positive rate drops to around 15%. Because bilateral inguinal lymph node dissection carries a significant risk of morbidity and death, many surgeons have advocated that inguinal dissection be performed only for patients with palpable lymph nodes several weeks after primary surgery, allowing the inflammatory reactions in these nodes to subside. Alternately, biopsy of sentinel lymph nodes has been suggested to detect inguinal metastasis, followed by inguinal dissection in patients with metastasis.[245-252]

Exophytic penile carcinoma forms a large polypoid mass, and microscopically most are well-differentiated squamous cell carcinoma with extensive keratinization and fingerlike projections invading the stroma. The ulcerating type of penile carcinoma that tends to originate on the glans penis grows invasively and is poorly to moderately differentiated. It has a higher incidence of lymph node metastases than the exophytic type.

Penile cancer initially spreads locally, destroying the prepuce and penile shaft.[207] Urethral involvement may occur with fistula formation. Buck's fascia, which is rich in elastic fibers, forms an initial barrier against tumor invasion. However, with progression, penetration of Buck's fascia and the corpus cavernosum occurs. Despite the rich vascularity of the corpus cavernosum, hematogenous spread is uncommon. Distant metastasis usually occurs through lymphatics, and the inguinal lymph nodes are generally the first involved. The lymphatics of the penis are richly anastomosing channels that cross the midline along the shaft and at the penile base. Therefore, metastasis may be to either side or both sides. The number of lymph nodes containing metastases correlates with prognosis.[253] Infection of the primary tumor can cause inguinal lymph node enlargement without metastases; therefore, sentinel node biopsy is commonly performed to stage the tumor accurately.

The extent of penile shaft involvement and the growth pattern of squamous cell carcinoma correlate with the frequency of lymph node metastases. Patients with tumors of the shaft and those with ulcerating growth pattern have a greater likelihood of metastasis. The size of the primary tumor, the grade, and the length of the delay in diagnosis have not correlated with the incidence of lymph node metastasis.[235,240,253,254] Palpable inguinal lymphadenopathy is present at diagnosis in 58% of patients.[207] Of these patients less than 50% have metastases; the others have inflammatory lymphadenopathy resulting from infection of the primary tumor. About 20% of patients with nonpalpable lymph nodes have metastases.[207] Presentation with distant metastases is rare in the absence of regional lymph node metastasis. Hematogenous dissemination is rare; less than 2% of patients with penile carcinoma have distant visceral metastases at the time of diagnosis. However, hepatic, pulmonary, and osseous metastases can occur in untreated cases.[254,255]

The most widely used clinical staging systems are Jackson's staging system (Table 13-4)[256] and the staging system of the American Joint Committee on Cancer (see box on page 703).[257] Grade and stage are the most reliable prognostic factors for penile carcinoma. Stage is the more important of the two. Patients have short survivals when there is spread to inguinal or iliac lymph nodes or distant metastases. Histologic grade correlates well with the clinical stage. Patients with well-differentiated tumors have a favorable prognosis, and more than 80% are long-term survivors. Patients with poorly differentiated tumors tend to have advanced stage and a poor prognosis.

TNM: THE STAGING SYSTEM OF THE AMERICAN JOINT COMMITTEE ON CANCER

Primary Tumor (T)

- TX Primary tumor cannot be assessed.
- T0 No evidence of primary tumor
- Tis Carcinoma in situ
- Ta Noninvasive verrucous carcinoma
- T1 Tumor invades subepithelial connective tissue.
- T2 Tumor invades the corpus spongiosum or cavernosum.
- T3 Tumor invades the urethra or prostate.
- T4 Tumor invades other adjacent structures.

Regional Lymph Nodes (N)

- NX Regional lymph node cannot be assessed.
- N0 No regional lymph node metastasis
- N1 Metastasis in a single superficial inguinal lymph node
- N2 Metastasis in multiple or bilateral superficial inguinal lymph node
- N3 Metastasis in deep inguinal or pelvic lymph node(s), unilateral or bilateral

Distant Metastasis (M)

- MX Presence of distant metastasis cannot be assessed.
- M0 No distant metastasis
- M1 Distant metastasis

From Beahrs OH, Henson DE, Hutter RVP et al: American Joint Committee on Cancer: manual for staging of cancer, ed 4, Philadelphia, 1992, Lea & Febiger.

Almost 50% of tumors originating on the shaft are poorly differentiated, whereas only 10% of tumors arising in the prepuce are high grade.[258]

The utility of DNA flow cytometric analysis in penile cancers is unclear.[259-262] Yu et al[259] reported that patients with diploid cancer had a better survival rate than those with aneuploid cancers, and low S-phase fractions were associated with favorable outcomes. The incidence of aneuploidy rises with increasing stage. Yu et al[259] also reported that all patients who appeared cured had diploid tumors whereas 80% of patients dying of cancer had aneuploid tumors. Gustafson et al[260] reported similar results; they found that low-grade malignancies were predominantly diploid whereas high-grade malignancies were not. Death from cancer occurred in only 1 of 14 patients with diploid cancer but occurred in 4 of 12 patients with nondiploid cancers.[260] Therefore, a better estimate of prognosis can be made by considering both the grade and ploidy of the tumor.

Variants of squamous cell carcinoma. Verrucous carcinoma. Since its first description in the oral cavity, verrucous carcinoma has been recognized in a variety of organs including the larynx, vulva, vagina, anus, and penis. Verrucous carcinoma of the penis accounts for 5% to 16% of penile malignancies.[263] It is commonly seen in middle-aged men.[263-269] Typically it is a large, fungating, frequently ulcerated warty lesion that burrows through the normal tissues (Fig. 13-33). Most arise on the coronal sulcus and spread to the glans and preputial skin. Microscopically, verrucous carcinoma is a well-differentiated squamous cell carcinoma with exophytic and endophytic papillary growth (Fig. 13-34). Characteristically, the tumor shows a broad-based

A

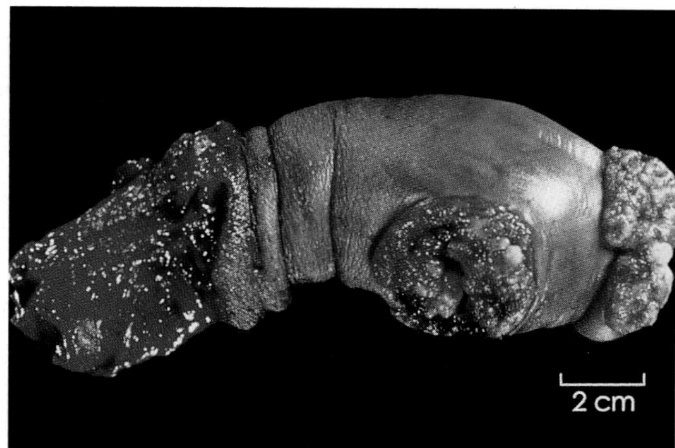

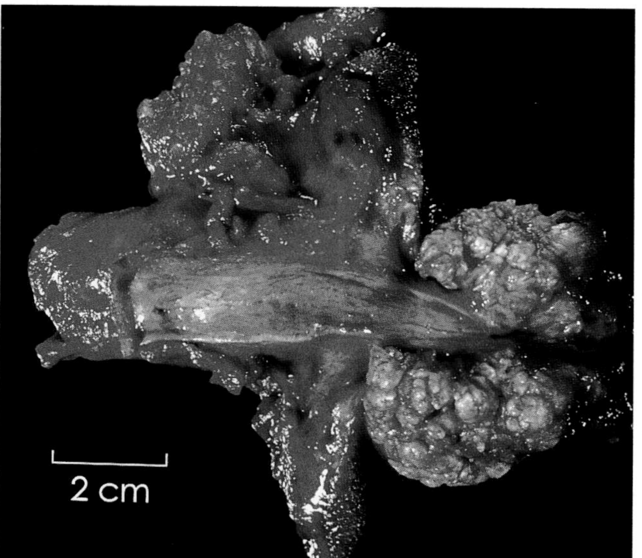

B

13-33. **A**, Verrucous carcinoma has grown out of the preputial orifice and eroded through the prepuce. **B**, Dissection reveals that verrucous carcinoma has grown extensively in the glans and prepuce, obliterating the preputial space. *(From Fletcher CDM: Diagnostic histopathology of tumors, Edinburgh, 1995, Churchill Livingstone.)*

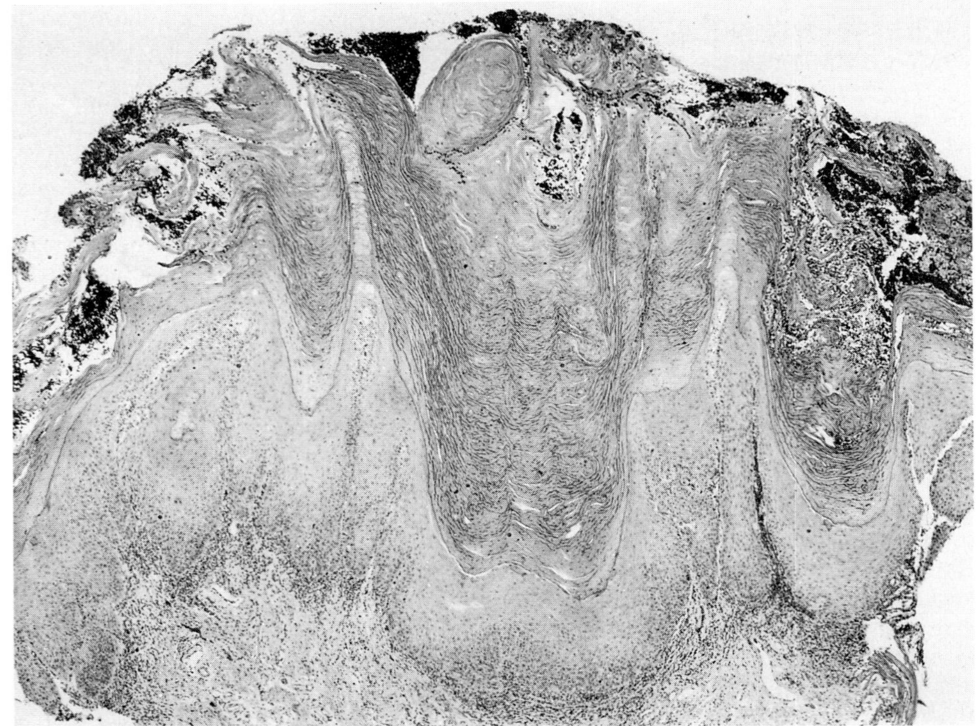

13-34. Verrucous carcinoma with marked hyperkeratosis and regular border with the dermis.

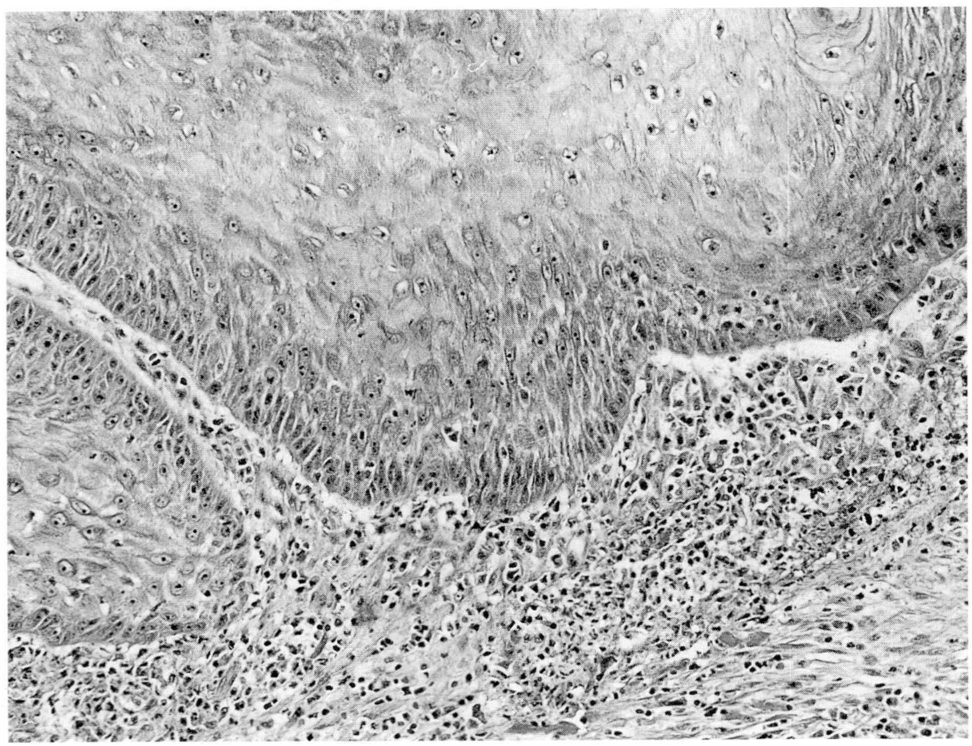

13-35. Deep margin of verrucous carcinoma showing lack of infiltration. Note the lack of nuclear atypia.

TABLE 13-5.
HISTOPATHOLOGIC FEATURES OF VERRUCOUS CARCINOMA

Morphologic Features	Frequency
Club-shaped, hyperplastic rete ridges	+++
Pushing deep margins	+++
Well-differentiated squamous epithelium	+++
Polygonal squamous cells with glassy cytoplasm	+++
Intercellular bridges	+++
Centrally located vesicular nuclei	+++
Central single nucleolus	+++
Well-formed intercellular edema	+++
Individual cell necrosis	+++
Hyperkeratosis	+++
Parakeratosis	+++
Keratin-filled clefts	+++
Cystic degeneration of rete ridges	+++
Heavy subepithelial inflammatory cell infiltrates	++
Intact basement membrane	++
Crust formation	++
Epithelial abscesses	++
Koilocyte-like cells	++
Superficial fibrovascular cores	++
Keratohyaline granules	+
Dermal abscesses	+
Anaplastic foci (hybrid verrucous and regular)	+
True koilocytes	-
True fibrovascular cores	-

"pushing" pattern of infiltration. Cytologic atypia is minimal, and mitotic figures are very rare and usually confined to the deeper portion of the tumor (Fig. 13-35). Vacuolated koilocyte-like change can often be seen in the superficial layers, but true koilocytosis with enlarged atypical and/or wrinkled nuclei and well-defined perinuclear halos is not seen (Table 13-5).[268]

Verrucous carcinoma tends to grow locally and does not metastasize. If inadequately treated, multiple recurrences are possible. The main differential diagnoses include condyloma acuminatum and the usual type of keratinizing squamous cell carcinoma. When the lesion is large, giant condyloma of Buschke-Löwenstein enters into the differential diagnosis. Whether verrucous carcinoma and giant condyloma of Buschke-Löwenstein are the same or different entities remains controversial. The consistent absence of human papillomaviruses 6, 11, 16, 18, and 31 in verrucous carcinoma suggests a fundamental difference between verrucous carcinoma and giant condyloma.[268] Masih et al[268] reported the uniform absence of the common genital human papillomaviruses in their cases of verrucous carcinoma and concluded that verrucous carcinoma is a distinct clinicopathologic entity that does not have a place in the morphologic spectrum of condyloma acuminatum and giant condyloma. Furthermore, penile giant condyloma of Buschke-Löwenstein has been shown to contain the same human papillomaviruses as condyloma acuminatum, with similar frequency.[270,271] On the other hand, some investigators have demonstrated human papillomaviruses 6 and 11 as well as preexisting condyloma acuminatum in some cases of verrucous carcinoma, suggesting a viral etiology.[219,267,269] The lack of cytologic atypia, mitotic figures, and infiltrative growth pattern are helpful in differentiating verrucous carcinoma from the usual type of squamous cell carcinoma.

About 25% of cases of penile verrucous carcinoma show microscopic foci of cellular anaplasia, higher mitotic activity, and ruptured basement membranes.[263,268] These tumors have been called *hybrid squamous-verrucous carcinoma* and similar tumors have been described in the oral cavity.[272] Hybrid squamous-verrucous carcinoma and verrucous carcinoma are similar with regard to patient age, location, and outcome after similar treatments, although the data on hybrid squamous-verrucous carcinoma are limited.[263,268] DNA ploidy and cell-cycle analysis done by Masih et al[268] showed that both verrucous carcinoma and hybrid squamous-verrucous carcinoma have diploid cell populations with similar proliferative indices.

Clinical outcome for patients with verrucous carcinoma varies according to the type of treatment. Partial or radical penectomy reduces the recurrence rate to 33%, compared with a recurrence rate of 80% for patients treated with local excision.[263,268,269] Therefore, partial or total penectomy is recommended. Radiation therapy should be avoided because it has been associated with dedifferentiation of verrucous carcinoma.[263,268,269,273]

Spindle cell (sarcomatoid) squamous cell carcinoma. Although spindle-cell squamous cell carcinoma is common in the oral cavity, upper respiratory tract, and esophagus, only a few cases have arisen on the penis.[274,275] In the reported cases, the cancer tended to form polypoid masses on the glans penis. Histologically, it is composed predominantly of spindle cells with focal squamous differentiation (Fig. 13-36). Marked nuclear pleomorphism and numerous mitotic figures are common in the spindle component. Although some reports suggest that spindle cell squamous cell carcinoma grows locally and has a favorable prognosis, Manglani et al[274] reported a case that had a very aggressive clinical course. Because of the limited number of reported cases, the prognostic significance of this variant of squamous cell carcinoma remains unclear. If they are analogous to spindle cell carcinomas of other organs, it is likely that they are aggressive tumors.

Basal cell carcinoma. Although basal cell carcinoma is the most common malignant skin tumor elsewhere on the body, it is rare in penile or scrotal skin.[276-279] Basal cell carcinoma may involve any portion of the penis but most often involves the shaft (56%), followed by the glans (30%) and prepuce (14%).[278,279] Patients range in age from 37 to 79 years.[278,279] Most reported patients have been white except for one Japanese patient reported in the literature.[279] Grossly, basal cell carcinoma is a small, irregular,

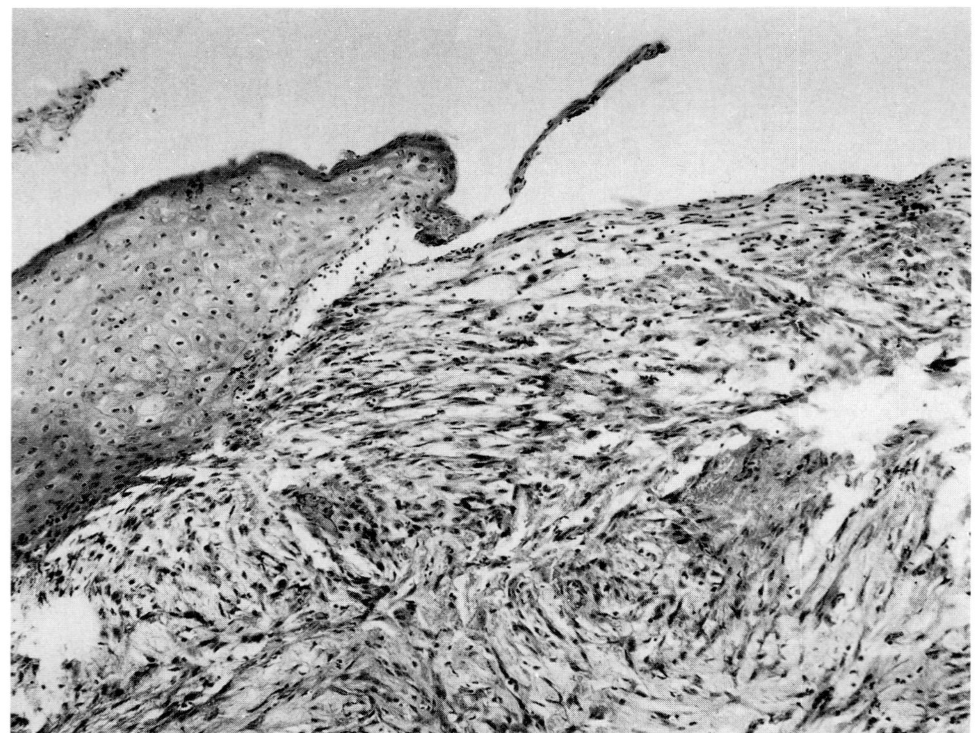

13-36. Spindle cell squamous cell carcinoma.

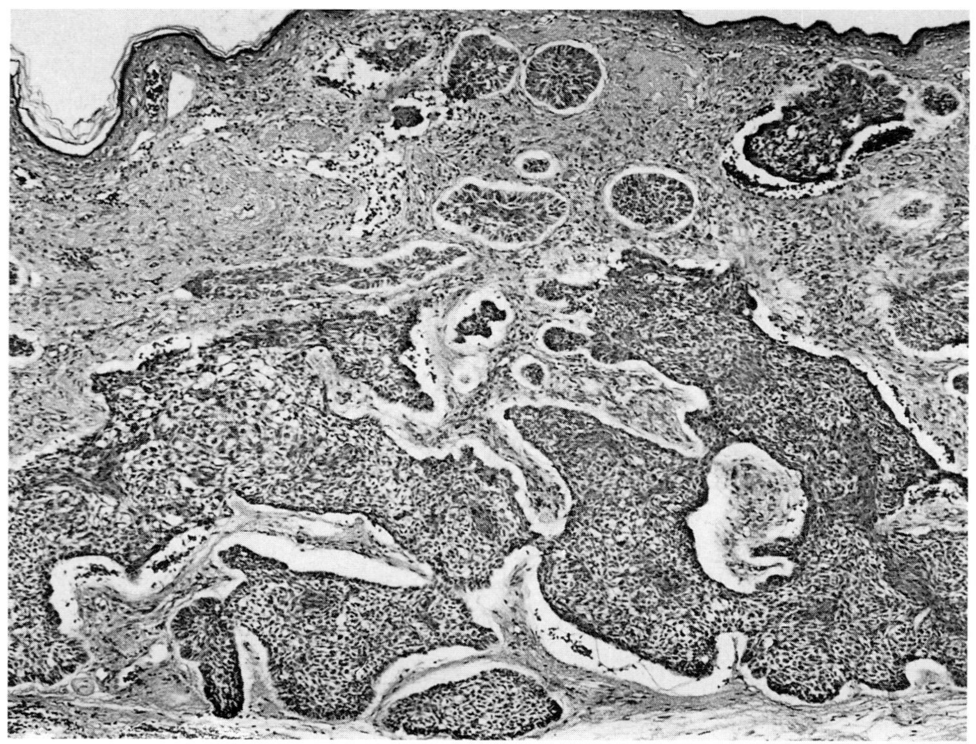

13-37. Basal cell carcinoma.

ulcerated mass. Histologically, it shows nests of small, uniform basaloid cells that have peripheral palisading (Fig. 13-37). The cells tend to form nests of bulbous fingerlike buds that extend from the epidermis. The cells lack intercellular bridges and the nuclei show little variation of size, shape, or intensity of staining and lack abnormal mitotic figures. The stroma adjacent to the tumor often shows a proliferation of "young" fibroblasts or it may appear mucinous. Frequently, the stroma retracts about the islands of basal cell carcinoma, resulting in peritumoral lacunae or cleftlike spaces. The clinical course of penile basal cell carcinoma tends to be indolent, and local excision is usually curative.

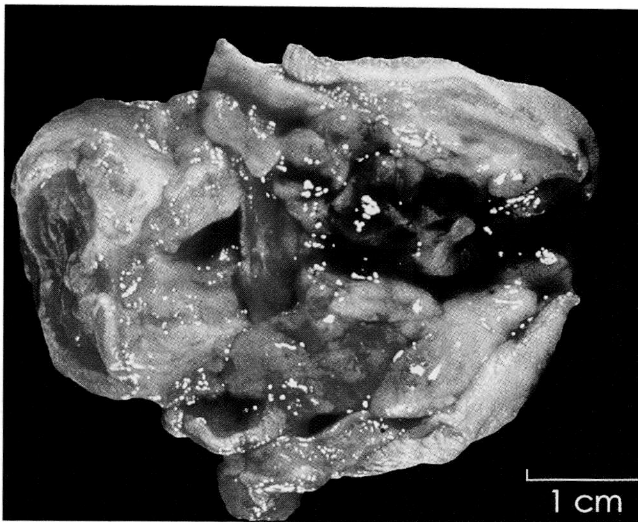

13-38. Malignant melanoma arising in the glans penis.

Malignant melanoma. Fewer than 100 cases of malignant melanoma of the penis have been reported, accounting for less than 1% of all penile cancers.[280-285] Most occur in white men in their fifth and sixth decades of life, a decade older than is typical for most cutaneous melanomas.[286] In contrast to squamous cell carcinoma, penile malignant melanoma is rare in men of African ancestry. In the majority of cases, melanoma arises on the glans (Fig. 13-38).[45]

Patients present with a black, brown, or blue variegated papule or ulcerated plaque. The histologic findings are identical to those of malignant melanoma arising in other mucosal or cutaneous sites (Fig. 13-39).[45] Different histologic subtypes of malignant melanoma, including nodular, superficial spreading, and acral lentiginous types, have been reported.[284-287]

Stage I melanoma is confined to the penis; stage II melanoma is metastatic to regional lymph nodes; stage III melanoma has distant metastases. The prognosis of penile malignant melanoma depends on the depth of invasion and the stage. Penile melanoma with a thickness of 0.75 mm or less has an excellent prognosis, while a depth of invasion of 1.5 mm or greater carries an extremely poor prognosis because of the high frequency of metastasis.[45] Overall, 50% of patients have lymph node metastases at the time of diagnosis.[45] Prophylactic superficial lymph node dissection has

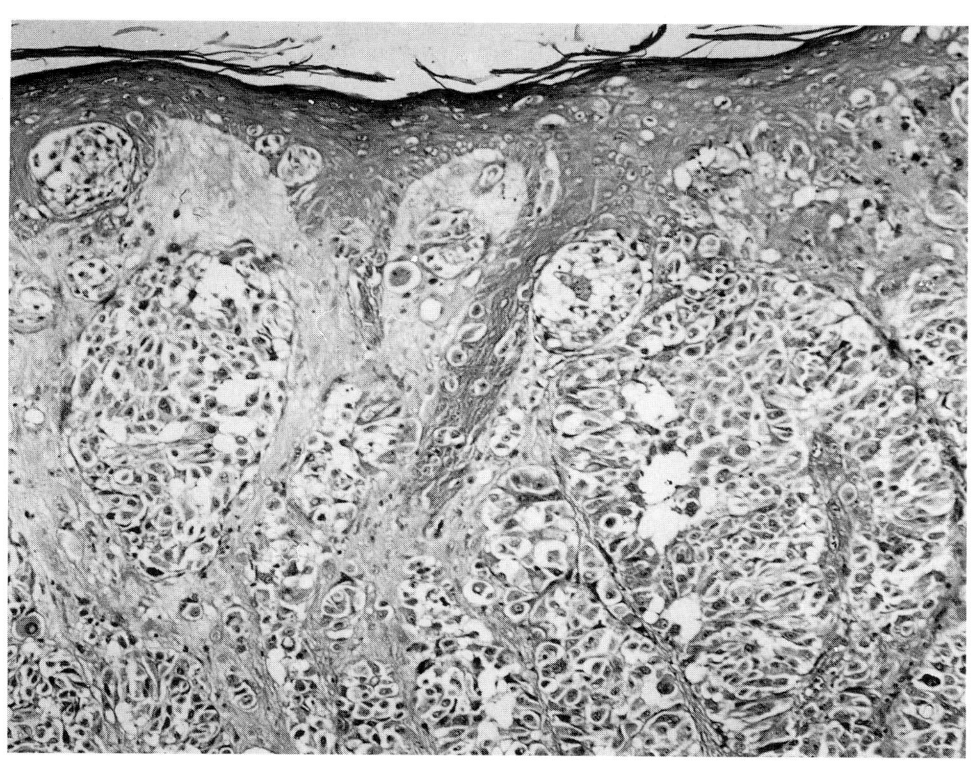

13-39. Nests of malignant melanoma cells undermine the epidermis.

been recommended as an adjunct to penectomy for stage I penile malignant melanoma more than 1.5 mm thick. Bilateral inguinal lymph node dissection is standard for stage II penile malignant melanoma.

Malignant melanoma of soft parts (clear cell sarcoma) is an uncommon neoplasm occurring most frequently in the tendons and aponeuroses of the extremities. This type of melanoma also has arisen in the penis.[288]

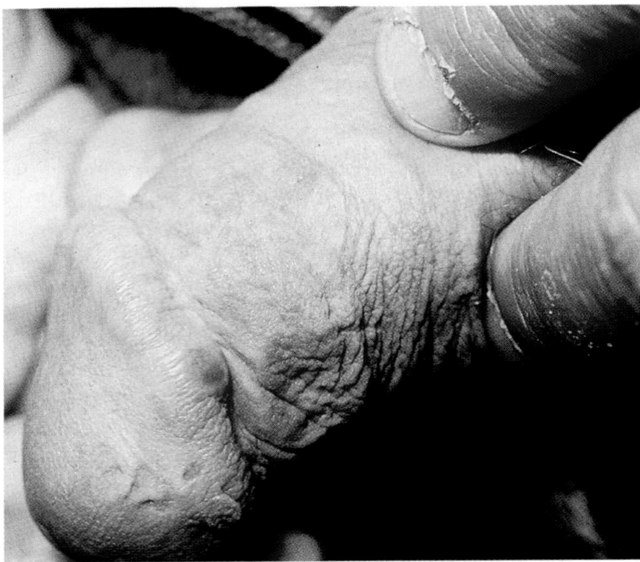

13-40. Kaposi's sarcoma presenting as a small purple nodule on the corona of the glans penis. *(Courtesy of Dr. A Hood, Indiana University, Indianapolis.)*

Sarcomas. Sarcomas as a group are the second most common type of penile cancer, after squamous cell carcinoma. Sarcomas of the penis are rare and account for less than 5% of all penile malignancies. Sarcomas have been reported in men of all ages, with a peak occurrence in the fifth and sixth decades of life, except for rhabdomyosarcoma, which is most common in children. With the exception of Kaposi's sarcoma, which most commonly arises on the glans penis, sarcomas are most frequently located on the penile shaft.

Vascular sarcomas, including Kaposi's sarcoma, epithelioid hemangioendothelioma, and angiosarcoma are the most common penile sarcomas. Sarcomas of myogenic, neurogenic, and fibrous origin also occur.[289] The histologic features of these lesions are similar to those of their counterparts arising at other locations.

AIDS–related Kaposi's sarcoma of the penis is increasing in frequency.[290-292] Approximately 20% of male AIDS patients with Kaposi's sarcoma have lesions on the penis, and as many as 3% of AIDS patients initially present with penile Kaposi's sarcoma (Fig. 13-40). The penis is rarely the first site of involvement of Kaposi's sarcoma, and its occurrence there is usually associated with other systemic lesions. The first case of Kaposi's sarcoma involving the penis was reported in 1986 by Saftel et al.[293] The tumors usually involve the skin of the shaft or the glans. When it involves the glans or corpus spongiosum, Kaposi's sarcoma may cause ure-

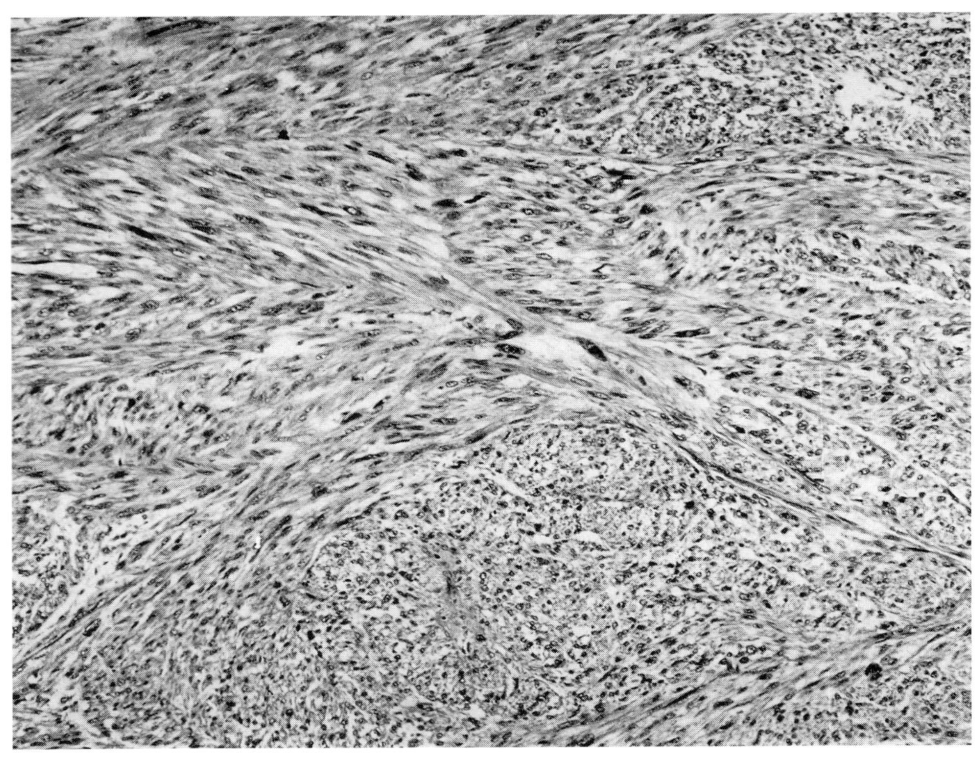

13-41. Leiomyosarcoma.

thral obstruction. Local excision can be effective for small localized lesions, but radiation therapy is also successful.[294,295]

Rarely, vascular sarcomas arise in the corpora cavernosa; about 35 cases have been reported.[296] The majority are hemangioendotheliomas and tend to be indolent. Epithelioid hemangioendotheliomas are composed of anastomosing networks of irregularly shaped vascular spaces lined by plump, often piled-up, endothelial cells with low-grade morphology.[297-299] High-grade tumors with solid masses of anaplastic tumor cells, hemorrhage, and necrosis have also been reported. These may metastasize to lymph nodes or hematogenously to distant sites such as lung, liver, and bone.

Leiomyosarcoma of the penis usually occurs in the fifth to seventh decades of life. Superficial leiomyosarcoma is thought to arise from the smooth muscle of the glans penis or the dermis of the shaft and usually forms subcutaneous nodules. Patients with superficial leiomyosarcoma tend to do well with local excision, but the tumor may recur locally. Deep leiomyosarcoma (Fig. 13-41) is less common, arising from the smooth muscle of the corpora cavernosa and tending to invade the urethra and metastasize early. Because of its tendency for widespread metastases, deep leiomyosarcoma of the penis carries a poor prognosis despite radical surgery.[300-302]

Fibrosarcoma can be superficial or deep and usually presents as a slowly growing, firm, nontender mass on the dorsum of the penile shaft or glans. Fibrosarcoma shares many clinical and gross features with leiomyosarcoma.[303] Immunohistochemical stains (for cytokeratin, smooth muscle actin, desmin, and vimentin) and the absence of overlying in situ carcinoma may be helpful to confirm their mesenchymal nature and rule out spindle cell squamous cell carcinoma. Malignant fibrous histiocytoma is rare in the penis, with only two cases reported in the literature, one of which was inflammatory malignant fibrous histiocytoma.[304,305]

Rhabdomyosarcoma has been reported in the penis, particularly on the shaft near the root. Most reported cases of rhabdomyosarcoma have arisen in children and were embryonal rhabdomyosarcoma.[306,307]

Eight cases of epithelioid sarcoma of the penis have been reported.[308,309] The patients ranged in age from 23 to 43 years (mean, 32 years). The penile lesions present as single or multiple, firm, slowly growing, painless subcutaneous nodules. The masses may produce surface ulceration and cause erectile pain or dysuria. Therefore, epithelioid sarcoma may mimic Peyronie's disease, urethral stricture, or ulcerating squamous carcinoma. Radical excision is the preferred method of treatment, although local excision combined with radiation therapy has been used with success. Epithelioid sarcoma is a slow-growing but aggressive tumor in the penis, as it is elsewhere in the body. Regardless of therapy, up to 80% of lesions recur locally. Metastases to the lung have been reported in two cases of the penile epithelioid sarcoma, but most reports lack long-term follow-up.

Other soft tissue sarcomas, including hemangiopericytoma and malignant schwannoma, have been reported to arise on the penis.

Benign mesenchymal neoplasms, such as hemangioma, lymphangioma, glomus tumor, neurofibroma, schwannoma, and granular cell tumor have been reported in the penis. The reported incidence of mesenchymal neoplasms is approximately equally divided between benign and malignant lesions.[258]

Primary lymphoma of the penis is rare, with only six reported cases. It has been suggested that this presentation is always a manifestation of occult nodal disease or a complication of late nodal lymphoma because there is no lymphoid tissue in the penis.[310,311]

Metastases to the penis. Although the penis has a rich and complex vascular circulation interconnected to the pelvic organs, metastases to the penis are rare and usually represent a late manifestation of systemic metastasis. In 1985 Powell et al[312] reviewed the literature and found only 219 cases. In a subsequent review, Perez-Mesa and Oxenhandler[313] reported six additional cases. In all reported series the most common primary site was the prostate, followed by the bladder, the rectosigmoid, and the kidney.[312-316] Less common primary sites include the testes, ureters, and nonpelvic organs such as the lung, pancreas, nasopharynx, larynx, and bone.[312-319]

The most common site for metastatic deposits is the corpus cavernosum.[314] Clinically, metastases usually present as multiple, palpable, painless nodules that may involve the skin and ulcerate, mimicking a syphilitic chancre. In 50% of patients, diffuse involvement of the corpus cavernosum causes priapism.[314] Hematuria and dysuria also can occur. In the great majority of cases, penile metastases occur in the terminal stage of a known cancer and pose no diagnostic difficulty. Rarely, penile metastases may be the primary presentation of an occult cancer.[320,321] Metastases to the penis should be suspected in any patient with a known cancer who has an onset of priapism or an unusual penile lesion.

The prognosis is poor for patients with metastases to the penis; Paquin and Rowland[322] reported that 95% of patients died within weeks to months of diagnosis. Similarly, Mukamel et al[323] reported that 71% of patients died within 6 months of diagnosis, and they have suggested that total penectomy may be indicated for relief of pain or severe urinary symptoms if metastases are confined to the penis without extension to the pelvis or pelvic diaphragm.

DISEASES OF THE SCROTUM

NON-NEOPLASTIC DISEASES

Fournier's gangrene

Fournier's gangrene is an idiopathic form of necrotizing fasciitis of the subcutaneous tissue and skeletal muscle of the genitals and perineum, particularly that of the scrotum.[324,325] The lesions begin as reddish plaques with necrosis (Fig. 13-42) and are accompanied by severe systemic symptoms including pain and fever. The lesions progress to develop localized edema, become insensitive, and form blisters that overlie an area of cellulitis. Most cases have accompanying scrotal emphysema. Without

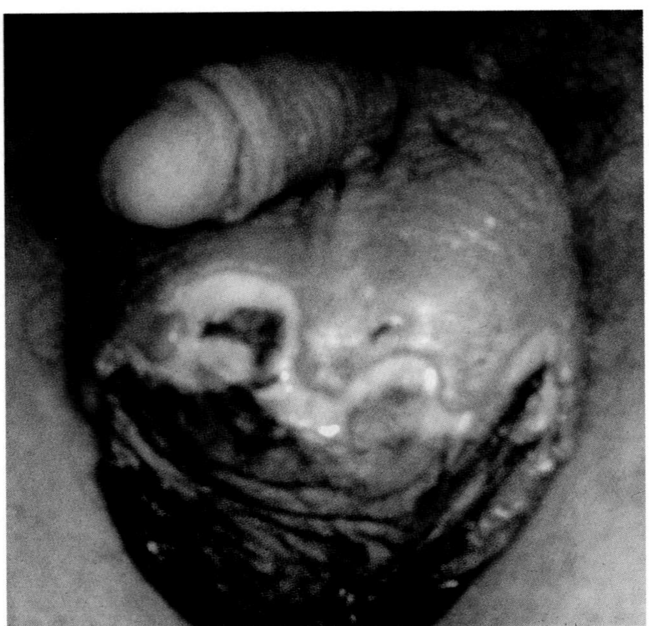

13-42. Fournier's gangrene. *(Courtesy of Dr. Hans Stricker, Henry Ford Hospital, Detroit, MI.)*

prompt diagnosis and aggressive treatment, ulceration and gangrene ensue.

Fournier's gangrene probably results from infection by staphylococcal or streptococcal species, which may be pure or, more commonly, are mixed with other gram-negative bacilli and anaerobic bacteria. Diabetes, alcoholism, immunosuppression, recent surgical intervention, trauma, and morbid obesity are predisposing factors but are not necessary for development of Fournier's gangrene.[325] Fournier's gangrene is a serious, life-threatening condition that requires vigorous and prompt therapy.[324,326] Clinically, the infection resembles clostridial gas gangrene, and in the past frozen sections were performed to detect gas bubbles. Today most experts believe that this does not yield clinically significant information and is unnecessary. Definitive treatment includes wide débridement, intravenous broad-spectrum antibiotics, and skin grafting.[326]

A necrotizing inflammatory process that is clinically similar to Fournier's gangrene but involves the glans penis is called *Corbus' disease* or *gangrenous balanitis*.[327-329] This condition is caused by anaerobic bacteria and can cause total necrosis of the glans penis. Gangrene of the penis may also be caused by constricting bands from external urinary drainage devices[330] and other constricting injuries.[331]

Hidradenitis suppurativa

Hidradenitis suppurativa is a chronic, suppurative inflammatory disease that is part of the follicular occlusion triad: hidradenitis suppurativa, acne conglobata, and perifollicular capitis.[332] First described by Verneuil in 1854, hidradenitis suppurativa is included with other lesions of the triad because of histologic and pathogenetic similarities.[333]

The term *hidradenitis suppurativa* is a misnomer since it is an inflammatory process of apocrine and eccrine glands that are obstructed by follicular hyperkeratosis. Thus, follicular hyperkeratosis is the root cause of the rupture of dilated pilosebaceous structures, which extrudes keratin and apocrine and eccrine products and commensal bacteria into the dermis, inciting the acute necrotizing and granulomatous reaction with abscess formation that extends into the deep connective tissue and upward onto the epidermis as sinus tracts in the lesions, typically seen by surgical pathologists.

The causes for the obstructing follicular hyperkeratosis are not fully understood, but may include genetic, hormonal, mechanical, and environmental factors.[334,335] Females with androgenic disturbances, obese patients, and patients with intertrigo are especially predisposed to hidradenitis suppurativa. Puberty also is a risk factor. Cultures are often negative, but superinfection is usually due to staphylococci, streptococci, or a mixture of bacteria, including anaerobes and actinomyces species.[336]

Clinically, the lesions begin as tender erythematous papules and progress to form fluctuant nodules which may have draining sinuses. Coalescence of adjacent involved follicles forms large plaques. The axilla is the most common site, but hidradenitis suppurativa also occurs in the skin of the groin, perianal, areolar, and periumbilical regions. Treatment is difficult, and antibiotics and intralesional steroid injections may be ineffective. Incision and drainage or localized excision is frequently necessary.[337]

Idiopathic scrotal calcinosis

Scrotal calcinosis occurs in two settings: calcification of preexisting epidermal or pilar cysts and calcification of dermal connective tissue in the absence of cysts (idiopathic scrotal calcinosis).[338,339] A hypothesis for the latter form favors origin from eccrine duct milia because of immunohistochemical positivity for carcinoembryonic antigen, a marker for eccrine sweat glands.[340]

Patients are usually young men, but children and older men have also been affected. They usually have multiple (up to 50) long-standing firm-to-hard nodules varying in size from a few millimeters up to 3 cm. The overlying skin is usually intact but may ulcerate, releasing cheesy material. Occasionally, a single hard nodule may be present.[341]

Histologically, the lesions lie within the dermis and contain granules and globules of hematoxylinophilic calcific material. They may or may not be accompanied with giant cell granulomatous inflammation and include recognizable cyst wall (Fig. 13-43). It is plausible that idiopathic scrotal calcinosis represents an end-stage phenomenon of numerous "old" epidermal cysts that over time have lost their cyst walls.[342-345] Treatment may be unnecessary for asymptomatic lesions, but surgery may be necessary for infected, recurrent, or extensive lesions.

Lipogranuloma

Lipogranuloma (also known as paraffinoma, sclerosing lipogranuloma, and Tancho's nodules) may involve the penile or scrotal skin. In penile lipogranuloma the lesion is usually due to hypodermic injection of substances such as paraffin, silicone, oil, or wax into the penis for penile

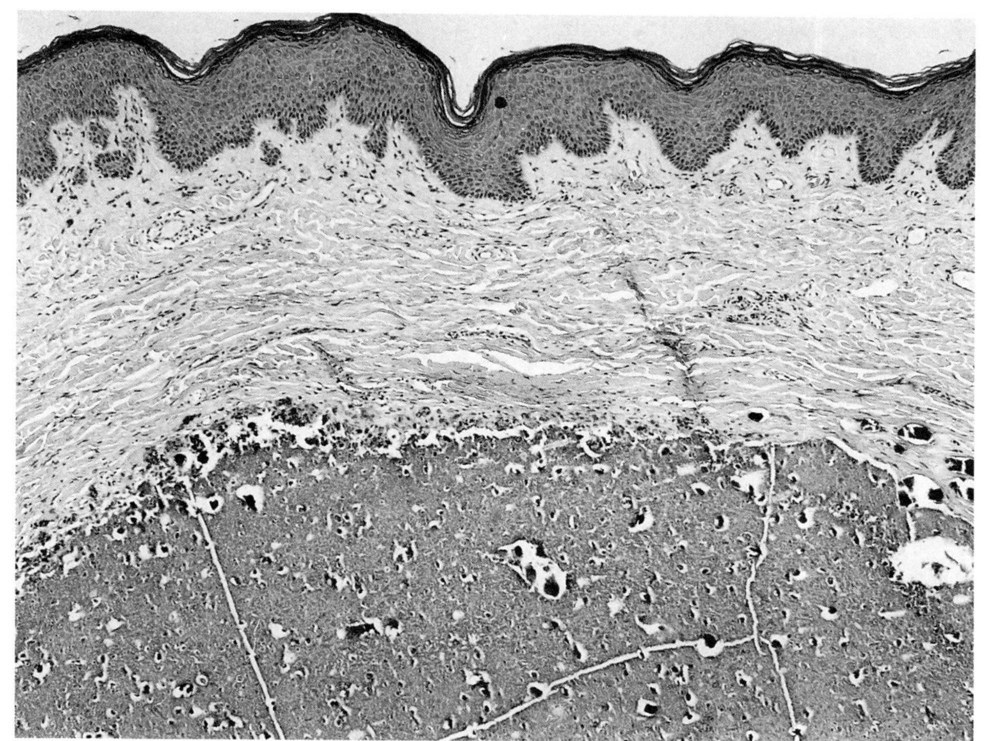

13-43. Scrotal calcinosis.

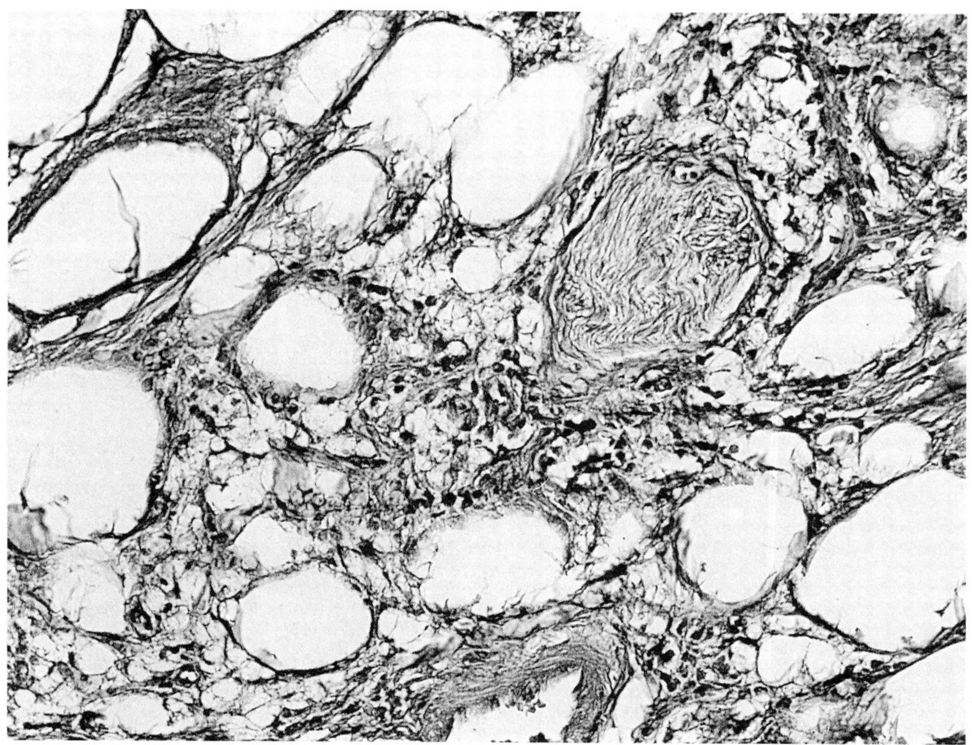

13-44. Scrotal lipogranuloma.

enlargement or sexual gratification.[346-351] In the scrotum, besides injection of foreign material, trauma, cold weather, and topical application of ointment (suggesting percutaneous absorption) have also been implicated.[347,348,352] Most lesions are seen in men less than 40 years old who complain of a localized plaque or mass which may be tender and indurated and as large as several centimeters in diameter. Biopsy is necessary, especially in the absence of clinical history of injection of exogenous material.

Microscopically, the lesion consists of lipid vacuoles embedded in a sclerotic stroma, usually accompanied by a histiocytic or foreign-body granulomatous infiltrate with or without eosinophils (Fig. 13-44).[352] The differential diagnosis includes signet ring cell carcinoma and malakoplakia. The diagnosis of lipogranuloma may be confirmed by histochemical stains for lipid.

Epidermal cyst

Epidermal cysts (keratinous cysts) are common in the scrotum.[45,353] They present as single or multiple rubbery-firm subdermal or intradermal nodules. Typically they contain gray-white cheesy material.[353] They are lined by keratinizing squamous epithelium.

Fat necrosis

Fat necrosis of the scrotum usually occurs in children and adolescents,[354] appearing as firm nodules in the lower portion of the scrotal wall. Two thirds of patients have bilateral nodules.[354] The lesion may develop when scrotal fat crystallizes following exposure to cold.

NEOPLASTIC DISEASES

Benign and malignant neoplasms of the scrotum are rare and most arise from the skin and adnexal structures.[45] Hemangioma, leiomyoma, and angiokeratoma are the most common benign scrotal neoplasms.[45,355] Squamous cell carcinoma is the most common scrotal cancer.[356-363] Recently, a case of aggressive angiomyxoma was reported in the scrotum.[364]

Squamous cell carcinoma

Scrotal squamous cell carcinoma was the first cancer linked to occupational exposure to a carcinogen. In the eighteenth century, men exposed to soot and dust (for example, chimney sweeps and cotton factory workers) had an increased incidence of scrotal squamous cell carcinoma. Pott[365] described this association, and the tumor was subsequently referred to as Pott's cancer or chimney sweep's cancer. Squamous cell carcinoma of the scrotum also occurs in men with other occupations, such as tar workers, paraffin and shale oil workers, machine operators in the engineering industry, petroleum wax pressmen, workers in the screw-making industry, and automatic lathe operators.[361] Later, 3'4'-benzpyrene was discovered to be the causative agent.[366] Andrews et al[361] reported several risk factors for the development of squamous cell carcinoma of the scrotum, including a history of psoriasis treated with coal tar or arsenic, condyloma acuminatum, and multiple cutaneous epitheliomas.

Squamous cell carcinoma is the most common malignant tumor of the scrotum, but the incidence of squamous cell carcinoma of the scrotum is much lower than that of penile carcinoma.[356-363] Since the first report of 18 cases in the United States, more than 100 cases have been reported. Squamous carcinoma of the scrotum most frequently presents as a solitary lesion. The early lesion is a slowly growing pimple, wart, or nodule, usually on the anterolateral aspect of the scrotum. These lesions later ulcerate and have raised, rolled edges with variable amounts of seropurulent discharge. Invasion of the scrotal contents or the penis has been observed in patients with advanced lesions. Some authors have suggested that scrotal cancer is uncommon among black men; however, because of the relatively small number of cases in each reported series, the racial distribution has not been established.[356-363]

Squamous cell carcinoma of the scrotum occurs primarily during the sixth and seventh decades of life.[356,361,362] The left scrotum is more frequently affected than the right,[361,362] and this predominance seems to reflect the site of exposure to carcinogens. When occupational exposure is excluded, the sides are equally frequently affected. Ipsilateral inguinal lymphadenopathy is observed at the time of initial presentation in 50% of patients.[359,361]

Microscopically, squamous cell carcinoma of the scrotum is similar to that of the penis. It is usually well differentiated to moderately differentiated and keratinization is common. The surrounding epidermis shows hyperkeratosis, acanthosis, and dyskeratosis. There is a strong correlation between stage and survival, but grade does not appear to add prognostic information, although most studies are limited by small sample size.

The differential diagnosis of scrotal squamous cell carcinoma includes a wide variety of lesions, ranging from nevus, epidermal cyst, eczema, psoriasis, folliculitis, syphilis, tuberculous epididymitis, and periurethral abscess to benign and malignant neoplasms such as hemangioma, lymphangioma, basal cell carcinoma, malignant melanoma, Paget's disease, and various sarcomas.[367]

TABLE 13-6.
STAGING SYSTEM FOR SCROTAL CARCINOMA

Stage	Description
A1	Localized to scrotal wall
A2	Locally extensive tumor invading adjacent structure (testis, spermatic cord, penis, pubis, perineum)
B	Metastatic disease involving inguinal lymph nodes only
C	Metastatic disease involving pelvic lymph nodes without evidence of distant spread
D	Metastatic disease beyond the pelvic lymph nodes involving distant organs

From Lowe FC: Squamous cell carcinoma of the scrotum, J Urol 130:423-427, 1983.

The staging system for the scrotum was proposed by Lowe (Table 13-6).[359] The prognosis is poor for patients with squamous cell carcinomas of the scrotum; the 5-year survival rate is 30% to 52%. Ray and Whitmore[357] reported a 70% 5-year survival rate for patients with stage A carcinoma and 44% for patients with stage B carcinoma. Patients with stage C or stage D cancer have little chance for long-term survival.[367]

Basal cell carcinoma

Basal cell carcinoma of the scrotum is rare, accounting for less than 10% of scrotal malignancies.[360,368-371] The average age of patients is 65 years, with an age range of 42 to 82 years.[370] Clinically, the lesions present as painless plaques or ulcerated nodules. There is a predilection for basal cell carcinoma to occur on the left side of the scrotum.[369] Unlike squamous cell carcinoma, there is no known occupational risk factor or carcinogen. Human papillomavirus infection does not appear to play a role. It is possible that basal cell carcinoma of the scrotum is more likely to metastasize than basal cell carcinoma of other sites.[370]

Paget's disease

Extramammary Paget's disease rarely involves the penile or scrotal skin.[372-376] Most cases are associated with an underlying carcinoma (either adnexal or visceral), including carcinoma of the urinary bladder, prostate, and urethra. Penile and scrotal Paget's disease most often occurs during the sixth and seventh decades of life, usually presenting as a scaly, eczematous lesion. Microscopically, it consists of an intraepithelial proliferation of atypical cells with vacuolated cytoplasm and large vesicular nuclei (Fig. 13-45). The atypical cells tend to cluster at the tips of the rete ridges. Hyperkeratosis, parakeratosis, and papillomatosis are common. The intraepithelial neoplastic cells contain intracytoplasmic neutral and acidic mucopolysaccharides, which can be demonstrated by periodic acid–Schiff, mucicarmine, alcian blue, and aldehyde fuscin stains. The differential diagnosis includes squamous cell carcinoma in situ and malignant melanoma. Because intracytoplasmic mucin is not a feature of melanoma or squamous carcinoma in situ, mucin stains are helpful in establishing the diagnosis. Immunoperoxidase staining for carcinoembryonic antigen, S-100 protein, and HMB-45 also may be helpful because the cells of Paget's disease often contain carcinoembryonic antigen whereas melanoma cells are negative, and melanoma cells usually are positive for either S-100 protein or HMB-45 whereas the cells of Paget's disease are negative for these reactions.[377]

Sarcoma

Sarcoma of the scrotum, excluding extension of sarcoma from the spermatic cord, is extremely rare.[378] The most common type is leiomyosarcoma, which arises from the dartos muscle; fewer than 20 cases have been reported.[378-381] The age at presentation ranges from 35 to 89 years. A case of radiation-induced leiomyosarcoma was reported in the scrotum.[379] Only five patients have a long-term follow-up, and four of the five eventually developed distant metastases.[378] Scrotal leiomyosarcoma

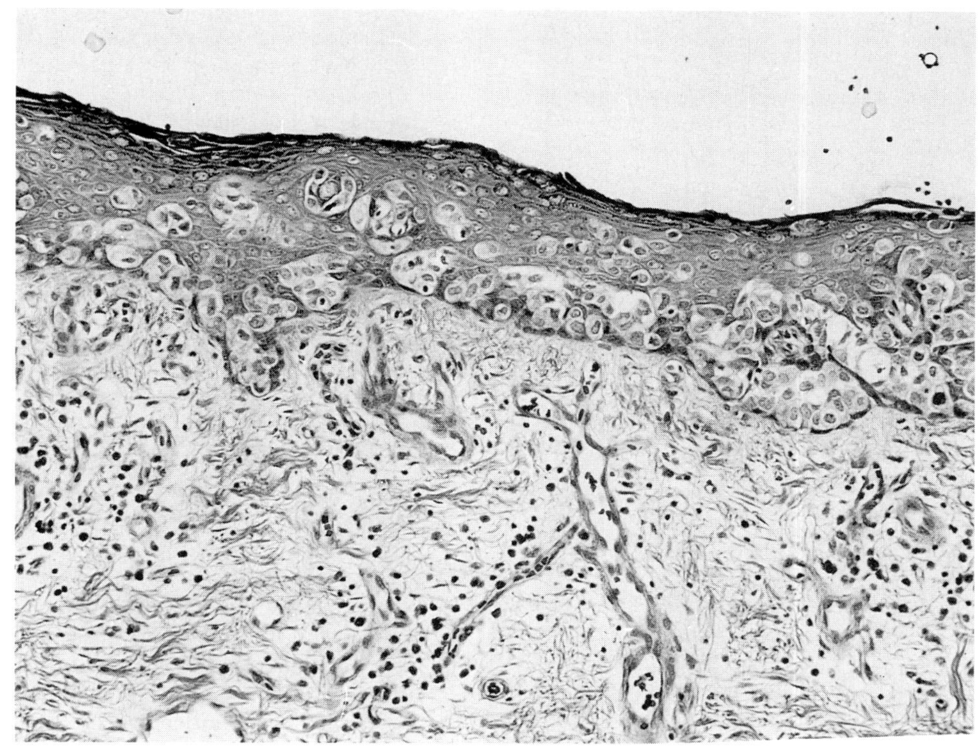

13-45. Paget's disease.

appears to behave similarly to subcutaneous leiomyosarcoma. Lymphatic metastases are rare, but long-term follow-up is necessary because of the possibility of late visceral metastases or recurrence. Recently, a case with combined features of liposarcoma and leiomyosarcoma was reported in the scrotum.[382] A case of malignant fibrous histiocytoma arising from the scrotal wall has also been reported.[383]

REFERENCES

1. Dees JE: Congenital epispadias with incontinence, J Urol 62:513-522, 1949.
2. Kramer SA, Kelalis PP: Assessment of urinary continence in epispadias: review of 94 patients, J Urol 128:290-293, 1982.
3. Campbell M: Epispadias: a report of 15 cases, J Urol 67:988-999, 1952.
4. Arap S, Nahas WC, Giron AM et al: Incontinent epispadias: surgical treatment of 38 cases, J Urol 140:577-581, 1988.
5. Duckett JW: Hypospadias. In Walsh PC, Retik AB, Stamey TA et al, eds: Campbell's urology, ed 6, Philadelphia, 1992, WB Saunders.
6. Juskiewenski S, Vaysse P, Guitard J et al: Traitement des hypospadias anterieurs: place de la balanoplastie, J Urol (Paris) 89:153-156, 1983.
7. Sweet RA, Schrott HG, Kurland R et al: Study of the incidence of hypospadias in Rochester, Minnesota, 1940–1970, and a case-control comparison of possible etiologic factors, Mayo Clin Proc 49:52-59, 1974.
8. Sheldon TB, Noe HN: The role of excretory urography in patients with hypospadias, J Urol 135:97-100, 1985.
9. Gonzales JR: Micropenis, AUA Update Series 2:1, 1983.
10. Lee PA, Mazur T, Danish R et al: Micropenis: I. Criteria, etiologies and classification, Johns Hopkins Med J 146:156-163, 1980.
11. Marizels M, Zaontz M, Donovan J et al: Surgical correction of the buried penis: description of a classification system and technique to correct the diagnosis, J Urol 136:268-271, 1986.
12. Skoog SJ, Belman AB: Aphallia: its classification and management, J Urol 141:589-592, 1989.
13. Gilbert J, Clark RD, Koyle MA: Penile agenesis: a fatal variation of an uncommon lesion, J Urol 143:338-339, 1990.
14. Hollowell JG, Witherington R, Ballagas AJ et al: Embryologic considerations of diphallus and associated anomalies, J Urol 117:728-732, 1977.
15. Kapoor R, Saha MM: Complete duplication of the bladder, urethra and external genitalia in a neonate: a case report, J Urol 137:1243-1244, 1987.
16. Kaplan GW, Brock WA: The etiology of chordee, Urol Clin North Am 8:383-387, 1981.
17. Gelbard MK, Dorey F, James K: The natural history of Peyronie's disease, J Urol 144:1376-1379, 1990.
18. Yamaguchi T, Hamasuna R, Hasui Y et al: 47,XXY/48,XXY, +21 chromosomal mosaicism presenting as hypospadias with scrotal transposition, J Urol 142:797-801, 1989.
19. Cohen-Addad N, Zarafu IW, Hanna MK: Complete penoscrotal transposition, Urology 26:149-152, 1985.
20. Elder JS, Jeffs RD: Suprainguinal ectopic scrotum and associated anomalies, J Urol 127:336-338, 1982.
21. Lowe FC, Brendler CB: The urologic examination and diagnostic techniques. In Walsh PC, Retik AB, Stamey TA et al, eds: Campbell's urology, ed 6, Philadelphia, 1992, WB Saunders.
22. Schellhammer PF, Jordan GH, Scholossberg SM: Tumors of the penis. In Walsh PC, Retik AB, Stamey TA et al, eds: Campbell's urology, ed 6, Philadelphia, 1992, WB Saunders.
23. Robson WL, Leung AK: The circumcision question, Postgrad Med 91:237-242, 1992.
24. Clemmensen OJ, Krogh J, Petri M: The histologic spectrum of prepuces from patients with phimosis, Am J Dermatopathol 10:104-108, 1988.
25. Gozal D: Paraphimosis apparently associated with Plasmodium falciparum infection, Tran R Soc Trop Med Hyg 85:443, 1991.
26. Romero-Perez P, Amat-Cecilia M, Amdrada-Becerra E: Metastasis in the glans of prostatic adenocarcinoma. Apropos of a case, Actas Urol Esp 15:284-287, 1991.
27. Reddy CRRM, Devendranath V, Pratap S: Carcinoma of penis—role of phimosis, Urology 24:85-88, 1984.
28. Brinton LA, Li JY, Rong SD et al: Risk factors for penile cancer: results from a case-control study in China, Int J Cancer 47:504-509, 1991.
29. Escala JM, Rickwood AM: Balanitis, Br J Urol 63:196-197, 1989.
30. Vohra S, Badlani G: Balanitis and balanoposthitis, Urol Clin North Am 19:143-147, 1992.
31. Lynch PJ: Cutaneous diseases of the external genitalia. In Walsh PC, Retik AB, Stamey TA et al, eds: Campbell's urology, ed 6, Philadelphia, 1992, WB Saunders.
32. Abdullah AN, Drake SM, Wade AA et al: Balanitis (balanoposthitis) in patients attending a department of genitourinary medicine, Int J STD AIDS 3:128-129, 1992.
33. Zoon JJ: Balanophosthite chronique circonscrite benigne plasmocytes, Dermatologica 105:1-7, 1952.
34. Jolly BB, Krishnamurty S, Vaidyanathan S: Zoon's balanitis, Urol Int 50:182-184, 1993.
35. Arango-Toro O, Rosales-Bordes A, Vese-Llanes J et al: Plasmacellular balanoposthitis of Zoon, Arch Esp Urol 43:337-339, 1990.
36. Souteyrand P, Wong E, MacDonald DM: Zoon's balanitis (balanitis circumscripta plasmacellularis), Br J Dermatol 105:195-199, 1981.
37. Brodin M: Balanitis circumscripta plasmacellularis, J Am Acad Dermatol 2:33-35, 1980.
38. Baldwin HE, Geronemus RG: The treatment of Zoon's balanitis with the carbon dioxide laser, J Dermatol Surg Oncol 15:491-494, 1989.
39. Rowell NR: Lupus erythematosus, scleroderma and dermatomyositis. The "collagen" or "connective-tissue" diseases. In Rook A, Wilkinson DS, Ebling FJG et al, eds: Textbook of dermatology, ed 4, Oxford, 1986, Blackwell Scientific Publications.
40. Datta C, Dutta SK, Chaudhuri A: Histopathological and immunological studies in a cohort of balanitis xerotica obliterans, J Indian Med Assoc 91:146-148, 1993.
41. Post B, Janner M: Lichen sclerosus et atrophicus penis, Z Hautkr 50:675-681, 1975.
42. Harrington CI, Dunsmore IR: An investigation into the incidence of autoimmune disorders in patients with lichen sclerosus et atrophicus, Br J Dermatol 104:563-566, 1981.

43. Thomas RHM, Ridley CM, Black MM: The association of lichen sclerosus et atrophicus related disease in males, Br J Dermatol 109:661-664, 1983.
44. Harrington CI, Gelsthorpe K: The association between lichen sclerosus et atrophicus and HLA-B40, Br J Dermatol 104:561-562, 1981.
45. Hewan-Lowe K, Moreland A, Finnerty DP: Penis and scrotum, tumors and related disorders. In Someren A, ed: Urologic pathology with clinical and radiologic correlations, New York, 1990, Macmillan.
46. Gottschalk HR, Cooper ZK: Lichen sclerosus et atrophicus with bullous lesions and extensive involvement, Arch Dermatol 55:433-440, 1947.
47. Dore B, Grange P, Irani J et al: Atrophicus sclerosis lichen and cancer of the glans, J Urol (Paris) 95:415-418, 1989.
48. Campus GV, Alia F, Bosincu L: Squamous cell carcinoma and lichen sclerosus et atrophicus of the prepuce, Plast Reconstr Surg 89:692-694, 1992.
49. Pride HB, Miller OF, Tyler WB: Penile squamous cell carcinoma arising from balanitis xerotica obliterans, J Am Acad Dermatol 29:469-473, 1993.
50. Perry HO, Mayne JG: Psoriasis and Reiter's syndrome, Arch Dermatol 92:129-136, 1965.
51. Keat A: Reiter's syndrome and reactive arthritis in perspective, N Engl J Med 309:1606-1615, 1983.
52. Calin A: Reiter's syndrome. In Kelly WN, Harris ED Jr, Ruddy S et al, eds: Textbook of rheumatology, ed 3, Philadelphia, 1989, WB Saunders.
53. Good AE, Schultz JS: Reiter's syndrome following *Shigella flexneri* 2a, Arthritis Rheum 20:100-104, 1977.
54. Keat A, Rowe I: Reiter's syndrome and associated arthritides, Rheum Dis Clin North Am 17:25-42, 1991.
55. Cuttica RJ, Scheines EJ, Garay SM et al: Juvenile onset Reiter's syndrome. A retrospective study of 26 patients, Clin Exp Rheumatol 10:285-288, 1992.
56. Rehman MU, Cantwell R, Johnson CC et al: Inapparent genital infection with *Chlamydia trachomatis* and its potential role in the genesis of Reiter's syndrome, DNA Cell Biol 11:215-219, 1992.
57. Tuncer T, Arman MI, Akyokus A et al: HLA B27 and clinical features in Reiter's syndrome, Clin Rheumatol 11:239-242, 1992.
58. Hansfield HH, Pollock PS: Arthritis associated sexually transmitted diseases. In Holmes KK, Mardh P, Sparling PF et al, eds: Sexually transmitted diseases, ed 2, New York, 1990, McGraw-Hill.
59. Lever WF, Schaumburg-Lever G: Noninfectious erythematous, papular and squamous diseases. In Lever WF, Schaumburg-Lever G, eds: Histopathology of the skin, ed 7, Philadelphia, 1989, JB Lippincott.
60. Wilson SK, Delk JR: A new treatment for Peyronie's disease: modeling the penis over an inflatable penile prosthesis, J Urol 152:1121-1123, 1994.
61. Enzinger FM, Weiss SW: Fibromatoses. In Enzinger FM, Weiss SW, eds: Soft tissue tumors, ed 3, St. Louis, 1995, Mosby–Year Book.
62. Smith BH: Subclinical Peyronie's disease, Am J Clin Pathol 52:385-390, 1969.
63. Neyberg LM, Bias WB, Hochberg MC et al: Identification of an inherited form of Peyronie's disease with autosomal dominant inheritance and association with Dupuytren's contracture and histocompatibility B7 cross reacting antigens, J Urol 128:48-51, 1982.
64. Vande Berg JS, Devine CJ, Horton CE et al: Peyronie's disease: an electron microscopic study, J Urol 126:333-336, 1981.
65. Hinman F Jr: Etiologic factors in Peyronie disease, Urol Int 35:407-413, 1980.
66. Kaufman JJ: Peyronie's: its cause, Scand J Urol Nephrol 138(suppl):219, 1991.
67. Rompel R, Weidner W, Mueller-Eckhardt G: HLA association of idiopathic Peyronie's disease: an indication of autoimmune phenomena in etiopathogenesis? Tissue Antigens 38:104-106, 1991.
68. Bivens CH, Maracek RL, Feldman JM: Peyronie's disease—a presenting complaint of the carcinoid syndrome, N Engl J Med 289:844-846, 1973.
69. Guerneri S, Stioui S, Mantovani F et al: Multiple clonal chromosome abnormalities in Peyronie's disease, Cancer Genet Cytogenet 52:181-185, 1991.
70. Chiang PH, Chiang CP, Shen MR et al: Study of the changes in collagen of the tunica albuginea in venogenic impotence and Peyronie's disease, Eur Urol 21:48-51, 1992.
71. McRoberts JW: Peyronie's disease, Surg Gynecol Obstet 129:1291-1294, 1969.
72. Montorsi F, Guazzoni G, Bergamaschi F et al: Patient-partner satisfaction with semirigid penile prostheses for Peyronie's disease: a 5-year followup study, J Urol 150:1819-1821, 1993.
73. Gelbrad MK: Dystrophic penile calcification in Peyronie's disease, J Urol 139:738-740, 1988.
74. Champion RH, Wegrzyn J: Congenital os penis, J Urol 91:663, 1964.
75. Hoeg OM: Human penile ossification. A case report, Scand J Urol Nephrol 20:231-232, 1986.
76. Goldstein I, Krane RJ: Diagnosis and therapy of erectile dysfunction. In Walsh PC, Retik AB, Stamey TA et al, eds: Campbell's urology, ed 6, Philadelphia, 1992, WB Saunders.
77. Petrou AP, Barrett DM: The use of penile prosthesis in erectile dysfunction, Semin Urol 8:138-152, 1990.
78. Kessler R: Surgical experience with the inflatable penile prosthesis, J Urol 124:611-613, 1980.
79. Kasebayashi Y, Hayashi Y, Hirao K et al: A case of penile cavernitis following a penile prosthesis implantation, Hinyokika Kiyo 37:1555-1557, 1991.
80. Fulow WL, Goldwasser B, Gundian JC: Implantation of model AMS 700 penile prosthesis: long-term results, J Urol 139:741-742, 1988.
81. Pohl J, Pott B, Kleinhans G: Priapism: a three-phase concept of management according to aetiology and prognosis, Br J Urol 58:113-118, 1986.
82. Hinman F Jr: Priapism: reasons for failure of therapy, J Urol 83:420-428, 1960.
83. Spycher MA, Hauri D: The ultrastructure of the erectile tissue in priapism, J Urol 135:142-150, 1986.
84. Winter CC, McDowell G: Experience with 105 patients with priapism: update review of all aspects, J Urol 140:980-983, 1988.
85. Rosebury T: Microbes and morals. Viking, 1971, New York.

86. Judson FN: Gonorrhea, Med Clin North Am 74:1353-1366, 1990.
87. Hawley HB: Gonorrhea. Finding and treating a moving target, Postgrad Med 94:105-111, 1993.
88. Ramon QD, Betlloch MI, Jimenez MR: Gonococcal infection of the penile median raphe, Int J Dermatol 26:242-243, 1987.
89. Katsman L: Gonorrheal abscess of the penis, Vestn Dermatol Venerol 5:64-65, 1980.
90. Gaffoor PM, Bayyari KH: Gonococcal tysonitis: an unusual penile infection, Indian J Dermatol 34:90-91, 1989.
91. Webster LA, Berman SM, Greenspan JR: Surveillance for gonorrhea and primary and secondary syphilis among adolescents, United States—1981–1991, MMWR CDC Surveill Summ 43:1-11, 1993.
92. Sparling PF: Natural history of syphilis. In Holmes KK, Mardh P, Sparling PF, eds: Sexually transmitted diseases, New York, 1990, McGraw-Hill.
93. Hutchinson CM, Hook EW III: Syphilis in adults, Med Clin North Am 74:1389-1416, 1990.
94. Tramont EC: Syphilis in HIV-infected persons, AIDS Clin Rev, 61-72, 1993-1994.
95. Mencus A, Antal GM: The endemic treponematoses: not yet eradicated, World Health Stat Q 45:228-237, 1992.
96. Pariser H: Syphilis, Prim Care 16:603-619, 1989.
97. Jeerapaet P, Ackerman AB: Histologic patterns of secondary syphilis, Arch Dermatol 107:373-377, 1973.
98. Abell E, Marks R, Wilson-Jones E: Secondary syphilis: a clinicopathological review, Br J Dermatol 93:53-61, 1975.
99. Cochran RIE, Thomson J, Fleming KA et al: Histology simulating reticulosis in secondary syphilis, Br J Dermatol 95:251-254, 1976.
100. Poulsen A, Kobayasi T, Secher L et al: Treponema pallidum in macular and papular secondary syphilis skin eruptions, Acta Derm Venereol 66:251-258, 1986.
101. Nahmias AJ, Roizman D: Infection with herpes simplex virus 1 and 2, N Engl J Med 29:667-719, 1973.
102. Rudlinger R, Norval M: Herpes simplex virus infections: new concepts in an old disease, Dermatologica 178:1-5, 1989.
103. Corey L: Herpes simplex virus infections during the decade since the licensure of acyclovir, J Med Virol 1(suppl):7-12, 1993.
104. Arbesfeld DM, Thomas I: Cutaneous herpes simples virus infections, Am Fam Physician 43:1655-1664, 1991.
105. Ashley RL: Laboratory techniques in the diagnosis of herpes simplex infection, Genitourin Med 69:174-183, 1993.
106. McSorley J, Shapiro L, Brownstein MH et al: Simplex and varicella-zoster: comparative cases, Int J Dermatol 13:69-75, 1974.
107. Whitley RJ: Neonatal herpes simplex virus infections, J Med Virol 1(suppl):13-21, 1993.
108. Favre M, Hellerstrom S: The epidemiology, aetiology and prophylaxis of lymphogranuloma inguinale, Acta Derm Venereol 34(suppl):1-9, 1954.
109. Burgoyne RA: Lymphogranuloma venereum, Prim Care 17:153-157, 1990.
110. Heaton ND, Yates-Bell A: Thirty-year follow-up of lymphogranuloma venereum, Br J Urol 70:693-694, 1992.
111. Faro S: Lymphogranuloma venereum, chancroid, and granuloma inguinale, Obstet Gynecol Clin North Am 16:517-530, 1989.
112. Sheldon WH, Heyman A: Lymphogranuloma venereum, Am J Pathol 23:653-664, 1947.
113. Schubiner HH, LeBar WD, Joseph S et al: Evaluation of two rapid tests for the diagnosis of *Chlamydia trachomatis* genital infections, Eur J Clin Microbiol Infect Dis 11:553-556, 1992.
114. Bassa AG, Hoosen AA, Moodley J et al: Granuloma inguinale (donovanosis) in women. An analysis of 61 cases from Durban, South Africa, Sex Transm Dis 20:164-167, 1993.
115. Richens J: The diagnosis and treatment of donovanosis (granuloma inguinale), Genitourin Med 67:441-452, 1991.
116. Sayal SK, Kar PK, Anand LC: A study of 255 cases of granuloma inguinale, Indian J Dermatol 32:91-97, 1987.
117. Sehgal VN, Sharma HK: Donovanosis, J Dermatol 19:932-46, 1992.
118. Beerman H, Sonck CE: The epithelial changes in granuloma inguinale, Am J Syph 36:501-510, 1952.
119. Fritz GS, Hubler WR, Dodson RF et al: Mutilating granuloma inguinale, Arch Dermatol 111:1464-1465, 1975.
120. Davis CM, Collins C: Granuloma inguinale: an ultrastructural study of *Calymmatobacterium granulomatis*, J Invest Dermatol 53:315-321, 1969.
121. Barnes R, Masood S, Lammert N et al: Extragenital granuloma inguinale mimicking a soft-tissue neoplasm: a case report and review of the literature, Hum Pathol 21:559-561, 1990.
122. Van-Dyck E, Piot P: Laboratory techniques in the investigation of chancroid, lymphogranuloma venereum and donovanosis, Genitourin Med 68:130-133, 1992.
123. Freinkel AL, Dangor Y, Koornhof HJ et al: A serological test for granuloma inguinale, Genitourin Med 68:269-272, 1992.
124. Ducrey A: Experimentelle Untersuchungen uber den Ansteckungsstoff des weichen Schankers und uber die Bubonen, Monatsh f prakt Dermat Hamb 9:387-405, 1889.
125. Schmid GP, Sanders LL Jr, Blount JH et al: Chancroid in the United States: reestablishment of an old disease, JAMA 258:3265-3268, 1987.
126. Jordan WC: Chancroid: a review for the family practitioner, J Natl Med Assoc 83:724-726, 1991.
127. Margolis RJ, Hood AF: Chancroid: diagnosis and treatment, J Am Acad Dermatol 6:493-499, 1982.
128. Gaisin A, Heaton CL: Chancroid: alias the soft chancre, Int J Dermatol 14:188-197, 1975.
129. Jones CC, Rosen T: Cultural diagnosis of chancroid, Arch Dermatol 127:1823-1827, 1991.
130. Chui L, Albritton W, Paster B et al: Development of the polymerase chain reaction for diagnosis of chancroid, J Clin Microbiol 31:659-664, 1993.
131. Jessamine PG, Plummer FA, Ndinya-Achola JO et al: Human immunodeficiency virus, genital ulcers and the male foreskin: synergism in HIV-1 transmission, Scand J Infect Dis 69(Suppl):181-186, 1990.
132. Simonsen JN, Cameron DW, Yakinya MN et al: Human immunodeficiency virus infection in men with sexually transmitted diseases, N Engl J Med 319:274-278, 1988.
133. Lynch PJ: Cutaneous diseases of the external genitalia. In Walsh PC, Retik AB, Stamey TA et al, eds: Campbell's urology, ed 6, Philadelphia, 1992, WB Saunders.
134. Burchard KW: Fungal sepsis, Infect Dis Clin North Am 6:677-692, 1992.

135. Humayun H, Maliwan N: Emphysematous genital infection caused by candida albicans, J Urol 128:1049-1054, 1982.
136. Heilesen B: Studies on *Acarus scabiei* and scabies, Acta Derm Venereol 26(Suppl):1-370, 1946.
137. Barrett NG, Morse DL: The resurgence of scabies, Commun Dis Rep CDR Rev 3:32-34, 1993.
138. Fernandez N, Torres A, Ackerman AB: Pathological finding in human scabies, Arch Dermatol 113:320-324, 1977.
139. Hejazi N, Mehregan AH: Scabies. Histological study of inflammatory lesions, Arch Dermatol 111:37-39, 1975.
140. Orkin M, Maibach HI: This scabies pandemic, N Engl J Med 289:496-498, 1978.
141. Yang SA, Lu CF, Kuo MC et al: Clinical and scanning electron microscopic studies on Norwegian scabies infection, Kao Hsiung I Hsueh Ko Hsueh Tsa Chih 8:569-575, 1992.
142. Estes SA, Estes J: Therapy of scabies: nursing homes, hospitals, and the homeless, Semin Dermatol 12:26-33, 1993.
143. Billstein SA, Mattaliano VJ Jr: The nuisance sexually transmitted diseases: molluscum contagiosum, scabies, and crab lice, Med Clin North Am 74:1487-1505, 1990.
144. Levine GI: Sexually transmitted parasitic diseases, Prim Care 18:101-128, 1991.
145. Hutchinson DB, Farquhar JA: Trimethoprim-sulfamethoxazole in the treatment of malaria, toxoplasmosis, and pediculosis, Rev Infect Dis 4:419-425, 1982.
146. Porter CD, Blake NW, Cream JJ et al: Molluscum contagiosum virus, Mol Cell Biol Hum Dis Ser 1:233-257, 1992.
147. Epstein WL: Molluscum contagiosum, Semin Dermatol 11:184-189, 1992.
148. Lutzner MA: Molluscum contagiosum, verruca and zoster viruses, Arch Dermatol 23:436-444, 1963.
149. Mescon H, Gray M, Moretti G: Molluscum contagiosum, J Invest Dermatol 23:293-308, 1954.
150. Henao M, Freeman RG: Inflammatory molluscum contagiosum, Arch Dermatol 90:479-482, 1964.
151. Golledge CL, Phillips G: *Corynebacterium minutissimum* infection, J Infect 23:73-76, 1991.
152. Sarkany I, Taplin D, Blank H: Incidence and bacteriology of erythrasma, Arch Dermatol 85:578-582, 1962.
153. Montes LF, Black SH, McBride ME: Bacterial invasion of the stratum corneum in erythrasma. Ultrastructural evidence for a keratolytic action exerted by *Corynebacterium minutissimum*, J Invest Dermatol 49:474-485, 1967.
154. Saffrin S: Treatment of acyclovir-resistant herpes simplex virus infections in patients with AIDS, J Acquir Immune Defic Syndr 5(suppl)1:S29-S32, 1992.
155. Coleman DC, Bennett DE, Sullivan DJ et al: Oral candida in HIV infection and AIDS: new perspectives/new approaches, Crit Rev Microbiol 19:61-82, 1993.
156. Schwartz JJ, Myskowski PL: Molluscum contagiosum in patients with human immunodeficiency virus infection. A review of twenty-seven patients, J Am Acad Dermatol 27:583-588, 1992.
157. Orkin M: Scabies in AIDS, Semin Dermatol 12:9-14, 1993.
158. Brancato L, Itescu S, Skovron ML et al: Aspects of the spectrum, prevalence and disease susceptibility determinants of Reiter's syndrome and related disorders associated with HIV infection, Rheumatol Int 9:137-141, 1989.
159. Kaplan MH, Sodick N, McNutt NS et al: Dermatologic findings and manifestations of acquired immunodeficiency syndrome (AIDS), J Am Acad Dermatol 16:485-506, 1987.
160. Overly WL, Jakubek DJ: Multiple squamous cell carcinomas and HIV infections, Ann Intern Med 106:334, 1987 (letter).
161. Milburn PB, Brandsma JL, Goldsman CI et al: Disseminated warts and evolving squamous cell carcinoma in a patient with AIDS, J Am Acad Dermatol 19:401-405, 1988.
162. Croxson T, Chabow AB, Rorat E et al: Intraepithelial carcinoma of the anus in homosexual men, Dis Colon Rectum 27:325-330, 1984.
163. Gelquin J, Weiss L, Kazatchkine MD: Genital and oral erosions induced by foscarnet, Lancet 335:287, 1990.
164. Fegueux S, Salmon D, Picard C et al: Penile ulceration with foscarnet, Lancet 335:547, 1990.
165. Rosenberg SK, Reid R: Sexually transmitted papilloma viral infections in the male. I. Anatomic distribution and clinical features, Urology 29:488-492, 1987.
166. Chuang T-Y: Condyloma acuminata (genital warts). An epidemiologic view, J Am Acad Dermatol 16:376-384, 1987.
167. Chuang T-Y, Perry HO, Kurland LT et al: Condyloma acuminatum in Rochester, Minn, 1950–1978. I: epidemiology and clinical features, Arch Dermatol 120:469-475, 1984.
168. Syrjanen K, Syrjanen S: Epidemiology of human papillomavirus infections and genital neoplasia, Scand J Infec Dis 69(Suppl):7-17, 1990.
169. Barrasso R, De Brux J, Croissant O et al: High prevalence of papilloma virus-associated penile intraepithelial neoplasia in sexual partners of women with cervical intraepithelial neoplasia, N Engl J Med 317:916-923, 1987.
170. Schackner L, Hankin DE: Assessing child abuse in childhood condyloma acuminatum, J Am Acad Dermatol 123:157-160, 1985.
171. Oriel JD: Natural history of genital warts, Br J Venereal Dis 47:1-13, 1971.
172. Margolis S: Genital warts and molluscum contagiosum, Urol Clin North Am 11:163-170, 1984.
173. Goette DK: Review of erythroplasia of Queyrat and its treatment, Urology 8:311-315, 1976.
174. Del Mistro A, Braunstein JD, Halwer M et al: Identification of human papilloma virus types in male urethral condylomata acuminata by in situ hybridization, Hum Pathol 18:936-940, 1987.
175. O'Brien WM, Jenson AB, Lancaster WD et al: Human papillomavirus typing of penile condyloma, J Urol 141:863-865, 1989.
176. Nuovo GJ, Hochman HA, Eliezri HA et al: Detection of Human papillomavirus DNA in penile lesions histologically negative for condylomata. Analysis by in-situ hybridization and the polymerase chain reaction, Am J Surg Pathol 14:829-836, 1990.
177. Weaver MG, Abdul-Karim FM, Dale G et al: Detection and localization of human papillomavirus in penile condylomas and squamous cell carcinomas using in-situ hybridization with biotinylated DNA viral probes, Mod Pathol 2:94-100, 1989.
178. Glicksman JM, Freeman RG: Pearly penile papules. A statistical study of incidence, Arch Dermatol 93:56-59, 1966.
179. Johnson BL, Baxter DL: Pearly penile papules, Arch Dermatol 90:166-167, 1964.
180. Tannenbaum MH, Becker SW: Papillae of the corona of the glans penis, J Urol 93:391-395, 1965.

181. Lever WF, Schaumburg-Lever G: Tumors of the epidermal appendages. In Lever WF, Schaumburg-Lever G, eds: Histopathology of the skin, New York, 1983, JP Lippincott.
182. Cole LA, Helwig EB: Mucoid cysts of the penile skin, J Urol 115:397-400, 1976.
183. Golitz LE, Robin M: Median raphe canals of the penis, Cutis 27:170-172, 1981.
184. Asarch RG, Golitz LE, Sausker WF et al: Median raphe cysts of the penis, Arch Dermatol 115:1084-1086, 1979.
185. Gray MR, Ansell ID: Pseudo-epitheliomatous hyperkeratotic and micaceous balanitis: evidence for regarding it as pre-malignant, Br J Urol 66:103-104, 1990.
186. Lortat-Jacob E, Civatte J: Balanite pseudoépitheliomateuse kératosique et micacée, Bull Soc Franc Dermatol Syph 68:164-167, 1961.
187. Rosai J: Penis and scrotum. In Rosai J, ed: Ackerman's surgical pathology, ed 7, St. Louis, 1996, Mosby–Year Book.
188. Kaye V, Zhang G, Dehner LP et al: Carcinoma in situ of penis: is distinction between erythroplasia of Queyrat and Bowen's disease relevant, Urology 36:479-482, 1990.
189. Aynaud O, Ionesco M, Barrasso R: Penile intraepithelial neoplasia: specific clinical features correlate with histologic and virologic findings, Cancer 74:1762-1767, 1994.
190. Gerber GS: Carcinoma in situ of the penis, J Urol 151:829-833, 1994.
191. Queyrat L: Erythroplasie du gland, Bull Soc Franc Dermatol Syph 22:378-382, 1911.
192. Graham JH, Helwig EB: Erythroplasia of Queyrat: a clinicopathologic and histochemical study, Cancer 32:1396-1414, 1973.
193. Andersson L, Johnsson G, Brehmer-Andersson E: Erythroplasia of Queyrat-carcinoma in situ, Scand J Urol Nephrol 1:303-306, 1967.
194. Mostofi FK, Price EB Jr: Tumors of the penis and scrotum. In Mostofi FK, Price EB Jr, eds: Tumors of the male genital system. Atlas of tumor pathology, Washington, DC, 1973, Armed Forces Institute of Pathology.
195. Haneke E: Skin diseases and tumors of the penis, Urol Int 37:172-182, 1982.
196. Patterson JW, Kao GF, Graham JH et al: Bowenoid papulosis: a clinicopathologic study with ultrastructural observations, Cancer 57:823-836, 1986.
197. Graham JH, Helwig EB: Bowen's disease and its relationship to systemic cancer, Arch Dermatol 83:738-758, 1961.
198. Chuang TY, Tse J, Reizner GT: Bowen's disease (squamous cell carcinoma in-situ) as a skin marker for internal malignancy: a case control study, Am J Prev Med 6:238-243, 1990.
199. Callen JP, Headington JT: Bowen's and non-Bowen's squamous intraepithelial neoplasia of the skin: relationship to internal malignancy, Arch Dermatol 116:422-426, 1980.
200. Wade TR, Kopf AW, Ackerman AB: Bowenoid papulosis of the penis, Cancer 42:1890-1903, 1978.
201. Taylor DR Jr, South DA: Bowenoid papulosis: a review, Cutis 27:92-98, 1981.
202. Eisen RF, Bhawan J, Cahn TH: Spontaneous regression of bowenoid papulosis of the penis, Cutis 32:269-272, 1983.
203. Chesney TM, Murphy WM: Diseases of the penis and scrotum. In Murphy WM, ed: Urological pathology, Philadelphia, 1989, WB Saunders.
204. Zachow KR, Ostrow RS, Bender M et al: Detection of human papillomavirus DNA in anogenital neoplasias, Nature 300:771-773, 1982.
205. Zelickson AS, Prawer SE: Bowenoid papulosis of the penis, demonstration of intranuclear viral-like particles, Am J Dermatopathol 2:305-308, 1980.
206. Barnes RD, Sarembock LA, Abratt RP et al: Carcinoma of penis, J R Coll Surg Edinb 34:44-46, 1989.
207. Sufrin G, Huben R: Benign and malignant lesions of the penis. In Gillenwater JY, Grayhack JT, Howards SS et al, eds: Adult and pediatric urology, ed 3, St. Louis, 1995, Mosby–Year Book.
208. Persky L, deKernion J: Carcinoma of the penis, CA Cancer J Clin 36:258-273, 1986.
209. Dodge OG, Linsell CA: Carcinoma of the penis in Uganda and Kenya Africans, Cancer 16:1255-1263, 1963.
210. Riveros M, Lebron R: Geographic pathology of cancer of penis, Cancer 16:798-811, 1963.
211. Brinton LA, Li JY, Rong SD et al: Risk factors for penile cancer: results from a case-control study in China, Int J Cancer 47:504-509, 1991.
212. Bissada NK, Morcos RR, El-Senoussi M: Post-circumcision carcinoma of the penis: clinical aspects, J Urol 135:283-285, 1986.
213. Leiter E, Lefkovitis AM: Circumcision and penile cancer, N Y State J Med 75:1520-1525, 1975.
214. Dagher R, Selzer ML, Lapides J: Carcinoma of the penis and the anti-circumcision crusade, J Urol 110:79-80, 1980.
215. Apt A: Circumcision and prostatic cancer, Acta Med Scand 178:493-504, 1965.
216. Jensen MS: Cancer of the penis in Denmark 1942 to 1962 (511 cases), Dan Med Bull 24:66-72, 1977.
217. Reddy CRRM, Devendranath V, Pratap S: Carcinoma of penis—role of phimosis, Urology 24:85-88, 1984.
218. Koutsky LA, Wolner-Hanssen P: Genital papillomavirus infections: current knowledge and future prospects, Obstet Gynecol Clin North Am 16:541-564, 1989.
219. Loning T, Riviere A, Henke RP et al: Penile/anal condylomas and squamous cell cancer. A HPV DNA hybridization study, Virchows Arch A Pathol Anat Histopathol 413:491-498, 1988.
220. McCance DJ, Kalache A, Ashdown K et al: Human papillomavirus types 16 and 18 in carcinomas of penis from Brazil, Int J Cancer 37:55-59, 1986.
221. Broker TR, Chin MT, Dong G et al: Papillomavirus transcriptional regulation in human genital neoplasia. Proceedings of the annual meeting of the American Association of Cancer Research, 31:488-490, 1990 (abstract).
222. Masih AS, Stoler MH, Farrow GM et al: Human papillomavirus in penile squamous cell lesions: a comparison of an isotopic RNA and two commercial nonisotopic DNA in situ hybridization methods, Arch Pathol Lab Med 117:302-307, 1993.
223. Scinicariello F, Rady P, Saltzstein D et al: Human papillomavirus 16 exhibits a similar integration pattern in primary squamous cell carcinoma of the penis and in its metastasis, Cancer 70:2143-2148, 1992.
224. Starkar FH, Miles BJ, Plieth DM et al: Detection of human papillomavirus in squamous neoplasm of the penis, J Urol 147:389-392, 1992.

225. Wiener JS, Effert PJ, Humphrey PA et al: Prevalence of human papillomavirus types 16 and 18 in squamous cell carcinoma of the penis: a retrospective analysis of primary and metastatic lesions by differential polymerase chain reaction, Int J Cancer 50:694-701, 1992.
226. Graham S, Priore R, Graham M et al: Genital cancer in wives of penile cancer patients, Cancer 44:1870-1874, 1979.
227. Maiche AG, Pyrhonen S: Risk of cervical cancer among wives of men with carcinoma of the penis, Acta Oncol 29:569-571, 1990.
228. Villa LL, Lopes A: Human papillomavirus DNA sequences in penile carcinomas in Brazil, Int J Cancer 37:853-855, 1986.
229. Zur Hausen H: Papillomaviruses in human cancers, Mol Carcinog 1:147-150, 1988.
230. Obalek S, Jablonska S, Beaudenon S et al: Bowenoid papulosis of the male and female genitalia: risk of cervical neoplasia, J Am Acad Dermatol 14:433-444, 1986.
231. Solivan GA, Smith KJ, James WD: Cutaneous horn of the penis: its association with squamous cell carcinoma and HPV-16 infection, J Am Acad Dermatol 23:969-972, 1990.
232. Rosemberg SK, Herman G, Elfont E: Sexually transmitted papillomaviral infection in the males. VII: Is cancer of penis sexually transmitted? Urology 37:437-440, 1991.
233. Stern RS, Members of the Photochemotherapy Follow-up Study: Genital tumors among men with psoriasis exposed to psoralens and ultraviolet A radiation (PUVA) and ultraviolet B radiation, N Engl J Med 332:1093-1097, 1990.
234. Droller MJ: Carcinoma of penis: an overview, Urol Clin North Am 7:783-784, 1980.
235. Fraley EE, Zhang G, Sazama R et al: Cancer of the penis. Prognosis and treatment plans, Cancer 55:1618-1624, 1985.
236. Jones WG, Hamers H, Van Den Bogaert W: Penis cancer. A review by the joint radiotherapy committee of the European Organization for Research and Treatment of Cancer (EORTC) genitourinary and radiotherapy groups, J Surg Oncol 40:227-231, 1989.
237. Fossa SD, Hall KS, Johannessen NB et al: Cancer of the penis, Eur Urol 13:372-377, 1987.
238. Narayana AS, Olney LE, Loening SA et al: Carcinoma of the penis, Cancer 49:2185-2191, 1982.
239. Merrin CE: Cancer of the penis, Cancer 45:1973-1979, 1980.
240. Burgers JK, Badalament RA, Drago JR: Penile cancer: clinical presentation, diagnosis, and staging, Urol Clin North Am 19:247-256, 1992.
241. Derrick FC Jr, Lynch KM Jr, Kretkowski RC et al: Epidermoid carcinoma of the penis: computer analysis of 87 cases, J Urol 110:303-305, 1973.
242. Lucia MS, Miller GJ: Histopathology of malignant lesions of the penis, Urol Clin North Am 19:227-246, 1992.
243. Maiche AG, Pyrhonen S, Karkinen M: Histological grading of squamous cell carcinoma of the penis. A new grading system, Br J Urol 67:522-526, 1991.
244. Cubilla AL, Barreto J, Caballero C et al: Pathologic features of epidermoid carcinoma of the penis: a prospective study of 66 cases, Am J Surg Pathol 17:753-763, 1993.
245. Ornellas AA, Seixas ALC, de Moraes JR: Analysis of 200 lymphadenectomies in patients with penile carcinoma, J Urol 146:330-332, 1991.
246. Srinivas V, Joshi A, Agarwal B et al: Penile cancer—the sentinel lymph node controversy, Urol Int 47:108-109, 1991.
247. Horenblas S, van Tinteren H, Delemarre JFM et al: Squamous cell carcinoma of the penis. III. Treatment of regional lymph nodes, J Urol 149:492-497, 1993.
248. Young MJ, Reda DJ, Waters WB: Penile carcinoma: a twenty-five-year experience, Urology 38:529-532, 1991.
249. Maiche AG, Pyrhonen S: Clinical staging of cancer of the penis: by size? by localization? or by depth of infiltration? Eur Urol 18:16-22, 1990.
250. Fraley EE, Zhang G, Manivel C et al: The role of ilioinguinal lymphadenectomy and significance of histological differentiation in treatment of carcinoma of the penis, J Urol 142:1478-1482, 1989.
251. Ayyappan K, Ananthakrishnan N, Sankaran V: Can regional lymph node involvement be predicted in patients with carcinoma of the penis? Br J Urol 73:549-553, 1994.
252. Horenblas S, van Tinteren H: Squamous cell carcinoma of the penis. IV. Prognostic factors of survival: analysis of tumor, nodes and metastasis classification system, J Urol 151:1239-1243, 1994.
253. Pow-Sang JE, Benavente V, Pow-Sang JM et al: Bilateral inguinal lymph node dissection in the management of cancer of the penis, Sem Surg Oncol 6:241-242, 1990.
254. Schellhammer PF, Jordan GH, Schlossberg SM: Tumors of the penis. In Walsh PC, Retik AB, Stamey TA et al, eds: Campbell's urology, ed 6, Philadelphia, 1992, WB Saunders.
255. Johnson DE, Fuerst DE, Ayala AG: Cancer of the penis: experience with 153 cases, Urology 1:404-408, 1973.
256. Jackson SM: The treatment of carcinoma of the penis, Br J Surg 53:33-35, 1966.
257. Beahrs OH, Henson DE, Hutter RVP et al: American Joint Committee on Cancer: manual for staging of cancer, ed 4, Philadelphia, 1992, JB Lippincott.
258. Nitti VW, Macchia RJ: Neoplasms of the penis. In Hashmat AI, Das S, eds: The penis, Philadelphia, 1993, Lea and Febiger.
259. Yu DS, Chang SY, Ma CP: DNA ploidy, S-phase fraction and cytomorphometry in relation to survival of human penile cancer, Urol Int 48:265-269, 1992.
260. Gustafsson O, Tribukait B, Nyman CR et al: DNA pattern and histopathology of penis. A prospective study, Scand J Urol Nephrol Suppl 110:219-222, 1988.
261. Hoofnagle RF, Mahin EJ, Lamm DL et al: Deoxyribonucleic acid flow cytometry of squamous cell carcinoma of the penis, J Urol 143:352A, 1990.
262. Pettaway CA, Stewart D, Vuitch F et al: Penile squamous carcinoma. DNA flow cytometry versus histopathology for prognosis, J Urol 145:367A, 1991.
263. Johnson DE, Lo RK, Srigley J et al: Verrucous carcinoma of the penis, J Urol 133:216-218, 1985.
264. McKee PH, Lowe D, Haigh RJ: Penile verrucous carcinoma, Histopathology 7:897-906, 1983.
265. Kraus FT, Perez-Mesa C: Verrucous carcinoma. Clinical and pathologic study of 105 cases involving oral cavity, larynx, and genitalia, Cancer 19:26-38, 1966.
266. Yeager JK, Findlay RF, McAleer IM: Penile verrucous carcinoma, Arch Dermatol 126:1208-1210, 1990.
267. Blessing K, McLaren K, Lessells A: Viral etiology for verrucous carcinoma, Histopathology 10:1101-1102, 1986.

268. Masih AS, Stoler MH, Farrow GM et al: Penile verrucous carcinoma: a clinicopathologic, human papillomavirus typing and flow cytometric analysis, Mod Pathol 5:48-55, 1992.
269. Noel JC, Vandenbossche M, Peny MO et al: Verrucous carcinoma of the penis: importance of human papillomavirus typing for diagnosis and therapeutic decision, Eur Urol 22:83-85, 1992.
270. de Villiers EM, Schneider A, Gross G et al: Analysis of benign and malignant urogenital tumors for human papillomavirus infection by labelling cellular DNA, Med Microbiol Immunol 174:281-286, 1986.
271. Gissmann L, de Villiers EM, zur Hausen H: Analysis of human genital warts (condylomata acuminata) and other genital tumors for human papillomavirus type 6 DNA, Int J Cancer 29:143-146, 1982.
272. Medina JE, Dichtel W, Luna MA: Verrucous-squamous carcinomas of the oral cavity: a clinicopathologic study of 104 cases, Arch Otolaryngol Head Neck Surg 110:437-440, 1984.
273. Fukunaga M, Yokoi K, Miyazawa Y et al: Penile verrucous carcinoma with anaplastic transformation following radiotherapy, Am J Surg Pathol 18:501-505, 1994.
274. Manglani KS, Manaligod JR, Biswamay R: Spindle cell carcinoma of the glans penis: a light and electron microscopic study, Cancer 46:2266-2272, 1980.
275. Wood EW, Gardner WA Jr, Brown FM: Spindle cell squamous carcinoma of the penis, J Urol 107:990-991, 1972.
276. Rahbari H, Mehregan AH: Basal cell epitheliomas in usual and unusual sites, J Cutan Pathol 6:425-431, 1979.
277. Hall TC, Britt DB, Woodhead DM: Basal cell carcinoma of the penis, J Urol 99:314-315, 1968.
278. McGregor DH, Tanimura A, Weigel JW: Basal cell carcinoma of penis, Urology 20:320-323, 1982.
279. Goldminz D, Scott G, Klaus S: Penile basal cell carcinoma. Report of a case and review of the literature, J Am Acad Dermatol 20:1094-1097, 1989.
280. Stillwell TJ, Zincke H, Gaffey TA et al: Malignant melanoma of the penis, J Urol 140:72-75, 1988.
281. Oldbring J, Mikulowski P: Malignant melanoma of the penis and male urethra. Report of nine cases and review of the literature, Cancer 59:581-587, 1987.
282. Begun FP, Grossman HB, Diokno AC et al: Malignant melanoma of the penis and male urethra, J Urol 132:123-125, 1984.
283. Manivel JC, Fraley EE: Malignant melanoma of the penis and male urethra: 4 case reports and literature review, J Urol 139:813-816, 1988.
284. Johnson DE, Ayala AG: Primary melanoma of the penis, Urology 2:174-177, 1973.
285. Rashid AMH, Williams RM, Horton LWL: Malignant melanoma of penis and male urethra: is it a difficult tumor to diagnose? Urology 41:470-471, 1993.
286. Konigsberg HA, Gray GF: Benign melanosis and malignant melanoma of penis and male urethra, Urology 7:323-326, 1976.
287. Jaeger N, Wirtler H, Tschubel K: Acral lentiginous melanoma of penis, Eur Urol 8:182-184, 1982.
288. Saw D, Tse CH, Chan J et al: Clear cell sarcoma of the penis, Hum Pathol 17:423-425, 1986.
289. Dehner LP, Smith BH: Soft tissue tumors of the penis. A clinicopathologic study of 46 cases, Cancer 25:1431-1447, 1970.
290. Casado M, Jimenez F, Borbujo J et al: Spontaneous healing of Kaposi's angiosarcoma of the penis, J Urol 139:1313-1315, 1988.
291. Lowe FC, Lattimer G, Metroka CE: Kaposi's sarcoma of the penis in patients with acquired immunodeficiency syndrome, J Urol 142:1475-1477, 1989.
292. Bayne P, Wise G: Kaposi sarcoma of penis and genitalia: a disease of our times, Urology 31:22-25, 1988.
293. Saftel AD, Sadick NS, Waldbaum RS: Kaposi's sarcoma of the penis in a patient with the acquired immunodeficiency syndrome, J Urol 136:673-675, 1986.
294. Vapnek JM, Quivey JM, Carroll PR: Acquired immunodeficiency syndrome-related Kaposi's sarcoma of the male genitalia: management with radiation therapy, J Urol 146:333-336, 1991.
295. Lands RH, Ange D, Hartman DL: Radiation therapy for classic Kaposi's sarcoma presenting only on the glans penis, J Urol 147:468-470, 1992.
296. Rasbridge SA, Parry JRW: Angiosarcoma of the penis, Br J Urol 63:440-441, 1989.
297. Weiss SW, Enzinger FM: Epithelioid hemangioendothelioma: a vascular tumor often mistaken for a carcinoma, Cancer 50:970-981, 1982.
298. Deutsch M, Lee RLS, Mercado R: Hemangioendothelioma of the penis with late appearing metastases: report of a case with review of the literature, J Surg Oncol 5:27-34, 1973.
299. Calonje E, Fletcher CDM, Wilson-Jones E et al: Retiform hemangioendothelioma: a distinctive form of low-grade angiosarcoma delineated in a series of 15 cases, Am J Surg Pathol 18:115-125, 1994.
300. Isa SS, Almaraz R, Magovern J: Leiomyosarcoma of the penis: case report and review of the literature, Cancer 54:939-942, 1984.
301. Valadez RA, Waters WB: Leiomyosarcoma of penis, Urology 27:265-267, 1986.
302. Pow-sang MR, Orihuela E: Leiomyosarcoma of the penis, J Urol 151:1643-1645, 1994.
303. Wilson LS, Lockhart JL, Bergman H et al: Fibrosarcoma of the penis. Case report and review of the literature, J Urol 129:606-607, 1983.
304. Parsons MA, Fox M: Malignant fibrous histiocytoma of the penis, Eur Urol 14:75-76, 1988.
305. Fletcher CDM, Lowe D: Inflammatory fibrous histiocytoma, Histopathology 8:1079-1084, 1984.
306. Dalkin B, Zaontz MR: Rhabdomyosarcoma of the penis in children, J Urol 141:908-909, 1989.
307. Pak K, Sakaguchi N, Takayama H et al: Rhabdomyosarcoma of the penis, J Urol 136:438-439, 1986.
308. Huang DJ, Stanisic TH, Hansen KK: Epithelioid sarcoma of the penis, J Urol 147:1370-1372, 1992.
309. Gower RL, Pambakian H, Fletcher CDM: Epithelioid sarcoma of the penis: a rare tumour to be distinguished from squamous carcinoma, Br J Urol 59:592-593, 1987.
310. Gonzalez-Campora R, Nogales FF, Lerma E et al: Lymphoma of the penis, J Urol 126:270-271, 1981.
311. Yu GSM, Nseyo UO, Carson JW: Primary penile lymphoma in a patient with Peyronie's disease, J Urol 142:1076-1077, 1989.
312. Powell BL, Craig JB, Muss HB: Secondary malignancies of the penis and epididymis: a case report and review of the literature, J Clin Oncol 3:110-116, 1985.

313. Perez-Mesa C, Oxenhandler R: Metastatic tumors of the penis, J Surg Oncol 42:11-15, 1989.
314. Haddad FS: Penile metastases secondary to bladder cancer. Review of the literature, Urol Int 39:125-142, 1984.
315. Robey EL, Schellhammer PF: Four cases of metastases to the penis and review of the literature, J Urol 132:992-994, 1984.
316. Khubchandani M: Metachronous metastasis to the penis from carcinoma of the rectum. Report of a case, Dis Colon Rectum 29:52-54, 1986.
317. Hashimoto H, Saga Y, Watabe Y et al: Case report: secondary penile carcinoma, Urol Int 44:56-57, 1989.
318. Ordonez NG, Ayala AG, Bracken RB: Renal cell carcinoma metastatic to penis, Urology 19:417-419, 1982.
319. Perez LM, Shumway RA, Carson CC et al: Penile metastasis secondary to supraglottic squamous cell carcinoma: review of the literature, J Urol 147:157-160, 1992.
320. Adjiman S, Flam TA, Zerbib M et al: Delayed nonurothelial metastatic lesions to the penis. A report of two cases, Eur Urol 16:391-392, 1989.
321. Powell FC, Venencie PY, Winkelmann RK: Metastatic prostate carcinoma manifesting as penile nodules, Arch Dermatol 20:1604-1606, 1984.
322. Paquin AJ, Roland SI: Secondary carcinoma of the penis: a review of the literature and a report of nine new cases, Cancer 9:626-632, 1956.
323. Mukamel E, Farrer J, Smith RB et al: Metastatic carcinoma to penis: when is total penectomy indicated? Urology 29:15-18, 1987.
324. Paty R, Smith AD: Gangrene and Fournier's gangrene, Urol Clin North Am 19:149-162, 1992.
325. Ecker KW, Derouet H, Omlor G et al: Fournier's gangrene, Chirurg 64:58-62, 1993.
326. de Roos WK, van Lanschot JJ, Bruining HA: Fournier's gangrene: the need for early recognition and radical surgical debridement, Neth J Surg 43:184-188, 1991.
327. Corbus BC, Harris FG: Erosive and gangrenous balanitis. The fourth venereal disease, JAMA 52:1474-1477, 1909.
328. Barile MF, Blumberg JM, Kraul CW et al: Penile lesions among U.S. Armed Forces personnel in Japan. The prevalence of herpes simplex and the role of pleuropneumonia-like organisms, Arch Dermatol 86:273-281, 1962.
329. Schneider PR, Russell RC, Zook EG: Fournier's gangrene of the penis: a report of two cases, Ann Plast Surg 17:87-90, 1986.
330. Jayachandran S, Mooppan UMM, Kim H: Complications from external (condom) urinary drainage devices, Urology 25:31-34, 1985.
331. Sheinfeld J, Cos LR, Etruck E et al: Penile tourniquet injury due to a coil of hair, J Urol 133:1042-1043, 1985.
332. Lane JE: Hidrosadenitits axillaris of Verneuil, Arch Dermatol Syphilol 28:609-614, 1933.
333. Brunsting HA: Hidradenitis and other variants of acne, Arch Dermatol Syphilol 65:303-315, 1952.
334. Shelly WB, Cahn MM: The pathogenesis of hidradenitis suppurativa in man, Arch Dermatol 72:562-565, 1955.
335. Curry SS, Gaither DH, King LE Jr: Squamous cell carcinoma arising in dissecting perifolliculitis of the scalp, J Am Acad Dermatol 4:673-678, 1981.
336. Moyer DG, Williams RM: Perifolliculitis capitis abscedens et suffodiens, Arch Dermatol 85:378-384, 1962.
337. Banerjee AK: Surgical treatment of hidradenitis suppurativa, Br J Surg 79:863-866, 1992.
338. Shapiro L, Platt N, Torres-Rodriguez VM: Idiopathic calcinosis of the scrotum, Arch Dermatol 102:199-204, 1970.
339. Swinehart JM, Golitz LE: Scrotal calcinosis. Dystrophic calcification of epidermoid cysts, Arch Dermatol 118:985-988, 1982.
340. Dare AJ, Axelsen RA: Scrotal calcinosis: origin from dystrophic calcification of eccrine duct milia, J Cutan Pathol 15:142-149, 1988.
341. Kaskas M, Dabrowski A, Sabbah M et al: Idiopathic calcinosis of the scrotum. Apropos of a case. Review of the literature, J Urol (Paris) 97:287-290, 1991.
342. Song DH, Lee KH, Kang WH: Idiopathic calcinosis of the scrotum: histopathologic observations of fifty-one nodules, J Am Acad Dermatol 19:1095-1101, 1988.
343. Akosa AB, Gilliland EA, Ali MH et al: Idiopathic scrotal calcinosis: a possible aetiology reaffirmed, Br J Plast Surg 42:324-327, 1989.
344. Fetsch JF, Montgomery EA, Meis JM: Calcifying fibrous pseudotumor, Am J Surg Pathol 17:502-508, 1993.
345. Malcolm A: Idiopathic calcinosis of the scrotum, Br J Urol 54:190, 1982.
346. Smetana HF, Bernhard W: Sclerosing lipogranuloma, Arch Pathol 50:296-325, 1950.
347. Oertel YC, Johnson FB: Sclerosing lipogranuloma of male genitalia. Review of 23 cases, Arch Pathol 101:321-326, 1977.
348. Matsuchima M, Tajima M, Maki A et al: Primary lipogranuloma of the male genitalia, Urology 31:75-77, 1988.
349. Steward RC, Beason ES, Hayes CW: Granulomas of the penis from self-injection with oils, Plast Reconstr Surg 64:108-111, 1979.
350. Matsuda T, Shichiri Y, Hida S et al: Eosinophilic sclerosing lipogranuloma of the male genitalia not caused by exogenous lipids, J Urol 140:1021-1024, 1988.
351. Gilmore JAI, Weingad DA, Burgdorf WHC: Penile nodules in Southeast Asian men, Arch Dermatol 119:446-447, 1983.
352. Takihara H, Takahashi M, Ueno T et al: Sclerosing lipogranuloma of the male genitalia: analysis of the lipid constituents and histological study, Br J Urol 71:58-62, 1993.
353. Yamamoto S, Maekawa T, Kumata N et al: Giant epidermoid cyst of the scrotum, Hinyokikakiyo 38:1273-1276, 1992.
354. Hollander JB, Begun FP, Lee RD: Scrotal fat necrosis, J Urol 134:150-151, 1985.
355. Gioglio L, Porta C, Moroni M et al: Scrotal angiokeratoma (Fordyce): histopathological and ultrastructural findings, Histol Histopathol 7:47-55, 1992.
356. McDonald MW: Carcinoma of scrotum, Urology 19:269-274, 1982.
357. Ray B, Whitmore WF: Experience with carcinoma of the scrotum, J Urol 117:741-745, 1977.
358. Gerber WL: Scrotal malignancies: the University of Iowa experience and review of the literature, Urology 26:337-342, 1985.
359. Lowe FC: Squamous cell carcinoma of the scrotum, J Urol 130:423-427, 1983.
360. Parys BT, Hutton JL: Fifteen-year experience of carcinoma of the scrotum, Br J Urol 68:414-417, 1991.

361. Andrews PE, Farrow GM, Oesterling JE: Squamous cell carcinoma of the scrotum: long-term followup of 14 patients, J Urol 146:1299-1304, 1991.
362. Gross DJ, Schosser RH: Squamous cell carcinoma of the scrotum, Cutis 47:402-404, 1991.
363. Burmer GC, True LD, Krieger JN: Squamous cell carcinoma of the scrotum associated with human papillomaviruses, J Urol 149:374-377, 1993.
364. Tsang WY, Chan JK, Lee KC et al: Aggressive angiomyxoma occurring in men, Am J Surg Pathol 16:1059-1065, 1992.
365. Pott P: Cancer scroti. In Hawes L, Clarke W, Collins R, eds: Chirurgical works, London, 1775, Longman.
366. Waldron HA: On the history of scrotal cancer, Ann R Coll Surg Engl 65:420-422, 1983.
367. Lowe FC: Squamous cell carcinoma of the scrotum, Urol Clin North Am 19:397-405, 1992.
368. Grossman HB, Sogani PC: Basal cell carcinoma of scrotum, Urology 17:241-242, 1981.
369. Greider HE, Vernon SD: Basal cell carcinoma of the scrotum. A case report and literature review, J Urol 127:145-146, 1982.
370. Nahass GT, Blauvelt A, Leonardi CL et al: Basal cell carcinoma of the scrotum, J Am Acad Dermatol 26:574-578, 1992.
371. Parys BT: Basal cell carcinoma of the scrotum. A rare clinical entity, Br J Urol 68:434-435, 1991.
372. Hoch WH: Adenocarcinoma of the scrotum (extramammary Paget's disease). A case report and review of the literature, J Urol 132:137-139, 1984.
373. Mitsudo S, Nakanishi I, Koss L: Paget's disease of the penis and adjacent skin. Its association with fatal sweat gland carcinoma, Arch Pathol Lab Med 105:518-520, 1981.
374. Helwig EB, Graham JH: Anogenital extramammary Paget's disease. A clinicopathological study, Cancer 16:387-403, 1963.
375. Perez MA, Larossa DD, Tomaszewski JE: Paget's disease primarily involving the scrotum, Cancer 63:970-975, 1989.
376. Takahashi Y, Komeda H, Horie M et al: Paget's disease of the scrotum, Hinyokikakiyo 34:1069-1072, 1988.
377. Ordonez NG, Awalt H, Mackay B: Mammary and extramammary Paget's disease: an immunohistochemical and ultrastructural study, Cancer 59:1173-1183, 1987.
378. Moon TD, Sarma DP, Rodriguez FH: Leiomyosarcoma of the scrotum, J Am Acad Dermatol 20:290-292, 1989.
379. Dalton DP, Rushovich AM, Victor TA, Larson R: Leiomyosarcoma of the scrotum in a man who had received scrotal irradiation as a child, J Urol 139:136-138, 1988.
380. Washecka RM, Sidhu G, Surya B: Leiomyosarcoma of scrotum, Urology 34:144-146, 1989.
381. Naito S, Kaji S, Kumazawa J: Leiomyosarcoma of the scrotum. Case report and review of literature, Urol Int 43:242-244, 1988.
382. Suster S, Wong TY, Moran CA: Sarcomas with combined features of liposarcoma and leiomyosarcoma. Study of two cases of an unusual soft-tissue tumor showing dual lineage differentiation, Am J Surg Pathol 17:905-911, 1993.
383. Watanabe K, Ogawa A, Komatsu H et al: Malignant fibrous histiocytoma of the scrotal wall: a case report, J Urol 140:151-152, 1988.

Chapter 14

ADRENAL GLANDS

ERNEST E. LACK, M.D.
JOHN A. BRYAN, M.D.
MICHAEL LEWIN-SMITH, M.D.

EMBRYOLOGY AND NORMAL GROSS ANATOMY

ADRENAL CORTEX

The primordium of the adrenal cortex becomes evident at Carnegie stage 14 (approximately 5 mm to 7 mm and 32 days) just lateral to the base of the dorsal mesentery near the cranial end of the mesonephros.[1,2] The adrenal cortical primordia are of mesodermal origin, and during development in the late embryo and fetus, the portion of the developing cortex that occupies the greatest volume is referred to as the fetal or provisional cortex. This layer of cortex comprises about 80% of the newborn adrenal gland, and undergoes marked regression in the first weeks of life; this is shown graphically in Figure 14-1, in which the combined weight of the adrenal glands decreases by almost 50% by the ninth to fourteenth week following birth.[3] The adult or definitive cortex forms a much thinner outer zone beneath the adrenal capsule and ultimately becomes the trilayered adrenal cortex of the adult. There is convincing evidence for centripetal migration or displacement of adrenal cortical cells in experimental animals, thus supporting the original cell migration theory of Gottschau, which proposed that migrating adrenal cortical cells were capable of producing all of the major adrenal cortical hormones.[3]

On gross examination, the late fetal or neonatal adrenal gland is relatively soft, and in transverse sections there may be rather dark coloration of the fetal zone, which at this stage is quite broad. This dark appearance, shown in Figure 14-2, may be misinterpreted as adrenal hemorrhage or apoplexy. The adrenal glands in newborns have smoother external surfaces than the adrenal glands in adults. In the adult, the right adrenal gland is roughly pyramidal, and the left is more elongate (Fig. 14-3). Inspection of the intact capsular surface of the gland following removal of periadrenal connective tissue and fat may reveal small capsular extrusions of cortex; some of these are directly connected with the underlying cortex,

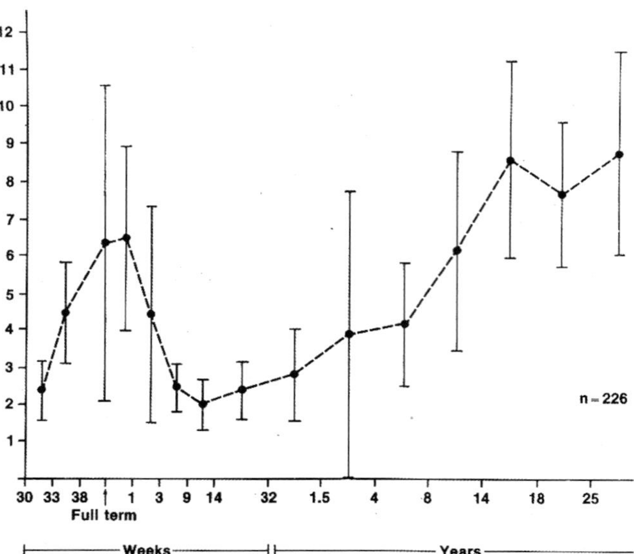

14-1. Average combined weight of the adrenal glands from 226 autopsies by age. Note the marked reduction in combined weight in the first few weeks of life caused by regression of the fetal (provisional) cortex. *(From Lack EE, Kozakewich HPW: Embryology, developmental anatomy, and selected aspects of non-neoplastic pathology. In Lack EE, ed: Pathology of the adrenal glands, New York, 1990, Churchill Livingstone.)*

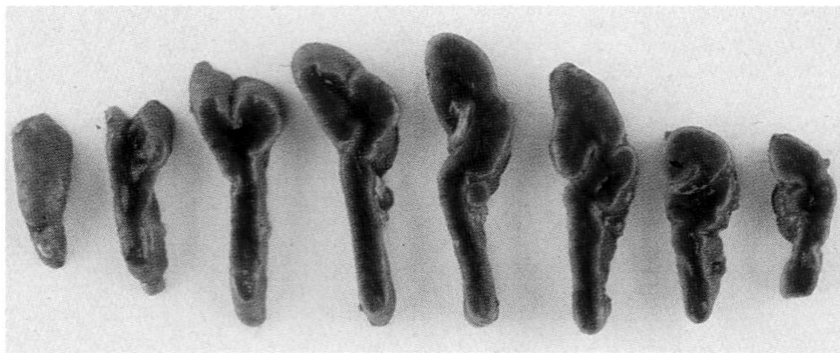

14-2. Adrenal gland from a newborn infant. Note dark congested fetal (provisional) cortex and thin rim of pale adult (definitive) cortex. Cortical extrusion is also present centrally.

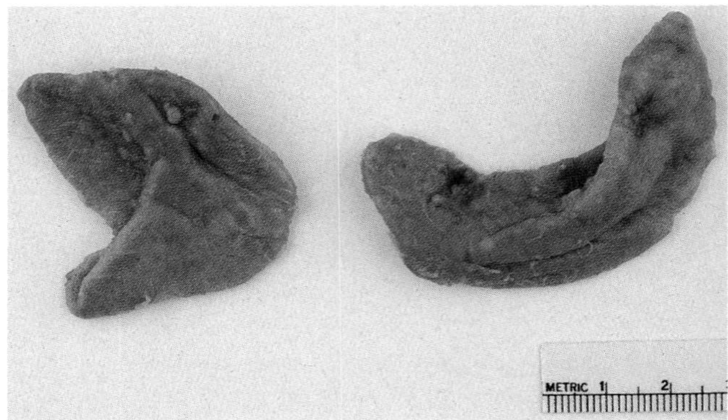

14-3. Normal adrenal glands from an adult. The right is roughly pyramidal (*left side of photo*), while the left is elongate (*right side of photo*). Longitudinal ridge (crista) is flanked by lateral extensions (alae).

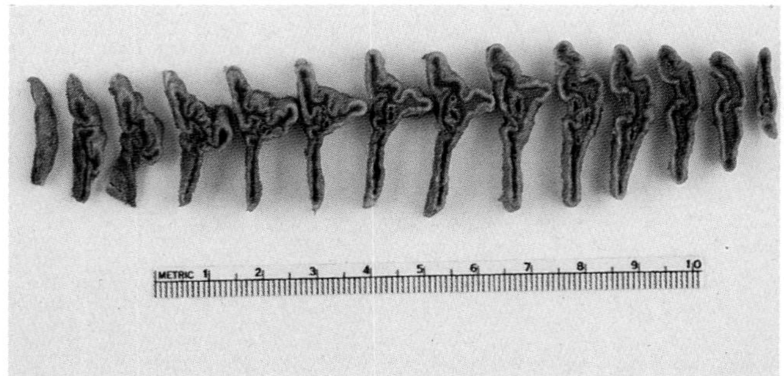

14-4. Normal adrenal from an adult. An incomplete cuff of cortical cells is present around a central adrenal vein in the medulla. The adrenal vein is present on the ventral surface toward the head of the gland. The dorsal ridge (crista) is flanked by lateral and medial extensions (alae). Medullary tissue is concentrated in the body and head and appears gray, in contrast to the bright yellow cortex.

but others seem to lie free on the capsular surface or unattached in periadrenal fat. Transverse sections of adrenal gland in the adult reveal a bright yellow, relatively uniform cortex with a gray-white medulla that is concentrated in the head and body of the gland (Fig. 14-4). A cuff of cortical cells may be noted partially or entirely surrounding larger tributaries of the adrenal vein. The dorsal surface of the adrenal gland has a longitudinal ridge or crista that is flanked by medial and lateral extensions or alae (wings). The anterior (or ventral) surface of the adrenal gland is relatively smooth, and it is from this surface of the gland that the adrenal veins exit and drain into the inferior vena cava on the right side and the renal vein on the left. The orientation of the adrenal gland in vivo differs from that depicted in gross photographs of specimens in surgical or autopsy material. As seen in Figure 14-5, the glands are oriented in a more vertical axis with the ridge (or crista) projecting posteriorly and flanked by medial and lateral alae. The thickness of the adult cortex is 2 mm or greater throughout most of the gland, although there may be some variability from area to area, and cortical nodularity may complicate the morphology.[3]

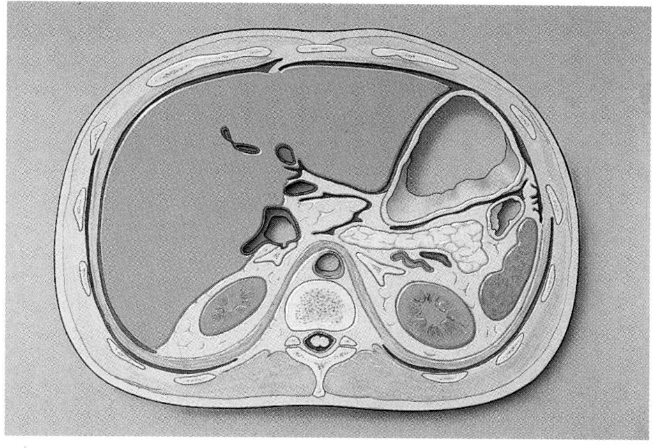

14-5. Diagram of transverse cut of abdomen in an adult showing orientation of the adrenal glands and relation with kidneys. Ventral aspect of both glands is relatively flat while dorsal surface has longitudinal ridge (crista). Lateral extensions (alae) are often referred to as medial and lateral limbs on computed tomographic scan.

ADRENAL MEDULLA

Chromaffin tissue of the adrenal medulla in the fetal and newborn adrenal gland is inconspicuous on gross examination of transverse sections of the gland. In the adult, however, chromaffin tissue is concentrated in the body and head of the gland, with the latter regions being directed inferomedially in vivo.[3,4] As seen in Figure 14-6, the ratio of area occupied by cortex relative to that of medulla decreases considerably from the tail to the body and head of the gland. The normal overall ratio of cortex to medulla is about 10 to 1. The distribution and amount of chromaffin tissue within the gland, as well as other factors such as adrenal weight, may be important in determining whether there is adrenal medullary hyperplasia.[4] Another consideration is morphologic abnormalities of the adrenal cortex, which can affect the overall ratio, such as adrenal cortical atrophy. The adrenal medulla is composed of chromaffin cells derived from primitive sympathicoblasts of neural crest origin that migrate into the dorsomedial aspect of the adrenal primordium and become apparent at Carnegie stages 16 and 17 (approximately 11 mm to 14 mm and 41 days).[1,2] Most of the developing chromaffin tissue in fetal life is extraadrenal, with the largest collections of cells in the paraaortic region, near the origin of the superior mesenteric and renal arteries down to the aortic bifurcation; these chromaffin structures were first characterized in the human fetus by Zuckerkandl[5] in 1901, who referred to them as the *aortic bodies*.

MICROSCOPIC ANATOMY

At birth, the thin rim of adult (definitive) cortex imperceptibly blends into cells of the fetal (provisional) cortex. The definitive cortex apparently begins to grow soon after birth,[6] with zonation into the zona glomerulosa and zona fasciculata first appears at 2 to 4 weeks. According to some investigators, the zona reticularis

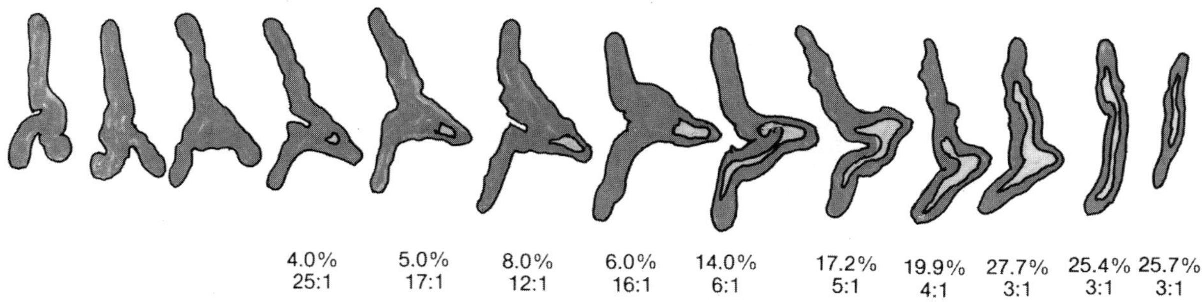

14-6. Schematic drawing of transverse sections of adrenal gland from an adult. Chromaffin tissue is concentrated in the body and head. Figures indicate percentage of cross sectional area occupied by medulla (*top row*) and ratio of areas of cortex to medulla (*bottom row*).

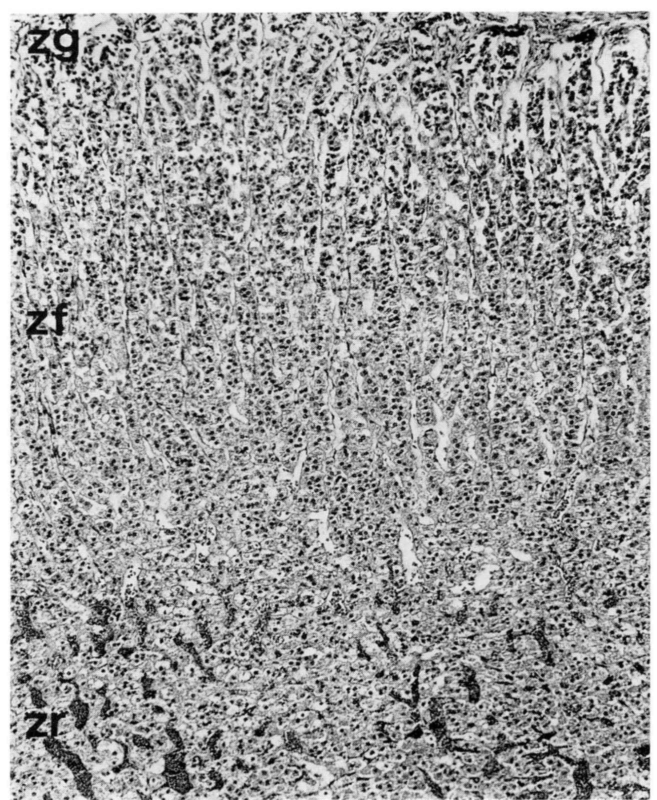

14-7. Normal adult adrenal cortex. Zona glomerulosa (*zg*) is at top of field beneath adrenal capsule and forms a thin, discontinuous layer of cells. Most of cortex is occupied by radial interconnecting cords of zona fasciculata (*zf*), which contain cells with pale-staining, lipid-rich cytoplasm. Zona reticularis (*zr*) has interconnecting short cords of cells with compact, eosinophilic cytoplasm and congested microvasculature.

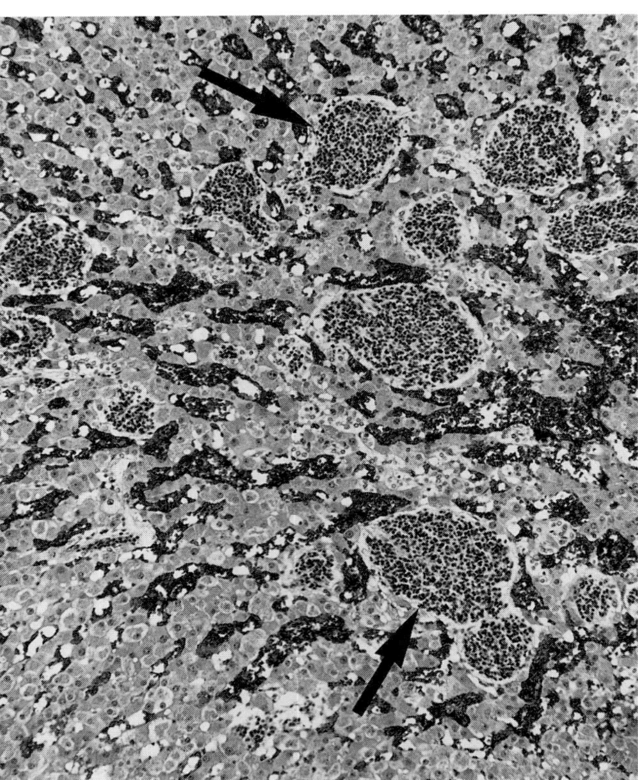

14-8. Neuroblastic nodules in provisional zone of a 16-week fetal adrenal gland (*arrows*).

appears at about 4 years,[6] but others contend that it appears before 1 year.[7] The zona glomerulosa contains cells with dark round nuclei and relatively scant cytoplasm arranged in interlacing cords and spherules; this zone is normally thin, ill-defined, and may appear discontinuous in the normal adult gland (Fig. 14-7). This layer blends imperceptibly into the zona fasciculata, which constitutes most of the adult cortex, and consists of long columns of large cells with pale finely vacuolated cytoplasm in the unstressed gland. The transition between the innermost zona fasciculata and the zona reticularis contains cells with more compact eosinophilic cytoplasm separated by thin-walled sinusoids and irregular short cords of cells. Reticularis cells may contain prominent granular pigment representing lipofuscin. Chromaffin cells of the adrenal medulla are polyhedral and arranged in short anastomosing cords or nests with a prominent vascular network, or there may be a more solid or diffuse arrangement of cells. Adrenal chromaffin cells secrete predominantly epinephrine, with lesser amounts of norepinephrine.[4] In the fetal and neonatal adrenal, one may encounter small nests of primitive neuroblastic cells (Fig. 14-8), which may be a part of normal developmental anatomy[3,4] (see discussion under *In situ* neuroblastoma later in this chapter).

The zona glomerulosa is the site of aldosterone production and is responsive to stimulation by angiotensin as well as adrenocorticotrophic hormone. The zona fasciculata produces corticosteroids such as cortisol, while the zona reticularis is responsible for sex steroid production. Longitudinal pillars of smooth muscle are found predominantly in the head of the adrenal gland around tributaries of the adrenal vein and are thought to act as "sluice gates" that retard the flow of blood from the medullary venous sinuses and plexus reticularis during muscle contraction.[8] The muscular bundles may help to regulate medullary blood flow and may influence the degree of congestion in the zona reticularis and zona fasciculata of the adjacent cortex.

EXAMINATION

Examination of the intact adrenal gland is best accomplished by careful removal of as much investing connective tissue and fat as possible in order to obtain an accurate weight. The weight of the cleanly dissected gland often provides valuable information regarding adrenal cortical or medullary pathology. In the study by Stoner et al,[6] the average combined weight of the adrenal glands at birth was 10 g (range, 2 to 17 g), whereas the average weight was 6 g at 7 days of age and 5 g at 2 weeks of age. Quinan and Berger[9] studied the adult adrenal, concentrating on ostensibly healthy subjects who had died suddenly, and found that the average weight of each gland was 4.15 g without significant difference between the sides. Studzinski et al[10] examined surgically removed adrenal glands from women with breast cancer and reported an average adrenal weight of 4 g, with little variation (standard deviation, 0.8 g). Adrenal glands obtained at autopsy from individuals who had not died suddenly or unexpectedly tended to be heavier, with an average weight of 6 g; this difference was attributed to the stress of illness and the trophic influence of endogenous adrenocorticotrophic hormone.[10] Using these data, each normal adrenal gland should weigh less than 6 g, provided excess periadrenal fat and connective tissue are carefully removed.

CONGENITAL ANOMALIES

ADRENAL APLASIA AND HYPOPLASIA

Complete bilateral adrenal aplasia is rare, and may occur in a familial setting.[11] There are four forms of congenital adrenal hypoplasia: (1) a sporadic form associated with hypopituitarism; (2) an autosomal recessive form; (3) an X-linked cytomegalic form associated with hypogonadotropic hypogonadism; and (4) a form associated with glycerol kinase deficiency.[12] The hereditary form of congenital adrenal hypoplasia is divided into a miniature type, which affects both sexes and causes extremely small adrenal glands with normal architecture, and the more common cytomegalic type, which has an X-linked pattern of inheritance.[3] In the cytomegalic type, affected males have small adrenal glands that are architecturally abnormal and contain scattered cytomegalic cells that are sometimes vacuolated and may contain intranuclear pseudoinclusions. The onset of adrenal cortical insufficiency is variable and depends chiefly on the endocrine reserve of the existing adrenal cortex. Affected infants may present in the newborn period with weight loss, vomiting, dehydration, and a tendency toward severe salt-loss. Prompt recognition of this rare adrenoprival condition results in improved survival. Male patients with the X-linked cytomegalic form of adrenal hypoplasia typically have hypogonadotropic hypogonadism in adolescence, which is probably of hypothalamic origin with prenatal onset and may be caused by a deficiency of gonadotropin-releasing hormone.[13] Adrenal insufficiency has also been reported in several other conditions, including familial glucocorticoid deficiency, glycerol kinase deficiency, and selective hypoaldosteronism.[3]

ADRENAL HETEROTOPIA

During embryologic development, the adrenal primordium is in close proximity to the urogenital ridge, accounting for the accessory and heterotopic adrenal tissue that may occur in sites in the upper abdomen and along lines of descent of the gonads.[3] Heterotopic adrenal tissue has been described in up to 32% of patients in the region of the celiac axis, and at this site, about half of the lesions contained both cortex and medulla.[14] Accessory adrenal tissue in sites further from the upper abdomen usually consists of cortical tissue alone, without the distinctive zones of the normal adult adrenal gland. Other sites of heterotopia include the broad ligament near the ovary (23%),[15] kidney (6%, usually subcapsular),[16] along the spermatic cord (3.8% to 9.3%; higher incidence observed for males undergoing surgery for an undescended testis),[17] the testicular adnexa (7.5%),[18] and other rarely described sites that defy ready embryologic explanation such as placenta,[19] lung,[20,21] and an intracranial intradural location.[22] Only rarely have intratesticular[23] or intraovarian[24] cortical rests occurred within the substance of the gonads. There have been a few reports of adrenal cortical or hyperplastic nodules arising from accessory adrenal tissue in the broad ligament,[25] spermatic cord, hepatic parenchyma,[26] and the spinal canal.[27]

Union or adhesion of the adrenal gland to kidneys or liver has also been reported, with the distinction being whether a continuous connective tissue capsule separates the two organs.[28] Adrenal fusion is a rare anomaly in which the adrenal glands are fused in the midline, and may be associated with other congenital midline defects such as spinal dysraphism or indeterminant visceral situs.[3] Abnormal adrenal shape has also been reported in some cases of renal agenesis where the glands may be ovoid with smoother contours.[3]

ADRENAL CYTOMEGALY

Congenital adrenal cytomegaly is usually an incidental finding in an adrenal gland that otherwise appears grossly normal. It has been reported in about 3% of newborn autopsies and 6.5% of premature stillborns.[29] The cytomegaly affects cells of the fetal (provisional) cortex, and may be bilateral or unilateral, focal or diffuse. The cytomegalic cell has an enlarged hyperchromatic nucleus and increased volume of cytoplasm. Nuclei may be markedly pleomorphic and occasionally contain intranuclear "pseudoinclusions," which are indentations of the nucleus with invagination of cytoplasm; despite the marked nuclear abnormalities, mitotic figures are characteristically absent.

Adrenal cytomegaly is a characteristic component of the Beckwith-Wiedemann syndrome (Fig. 14-9),[30-32] sometimes called the *EMG syndrome*, which refers to a major triad of findings—*e*xomphalos, *m*acroglossia, and *g*igantism.[3] The estimated frequency of this disorder is one in 13,000 births; most reported cases are sporadic, although some seem to have a mendelian pattern of inheritance.[3] The adrenal glands in this disorder are enlarged, with combined weights as high as 16 g. The adrenal cytomegaly is usually marked and is typically bilateral and diffuse. Curiously, adrenal chromaffin tissue may be hyperplastic or inappropriately mature.[4,32] There may be visceromegaly affecting the kidneys and pancreas, and some infants develop severe neonatal hypoglycemia, which may prove fatal. There is also an increased incidence of malignant tumors in this disorder, usually Wilms' tumor or adrenal cortical carcinoma, but other neoplasms have also been reported, including neuroblastoma and pancreatoblastoma.[3] The presence of hemihypertrophy in children predicts greater risk for the development of a malignant neoplasm.

ADRENOLEUKODYSTROPHY

Adrenoleukodystrophy occurs in multiple forms. The neonatal form usually has an autosomal recessive inheritance, and the childhood form is an X-linked disorder; an adult variant of adrenoleukodystrophy known as *adrenomyeloneuropathy* is recognized in which there is progressive spastic paraparesis and distal polyneuropathy with onset usually in the second or third decade of life.[3] Adrenoleukodystrophy or adrenomyeloneuropathy should be considered in the differential diagnosis of boys or young men who present with unexplained adrenal cortical insufficiency because neurologic symptoms may not be evident at the time of presentation. Adrenoleukodystrophy is a peroxisomal disorder resulting from diminished capacity to oxidize branched or very long chain fatty acids of 24 to 30 carbon atoms. This lipid material accumulates in tissue as cholesterol esters that may exert a toxic effect on cells, with crystallization of lamellae and disruption of cell membranes.[3] This mechanism may account for the pathogenesis of adrenal cortical insufficiency and degeneration of white matter, particularly involving the posterior cerebrum, cerebellum, and descending corticospinal tracts.

Adrenal glands in adrenoleukodystrophy are often quite small. There is thinning of adrenal cortex with characteristic enlargement of cortical cells with abundant "ground glass" or "waxy" cytoplasm;[33] these cells have been called *balloon cells*, and may have a fibrillar or striated appearance caused by lipid material being extracted during routine processing. On ultrastructural examination bilamellar and lamellar lipid inclusions can be seen, which are virtually pathognomonic for the disorder. The adrenal cortical insufficiency in this disorder is primary and not caused by pituitary or hypothalamic dysfunction.

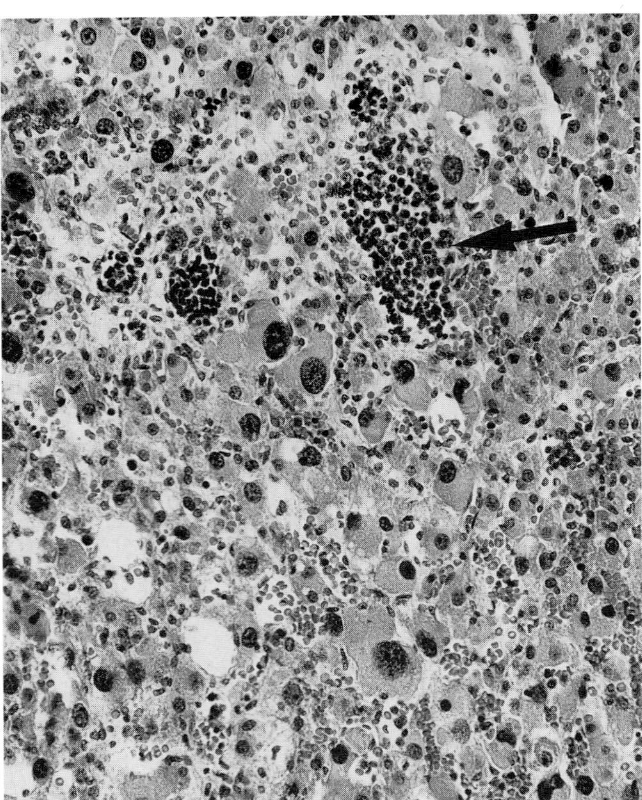

14-9. Adrenal in Beckwith-Wiedemann syndrome. Provisional zone of fetal adrenal gland shows prominent cytomegaly with cells having greatly enlarged hyperchromatic nuclei. Small nests of neuroblastic cells are also evident (*arrow*).

CONGENITAL ADRENAL HYPERPLASIA

Congenital adrenal hyperplasia (adrenogenital syndrome) is a rare autosomal recessive disorder caused by a deficiency of one of five different enzymes in the steroid biosynthetic pathway of the adrenal cortex.[3] The first unmistakable and thorough description of congenital adrenal hyperplasia was by the Italian anatomist de Crecchio[34] in 1865, who dissected the cadaver of an apparent male of about 40 years of age who had bilateral cryptorchidism and partial hypospadias; further examination, however, revealed a vagina, uterus, fallopian tubes, ovaries, and very large adrenal glands. The subject was also said to have had frequent diarrhea and vomiting, and in his final days had extreme weakness and exhaustion, which almost certainly represented an Addisonian crisis.

The most common cause of congenital adrenal hyperplasia is 21-hydroxylase deficiency, which accounts for about 90% to 95% of cases.[35,36] This deficiency has been divided into a classic form, with an incidence of 1 in 5,000 to 1 in 15,000 live births in most white populations; a nonclassic form, which is among the most frequent of autosomal recessive disorders in the white population; and a cryptic form in which patients are asymptomatic despite having the same biochemical abnormality.[35] Mutations in the encoding gene have been confirmed as the basis of endocrine disease in all adrenal steroidogenic enzymes required for synthesis of cortisol except cholesterol desmolase.[36] In 21-hydroxylase deficiency, there is insufficient production of cortisol resulting in a lack of negative feedback at the pituitary/hypothalamic level and secondary trophic stimulation of the adrenal glands by increased adrenocorticotrophic hormone levels. In about two thirds of cases of the classic disorder, biosynthesis of aldosterone is also affected, leading to "salt wasting"; if unrecognized or severe enough, this may result in death in the first few weeks of life.[3] The remaining one third of cases have "simple virilizing disease" without significant impairment of aldosterone biosynthesis. Because of the enzymatic block, precursor steroids accumulate and are diverted into the sex steroid pathway with increased androgen production. The development of external genitalia is under the control of androgens in utero; because of this, affected females usually have ambiguous genitalia with clitoromegaly and fusion of the labioscrotal folds, although the internal female organs develop normally. The ambiguous genitalia in the female may be so extreme that the child is incorrectly assumed to be male. Affected males usually appear normal at birth.

About 5% to 8% of cases of congenital adrenal hyperplasia are caused by the classic form of 11-ß-hydroxylase deficiency.[35] Other enzymatic defects causing congenital adrenal hyperplasia include deficiency of 3-ß-hydroxysteroid dehydrogenase, 17-α-hydroxylase, and the rare deficiency of cholesterol desmolase, the enzyme involved in early steroidogenesis.

Pathology of adrenal glands in congenital adrenal hyperplasia

Today, it is relatively uncommon to find adrenal glands of patients who died of unrecognized or untreated congenital adrenal hyperplasia. Grossly, the adrenal glands are enlarged, often with a convoluted or cerebriform surface with excess cortical plications and folding. The glands frequently have a light brown color reminiscent of the zona reticularis, resulting from the sustained trophic effect of adrenocorticotrophic hormone and conversion of lipid-rich, pale-staining cells to cortical cells with lipid-depleted compact eosinophilic cytoplasm. In children, the weight of each adrenal gland may be 10 to 15 g, whereas in older individuals, each adrenal gland may weigh 30 to 35 g.[3] Cholesterol desmolase deficiency is also called *congenital lipoid hyperplasia* because there is accumulation of cholesterol and cholesterol esters, which gives the gland a bright-yellow or white appearance on cross section.

Testicular tumors in congenital adrenal hyperplasia

Occasionally, male patients with congenital adrenal hyperplasia, particularly the salt-losing form of 21-hydroxylase deficiency, develop one or more testicular tumors in adolescence or young adulthood. The tumors are often bilateral (83%) and may cause testicular pain and tenderness.[37] Several reports in the literature clearly document that the tumors are adrenocorticotrophic hormone-dependent, as evidenced by reduction of testicular size and associated symptoms with suppressive doses of dexamethasone, and recrudescence of testicular enlargement with adrenocorticotrophic hormone stimulation. Laboratory testing has also demonstrated adrenocorticotrophic hormone-dependent steroidogenesis by the tumors.[38]

The tumors may be 2 cm to 10 cm in diameter in older patients. Most of the smaller tumors appear to be located in the hilum of the testis, but with larger tumors the precise sight of origin is difficult to determine.[37] On cross section, the tumors often have a lobulated appearance with bulging, tan to dark brown nodules; the histologic appearance resembles that of a Leydig cell tumor, although crystalloids of Reinke are absent. Nuclei are usually round to oval with a single prominent nucleolus, which may be central or somewhat eccentric. Cells have granular, pink cytoplasm with relatively distinct cell borders. The cells are usually arranged in sheets or small nests with intersecting fibrous bands, and reticulin stains often demonstrate an intimate pattern of isolation of individual and small clusters of cells.

Virtually identical testicular tumors of this type have been reported in male patients with Nelson's syndrome;[39] rarely, a female patient with Nelson's syndrome may develop similar adrenal rest tumors in the region of the ovaries[25] where heterotopic adrenal cortical tissue occasionally is found. The histogenesis of these interesting testicular tumors is not clear; possibilities include origin from Leydig cells, adrenal cortical rests, or multipotent testicular stromal cells capable of differentiation into either Leydig or adrenal cortical cells depending upon the hormonal milieu. It is unclear whether these tumors are neoplasms or hyperplastic masses. In favor of hyperplasia are their adrenocorticotrophic hormone-dependence, bilaterality, and the fact that malignant progression has never occurred.

Other tumors associated with congenital adrenal hyperplasia

Rare cases of adrenal cortical adenoma and carcinoma have been reported in patients with congenital adrenal hyperplasia.[3,40] It has been suggested that persistent adrenocorticotrophic hormone stimulation may result in neoplastic transformation of some adrenal cortical cells, but this is unproven. Other tumors have been reported in association with congenital adrenal hyperplasia, including osteosarcoma and Ewing's sarcoma,[41] but their relationship with congenital adrenal hyperplasia and the underlying biochemical abnormality is unclear.

STRESS-RELATED CHANGES OF THE ADRENAL GLAND

One of the most common histologic changes observed in the adrenal gland of patients under stress is conversion of lipid-rich, pale-staining cortical cells of the zona fasciculata to cells with compact, lipid-depleted eosinophilic cytoplasm. This is particularly common in acquired immunodeficiency syndrome (AIDS) (Fig. 14-10). Another abnormality reported in stress-related conditions is degeneration of the outer zona fasciculata, initially described as

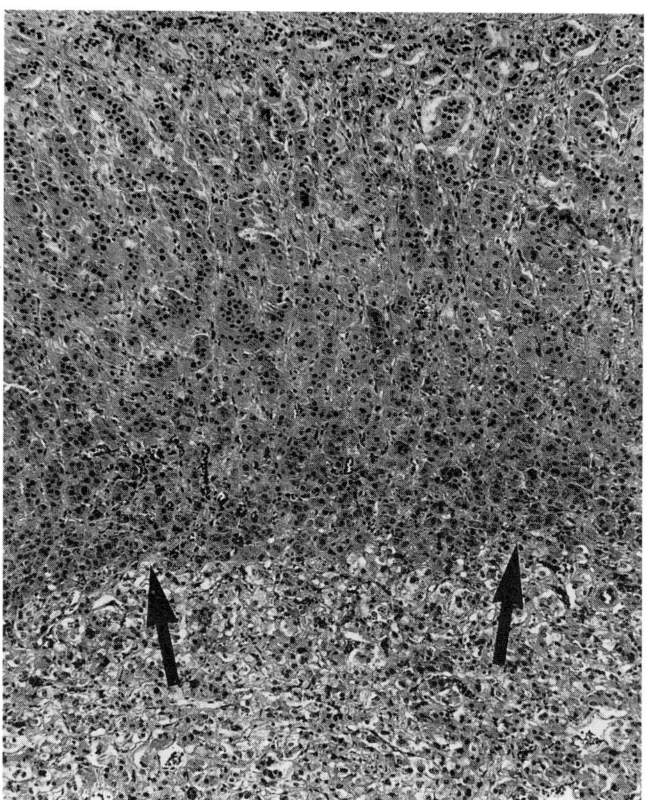

14-10. Adrenal gland of an adult who died of AIDS. The cortex showed severe lipid depletion, characterized by numerous cells with compact eosinophilic cytoplasm. The corticomedullary junction is indicated by arrows.

"tubular degeneration"; this abnormality appears with scattered necrosis of cortical cells, shedding of vacuolated cytoplasm, and exudation of fluid into cords of cortical cells in the outer zona fasciculata.[42] A peculiar vacuolization of the fetal adrenal cortex has been described in infants with erythroblastosis fetalis, and nearly identical changes have been observed in thalassemia major.[3] A relationship with intrauterine stress and hypoxia has been suggested. A pattern of focal lipid depletion has also been reported as lipid reversion, which suggests recovery from stress and replenishment of lipid in cells of the inner zona fasciculata. In areas of lipid reversion, the outer aspect of the adrenal cortex contains little or no lipid, although lipid is prominent in the inner zona fasciculata.[7]

OTHER ABNORMALITIES

There may be conspicuous iron accumulation in the form of hemosiderin within cells of the outer cortex, particularly the zona glomerulosa, in conditions such as primary hemochromatosis and transfusion hemosiderosis.[3] In some cases, there may be associated hypothalamic-pituitary dysfunction caused by excess iron deposition, which may result in endocrine insufficiency of gonads, thyroid, and adrenal glands. A variety of drugs and cytotoxic agents also have direct anti-adrenal activity; examples include dichlorodiphenyltrichloroethane (DDT) and its derivative o,p'DDD, which has been used for palliative treatment of patients with adrenal cortical carcinoma because of its adrenolytic effect on normal and neoplastic cortical cells. Another agent with anti-adrenal activity is ketoconazole, a broad-spectrum antifungal drug that blocks adrenal steroid synthesis.[3] Linear hyaline fibrosis has also been reported in the zona reticularis following radiation, probably because of structural damage of the vascular plexus of the reticular zone.[43]

Anencephaly is a severe developmental defect of anterior neural tube structures with agenesis of much of the brain and cranial vault. The pituitary gland is difficult to find grossly, but in histologic sections is often identified, although reduced in amount. The adrenal glands are often extremely small in this disorder, with an average combined weight in one study of 1.8 g, but a significant number weighed less than 1 g.[44] The fetal cortex is often normal in size and structure until approximately 20 weeks of gestation, after which it progressively involutes, similar to changes that normally occur following birth; chromaffin tissue may appear relatively prominent.

NON-NEOPLASTIC DISEASES

INFLAMMATION AND INFECTION

Nonspecific adrenalitis

Focal chronic adrenalitis is common, and has been found in up to 48% of autopsies, appearing as small aggregates of lymphocytes admixed with plasma cells adjacent to veins or venules in the cortical-medullary junction.[45] Focal chronic adrenalitis of this type is not considered to be a primary adrenal disorder, but represents a nonspecific inflammatory reaction, possibly related to inflammation in neighboring organs such as chronic pyelonephritis. Autoantibodies may be directed against adrenal medullary or chromaffin cells in type 1 (insulin-dependent) diabetes mellitus, and this organ-specific autoimmunity might be related to diabetic autonomic neuropathy.[4]

Herpetic adrenalitis

Members of the herpesvirus group may infect the adrenal gland, including herpes simplex, cytomegalovirus, and varicella-zoster virus. A characteristic pattern of herpetic adrenalitis occurs with disseminated herpes simplex infection in newborns, called *neonatal hepatoadrenal necrosis*; it was first described by Haas in 1935.[46] The foci of herpes simplex infection or varicella-zoster infection tend to be circumscribed, small "punched-out" areas of coagulative necrosis, with scant inflammation. The necrosis within the cortex may become widespread and confluent.[3] Eosinophilic Cowdry type A intranuclear inclusions are the diagnostic hallmark, usually occurring in cells bordering the zones of necrosis. It may not be possible to distinguish varicella-zoster infection from herpes simplex by routine light microscopy.

Disseminated cytomegalovirus infection in the newborn involves a wide variety of organs and tissues, including the adrenal gland. Some infants may have multiple mobile blue-gray subcutaneous nodules caused by dermal

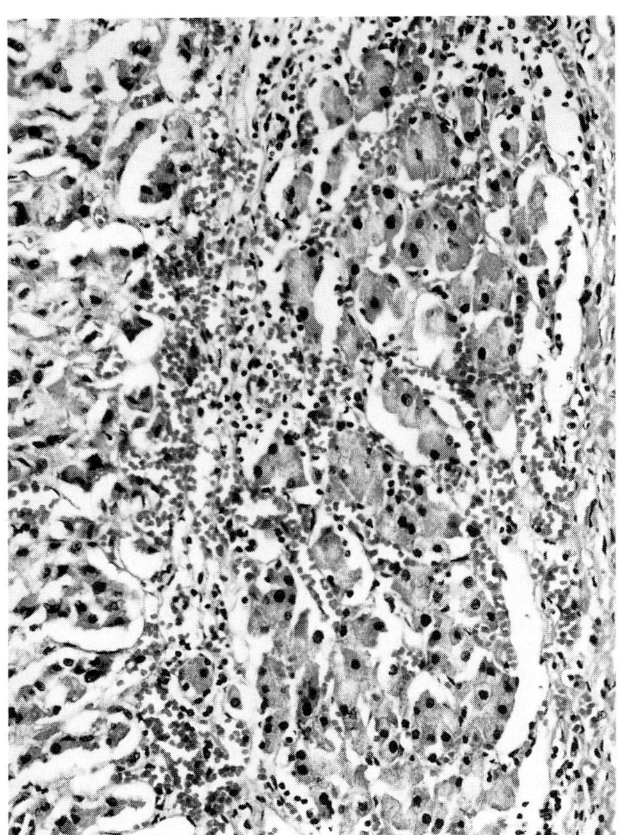

14-11. Primary idiopathic or autoimmune form of Addison's disease. Atrophic adrenal cortex (*right side*) contains cells with compact, eosinophilic cytoplasm. Medulla is present at left.

erythropoiesis. The appearance of the pigmented nodules may be striking, giving the infant an appearance described as a "blueberry muffin."[3] The viral cytopathic effect in cytomegalovirus adrenalitis is virtually pathognomonic, with sharply defined large amphophilic intranuclear inclusions with characteristic halos and small, granular basophilic granules within the cytoplasm. Cytomegalovirus adrenalitis is relatively common in patients with AIDS; death is attributed in part in some cases to adrenal cortical insufficiency. In one study, about 50% of patients with AIDS had evidence of cytomegalovirus infection at autopsy, and the adrenal glands were most commonly involved (75%), with cortical or medullary necrosis.[47] Necrosis of the medulla caused by cytomegalovirus infection may be greater than that of the cortex, and it is useful to note that there is no deficiency syndrome caused by destruction of the adrenal medulla. Cytomegalovirus infection of the adrenal in AIDS may result in latent or overt cortical insufficiency, requiring prophylactic treatment with corticosteroids.[48]

CHRONIC ADRENAL CORTICAL INSUFFICIENCY (ADDISON'S DISEASE)

Idiopathic or autoimmune Addison's disease

The most common type of Addison's disease is idiopathic or autoimmune, and is regarded as an organ-specific autoimmune form of adrenalitis. One proposed mechanism is aberrant expression of class II major histocompatibility antigens by target cells and presentation of adrenal-specific autoantigen to T-helper lymphocytes, which, in turn, initiates an autoimmune response.[3] It is uncertain whether class II antigen expression is a primary event or mediated by lymphokines, which are related to the inflammatory infiltrate. The adrenal in this disorder may be greatly reduced in size and volume, making gross identification difficult at autopsy unless numerous tissue blocks from the suprarenal bed are examined. The adrenal cortex has a large endocrine reserve, and it is estimated that up to 90% or more of the cortex must be ablated before functional impairment is apparent.[3] In some cases, intercurrent illness, infection, or surgery may precipitate an Addisonian crisis. The residual cortex is often thin and discontinuous with scattered islands of cortical cells (Fig. 14-11) admixed with lymphocytes, plasma cells, and occasional lymphoid follicles, sometimes with reactive germinal centers. Cortical cells may be enlarged with ample compact, eosinophilic cytoplasm, and occasional nuclear alteration, including "pseudoinclusions." On occasion, residual cortex may be difficult to identify and there may be little or no inflammation.

Autoimmune polyendocrinopathy-candidiasis-ectodermal dystrophy is an autosomal recessive disorder with

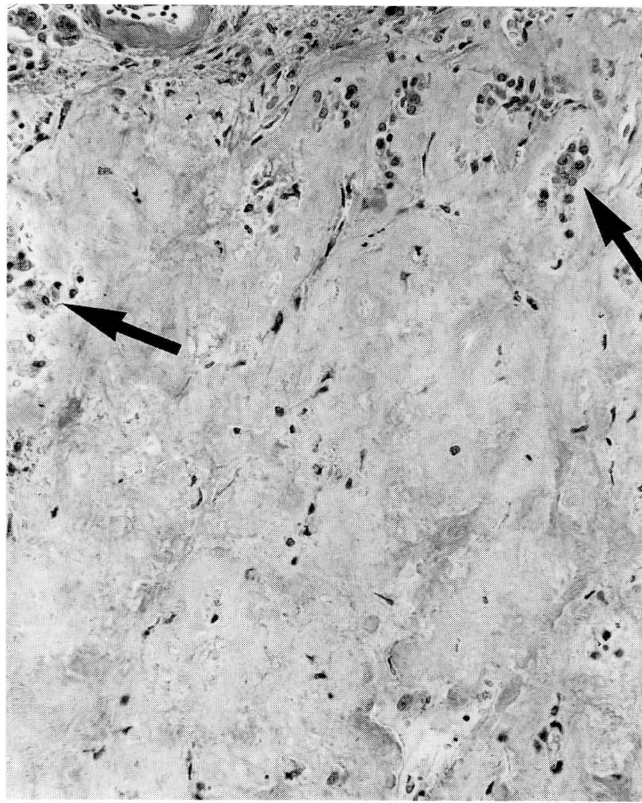

14-12. Amyloidosis of adrenal cortex. Only small nests of cortical cells remain (*arrows*).

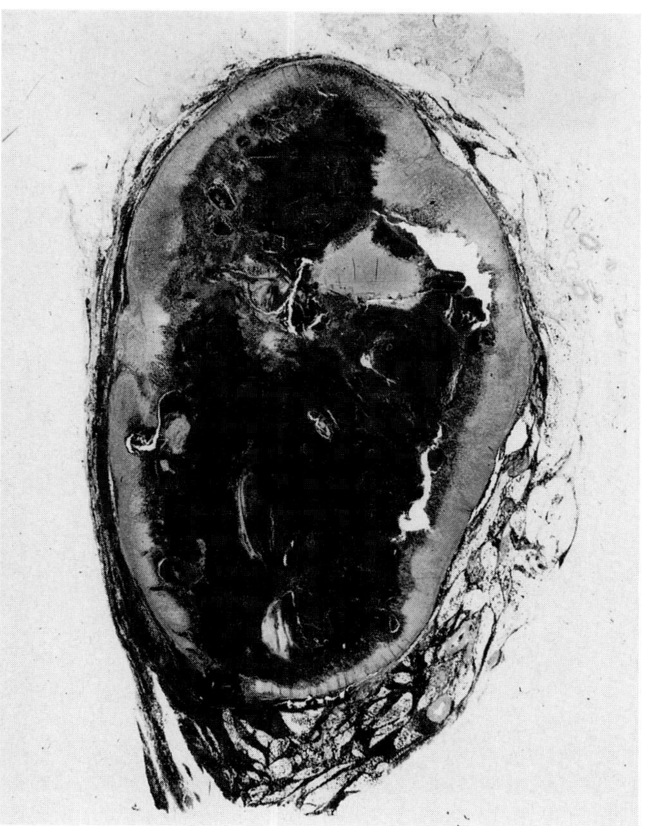

14-13. Adrenal in Waterhouse-Friederichsen syndrome. Extensive necrosis and hemorrhage were present in the gland and extended into periadrenal connective tissue. *(From Lack EE, Kozakewich HPW: Pathology. In Javadpour N, ed: Principles and management of adrenal cancer, Berlin, 1987, Springer-Verlag.)*

endocrine insufficiency involving various organs, including the adrenal cortex. This disorder has also been called *autoimmune polyglandular disease type I* and has a variety of manifestations.[49] The combination of nontuberculous Addison's disease and thyroid insufficiency is called Schmidt's syndrome.[50]

Adrenal tuberculosis

Adrenal tuberculosis once was the leading cause of Addison's disease. According to the review by Guttman[51] of cases between 1900 and 1929, 70% resulted from tuberculosis, and 19% were caused by primary or idiopathic atrophy. The endemic nature of bovine tuberculosis in the early decades of this century is reflected in the comment by Dunlop,[52] who characterized cream on top of the milk in those days as often being composed of "tuberculous pus." The tuberculous adrenal is often enlarged, with extensive areas of caseous necrosis. A classic granulomatous reaction with numerous epithelioid histiocytes is present typically in extra-adrenal sites but not the adrenal, suggesting that the locally high levels of adrenal corticosteroids dampen the host inflammatory response.[3]

Histoplasmosis and other fungal infections

Disseminated histoplasmosis is a recognized cause of Addison's disease. In a study of almost 100 cases, 7% of patients had chronic adrenal cortical insufficiency.[53] Similar to tuberculosis, extensive caseous necrosis is a common finding, although a granulomatous response is the exception rather than the rule. Perivasculitis involving extracapsular adrenal vessels may lead to extensive infarction and caseous necrosis, resulting in loss of adrenal parenchyma and development of Addison's disease. Other mycotic infections causing Addison's disease are less frequent, including North American blastomycosis, South American blastomycosis, and coccidioidomycosis.[3]

Amyloidosis

The adrenal may be involved in primary and secondary (AA) forms of amyloidosis. In primary amyloidosis, there tends to be involvement of arterioles, whereas in the secondary form there is usually extensive involvement of the cortex by the characteristic homogeneous eosinophilic material, resulting in severe atrophy and distortion of cells in the zona fasciculata and zona reticularis (Fig. 14-12).

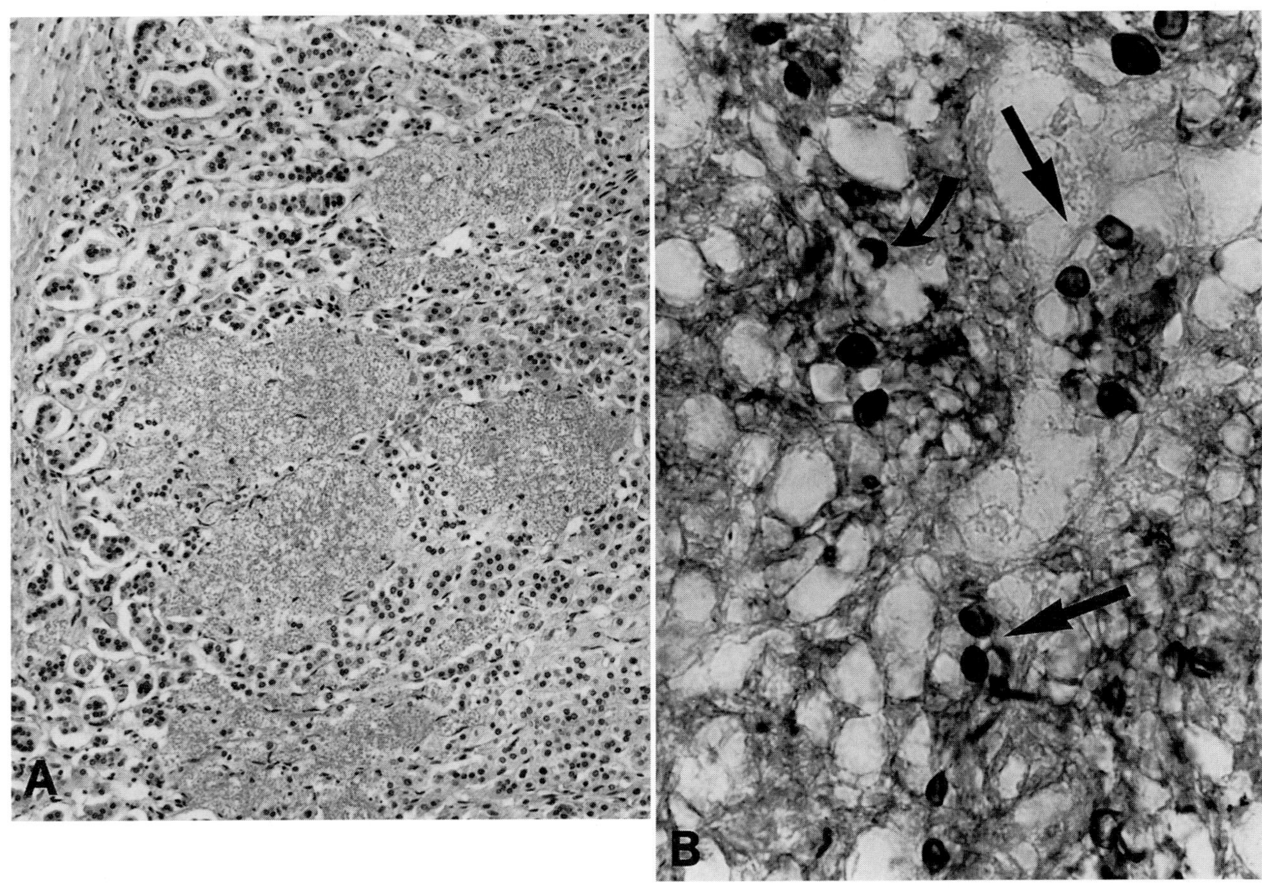

14-14. **A**, Adrenal gland extensively involved by *Pneumocystis carinii* infection in a patient with AIDS. Note characteristic "foamy" exudate in cortex. Adrenal capsule is on left side. **B** Gomori methenamine silver stain shows several *Pneumocystis carinii* organisms (*straight arrows*), some with cup-shaped indentations when viewed in profile (*curved arrow*).

ACUTE ADRENAL CORTICAL INSUFFICIENCY

Acute adrenal cortical insufficiency can occur in the setting of systemic infection with Waterhouse-Friederichsen syndrome, but seldom is it documented by laboratory or biochemical studies. Waterhouse-Friederichsen syndrome is seen classically in meningococcemia, but occasionally other bacteria, such as *Streptococcus pneumoniae* are causative. The course of the disease is usually fulminant, with fatal outcome within 48 hours of onset, accompanied by mucocutaneous petechial hemorrhages and vascular collapse. The adrenal is usually intensely hemorrhagic, with confluent areas of coagulative necrosis, often associated with small fibrin deposits within sinusoids; occasionally, there is more extensive hemorrhage, with expansion of the gland and periadrenal hemorrhage (Fig. 14-13).

RARE INFECTIONS

Rarely the adrenal is involved by other infectious agents such as *Pneumocystis carinii* (Fig. 14-14), usually in patients with AIDS.[54] Malakoplakia of the adrenal gland has also been reported.[55] Echinococcal cyst of the adrenal gland is usually an incidental autopsy finding.[56]

ADRENAL CORTICAL HYPERPLASIA

NODULAR ADRENAL GLAND

Cortical nodularity in the adrenal poses significant diagnostic problems for the pathologist at the autopsy table and in surgical material. Nodularity usually occurs in individuals without biochemical or clinical signs or symptoms of adrenal cortical hyperfunction. By definition, hyperplasia refers to an increase in the number of cells in tissue or in an organ, which in the adrenal cortex results in diffuse, symmetric thickening with or without cortical nodules (Fig. 14-15). The spectrum of diffuse and nodular adrenal cortical hyperplasia is broad. The incidence of cortical nodularity with eucorticalism can be analyzed from material obtained at autopsy or in patients who are discovered to have cortical nodules in vivo.

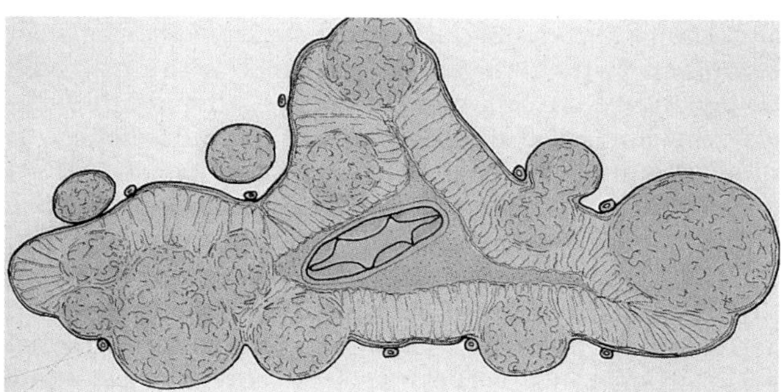

14-15. Schematic view of nodular adrenal gland in transverse section. Accessory nodules of cortical cells may be seen lying free within periadrenal fat, on the capsular surface, or attached to underlying cortex (capsular extrusion). A dominant macronodule within cortex can simulate a neoplasm. Multiple small capsular arterioles are present on surface of gland. Central adrenal vein in medullary compartment has discontinuous bundles of smooth muscle allowing close contact of chromaffin cells or cortical cells with vascular lumen. Occasionally one may see a mushroom-like intravascular protrusion by cortical or medullary cells.

Nodular adrenal gland at autopsy

Incidence, size, and functional features. Early studies of adrenal cortical nodularity at autopsy considered any solitary adrenal cortical nodule greater than 3 mm to 5 mm in diameter to be a nonfunctional adenoma.[3] Several studies have shown that the incidence of cortical nodularity increases with age,[57] and may be associated with hypertension[57] and diabetes mellitus.[58] The early study by Spain and Weinsaft[59] identified solitary adrenal cortical adenomas in 29% of elderly women. Another autopsy study reported a cortical adenoma 1.5 cm or more in size in up to 20% of hypertensive individuals compared with only 1.8% of normotensive patients.[60] In two of the largest studies of adrenal cortical adenomas detected at autopsy, the frequency was 1.5% to 2.9% of cases in a study population of over 16,000.[61,62] The study by Dobbie[57] showed that incidental adrenal cortical nodules may be present in virtually every region of the cortex, with the degree of nodularity varying widely from gland to gland. Adrenal nodularity was almost always bilateral, and, in some cases, there was significant disparity in the weights of the glands from an individual patient. Some nodules are as large as 3 cm in diameter and may display lipomatous or myelolipomatous metaplasia. Occasionally, degenerative features are noted such as fibrosis or microcystic change. Most cortical nodules are less than 1 cm in diameter. In Dobbie's study,[57] some nodules were related to capsular arteriopathy, which, in turn, was related to aging. For many of these cortical nodules it seems inappropriate to use the term *adenoma*, which implies a true neoplasm. Cortical hyperplasia implies some degree of cortical hyperfunction in addition to the increase in cortical tissue volume.

The pathogenesis of *nonhyper*functional cortical nodules is uncertain. There is a significant correlation between adrenal capsular arteriopathy and cortical nodularity;[57] hyalinization and intimal proliferation with luminal obstruction may be an important etiologic factor, resulting in localized cortical ischemia with secondary regenerative change and hyperplasia and subsequent formation of one or more cortical nodules. Based on this hypothesis, most cortical nodules can be regarded as secondary to hypertension rather than a cause of it. Other investigators have logically questioned the validity of this theory.

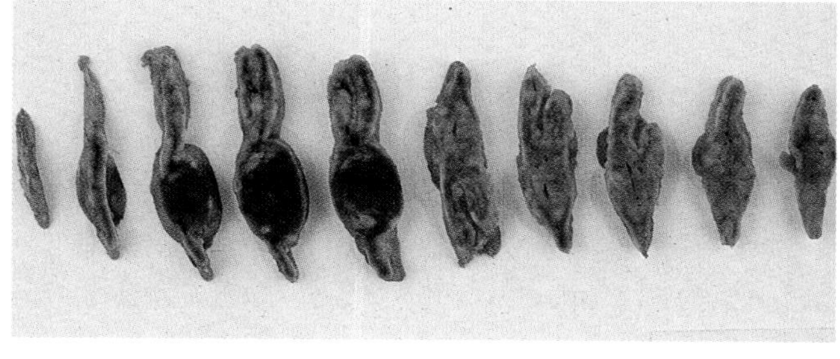

14-16. Incidental pigmented adrenal cortical nodule. Adjacent cortex contained numerous small pale-yellow nodules.

Incidental pigmented cortical nodule. Incidental pigmented nodules of adrenal cortex vary from 0.1 cm to 1.5 cm in diameter, and are usually located in the zona reticularis, often with expansion and distortion of the adjacent cortex or medulla (Fig. 14-16). The frequency of grossly identifiable pigmented nodules at autopsy varies according to the method of adrenal sectioning, the number of sections examined, and the level of interest of the pathologist searching for lesions. Retrospective study of autopsy material shows pigmented adrenal cortical nodules in 2.2% to 10.4% of cases.[63,64] When the glands are thinly sectioned, nodules are detected in 37% of cases.[63] The pigmented nodule is usually solitary but may be multiple, and in 11% of cases the nodules are bilateral. Histologically, the cells have compact eosinophilic cytoplasm with variable amounts of intracellular granular brown pigment, which has staining characteristics similar to lipofuscin (Fig. 14-17). A recent study suggested the presence of neuromelanin.[64]

Incidental cortical nodules discovered in vivo

Incidence. The increasing use of sensitive imaging studies such as computed tomography has identified many adrenal masses in asymptomatic patients. The prevalence of these asymptomatic adrenal masses varied from 0.6% to 1.3% in three combined series in which computed tomography scans were performed on over 5,000 patients.[65-67] The average size of the incidental adrenal nodules in one study was 2.8 cm, but some reached 5 cm in diameter. In a study of incidentally discovered adrenal cortical nodules in patients with known malignancies the average diameter was 2.4 cm, with a range of 1.5 cm to 4 cm.[68]

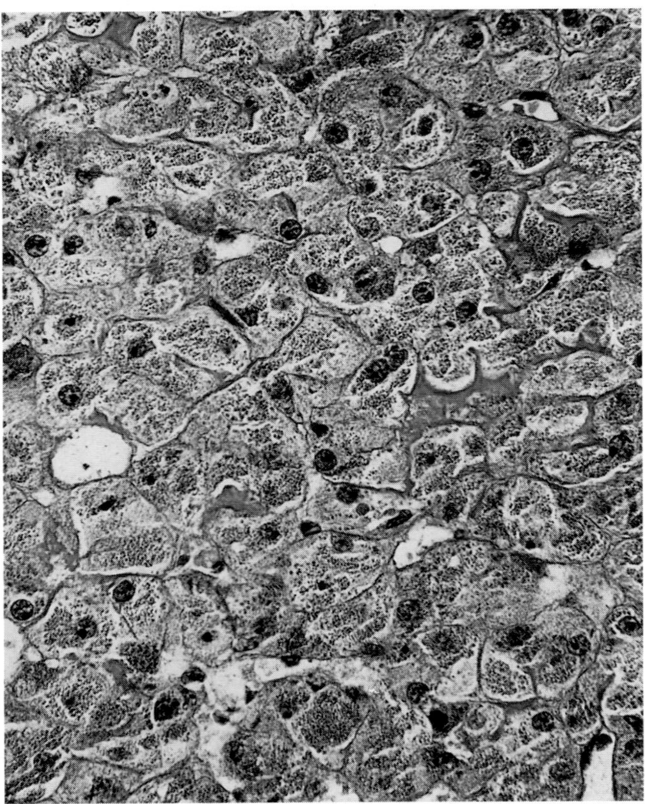

14-17. Incidental pigmented adrenal cortical nodule. Cells contain abundant granular lipofuscin pigment. Nuclei are uniform and many contain small central to eccentric nucleoli.

Functional status. Magnetic resonance imaging may provide some information in tissue characterization of adrenal masses; T_2-weighted pulse sequences provide some specificity in separating *nonhyper*functioning cortical adenomas, which have low signal intensity, from metastases with intermediate signal intensity and pheochromocytomas, which tend to have high signal intensity.[69] Magnetic resonance imaging does not allow distinction between *functional* and *nonfunctional* (or *nonhyper*functional) cortical adenomas, or small adrenal cortical carcinomas that lack necrosis and other secondary changes. Adrenal cortical scintigraphy with a radioiodinated cholesterol precursor often shows tracer uptake, indicating cortical steroid synthesis.[70-73] Various enzymes in cortical steroid synthesis are present, according to immunohistochemical staining, indicating that the nodules have the capacity for corticosteroidogenesis, although not in sufficient amounts to elicit signs or symptoms of endocrine hyperfunction or abnormal biochemical findings to alter the hypothalamic-pituitary-adrenal axis.[74] Many incidental cortical nodules (or adenomas), therefore, are considered *nonhyper*functional rather than *non*functional, without excess production of adrenal cortical steroids. Cortical nodularity in this setting has been compared with nodular euthyroid (nontoxic) goiter.

Approach to nodular adrenal discovered in vivo. The incidentally discovered benign *nonhyper*functioning adrenal cortical nodule or adenoma is a diagnostic challenge in a patient without a known malignancy. Fine needle aspiration under computed tomography or ultrasound guidance may provide valuable information,[75] particularly in cases in which it is not possible to reliably distinguish metastasis from adrenal cortical nodule or neoplasm with computed tomography. Occasionally, aspiration yields cells with bare nuclei stripped of cytoplasm, which might be confused with small cell malignancy. Correlation of cytologic findings with imaging results, clinical findings, and endocrinologic data is often essential. Adrenal cortical carcinoma should be considered in the differential diagnosis. If the prevalence of biochemically silent adrenal cortical carcinoma is 1 in 250,000 population, it is estimated that over 60 operations would have to be performed in patients with an adrenal mass 6 cm in diameter to remove one adrenal cortical carcinoma.[76] The size of the adrenal mass alone assumes importance as a distinguishing feature in decision making, although the reported cut point for size varies from 3 to 5 cm or more.[77-81] Bravo,[81] using 6 cm as the cut point, recommended the following: (1) the tumor should be resected if more than 6 cm in diameter and functional, or less than 6 cm and nonfunctional, but only if the magnetic resonance imaging–T_2-weighted signal intensity is greater than 3 (adrenal versus liver); (2) fine needle aspiration for nonfunctional tumors less than 6 cm with magnetic resonance imaging–T_2 signal intensity greater than 1.4 but less than 3; and (3) nonfunctional tumors less than 6 cm with magnetic resonance imaging–T_2 signal intensity < 1.4 should be evaluated yearly and resected if size increases by 1.0 cm per year.

ADRENAL CORTICAL HYPERFUNCTION WITH HYPERCORTISOLISM

There are several basic noniatrogenic causes of Cushing's syndrome (Fig. 14-18). The three most common causes are: (1) pituitary-dependent adrenocorticotrophic hormone overproduction, commonly referred to as Cushing's disease, which accounts for about 60% to 70% of cases in adults; (2) adrenal cortical neoplasm with autonomous overproduction of cortisol, which accounts for 17% to 25% of cases in adults; and (3) ectopic production of adrenocorticotrophic hormone (15% to 16% of cases), or rarely ectopic production of corticotropin-releasing factor.[82-85] In childhood, Cushing's syndrome is most often caused by a cortisol-producing cortical neoplasm, particularly in the very young,[86] whereas older children are more likely to have a pituitary-dependent form of hypercortisolism (Cushing's disease). Most patients with a pituitary-dependent form of hypercortisolism caused by adrenocorticotrophic hormone overproduction have a pituitary microadenoma or macroadenoma.[87-89] In some cases, a pituitary tumor is not detected, and the disease may result from hyperplasia of adrenocorticotrophic hormone–producing cells or abnormal hypothalamic regulation with secondary adrenocorticotrophic hormone hypersecretion.

Pituitary-dependent hypercortisolism (Cushing's disease)

Diffuse and micronodular adrenal cortical hyperplasia. With the high success rate of transsphenoidal adenomectomy for adrenocorticotrophic hormone–producing pituitary neoplasms,[87] the pathologist rarely has the opportunity to examine adrenal glands in this disorder that have been surgically removed. Bilateral adrenalectomy is usually done only after failed resection

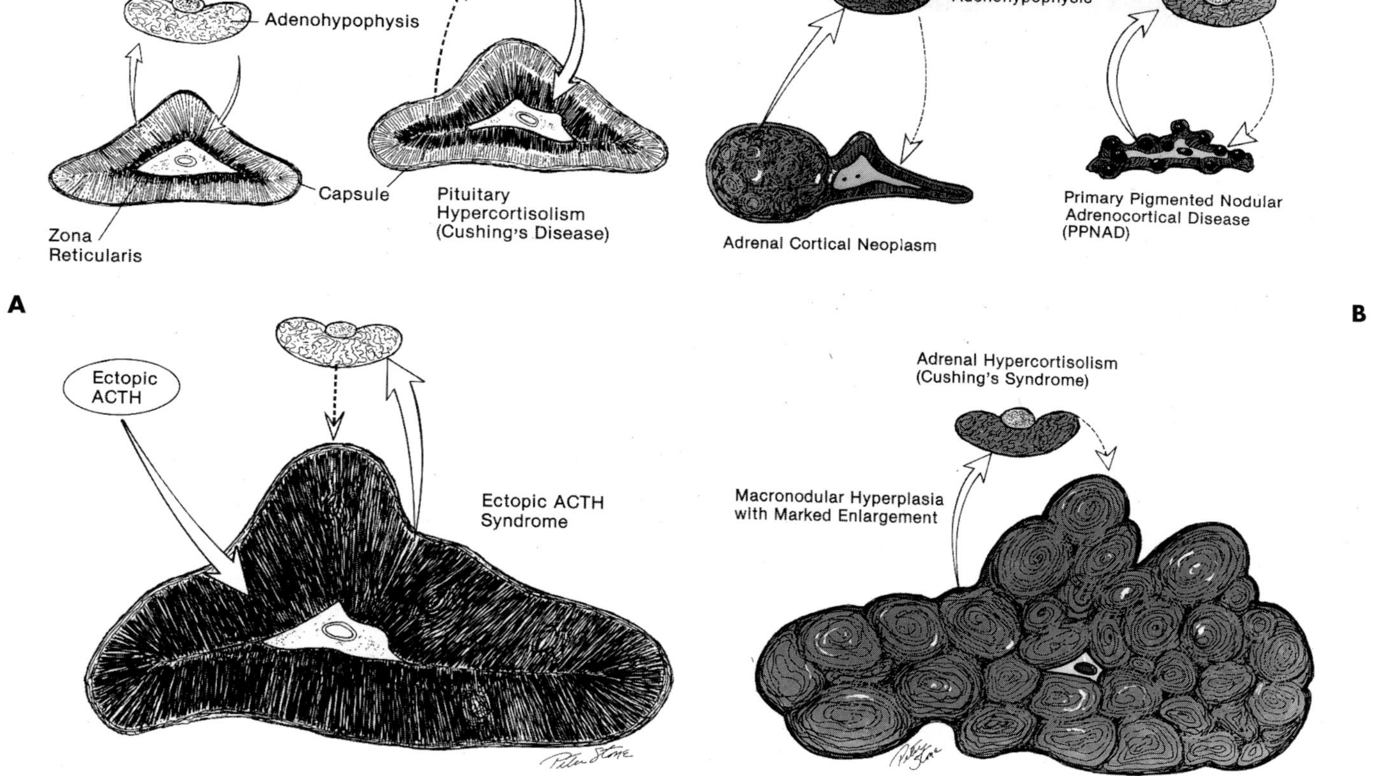

14-18. **A**, Normal hypothalamic-pituitary-adrenal axis (*upper left*). Pituitary (or adrenocorticotrophic hormone)-dependent hypercortisolism (*upper right*) is characteristic of Cushing's disease. Ectopic adrenocorticotrophic hormone syndrome (*lower half*) with enlarged, dark adrenal gland caused by trophic influence of adrenocorticotrophic hormone with predominance of cells with compact, lipid-depleted cytoplasm. **B**, Noniatrogenic causes of Cushing's syndrome. Cortisol-secreting cortical neoplasm (*upper left*) with autonomous hyperfunction and feedback inhibition of adrenocorticotrophic hormone release from adenohypophysis. Rare examples of Cushing's syndrome are caused by primary pigmented nodular adrenocortical disease (*upper right*) and macronodular hyperplasia with marked adrenal enlargement (*lower half*).

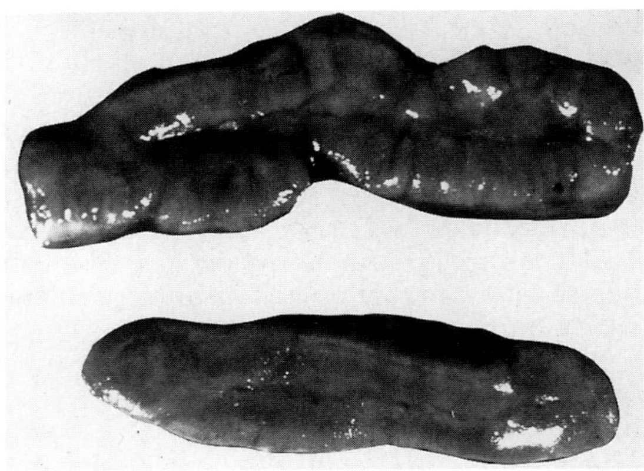

14-19. Transverse sections of a 3.5 g adrenal gland with mild nodularity surgically resected from an 8-year-old boy with Cushing's disease. Patient underwent several attempts at transsphenoidal pituitary resection. Patient was also treated with radiation (4,800 cGy), but tumor recurred on several occasions. Nelson's syndrome subsequently developed with radiologically detectable changes in the sella.

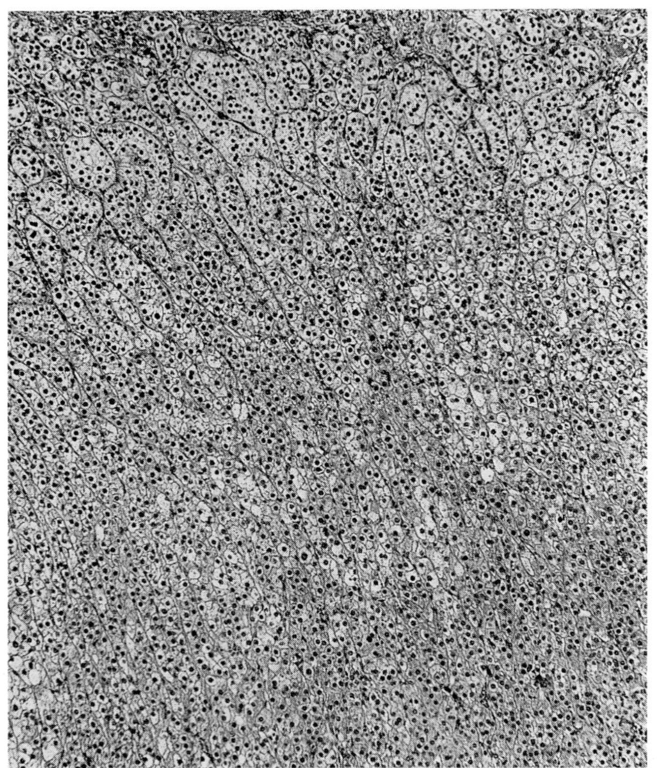

14-20. Adrenal in Cushing's disease caused by an adrenocorticotrophic hormone-producing pituitary adenoma. Cortex is hyperplastic with conversion of many cells throughout zona fasciculata into reticularis-type cells with compact, eosinophilic cytoplasm caused by lipid depletion.

of a pituitary adenoma. The pathologic alterations in the adrenal may be so subtle that the gland might be regarded as "normal" if not correlated with clinical and biochemical data.[3,40] The size and weight of the mildly stimulated gland may be only slightly increased, usually

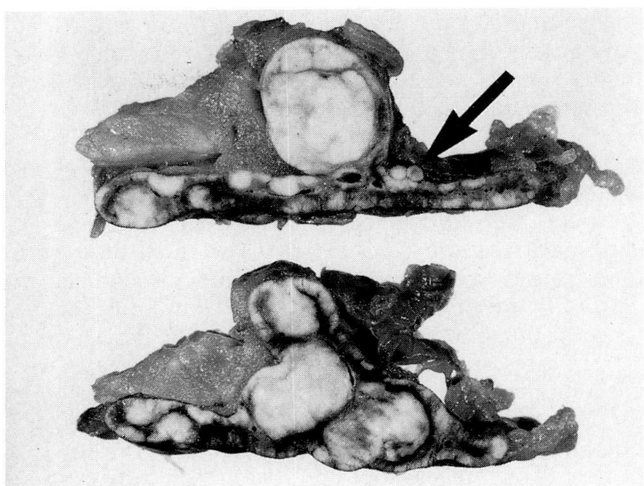

14-21. Macronodular adrenal cortical hyperplasia in a patient with multiple endocrine neoplasia syndrome type I who developed Cushing's syndrome caused by a presumed adrenocorticotrophic hormone-producing pituitary adenoma. Multiple pale cortical nodules range up to 1.5 cm in diameter, including small capsular extrusions (*arrow*). *(Modified from Lack EE, Travis WD, Oertel JE: Adrenal cortical nodules, hyperplasia, and hyperfunction. In Lack EE, ed: Pathology of the adrenal glands, New York, 1990, Churchill Livingstone.)*

between 6 and 12 g; the average weight in a recent study was 8.2 g.[90]

On transverse sectioning, the adrenal gland may have a somewhat rounded contour, and the larger glands may demonstrate a mild degree of nodularity (Fig. 14-19) with nodules up to 3 mm in diameter randomly distributed throughout the cortex. Capsular extrusions may appear accentuated, including the cuff of cortical cells around tributaries of the central adrenal vein. The microscopic hallmark of adrenocorticotrophic hormone stimulation in Cushing's disease is conversion of lipid-rich, pale-staining cortical cells in the inner one third to one half of the cortex into cells with compact eosinophilic cytoplasm, similar to the zona reticularis (Fig. 14-20). The net effect is what appears to be a greatly expanded zona reticularis except for the absence of lipochrome pigment in the outer part, which actully is zona fasciculata.[3,40] The extent to which vacuolated, lipid-rich cells are converted into compact, lipid-depleted cells is variable under the influence of a variety of physiologic factors.[3] The zona glomerulosa may be even more difficult to identify because of expansion of the zona fasciculata. Some cortical cells may extend irregularly into periadrenal adipose tissue or intermingle in irregular nests with chromaffin cells. Some of these changes may be subtle, particularly in the mildly stimulated glands, and correlation with clinical and biochemical data is crucial.[3,40]

Macronodular hyperplasia. Macronodular hyperplasia is present in about 20% of cases of hyperplasia with Cushing's disease,[3] but this is variable.[91] The morphology may be more confusing than that of diffuse or micronodular hyperplasia. Nodules up to 2 cm in diameter or larger (Fig. 14-21) protrude from one or more sides of the gland; they may also be situated deep within the adrenal, identifiable only when the gland is sectioned in the transverse plane. Smals et al[90] used the designation macronodular hyperplasia for grossly visible nodules 0.5 cm or greater in diameter, with some nodules up to 5 cm in diameter. Separation of micronodular and macronodular hyperplasia is difficult, and there is a morphologic continuum between the two processes, making this distinction arbitrary.

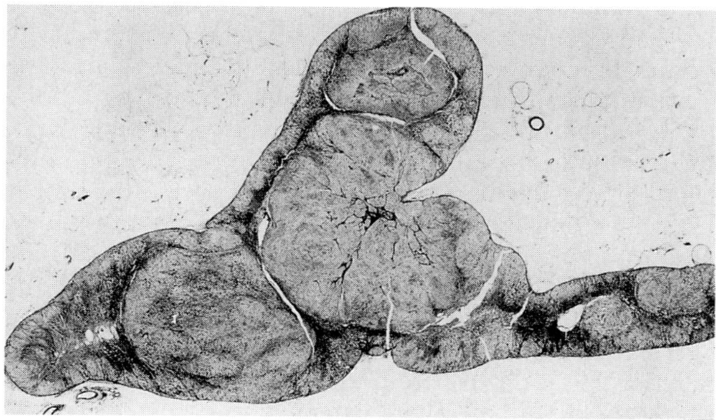

14-22. Pituitary-dependent macronodular adrenal cortical hyperplasia (same as Fig. 14-21). Irregular expansile cortical nodules blend with adjacent hyperplastic cortex. Adrenal medulla was difficult to identify in random transverse sections of the gland. *(From Lack EE, Travis WD, Oertel JE: Adrenal cortical nodules, hyperplasia, and hyperfunction. In Lack EE, ed: Pathology of the adrenal glands, New York, 1990, Churchill Livingstone.)*

Macronodular hyperplasia is characterized by disparity in size and weight between the adrenals. In the study by Smals et al,[90] the female to male ratio for macronodular hyperplasia was 5:1, identical to that for diffuse and micronodular hyperplasia. However, there are several important differences between micronodular and macronodular hyperplasia. The average age of patients with macronodular hyperplasia (44 years) is considerably older than those with diffuse and micronodular hyperplasia (31 years), and disease duration is longer with macronodular hyperplasia (8 years vs. 2 years). The average adrenal in macronodular hyperplasia weighs 16 g, nearly twice the observed weight in diffuse and micronodular hyperplasia.[90] As noted by Cohen et al,[92] the medullary compartment may be compressed by the prominent cortical nodules, and in many sections may be difficult to recognize (Fig. 14-22). There may be foci of lipomatous or myelolipomatous metaplasia.

Ectopic adrenocorticotrophic hormone syndrome with secondary hypercortisolism. About 15% of cases of Cushing's syndrome in adults result from ectopic production of adrenocorticotrophic hormone[93] by bronchial carcinoid tumor, bronchogenic small cell carcinoma, pancreatic islet cell tumor, medullary thyroid carcinoma, or pheochromocytoma or other rare neoplasms. Ectopic production of corticotropin releasing factor may occur, and may be accompanied by ectopic adrenocorticotrophic hormone secretion.[3,40] Nearly all normal tissues are capable of producing small amounts of the inactive precursor of adrenocorticotrophic hormone, probably pro-opiomelanocortin, and cancers may

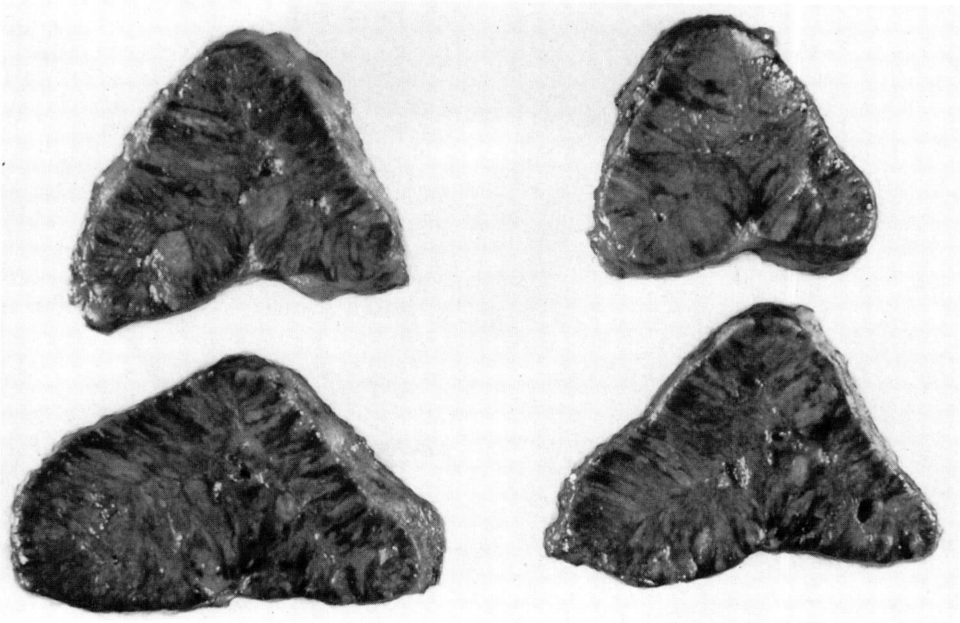

14-23. Ectopic adrenocorticotrophic hormone syndrome caused by a bronchial carcinoid tumor that was occult for several years. Right adrenal gland weighed 12 g and left adrenal gland weighed 11 g. Dark appearance on cross section is caused by intense stimulation by adrenocorticotrophic hormone with conversion of lipid-rich cortical cells to lipid-depleted cells with compact, eosinophilic cytoplasm. *(From Lack EE, Travis WD, Oertel JE: Adrenal cortical nodules, hyperplasia, and hyperfunction. In Lack EE, ed: Pathology of the adrenal glands, New York, 1990, Churchill Livingstone.)*

overproduce this substance, although few convert it into adrenocorticotrophic hormone; in this regard, ectopic adrenocorticotrophic hormone production may not be "ectopic."[94] Correct identification of the source of adrenocorticotrophic hormone secretion is essential in order to avoid unnecessary pituitary surgery.[95] In ectopic adrenocorticotrophic hormone syndrome serum levels are usually quite elevated, sometimes over 250 pg/ml, whereas in Cushing's disease adrenocorticotrophic hormone levels are rarely over 200 pg/ml, and are commonly in the upper range of normal or only slightly elevated.[40] Some patients with aggressive fast growing tumors such as bronchogenic small cell carcinoma lack signs and symptoms of Cushing's syndrome, with the clinical findings dominated by electrolyte disturbances and cachexia. Some slow growing neoplasms such as bronchial carcinoid tumor may be associated with marked changes of Cushing's syndrome, although the primary tumor remains occult, sometimes for years.[96]

Grossly, the adrenal glands are often symmetrically enlarged with rounded contours, and frequently weigh 10 to 15 g each; occasionally, the individual adrenal may weigh more than 20 g, or rarely 30 g.[3,40] In this setting the adrenal glands are under intense and persistent trophic stimulation by adrenocorticotrophic hormone, and the glands on transverse sectioning may be tan to brown because of conversion of lipid-rich, pale-staining cortical cells to cells with more compact eosinophilic cytoplasm (Fig. 14-23). The cortex is enlarged to 0.3 to 0.4 cm in thickness, but in some cases may be even wider. There is typically diffuse cortical hyperplasia, but sometimes there may be vague nodularity (Fig. 14-24).

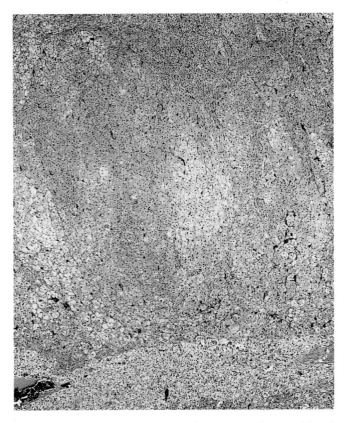

14-24. Ectopic adrenocorticotrophic hormone syndrome. Adrenal cortex is markedly hyperplastic with columns and cords of lipid-depleted cells. Faint nodularity was evident in some areas.

Primary pigmented nodular adrenocortical disease. Primary pigmented nodular adrenocortical disease is a rare form of pituitary- or adrenocorticotrophic hormone-independent hypercortisolism, referred to by a wide variety of terms that reflect the uncertainty regarding pathogenesis and etiology.[3,40] The disorder typically occurs in younger patients, typically females, and the associated Cushing's syndrome may be severe, with bone pain and pathologic fractures.[97] A variety of endocrinologic studies, including dynamic endocrine testing, indicate a primary adrenal source for the hypercortisolism.[98] Imaging studies of the sella and pituitary fossa reveal no abnormalities, and selective venous sinus sampling of the inferior petrosal sinus excludes pituitary origin for the adrenocorticotrophic hormone.

The adrenal glands in primary pigmented nodular adrenocortical disease are normal on computed tomography scan, but unilateral or bilateral nodularity may be present, including macronodules greater than 1 cm in diameter.[40] The weight of each adrenal varies from 0.9 to 13.4 g, with an average combined weight of 9.6 g; the gland is usually normal in size.[98] Small pigmented micronodules, 1 to 3 mm in diameter, may be seen through the intact capsular surface of the gland, but transverse sections usually reveal the pigmented nodules to better advantage (Fig. 14-25). Complete removal of the investing connective tissue and fat may be impeded by these small nodules when they protrude through the capsule or extend into the periadrenal fat. The pigmented nodules are light gray, gray-brown, dark brown, or jet black. The term micronodular is somewhat arbitrary, because many of the intensely pigmented nodules are grossly apparent, even when they are less than 1 mm in diameter.

The histologic features of the pigmented nodules may be less striking than the gross features (Fig. 14-26). The pigmented nodules are usually round to oval and are present within the zona reticularis or they interface with the adjoining medulla. Their configuration varies from hourglass and strings of beads to links of sausages. They are

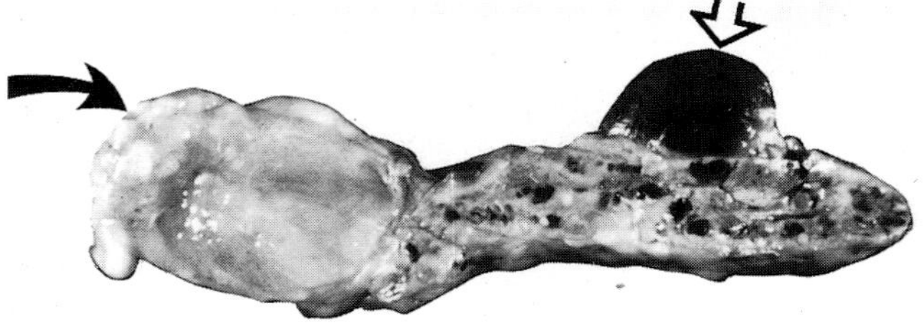

14-25. Primary pigmented nodular adrenocortical disease. Transverse section of adrenal gland shows numerous dark pigmented nodules, one nearly 1 cm in diameter (*open arrow*). Another nodule (*curved arrow*) is pale-yellow and has small foci of necrosis. Patient was a member of a family with the complex of myxomas, spotty pigmentation, and endocrine overactivity.

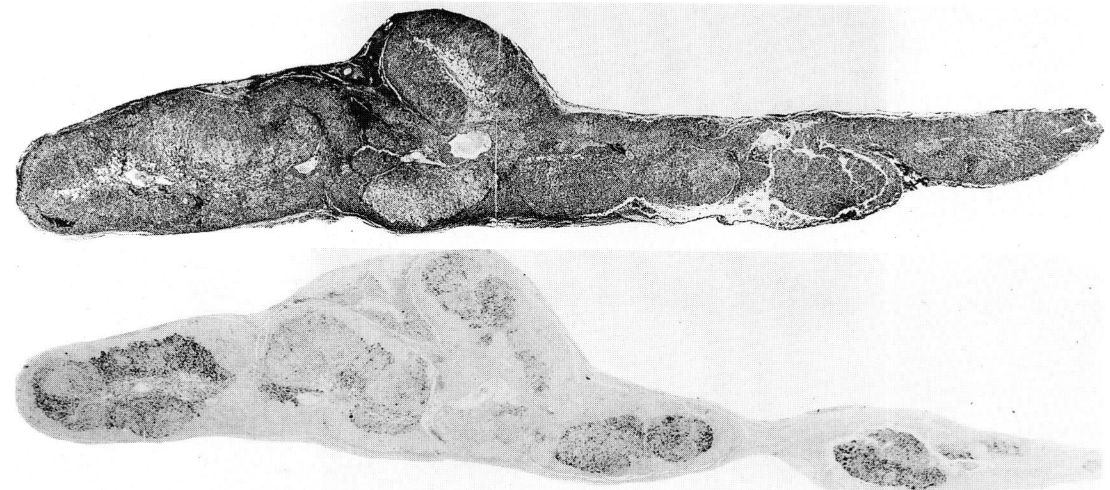

14-26. **A**, Primary pigmented nodular adrenocortical disease. Numerous pigmented nodules were apparent in transverse section of gland, but were much more clearly delineated on gross examination. **B**, Pigmented nodules contain cells that are argentaffin-positive causing them to stand out in contrast to remaining gland. Some areas show marked atrophy of internodular cortex.

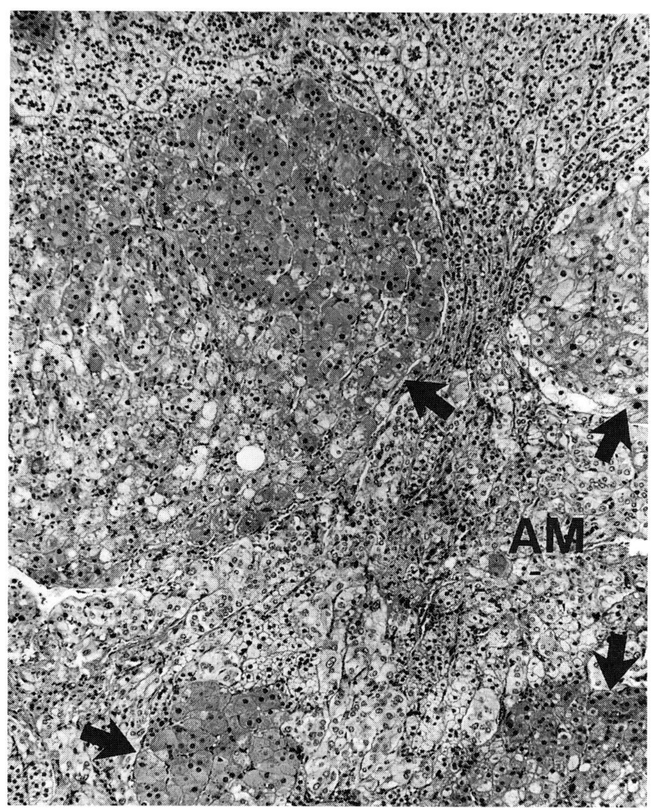

14-27. Several pigmented micronodules in primary pigmented nodular adrenocortical disease (*arrows*) are located in inner aspect of cortex and impinge on the medulla (*AM*).

typically unencapsulated, but have expansile borders, and may cause distortion or compression of adjacent uninvolved cells (Fig. 14-27). Occasionally, there is intraluminal projection of a small pigmented nodule into tributaries of the central adrenal vein at sites with interrupted bundles of smooth muscle. In most nodules, the cells contain compact eosinophilic cytoplasm with variable amounts of coarse granular pigment, which usually has the staining characteristics of lipofuscin. Some nodules contain cells with pale-staining lipid-rich cytoplasm, and, occasionally, cells may be large with a ballooned appearance. Sparse lymphocytic infiltrates have rarely been noted around vessels or actually within the nodules, and occasionally one may see a lipomatous or even myelolipomatous metaplastic component.[40]

The etiology and pathogenesis of primary pigmented nodular adrenocortical disease are unknown, but several theories have been proposed:[98]

1. hamartomous malformation or dysplasia of the cortex
2. primary abnormality of the zona reticularis
3. occult adrenocorticotrophic hormone–producing pituitary adenoma with adrenal cortical nodules becoming functionally autonomous
4. embryonic developmental error in the cortex at the adrenarche
5. block in evolution of zona fasciculata cells into cells of zona reticularis, with accumulation of autonomous cells at the interface
6. organ-specific autoimmune hypercortisolism (Cushing's syndrome)

The autoimmune theory of hypercortisolism is based on reports of circulating adrenal stimulating immunoglobulin in this disorder[99]; the adrenal stimulating immunoglobulin is presumably directed against adrenocorticotrophic hormone receptors or receptor binding sites. Further study should determine whether primary pigmented nodular adrenocortical disease is an autoimmune disorder or one in which the circulating adrenal stimulating immunoglobulin is merely an epiphenomenon. A recent immunohistochemical study of primary pigmented nodular adrenocortical disease revealed intense immunoreactivity for all enzymes involved in steroidogenesis in cells of the cortical nodules, particularly those with abundant eosinophilic cytoplasm, unlike cells of the internodular cortex.[100]

The treatment of choice for primary pigmented nodular adrenocortical disease is bilateral adrenalectomy,[101] with the removal of both adrenal glands even if they appear normal or small. In some cases, subtotal resection may be possible, although about one third of the patients initially treated by unilateral or subtotal adrenalectomy require completion of total adrenalectomy because of persistence or recurrence of Cushing's syndrome.[98] It is important to note that Nelson's syndrome has not been reported following bilateral adrenalectomy in patients with primary pigmented nodular adrenocortical disease.

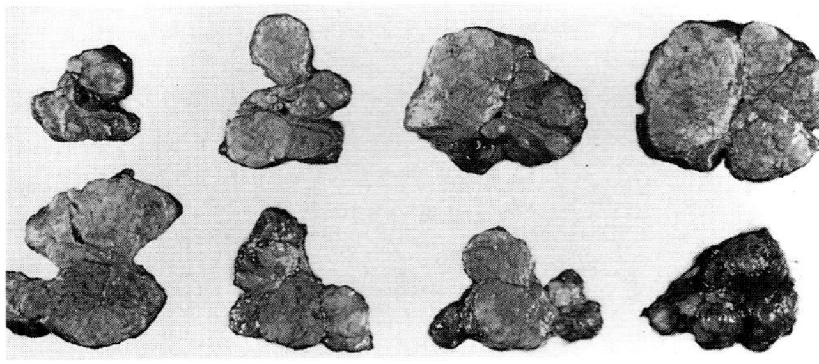

14-28. Macronodular adrenal cortical hyperplasia with marked adrenal enlargement. Transverse sections of one adrenal gland are displayed. Combined weight of both glands was about 90 g.

Complex of myxomas, spotty pigmentation, and endocrine overactivity. This is a complex array of diverse abnormalities, which, in the review by Carney et al,[102] included cardiac myxoma (72%), spotty mucocutaneous pigmentation (65%), testicular tumors, particularly large cell calcifying Sertoli cell tumor (56% of males), primary pigmented nodular adrenocortical disease (45%), cutaneous myxoma (45%), mammary myxoid fibroadenoma (30% of females), and other abnormalities such as growth hormone-secreting pituitary tumor and psammomatous melanotic schwannoma.[3,40,102] The disorder has an autosomal dominant inheritance. If a patient has two or more elements of this complex, particularly primary pigmented nodular adrenocortical disease, bilateral large cell calcifying Sertoli cell tumor of testis, or mucocutaneous pigmentation, investigation for cardiac myxoma (which may be multiple) is recommended for early detection and treatment.

Macronodular hyperplasia with marked adrenal enlargement

Macronodular hyperplasia with marked adrenal enlargement is a rare primary autonomous form of adrenal hypercortisolism that is adrenocorticotrophic hormone and pituitary independent.[3,40] Careful endocrinologic investigation, including dynamic testing, reveals elevated plasma cortisol levels, undetectable adrenocorticotrophic hormone levels, and loss of diurnal rhythmicity. There is

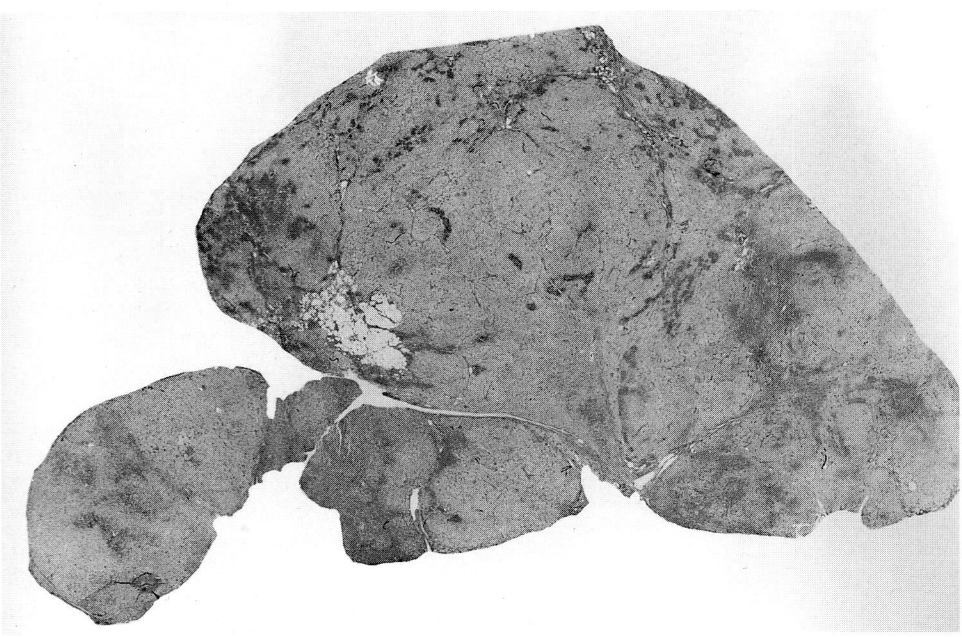

14-29. Macronodular adrenal cortical hyperplasia with marked adrenal enlargement. Note multiple irregular nodules of hyperplastic adrenal cortex as well as small area of metaplastic fat. Most hyperplastic cells had lipid-rich, pale-staining cytoplasm.

no detectable abnormality of the sella or pituitary fossa, including one patient who was reinvestigated almost 26 years later.[103] An unusual case of adrenocorticotrophic hormone-independent macronodular hyperplasia with marked adrenal enlargement occurred in a male patient who presented with feminization and Cushing's syndrome; the combined adrenal glands weighed 86 g.[40] The average patient age is about 50 years, with slight male predominance, and the duration of Cushing's syndrome ranged from about 1 to 10 years in one study.[103]

The adrenal glands in macronodular hyperplasia with marked adrenal enlargement are significantly enlarged and simulate an adrenal neoplasm.[40] The combined weight ranges from 60 g to 180 g, with an extraordinary degree of nodular cortical hyperplasia; the nodules in one study ranged in size from 0.2 to 3.8 cm (Fig. 14-28).[103] The nodules are yellow or golden-yellow, typically unencapsulated, and blend in imperceptibly with the hyperplastic cortex. The medullary compartment may be distorted and difficult to recognize in random sections of the gland, similar to macronodular hyperplasia. Cortical cells have a variable amount of finely vacuolated, lipid-rich pale-staining cytoplasm (Fig. 14-29). There may be scattered cells with compact eosinophilic cytoplasm. Rarely cells with large ballooned vacuolated cytoplasm are present, and occasionally one may see lipomatous or myelolipomatous metaplasia. There is weak immunoreactivity in macronodular hyperplasia with marked adrenal enlargement for 3-ß-hydroxysteroid dehydrogenase and other enzymes involved in steroidogenesis, whereas strong staining is noted in adrenal cortical adenoma[104] and primary pigmented nodular adrenocortical disease.[100] In situ hybridization study of P-450c17 has also been used to localize the site of steroidogenesis, and results suggest that the degree of corticosteroidogenesis by individual cortical cells is low and that a significant increase in cell number is necessary before excessive cortisol production occurs with production of Cushing's syndrome.[105] As indicated in Figure 14-30, a possible relationship between macronodular hyperplasia with marked adrenal enlargement and macronodular hyperplasia of Cushing's disease can not be definitively established in most cases. The treatment proposed for this rare disorder is bilateral adrenalectomy. As in macronodular hyperplasia in Cushing's disease, the clinical and biochemical features may be misleading and suggest an underlying adrenal cortical neoplasm.

MULTIPLE ENDOCRINE NEOPLASIA TYPE I

Multiple endocrine neoplasia type I (Wermer's syndrome)[106] occurs as an autosomal dominant trait with somewhat variable expression or in sporadic form or affects family members in whom manifestations are detectable only after close scrutiny. The genetic defect is located on chromosome 11q13.[107] In a review by Ballard et al,[108] adrenal findings at autopsy included cortical adenoma, "miliary" adenoma, hyperplasia, multiple adenomas, and nodular hyperplasia, but only 1 of 31 patients had clinical hypercorticalism. Cushing's disease may occur in multiple endocrine neoplasia type I, but it is rare (see Fig. 14-21, 14-22).[109]

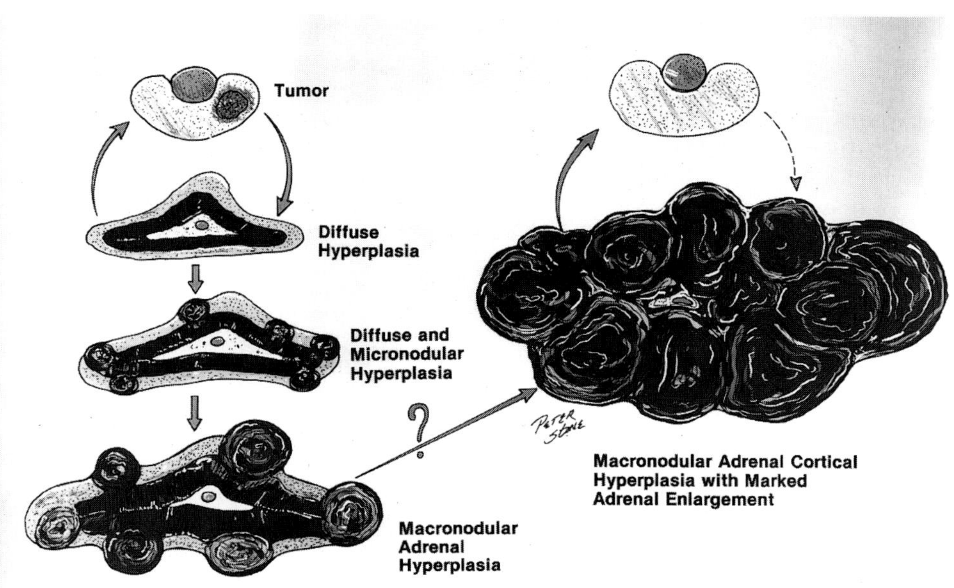

14-30. Schematic diagram of progression of pituitary (or adrenocorticotrophic hormone)-dependent Cushing's disease into micronodular and macronodular adrenal cortical hyperplasia. Macronodular adrenal cortical hyperplasia with marked adrenal enlargement appears to be a primary form of adrenal hypercortisolism (Cushing's syndrome) by sensitive imaging and biochemical studies. Relationship with macronodular adrenal hyperplasia (*lower left*) is uncertain.

OTHER RARE CAUSES OF CUSHING'S SYNDROME

There are several other rare causes of Cushing's syndrome that are reviewed elsewhere.[40] These include McCune-Albright syndrome (triad of café au lait spots, polyostotic fibrous dysplasia, and sexual precocity), hyperfunction of various endocrine glands (e.g., hypercortisolism) caused by a somatic mutation with activation of a signal transduction pathway generating cAMP,[110,111] and food-dependent Cushing's syndrome caused by abnormal responsiveness of the adrenal glands to physiologic secretion of gastric inhibitory polypeptide.[112,113]

ADRENAL CORTICAL HYPERPLASIA WITH HYPERALDOSTERONISM

Up to 35% of cases of primary hyperaldosteronism are idiopathic, with bilateral hyperplasia of zona glomerulosa,[114] but a higher incidence is noted in milder forms of the disorder.[115] Patients are usually managed medically; adrenalectomy is reserved for patients with an aldosterone producing adenoma because of a more predictable response in terms of amelioration or normalization of systemic hypertension.[40] The cause of this disorder is uncertain, but may be due to an aldosterone-stimulating factor from the anterior pituitary.[116,117]

ADRENAL CORTICAL HYPERPLASIA WITH EXCESS SEX STEROID SECRETION

This disorder is limited to cases of congenital adrenal hyperplasia.

ADRENAL MEDULLARY HYPERPLASIA

Adrenal medullary hyperplasia is inherited or occurs sporadically. The inherited form usually arises in the setting of multiple endocrine neoplasia syndromes type 2a and 2b, and is diffuse or nodular, and often multicentric and bilateral.[118,119] Sporadic adrenal medullary hyperplasia is now accepted as an entity, occurring in patients with symptoms of pheochromocytoma, including paroxysmal or sustained hypertension, headaches, palpitations, and diaphoresis; surgical exploration fails to reveal a catecholamine-secreting tumor. Adrenal medullary hyperplasia in this setting is in the differential diagnosis of "pseudopheochromocytoma." Adrenal medullary hyperplasia has also been reported in patients with cystic fibrosis and the Beckwith-Wiedemann syndrome.[4,32,40]

In multiple endocrine neoplasia syndrome types 2a and 2b, one of the earliest manifestations of adrenal medullary hyperfunction is an elevated ratio of epinephrine to norepinephrine in the urine.[118] One suggested treatment for such patients is bilateral total adrenalectomy. Involvement of the adrenal glands by adrenal medullary hyperplasia may be symmetric or asymmetric. The distinction between adrenal medullary hyperplasia and pheochromocytoma in multiple endocrine neoplasia type 2 is arbitrary. Carney et al[119] adopted a cut point of 1 cm diameter to separate adrenal medullary hyperplasia and pheochromocytoma. Nodules larger than 1 cm are considered pheochromocytoma. This size was chosen because it was the lower extreme in the range of size of pheochromocytomas reported in the first series Atlas of Tumor Pathology on the adrenal. Histologically, adrenal medullary hyperplasia consists of expansile nodular growth of the medulla with distortion of the adjacent cortex or adjacent normal-appearing medulla. There may be numerous extensively vacuolated cells, as well as intracytoplasmic hyaline globules, some of which appear to be present in the extracellular space. Mitotic figures may be present, but are usually not numerous, and there may be some nuclear pleomorphism. In a recent study of adrenal medullary hyperplasia and pheochromocytoma, DNA content was found to be diploid or euploid in normal and hyperplastic glands, while 87% of clinically benign pheochromocytomas (33 of 38 cases) and all five malignant pheochromocytomas had nondiploid or aneuploid DNA histograms.[120]

ADRENAL CYST

Nonneoplastic adrenal cysts are uncommon, usually occurring in the fifth and sixth decades, although cases have been reported from birth to 76 years.[121] There is a predilection for women, with a female:male ratio of about 3:1.[122] Adrenal cysts are usually small and discovered incidentally at autopsy. Rarely, they may be extremely large, containing several liters of fluid and compressing the abdominal contents. Adrenal cysts are classified as parasitic (7% of cases, usually echinococcal), epithelial (9%), endothelial (45%), and pseudocyst (39%).[121] Epithelial cysts are subdivided into three categories: (1) true glandular or retention cysts; (2) embryonal cysts lined by cylindrical epithelium derived from displaced urogenital tissue that has undergone cystic transformation; and (3) cystic change within an adrenal adenoma, carcinoma, or pheochromocytoma.[123] It has also been proposed that an epithelial lined adrenal cyst rarely may develop from entrapped mesothelium.[124]

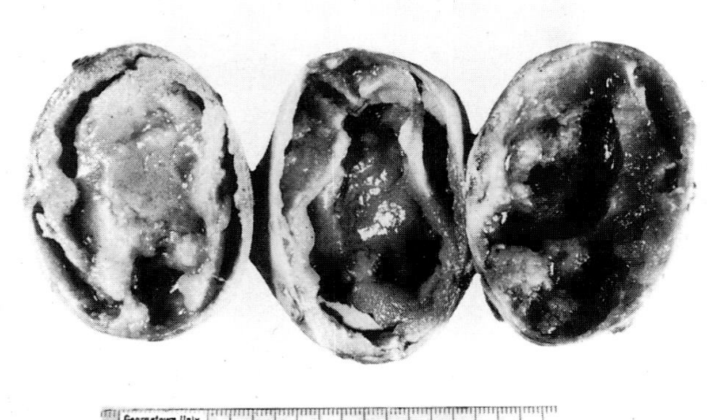

14-31. Adrenal pseudocyst on cross section contains grumous, soft, pale-tan debris. Dystrophic calcification was present in wall of cyst.

Adrenal pseudocysts are the most common type of adrenal cyst seen at surgery and often appear as a large unilocular cyst with an irregular lining, containing red-brown bloody fluid (Fig. 14-31). Some adrenal pseudocysts probably arise by hemorrhage into normal or pathologic adrenals; a small number result from hemorrhage into an underlying tumor.[121,123] Immunohistochemical studies show a vascular endothelial lining in some adrenal pseudocysts.[125,126] Some hemorrhagic cysts may also arise when hemorrhage occurs in a preexisting vascular malformation.[126] There may be entrapment of nests of cortical cells by extravasated blood, and this hemorrhagic cyst should be distinguished from necrotic adrenal cortical neoplasm.[126] Breast carcinoma has initially presented as metastasis to an adrenal cyst, and mature adipose tissue and myelolipomatous metaplasia have also been described within adrenal pseudocysts.[127]

Microscopic cysts are a frequent histologic finding in the permanent cortex of fetal and premature adrenal glands, being reported in up to 62% of stillbirths under 35 weeks gestational age.[128] A significant correlation with short gestation and short survival after birth has been reported.[129] Three possible pathogenetic mechanisms have been proposed:

1. an intrinsic developmental process
2. infection
3. generalized reaction to stress

MYELOLIPOMA

Adrenal myelolipoma is a benign tumefactive lesion consisting of mature adipose tissue admixed with a variable amount of hematopoietic elements. This lesion occurs most frequently in the adrenal gland, although it also occurs in extra-adrenal sites[130] including stomach, liver,[131] mediastinum, and the presacral region.[40,123] The etiology is unknown, although some data suggest that it arises under hormonal influence by metaplasia of adrenal cortical or stromal cells.[123] Intraadrenal fat and hematopoietic tissue have been induced experimentally by injecting crude pituitary adrenocorticotrophic hormone extract into adrenal glands,[132] and myelolipomatous foci may be seen in patients with excess cortical activity such as hyperfunctioning adrenal cortical adenoma or adrenal cortical hyperplasia. Others have suggested that myelolipoma derives from emboli from the bone marrow or from embryonic rests of hematopoietic tissue.[123]

The incidence at autopsy is 0.01% to 0.2%, and it is most common in persons over 40 years of age, with a roughly equal sex predilection.[133] Most patients are asymptomatic, and most cases of myelolipoma are discovered incidentally. When patients are symptomatic, it is usually because of the large size of the myelolipoma, resulting in abdominal or flank pain, dysuria, hematuria, or rarely, catastrophic spontaneous retroperitoneal hemorrhage.[134] It may occur in patients with concurrent endocrinologic disorders, such as Cushing's disease,[135] Cushing's syndrome,[136] Conn's syndrome,[137] Addison's disease, and congenital adrenal hyperplasia.[40,133]

Grossly, myelolipoma forms a soft, well-circumscribed mass that is variegated yellow to red-brown (Fig. 14-32).

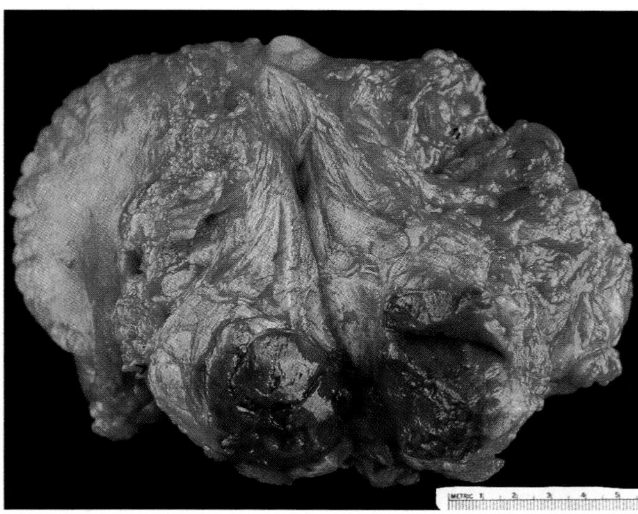

14-32. Juxta-adrenal myelolipoma on cross section appears red-brown because of abundant hematopoietic elements. Lesion measures about 3.5 cm in diameter and is partially enveloped by adipose tissue.

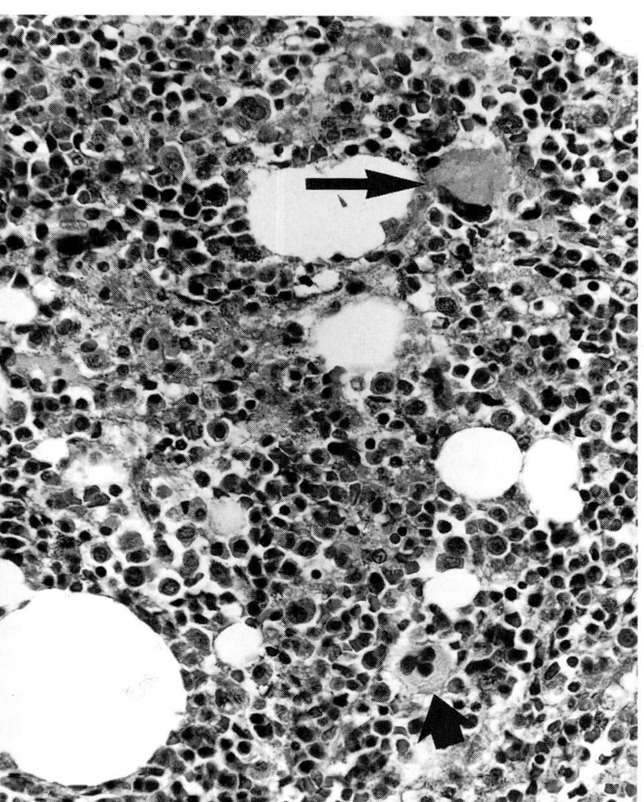

14-33. Myelolipoma consists of fat mixed with hematopoietic elements including megakaryocytes (*arrows*).

It ranges in size from a few millimeters up to 34 cm. Microscopically, there is hematopoietic tissue comprising various combinations of the three cell lines, with an admixture of mature fatty tissue (Fig. 14-33). Bony trabeculae, hemorrhage, and fibrosis are occasionally seen. Myelolipoma is detected more frequently with the advent of computed tomography and magnetic resonance imaging; fine needle aspiration biopsy has proved useful in preoperative diagnosis.[138] Treatment varies from radiographic surveillance for small lesions in asymptomatic patients to surgical excision of large or symptomatic lesions.

ADRENAL HEMORRHAGE

Adrenal hemorrhage can complicate cardiac disease, thromboembolic disease, sepsis, postoperative or postpartum state, or coagulopathy (e.g., heparin administration).[3] Patients may become symptomatic with abdominal or lower chest pain and fever. Newborn infants may also present with manifestations of adrenal hemorrhage or hematoma formation.[3,123] Occasionally, adrenal hemorrhage is bilateral and massive.[139]

ADRENAL NEOPLASMS

ADRENAL CORTICAL NEOPLASMS

Adrenal cortical adenoma with Cushing's syndrome

Adrenal cortical adenoma is usually small, weighing less than 50 g. The tumors had an average weight in one series of 36 g (range, 12.5 g to 126 g).[140] On transverse section, it usually appears as a sharply circumscribed or encapsulated mass.[40,141] Almost all tumors are unilateral and solitary, although there are rare exceptions.[142,143] Adenomas may be yellow or golden-yellow throughout, or have irregular mottling or diffuse dark brown areas (Fig. 14-34). The color of the tumor depends on a number of factors including the presence of congestion or hemorrhage and the content of neutral lipid and lipofuscin.[40,141,144]

Although many tumors appear grossly encapsulated, histologic study reveals a relatively smooth expansile border without a true capsule. Compression of the adjacent parenchyma and connective tissue, including the expanded adrenal capsule itself, creates a "pseudocapsule." Adenomas usually consist of cells with relatively abundant pale lipid-rich cytoplasm resembling the zona fasciculata, but there may be cells with more compact eosinophilic cytoplasm. Architecturally, the cells are arranged in short trabeculae, blunt cords, or a nesting or alveolar pattern (Fig. 14-35). Nuclei are usually vesicular, with a single, small nucleolus. There may be nuclear enlargement and pleomorphism, but these are usually focal and mild to moderate in degree (Fig. 14-36). Also, there may be foci of lipomatous or myelolipomatous metaplasia. Endocrinologic data and clinical information are often essential to distinguish an adrenal cortical neoplasm associated with Cushing's syndrome from an incidental *nonhyper*functioning macronodule or an adenoma associated with a different endocrine syndrome.[40,141] An important clue to the presence of Cushing's syndrome is cortical atrophy in the attached adrenal or the contralateral gland. Ultrastructural study

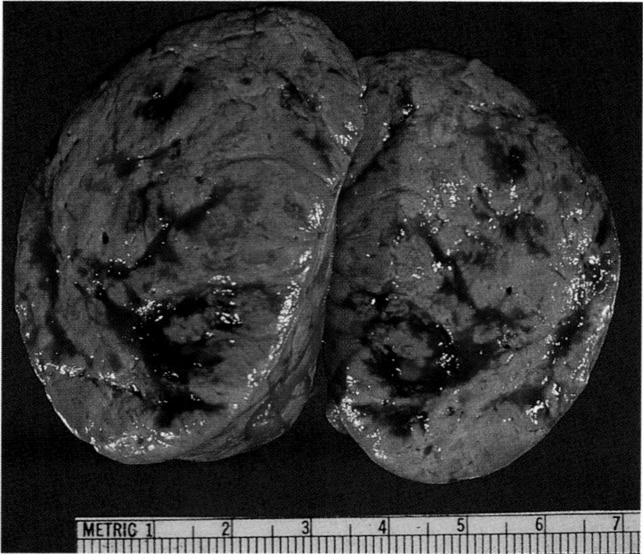

14-34. Adrenal cortical adenoma with Cushing's syndrome.

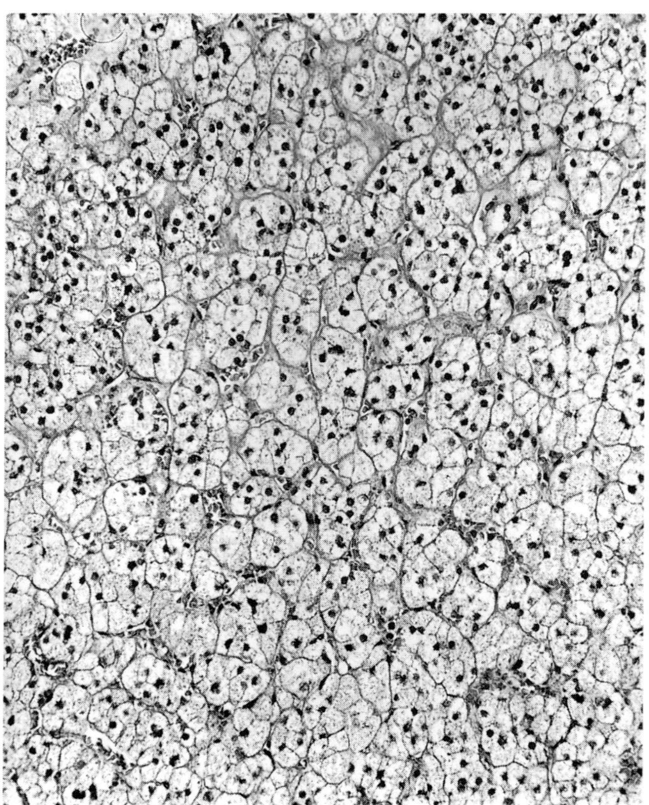
14-35. Adrenal cortical adenoma in Cushing's syndrome. Cells are arranged in alveoli or short cords.

reveals abundant intracytoplasmic lipid in most cases (Fig. 14-37). Mitochondria may have tubulovesicular cristae, similar to normal cells of zona fasciculata, or may have lamellar cristae characteristic of zona reticularis. Smooth endoplasmic reticulum is usually abundant.

Adrenal cortical adenoma with primary hyperaldosteronism (Conn's syndrome)

Clinical features. It has been estimated that 65% to 85% of cases of primary hyperaldosteronism are caused by an aldosterone-secreting cortical adenoma, but recent data indicate that idiopathic bilateral hyperplasia may be a more frequent cause, particularly if the mild examples are included. The aldosterone-secreting adenoma is an important surgical lesion because it is a curable form of systemic hypertension. The prevalence of an aldosterone-secreting adenoma in the hypertensive population ranges from 0.5% to 8%,[141] although Conn[145] suggested that primary hyperaldosteronism may be the cause of up to 20% of all cases of essential hypertension based upon the incidence of solitary "adenoma" 1.5 cm or greater in diameter reported in hypertensive individuals at autopsy (20%).[60] However, incidental cortical nodules are common in patients 50 to 80 years of age, as well as in those with hypertension.[57] It is uncertain whether hypertension results from the incidental nodule or is a cause of it, perhaps related to capsular arteriopathy. This controversy can be forever rekindled however because one can postulate that over time there may be conversion of glomerulosa-type cells within these incidental nodules to cells having different functional characteristics; when the incidental "adenoma" is discovered, the patient may already have established systemic hypertension without the expected biochemical profile of an aldosterone-secreting adenoma.[141]

Pathology. Aldosterone-secreting adrenal cortical adenoma (aldosteronoma) is usually solitary, small, and measures only a few centimeters in diameter; many are less than 2 cm in diameter,[141] although most are large enough to be visible on abdominal computed tomography scan. Grossly, the tumor may project from one portion of the gland, although it may be difficult to appreciate in the intact gland without transverse sectioning. The tumor is often homogeneous and diffusely bright yellow-orange and may be sharply demarcated from the adjacent cortex, simulating encapsulation (Fig. 14-38). Architectural patterns include alveolar or nesting arrangement, short cords or trabeculae of cells (Fig. 14-39).

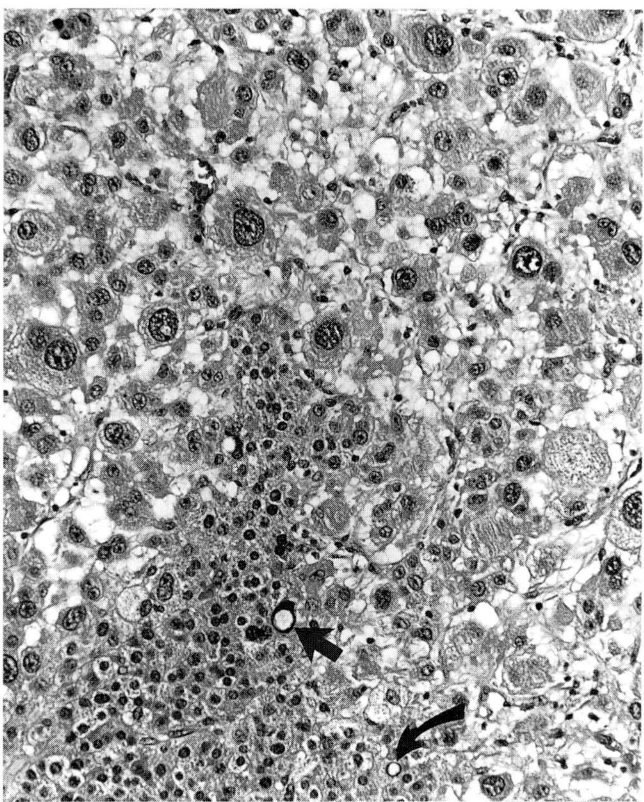

14-36. Adrenal cortical adenoma in Cushing's syndrome. Note focally marked variability in nuclear size and hyperchromasia. Many cells in this field have compact, eosinophilic cytoplasm and several have nuclear "pseudoinclusions" (*arrows*).

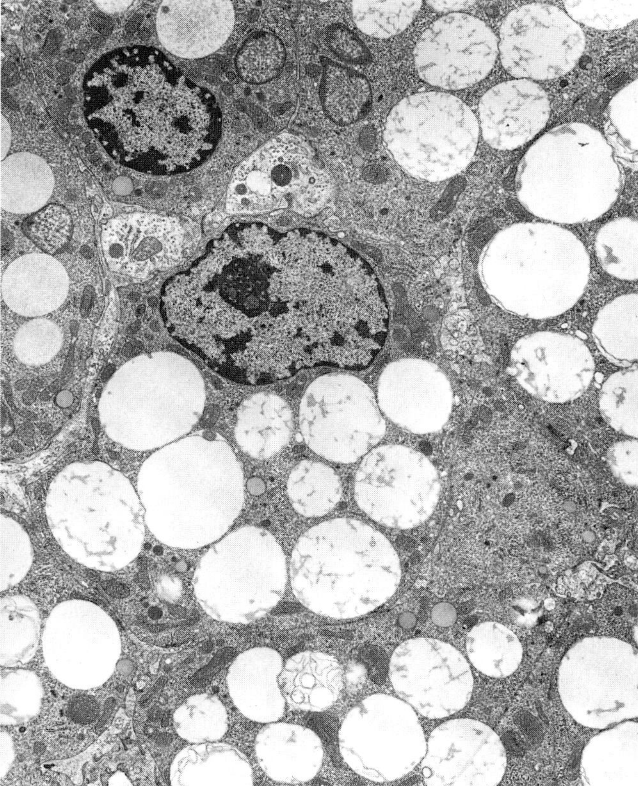

14-37. Adrenal cortical adenoma in Cushing's syndrome. Cells contain large lipid globules and prominent smooth endoplasmic reticulum. (x 3,500) *(From Lack EE, Travis WD, Oertel JE: Adrenal cortical neoplasms. In Lack EE, ed: Pathology of the adrenal glands, New York, 1990, Churchill Livingstone.)*

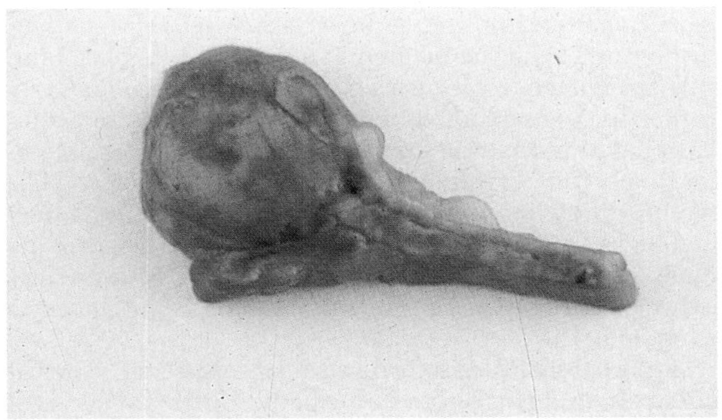

14-38. Aldosterone-secreting adrenal cortical adenoma. Tumor was 1 cm in diameter and yellow-orange on cross section.

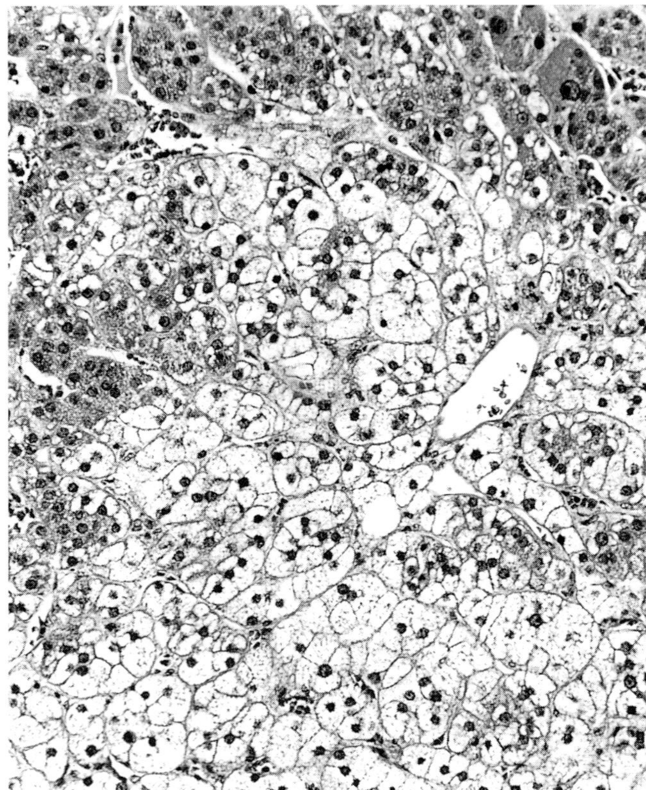

14-39. Aldosterone-producing adrenal cortical adenoma. Most cells have lipid-rich finely vacuolated cytoplasm.

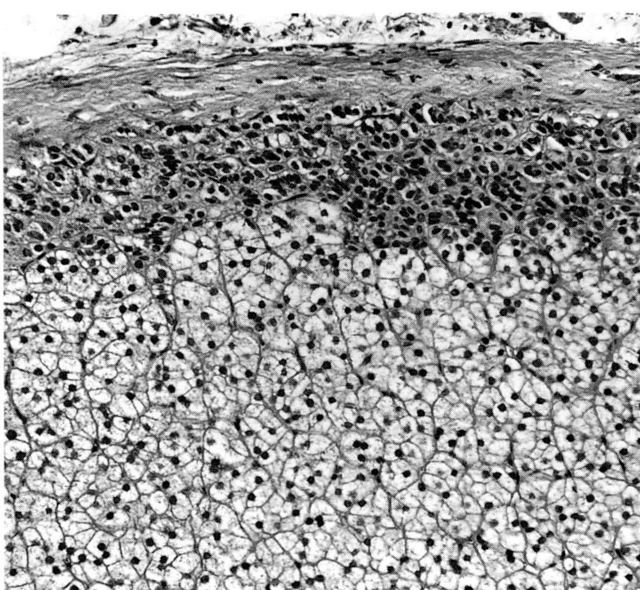

14-40. Hyperplasia of zona glomerulosa is apparent as a continuous band of cells beneath the capsule. Numerous foci such as this may be present in the cortex adjacent to aldosterone-secreting adenoma.

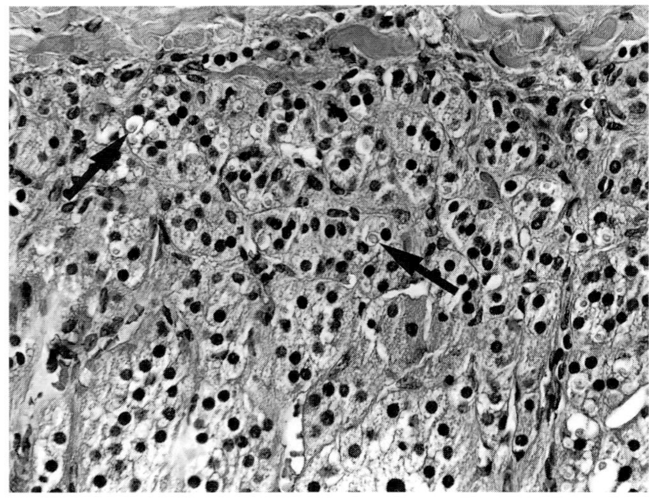

14-41. Spironolactone bodies (*arrows*) appear as single scroll-like, eosinophilic inclusions within zona glomerulosa cells. Many are surrounded by a clear space.

Four types of cells have been described by light microscopic examination, often with multiple types within the same tumor.[7] The most common cell type is large, with pale-staining lipid-rich cytoplasm resembling those of the zona fasciculata. A second cell type appears as clusters of smaller cells resembling those of the zona glomerulosa, with a high nuclear to cytoplasmic ratio and a small amount of vacuolated cytoplasm. The third cell type consists of scattered cells with compact eosinophilic cytoplasm similar to cells of the zona reticularis. The fourth cell type, "hybrid" cells, has morphologic features between zona glomerulosa–type and zona fasciculata–type cells. The attached or contralateral adrenal often shows hyperplasia of the zona glomerulosa with a broad focal or discontinuous zone beneath the capsule (Fig. 14-40), sometimes with small tongues of glomerulosa-type cells extending inward from the capsule. The term *hybrid* refers to the capacity of the cell to synthesize cortical steroids, which are normally produced by the zona glomerulosa (aldosterone) or the zona fasciculata (cortisol). Aldosterone-secreting adenomas may originate from hybrid cells or zona fasciculata–type cells. This would account for the functional behavior of tumor cells in vivo, as evi-

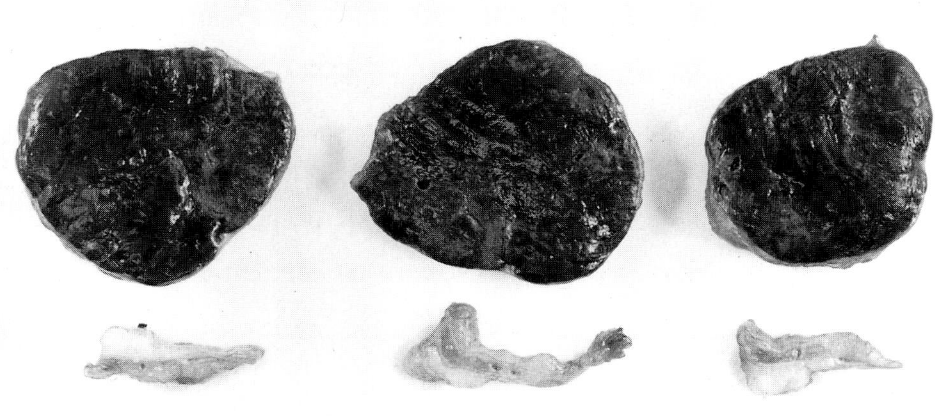

14-42. Pigmented (black) adrenal cortical adenoma with Cushing's syndrome. The tumor is 3.5 cm in diameter. Sectioned surfaces of tumor are diffusely black with vague lobulation. Residual adrenal gland (*lower row*) shows marked cortical atrophy.

denced by modulation of aldosterone secretion by adrenocorticotrophic hormone, lack of responsiveness to angiotensin II (the dominant secretagogue and trophic hormone for the glomerulosa-type cells under normal conditions), secretion of the hybrid steroids in large quantities, and the ability of the cells to produce cortisol in vitro and sometimes in large quantities in vivo.[146] Ultrastructurally, these cells show morphologic heterogeneity[40,140,147] including round to elongate mitochondria with cristae that are short and tubular, vesicular, or lamellar or shelflike, typical of zona glomerulosa–type cells.

Spironolactone bodies. Lightly eosinophilic, scroll-like intracytoplasmic inclusions have been described in zona glomerulosa–type (non-neoplastic or neoplastic) cells in patients treated with the aldosterone antagonist spironolactone (Aldactone) (Fig. 14-41).[40,141,148] Ultrastructural study suggests origin from tightly packed tubules of endoplasmic reticulum.[149] These inclusion-like structures are called *spironolactone bodies*. They typically range in size from 2 to 12 µm, but most are equal in size or slightly larger than the adjacent nucleus. These structures may be highlighted with Luxol fast blue stain because of their rich phospholipid content.[40,141] Although the specificity of these inclusions has been questioned, they are generally regarded as rather specific markers for spironolactone administration. In one study, the number of spironolactone bodies within cells of the aldosterone-secreting adenoma correlated positively with the proportion of glomerulosa-type cells.[150]

Functional pigmented (black) adrenal cortical adenoma

Pigmented (black) adrenal cortical adenoma is characterized by diffuse black pigmentation on cross section (Fig. 14-42), although there may be some areas that are dark-brown or yellow-brown.[151] Pigmented adrenal cortical adenoma is usually diagnosed in the third to the fifth

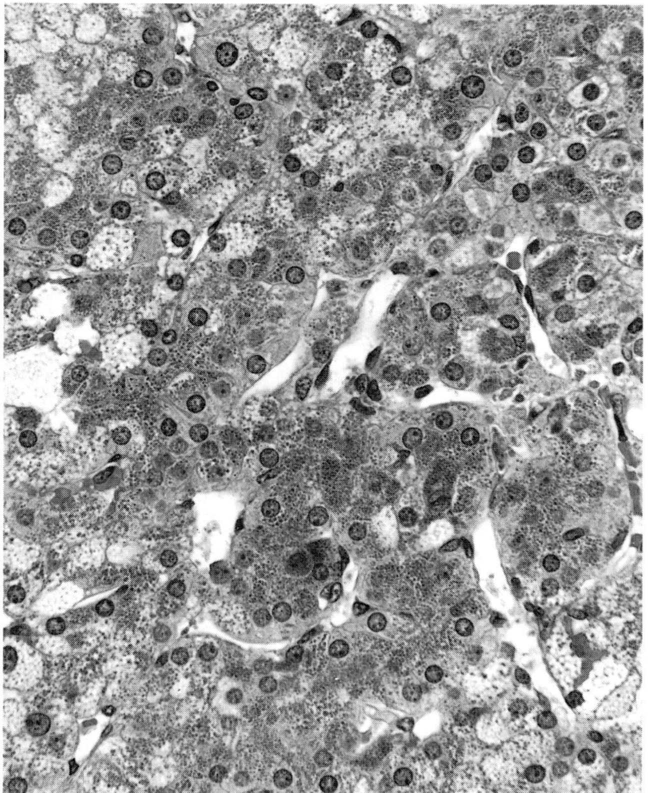

14-43. Pigmented (black) adenoma causing Cushing's syndrome. Tumor cells form nests and short cords and have abundant intracytoplasmic granular lipofuscin pigment.

decades of life, with distinct predilection for females.[141] This tumor is most often associated with Cushing's syndrome, although it has also been reported with primary hyperaldosteronism.[40,141] Microscopically, the architectural patterns are similar to other adenomas. The histologic hallmark is the conspicuous brown or golden-brown granular pigment in the cytoplasm (Fig. 14-43), which has the staining characteristics of lipofuscin. A recent study, however, suggested that some of the pigment may be neuromelanin.[64] As with other adenomas, these may be areas of lipomatous or myelolipomatous metaplasia.[40] Ultrastructurally, the cells contain relatively few lipid globules, but have a variable number of electron-dense granules that are often associated with small lipid vacuoles (Fig. 14-44) characteristic of lipfuscin.[40,141] There are no melanosomes or premelanosomes.

Adrenal cortical neoplasms with virilization or feminization

Adrenal cortical neoplasms associated with virilization or feminization are clinically important because of the potential for malignant behavior. Many have unfavorable gross or microscopic findings such as large size and areas of necrosis. A recent review of adult females with virilizing adrenal cortical tumors found that at least 17% were clinically malignant;[152] an even greater proportion of feminizing adrenal cortical neoplasms were malignant.[153]

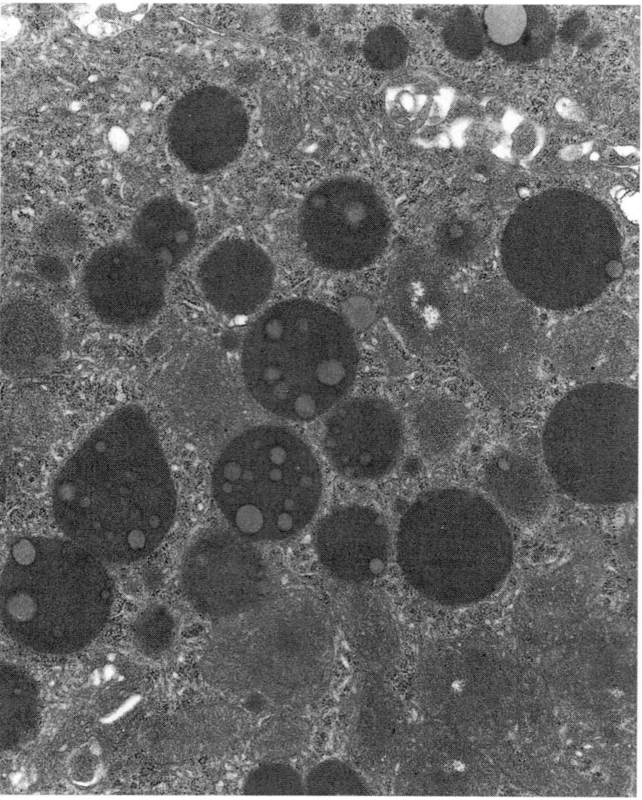

14-44. Black adenoma of adrenal gland from a patient with Cushing's syndrome. Note numerous electron-dense structures, some containing small lipid droplets. (x 17,000)

Histologically, there is often a predominance of compact cells with eosinophilic cytoplasm, but this histologic pattern is not specific. Virilization has also been reported with tumors classified as Leydig cell adenoma of adrenal gland, which contain Reinke crystalloids, a pathognomonic feature of Leydig (or hilus) cells.[154] Rarely, Leydig cells are present in the adrenal cortex, probably because of the close embryologic relation between developing adrenal primordia and gonads.[155]

Adrenal cortical oncocytoma

Rarely adrenal cortical neoplasms are composed of cells with abundant, finely granular, eosinophilic cytoplasm typical of oncocytoma (Fig. 14-45).[156-159] Some of these tumors contain low levels of enzyme activity in cortical steroidogenesis and are considered nonfunctional.[158] Although a number of tumors classified as oncocytoma have had a benign clinical course, an occasional case has proved to be malignant.[160]

Adrenal cortical carcinoma

Incidence and clinical features. Adrenal cortical carcinoma is rare, annually occurring in about two persons per million population in the United States.[161] A number of large series of adrenal cortical carcinoma have been reported in the last few decades, mainly in adult patients. There is a slight female predominance and the peak incidence is in the fifth to seventh decades of life, although there is a second peak in childhood.[162] Presenting signs and symptoms include abdominal pain, palpable mass, fatigue, weight loss, and, in 10% to 20% of patients, intermittent low-grade fever that may be caused by tumor necrosis.[40,141] Regional or distant metastases occur in 25% or more of patients.[40,141,163] Because adrenal cortical carcinomas usually are inefficient producers of steroids, clinical evidence of excess hormone secretion usually does

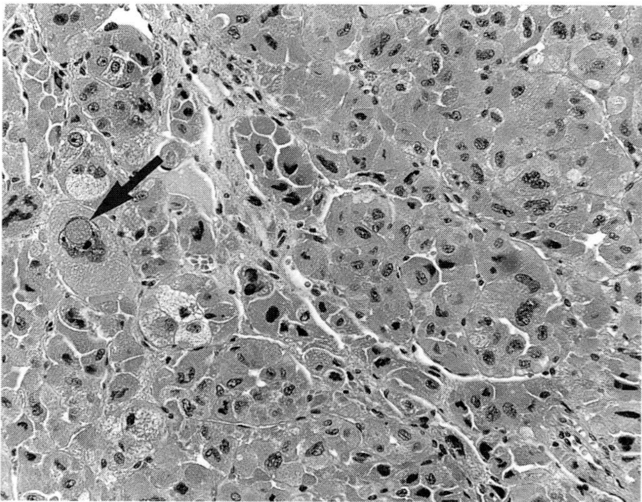

14-45. Incidental nonhyperfunctional adrenal cortical adenoma is composed of cells with abundant, granular eosinophilic cytoplasm (oncocytoma). Nuclei are moderately pleomorphic and hyperchromatic with occasional nuclear "pseudoinclusions" (*arrow*). Tumor weighed less than 15 g.

not become apparent until the tumor is large. Some tumors, therefore, are classified clinically as functionally inactive. When an endocrine syndrome is present, it may be pure, but in some cases is part of a mixed endocrine picture, such as Cushing's syndrome and virilization. Purely virilizing adrenal cortical carcinoma is uncommon in adults, and feminizing adrenal cortical carcinoma is rare. Primary hyperaldosteronism caused by adrenal cortical carcinoma is relatively uncommon.[40,141]

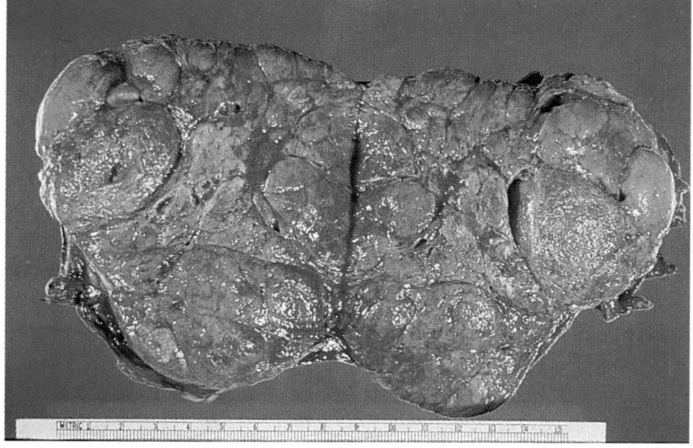

14-46. Adrenal cortical carcinoma. Tumor weighed over 1,000 g.

Pathology. Adrenal cortical carcinoma is usually large, and careful gross examination may often suggest malignancy. The average recorded weight in several series ranged from 705 to 1210 g.[40] Tang and Gray[164] reported that all adrenal cortical tumors over 95 g were malignant, whereas tumors weighing less than 50 g were benign. However, weight alone is not reliable as a distinguishing characteristic, because some small adrenal cortical carcinomas have metastasized, including tumors weighing 40 g or less.[40,141,165] Also, some cortical neoplasms weighing more than 1000 g do not show evidence of malignancy. Adrenal cortical carcinoma may be so large that the adrenal is displaced and difficult to find, and there may be areas of necrosis, hemorrhage, and cystic change.[40,141] Larger tumors are often coarsely lobulated with intersecting fibrous bands. The tumor is usually yellow, yellow-orange (Fig. 14-46), or tan-brown.

Adrenal cortical carcinoma has a variety of architectural patterns, including trabecular, alveolar (nesting), and solid (diffuse) patterns. The most characteristic pattern is a trabecular arrangement of cells with broad anastomosing columns separated by delicate elongate vascular spaces (Fig. 14-47). Some of the trabeculae, when cut in cross section or oblique planes, appear as free floating

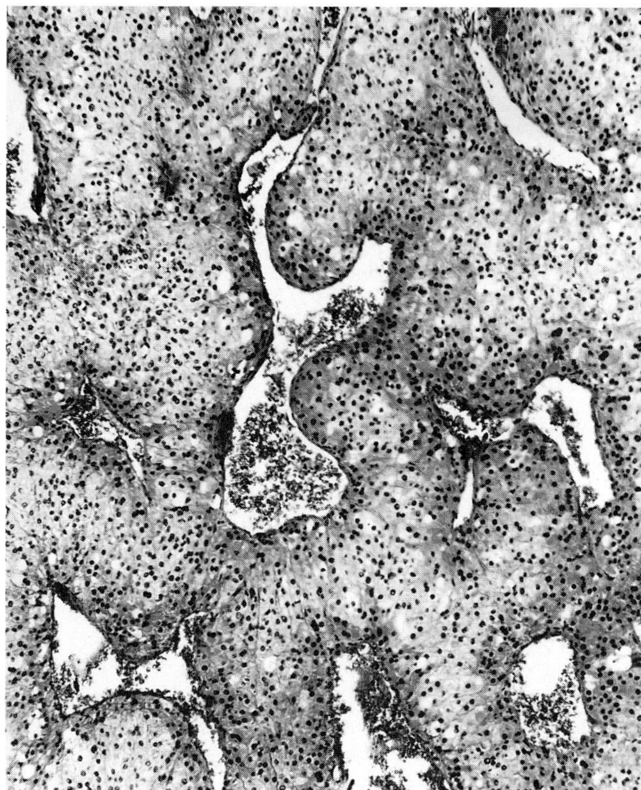

14-47. Adrenal cortical carcinoma. Tumor has broad anastomosing trabeculae and gaping sinusoids with delicate endothelium. Tumor cells have compact, eosinophilic cytoplasm and small, uniform nuclei. Patient died of metastases within a year following diagnosis, and at autopsy had massive invasion of inferior vena cava.

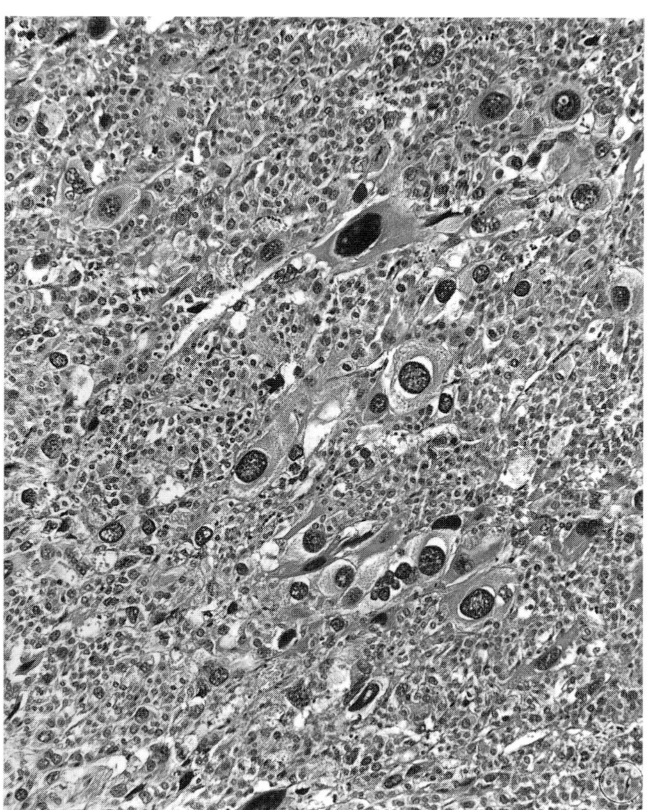

14-48. Adrenal cortical carcinoma. Tumor cells have marked nuclear pleomorphism and hyperchromasia.

islands of tumor cells. Rarely, a pseudoglandular arrangement of cells may be seen, or the tumor may have a myxoid appearance.[40,141] Most tumor cells in adrenal cortical carcinoma have compact, eosinophilic cytoplasm that is poor in lipid. Foci of vascular invasion usually appear as unattached plugs of tumor within vascular spaces. Nuclear pleomorphism and hyperchromasia can be spectacular in adrenal cortical carcinoma (Fig. 14-48), but nuclear atypia alone is not a reliable indicator of malignancy.[40,141] Mitotic figures may be numerous in adrenal cortical carcinoma, and are rare in adenoma and adrenal hyperplasia. In the study by Weiss, only two nonmetastasizing adrenal cortical tumors contained fewer than 3 mitotic figures per 50 high power fields (hpf), whereas 78% of adrenal cortical carcinoma cases contained more than five mitotic figures per hpf, and 17% had more than 50 per 50 hpf.[166]

An unusual feature of adrenal cortical carcinoma (and some adenomas) is the presence of intracytoplasmic hyaline globules, similar to those commonly seen in pheochromocytomas.[167] An alveolar growth pattern and cells with compact, eosinophilic cytoplasm and intracytoplasmic globules in adrenal cortical carcinoma may be mistaken for pheochromocytoma. Another pitfall in the diagnosis of adrenal cortical neoplasms is immunoreactivity for synaptophysin, a marker that is used for documenting neuroendocrine differentiation.[168,169] Ultrastructurally, intracytoplasmic lipid vacuoles are often sparse or absent and cellular organelles may be moderate or few in number.[170] There may be flattened cisternae of rough endoplasmic reticulum in stacks or short parallel lamellae. Smooth endoplasmic reticulum may form an intricate anastomosing network.

Clinical behavior. A number of studies have proposed histologic criteria to predict malignant behavior. Hough et al[171] reported that the stongest predictors were broad fibrous bands, diffuse growth pattern, and vascular invasion. Weiss[166] analyzed the predictive value of nine histologic parameters and found that recurrence or metastasis occured only in tumors with a mitotic rate greater than five per hpf, atypical mitotic figures, and invasion of venous structures. Van Slooten et al[172] used a histologic index based on seven histologic parameters to predict outcome. Despite these findings, it is clear that a small but significant number of adrenal cortical neoplasms have unpredictable clinical behavior, and long-term follow-up in troublesome cases is the final arbiter in diagnosis.[141] Mitotic rate has been used to separate low-grade and high-grade adrenal cortical carcinoma; the median survival for patients with low-grade adrenal cortical carcinoma ($\leq$ 20 mitotic figures per 50 hpf) was 58 months compared with 14 months for high-grade tumors (> 20 mitotic figures per 50 hpf).[173] DNA ploidy analysis has also been used to predict outcome but the results have been controversial.[40,141,174-177] According to some investigators, the greatest value of DNA ploidy analysis may be predictive of outcome in patients undergoing potentially curative surgical resection.[178]

The pattern of metastasis of adrenal cortical carcinoma reflects both lymphatic and hematogenous dissemination. The sites of metastases in patients dying of adrenal cortical carcinoma included liver (92%), lung (78%), retroperitoneum (48%), intra-abdominal lymph nodes (32%), intrathoracic lymph nodes (26%), and other sites such as bone.[141]

Cytologic features and immunohistochemistry. Percutaneous fine needle aspiration may be helpful in the preoperative diagnosis of adrenal cortical carcinoma, but extreme caution must be exercised in trying to differentiate adrenal cortical carcinoma from a benign adrenal cortical neoplasm on cytologic features alone.[40,141] Careful correlation with clinical and endocrinologic data is needed, combined with a knowledge of other factors such as tumor size and imaging characteristics.

The differential diagnosis of adrenal cortical carcinoma may be aided by special stains, including immunohistochemistry. Adrenal cortical carcinoma does not have a pathognomonic immunohistochemical profile. Several studies indicate that most tumors are positive for vimentin and negative for epithelial markers such as cytokeratin.

Other adrenal cortical neoplasms

Several examples of adrenal carcinosarcoma have been reported in adults, consisting of mixtures of sarcomatous elements and adrenal cortical carcinoma.[179-181] An example of virilizing adrenocortical blastoma was reported in an infant who had an elevated serum level of alpha-fetoprotein.[182]

ADRENAL MEDULLARY NEOPLASMS

Pheochromocytoma

Incidence and clinical features. Pheochromocytoma is an uncommon tumor in surgical pathology practice, with an estimated average annual incidence of eight per million person years (excluding familial cases).[183] It has been suggested that for every pheochromocytoma diagnosed during life, there are two that remain undiscovered, but recent data show more of them diagnosed during life, probably reflecting increased clinical awareness, heightened diagnostic acumen, and more sensitive laboratory testing. Pheochromocytoma has been referred to as the "10% tumor"—10% bilateral, 10% extra-adrenal, 10% malignant, and 10% occurring in childhood, but this is only an approximation that must be correlated with other factors such as tumor location, patient age, and familial predisposition.[4,184] About 95% of cases of sporadic pheochromocytoma in adults are solitary, 5% are bilateral, and 5% to 10% are extra-adrenal in location. Over 50% of cases of familial pheochromocytoma are bilateral, and the tumor may be multicentric within the adrenal gland.[4,184] In childhood, there is an increased incidence of bilateral pheochromocytoma, as well as multicentric and extra-adrenal tumors. The peak incidence is in the fifth decade of life, but pheochromocytoma can occur at virtually any age. Most clinical series report a roughly equal sex incidence.

Pathology. Sporadic pheochromocytoma usually forms a unicentric spherical or oval mass that is often sharply circumscribed and may appear encapsulated. Histologic sections taken at the periphery of the tumor often show a fibrous pseudocapsule or no capsule at all.

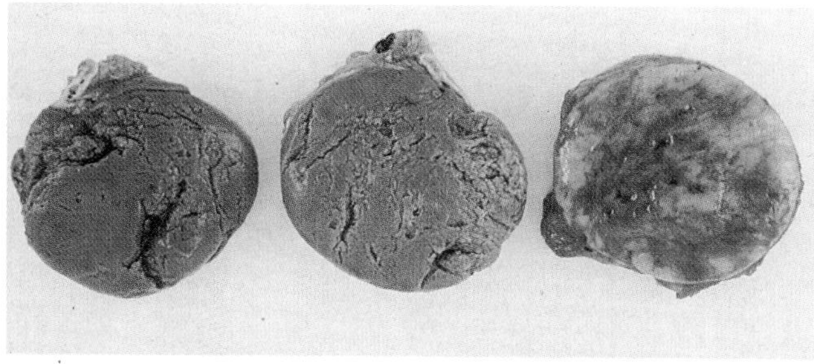

14-49. Pheochromocytoma. Cross section of 3.5 cm tumor on right is fleshy, pale tan with mottled areas of congestion. Two other portions of the same tumor had been fixed in Zenker's solution and show a positive chromaffin reaction with a mahogany brown color.

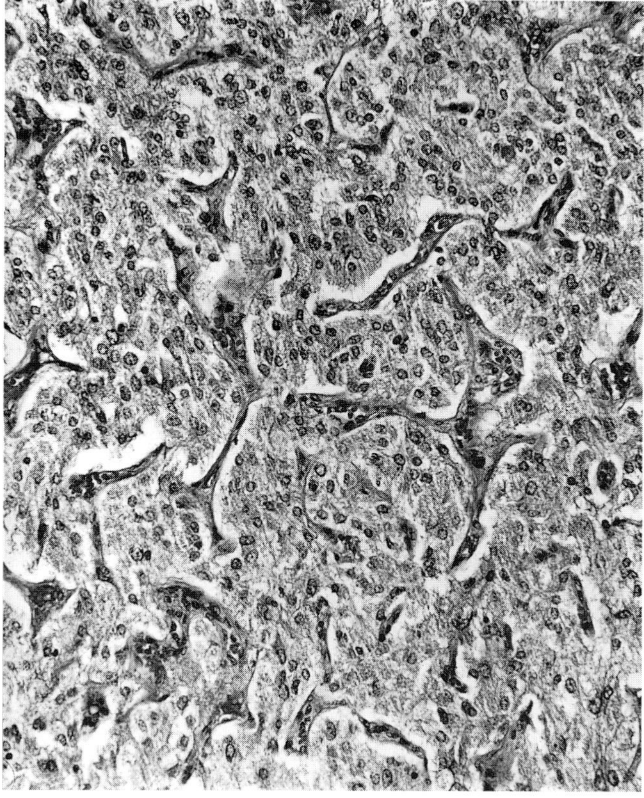

14-50. Pheochromocytoma. Prominent trabecular pattern with anastomosing cords of cells.

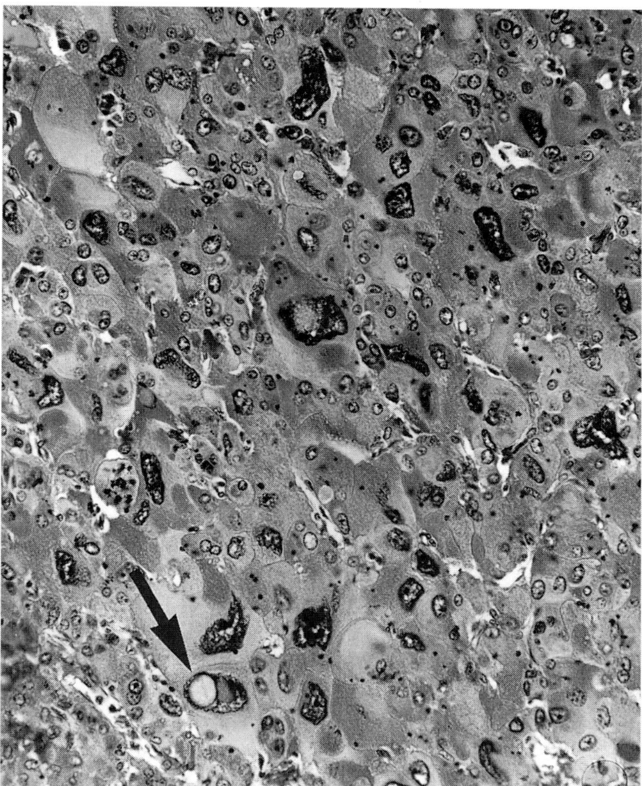

14-51. Pheochromocytoma with solid or diffuse growth pattern. Cells have abundant amphophilic cytoplasm. Note marked nuclear pleomorphism and hyperchromasia as well as nuclear "pseudoinclusion" (*arrow*).

Most pheochromocytomas are 3 to 5 cm in diameter, with an average weight in several large series ranging from 73 to 156.5 g.[4,184] The average weight of clinically malignant tumors tends to be greater than benign tumors. Pheochromocytoma is usually resiliently firm, with a glistening gray-white surface (Fig. 14-49), which may be altered by degenerative changes such as congestion, hemorrhage, or necrosis, and some tumors undergo cystic change that may be marked. Rarely, pheochromocytoma grows into the inferior vena cava, and may extend on into the right atrium, mimicking renal cell carcinoma.[4,184]

Pheochromocytoma usually has an alveolar or trabecular pattern (Fig. 14-50), and the two patterns may be mixed. Occasionally, tumor cells are arranged in a predominantly solid or diffuse pattern (Fig. 14-51). The spindle cell pattern is uncommon and rarely is the dominant feature within the neoplasm. There may be a compressed fibrous pseudocapsule between the pheochromocytoma and adjacent cortex, but sometimes there is no intervening fibrous connective tissue (Fig. 14-52). There may even be intermingling with non-neoplastic cortical cells at the periphery. Alterations in the supporting stroma, including sclerosis, edema, and changes in the vasculature, which could create diagnostic confusion, may also be present. A recent study reported amyloid in 14 of 20 cases of pheochromocytoma (70%), but no electron microscopic illustrations were provided.[185]

The cytoplasm of pheochromocytoma cells is often lightly eosinophilic and finely granular, but it may be basophilic or lavender. Nuclear "pseudoinclusions" have been reported in about one third of pheochromocytoma[4,184] and typically appear as sharply defined round to oval structures that contain cytoplasm having the same staining intensity as the remainder of the cell, although they sometimes appear pale or empty (see Fig. 14-51). These are invaginations of cytoplasm (Fig. 14-53). Some tumors contain cells with prominent nuclear hyperchromasia and pleomorphism, but this is not useful in predicting clinical behavior. Cytoplasmic hyaline globules can be found in some pheochromocytomas and are

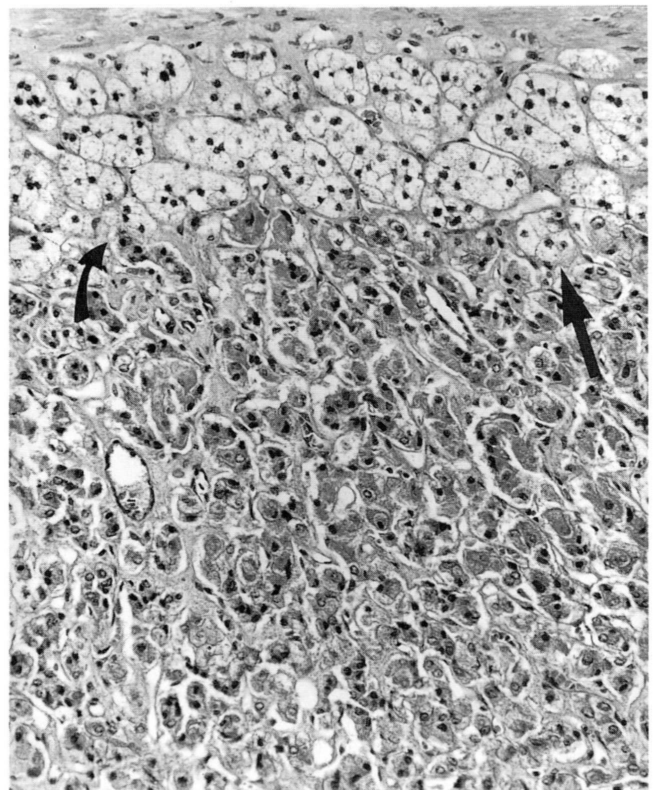

14-52. Pheochromocytoma with an alveolar or nesting pattern. Section taken through periphery of tumor shows junction with residual cortex (*arrows*) and lack of encapsulation.

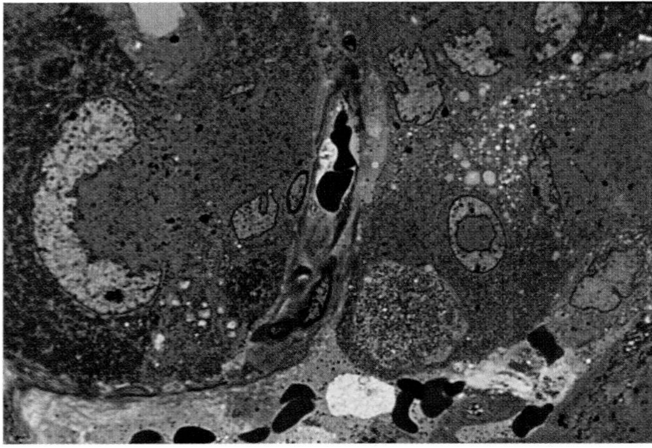

14-53. Pheochromocytoma. Nuclear "pseudoinclusion" is present in right side of field viewed en face. Nucleus of tumor cell on left side shows a deep indentation with jagged border that represents a "pseudoinclusion" viewed in profile. (Toluidine blue stain x 1,000.)

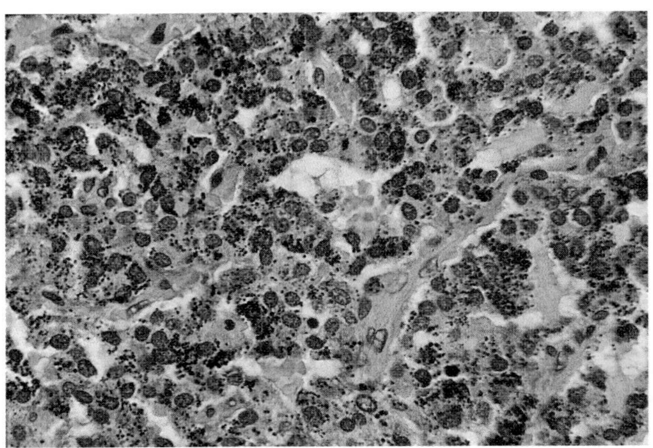

14-54. Pigmented pheochromocytoma with abundant granular pigment that is consistent with lipofuscin. Ultrastructural study revealed no melanosomes or premelanosomes. A heavily pigmented tumor such as this may be mistaken for a pigmented black adenoma or malignant melanoma.

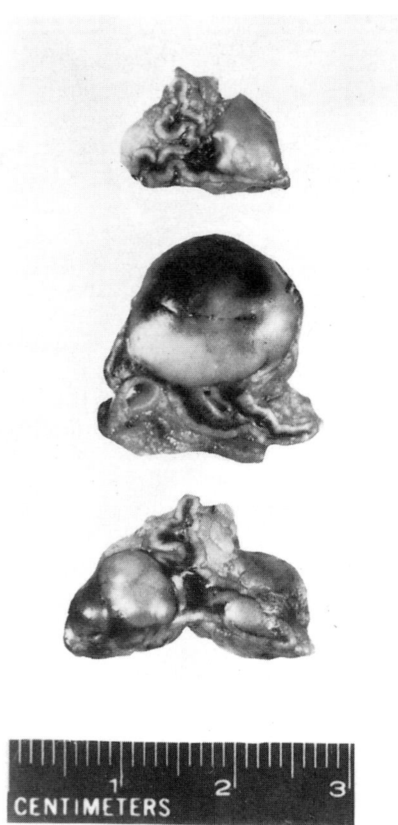

14-55. Multifocal nodular hyperplasia of adrenal medulla with early pheochromocytomas in multiple endocrine neoplasia syndrome type 2a (Sipple's syndrome). The adrenal glands had similar gross appearances. Transverse sections of left adrenal gland show multiple nodules expanding the medullary compartment with the largest nodule 1.5 cm in diameter. *(From Lack EE: Pathology of adrenal and extra-adrenal paraganglia, Vol 29, Major problems in pathology, Philadelphia, 1994, WB Saunders.)*

characteristically PAS-positive and resistant to diastase digestion. The globules are slightly refractile, identical to those seen in medullary chromaffin cells. These globules are detected in almost 50% of cases of sympathoadrenal paraganglioma[186] and are probably related to secretory activity. In some tumors, the cytoplasm is deeply eosinophilic and copious, reminiscent of oncocytic changes. Lipid degeneration gives the cytoplasm a clear vacuolated appearance and can mimic an adrenal cortical neoplasm.[187,188] Some pheochromocytomas contain scattered cells resembling neuronal or ganglion cells with tapering cytoplasmic processes and peripheral aggregation of basophilic material resembling Nissl substance. Periadrenal brown fat may be associated with pheochromocytoma,[189] but its incidence and functional importance are uncertain.[190] Pigmented pheochromocytoma and extraadrenal paraganglioma are extremely rare.[40,191] These tumors may have a jet-black gross appearance caused by an abundance of intracytoplasmic granules of lipofuscin (Fig. 14-54). The differential diagnosis of pigmented (black) adrenal neoplasms includes cortical adenoma, pheochromocytoma, and malignant melanoma (primary or secondary).

Pheochromocytoma in multiple endocrine neoplasia. Multiple endocrine neoplasia syndrome type 2a (Sipple's syndrome) is an autosomal dominant disorder with a high degree of penetrance including various combinations of pheochromocytoma, medullary thyroid carcinoma, and parathyroid hyperplasia. Multiple endocrine neoplasia syndrome type 2b also has an autosomal dominant mode of inheritance, but many patients appear to have the isolated or sporadic form of the disorder. It is possible that clinically aggressive medullary thyroid carcinoma that occurs in this setting causes death at an early age without the patient being able to pass the syndrome on to a future generation.[4] Some cases may be truly sporadic as the result of gene mutations. The pheochromocytomas in multiple endocrine neoplasia types 2a and 2b are frequently multicentric (Fig. 14-55) and bilateral (Fig. 14-56), and in some cases where residual chromaffin tissue is recognizable there may be extratumoral adrenal medullary hyperplasia.[192] Gross morphologic features may be sufficiently distinctive that the surgical pathologist should be alerted to the possibility of the associated syndrome.[4]

The phenotypic expression of multiple endocrine neoplasia type 2b is very distinctive. Medullary thyroid carcinoma in this syndrome is usually aggressive, and recurrence and metastasis pose the most pernicious component.[4] Pheochromocytoma is often preceded by adrenal medullary hyperplasia.[118,119] There is a low incidence of clinical and biochemical hyperfunction of parathyroid glands in contrast to multiple endocrine neoplasia type 2a.[4] There is very characteristic mucosal neuromatous proliferation involving lips, tongue (Fig. 14-57), oral mucosa, and conjunctivae; ganglioneuromatosis may involve the upper aerodigestive tract and lower gastrointestinal tract. This may lead to a variety of intestinal manifestations, including motility disorders and megacolon mimicking Hirschsprung's disease.[4] Other findings include ocular abnormalities such as thickened corneal nerves, conjunctival and eyelid neuromas, and rarely failing vision. Various neuromuscular abnormalities have been described, such as marfanoid habitus, elongated facies, dolichocephaly, laxity of joints, lordosis, kyphosis, pes cavus, and

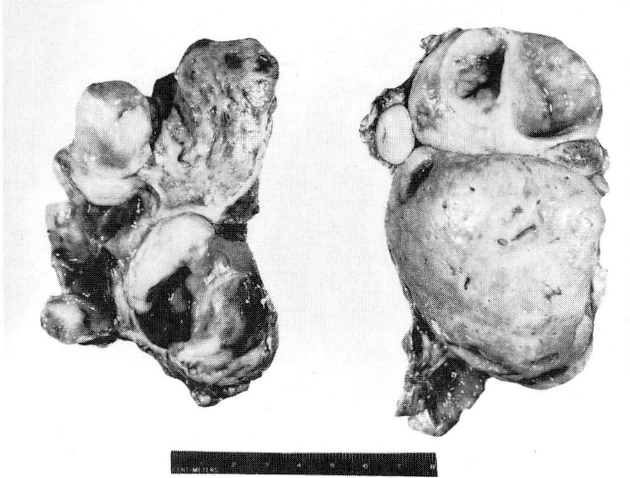

14-56. Bilateral pheochromocytomas in multiple endocrine neoplasia syndrome type 2a. The tumors weighed 168 and 220 g.

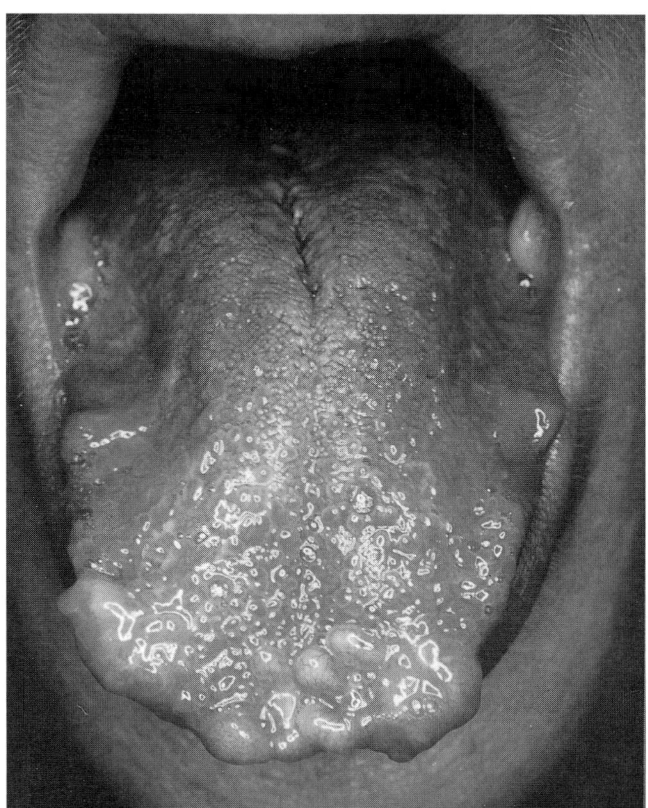

14-57. Patient with multiple endocrine neoplasia syndrome type 2b. Tongue is studded with neuromas, particularly along lateral borders and tip. *(From Lack EE: Adrenal medullary hyperplasia and pheochromocytoma. In Lack EE ed: Pathology of the adrenal glands, New York, 1990, Churchill Livingstone.)*

cox valga. The gastrointestinal manifestations in multiple endocrine neoplasia type 2b are very important to recognize because they form a prominent component of the syndrome, often antedating the endocrine neoplasms.[193]

Composite pheochromocytoma. The term *composite pheochromocytoma* refers to pheochromocytomas in which there is a component that resembles neuroblastoma, ganglioneuroblastoma (Fig. 14-58), ganglioneuroma, or malignant peripheral nerve sheath tumor (malignant schwannoma).[4] A few have secreted vasoactive intestinal peptide, causing the watery diarrhea syndrome. The capacity for synthesis and secretion of vasoactive intestinal peptide is associated with neuronal or ganglionic phenotype. Neoplastic chromaffin cells in vitro may exhibit intense neuritic outgrowth of cell processes, indicative of one of several neuronal characteristics. The existence of composite pheochromocytoma with neural and endocrine features in vivo is ample testimony to the close morphologic and functional kinship of the nervous system and the endocrine system.[4]

Pseudopheochromocytoma. The term *pseudopheochromocytoma* refers to the unusual circumstance of a patient with signs or symptoms of a pheochromocytoma, but on surgical exploration no neoplasm is found. Examples include adrenal medullary hyperplasia, adrenal myelolipoma, renal cyst, coarctation of abdominal aorta, and astrocytoma.[4] Rarely, patients may develop signs and symptoms suggesting pheochromocytoma following surreptitious administration of epinephrine or other agents that produce provocative clinical manifestations.[4]

Immunohistochemistry and other features. The catecholamine synthesizing enzymes, tyrosine hydroxylase, dopamine-ß-hydroxylase, and phenylethanolamine N-methyltransferase have been identified in pheochromocytoma, and correlate with the functional capacity of this tumor to produce norepinephrine and epinephrine.[4] The ratio of epinephrine to norepinephrine in the normal adrenal medulla is about 4 to 1, whereas in pheochromocytomas norepinephrine predominates.[4] The immunohistochemical profile of pheochromocytoma is quite broad;[194] it typically contains neuron-specific enolase and other neuroendocrine markers, such as chromogranin A and synaptophysin. Pheochromocytoma can also express a broad array of other regulatory peptides and hormones, including enkephalins, somatostatin, vasoactive intestinal peptide, substance P, adrenocorticotrophic hormone, and calcitonin.[194] Rare cases are associated with paraneoplastic

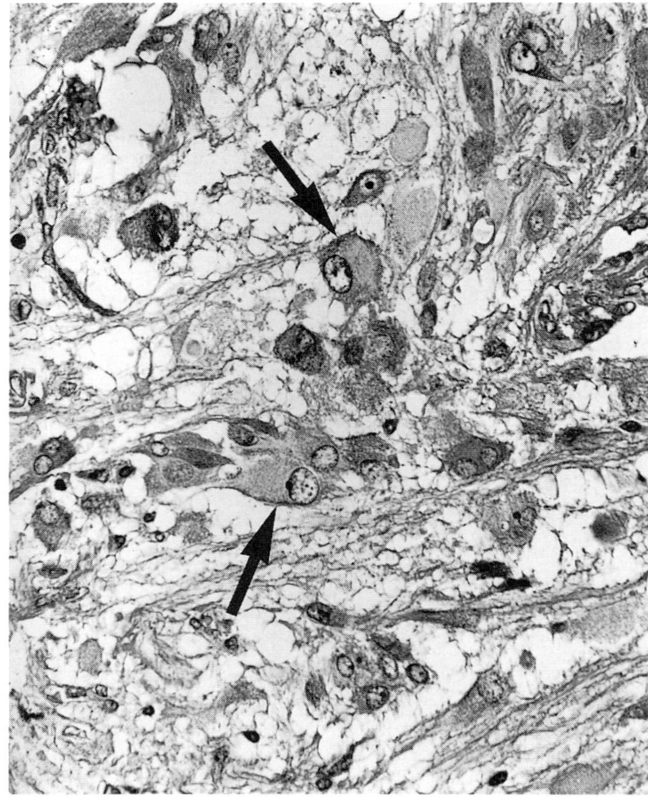

14-58. Composite pheochromocytoma. Cells (*arrows*) have neuronal or ganglionic features with eccentric, prominent nuclei, abundant cytoplasm with distinct borders and tapering extensions, and some have peripheral granular cytoplasmic basophilia consistent with Nissl substance. Note the prominent fibrillar matrix resembling neuropil. Other areas have typical morphology of a pheochromocytoma.

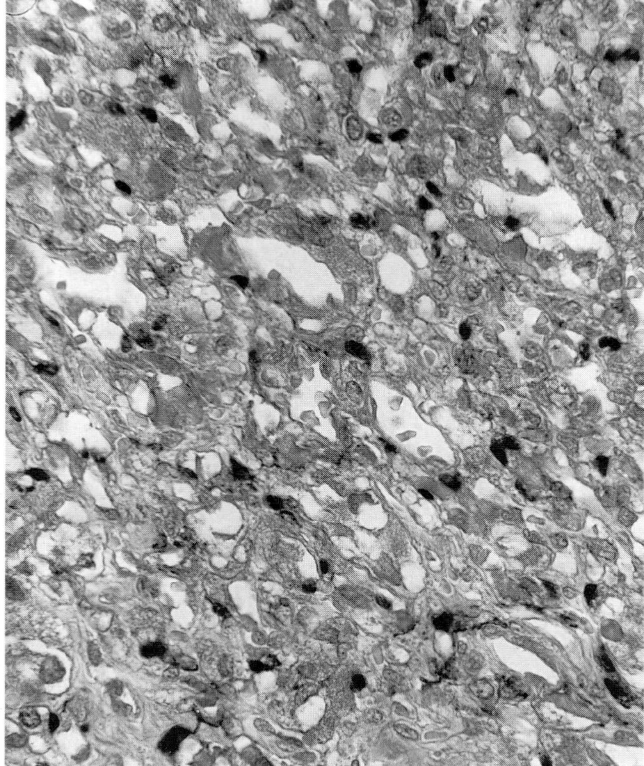

14-59. Pheochromocytoma. Sustentacular cells are demonstrated by immunostaining for S-100 protein, which highlights nuclei and slender cytoplasmic extensions. These cells are located at the periphery of nests and cords of pheochromocytoma cells.

syndrome caused by the secretion of one of the neuropeptides such as vasoactive intestinal peptide with watery diarrhea syndrome and adrenocorticotrophic hormone with Cushing's syndrome.[4]

The ultrastructural hallmark of pheochromocytoma is the presence of dense-core neurosecretory-type granules, which have variable distribution and density within neoplastic cells.[195] Sparse numbers of granules in some cells may help to explain a low to absent intensity of immunostaining for neuroendocrine markers such as chromogranin A. Sustentacular cells are also present in pheochromocytoma, appearing as S-100 protein immunoreactive cells at the periphery of cords and clusters of neoplastic chromaffin cells (Fig. 14-59). Tannenbaum[196] found that granule morphology correlated with catecholamine content as determined biochemically. Two distinct types of granules are recognized; one was associated with norepinephrine storage and had a distinct prominent, eccentric halo or electron lucent space adjacent to the dense core, and the other was associated with epinephrine storage and the granules were more uniform (Fig. 14-60). Given the wide array of neuropeptides and hormones in pheochromocytoma, this distinction based solely on granule morphology is no longer tenable.[4,184] Some granules, in fact, may be quite pleomorphic and may contain more than one peptide.

Fine needle aspiration of pheochromocytoma may create problems in cytologic interpretation, and malignant diagnoses rendered solely on the basis of cytologic and nuclear atypia may be erroneous.[4] Occasional complications have also been reported, including catecholamine crisis with marked alteration in blood pressure, sometimes with uncontrollable intraabdominal hemorrhage.[4] In smear and imprint preparations of pheochromocytoma, nuclei may appear suspended in a syncytium of ill-defined cytoplasm, and there may be considerable variation in nuclear size and shape (Fig. 14-61). Other cytologic features include intranuclear "pseudoinclusions" and enlarged hyperchromatic nuclei, sometimes stripped of cell cytoplasm.[4]

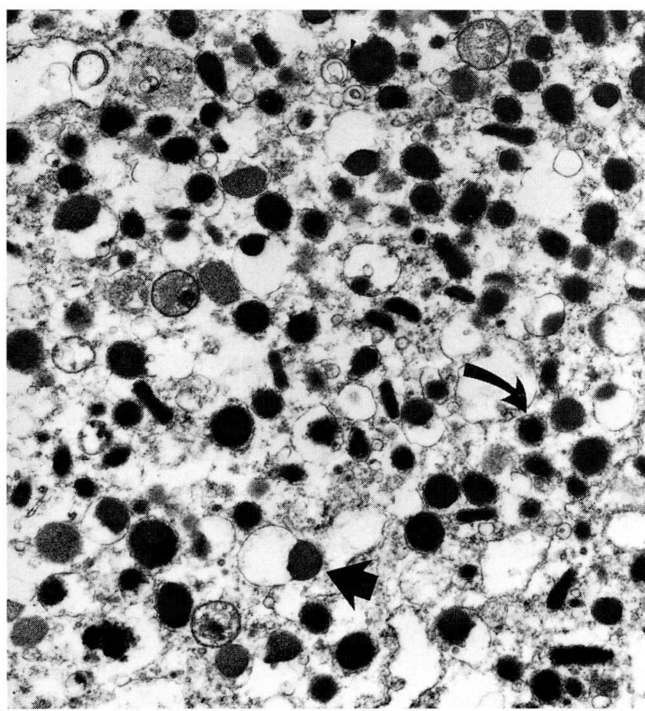

14-60. Pheochromocytoma. Electron micrograph shows numerous dense-core neurosecretory granules; some granules have an investing membrane with uniform thin halo (*curved arrow*) while other granules have an eccentric dense core with wide asymmetric halo (*straight arrow*). Other neurosecretory granules are pleomorphic. (x 15,000)

Clinical behavior. The incidence of clinically malignant adrenal pheochromocytoma is relatively low, and it is important to consider these separately from extra-adrenal paraganglioma which have a significantly higher incidence of malignant behavior.[4] Early reviews cite a frequency of malignant behavior in adrenal pheochromocytoma of 2.4% to 2.8% in adults,[197-199] while 2.4% were malignant in children.[198] Recent studies show an incidence of malignancy ranging from 7% to 14%.[4] It is notoriously difficult on gross and histologic evaluation to predict which tumors are malignant. The histology of benign and malignant pheochromocytoma overlaps to such an extent that the most important criterion acceptable for malignancy is the presence of metastases in sites where non-neoplastic chromaffin tissue is not normally found.[200] Flow cytometry studies suggest that ploidy may be an independent prognostic factor: none of the patients with diploid tumors died of pheochromocytoma.[201,202] Aneuploid histograms have been reported in pheochromocytoma, which are clinically benign or cured by surgery. A low proportion (or absence) of S-100 protein immunoreactive cells has also been correlated with malignant behavior of paraganglioma,[203,204] but it may not be a reliable discriminator in the evaluation of individual cases.[205]

Neuroblastoma and ganglioneuroblastoma

Incidence and age distribution. Neuroblastoma rates fourth in frequency of malignant tumors in patients under 15 years of age, exceeded only by

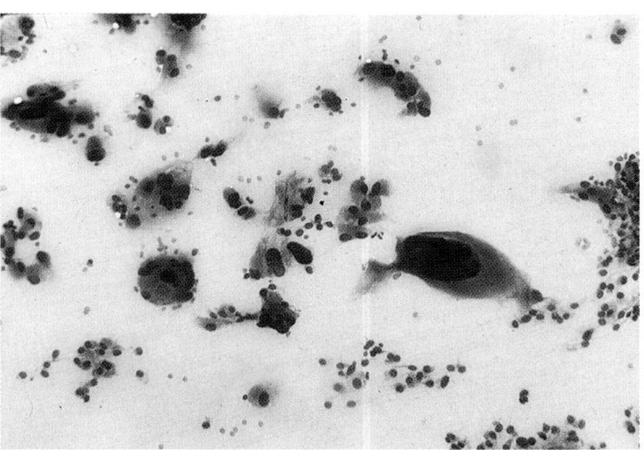

14-61. Pheochromocytoma. Touch imprint smear of resected tumor shows marked variation in nuclear size, which might lead to a presumptive diagnosis of malignancy. (Diff Quik stain)

leukemia, malignant lymphoma, and brain tumors.[4] The incidence of neuroblastoma is estimated at 8.7 per million and ganglioneuroblastoma is 1.8 per million population per year.[4] There are no apparent sex-related differences in incidence rates. In a series of 118 patients from Boston Children's Hospital, 88% were 5 years of age or younger at diagnosis, with a median age of 21 months.[206] Neuroblastoma and ganglioneuroblastoma are rare in the second decade of life, and exceedingly rare in adults. Occasionally, neuroblastoma appears in multiple members of a family, and some data suggest an autosomal dominant pattern of inheritance, but there are obvious difficulties in determining the incidence and penetrance of an inherited susceptibility because of the capacity for regression or spontaneous maturation, as well as early death and long-term treatment complications that prevent reproduction and evaluation of multiple pedigrees.[207,208] Neuroblastoma and ganglioneuroblastoma may be associated with watery diarrhea syndrome caused by vasoactive intestinal peptide production, Cushing's syndrome, opsoclonus/myoclonus, and alopecia. Heterochromia iridis has also been reported with mediastinal and cervical neuroblastoma and ganglioneuroma.[4,209]

Screening programs for neuroblastoma. The first screening for neuroblastoma began in Japan in 1974, and others have followed.[4,210] Screening in Japan has resulted in an increased annual detection rate for these tumors (93 per million) compared with the baseline rate of 13.3 per million. Children are screened at 6 months of age with a qualitative vanillylmandelic acid spot test. The prognosis for children with neuroblastoma detected by screening is favorable because of low clinical stage and early age at diagnosis, both independent prognostic factors.[4] Most children are considered to be in a low-risk subgroup with potential for spontaneous regression, thus accounting for the substantial increase of newly diagnosed cases of neuroblastoma through screening.[211]

Anatomic distribution of primary tumors. The distribution of neuroblastoma and ganglioneuroblastoma parallels that of the sympathetic nervous system with tumors arising anywhere from the neck to the pelvis. The anatomic distribution of primary tumors in a report of 118 patients was as follows: intraabdominal (67.8%), with most arising in the adrenal glands (38.1%) and 29.7% being nonadrenal; intrathoracic (20.3%); cervical (3.4%); pelvic (3.4%); and in 5.1%, precise anatomic origin was undetermined.[206] Patients with neuroblastoma and ganglioneuroblastoma may have spinal cord compression caused by extradural intraspinal ("dumbbell") configuration of the tumor; similar spinal cord compression may be occasionally seen with ganglioneuroma.[4]

TABLE 14-1.
STAGING SYSTEM PROPOSED BY THE INTERNATIONAL STAGING SYSTEM WORKING PARTY WITH INCIDENCE AND SURVIVAL ACCORDING TO STAGE OF TUMOR AT DIAGNOSIS

	Staging Criteria	Incidence	Survival at 5 Years
Stage 1	Localized tumor confined to the area of origin, complete gross excision, with or without microscpoic residual disease; identifiable ipsilateral and contralateral lymph nodes negative microscopically	5%	90% or greater
Stage IIa	Unilateral tumor with incomplete, gross excision; identifiable ipsilateral and contralateral lymph nodes negative microscopically	10%	70-80%
Stage IIb	Unilateral tumor with complete or incomplete gross excision; with positive ipsilateral regional lymph nodes; identifiable contralateral lymph nodes negative microscopically		
Stage III	Tumor infiltrating across the midline with or without regional lymph node involvement; or, midline tumor with bilateral regional lymph node involvement	25%	40-70% (depending on completeness of surgical resection)
Stage IV	Dissemination of the tumor to distant lymph nodes, bone, bone marrow, liver and/or other organs (except as defined in stage IV-S)	60%	More than 60% if age at diagnosis is younger than 1 year; 20% if age at diagnosis is older than 1 year and under 2 years; 10% if age at diagnosis is over 2 years.
Stage IVS	Localized primary tumor as defined for stage I or II with dissemination limited to liver, skin, and/or bone marrow	5%	More than 80%

From Philip T: Overview of current treatment of neuroblastoma, Am J Pediatr Hematol/Oncol 14:97-102, 1992.

Staging classification and prognosis. The staging classification proposed by Evans et al has been popular for decades and continues to provide valuable prognostic information.[4,212] An interim working staging system has also been proposed and incidence as well as survival data are shown in Table 14-1 based on stage at diagnosis.[213] From 60% to 70% of patients with neuroblastoma and ganglioneuroblastoma have metastases at the time of presentation (i.e., stages IV and IV-S), while 30% to 40% of patients have localized disease (stages I, II, and III).[4] Children with a tumor primary in the cervical, intrathoracic, or pelvic areas have a better prognosis stage-for-stage compared with patients with intraabdominal primaries, but a disproportionate number may have low-stage tumor or are less than 2 years of age and frequently less than 1 year of age at diagnosis.[4] Other staging classifications of neuroblastoma and ganglioneuroblastoma have been proposed. The international staging system yields an incidence and 5 year survival (see Table 14-1).[213]

In situ neuroblastoma. The term *in situ* neuroblastoma refers to a small nodule of cells within the adrenal that is histologically indistinguishable from childhood neuroblastoma, without evidence of tumor elsewhere in the body.[214] In the series by Beckwith and Perrin,[214] the nodules ranged in size from 0.7 to 9.5 mm in diameter. The incidence is estimated to be 1 per 224 infants. In situ neuroblastoma is about 45 times more common than clinical neuroblastoma. The obvious conclusion, if these lesions are indeed neoplastic, is that many undergo spontaneous involution or maturation, or remain clinically occult. It may be difficult to distinguish nodules of neuroblastic cells that are a normal part of the embryologic development of the adrenal gland (see Figure 14-8) from in situ neuroblastoma.[4,209,215]

Stage IV-S neuroblastoma. Stage IV-S (S = special) neuroblastoma refers to a distinct group of patients with neuroblastoma metastatic to liver, skin, or bone marrow without radiologic or other evidence of bone metastases.[4,209,216] These children usually have a small adrenal primary, but in a minority of cases no primary can be identified.[217] The patients are usually young with a median age of about 3 months. The prognosis is good with survival rates of 80% or more, and many of the tumors undergo spontaneous regression. There is a small subset of children with stage IV-S neuroblastoma whose

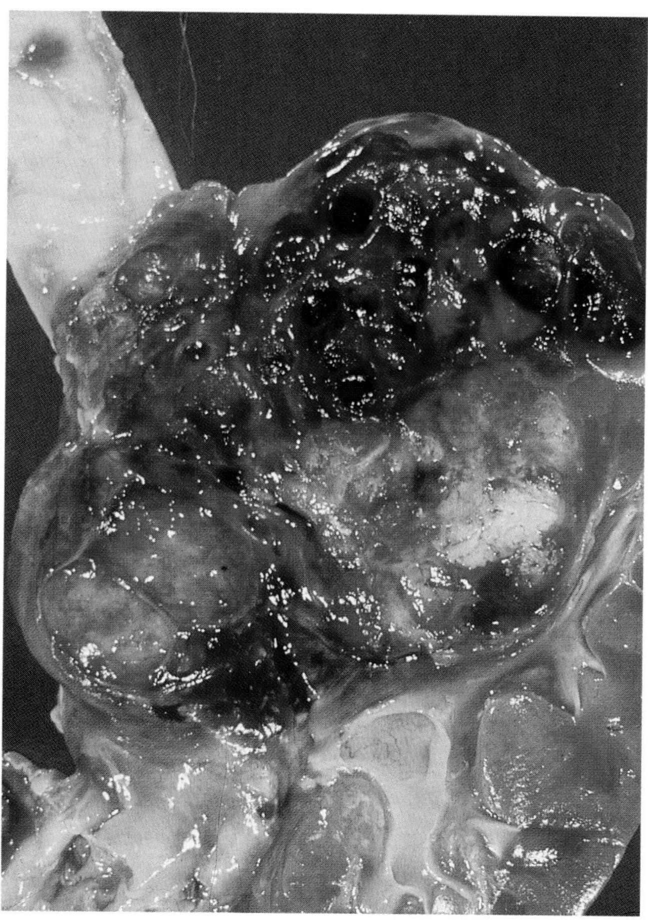

14-62. Neuroblastoma at autopsy virtually replaces entire adrenal gland and compresses adjacent kidney. Cut surface of tumor has coarse lobulations and is hemorrhagic.

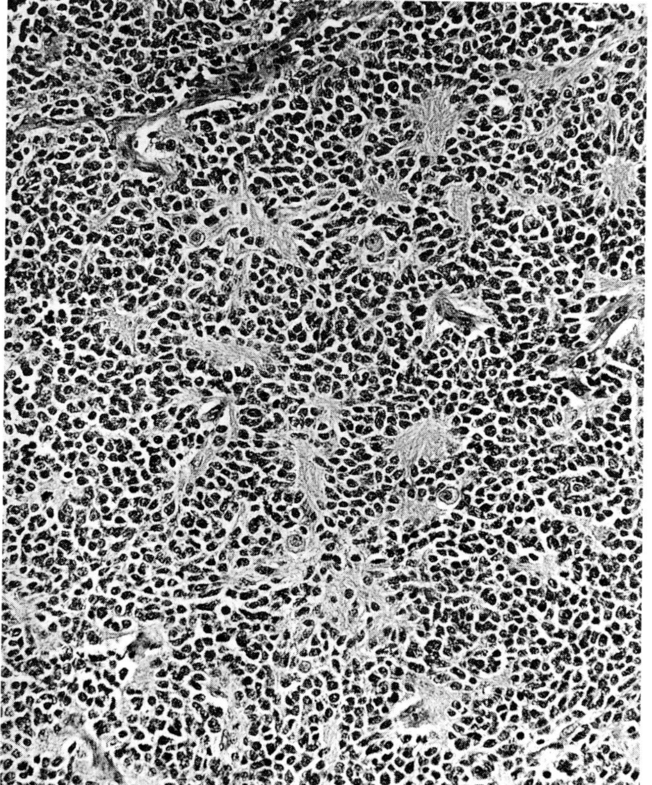

14-63. Neuroblastoma (stroma-poor in the Shimada classification). The cells are closely packed with indistinct cellular borders. Note the Homer Wright rosettes. Some fibrillar material forms perivascular pseudorosettes.

tumor is diagnosed in the first 6 weeks of life with marked abdominal distention caused by massive liver involvement by neuroblastoma. The outlook for these patients is less favorable because massive enlarging hepatomegaly may cause secondary complications such as compromise in cardiorespiratory function.[218] Some authors speculate that stage IV-S neuroblastoma is a mass of hyperplastic nodules of mutated cells that lack the genetic events for transformation into overtly malignant tumor such as neuroblastoma.[219]

Pathology. Gross pathology. Neuroblastoma and ganglioneuroblastoma usually present as a solitary unicentric mass or confluent mass of nodules. Rarely, the tumors grow into the inferior vena cava and measure up to 10 cm or larger.[4,209] On cross section, they are variable in appearance and consistency depending upon the amount of immature neuroblastic tissue. Usually, the tumors have coarse lobulations with areas of hemorrhage and necrosis (Fig. 14-62). Viable tumors may appear pale-gray and have a soft encephaloid consistency.

Microscopic pathology. Neuroblastoma and ganglioneuroblastoma often have a lobular growth pattern with delicate, incomplete fibrovascular septa but some cases have a diffuse or solid pattern. There is a continuum in the morphologic appearance of neuroblastoma and ganglioneuroblastoma.[4,220] Within this morphologic spectrum there may be patterns merging imperceptibly with ganglioneuroblastoma, which are well-differentiated (Shimada stroma predominant, well-differentiated category) and simulate mature ganglioneuroma; at the other end of the spectrum, the tumor pattern is that of undifferentiated neuroblastoma.[4,209,221] Typical Homer Wright rosettes can be found in some tumors (Fig. 14-63),[222] and there may be broad matted tangles of neuritic processes. The degree of ganglion cell differentiation varies from tumor to tumor, and even within the same tumor. The nuclei of neuroblastoma often have a stippled or dispersed "salt and pepper" pattern of nuclear chromatin (Fig. 14-64). Anaplastic neuroblastoma has marked cellular and nuclear pleomorphism,[223] but this finding has no apparent impact on survival after controlling for stage.[224]

Morphologic evidence of ganglion cell differentiation includes nuclear enlargement, increased amount of eosinophilic cytoplasm, distinct cell borders, prominent nucleolus, and peripheral granular material within the cytoplasm that represents Nissl substance (Fig. 14-65). A variety of stromal alterations may be seen in neuroblastoma and ganglioneuroblastoma, including hemorrhage, necrosis, dystrophic calcification, and marked cystic degeneration.[4,209] Cystic neuroblastoma may simulate adrenal cyst or hematoma. Immunostaining for S-100 protein highlights slender, dendritic cells near fibrovascular septa, which represent satellite cells or indicate differentiation into Schwann cells. Large numbers of S-100 protein immunoreactive cells in undifferentiated neuroblastoma are associated with a good prognosis;[225] conversely, large numbers of ferritin-positive cells are associated with a poor prognosis.[4] Ultrastructural characteristics of neuroblastoma and ganglioneuroblastoma include neuritic extensions with neurofilaments, neurotubules, and dense-core neurosecretory granules, which are usually sparse in number (Fig. 14-66).[195]

Grading. A variety of grading systems have been proposed for childhood neuroblastoma and ganglioneuroblastoma. Beckwith and Martin[226] recognized four grades of differentiation; grade I has the highest level of ganglion cell differentiation with good survival, and grade IV is undifferentiated with poor survival. Other grading sys-

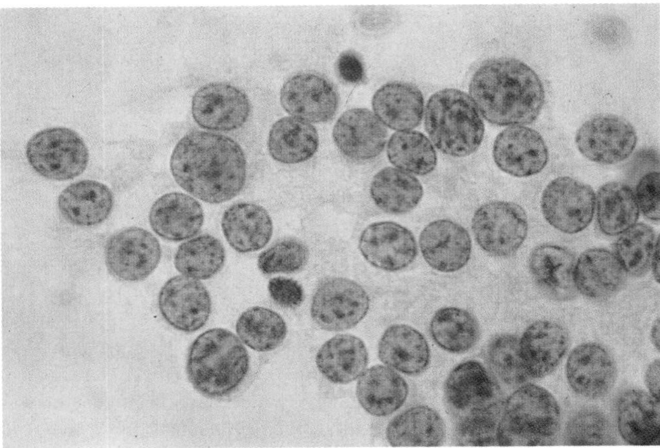

14-64. Touch imprint of neuroblastoma (stroma-poor in the Shimada classification). Nuclei have dispersed chromatin ("salt and pepper" nuclei), and are separated by pale pink cytoplasm with indistinct borders.

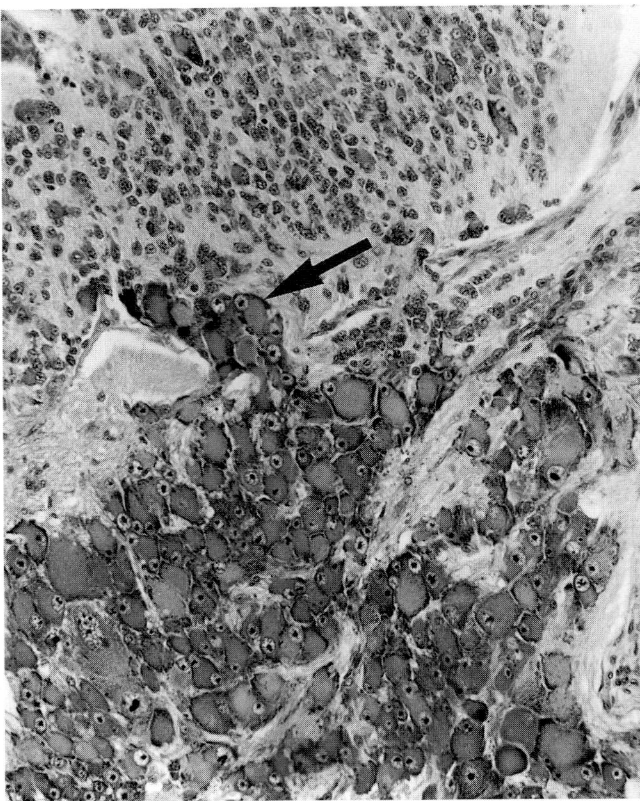

14-65. Ganglioneuroblastoma with well-developed ganglion cells (*arrow*).

tems employed three levels of differentiation.[4,227] In 1984, Shimada et al[228] introduced age-linked grading of neuroblastoma, based on the patient's age at diagnosis, degree of maturation or percent of differentiating elements, and the mitosis-karyorrhexis index. The stroma-rich category shows extensive growth of Schwannian and other supporting elements with three groups (Fig. 14-67): the well differentiated and intermixed groups have a favorable prognosis (92% to 100% 5 year survival), and the nodular group has an unfavorable prognosis (18% survival). The stroma-poor category has two groups (Fig. 14-68): the favorable stroma-poor group has a 5 year survival of 84%, and the unfavorable stroma-poor group has a 5 year survival of 4.5%. Several studies have supported the utility of the Shimada grading system.[229,230]

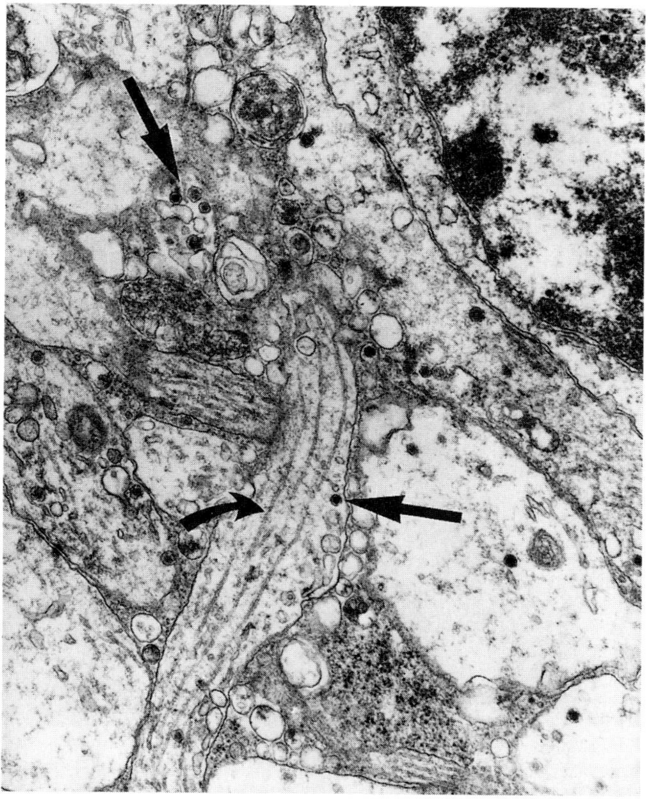

14-66. Neuroblastoma. Neuritic processes contain microtubules (*curved arrow*) and sparse numbers of dense core neurosecretory granules (*straight arrows*). (x 27,000)

A new histologic grading system was proposed by Joshi et al[231] in which the grade of the neoplasm was based on the mitotic rate or presence of calcification. Two risk groups were defined: the low-risk group consisted of patients in both age groups (< 1 year and > 1 year) with grade 1 tumors (i.e., low mitotic rate [< 10 per 10 hpf], calcifications present) and patients less than 1 year of age with grade 2 tumors (low mitotic rate or calcification present), and the high-risk group consisted of patients greater than 1 year of age with grade 2 tumors and patients in both age groups with grade 3 tumors (high mitotic rate [> 10 per 10 hpf], no calcification). A high degree of concordance was seen between the low-risk and high-risk groups (84%) and the favorable and unfavorable histology groups in the Shimada classification. The survival curves, therefore, are very similar.[231]

Clinical behavior. A fascinating aspect of these neoplasms is occasional spontaneous regression or maturation into fully mature ganglioneuroma.[4,232] The concept of Collins' law[233] has been applied to children with neuroblastoma, which gives a rough approximation of the doubling time of a tumor measured as a period of risk that is equal to the patients age at diagnosis plus 9 months. According to this concept, a child with neuroblastoma who has not been cured of the tumor will relapse within this time span; older children, therefore, must theoretically be followed for a much longer period of time because of the expanded period of risk. Two syndromes of metastatic neuroblastoma can be found in the early literature; the Pepper syndrome with prominent hepatic metastases and the Hutchison syndrome with skull metastases presenting at a somewhat later age.[234] The cases described as Pepper in 1901 probably correspond to stage IV-S neuroblastoma.[4]

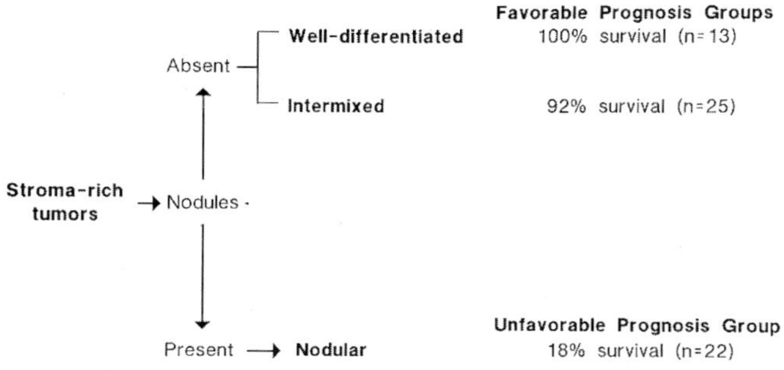

14-67. Stroma-rich neuroblastoma according to the Shimada age-linked classification. Survival data are indicated for the favorable and unfavorable groups. *(From Lack EE: Pathology of adrenal and extra-adrenal paraganglia, Vol 29, Major problems in pathology, Philadelphia, 1994, WB Saunders.)*

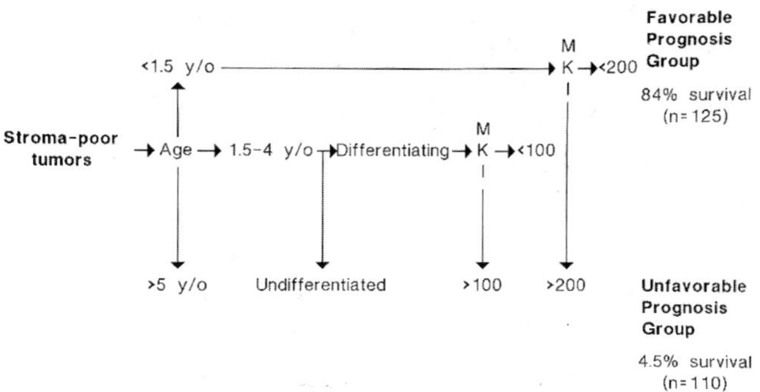

14-68. Stroma-poor neuroblastoma according to the Shimada age-linked classification. Favorable and unfavorable prognosis groups are indicated along with survival data. *(From Lack EE: Pathology of adrenal and extra-adrenal paraganglia, Vol 29, Major problems in pathology, Philadelphia, 1994, WB Saunders.)*

Because there is no correlation between the laterality of the adrenal tumor and the pattern of metastases, the concept of these syndromes is obsolete. Metastatic spread of neuroblastoma and ganglioneuroblastoma occurs by both hematogenous and lymphatic routes, with involvement of sites such as bone and lymph nodes. Cranial involvement by metastatic neuroblastoma is usually confined to calvarial bone, leptomeninges, and dura with intrinsic involvement of brain parenchyma being very rare.[4]

Ganglioneuroma

Ganglioneuroma consists of mature or mildly dysmorphic ganglion cells set in an abundant mixture of mature Schwann cells.[4] This benign tumor is usually located in the posterior mediastinum; it may also be seen in the retroperitoneum; it is relatively uncommon in the adrenal gland.[4] Ganglioneuroma typically presents as a circumscribed tumor that is firm, rubbery, and gray-white to tan-yellow (Fig. 14-69). Grossly, ganglioneuroma may have a trabecular or whorled appearance reminiscent of leiomyoma. Larger tumors may have degenerative features such as hemorrhage and cystic change. Histologically, there is often considerable variation in the distribution and density of ganglion cells; areas with a paucity or absence of ganglion cells may be mistaken for a neurofibroma. Ganglion cells may be exceedingly well differentiated with Nissl substance, and complete or partial collarette of cells resembling satellite cells, and some ganglion cells, may contain granular tan to brown pigment (Fig. 14-70).

Whether ganglioneuroma arises de novo or by maturation (differentiation) of a preexisting neuroblastoma or ganglioneuroblastoma remains controversial. Transformation of ganglioneuroma to malignant peripheral nerve sheath tumor (malignant schwannoma) has been rarely observed.[4,40] In some cases, malignant schwannoma has arisen de novo without any history of chemotherapy, radiation treatment, or von Recklinghausen's disease, but other cases have developed following radiation therapy. There have also been a few examples of adrenal ganglioneuroma with hilus or Leydig cells containing typical crystalloids of Reinke;[235] the tumor reported by Aguirre and Sculley[236] was associated with masculinization.

OTHER ADRENAL TUMORS

Malignant lymphoma

Malignant lymphoma secondarily involving the adrenal usually occurs in the setting of widespread high stage tumor, with an incidence of 18% to 25% of fatal cases.[4,123] Bilateral adrenal involvement is present in 9% of cases of Hodgkin's disease and 18% of non-Hodgkin's malignant lymphoma.[123] Malignant lymphoma rarely presents primarily in the adrenal without detectable extraadrenal involvement. Addison's disease may rarely result from massive involvement of the adrenal glands by malignant lymphoma, and the adrenal cortical insufficiency may resolve following treatment with combination chemotherapy.[40,123] Adrenal insufficiency has also been reported with a form of malignant lymphoma with prominent vascular involvement, previously referred to as malignant lymphomatosis or malignant angioendotheliomatosis. Plasmacytoma presenting primarily in the adrenal gland is extremely unusual[237] and may represent the early stage of malignant lymphoma with plasmacytoid features.[123]

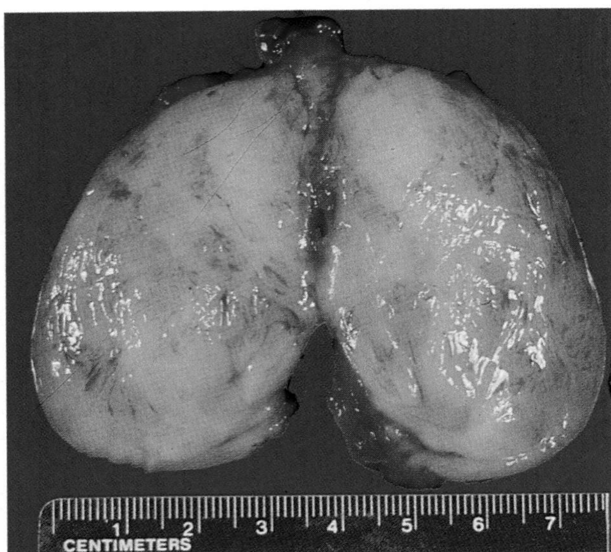

14-69. Ganglioneuroma is homogeneous pale tan on cross section. The tumor was 7 cm x 5 cm x 4 cm.

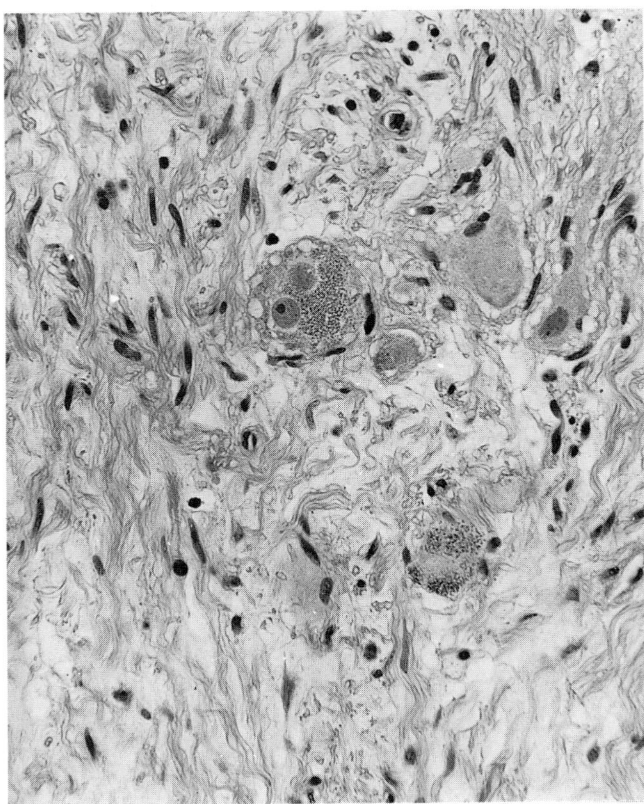

14-70. Ganglioneuroma. Ganglion cells mingle with Schwann cells. Some ganglion cells contain granular neuromelanin pigment.

Mesenchymal tumors

Vascular neoplasms. Primary angioformative neoplasms of the adrenal glands are extremely unusual. Adrenal hemangioma may be found incidentally at autopsy, but several cases have been detected during life as a surgical lesion. Visceral hemangioma may also occur in the setting of hereditary hemorrhagic telangiectasia (Rendu-Osler-Weber syndrome), but adrenal involvement is very rare.[123] Adrenal hemangioma is usually of the cavernous type although capillary hemangioma has also been reported. Angiosarcoma may occur in the adrenal gland and may have epithelioid features[238] that include the presence of epithelial-specific immunohistochemical markers such as cytokeratin.[239]

Smooth muscle neoplasms. Both leiomyoma and leiomyosarcoma occur rarely in the adrenal, with histologic features similar to smooth muscle neoplasms occurring in other sites.[40,240]

Other rare soft tissue tumors. Neurilemoma and neurofibroma arising in the adrenal gland are extremely unusual.[40] Malignant peripheral nerve sheath tumor (malignant schwannoma) has also been reported,[241] and, in one case, was part of a composite pheochromocytoma.[40]

Malignant melanoma

Primary melanoma of the adrenal gland is extremely rare and highly malignant, usually occurring in middle-aged individuals.[40] Origin of a malignant melanoma within the adrenal is reasonable given the common embryogenesis of adrenal chromaffin cells and melanocytes from the neuroectoderm. It may be very difficult to exclude the possibility of primary mucocutaneous malignant melanoma that has metastasized to the adrenal. A recent review of primary melanoma of the adrenal gland reveals only six cases reported since 1946; the tumors were regarded as melanotic pheochromocytoma and not true melanocytic neoplasms.[242] Pigmented pheochromocytoma has been rarely reported, but does not contain true melanosomes or premelanosomes.[40]

Other unusual tumors and tumor-like lesions

Ovarian thecal metaplasia is an incidental microscopic lesion composed of plump spindle cells. It is typically wedge-shaped and attached to the adrenal capsule, and may contain small nests of cortical cells.[3,40] Foci measure up to 2 mm in size and may be multiple.[243] Most cases occur in females, but rare cases have been seen in male patients. Macroscopic tumefactive spindle cell lesions of the adrenal glands have been described in two individuals, one male and one female, and S-100 protein immunoreactivity suggested they originated from Schwann cells.[244] A case of granulosa cell tumor of the adrenal gland has also been reported.[245] Leydig cells have also been described in the adrenal gland as an incidental finding, a component of adrenal ganglioneuroma, or rarely a pure adrenal Leydig cell adenoma. Adenomatoid tumor of the adrenal gland also occurs, with formation of tubular or glandlike spaces, and probably is mesothelial in origin.[246]

TUMORS METASTATIC TO ADRENAL GLAND

The adrenal gland is the fourth most common site of metastatic cancer, following lung, liver, and bone; per unit weight, it is more frequently involved than the other sites (Fig. 14-71),[40,123] probably because the adrenal vascular supply has a high flow volume and sinusoidal vascular pattern. Metastases to the adrenal most commonly originate in the lung (Fig. 14-72) and breast, but other primary sites include kidney, stomach, pancreas, and skin (malignant melanoma). Rarely, metastases to the adrenal are massive, resulting in cortical insufficiency (Addison's disease).[40,123] Computed tomography or ultrasound guided fine needle aspiration biopsy may be useful in documenting the presence of adrenal metastases. Metastases to the adrenal can simulate poorly differentiated adrenal cortical carcinoma.

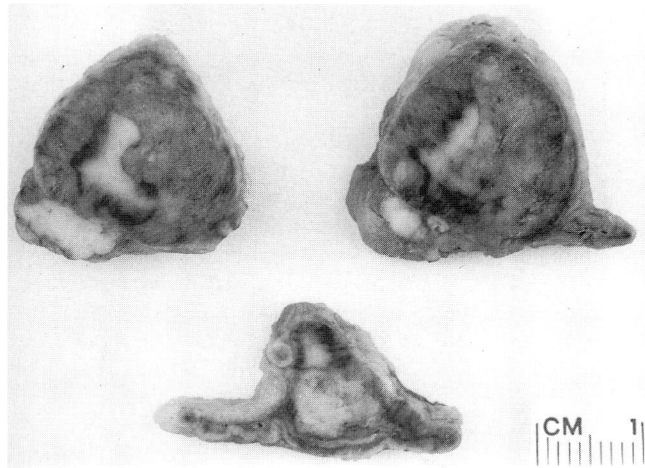

14-71. Bronchial carcinoma metastatic to adrenal gland has a variegated color with geographic zones of necrosis with hyperemic borders.

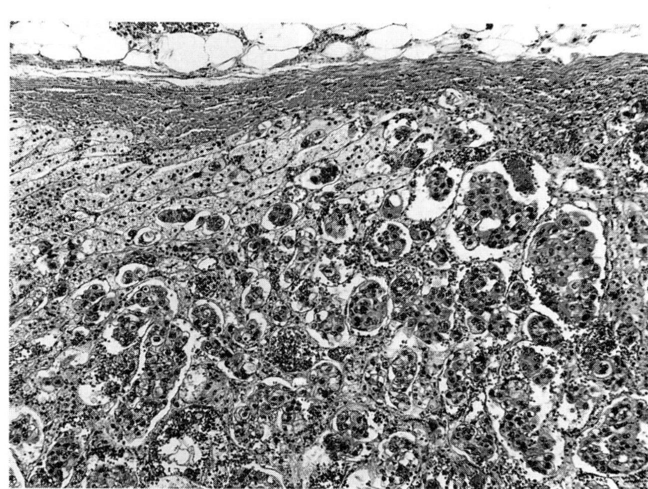

14-72. Bronchogenic adenocarcinoma metastatic to adrenal gland.

REFERENCES

1. Crowder R: The development of the adrenal gland in man, with special reference to origin and ultimate location of cell types and evidence in favor of the "cell migration" theory, Contrib Embryol Carneg Instu 36:193-210, 1957.
2. O'Rahilly R: The timing and sequence of events in the development of the human endocrine system during the embryonic period proper, Anat Embryol 166:439-451, 1983.
3. Lack EE, Kozakewich HPW: Embryology, developmental anatomy and selected aspects of non-neoplastic pathology. In Lack EE, ed: Pathology of the adrenal glands, New York, 1990, Churchill Livingstone.
4. Lack EE: Pathology of adrenal and extra-adrenal paraganglia, Vol 29 in Major problems in pathology, Philadelphia, 1994, WB Saunders.
5. Zuckerkandl E: Ueber Nebenorgane des sympathicus im Retroperitonaealraum des Menschen, Verh Dtsch Anat Ges 15:95-107, 1901.
6. Stoner HB, Whiteley HJ, Emery JL: The effect of systemic disease on the adrenal cortex of the child, J Pathol Bacteriol 66:171-183, 1953.
7. Symington T: Functional pathology of the human adrenal gland, Baltimore, 1969, Williams and Wilkins.
8. Dobbie JW, Symington T: The human adrenal gland with special reference to the vasculature, J Endocrinol 34:479-489, 1966.
9. Quinan C, Berger AA: Observations on human adrenals with special reference to the relative weight of the normal medulla, Ann Int Med 6:1180-1192, 1933.
10. Studzinski GP, Hay DCF, Symington T: Observations on the weight of the human adrenal gland and the effect of preparations of corticotropin of different purity on the weight and morphology of the human adrenal gland, J Clin Endocrinol Metab 23:248-254, 1963.
11. Pakravan P, Kenny FM, Depp R et al: Familial congenital absence of adrenal glands: evaluation of glucocorticoid, mineralocorticoid, and estrogen metabolism in the perinatal period, J Pediatr 84:74-78, 1974.
12. Wise JE, Metalon R, Morgan AM et al: Phenotypic features of patients with congenital adrenal hypoplasia and glycerol kinase deficiency, Am J Dis Child 141:744-747, 1987.
13. Kruse K, Sippell WG, Schnakenburg KV: Hypogonadism in congenital adrenal hypoplasia: evidence for a hypothalamic origin, J Clin Endocrinol Metab 58:12-17, 1984.
14. Graham LS: Celiac accessory adrenal glands, Cancer 6:149-152, 1953.
15. Falls JL: Accessory adrenal cortex in the broad ligament: incidence and functional significance, Cancer 8:143-150, 1955.
16. Apitz K: Die geschwülste und gewebsmissbildungen der Nierenrinde. I. Die intrarenalen Nebenniereninseln, Virchows Arch [Pathol Anat] 311:285-305, 1944.
17. Mares AJ, Shkolni, A, Sacks M et al: Aberrant (ectopic) adrenocortical tissue along the spermatic cord, J Pediatr Surg 15:289-292, 1980.
18. Dahl EV, Bahn RC: Aberrant adrenal cortical tissue near the testis in human infants, Am J Pathol 40:587-598, 1962.
19. Labarrere CA, Caccamo D, Telenta M et al: A nodule of adrenocortical tissue within a human placenta: light microscopic and immunocytochemical findings, Placenta 5:139-144, 1984.
20. Bozic C: Ectopic fetal adrenal cortex in the lung of a newborn, Virchows Arch A Path Anat Histol 363:371-374, 1974.
21. Armin A, Castelli M: Congenital adrenal tissue in the lung with adrenal cytomegaly, Am J Clin Pathol 82:225-228, 1984.
22. Weiner MF, Dallgard SA: Intracranial adrenal gland, Arch Pathol 67:228-233, 1959.
23. Roosen-Runge EC, Lund J: Abnormal sex cord formation and an intratesticular adrenal cortical nodule in a human fetus, Anat Rec 173:57-68, 1972.
24. Symonds DA, Driscoll SG: An adrenal cortical rest within the fetal ovary: report of a case, Am J Clin Pathol 60:562-564, 1973.
25. Verdonk C, Guerin C, Lufkin E et al: Activation of virilizing adrenal rest tissues by excessive ACTH production. An unusual presentation of Nelson's syndrome, Am J Med 73:455-459, 1982.
26. Contreras P, Altieri E, Liberman C et al: Adrenal rest tumor of the liver causing Cushing's syndrome: treatment with ketoconazole preceding an apparent surgical cure, J Clin Endocrinol Metab 60:21-28, 1985.
27. Kepes JJ, O'Boynick P, Jones S et al: Adrenal cortical adenoma in the spinal canal of an 8-year-old girl, Am J Surg Pathol 14:481-484, 1990.
28. Dolan MF, Janovski NA: Adreno-hepatic fusion, Arch Pathol 86:22-24, 1968.
29. Craig JM, Landing BH: Anaplastic cells of fetal adrenal cortex, Am J Clin Pathol 21:940-949, 1951.
30. Beckwith JB: Extreme cytomegaly of the adrenal fetal cortex, omphalocele, hyperplasia of kidneys and pancreas, and Leydig cell hyperplasia another syndrome? Presented at Annual Meeting of Western Society for Pediatric Research, Los Angeles, Nov 11, 1963.
31. Wiedemann H-R: Complexe malformatif familial avec hernie umbilicale et macroglossie, un "syndrome nouveau," J Genet Hum 13:223-232, 1964.
32. Beckwith JB: Macroglossia, omphalocele, adrenal cytomegaly, gigantism and hyperplastic visceromegaly, Birth Defects, Original Article Series 5:188-196, 1969.
33. Powers JM, Schaumberg HH: The adrenal cortex in adrenoleukodystrophy, Arch Pathol 96:305-310, 1973.
34. de Crecchio L: Sopra un caso di apparenzi virili in una donna, Morgagni 7:154-188, 1865.
35. White PC, New MI, Dupont B: Congenital adrenal hyperplasia, New Engl J Med 316:1519-1524, 316:1580-1586, 1987.
36. Kalaitzoglou G, New MI: Congenital adrenal hyperplasia. Molecular insights learned from patients, Receptor 3:211-222, 1993.
37. Rutgers JL, Young RL, Scully RE: The testicular "tumor" of the adrenogenital syndrome. A report of six cases and review of the literature on testicular masses in patients with adrenocortical disorders, Am J Surg Pathol 12:503-513, 1988.
38. Radfar N, Bartter FC, Easley R et al: Evidence for endogenous LH suppression in a man with bilateral testicular tumors and congenital adrenal hyperplasia, J Clin Endocrinol Metab 45:1194-1204, 1977.
39. Johnson RE, Scheithauer B: Massive hyperplasia of testicular adrenal rests in a patient with Nelson's syndrome, Am J Clin Pathol 77:501-507, 1982.
40. Lack EE: Tumors of adrenal glands and extra-adrenal paraganglia, 3rd series Atlas of tumor pathology. Washington, DC, Armed Forces Institute of Pathology (in press).

41. Duck SC: Malignancy associated with congenital adrenal hyperplasia, J Pediatr 99:423-424, 1981.
42. Rich AR: A peculiar type of adrenal cortical damage associated with acute infection, and its possible relation to circulatory collapse, Bull Johns Hopkins Hosp 74:1-15, 1944.
43. Sommers SC, Carter ME: Adrenocortical postirradiation fibrosis, Arch Pathol 99:421-423, 1975.
44. Benirschke K: Adrenals in anencephaly and hydrocephaly, Obstet Gynecol 8:412-425, 1956.
45. Griffel B: Focal adrenalitis. Its frequency and correlation with similar lesions in the thyroid and kidney, Virchows Arch A Path Anat Histol 364:191-198, 1974.
46. Hass GM: Hepato-adrenal necrosis with intranuclear inclusion bodies: report of a case, Am J Pathol 11:127-142, 1935.
47. Klatt EC, Shibata D: Cytomegalovirus infection in the acquired immunodeficiency syndrome. Clinical and autopsy findings, Arch Pathol Lab Med 112:540-544, 1988.
48. Donovan DS Jr, Dluhy RG: AIDS and its effect on the adrenal gland, The Endocrinologist 1:227-232, 1991.
49. Ahonen P, Myllärniemi S, Sipilä I et al: Clinical variation of autoimmune polyendocrinopathy-candidiasis-ectodermal dystrophy (APECED) in a series of 68 patients, N Engl J Med 322:1829-1836, 1990.
50. Schmidt MB: Eine biglanduläre Erkrankung (Nebennieren und Schilddrüse) bei morbus Addisonii, Verh Dtsch Ges Pathol 21:212-221, 1926.
51. Guttman PH: Addison's disease. A statistical analysis of five hundred and sixty-six cases and a study of the pathology, Arch Pathol 10:742-785, 1930.
52. Dunlop D: Eighty-six cases of Addison's disease, Br Med J Oct 12:887-891, 1963.
53. Goodwin RA Jr, Shapiro JL, Thurman GH et al: Disseminated histoplasmosis: clinical and pathologic correlations, Medicine 59:1-33, 1980.
54. Cote RJ, Rosenblum M, Telzak EE: Disseminated Pneumocystis carinii infection causing extrapulmonary organ failure: clinical, pathologic, and immunohistochemical analysis, Modern Pathol 3:25-30, 1990.
55. Benjamin E, Fox H: Malakoplakia of the adrenal gland, J Clin Pathol 34:606-611, 1981.
56. Bartsch G, Bodner E, Buchsteiner R et al: Echinococcal cyst of the adrenal gland, Eur Urol 1:240-242, 1975.
57. Dobbie JW: Adrenocortical nodular hyperplasia: the ageing adrenal, J Pathol 99:1-18, 1969.
58. Hedeland H, Östberg G, Hökfelt B: On the prevalence of adrenocortical adenomas in an autopsy material in relation to hypertension and diabetes, Acta Med Scand 184:211-214, 1968.
59. Spain DM, Weinsaft P: Solitary adrenal cortical adenoma in elderly female. Frequency, Arch Pathol 78:231-233, 1964.
60. Shamma AH, Goddard JW, Sommers SC: A study of the adrenal status in hypertension, J Chronic Dis 8:587-595, 1958.
61. Russi S, Blumenthal HT, Gray SH: Small adenomas of the adrenal cortex in hypertension and diabetes, Arch Intern Med 76:284-291, 1945.
62. Commons RR, Callaway CP: Adenomas of the adrenal cortex, Arch Intern Med 81:37-41, 1948.
63. Robinson MJ, Pardo V, Rywlin AM: Pigmented nodules (black adenomas) of the adrenal. An autopsy study of incidence, morphology and function, Hum Pathol 3:317-325, 1972.
64. Damron TA, Schelper RL, Sorensen L: Cytochemical demonstration of neuromelanin in black pigmented adrenal nodules, Am J Clin Pathol 87:334-341, 1987.
65. Glazer HS, Weyman PJ, Sagel SS et al: Non-functioning adrenal masses: incidental discovery on computed tomography, AJR 139:81-85, 1982.
66. Prinz RA, Brooks MH, Churchill R et al: Incidental asymptomatic adrenal masses detected by computed tomographic scanning, JAMA 248:701-704, 1982.
67. Abecassis M, McLoughlin MJ, Longer B et al: Serendipitous adrenal masses: prevalance, significance and management, Am J Surg 149:783-788, 1985.
68. Francis IR, Smid A, Gross MD et al: Adrenal masses in oncologic patients: functional and morphologic evaluation, Radiology 166:353-356, 1988.
69. Keiser HR, Doppman JL, Robertson CN et al: Diagnosis, localization, and management of pheochromocytoma. In Lack EE, ed: Pathology of the adrenal glands, New York, 1990, Churchill Livingstone.
70. Beierwaltes WH, Sturman MF, Ryo U et al: Imaging functional nodules of the adrenal glands with I 131-19 iodocholesterol, J Nucl Med 15:246-251, 1974.
71. Rizza RA, Wahner HW, Spelsberg TC et al: Visualization of nonfunctional adrenal adenomas with iodocholesterol: possible relationship to subcellular distribution of tracer, J Nucl Med 19:458-463, 1978.
72. Gross MD, Valk TW, Freitas JE et al: The relationship of adrenal iodomethylnorcholesterol (NP-59) uptake to indices of adrenal cortical function in Cushing's syndrome, J Clin Endocrinol Metab 52:1062-1066, 1981.
73. Gross MD, Wilton GP, Shapiro B et al: Functional and scintigraphic evaluation of the silent adrenal mass, J Nucl Med 28:1401-1407, 1987.
74. Suzuki T, Sasano H, Sawai T et al: Small adrenocortical tumors without apparent clinical endocrine abnormalities. Immunolocalization of steroidogenic enzymes, Pathol Res Pract 188:883-889, 1992.
75. Krestin GP, Friedmann G, Fishbach R et al: Evaluation of adrenal masses in oncologic patients: dynamic contrast-enhanced MR vs CT, J Comput Assist Tomogr 15:104-110, 1991.
76. Copeland PM: The incidentally discovered adrenal mass, Ann Int Med 98:940-945, 1983.
77. Ross NS, Aron DC: Hormonal evaluation of the patient with an incidentally discovered adrenal mass, N Engl J Med 323:1401-1405, 1990.
78. Nadler JL, Rabin R: Evaluation and management of the incidentally discovered adrenal mass, The Endocrinologist 1:5-9, 1991.
79. Roubidoux M, Dunnick NR: Adrenal cortical tumors, Bull NY Acad Med 67:119-130, 1991.
80. Case Records of the Massachusetts General Hospital. Case 6-1991, N Engl J Med 324:400-408, 1991.
81. Bravo EL: Pheochromocytoma: new concepts and future trends, Kidney Int 40:544-556, 1991.
82. Orth DN, Liddle GW: Results of treatment in 108 patients with Cushing's syndrome, N Engl J Med 285:243-247, 1971.
83. Liddle GW: Cushing's syndrome, Ann NY Acad Sci 297:594-602, 1977.
84. Gold EM: The Cushing syndromes: changing views of diagnosis and treatment, Ann Intern Med 90:829-844, 1979.

85. Carpenter PC: Cushing's syndrome: update of diagnosis and management, Mayo Clin Proc 61:49-58, 1986.
86. Mandel S: Cushing's syndrome in infancy, The Endocrinologist 4:28-32, 1994.
87. Klibanski A, Zervas NT: Diagnosis and management of hormone-secreting pituitary adenomas, N Engl J Med 324:822-831, 1991.
88. Oldfield EH, Doppman JL, Nieman LK et al: Petrosal sinus sampling with and without corticotropin-releasing hormone for the differential diagnosis of Cushing's syndrome, N Engl J Med 325:897-905, 1991.
89. Miller J, Crapo L: The biochemical diagnosis of hypercortisolism, The Endocrinologist 4:7-16, 1994.
90. Smals AGH, Pieters GFFM, van Haelst UJG et al: Macronodular, adrenocortical hyperplasia in longstanding Cushing's disease, J Clin Endocrinol Metab 58:25-31, 1984.
91. Doppman JL, Miller DL, Dwyer AJ et al: Macronodular adrenal. hyperplasia in Cushing's disease, Radiology 166:347-352, 1988.
92. Cohen RB, Chapman WB, Castleman B: Hyperadrenocorticism (Cushing's disease): a study of surgically resected adrenal glands, Cancer 35:537-561, 1959.
93. Grua JR, Nelson DH: ACTH-producing tumors, Endocrinol Metab Clin N Am 20:319-362, 1991.
94. Odell WD: Ectopic ACTH secretion. A misnomer, Endocrinol Metab Clin N Am 20:371-379, 1991.
95. Doppman JL: The search for occult ectopic ACTH-producing tumors, The Endocrinologist 2:41-46, 1992.
96. Leinung MC, Young WF Jr, Whitaker MD et al: Diagnosis of corticotropin-producing bronchial carcinoid tumors causing Cushing's syndrome, Mayo Clin Proc 65:1314-1321, 1990.
97. Shenoy BV, Carpenter PC, Carney JA: Bilateral primary pigmented nodular adrenocortical disease. Rare cause of the Cushing's syndrome, Am J Surg Pathol 8:335-344, 1984.
98. Carney JA, Young WF Jr: Primary pigmented nodular adrenocortical disease and its associated conditions, The Endocrinologist 2:6-21, 1992.
99. Wulffraat NM, Drexhagge HA, Wiersinga WM et al: Immunoglobulins of patients with Cushing's syndrome due to pigmented adrenocortical micronodular dysplasia stimulate in vitro steroidogenesis, J Clin Endocrinol Metab 66:301-307, 1988.
100. Sasano H, Miyazaki S, Sawai T et al: Primary pigmented nodular adrenocortical disease (PPNAD): immunohistochemical and in situ hybridization analysis of steroidogenic enzymes in eight cases, Modern Pathol 5:23-29, 1992.
101. Grant CS, Carney JA, Carpenter PC et al: Primary pigmented nodular adrenocortical disease: diagnosis and treatment, Surgery 100:1178-1184, 1986.
102. Carney JA, Gordon H, Carpenter PC et al: The complex of myxomas, spotty pigmentation, and endocrine overactivity, Medicine 64:270-283, 1985.
103. Doppman JL, Nieman LK, Travis WD et al: CT and MR imaging of massive macronodular adrenocortical disease: a rare cause of autonomous primary adrenal hypercortisolism, J Comput Assist Tomogr 15:773-779, 1991.
104. Aiba M, Hirayama A, Iri H et al: Adrenocorticotropic hormone-independent bilateral adrenocortical macronodular hyperplasia as a distinct subtype of Cushing's syndrome. Enzyme histochemical and ultrastructural study of four cases with a review of the literature, Am J Clin Pathol 96:334-340, 1991.
105. Sasano H, Suzuki T, Nagura H: ACTH-independent macronodular adrenocortical hyperplasia: immunohistochemical and in situ hybridization studies of steroidogenic enzymes, Modern Pathol 7:215-219, 1994.
106. Wermer P: Genetic aspects of adenomatosis of endocrine glands, Am J Med 16:363-371, 1954.
107. Skogseid B, Larsson C, Lindgren P-G et al: Clinical and genetic features of adrenocortical lesions in multiple endocrine neoplasia type 1, J Clin Endocrinol Metab 75:76-81, 1992.
108. Ballard HS, Frame B, Hartsock RJ: Familial multiple endocrine adenoma—peptic ulcer complex, Medicine 43:481-516, 1964.
109. Miyagawa K, Ishibashi M, Kasuga M et al: Multiple endocrine neoplasia type I with Cushing's disease primary hyperparathyroidism and insulin-glucagonoma, Cancer 61:1232-1236, 1988.
110. Weinstein LS, Shenker A, Gejman PV et al: Activating mutations of the stimulatory G protein in McCune-Albright syndrome, N Engl J Med 325:1688-1695, 1991.
111. Bertagna X: New causes of Cushing's syndrome, N Engl J Med 327:1024-1025, 1992.
112. Reznik Y, Allali-Zerah V, Chayvialle JA et al: Food-dependent Cushing's syndrome mediated by aberrant adrenal sensitivity to gastric inhibitory polypeptide, N Engl J Med 327:981-986, 1992.
113. Lacroix A, Bolté E, Tremblay J et al: Gastric inhibitory polypeptide-dependent cortisol hypersecretion—a new cause of Cushing's syndrome, N Engl J Med 327:974-980, 1992.
114. Neville AM, O'Hare MJ: Histopathology of the human adrenal cortex, Clin Endocrinol Metab 14:791-820, 1985.
115. Young WF Jr, Hogan MJ, Klee GG et al: Primary aldosteronism: diagnosis and treatment, Mayo Clin Proc 65:96-110, 1990.
116. Carey RM, Sen S, Doland LM et al: Idiopathic hyperaldosteronism: a possible role for aldosterone-stimulating factor, N Engl J Med 311:94-100, 1984.
117. Gill JR Jr: Hyperaldosteronism. In Becker KL, ed: Principles and practice of endocrinology and metabolism, Philadelphia, 1990, JB Lippincott.
118. DeLellis RA, Wolfe HJ, Gagel RT et al: Adrenal medullary hyperplasia. A morphometric analysis in patients with familial medullary thyroid carcinoma, Am J Pathol 83:177-190, 1976.
119. Carney JA, Sizemore GW, Sheps SG: Adrenal medullary disease in multiple endocrine neoplasia, type 2. Pheochromocytoma and its precursors, Am J Clin Pathol 66:279-290, 1976.
120. Padberg B-C, Garbe E, Achilles E et al: Adrenomedullary hyperplasia and phaeochromocytoma. DNA photometric findings in 47 cases, Virchows Archiv A Pathol Anat 416:443-446, 1990.
121. Foster DG: Adrenal cysts. Review of the literature and report of case, Arch Surg 92:131-143, 1966.
122. Abeshouse GA, Goldstein RB, Abeshouse BS: Adrenal cysts: review of the literature and report of three cases, J Urol 81:711-719, 1959.
123. Travis WD, Oertel JE, Lack EE: Miscellaneous tumors and tumefactive lesions of the adrenal gland. In Lack EE, ed: Pathology of the adrenal glands, New York, 1990, Churchill Livingstone.

124. Medeiros LJ, Weiss LM, Vickery AL: Epithelial-lined (true) cyst of the adrenal gland: a case report, Hum Pathol 20:491-492, 1989.
125. Groben PA, Roberson JB, Anger SR et al: Immunohistochemical evidence for the vascular origin of primary adrenal pseudocysts, Arch Pathol Lab Med 110:121-123, 1986.
126. Gaffey MJ, Mills SE, Fechner RE et al: Vascular adrenal cysts. A clinicopathologic and immunohistochemical study of endothelial and hemorrhagic (pseudocystic) variants, Am J Surg Pathol 13:740-747, 1989.
127. Gaffey MJ, Mills SE, Medeiros LJ et al: Unusual variants of adrenal pseudocysts with intracystic fat, myelolipomatous metaplasia, and metastatic carcinoma, Am J Clin Pathol 94:706-713, 1990.
128. Oppenheimer EH: Cyst formation in the outer adrenal cortex: studies in the human fetus and newborn, Arch Pathol 87:653-659, 1969.
129. Rodin AE, Hsu FL, Whorton EB: Microcysts of the permanent adrenal cortex in perinates and infants, Arch Pathol Lab Med 100:499-502, 1976.
130. Hunter SB, Schemankewitz EH, Patterson C et al: Extra-adrenal myelolipoma. A report of two cases, Am J Clin Pathol 97:402-404, 1992.
131. Nishizaki T, Kanematsu T, Matsumata T et al: Myelolipoma of the liver. A case report, Cancer 63:930-934, 1989.
132. Seyle S, Stone H: Hormonally induced transformation of adrenal into myeloid tissue, Am J Pathol 26:211-233, 1950.
133. Plaut A: Myelolipoma in the adrenal cortex (myeloadipose structures), Am J Pathol 34:487-515, 1958.
134. Del Gaudio A, Solidaro G: Myelolipoma of the adrenal gland: report of two cases with a review of the literature, Surgery 99:293-301, 1986.
135. Bennett BD, McKenna T, Hough AJ et al: Adrenal myelolipoma associated with Cushing's disease, Am J Clin Pathol 73:443-447, 1980.
136. Vyberg M, Sestoft L: Combined adrenal myelolipoma and adenoma associated with Cushing's syndrome, Am J Clin Pathol 86:541-545, 1986.
137. Whaley D, Becker S, Presbrey T et al: Adrenal myelolipoma associated with Conn's syndrome: CT evaluation, J Comput Assist Tomogr 9:959-960, 1985.
138. DeBlois GG, DeMay RM: Adrenal myelolipoma diagnosed by computed tomography-guided fine needle aspiration, Cancer 55:848-850, 1985.
139. Rao RH, Vagnucci AH, Amico JA: Bilateral massive adrenal hemorrhage: early recognition and treatment, Ann Int Med 110:227-235, 1989.
140. Bertagna C, Orth DN: Clinical and laboratory findings and results of therapy in 58 patients with adrenocortical tumors admitted to a single medical center (1951-1978), Am J Med 71:855-875, 1981.
141. Lack EE, Travis WD, Oertel JE: Adrenal cortical neoplasms. In Lack EE, ed: Pathology of the adrenal glands, New York, 1990, Churchill Livingstone.
142. Aiba M, Kawakami M, Ito Y et al: Bilateral adrenocortical adenomas causing Cushing's syndrome. Report of two cases with enzyme histochemical and ultrastructural studies and a review of the literature, Arch Pathol Lab Med 116:146-150, 1992.
143. Kato S, Masunaga R, Kawabe T et al: Cushing's syndrome induced by hypersecretion of cortisol from only one of bilateral adrenocortical tumors, Metabolism 41:260-263, 1992.
144. O'Leary TJ, Liotta LA, Gill JR: Pigmented adrenal nodules in Cushing's syndrome, Arch Pathol Lab Med 106:257, 1982.
145. Conn JW: Plasma renin activity in primary aldosteronism. Importance in differential diagnosis and in research of essential hypertension, JAMA 190:222-225, 1964.
146. Ganguly A: Cellular origin of aldosteronomas, Clin Investig 70:392-395, 1992.
147. Eto T, Kumamoto K, Kawasaki T et al: Ultrastructural types of cells in adrenal cortical adenoma with primary aldosteronism, J Pathol 128:1-6, 1979.
148. Janigan DT: Cytoplasmic bodies in the adrenal cortex of patients treated with spironolactone, Lancet 1:850-852, 1963.
149. Jenis EH, Hertzog RW: Effect of spironolactone on the zona glomerulosa of the adrenal cortex: light and electron microscopy, Arch Pathol 88:530-539, 1969.
150. Cohn D, Jackson RV, Gordon RD: Factors affecting the frequency of occurrence of spironolactone bodies in aldosteronomas and non-tumorous cortex, Pathology 15:273-277, 1983.
151. Komiya I, Takasu N, Aizawa T et al: Black (or brown) adrenal cortical adenoma: its characteristic features on computed tomography and endocrine data, J Clin Endocrinol Metab 61:711-717, 1985.
152. Mattox JH, Phelan S: The evaluation of adult females with testosterone producing neoplasms of the adrenal cortex, Surg Gynecol Obstet 164:98-101, 1987.
153. Gabrilove JL, Sharma DC, Wotiz HH et al: Feminizing adrenocortical tumors in the male. A review of 52 cases including a case report, Medicine 44:37-79, 1965.
154. Pollock WJ, McConnell CF, Hilton C et al: Virilizing Leydig cell adenoma of adrenal gland, Am J Surg Pathol 10:816-822, 1986.
155. Lack EE, Nauta RJ: Intracortical Leydig cells in a patient with an aldosterone-secreting adrenal cortical adenoma, J Urol Pathol 1:411-418, 1993.
156. Kakimoto S, Yushita Y, Sanefuji T et al: Nonhormonal adrenocortical adenoma with oncocytoma-like appearance, Hinyokika Kiyo 32:757-763, 1986.
157. Erlandson RA, Reuter VE: Oncocytic adrenal cortical adenoma, Ultrastr Pathol 15:539-547, 1991.
158. Sasano H, Suzuki T, Sano T et al: Adrenocortical oncocytoma. A true nonfunctioning adrenocortical tumor, Am J Surg Pathol 15:949-956, 1991.
159. Nguyen G-K, Vriend R, Ronaghan D et al: Heterotopic adrenocortical oncocytoma. A case report with light and electron microscopic studies, Cancer 70:2681-2684, 1992.
160. El-Naggar AK, Evans DB, MacKay B: Oncocytic adrenal cortical carcinoma, Ultrastr Pathol 15:549-556, 1991.
161. Hutter AM, Kayhoe DE: Adrenal cortical carcinoma. Clinical features of 138 patients, Am J Med 41:572-580, 1966.
162. Wooten MD, King DK: Adrenal cortical carcinoma. Epidemiology and treatment with mitotane and a review of the literature, Cancer 72:3145-3155, 1993.
163. King DR, Lack EE: Adrenal cortical carcinoma. A clinical and pathologic study of 49 cases, Cancer 44:239-244, 1979.
164. Tang CK, Gray GF: Adrenocortical neoplasms. Prognosis and morphology, Urology 5:691-695, 1975.
165. Gandour MJ, Grizzle WE: A small adrenocortical carcinoma with aggressive behavior. An evaluation of criteria for malignancy, Arch Pathol Lab Med 110:1076-1079, 1986.
166. Weiss LM: Comparative histologic study of 43 metastasizing and nonmetastasizing adrenocortical tumors, Am J Surg Pathol 8:163-169, 1984.

167. Lack EE, Mulvihill JJ, Travis WD et al: Adrenal cortical neoplasms in the pediatric and adolescent age group. Clinicopathologic study of 30 cases with emphasis on epidemiological and prognostic factors, Pathol Annu 27:1-53, 1992.
168. Miettinen M: Neuroendocrine differentiation in adrenocortical carcinoma. New immunohistochemical findings supported by electron microscopy, Lab Invest 66:169-174, 1992.
169. Schröder S, Padberg B-C, Achilles E et al: Immunocytochemistry in adrenocortical tumors: a clinicopathological study of 72 neoplasms, Virchows Archiv A Pathol Anat 420:65-70, 1992.
170. Mackay B, El-Naggar A, Ordonez NG: Ultrastructure of adrenal cortical carcinoma, Ultrastr Pathol 18:181-190, 1994.
171. Hough AJ, Hollifield JW, Page DL et al: Prognostic factors in adrenal cortical tumors. A mathematical analysis of clinical and morphologic data, Am J Clin Pathol 72:390-399, 1979.
172. Van Slooten H, Schaberg A, Smeenk D et al: Morphologic characteristics of benign and malignant adrenocortical tumors, Cancer 55:766-773, 1985.
173. Weiss LM, Medeiros LJ, Vickery AL Jr: Pathologic features of prognostic significance in adrenal cortical carcinoma, Am J Surg Pathol 13:202-206, 1989.
174. Cibas ES, Medeiros LJ, Weinberg DS et al: Cellular DNA profiles of benign and malignant adrenocortical tumors, Am J Surg Pathol 14:948-955, 1990.
175. Camuto P, Citrin D, Schinella R et al: Adrenal cortical carcinoma: flow cytometric study of 22 cases on ECOG study, Urology 37:380-384, 1991.
176. Zerbini C, Kozakewich HPW, Weinberg DS et al: Adrenocortical neoplasms in childhood and adolescence: analysis of prognostic factors including DNA content, Endocr Pathol 3:116-128, 1992.
177. Bugg MF, Ribeiro RC, Roberson PK et al: Correlation of pathologic features with clinical outcome in pediatric adrenocortical neoplasia: a study of a Brazilian population, Am J Clin Pathol 101:625-629, 1994.
178. Hosaka Y, Rainwater LM, Grant CS et al: Adrenocortical carcinoma: nuclear deoxyribonucleic acid ploidy studies by flow cytometry, Surgery 102:1027-1034, 1987.
179. Decorato JW, Gruber H, Petti M et al: Adrenal carcinosarcoma, J Surg Oncol 45:134-136, 1990.
180. Fischler DF, Nunez C, Levin HS et al: Adrenal carcinosarcoma presenting in a woman with clinical signs of virilization. A case report with immunohistochemical and ultrastructural findings, Am J Surg Pathol 16:626-631, 1992.
181. Barksdale SK, Marincola FM: Carcinosarcoma of the adrenal cortex presenting with minerolocorticoid excess, Am J Surg Pathol 17:941-945, 1993.
182. Molberg K, Vuitch F, Stewart D et al: Adrenocortical blastoma, Hum Pathol 23:1187-1190, 1992.
183. Beard CM, Sheps SG, Kurland LT et al: Occurrence of pheochromocytoma in Rochester, Minnesota, 1950 through 1979, Mayo Clin Proc 58:802-804, 1983.
184. Lack EE: Adrenal medullary hyperplasia and pheochromocytoma. In Lack EE, ed: Pathology of the adrenal glands, New York, 1990, Churchill Livingstone.
185. Steinhoff MM, Wells SA Jr, DeSchryver-Kecskemeti K: Stromal amyloid in pheochromocytomas, Hum Pathol 23:33-36, 1992.
186. Linnoila RI, Keiser HR, Steinberg SM et al: Histopathology of benign versus malignant sympathoadrenal paragangliomas. Clinicopathologic study of 120 cases including unusual histologic features, Hum Pathol 21:1168-1180, 1990.
187. Ramsay JA, Asa SL, van Nostrand AWP et al: Lipid degeneration in pheochromocytomas mimicking adrenal cortical tumors, Am J Surg Pathol 11:480-486, 1987.
188. Unger PD, Cohen JM, Thung SN et al: Lipid degeneration in a pheochromocytoma histologically mimicking an adrenal cortical tumor, Arch Pathol Lab Med 114:892-894, 1990.
189. Melicow MM: Hibernating fat and pheochromocytoma, Arch Pathol 63:367-372, 1957.
190. Medeiros LJ, Katsas GG, Balogh K: Brown fat and adrenal pheochromocytoma. Association or coincidence? Hum Pathol 16:970-972, 1985.
191. Chetty R, Clark SP, Taylor DA: Pigmented pheochromocytomas of the adrenal medulla, Hum Pathol 24:420-423, 1993.
192. Webb TA, Sheps SG, Carney JA: Differences between sporadic pheochromocytoma and pheochromocytoma in multiple endocrine neoplasia, type 2, Am J Surg Pathol 4:121-126, 1980.
193. Carney JA, Go VLW, Sizemore GW et al: Alimentary-tract ganglioneuromatosis. A major component of the syndrome of multiple endocrine neoplasia, type 2b, N Engl J Med 295:1287-1291, 1976.
194. Linnoila RI, Lack EE, Steinberg SM et al: Decreased expression of neuropeptides in malignant paragangliomas: an immunohistochemical study, Hum Pathol 19:41-50, 1988.
195. Erlandson RA: Diagnostic transmission electron microscopy of tumors, New York, 1994, Raven Press.
196. Tannenbaum M: Ultrastructural pathology of adrenal medullary tumors, Pathol Annu 5:145-171, 1970.
197. Symington T, Goodall AL: Studies in pheochromocytoma. I. Pathological aspects, Glas Med J 34:75-96, 1953.
198. Hume DM: Pheochromocytoma in the adult and in the child, Am J Surg 99:458-496, 1960.
199. Melicow MM: One hundred cases of pheochromocytoma (107 tumors) at the Columbia-Presbyterian Medical Center 1926-1976. A clinicopathological analysis, Cancer 40:1987-2004, 1977.
200. Neville AM: The adrenal medulla. In Symington T, ed: Functional pathology of the human adrenal gland, Baltimore, 1969, Williams and Wilkins.
201. Hosaka Y, Rainwater LM, Grant CS et al: Pheochromocytoma: nuclear deoxyribonucleic acid patterns studied by flow cytometry, Surgery 100:1003-1010, 1986.
202. Nativ O, Grant CS, Sheps SG et al: The clinical significance of nuclear DNA ploidy pattern in 184 patients with pheochromocytoma, Cancer 69:2683-2687, 1992.
203. Kliewer KE, Wen D-R, Cancilla PA et al: Paragangliomas: assessment of prognosis by histologic, immunohistochemical, and ultrastructural techniques, Hum Pathol 20:29-39, 1989.
204. Kliewer KE, Cochran AJ: A review of the histology, ultrastructure, immunohistology, and molecular biology of extra-adrenal paragangliomas, Arch Pathol Lab Med 113:1209-1218, 1989.
205. Linnoila RI, Becker RL Jr, Steinberg SM et al: The role of S-100 protein containing cells in the prognosis of sympathoadrenal paragangliomas, Modern Pathol 6:39A, 1993.
206. Rosen EM, Cassady JR, Frantz CN et al: Neuroblastoma: the Joint Center for Radiation Therapy/Dana-Farber Cancer Institute/Children's Hospital experience, J Clin Oncol 2:719-732, 1984.

207. Kushner BH, Gilbert F, Helson L: Familial neuroblastoma: case reports, literature review and etiologic considerations, Cancer 57:1887-1893, 1986.
208. Brodeur GM: Molecular biology and genetics of human neuroblastoma. In Pochedly C, ed: Neuroblastoma: tumor biology and therapy, Boca Raton, 1990, CRC Press.
209. Lack EE, Kozakewich HPW: Adrenal neuroblastoma, ganglioneuroblastoma, and related tumors. In Lack EE, ed: Pathology of the adrenal glands, New York, 1990, Churchill Livingstone.
210. Sawada T: Past and future of neuroblastoma screening in Japan, Am J Ped Hematol Oncol 14:320-326, 1992.
211. Hachitanda Y, Ishimoto K, Naito M et al: 100 neuroblastomas detected through mass screening system in Japan, Modern Pathol 6:4P(19), 1993.
212. Bowman LC, Santana VM, Green AA et al: Staging systems in neuroblastoma: which is best? J Clin Oncol 9:189-193, 1991.
213. Philip T: Overview of current treatment of neuroblastoma, Am J Pediatr Hematol Oncol 14:97-102, 1992.
214. Beckwith JB, Perrin EV: In situ neuroblastomas: a contribution to the natural history of neural crest tumors, Am J Pathol 43:1089-1104, 1963.
215. Turkel SB, Itabashi HH: The natural history of neuroblastic cells in the fetal adrenal gland, Am J Pathol 76:225-236, 1974.
216. Evans AE, D'Angio GJ, Randolph J: A proposed staging for children with neuroblastoma: Children's Cancer Study Group A, Cancer 27:374-378, 1971.
217. Evans AE, Baum E, Chard R: Do infants with stage IV-S neuroblastoma need treatment? Arch Dis Child 56:271-274, 1981.
218. Stephenson SR, Cook BA, Mease AD et al: The prognostic significance of age and pattern of metastases in stage IV-S neuroblastoma, Cancer 58:372-375, 1986.
219. Knudson AG Jr, Meadows AT: Regression of neuroblastoma IV-S: a genetic hypothesis, N Engl J Med 302:1254-1256, 1980.
220. Adam A, Hochholzer L: Ganglioneuroblastoma of the posterior mediastinum, Cancer 47:373-381, 1981.
221. Triche TJ: Differential diagnosis of neuroblastoma and related tumors. In Lack EE, ed: Pathology of the adrenal glands, New York, 1990, Churchill Livingstone.
222. Wright JH: Neurocytoma or neuroblastoma, a kind of tumor not generally recognized, J Experim Medicine 12:556-561, 1910.
223. Cozzutto C, Carbone A: Pleomorphic (anaplastic) neuroblastoma, Arch Pathol Lab Med 112:621-625, 1988.
224. Chatten J: Anaplastic neuroblastoma, Arch Pathol Lab Med 113:9-10, 1989.
225. Shimada H, Aoyama C, Chiba T et al: Prognostic subgroups for undifferentiated neuroblastoma: immunohistochemcial study with anti-S-100 protein antibody, Hum Pathol 16:471-476, 1985.
226. Beckwith JB, Martin RF: Observations on the histopathology of neuroblastomas, J Pediatr Surg 3:106-110, 1986.
227. Hughes M, Marsden HB, Palmer MK: Histologic patterns of neuroblastoma related to prognosis and clinical staging, Cancer 34:1706-1711, 1974.
228. Shimada H, Chatten J, Newton WA Jr et al: Histopathologic prognostic factors in neuroblastic tumors: definition of subtypes of ganglioneuroblastoma and an age-linked classification of neuroblastomas, JNCI 73:405-416, 1984.
229. Chatten J, Shimada H, Sather HN et al: Prognostic value of histopathology in advanced neuroblastoma: a report from the Children's Cancer Study Group, Hum Pathol 19:1187-1198, 1988.
230. Joshi VV, Chatten J, Sather HN et al: Evaluation of the Shimada classification in advanced neuroblastoma with a special reference to the mitosis-karyorrhexis index: a report from the Children's Cancer Study Group, Modern Pathol 4:139-147, 1991.
231. Joshi VV, Cantor AB, Altschuler G et al: Age-linked prognostic categorization based on a new histologic grading system of neuroblastomas: a clinicopathologic study of 211 cases from the Pediatric Oncology Group, Cancer 69:2197-2211, 1992.
232. Cushing H, Wolbach SB: The transformation of a malignant paravertebral sympathicoblastoma into a benign ganglioneuroma, Am J Pathol 3:203-216, 1927.
233. Collins VP: Wilms' tumor: its behavior and prognosis, J La State Med Soc 107:474-480, 1955.
234. Willis RA: The spread of tumors in the human body, 3rd ed, London, 1973, Butterworth & Co. Ltd.
235. Scully RE, Cohen RB: Ganglioneuroma of adrenal medulla containing cells morphologically identical to hilus cells (extraparenchymal Leydig cells), Cancer 14:421-425, 1961.
236. Aguirre P, Scully RE: Testosterone-secreting adrenal ganglioneuroma containing Leydig cells, Am J Surg Pathol 7:699-705, 1983.
237. Page DL, DeLellis RA, Hough AJ: Tumors of the adrenal. In Atlas of tumor pathology, AFIP 2nd series, fascicle 23, Washington, DC, 1986, Armed Forces Institute of Pathology.
238. Livaditou A, Alexiou G, Floros D et al: Epithelioid angiosarcoma of the adrenal gland associated with chronic arsenical intoxication? Pathol Res Pract 187:284-289, 1991.
239. Ben-Izhak O, Auslander L, Rabinson S et al: Epithelioid angiosarcoma of the adrenal gland with cytokeratin expression. Report of a case with accompanying mesenteric fibromatosis, Cancer 69:1808-1812, 1992.
240. Lack EE, Graham CW, Azumi N et al: Primary leiomyosarcoma of adrenal gland. Case report with immunohistochemical and ultrastructural study, Am J Surg Pathol 15:899-905, 1991.
241. Ayala GE, Ettinghausen SE, Epstein AH et al: Primary malignant peripheral nerve sheath tumor of the adrenal gland. Case report and literature review, J Urol Pathol 2:265-272, 1994.
242. Dao AH, Page DL, Reynolds VH et al: Primary malignant melanoma of the adrenal gland. A report of two cases and review of the literature, Am Surg 56:199-203, 1990.
243. Fidler WJ: Ovarian thecal metaplasia in adrenal glands, Am J Clin Pathol 67:318-323, 1977.
244. Carney JA: Unusual tumefactive spindle cell lesions in the adrenal glands, Hum Pathol 18:980-985, 1987.
245. Orselli RC, Bassler TJ: Theca granulosa tumor arising in the adrenal, Cancer 31:474-477, 1973.
246. Travis WD, Lack EE, Azumi N et al: Adenomatoid tumor of the adrenal gland with ultrastructural and immunohistochemical demonstration of a mesothelial origin, Arch Pathol Lab Med 114:722-724, 1990.

INDEX

Note: Page numbers in *italics* indicate illustrations; **boldface** page numbers indicate tables.

J

K

N